Continued on back endsheets.

CAMPBELL'S
OPERATIVE
ORTHOPAEDICS

The following handheld software also is available to accompany your *Campbell's Operative Orthopaedics*, tenth edition. Each PDA contains 75 to 150 operative procedures that have been written in bulleted format.

Canale: PDA Series
Techniques in Operative Orthopaedics: PDA Set
ISBN Retail: 0-323-02289-8

Canale: PDA Series
Techniques in Operative Orthopaedics: Adult Reconstruction
ISBN Retail: 0-323-02275-8
Download: 0-323-02276-6

Canale: PDA Series
Techniques in Operative Orthopaedics: Congenital Anomalies and Pediatrics
ISBN Retail: 0-323-02277-4
Download: 0-323-02278-2

Canale: PDA Series
Techniques in Operative Orthopaedics: Spine
ISBN Retail: 0-323-02279-0
Download: 0-323-02280-4

Canale: PDA Series
Techniques in Operative Orthopaedics: Sports Medicine and Arthroscopy
ISBN Retail: 0-323-02269-3
Download: 0-323-02270-7

Canale: PDA Series
Techniques in Operative Orthopaedics: Hand
ISBN Retail: 0-323-02267-7
Download: 0-323-02268-5

Canale: PDA Series
Techniques in Operative Orthopaedics: Ankle and Foot
ISBN Retail: 0-323-02273-1
Download: 0-323-02274-X

Canale: PDA Series
Techniques in Operative Orthopaedics: Trauma
ISBN Retail: 0-323-02271-5
Download: 0-323-02272-3

Volume Two

TENTH EDITION

CAMPBELL'S
OPERATIVE
ORTHOPAEDICS

Edited by

S. TERRY CANALE, MD

Professor and Chairman, Department of Orthopaedic Surgery
University of Tennessee–Campbell Clinic;
Chief of Pediatric Orthopaedics
Le Bonheur Children's Medical Center
Memphis, Tennessee

Editorial Assistance by

KAY DAUGHERTY and LINDA JONES

Art coordination by

BARRY BURNS

With over 9000 illustrations

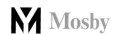 Mosby

An Affiliate of Elsevier Science
St. Louis   London   Philadelphia   Sydney   Toronto

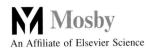
Mosby

An Affiliate of Elsevier Science

The Curtis Center
Independence Square West
Philadelphia, Pennsylvania 19106

Notice

Medicine is an ever-changing field. Standard safety precautions must be followed, but as new research and
clinical experience broaden our knowledge, changes in treatment and drug therapy may become necessary
or appropriate. Readers are advised to check the most current product information provided by the
manufacturer of each drug to be administered to verify the recommended dose, the method and duration of
administration, and contraindications. It is the responsibility of the licensed prescriber, relying on experience
and knowledge of the patient, to determine dosages and the best treatment for each individual patient. Neither
the publisher nor the author assumes any liability for any injury and/or damage to persons or property arising
from this publication.

Previous editions copyrighted 1939, 1949, 1956, 1963, 1971, 1980, 1987, 1992, 1998

International Standard Book Number 0-323-01240-X

Publishing Director: Richard H. Lampert
Development Director: Kathryn H. Falk
Publishing Services Manager: Patricia Tannian
Project Manager: John Casey
Design Manager: Gail Morey Hudson
Cover Design: Renée Duenow

GW/MVY

Printed in the United States of America

Last digit is the print number: 9 8 7 6 5 4 3 2 1

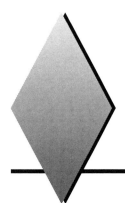

Contributors

FREDERICK M. AZAR, MD
Assistant Professor and Residency Program Director
Department of Orthopaedic Surgery
University of Tennessee–Campbell Clinic
Memphis, Tennessee

JAMES H. BEATY, MD
Professor, Department of Orthopaedic Surgery
University of Tennessee–Campbell Clinic;
Chief of Staff, Campbell Clinic
Memphis, Tennessee

JAMES H. CALANDRUCCIO, MD
Assistant Professor, Department of Orthopaedic Surgery
University of Tennessee–Campbell Clinic
Memphis, Tennessee

S. TERRY CANALE, MD
Professor and Chairman, Department of Orthopaedic Surgery
University of Tennessee–Campbell Clinic;
Chief of Pediatric Orthopaedics
Le Bonheur Children's Medical Center
Memphis, Tennessee

PETER G. CARNESALE, MD
Associate Professor Emeritus
Department of Orthopaedic Surgery
University of Tennessee–Campbell Clinic
Memphis, Tennessee

KEVIN B. CLEVELAND, MD
Instructor, Department of Orthopaedic Surgery
University of Tennessee–Campbell Clinic
Memphis, Tennessee

ANDREW H. CRENSHAW, Jr., MD
Assistant Professor, Department of Orthopaedic Surgery
University of Tennessee–Campbell Clinic
Memphis, Tennessee

JOHN R. CROCKARELL, Jr., MD
Assistant Professor, Department of Orthopaedic Surgery
University of Tennessee–Campbell Clinic
Memphis, Tennessee

GREGORY DABOV, MD
Instructor, Department of Orthopaedic Surgery
University of Tennessee–Campbell Clinic
Memphis, Tennessee

A.U. (DAN) DANIELS, MD
Professor Emeritus, Department of Orthopaedic Surgery
University of Tennessee–Campbell Clinic
Memphis, Tennessee

JEFFREY A. DLABACH, MD
Instructor, Department of Orthopaedic Surgery
University of Tennessee–Campbell Clinic
Memphis, Tennessee

BARRY L. FREEMAN III, MD
Professor, Department of Orthopaedic Surgery
University of Tennessee–Campbell Clinic
Memphis, Tennessee

JAMES L. GUYTON, MD
Assistant Professor, Department of Orthopaedic Surgery
University of Tennessee–Campbell Clinic
Memphis, Tennessee

JAMES W. HARKESS, MD
Assistant Professor, Department of Orthopaedic Surgery
University of Tennessee–Campbell Clinic
Memphis, Tennessee

ROBERT K. HECK, Jr., MD
Instructor, Department of Orthopaedic Surgery
University of Tennessee–Campbell Clinic
Memphis, Tennessee

CHRISTOPHER HENDRIX, DPM
Staff, Campbell Clinic
Memphis, Tennessee

MARK T. JOBE, MD
Assistant Professor, Department of Orthopaedic Surgery
University of Tennessee–Campbell Clinic
Memphis, Tennessee

DAVID G. LaVELLE, MD
Associate Professor, Department of Orthopaedic Surgery
University of Tennessee–Campbell Clinic
Memphis, Tennessee

MARVIN R. LEVENTHAL, MD
Associate Professor, Department of Orthopaedic Surgery
University of Tennessee–Campbell Clinic
Memphis, Tennessee

DOUGLAS A. LINVILLE, MD
Associate Professor, Department of Orthopaedic Surgery
University of Tennessee–Campbell Clinic
Memphis, Tennessee

SANTOS F. MARTINEZ, MD
Physical Medicine and Rehabilitation
Campbell Clinic
Memphis, Tennessee

ROBERT H. MILLER III, MD
Assistant Professor, Department of Orthopaedic Surgery
University of Tennessee–Campbell Clinic
Memphis, Tennessee

G. ANDREW MURPHY, MD
Instructor, Department of Orthopaedic Surgery
University of Tennessee–Campbell Clinic;
Co-Director, Campbell Clinic Foot and Ankle
    Surgery Fellowship
Memphis, Tennessee

ASHLEY L. PARK, MD
Clinical Assistant Professor, Department of Internal Medicine
Division of Rehabilitation Medicine
University of Tennessee College of Medicine;
Staff, Campbell Clinic
Memphis, Tennessee

EDWARD A. PEREZ, MD
Instructor, Department of Orthopaedic Surgery
University of Tennessee–Campbell Clinic
Memphis, Tennessee

BARRY B. PHILLIPS, MD
Assistant Professor, Department of Orthopaedic Surgery
University of Tennessee–Campbell Clinic
Memphis, Tennessee

ROBERT M. PICKERING, MD
Assistant Professor, Department of Orthopaedic Surgery
University of Tennessee–Campbell Clinic
Memphis, Tennessee

E. GREER RICHARDSON, MD
Professor, Department of Orthopaedic Surgery
University of Tennessee–Campbell Clinic;
Co-Director, Campbell Clinic Foot and Ankle
    Surgery Fellowship
Memphis, Tennessee

WILLIAM C. WARNER, Jr., MD
Associate Professor, Department of Orthopaedic Surgery
University of Tennessee–Campbell Clinic;
Chief, Mississippi Children's Special Services
Le Bonheur Children's Hospital
Memphis, Tennessee

A. PAIGE WHITTLE, MD
Assistant Professor, Department of Orthopaedic Surgery
University of Tennessee–Campbell Clinic;
Chief of Orthopaedics
Veterans Administration Hospital
Memphis, Tennessee

KEITH D. WILLIAMS, MD
Assistant Professor, Department of Orthopaedic Surgery
University of Tennessee–Campbell Clinic
Memphis, Tennessee

DEXTER H. WITTE, MD
Clinical Assistant Professor of Radiology
Department of Orthopaedic Surgery
University of Tennessee–Campbell Clinic
Memphis, Tennessee

GEORGE W. WOOD II, MD
Professor, Department of Orthopaedic Surgery
University of Tennessee–Campbell Clinic;
Chief of Orthopaedic Trauma, Regional Medical Center
Memphis, Tennessee

PHILLIP E. WRIGHT II, MD
Professor, Director, Hand Fellowship
Department of Orthopaedic Surgery
University of Tennessee–Campbell Clinic
Memphis, Tennessee

In fond memory of

Dr. Alvin J. Ingram and **Dr. Fred P. Sage**

two of the "giants" of orthopaedic surgery on whose shoulders we stand.

To my wife

Martha (Sissie) Canale

without whose support and encouragement
this book would not have been possible.

Willis C. Campbell, M.D.
1880-1941

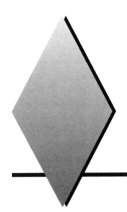

Preface

Almost 75 years ago Willis Cahoon Campbell wrote his *Textbook on Orthopaedic Surgery*. The first edition of *Campbell's Operative Orthopaedics* was published in 1939. We are now celebrating the tenth edition of the text.

The growth of the field of orthopaedic surgery has been paralleled by the growth of *Campbell's Operative Orthopaedics*. The enormous advances in our understanding of orthopaedic conditions and in the devices and techniques used to treat them were made possible by pioneer physicians in orthopaedics, many of whom also were contributors to earlier editions of *Campbell's Operative Orthopaedics*. Although Campbell alone wrote and edited the first edition, he soon had admirable help from partners such as Speed, Knight, Smith, Boyd, and Crenshaw and also from others outside the Campbell Clinic such as Smith-Peterson, Aufranc, Bateman, and Slocum. This tenth edition is deeply indebted to all those past and present contributors to this text.

All of us in the field of orthopaedic surgery can be proud because of the significant advances and contributions made in the areas of arthroscopy and arthroplasty and in the subspecialties of sports medicine, hand, foot, pediatrics, joint reconstruction, and rehabilitation. The inventions and innovations in each of these areas have lessened the burden of disease on our patients and will do so even more in the future. As a result of the ever-expanding knowledge and experience of orthopaedic surgeons, in past editions and especially in this edition, *Campbell's Operative Orthopaedics* has tried to describe the most useful of these operative advances. We have not aspired to be the first to "pick up the sword," nor have we wanted to be the last to "drop the shield." We have attempted to include the mainstream, proven techniques, along with some of the promising cutting-edge techniques and even some of the older techniques that may be applicable to areas of the world where the latest technology is unavailable.

In keeping up with the times and changing technology, this edition includes a CD-ROM with videos that demonstrate commonly performed orthopaedic operations. Also, the content of the four-volume set is available both in print and on a CD-ROM. Finally, key techniques in *Campbell's Operative Orthopaedics* are available in seven handheld (PDA) modules: adult reconstruction, congenital anomalies and pediatrics, spine, sports medicine and arthroscopy, hand, ankle and foot, and trauma.

Several other new features have been added to this edition. Techniques are numbered within each chapter, and all techniques in each volume are listed on the front and back endsheets for quick reference. Key references in the exhaustive reference lists are highlighted in boldface type. CD-ROM icons within the text indicate that the technique being described also is demonstrated on the video CD.

The publishing of a new edition of *Campbell's Operative Orthopaedics* every 6 or 7 years means that the minute one edition is completed, even while the presses are still hot, we start working on the next edition. People often ask me how we can turn out almost 5000 pages of text with nearly 10,000 illustrations every 5 or 6 years. My answer is easy and can be summed up in four words: Kay, Linda, Barry, and Joan. Without the hard work of Kay Daugherty, Linda Jones, Barry Burns, and Joan Crowson, this book would not be 75 years old.

S.T. Canale

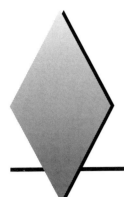

Contents

CAMPBELL'S
OPERATIVE
ORTHOPAEDICS

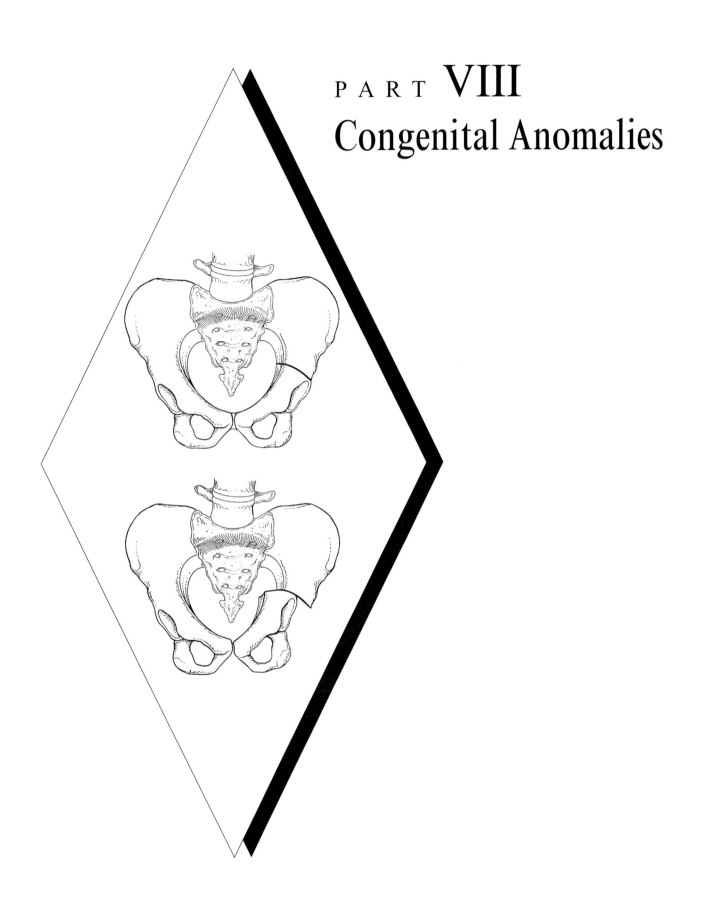

PART VIII
Congenital Anomalies

Congenital Anomalies of Lower Extremity

James H. Beaty

Congenital anomalies of the foot and lower extremity are described in this chapter. Congenital anomalies of the hip and pelvis are described in Chapter 27 and those of the trunk and upper extremities in Chapter 28. Congenital anomalies of the spine are discussed in Chapters 37 and 38, and those of the hand in Chapter 76. Many of the operative techniques described here are useful for other conditions and are found in the references in other chapters.

The most common anomaly of the toes is *polydactyly,* that is, the presence of supernumerary digits; others are *syndactyly* (webbed toes), *macrodactyly* (enlarged toes), and *congenital contracture or angulation.* Any of these conditions may require surgery. When surgery is contemplated for anomalies of the toes, several factors must be considered, including cosmesis,

pain, and difficulty in fitting shoes. A satisfactory clinical result should correct all of these problems.

Polydactyly

Polydactyly of the toes may occur in established genetic syndromes but occurs most commonly as an isolated trait with an autosomal dominant inheritance pattern and variable expression. The overall incidence of polydactyly is approximately 2 cases per 1000 live births. Surgical treatment of polydactyly is amputation of the accessory digit. Preoperative roentgenograms should be obtained to detect any extra metatarsal articulating with the digit, which should be

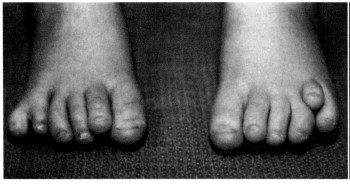
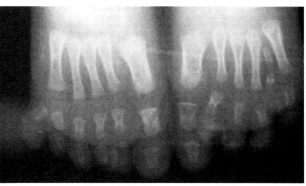

Fig. 26-1   A, Bilateral polydactyly in 6-month-old child. **B,** Accessory metatarsal of left foot can be seen on roentgenogram.

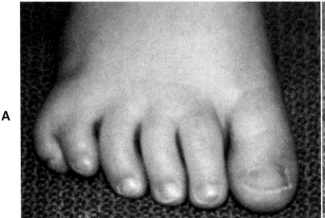
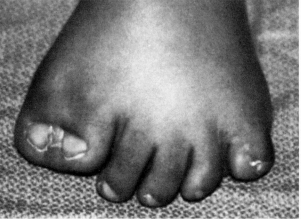

Fig. 26-2   Polydactyly-syndactyly. A, Simple type, right fifth toe with syndactyly of web space. **B,** Complex type, left great toe and fifth toe with bony and soft tissue syndactyly.

amputated with its associated digit (Fig. 26-1). Occasionally, a combined polydactyly-syndactyly deformity requires more complex surgical correction (Fig. 26-2), such as resection of the more peripheral digit using residual skin for coverage or the Bilhaut-Cloquet procedure.

Venn-Watson classified polydactyly and directed attention to the difference between preaxial and postaxial types (Fig. 26-3). In preaxial polydactyly the most medial great toe usually is excised. The remaining great toe should have a careful repair of the capsule if necessary to prevent residual hallux varus; Kirschner wire fixation is used for 4 to 6 weeks. The technique for postaxial polydactyly is described below.

◆ AMPUTATION OF EXTRA TOE

TECHNIQUE 26-1
At the base of the toe to be amputated, make an oval or racquet-shaped incision through the skin and fascia (Fig. 26-4). Draw the tendons distally as far as possible and divide them. Incise the capsule of the metatarsophalangeal

joint transversely, dissect it from the metatarsal, and disarticulate the joint. With an osteotome or bone-cutting forceps, sharply resect any bone that may have protruded from the metatarsal head to support the articular surface of the amputated phalanx. If the roentgenogram has revealed an extra metatarsal, resect it after continuing the incision proximally on the lateral or dorsal aspect of the foot.

Syndactyly

Syndactyly of the toes rarely interferes with function, and surgery is indicated primarily for cosmetic reasons; the same technique is used as for the fingers (see Chapter 76).

Macrodactyly

Macrodactyly occurs when one or more toes or fingers have hypertrophied and are significantly larger than the surrounding

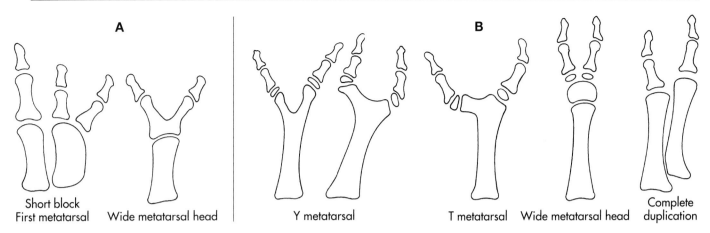

Fig. 26-3   Venn-Watson classification of polydactyly. **A,** Preaxial polydactyly. **B,** Postaxial polydactyly. (Redrawn from Venn-Watson EA: *Orthop Clin North Am* 7:909, 1976.)

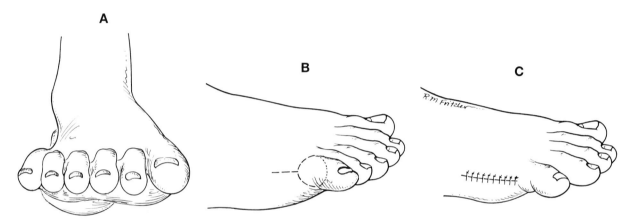

Fig. 26-4   Polydactyly. **A,** Front view of foot. **B,** Outline of incision passing through web space between fifth and sixth toes and extending in racquet-shaped incision along lateral border of foot. **C,** Surgical excision of supernumerary digit.

toes or fingers. The most common associated conditions are neurofibromatosis and hemangiomatosis. Surgery is indicated to relieve functional symptoms, primarily pain or difficulty in fitting shoes. The cosmetic goal is to alter the grotesque appearance of the toes and foot and to achieve a foot similar in size to the opposite foot (Fig. 26-5).

Many operative procedures have been described for the treatment of macrodactyly, including reduction syndactyly, soft tissue debulking combined with ostectomy or epiphysiodesis, toe amputation, and ray amputation. Soft tissue debulking combined with ostectomy or epiphysiodesis can be used in the initial treatment of a single digit with macrodactyly; unfortunately, the recurrence rate with this technique is virtually 100%. Grogan et al. reported that their best results were obtained with ray amputation, phalangeal epiphysiodesis, and debulking in 10 patients with congenital lipofibromatosis and macrodactyly of the foot. Syndactylization and phalangeal resection were not as successful. They recommended ray resection, combined with debulking repeated as necessary. Kotwal and Farooque de-

scribed a staged procedure in which defatting was done on one side of digit, usually the convex, to reduce the thickness by 10% to 20% (Fig. 26-6). Three months later, defatting was done on the other side, along with shortening of the bone. In their technique an entire phalanx was removed, the capsules of the adjacent joints were sutured, and a Kirschner wire was inserted for stabilization. At an average follow-up of 9 years, 12 of 21 patients had good results (reduction by 50% or more), 7 had satisfactory results (reduction by 25% to 50% but with angular deformity), and 2 had poor results (cosmetically unacceptable, requiring amputation).

When enlargement of the toe or forefoot is less severe, epiphysiodesis of the phalangeal physes is recommended when the toe reaches adult size; debulking is repeated as necessary. Topleski et al. reported that in 9 of 11 macrodactylic toes treated with open epiphysiodesis and debulking the overall length of the proximal phalanx did not change in the average 2-year follow-up after surgery. The average age at the time of surgery was 3.7 years (11 months to 6.5 years). Ray amputation

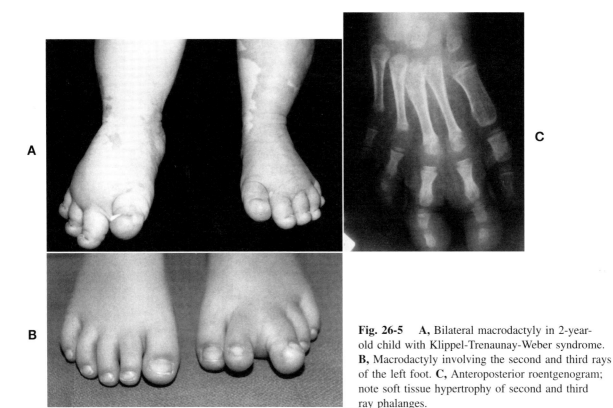

Fig. 26-5   A, Bilateral macrodactyly in 2-year-old child with Klippel-Trenaunay-Weber syndrome. **B,** Macrodactyly involving the second and third rays of the left foot. **C,** Anteroposterior roentgenogram; note soft tissue hypertrophy of second and third ray phalanges.

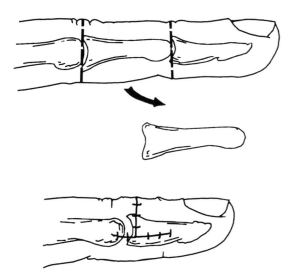

Fig. 26-6   Bone shortening with removal of whole phalanx for macrodactyly. (From Kotwal PP, Farooque M: Macrodactyly, *J Bone Joint Surg* 80B:651, 1998.)

is indicated in patients with massive enlargement of the bone and soft tissues. Ray amputation is also the procedure of choice for severe recurrence after reduction syndactyly or soft tissue debulking. Hallux valgus may occur after resection of the second ray and occasionally requires surgical correction during adolescence.

◆ RAY REDUCTION

TECHNIQUE 26-2
Outline dorsal skin incisions along the ray to be reduced, with a single long incision or multiple small incisions along the metatarsal and phalanges. Debulk any fibrofatty tissue, taking care to protect the digital neurovascular bundles. Osteotomize the metatarsal neck and shorten the metatarsal by removing a segment of sufficient length to match this metatarsal to the others. Fuse the physis at the level of the metatarsal head. If necessary, repeat this process for any phalanges until the ray has been shortened to normal length. Insert a smooth, longitudinal Kirschner wire from the tip of the toe to the base of the metatarsal to align the ray. Secure hemostasis and close the wound with interrupted sutures and apply a short leg cast.

AFTERTREATMENT. The Kirschner wire is removed at 6 weeks, and a short leg walking cast is worn for 6 more weeks.

◆ RAY AMPUTATION

TECHNIQUE 26-3
Outline the ray to be amputated with skin flaps to include amputation from the tip of the toe to the base of the

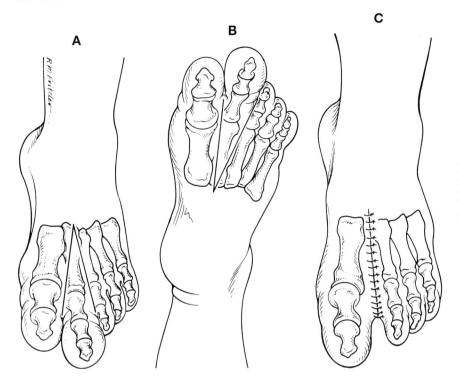

Fig. 26-7   Ray amputation for macrodactyly. **A,** Incision on dorsal surface of foot. **B,** Plantar incision. **C,** Closed incision after amputation.

metatarsal. Make dorsal and plantar incisions starting over the metatarsophalangeal joint, with connecting incisions in the web space of adjacent toes. Continue the incisions proximally, both dorsally and plantarward, to the base of the metatarsal to be resected (Fig. 26-7). Amputate the metatarsal and its associated phalanges, as well as any surrounding hypertrophied soft tissue. Take care to protect the neurovascular bundles that supply adjacent toes. After adequate resection of tissue, close the wound with interrupted sutures in the usual manner.

AFTERTREATMENT. A short leg cast is applied to protect the wound until healing occurs at 6 to 12 weeks.

◆ Cleft Foot (Partial Adactyly)

Cleft foot (lobster foot) is an anomaly in which a single cleft extends proximally into the foot, sometimes even as far as the midfoot. Generally one or more toes and parts of their metatarsals are absent, and often the tarsals are abnormal. Although the deformity varies in degree and type, the first and fifth rays usually are present (Fig. 26-8). If a metatarsal is partially or completely absent, its respective toe is always absent. Based on a study of the roentgenographic characteristics of 173 cleft feet (128 from the literature), Blauth and Borisch classified the deformities into six types based on the number of metatarsal bones present. Types I and II are cleft feet with minor deficiencies, both having five metatarsals. The metatarsals are all normal in type I and partially hypoplastic in type II. The number of identifiable metatarsals decreases progressively: type III, four metatarsals; type IV, three metatarsals; type V, two metatarsals; and type VI, one metatarsal.

Abraham et al. described a simplified clinical classification on which they based treatment recommendations (Fig. 26-9). Type I has a central ray cleft or deficiency (usually second or third rays or both) extending up to the mid-metatarsal level without splaying of medial or lateral rays. For this type of cleft foot, they recommended soft tissue syndactylism with partial hallux valgus correction if needed. Type II has a deep cleft up to the tarsal bones with forefoot splaying, for which they recommended soft tissue syndactylism, with first-ray osteotomy if needed, before the age of 5 years. Type III is a complete absence of the first through third or fourth rays, for which they did not recommend surgery. They reported satisfactory results (no additional surgery, no recurrence of the cleft, normal painless shoe wear, and satisfied patient) after 23 of 24 surgical procedures (Fig. 26-10); 6 of 9 untreated feet (6 type I, 2 type II, and 1 type III) also had satisfactory results. Abraham et al. recommended syndactylism for all type II cleft feet in the first 3 years of life while the forefoot is still supple. All of their patients older than 5 years with type II deformities had first ray amputation.

Any surgery for cleft foot should improve function and appearance. When the cleft extends proximally between the metatarsals, the skin of the apposing surfaces within the cleft is excised, but dorsal and plantar flaps are left that will close the cleft when sutured together. If a metatarsal has no corresponding toe, it is resected and the cleft is closed as just described

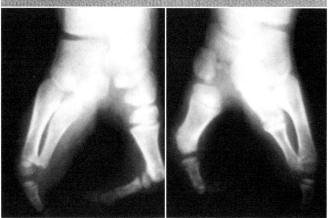

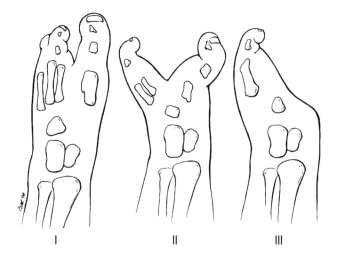

Fig. 26-8 **A,** Bilateral cleft foot in 4-year-old boy. **B,** Antero-posterior view; note angular deformity of metatarsophalangeal joints of great toe and fifth toe.

Fig. 26-9 Clinical classification of cleft foot deformity (see text). (From Abraham E, Waxman B, Shirali S, Durkin M: *J Pediatr Orthop* 19:404, 1999.)

(Fig. 26-11). Any bony or joint deformity of the first or fifth ray should be corrected at the time of surgery. This may require capsulotomies and osteotomies of any retained rays. If pin fixation is used, the pins and short leg cast are removed 6 weeks after surgery, and a short leg walking cast may be worn for an additional 4 to 6 weeks.

Wood, Pepper, and Shook reported good cosmetic and functional results in seven patients after a simplified cleft closure using rectangular flaps. According to them, this technique is easier than techniques using multiple triangular flaps and produces superior cosmetic results. They recommend correction of the cleft foot as early as 6 months of age because of fewer anesthesia risks, minimal growth deformities, and malleability of the soft tissues.

TECHNIQUE 26-4 *(Wood, Pepper, Shook)*

At least two metatarsals must be present for good cleft closure. On the lateral side, or fifth ray, raise a rectangular flap, starting from the plantar surface of the foot to the

continued

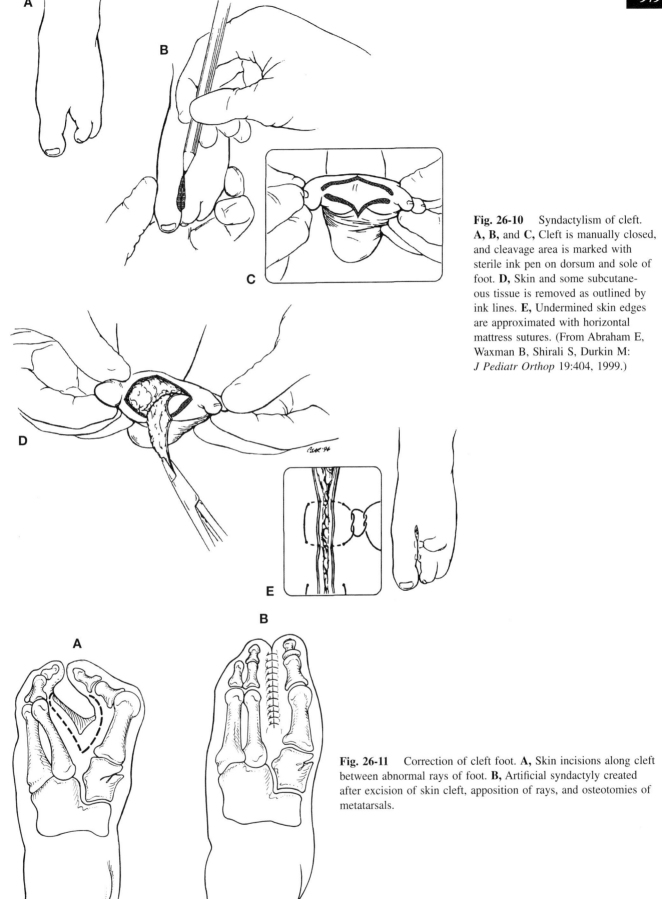

Fig. 26-10 Syndactylism of cleft. **A, B,** and **C,** Cleft is manually closed, and cleavage area is marked with sterile ink pen on dorsum and sole of foot. **D,** Skin and some subcutaneous tissue is removed as outlined by ink lines. **E,** Undermined skin edges are approximated with horizontal mattress sutures. (From Abraham E, Waxman B, Shirali S, Durkin M: *J Pediatr Orthop* 19:404, 1999.)

Fig. 26-11 Correction of cleft foot. **A,** Skin incisions along cleft between abnormal rays of foot. **B,** Artificial syndactyly created after excision of skin cleft, apposition of rays, and osteotomies of metatarsals.

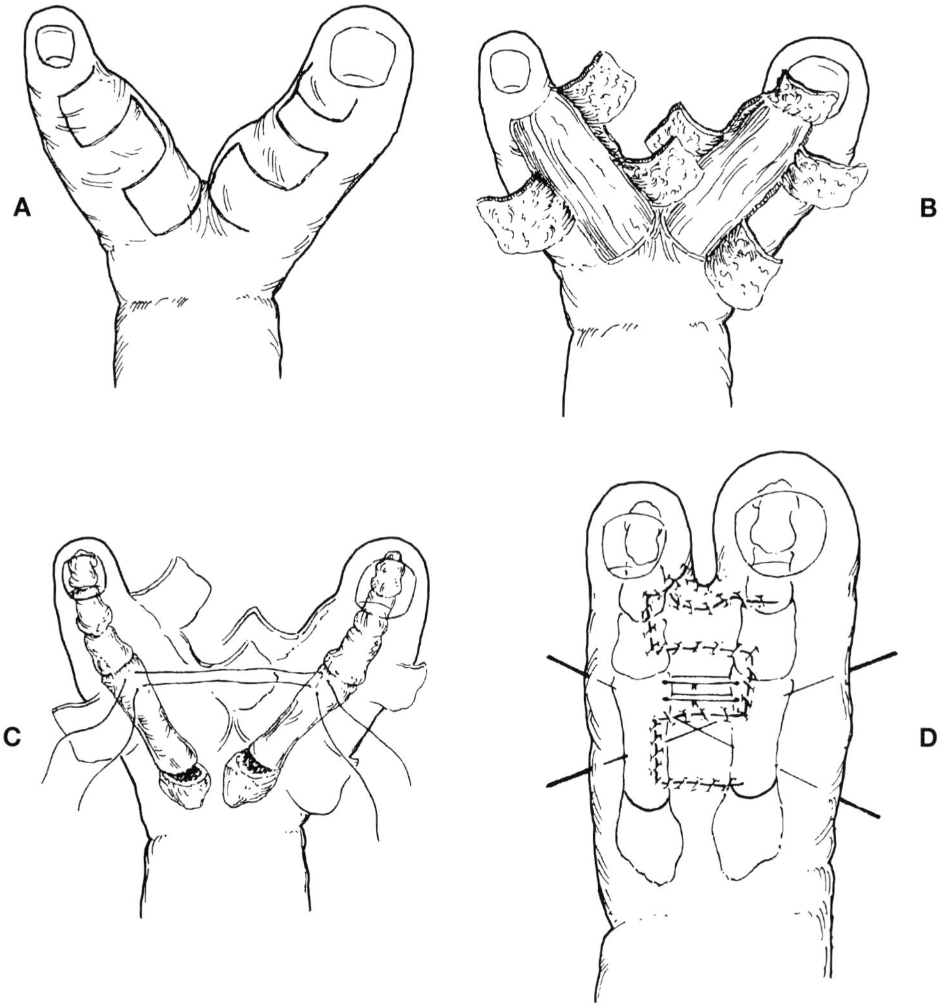

Fig. 26-12 Cleft-foot closure (see text). **A,** Rectangular flaps are raised on both rays. **B,** Flaps are raised until skin of entire cleft is removed. At distal tip of longer toe, flap is raised to suture to adjacent toe to make wide toe web. **C,** If toes spring apart, closing wedge osteotomy is made at base of each metatarsal to centralize bones. **D,** Kirschner wires are inserted to maintain position. (From Wood VE, Peppers TA, Shook J: *J Pediatr Orthop* 17:501, 1997.)

dorsum (Fig. 26-12, *A*). This does not include fascia but includes a fairly thick flap with fat. Exactly opposite this flap on the medial side, or first ray, raise a rectangular flap starting on the dorsum of the foot to the plantar aspect. Repeat this two or three times until the skin of the entire cleft is removed (Fig. 26-12, *B*). At the longest toe, raise a distally based flap for suturing to the adjacent toe to make a wide web. If the toes spring apart, make a closing wedge osteotomy at the base of each metatarsal to centralize the toes (Fig. 26-12, *C*) and stabilize the osteotomies with Kirschner wires (Fig. 26-12, *D*). To further stabilize the intermetacarpal distance and unload tension on the surgical flaps, reconstruct the intermetacarpal ligament with either local ligamentous tissue, joint capsule, or tendon obtained from the cleft foot or with autograft plantaris tendon or fascia lata. Close the wound in routine fashion and apply a cast.

AFTERTREATMENT. At 3 weeks, weight-bearing in a walking cast is allowed. At 6 weeks, the cast is discontinued and the Kirschner wires are removed.

Contracture or Angulation of Toes

Congenital contracture, angulation, or subluxation of the fifth toe is a fairly common familial deformity but rarely causes symptoms. The anomaly is rarely disabling, and surgery usually is indicated only to improve function of the foot. The direction of angulation of the fifth toe determines the operative procedure (Fig. 26-13). Surgical procedures for the correction of an angulated toe include soft tissue correction alone, soft tissue correction with proximal phalangectomy, and amputation. Black et al. reported good results in 34 of 36 (94%) Butler arthroplasties done for correction of a dorsally overriding fifth toe.

One complication of the Butler arthroplasty is the potential for vascular damage caused by excessive tension on the neurovascular bundle. This complication can be prevented by (1) avoiding any tension on the neurovascular bundle, (2) taking care not to manipulate or exert traction on the toe, and (3) avoiding the use of circumferential taping or rigid splinting.

◆ ARTHROPLASTY OF FIFTH METATARSOPHALANGEAL JOINT

TECHNIQUE 26-5 *(Butler)*

After preparing and draping the foot and applying a tourniquet, make a double racquet incision, with the dorsal handle following the extensor longus tendon and the plantar handle inclined laterally to provide a circumferential incision (Fig. 26-14, *A*). To expose the contracted extensor tendon, elevate skin flaps by blunt dissection, taking care to protect the neurovascular bundle (Fig. 26-14, *B*). Transect the extensor tendon to the fifth toe and divide the dorsal aspect of the metatarsophalangeal joint capsule (Fig. 26-14, *C*). The toe should now partially rotate downward and laterally into the correct position. In long-

continued

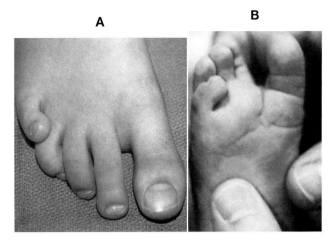

Fig. 26-13 Congenital contracture of fifth toe. **A,** Dorsal overlapping of fifth toe over fourth toe. **B,** Fifth toe shows plantar flexion and medial contracture beneath fourth toe.

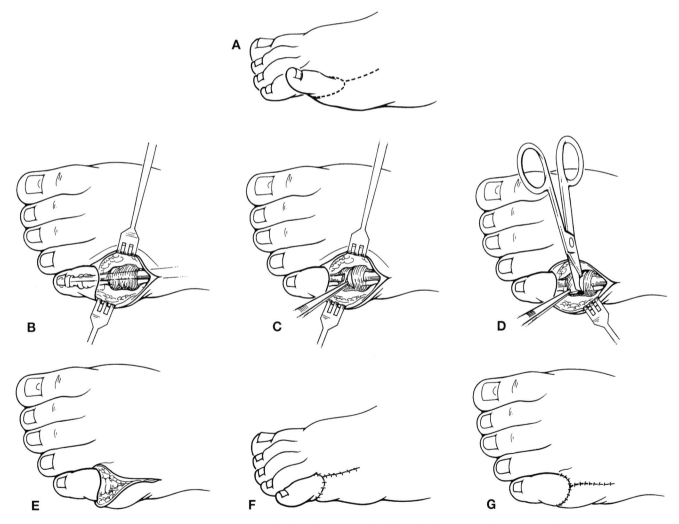

Fig. 26-14 Butler arthroplasty. **A,** Double racquet incision. **B,** Exposure of extensor tendon. **C,** Transection of extensor tendon. **D,** Separation of adherent capsule. **E,** Corrected position of toe. **F** and **G,** Skin closure. (Redrawn from Black GB, Grogan DP, Bobechko WP: *J Pediatr Orthop* 5:438, 1985.)

standing deformities, the plantar aspect of the capsule is adherent and prevents full reduction of the proximal phalanx on the metatarsal during derotation of the toe. If necessary, separate the adherent plantar capsule by blunt dissection and divide it transversely to allow the toe to lie freely in a fully corrected position (Fig. 26-14, *D* and *E*). Close the skin with multiple interrupted sutures and apply a light dressing to the suture line (Fig. 26-14, *F* and *G*). No splint or cast is necessary.

AFTERTREATMENT. A short leg cast or postoperative surgical shoe may be worn, with a light dressing only over the fifth toe. Protected activity is allowed as tolerated.

Congenital Hallux Varus

Congenital hallux varus is a deformity in which the great toe is angled medially at the metatarsophalangeal joint. It should not be confused with varus deformity of the first metatarsal (metatarsus primus varus) in which the metatarsophalangeal joint is not deformed. The varus deformity of the toe can vary in severity from only a few degrees to as much as 90 degrees.

Congenital hallux varus usually is unilateral and is associated with one or more of the following: (1) a short, thick first metatarsal, (2) accessory bones or toes, (3) varus deformity of one or more of the four lateral metatarsals, and (4) a firm fibrous band that extends from the medial side of the great toe to the base of the first metatarsal (Fig. 26-15).

The explanation for this anomaly is that two great toes

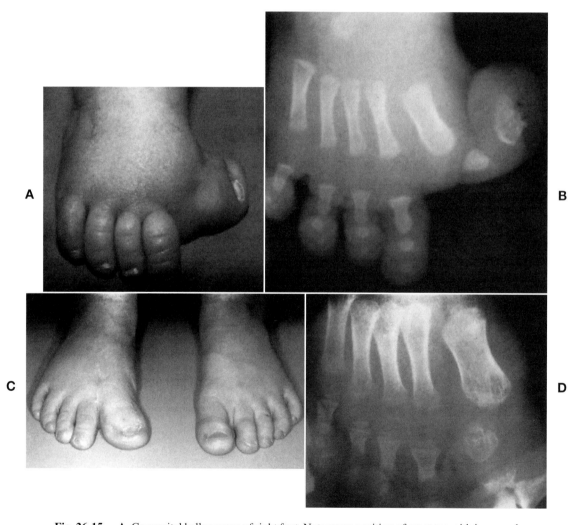

Fig. 26-15 **A,** Congenital hallux varus of right foot. Note varus position of great toe with increased web space between great and second toes. **B,** Anteroposterior roentgenogram; note short first metatarsal and accessory distal phalanx. Clinical (**C**) and roentgenographic (**D**) appearance after surgical correction.

originate in utero but the medial or accessory one fails to develop. Later, the rudimentary medial toe, together with the band of fibrous tissue, acts like a taut bowstring and gradually pulls the more fully developed great toe into a varus position.

The proper treatment for congenital hallux varus depends on the severity of the deformity and the rigidity of the contracted soft structures. The Farmer technique is effective in correcting mild or moderate deformity. The operation of Kelikian et al. is also satisfactory for severe deformity with an excessively short first metatarsal (Fig. 26-16). If the deformity is complicated by traumatic arthritis of the metatarsophalangeal joint, arthrodesis of this joint (Chapter 78) is indicated. In rare cases, if the deformity is too severe either to be corrected or to undergo arthrodesis, amputation is indicated.

◆ CREATION OF SYNDACTYLY OF GREAT TOE AND SECOND TOE FOR HALLUX VARUS

TECHNIQUE 26-6 *(Farmer)*

Raise a broad Y-shaped flap of skin and subcutaneous tissue from the dorsal surface of the web between the first and second toes (Fig. 26-17); base the flap dorsally in the space between the first and second metatarsals and include in it the skin contiguous with the web distally along the two toes for one third of their length. From the medial edge of the base of the flap, curve the incision medially and slightly distally across the medial aspect of the first metatarsophalangeal joint. Deepen this incision transversely through the medial part of the capsule of the first metatarsophalangeal joint.

Next, move the great toe laterally against the second toe and create a syndactyly between these two toes by suturing the apposing skin edges together. A smooth longitudinal Kirschner wire can be inserted from the tip of the great toe into the first metatarsal to align the great toe in a neutral position. Excise any accessory phalanx or hypertrophic soft tissue from the great toe through a separate dorsomedial incision. Now swing the Y-shaped flap of skin and subcutaneous tissue medially and suture it in place to cover the defect in the skin on the dorsal and medial aspects of the first metatarsophalangeal joint.

In an alternative technique described by Farmer, the Y-shaped flap of skin and subcutaneous tissue is raised from the plantar surface of the foot (Fig. 26-18), and the rest of the procedure is the same as described above, with the flap swung medially to cover the defect in the skin at the first metatarsophalangeal joint. Any defect that cannot be closed by the flap is either left open to heal secondarily or is covered by a full-thickness skin graft.

AFTERTREATMENT. The foot is immobilized in a cast. At 6 weeks the cast and pins are removed, and full activities are allowed.

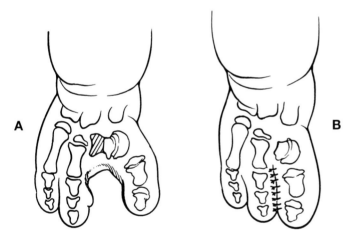

Fig. 26-16 Kelikian procedure for congenital hallux varus. **A,** Preoperative appearance of foot. **B,** After artificial syndactyly.

Congenital Metatarsus Adductus

Metatarsus adductus, which consists of adduction of the forefoot in relation to the midfoot and hindfoot, is a fairly common anomaly, often causing in-toeing in children. It can occur as an isolated anomaly or in association with clubfoot. Of those individuals with metatarsus adductus, 1% to 5% also have developmental dysplasia of the hip or acetabular dysplasia.

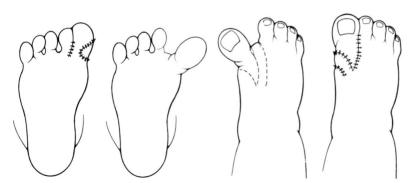

Fig. 26-17 Farmer procedure for congenital hallux varus (see text).

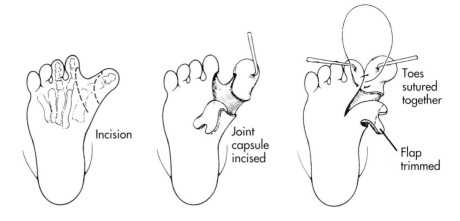

Fig. 26-18 Alternative Farmer procedure for congenital hallux varus (see text).

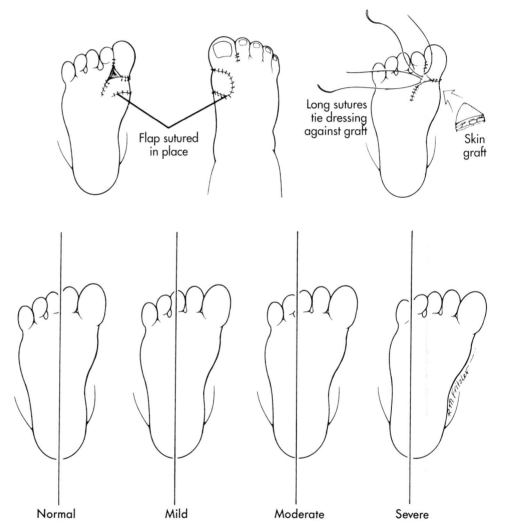

Fig. 26-19 Heel bisector defines relationship of heel to forefoot from left to right: normal (bisecting second and third toes), mild metatarsus adductus (bisecting third toe), moderate metatarsus adductus (bisecting third and fourth toes), and severe metatarsus adductus (bisecting fourth and fifth toes). (Redrawn from Bleck EE: *J Pediatr Orthop* 3:2, 1983.)

Clinically, metatarsus adductus can be classified as mild, moderate, or severe, as described by Bleck (Fig. 26-19). In the mild form the forefoot can be clinically abducted to the midline of the foot and beyond (Fig. 26-20, *A*). The moderate form has enough flexibility to allow abduction of the forefoot to the midline but usually not beyond (Fig. 26-20, *B*). In rigid metatarsus adductus, the forefoot cannot be abducted at all. There also may be a transverse crease on the medial border of the foot or an enlargement of the web space between the great and second toes (Fig. 26-21). In general, mild metatarsus adductus will resolve without treatment. Moderate or severe metatarsus adductus is best treated initially by serial stretching

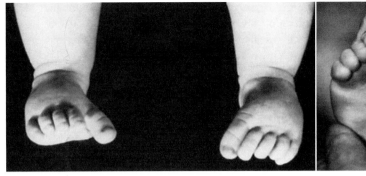
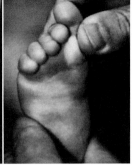

Fig. 26-20 Congenital metatarsus adductus. **A,** Mild. **B,** Moderate.

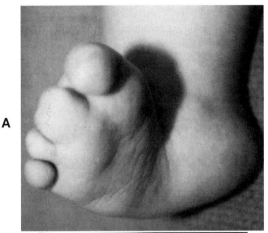

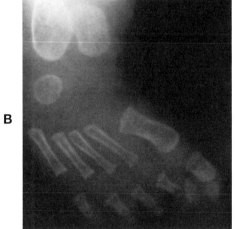

Fig. 26-21 Congenital metatarsus adductus. **A,** Severe; note deep medial transverse crease. **B,** Severe adduction as seen on roentgenogram.

and casting for 6 to 12 weeks or until the foot is clinically flexible. Katz et al. reported correction of metatarsus adductus in 65 infants with moderate (37 feet) or severe (48 feet) deformities after treatment with below-knee plaster casting.

Metatarsus adductus may be seen as a residual deformity in patients previously treated for congenital clubfoot, either surgically or nonsurgically. This residual metatarsus adductus can be rigid, indicating a fixed positioning of the forefoot on the midfoot and hindfoot, or it can be dynamic, caused by imbalance of the tibialis anterior tendon during gait. The rigidity or flexibility of the forefoot should be determined before undertaking any surgical correction in an older child.

Late sequelae of metatarsus adductus may include an increased risk of stress fractures of the lateral metatarsal bones. Theodorou et al. documented an association between metatarsus adductus deformity and lateral metatarsal stress fractures in 11 patients aged 25 to 61 years, which they attributed to altered biomechanics that placed greater loads across the lateral aspect of the foot.

TREATMENT

In a young child surgery is not indicated until conservative treatment has failed. Once a child passes the appropriate age for serial stretching and casting, surgery becomes a reasonable option. The indications for surgery include pain, objectionable appearance, or difficulty in fitting shoes because of residual forefoot adduction.

Numerous soft tissue and bony procedures have been described for correction of metatarsus adductus. We prefer to tailor the surgery to the age and deformity of the particular child (Box 26-1).

Heyman, Herndon, and Strong described mobilization of the tarsometatarsal and intermetatarsal joints by capsular release for correction of severe metatarsus adductus. This procedure occasionally is indicated in preschool children. Potential complications of the procedure include subluxation of the bases of the metatarsals and injury to the small joints of the midfoot and forefoot.

In 1970 Kendrick et al. reviewed 80 feet treated by capsular releases at the metatarsal bases (Heyman-Herndon-Strong procedure), and the result was good or excellent in 92%. They recommended the operation for children 3 to 8 years of age. Stark, Johnson, and Winter, however, reviewed results in 32 patients and found a 41% overall failure rate and a 51% incidence of painful dorsal prominence at the surgical scar. Asirvatham and Stevens reported treatment of 29 resistant forefoot adduction deformities (12 metatarsus adductus, 17 skew foot) with medial capsulotomy and abductor hallucis lengthening at an average age of 3.6 years. At a mean 3.6-year follow-up, all had improved talus–first metatarsal angles; 2

children complained of pain and 1 had persistent difficulty with shoe fitting.

In children 4 years old and older with a residual rigid metatarsus adductus, multiple metatarsal osteotomies are preferred. Berman and Gartland described dome-shaped osteotomies made at the bases of the metatarsals for this situation. Full correction also may require small lateral closing wedge osteotomies. Anderson and Schoenecker and McHale and

Lenhart described opening wedge osteotomy of the medial cuneiform, combined with closing wedge osteotomy of the cuboid, as another option for surgical correction of complex midfoot deformities.

Rarely, in children with dynamic metatarsus adductus from imbalance of the tibialis anterior tendon, especially after treatment for congenital clubfoot, either a split transfer of the tibialis anterior tendon or transfer of the entire tendon to the middle cuneiform is appropriate if symptoms are sufficient to require surgery, but this is infrequently indicated in neurologically normal children.

◆ Dome-Shaped Osteotomies of Metatarsal Bases

Berman and Gartland recommended dome-shaped osteotomies for all five metatarsal bases for resistant forefoot adduction in children 4 years of age and older (Fig. 26-22).

For a mature foot with uncorrected metatarsus adductus, or if all the medial soft tissue structures are contracted, they recommended a laterally based closing wedge osteotomy through the bases of the metatarsals. Correcting the alignment without shortening the lateral border of the foot can cause excessive tension on the skin on the medial border or on the neurovascular bundle posterior to the medial malleolus. Steinmann pins inserted parallel to the medial and lateral

---

BOX 26-1 • Treatment of Metatarsus Adductus

None: mild deformities resolve
Serial stretching and casting: rarely for moderate and severe deformities
Surgery: severe deformity uncorrected by conservative treatment
    Pain
    Objectionable appearance
    Difficulty in fitting shoes
2-4 yr   Tarsometatarsal capsulotomies (Heyman, Herndon, and Strong)
≥4 yr   Multiple metatarsal osteotomies (Berman and Gartland)
       Medial cuneiform, lateral cuboid double osteotomy

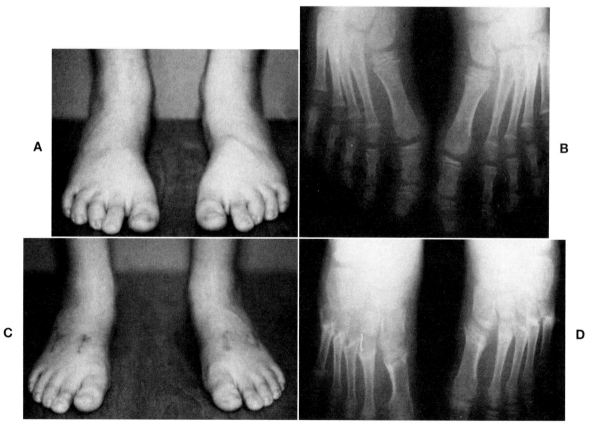

Fig. 26-22 **A** and **B,** Rigid metatarsus adductus in 8-year-old child. **C** and **D,** After multiple metatarsal osteotomies.

borders of the foot usually are necessary to hold the foot in the corrected position until the osteotomies have healed. Without internal fixation the tight structures on the medial side may cause recurrence of deformity.

TECHNIQUE 26-7 *(Berman and Gartland)*

Approach all five metatarsal bases dorsally. Make two longitudinal dorsal incisions, one between the first and second metatarsals and the other overlying the fourth. Protect the extensor tendons and superficial nerves and preserve the superficial veins as much as possible. Next, expose subperiosteally the proximal metaphysis of each metatarsal and with a small power drill make a dome-shaped osteotomy in each with the apex of the dome proximally (Fig. 26-23). Avoid the physis at the base of the first metatarsal. If adequate correction cannot be obtained by these osteotomies, resect small wedges of bone based laterally at the osteotomies as needed. Align the metatarsals and transfix the foot in the corrected position with small, smooth Steinmann pins inserted proximally through the shafts of the first and fifth metatarsals and across the osteotomies in these bones. Prevent dorsal or volar angulation and overriding of the fragments. Before closing the wound, check the placement of the pins, position of the osteotomies, and forefoot alignment by roentgenograms (Fig. 26-24). The anteroposterior talus–first metatarsal angle should be corrected to 0 to 10 degrees.

AFTERTREATMENT. A short leg cast is applied with the foot in the corrected position. At 6 weeks the cast and pins are removed and weight-bearing is begun, commonly in a walking cast for 3 to 6 weeks.

◆ Cuneiform and Cuboid Osteotomies

McHale and Lenhart recommended opening wedge osteotomy of the medial cuneiform and closing wedge osteotomy of the cuboid for correction of deformities in the midfoot with severe shortening of the medial column ("bean-shaped" foot).

TECHNIQUE 26-8 *(McHale and Lenhart)*

With the anesthetized patient supine, make a small longitudinal incision over the cuboid (Fig. 26-25, *A*). Remove a 7- to 10-mm wedge with its base in a dorsolateral position (Fig. 26-25, *B*). Approach the medial cuneiform by using part of the distal extension of the medial incision (Fig. 26-25, *A*) or a 2-cm incision medially over the medial cuneiform. Make the osteotomy in the cuneiform, leaving the anterior tibialis attached to the distal piece of bone. Spread the medial cuneiform osteotomy with a vertebral lamina spreader and insert the wedge of bone removed from the cuboid, with the base of the wedge straight medially (Fig. 26-25, *C*). Check clinical correction of the deformity (Fig. 26-25, *D*). If the lateral border of the foot still appears prominent (midfoot supination has not been corrected), remove a larger wedge of bone from the cuboid. Use two

continued

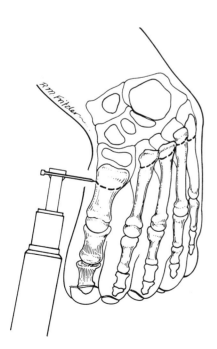

Fig. 26-23 Berman and Gartland technique for metatarsal osteotomies. Dome-shaped osteotomy is completed at base of each metatarsal.

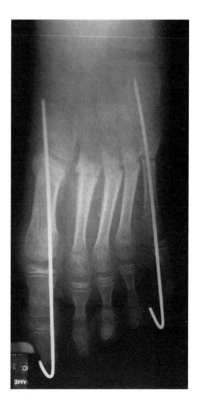

Fig. 26-24 Completed osteotomies with Steinmann pins inserted to hold corrected position.

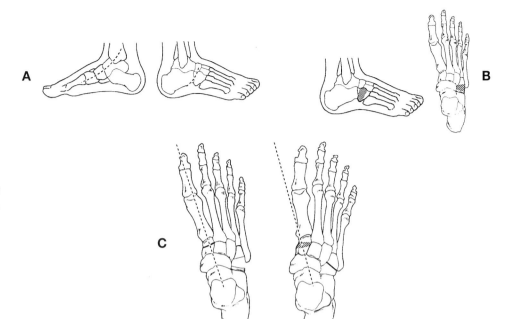

Fig. 26-25   Osteotomies of medial cuneiform and cuboid for correction of residual deformity. **A,** Lateral and medial incisions. **B,** Removal of dorsolateral wedge from cuboid. **C,** Placement of wedge in osteotomy in medial cuneiform. (Redrawn from McHale KA, Lenhart MK: *J Pediatr Orthop* 11:374, 1991.)

smooth Kirschner wires to fix the foot in the corrected position. Insert one pin through the cuboid, starting in the calcaneus and exiting through the base of the fifth metatarsal. Place the other pin through the first web space, through the medial cuneiform and tarsal navicular, and into the talus. Confirm the position of the pins and the correction of the bony deformity with roentgenograms. After correct positioning of the foot, the lateral three toes may remain in passively uncorrectable flexion. If so, perform simple flexor tenotomy. Close the wounds and apply a short leg cast with thick cotton padding to allow for swelling.

AFTERTREATMENT. At 2 weeks the wounds are checked, and a more form-fitting, non-weight-bearing cast is applied. The pins are removed at 6 weeks, and a weight-bearing cast is applied. This cast is worn until bony union is evident on roentgenograms, usually at 8 to 12 weeks.

Congenital Clubfoot (Talipes Equinovarus)

The incidence of congenital clubfoot is approximately 1 in every 1000 live births. Although most cases are sporadic occurrences, families have been reported with clubfoot presenting as an autosomal dominant trait with incomplete penetrance. Bilateral deformities occur in 50% of patients.

Several theories have been proposed regarding the cause of clubfoot. One is that a primary germ plasm defect in the talus causes continued plantar flexion and inversion of this bone, with subsequent soft tissue changes in the joints and musculotendinous complexes. Another theory is that primary soft tissue abnormalities within the neuromuscular units cause secondary bony changes. Clinically, children with clubfoot have a hypotrophic anterior tibial artery in addition to the obvious atrophy of the musculature about the calf. Several authors have documented abnormal distribution of type I and type II muscle fibers in clubfeet. The abnormal foot may be as much as one half to one size smaller in both length and width.

The pathological changes caused by congenital clubfoot must be understood if the anomaly is to be treated effectively. The three basic components of clubfoot are equinus, varus, and adduction deformities. However, the deformity varies in severity; the entire foot may be in an equinus and varus position with the forefoot adducted and a cavus deformity present, or the condition may be much less severe, with the foot being in only a mild equinus and varus position (Fig. 26-26). Clubfoot is accompanied by internal tibial torsion. The ankle, midtarsal, and subtalar joints all are involved in the pathological process.

In the early 1970s Turco attributed the deformity to medial displacement of the navicular and calcaneus around the talus, and his observations at surgery have helped to more clearly delineate the bony deformities in clubfoot. According to Turco, the talus is forced into equinus by the underlying calcaneus and navicular, while the head and neck of the talus are deviated medially. The calcaneus is inverted under the talus, with the posterior end displaced upward and laterally and the anterior end displaced downward and medially.

McKay added an awareness of the three-dimensional aspect of bony deformity of the subtalar complex in clubfoot. According to his description, the relationship of the calcaneus

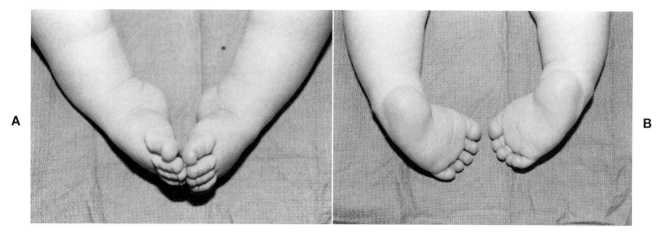

Fig. 26-26   Bilateral congenital clubfoot in newborn. **A,** Anterior view: adduction and supination of forefoot and equinus of hindfoot. **B,** Posterior view: inversion, plantar flexion, and internal rotation of calcaneus, as well as cavus deformity with transverse plantar crease.

to the talus is characterized by abnormal rotation in the sagittal, coronal, and horizontal planes. As the calcaneus rotates horizontally while pivoting on the interosseous ligament, it slips beneath the head and neck of the talus anterior to the ankle joint and the calcaneal tuberosity moves toward the fibular malleolus posteriorly. Thus the proximity of the calcaneus to the fibula is primarily caused by horizontal rotation of the talocalcaneal joint rather than by equinus alone. The heel appears to be in varus because the calcaneus rotates through the talocalcaneal joint in a coronal plane as well as horizontally. The talonavicular joint is in an extreme position of inversion as the navicular moves around the head of the talus. The cuboid is displaced medially on the calcaneus.

Herzenberg et al. demonstrated with three-dimensional computer modeling that in a clubfoot the talar neck is internally rotated relative to the ankle mortise, but the talar body is externally rotated in the mortise. They also showed the calcaneus to be significantly internally rotated with the sloped articular facet of the calcaneocuboid joint causing additional internal rotation of the midfoot.

Contractures or anomalies of the soft tissues exert further deforming forces and resist correction of bony deformity and realignment of the joints. Talocalcaneal joint realignment is opposed by the calcaneofibular ligament, the superior peroneal retinaculum (calcaneal fibular retinaculum), the peroneal tendon sheaths, and the posterior talocalcaneal ligament. Resisting realignment of the talonavicular joint are the tibialis posterior, the deltoid ligament (tibial navicular), the calcaneonavicular ligament (spring ligament), the entire talonavicular capsule, the dorsal talonavicular ligament, the bifurcated (Y) ligament, the inferior extensor retinaculum, and occasionally the cubonavicular oblique ligament. Internal rotation of the calcaneocuboid joint causes contracture of the bifurcated (Y) ligament, the long plantar ligament, the plantar calcaneocuboid ligament, the navicular cuboid ligament, the inferior extensor retinaculum (cruciate ligament), the dorsal calcaneocuboid ligament, and occasionally the cubonavicular ligament.

The metatarsals often are also deformed. They may deviate at their tarsometatarsal joints, or these joints may be normal and the shafts of the metatarsals themselves may be adducted.

If the clubfoot is allowed to remain deformed, many other late adaptive changes occur in the bones. These changes depend on the severity of the soft tissue contractures and the effects of walking. In untreated adults, some of the joints may spontaneously fuse, or they may develop degenerative changes secondary to the contractures.

The initial examination of the foot and the progress of treatment should depend on both clinical judgment and roentgenographic examination. A standard roentgenographic technique is essential, and the technician should be carefully instructed in its use.

ROENTGENOGRAPHIC EVALUATION

Roentgenograms should be included as part of the evaluation of clubfoot, before, during, and after treatment. In a nonambulatory child, standard roentgenograms include anteroposterior and stress dorsiflexion lateral roentgenograms of both feet. Anteroposterior and lateral standing roentgenograms may be obtained for an older child.

Important angles to consider in the evaluation of clubfoot are the talocalcaneal angle on the anteroposterior roentgenogram, the talocalcaneal angle on the lateral roentgenogram, and the talus–first metatarsal angle (Fig. 26-27). The anteroposterior talocalcaneal angle in normal children ranges from 30 to 55 degrees (Box 26-2). In clubfoot this angle progressively decreases with increasing heel varus. On the dorsiflexion lateral roentgenogram, the talocalcaneal angle in a normal foot varies from 25 to 50 degrees; in clubfoot this angle progressively decreases with the severity of the deformity to an angle of zero. The tibiocalcaneal angle in a normal foot is 10 to 40 degrees on the stress lateral roentgenogram. In clubfoot this angle generally is negative, indicating equinus of the calcaneus in relation to the tibia. Finally, the talus–first metatarsal angle is a

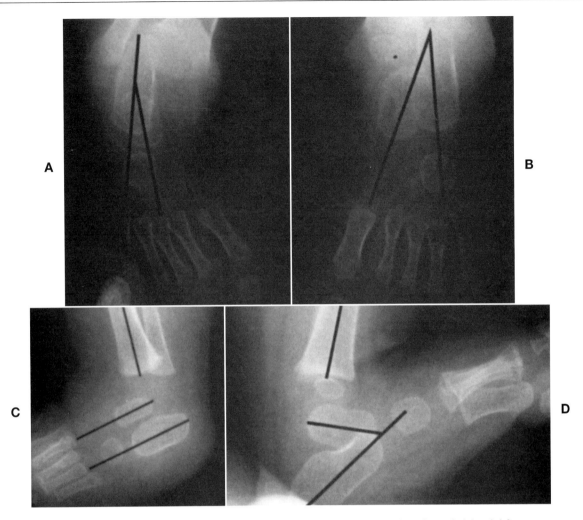

Fig. 26-27 Roentgenographic evaluation of clubfoot. **A,** Anteroposterior view of right clubfoot with decrease in talocalcaneal angle and negative talus–first metatarsal angle. **B,** Talocalcaneal angle on anteroposterior view of normal left foot. **C,** Talocalcaneal angle of zero and negative tibiocalcaneal angle on dorsiflexion lateral view of right clubfoot. **D,** Talocalcaneal and tibiocalcaneal angles on dorsiflexion lateral view of normal left foot.

BOX 26-2 • Normal Range of
Roentgenographic Angles
for Comparison to Clubfoot

Talocalcaneal angle
  Anteroposterior view: 30 to 55 degrees
  Dorsiflexion lateral view: 25 to 50 degrees
Tibiocalcaneal angle
  Stress lateral view: 10 to 40 degrees
Talus–first metatarsal angle
  Anteroposterior view: 5 to 15 degrees

---

roentgenographic measurement of forefoot adduction. This is useful in the treatment of metatarsus adductus alone but is equally important in the treatment of clubfoot to evaluate the position of the forefoot. In a normal foot, this angle is 5 to 15 degrees on the anteroposterior view; in clubfoot, it usually is negative, indicating adduction of the forefoot.

Because these roentgenographic angles often are used as criteria for evaluating outcome, it is helpful to know which angles normally change with age and to what extent. The authors measured nine commonly used angles (Fig. 26-28) on 165 roentgenograms of the normal feet in 63 patients with unilateral clubfoot. Anteroposterior and lateral views were made at the first visit, interval follow-up, and last visit, with an average follow-up of 6 years. Foot angles at the first and last visits were compared (Table 26-1). The talocalcaneal and talus–first metatarsal angles and talocalcaneal index decreased significantly (p <0.001), with a decrease of approximately 1 degree per year, reflecting changes in hindfoot valgus and forefoot abduction with normal growth. The anteroposterior calcaneus–second metatarsal angle and the lateral talocalcaneal, talus–first metatarsal, and calcaneus–first metatarsal angles decreased slightly. In contrast, the lateral tibiocalcaneal and tibiotalar angles increased with age (Fig. 26-29).

Joseph et al. measured talocalcaneal angles on anteroposterior, stress dorsiflexion, and plantarflexion lateral roentgeno-

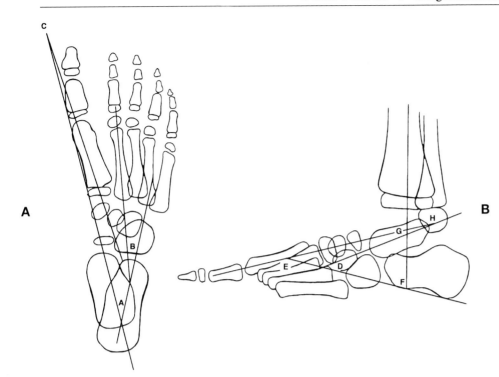

Fig. 26-28 Nine angles commonly used for evaluation of clubfoot deformity. **A,** On anteroposterior roentgenogram: *A,* anteroposterior calcaneal angle; *B,* calcaneus–second metatarsal angle; *C,* anteroposterior talus–first metatarsal angle. **B,** On lateral roentgenogram: *D,* lateral talocalcaneal angle; *E,* calcaneus–first metatarsal angle; *F,* tibiocalcaneal angle; *G,* tibiotalar angle; *H,* lateral talus–first metatarsal angle. The talocalcaneal angle is the sum and *A* and *D.*

Table 26-1 Progression of Foot Angles in Normal Feet Over Average 6-Year Follow-up

Angle	Average First Visit (degrees)	Average Last Visit (degrees)
ANTEROPOSTERIOR VIEW		
Talocalcaneal	36.3	27.4
Calcaneal–second metatarsal	14.4	12.3
Talus–first metatarsal	16.9	8.1
LATERAL VIEW		
Talocalcaneal	46	44.2
Calcaneal–first metatarsal	150	148
Tibiocalcaneal	61.5	73.2
Talus–first metatarsal	16.3	12.1
Talocalcaneal index	83	71.6

grams of 75 normal feet and 145 clubfeet and found considerable overlap in the ranges of normal and clubfeet for all angles measured. In a mathematical model to predict the probability of clubfoot correction, a difference of 20 degrees between the lateral talocalcaneal angles measured on the stress dorsiflexion and plantarflexion views indicated a 93% probability that the hindfoot deformity had been adequately corrected.

Roentgenographic findings correlate well with the clinical appearance of the foot and with the result after nonsurgical and surgical treatment. Adequate roentgenograms should be obtained during treatment to ensure that the foot is corrected not only clinically but also roentgenographically. If the deformity is unilateral, the normal foot can be used as a control to determine roentgenographic correction.

MRI and CT scanning have been recommended for preoperative and postoperative evaluation of clubfoot deformities, but we have not found these necessary for most patients.

Classification

Comparison of results of clubfoot treatment is hampered by the lack of a widely used, uniform classification system to describe the initial severity of the deformity and the outcome after treatment. A number of mostly clinical classification schemes have been proposed, including those by Carroll, Goldner, and Catterall. Two of the more recent classifications by Pirani et al. and Dimeglio et al. are based solely on physical examination and require no roentgenographic measurements or other special studies. Flynn et al. compared the two systems in the evaluation of 55 clubfeet by two orthopaedic surgeons and found that both had very good interobserver reliability after the initial learning phase. Although reliability for both systems has been demonstrated, effectiveness has not. Longer follow-up and larger numbers of patients are necessary to determine if these classifications can identify early those feet that will require surgical treatment and perhaps identify factors that are predictive of recurrence. A standardized system for scoring severity of the pretreatment deformity and the outcome after treatment would allow more accurate evaluation and comparison of different treatment methods.

NONOPERATIVE TREATMENT

The initial treatment of clubfoot is nonoperative. Various treatment regimens have been proposed, including the use of corrective splinting, taping, and casting. Treatment consists of

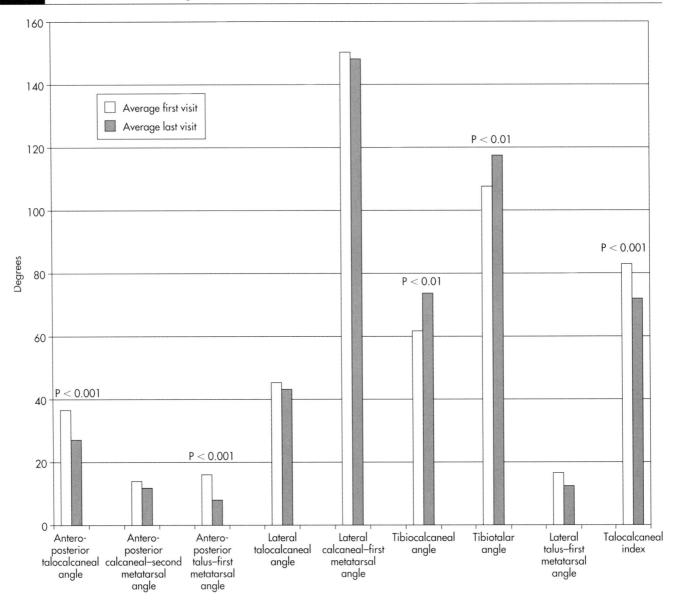

Fig. 26-29   Graph illustrating average angle values of normal foot in children with unilateral clubfoot; note that all angles decrease with age, except tibiocalcaneal and tibiotalar angles.

weekly serial manipulation and casting during the first 6 weeks of life, followed by manipulation and casting every other week until the foot is clinically and roentgenographically corrected. With experience, the clinician is able to predict which feet will respond to nonsurgical treatment. The more rigid the initial deformity, the more likely that surgical treatment will be required.

The order of correction by serial manipulation and casting should be as follows: first, correction of forefoot adduction; next, correction of heel varus; and finally, correction of hindfoot equinus. Correction should be pursued in this order so that a rocker-bottom deformity will be prevented by dorsiflexing the foot through the hindfoot rather than the midfoot. The casting program initially outlined by Kite and modified by Lovell and Hancock has been successful. The success rate of serial manipulation and casting, as reported in the literature, ranges from 15% to 80%. Yamamoto et al. used a modified Denis-Browne splint after manipulation and casting for treatment of 113 clubfeet in 76 children. Surgery was eventually required in 41 feet (36%). Of 69 feet without surgery, 66 (85%) had excellent or good results at an average 12-year follow-up. Including the 41 feet with surgical treatment, the success rate was 60%: 100% in mild deformed feet, 70% in moderately deformed feet, and 42% in severely deformed feet. There has been a renewed interest in recent years in the Ponseti casting technique, and a number or centers now believe that most clubfeet can be treated by Ponseti casting rather than surgery. Our experience has been that correction occurs in approximately 5% of children with serial casting alone. If a rocker-bottom deformity does occur, the forefoot can be placed back in plantar flexion and casting can be resumed. Surgery frequently is necessary in this situation.

If the clubfoot is corrected by the time the child is 6 months of age, this should be documented by both the clinical appearance and repeated anteroposterior and dorsiflexion

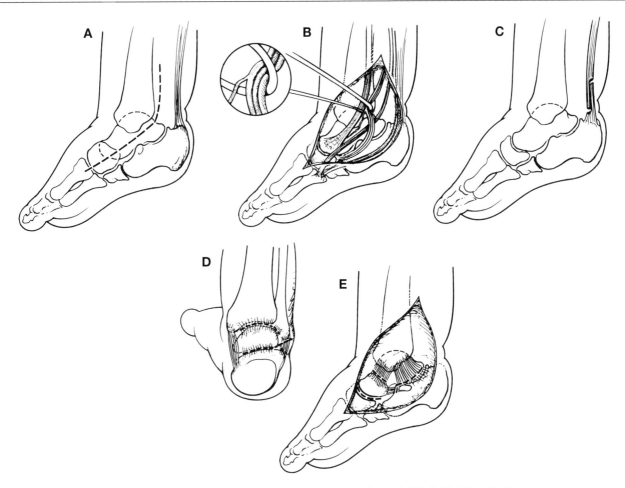

Fig. 26-30   Turco procedure for posteromedial clubfoot release. **A,** Medial incision. **B,** Exposure and lengthening of posterior tibial, flexor digitorum longus, and flexor hallucis longus tendons. *Inset,* Mobilization of neurovascular bundle. **C,** Z-plasty lengthening of tendo calcaneus. **D,** Incision of posterior capsule of ankle joint. **E,** Release of talonavicular joint and spring ligament, medial subtalar ligaments, and interosseous ligament.

lateral stress roentgenograms. The foot can be placed in an ankle-foot orthosis that can be used part-time on children with compliant families.

OPERATIVE TREATMENT

Surgery in clubfoot is indicated for deformities that do not respond to conservative treatment by serial manipulation and casting. Often in children with a significant rigid clubfoot deformity, the forefoot has been corrected by conservative treatment but the hindfoot remains fixed in both varus and equinus or the deformity has recurred. Surgery in the treatment of clubfoot must be tailored to the age of the child and to the deformity to be corrected.

In rare cases, for mild deformities with no severe internal rotational deformity of the calcaneus that requires extensive posterolateral release, the treatment of choice is a one-stage surgical release, such as the posteromedial release described by Turco (Fig. 26-30). A more extensive release that includes the posterolateral ligament complex most often is required for severe posterolateral deformity. The procedure described by McKay takes into consideration the three-dimensional defor-

mity of the subtalar joint and allows correction of the internal rotational deformity of the calcaneus and release of the contractures of the posterolateral and posteromedial foot. A modified McKay procedure through a transverse circumferential (Cincinnati) incision is our preferred technique for the initial surgical management of most clubfeet.

For severe deformities, Carroll uses two separate incisions, a curvilinear medial incision and a posterolateral incision (Fig. 26-31), to allow adequate exposure for plantar, lateral, medial, and posterior releases. The correction of the pathological condition is almost identical in the McKay and Carroll techniques; the choice of one or two incisions depends on the surgeon's preference.

Manzone found no significant differences in roentgenographic or functional results in 15 clubfeet treated with posteromedial release and 15 similar clubfeet treated with complete circumferential release. Haasbeck and Wright, however, found that an average of 28 years after surgery patients who had comprehensive (Carroll) release had fewer operations, more complete correction of heel varus, and improved subtalar motion compared to those with posteromedial release.

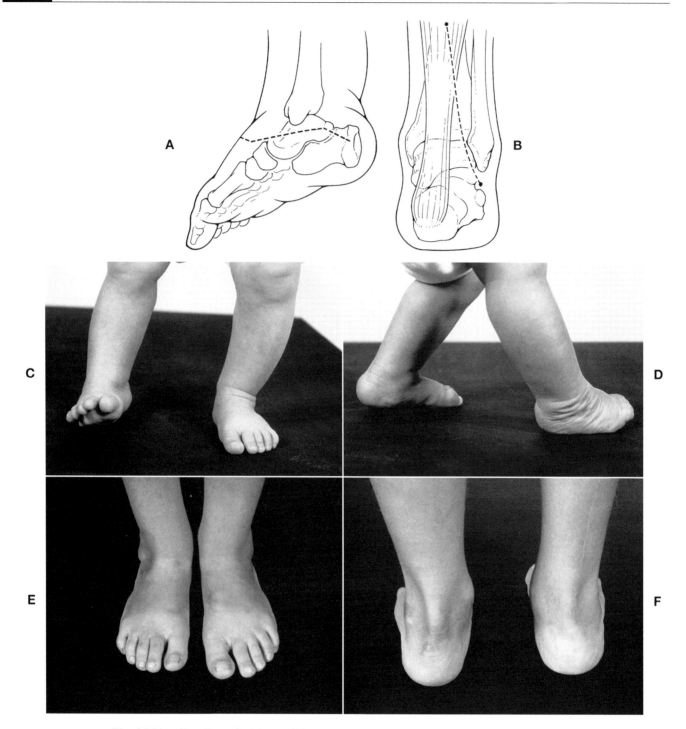

Fig. 26-31 Carroll two-incision technique. **A,** Medial incision; center of heel, front of medial malleolus, and base of first ray form a triangle. Incision *(dotted line)* parallels base of triangle but curves plantarward proximally and anteriorly distally. **B,** Posterolateral incision runs obliquely from midline of distal calf posteriorly to point midway between tendo calcaneus and lateral malleolus. **C** and **D,** Right clubfoot preoperatively. **E** and **F,** After surgical correction. (Courtesy of Norris Carroll, MD.)

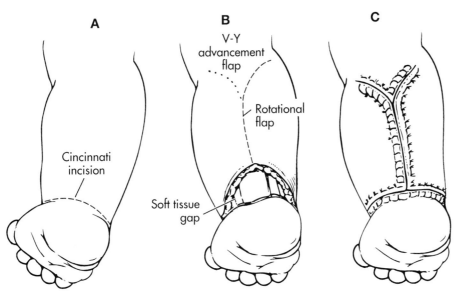

Fig. 26-32 V-Y advancement flap for closure of Cincinnati incision. **A,** Typical incision. **B,** Wound gapping after full correction of clubfoot; potential flaps are outlined. **C,** Completed V-Y advancement flaps with foot in full correction. (Redrawn from Lubicky JP, Altiok H: Regional fasciocutaneous flap closure for clubfoot surgery, *J Pediatr Orthop* 21:50, 2001.)

General principles for any one-stage extensile clubfoot release include (1) release of the tourniquet at the completion of the procedure, obtaining hemostasis by electrocautery and (2) careful subcutaneous and skin closure, with the foot in plantar flexion, if necessary, to prevent tension on the skin. The foot can be placed in a fully corrected position 2 weeks after surgery at the first postoperative cast change. Surgery can be done with the child supine or prone, at the discretion of the surgeon.

Posteromedial Release
◆ Transverse Circumferential (Cincinnati) Incision
One option for posteromedial or posterolateral release is the use of the transverse circumferential incision, also known as the *Cincinnati incision.* This incision provides excellent exposure of the subtalar joint and is useful in patients with a severe internal rotational deformity of the calcaneus. One potential problem with this incision is tension on the suture line when attempting to place the foot in dorsiflexion to apply the postoperative cast. To avoid this, the foot can be placed in plantar flexion in the immediate postoperative cast and then in dorsiflexion to the corrected position at the first cast change when the wound has healed at 2 weeks. This cast change frequently requires sedation or outpatient general anesthesia.

Lubicky and Altiok described the use of a fasciocutaneous flap closure in nine clubfeet that were treated with comprehensive posteromedial-lateral release through a Cincinnati incision (Fig. 26-32). The rotation of V-Y flaps allowed complete wound closure without any skin tension. All incisions healed without problems. Although such flap closure is infrequently needed, this method appears safe and simple to use if primary skin closure is difficult with the foot in a fully corrected position.

TECHNIQUE 26-9 *(Crawford, Marxen, and Osterfeld)*
Begin the incision on the medial aspect of the foot in the region of the naviculocuneiform joint (Fig. 26-33, *A*). Carry the incision posteriorly, gently curving beneath the distal

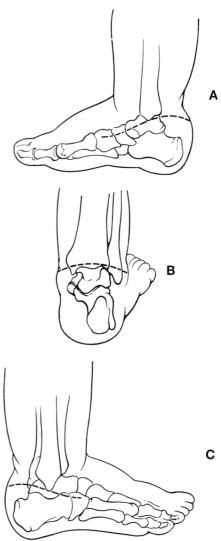

Fig. 26-33 Transverse circumferential (Cincinnati) incision as described by Crawford et al. **A,** Medial view. **B,** Posterior view. **C,** Lateral view. (Redrawn from Crawford AH, Marxen JL, Osterfeld DL: *J Bone Joint Surg* 64A:1355, 1982.)

continued

end of the medial malleolus and then ascending slightly to pass transversely over the tendo calcaneus approximately at the level of the tibiotalar joint (Fig. 26-33, *B*). Continue the incision in a gentle curve over the lateral malleolus and end it just distal and slightly medial to the sinus tarsi (Fig. 26-33, *C*). Extend the incision distally either medially or laterally, depending on the requirements of the operation.

◆ Extensile Posteromedial and Posterolateral Release (Modified McKay Procedure)

TECHNIQUE 26-10

Incise the skin through a transverse circumferential (Cincinnati) incision, preserving if possible the veins on the lateral side and protecting the sural nerve. Then dissect the subcutaneous tissue up and down the tendo calcaneus to lengthen the tendon at least 2.5 cm in the coronal plane. Incise the superior peroneal retinaculum off the calcaneus at the point where it blends with the sheath of the tendo calcaneus. Dissecting carefully, separate the calcaneofibular and posterior calcaneotalar ligaments, the thickened superior peroneal retinaculum, and the peroneal tendon sheath. Cut off the calcaneofibular ligament close to the calcaneus (this ligament is short and thick and attached very close to the apophysis). Elevate the peroneal tendon sheaths and the superior peroneal retinaculum from the lateral side of the calcaneus, using sharp dissection but taking care not to cut the peroneal tendons.

Incise the lateral talocalcaneal ligament and the lateral capsule of the talocalcaneal joint from their attachment to the calcaneocuboid joint to the point where they enter the sheath of the flexor hallucis longus tendon posteriorly. In more resistant clubfeet, the origin of the extensor digitorum brevis, cruciate crural ligament (inferior extensor retinaculum), dorsal calcaneocuboid ligament, and, occasionally, cubonavicular oblique ligament must be dissected off the calcaneus to allow the anterior portion of the calcaneus to move laterally.

On the medial side dissect free the neurovascular bundle (medial and lateral plantar nerves and associated vascular components) into the arch of the foot, taking special care to preserve the medial calcaneal branch of the lateral plantar nerve. Protect and retract the neurovascular bundle with a small Penrose drain. Complete dissection of the medial and lateral neurovascular bundle throughout the arch of the foot.

Enter the compartment of the medial plantar neurovascular bundle and follow it into the arch of the foot well beyond the cuneiforms, taking down the master knot of Henry. Elevate the abductor hallucis muscle and the sheaths of the posterior tibial tendon and the flexor hallucis longus and flexor digitorum longus tendons. Section the narrow strip of fascia between the medial and lateral branches of the plantar nerve to allow the abductor hallucis to slide distally.

Enter the sheath of the posterior tibial tendon just posterior to and above the medial malleolus. Split the sheath and superficial deltoid ligament up the tibia until the muscle can be identified. Then lengthen the tendon by Z-plasty at least 2.5 cm proximal from the medial malleolus to the maximal distance allowed by the incision. Starting from the point at which the flexor digitorum longus and the flexor hallucis longus tendons cross, sharply dissect both sheaths from the sustentaculum tali, moving in a proximal direction until the talocalcaneal joint is entered.

Continue the dissection down and around the navicular, holding the distal segment of the lengthened posterior tibial tendon attached to the bone. Open the talonavicular joint by pulling on the remaining posterior tibial tendon attachment and carefully cut the deltoid ligament (medial tibial navicular ligament), talonavicular capsule, dorsal talonavicular ligament, and plantar calcaneonavicular (spring) ligament close to the navicular. Enter and carefully expose by blunt dissection and retraction the interval between the dorsal aspect of the talonavicular joint and the extensor tendons and neurovascular bundle on the dorsum of the foot. Be sure not to dissect or disturb the blood supply to the dorsal aspect of the talus.

Follow through with the dissection, incising the capsule of the talonavicular joint all the way around medially, inferiorly, superiorly, and laterally. Inferior and lateral to the joint is the bifurcated (Y) ligament; incise both ends of this ligament to correct the horizontal rotation of the calcaneus. Complete the release of the talocalcaneal joint ligaments and capsule by incising the remaining medial and posteromedial capsule and superficial deltoid ligament attached to the sustentaculum tali. Do not incise the three talocalcaneal ligaments (interosseous ligaments) at this point. Retract the lateral plantar nerve, detach the origin of the quadratus plantae muscle using a periosteal elevator on the medial inferior surface of the calcaneus, and expose the long plantar ligament over the plantar calcaneocuboid ligament and the peroneus longus tendon.

At this point, the talus should roll back into the ankle joint, exposing at least 1.5 cm of hyaline cartilage on its body. If this does not happen, incise the posterior talofibular ligament. If the talus still does not roll back into the ankle joint, cut the *posterior portion only* of the deep deltoid ligament.

Now the decision must be made as to the necessity of dividing the interosseous talocalcaneal ligament to correct the horizontal rotational abnormality through the talocalcaneal joint. This decision depends on the completeness of the correction and the mobility of the subtalar complex, as determined by the position of the foot. Line up the medial side of the head and neck of the talus with the medial side of the cuneiforms and medially push the calcaneus posterior to the ankle joint while pushing the foot as a whole in a posterior direction. Then examine the angle made by the intersection of the bimalleolar ankle plane with the horizontal plane of the foot; if the angle is 85 to 90 degrees, the ligament need not be cut. However, in children older than 1 year of age such an incision generally is necessary because the ligament usually has become broad and thick, preventing derotation of the talocalcaneal joint.

After the foot has been satisfactorily corrected, pass a 0.062-inch Kirschner wire through the talus from the posterior aspect to the middle of the head. Positioning the pin in a slightly lateral direction in the head of the talus is beneficial in older children with more pronounced medial deviation of the talar head and neck because it allows lateral displacement of the navicular and cuneiforms on the head of the talus to eliminate forefoot adduction. Pass the pin through the talonavicular joint and cuneiforms and out the forefoot on either the medial or lateral side of the first metatarsal. While an assistant inserts the pin, mold the forefoot out of adduction. Cut off the end of the pin close to the body of the talus and then use a drill anteriorly to advance the pin out the forefoot until it becomes buried in the posterior body of the talus.

To correct rotation of the calcaneus beneath the talus, push the calcaneocuboid joint anterior to the ankle joint in a lateral direction while pushing the calcaneus posterior to the ankle joint in a medial and plantar direction. Check for

proper positioning of the foot: the longitudinal plane of the foot is 85 to 90 degrees to the bimalleolar ankle plane, and the heel under the tibia is in slight valgus. If the talocalcaneal ligament has been divided, insert a pin through the calcaneus, burying it deep in the talus from the plantar surface. Be careful not to penetrate the ankle joint.

Suture all tendons snugly with the foot in a maximum of 20 degrees of dorsiflexion. After suturing the tendons, pull the sheaths of the flexor hallucis longus and flexor digitorum longus tendons down over them. Reposition the lengthened posterior tibialis tendon in its sheath and repair the sheath beneath the medial malleolus. With the fibrofatty tissue left attached to the calcaneus anterior to the tendo calcaneus, cover the lateral aspect of the ankle joint. Keep the peroneal tendons and sheaths from subluxating around the fibula by suturing the sheaths of the peroneal tendons to the fibrofatty flap. Close the subcutaneous tissue and skin with interrupted sutures.

Apply nonadherent dressing and then, very loosely, one or two layers of cast padding. With the knee bent approximately 90 degrees, roll strips of pound cotton 3 to 4 inches wide around the foot, up the calf, and over the thigh. Apply light pressure with loosely woven gauze and roll on another layer of cast padding. Holding the foot in a neutral or slightly plantar-flexed position, apply a few rolls of plaster from the toes to midthigh (Fig. 26-34).

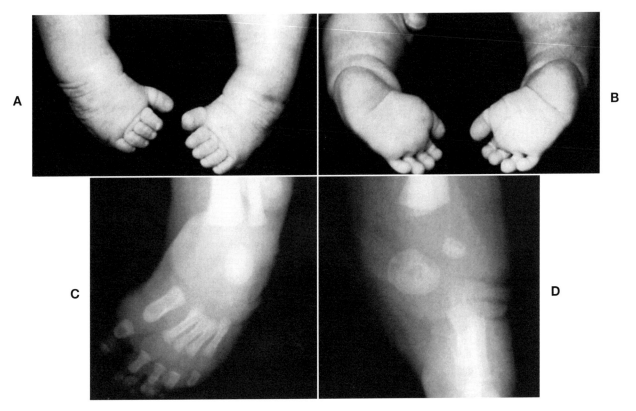

Fig. 26-34   Bilateral clubfoot deformities before modified McKay procedure. **A** and **B,** Clinical appearance. **C,** Roentgenographic appearance on anteroposterior view. **D,** Dorsiflexion, lateral view.

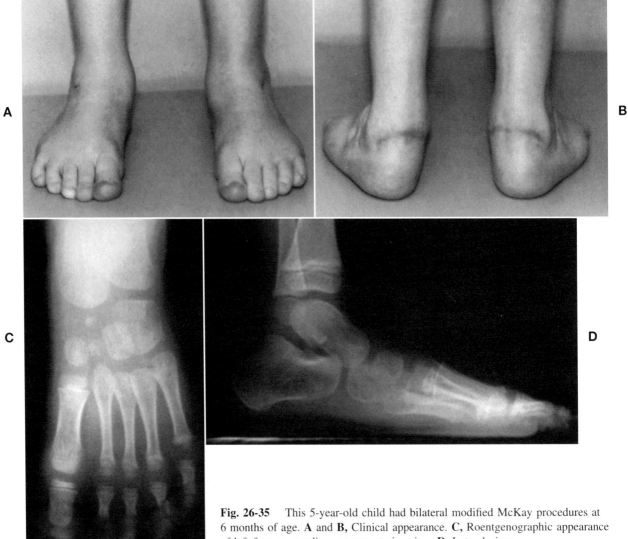

Fig. 26-35   This 5-year-old child had bilateral modified McKay procedures at 6 months of age. **A** and **B,** Clinical appearance. **C,** Roentgenographic appearance of left foot on standing anteroposterior view. **D,** Lateral view.

AFTERTREATMENT. A long leg cast is applied with the foot in plantar flexion. At 2 weeks the cast is changed, and the foot is placed in the corrected position. This can be done with sedation or general anesthesia as an outpatient procedure. At 6 weeks the cast is changed again, and the pins are removed (Fig. 26-35). All casts are discontinued at 10 to 12 weeks after surgery.

◆   ◆   ◆

Special attention should be given to two specific problems in clubfoot. The first is residual hindfoot equinus in children 6 to 12 months of age who have obtained adequate correction of forefoot adduction and hindfoot varus. This equinus can be corrected adequately by tendo calcaneus lengthening and posterior capsulotomy of the ankle and subtalar joints without an extensive one-stage posteromedial release. The physical examination and roentgenograms must be reviewed carefully to be certain that a more extensive release is not required instead of a limited procedure that corrects only hindfoot equinus. The heel varus and internal rotation must have been corrected

adequately if tendo calcaneus lengthening and posterior capsulotomy alone are to be used.

The second specific problem is dynamic metatarsus adductus caused by overpull of the tibialis anterior tendon in older children who have had correction of clubfoot. In the rare child with symptoms, the treatment of choice is transfer of the tibialis anterior tendon, either as a split transfer or as a transfer of the entire tendon to the middle cuneiform. The forefoot must be flexible for a tendon transfer to succeed. This treatment rarely is indicated in neurologically normal children.

◆ Tendo Calcaneus Lengthening and Posterior Capsulotomy

TECHNIQUE 26-11

Make a straight longitudinal incision over the medial aspect of the tendo calcaneus, beginning at its most distal point and extending proximally to 3 cm above the level of the ankle joint. Carry sharp dissection through the subcutaneous tissue. Identify the tendo calcaneus and make an incision through the peritenon medially. Dissect the tendo calcaneus circumferentially to expose it for a length of 3 to 4 cm. Perform a tenotomy of the plantaris tendon if it is present. Identify medially the tendons of the flexor hallucis longus, flexor digitorum communis, and tibialis posterior, as well as the neurovascular bundle; protect these with Penrose drains. Perform a Z-plasty to lengthen the tendo calcaneus by releasing the medial half distally and the lateral half proximally for a distance of 2.5 to 4 cm (Fig. 26-36).

Gently debride pericapsular fat at the level of the subtalar joint. Identify the posterior aspect of the ankle joint by gentle plantar flexion and dorsiflexion of the foot. If the ankle joint cannot be easily identified, make a small vertical incision in the midline until synovial fluid exudes from the joint. Then perform a transverse capsulotomy at the most medial aspect, stopping at the sheath of the tibialis posterior tendon and the most lateral articulation of the tibiofibular joint. Take care not to divide the tibialis posterior tendon sheath and its underlying deep deltoid ligament.

If posterior subtalar capsulotomy is required, enter the subtalar joint at the most proximal aspect of the sheath of the flexor hallucis longus tendon and extend the capsulotomy medially and laterally as necessary. Place the foot in 10 degrees of dorsiflexion and approximate the tendo calcaneus to assess tension. Then place the foot in plantar flexion and repair the tendo calcaneus at the appropriate length. Deflate the tourniquet, obtain hemostasis with electrocautery, and close the wound in layers. Apply a long leg, bent-knee cast with the foot in 5 degrees of dorsiflexion.

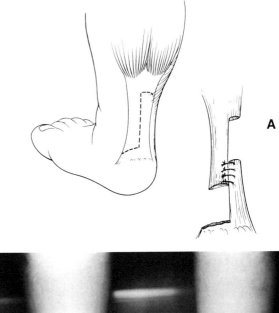

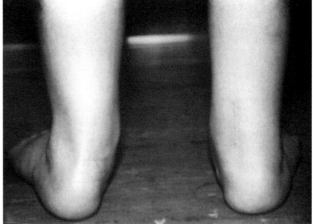

Fig. 26-36   **A,** Tendo calcaneus lengthening. **B,** Clinical appearance after lengthening in right foot.

AFTERTREATMENT. The cast is removed 6 weeks after surgery. Postoperative bracing with either an ankle-foot orthosis or a short leg Phelps brace can be used for 6 to 9 months longer.

RESISTANT CLUBFOOT

Treatment of residual or resistant clubfoot in an older child is one of the most difficult problems in pediatric orthopaedics. The deformity may take many forms, and there are no clear-cut guidelines for treatment. Each child must be carefully evaluated to determine what treatment will best correct his or her particular functional impairment. Thorough physical examination should include careful assessment of the forefoot and hindfoot. Residual forefoot deformity should be determined to be either dynamic (with a flexible forefoot) or rigid. The amount of inversion and eversion of the calcaneus should be determined, as well as dorsiflexion and plantar flexion of the ankle. Any prior surgical procedures causing significant scarring about the foot or loss of motion should be noted. Standing anteroposterior and lateral roentgenograms should be obtained to assess anatomical measurements; if the clubfoot deformity is unilateral, the opposite foot can be used as a control for measurements. All possible etiologies of the persistent deformity, including underlying neuropathy, abnormal growth of the bones, or muscle imbalance, should be investigated. In a group of 159 clubfeet that required reoperation for residual deformities, Tarraf and Carroll found that the most common persistent deformities were forefoot adduction and supination (95 of feet) and that these deformities resulted from undercorrection at the time of the primary operation. Undercorrection resulted from failure to release the calcaneocuboid joint and plantar fascia and failure to recognize residual forefoot adduction on intraoperative roentgenograms.

Incomplete correction may not be obvious at the time of surgery, but it becomes apparent with growth as the persistent deformities become more evident. Clubfoot that appears by clinical and roentgenographic evaluation to be uncorrected may not always require surgery. The functional ability of the child, the severity of symptoms associated with the deformity, and the likelihood of progression if the deformity is left untreated must be considered when treatment decisions are being made.

The basic surgical correction of resistant clubfoot includes both soft tissue release and bony osteotomies. The appropriate procedures and combination of procedures depend on the age

Table 26-2 Treatment of Resistant Clubfoot

Deformity	Treatment
Metatarsus adductus	>5 yr: metatarsal osteotomy
Hindfoot varus	<2-3 yr: modified McKay procedure
	3-10 yr
	Dwyer osteotomy (isolated heel varus)
	Dillwyn-Evans procedure (short medial column)
	Lichtblau procedure (long lateral column)
	10-12 yr: triple arthrodesis
Equinus	Tendo calcaneus lengthening plus posterior capsulotomy of subtalar joint, ankle joint (mild to moderate deformity)
	Lambrinudi procedure (severe deformity, skeletal immaturity)
All three deformities	>10 yr: triple arthrodesis

of the child, the severity of the deformity, and the pathological processes involved. General guidelines for use in decision making are outlined in Table 26-2.

In general, the older the child, the more likely it is that combined procedures will be required. Children 2 to 3 years of age may be candidates for the modified McKay procedure (p. 996), but if previous soft tissue release has caused stiffness of the subtalar joint, avascular necrosis of the talus, or severe skin contractures, osteotomies are a better choice. Children over 5 years of age almost always require osteotomies for correction of resistant deformity; children between 1 year and 5 years of age constitute a gray area in which treatment guidelines are unclear and careful judgment is required. The separate components of the residual deformity must be assessed accurately and treatment directed appropriately. Common components of resistant clubfoot deformity are adduction or supination, or both, of the forefoot, a short medial column or long lateral column of the foot, internal rotation and varus of the calcaneus, and equinus.

Correction of the forefoot with residual adduction or supination or both is similar to correction of isolated metatarsus adductus by multiple metatarsal osteotomies or by combined medial cuneiform and lateral cuboid osteotomies, when the deformity is in the forefoot. Kuo et al. reported good results in 71 feet with residual dynamic forefoot supination and adduction deformities after anterior tibial tendon transfers. Because dynamic supination and adduction often are caused by overactivity of the anterior tibial tendon and underactivity of the peroneal tendon, Kuo et al. suggested that a tendon-balancing procedure is the most reasonable solution. Ezra et al. also reported good results after transfer of the anterior tibial tendon in 27 previously treated clubfeet with residual dynamic supination deformities.

Evaluation of the hindfoot should determine whether the deformity is caused by isolated heel varus, a long lateral column of the foot, or a short medial column. In children younger than 2 or 3 years of age who have had no previous surgery, residual heel varus may be corrected by extensive subtalar release, but children 3 to 10 years of age who have residual soft tissue and bony deformities usually require combined procedures.

In a consecutive prospective group of 60 children (103 surgically treated clubfeet), Stevens and Otis found ankle valgus ranging from 5 degrees to 25 degrees in 40 patients (67%). They warned that ankle valgus must be differentiated from hindfoot valgus because the methods and timing of surgical correction are different. For symptomatic ankle valgus, they recommended percutaneous medial malleolar epiphysiodesis using a 4.5-mm cannulated cortical screw and reported that this did not cause physeal closure in any of their patients.

For isolated heel varus with mild supination of the forefoot, a Dwyer osteotomy with a lateral closing wedge osteotomy of the calcaneus can be performed. Opening wedge osteotomy of the calcaneus occasionally is followed by sloughing of tight skin along the incision over the calcaneus. Consequently, although some height of the calcaneus is lost after a lateral closing wedge osteotomy, most authors now prefer lateral closing wedge osteotomy with Kirschner wire fixation, if necessary. The ideal age for the operation is 3 to 4 years, but there is really no upper age limit.

If the hindfoot deformity includes heel varus and residual internal rotation of the calcaneus with a long lateral column of the foot, the Lichtblau procedure may be appropriate. This procedure corrects the long lateral column of the foot by a closing wedge osteotomy of the lateral aspect of the calcaneus or by cuboid enucleation. The best results with this procedure are obtained in children 3 years of age or older in whom the calcaneus and lateral column are long relative to the talus. Potential complications include the development of a "Z"-foot, or "skew"-foot, deformity.

Schaefer and Hefti reported that no further surgery was required in 22 idiopathic clubfeet with residual adductus deformity treated with combined cuboid-cuneiform osteotomy. Adductus of the forefoot, as measured by the calcaneal-second metatarsal angle, improved from an average of 20.7 degrees preoperatively to 8.9 degrees postoperatively.

Residual heel equinus can be corrected by tendo calcaneus lengthening and posterior ankle and subtalar capsulotomies in a younger child with a mild deformity. In rare cases an isolated, fixed equinus deformity in an older child will require a Lambrinudi arthrodesis.

Lehman et al. reported good long-term results (5 to 14 years) in 26 of 27 feet with recurrent clubfoot deformities treated with complete soft tissue release and calcaneocuboid fusion. They suggested that in patients aged 4 to 8 years this will not cause overcorrection and will produce a flexible, functional foot, thereby possibly avoiding the need for later triple arthrodesis.

Wei, Sullivan, and Davidson described talonavicular arthrodesis for residual midfoot deformities in 16 patients with 19 previously corrected clubfeet; 8 feet in 7 patients also required lateral column shortening with a calcaneal wedge osteotomy. The average patient age at the time of surgery was 11 years (4 to 20 years). At 4 years after surgery, the 15 patients available for follow-up (17 feet) all reported improvement in symptoms.

If all three deformities are present in a child older than 10 years of age, triple arthrodesis may be appropriate. Internal tibial torsion occasionally occurs with resistant clubfoot deformity but rarely requires derotational osteotomy. Before tibial osteotomy is considered, it must be determined absolutely that the pathological condition is confined to the tibia and is not a resistant deformity in the foot.

Correction using the Ilizarov device, with or without bony procedures, may be appropriate for children with severe soft tissue and bony deformities. Wallander et al. reported use of the Ilizarov device in 10 feet in 7 patients with persistent deformities after clubfoot surgery. At an average follow-up of 40 months, 6 of the 7 patients and their parents were satisfied with the results; however, persistent reduction of ankle joint motion, limited walking capacity, and intermittent pain were common. Thirteen of the 17 feet treated by Bradish and Noor with gradual distraction and realignment had excellent or good results at an average of 3 years after surgery.

◆ Osteotomy of Calcaneus for Persistent Varus Deformity of Heel

In 1963 Dwyer reported osteotomy of the calcaneus for relapsed clubfoot using an opening wedge osteotomy medially to increase the length and height of the calcaneus. The osteotomy is held open by a wedge of bone taken from the tibia.

TECHNIQUE 26-12 *(Dwyer, Modified)*

Expose the calcaneus through a lateral incision over the calcaneus, cuboid, and base of the fifth metatarsal. Strip the lateral surface of the bone subperiosteally and with a wide osteotome resect a wedge of bone based laterally large enough, when removed, to permit correction of the heel varus. Take care not to injure the peroneal tendons. Remove the wedge of bone, place the heel into the corrected position, and close the incision with interrupted sutures. If necessary, fix the osteotomy with a Kirschner wire. Apply a short leg cast with the foot in the corrected position.

AFTERTREATMENT. The Kirschner wire is removed at 6 weeks, and casting is discontinued at 3 months.

◆ Medial Release with Osteotomy of Distal Calcaneus (Lichtblau Procedure)

An alternative to calcaneocuboid arthrodesis is lateral closing wedge osteotomy of the calcaneus, as described by Lichtblau (Fig. 26-37). This procedure may prevent the long-term stiffness of the hindfoot seen with the Dillwyn-Evans procedure.

TECHNIQUE 26-13 *(Lichtblau)* (Fig. 26-38)

If soft tissue release medially is required, make an incision on the medial aspect of the foot beginning about 1 cm below the medial malleolus, crossing the tuberosity of the navicular, and sloping downward to the base of the first metatarsal. Identify and free the superior border of the abductor hallucis muscle and reflect it plantarward. Isolate the tibialis posterior tendon at its insertion on the beak of the navicular, dissect it from its sheath, and perform a Z-plasty about 1 cm from its insertion. Allow the proximal end of the tendon to retract, using the distal end as a guide to the talonavicular joint. Resect the tendon sheath overlying the joint and open it generously on its medial, dorsal, and plantar aspects. Open the flexor tendon sheaths and lengthen them by Z-plasty technique.

Now make a lateral incision 4 cm long centered over the calcaneocuboid joint. Dissect the origin of the extensor digitorum brevis muscle from the calcaneus and reflect it distally to permit exposure and opening of the calcaneocuboid joint. Identify the distal end of the calcaneus and perform a wedge-shaped osteotomy, removing about 1 cm of the distal and lateral border of the calcaneus and 2 mm of the distal and medial border. Take care to leave the articular surface of the calcaneus intact. Bring the cuboid into contact with the distal end of the calcaneus at the osteotomy site and evaluate the amount of correction of the varus deformity. If the cuboid cannot be closely approximated to the calcaneus, resect more of the calcaneus. A smooth Kirschner wire can be inserted across the calcaneocuboid joint to fix the osteotomy. Repair all soft tissues and close the subcutaneous tissue and skin. Apply a long leg cast with the foot in the corrected position.

AFTERTREATMENT. Three weeks after surgery the long leg cast is changed to a short leg cast that is worn for 6 more weeks. The pin is removed at 8 to 12 weeks.

Triple Arthrodesis and Talectomy for Uncorrected Clubfoot

Triple arthrodesis and talectomy generally are salvage operations for uncorrected clubfoot in older children and adolescents. Galdino et al., however, reported excellent or good results in 68% of 19 triple arthrodeses in children 10 years of age or younger (the average age at surgery was 8.4 years) who had severe hindfoot deformity after failure of soft tissue release (Figs. 25-39 and 25-40). Nonunion occurred in 7% of joints, and fair and poor results were caused primarily by residual rather than recurrent deformity. They believe that triple arthrodesis is functionally and cosmetically superior to talectomy. Triple arthrodesis corrects the severely deformed foot by a lateral closing wedge osteotomy through the subtalar and midtarsal joints. Functional results generally are improved despite postoperative joint stiffness. Talectomy should be reserved for severe, untreated clubfoot, for previously treated

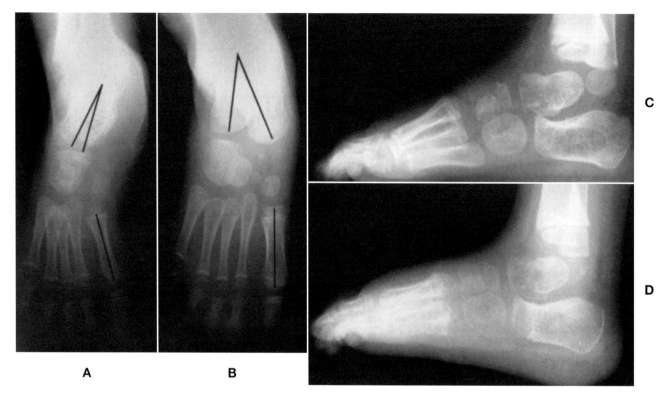

Fig. 26-37   Severe residual clubfoot deformity in 5-year-old child on anteroposterior (**A**) and lateral (**C**) roentgenograms. **B** and **D,** After Lichtblau procedure.

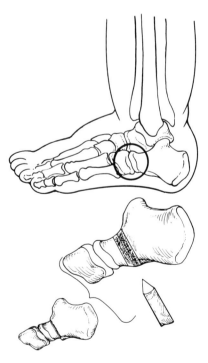

Fig. 26-38   Lichtblau procedure (see text).

clubfoot that is uncorrectable by any other surgical procedures, and for neuromuscular clubfoot.

◆ Triple Arthrodesis

TECHNIQUE 26-14

Make an incision along the medial side of the foot parallel to the inferior border of the calcaneus. Free the attachments of the plantar fascia and of the short flexors of the toes from the plantar aspect of the calcaneus. Then, by manipulation, correct the cavus deformity as much as possible. Next, through an oblique anterolateral approach, expose the midtarsal and subtalar joints (Fig. 26-41). Then resect a laterally based wedge of bone that includes the midtarsal joints. Resect enough bone to correct the varus and adduction deformities of the forefoot.

Next, through the same incision, resect a wedge of bone, again laterally based, that includes the subtalar joint. Resect enough bone to correct the varus deformity of the calcaneus. If necessary, include in the wedge the navicular and most of the cuboid and lateral cuneiform, as well as the anterior part of the talus and calcaneus, and in the second wedge much of

continued

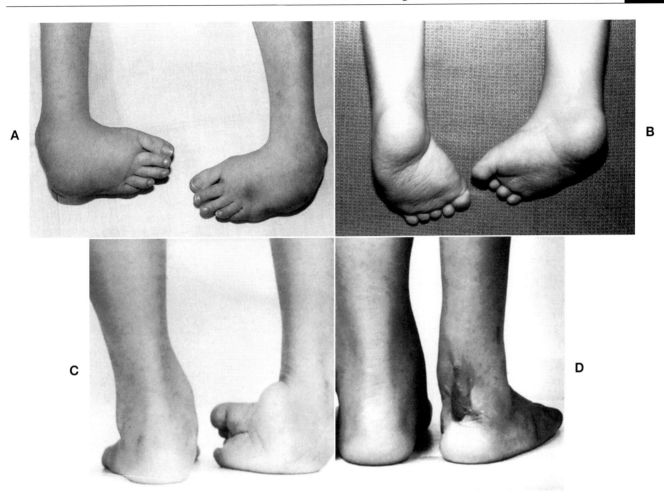

Fig. 26-39   A, Untreated clubfoot in 14-year-old girl. **B,** Bilateral recurrent clubfoot in 2-year-old child after undercorrection at 6 months of age. **C,** Uncorrected clubfoot in 10-year-old girl. **D,** After posteromedial release and triple arthrodesis. (**C** and **D** from Galindo MJ Jr, Siff SJ, Butler JE, et al: *Foot Ankle* 7:319, 1987.)

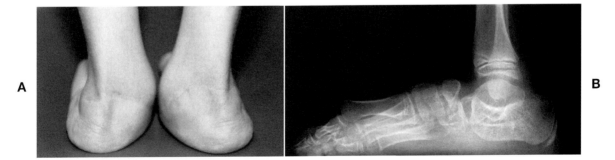

Fig. 26-40   A, Overcorrected clubfoot in 12-year-old boy, showing hindfoot valgus, dorsal dislocation of navicular on talus, and dorsal bunion deformity. **B,** Standing lateral roentgenogram.

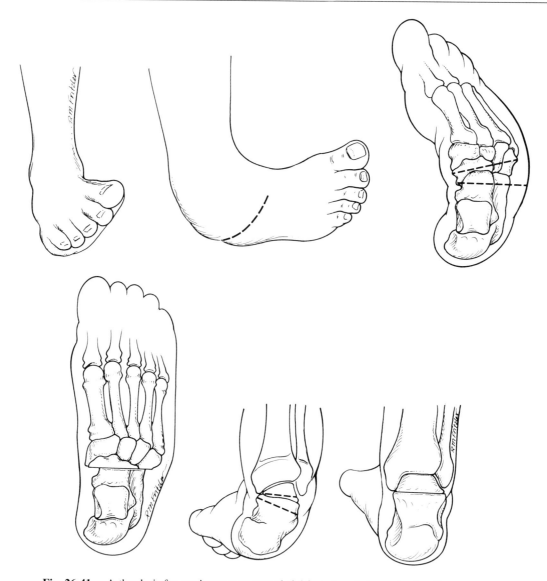

Fig. 26-41   Arthrodesis for persistent or untreated clubfoot. Area between broken lines represents amount of bone removed from midtarsal region and subtalar joint in moderate fixed deformity. In severe deformity, wedge may include large part of talus and calcaneus and even part of cuneiforms.

the superior part of the calcaneus and the inferior part of the talus. Finally, lengthen the tendo calcaneus by Z-plasty and perform a posterior capsulotomy of the ankle joint. By manipulating the ankle, correct the equinus deformity. Hold the correct position with a Kirschner wire inserted through the calcaneocuboid and talonavicular joints or with staple fixation.

AFTERTREATMENT. With the foot in the corrected position and the knee flexed 30 degrees, a long leg cast is applied from the base of the toes to the groin. The Kirschner wire and cast are removed at 6 weeks. A short leg walking cast is worn for 4 more weeks.

◆ ◆ ◆

Trumble et al. described a talectomy for clubfoot deformity in patients with myelomeningocele, but the technique can be modified for treatment of a severe, resistant, idiopathic clubfoot deformity.

◆ **Talectomy**

TECHNIQUE 26-15 *(Trumble et al.)*
Expose the talus through an incision parallel to the inferior border of the calcaneus (Fig. 26-42, *A*). If additional soft tissue release is required, talectomy can be done after circumferential release (p. 995). Carry the dissection to the

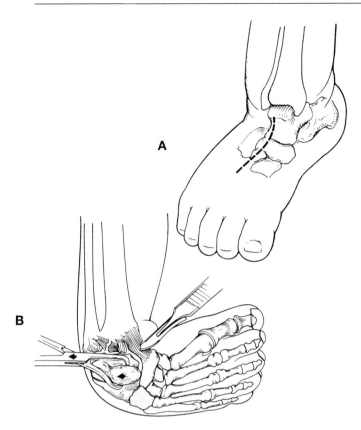

Fig. 26-42   Talectomy. **A,** Anterolateral skin incision. **B,** Total talectomy.

prominent lateral articular margin of the navicular in the interval between the extensor digitorum longus and peroneus tertius tendons. Invert and plantar flex the forefoot. Place a towel clip around the neck of the talus and deliver it into the wound; dissect all of its ligaments (Fig. 26-42, *B*). Be sure to excise the talus intact because retained remnants of cartilage may interfere with proper positioning of the foot; these remnants also may grow and cause later deformity and loss of correction. Derotate the forefoot and displace the calcaneus posteriorly into the ankle mortise until the navicular abuts the anterior edge of the tibial plafond. The exposed articular surface of the tibial plafond should be opposite the middle articular facet of the calcaneus. If necessary to obtain adequate posterior displacement, excise the tarsal navicular. Section both the deltoid and lateral collateral ligaments of the ankle. Correct equinus deformity of the hindfoot by sectioning the tendo calcaneus and allowing its proximal end to retract.

In feet with uncorrected, severe equinovarus deformity, the dome of the talus may be extruded anterior to its normal

relationship in the ankle mortise. Adaptive narrowing of the mortise may require release of the anterior and posterior tibiofibular ligaments of the syndesmosis to allow proper posterior positioning of the calcaneus.

In the proper plantigrade position, the long axis of the foot should be aligned at a right angle to the bimalleolar axis of the ankle, not to the axis of the knee joint. This usually requires 20 to 30 degrees of external rotation of the foot. When the proper position has been achieved, insert one or two Steinmann pins from the heel through the calcaneus and into the distal tibia. Apply a long leg cast with the knee flexed to 60 degrees.

AFTERTREATMENT. The Steinmann pins are removed at 6 weeks and a below-the-knee, weight-bearing cast is applied. This is worn for 12 more weeks.

Dorsal Bunion

Dorsal bunions that develop after clubfoot surgery have been attributed to muscle weakness or imbalance. McKay reported dorsal bunions in 11 children after posteromedial release for clubfoot and attributed the deformity to weakness of the triceps surae. The bunion develops as the patient tries to push off with the toe flexors to compensate for the tricep's weakness. Another suggested factor is imbalance between the anterior tibialis muscle and an impaired peroneus longus muscle. Most authors recommend transfer of the flexor hallucis longus to the neck of the first metatarsal, combined with bony correction by plantar closing wedge osteotomy of the first metatarsal (Fig. 26-43).

◆ First Metatarsal Osteotomy and Tendon Transfer for Dorsal Bunion

TECHNIQUE 26-16 *(Smith and Kuo)*

Through a medial incision, expose the first metatarsal and perform a proximal plantar closing wedge osteotomy. Bring the metatarsal into alignment with the forefoot by plantar flexion and insert a Kirschner wire for fixation. Carry the incision distally or make a second incision at the metatarsophalangeal joint to allow identification and transection of the flexor hallucis longus tendon. Drill a hole in the distal first metatarsal neck in a dorsal-to-plantar direction. Pass the flexor hallucis tendon through the hole and suture it back on itself. Close the wounds and apply a short leg, non-weight-bearing cast.

AFTERTREATMENT. Non-weight-bearing is continued in the cast for 6 weeks, after which the Kirschner wire is removed. A walking cast is then worn for 4 weeks. Full activity usually can be resumed at 3 to 4 months.

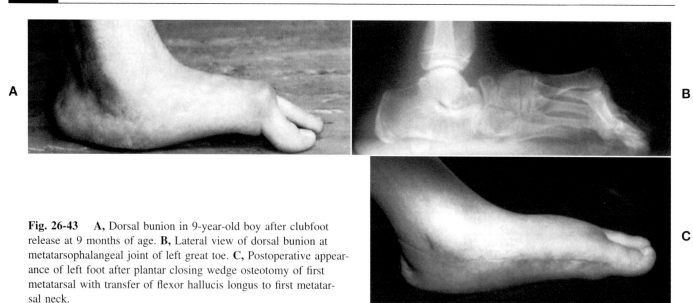

Fig. 26-43 **A,** Dorsal bunion in 9-year-old boy after clubfoot release at 9 months of age. **B,** Lateral view of dorsal bunion at metatarsophalangeal joint of left great toe. **C,** Postoperative appearance of left foot after plantar closing wedge osteotomy of first metatarsal with transfer of flexor hallucis longus to first metatarsal neck.

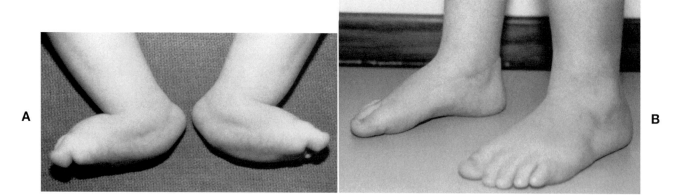

Fig. 26-44 **A,** Bilateral congenital vertical talus in 14-month-old child. **B,** At 6 years of age, after bilateral operative correction at age 14 months in which transverse circumferential approach was used.

Congenital Vertical Talus

Congenital vertical talus, rocker-bottom flatfoot, or congenital rigid flatfoot must be distinguished from flexible pes planus commonly seen in infants and children. Congenital vertical talus may be associated with a number of neuromuscular disorders, such as arthrogryposis and myelomeningocele, but it also may occur as an isolated congenital anomaly.

CLINICAL AND ROENTGENOGRAPHIC FINDINGS

Congenital vertical talus usually can be detected at birth by the presence of a rounded prominence of the medial and plantar surfaces of the foot produced by the abnormal location of the head of the talus (Fig. 26-44). The talus is so distorted plantarward and medially as to be almost vertical. The calcaneus also is in an equinus position but to a lesser degree.

The forefoot is dorsiflexed at the midtarsal joints, and the navicular lies on the dorsal aspect of the head of the talus. The sole is convex, and there are deep creases on the dorsolateral aspect of the foot anterior and inferior to the lateral malleolus.

As the foot develops and weight-bearing is begun, adaptive changes occur in the tarsals. The talus becomes shaped like an hourglass but remains in so marked an equinus position that its longitudinal axis is almost the same as that of the tibia, and only the posterior third of its superior articular surface articulates with the tibia. The calcaneus remains in an equinus position also and becomes displaced posteriorly, and the anterior part of its plantar surface becomes rounded. Callosities develop beneath the anterior end of the calcaneus and along the medial border of the foot superficial to the head of the talus. When full weight is borne, the forefoot becomes severely abducted and the heel does not touch the floor. Adaptive changes, of course, occur in the soft structures. All the capsules, ligaments, and

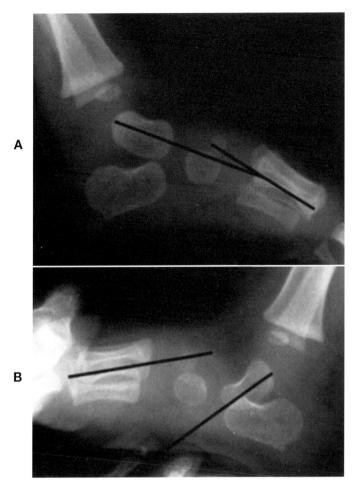

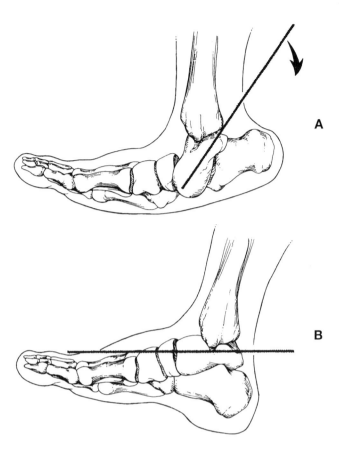

Fig. 26-45   Plantar flexion lateral stress roentgenograms in diagnosis of congenital vertical talus. **A,** In normal foot, long axis of first metatarsal passes plantarward to long axis of talus. **B,** In congenital vertical talus, long axis of first metatarsal remains dorsal to long axis of talus, indicating dorsal dislocation of midfoot and forefoot. Note equinus deformity of calcaneus.

Fig. 26-46   Single-stage correction of congenital vertical talus. **A,** Threaded Kirschner wire is placed axially in vertical talus from posterior and is used as "joystick" to manipulate talus into reduced position. **B,** Wire is advanced across talonavicular joint. (From Kodros SA, Dias LS: Single-stage surgical correction of congenital vertical talus, *J Pediatr Orthop* 19:42, 1999.)

tendons on the dorsum of the foot become contracted. The tendons of the tibialis posterior and peroneus longus and brevis may come to lie anterior to the malleoli and act as dorsiflexors rather than plantar flexors.

Congenital vertical talus can be difficult to distinguish from severe pes planus, although the two can be differentiated by the use of appropriate roentgenograms. Routine roentgenograms should include anteroposterior and plantar flexion lateral views; the latter will confirm the diagnosis of congenital vertical talus (Fig. 26-45).

TREATMENT

Congenital vertical talus is difficult to correct and tends to recur. Gentle manipulations, however, followed by immobilization in a cast are beneficial in that the skin, the fibrous tissue structures, and the tendons on the anterior aspect of the foot and ankle are stretched. Reduction of the talonavicular joint rarely

is possible by conservative means alone; consequently, open reduction usually is necessary.

The exact surgery indicated is determined by the age of the child and the severity of the deformity. Children 1 to 4 years old generally are best treated by open reduction and realignment of the talonavicular and subtalar joints. Occasionally, in children 3 years of age or older who have a severe deformity, navicular excision is required at the time of open reduction. Children 4 to 8 years old can be treated by open reduction and soft tissue procedures combined with extraarticular subtalar arthrodesis. Children 12 years old or older are best treated by triple arthrodesis for permanent correction of the deformity.

Kodros and Dias (1999) reported 31 good and 11 fair results in 42 feet treated with a single-stage procedure in which a threaded Kirschner wire is used as a "joystick" to manipulate the talus into correct position. The corrected position is held with threaded Kirschner wires across the talonavicular and subtalar joints (Fig. 26-46). The only complications reported

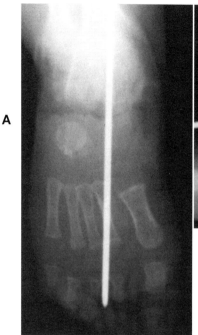
A

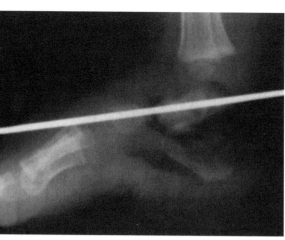
B

Fig. 26-47 Intraoperative roentgenograms after correction of congenital vertical talus through transverse circumferential approach. **A,** Anteroposterior view shows correction of talocalcaneal and talus–first metatarsal angles. **B,** Lateral view shows corrected position of talus and reduction of navicular and forefoot after fixation with single Steinmann pin.

were mild pain in 3 feet and 1 superficial pin site infection. At an average of 7 years after surgery, 10 feet had required subsequent operations; 6 of these were in patients who had neural tube defects.

For a young child with a mild or moderate deformity, the technique of Kumar, Cowell, and Ramsey is recommended. For an older child with a more severe or a recurrent deformity, open reduction and a Grice extraarticular subtalar fusion are recommended by Coleman et al. For a child 12 years old or older with functional symptoms, a triple arthrodesis is preferred.

◆ **Open Reduction and Realignment of Talonavicular and Subtalar Joints**

TECHNIQUE 26-17 *(Kumar, Cowell, and Ramsey)*

Make the first of three incisions on the lateral side of the foot, centered over the sinus tarsi or use the transverse circumferential (Cincinnati) approach (see Fig. 26-33), which we prefer. Avoid entering the sinus tarsi laterally. Expose the extensor digitorum brevis and reflect it distally to expose the anterior part of the talocalcaneal joint. Next, identify the calcaneocuboid joint and release all tight structures around it, including the calcaneocuboid ligament.

Make the second incision on the medial side of the foot, centered over the prominent head of the talus. This exposes the head of the talus and medial part of the navicular. The tibialis anterior tendon also is exposed; if the tendon is contracted, lengthen it by Z-plasty. Release all tight structures on the medial and dorsal aspects of the head of the talus and the navicular. Free also the anterior part of the talus from its ligamentous attachments to the navicular and calcaneus. This includes releasing the dorsal talonavicular ligament, the plantar calcaneonavicular ligament, and the anterior part of the superficial deltoid ligament. If necessary, divide part of the talocalcaneal interosseous ligament so that the talus can be easily maneuvered into position by a blunt instrument. If the peroneal, extensor hallucis longus, and extensor digitorum longus tendons remain contracted, expose and lengthen them by Z-plasty.

Make a third incision 2 inches long on the medial side of the tendo calcaneus. Lengthen this tendon by Z-plasty and, if necessary, perform a capsulotomy of the posterior ankle and subtalar joints. The talus and calcaneus can now be placed in the corrected position and the forefoot reduced on the hindfoot. Pass a smooth Steinmann pin through the navicular and into the neck of the talus to maintain the reduction. Obtain anteroposterior and lateral roentgenograms to confirm reduction of the vertical talus (Fig. 26-47). Make an attempt to reconstruct the talonavicular ligament and close the wound in layers. Apply a long leg cast with the knee flexed and the foot in proper position.

AFTERTREATMENT. At 8 weeks the cast and Steinmann pin are removed. A new long leg cast is applied, and this type of cast is worn for 1 month. A short leg cast is worn for an additional month. The foot then is supported in an ankle-foot orthosis for another 3 to 6 months.

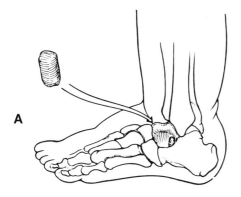
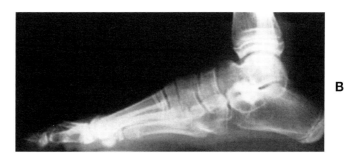

Fig. 26-48   Grice-Green subtalar fusion. **A,** Preparation of graft bed and placement of graft in lateral aspect of subtalar joint. **B,** Lateral view of 10-year-old patient who had open reduction and Grice-Green fusion for congenital vertical talus at 3 years of age.

◆ Open Reduction and Extraarticular Subtalar Fusion

Coleman et al. described open reduction and extraarticular subtalar fusion in older children with severe deformities. This technique combines the procedure of Kumar et al. with a Grice-Green fusion performed 6 to 8 weeks afterward. Dennyson and Fulford modified this technique by using screw fixation across the talocalcaneal joint.

TECHNIQUE 26-18 (Grice-Green)

Make a short curvilinear incision on the lateral aspect of the foot directly over the subtalar joint. Carry the incision down through the soft tissues to expose the cruciate ligament overlying the joint. Split this ligament in the direction of its fibers and dissect the fatty and ligamentous tissues from the sinus tarsi. Dissect the short toe extensors from the calcaneus and reflect them distally. The relationship of the calcaneus to the talus now can be determined and the mechanism of the deformity demonstrated. Place the foot in equinus and then invert it to position the calcaneus beneath the talus. A severe, long-standing deformity may require division of the posterior capsule of the subtalar joint or removal of a small piece of bone laterally from beneath the anterosuperior articular surface of the calcaneus. Insert an osteotome or broad periosteal elevator into the sinus tarsi and block the subtalar joint to evaluate the stability of the graft and its proper size and position. Prepare the graft beds by removing a thin layer of cortical bone from the inferior surface of the talus and superior surface of the calcaneus (Fig. 26-48).

Make a linear incision over the anteromedial surface of the proximal tibial metaphysis, incise the periosteum, and take a block of bone large enough for two grafts (usually 3.5 to 4.5 cm long and 1.5 cm wide). As an alternative to tibial bone, a short segment of the distal fibula or a circular segment of the iliac crest can be used. Cut the grafts to fit the prepared beds. Use a rongeur to shape the grafts so that they can be countersunk into cancellous bone to prevent lateral displacement. With the foot held in a slightly overcorrected

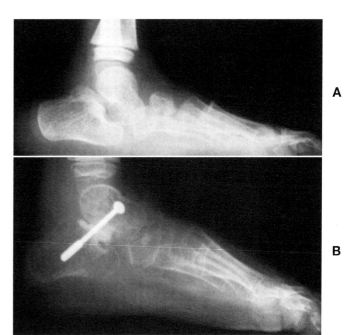

Fig. 26-49   **A,** Congenital vertical talus in 6-year-old child. **B,** Corrected position of talus fixed with screw through neck of talus into calcaneus, as described by Dennyson and Fulford. Bone graft in middle and posterior aspects of subtalar joint.

position, place the grafts in the sinus tarsi. Evert the foot to lock the grafts in place. If a segment of the fibula or iliac crest is used, a smooth Kirschner wire can be used to hold the graft in place for 12 weeks or a screw can be inserted anteriorly from the talar neck into the calcaneus, as described by Dennyson and Fulford, for rigid fixation (Fig. 26-49). The foot now should be stable enough to allow correction of equinus deformity by tendo calcaneus lengthening if necessary. Apply a long leg cast with the knee flexed, the ankle in maximal dorsiflexion, and the foot in the corrected position.

AFTERTREATMENT. The long leg cast is worn for 12 weeks, and weight-bearing is not allowed. The Kirschner wire then is removed, and a short leg walking cast is worn for 4 more weeks.

Triple Arthrodesis

Older children with uncorrected vertical talus who have pain or difficulty with shoe wear can be treated with triple arthrodesis. The procedure generally requires medial and lateral incisions and adequate osteotomies to place the foot in a plantigrade position, a technique similar to that used for correction of a severe tarsal coalition deformity (Chapter 79).

Congenital Angular Deformities of Leg

Congenital angular deformities of the leg are primarily of two kinds: those in which the apex of the angulation is anterior, and those in which it is posterior. In both the tibia often is bowed not only anteriorly or posteriorly but also medially or laterally; Badgley, O'Connor, and Kudner suggested the term *congenital kyphoscoliotic tibia* for both these deformities. Anterior bowing of the tibia is commonly associated with neurofibromatosis.

Posterior angular deformities of the tibia tend to improve with growth (Fig. 26-50). A limb-length discrepancy also may be present, ranging from several millimeters to several

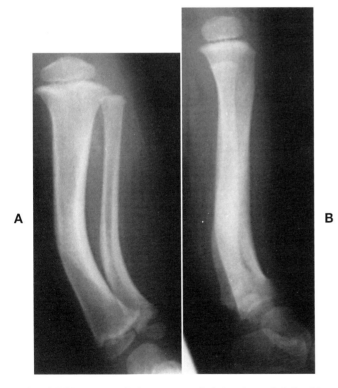

Fig. 26-50 Congenital posteromedial bowing of left tibia. **A,** Anteroposterior view. **B,** Lateral view.

centimeters. Children with these deformities should be examined yearly for any potential limb-length discrepancy that may require limb equalization, usually by an appropriately timed epiphysiodesis or limb lengthening in severe deformities.

Anterior angular deformities of the tibia are more worrisome because of their potential association with congenital pseudarthrosis of the tibia. Occasionally these tibiae maintain a normal medullary canal and show no evidence of narrowing or of the sclerotic "high-risk tibia." If any indication of narrowing of the medullary canal is present or develops in an anteriorly bowed tibia, the limb should be braced until skeletal maturity is reached.

Unilateral anterior bowing of the tibia with duplication of the great toe has been described as a distinct syndrome. In the children with this rare syndrome reported by Karden et al., Adamsbaum et al., Kitoh et al., and Weaver et al., the tibial bowing resolved spontaneously. Weaver et al. emphasized that this syndrome should be considered in the differential diagnosis of anterolateral tibial bowing and should not be mistaken for congenital pseudarthrosis. Associated conditions, in addition to duplication of the great toe, included shortening of the tibia that resulted in significant leg-length discrepancy, clinodactyly, and anomalous maturation of the carpal bones and metacarpals.

Congenital Pseudarthrosis of Fibula and Tibia

Congenital pseudarthrosis is a specific type of nonunion that at birth is either present or incipient. Its cause is unknown, but it occurs often enough in patients with either neurofibromatosis or related stigmata to suggest that neurofibromatosis, if not the cause of congenital pseudarthrosis, is closely related to it. Congenital pseudarthrosis most commonly involves the distal half of the tibia and often that of the fibula in the same limb.

FIBULA

Congenital pseudarthrosis of the fibula often precedes or accompanies the same condition in the ipsilateral tibia. Several grades of severity of this pseudarthrosis are seen: bowing of the fibula without pseudarthrosis, fibular pseudarthrosis without ankle deformity, fibular pseudarthrosis with ankle deformity, and fibular pseudarthrosis with latent pseudarthrosis of the tibia. Sometimes it even develops between the time of successful bone grafting of a pseudarthrosis of the tibia and skeletal maturity. Then, because the lateral malleolus becomes displaced proximally, a progressive valgus deformity of the ankle develops.

Until skeletal maturity is reached, the ankle can be stabilized by an ankle-foot orthosis. At maturity any significant deformity can be treated by supramalleolar osteotomy made through essentially normal bone, and union of the osteotomy can be expected. Langenskiöld, however, has devised an operation for children to prevent this valgus deformity or halt its progression.

He creates a synostosis between the distal tibial and fibular metaphyses. Because in congenital pseudarthrosis securing union by bone grafting may be as difficult in the fibula as in the tibia, an operation that prevents the ankle deformity without grafting in fibular pseudarthrosis is useful (Fig. 26-51).

◆ Tibiofibular Synostosis

TECHNIQUE 26-19 *(Langenskiöld)*

Make a longitudinal incision anteriorly over the distal fibula. Divide the fibula 1 to 2 cm proximal to the level of the distal tibial physis and excise the cone-shaped part of the distal fibular shaft. In the lateral surface of the tibia, at the level of the cut surface of the fibula, and at the attachment of the interosseous membrane, make a hole as wide as the diameter of the fibula. Then, proximal to the hole, remove the periosteum and interosseous membrane from the tibia over an area of several square centimeters. From the ilium obtain a bone graft the same width as that of the hole in the tibia and long enough to extend from the lateral surface of the fibula into the spongy bone of the tibial metaphysis. Insert the graft perpendicular to the long axis of the limb so that it rests on the cut surface of the fibula and extends into the slot in the tibial cortex. Then pack spongy iliac bone in the angle between the proximal surface of the graft and the lateral surface of the tibia. Apply a cast from below the knee to the base of the toes.

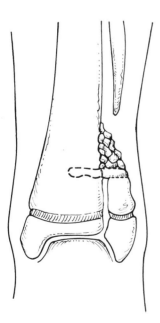

Fig. 26-51 Langenskiöld technique for creating synostosis between distal tibial and fibular metaphyses to prevent valgus deformity of ankle in congenital pseudarthrosis of fibula (see text). (Redrawn from Langenskiöld A: *J Bone Joint Surg* 49A:463, 1967.)

AFTERTREATMENT. At 2 months full weight-bearing in the cast is allowed, and at 4 months the cast is discontinued.

TIBIA

Congenital pseudarthrosis of the tibia is rare, with an incidence of approximately 1 in 250,000 live births. Most large series report 50% to 90% association of this disorder with the stigmata of neurofibromatosis, including skin and osseous lesions. In a large multicenter study from the European Pediatric Orthopaedic Society, 186 (55%) of 340 patients had symptoms of neurofibromatosis.

Classification

Congenital pseudarthrosis of the tibia has been classified by Boyd into the following six types: *Type I* pseudarthrosis occurs with anterior bowing and a defect in the tibia present at birth. Other congenital deformities also may be present, and these may affect the management of the pseudarthrosis.

Type II pseudarthrosis occurs with anterior bowing and an hourglass constriction of the tibia present at birth. Spontaneous fracture, or fracture following minor trauma, commonly occurs before 2 years of age. This is the so-called high-risk tibia. The tibia is tapered, rounded, and sclerotic, and the medullary canal is obliterated. This type is the most common, is often associated with neurofibromatosis, and has the poorest prognosis. Recurrence of the fracture is common during the growth period but decreases in frequency with age and generally ceases to occur after skeletal maturation (Fig. 26-52).

Type III pseudarthrosis develops in a congenital cyst, usually near the junction of the middle and distal thirds of the tibia. Anterior bowing may precede or follow the development of a fracture. Recurrence of the fracture after treatment is less common than in type II, and excellent results after only one operation have been reported to last well into adulthood (Fig. 26-53).

Type IV pseudarthrosis originates in a sclerotic segment of bone in the classic location without narrowing of the tibia. The medullary canal is partially or completely obliterated. An "insufficiency" or "stress" fracture develops in the cortex of the tibia and gradually extends through the sclerotic bone. With completion of the fracture, healing fails to occur and the fracture widens and becomes a pseudarthrosis. The prognosis for this type is generally good, especially when it is treated before the "insufficiency" fracture becomes complete (Fig. 26-54).

Type V pseudarthrosis of the tibia occurs with a dysplastic fibula. A pseudarthrosis of the fibula or tibia or both may develop. The prognosis is good if the lesion is confined to the fibula. If the lesion progresses to a tibial pseudarthrosis, the natural history usually resembles that of type II.

Type VI pseudarthrosis occurs as an intraosseous neurofibroma or schwannoma that results in a pseudarthrosis. This is extremely rare. The prognosis depends on the aggressiveness and treatment of the intraosseous lesion.

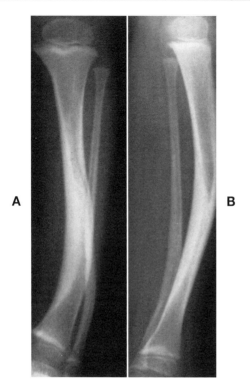

Fig. 26-52   Type II congenital pseudarthrosis of tibia. **A,** Antero-posterior view of left tibia. **B,** Lateral view. Note anterior bowing and narrow, sclerotic medullary canal.

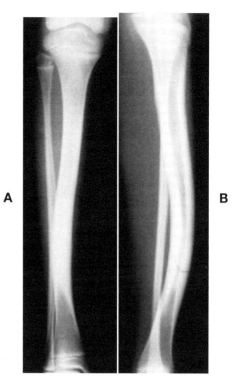

Fig. 26-54   Type IV congenital pseudarthrosis of tibia. **A,** An-teroposterior view of right tibia. **B,** Lateral view. Note fracture in anterior cortex in distal third of tibia.

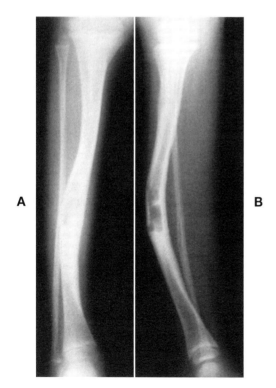

Fig. 26-53   Type III congenital pseudarthrosis of tibia. **A,** An-teroposterior view of right tibia. **B,** Lateral view. Note cyst formation in middle third of tibia with anterior bowing and narrow medullary canal distal to cyst.

Treatment

Treatment of congenital pseudarthrosis of the tibia depends on the age of the patient and the type of pseudarthrosis. A true congenital pseudarthrosis of the tibia will not heal when treated by casting alone. The decision must be made whether to attempt to secure union or if amputation is the treatment of choice. Factors favoring amputation include anticipated short-ening of more than 2 or 3 inches (5 to 7.5 cm), a history of multiple failed surgical procedures, and stiffness and decreased function of a limb that would be more useful after an amputation and fitting with a prosthesis.

For the tibia with a cyst in the medullary canal (type III), prophylactic curettage and autogenous iliac bone grafting are recommended. The limb is immobilized in plaster until the graft has united, and then a patellar tendon–bearing brace is worn until skeletal maturity is reached.

A tibia with anterior bowing and a narrow, sclerotic canal (type II or the high-risk tibia) often fractures during the first 2 years of life. Initially, bracing may be beneficial for an anterolaterally bowed tibia with a narrow canal in which a fracture has not developed. Grill et al., in a report from the European Paediatric Orthopaedic Society, noted that conserva-tive treatment may have a place in the treatment of congenital pseudarthrosis of the tibia. They found that the use of a stable and well-adjusted KAFO with an anterior shield in the pre-pseudarthrotic stage delayed fracture and pseudarthrosis and allowed patients to reach an older age before undergoing surgical treatment. They believed this important because they found better healing rates in children who were older than 3 years of age at the time of surgery than in younger children. Once a fracture does occur, the treatment is surgery.

Established congenital pseudarthrosis of the tibia has been treated in the past by bone grafting or amputation. Osseous union probably is more difficult to obtain in this condition than in any other. Boyd and Sage reviewed the English literature in 1958 and found that primary union was obtained in approximately 56% of 91 patients treated with 23 different surgical procedures. Morrissy, Riseborough, and Hall reported union in fewer than 50% of 40 patients treated with 172 bone-grafting procedures, and Murray and Lovell reported successful treatment in only 31% of 36 pseudarthroses after a total of 85 grafting procedures. In a long-term follow-up study, Crossett et al. reported good or fair results in 52% of 25 patients treated with 96 surgical procedures. Traub, O'Connor, and Masso reported that of 30 patients with 33 involved tibiae, 14 patients (15 limbs) required amputation despite multiple attempts to obtain union (average 4.7 procedures). Patients in whom union was obtained had an average of 2.8 surgical procedures. Traub et al. identified several factors that correlated with poor results: neurofibromatosis, dysplastic lesions, and multiple surgical procedures. They cautioned that even when union is obtained, leg-length discrepancy and malalignment may require surgical correction.

The age of the patient, the difficulty in obtaining union, and, should union be obtained, the anticipated residual shortening and other deformities of the tibia must all be considered. In an infant or young child, bone grafting is indicated as early as feasible. Even though the likelihood of obtaining union increases with increasing age, especially after puberty, the longer grafting is delayed, the shorter and more poorly developed the leg will be. When union is obtained in a young child, weight-bearing in a brace results in more normal development of the limb. The child's parents should be told that treatment often consists of several operations and that even then amputation may be necessary later because of failure to obtain union. If grafting is indicated but for some reason must be delayed, the limb should be braced to prevent increased angulation at the pseudarthrosis. In an older child, bone grafting is indicated unless shortness or other deformity of the limb is such that function would be better after amputation and fitting with a prosthesis. McElvenny first called attention to the heavy cuff of tissue surrounding the bone at the pseudarthrosis, and he reasoned that the presence of this tissue, whether congenital or a result of a fracture, may decrease bone production and consequently healing. Any operation for congenital pseudarthrosis should include complete excision of this tissue.

Bone-grafting procedures remain the mainstay of treatment for congenital pseudarthrosis of the tibia. Although many techniques have been described, the most commonly used in recent years is the intramedullary rodding technique described by Anderson, Schoenecker, Sheridan, and Rich. They reported union of an established congenital pseudarthrosis of the tibia in

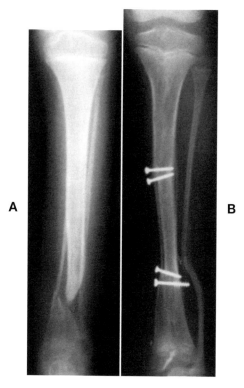

Fig. 26-55 Congenital pseudarthrosis of tibia treated with vascularized fibular bone graft. **A,** Preoperative roentgenogram of tibia with established distal pseudarthrosis after multiple failed surgical procedures. **B,** Three years after repair with vascularized fibular graft.

9 of 10 patients; 1 patient required additional bone grafting before union occurred. Although refractures occurred in 5 patients, 3 of whom required additional procedures, at an average follow-up of 6 years all 10 patients were able to walk without pain. In their study of 18 patients with congenital pseudarthrosis of the tibia, Baker, Cain, and Tullos reported that the best results (union in 7 of 8 patients) were obtained with intramedullary rod fixation, bone grafting, and the use of an osteostimulator, as described by Paterson and Simonis, followed by intramedullary fixation and bone grafting (union in 3 of 5 patients). Of a total of 36 operations done to obtain union in these patients, only 9 (2 of 23) of those without intramedullary fixation were successful.

A more recent technique is the free vascularized bone graft with either fibular or iliac crest grafts (Fig. 26-55). Weiland et al. reported eventual union in 18 of 19 pseudarthroses of the tibia treated with free vascularized fibular bone grafts; however, there were 5 nonunions after the index operation, and 9 bone-grafting procedures were needed in those 5 patients. Heikkinen et al. reported bony union and ability to walk without external support at 14-year follow-up of 10 patients treated with resection of the pseudarthrosis and reconstruction with a free vascularized graft. Other authors have reported good results with this technique in small series of patients; however, the procedure requires experience with microvascular techniques.

Good preliminary results were reported with the Ilizarov technique, but problems have included difficulty transporting the proximal tibia, "docking" malalignment, and poor quality of regenerated bone, leading to refracture. In a multicenter study conducted by the European Paediatric Orthopaedic Society (Grill et al.), however, the Ilizarov technique was shown to be the optimal method of treatment, with a fusion rate of 75.5% and the best correction of additional deformities. The authors also noted that of 120 patients reported in the literature, the Ilizarov technique obtained satisfactory healing in 94 (78%). The findings from this study of 340 patients who underwent 1287 procedures for congenital pseudarthrosis of the tibia identified the goals of treatment of the biological problems: (1) resection of the pseudarthrosis to provide stability, the basic requirement for bony consolidation, (2) correction of length discrepancy and axial deformity, (3) achievement of fusion, and (4) correction of additional problems around the main deformity such as alignment, leg-length discrepancy, and ankle valgus. The authors concluded that plating and rodding failed to provide adequate stability for the pseudarthrosis to heal and that when this kind of fixation was used, too little of the pseudarthrotic bone was resected. In addition, that suggested that neither plating, rodding, nor vascularized fibular transfer provides correction of shortening and valgus ankle deformity. They listed as advantages of the ring fixator that it (1) provides excellent stability, (2) allows complete resection of the pseudarthrotic area regardless of the size of the resected segment because the device allows lengthening or segmental bone transport, (3) enables weight bearing during the whole time of treatment,

which stimulates healing of bone and soft tissues, (4) also can be used to transport the fibula distally, and (5) does not prohibit other treatment methods if this method fails. Disadvantages are that it is time consuming, is not easy to perform, and, in some cases, can lead to varying degrees of complications such as pin track infections, fracture, ankle valgus, and ankle stiffness. The consensus was that surgery should not done in children younger than 3 years of age and, if possible, surgery should be postponed until the age of 5 years.

For most established pseudarthroses, initial treatment should be intramedullary rodding and bone grafting. Vascularized fibular grafts may be indicated for pseudarthroses with gaps of more than 3 cm and for those in which multiple surgical procedures have failed. The Boyd dual onlay bone graft is indicated only for type IV pseudarthrosis.

◆ **Insertion of Williams Intramedullary Rod and Bone Grafting**

TECHNIQUE 26-20 *(Anderson et al.)* (Fig. 26-56)
Position the patient supine on a radiolucent operating table and apply a tourniquet to the thigh. Expose the ipsilateral iliac crest and harvest as much cancellous bone and bone from the outer table as can be obtained safely. Approach the tibia through an anterior incision that is centered over the pseudarthrosis and just lateral to the tibial crest. Divide the deep fascia of the anterior compartment at this level. Subperiosteally, expose the normal bone of the tibial shaft

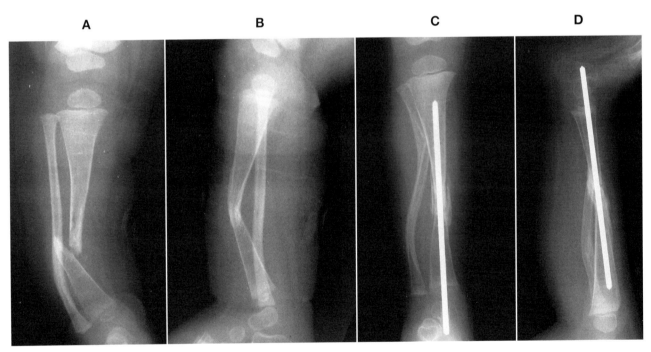

Fig. 26-56 Insertion of Peter Williams rod for congenital pseudarthrosis of tibia, as described by Anderson et al. **A,** Anteroposterior view of type II congenital pseudarthrosis of tibia in 16-month-old child. **B,** Lateral view. **C,** Postoperative anteroposterior view. **D,** Postoperative lateral view.

just proximal and distal to the pseudarthrosis. Completely excise the bone and fibrous tissue at the pseudarthrosis until normal medullary bone of both tibial fragments is exposed. Resection generally results in tibial shortening of 1 to 3 cm. Ream the medullary canals of both tibial fragments with a drill or small curet, or both.

The Williams device consists of an in-dwelling rod and an insertion rod. The in-dwelling rod is smooth and cylindrical and varies in diameter. The proximal end is machined to a diamond tip, and the distal blunt end is threaded internally for approximately 15 mm so that a second (insertion) rod of equal outside diameter can be attached to it temporarily. The insertion rod is machined proximally so that its external threads screw into the distal end of the in-dwelling rod, and it is machined distally to a diamond tip. To determine the rod length needed, make a lateral roentgenogram to determine the expected length of the leg after the affected bone and fibrous tissues have been removed and the angular deformity has been corrected.

Drive the coupled rods into the distal part of the tibia at the site of the osteotomy, across the ankle and subtalar joints, and out the sole through the heel pad. When the rod is placed across the ankle joint, it is important to correct valgus deformity of the ankle and dorsiflexion deformity of the foot, which are the inevitable consequences of weight-bearing on an anterolaterally bowed tibia. Fluoroscopy is helpful during this part of the procedure.

Approximate the tibial fragments and drive the rod retrograde into the region of the proximal tibial metaphysis, nearly to the tibial physis but not encroaching on it. Unscrew the insertion rod a single full turn and verify the junction of the rod on a lateral roentgenogram. Fully disassemble (unscrew) the insertion rod and remove it, leaving the distal end of the implanted rod in the calcaneus.

Pack the autologous corticocancellous bone strips from the iliac crest around the osteotomy and secure them with circumferential sutures of fine stainless steel or, as have been used more recently, absorbable sutures. Close the subcutaneous tissue and skin and apply a single hip spica cast.

AFTERTREATMENT. The duration of immobilization and the type of cast are determined by the amount of healing noted on clinical and roentgenographic examinations. When healing is sufficient, the hip spica cast is discontinued and an above-the-knee cast is applied. Removal of the cast and institution of progressive weight-bearing usually are possible between 3 and 9 months after surgery. A knee-ankle-foot orthosis or patellar tendon–bearing brace is worn until skeletal maturity is reached.

Complications
Stiffness of the Ankle and Hindfoot. A stiff ankle should be expected until the distal tip of the rod is proximal to the ankle joint after longitudinal growth of the distal end of the tibia. Even if stiffness persists, it rarely hampers functional results.

Refracture. Refracture is common in patients with pseudarthroses, despite apparently solid clinical and roentgenographic union. Refracture can be managed with casting or removal and replacement of the intramedullary rod with additional bone grafting. Because of the likelihood of refracture, removal of the rod after union is not recommended until skeletal maturity has been reached.

Valgus Ankle Deformity. The distal tibial fragment must be fixed so that valgus deformity of the ankle is corrected at the time of placement of the intramedullary rod. Intraoperative fluoroscopy is useful for monitoring this procedure. Long-term bracing is mandatory during the growth years to minimize progressive valgus ankle deformity, or surgical treatment with the Langenskiöld procedure may be indicated.

Tibial Shortening. Tibial shortening should be anticipated in almost all these children. The maximal projected shortening in the patients of Anderson et al. was 4 cm. In selected patients, tibial shortening can be treated by a well-timed contralateral epiphysiodesis or limb lengthening of the proximal tibia.

The Boyd dual onlay bone graft (Fig. 26-57) is the treatment of choice only in patients with "stress" (type IV) fractures that

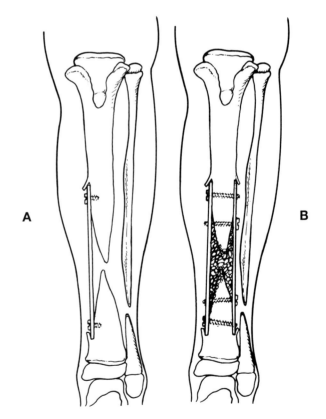

Fig. 26-57   Boyd dual onlay bone graft for congenital pseudarthrosis of tibia. **A,** First graft temporarily held in position by two short screws. **B,** Medial and lateral grafts fixed with transfixing screws. Resected pseudarthrosis filled with cancellous grafts.

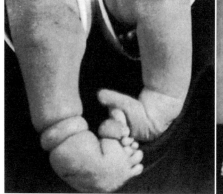 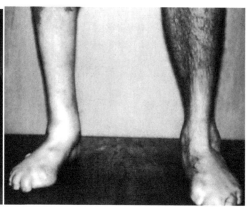

Fig. 26-58   **A,** Congenital constriction of right leg and great toe and bilateral clubfoot. **B,** Adult with loss of several toes caused by congenital constrictions.

proceed to pseudarthrosis but do not have a wide gap between the bone ends. Intramedullary nailing with bone grafting, with or without electrical stimulation, is recommended for an established pseudarthrosis. The vascularized graft or the Ilizarov technique may be useful initially in severe cases with significant shortening and a wide nonunion or in patients in whom medullary nailing and standard bone grafting procedures fail.

Constrictions of Leg

A congenital circumferential constriction, or "Streeter" band of the soft tissues of the leg, is rare. It is seen at birth as a depression in the soft tissues completely encircling the limb (Fig. 26-58). Often the foot also is deformed, the deep fascia may be affected, and usually the lymphatic vessels and superficial circulation are partially obstructed. Distal to the constriction is a persistent pitting edema that can be cured only by excising the constriction and, in most instances, the edematous tissues distal to it. Fractures of the tibia and fibula at the level of the constriction have been reported. In marked contrast to congenital pseudarthrosis, after successful treatment of the constriction, the fractures heal promptly without surgery.

Traditionally, constriction bands have been released in two or three stages to prevent vascular compromise of the distal part of the extremity. More recently, however, several authors have reported good results with one-stage release. Greene recommended a one-stage operation for all circumferential constriction bands, superficial or deep. The advantages of a one-stage release include easier postoperative care, especially in infants, and avoidance of a second or third operation with additional periods of anesthesia.

The association of congenital constricting bands with clubfoot was reported by Cowell and Hensinger, Allington et al., and Gomez, among others. The prevalence of clubfoot in patients with congenital constricting bands ranges from 12% to 56%.

Hennigan and Kuo divided 135 constriction bands in 73 patients into four zones (Fig. 26-59). Most (50%) were in zone 2, between the knee and ankle. They also classified the bands

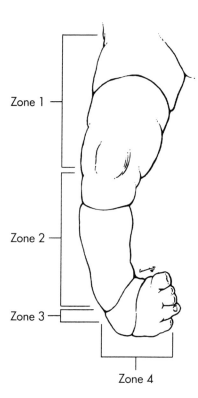

Fig. 26-59   Zones of constricting bands described by Hennigan and Kuo (see text). (From Hennigan SP, Kuo KN: Resistant talipes equinovarus associated with congenital constriction band syndrome, *J Pediatr Orthop* 20:240, 2000.)

according to severity: grade 1 bands involved subcutaneous tissue, grade 2 bands extended to the fascia, grade 3 bands extended to the fascia and required release, and grade 4 bands were congenital amputations. In their series, 45% were grade 4, 33% were grade 3, 19% were grade 2, and 3% were grade 1. The prevalence of clubfoot deformity was 47% (34 of 73 patients); 28 of the 73 children (38%) had at least one ipsilateral constricting band and a clubfoot deformity (37 clubfeet). Twenty-six clubfeet were not associated with any documented neurological deficit, and 11 were associated with a documented neurological deficit. All neurological deficits were in children with grade 3 bands in zone 2, and clubfoot in these children required numerous and more extensive surgeries, with poorer results, than those in children with no neurological deficits. These authors suggested early complete soft tissue release, along with consideration of tendon transfers, and noted that bony surgery eventually will be necessary and prolonged bracing will be needed to prevent recurrence.

◆ ONE-STAGE RELEASE OF CIRCUMFERENTIAL CONSTRICTING BAND

TECHNIQUE 26-21 *(Greene)*

Excise a 1- to 2-mm margin of normal skin and subcutaneous tissue to minimize the risk of recurrence. Resect all constricted fascia and muscle that have been converted to dense fibrous connective tissue. After resection of the tissue within the constriction band, identify the vascular and neurological structures proximal and distal to the band by careful dissection as the skin and subcutaneous tissue are undermined. If subcutaneous tissue is excessive, especially on the dorsum of the fingers, debulking should be done. Close the skin with multiple Z-plasties, fashioning fairly large flaps at an angle of 60 degrees.

TECHNIQUE 26-22 (Peet)

Remove the entire constriction by circumferential excision of the skin and subcutaneous tissue down to the deep fascia (Fig. 26-60). If the limb tapers, curve the distal incision in a serpentine line so that its length is about the same as that of the proximal one. Then undermine the skin and subcutaneous tissue on each side of the excised area. Approximate the deep tissues with interrupted sutures. Approximate the skin edges with interrupted mattress sutures except in one area; in this area lengthen the edges of the skin with one or more Z-plasties, the limbs of which are approximately 2 cm long. Raise and transpose the triangular flaps and suture them in position with small interrupted sutures.

AFTERTREATMENT. A pressure bandage is applied from proximal to the area of surgery to the distal end of the limb. With young children a cast or plaster splint is applied and worn for 2 to 3 weeks until the incision has healed.

Congenital Hyperextension and Dislocation of Knee

Congenital hyperextension of the knee is only the lowest grade of an abnormality that is divided into three grades according to severity. These are grade 1, congenital hyperextension; grade 2, congenital hyperextension with anterior subluxation of the tibia

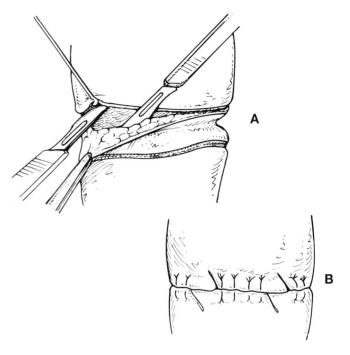

Fig. 26-60 Congenital constriction. **A,** Excision of constricture and undermining of skin edges. **B,** Skin edges have been sutured except in two areas in which Z-plasty incisions have been made. (Redrawn from Peet EW. In Rob C, Smith R, eds: *Operative surgery*, part 10, London, 1959, Butterworth.)

on the femur; and grade 3, congenital hyperextension with anterior dislocation of the tibia on the femur (Fig. 26-61).

Congenital hyperextension or dislocation of the knee usually is associated with skeletal abnormalities elsewhere in the extremity. In a study of 155 children with congenital dislocation of the knee, Katz, Grogono, and Soper found other musculoskeletal abnormalities in 82; 45 had congenital dislocation of the hip. In their study of 15 knees with congenital hyperextension and anterior subluxation of the tibia, Curtis and Fisher found an abnormality of the hip in 11 patients. Johnson, Audell, and Oppenheim found other abnormalities in 88% of their 17 patients, and Nogi and MacEwen reported congenital hip dysplasia in 8 of 17 patients (Fig. 26-62).

Katz et al. found the cruciate ligaments in five knees to be either markedly attenuated or absent, and they postulated that the basic defect in congenital dislocation of the knee is absence or hypoplasia of these ligaments. Other investigators, however, consider these findings a result of the dislocation.

The pathological condition usually varies with the severity of the deformity, but always the anterior capsule of the knee and the quadriceps mechanism are contracted. As the severity of the anterior displacement of the tibia increases, other findings include intraarticular adhesions and other abnormalities within the joint and hypoplasia or absence of the patella. Curtis and Fisher noted fibrosis and loss of bulk of the vastus lateralis muscle. Further, the suprapatellar pouch was obliterated by the adherent quadriceps tendon, and in more than half of the knees the patella was displaced laterally. In severe anterior dislocation

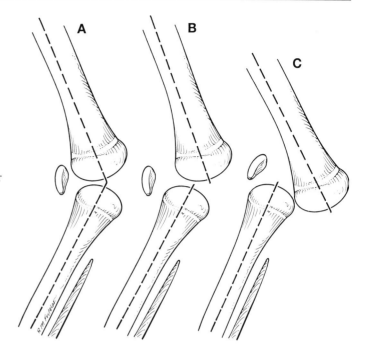

Fig. 26-61   **A,** Congenital hyperextension. **B,** Subluxation of knee. **C,** Dislocation of knee. (Redrawn from Curtis BH, Fisher RL: *J Bone Joint Surg* 51A:225, 1969.)

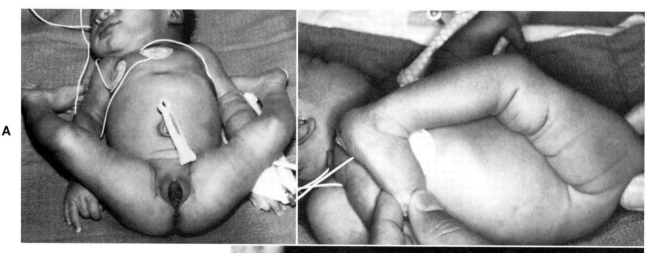

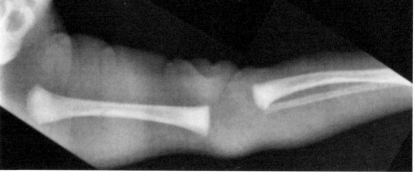

Fig. 26-62   Congenital dislocation of knee. **A,** Newborn with bilateral dislocations. **B,** Note prominence of femoral condyles posterior to anteriorly dislocated tibia and fibula. **C,** Anterior displacement of tibia and fibula is evident on lateral roentgenogram. (Courtesy Jay Cummings, MD.)

the collateral ligaments coursed anteriorly from their femoral attachments, and the hamstring muscles in some patients were subluxated anteriorly to function as extensors of the knee in this deformed position.

The treatment of congenital hyperextension of the knee depends on the severity of the subluxation or dislocation and the age of the patient. In the newborn with mild to moderate hyperextension or subluxation, conservative treatment methods such as the use of the Pavlik harness for posturing of the knee in a continued position and serial casting to increase knee flexion are most likely to succeed. Ko, Shih, and Wenger reported treating 24 congenital knee dislocations in 17 patients from 10 minutes to 26 days old with immediate reduction, serial casting, or traction. At an average follow-up of almost 5 years, excellent or good results were obtained in all patients who had no associated anomalies.

Roach and Richards proposed two criteria for successful nonoperative treatment of congenital knee dislocation: roentgenographic evidence of reduction and knee flexion to 90 degrees or more. According to most authors, nonoperative treatment can be continued for up to 3 months.

In children who do not respond to conservative measures, the use of skeletal traction for correction is an option, but the deformity is difficult to correct with this method. In older children with moderate or severe subluxation or dislocation, surgery is indicated. In a child with both congenital dislocation of the knee and congenital dislocation of the hip, surgical correction of the knee first is advisable.

Curtis and Fisher described a procedure for correction of congenital dislocation of the knee that is recommended for children between the ages of 6 and 18 months. The technique combines anterior capsular release, lengthening of the quadriceps mechanism, and release of intraarticular adhesions. Occasionally, the articular surfaces of the knee remain abnormal if the deformity recurs. Ideally, a functional range of motion can be obtained. In rare cases osteotomy of the femur or tibia may be required in an older child.

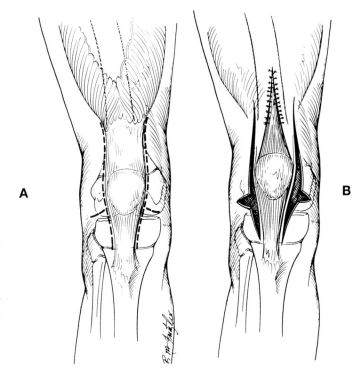

Fig. 26-63 Curtis and Fisher technique for congenital dislocation of knee. **A,** Lines of incision to release anterior capsule medially and laterally, as well as medial and lateral retinaculum of quadriceps mechanism. **B,** Correction after soft tissue release and lengthening of rectus femoris muscle.

◆ CAPSULAR RELEASE AND QUADRICEPS LENGTHENING FOR CORRECTION OF CONGENITAL KNEE DISLOCATION

TECHNIQUE 26-23 *(Curtis and Fisher)*

Make a long anterior midline incision starting superomedially at the level of the middle third of the femur and extending inferolaterally to the tibial tuberosity. Expose the anterior thigh muscles and divide the quadriceps mechanism superior to the patella by either an inverted V-shaped incision (Fig. 26-63) or a Z-plasty. The former incision provides a tongue of tissue superior to the patella that is suitable for attachment of the proximal muscle mass after the extensor mechanism has been lengthened. Next, divide the anterior capsule transversely and extend the incision posteriorly to the tibial and fibular collateral ligaments. Mobilize and displace these ligaments posteriorly as the knee is flexed. If the patella is displaced laterally, release the lateral part of the patellar tendon and the vastus lateralis so that the patella can be moved to its proper location on the femoral condyles. Release any tight iliotibial band and lengthen the fibular collateral ligament if needed. Mobilize all normal-appearing quadriceps muscle and align it in the long axis of the femur to exert a direct pull on the patella. Suture the lengthened quadriceps mechanism with repair of the vastus medialis muscle to the lengthened rectus femoris.

Evaluate tracking of the patella from extension to 90 degrees of flexion. Close the wound and apply a long leg cast with the knee flexed 30 degrees.

AFTERTREATMENT. If the anterior skin is under excessive tension, the cast can be changed at 2 weeks with the use of outpatient anesthesia. At 4 to 6 weeks the cast is removed, and active and passive exercises are begun. In older patients, continuous passive motion can be used to regain motion during the first 3 to 6 weeks after surgery, and a long leg brace is worn for 6 to 12 months to prevent hyperextension of the knee.

Congenital Dislocation of Patella

Congenital dislocation of the patella often is familial and bilateral. Occasionally it is accompanied by other abnormalities, especially arthrogryposis multiplex congenita and Down syndrome. It is persistent and irreducible and usually accompanied by abnormalities of the quadriceps mechanism. The vastus lateralis may be absent or severely contracted, and the patella may be dislocated laterally and attached to the anterior aspect of the iliotibial band. Often the patella is small and misshapen and in an abnormal location in the quadriceps mechanism. Genu valgum and external rotation of the tibia on the femur commonly develop. The capsule on the medial side of the knee is stretched, the lateral femoral condyle is flattened, or the insertion of the patellar tendon is located more laterally than normally.

Eilert noted that two clinical syndromes have been described in the literature: congenital dislocation of the patella or fixed lateral dislocation of the patella and habitual dislocation of the patella, which he suggested should be more accurately termed "obligatory dislocation" of the patella. These two syndromes have different clinical presentations (Table 26-3), and the timing of surgical correction is different.

The diagnosis of congenital dislocation of the patella is difficult to make before the patient is 3 to 4 years old because of lack of ossification of the patella. MRI can show the cartilaginous patella lying lateral to the femur and can confirm the diagnosis when congenital lateral patellar dislocation is suspected. Several authors have described the use of ultrasound to define the position of the cartilaginous patella. Because the severity of the deformity is directly related to the length of time that the deformity is allowed to remain uncorrected, surgery can be done as soon as the diagnosis is made to try to prevent a valgus, flexion, external rotation deformity of the knee (Fig. 26-64).

In a group of 35 patients with congenital or habitual dislocation of the patella, Gao, Lee, and Bose found the underlying pathological condition to be contracture of the quadriceps mechanism in all; the contractures were more severe in those with congenital dislocations. Operative techniques vary according to the extent and degree of these operative findings. The primary objective is release of the contracted structures on the lateral side of the patella (the lateral capsule, iliotibial band, and lateral portion of the quadriceps) to allow reduction of the patella. Medial plication of the lax capsule is necessary to stabilize the reduced patella. In most patients, especially younger children, extensive lateral release and capsular plication are sufficient to obtain patellofemoral congruency. In older children, advancement of the vastus medialis often is necessary to tighten the muscle and improve muscle action.

Gao et al. obtained satisfactory results in 88 of patients with extensive lateral release, medial plication, and transfer of the lateral half of the patellar tendon. Langenskiöld and Ritsilä reported successful treatment of 18 congenitally dislocated knees with lateral release and medial transfer of the patellar tendon. Gordon and Schoenecker treated 10 patients with 13 involved knees using lateral release and VMO advancement and entire patellar transfer in skeletally immature patients and medial transfer of the tibial tubercle in skeletally mature patients. At an average 5-year follow-up, all patients reported relief of pain and a marked increase in activity tolerance.

Table 26-3 Two Types of Congenital Dislocation of the Patella

Persistent Dislocation	Obligatory Dislocation
Patella is dislocated lateral and persistent in that location	Patella dislocates and reduces spontaneously with flexion and extension of knee joint
Often obvious in infancy	Usually present at 5 to 10 years of age
Frequently associated with generalized syndrome	Usually isolated anomaly
Knee flexion contracture is present	Range of knee motion usually normal
Nearly always produces functional disability	May be well tolerated with little functional disability
Early surgical correction	Surgical correction can be delayed until patient is symptomatic

Adapted from Eilert RE: *Clin Orthop* 389:22, 2001.

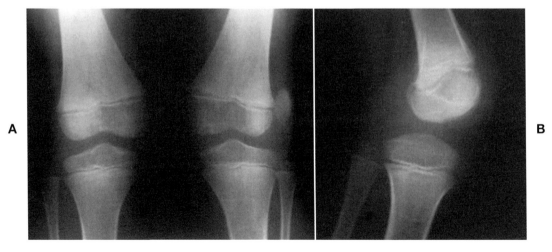

Fig. 26-64 Untreated congenital dislocation of left patella in 5-year-old boy. **A,** Anteroposterior view shows fixed lateral dislocation. **B,** On lateral view, patella appears absent because of superimposed femoral condyles.

◆ LATERAL RELEASE AND MEDIAL PLICATION AND PATELLAR TENDON TRANSFER

TECHNIQUE 26-24 *(Beaty; Modified from Gao et al. and Langenskiöld)*

Make a midline incision from the distal aspect of the femur to the tibial tuberosity. Perform full-thickness skin dissection over the patella to expose the medial and lateral aspects of the knee joint and the quadratus femoris muscle. Release the vastus lateralis from its most proximal muscle origin in the quadratus femoris to the level of the joint. This may require release of the iliotibial band laterally to the intermuscular septum. Because a midline surgical incision over the patella tends to heal with more proliferative scarring in children than adults, Eilert suggested making the surgical incision over the anterolateral knee so that the scar is not under direct pressure against the patella. The incision must be long enough to expose a sufficient portion of the quadriceps muscle so that it can be realigned, and in an infant with congenital patellar dislocation, the incision may extend halfway up the thigh.

Occasionally the rectus femoris must be dissected and lengthened by a Z-plasty. Incise the vastus medialis obliquus from its origin proximally and distally from the patella, the medial capsule, and the patellar tendon. Reduce the patella into the femoral groove. Reattach laterally and distally the vastus medialis obliquus to the patellar tendon and medial retinaculum to secure the patella in the femoral groove. Once the initial suture has been placed distally, move the knee through a gentle range of motion to assess reduction and tracking of the patella in the femoral groove. If the tension is too tight on the vastus medialis obliquus, remove the suture and transfer the muscle slightly proximally. If the tension is too lax, attach the vastus medialis obliquus farther distally and laterally.

Occasionally the patella is so unstable that the gracilis or semitendinous tendon must be divided at the musculotendinous junction and then transferred into the patella as a checkrein for added stability. The vastus medialis obliquus is then sutured to the remaining retinaculum of the patella and the quadratus femoris. Continue the repair of the vastus medialis obliquus proximally and distally. Move the knee again through a range of motion to ensure reduction of the patella in the femoral groove and normal tracking during flexion and extension. Deflate the tourniquet and obtain hemostasis with electrocautery. Insert a drain deep into the wound and close the subcutaneous tissue and skin. Apply a long leg cast with the knee in 30 degrees of flexion.

AFTERTREATMENT. The cast is removed approximately 6 weeks after surgery, and both active and passive range-of-motion exercises are begun.

Congenital Deficiencies of Long Bones*

The first scientific approach to the problem of congenital long bone deficiencies was devised by Frantz and O'Rahilly in 1961. Their widely used classification system described deficiencies as terminal or intercalary. In terminal deficiencies, there is an amputation with no body parts distal to the site (Fig. 26-65, *A*). In intercalary deficits, a middle segment is missing, but the distal segments are present (Fig. 26-65, *B*). Terminal and intercalary deficiencies are further defined as transverse or longitudinal. For example, the complete absence of a hand at the wrist is a terminal transverse deficiency. A complete hand without a radius or ulna is an intercalary transverse deficiency. An example of a terminal longitudinal deficiency is fibular hemimelia in which the lateral two rays also are missing. Fibular hemimelia in which the foot is normal is an intercalary longitudinal deficiency.

In 1964 Swanson, in conjunction with the American Society for Surgery of the Hand and the Federation of Societies for Surgery of the Hand, devised a more specific classification scheme. Although this system was devised originally for upper extremity deficiencies, it is applicable to the lower extremities as well. Like its predecessors, the Swanson classification scheme aids in taxonomy but not in treatment planning. Regardless of taxonomy, each child must be evaluated carefully because no two children are exactly alike.

TIBIAL HEMIMELIA

Since the disorder was first described by Otto in 1941, tibial hemimelia has been known by a variety of names, including *congenital longitudinal deficiency of the tibia, congenital dysplasia of the tibia, paraxial tibial hemimelia, tibial dysplasia,* and *congenital deficiency or absence of the tibia.* This condition actually represents a spectrum of deformities, ranging from total absence of the tibia (the most severe form) to mild hypoplasia of the tibia (the least severe form). The incidence has been estimated at 1 in 1 million live births, and the condition may be bilateral in as many as 30% of patients. It usually occurs sporadically, although familial cases with either autosomal dominant or recessive transmission patterns have been reported. At least four distinct syndromes have tibial hemimelia as a component: polydactyly–triphalangeal thumb syndrome (Werner syndrome), tibial hemimelia diplopodia, tibial hemimelia–split hand/foot syndrome, and tibial hemimelia–micromelia–trigonal brachycephaly syndrome. Although the exact cause is unknown, Sweet and Lane described a murine model for tibial

---

*Much of the information and many illustrations in this section are taken from the work of Dr. John E. Herzenberg in Chapter 5, Congenital Limb Deficiency and Limb Length Discrepancy, in Canale ST, Beaty JH: *Operative pediatric orthopaedics,* ed 2, St Louis, 1995, Mosby.

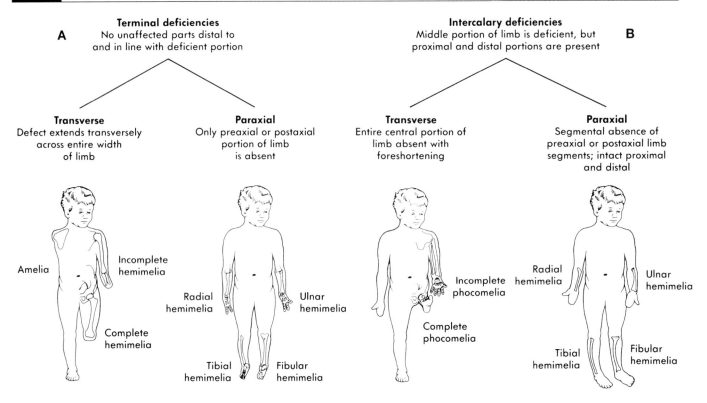

A

Terminal deficiencies
No unaffected parts distal to
and in line with deficient portion

Transverse
Defect extends transversely
across entire width
of limb

Paraxial
Only preaxial or postaxial
portion of limb
is absent

Amelia

Incomplete
hemimelia

Complete
hemimelia

Radial
hemimelia

Ulnar
hemimelia

Tibial
hemimelia

Fibular
hemimelia

B

Intercalary deficiencies
Middle portion of limb is deficient, but
proximal and distal portions are present

Transverse
Entire central portion of
limb absent with
foreshortening

Paraxial
Segmental absence of
preaxial or postaxial limb
segments; intact proximal
and distal

Incomplete
phocomelia

Complete
phocomelia

Radial
hemimelia

Ulnar
hemimelia

Tibial
hemimelia

Fibular
hemimelia

Fig. 26-65 Frantz-O'Rahilly classification of congenital limb deficiencies. **A,** Terminal deficiencies. **B,** Intercalary deficiencies. (Modified from Hall CB, Brooks MB, Dennis JF: *JAMA* 181:590, 1962.)

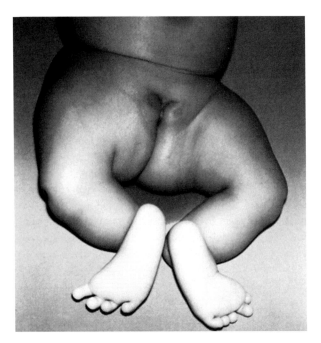

Fig. 26-66 Bilateral tibial hemimelia in 3-month-old girl; note absence of great toe on right foot, severe varus deformities of feet, and fixed knee flexion contractures.

hemimelia in which the dominant mutation resides on the X chromosome.

The involved leg is short, and the fibular head is palpable if it is proximally displaced. The foot is held in severe equinovarus, and the hindfoot is stiff (Fig. 26-66). In older children, the proximal tibial anlage may be palpable, even if it is not roentgenographically visible. The knee is generally flexed and, in more severe deformities, quadriceps insufficiency causes a lack of knee extension. Careful clinical evaluation of the quadriceps extensor mechanism is important, because this has significant prognostic value regarding the potential for reconstruction of the knee. Femoral hypoplasia may be seen.

Classification

The most widely used classification scheme for tibial hemimelia is that of Jones, Barnes, and Lloyd-Roberts (Fig. 26-67), which is based on the early roentgenographic presentation; treatment recommendations are given for each type.

In type 1A deformity there is a complete roentgenographic absence of the tibia and a hypoplastic distal femoral epiphysis (compared to the normal side; Fig. 26-68). In type 1B deformity there also is no roentgenographic evidence of a tibia, but the distal femoral epiphysis appears more normal in size and shape.

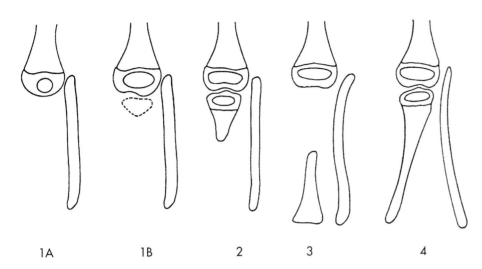

1A   1B   2   3   4

Fig. 26-67 Classification of tibial hemimelia. In type 1A, fibula is dislocated proximally, tibia is not roentgenographically evident, and distal femoral epiphysis is smaller than on normal side. In type 1B, fibula is dislocated proximally, and proximal tibial anlage may be visible at birth on ultrasound or magnetic resonance imaging studies but not on plain roentgenograms. Type 2 deformity has proximal dislocation of fibula and roentgenographically visible proximal tibia with normal-appearing knee joint. In type 3 deformity, fibula is dislocated proximally, distal tibia is roentgenographically visible, but proximal tibia is not seen. In the rare type 4 deformity, fibula has migrated proximally, with diastasis of distal tibiofibular joint. (Modified from Jones E, Barnes J, Lloyd-Roberts GC: *J Bone Joint Surg* 60B:31, 1978.)

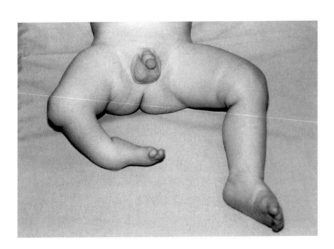

Fig. 26-68 Congenital tibial hemimelia type 1A.

This difference is critical because the type 1B deformity has a proximal tibial cartilaginous anlage that can be expected to ossify with time. Modern imaging techniques, such as arthrography, ultrasound, and MRI, have shown this cartilaginous anlage in type 1B deformities (Fig. 26-69). In time the proximal tibial anlage of a type 1B deformity may ossify to become a type 2 lesion.

In type 2 deformity a proximal tibia of varying size is present at birth. The fibula usually is normal in size, but the head is proximally dislocated (see Fig. 26-69, *A*).

Type 3 deformity, in which the proximal tibia is not roentgenographically visible, is rare. The distal tibial epiphysis sometimes is visible, along with a mature distal metaphysis; however, there may be only a diffuse calcified density within the distal tibial anlage. The distal femoral epiphysis usually is well formed, but the upper end of the fibula is proximally dislocated. Although the distal femoral epiphysis usually is of normal size, the knee generally is unstable.

In the rare type 4 deformity, the tibia is shortened and there is a proximal migration of the fibula with distal tibial fibular diastasis (Fig. 26-70). This also has been called *congenital diastasis of the ankle joint* and *congenital tibiofibular diastasis.*

In tibial hemimelia the superficial peroneal nerve may terminate at the level of the ankle. Leg muscles that normally insert on the plantar surface of the foot tend to blend into a common tendon sheet. The talus and calcaneus frequently are congenitally fused. The anterior tibial artery is absent, and the plantar arterial arch is incomplete. Similar vascular findings in clubfoot and fibular hemimelia suggest reduced vascular flow as a cause. Associated anomalies generally are most severe when the tibia is least developed. In type 4 deformities, the distal tibial epiphysis may be absent.

Treatment

As with all congenital lower limb deficiencies, the goal of treatment is a functional limb equal in length to the normal limb. The type of surgical treatment depends on the roentgenographic classification and clinical appearance. For severe deficiencies, amputation and prosthetic rehabilitation are the most practical means of treatment. Type 1A deformities are most frequently treated with knee disarticulation; however, type 1B deformities often can be reconstructed to yield a functional knee joint.

The two options for treatment of type 1A deformities are knee disarticulation or knee reconstruction (with or without foot amputation). The easiest and frequently most effective

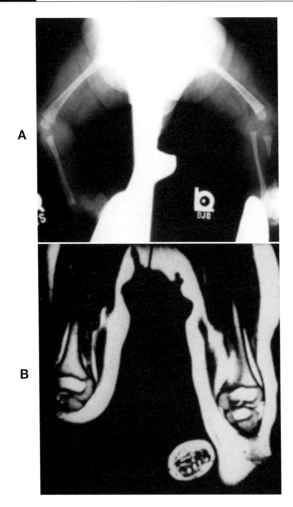

Fig. 26-69 **A,** Bilateral tibial hemimelia in newborn. Note presence of proximal tibial remnant on left and absence of remnant on right. Distal femoral epiphyses are equally well developed. Thus left side is type 2 deformity and right side is type 1B deformity. **B,** Magnetic resonance imaging of same patient shows proximal tibial anlage on both sides; left side has bony epiphysis, whereas right side is purely cartilaginous. Flexion contractures of both knees in these coronal images obscure lower legs.

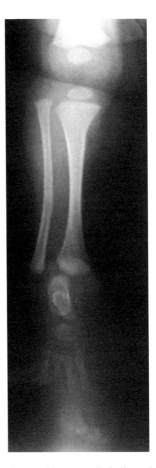

Fig. 26-70 Newborn with congenital diastasis of ankle representing type 4 tibial hemimelia; note absence of first ray.

option is knee disarticulation followed by fitting with an above-knee prosthesis. This provides a definitive solution with one operation. Knee disarticulation is preferred over above-knee amputation because above-knee amputation for type 1A deformity may result in skin problems from bony stump overgrowth. Because the ultimate femoral growth often is diminished, the end result of a knee disarticulation may be a functional above-knee amputation level. Children treated in this manner are almost uniformly active, functional prosthetic users. Attempts to correct the equinovarus and absent knee joint frequently result in repeated operations and eventual failure. It may be reasonable to preserve the foot in bilateral deformities, since limb-length discrepancy is not a consideration, but attempts to reconstruct the knee in conjunction with foot amputation have produced mixed results.

Brown described reconstruction of type 1A tibial hemimelia in two patients in whom the fibula was surgically transferred into the intercondylar notch to create a tibia (Fig. 26-71). In 1972 Brown and Pohnert reported 40 patients treated with this procedure, of whom 22 were functioning satisfactorily and 18 required secondary revision procedures for flexion deformities of the knee. Brown redefined his indications to include a child under 1 year of age (preferably under 6 months) with the physical potential to walk, a functioning quadriceps mechanism, and full passive extension of the knee.

Subsequent authors have reported failure of the procedure to reliably obtain good results. In reports by Jayakumar and Eilert, Schoenecker et al., and Loder and Herring, poor results ranged from 50% to 100%, with most patients requiring further surgery because of knee joint instability or stiffness. The success of the Brown procedure depends on the presence of a functioning quadriceps mechanism, the absence of flexion contracture, and an intact proximal tibial anlage, which are more likely indications for tibiofibular synostosis.

In type 1B and type 2 deformities a functional knee joint exists, and knee disarticulation is not required if the quadriceps

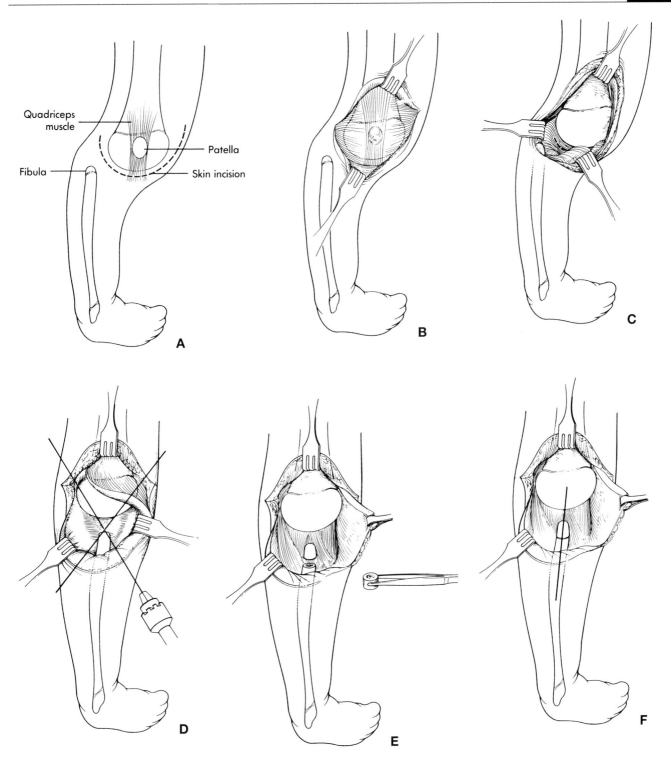

Fig. 26-71 Brown procedure. **A,** Incision begins anterolaterally, extends inferiorly, and ends anteromedially. **B** and **C,** Interposed tissues between displaced proximal fibula and distal femur must be completely sectioned. **D,** Fibula is then brought down underneath femur and held with crossed Kirschner wires or medullary wire. **E** and **F,** If fibula cannot be brought to level of intercondylar notch, segmental resection can be performed and fixed with medullary Kirschner wire. (Modified from Brown FW: *J Bone Joint Surg* 47A:695, 1965.)

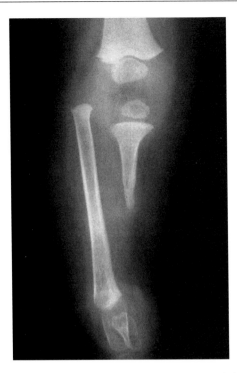

Fig. 26-72 Type 2 tibial hemimelia in 18-month-old child who underwent transfer of fibula to tibia. Because periosteal sleeve was left intact, connection between transferred distal fibula and original proximal fibula reformed. Syme amputation may be considered as a second stage.

mechanism is present and functional. A proximal tibiofibular synostosis combined with a Syme amputation or distal reconstruction is the treatment of choice (Fig. 26-72). Making a synostosis between the fibula and tibia creates a more uniform, in-line, weight-bearing mechanical axis. When the fibula is not transferred to the tibia, a peculiar, curved, hypertrophied fibula develops, causing a secondary deformity. Fusing the fibula underneath the tibia encourages its transformation into a more tibia-like bone. The Syme amputation is preferred to a through-bone amputation to prevent transdiaphyseal problems of bony stump overgrowth and to preserve maximal length of the stump.

Attempts have been made to treat tibial hemimelia with surgical equalization of leg length, production of a plantigrade foot, and creation of a stable knee. However, traditional leg-lengthening procedures, soft tissue reconstruction, and casting have not reliably achieved these goals in patients with tibial hemimelia. For this reason, the treatment pendulum has swung toward early amputation and prosthetic rehabilitation. With the introduction to North America of the Ilizarov method of extremity reconstruction, the pendulum is swinging back toward restoration of leg length, production of a plantigrade foot, and achievement of a stable knee with a functional range of motion for type 2 and type 4 lesions. However, the primary treatment remains early amputation and prosthetic rehabilitation for type 1A and type 3 deformities.

Other ingenious procedures have been used for reconstruc-

tion in children with tibial hemimelia. With ipsilateral femoral deficiency, arthrodesis of the fibula to the distal femur can be performed or, in younger children, chondrodesis, aligning the fibula directly with the femur and the intercondylar notch. Combining this with a Syme amputation significantly lengthens the effective lever arm of the femur.

Although Syme and Boyd amputations have been the accepted treatments to make prosthetic rehabilitation easier, other alternatives have been described. If a family is absolutely opposed to amputation of the foot, an acceptable alternative is reconstruction of the foot and ankle complex by implanting the distal fibula into the talus in an extreme equinus position to increase the length of the limb (Fig. 26-73, A). Prostheses can be constructed to take advantage of this extra length while accommodating the foot.

In type 1B deficiencies, a knee joint exists even if it cannot be seen on roentgenograms, and functional reconstruction may be possible, as in type 2 deficiencies. In both types a proximal tibial segment is present. The recommended treatment is transection of the proximal fibula at the level of the distal tip of the proximal tibial remnant and transfer of the distal fibula to fuse with the tibial remnant. Putti used a side-to-side configuration (Fig. 26-73, B and C), but most authors now prefer end-to-end alignment between the tibial remnant and the fibula. Although it would seem preferable to wait until the proximal tibial anlage ossifies, Jones, Barnes, and Lloyd-Roberts reported that stability can be achieved even when the proximal tibia is purely cartilaginous. At a second stage, amputation of the foot is done to make prosthetic rehabilitation easier. Retention of the foot during the proximal tibial reconstruction is helpful because it serves as a fixation point for a long leg cast.

Newer techniques of limb reconstruction, such as those described by Ilizarov, may allow equalization of limb lengths in severe tibial hemimelia, even when associated with severe equinovarus deformity, but currently the best results are obtained with foot amputation and prosthetic limb equalization in type 1B or type 2 deficiency. Some authors recommend knee disarticulation even in type 2 deficiencies if severe knee flexion contractures are present before surgery. Proximal tibiofibular synostosis is not absolutely indicated for all type 2 deformities; the literature contains reports of satisfactory prosthetic rehabilitation after Syme amputation alone; however, if the fibula is transferred under the tibial remnant, it can be expected to reliably remodel and eventually form into a large, tibia-like bone.

Type 3 deficiencies are extremely rare and in the limited reports available have been treated with amputations of the foot at either the Syme or Chopart level. In these patients, the knee joint generally is stable and the fibula is proximally displaced. These patients function well as below-knee amputees. In some patients, tibiofibular synostosis may be possible.

For patients with type 4 deficiencies, treatment must be individualized. Syme amputation provides excellent function. Customized reconstruction of the ankle joint to retain the foot and ankle has also been described. Most patients can be treated

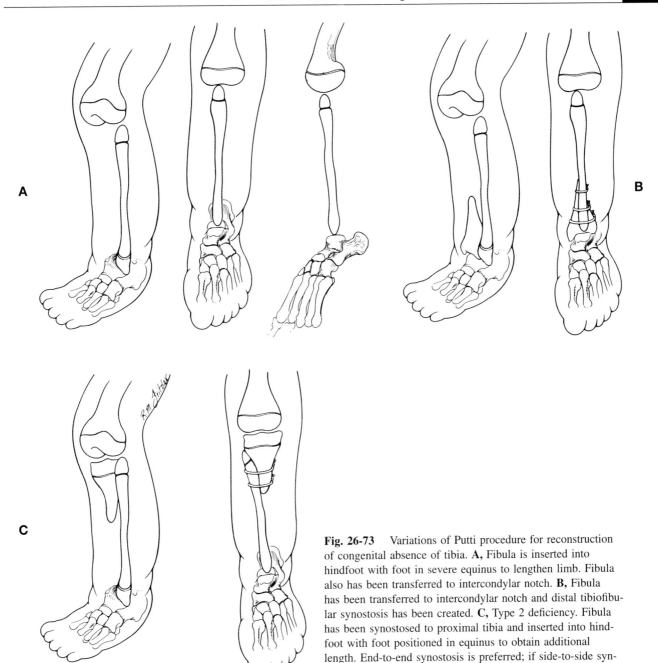

Fig. 26-73 Variations of Putti procedure for reconstruction of congenital absence of tibia. **A,** Fibula is inserted into hindfoot with foot in severe equinus to lengthen limb. Fibula also has been transferred to intercondylar notch. **B,** Fibula has been transferred to intercondylar notch and distal tibiofibular synostosis has been created. **C,** Type 2 deficiency. Fibula has been synostosed to proximal tibia and inserted into hindfoot with foot positioned in equinus to obtain additional length. End-to-end synostosis is preferred; if side-to-side synostosis is performed, transverse screw can be used for fixation.

with combinations of distal tibiofibular synostosis and distal fibular epiphysiodesis. Equinovarus deformities of the foot, if present, require soft tissue releases.

◆ Distal Fibulotalar Arthrodesis

TECHNIQUE 26-25
Place the patient supine on the operating table. Approach the distal fibulotalar articulation anterolaterally to expose both bones. Dissect soft tissue to allow central placement of the body of the talus onto the distal end of the fibula. Create a trough through the dome of the talus into which the distal fibula is placed plantigrade and in neutral alignment with the foot. If necessary, fix the fibulotalar articulation with longitudinal and crossed Kirschner wires. Remove the cartilage from the distal fibular epiphysis and from the dome of the talus to allow bone-to-bone contact. Close the wound and apply a long leg, bent-knee cast.

AFTERTREATMENT. The cast is worn until the arthrodesis has united, usually at 12 to 16 weeks.

◆ Proximal Tibiofibular Synostosis

TECHNIQUE 26-26 (see Fig. 26-72)

Make an anterolateral incision beginning at the proximal tibia and extending distally and anteriorly to the middle third of the tibia. Identify and protect the peroneal nerve. Dissect a sufficient portion of the anterior compartment musculature from the proximal medial tibia to expose the proximal tibial cartilaginous anlage (in type 1B deficiency) or the bony proximal tibia (in type 2 deficiency). Leave the proximal attachments of the fibula intact, but perform a subperiosteal dissection of the fibula. At an appropriate point opposite the distal end of the proximal tibial anlage, perform an osteotomy of the fibula. Drill a Steinmann pin of appropriate size distally through the medullary canal of the fibula out the plantar aspect of the foot. Reduce the fibula on the proximal tibia and drive the medullary pin retrograde into the proximal tibial remnant. If necessary, pass the pin into the distal femur for stability. Distally, bend the pin 90 degrees and cut it off below the level of the skin to be removed 6 to 8 weeks later. Immobilize the leg in a cast.

At a later date, the foot may be amputated. In some patients the foot may be salvaged with a combination of soft tissue release, Ilizarov technique, and talectomy or arthrodesis as needed. The tip of the proximal tibial remnant should be sectioned sufficiently to create a wide surface for either chondrodesis or synostosis with the fibula. The periosteum of the fibula should be sutured to the proximal tibial remnant, if possible, to prevent reformation of the fibula to its proximal remnant.

FIBULAR HEMIMELIA

Fibular hemimelia, also known as *congenital absence of the fibula, congenital deficiency of the fibula, paraxial fibular hemimelia,* and *aplasia or hypoplasia of the fibula,* is the most common long bone deficiency (followed by aplasia of the radius, femur, tibia, ulna, and humerus). Whether vascular dysgenesis and relative ischemia affect the developing mesenchyme and cause the skeletal dysplasia seen in fibular hemimelia is still conjectural. There are no clear genetic or toxic pathogenetic mechanisms. Fibular hemimelia consists of a spectrum of anomalies, the least severe being mild fibular shortening and the most severe being total absence of the fibula associated with defects in the foot, tibia, and femur. Because of the myriad anomalies associated with even mild fibular deficiency, Stevens and Arms suggested that *postaxial hypoplasia* is a more descriptive designation for this condition.

The clinical presentation depends on the specific classification and associated anomalies. Generally, there is leg-length

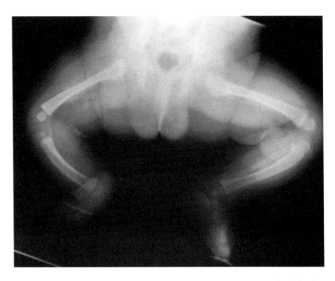

Fig. 26-74   Roentgenogram of infant with classic fibular hemimelia. Femur and tibia are both short, and foot is in valgus with absent lateral rays.

discrepancy with equinovalgus deformity of the foot, flexion contracture of the knee, femoral shortening, instability of the knee and ankle, and a stiff hindfoot with absent lateral rays (Fig. 26-74). Although equinovalgus is by far the most common foot deformity, equinovarus and calcaneovalgus also have been reported. Clinical problems are leg-length inequality and foot and ankle instability. In bilateral involvement, the leg-length discrepancy generally is manifested as disproportionate dwarfism because both sides usually are affected to a similar degree.

Classification

A useful classification scheme has been proposed by Achterman and Kalamchi (Fig. 26-75), who distinguished a type 1 deformity (hypoplasia of the fibula) from a type 2 deformity (complete absence of the fibula). Type 1 deformities are further subdivided into types 1A and 1B. In type 1A, the proximal fibular epiphysis is distal to the proximal tibial epiphysis and the distal fibular epiphysis is proximal to the talar dome. In type 1B, the deficiency of the fibula is more severe, with 30% to 50% of the length missing and no distal support for the ankle joint (Fig. 26-76). Abnormalities of the femur are common, as is hypoplasia of the patella and lateral femoral condyle. The cruciate ligaments also are clinically unstable. Angulation of the tibia is found most often in patients with type 2 deficiencies. Ball-and-socket ankle joints are present in most patients with type 1A deficiencies, and more severe foot and ankle problems are found in those with type 2 deformities. However, some patients with type 2 deformities have relatively stable ankle joints despite the absence of a fibula, and others have complete instability of the tibiotalar articulation. Tarsal coalitions and absence of the lateral rays are common.

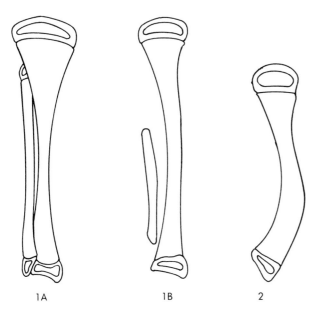

1A   1B   2

Fig. 26-75 Achterman and Kalamchi classification of fibular hemimelia. Type 1A: proximal fibular epiphysis is more distal, and distal fibular epiphysis is more proximal than normal. Type 1B: more severe deficiency of fibula with at least 30% to 50% of fibula missing and no distal support to ankle joint. Type 2: complete absence of fibula with bowing and shortening of tibia. (Modified from Achterman C, Kalamchi A: *J Bone Joint Surg* 61B:133, 1979.)

Treatment

At the initial evaluation the physician should attempt to predict the ultimate limb-length discrepancy, based on the current percentage of shortening. The percentage of shortening tends to remain constant throughout growth. For an anticipated mild leg-length discrepancy, the goals of treatment are equalization of limb length and correction of the foot deformity. Shoe lifts are prescribed during the growth period, and epiphysiodesis of the normal leg is performed at the appropriate time so that leg lengths are equal at the end of skeletal growth. If contralateral epiphysiodesis or shortening would result in unacceptable overall diminution of height, the physician is faced with a difficult decision: either the short leg is lengthened, or the foot is amputated and length is equalized with a prosthesis. Several studies have examined the validity of predicting leg-length inequality. Kruger and Talbott found that more severe shortening was associated with more normal feet; other series have found just the opposite. Generally, because the percentage of shortening seen in an infant remains relatively constant throughout childhood, reasonable predictions of final leg-length discrepancy can be made based on very early roentgenograms. If the predicted discrepancy is more than can be corrected with limb equalization procedures, a Syme amputation and prosthetic rehabilitation are recommended. Early amputation aids psychological acceptance of amputation for both the parents and the child. Choi, Kumar, and Bowen recommend early foot amputation if the end of the foot is above

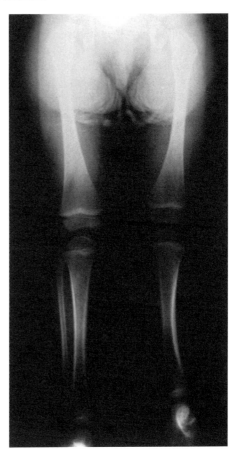

Fig. 26-76 Achterman and Kalamchi type 1B fibular hemimelia with very hypotrophic, faintly visible fibula, mild shortening of femur, and moderate shortening of tibia.

the level of the distal third of the tibia on the normal side. However, Ilizarov methods have salvaged feet with greater amounts of shortening. Stevens and Arms recommended combining limb lengthening with hemiepiphysiodesis of the distal femur or ankle or both to correct valgus alignment. They also suggest that adjunctive contralateral epiphysiodesis might be preferable to repeated limb lengthening, emphasizing the multiple procedures that may be required for associated deformities. Some authors recommend reconstruction of the ankle joint with soft tissue procedures or bony reconstruction of a stable ankle mortise. Thomas and Williams recommended Gruca's tibial osteotomy to reconstruct the ankle joint even when eventual amputation is recommended because this allows the child to spend the major portion of the growing and developmental years without having to rely on prostheses. Other authors, however, have found that children undergoing amputation in late childhood or early adolescence frequently stated that they wished they had had definitive amputation much earlier. Therefore the Gruca procedure rarely is indicated and should be used only when the foot is to be salvaged and the ankle requires stabilization.

For more severe deformities of the foot, multiple soft tissue releases have not reliably obtained a plantigrade foot. More severe foot deformities also may be accompanied by more severe degrees of limb shortening. Faced with the prospect of multiple and unpredictable surgeries to correct both limb-length discrepancy and foot deformities, early amputation and prosthetic reconstruction usually are considered the best options.

Choi et al. (2000) noted that the distal tibial epiphysis in patients with fibular hemimelia often is wedge-shaped, and they found that the severity of the wedging was predictive of the severity of foot deformity after tibial lengthening. In 44 patients who had tibial lengthening because of partial or total absence of the fibula, they identified three types of wedge-shaped epiphyses and related these to the prognosis of foot deformity after lengthening. In patients with mildly wedged epiphyses (type I), varying degrees of mild growth retardation and minimal foot deformity should be anticipated; in those with moderately wedged epiphyses (type II), worsened asymmetrical growth retardation and progressive foot deformity should be expected; and in those with severely wedged epiphyses (type III), severe growth retardation and severe foot deformities should be expected.

The maximal amount of limb-length discrepancy that can be corrected with a lengthening procedure has been variously described. Kawamura et al. stated that lengthening of more than 10% of the length of the involved bone is inadvisable, but greater lengthenings are now routinely being performed, especially with the Ilizarov technique. Currently, the Syme amputation and prosthetic fitting are recommended when limb-length discrepancy is predicted to be more than 12 to 15 cm and the foot is deformed. The advantages of early amputation include fewer hospitalizations and surgical procedures. Children who undergo amputation at an early age show excellent emotional adaptation to their disability and have good functional results. Naudie et al. reported that 12 patients (13 limb segments) with early amputation and prosthetic fitting had fewer hospital admissions, clinical visits, and periods of absence from school than 10 patients who had Ilizarov tibial lengthenings. McCarthy et al. compared outcomes at approximately 7-year follow-up in 15 patients who had early amputation to those in 10 patients who had tibial lengthening and found that patients who had amputations were able to perform more activities, had less pain, were more satisfied, had a lower complication rate, and had undergone fewer surgical procedures than those with lengthenings.

Various reconstructive procedures have been described. For equinovalgus deformity, both posterior and lateral releases are required. The tendo calcaneus, as well as the fibrocartilaginous anlage of the absent fibula, must be released. In older children ankle valgus can be corrected with a dome or varus supramalleolar osteotomy. Varus osteotomy shortens the limb somewhat but also eliminates the medial prominence associated with a simple closing wedge osteotomy (Fig. 26-77). A Wiltse osteotomy corrects the translational deformity (Fig. 26-78).

At the time of the Syme amputation, any residual bowing of

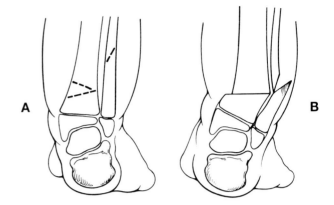

Fig. 26-77   **A,** Closing wedge technique can result in translation deformity with prominent medial malleolus **(B).**

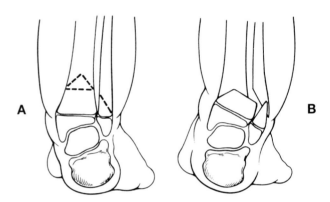

Fig. 26-78   Wiltse varus osteotomy for valgus ankle deformity. This osteotomy corrects translation that occurs during closing wedge osteotomy, **A,** Translatory shift occurs because deformity is present in ankle joint, and osteotomy is done more proximally in metaphysis. **B,** Translating distal fragment laterally results in more natural contour of ankle.

the tibia can be corrected with an osteotomy. Although a Boyd amputation offers greater length than a Syme procedure, it should be used cautiously in very young children because the Boyd amputation leaves a remnant of calcaneus that can migrate posteriorly (Fig. 26-79). Prophylactic sectioning of the tendo calcaneus should be considered when amputation is performed for congenital limb deficiencies.

◆ Varus Supramalleolar Osteotomy of the Ankle

TECHNIQUE 26-27 *(Wiltse)*

Make an anterior approach to the distal tibia and a lateral approach to the distal fibula. Create a triangular osteotomy, removing a segment of bone that can be used for bone grafting (see Fig. 26-78, *A*). Make the base of the triangle parallel to the floor but not parallel to the ankle joint. Make an oblique osteotomy of the distal fibula. Displace the distal segments proximally and laterally to avoid excessive

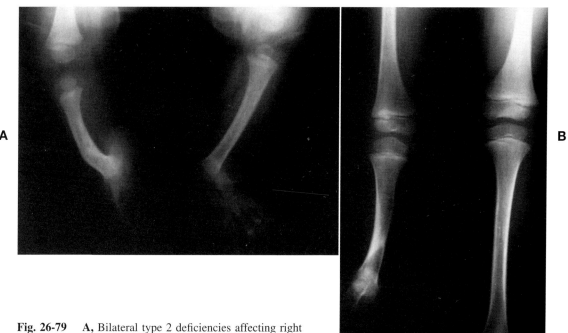

Fig. 26-79   A, Bilateral type 2 deficiencies affecting right side more severely than left side: four rays on left foot and only three on right. **B,** After Boyd amputation on right and foot centralization on left. (Courtesy Robert N Hensinger, MD.)

prominence of the medial malleolus (see Fig. 26-78, *B*). Fix the osteotomy with Steinmann pins and apply a long leg cast.

AFTERTREATMENT. Weight-bearing is not allowed until the osteotomies have healed adequately.

PROXIMAL FEMORAL FOCAL DEFICIENCY

Like many other congenital longitudinal and transverse deficiencies, proximal femoral focal deficiency (PFFD) includes a broad spectrum of defects. Mild forms result in minor hypoplasia of the femur, whereas severe involvement may result in complete agenesis of the femur (Fig. 26-80). Most commonly, PFFD consists of a partial skeletal defect in the proximal femur with a variably unstable hip joint, shortening, and associated other anomalies. Most patients with PFFD, especially those with bilateral involvement, have associated anomalies, the most common of which are fibular hemimelia and agenesis of the cruciate ligaments of the knee. A variety of other congenital anomalies have been reported in association with PFFD, including clubfoot, congenital heart anomalies, spinal dysplasia, and facial dysplasias. Grogan, Holt, and Ogden examined 26 amputation specimens and found talocalcaneal coalitions in 14 (54%): 1 in 9 patients who had PFFD alone, 6 in 8 who had fibular hemimelia alone, and 7 in 9 who had both PFFD and fibular hemimelia.

The incidence of PFFD has been reported to be 1 per 50,000 live births. Maternal diabetes has been implicated in femoral hypoplasia.

Classification

Aitken's four-part classification scheme (classes A, B, C, and D) is one of the earliest attempts to provide a systematic taxonomy of this condition (Fig. 26-81). In class A (Fig. 26-81, *A*) there is a normal acetabulum and femoral head with shortening of the femur and absence of the femoral neck on early roentgenograms. With age, the cartilaginous neck ossifies, although this frequently is associated with a pseudarthrosis. This may heal, but the usual roentgenographic picture shows severe coxa vara with significant shortening of the limb. Class B is similar to class A in that an acetabulum and femoral head are present; however, there is no bony connection between the proximal femur and the femoral head, and a pseudarthrosis is present (Fig. 26-81, *B*). In class C (Fig. 26-81, *C*) there is further degradation in the formation of the hip, characterized by a dysplastic acetabulum, absent femoral head, and short femur. A small, separate ossific tuft can be seen at the proximal end of the femur. In class D the acetabulum, femoral head, and proximal femur are totally absent (Fig. 26-81, *D*) and, unlike in class C, there is no ossified tuft capping the proximal femur. Class D patients often have bilateral anomalies.

Other authors have expanded the definition of PFFD to include lesser expressions of femoral malformation. In his evaluation of 125 patients with PFFD, Pappas described nine classes that ranged in severity from complete absence of the proximal femur (class I) to mild femoral aplasia (class IX). The Pappas class II corresponds to the Aitken class D, the Pappas

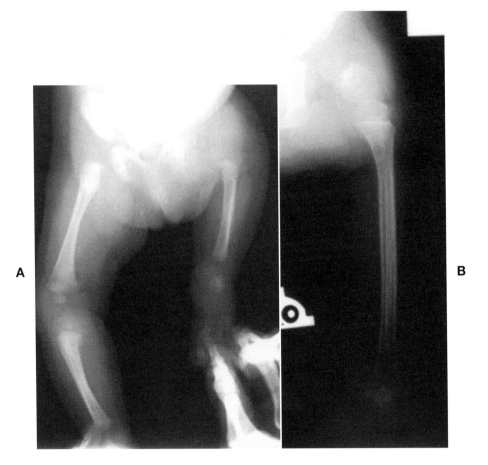

Fig. 26-80 **A,** Infant with severe proximal femoral focal deficiency. In addition to absent femur, tibia is short, and lateral ray is absent. **B,** At 5 years of age, after Boyd amputation. Note that distal femoral epiphysis is seen, but there is no femoral shaft or head. Acetabulum shows no sign of development. Cartilaginous anlage of distal femoral epiphysis was present at birth but not yet roentgenographically evident.

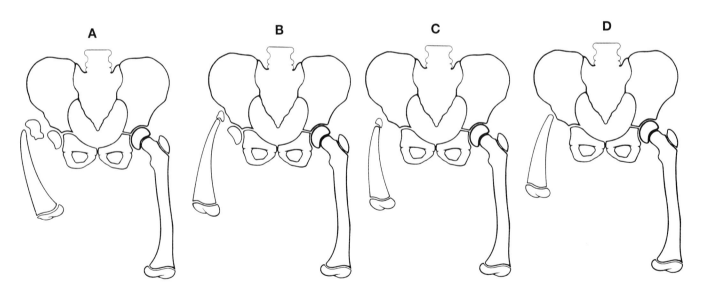

Fig. 26-81 Aitken classification scheme for proximal femoral focal deficiency. **A,** In class A, hip joint appears formed, but femoral neck is absent on early roentgenograms and femur is shortened. **B,** In class B, femoral head is more rudimentary and deficiency of proximal femoral shaft is more significant. Pseudarthrosis between femoral shaft and head is always present. **C,** In class C, femoral head is absent, acetabulum is shallow, and proximal femur is represented only by small tufts. **D,** In class D, femoral head and acetabulum are absent and deficiency of femoral shaft is more significant. (From Aitken GT: *Instr Course Lect* 24:81, 1975.)

class III corresponds to the Aitken class B, and the Pappas classes IV and V may be correlated with the Aitken class A (Table 26-4). Kalamchi et al. developed a simplified classification scheme for congenital deficiency of the femur that included five groups: group I, short femur and intact hip joint; group II, short femur and coxa vara of the hip; group III, short femur but well-developed acetabulum and femoral head; group IV, absent hip joint and dysplastic femoral segment; and group V, total absence of the femur.

In their review of 69 patients, Gillespie and Torode found that two major groups could be identified for treatment purposes. Group I patients had a hypoplastic femur in which both the hip and knee were reconstructible and leg equalization was sometimes possible. Group II patients exhibited a "true" PFFD in which the hip joint was markedly abnormal. Although some of these patients had tenuous connections between the femoral head and the proximal femur, the alignment and surrounding musculature were markedly abnormal. Also, these legs were too shortened, rotated, and marred by flexion contractures of the hip and knee to be reconstructible. These patients required only those reconstructive procedures that make prosthetic fitting easier.

Treatment

The major problems are limb-length inequality and variable inadequacy of the proximal femoral musculature and hip joint. Treatment is highly individualized and ranges from amputation and prosthetic rehabilitation to limb salvage, lengthening, and hip reconstruction. The natural history of the particular variant and the limitations of surgical reconstruction must be considered.

Often no surgical reconstruction of any kind is indicated. Bilateral PFFD is best treated nonoperatively (Fig. 26-82). These patients can walk well without prostheses, but for social or cosmetic reasons extension prostheses may be provided. The patients learn to accept their short stature and are quite functional. Foot surgery may be required to correct other anomalies. Limb lengthening is not indicated in these patients because extreme lengthening would be necessary, and the hips are unstable. Knee fusion is not indicated because the knee functions in conjunction with the hip pseudarthrosis to provide useful motion.

Stability of the hip is important in determining treatment. For patients with both a femoral head and an acetabulum (Aitken classes A and B), many authors have recommended surgery to establish continuity between the femoral head and the femur, but this may be technically difficult if there is little bone stock to work with in the proximal femur. For this reason, surgery is best delayed until ossification of the femoral head and proximal metaphysis is adequate. In some patients the femur is so short that a simultaneous knee fusion is performed, creating a one-bone leg (Fig. 26-83). With limited bone stock for proximal fixation, autogenous bone grafts should be added to the pseudarthrosis site. Although the roentgenographic picture may be improved with correction of the proximal pseudarthrosis, it remains to be shown that function is

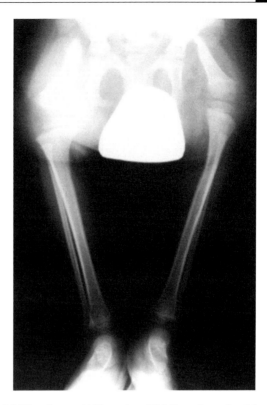

Fig. 26-82 Severe (Aitken class D) bilateral proximal femoral focal deficiency in 3-year-old boy; note total lack of formation of acetabulum.

improved. In fact, many patients treated nonoperatively have good motion and reasonably good function. Stabilizing the proximal pseudarthrosis may diminish the overall range of motion of the hip. For less severe PFFD (Pappas classes VII, VIII, and IX), hip reconstruction is limited to osteotomies that improve biomechanical alignment. Care must be taken not to damage the proximal femoral physis in these children, who already have problems with diminished growth of the femur.

Bowen et al. emphasized the importance of avoiding hip subluxation and dislocation during femoral lengthening in patients with unilateral femoral shortening. In their report of 44 patients, they identified several factors that predict progressive subluxation or dislocation of the hip during femoral lengthening: (1) type of deformity (Kalamchi classification), (2) the combined abnormality of coxa vara plus the varus bow of the femoral shaft, and (3) acetabular dysplasia present before lengthening. No hip abnormalities occurred after lengthening in patients with Kalamchi type I or II deficiencies, but progressive subluxation or dislocation of the hip occurred in those with type IIIA femurs with a combined coxa vara plus varus bow of the femoral shaft of less than 115 degrees and an acetabular index of more than 25 degrees. They recommended correction of the varus bow of the femur and the neck-shaft angle to 120 degrees and the acetabular index to less than 25 degrees before lengthening of type IIIA femurs.

For more severe deformities in which there is no femoral head or acetabulum (Aitken classes C and D or Pappas classes

Table 26-4 Nine Pappas Classes of Congenital Abnormalities of the Femur

	Class I	Class II (Aitken D)	Class III (Aitken B)	Class IV (Aitken A)
Femoral shortening (%)	—	70-90	45-80	40-67
Femoral-pelvic abnormalities	Femur absent Ischiopubic bone structures underdeveloped and deficient Lack of acetabular development	Femoral head absent Ischiopubic bone structures delayed in ossification	No osseous connection between femoral shaft and head Femoral head ossification delayed Acetabulum may be absent Femoral condyles maldeveloped Irregular tuft on proximal end of femur (rare)	Femoral head and shaft joined by irregular calcification in fibrocartilaginous matrix
Associated abnormalities	Fibula absent	Tibia shortened Fibula, foot, knee joint, and ankle joint abnormal	Tibia shortened 0%-40% Fibula shortened 5%-100% Patella absent or small and high riding Knee joint instability common Foot malformed	Tibia shortened 0%-20% Fibula shortened 4%-60% Knee joint instability frequent Foot small with infrequent malformations
Treatment objectives	Prosthetic management	Pelvic-femoral stability through prosthetic management	Union between femoral shaft and hip for stability Prosthetic management	Union between femoral head, neck, and shaft Prosthetic management

From Pappas AM: *J Pediatr Orthop* 3:45, 1983.

II and III), most authors recommend that no attempt be made at hip reconstruction, although there are notable exceptions. King recommended iliofemoral fusion, which requires a simultaneous Chiari osteotomy to create a suitable bony bed to receive the small femoral remnant, allowing the knee joint to assume the function of the hip joint. Fixsen and Lloyd-Roberts also used this technique, with additional bone graft to ensure fusion. Although this technique eliminates the hip instability, it may severely limit mobility of the limb. Even with a certain amount of instability, the knee generally functions as a hinge, providing flexion and extension only. Rotation and abduction are lost after iliofemoral arthrodesis. Steel et al. reported four patients with iliofemoral fusions for Aitken class C or D deficiencies and argued that untreated patients have progressive instability and proximal migration of the femur, which interfere with the fitting and functioning of a prosthesis. Steel's technique includes

Class V (Aitken A)	Class VI	Class VII	Class VIII	Class IX
48-85	30-60	10-50	10-41	6-20
Femur incompletely ossified, hypoplastic, and irregular Midshaft of femur abnormal	Distal femur short, irregular, and hypoplastic Irregular distal femoral diaphysis	Coxa vara Hypoplastic femur Proximal femoral diaphysis irregular with thickened cortex Lateral femoral condyle deficiency common Valgus distal femur	Coxa valga Hypoplastic femur Femoral head and neck smaller Proximal femoral physis horizontal Abnormality of femoral condyles common, with associated bowing of shaft and valgus of distal femur	Hypoplastic femur
Tibia shortened 4%-27% Fibula shortened 10%-100% Knee joint instability common Severe malformations of foot common	Single-bone lower leg Patella absent Foot malformed	Tibia shortened <10%-24% Fibula shortened <10%-100% Lateral and high-riding patella common	Tibia shortened 0%-36% Fibula shortened 0%-100% Lateral and high-riding patella common Foot malformed	Tibia shortened 0%-15% Fibula shortened 3%-30% Additional ipsilateral and contralateral malformations common
Prosthetic management	Prosthetic management	Extremity length equality Improved alignment of (a) proximal and (b) distal femur	Extremity length equality Improved alignment of (a) proximal and (b) distal femur	Extremity length equality

closing wedge osteotomies to eliminate the anterior bowing and to fuse the femur to the ilium so that the shaft is pointed as anteriorly as possible. This allows the knee joint to extend fully to simulate the 90 degrees of hip flexion required for sitting and to flex 90 degrees to simulate the neutral position of the hip for walking.

Surgical limb lengthening, with or without contralateral shortening, should be considered only if the femur is intact. In 1982 Herring and Coleman suggested 10 to 12 cm as the maximal amount of lengthening possible in a single long bone with congenital deficiency and, combined with contralateral shortening, 17 cm as the maximal amount of inequality that could be corrected. They recommended limb lengthening only in the femur with over 60% of predicted femoral length or less than 17 cm of projected shortening; other prerequisites for lengthening were hip stability and a stable, plantigrade foot.

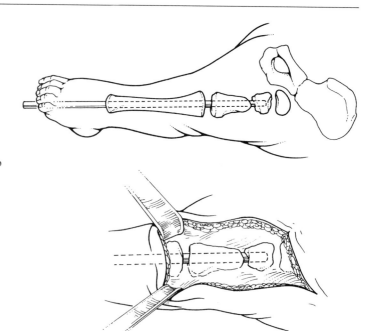

Fig. 26-83   When proximal femur is small, with pseudar-throsis between femoral neck and shaft, it can be stabilized to create better lever arm. Simultaneous knee arthrodesis can be performed to create one-bone leg. If possible, medullary fixation should stop just short of proximal femoral epiphysis.

Gillespie and Torode, using Wagner's technique of leg lengthening, suggested that lengthening be considered for femurs that are at least 60% of normal length. Because of failures and complications, several authors, including Dahl et al., Karger et al., and Stanitski et al., suggested that maximal lengthening should be 10% to 25% of the initial segment length. The Ilizarov method of lengthening, using circular external fixators, has extended these limits. The Ilizarov device allows extension proximally or distally with hinges to prevent knee and hip subluxation. Yun, Severino, and Reinker reported Ilizarov lengthenings in 35 bone segments (18 femurs, 11 tibias, 5 forearms, and 1 humerus) in 31 patients with an average age of 12 years. Their average initial goal was lengthening of 35% (20% to 63%); an average 33% lengthening (16% to 77%) was obtained, which was within 2.5 cm of the stated goal in 31 of the 35 procedures. No statistically significant difference was found among success rates according to bone type, age, etiology, or preoperative complexity. Lengthening was significantly more successful with initial goals of 55% or less.

Regardless of technique, limb lengthening in patients with PFFD is difficult, with the ever-present danger of knee and hip subluxation. For predicted discrepancies greater than 12 to 14 cm, lengthening can be performed in stages: one at 4 or 5 years of age, a second at age 8 or 9 years, and a third during adolescence. Depending on the predictions of the patient's overall height based on the normal leg, a contralateral epiphysiodesis may be indicated.

If limb lengthening is not feasible, various approaches are available to make prosthetic rehabilitation easier. Most children with PFFD can learn to walk without a prosthesis, but a prosthesis helps equalize leg lengths. An extension prosthesis is acceptable for a small child, but when the child becomes a teenager, a more cosmetically pleasing prosthesis can be fitted

after amputation of the foot. Amputation of the foot should be performed between 1 and 2 years of age, before the parents and child become psychologically attached to the concept of having a foot and an extension prosthesis.

An alternative approach is to use the prosthesis to mold the foot into equinus so that it fits into an above-knee amputation prosthetic socket. The socket is fashioned to include the entire femur. Later an arthrodesis can be performed, if necessary, to make prosthetic fitting easier. It is possible, however, that some knee motion within the stump of the prosthesis may serve as a protective mechanism for the abnormal proximal hip. If a knee arthrodesis is performed, the potential benefits in gait and prosthetic fitting may be outweighed by the increased stress placed on the proximal femur and proximal hip articulation and pseudarthrosis, if present.

Currently, knee arthrodesis with foot amputation, rather than limb lengthening, is the preferred treatment for significant deformities (Fig. 26-84). Ankle disarticulation, Syme amputation, or Boyd amputation can be used. The heel pad is stabilized by either the Syme or Boyd amputation, an advantage over simple ankle disarticulation. The Boyd amputation saves the entire calcaneus and provides a slightly more bulbous stump and additional length. However, if the combined length of the tibia, femoral remnant, and foot is greater than the femur on the opposite side, taking into account potential growth, then there is no advantage in the small increase and additional length provided by the Boyd amputation. It is possible to fuse the knee over an intramedullary Rush rod and still allow longitudinal growth of the distal femoral and proximal tibial physes.

Prosthetic reconstruction can be made easier in severe cases by a Syme amputation. The child is observed with serial scanograms until sufficient data have been collected to construct a working Moseley straight-line graph; then further surgery can be planned. If knee arthrodesis is selected to

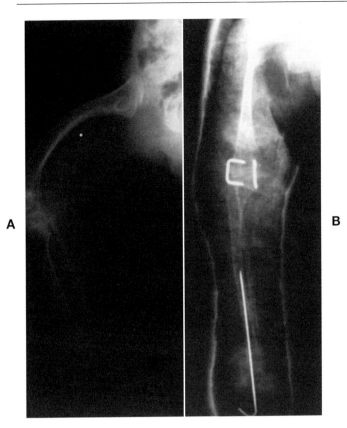

Fig. 26-84   **A,** Proximal femoral focal deficiency in 7-year-old child; femur is severely shortened, and tibia is relatively hypoplastic. **B,** After Boyd ankle amputation, stabilization with medullary Steinmann pin, and staple arthrodesis of knee joint, patient can be rehabilitated as after knee disarticulation.

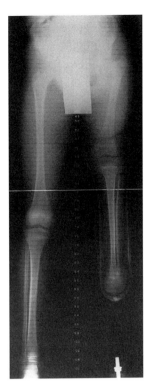

Fig. 26-85   Twelve-year-old child with previous Boyd amputation but no knee arthrodesis. Prosthetic management is that of below-the knee amputation, but result is cosmetically poor because of very long "tibia."

improve fitting of a prosthesis and gait, the physes around the knee can be epiphysiodesed if necessary to ensure that the prosthetic knee will be at the same level as the contralateral normal knee when the child reaches skeletal maturity. Precise predictions are not necessary because small amounts of additional shortening in the involved leg can be readily accommodated by the prosthesis. If, however, the involved femorotibial unit is longer than the contralateral normal femur, the prosthetic knee must be placed in either a very proximal or a very distal position, which is less cosmetically desirable (Fig. 26-85). Although this can be treated with a leg-shortening procedure at skeletal maturity, a simpler preventive procedure, such as a well-timed epiphysiodesis during the growing years, is preferable.

◆ Rotation Plasty

Van Nes described his below-knee rotation plasty in 1950, although it was originally performed by Borggreve some 20 years before. The operation was modified by Kostuik et al. and later by Gillespie and Torode to make it more suitable for reconstruction in PFFD. This reconstruction should be considered in patients who, because of significant femoral shortening, are not candidates for femoral lengthening. The procedure combines arthrodesis of the knee with rotation of the distal tibia 180 degrees externally so that the ankle joint becomes a functional knee joint: ankle plantar flexion becomes "knee" extension and ankle dorsiflexion becomes "knee" flexion. A reasonably stable hip joint and a well-functioning ankle are required for this technique. Unfortunately, many patients with PFFD also have fibular hemimelia, with a poorly functioning ankle joint. An arc or ankle motion of at least 90 degrees is required for rotation plasty reconstruction to be beneficial. The femur, knee, and tibia should equal the length of the opposite femur, but this usually is not the case, so ipsilateral knee epiphysiodesis is done to equalize the reconstructed femoral unit and the contralateral normal femur.

Some significant problems must be discussed with the patient and parents before undertaking this type of reconstruction. First, the appearance of the leg, with the foot rotated backward (Fig. 26-86), can be psychologically disturbing; great care should be taken in the preoperative consultation to make this clear. It is helpful to have another patient who has already undergone the procedure demonstrate how the prosthesis functions. If such a patient is not available, the family should be shown photographs and drawings of a rotation plasty. Another problem, especially in young children, is derotation of the surgically rotated foot. Of 20 patients with Van Nes rotation

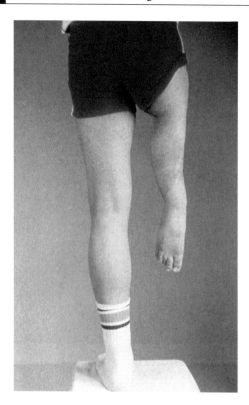

Fig. 26-86   Appearance of limb after Van Nes rotation plasty.

plasties reported by Kostuik et al., 12 required a subsequent derotation and half of those required a second derotation operation. They recommend that this reconstruction be deferred until the age of 12 years. Torode and Gillespie modified the procedure to limit the amount of derotation. Alman, Krajbich, and Hubbard compared the results of rotation plasty in nine patients to the results of Syme amputation in seven patients at an average follow-up of almost 10 years. They found no difference in gross motor function or perceived physical appearance between the two groups, but rotation plasty had resulted in a slightly more (10%) energy-efficient gait than had Syme amputation. Hillman et al. reported EMG and gait analyses of 43 patients ranging in age from 7 to 63 years who had rotationplasty for treatment of femoral or tibial bone tumors. All patients had good functional results, although older patients generally had lower functional scores, shorter walking distances, and worse gait patterns. Younger patients were better able to adapt to the altered anatomical and functional situation and to develop good function. Fowler et al. compared gait mechanics in patients with Syme amputations to those in patients with Van Nes rotational osteotomies and found that those with Van Nes procedures had more efficient gait mechanics and reduced energy expenditure compared to those with amputation.

TECHNIQUE 26-28 *(Van Nes)* (Fig. 26-87)

Position the patient supine and drape the entire limb free so that the skin is exposed from the toes to the iliac crest. Place a small towel under the sacrum. Begin the incision proximal and lateral to the knee and extend it across the knee distally along the subcutaneous crest of the tibia. Elevate the flaps medially and laterally to expose the knee capsule and patellar tendon. Divide the patellar tendon and open the knee capsule transversely. Apply traction on the capsule proximally and distally to expose the knee joint fully by dividing the collateral ligaments and the anterior, medial, and lateral capsule. On the medial side, carefully dissect out the insertion of the adductor magnus up to the level of the femoral artery. Divide the adductor magnus to enable the artery to derotate anteriorly and to limit postoperative derotation. Trace the femoral artery distally and posteriorly as it becomes the popliteal artery. Divide the medial hamstring muscles at their insertion. On the lateral side, carefully dissect out the peroneal nerve. If the fibula is deficient, the anatomical relationship between the peroneal nerve and the proximal fibular head may be abnormal. To prevent damage to the peroneal nerve, trace the nerve proximally to its point of origin on the sciatic nerve. Release any fascial attachments distally over the peroneal nerve.

After the major neurovascular structures have been completely identified and protected, divide the posterior knee capsule and section the origins of the gastrocnemius heads. The only remaining attachments from the femur to the tibia are the skin, subcutaneous tissues, and neurovascular structures. Release the lateral hamstrings. With an osteotome or oscillating saw, remove the articular cartilage of the proximal tibia down to the level of the proximal tibial epiphysis. Do not damage the proximal tibial physis.

If the leg needs to be shortened, shorten the femur by removing both the distal femoral epiphysis and physis. Next, insert an intramedullary Rush rod through the distal femur proximally, exiting through the piriformis fossa into the buttock. If necessary, ream the femur with a drill to prevent comminution during nail insertion. Make a small incision in the buttock where the nail exits. Then remove the nail and reinsert it from proximal to distal through the femur and into the tibia, stopping short of the distal tibial physis. While the nail is being inserted, rotate the tibia externally to relax the peroneal nerve. Gently transfer the femoral popliteal artery anteriorly through the adductor hiatus. If the leg cannot be comfortably rotated through the knee resection, obtain additional rotation through a separate osteotomy in the midshaft of the tibia, which also will be stabilized by the intramedullary nail. Additional shortening can be performed through the tibia if necessary. In such instances a fibular osteotomy also is performed. Attempt to rotate the extremity 180 degrees. If the rotation places too much torque on the vascular structures and the distal pulses are lost, derotate the leg through the knee until the pressure on the vessels is relieved. Close the wounds and apply a spica cast that maintains rotation.

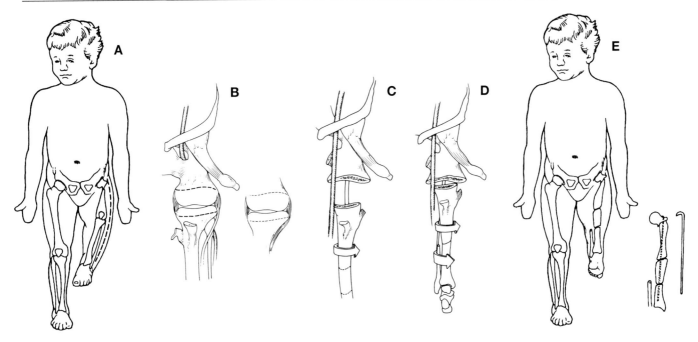

Fig. 26-87 Van Nes rotation plasty. Preoperatively, ankle joint of shortened extremity is approximately at level of opposite knee joint. **A,** Long incision on lateral aspect of leg, extending from hip to midshaft of tibia. **B,** Quadriceps and sartorius tendons are taken down distally to expose adductor hiatus and femoral artery; peroneal nerve is dissected free. **C,** After resection of knee joint and freeing of femoral-popliteal artery, tibia is externally rotated 140 degrees. **D,** Further rotation of 40 degrees more is possible after tibial osteotomy, allowing stretch on soft tissues to spread over greater distance. External rotation is preferred to internal rotation to prevent stretching of peroneal nerve. **E,** Fixation with medullary Rush rod. (Modified from Torode IP, Gillespie R: *J Bone Joint Surg* 65B:569, 1983.)

AFTERTREATMENT. If derotation of the foot was required to relieve vascular pressure, then the foot is rotated serially using successive hip spica casts to turn the foot on the axis of the intramedullary nail. When the osteotomies have healed, the child is fitted with a modified below-knee prosthesis. Although it is possible to amputate the toes to make the foot look more like a below-knee stump and less like a "backward" foot, most patients decline this option.

Amputations

Although most of the basic surgical principles of amputation in adults apply to children, there are important differences. Most amputations in children are performed for congenital conditions. Either the child is born without a portion of the limb, or an amputation is performed to make reconstruction and prosthetic rehabilitation easier in a deficient limb. Trauma accounts for most acquired amputations in children. Unlike typical adult dysvascular patients, children may tolerate skin grafts over stumps and, to a certain extent, tension at the suture line. Most revision surgery in children with congenital amputations involves the lower extremity. Revision amputation surgery in upper extremity limb deficiencies rarely is required.

Prosthetic fitting after amputation in children should begin after complete wound healing and standard stump preparation. A rigid postoperative plaster dressing that is bivalved to allow for swelling is preferred. Once the wounds are sufficiently healed, stump wrapping with elastic bandages is begun to prepare the stump for a prosthesis. Phantom pain and phantom sensations are problems in child amputees, especially after tumor surgery. Neuroma formation is rare, but gentle handling of the nerves and sectioning with a sharp knife without applying excessive traction on the nerves should be routine in all amputation surgery in children.

In planning amputation surgery, maximal length should be preserved to provide maximal lever arm strength for powering a prosthesis. Physes should be preserved whenever possible to ensure continued growth of the limb. This is especially true for the physes around the knee, which provide most of the growth in the lower extremity, and the physes around the shoulder and wrist, which provide most of the longitudinal growth of the upper extremity. Although amputation through a long bone in a growing child can result in appositional terminal overgrowth, this is not an adequate reason for sacrificing length. In below-knee amputations in young children, it is highly likely that the fibula, and to a lesser extent the tibia, will overgrow, but this can be satisfactorily remedied by revision surgery. Although knee disarticulation would prevent overgrowth, it is far more important to preserve the knee joint to power a below-knee prosthesis than to prevent overgrowth of the stump. Even short below-knee segments should be preserved if

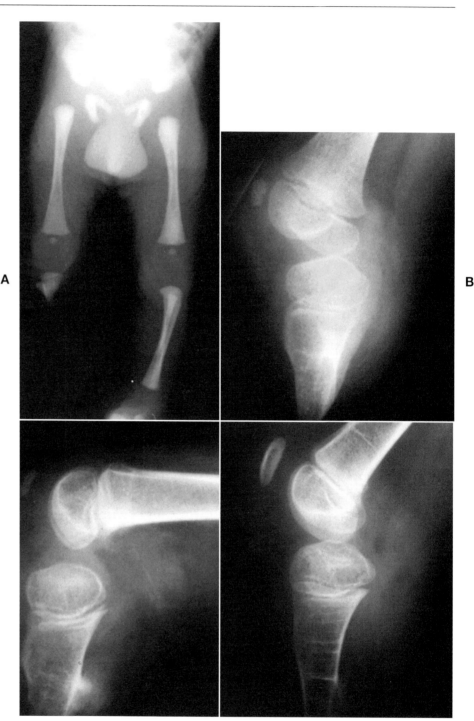

Fig. 26-88   A, Newborn with congenital amputation through proximal tibia. **B,** At 5 years of age, continued growth of distal stump and penciling resulted in protrusion of bone from skin. (Courtesy Robert N. Hensinger, MD.)

possible in growing children. Loder and Herring found that the gait characteristics of children with knee disarticulations were not a problem for moderate activities, but the inability to run well placed significant limitations on sports activities. Because the proximal tibial physis contributes most of the growth of the tibia, an initially short stump has the potential to become a longer, more functional stump. Further, in older children, it is possible to lengthen a short below-knee stump using the Ilizarov technique to provide a more functional stump in selected patients.

Terminal overgrowth has been reported most frequently in the humerus, followed by the fibula, tibia, and femur. Because it appears to be caused by appositional periosteal bone formation distally and not by epiphyseal growth proximally (Fig. 26-88), epiphysiodesis does not prevent stump overgrowth. A variety of techniques have been devised to prevent stump overgrowth, but none has been completely successful. Small bone spurs that form at the edge of the transected bone do not constitute true overgrowth and rarely require surgical removal. Stump overgrowth occurs in both congenital and traumatic amputations.

Another unusual problem, unique to growing children with

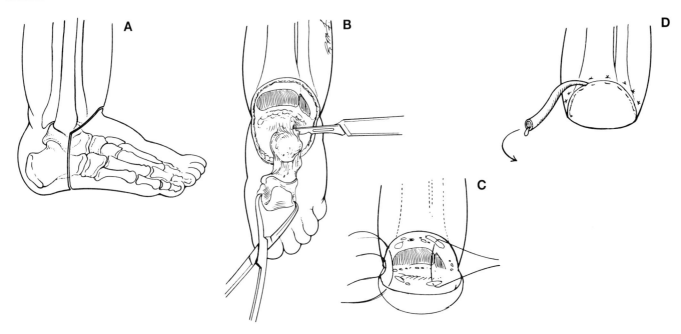

Fig. 26-89   Syme amputation. **A,** Fish-mouth incision. **B,** Enucleation of talus and calcaneus. **C,** Plantar flap sutured to distal tibia. **D,** Completed closure with drain in place.

below-knee amputations, was described by Mowery, Herring, and Jackson. They found patellar dislocations to be a common problem in adolescents, and in all patients they found patella alta, presumably caused by the force of the patellar tendon–bearing prosthesis against the lower surface of the patella. They postulated that this elongation of the patellar tendon might be prevented by earlier modification of the prosthesis to distribute the force around a greater area rather than concentrating it on the patellar tendon.

Ankle Disarticulation

Although standard amputation techniques are described in Chapter 10, important variations of amputations about the ankle exist for reconstruction in children with congenital limb deficiencies. The two most common reconstructive amputations performed for these children are the Syme and Boyd procedures. The Syme amputation is a modified ankle disarticulation. The Boyd procedure amputates all of the foot bones, except the calcaneus, and fuses the calcaneus to the distal tibia.

Many studies have documented excellent results with both procedures, yet the literature seems to favor a well-performed Boyd amputation over a Syme amputation. The problems encountered in Syme amputations in children have been overgrowth of retained calcaneus apophyses, heel pad migration, and formation of exostoses. The advantages of the Boyd operation are the additional length gained and the prevention of the posterior displacement of the heel pad, which occurs in many patients with Syme amputations. However, in the Boyd amputation it is important to align the calcaneus properly. If the calcaneus is not aligned correctly, it angulates into equinus and interferes with weight-bearing.

A problem common to both the Syme and the Boyd amputations is the flare of the distal tibial metaphysis, which gives a bulbous shape to the distal stump and necessitates a special prosthesis with a removable medial window. However, in children with congenital limb deficiencies such as tibial or fibular hemimelia, the distal ankle is relatively hypoplastic, so a bulbous stump usually is not a problem. A common problem in the Syme amputation is posterior migration of the heel pad despite attempts to anchor the heel pad distally. The Boyd amputation obviates this problem by producing an arthrodesis of the calcaneus to the distal tibia, although this may be difficult to achieve in very young children whose calcaneus is largely cartilaginous.

◆ Syme Amputation

TECHNIQUE 26-29
Make a fish-mouth incision beginning at the lateral malleolus, extending over the dorsum of the foot, and ending 1 cm distal to the medial malleolus (Fig. 26-89, *A*). The plantar portion should extend distally enough to allow adequate skin closure anteriorly. Place the foot in as much equinus as possible to expose the anterior ankle capsule and divide it. Next, divide the deltoid ligament between the talus and the medial malleolus but do not damage the nearby posterior tibial vessels. Section the lateral ligament between the calcaneus and fibula. Grasp the talus with a large clamp and further force it into equinus to permit dissection of the posterior ankle capsule. Make a subperiosteal dissection of the posterior aspect of the calcaneus through the ankle joint.

continued

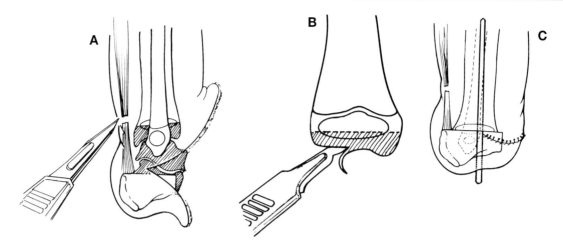

Fig. 26-90 Boyd amputation. **A,** Fish-mouth incision; shaded areas represent resected bone. **B,** Cartilage of distal tibia is removed by shaving gradually until bony epiphysis is reached; calcaneus is shifted anteriorly, and tendo calcaneus is sectioned to prevent it from migrating proximally. **C,** Fixation with smooth medullary pin aids fusion of calcaneus to distal tibial epiphysis.

Cut the tendo calcaneus at its point of insertion into the calcaneus but do not "button hole" through the skin. Place further traction on the hindfoot and further hyperflexion into equinus and dissect the soft tissues with a periosteal elevator and a knife, making sure to stay in the subperiosteal plane to avoid damaging the heel pad. Continue the dissection until the entire calcaneus has been excised (Fig. 26-89, *B*). To anchor the heel pad, drill holes in the anterior aspect of the distal tibia and use stout sutures from the distal aspect of the heel pad, anchoring it in the aponeurosis of the distal tibia (Fig. 26-89, *C*). In children it is not necessary to remove the cartilage of the distal tibia, but if desired the flare of the medial malleolus and distal fibula can be trimmed to create a more even weight-bearing surface. Pull the flexor tendons distally, transect them, and allow them to retract. Ligate the posterior and anterior tibial arteries as far distally as possible to prevent ischemic necrosis of the flaps. Insert suction drains in the wound and close the skin in layers (Fig. 26-89, *D*). Apply a rigid plaster dressing to diminish pain after surgery; bivalve the cast to allow for swelling.

AFTERTREATMENT. Weight-bearing on the stump in a cast is delayed until the wound has adequately healed.

♦ **Boyd Amputation**

TECHNIQUE 26-30
Make a fish-mouth incision as described for the Syme amputation. Elevate the skin flaps proximally and amputate the forefoot through the midtarsal joints. Excise the entire talus, using sharp dissection. With an oscillating saw

or osteotome, transect the distal end of the calcaneus (Fig. 26-90, *A*). In a similar manner remove the articular surface of the subtalar joint on the calcaneus perpendicular to the long axis of the tibia. Resect an adequate amount of the distal tibial articular cartilage so that the bony epiphysis of the distal tibia is exposed (Fig. 26-90, *B*). Shape the calcaneus to fit accurately against the surface of the distal tibial epiphysis. Stabilize this with a smooth Steinmann pin that enters the heel pad and provides fixation to the tibia by crossing the distal tibial physis into the metaphysis. Occasionally the tendo calcaneus must be severed to allow accurate positioning of the calcaneus. It is important to shift the calcaneus anteriorly before fixing it with the Steinmann pin (Fig. 26-90, *C*). Section the medial and lateral plantar nerves and allow them to retract. Section the posterior and anterior tibial arteries as far distally as possible to prevent wound necrosis. Close the wound over drains and apply a plaster cast. A hip spica cast may be necessary for young children.

AFTERTREATMENT. The pin usually can be removed at 6 weeks, and a new cast is applied and worn for an additional 6 weeks. After this the stump usually has healed sufficiently for prosthetic rehabilitation.

Limb-Length Discrepancy

Limb-length equality in the lower extremity is not simply a cosmetic concern, it also is a functional concern. The short-leg gait is awkward, increases energy expenditure because of the excessive vertical rise and fall of the pelvis, and may result in back pain from long-standing significant discrepancies. In a study of 23 young adults with untreated limb-length discrepancy of 1.2 to 5.2 cm, Papaioannou et al. found compensatory scoliosis and decreased spinal mobility but no back pain. Giles and Taylor, and Friberg studied much larger groups of patients and concluded that significant limb-length discrepancy causes low back pain and that the pain is diminished by limb equalization.

Limb-length inequality may result from trauma or infection that damages the physis, from asymmetrical paralytic conditions (e.g., poliomyelitis or cerebral palsy), or from tumors or tumorlike conditions that affect bone growth by stimulating asymmetrical growth, such as occurs with juvenile rheumatoid arthritis or postfracture hypervascularity. Idiopathic unilateral hypoplasia and hyperplasia are other common causes of limb-length discrepancy.

The treatment of limb-length discrepancy must be tailored to the specific conditions and needs of the individual patient. Treatment plans can be formulated only after a careful evaluation that includes assessment of the chronological and skeletal ages of the patient, the current and predicted discrepancy in the limb lengths, the predicted adult height, the cause of the discrepancy, the functional status of the joints, and the social and psychological background of the patient and family.

CLINICAL ASSESSMENT

The simplest means of measuring limb-length discrepancy is to place wooden blocks of known heights under the short leg until the pelvis is level; however, asymmetrical pelvic development or pelvic obliquity can cause miscalculation. Measurement also can be made from the anterosuperior iliac spine to the medial malleolus. Clinical evaluation should include assessment for any rotational and angular deformities, foot height differences, scoliosis, pelvic obliquity, and joint mobility and function. In certain paralytic conditions, particularly spastic diplegia, mild shortness of the paralytic side actually can improve gait by allowing the paralytic foot to clear the floor more easily during the swing phase of gait. Flexion contractures of the knee and hip make the limb appear shorter than it really is, both on clinical and roentgenographic examinations.

The goals of treatment are a balanced spine and pelvis, equal limb lengths, and a correct mechanical weight-bearing axis. In patients with rigid scoliosis and an oblique lumbosacral take-off, some degree of limb-length discrepancy may be desirable to preserve a balanced spine.

Roentgenographic measurements are important for accuracy because clinically palpable landmarks may be inaccurate. Two commonly used roentgenographic techniques for measuring limb-length discrepancy are the standing orthoroentgenogram and the scanogram. Both techniques involve placing a radiopaque ruler behind the limbs. The orthoroentgenogram is made on a long cassette that includes the hip, knee, and ankle on a single exposure. A magnification marker placed on the leg at the level of the bone minimizes magnification error. The scanogram uses separate exposures of the hip, knee, and ankle,

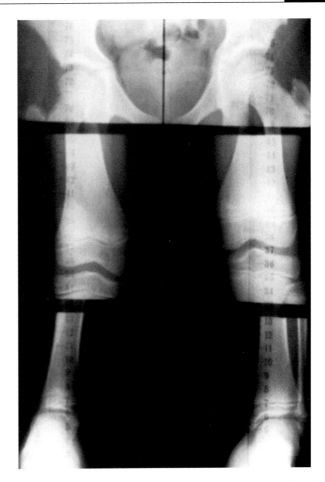

Fig. 26-91   Scanogram obtained for evaluation of limb length discrepancy in 12-year-old boy with fibular hemimelia on right.

so there is little parallax error (Fig. 26-91). However, it does require that the child remain still for all three exposures. Standing orthoroentgenograms offer the additional benefit of showing limb alignment. It is imperative that the legs be positioned with the patellae facing forward. A view of the left wrist is obtained to estimate skeletal age from the Greulich and Pyle atlas; however, this is not necessary for children younger than 5 years of age because the skeletal and chronological ages are not significantly different in these children.

Computed tomography (CT) scanograms have been proposed as an improvement over standard scanograms because the radiation exposure is less and accuracy is not compromised. On lateral CT scanograms, accurate measurement can be made of even the limb with a flexion deformity, as shown by Huurman et al. On biplanar CT scanograms, as proposed by Carey et al., foot height also can be measured.

Two techniques are widely used to predict growth and to help the surgeon decide the timing of limb equalization procedures. One is the Green-Anderson growth-remaining chart. Proper use of this chart requires the clinician to estimate the percentage of growth inhibition for the patient by taking two interval measurements separated by at least 3 months. The growth difference between the involved limb and the normal

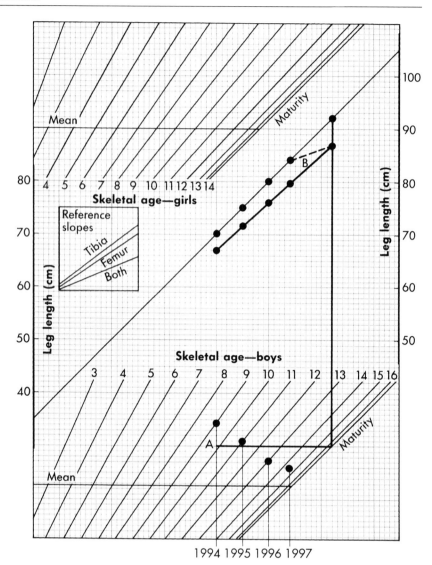

Fig. 26-92 Moseley straight-line graph. Example shown is boy with idiopathic hemiatrophy observed clinically for 4 consecutive years. In 1994 longer leg measured 70 cm, shorter leg was 67 cm, and bone age was 9 years. Additional scanograms and bone age roentgenograms are plotted as shown. Note horizontal straight line (A) extending to maturity line with equal number of skeletal ages above and below line. At skeletal maturity, longer leg is projected to measure 92 cm and shorter leg, 87 cm. Dotted line (B) represents projected growth of longer leg if epiphysiodeses of distal femur and proximal tibia are performed when longer leg reaches 84 cm in length, thus obtaining limb equalization by skeletal maturity.

limb is multiplied by 100, and that result is divided by the growth of the normal limb. Moseley simplified the Green-Anderson chart by mathematically manipulating the original data to allow it to fit on a straight-line graph that is both visually graphic and easier to apply (Fig. 26-92). It avoids the need for mathematical calculations of growth inhibition and provides a ready prediction of the results of epiphysiodesis, lengthening, and shortening (Box 26-3). Reference slopes are provided for predicting future limb growth after epiphysiodesis of the distal femur, the proximal tibia, or both. The difference between the slopes of the normal leg and the short leg is the growth inhibition. Lengthening of the short leg in a growing child can be depicted by a sharp vertical rise, followed by a continued gradual slope equivalent to the slope of growth before lengthening (Fig. 26-93).

One criticism of the Green-Anderson tables and the Moseley straight-line graph for limb-length discrepancy is that they do not include an estimation for foot height. For example, a discrepancy of 4 cm by roentgenographic scanograms may be

5 cm by the clinical block technique if the short leg also has a small foot and ankle unit.

Pritchett devised new straight-line graphs based on more recent growth data from the Denver Child Research Council. Pritchett points out that growth rates are not constant throughout childhood. Of special importance is Pritchett's observation that growth of the distal femoral and proximal tibial physes slows down by half in the last 2 years of growth. Although Pritchett's modifications may be more accurate than Moseley's original technique, his graph is not as widely accepted because it requires the use of additional clear acetate overlay lines.

There are some fundamental problems with both the Green-Anderson and Moseley methods. The original data for growth and height may not be applicable to modern children. The skeletal age according to Greulich and Pyle's atlas is at best an approximation. Human growth is not always mathematically predictable because it is influenced by nutritional, metabolic, hormonal, and socioeconomic factors. Shapiro identified five

---

BOX 26-3 • Instructions for Using Moseley Straight-Line Graph for Leg-Length Inequality

---

DEPICTION OF PAST GROWTH

At each office visit, obtain three values:

Length of the normal leg measured by orthoroentgenogram from the most superior part of the femoral head to the middle of the articular surface of the tibia at the ankle

Length of the short leg

Roentgenographic estimate of skeletal age

Place the point for the normal leg on the normal leg line of the appropriate length.

Draw a vertical line through that point the entire height of the graph and through the skeletal age "scalar" area of either boys or girls; this line represents the current skeletal age.

Place the point for the short leg on the current skeletal age line of the correct length.

Mark the point where the current skeletal age line intersects that sloping "scalar" in the skeletal age area that corresponds to the roentgenographic estimate of skeletal age.

Plot successive sets of three points in the same fashion.

Draw the straight line that best fits the points plotted previously for successive lengths of the short leg.

Discrepancy is represented by the vertical distance between two growth lines.

Inhibition is represented by the difference in the slope between the two growth lines, taking the slope of the normal leg as 100.

PREDICTION OF FUTURE GROWTH

Extend to the right the growth line of the short leg.

Draw the horizontal straight line that best fits the points plotted previously in the skeletal age area.

Growth percentile is represented by the position of that horizontal line and indicates whether the child is taller or shorter than the mean.

Skeletal age scale is represented by the intersections of this horizontal line with the scalars in the skeletal age area. The maturity point is the intersection of the line with the maturity scale.

Through the maturity point draw a vertical line. This line represents maturity and the cessation of growth. Its intersection with the growth lines of the two legs represents their anticipated lengths at maturity.

In keeping a child's graph up to date it is recommended that these lines be drawn in pencil. The addition of further data makes this method more accurate and may require slight changes in the positions of these lines.

EFFECT OF SURGERY

Epiphysiodesis

Ascertain the length of the normal leg just before surgery and mark that point on the normal leg line.

From that point draw a line parallel to the reference point for the particular physis fused. This is the new growth line for the normal leg. (Contribution of physes to total growth of leg: distal femur, 37%; proximal tibia, 28%; both, 65%.)

The percentage decrease in slope of the new growth line (taking the previous slope as 100%) exactly represents the loss of the contribution of the fused physis or physes.

Lengthening

Draw the growth line for the lengthened leg exactly parallel to the previous growth line but displaced upward by a distance exactly equal to the length increase achieved. Since the physes are not affected, neither is the growth rate, and the slope of the line is therefore unchanged.

TIMING OF SURGERY

Epiphysiodesis

Project the growth line of the short leg to intersect the maturity line, taking into account the effect of a lengthening procedure if necessary.

From the intersection with the maturity line draw a line whose slope is equal to the reference slope for the proposed surgery.

The point at which this line meets the growth line of the normal leg indicates the point at which surgery should be done. Note that this point is defined not in terms of the calendar, but in terms of the length of the normal leg.

Lengthening

Since lengthening procedures do not affect the rate of growth, the timing of this procedure is not critical and is governed by clinical considerations.

POSTSURGICAL FOLLOW-UP

Draw the new growth line of the normal leg as explained under Effect of Surgery.

Data are plotted exactly as before except that the length of the short leg is plotted first and is placed on the growth line previously established for the short leg.

---

distinct patterns of limb-length discrepancy in a review of more than 800 children, implying that growth inhibition may differ in certain etiologies of limb-length discrepancy, making standard growth prediction charts inaccurate. For example, limb-length discrepancy in some children with juvenile rheumatoid arthritis and Perthes disease may follow an upward slope–downward slope pattern in which the discrepancy corrects itself. In overgrowth after a femoral fracture, the pattern of growth may level off, and after a short period the discrepancy remains constant. Despite these atypical patterns, most leg-length discrepancies follow the traditional growth prediction curves.

Simpler methods of predicting growth are available. The Menelaus method is convenient because it requires no special charts or graphs and relies on chronological age rather than skeletal age. Menelaus assumes that in adolescents over 9 years of age, the distal femur grows ⅜ inch per year, the proximal tibia grows ¼ inch per year, and growth ceases at age 14 years in girls and at age 16 years in boys. Using his technique, Menelaus achieved a final limb-length discrepancy of less than ¾ inch in 94 of patients who underwent epiphysiodesis. In summary, all the methods are, at best, approximations. A final clinical discrepancy of 1 to 1.5 cm after treatment should be considered an excellent outcome.

Paley, Bhave, Herzenberg, and Bowen developed a "multiplier" method for predicting limb-length discrepancy at skeletal maturity. Using available databases, they divided

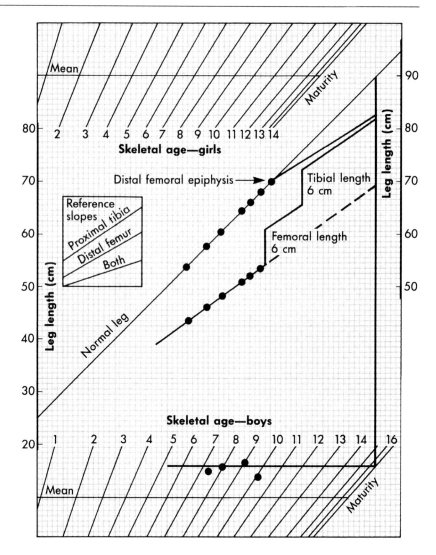

Fig. 26-93 Moseley graph of patient with congenitally short femur and fibular hemimelia demonstrates plan of femoral lengthening, tibial lengthening, and distal femoral epiphysiodesis. (From Moseley CF: *J Bone Joint Surg* 59A:174, 1977.)

femoral and tibial lengths at skeletal maturity by femoral and tibial lengths at each age for each percentile group. The resultant number was called the *multiplier.* This multiplier is used in formulae to predict limb-length discrepancy and the amount of growth remaining and to calculate the timing of epiphysiodesis. According to these authors, the multiplier method allows for a quick calculation of predicted limb-length discrepancy at skeletal maturity, without the need to plot graphs, and is based on as few as one or two measurements. A simple chart of multipliers and several formulae are all that is required (Table 26-5; see also Box 26-3). The multiplier method can be applied to total limb-length discrepancy, including femoral, tibial, and foot-height differences. Clinical data in their study confirmed that the multiplier method correlated closely with the Moseley method. In a group of patients with limb-lengthenings, there was no difference in the accuracy of the two methods; in a group with epiphysiodeses, the multiplier method was more accurate.

TREATMENT

Four types of treatment are available for limb-length equalization: shoe lift or prosthetic conversion, epiphysiodesis of the long leg, shortening of the long leg (in patients too old for epiphysiodesis), and lengthening of the short leg. Judicious combinations of ipsilateral lengthening and contralateral epiphysiodesis can be used for significant discrepancies to reduce the amount of lengthening required.

For small discrepancies of 1.5 cm or less, no treatment is necessary. If a patient desires, a 1-cm shoe lift can be provided to wear inside the shoe. The lift need not compensate for the entire discrepancy, since people rarely stand erect with both knees and hips straight, and many people have small (1 cm) differences that are functionally insignificant. The degree of discrepancy that can be compensated for with an internal shoe lift is limited, however, and for differences of 2 to 4 cm a lift on the outside of the shoe is necessary, although it can taper

> **Table 26-5** Lower-Limb Multipliers for Boys and Girls

Age (yr + mo)	Multiplier	
	Boys	**Girls**
Birth	5.080	4.630
0 + 3	4.550	4.155
0 + 6	4.050	3.725
0 + 9	3.600	3.300
1 + 0	3.240	2.970
1 + 3	2.975	2.750
1 + 6	2.825	2.600
1 + 9	2.700	2.490
2 + 0	2.590	2.390
2 + 3	2.480	2.295
2 + 6	2.385	2.200
2 + 9	2.300	2.125
3 + 0	2.230	2.050
3 + 6	2.110	1.925
4 + 0	2.000	1.830
4 + 6	1.890	1.740
5 + 0	1.820	1.660
5 + 6	1.740	1.580
6 + 0	1.670	1.510
6 + 6	1.620	1.460
7 + 0	1.570	1.430
7 + 6	1.520	1.370
8 + 0	1.470	1.330
8 + 6	1.420	1.290
9 + 0	1.380	1.260
9 + 6	1.340	1.220
10 + 0	1.310	1.190
10 + 6	1.280	1.160
11 + 0	1.240	1.130
11 + 6	1.220	1.100
12 + 0	1.180	1.070
12 + 6	1.160	1.050
13 + 0	1.130	1.030
13 + 6	1.100	1.010
14 + 0	1.080	1.000
14 + 6	1.060	NA*
15 + 0	1.040	NA
15 + 6	1.020	NA
16 + 0	1.010	NA
16 + 6	1.010	NA
17 + 0	1.000	NA

MULTIPLIER METHOD FOR PREDICTING LOWER-LIMB-LENGTH DISCREPANCIES

Congenital Limb-Length Discrepancy

$$\Delta_m = \Delta \times M$$

This formula can be used to determine limb-length discrepancy in patients with congenital short femur, fibular hemimelia, hemihypertrophy, or hemiatrophy.

Developmental Limb-Length Discrepancy

$$\Delta_m = \Delta + (I \times G)$$

where $I = 1 - (S - S')/(L - L')$ and $G = L(M - 1)$. This formula can be used to determine the limb-length discrepancy in patients with Ollier disease, poliomyelitis, or growth arrest. It also can be used to determine the discrepancy in patients with a congenital discrepancy. It also is useful in predicting the growth-remaining discrepancy in patients who have already undergone one or more limb-lengthening procedures.

Length at Skeletal Maturity

$$L_m = L \times M$$

This formula can be used to determine the length of the femur, tibia, femur and tibia, or entire lower limb, including the foot height. It applies equally to the short and long limbs.

Timing of Epiphysiodesis

$$L_\epsilon = L_m - G_\epsilon$$

and

$$M_\epsilon = L_m/L_\epsilon.$$

Look in the multiplier table for the value of M_ϵ and determine which age corresponds to this multiplier value. This is the age of the patient at the time of epiphysiodesis.

G, amount of growth remaining; I, amount of growth inhibition; L, current length of long limb; L', length of long limb as measured on previous radiographs (preferably made at least 6 or 12 months before current radiographs); L_m, length of femur or tibia at skeletal maturity; M, multiplier; S, current length of short limb; S', length of short limb as measured on previous radiographs (preferably made at least 6 or 12 months before current radiographs); Δ, current limb-length discrepancy; Δ_m, limb-length discrepancy at skeletal maturity; ϵ, desired correction following epiphysiodesis; G_ϵ, amount of femoral or tibial growth remaining at age of epiphysiodesis ($G_\epsilon = \epsilon/0.71$ for femur and $\epsilon/0.57$ for tibia); L_ϵ, desired length of bone to undergo epiphysiodesis at time of epiphysiodesis; M_ϵ, multiplier at age of epiphysiodesis.

From Paley D, Bhave A, Herzenberg JE, Bowen JR: *J Bone Joint Surg* 82A:1432, 2000.
*NA, Not applicable.

toward the front of the shoe. For small discrepancies a heel lift can be used, and for larger differences, a full-sole lift. To limit the amount of external lift, the shoemaker can shave down the heel on the long leg shoe by 1 cm. A shoe lift can be used for large discrepancies if the patient declines shortening or lengthening. Lifts of 5 to 10 cm, however, are unsightly and unstable and may require additional uprights or an ankle-foot orthosis to help support the ankle.

Many children reject shoe lifts upon reaching adolescence, preferring instead to walk with compensatory mechanisms, including ankle equinus, pelvic tilt, and contralateral knee flexion. Extension prostheses are "modified shoe lifts" in that the foot is not amputated. Instead, the foot is forced into an equinus position and is fitted into a custom prosthesis that has a prosthetic foot distal to the natural foot. Conversion with a Syme or Boyd amputation, however, is preferred to make prosthetic fitting easier.

OPERATIVE TREATMENT

Theoretically, lengthening of the short limb is the optimal treatment, but technical difficulty and frequent complications of lengthening procedures have made epiphysiodesis a more attractive option for small discrepancies. For growing children, epiphysiodesis is a relatively simple procedure with reasonably low morbidity and fast recovery. In adolescents too old for effective epiphysiodesis, limb shortening is accurate, safe, and simple, with a complication rate only slightly higher than epiphysiodesis. Joint stiffness after shortening is rare because the muscles are made somewhat slack by shortening of the limb, unlike lengthening, which frequently results in permanent joint stiffness and subluxation.

Shortening has several disadvantages: (1) the normal limb is operated on rather than the pathological limb, and if there is a deformity in the short limb, a second operation may be necessary to correct that deformity; (2) as shown by Wagner, the resulting body proportions may be cosmetically displeasing after shortening; (3) the degree of shortening possible is limited because of the inability of the muscles to adapt to shortening of more than 5 cm; and (4) the final height after shortening or epiphysiodesis may be unacceptably low.

Based on skeletal age, an estimation of predicted adult height can be made with the Bayley-Pinneau tables using the Green-Anderson assumption that skeletal age correlates with the percentage of mature height. These tables take into account the child's current height, chronological age, and skeletal age. An estimation of adult height is helpful in determining if lengthening is appropriate. For example, in an adolescent boy with a predicted height of 5 feet and 11 inches, shortening by 2 inches is not as unacceptable as it would be if the predicted height were 5 feet 2 inches.

Advances in technology, including Russian and Italian systems of distraction osteogenesis, represent improvements over the Wagner method of lengthening and have had promising results, but long-term results are still forthcoming.

◆ Epiphysiodesis

Phemister described epiphysiodesis in 1933, and his original technique, with minor modifications, has been widely used for limb-length equalization. Most authors recommend epiphysiodesis when 2 to 5 cm of shortening is required; however, Menelaus and others recommended epiphysiodesis for discrepancies of up to 8 to 10 cm to avoid the complications of limb lengthening.

Phemister removed a rectangular piece of the lateral cortex

on either side of the epiphysis and reinserted it in a reversed position. White developed special hollow chisels to remove a square block of bone and curetted the physeal cartilage deep in the hole before replacing the bone block in a reversed position. A newer technique of epiphysiodesis involves the use of percutaneous instrumentation to obliterate the physis through small, cosmetically pleasing incisions. Experimental evidence reported by Canale et al. and by Ogilvie indicate that the physis can be effectively obliterated by this technique. Early clinical results from Canale et al., Ogilvie, and Bowen and Johnson support these findings. More recently, Horton and Onley reported 42 percutaneous epiphysiodeses in 26 patients, all of which achieved physeal arrest without angular deformity, neurovascular complications, or fractures. Angled curets can be used instead of high-speed burrs to scrape the epiphyseal cartilage.

Metaizeau et al. describe a technique for percutaneous epiphysiodesis using transphyseal screws (PETS). In 32 patients with leg-length discrepancies, PETS reduced the final discrepancy to less than 1 cm in 82% and to 5 mm or less in 56%. In 9 patients with angular deformities, a preoperative average of 7 degrees genu valgum in 6 patients was reduced to 1.4 degrees, and 3 genu varum deformities of 6, 7, and 12 degrees were corrected to 1 degree of valgus, 0 degrees, and 2 degrees of varus, respectively. Metaizeau et al. cited as advantages of PETS simplicity of the technique, short operating time, rapid postoperative rehabilitation, and reversibility.

TECHNIQUE 26-31 *(Métaizeau et al.)*

Prepare and drape the entire lower limb from groin to foot. Through a small stab incision over the lateral aspect of the distal femoral metaphysis, drill a hole directed obliquely downward and medially. Aiming slightly posterior to the mid-coronal plane of the femur, advance the drill past the anatomical axis to cross the physis at the junction of its middle and inner thirds and stop just short of the articular surface of the medial femoral condyle. Insert a cancellous screw with long threads; a cancellous screw with short threads and a washer can be used. Insert the second screw from the medial aspect, symmetrically to the first screw in relation to the anatomical axis of the distal femur, but slightly anterior to the mid-coronal plane so as to avoid the first screw (Fig. 26-94).

An alternative construct consists of two more vertically oriented screws that cross neither each other nor the anatomical axis of the distal femur. Instead, they traverse the physis, one at either end of its middle third, for a more even distribution of arresting forces (Fig. 26-95). This technique looks easier in theory than it does in practice. Correct placement of the screws is not always easy to achieve, because the thickness of the soft tissues determines whether adequate vertical inclination of the drill can be obtained in relation to the long axis of the limb.

Begin insertion of the lateral tibial screw just posterior to the tibial crest to avoid the muscles of the anterior

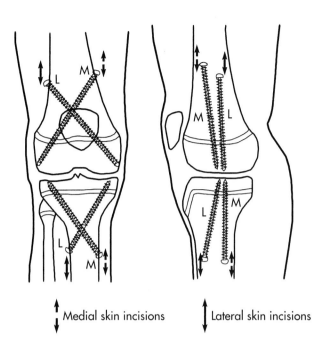

Fig. 26-94 Percutaneous epiphysiodesis using transphyseal screws (PETS). Paired crossed transphyseal screws across distal femoral and proximal tibial physes. *M,* Medial screws; *L,* lateral screws. (From Métaizeau JP, Wong-Chung J, Bertrand H, Pasquier P: *J Pediatr Orthop* 18:363, 1998.)

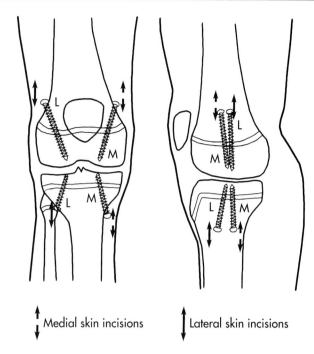

Fig. 26-95 Percutaneous epiphysiodesis using transphyseal screws (PETS). Nonintersecting transphyseal screws. Each pair crosses a physis, one screw at either end of its middle third. *M,* Medial screws; *L,* lateral screws. (From Métaizeau JP, Wong-Chung J, Bertrand H, Pasquier P: *J Pediatr Orthop* 18:363, 1998.)

compartment of the leg. Direct it medially, upward and slightly posteriorly, to cross the physis at the junction of its middle and medial thirds (see Fig. 26-94). Again, an alternative construct can be used in which screws do not cross each other or the anatomical axis of the tibia (see Fig. 26-95).

After insertion of all screws, fully flex the knee to free any adhesions between screws and the quadriceps apparatus.

Proximal fibular epiphysiodesis is done only if more than 2 cm of tibial correction is needed. Percutaneous insertion of a screw across the proximal fibular epiphysis is dangerous. A short incision is required to identify and protect the peroneal nerve. Open curettage also can be done through a small anterior approach.

◆ ◆ ◆

Phemister's open technique can be accomplished without intraoperative fluoroscopy and thus may be more appropriate when "high-tech" percutaneous methods cannot be performed. An alternative method of epiphysiodesis is physeal stapling, but this technique is largely reserved for hemiepiphysiodesis in angular corrections.

Regardless of the technique used, careful timing and consideration of the final height of the knee are important. For discrepancies involving the femur and tibia, epiphysiodesis of both may be required to ensure that the knees and pelvis

will be level. Operative complications are uncommon; reported complications include cutaneous nerve entrapment, infection, asymmetrical growth arrest, undercorrection, and overcorrection.

◆ **Physeal Exposure Around the Knee**

TECHNIQUE 26-32 *(Abbott and Gill, Modified)*
Flex the knee 30 degrees to relax the hamstring muscles and make a lateral incision 6.5 cm proximal to the lateral femoral condyle, continuing distally between the biceps tendon and iliotibial band to the fibular head and then extending anteriorly over the lateral aspect of the tibia. Enter the interval between the lateral intermuscular septum and the vastus lateralis. Cauterize the superior geniculate arteries. Make a vertical incision in the periosteum over the physis and identify the thin "white line" of cartilage.

Protect the peroneal nerve behind the fibular head and incise the periosteum over the anterior aspect of the fibular head. Reflect the anterior compartment muscles off the tibia distally to expose the proximal tibial physis. On the medial side make a curved incision starting at the adductor tubercle and continuing first posteriorly and then anteriorly along the sartorius tendon. Ligate the geniculate arteries. Open the periosteum of the distal femur between the vastus medialis and intermedius muscles. Keep the dissection subperiosteal

continued

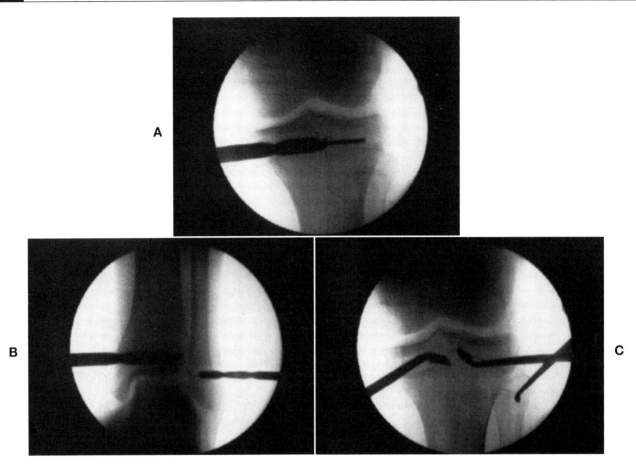

Fig. 26-96   **A,** Insertion of cannulated reamer over guide pin in proximal tibia. **B,** Percutaneous drilling of distal tibial and fibular physes. **C,** Alternative method of using curets inserted through drill holes in cortex.

to avoid entering the knee joint. Over the proximal tibia retract the pes anserinus tendon posteriorly, ligate the geniculate arteries, and make a vertical incision to aid in subperiosteal exposure to locate the physis.

Four short (2.5-cm) incisions can be used rather than two long ones to improve cosmesis. Dissection of the peroneal nerve is not mandatory. Fluoroscopy or image intensification, using needles to locate the physes, is helpful in placing the incisions. Preoperative roentgenograms showing the relation of the distal femoral physis to the patella also aid placement of the incision.

◆ **Percutaneous Epiphysiodesis**

TECHNIQUE 26-33 *(Canale et al.)*

After administration of general anesthesia, place the patient supine on the operating table. Prepare the limb in the standard fashion and drape it free. A tourniquet can be used

if desired. Place a hemostat on the lateral aspect of the leg to locate the lateral portion of the distal femoral physis. After it has been located with image intensification, make small medial and lateral stab wounds approximately 1.5 cm long. Place a smooth Steinmann pin or Kirschner wire into the physis and drill it into the side of the distal femoral physis. Confirm correct positioning of the pin on both anteroposterior and lateral image intensification views. Rotate the image intensifier rather than the leg because rotation of the leg causes the iliotibial band and medial musculature to tighten and interfere with placement of instruments. Place a cannulated reamer over the guide pin (Fig. 26-96, *A*) and drill into the physis approximately halfway across; verify this with image intensification. After removal of the reamer, introduce a high-speed pneumatic drill with a dental burr. Take care to protect the skin during drilling to prevent heat necrosis of the skin; using a guard for the dental burr is helpful. As an alternative, use angled and straight curets to remove the physis (Fig. 26-96, *B*). Ream the physis proximally and distally, anteriorly and posteriorly, especially at the periphery, to create a "bull's-eye" effect in the center of the physis at the lateral periphery.

It is not necessary to remove the entire physis. A lucent area or blackout effect will be noted on image intensification where the physis and surrounding bone have been removed. If the bull's-eye effect is not achieved, use a curet or larger reamer (such as from an adult compression hip screw set) and repeat the procedure on the medial side with frequent image intensification evaluation. Often the medial and lateral defects can be connected. Thoroughly irrigate to remove all loose pieces of cartilage and cancellous bone. Close the wounds with subcutaneous sutures and apply a sterile dressing.

The same technique is used in the proximal tibial physis, except that the tibial physis is more undulating than the femoral and requires more careful drilling (Fig. 26-96, *B*). Epiphysiodesis of the proximal fibular physis may not be necessary, especially if the desired growth arrest in the proximal tibia is less than 2.5 cm. Perform proximal fibular epiphysiodesis with a small Steinmann pin, a small cannulated reamer, and a hand drill or curet under direct vision through a small separate incision. Because of the possibility of mechanical or thermal damage to the peroneal nerve, take great care in this area.

As a modification of this technique, a radiolucent imaging table can be used instead of a fracture table. Use a tourniquet and make the stab wound large enough to insert a ¼-inch drill bit to broach the cortex. Curet the physis with angled and straight curets, using the image intensifier as needed (Fig. 26-96, *C*).

In the proximal tibia it is important to palpate the fibular head, make the incision over the physis under image control, and stay anterior. A drill is not required to broach the proximal fibular cortex; a small, straight curet works well and does not risk injury to the peroneal nerve.

AFTERTREATMENT. Immediate weight-bearing in a soft knee immobilizer is allowed. The immobilizer is worn for approximately 2 to 3 weeks. If both femoral and tibial epiphysiodeses have been done, a knee immobilizer is worn for 10 to 14 days, and then active range-of-motion exercises are begun. Crutches are used for guarded weight-bearing for the first 4 weeks.

Limb Shortening

Shortening usually is reserved for skeletally mature patients who can accept the loss of stature necessary to equalize limb lengths. When planning surgery, both ultimate length and alignment should be considered. Wagner outlined the standard approach to limb shortening, but improvements have been made in femoral shortening techniques, such as a closed technique for diaphyseal shortening described by Winquist, Hansen, and Pearson. In the femur, 5 to 6 cm is the maximal length that can be removed without seriously affecting muscle

function; in the tibia, the maximum probably is 2 to 3 cm, although Menelaus reported resection of 5.1 cm of the tibia in one patient.

In general, femoral shortening is tolerated better than tibial shortening because the soft tissue muscular envelope is much larger, making skin closure easier, offering a better cosmetic result, and ensuring prompt union of the osteotomy. However, if the discrepancy is largely confined to the tibia, tibial shortening is preferred to make the knee heights level.

Wagner recommends metaphyseal osteotomy if angular or rotational correction is required and diaphyseal osteotomy if shortening alone is necessary. Proximal metaphyseal osteotomy of the femur has fewer complications than distal osteotomy, which may compromise knee motion. Additionally, proximal femoral shortening has less negative effect on the strength of the quadriceps. Distal femoral metaphyseal osteotomy should be avoided unless necessary for correction of angular deformity. The development of interlocking intramedullary fixation has made diaphyseal shortening preferable to metaphyseal osteotomy in the femur, even if rotational correction is needed. Intramedullary nailing of femoral fractures in adolescents has been implicated in avascular necrosis of the femoral head. Shortening over an intramedullary rod should be delayed until complete skeletal maturity has been reached, or the entry portal of the nail should be the greater trochanter instead of the piriformis fossa.

♦ Proximal Femoral Metaphyseal Shortening

TECHNIQUE 26-34 *(Wagner)* (Fig. 26-97)
Before surgery, plan the osteotomy to provide the needed angular correction, using tracing paper to outline the osteotomy cuts. Through a proximal lateral incision, split the fascia lata and elevate the vastus lateralis and the periosteum. Fashion an insertion site for the right-angle blade plate or hip screw according to the preoperative plan. Mark the bone to control rotation and remove the proscribed segment with an oscillating saw. Leave a spike of medial cortex and lesser trochanter intact to act as a buttress. Remove the segment, and bring the distal fragment into direct apposition with the proximal segment. Apply the osteosynthesis plate and insert the screws to create compression across the osteotomy.

♦ Distal Femoral Metaphyseal Shortening

TECHNIQUE 26-35 *(Wagner)* (Fig. 26-98)
Before surgery, make a careful plan on tracing paper, outlining the planned resection and angular correction. Make a lateral incision through the fascia lata and elevate the vastus lateralis anteriorly, avoiding the knee joint. Use the blade plate seating device to prepare the entrance for the

continued

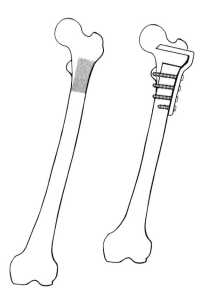

Fig. 26-97   Wagner technique for proximal femoral metaphyseal shortening. (Modified from Wagner H. In Hungerford DS, ed: *Progress in orthopaedic surgery,* Berlin, 1977, Springer-Verlag.)

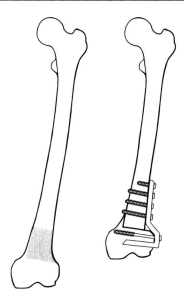

Fig. 26-98   Wagner technique for distal femoral metaphyseal shortening. (Modified from Wagner H. In Hungerford DS, ed: *Progress in orthopaedic surgery,* Berlin, 1977, Springer-Verlag.)

blade plate. With an oscillating saw, make the proximal osteotomy and then the distal osteotomy. For added stability, try to preserve a medial spike of bone with the distal fragment. Impact the two fragments and apply the blade under compression or insert a distal femoral sliding screw and fixation plate device.

◆ Proximal Tibial Metaphyseal Shortening

TECHNIQUE 26-36 *(Wagner)* (Fig. 26-99)
Through a lateral incision, resect a portion of the fibula at the junction of the proximal and middle thirds. Make a separate anterior incision to expose the proximal tibia subperiosteally. Resect the desired amount of bone (no more than 4 cm, except in unusual circumstances) below the tibial tuberosity with an oscillating saw. Hold the two bone ends under compression with a T-plate. Perform a prophylactic fasciotomy. Wound closure may be difficult because of the nature of the skin about the proximal tibia.

◆ Tibial Diaphyseal Shortening

TECHNIQUE 26-37 *(Broughton, Olney, and Menelaus)*
Make a longitudinal incision over the anteromedial surface of the tibia. Perform a subperiosteal dissection and make a step-cut osteotomy, removing the desired amount of bone

and allowing for 5 to 7.5 cm of overlap after shortening. Through a separate incision remove an equivalent amount of bone from the midshaft of the fibula (Fig. 26-100, *A*). Shorten the leg and fix the step-cut osteotomy with two lag screws (Fig. 26-100, *B*) or, in mature patients, with an intramedullary nail (Fig. 26-101). This is the only technique indicated in skeletally immature patients.

◆ Closed Femoral Diaphyseal Shortening

TECHNIQUE 26-38 *(Winquist, Hansen, and Pearson)*
Position the patient on a fracture table in the supine "scissor" position. Use the standard techniques for closed medullary nailing (Chapter 51) and ream to the desired width in 0.5-mm increments. Consider venting the distal metaphyseal-diaphyseal junction with a 4.8-mm cannulated drill bit to prevent fat embolism. Adjust the saw for the appropriate depth according to the preoperative plan and insert the saw until, with the blade fully retracted, the measuring device is seated firmly against the greater trochanter. While an assistant applies pressure to hold the measuring device in place for both the proximal and distal cuts, deploy the saw blade in increments, making complete revolutions (Fig. 26-102, *A*). If necessary, back up one index notch to repeat the cuts if the blade is getting stuck. Slowly continue cutting until the final index mark is reached, at which point the blade is fully deployed. The most difficult area to cut is posteriorly in the linea aspera. If necessary,

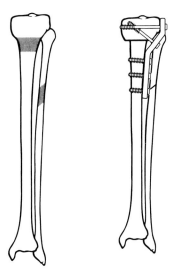

Fig. 26-99 Wagner technique for proximal tibial metaphyseal shortening. (Modified from Wagner H. In Hungerford DS, ed: *Progress in orthopaedic surgery,* Berlin, 1977, Springer-Verlag.)

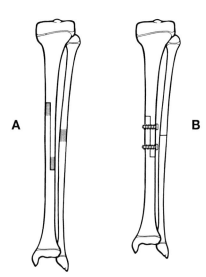

Fig. 26-100 Technique for tibial diaphyseal shortening in skeletally immature patients. (Modified from Broughton NS, Olney BW, Menelaus NB: *J Bone Joint Surg* 71B:242, 1989.)

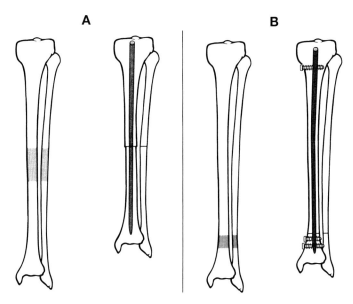

Fig. 26-101 **A,** Diaphyseal shortening with medullary fixation. **B,** Distal tibial shortening with locked intramedullary nail. (Modified from Wagner H. In Hungerford DS, ed: *Progress in orthopaedic surgery,* Berlin, 1977, Springer-Verlag.)

complete the cut percutaneously with a thin osteotome. The next larger size blade and cam can be inserted to get a larger cutting diameter, but this can be difficult if the canal is not reamed widely enough.

After completing the first cut, retract the blade fully. Remove the foot from the fracture table and angulate the distal femur 60 to 70 degrees in all directions to complete the osteotomy; then replace the traction. Advance the measuring device handle distally while holding the locking nut in place. The distance that develops between these two components should equal the amount of femur to be

resected. Spin the locking nut distally to lock the measuring device handle. With an assistant holding the measuring device firmly against the greater trochanter, make the second (proximal) osteotomy in the same fashion as the first. After completing the second osteotomy, retract the blade fully and remove the saw. The resected bone should be subtrochanteric rather than diaphyseal to lessen the effect on the quadriceps mechanism.

Insert an internal chisel of appropriate size, hook the medial aspect of the intercalary segment, and pound on the handle backward with a tuning-fork hammer to split the

continued

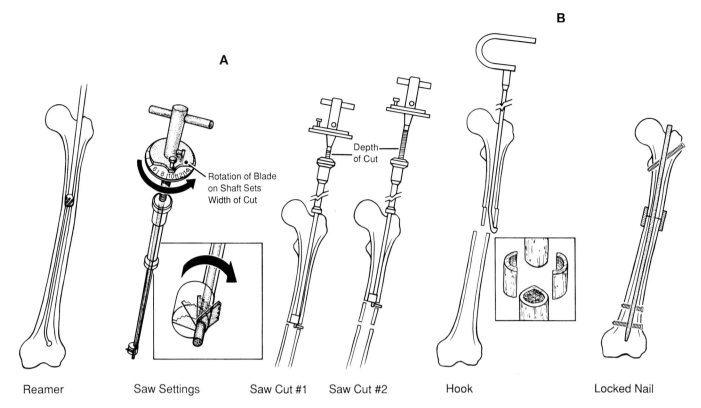

Reamer   Saw Settings   Saw Cut #1   Saw Cut #2   Hook   Locked Nail

Fig. 26-102 Closed femoral diaphyseal shortening, as described by Winquist et al. (see text). **A,** Medullary canal is reamed with standard cannulated reamer. Special medullary saw is inserted into reamed canal. One or two rotations are made with saw at each setting, and saw is progressively opened until blade is completely exposed. **B,** After both saw cuts have been made, intercalary segment is split using back-cutting chisel. Rotational alignment and distraction can be controlled with locked medullary nail.

bone (Fig. 26-102, *B*). Repeat this maneuver at least one more time on the lateral segment. Use the hook of the chisel to push the fragments away from the canal. Have the unscrubbed surgeon again remove the foot from the fracture table and impact the osteotomy, displacing the segmental fragments to either side, using the chisel to manipulate the fragments if necessary. In some cases splitting of the "napkin ring" resected bone piece is unsuccessful. Should this occur, make a small lateral incision to remove the intercalary segment. Pass a nail-driving guide wire across the osteotomy and insert an appropriate-sized nail for fixation while the unscrubbed surgeon maintains rotational alignment. Lock the nail proximally and distally for rotational control and to prevent inadvertent lengthening postoperatively (Fig. 26-103). Steinmann pins can be inserted into the lateral aspect of the femoral condyle and the greater trochanter just before the first osteotomy to serve as references for rotational alignment control. Check rotational alignment before leaving the operating room.

AFTERTREATMENT. A knee splint is used to stabilize the shortened quadriceps mechanism, and a vigorous strengthening program is begun. Rehabilitation is faster if the patient has participated in a quadriceps- and hamstring-strengthening program before surgery. Rotation or distraction at the osteotomy site may occur if a locked nail is not used.

Limb Lengthening

A limb-lengthening program requires a patient and family fully committed to maximal participation in an extended project. The success of limb lengthening depends largely on the patient's efforts in physical therapy and the care of the external fixator. Although technical improvements have reduced the frequency with which major complications associated with limb lengthening occur, the process remains difficult and should be performed by surgeons with appropriate experience.

Shortening procedures are preferable for many patients who are candidates for limb lengthening. Patients who are unable to participate in frequent follow-up or who do not have the support to care for the fixator properly and to undergo vigorous physical therapy are best treated by means other than lengthening. Candidates for limb lengthening and their parents benefit from meeting other patients in various stages of the lengthening process.

Acute long bone lengthening seldom is indicated; however, Salter described acute distraction and interposition grafting

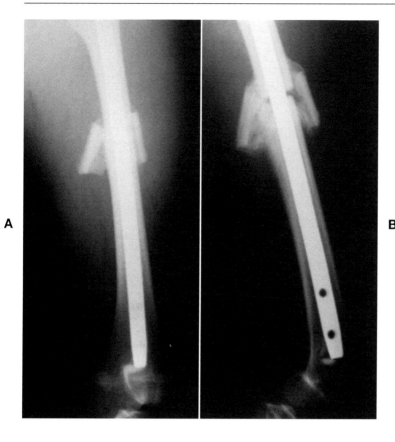

Fig. 26-103   **A,** This 16-year-old girl underwent 4-cm closed femoral shortening. Shortly after surgery, intercalary fragment is seen around site of osteotomy, acting as bone graft. **B,** Eight weeks later, osteotomy has healed. Note at least 4 mm of distraction occurred after osteotomy. Locking of nail is recommended to preserve alignment and length, if necessary.

through the innominate bone. Millis and Hall reported a modification of this technique; they achieved an average lengthening of 2.3 cm in 20 patients with acetabular dysplasia with femoral shortening, pure limb-length inequality, decompensated scoliosis, and primary intrapelvic asymmetry. This technique may be useful in patients who also require acetabular reconstruction, but epiphysiodesis or gradual distraction lengthening techniques are more reliable alternatives for isolated limb-length discrepancy.

◆ Transiliac Lengthening

TECHNIQUE 26-39 *(Millis and Hall)*
Use the anterior ilioinguinal approach to the pelvis described for the Salter innominate osteotomy (Chapter 27). Use a Gigli saw to make the osteotomy from the sciatic notch to the anteroinferior iliac spine (Fig. 26-104, *A*). Insert a lamina spreader into the anterior aspect of the osteotomy. Have an assistant apply caudally directed pressure on the iliac crest to prevent displacement of the proximal fragment by shear force through the sacroiliac joint while another assistant applies traction to the femur, keeping the knee flexed to relax the sciatic nerve. Fashion a full-thickness block of iliac crest into a trapezoid. The height of the graft directly superior to the acetabulum determines the amount of lengthening. Wedge the iliac graft into the dis-

traction site (Fig. 26-104, *B*) and hold it with two large, threaded Steinmann pins that transfix the proximal fragment, the graft, and the distal supraacetabular fragment (Fig. 26-104, *C*).

AFTERTREATMENT. Traction is applied for 5 days. Range-of-motion exercises are begun at 3 days, and touchdown weight-bearing is allowed at 7 days. Full weight-bearing is delayed until graft incorporation is evident on roentgenograms, usually at 3 to 6 months.

Lengthening by Slow Distraction. Osteotomy followed by gradual distraction of the bone fragments with a mechanical apparatus has been the basic procedure for limb lengthening since Putti's report of the technique in 1921. Osteotomy and fixation techniques have been modified by several authors, but disturbingly high complication rates (Fig. 26-105) were reported with all methods, including deep infection, nonunion, fracture after plate removal, malunion, and nerve palsy. Wagner introduced a low-profile, mobile, monolateral fixator that improved results, and DeBastiani designed a similar but more versatile fixator (Orthofix). In the early 1950s Ilizarov devised a thin-wire, circular external fixator for fracture fixation and found that slow distraction with the device caused regeneration of bone in the distraction gap. For lengthening procedures, he used a percutaneous "corticotomy" in which the accessible

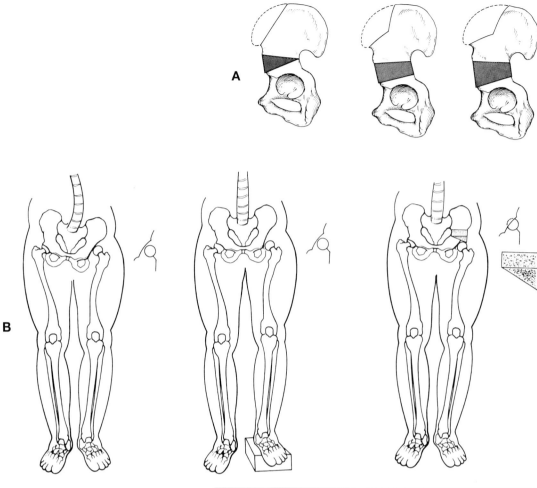

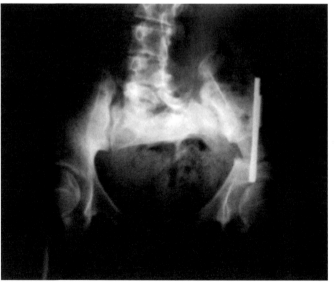

Fig. 26-104   A, Acute transiliac lengthening accomplished by modification of Salter technique. Instead of triangular graft, square or trapezoidal graft is used. The larger the graft, the more lengthening is achieved. **B,** Acetabular dysplasia and mild limb-length inequality. Pelvic obliquity results in compensatory scoliosis. In middle figure, block has been placed beneath shorter leg. Although this balances pelvis and straightens spine, it causes acetabulum to be even more vertical. On right, transiliac lengthening has been performed to improve femoral acetabular coverage and regain length. **C,** Transiliac lengthening with trapezoidal graft. (**A** and **B** modified from Mills MB, Hall JE: *J Bone Joint Surg* 61A:1182, 1979.)

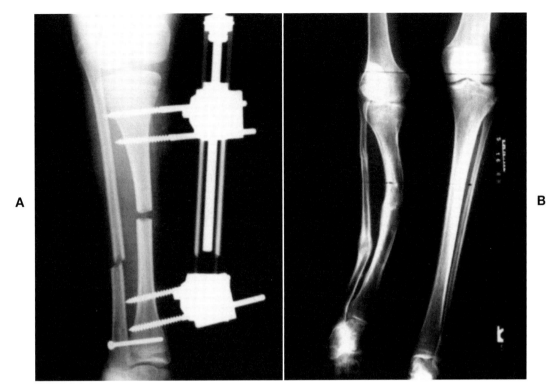

Fig. 26-105   A, Wagner lengthening procedure in adolescent with tibial hemimelia. **B,** Follow-up 4 years later shows results of several complications encountered during and after lengthening. Tibia, which fractured after removal of plate, has healed in valgus alignment, foot is in severe equinus, and leg-length discrepancy persists.

cortices of a long bone are cut with a 5-mm osteotome through a 10-mm skin incision (Fig. 26-106), avoiding as much as possible penetration of the medullary canal. After 5 to 7 days, distraction is begun at the rate of 0.25 mm four times each day. The thin wires (1.8 or 1.5 mm) are tensioned up to 130 kg to provide adequate stiffness for bone segment stability. Simultaneous or sequential correction of axial, translational, and rotational deformities is possible. In children, the fixator is worn approximately 1 month for each centimeter of lengthening, and in adults, for about 1.5 months for each centimeter. This lengthy period of fixator wear is one of the major disadvantages of Ilizarov's technique. The Ilizarov apparatus was modified by Catagni et al., who replaced the semicircular rings with 90-degree and 120-degree arches that attach to bone with standard 5-mm or 6-mm half-pins. Green further modified the Ilizarov apparatus to facilitate half-pin fixation on the rings. Monticelli and Spinelli combined heavy transfixation pins with thin, tensioned wires on modified rings.

Paley classified complications of limb lengthening as *problems*, *obstacles*, and *complications*. A problem, such as a minor pin track infection, can be dealt with in an outpatient setting. An obstacle requires a secondary procedure, such as repeat corticotomy, for permanent consolidation of the lengthening gap. Neither problems nor obstacles necessarily prevent a good result. A complication is an unexpected sequel that compromises the final result. A minor complication, such as residual equinus contracture, can be treated surgically to improve the result. A major complication, such as a permanent nerve palsy, might not be improved by surgery.

The classic Wagner method of open osteotomy, immediate diastasis, and 1 mm per day of lengthening followed by plate fixation and bone grafting is largely of historical interest. Newer techniques of percutaneous corticotomy and distraction osteogenesis are now standard. Two basic types of external fixators are available for limb lengthening after percutaneous corticotomy: large half-pin monolateral devices and circular devices that attach with combinations of wires and half-pins. The monolateral devices are relatively simple to apply but are limited in correcting angular and rotational deformities and do not effect simultaneous correction of complex deformities. The original Wagner device is adjustable in only two planes and the Hoffman modification in one additional plane. DeBastiani's device (Orthofix) has modular components that allow certain simple angular corrections. The Ilizarov device is extremely modular and can be adapted with extensions and hinges to lengthen and correct angular and translational deformities simultaneously. Rotational deformities can be corrected either at the time of fixator application or later by applying outriggers to the rings. The circular devices are more difficult to apply than the monolateral fixators, and extensive training and experience are recommended before using them. For detailed descriptions of the components of these fixators, preoperative planning, and frame construction and application, see Chapter 51.

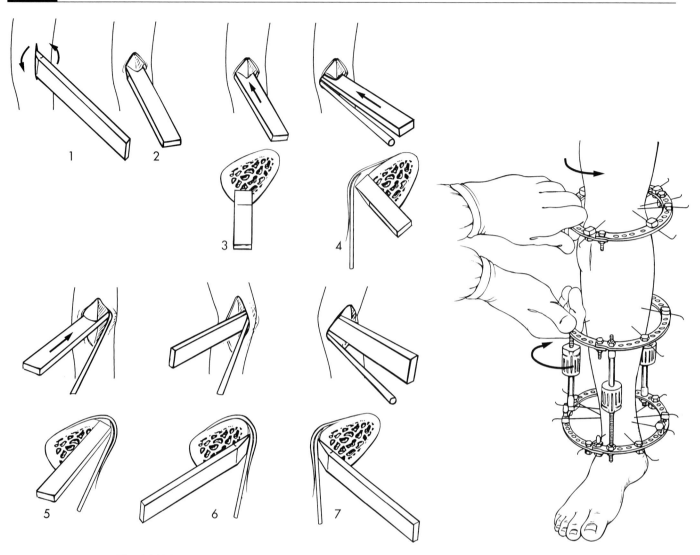

Fig. 26-106   Percutaneous tibial corticotomy, modified from Ilizarov. Entire tibia is cut through 1.5-cm incision centered over anterior crest. Small elevator lifts periosteum on medial and lateral cortices; 5-mm osteotome is used to cut first medial and then lateral cortex. Osteotome is reinserted in medial cortex and twisted 90 degrees to help fracture posterior cortex. This maneuver is repeated along lateral cortex. If necessary, Ilizarov rings can be used to complete posterior aspect of corticotomy by externally rotating distal segment. (Redrawn from Paley D, Catagni MA, Argnani F, et al: *Clin Orthop* 241:146, 1989.)

◆ **Tibial Lengthening**

TECHNIQUE 26-40 *(Wagner)* (Fig. 26-107)
Position the patient supine on a radiolucent table. Expose the distal lateral fibula and insert one or two cortical screws 1.5 cm apart to transfix the fibula to the tibia to prevent proximal migration of the fibula during lengthening. Transect the fibula just proximal to the upper screw. Next, insert the proximal and distal four parallel Schanz screws anteromedially through stab incisions in the subcutaneous border of the tibia, parallel to the plane of the knee joint. Make an anterior incision and dissect subperiosteally to expose the midshaft of the tibia. Make a transverse

osteotomy with an oscillating saw and incise the periosteum. Close the wounds over drains and attach the distraction device. Lengthen the tendo calcaneus if the amount of lengthening is to be substantial.

AFTERTREATMENT. Distraction is continued 1.5 mm daily (about 1 cm per week). Partial weight-bearing with crutches and vigorous physical therapy are begun as soon as possible. Dry bandages are used to protect the pin sites, and antibiotic solution is used as necessary. After the desired length has been obtained, an osteosynthesis plate is applied over the anterolateral surface of the tibia. If callus is insufficient, autologous

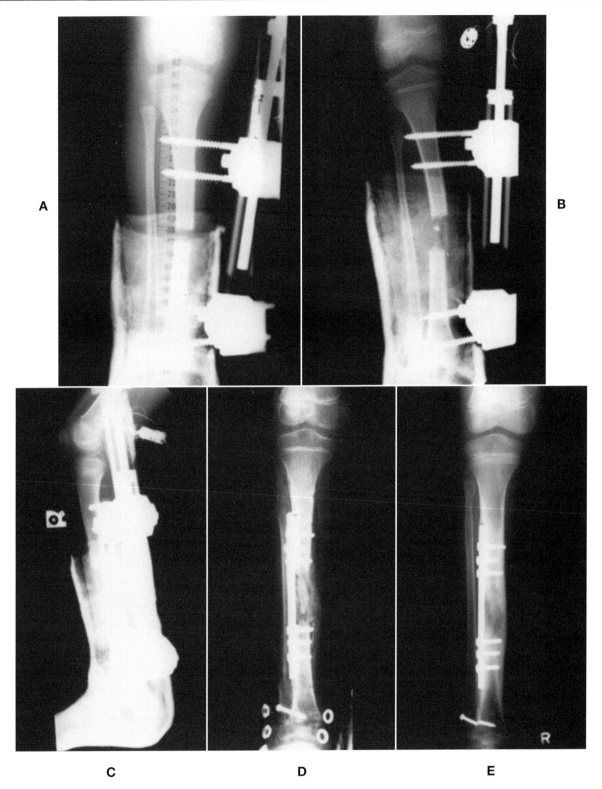

C   D   E

Fig. 26-107   A, Wagner tibial lengthening immediately after surgery, with 1.2-cm initial diastasis. **B,** After gradual lengthening, note beginning of valgus deformation. Fibula underwent spontaneous epiphysiolysis in response to lengthening. **C,** During lengthening; note short leg cast applied around fixator to keep foot from developing equinus. **D,** At end of lengthening, after application of Wagner plate, bone grafting, and removal of fixator; note new bone formation in proximal fibula after epiphysiolysis. **E,** Six months later, incorporation of bone graft and neocorticalization; proximal fibular epiphysis appears intact despite having undergone epiphysiolysis. (Courtesy Thomas F Kling, MD.)

corticocancellous bone graft is added. Protected weight-bearing is continued, and the plate is removed when the tibia has healed completely and the medullary canal is reconstituted.

Coleman and Stevens modified Wagner's procedure by making an oblique osteotomy of the fibula and fixing the distal tibia and fibula with only one screw, by routinely performing an anterior compartment fasciotomy, and by decompressing the peroneal nerve prophylactically in congenital deformities.

TECHNIQUE 26-41 (DeBastiani et al.)

Place the patient supine on a radiolucent table. Resect 2 cm of the distal fibula through a lateral approach. Use the mated Orthofix drills, drill guides, and screw guides to insert the conical, self-tapping cortical and cancellous screws. Insert a cancellous screw 2 cm distal to the medial aspect of the knee, parallel to the knee joint. Place the appropriate rigid template parallel to the diaphysis of the tibia and insert the distalmost screw. Next, go to the proximal part of the template and insert the next screw in the fourth template hole distal to the upper screw. The last screw to be placed is in the distal template, in the hole farthest away from the distalmost screw. Remove the template and perform a corticotomy just distal to the tibial tuberosity.

Incise the anterior skin and periosteum longitudinally. Under direct vision, drill a series of unicortical holes in the tibia. Set the drill stop at 1 cm to prevent penetration of the marrow. Use a thin osteotome to connect the drill holes and to divide along the posteromedial and posterolateral cortices as much as can be done safely. Flex the tibia at the corticotomy to crack the posterior aspect of the tibia. Apply the Orthofix lengthener. If the fracture fixation device is used, fix the ball joint rigidly with a small amount of methylmethacrylate. Suture the periosteum and close the skin over drains.

AFTERTREATMENT. Partial weight-bearing and physical therapy are begun immediately. Distraction is delayed until callus is visible on roentgenograms, usually by 10 to 15 days. Distraction is begun at 0.25 mm every 6 hours but can be reduced if pain or muscle contraction occurs. Roentgenograms are made 1 week after distraction begins to ensure a complete corticotomy and are made at 4-week intervals thereafter. If the regenerated callus is of poor quality, distraction is stopped for 7 days. Recompression is indicated for gaps in the callus and for evidence of excessive neurovascular distraction. When the desired length is obtained, the body-locking screw mechanism is tightened and the distraction mechanism is removed from the fixator. Full weight-bearing is allowed until good callus consolidation is seen, and then the body-locking screw is unlocked to allow dynamic axial compression. The fixator is removed when corticalization is complete. If stability is confirmed, the screws are removed. If there is any doubt as to stability of the bone, the fixator is replaced for an additional period.

TECHNIQUE 26-42 (Ilizarov, Modified)
(Fig. 26-108)

Frame preconstruction involves assembling a frame consisting of four equal Ilizarov rings sized to the patient; use the smallest-diameter rings that leave sufficient space for swelling after surgery. There should be one fingerbreadth of space between the proximal ring and the tibial tuberosity and two fingerbreadths posteriorly at the largest diameter of the posterior calf muscles. The most proximal ring can be a ⅝-inch ring to allow more knee flexion after surgery, especially if the ipsilateral femur is to be lengthened at the same time, because full rings would touch each other with relatively little knee flexion. Connect the upper two rings with 20-mm threaded, hexagonal sockets for better stability. In small patients there may be room proximally for only one ring and a drop wire (Fig. 26-109). The distal two rings can be spaced farther apart than the top two rings for better stability, but for significant lengthening it is better to have the distal two-ring construct relatively farther away from the intended proximal metaphyseal corticotomy site; such an arrangement maximizes the amount of soft tissue available for stretching, contributing to the overall lengthening. For initial preconstruction, use only two connections between each pair of rings, one anteriorly and one directly posteriorly. Plan the frame so that the central connection bolts are centered directly over the tibial tuberosity and the anterior crest of the tibia. Assemble all rings symmetrically. To compensate for the anterior and valgus angulation that often occurs during tibial lengthening, some surgeons connect the upper two-ring set to the lower set with anterior and posterior threaded rods attached to the lower of the proximal two rings with conical washer couples. These allow a tilt of up to 7 degrees to be built into the system. Adjust the frame so that the proximal rings are higher anteriorly and medially. The frame is applied in this "cockeyed" position, but after the corticotomy is made, the conical washer bolts are removed and all four rings are brought into parallel alignment, placing the tibia in about 5 degrees of prophylactic recurvatum and varus.

More often, a symmetrically aligned frame is used without any prophylactic positioning. Instead, careful attention is paid to the follow-up roentgenograms during lengthening. If axial deviations are found at the end of lengthening, corrective hinges are placed onto the ring to obtain proper alignment.

For frame application, position the patient on a radiolucent table and apply a tourniquet to the upper thigh. Through a lateral incision, expose the midfibula by subperiosteal dissection and transect it with an oscillating saw. Release the tourniquet and close the fibular wound in layers. Under fluoroscopic control, insert a reference wire from medial to lateral, perpendicular to the long axis of the tibia (for a normally aligned leg), just below the proximal tibial physis. Use 1.8-mm wires in large children and

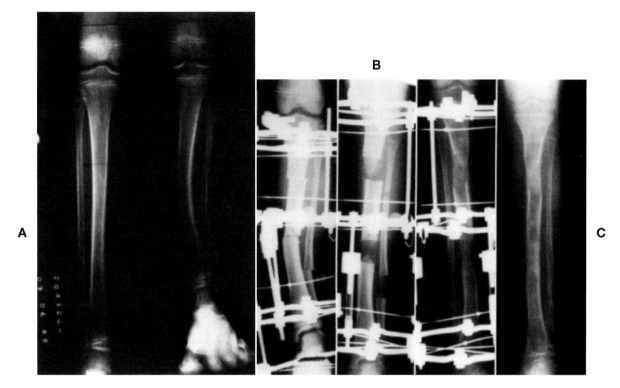

Fig. 26-108   **A,** Congenital posteromedial bowing of tibia in 11-year-old girl. Although deformity largely corrected spontaneously, child is left with 6 cm of shortening and valgus angulation in midshaft of tibia. **B,** Double-level tibial lengthening. Lower corticotomy is made at apex of angular deformity in midshaft, and upper corticotomy could have been made more proximally in metaphyseal region. After distraction with appropriately placed hinge, more distal corticotomy not only opens up for elongation but also corrects valgus deformity. **C,** Final result after removal of fixator shows excellent regenerated bone in gaps. This 6-cm lengthening required 4½ months in fixator. Premature consolidation of proximal fibular osteotomy resulted in spontaneous proximal fibular epiphysiolysis.

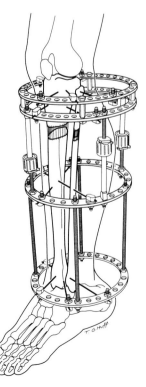

Fig. 26-109   Typical Ilizarov frame for moderate tibial lengthening. In skeletally immature child with intact physes, proximal segment would not have enough room for two rings. Single ring distal to proximal tibial epiphysis is used with drop wire for additional segmental stabilization of proximal segment. For significant amount of lengthening, third ring can be placed more distally to allow greater mass of soft tissue for recruitment into lengthening process.

adolescents and 1.5-mm wires in smaller children. Attach the preassembled frame to this reference wire. Place another wire from the fibula to the tibia just proximal to the distal tibial physis. Use the standard Ilizarov principles of wire insertion and fixation at all times (Chapter 51). Wires should be pushed or gently tapped through the soft tissues rather than drilled, especially when exiting close to neurovascular structures. When passing wires through the anterior compartment muscles, hold the foot dorsiflexed for the same reason. Incise the skin to allow passage of olive wires. Never pull or bend a wire to the ring. Instead, build up to the wire with washers or posts as necessary to avoid undue torque and undesirable moments on the tibia. Tension the wires to 130 kg unless the wire is suspended off a ring, in which case 50 to 60 kg of tension is used to prevent warping of the ring. It is best to use two wire tensioners to tighten two wires simultaneously on the same ring, if possible, to prevent warping of the ring. After tensioning and securing the wires, cut the ends long (about 4 cm) and curl the ends of the wire directly over the wire-fixation bolt to allow later retensioning, if necessary. Bend the cut wire points into available ring holes so that they will not injure the patient or staff members.

Once the first two wires have been attached to the frame and tensioned, the frame can act as a drill guide for placement of the remaining wires. The wires in the first ring are the initial transverse reference wire and a medial face wire that is parallel to the medial surface of the tibia. Place a third wire from the fibular head into the tibia to prevent dissociation of the proximal tibiofibular joint during lengthening. This wire does not risk damage to the peroneal nerve if the fibular head is readily palpable. Do not use an olive wire because it would compress the proximal tibiofibular joint. Ideally, this wire should be proximal to the proximal fibular physis. In the second ring, place a transverse wire and another medial face wire, avoiding the pes anserinus tendons, if possible. Because there is a strong tendency to valgus during proximal tibial lengthening, place olive wires on the top and bottom rings laterally and on the middle two rings medially to function as fulcrums for bending the tibia into varus. Half-pins (5 mm or 6 mm) are now used more frequently, especially in the diaphysis.

For corticotomy, remove the two threaded rods connecting the proximal fixation block with the distal fixation block. Make a 2-cm incision over the crest of the tibia just below the tibial tuberosity. Incise the periosteum longitudinally and insert a small periosteal elevator. Elevate a narrow portion of periosteum the width of the small periosteal elevator along the medial and lateral surfaces of the tibia. Insert a 1.2-cm (½ inch) osteotome transversely into the thick anterior cortex. Use a 5-mm (¼ inch) osteotome to score the medial side and then the lateral side. The periosteal elevator can be placed flush along the bone to act as a directional guide for the osteotome. The corticotomy is guided both by feel and by hearing the sound change when the osteotome exits the back cortex. On the medial side, no important structures are at risk; on the lateral cortex, the tibialis posterior muscle belly is between the tibia and the deep neurovascular structures. After cutting the medial and lateral cortices, withdraw the osteotome and reinsert it along the medial cortex. Turn the osteotome 90 degrees to spread the cortices and crack the posterior cortex. Repeat this maneuver at the lateral cortex, if needed. Although Ilizarov recommended not violating the medullary canal, most Western surgeons have adopted DeBastiani's method of making several front-to-back drill holes to weaken the posterior cortex. The corticotomy also can be completed by externally rotating the distal tibia, but do not internally rotate the tibia for fear of stretching the peroneal nerve.

For proximal or distal tibial metaphyseal "corticotomies," a Gigli saw makes a smooth osteotomy without risk of fracture into adjacent pin sites. The Gigli saw method requires two transverse incisions, one anteriorly and one posteromedially. Subperiosteal dissection with a small elevator is done on all three sides of the tibia. Right-angle and curved clamps are used to pass a heavy suture, which is then tied to the Gigli saw. The suture can be passed before frame application and the Gigli saw after completion of the fixation. When activating the saw, assistants must retract the skin edges. Care is taken to protect the medial face periosteum at the final part of the osteotomy.

For frame assembly, reduce the fracture and insert four distraction rods or graduated telescopic rods, approximately 90 degrees apart, between the middle two rings. Close the corticotomy site, over a drain if necessary, and apply compressive dressings. Dress the wire sites with foam sponges held in place by plastic clips or rubber stoppers. If rubber stoppers are used, put them on before fixing the wires to the rings.

AFTERTREATMENT. Physical therapy and crutch walking with partial weight-bearing are begun immediately. Distraction is delayed for 5 to 7 days. In children the distraction rate is 0.25 mm four times per day. The patient and family are taught to care for the pins before discharge from the hospital, usually 5 to 7 days after surgery. Roentgenograms are made 7 to 10 days after distraction is begun to document separation at the corticotomy site. Regenerated bone should be seen in the gap by 4 to 6 weeks, although linear streaks of regenerated bone usually are visible before then, especially in younger children. If the regenerated bone formation is insufficient, the rate of distraction should be slowed, stopped, or in some instances temporarily reversed. Weight-bearing and functional activity of the limb aid in maturation of the regenerated bone. Ultrasonography can detect cyst formation, which, if extensive, ultimately requires cancellous autogenous bone grafting. During distraction, knee flexion contractures and ankle equinus contractures can be prevented with prophylactic splints and orthoses. The fixator is removed when there is evidence of corticalization of the regenerated bone and the patient is able to walk without aids.

◆ ◆ ◆

For significant lengthening, especially when ankle mobility is abnormal before surgery, the foot can be fixed into the lengthening device by inserting an olive wire from each side of the calcaneus at divergent angles to one another. These are attached to an appropriate-sized half ring. This half ring must be within 2 cm of the back of the heel to capture the obliquely placed wires anteriorly. The heel ring is connected to the lowest ring of the lengthening frame with short plates and threaded rods. The heel ring and wires can be removed after lengthening is complete to prevent subtalar stiffness. A custom orthosis can be constructed to accommodate the foot construct.

For lengthening of more than 6 cm, double-level lengthening speeds the process and reduces the time in fixation by about 40%. In this modification, three rings are used, with a drop wire off each ring to give "bilevel" fixation at each segment (see Fig. 26-108). The fibula should have one wire transfixing it at each of the three rings. Two fibular osteotomies and two corticotomies are required, one of each just below the proximal ring and one of each just above the distal ring. A heel ring and wires are added to prevent equinus of the ankle. The bottom two rings can be connected to provide a stable handle on the distal segments to complete the proximal corticotomy, and the top two rings can be connected to complete the distal corticotomy.

If a fixed knee contracture develops during lengthening, the physical therapy treatments should be done more often. If the knee contracture does not respond to physical therapy and splinting, the frame can be extended proximally to the thigh with a cuff cast incorporating a ring and a hinge incorporated at the approximate axis of rotation of the knee. The device can then be used to slowly distract and correct the knee contracture.

To correct other deformities of the tibia while lengthening, the Ilizarov frame can be modified with hinges to effect angular and translational correction simultaneously. Internal rotation can be corrected distally by osteotomy at the time of fixator application. Proximally, internal rotation should be corrected gradually after lengthening is complete but before the regenerated bone is solid. Use of the Ilizarov device for multiplane corrections should be attempted only by surgeons with experience in these techniques.

◆ **Femoral Lengthening**

TECHNIQUE 26-43 *(Wagner)*

Place the patient supine on a radiolucent table with a bolster under the ipsilateral buttock. With image intensifier assistance, insert the two most proximal pins at the level of the lesser trochanter, perpendicular to the anatomical axis of the femur, and insert the two most distal pins at the level of

the superior pole of the patella. Predrill the 6.5-mm self-tapping Schanz pins with a 3.2-mm drill bit and insert them in a plane perpendicular to the long axis of the femur, using a drill guide. The two-pin groupings should be made in the same plane. Expose the midshaft of the femur subperiosteally through a posterolateral approach to the interval between the vastus lateralis and the biceps femoris. Make a transverse osteotomy of the femur with an oscillating saw and close the wound over drains. Attach the distraction device to the Schanz pins, leaving 2 cm of clearance to allow for swelling of the lateral thigh. Wagner originally recommended 5 mm of acute distraction to prevent painful contact between the bone fragments, but this is rarely done now.

AFTERTREATMENT. Distraction is continued by turning the knob of the device one complete turn daily. This lengthens the femur by 1.5 mm. The distraction can be divided if one complete turn is too painful. Partial weight-bearing with forearm crutches is encouraged, and vigorous physical therapy of the hip and knee is mandatory. Varus and anterior angulation can be corrected by adjusting the linkage between the Schanz pins and the lengthener. Daily pin care is necessary to prevent pin sepsis. If the skin becomes very tented over the pins, it should be incised, using local anesthesia. The hamstrings and adductors can be lengthened if necessary. After the desired length has been achieved, a plate and, if necessary, autologous iliac crest bone graft are applied (Fig. 26-110). After the plate and bone graft have been applied and the skin has been closed over a drain, the fixator is removed. Weight-bearing is gradually increased. The plate is removed once reconstitution of the femur and medullary canal is normal.

◆ ◆ ◆

The Hoffman modification of the Wagner device allows rotation in three planes and is somewhat easier to apply (Fig. 26-111). A 4.5-mm drill bit is used to predrill the holes for a 6-mm half-pin. Dick and Tietjen recommended transection of the periosteum and acute distraction of 10 mm, followed by daily distraction of 1 to 2 mm. They also suggested excising a tract of iliotibial band and intermuscular septum. Tenotomy of the adductors may reduce varus deviation during lengthening. Special plates, which have no screw holes in the area of the lengthening gap, have been designed to prevent plate breakage.

Coleman and Stevens recommended plate removal in two stages to prevent fracture through the stress-shielded bone or screw holes. At the first stage, half the screws are removed completely, and the remaining half are loosened by one or two turns and are removed with the plate 6 to 12 months later.

TECHNIQUE 26-44 *(DeBastiani et al.)*

Place the patient supine on a radiolucent table. Use the mated drills, drill guides, and screw guides to insert the

continued

A   B   C

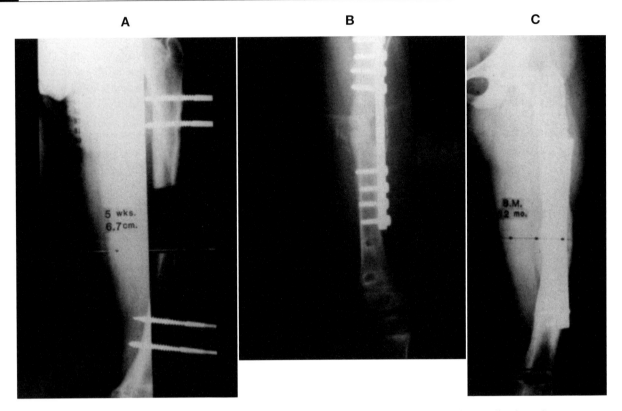

Fig. 26-110   **A,** Wagner apparatus used for 6.7-cm femoral lengthening. **B,** After application of Wagner plate and bone graft and immediately after removal of external fixator. **C,** One year after lengthening, hypertrophy of callus is seen.

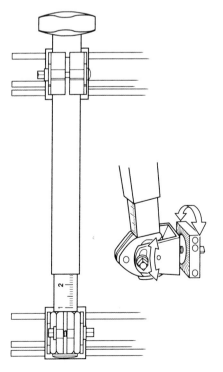

Fig. 26-111   Hoffman modification of Wagner device allows rotation in three planes.

conical self-tapping cortical and cancellous screws. Insert a cortical screw at the level of the lesser trochanter, perpendicular to the shaft of the femur. Attach the rigid template and insert the distalmost screw, being careful to line the template up parallel to the shaft of the femur. Return to the proximal end of the template and insert the next screw in the fourth template hole distal to the upper screw. The last screw to be placed is in the distal template, in the hole farthest away from the distalmost screw. Remove the template and perform a corticotomy 1 cm distal to the proximal two screws (just distal to the iliopsoas insertion). Incise the anterior thigh skin longitudinally and dissect bluntly between the sartorius muscle and the tensor fasciae latae muscle and through the substance of the vastus intermedius and rectus femoris muscles. Incise the periosteum longitudinally and elevate it laterally and medially. Under direct vision, drill a series of 4.8-mm unicortical holes in the visible aspect of the anterior two thirds of the circumference of the femur (Fig. 26-112, *A*). Set the drill stop at 1 cm to prevent penetration of the marrow. Use a thin osteotome to connect the drill holes without violating the marrow. Flex the femur at the corticotomy to crack the

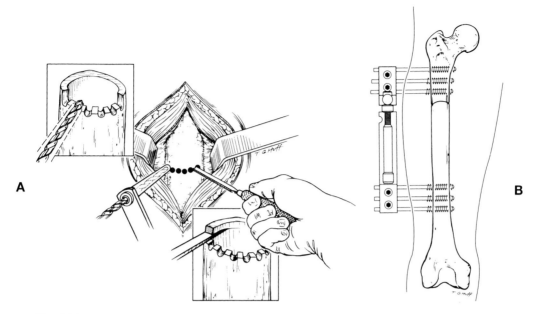

Fig. 26-112   **A,** DeBastiani technique for corticotomy. Using limited open exposure and Orthofix drill, multiple holes are drilled in anterior half of bone. These are connected with 5-mm osteotome, which also is used to complete corticotomy posteriorly. **B,** Orthofix device for femoral lengthening. To control varus deviation, three screws are used proximally and three distally, or frame can be applied with prophylactic valgus built into construct. (**B** modified from Aldegheri R, Renz-Brivio L, Agostini S: *Clin Orthop* 141:137, 1989.)

posterior cortex, completing the corticotomy. Do not use the Orthofix pins as handles to complete the corticotomy, or they may loosen. Reduce the fracture and apply the Orthofix lengthener. If the Orthofix fracture-fixation device is used, fix the ball joint rigidly with a small amount of methylmethacrylate. The Orthofix slide-lengthening device can be used with or without swivel clamps. If swivel clamps are used, blocking them with methylmethacrylate should be considered. The slide lengthener is especially useful for double-level lengthening.

Price recommends acute valgus of a few degrees for subtrochanteric lengthening to help prevent the common problem of varus at this level. Adductor tenotomy also is advised. Suture the periosteum and close the skin over drains. The use of six pins has been recommended for femoral lengthening to gain stability and to resist a tendency for varus deviation (Fig. 26-112, *B*).

AFTERTREATMENT. Aftertreatment is the same as that for tibial lengthening (p. 1058).

TECHNIQUE 26-45 *(Ilizarov, Modified)*

Frame preconstruction includes the following considerations. The standard femoral lengthening frame consists of a proximal fixation block made of two arcs, a distal fixation block made of two identically sized rings, and an "empty"

middle ring (usually one size larger than the distal rings) to link the two fixation blocks. Preconstruct the frame before surgery to reduce the time spent in the operating room. Use the smallest-diameter rings that leave sufficient space for swelling after surgery because smaller rings give a more mechanically stable construct. There should be one finger-breadth of space between the distal ring and the anterior thigh and two fingerbreadths posteriorly at the largest diameter of the posterior calf muscles. The distalmost ring can be a ⅝-inch ring to allow more knee flexion after surgery. This is especially important if there is to be a simultaneous lengthening of the ipsilateral tibia with proximal tibial rings. (Full rings would touch each other after relatively little knee flexion, limiting knee mobility.) Connect the bottom two rings initially with two 20- or 40-mm threaded hexagonal sockets for better stability, one positioned directly anteriorly and one directly posteriorly. With the newer carbon fiber rings, it is possible to "cut out" the back portion of the distal ring as needed to improve knee flexion and prevent impingement against a tibial construct. Appropriate reinforcement to the nearest ring is required before the carbon fiber ring is cut. In small patients there may be room distally for only one ring and a drop wire. Plan the frame so that the central connection bolts are centered directly over the anterior and posterior midlines. Choose two parallel arcs to match the contour of the proximal lateral thigh, usually a 90-degree arc most proximally and a

continued

120-degree arc below it; this causes less impingement of the proximal end of the fixator against the lower abdomen and pelvis during hip flexion. Connect the two arcs with two 40-mm hexagonal sockets. The reach of the 120-degree arc can be extended by attaching two oblique supports off the first and last holes on the arc. Attach the oblique support to the empty middle ring, which will not hold any wires but will allow a more even 360-degree push-off between the distal and proximal fixation blocks. Connect the empty middle ring to the distal fixation block with two threaded rods, one placed anteriorly and one medially, to align the empty ring with the distal ring block anteriorly and medially where the soft tissue sleeve of the thigh is minimal, and the larger, empty ring laterally and posteriorly where extra skin clearance is required. Later it may be necessary to build out from the distal block laterally and posteriorly with short connection plates to have additional threaded rods or graduated telescopic rods in these locations.

For placement of reference wires, position the patient supine with a folded sheet under the ipsilateral buttock. A radiolucent table that splits at the lower extremities, allowing removal of the part of the table under the involved leg, is helpful. Place the foot on a Mayo stand or other small table to permit flexion and extension of the knee and hip to allow assessment of acceptable placement of the wires in the soft tissues around the knee. Use fluoroscopy to guide insertion of the distal reference wire. In the distal femur, use 1.8-mm wires, and in the proximal femur, use 5-mm conical self-drilling, self-tapping screws. If preferred, other heavy-gauge half-pins, especially those designed to be predrilled, can be substituted. When using conical pins, be careful not to back them out once they have been inserted or they will loosen. Under fluoroscopic control, insert as the distal reference wire an olive wire from lateral to medial, almost perpendicular to the mechanical axis of the femur, parallel to the knee joint but slightly higher on the medial side at the level of the adductor tuberosity. For the proximal reference pin, insert a half-pin just distal to the level of the greater trochanter, parallel to an imaginary line drawn from the tip of the greater trochanter to the center of the femoral head, normally within 3 degrees of parallel to the axis of the knee joint. The distal reference wire should be perpendicular to the mechanical axis of the femur, not perpendicular to the anatomical axis (Fig. 26-113, A). This is important because lengthening should take place along the mechanical axis rather than the shaft axis. Failure to adhere to this principle disrupts the normal mechanical axis and causes medialization of the knee (Fig. 26-114).

Secure the preassembled frame to the top reference pin and bottom reference wire and ensure that clearance between the skin and the frame is adequate and that all connections are tight. Tension the wires to 130 kg of force after fixing the olive end of the wire to the distal ring. Ensure adequate soft tissue clearance and then use the frame as a guide to insert the proximal half-pin secured with either a monopin fixation clamp or a buckle clamp (see Fig. 26-113, B and C). For fixation, insert two oblique smooth wires on the distal ring and one medial olive wire and an oblique smooth wire on the ring above. Some important technical points must be remembered while inserting the wires. When inserting a wire from the anterior to the posterior thigh, first flex the knee 45 degrees as the wire penetrates the anterior skin. Then flex the knee 90 degrees as the wire penetrates the quadriceps muscle. Then drill the wire through the femur just to the opposite cortex. Tap the wire through the soft tissue, keeping the knee fully extended as the wire traverses the hamstrings; flex the knee to 45 degrees as the wire exits the skin. After each wire has been inserted, move the knee from full extension to 90 degrees of flexion. The wire should "float" in the soft tissue and should not be pulled by the muscle or cause tenting of the skin. This technique of wire placement helps minimize skin irritation and joint contractures. If a wire does not exit directly in the plane of the ring, build the ring up to the level of the wire with washers or posts. Do not bend the wire in any plane to make it lie closer to the ring. In the proximal arc, add one more pin anteriorly, on the opposite side of the arc, to avoid the reference pin. Do not insert this pin any more medially than the anterosuperior iliac spine, or the femoral nerve will be at risk. On the second arc, place two additional pins, one on each side of the arc, in the oblique plane between the two top pins. The ideal mechanical placement of wires and pins should approach 90 degrees when viewed axially, within anatomical limits. A 90-degree fixation spread within a given ring or fixation block resists bending moments in a more uniform manner. Olive wires add mechanical strength to the construct but should not be overused. The olive wires function as fulcrums, acting on the bone to resist or correct axial deviation. Lengthening around the knee tends to angulate into valgus, whereas lengthening near the ankle and hip tends to angulate into varus. All sites are prone to anterior angulation. The olive wires in the femoral construct are placed strategically to resist valgus angulation. An additional olive wire can be placed opposite the lateral olive wire of the distal ring to lock the distal ring into place, if desired. More recently, an alternative method of distal ring fixation has been used, consisting of one transverse reference wire and two half-pins, one posteromedial and one posterolateral.

For corticotomy, remove the anterior and medial connecting rods from between the empty ring and the distal fixation block. Make a ½-inch incision in the lateral skin just proximal to the distal fixation block. Incising the fascia lata transversely makes the lengthening process easier and diminishes the tendency for valgus angulation. Dissect bluntly down to the femur with Mayo scissors and insert a small, sharp periosteal elevator down to the lateral cortex of the femur. With a knife, make a longitudinal incision

continued

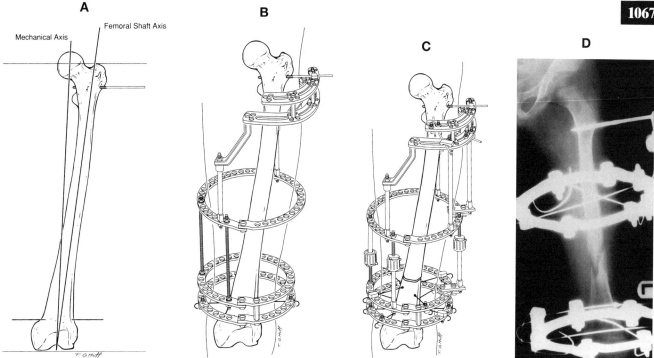

Fig. 26-113 Application of Ilizarov frame (see text). **A,** Frame is applied perpendicular to mechanical axis, not femoral shaft axis. Distally, reference wire is placed parallel to femoral condyles. Proximally, reference pin is drilled perpendicular to mechanical axis. **B,** Ilizarov femoral lengthening frame is constructed on proximal and distal reference pins. Middle ring is larger in diameter than distal two rings to accommodate conical shape of thigh. **C,** Completed femoral frame. Graduated telescopic distractors are placed in alternating up-down position for greater stability. Olive wires add greater stability to construct. "Empty" middle ring serves as even push-off point. **D,** Modified Ilizarov frame in place after femoral corticotomy for lengthening.

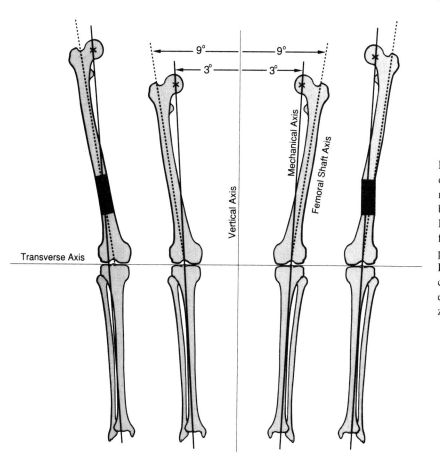

Fig. 26-114 Difference between lengthening of femoral shaft axis and lengthening of mechanical axis of femur. *Left,* Femur has been lengthened along femoral shaft axis. Knee is moved medially so that line drawn from center of femoral head to center of ankle passes lateral to intercondylar notch. *Right,* Lengthening has been done parallel to mechanical axis, allowing axis to remain properly aligned; however, this does give slight zigzag appearance to femur.

through the periosteum and then use the elevator to strip a thin, 1-cm wide section of periosteum anterior and posterior, as much as can be reached. Transect the lateral cortex with a ½-inch osteotome; then cut the anterior and posterior cortices, including the linea aspera, with a ¼-inch osteotome. Do not violate the medullary canal. To prevent medial cortex comminution and fracture extension into the distal wires, predrill three 3.2-mm holes in the medial cortex, inserting the drill from the lateral wound. Fracture the most medial cortex by bending the femur. Be sure the fragments demonstrate enough motion to indicate complete corticotomy but do not widely displace them. Reduce the fracture and align the proximal and distal fixation blocks parallel to each other. Use four upright, threaded rods or short, graduated, telescopic tubes to connect the distal fixation block to the empty ring (see Fig. 26-113, *C*). Complete the frame by adding components until there are four connectors between every arc or ring in the frame (see Fig. 26-113, *D*). Close the skin over a drain if needed and apply a pressure dressing to the lateral wound. Dress the wire and pin sites with sponges. Apply rubber stoppers to each wire and pin site before attaching them to the frame. The stoppers help maintain slight pressure on the pin dressings and minimize pin-skin interface motion, which is a prelude to pin site infection. Wrap the proximal four pins tightly with stretch gauze to minimize skin motion over these pins.

AFTERTREATMENT. Physical therapy and protected weight-bearing with crutches are begun immediately. Knee flexion of at least 45 to 75 degrees is encouraged, but the knee is splinted in extension at night. Lengthening is begun at 4 to 6 days after surgery, depending on the age of the child, and progresses at a rate of 0.25 mm four times daily. The patient and family are taught how to lengthen before discharge from the hospital, and a record of lengthening should be maintained. Although lengthening at precisely every 6 hours is desirable, it is far more practical to lengthen at breakfast, lunch, dinner, and bedtime. A preoperative lateral view of the knee is essential to help judge early signs of subluxation, especially during large lengthenings in patients with congenital deficiencies of the femur. Roentgenograms should be made 7 to 10 days after lengthening is begun to ensure distraction of the corticotomy. If insufficient regenerated bone is present after 4 to 6 weeks, the rate of distraction can be adjusted.

Once the desired length has been achieved, the fixator is kept in place until there is corticalization of the regenerated bone. Some surgeons "train" the regenerated bone before fixator removal by placing it under slight compression or by retensioning the wires. Weight-bearing and fixator stability are critical factors in producing healthy regenerated bone. At the time of fixator removal, the knee can be manipulated if necessary but only before removal of the device. Protected weight-bearing and vigorous physical therapy are continued,

and activity is gradually increased. When lengthening is complete, knee motion typically is limited to about 40 degrees, but after the frame is removed, motion usually is regained at the rate of 10 to 15 degrees a month.

The Ilizarov frame and application can be modified to correct deviation of the mechanical axis or deformity of the proximal femur. Hinges can be placed at the lengthening corticotomy site to effect angular correction. Proximal deformities can be immediately corrected by percutaneous osteotomy between the two proximal arcs. The arcs are initially angulated relative to one another, the osteotomy is performed, and the arcs are immediately brought into parallel alignment to effect the desired correction. Rotational corrections are best done acutely through a proximal (subtrochanteric) osteotomy at the time of initial frame application.

Complications of Lengthening. All types of limb-lengthening devices and techniques have some complications in common, but certain complications are more or less likely to occur with a given device.

Pin Track Infection. The most common problem is pin track infection, which can be minimized by careful pin insertion. Thin wires should be inserted through the skin directly at the level that the wire will enter bone to prevent tenting of the skin. At the end of the procedure, moving the nearby joints through a full range of motion will identify skin tenting over wires, and the sites can be released with a scalpel. The thin transfixion wires may cause fewer problems than the large half-pins, but skin and muscle motion over any wire or pin should be minimized by special dressing techniques. For thin-wire fixators, commercially available 1-inch foam cubes with a slit are placed around the pin site. The slit is then stapled to hold the cube in place. Finally, a clip or previously applied rubber stopper is lowered onto the foam to apply mild pressure on the skin. Excessive pressure, however, should be avoided because it can cause ulcerations, especially over bony prominences. For large pins, especially in the thigh, surgical gauze can be wrapped snugly around two or more neighboring pins to apply pressure to the skin around the pins. All wire and pin care should include daily sterilization with an antiseptic, such as povidone-iodine (Betadine) or chlorhexidine gluconate (Hibistat), but only a small amount (1 ml per pin) should be used to avoid skin irritation. If the skin becomes irritated, the solution can be diluted or a nonirritating antibiotic ointment, such as polymyxin B sulfate–neomycin sulfate (Neosporin), can be used.

At the first sign of pin track infection, broad-spectrum antibiotics should be given, local pin care should be intensified, and the pin site should be incised to promote drainage if necessary. If the infection does not improve with these measures, the pin may have to be removed. If pin removal jeopardizes the stability of the frame, a replacement pin should be inserted. With the Ilizarov apparatus this is relatively simple: a wire can be placed in a nearby hole or dropped off the ring on a post to avoid the infected pin site. With monolateral fixators, insertion of a replacement pin away from the infected site is more difficult. The Orthofix supplemental screw device can be useful for inserting additional half-pins off-axis. Severe infection usually requires curettement of the pin track and bone.

Muscular Problems. The most difficult complications that occur during lengthening are related to the muscles. In theory the bones can be lengthened by any amount, but the muscles have a limited ability to stretch. Typically, the muscles that cause the most problems are the triceps surae during tibial lengthening and the quadriceps during femoral lengthening. Knee flexion contracture is common during tibial lengthening and can be prevented with prophylactic splinting, especially at night. Custom orthoses or commercially available Dynasplints are helpful, and vigorous, frequent physical therapy also is critical. Prophylactic treatment should be begun within 1 week of the original surgery. For tibial lengthenings of more than 4 to 5 cm, the foot should be fixed in neutral position by applying a posterior plaster splint for monolateral fixators or by placing two wires in the heel and connecting them to a ring attached to the frame of a thin-wire circular fixator. The heel pins should be removed as soon as possible after lengthening is complete (provided the knee is not contracted) to allow the subtalar and ankle joints to regain motion. Lengthening of the tendo calcaneus should be considered if residual contracture persists. Any preoperative contracture of the tendo calcaneus should be corrected before or during tibial lengthening.

Joint Problems. Joint subluxation or dislocation has been reported during femoral lengthening, especially if either the hip or knee joint is unstable before surgery (as is frequently the case in patients with PFFD). In patients with congenital deformities, prophylactic tenotomies of the rectus femoris proximally, the adductors, and sometimes the hamstrings can be useful. For hips with varus deformities, corrective valgus osteotomy should be delayed until after lengthening. As a general rule, the hip roentgenogram should show a center-edge angle of at least 15 to 20 degrees before femoral lengthening is considered; otherwise, a preliminary pelvic osteotomy may be necessary. The cruciate ligaments generally are deficient in patients with PFFD, making knee subluxation more likely, and prophylactic fixation of the knee joint with a mobile hinge is possible with the Ilizarov apparatus. A posteriorly dislocated tibia can be slowly pulled anteriorly with a mobile Ilizarov hinge on a rail to reduce the dislocation and allow knee motion. With the monolateral fixators, these options are not available. For hip subluxation, traction and bed rest usually are sufficient.

Neurovascular Problems. Neurovascular complications usually are related to faulty pin placement but may result from stretching during lengthening. If the rate of distraction is 1 mm per day, then neurovascular tissues almost always are able to stretch to accommodate the lengthening. Decreasing or temporarily stopping the distraction usually is sufficient. If a cutaneous nerve is tented over a wire or pin, removal of the pin is indicated. Peroneal nerve dysfunction that occurs during tibial lengthening should be treated by nerve decompression at the fibular head, extending proximally 5 to 7 cm and distally into the anterior compartment. Hypertension rarely is seen with slow, gradual distraction.

Bony Problems. Bony complications of distraction osteogenesis include premature consolidation and delayed consolidation. In Wagner lengthening, common problems are deep infection, pseudarthrosis, plate breakage, and malunion. With distraction osteogenesis by either the Ilizarov or DeBastiani technique, delayed or premature consolidation usually can be resolved without compromising a satisfactory result. Premature consolidation is caused by an excessive latency period. For femoral lengthening in children, a latency period of 5 days is recommended and for tibial lengthening, 7 days. For older patients and those with compromised vascularity to the limb, longer latency periods may be appropriate. Premature consolidation of the fibula in tibial lengthenings can be prevented by using a standard open osteotomy of the fibula instead of a corticotomy. In some reports of premature consolidation, patients reported successively difficult lengthening until finally a "pop" was felt, followed by brief but intense pain, indicating spontaneous rupture through the consolidated regenerated bone. The bone ends should be brought back to the level of apposition before the rupture and, after a brief latency period, lengthening is resumed. Failure to "back up" can result in cyst formation and nonunion.

Delayed consolidation is more common with diaphyseal lengthening than with metaphyseal corticotomy. Contributing factors include frame instability, overly vigorous corticotomy with excessive periosteal stripping, and a distraction rate that is too rapid, especially after too brief a latency period. Gigli saw osteotomies in thick diaphyseal cortical bone can lead to delayed healing. Underlying medical or nutritional problems and lack of exercise are other contributing factors. In addition to correcting these factors, distraction can be slowed or stopped, the bone can be compressed, or it can be alternatively compressed and lengthened. Walking and normal use of the limb should always be encouraged. In adults and older children, the best regenerated bone develops in those who are active and use analgesics sparingly. Autologous cancellous bone grafting of the gap is a final resort. Extra precautions should be taken during the preparation and draping of the fixator because the pin sites may harbor bacteria. With Wagner lengthening, bone grafting of the gap is expected, but it is easier to drape the monolateral fixators out of the sterile operative site. Malunion and axial deviation during lengthening have been discussed in previous sections describing techniques.

References

ANOMALIES OF TOES
Abraham E, Waxman B, Shirali S, Durkin M: Congenital cleft-foot deformity treatment, *J Pediatr Orthop* 19:410, 1999.

Allen BL Jr: Plantar-advancement skin flap for central ray resections in the foot: description of a technique, *J Pediatr Orthop* 17:785, 1997.

Black GB, Grogan DP, Bobechko WP: Butler arthroplasty for correction of the adducted fifth toe: a retrospective study of 36 operations between 1968 and 1982, *J Pediatr Orthop* 5:438, 1985.

Blauth W, Borisch NC: Cleft feet: Proposals for a new classification based on roentgenographic morphology, *Clin Orthop* 258:41, 1990.

Dennyson WG, Bear JN, Bholla KD: Macrodactyly in the foot, *J Bone Joint Surg* 59B:355, 1977.

Diamond LS, Gould VE: Macrodactyly of the foot: surgical syndactyly after wedge resection, *South Med J* 67:645, 1974.

Farmer AW: Congenital hallux varus, *Am J Surg* 95:274, 1958.

Greiss ME, Williams DH: Macrodystrophia lipomatosis in the foot: a case report and review of the literature, *Arch Orthop Trauma Surg* 110:220, 1991.

Grogan DP, Bernstein RM, Habal MB, Ogden JA: Congenital lipofibromatosis associated with macrodactyly of the foot, *Foot Ankle* 12:40, 1991.

Hamer AJ, Stanley D, Smith TW: Surgery for the curly toe deformity: a double-blind, randomised, prospective trial, *J Bone Joint Surg* 75B:662, 1993.

Hubbard AM, Davidson RS, Meyer JS, Mahboubi S: Magnetic resonance imaging of skewfoot, *J Bone Joint Surg* 78A:389, 1996.

Kalen V, Burwell DS, Omer GE: Macrodactyly of the hands and feet, *J Pediatr Orthop* 8:311, 1988.

Kelikian H, Clayton L, Loseff H: Surgical syndactylia of the toes, *Clin Orthop* 19:209, 1961.

Kotwal PP, Farooque M: Macrodactyly, *J Bone Joint Surg* 80B:651, 1998.

Kovalsky E, Guttmann GG: Early surgical correction of unilateral cleft foot deformity, *Orthopedics* 13:348, 1990.

Lapidus PW: Transplantation of the extensor tendon for correction of the overlapping fifth toe, *J Bone Joint Surg* 24:555, 1942.

Lenke LG, Schoenecker PL, Gilula LA: Imaging rounds no 105, *Orthop Rev* 20:295, 1991.

Leonard MH, Rising EE: Syndactylization to maintain correction of overlapping fifth toe, *Clin Orthop* 43:241, 1965.

Meyerding HW, Upshaw JE: Heredofamilial cleft foot deformity (lobster-claw or splitfoot), *Am J Surg* 74:889, 1947.

Nakamura K, Ohara K, Ohta E: A new surgical technique for postaxial polydactyly of the foot, *Plast Reconstr Surg* 97:133, 1996.

Thompson TC: Surgical treatment of disorders of the fore part of the foot, *J Bone Joint Surg* 46A:1117, 1964.

Topoleski TA, Ganel A, Grogan DP: Effect of proximal phalangeal epiphysiodesis in the treatment of macrodactyly, *Foot Ankle Int* 18:500, 1997.

Venn-Watson EA: Problems in polydactyly of the foot, *Orthop Clin North Am* 7:909, 1976.

Weaver KM, Henry GW, Reinker KA: Unilateral duplication of the great toe with anterolateral tibial bowing. *J Pediatr Orthop* 16:73, 1996.

Wood VE, Peppers TA, Shook J: Cleft-foot closure: a simplified technique and review of the literature. *J Pediatr Orthop* 17:501, 1997.

ANOMALIES OF FOOT

Congenital Metatarsus Adductus

Anderson D, Schoenecker P: Combined lateral column shortening and medial column lengthening in the treatment of severe forefoot adductus. Paper presented at the First International Congress on Clubfeet, Milwaukee, Sept 1990.

Asirvatham R, Stevens PM: Idiopathic forefoot-adduction deformity: medial capsulotomy and abductor hallucis lengthening for resistant and severe deformities, *J Pediatr Orthop* 17:496, 1997.

Berman A, Gartland JJ: Metatarsal osteotomy for the correction of adduction of the fore part of the foot in children, *J Bone Joint Surg* 53A:498, 1971.

Bleck EE: Metatarsus adductus: classification and relationship to outcomes of treatment, *J Pediatr Orthop* 3:2, 1983.

Heyman CH, Herndon CH, Strong JM: Mobilization of the tarsometatarsal and intermetatarsal joints for the correction of resistant adduction of the fore part of the foot in congenital clubfoot or congenital metatarsus varus, *J Bone Joint Surg* 40A:299, 1958.

Katz K, David R, Soudry M: Below-knee plaster cast for the treatment of metatarsus adductus, *J Pediatr Orthop* 19:49, 1999.

Kendrick RE, Sharma NK, Hassler WL, Herndon CH: Tarsometatarsal mobilization for resistant adduction of the fore part of the foot: a follow-up study, *J Bone Joint Surg* 52A:61, 1970.

Lichtblau S: Section of the abductor hallucis tendon for correction of metatarsus varus deformity, *Clin Orthop* 110:227, 1975.

Ponseti IV, Becker JR: Congenital metatarsus adductus: the results of treatment, *J Bone Joint Surg* 48A:702, 1966.

Stark JG, Johnson JE, Winter RB: The Heyman-Herndon tarsometatarsal capsulotomy for metatarsus adductus: results in 48 feet, *J Pediatr Orthop* 7:305, 1987.

Theodorou DJ, Theodorou SJ, Boutin RD, et al: Stress fractures of the lateral metatarsal bones in metatarsus adductus foot deformity: a previously unrecognized association, *Skeletal Radiol* 28:679, 1999.

Clubfoot

Addison A, Fixen JA, Lloyd-Roberts GC: A review of the Dillwyn Evans type collateral operation in severe clubfoot, *J Bone Joint Surg* 65B:12, 1983.

Allington NJ, Kumar SJ, Guille JT: Clubfeet associated with congenital constriction bands of the ipsilateral lower extremity, *J Pediatr Orthop* 15:599, 1995.

Anderson AF, Fowler SB: Anterior calcaneal osteotomy for symptomatic juvenile pes planus, *Foot Ankle* 4:274, 1984.

Aronson J, Puskarich CL: Deformity and disability from treated clubfoot, *J Pediatr Orthop* 10:109, 1990.

Atar D, Grant AD, Silver L, et al: The use of a tissue expander in clubfoot surgery: a case report and review, *J Bone Joint Surg* 72B:574, 1990.

Bensahel H, Catterall A, Dimeglio A: Practical applications in idiopathic clubfoot: a retrospective multicentric study in EPOS, *J Pediatr Orthop* 10:186, 1990.

Bényi P: A modified Lambrinudi operation for drop foot, *J Bone Joint Surg* 42B:333, 1960.

Bradish CF, Tan S: Residual bone cysts after Ilizarov treatment of relapsed clubfoot, *J Pediatr Orthop* 21:218, 2001.

Brougham DI, Nicol RO: Use of the Cincinnati incision in congenital talipes equinovarus, *J Pediatr Orthop* 8:696, 1988.

Carroll NC: Congenital clubfoot: pathoanatomy and treatment, *Instr Course Lect* 36:117, 1987.

Carroll NC: Controversies in the surgical management of clubfoot, *Instr Course Lect* 45:331, 1996.

Chang CH, Huang SC: Clubfoot deformity in congenital constriction band syndrome: manifestations and treatment, *J Formos Med Assoc* 97:328, 1998.

Cooper DM, Deitz FR: Treatment of idiopathic clubfoot: a thirty-year follow-up note, *J Bone Joint Surg* 77A:1477, 1995.

Crawford AH, Gupta AK: Clubfoot controversies: complications and causes for failure, *Instr Course Lect* 45:339, 1996.

Crawford AH, Marxen JL, Osterfeld DL: The Cincinnati incision: a comprehensive approach for surgical procedures of the foot and ankle in childhood, *J Bone Joint Surg* 64A:1355, 1982.

Cummings J, Lovell WW: Current concepts: operative treatment of congenital idiopathic clubfoot, *J Bone Joint Surg* 70A:1108, 1988.

Cummings RJ, Bashore CJ, Bookout CB, Elliott MJ: Avascular necrosis of the talus after McKay clubfoot release for idiopathic congenital clubfoot, *J Pediatr Orthop* 21:221, 2001.

DePuy J, Drennan JC: Correction of idiopathic clubfoot: a comparison of results of early versus delayed posteromedial release, *J Pediatr Orthop* 9:44, 1989.

Dillwyn-Evans D: Relapsed clubfoot, *J Bone Joint Surg* 43B:722, 1961.

Dimeglio A, Bensahel H, Souschet P, et al: Classification of clubfoot, *J Pediatr Orthop B* 4:129, 1995.

Dunn HK, Samuelson KM: Flat-top talus: a long-term report of twenty clubfeet, *J Bone Joint Surg* 56A:57, 1974.

Dwyer FC: Osteotomy of the calcaneum for pes cavus, *J Bone Joint Surg* 41B:80, 1959.

Dwyer FC: The treatment of relapsed club foot by the insertion of a wedge into the calcaneum, *J Bone Joint Surg* 45B:67, 1963.

Dwyer FC: The present status of the problem of pes cavus, *Clin Orthop* 106:254, 1975.

Fisher RL, Shaffer SR: An evaluation of calcaneal osteotomy in congenital clubfoot and other disorders, *Clin Orthop* 70:141, 1970.

Flynn JM, Donohoe M, Mackenzie WG: An independent assessment of two clubfoot-classification systems, *J Pediatr Orthop* 18:323, 1998.

Galdino MJ Jr, Siff SJ, Butler JE, et al: Triple arthrodesis in young children: a salvage procedure after failed releases in severely affected feet, *Foot Ankle* 7:319, 1987.

Garceau GJ, Palmer RM: Transfer of the anterior tibial tendon for recurrent club foot: a long-term follow-up, *J Bone Joint Surg* 49A: 207, 1967.

Ghali NN, Smith RB, Clayden AD, et al: The results of pantalar reduction in the management of congenital talipes equinovarus, *J Bone Joint Surg* 65B:1, 1983.

Gomez VR: Clubfeet in congenital annular constricting bands, *Clin Orthop* 323:155, 1996.

Grill F, Franke J: The Ilizarov distractor for the correction of relapsed or neglected clubfoot, *J Bone Joint Surg* 69B:593, 1987.

Haasbeek JF, Wright JG: A comparison of the long-term results of posterior and comprehensive release in the treatment of clubfoot, *J Pediatr Orthop* 17:29, 1997.

Herbsthofer B, Eckardt A, Rompe JD, Kullmer K: Significance of radiographic angle measurements in evaluation of congenital clubfoot, *Arch Orthop Trauma Surg* 117:324, 1998.

Hersh A, Fuchs LA: Treatment of the uncorrected clubfoot by triple arthrodesis, *Orthop Clin North Am* 4:103, 1973.

Herzenberg JE, Carroll NC, Christofersen MR, et al: Clubfoot analysis with three-dimensional computer modeling, *J Pediatr Orthop* 8:257, 1988.

Hoffmann AA, Constine RM, McBride GG, et al: Osteotomy of the first cuneiform as treatment of residual adduction of the fore part of the foot in club foot, *J Bone Joint Surg* 66A:985, 1984.

Howard CB, Benson MK: Clubfoot: its pathological anatomy, *J Pediatr Orthop* 13:654, 1993.

Hudson I, Catterall A: Posterolateral release for resistant clubfoot, *J Bone Joint Surg* 76B:281, 1994.

Irani RN, Sherman MS: The pathological anatomy of club foot, *J Bone Joint Surg* 45A:45, 1963.

Joseph B, Ajith K, Varghese RA: Evaluation of the hemi-Cincinnati incision for posteromedial soft tissue release in clubfoot, *J Pediatr Orthop* 20:524, 2000.

Joseph B, Bhatia M, Nair NS: Talocalcaneal relationship in clubfoot, *J Pediatr Orthop* 21:60, 2001.

Karski T, Wósko I: Experience in the conservative treatment of congenital clubfoot in newborns and infants, *J Pediatr Orthop* 9:134, 1989.

Kite JH: Principles involved in treatment of clubfoot, *J Bone Joint Surg* 21:595, 1939.

Kitziger K, Wilkins K: Absent posterior tibial artery in an infant with talipes equinovarus, *J Pediatr Orthop* 11:777, 1991.

Kranicz J, Than P, Kustos T: Long-term results of the operative treatment of clubfoot: a representative study, *Orthopedics* 21:669, 1998.

Kuo KN, Hennigan SP, Hastings ME: Anterior tibial tendon transfer in residual dynamic clubfoot deformity. *J Pediatr Orthop* 21:35, 2001.

Lambrinudi C: New operation on drop-foot, *Br J Surg* 15:193, 1927.

Lambrinudi C: A method of correcting equinus and calcaneus deformities at the sub-astragaloid joint, *Proc Roy Soc Med* 26:788, 1933.

LaReaux RL, Hosey T: Results of surgical treatment of talipes equino-valgus by means of navicular-cuneiform arthrodesis with midcuboid osteotomy, *J Foot Surg* 26:412, 1987.

Lehman WB, Atar D, Bash J, et al: Results of complete soft tissue clubfoot release combined with calcaneocuboid fusion in the 4-year to 8-year age group following failed clubfoot release, *J Pediatr Orthop B* 8:181, 1999.

Letts M, Davidson D: The role of bilateral talectomy in the management of bilateral rigid clubfeet, *Am J Orthop* 28:106, 1999.

Lichtblau S: A medial and lateral release operation for clubfoot: a preliminary report, *J Bone Joint Surg* 55A:1377, 1973.

Lloyd-Roberts GC, Swann M, Catterall A: Medial rotational osteotomy for severe residual deformity in clubfoot: a preliminary report on a new method of treatment, *J Bone Joint Surg* 56B:37, 1974.

Lovell WW, Hancock CI: Treatment of congenital talipes equinovarus, *Clin Orthop* 70:79, 1970.

Lubicky JP, Altiok H: Regional fasciocutaneous flap closure for clubfoot surgery, *J Pediatr Orthop* 21:50, 2001.

Macnicol MF, Nadeem RD, Forness M: Functional results of surgical treatment in congenital talipes equinovarus (clubfoot): a comparison of outcome measurements, *J Pediatr Orthop* 9:285, 2000.

Magone JB, Torch MA, Clark RN, Kean JR: Comparative review of surgical treatment of the idiopathic clubfoot by three different procedures at Columbus Children's Hospital, *J Pediatr Orthop* 9:49, 1989.

Manzone P: Clubfoot surgical treatment: preliminary results of a prospective comparative study of two techniques, *J Pediatr Orthop B* 8:246, 1999.

McHale KA, Lenhart MK: Treatment of residual clubfoot deformity—the "bean-shaped" foot—by open wedge medial cuneiform osteotomy and closing wedge cuboid osteotomy: clinical review and cadaver correlations, *J Pediatr Orthop* 11:374, 1991.

McKay DW: Dorsal bunions in children, *J Bone Joint Surg* 65A:975, 1983.

McKay DW: New concept of and approach to clubfoot treatment. I. Principles and morbid anatomy, *J Pediatr Orthop* 2:347, 1982.

McKay DW: New concept of and approach to clubfoot treatment. II. Correction of clubfoot, *J Pediatr Orthop* 3:10, 1983.

McKay DW: New concept of and approach to clubfoot treatment. III. Evaluation and results, *J Pediatr Orthop* 3:141, 1983.

Napiontek M: Transposed skin graft for wound closure after Cincinnati incision. Experience in seven patients with severe foot deformities, *Acta Orthop Scand* 67:280, 1996.

Otremski I, Salama R, Khermosh O, Weintroub S: Residual adduction of the forefoot: a review of the Turco procedure for congenital club foot, *J Bone Joint Surg* 69B:832, 1987.

Pirani S, Outerbridge H, Moran M, Sawatsky B: A method of evaluating the virgin clubfoot with substantial interobserver reliability. Presented at the annual meeting of the Pediatr Orthopaedic Society of North America, Miami, 1995.

Ponseti IV: Treatment of congenital clubfoot, *J Bone Joint Surg* 74A:448, 1992.

Ponseti IV: Common errors in the treatment of congenital clubfoot, *Int Orthop* 21:137, 1997.

Porter RW: Congenital talipes equinovarus. I. Resolving and resistant deformities, *J Bone Joint Surg* 69B:822, 1987.

Reimann I, Werner HH: Congenital metatarsus varus: on the advantages of early treatment, *Acta Orthop Scand* 46:857, 1975.

Rumyantsev NJ, Ezrohi VE: Complete subtalar release in resistant clubfeet: a critical analysis of results in 146 cases, *J Pediatr Orthop* 17:490, 1997.

Sangeorzan BJ, Mosca V, Hansen ST Jr: Effect of calcaneal lengthening on relationships among the hindfoot, midfoot, and forefoot, *Foot Ankle* 14:136, 1993.

Shapiro F, Glimcher MJ: Gross and histologic abnormalities of the talus in congenital clubfoot, *J Bone Joint Surg* 61A:522, 1979.

Silver CM, Simon SD, Litchman HM: Long-term follow-up observations on calcaneal osteotomy, *Clin Orthop* 99:181, 1974.

Simons GW: Complete subtalar release in club feet. I. A preliminary report, *J Bone Joint Surg* 67A:1044, 1985.

Simons GW: Complete subtalar release in club feet. II. Comparison with less extensive procedures, *J Bone Joint Surg* 67A:1056, 1985.

Smith PD, Kuo KN: Dorsal bunion after treatment for clubfoot, *Orthop Consult* 13:4, 1992.

Sodre H, Bruschini S, Mestriner LA, et al: Arterial abnormalities in talipes equinovarus as assessed by angiography and the Doppler technique, *J Pediatr Orthop* 10:101, 1990.

Stanitski CL, Ward WT, Grossman W: Noninvasive vascular studies in clubfoot, *J Pediatr Orthop* 12:514, 1991.

Stevens PM, Otis S: Ankle valgus and clubfeet, *J Pediatr Orthop* 19:515, 1999.

Tarraf YN, Carroll NC: Analysis of the components of residual deformity in clubfeet presenting for reoperation, *J Pediatr Orthop* 12:207, 1992.

Tayton K, Thompson P: Relapsing club feet: late results of delayed operation, *J Bone Joint Surg* 61B:474, 1979.

Thompson TC: Astragalectomy and the treatment of calcaneovalgus, *J Bone Joint Surg* 21:627, 1939.

Toohey JS, Campbell P: Distal calcaneal osteotomy in resistant talipes equinovarus, *Clin Orthop* 197:224, 1985.

Trumble T, Banta JV, Raycroft JF, Curtis BH: Talectomy for equinovarus deformity in myelodysplasia, *J Bone Joint Surg* 67A:21, 1985.

Turco VJ: Surgical correction of the resistant club foot: one-stage posteromedial release with internal fixation: a preliminary report, *J Bone Joint Surg* 53A:477, 1971.

Turco VJ: Resistant congenital clubfoot, *Instr Course Lect* 24:104, 1975.

Turco VJ: Resistant congenital clubfoot: one-stage posteromedial release with internal fixation, *J Bone Joint Surg* 61A:805, 1979.

Victoria-Diaz A, Victoria-Diaz J: Pathogenesis of idiopathic clubfoot, *Clin Orthop* 185:14, 1984.

Wallander H, Hansson G, Tjernstrom B: Correction of persistent clubfoot deformities with the Ilizarov external fixator. Experience in 10 previously operated feet followed for 2-5 years, *Acta Orthop Scand* 67:283, 1996.

Wesley MS, Barenfield PA: Mechanism of the Dwyer calcaneal osteotomy, *Clin Orthop* 70:137, 1970.

Wynne-Davies R: Talipes equinovarus: a review of eighty-four cases after completion of treatment, *J Bone Joint Surg* 46B:464, 1964.

Yamamoto H, Muneta T, Morita S: Nonsurgical treatment of congenital clubfoot with manipulation, cast, and modified Denis Browne splint, *J Pediatr Orthop* 18:538, 1998.

Zimny ML, Willig SJ, Roberts JM, et al: An electron microscopic study of the fascia from the medial and lateral sides of clubfoot, *J Pediatr Orthop* 5:577, 1985.

Congenital Vertical Talus

Becker-Andersen H, Reimann I: Congenital vertical talus: reevaluation of early manipulative treatment, *Acta Orthop Scand* 45:130, 1974.

Coleman SS, Martin AF, Jarrett J: Congenital vertical talus: pathogenesis and treatment, *J Bone Joint Surg* 48A:1442, 1966.

Coleman SS, Stelling FH III, Jarrett J: Congenital vertical talus: pathomechanics and treatment, *Clin Orthop* 70:62, 1970.

Dennyson WG, Fulford GE: Subtalar arthrodesis by cancellous grafts and metallic internal fixation, *J Bone Joint Surg* 58B:507, 1976.

Drennan JC: Congenital vertical talus, *Instr Course Lect* 45:315, 1996.

Green NA: One-stage release for congenital vertical talus. Paper presented at the meeting of the Pediatric Orthopaedic Society of North America, Hilton Head, SC, May 1989.

Grice DS: An extra-articular arthrodesis of the subastragalar joint for correction of paralytic flat feet in children, *J Bone Joint Surg* 34A:927, 1952.

Grice DS: Further experience with extraarticular arthrodesis of the subtalar joint, *J Bone Joint Surg* 37A:246, 1955.

Guttman G: Modification of the Grice-Green subtalar arthrodesis in children, *J Pediatr Orthop* 1:219, 1981.

Harrold AJ: Congenital vertical talus in infancy, *J Bone Joint Surg* 49B:634, 1967.

Harrold AJ: The problem of congenital vertical talus, *Clin Orthop* 97:133, 1973.

Jacobsen ST, Crawford AH: Congenital vertical talus, *J Pediatr Orthop* 3:306, 1983.

Jayakumar S, Cowell HR: Rigid flatfoot, *Clin Orthop* 122:77, 1977.

Kodros SA, Dias LS: Single-stage surgical correction of congenital vertical talus, *J Pediatr Orthop* 19:42, 1999.

Kumar SJ, Cowell HR, Ramsey PL: Foot problems in children. I. Vertical and oblique talus, *Instr Course Lect* 31:235, 1982.

McCall RE, Lillich JS, Harris JR, et al: The Grice extraarticular subtalar arthrodesis: a clinical review, *J Pediatr Orthop* 5:442, 1985.

Schrader LF, Gilbert RJ, Skinner SR, Ashley RK: Congenital vertical talus: surgical correction by a one-stage medial approach, *Orthopedics* 13:1233, 1990.

Scott SM, Janes PC, Stevens PM: Grice subtalar arthrodesis followed to skeletal maturity, *J Pediatr Orthop* 8:176, 1988.

Seimon LP: Surgical correction of congenital vertical talus under the age of 2 years, *J Pediatr Orthop* 7:405, 1987.

Stricker SJ, Rosen E: Early one-stage reconstruction of congenital vertical talus, *Foot Ankle Int* 18:535, 1997.

Tarsal Coalition

Conway JJ, Cowell HR: Tarsal coalition: clinical significance and roentgenographic demonstration, *Radiology* 92:799, 1969.

Cowell HR: Tarsal coalition: review and update, *Instr Course Lect* 31:264, 1982.

Cowell HR, Elener V: Rigid painful flatfoot secondary to tarsal coalition, *Clin Orthop* 177:54, 1983.

Danielson LG: Talocalcaneal coalition treated with resection, *J Pediatr Orthop* 7:513, 1987.

Gonzalez P, Kumar SJ: Calcaneonavicular coalition treated by resection and interposition of the extensor digitorum brevis muscle, *J Bone Joint Surg* 72A:71, 1990.

Harris RI: Rigid valgus foot due to talocalcaneal bridge, *J Bone Joint Surg* 37A:169, 1955.

Harris RI, Beath T: Etiology of peroneal spastic flatfoot, *J Bone Joint Surg* 30B:624, 1948.

Herzenberg JE, Goldner JL, Martinez S, et al: Computerized tomography of talocalcaneal tarsal coalition: a clinical and anatomic study, *Foot Ankle* 6:273, 1986.

Kumar SJ, Cowell HR, Ramsey PL: Foot problems in children. I. Vertical and oblique talus, *Instr Course Lect* 31:235, 1982.

Kumar SJ, Guille JT, Lee MS, et al: Osseous and nonosseous coalition of the middle facet of the talocalcaneal joint, *J Bone Joint Surg* 74A:519, 1992.

Mazzocca AD, Thompson JD, Deluca PA, Romness MJ: Comparison of the posterior approach versus the dorsal approach in the treatment of congenital vertical talus, *J Pediatr Orthop* 21:202, 2001.

Swiontkowski MF, Scranton PE, Hansen S: Tarsal coalitions: long-term results of surgical treatment, *J Pediatr Orthop* 3:287, 1983.

Takakura Y, Sugimoto K, Tanaka Y, et al: Symptomatic talocalcaneal coalition: its clinical significance and treatment, *Clin Orthop* 269: 249, 1991.

Warren MJ, Jeffree MA, Wilson DJ, et al: Computed tomography in suspected tarsal coalition: examination of 26 cases, *Acta Orthop Scand* 61:554, 1990.

CONGENITAL ANGULAR DEFORMITIES OF LEG AND CONGENITAL PSEUDARTHROSIS

Aegerter EE: The possible relationship of neurofibromatosis, congenital pseudarthrosis, and fibrous dysplasia, *J Bone Joint Surg* 32A:618, 1950.

Andersen KS: Congenital angulation of the lower leg and congenital pseudarthrosis of the tibia in Denmark, *Acta Orthop Scand* 43:539, 1972.

Anderson DJ, Schoenecker PL, Sheridan JJ, et al: Use of an intramedullary rod for the treatment of congenital pseudarthrosis of the tibia, *J Bone Joint Surg* 74A:161, 1992.

Badgley CE, O'Connor SJ, Kudner DF: Congenital kyphoscoliotic tibia, *J Bone Joint Surg* 34A:349, 1952.

Baker JK, Cain TE, Tullos HS: Intramedullary fixation for congenital pseudarthrosis of the tibia, *J Bone Joint Surg* 74A:169, 1992.

Boyd HB: Congenital pseudarthrosis: treatment by dual bone grafts, *J Bone Joint Surg* 23:497, 1941.

Boyd HB: Pathology and natural history of congenital pseudarthrosis of the tibia, *Clin Orthop* 166:5, 1982.

Boyd HB, Fox KW: Congenital pseudarthrosis: follow-up study after massive bone-grafting, *J Bone Joint Surg* 30A:274, 1948.

Boyd HB, Sage FP: Congenital pseudarthrosis of the tibia, *J Bone Joint Surg* 40A:1245, 1958.

Charnley J: Congenital pseudarthrosis of the tibia treated by the intramedullary nail, *J Bone Joint Surg* 38A:283, 1956.

Crossett LS, Beaty JH, Betz RR, et al: Congenital pseudarthrosis of the tibia: long-term follow-up study, *Clin Orthop* 245:16, 1989.

Dal Monte A, Donzelli O, Sudanese A, Baldini N: Congenital pseudarthrosis of the fibula, *J Pediatr Orthop* 7:14, 1987.

Dooley BJ, Menelaus MB, Paterson DC: Congenital pseudarthrosis and bowing of the fibula, *J Bone Joint Surg* 56B:739, 1974.

Dormans JP, Krajbich JI, Zuker RM, Demuynk M: Congenital pseudarthrosis of the tibia: treatment with free vascularized fibular grafts, *J Pediatr Orthop* 10:623, 1990.

Gilbert A, Brockman R: Congenital pseudarthrosis of the tibia: long-term follow-up of 29 cases treated by microvascular bone transfer, *Clin Orthop* 314:37, 1995.

Goldberg I, Maor P, Yosipovitch Z: Congenital pseudarthrosis of the tibia treated by a pedicled vascularized graft of the ipsilateral fibula: a case report, *J Bone Joint Surg* 70A:1396, 1988.

Gordon L, Weulker N, Jergensen H: Vascularized fibular grafting for the treatment of congenital pseudarthrosis of the tibia, *Orthopedics* 9:825, 1986.

Grogan DP, Love SM, Ogden JA: Congenital malformations of the lower extremities, *Orthop Clin North Am* 18:537, 1987.

Hefti F, Bollini G, Dungl P, et al: Congenital pseudarthrosis of the tibia: history, etiology, classification, and epidemiologic data, *J Pediatr Orthop B* 9:11, 2000.

Heikkinen ES, Poyhonen MH, Kinnunen PK, Seppanen UI: Congenital pseudarthrosis of the tibia: treatment and outcome at skeletal maturity in 10 children, *Acta Orthop Scand* 70:275, 1999.

Heyman CH, Herndon CH, Heiple KG: Congenital posterior angulation of the tibia with talipes calcaneus: a long-term report of eleven patients, *J Bone Joint Surg* 41A:476, 1959.

Hsu LCS, O'Brien JP, Yau ACMC, Hodgson AR: Valgus deformity of the ankle in children with fibular pseudarthrosis: results of treatment by bone-grafting of the fibula, *J Bone Joint Surg* 56A:503, 1974.

Ilizarov GA: The principles of the Ilizarov method, *Bull Hosp Jt Dis* 48:1, 1988.

Joseph B, Mathew G: Management of congenital pseudarthrosis of the tibia by excision of the pseudarthrosis, onlay grafting, and intramedullary nailing, *J Pediatr Orthop B* 9:16, 2000.

Karol LA, Haideri NF, Halliday SE, et al: Gait analysis and muscle strength in children with congenital pseudarthrosis of the tibia: the effect of treatment, *J Pediatr Orthop* 18:381, 1998.

Krida A: Congenital posterior angulation of the tibia: a clinical entity unrelated to congenital pseudarthrosis, *Am J Surg* 28:98, 1951.

Langenskiöld A: Pseudarthrosis of the fibula and progressive valgus deformity of the ankle in children: treatment by fusion of the distal tibial and fibular metaphyses: review of three cases, *J Bone Joint Surg* 49A:463, 1967.

Lawsing JF III, Puglisi A, Fielding JM, Liebler WA: Congenital pseudarthrosis of the tibia: successful one stage transposition of the fibula into the distal tibia: a case report, *Clin Orthop* 110:201, 1975.

Leung PC: Congenital pseudarthrosis of the tibia: three cases treated by free vascularized iliac crest graft, *Clin Orthop* 175:45, 1983.

Masserman RL, Peterson HA, Bianco AJ, Jr: Congenital pseudarthrosis of the tibia: a review of the literature and 52 cases from the Mayo Clinic, *Clin Orthop* 99:140, 1974.

McElvenny RT: Congenital pseudo-arthrosis of the tibia, *Q Bull Northwestern Univ Med School* 23:413, 1949.

McFarland B: Pseudarthrosis of the tibia in childhood, *J Bone Joint Surg* 33B:36, 1951.

Minami A, Ogino T, Sakuma T, et al: Free vascularized fibular grafts in the treatment of congenital pseudarthrosis of the tibia, *Microsurgery* 8:111, 1987.

Mooney JF III, Moore R, Sekiya J, Koman LA: Congenital pseudarthrosis of the tibia treated with a free vascularized fibular graft, *J South Orthop Assoc* 6:227, 1997.

Morrissy RT: Congenital pseudarthrosis of the tibia: factors that affect results, *Clin Orthop* 166:21, 1982.

Morrissy RT, Riseborough EJ, Hall JE: Congenital pseudarthrosis of the tibia, *J Bone Joint Surg* 63B:367, 1981.

Murray HH, Lovell WW: Congenital pseudarthrosis of the tibia: a long-term follow-up study, *Clin Orthop* 166:14, 1982.

Paley D, Catagni M, Arganani F, et al: Treatment of congenital pseudarthrosis of the tibia using the Ilizarov technique, *Clin Orthop* 280:81, 1992.

Paterson D: Treatment of nonunion with a constant direct current: a totally implantable system, *Orthop Clin North Am* 15:47, 1984.

Paterson DC, Simonis RB: Electrical stimulation in the treatment of congenital pseudarthrosis of the tibia, *J Bone Joint Surg* 67B:454, 1985.

Pho RW, Levack B, Satku K, et al: Free vascularized fibular graft in the treatment of congenital pseudarthrosis of the tibia, *J Bone Joint Surg* 67B:64, 1985.

Purvis GD, Holder JE: Dual bone graft for congenital pseudarthrosis of the tibia: variations of technic, *South Med J* 53:926, 1960.

Rathgeb JM, Ramsey PL, Cowell HR: Congenital kyphoscoliosis of the tibia, *Clin Orthop* 103:178, 1974.

Sharrard WJW: Treatment of congenital and infantile pseudarthrosis of the tibia with pulsing electromagnetic fields, *Orthop Clin North Am* 15:143, 1984.

Simonis RB, Shirali HR, Mayou B: Free vascularized fibular grafts for congenital pseudarthrosis of the tibia, *J Bone Joint Surg* 73B:211, 1991.

Sofield HA: Congenital pseudarthrosis of the tibia, *Clin Orthop* 76:33, 1971.

Sofield HA, Millar EA: Fragmentation realignment and intramedullary rod fixation of deformities of the long bones in children: a ten-year appraisal, *J Bone Joint Surg* 41A:1371, 1959.

Traub JA, O'Connor W, Masso PD: Congenital pseudarthrosis of the tibia: a retrospective review, *J Pediatr Orthop* 19:735, 1999.

Uchida Y, Kojima T, Sugioka Y: Vascularized fibular graft for congenital pseudarthrosis of the tibia: long-term results, *J Bone Joint Surg* 73B:846, 1991.

Umber JS, Moss SW, Coleman SS: Surgical treatment of congenital pseudarthrosis of the tibia, *Clin Orthop* 166:28, 1982.

Weiland AJ: Elective microsurgery for orthopaedic reconstruction. III. Vascularized bone transfers, *Instr Course Lect* 33:446, 1984.

Weiland AJ, Weiss AP, Moore JR, Tolo VT: Vascularized fibular grafts in the treatment of congenital pseudarthrosis of the tibia, *J Bone Joint Surg* 72A:654, 1990.

CONSTRICTIONS OF LEG

Askins G, Ger E: Congenital constriction band syndrome, *J Pediatr Orthop* 8:461, 1988.

Bourne MH, Klassen RA: Congenital annular constricting bands: review of the literature and a case report, *J Pediatr Orthop* 7:218, 1987.

Cozen L, Brockway A: Z-plasty procedure for release of constriction rings. In *Operative orthopedic clinics*, Philadelphia, 1955, JB Lippincott.

Greene WB: One-stage release of congenital circumferential constriction bands, *J Bone Joint Surg* 75A:650, 1993.

Hennigan SP, Kuo KN: Resistant talipes equinovarus associated with congenital constriction band syndrome, *J Pediatr Orthop* 20:240, 2000.

Peet EW: Congenital constriction bands. In Rob C, Smith R, eds: *Operative surgery*, part 10, Philadelphia, 1959, FA Davis.

Sarnat BG, Kagan BM: Prenatal constricting band and pseudoarthrosis of the lower leg, *Plast Reconstr Surg* 47:547, 1971.

Upton J, Tan C: Correction of constriction rings, *J Hand Surg* 16A:947, 1991.

CONGENITAL HYPEREXTENSION AND DISLOCATION OF KNEE

Bell MJ, Atkins RM, Sharrard WJW: Irreducible congenital dislocation of the knee: aetiology and management, *J Bone Joint Surg* 69B:403, 1987.

Bensahel H, Dal Monte A, Hjelmstedt A, et al: Congenital dislocation of the knee, *J Pediatr Orthop* 9:174, 1989.

Curtis BH, Fisher RL: Congenital hyperextension with anterior subluxation of the knee: surgical treatment and long-term observations, *J Bone Joint Surg* 51A:255, 1969.

Eilert RE: Dysplasia of the patellofemoral joint in children, *Am J Knee Surg* 12:114, 1999.

Ferris B, Aichroth P: The treatment of congenital knee dislocation: a review of nineteen knees, *Clin Orthop* 216:136, 1987.

Johnson E, Audell R, Oppenheim WL: Congenital dislocation of the knee, *J Pediatr Orthop* 7:194, 1987.

Katz MP, Grogono BJ, Soper KC: The etiology and treatment of congenital dislocation of the knee, *J Bone Joint Surg* 49B:112, 1967.

Ko JY, Shih CH, Wenger DR: Congenital dislocation of the knee, *J Pediatr Orthop* 19:252, 1999.

Lenke LG, Schoenecker PL, Gilula LA: Imaging rounds no 105, *Orthop Rev* 20:295, 1991.

Muhammad KS, Koman LA, Mooney JF III, Smith BP: Congenital dislocation of the knee: overview of management options, *J South Orthop Assoc* 8:93, 1999.

Niebauer JJ, King DE: Congenital dislocation of the knee, *J Bone Joint Surg* 42A:207, 1960.

Nogi J, MacEwen GD: Congenital dislocation of the knee, *J Pediatr Orthop* 2:509, 1982.

Roach JW, Richards BS: Instructional case: congenital dislocation of the knee, *J Pediatr Orthop* 8:226, 1988.

CONGENITAL DISLOCATION OF PATELLA

Eilert RE: Congenital dislocation of the patella, *Clin Orthop* 389:22, 2001.

Gao GX, Lee EH, Bose K: Surgical management of congenital and habitual dislocation of the patella, *J Pediatr Orthop* 10:255, 1990.

Ghanem I, Wattincourt L, Sering R: Congenital dislocation of the patella. I. Pathologic anatomy, *J Pediatr Orthop* 20:812, 2000.

Ghanem I, Wattincourt L, Sering R: Congenital dislocation of the patella. II. Orthopaedic management, *J Pediatr Orthop* 20:817, 2000.

Gordon JE, Schoenecker PL: Surgical treatment of congenital dislocation of the patella, *J Pediatr Orthop* 19:260, 1999.

Green JP, Waugh W: Congenital lateral dislocation of the patella, *J Bone Joint Surg* 50B:285, 1968.

Langenskiöld A, Ritsilä V: Congenital dislocation of the patella and its operative treatment, *J Pediatr Orthop* 12:315, 1992.

Lenke LG, Schoenecker PL, Gilula LA: Imaging rounds no 104, *Orthop Rev* 19:919, 1990.

McCall RE, Lessenberry HB: Case report: bilateral congenital dislocation of the patella, *J Pediatr Orthop* 7:100, 1987.

Stanisavljevic S, Zemenick G, Miller D: Congenital, irreducible, permanent lateral dislocation of the patella, *Clin Orthop* 116:190, 1975.

CONGENITAL LONG BONE DEFICIENCIES
General

Aitken GT: Amputation as a treatment for certain lower-extremity congenital anomalies, *J Bone Joint Surg* 41A:1267, 1959.

Day HJB: Nomenclature and classification in congenital limb deficiency. In Murdoch G, Donovan RG, eds: *Amputation surgery and lower limb prosthesis*, Oxford, England, 1988, Blackwell.

Frantz CH, O'Rahilly R: Congenital skeletal limb deficiencies, *J Bone Joint Surg* 43A:1202, 1961.

Herzenberg JE: Congenital limb deficiency and limb length discrepancy. In Canale ST, Beaty JH, eds: *Operative pediatric orthopaedics*, St Louis, 1992, Mosby.

Kalter H: Case reports of malformations associated with maternal diabetes: history and critique, *Clin Genet* 43:174, 1993.

Lenz W: Genetics and limb deficiencies, *Clin Orthop* 148:9, 1980.

O'Rahilly R: Morphological patterns in limb deficiencies and duplications, *Am J Anat* 89:135, 1951.

Swanson AB: A classification for congenital limb malformations, *J Hand Surg* 1:8, 1976.

Swanson, AB.: A classification for congenital limb malformations of the hand, *NJ Bull Acad Med* 10:166, 1964.

Tibial Hemimelia

Aitken GT: Amputation as a treatment for certain lower-extremity congenital anomalies, *J Bone Joint Surg* 41A:1267, 1959.

Aitken GT: Tibial hemimelia. A symposium on selected lower limb anomalies: surgical and prosthetic management, Washington, DC, 1971, National Academy of Sciences.

Aitken GT: The child amputee: an overview, *Orthop Clin North Am* 3:447, 1972.

Aitken GT: Congenital lower limb deficiencies, *Instr Course Lect* 24:81, 1975.

Bose K: Congenital diastasis of the inferior tibiofibular joint: report of a case, *J Bone Joint Surg* 58A:886, 1976.

Brown FW: Construction of a knee joint in congenital total absence of the tibia (paraxial hemimelia tibia): a preliminary report, *J Bone Joint Surg* 47A:695, 1965.

Brown FW, Pohnert WH: Construction of a knee joint in meromelia tibia (congenital absence of the tibia): a fifteen-year follow-up study, *J Bone Joint Surg* 54A:1333, 1972.

Christini P, Levy EJ, Facanha FA, et al: Fibular transfer for congenital absence of the tibia, *J Pediatr Orthop* 13:378, 1993.

de Sanctis N, Razzano E, Scognamiglio R, et al: Tibial agenesis: a new rationale in management of type II—report of three cases with long-term follow-up, *J Pediatr Orthop* 10:198, 1990.

Epps CH Jr, Tooms RE, Edholm CD, et al: Failure of centralization of the fibula for congenital longitudinal deficiency of the tibia, *J Bone Joint Surg* 73A:858, 1991.

Fernandez-Palazzi F, Bendahan J, Rivas S: Congenital deficiency of the tibia: a report on 22 cases, *J Pediatr Orthop* 7:298, 1998.

Garbarino JL, Clancy M, Harcke HT, et al: Congenital diastasis of the inferior tibiofibular joint: a review of the literature and report of two cases, *J Pediatr Orthop* 5:573, 1985.

Grissom LE, Harcke HT, Kumar SJ: Sonography in the management of tibial hemimelia, *Clin Orthop* 1:266, 1990.

Herring JA, Lloyd-Roberts G: Instructional case: management of tibial dysplasia, *J Pediatr Orthop* 1:339, 1981.

Igou RA Jr, Kruger LM: Fibula dimelia in association with ipsilateral proximal focal femoral deficiency, tibial deficiency, and polydactyly: a case report, *Clin Orthop* 258:237, 1990.

Jayakumar SS, Eilert RE: Fibular transfer for congenital absence of the tibia, *Clin Orthop* 139:97, 1979.

Jones E, Barnes J, Lloyd-Roberts GC: Congenital aplasia and dysplasia of the tibia with intact fibula: classification and management, *J Bone Joint Surg* 60B:31, 1978.

Kalamchi A, Dawe RV: Congenital deficiency of the tibia, *J Bone Joint Surg* 67B:581, 1985.

Kumar A, Kruger LM: Fibular dimelia with deficiency of the tibia, *J Pediatr Orthop* 13:203, 1993.

Lamb DW, Wynne-Davies R, Whitmore JM: Five-fingered hand associated with partial or complete tibial absence and pre-axial polydactyly: a kindred of 15 affected individuals in five generations, *J Bone Joint Surg* 65B:60, 1983.

Loder RT, Herring JA: Fibular transfer for congenital absence of the tibia: a reassessment, *J Pediatr Orthop* 7:8, 1987.

Miller LS, Armstrong PF: The morbid anatomy of congenital deficiency of the tibia and its relevance to treatment, *Foot Ankle* 3:396, 1992.

Otto AW: *Monstorum sexeentorum descripto anatomica sumptibus*, Breslau, 1841, Ferdinandi Hirt.

Putti V: Operative lengthening of the femur, *Surg Gynecol Obstet* 58:318, 1934.

Schoenecker PL, Capelli AM, Millar EA, et al: Congenital longitudinal deficiency of the tibia, *J Bone Joint Surg* 71A:278, 1989.

Simmons ED, Ginsburg GM, Hall JE: Brown's procedure for congenital absence of the tibia revisited, *J Pediatr Orthop* 16:85, 1996.

Sweet HO, Lane PW: X-linked polydactyly (Xpl): a new mutation in the mouse, *J Hered* 71:207, 1980.

Williams L, Wientroub S, Getty CJ, et al: Tibial dysplasia: a study of the anatomy, *J Bone Joint Surg* 65B:157, 1983.

Fibular Hemimelia

Achterman C, Kalamchi A: Congenital deficiency of the fibula, *J Bone Joint Surg* 61B:133, 1979.

Aldegheri R: Distraction osteogenesis for lengthening of the tibia in patients who have limb-length discrepancy or short stature, *J Bone Joint Surg* 81A:624, 1999.

Anderson L, Westin GW, Oppenheim WL: Syme amputation in children: indications, results, and long-term follow-up, *J Pediatr Orthop* 4:550, 1984.

Boakes JL, Stevens PM, Moseley RF: Treatment of genu valgus deformity in congenital absence of the fibula, *J Pediatr Orthop* 1:721, 1991.

Catagni MA: Management of fibular hemimelia using the Ilizarov method, *Instr Course Lect* 41:431, 1992.

Catagni MA, Bolano L, Cattaneo R: Management of fibular hemimelia using the Ilizarov method, *Orthop Clin North Am* 2:715, 1991.

Choi IH, Kumar SJ, Bowen JR: Amputation or limb-lengthening for partial or total absence of the fibula, *J Bone Joint Surg* 72A:1391, 1990.

Choi IH, Lipton GE, Mackenzie W, et al: Wedge-shaped distal tibial epiphysis in the pathogenesis of equinovalgus deformity of the foot and ankle in tibial lengthening for fibular hemimelia, *J Pediatr Orthop* 20:428, 2000.

Coventry MB, Johnson EW Jr: Congenital absence of the fibula, *J Bone Joint Surg* 34A:941, 1952.

Epps EH, Schneider PL: Treatment of hemimelias of the lower extremity, *J Bone Joint Surg* 71A:2, 1989.

Fulp T, Davids JR, Meyer LC, et al: Longitudinal deficiency of the fibula: operative treatment, *J Bone Joint Surg* 78A:674, 1996.

Herring JA: Symes amputation for fibular hemimelia: a second look in the Ilizarov era, *Instr Course Lect* 41:435, 1992.

Hootnick D, Boyd NA, Fixsen JA, Lloyd-Roberts GC: The natural history and management of congenital short tibia with dysplasia or absence of the fibula: a preliminary report, *J Bone Joint Surg* 59B:267, 1977.

Kawamura B, Hosono S, Takahashi T, et al: Limb lengthening by means of subcutaneous osteotomy, *J Bone Joint Surg* 50A:851, 1968.

Kruger LM: Recent advances in surgery of lower limb deficiencies, *Clin Orthop* 148:97, 1980.

Kruger LM, Talbott RD: Amputation and prosthesis as definitive treatment in congenital absence of the fibula, *J Bone Joint Surg* 43A: 625, 1961.

Kumar A, Kruger LM: Fibular dimelia with deficiency of the tibia, *J Pediatr Orthop* 13:203, 1993.

McCarthy JJ, Glancy CL, Chang FM, Eilert RE: Fibular hemimelia: comparison of outcome measurements after amputation and lengthening, *J Bone Joint Surg* 82A:1732, 2000.

Miller LS, Bell DF: Management of congenital fibular deficiency by Ilizarov technique, *J Pediatr Orthop* 12:651, 1991.

Naudie D, Hamdy RC, Fassier F, et al: Management of fibular hemimelia: amputation or limb lengthening, *J Bone Joint Surg* 79B:1040, 1997.

Pappas AM, Hanawalt BJ, Anderson M: Congenital defects of the fibula, *Orthop Clin North Am* 3:187, 1972.

Roux MO, Carlioz H: Clinical examination and investigation of the cruciate ligaments in children with fibular hemimelia, *J Pediatr Orthop* 19:247, 1999.

Serafin J: A new operation for congenital absence of the fibula: preliminary report, *J Bone Joint Surg* 49B: 59, 1967.

Sharma M, MacKenzie WG, Bowen JR: Severe tibial growth retardation in total fibular hemimelia after limb lengthening, *J Pediatr Orthop* 16:438, 1996.

Shatilov OE, Rozkov AV, Cheminova TV: Reconstructive surgery for fibular deficiency, *Prosthet Orthot Int* 15:137, 1991.

Thomas IH, Williams PF: The Gruca operation for congenital absence of the fibula, *J Bone Joint Surg* 69B:587, 1987.

Wiltse LL: Valgus deformity of the ankle: a sequel to acquired or congenital abnormalities of the fibula, *J Bone Joint Surg* 54A:595, 1972.

Proximal Femoral Focal Deficiency

Aitken GT: Proximal femoral focal deficiency: definition, classification, and management. In Aitken GT, ed: *Proximal femoral focal deficiency: a congenital anomaly*, Washington, DC, 1969, National Academy of Sciences.

Aitken GT: Congenital short femur with fibular hemimelia, *J Bone Joint Surg* 56A:1306, 1974.

Alman BA, Krajbich JI, Hubbard S: Proximal femoral focal deficiency: results of rotationplasty and Syme amputation, *J Bone Joint Surg* 77A:1876, 1995.

Amstutz HC, Wilson PD Jr: Dysgenesis of the proximal femur (coxa vara) and its surgical management, *J Bone Joint Surg* 44A:1, 1962.

Borggreve J: *Arch Orthop Chir* 28:175, 1930. (Cited in van Nes CP: Rotation-plasty for congenital defects of the femur, making use of the ankle of the shortened limb to control the knee joint of a prosthesis, *J Bone Joint Surg* 32B:12, 1950.)

Bowen JR, Kumar SJ, Orellana CA, et al: Factors leading to hip subluxation and dislocation in femoral lengthening of unilateral congenital short femur, *J Pediatr Orthop* 21:354, 2001.

Bryant DD III, Epps CH Jr: Proximal femoral focal deficiency: evaluation and management, *Orthopedics* 14:775, 1991.

Camera G, Dodero D, Parodi M, et al: Antenatal ultrasonographic diagnosis of a proximal femoral focal deficiency, *J Clin Ultrasound* 21:475, 1993.

Christini D, Levy EJ, Facanha FA, Kumar SJ: Fibular transfer for congenital absence of the tibia, *J Pediatr Orthop* 13:378, 1993.

Court C, Carlioz H: Radiological study of severe proximal femoral focal deficiency, *J Pediatr Orthop* 17:520, 1997.

Epps HE: Current concepts review: proximal femoral focal deficiency, *J Bone Joint Surg* 65A:867, 1983.

Fixsen JA, Lloyd-Roberts GC: The natural history and early treatment of proximal femoral dysplasia, *J Bone Joint Surg* 56B:86, 1974.

Fowler EG, Hester DM, Oppenheim WL, et al: Contrasts in gait mechanics of individuals with proximal femoral focal deficiency: Syme amputation versus Van Nes rotational osteotomy, *J Pediatr Orthop* 19:720, 1999.

Fowler E, Zernicke R, Setoguchi Y, Oppenheim W: Energy expenditure during walking by children who have proximal femoral focal deficiency, *J Bone Joint Surg* 78A:1857, 1996.

Gillespie R: Principles of amputation surgery in children with longitudinal deficiencies of the femur, *Clin Orthop* 256:29, 1990.

Gillespie R, Torode IP: Classification and management of congenital abnormalities of the femur, *J Bone Joint Surg* 65B:557, 1983.

Goddard NJ, Hashemi-Nejad A, Fixsen JA: Natural history and treatment of instability of the hip in proximal femoral focal deficiency, *J Pediatr Orthop* 4:145, 1995.

Grogan DP, Holt GR, Ogden JA: Talocalcaneal coalition in patients who have fibular hemimelia or proximal femoral focal deficiency: a comparison of radiographic and pathological findings, *J Bone Joint Surg* 76A:1363, 1994.

Hamal J, Winkelmann W, Becker W: A new modification of rotationplasty in a patient with proximal femoral focal deficiency Pappas type II, *J Pediatr Orthop B* 8:200, 1999.

Hamanishi C: Congenital short femur: clinical, genetic, and epidemiological comparison of the naturally occurring condition with that caused by thalidomide, *J Bone Joint Surg* 62B:307, 1980.

Hillmann A, Rosenbaum D, Schröter J, et al: Electromyographic and gait analysis of forty-three patients after rotationplasty, *J Bone Joint Surg* 82A:187, 2000.

Johansson E, Aparisi T: Missing cruciate ligament in congenital short femur, *J Bone Joint Surg* 65A:1109, 1983.

Johnson CE: Congenital short femur with coxa vara, *Orthopedics* 6:892, 1983.

Kalamchi A, Lowell HI, Kim KI: Congenital deficiency of the femur, *J Pediatr Orthop* 5:129, 1985.

King RE: Some concepts of proximal femoral focal deficiency. In Aitken GT, ed: *Proximal femoral focal deficiency: a symposium*, Washington, DC, 1969, National Academy of Sciences.

Koman LA, Meyer LC, Warren FH: Proximal femoral focal deficiency: a 50-year experience, *Dev Med Child Neurol* 24:344, 1982.

Kostuik JP, Gillespie R, Hall JE, Hubbard S: Van Nes rotational osteotomy for treatment of proximal femoral focal deficiency and congenital short femur, *J Bone Joint Surg* 57A:1039, 1975.

Kritter AE: Tibial rotation-plasty for proximal femoral focal deficiency, *J Bone Joint Surg* 59A:927, 1977.

Kruger LM, Stone PA: Suction-assisted lipectomy—an adjunct to orthopaedic treatment, *J Pediatr Orthop* 10:53, 1990.

Lange DR, Schoenecker PL, Baker CL: Proximal femoral focal deficiency: treatment and classification in forty-two cases, *Clin Orthop* 135:15, 1978.

Loder RT, Herring JA: Disarticulation of the knee in children: a functional assessment, *J Bone Joint Surg* 69A:1155, 1987.

Mowery CA, Herring JA, Jackson D: Dislocated patella associated with below-knee amputation in adolescent patients, *J Pediatr Orthop* 6:299, 1986.

Pappas AM: Congenital abnormalities of the femur and related lower-extremity malformations: classifications and treatment, *J Pediatr Orthop* 3:45, 1983.

Pirani S, Beauchamp RD, Li D, et al: Soft tissue anatomy of proximal femoral focal deficiency, *J Pediatr Orthop* 11:563, 1991.

Sanpera I Jr, Sparks LT: Proximal femoral focal deficiency: does a radiologic classification exist? *J Pediatr Orthop* 14:34, 1994.

Steel HH, Lin PS, Betz RR, et al: Iliofemoral fusion for proximal femoral focal deficiency, *J Bone Joint Surg* 69A:837, 1987.

Torode IP, Gillespie R: Rotationplasty of the lower limb for congenital defects of the femur, *J Bone Joint Surg* 65B:569, 1983.

Torode IP, Gillespie R: The classification and treatment of proximal femoral deficiencies, *Prosthet Orthot Int* 15:117, 1991.

Van Nes CP: Rotation-plasty for congenital defects of the femur, making use of the ankle of the shortened limb to control the knee joint of a prosthesis, *J Bone Joint Surg* 32B:12, 1950.

Westin GW, Gunderson FO: Proximal femoral focal deficiency: a review of treatment experiences. In Aitken GT, ed: *Proximal femoral focal deficiency: a congenital anomaly*, Washington, DC, 1969, National Academy of Sciences.

LIMB-LENGTH DISCREPANCY

Aaron AD, Eilert RE: Results of the Wagner and Ilizarov methods of limb lengthening, *J Bone Joint Surg* 78A:20, 1996.

Aaron A, Weinstein D, Thickman D, et al: Comparison of orthoroentgenography and computed tomography in the measurement of limb-length discrepancy, *J Bone Joint Surg* 74A:897, 1992.

Aldegheri R, Giampaolo T, Lavini F: Epiphyseal distraction: chondrodiastasis, *Clin Orthop* 241:117, 1989.

Aldegheri R, Giampaolo T, Lavini F: Epiphyseal distraction: hemichondrodiastasis, *Clin Orthop* 241:128, 1989.

Aldegheri R, Renzi-Brivio L, Agostini S: The callotasis method of limb lengthening, *Clin Orthop* 241:137, 1989.

Aldegheri R, Trivella G, Renzi-Brivio L, et al: Lengthening of the lower limbs in achondroplastic patients: a comparative study of four techniques, *J Bone Joint Surg* 70B:69, 1988.

Anderson M, Green WT, Messner MB: Growth and predictions of growth in the lower extremities, *J Bone Joint Surg* 45A:1, 1963.

Aronson J, Harrison BH, Stewart CL, Harp JH: The histology of distraction osteogenesis using different external fixators, *Clin Orthop* 241:106, 1989.

Aronson J, Harrison B, Boyd CM, et al: Mechanical induction of osteogenesis: the importance of pin rigidity, *J Pediatr Orthop* 8:396, 1988.

Bayley N, Pinneau SR: Tables for predicting adult height from skeletal age: revised for use with the Gruelich-Pyle hand standards, *J Pediatr* 49:423, 1952.

Beals RK: Hemihypertrophy and hemihypotrophy, *Clin Orthop* 166: 199, 1982.

Bell DF, Boyer MI, Armstrong PF: The use of the Ilizarov technique in the correction of limb deformities associated with skeletal dysplasia, *J Pediatr Orthop* 12:283, 1992.

Bjerkreim I: Limb lengthening by physeal distraction, *Acta Orthop Scand* 60:140, 1989.

Blair VP III, Walker ST, Sheridan JJ, Schoenecker PL: Epiphysiodesis: a problem of timing, *J Pediatr Orthop* 2:281, 1982.

Blane CE, Herzenberg JE, DiPietro MA: Radiographic imaging for Ilizarov limb lengthening in children, *Pediatr Radiol* 21:117, 1991.

Blount WP: A mature look at epiphyseal stapling, *Clin Orthop* 77:158, 1971.

Bonnard C, Favard L, Sollogoub I, et al: Limb lengthening in children using the Ilizarov method, *Clin Orthop* 293:83, 1993.

Bowen JR, Johnson WJ: Percutaneous epiphysiodesis, *Clin Orthop* 190:170, 1984.

Bowen JR, Levy EJ, Donohue M: Comparison of knee motion and callus formation in femoral lengthening with the Wagner or monolateral-ring device, *J Pediatr Orthop* 13:467, 1993.

Broughton NS, Olney BW, Menelaus MB: Tibial shortening for leg length discrepancy, *J Bone Joint Surg* 71B:242, 1989.

Canale ST, Christian CA: Techniques for epiphysiodesis about the knee, *Clin Orthop* 255:81, 1990.

Canale ST, Russell TA, Holcomb RL: Percutaneous epiphysiodesis: experimental study and preliminary clinical results, *J Pediatr Orthop* 6:150, 1986.

Carey RP, de Campo JF, Menelaus MB: Measurement of leg length by computerized tomographic scanography: brief report, *J Bone Joint Surg* 69B: 846, 1987.

Caton J: Leg lengthening with the Ilizarov technique: analysis and results of a multicenter study, *Rev Chir Orthop* 73(suppl 2):23, 1987.

Cattaneo R, Villa A, Catagni M, et al: Limb lengthening in achondroplasia by Ilizarov's method, *Int Orthop* 12:173, 1988.

Cattaneo R, Villa A, Catagni MA, et al: Lengthening of the humerus using the Ilizarov technique: description of the method and report of 43 cases, *Clin Orthop* 250:117, 1990.

Coglianese DB, Herzenberg JE, Goulet JA: Physical therapy management of patients undergoing limb lengthening by distraction osteogenesis, *J Orthop Sports Phys Ther* 17:124, 1993.

Coleman SS, Stevens PM: Tibial lengthening, *Clin Orthop* 136:92, 1978.

Dahl MT, Fischer DA: Lower extremity lengthening by Wagner's method and by callus distraction, *Orthop Clin North Am* 22:643, 1991.

Dal Monte A, Andrisano A, Manfrini M, Zucchi M: Humeral lengthening in hypoplasia of the upper limb, *J Pediatr Orthop* 5:202, 1985.

Dal Monte A, Donzelli O: Tibial lengthening according to Ilizarov in congenital hypoplasia of the leg, *J Pediatr Orthop* 7:135, 1987.

Dal Monte A, Donzelli O: Comparison of different methods of leg lengthening, *J Pediatr Orthop* 8:62, 1988.

DeBastiani G, Aldegheri R, Renzi-Brivio L, Trivella G: Limb lengthening by distraction of the epiphyseal plate: a comparison of two techniques in the rabbit, *J Bone Joint Surg* 68B:550, 1986.

DeBastiani G, Aldegheri R, Renzi-Brivio L, Trivella G: Limb lengthening by callus distraction (callotasis), *J Pediatr Orthop* 7:129, 1987.

Dewaele J, Fabry G: The timing of epiphysiodesis: a comparative study between the use of the method of Anderson and Green and the Moseley chart, *Acta Orthop Belg* 58:43, 1992.

Eldridge JC, Armstrong PF, Krajbich JI: Amputation stump lengthening with the Ilizarov technique: a case report, *Clin Orthop* 256:76, 1990.

Ensley NJ, Green NE, Barnes WP: Femoral lengthening with the Barnes device, *J Pediatr Orthop* 13:57, 1993.

Faber FW, Keessen W, van Roermund PM: Complications of leg lengthening: 46 procedures in 28 patients, *Acta Orthop Scand* 62:327, 1991.

Fjeld TO, Steen H: Growth retardation after experimental limb lengthening by epiphyseal distraction, *J Pediatr Orthop* 10:463, 1990.

Fleming B, Paley D, Kristiansen T, Pope M: A biomechanical analysis of the Ilizarov external fixator, *Clin Orthop* 241:95, 1989.

Friberg O: Clinical symptoms and biomechanics of lumbar spine and hip joint leg length inequality, *Spine* 8:643, 1983.

Galardi G, Comi G, Lozza L, et al: Peripheral nerve damage during limb lengthening: neurophysiology in five cases of bilateral tibial lengthening, *J Bone Joint Surg* 72B:121, 1990.

Garcia-Cimbrelo E, Olsen B, Ruiz-Yague M, et al: Ilizarov technique: results and difficulties, *Clin Orthop* 283:116, 1992.

Gil-Albarova J, de Pablos J, Franzeb M, et al: Delayed distraction in bone lengthening: improved healing in lambs, *Acta Orthop Scand* 63:604, 1992.

Giles LGF, Taylor JR: Low back pain associated with leg length inequality, *Spine* 6:510, 1981.

Green SA: Postoperative management during limb lengthening, *Orthop Clin North Am* 22:723, 1991.

Green SA: The Ilizarov method: Rancho technique, *Orthop Clin North Am* 22:677, 1991.

Green WT, Anderson M: Experiences with epiphyseal arrest in correcting discrepancies in length of the lower extremities in infantile paralysis: a method of predicting the effect, *J Bone Joint Surg* 29:659, 1947.

Greulich WW, Pyle SI: *Radiographic atlas of skeletal development of the hand and wrist*, ed 2, Stanford, Calif, 1959, Stanford.

Guarniero R, Barros Junior TE: Femoral lengthening by the Wagner method, *Clin Orthop* 250:154, 1990.

Guidera KJ, Hess WF, Highhouse KP, et al: Extremity lengthening: results and complications with the Orthofix system, *J Pediatr Orthop* 11:90, 1991.

Hamanishi C, Tanaka S, Tamura K: Early physeal closure after femoral chondrodiastasis, loss of length gain in five cases, *Acta Orthop Scand* 63:146, 1992.

Hamanishi C, Yasuwaki Y, Kikuchi H, et al: Classification of the callus in limb lengthening: radiographic study of 35 limbs, *Acta Orthop Scand* 63:430, 1992.

Herring JA, Coleman SS: Femoral lengthening, *J Pediatr Orthop* 2:432, 1982.

Herzenberg JE, Paley D: Leg lengthening in children, *Curr Opin Pediatr* 10:95, 1998.

Herzenberg JE, Waanders NA: Calculating rate and duration of distraction for deformity correction with the Ilizarov technique, *Orthop Clin North Am* 22:601, 1991.

Hood RW, Riseborough EJ: Lengthening of the lower extremity by the Wagner method: a review of the Boston Children's Hospital experience, *J Bone Joint Surg* 63A:1122, 1981.

Hrutkay JM, Eilert RE: Operative lengthening of the lower extremity and associated psychological aspects: the Children's Hospital experience, *J Pediatr Orthop* 10:373, 1990.

Huurman WW, Jacobsen FS, Anderson JC, Chu WK: Limb-length discrepancy measured with computerized axial tomographic equipment, *J Bone Joint Surg* 69A:699, 1987.

Ilizarov GA: The tension-stress effect on the genesis and growth of tissues. I. The influence of stability of fixation and soft tissue preservation, *Clin Orthop* 238:249, 1989.

Ilizarov GA: The tension-stress effect on the genesis and growth of tissues. II. The influence of rate and frequency of distraction, *Clin Orthop* 239:263, 1989.

Janovec M: Short humerus: results of 11 prolongations in 10 children and adolescents, *Arch Orthop Trauma Surg* 111:13, 1991.

Javid M, Shahcheraghi GH, Nooraie H: Ilizarov lengthening in centralized fibula, *J Pediatr Orthop* 20:160, 2000.

Johnston CE II, Bueche MJ, Williamson B, et al: Epiphysiodesis for management of lower limb deformities, *Instr Course Lect* 41:437, 1992.

Jones DC, Moseley CF: Subluxation of the knee as a complication of femoral lengthening by the Wagner technique, *J Bone Joint Surg* 67B:33, 1985.

Karger C, Guille JT, Bowen JR: Lengthening of congenital lower limb deficiencies, *Clin Orthop* 291:236, 1993.

Kawamura B, Hosono S, Takahashi T: The principles and technique of limb lengthening, *Int Orthop* 5:69, 1981.

Kempf I, Grosse A, Abalo C: Locked intramedullary nailing: its application to femoral tibial axial, rotational, lengthening, and shortening osteotomies, *Clin Orthop* 212:165, 1986.

Lamoureux J, Verstreken L: Progressive upper limb lengthening in children: a report of two cases, *J Orthop Pediatr* 6:481, 1986.

Lavini F, Renzi-Brivio L, de Bastiani G: Psychologic, vascular, and physiologic aspects of lower limb lengthening in achondroplastics, *Clin Orthop* 250:138, 1990.

Lee DY, Choi IH, Chung CY, et al: Triple innominate osteotomy for hip stabilisation and transiliac leg lengthening after poliomyelitis, *J Bone Joint Surg* 75B:858, 1993.

Lee DY, Choi IH, Chung CY, et al: A modified Wagner technique for femoral lengthening in skeletally mature patients with poliomyelitis, *Int Orthop* 17:154, 1993.

Lee DY, Choi IH, Chung CY, et al: Effect of tibial lengthening on the gastrocnemius muscle: a histopathologic and morphometric study in rabbits, *Acta Orthop Scand* 64:688, 1993.

Lee DY, Chung CY, Choi IH: Longitudinal growth of the rabbit tibia after callotasis, *J Bone Joint Surg* 75B:898, 1993.

Maffulli N, Pattinson RC, Fixsen JA: Lengthening of congenital limb length discrepancy using callotasis: early experience of the Hospital for Sick Children, *Ann R Coll Surg Engl* 75:105, 1993.

Malhis TM, Bowen JR: Tibial and femoral lengthening: a report of 54 cases, *J Pediatr Orthop* 2:487, 1982.

McCaw ST, Bates BT: Biomechanical implications of mild leg length inequality, *Br J Sports Med* 25:10, 1991.

McManus BF, O'Brien T: Leg lengthening by the transiliac method, *J Bone Joint Surg* 74B:275, 1992.

Menelaus MB: Correction of leg length discrepancy by epiphyseal arrest, *J Bone Joint Surg* 48B:336, 1966.

Métaizeau JP, Wong-Chung J, Bertrand H, Pasquier P: Percutaneous epiphysiodesis using transphyseal screws (PETS), *J Pediatr Orthop* 18:363, 1998.

Millis MB, Hall JE: Transiliac lengthening of the lower extremity: a modified innominate osteotomy for the treatment of postural imbalance, *J Bone Joint Surg* 61A:1182, 1979.

Monticelli G, Spinelli R: Distraction epiphysiolysis as a method of limb lengthening. I. Experimental study, *Clin Orthop* 154:254, 1981.

Monticelli G, Spinelli R: Distraction epiphysiolysis as a method of limb lengthening. III. Clinical applications, *Clin Orthop* 154:274, 1981.

Monticelli G, Spinelli R, Bonucci EL: Distraction epiphysiolysis as a method of limb lengthening. II. Morphologic investigations, *Clin Orthop* 154:262, 1981.

Moseley CF: A straight line graph of leg length discrepancies, *J Bone Joint Surg* 59A:174, 1977.

Moseley CF: A straight line graph for leg length discrepancies, *Clin Orthop* 126:33, 1978.

Moseley CF: Leg length discrepancy, *Orthop Clin North Am* 18:529, 1987.

Murray DW, Kambouroglou G, Kenwright J: One-stage lengthening for femoral shortening with associated deformity, *J Bone Joint Surg* 75B:566, 1993.

Nakamura E, Mizuta H, Sei A, et al: Knee articular cartilage injury in leg lengthening: histological studies in rabbits, *Acta Orthop Scand* 64:437, 1993.

Ogilvie JW: Epiphysiodesis: evaluation of a new technique, *J Pediatr Orthop* 6:147, 1986.

Osterman K, Merikanto J: Diaphyseal bone lengthening in children using Wagner device: long-term results, *J Pediatr Orthop* 11:449, 1991.

Paley D: Current techniques of limb lengthening, *J Pediatr Orthop* 8:73, 1988.

Paley D: Problems, obstacles and complications of limb lengthening by the Ilizarov technique, *Clin Orthop* 250:81, 1990.

Paley D, Bhave A, Herzenberg JE, Bowen JR: Multiplier method for predicting limb-length discrepancy, *J Bone Joint Surg* 82A:1432, 2000.

Paley D, Fleming BS, Catagni M, et al: Mechanical evaluation of external fixators used in limb lengthening, *Clin Orthop* 250:50, 1990.

Papaioannou T, Stokes I, Kenwright J: Scoliosis associated with limb-length inequality, *J Bone Joint Surg* 64A: 59, 1982.

Phemister DB: Operative arrestment of longitudinal growth of bones in the treatment of deformities, *J Bone Joint Surg* 15:1, 1933.

Porat S, Peyser A, Robin GC: Equalization of lower limbs by epiphysiodesis: results of treatment, *J Pediatr Orthop* 11:442, 1991.

Price CT: Metaphyseal and physeal lengthening, *Instr Course Lect* 38:331, 1989.

Price CT, Cole JD: Limb lengthening by callostasis for children and adolescents: early experience, *Clin Orthop* 250:105, 1990.

Pritchett JW: Lengthening the ulna in patients with hereditary multiple exostoses, *J Bone Joint Surg* 68A:561, 1986.

Putti V: Operative lengthening of the femur, *JAMA* 77:934, 1921.

Rainey RK: Operative femoral shortening by closed intramedullary technique, *Orthop Rev* 8:36, 1984.

Renzi-Brivio L, Lavini F, De Bastiani G: Lengthening in the congenital short femur, *Clin Orthop* 250:112, 1990.

Sabharwal S, Paley D, Bhave A, Herzenberg J: Growth patterns after lengthening of congenitally short lower limbs in young children, *J Pediatr Orthop* 20:137, 2000.

Saleh M, Milne A: Weight-bearing parallel-beam scanography for the measurement of leg length and joint alignment, *J Bone Joint Surg* 76B:156, 1994.

Salter RB: Innominate osteotomy in the treatment of congenital dislocation and subluxation of the hip, *J Bone Joint Surg* 43B:518, 1961.

Shapiro F: Developmental patterns in lower-extremity length discrepancies, *J Bone Joint Surg* 69A:684, 1987.

Siffert RS: Lower limb-length discrepancy, *J Bone Joint Surg* 68A:1101, 1987.

Stanitski DF: Limb-length inequality: assessment and treatment options, *J Am Acad Orthop Surg* 7:143, 1999.

Stephens DC: Femoral and tibial lengthening, *J Pediatr Orthop* 3:424, 1983.

Stevens PM, Arms D: Postaxial hypoplasia of the lower extremity, *J Pediatr Orthop* 20:166, 2000.

Tjernstrom B, Thoumas KA, Pech P: Bone remodeling after leg lengthening: evaluation with plain radiographs and computed tomography and magnetic resonance imaging scans, *J Pediatr Orthop* 12:751, 1992.

Velazquez RJ, Bell DF, Armstrong PF, et al: Complications of use of the Ilizarov technique in the correction of limb deformities in children, *J Bone Joint Surg* 75A:1148, 1993.

Villa A, Paley D, Catagni MA, et al: Lengthening of the forearm by the Ilizarov technique, *Clin Orthop* 250:125, 1990.

Wagner H: Operative lengthening of the femur, *Clin Orthop* 136:125, 1978.

Walker CW, Aronson J, Kaplan PA, et al: Radiologic evaluation of limb-lengthening procedures, *Am J Roentgenol* 156:353, 1992.

Westh RN, Menelaus MB: A simple calculation for the timing of epiphyseal arrest, *J Bone Joint Surg* 63B:117, 1981.

White SH, Kenwright J: The importance of delay in distraction of osteotomies, *Orthop Clin North Am* 22:569, 1991.

Winquist RA: Closed intramedullary osteotomies of the femur, *Clin Orthop* 212:157, 1986.

Winquist RA, Hansen ST Jr, Pearson RE: Closed femoral shortening, *J Bone Joint Surg* 57A:135, 1975.

Yadav SS: Double oblique diaphyseal osteotomy: a new technique for lengthening deformed and short lower limbs, *J Bone Joint Surg* 75B:962, 1993.

Yasui N, Kojimoto H, Shimizu H, et al: The effect of distraction upon bone, muscle, and periosteum, *Orthop Clin North Am* 22:563, 1991.

Young JW, Kostrubiak IS, Resnik CS, et al: Sonographic evaluation of bone production at the distraction site in Ilizarov limb-lengthening procedures, *Am J Roentgenol* 154:125, 1990.

Young NL, Davis RJ, Bell DF, et al: Electromyographic and nerve conduction changes after tibial lengthening by the Ilizarov method, *J Pediatr Orthop* 13:473, 1993.

Yun AG, Severino R, Reinker K: Attempted limb lengthenings beyond twenty percent of the initial bone length: results and complications, *J Pediatr Orthop* 20:151, 2000.

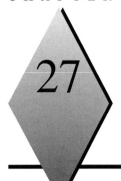

Congenital and Developmental Anomalies of Hip and Pelvis

27

James H. Beaty

Congenital and Developmental Dysplasia of Hip

Congenital dysplasia of the hip generally includes subluxation (partial dislocation) of the femoral head, acetabular dysplasia, and complete dislocation of the femoral head from the true acetabulum. In a newborn with true congenital dislocation of the hip the femoral head can be dislocated and reduced into and out of the true acetabulum. In an older child the femoral head remains dislocated and secondary changes develop in the femoral head and acetabulum.

Historically, the incidence of congenital dysplasia of the hip has been estimated to be approximately 1 in 1000 live births. Lehman et al., however, in a meta-analysis of the literature, estimated the incidence of developmental dysplasia of hip (DDH) revealed by physical examination done by pediatricians to be 8.6 per 1000; for orthopaedic screening, 11.5 per 1000; and for ultrasound examination, 25 per 1000. They also estimated the odds ratio for DDH and breech delivery (5:5), female sex (4:1), and positive family history (1:7). Bialik et al. reported that ultrasound screening of 18,060 hips detected 1001 that deviated from normal (incidence of 55.1 per 1000); however, only 90 hips remained abnormal at repeat examinations at 2 and 6 weeks, for a true DDH incidence of 5 per 1000. None of the other hips with "sonographic DDH" developed true DDH during 12-month follow-up. The left hip is more commonly involved than the right, and bilateral involvement is more common than involvement of the right hip alone.

Several risk factors should arouse suspicion of congenital dysplasia of the hip. The disorder is more common in females than in males, in many series as much as five times more common. Breech deliveries make up approximately 3% to 4% of all deliveries, and the incidence of congenital dysplasia of the hip is significantly increased in this patient population. MacEwen and Ramsey in a study of 25,000 infants found the combination of female infants and breech presentation to result in congenital dysplasia of the hip in 1 out of 35 such births. Congenital dysplasia of the hip is more common in firstborn children than in subsequent siblings. A family history of congenital dysplasia of the hip increases the likelihood of this condition to approximately 10%. Ethnic background plays some role, in that congenital dysplasia of the hip is more common in white children than in black children. Other reported examples include the high incidence among the Navajo Indians and the relatively low incidence among the Chinese. A strong association also exists between congenital dysplasia of the hip and other musculoskeletal abnormalities, such as congenital torticollis, metatarsus adductus, and talipes calcaneovalgus. In a study of 63 children younger than 6 months who had ultrasound scanning of bilateral sternocleido-mastoid muscles and bilateral hips, Tien et al. found the coexistence rate of congenital muscular torticollis and DDH to be 17%; if only those hips that required treatment were included, the rate was decreased to 8.5%. Walsh and Morrissy, in a review of 70 patients with congenital muscular torticollis, concluded that the rate of hip disease in children with torticollis is approximately 8%.

Several theories regarding the cause of congenital dysplasia of the hip have been proposed, including mechanical factors, hormone-induced joint laxity, primary acetabular dysplasia, and genetic inheritance. Breech delivery, with the mechanical forces of abnormal flexion of the hips, can easily be seen as a cause of dislocation of the femoral head. An increased incidence of congenital dysplasia of the hip has been reported in cultures that place infants in swaddling clothes with the hip in constant extension.

Several authors have proposed ligamentous laxity as a contributing factor in congenital dysplasia of the hip. The theory is that the influence of the maternal hormones that produce relaxation of the pelvis during delivery may cause enough ligamentous laxity in the child in utero and during the neonatal period to allow dislocation of the femoral head.

Wynne-Davies described a familial occurrence of a "shallow" acetabulum, defined as a "dysplasia trait," in proposing primary acetabular dysplasia as one of the risk factors for congenital dysplasia of the hip. The risk of a genetic influence was noted by Ortolani, who reported a 70% incidence of a positive family history in children with congenital dysplasia of the hip.

DIAGNOSIS AND CLINICAL PRESENTATION

The clinical presentation of congenital dysplasia of the hip varies according to the age of the child. In newborns (up to 6 months of age) it is especially important to perform a careful clinical examination because roentgenograms are not absolutely reliable in making the diagnosis of congenital dysplasia of the hip in this age group.

Several reports evaluated the use of ultrasound screening of newborns for early diagnosis of congenital dysplasia of the hip. The most comprehensive accounts of the anatomy of the infant hip by ultrasound are by Graf of Austria, who devised an ultrasonographic classification for hip dysplasia. Although ultrasound is noninvasive and relatively simple to use, a number of authors have emphasized that the examination is highly observer dependent and that it is easy to overdiagnose "dysplasia." The concern is that ultrasound diagnosis of dysplasia may result in unnecessary treatment.

Routine clinical screening should include both the Ortolani test and the provocative maneuver of Barlow. The Ortolani test is performed by gently abducting and adducting the flexed hip to detect any reduction into or dislocation of the femoral head from the true acetabulum. The provocative maneuver of Barlow detects any potential subluxation or posterior dislocation of the femoral head by direct pressure on the longitudinal axis of the femur while the hip is in adduction. Both these tests require a relaxed and pacified child (Fig. 27-1). However, a child may be born with acetabular dysplasia without dislocation of the hip, and the latter may develop weeks or months later. Westin et al. reported the late development of dislocation of the hip in children with normal neonatal clinical and roentgenographic examinations; they termed this *developmental dysplasia* as opposed to *congenital dysplasia* of the hip.

As the child reaches the age of 6 to 18 months, several factors in the clinical presentation change. Once the femoral head is dislocated and the ability to reduce it by abduction has disappeared, several other clinical signs become obvious. The first and most reliable is a decrease in the ability to abduct the dislocated hip because of a contracture of the adductor

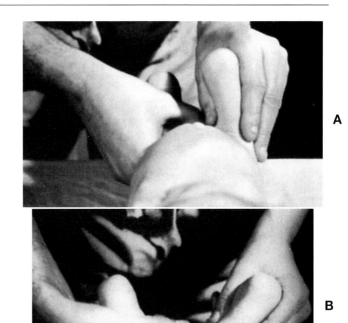

Fig. 27-1 Barlow (**A**) and Ortolani (**B**) maneuvers for routine screening of congenital dislocation of hip. Note that examiner gently stabilizes infant's left hip and lower extremity and places left hand around right thigh and index and middle fingers over greater trochanter.

musculature (Fig. 27-2, *A*). Castelein and Korte, however, found that in a group of 683 infants, limitation of abduction had a sensitivity for diagnosis of hip dysplasia of 69%, a specificity of 54%, a positive predictive value of 43%, and a negative predictive value of 78%. In 226 hips with sonographically proved dysplasia, 70 (31%) had no limitation of abduction, and in 457 hips without dysplasia, 210 (76%) had limited abduction. One hundred and thirty-six hips with limited abduction but normal sonograms were left untreated, and at an average 5-year follow-up all had developed normally. Asymmetrical skin folds (Fig. 27-2, *B*) are commonly mentioned as a sign to look for, but unfortunately this sign is not always reliable because normal children may have asymmetrical skin folds, and children with dislocated hips may have symmetrical folds. Ando and Gotoh, however, examined 2111 patients and found that 499 had abnormal inguinal folds; all patients determined to have complete dislocation or subluxation of the hip were among these 499. They recommended inguinal fold assessment as a useful adjunct to other screening methods for congenital dysplasia of the hip in 3- to 4-month-old infants and suggest that asymmetrical or abnormally long inguinal folds are indications for further evaluation. Omeroglu and Koparal found that the rate of DDH was nearly 16 times higher in hips with at least one abnormal clinical finding than in ones without any. Limitation of abduction and asymmetrical skin folds were the two most common findings.

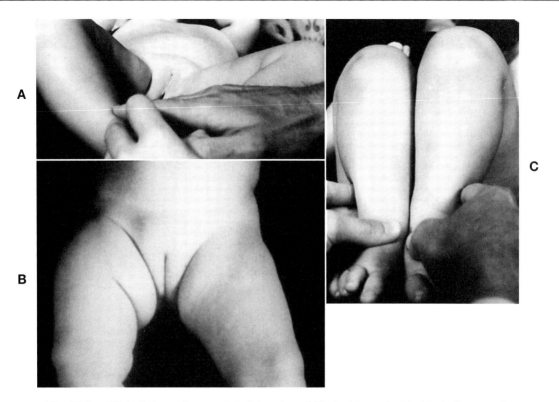

Fig. 27-2 Clinical signs of congenital dislocation of hip in 13-month-old girl. **A,** Decrease in abduction of right hip with adduction contracture. **B,** Asymmetrical skin fold with difference in levels of popliteal and gluteal skin clefts. **C,** Positive Galeazzi sign with apparent shortening of right lower extremity.

The Galeazzi sign is noted when the femoral head becomes displaced not only laterally but also proximally, causing an apparent shortening of the femur on the side of the dislocated hip (Fig. 27-2, *C*). Bilateral dislocations may appear symmetrically abnormal.

In a child of walking age with an undetected dislocated hip, families describe a "waddling" type of gait, indicating dislocation of the femoral head and a Trendelenburg gait pattern. Parents also may describe difficulty in abducting the hip during diaper changes.

Although roentgenograms are not always reliable in making the diagnosis of congenital dysplasia of the hip in newborns, screening roentgenograms may reveal any acetabular dysplasia or a teratological dislocation. As a child with a dislocated hip ages and the soft tissues become contracted, the roentgenograms become more reliable and helpful in the diagnosis and treatment (Fig. 27-3). The most commonly used lines of reference are the vertical line of Perkins and the horizontal line of Hilgenreiner, both used to assess the position of the femoral head. In addition, the Shenton line will be disrupted in an older child with a dislocated hip. Reference lines for the evaluation of the acetabulum include the acetabular index and the center edge (CE) angle of Wiberg. Normally the metaphyseal beak of the proximal femur lies within the inner lower quadrant of the reference lines noted by Perkins and Hilgenreiner. The acetabular index in a newborn generally is 30 degrees or less.

Any significant increase in this measurement may be a sign of acetabular dysplasia.

TREATMENT

The treatment of congenital or developmental dysplasia of the hip is age related and tailored to the specific pathological condition. Five treatment groups related to age have been designated: (1) newborn, birth to 6 months of age, (2) infant, 6 to 18 months of age, (3) toddler, 18 to 36 months of age, (4) child and juvenile, 3 to 8 years of age, and (5) adolescent and young adult, beyond 8 years of age.

Newborn (Birth to 6 Months of Age)

From birth to approximately 6 months of age, treatment is directed at stabilizing the hip that has a positive Ortolani or Barlow test or reducing the dislocated hip with a mild to moderate adduction contracture. A success rate of 85% to 95% has been reported in children treated in the Pavlik harness during the first few months of life. A multicenter study by Grill et al. for the European Paediatric Orthopaedic Society evaluated Pavlik harness treatment of 3611 hips in 2636 patients. They reported reduction rates of 92% overall and 95% in dysplastic hips. Taylor and Clarke, in a 6-year prospective study, reported treatment of DDH in 5.1 of 1000 live births. Of 370 hips identified as abnormal by ultrasound and treated with

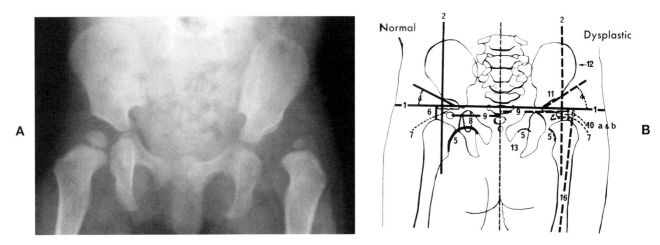

Fig. 27-3   A, Thirteen-month-old child with congenital dislocation of left hip. **B,** Roentgeno-graphic signs of congenital hip dislocation. *1,* Horizontal Y line (Hilgenreiner line). *2,* Vertical line (Perkins line). *3,* Quadrants (formed by lines *1* and *2*). *4,* Acetabular index (Kleinberg and Lieberman). *5,* Shenton line. *6,* Upward displacement of femoral head. *7,* Lateral displacement of femoral head. *8,* U figure of teardrop shadow (Kohler). *9,* Y coordinate (Ponseti). *10,* Capital epiphyseal dysplasia: (*a*) delayed appearance of center of ossification of femoral head, (*b*) irregular maturation of center of ossification. *11,* Bifurcation (furrowing of acetabular roof in late infancy (Ponseti). *12,* Hypoplasia of pelvis (ilium). *13,* Delayed fusion (ischiopubic juncture). *14,* Absence of shapely, defined, well-ossified acetabular margin, caused by delayed ossification of cartilage of roof of socket. *15,* Femoral shaft-neck angle. *16,* Adduction attitude of extremity. *17,* Development of epiphyses of other joints (knee, wrists, and lumbosacral spine). *18,* Radiolucent acetabular roof, limbus, joint capsule (arthrographic studies). (**B** from Hart V: *Congenital dysplasia of the hip joint and sequelae,* Springfield, Ill, 1952, Charles C Thomas.)

the Pavlik harness, 354 (95.7%) were successfully reduced; 16 required surgical treatment. Of those treated with the harness alone, only 1 (0.3%) had signs of mild avascular necrosis. As the child ages and soft tissue contractures develop, along with secondary changes in the acetabulum, the success rate of the Pavlik harness decreases. Attention to detail is required in the use of this harness because the potential complications include avascular necrosis of the femoral head.

When properly applied and maintained, the Pavlik harness is a dynamic flexion abduction orthosis that can produce excellent results in the treatment of dysplastic and dislocated hips in infants approximately 4 to 6 months of age. The harness is difficult to use in children who are crawling or who have soft tissue contractures. Once the diagnosis has been made, either clinically or roentgenographically, it is essential to evaluate carefully the direction of dislocation, the stability, and the reducibility of the hip before treatment. If a teratological dislocation is present, the Pavlik harness should not be used.

To determine whether pretreatment roentgenographic findings predicted treatment outcomes, Brien, Randolph, and Zahiri measured the superior gap (distance between the proximal metaphysis and Hilgenreiner's line) and the medial gap (distance between the femoral calcar and the lateral pelvic wall at that level) on the pretreatment roentgenograms of 67 dislocated hips in 53 infants (average age, 2.7 months) treated with abduction orthoses (Fig. 27-4). Splinting was successful in 22 hips (33%) and unsuccessful in 45 (67%); closed reduction

and casting was required in 30 of these 45 and open reduction in 15. From their data, these authors concluded that infants with evidence of hip dislocation on anteroposterior roentgenograms have a 92% failure rate if the superior gap is 3 mm or less and a 94% failure rate if the medial gap is 10 mm or more, regardless of the type of splint used. They suggested that splinting should not be used in infants with these roentgenographic measurements because failure is likely and earlier treatment with closed or open reduction might avoid delay in reduction and reduce the risk of femoral head avascular necrosis.

The Pavlik harness consists of a chest strap, two shoulder straps, and two stirrups. Each stirrup has an anteromedial flexion strap and a posterolateral abduction strap. The harness is applied with the child supine and in a comfortable undershirt. The chest strap is fastened first, allowing enough room for three fingers to be placed between the chest and the harness. The shoulder straps are buckled to maintain the chest strap at the nipple line. The feet are then placed in the stirrups one at a time. The hip is placed in flexion (90 to 110 degrees), and the anterior flexion strap is tightened to maintain this position. Finally, the lateral strap is loosely fastened to limit adduction, not to force abduction. Excessive abduction to ensure stability is not acceptable. The knees should be 3 to 5 cm apart at full adduction in the harness (Fig. 27-5).

The Barlow test should be performed within the limits of the harness to ensure adequate stability. The child is then placed

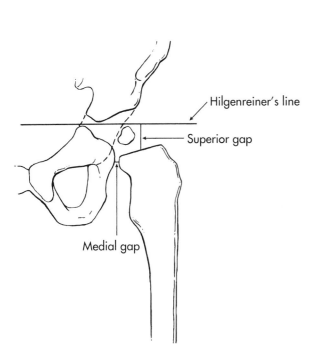

Fig. 27-4 Superior and medial gaps described by Brien et al. to predict treatment outcome. Superior gap is defined as distance between center of femoral head metaphysis and Hilgenreiner's line. Medial gap or lateralization is defined as distance between calcar of femur and lateral pelvic wall at that level. (From Brien EW, Randolph DA Jr, Zahiri CA: Radiographic analysis to determine the treatment outcome in developmental dysplasia of the hip, *Am J Orthop* 29:773, 2000.)

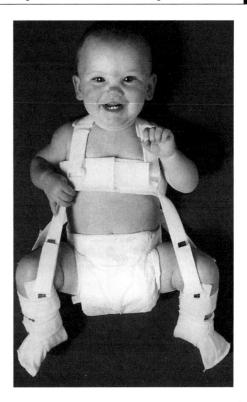

Fig. 27-5 Properly applied Pavlik harness (see text). (Courtesy Wheaton Brace, Carol Stream, Ill.)

prone and the greater trochanters are palpated; if asymmetry is noted, a persistent dislocation is present. A roentgenogram of the patient in the harness can help to confirm that the femoral neck is directed toward the triradiate cartilage (Fig. 27-6). After several weeks of harness wear, when the hip feels stable clinically, ultrasound is helpful to confirm reduction of the hip.

Four basic patterns of persistent dislocation have been observed after application of the Pavlik harness: *superior, inferior, lateral,* and *posterior.* If the dislocation is superior, additional flexion of the hip is indicated. If the dislocation is inferior, a decrease in flexion is indicated. A lateral dislocation in the Pavlik harness should be observed initially. As long as the femoral neck is directed toward the triradiate cartilage, as confirmed by roentgenogram or ultrasound, the head may gradually reduce into the acetabulum. A persistent posterior dislocation is difficult to treat, and Pavlik harness treatment frequently is unsuccessful. Posterior dislocation usually is accompanied by tight hip adductor muscles and may be diagnosed by palpation of the greater trochanter posteriorly.

If any of these patterns of dislocation or subluxation persist for more than 3 to 6 weeks, treatment in the Pavlik harness should be discontinued and a new program initiated; in most patients, this consists of optional traction, closed or open

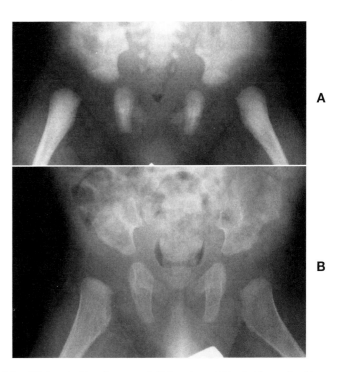

Fig. 27-6 **A,** Developmental dislocation of hip in 2-month-old boy. **B,** At 5 months of age after reduction in Pavlik harness.

reduction, and casting. The Pavlik harness should be worn full-time until stability is attained, as determined by negative Barlow and Ortolani tests. During this time the patient is examined once or twice a week, and the harness straps are adjusted to accommodate growth. The family is instructed in care of the child in the harness, including bathing, diapering, and dressing.

The duration of treatment depends on the patient's age at diagnosis and the degree of hip instability. For example, the duration of full-time harness wear for a patient with a dislocated hip is approximately equal to the age at which stability is attained plus 2 months. Weaning is then started by removing the harness for 2 hours each day. This time is doubled every 2 to 4 weeks until the device is worn only at night. Night bracing can be continued until the hip is normal roentgeno-graphically. Roentgenographic or ultrasound documentation can be used throughout the treatment period to verify the position of the hip. Roentgenograms are useful at the following times: immediately after the initiation of treatment, after any major adjustment in the harness, 1 month after weaning begins, at 6 months of age, and at 1 year of age.

Viere et al. reported that of 128 dislocations in 110 patients treated with the Pavlik harness, stable reduction was not obtained in 30 hips in 25 patients. Their statistically significant risk factors for Pavlik harness failure included absent Ortolani sign at initial evaluation (irreducible dislocation), bilateral hip dislocations, and delay of Pavlik harness treatment beyond 7 weeks of age. They concluded that failure of Pavlik harness management of congenital hip dislocation commonly indicates a need for open reduction and a more dysplastic acetabulum, which may lead to redislocation after closed reduction.

Suzuki and Yamamuro reported reduction in 94 of 233 dislocated hips with the use of the Pavlik harness; avascular necrosis occurred in 16 of the reduced hips. They observed that the more severe the dislocation, the higher the rates of both failed reduction and avascular necrosis, again emphasizing the need for gentle reduction and progression to further treatment when the harness fails. Inoue et al. cited an acetabular angle of 36 degrees or more and an age at initial application of 4 months or older as risk factors for a poor result after Pavlik harness treatment. Lerman et al., however, reported that age at diagnosis and initiation of treatment did not correlate with failure of Pavlik harness treatment. In their 93 patients, harness treatment failed in all 6 patients with irreducible hips and initial coverage of less than 20% (as determined by ultrasound). They suggested that patients with these two risk factors might be candidates for other treatment methods. The necessity for long-term follow-up of patients with Pavlik harness treatment was emphasized by Tucci et al., who found that 17% of hips demonstrated changes in the acetabulum at long-term follow-up despite normal roentgenograms at 3- and 5-year follow-up examinations.

Infant (6 to 18 Months of Age)

Once a child reaches crawling age (approximately 4 to 6 months), success with the Pavlik harness decreases signifi-

cantly. A child aged 6 to 18 months with a dislocated hip probably will require either closed manipulation or open reduction.

Children in this age group often are seen initially with a shortened extremity, limited passive abduction, and a positive Galeazzi sign. If the child is walking, a Trendelenburg gait may be present. Roentgenographic changes include delayed ossifi-cation of the femoral head, lateral and proximal displacement of the femoral head, and a shallow, dysplastic acetabulum.

With persistent dysplasia, the femoral head eventually moves superiorly and laterally with weight-bearing. The capsule becomes permanently elongated, and anteriorly the psoas tendon may obstruct reduction of the femoral head into the true acetabulum. The acetabular limbus may hypertrophy along the periphery of the acetabulum, and the ligamentum teres hypertrophies and elongates. The femoral head becomes reduced in size with posteromedial flattening, and coxa valga and excessive anteversion are noted. The true acetabulum is characteristically shallow and at surgery appears small because of the anterior capsular constriction and the hypertrophied limbus.

Treatment in this age group should follow a standard regimen, which includes adequate preoperative traction, adductor tenotomy, and closed reduction and arthrogram or open reduction in children with a failed closed reduction. Preoperative traction, adductor tenotomy, and gentle reduction with an acceptable "safe zone" are especially helpful in the prevention of avascular necrosis of the femoral head.

Krämer, Schleberger, and Steffen described a two-phase closed reduction technique that uses longitudinal skin traction followed by abduction splinting. They cited as advantages of this technique successful reduction with a nonaggressive method and a low incidence (3.4%) of femoral head avascular necrosis.

Preoperative Traction. The role of preliminary traction in reducing the incidence of avascular necrosis and in improving reduction is controversial. Disagreement exists about whether skin or skeletal traction should be used, whether home or in-hospital traction is preferable, about the amount of weight that should be used, the most beneficial direction of pull, and the duration of traction. In a survey of 335 members of the Pediatric Orthopaedic Society of North America, Fish, Herzenberg, and Hensinger found that 95% of respondents used traction, but opinions differed greatly regarding the use of preliminary traction in children of different ages, the use of home traction or hospital traction, the duration of traction, and the perceived benefits of traction.

Coleman questioned the efficacy of preliminary traction and discontinued its use. He reported no difference in the incidences of avascular necrosis in two groups of patients, one of which was treated with preliminary traction and one without traction. In a group of 47 congenitally dislocated hips, Kahle et al. found that either open or closed reduction was successful without preliminary traction in patients younger than 2 years of age, if the reduction could be obtained "without excessive force." Only two hips (4%) developed avascular necrosis, both in patients older than 1 year of age at the time of reduction.

Although controversial, if traction decreases the risk of avascular necrosis even slightly, the use of a home skin traction program in children with compliant and educated parents spares the expense of hospitalization and allows the child to stay in traction in a home environment. Skeletal traction is not indicated with the option of primary femoral shortening in older children. The objectives of traction or primary femoral shortening are to bring the laterally and proximally displaced femoral head down to and below the level of the true acetabulum to allow a more gentle reduction.

Adductor Tenotomy. A percutaneous adductor tenotomy under sterile conditions can be performed for a mild adduction contracture. For an adduction contracture of long duration, an open adductor tenotomy through a small transverse incision is preferable.

Closed Reduction. Gentle closed reduction is accomplished with the child under general anesthesia.

◆ Arthrography

The interposition of soft tissue in the acetabulum may be suggested by lateralization of the femoral head. Because the roentgenogram of the hip in an infant or young child cannot yield all the information desired in diagnosing or treating congenital dysplasia, arthrography is helpful in determining (1) whether mild dysplasia is present, (2) whether the femoral head is subluxated or dislocated, (3) whether manipulative reduction has been or can be successful, (4) to what extent any soft structures within the acetabulum may interfere with complete reduction of the dislocation, (5) the condition and position of the acetabular labrum (the limbus), and (6) whether the acetabulum and femoral head are developing normally during treatment. Because arthrograms are not always easy to interpret, the surgeon must be thoroughly familiar with the normal and abnormal signs they may reveal and with the technique of making arthrograms (Fig. 27-7).

An arthrogram of the hip is beneficial in all children, regardless of age, who are given a general anesthetic for closed reduction, unless closed reduction is obviously impossible. It is most helpful when manipulative reduction is unstable or when the femoral head is not concentrically seated within the acetabulum. Race and Herring emphasized the importance of confirming reduction by arthrography in 59 hips treated with closed reduction. Their results confirm that the most important factor that determines outcome of closed treatment of congenital hip dislocation is the quality of the initial reduction. In

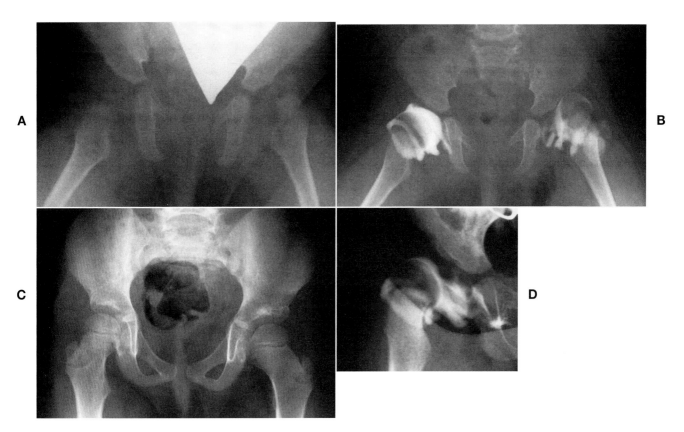

Fig. 27-7 A, Developmental dislocation of left hip in 5-month-old girl. **B,** Intraoperative arthrogram of irreducible left hip showing excessive pooling of dye. **C,** Same patient at age 4 years; note mild residual acetabular dysplasia of left hip. **D,** Arthrogram of right hip of 18-month-old girl with irreducible dislocation, capsular constriction, and hypertrophied labrum.

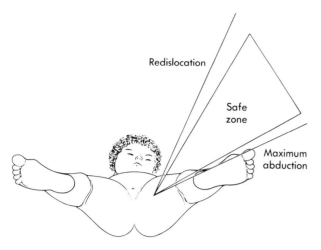

Fig. 27-8 "Safe zone" used to determine acceptability of closed reduction of congenital dislocation of hip.

hips with good or adequate reductions, 94% had good or acceptable results. Conversely, in those hips with poor reductions and those in which the quality of reduction could not be determined, only 21% had acceptable results. They also noted that as the quality of reduction declined, treatment time increased. Their criteria for accepting a reduction are a medial dye pool of 7 mm or less and maintenance of reduction in an acceptable "safe zone."

The use of image intensification in arthrography makes insertion of the needle much easier. The danger of damaging the articular surfaces by the needle is decreased, and the possibility of injecting the contrast medium directly into the ossific nucleus or the physis is prevented. When such equipment is not available, brief but careful use of an ordinary fluoroscope can aid in properly centering the needle.

The findings of the clinical examination and of arthrography at the time of attempted closed reduction determine if the hip will be stable or may require open reduction.

A clinical finding that usually indicates an acceptable closed reduction is the sensation of a "clunk" as the femoral head reduces in the true acetabulum. The "safe zone" concept of Ramsey, Lasser, and MacEwen can be used in determining the zone of abduction and adduction in which the femoral head remains reduced in the acetabulum. A wide safe zone (minimum of 20 degrees, preferably 45 degrees; Fig. 27-8) is desirable, and a narrow safe zone implies an unstable or unacceptable closed reduction. A careful clinical evaluation of the reduction should be made before and after adductor tenotomy and before the arthrogram, because once the hip capsule is distended with dye, clinical examination becomes more difficult.

Arthrography permits analysis of the cartilaginous anlage of the femoral head and acetabulum. Roentgenographic factors that help determine the success or failure of closed reduction include the amount of dye pooling in the medial joint space (preferably less than 5 to 7 mm) or an "hourglass" constriction obstructing reduction.

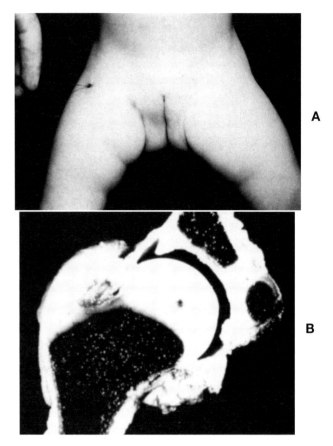

Fig. 27-9 **A,** Insertion of 22-gauge spinal needle one finger-breadth lateral to femoral artery and immediately inferior to anterosuperior iliac spine for arthrography. **B,** In necropsy specimen, areas of hip in which dye may be easily injected: beneath acetabular labrum, in medial or lateral capsular pouch, and at junction of ossified and cartilaginous portion of femoral head. (Courtesy John Ogden, MD.)

TECHNIQUE 27-1

Place the child supine after a general anesthetic has been administered. Perform sterile preparation and draping of the hip or hips. With a gloved fingertip locate the hip joint immediately inferior to the middle of the inguinal ligament and one fingerbreadth lateral to the pulsating femoral artery (Fig. 27-9). As an alternative, insert the needle medially, anterior to the adductor musculature. With the assistance of image intensification insert a 22-gauge needle, to which is attached a 5-ml syringe filled with normal saline solution, until it enters the hip joint; resistance will be met as the needle passes through the joint capsule. Next, inject the saline solution into the joint; this is easy at first but becomes more difficult as the joint becomes distended. Release the plunger of the syringe; if the joint has been successfully entered, the saline solution that is under pressure in it will reverse the plunger and fluid will escape into the syringe. Aspirate the saline solution from the joint and remove the syringe from the needle. Next, fill the syringe with 5 ml of a 25% strength Hypaque solution and inject 1 to 3 ml through the needle into the joint with image intensification. Rapidly withdraw the needle, and while the hip is still unreduced, have an arthrogram made. Before developing it, gently reduce the hip into a stable position and have a second arthrogram made. Maintain reduction until both arthrograms have been developed and studied.

When arthrograms are to be made of both hips, insert a needle into each, being sure that both are within the joints before either joint is injected. Inject both hips as described here and make arthrograms of both on the same cassette.

◆ Application of Hip Spica

After confirmation of a stable reduction, a hip spica cast is applied with the hip joint in 95 degrees of flexion and 40 to 45 degrees of abduction. Salter advocated this "human position" as best for maintaining hip stability and minimizing the risk of avascular necrosis. Kumar described an easily reproducible and simple technique for applying a hip spica cast. Fiberglass can be used in place of plaster, but the technique is described in its original form.

TECHNIQUE 27-2 *(Kumar)*

Place the anesthetized child on the spica frame. Abduct the hip to 40 to 45 degrees and flex it to about 95 degrees (Fig. 27-10, *A*). The amount of hip flexion and abduction required to keep the hip in the most stable position should be determined clinically and checked by roentgenograms.

After the correct position of flexion and abduction for stability is determined, place a small towel in front of the abdomen. Roll 2-inch (5 cm) Webril from the level of the nipples down to the ankles (Fig. 27-10, *B*). Pad around the bony points with 2-inch (5 cm) standard felt. Apply the first pad over the proximal end of the spica, near the nipple line (Fig. 27-10, *C*). Start a second piece of the same size felt at the level of the right groin and carry it posteriorly across the gluteal fold, over the right iliac crest, in front of the abdomen, over the lateral aspect of the left thigh, and then to the left inguinal area (Fig. 27-10, *C*). Apply a third piece of felt over the knee (Fig. 27-10, *D*) and a fourth piece above the ankle over the distal leg. Place similar pieces of felt over the opposite knee and leg.

Apply the plaster in two sections: a proximal section from the nipple line to the knees and a distal section from the knees to the ankles. Apply a single layer of 4-inch (10 cm) plaster roll from the nipple line to the level of the knees on both sides. Apply four or five plaster splints back to front from the nipple line to the back of the sacrum to reinforce the back of the cast. At the same time apply a short, thick splint over the anterolateral aspect of the inguinal area (Fig. 27-10, *E*). Apply another splint: starting

from the right inguinal area, carry it posteriorly across the gluteal region, the iliac crest, the front of the abdomen, and back the same way on the opposite thigh (Fig. 27-10, *E*). This is a reinforcing splint that attaches the thigh to the upper segment. Apply another long splint from the level of the knee across the anterolateral aspect of the inguinal area and up the chest wall (Fig. 27-10, *F*). This splint is one of the main anchors of the thigh to the body segment. Follow this by a roll of 4-inch (10 cm) plaster from the nipple line to the knees. This completes the proximal section of the spica. Next, complete the cast from the knees down to the ankles. Do this by applying on both sides a single roll of 3-inch (7.5 cm) plaster from the knee to the ankle level and reinforcing this by two splints over the medial and lateral aspects of the thigh, knee, and leg. Follow this by another roll of 3-inch (7.5 cm) plaster, then apply shoulder straps to prevent pistoning of the child in the cast (Fig. 27-10, *G*).

Since the cast is reinforced laterally around the hips, a wide segment can be removed from the front of the hips without weakening the cast. This permits better roentgenograms of the hips (Fig. 27-10, *G*).

The final view of the spica from inferiorly should appear as shown in Fig. 27-10, *H*, with about 40 to 45 degrees of abduction. The amount of abduction is determined by the position of hip stability. Once again we emphasize that excessive abduction should be avoided. We have found that the hips always are flexed less than they appear to be and are abducted more than they appear.

AFTERTREATMENT. Spica cast immobilization is continued for 4 months. The cast can be changed at 2 months with the patient under general anesthesia. Roentgenograms or arthrograms can be obtained to be sure that the femoral head is reduced anatomically into the acetabulum. Clinical and roentgenographic follow-up is essential until the hip is considered normal. Computed tomography (CT) scanning is useful in the postoperative assessment of reduction. In contrast to routine roentgenography, a cast does not alter the image of an axial CT scan (Fig. 27-11). Kawaguchi et al. recommended gadolinium-enhanced MR arthrography for evaluating reduction when conventional arthrography does not show complete concentric reduction and for confirming closed reduction immediately after manipulation. Compared with conventional arthrography and unenhanced MR arthrography, gadolinium-enhanced MR arthrography gives clearer views of all anatomical structures. Because of its high cost, MR arthrography probably should be reserved for instances in which conventional arthrograms show equivocal results. In this situation, MR arthrography can be helpful in making treatment decisions by delineating structures that may be impeding reduction.

Open Reduction. In children in whom efforts to reduce a dislocation without force have failed, open reduction is indicated to correct the offending soft tissue structures and to

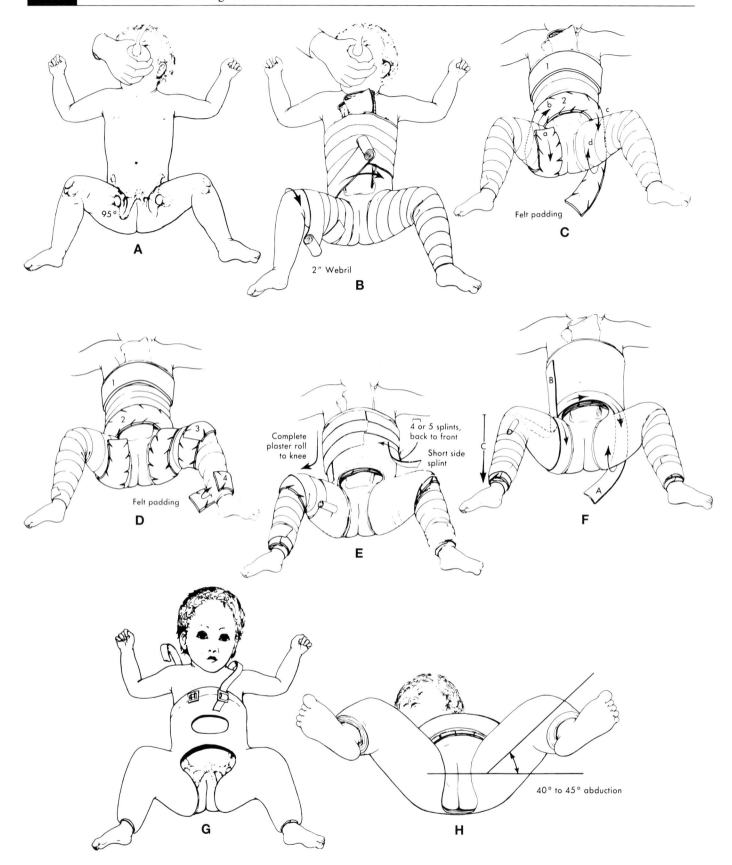

Fig. 27-10   Technique of application of spica cast for congenital dislocation of hip (see text). Note positioning of patient in "human" position. (From Kumar SJ: *J Pediatr Orthop* 1:97, 1981.)

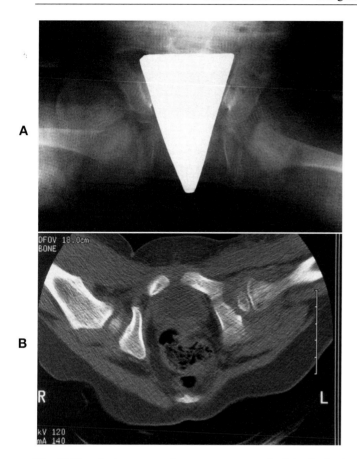

Fig. 27-11   **A,** Anteroposterior roentgenogram of pelvis obtained with patient in spica cast after closed reduction. Note difficulty in assessing position of femoral head. **B,** CT scan of pelvis to confirm bilateral reduction of femoral head into true acetabulum.

reduce the femoral head concentrically in the acetabulum. This surgical option is indicated by pathology rather than by age because open reduction may be required in children younger than 6 months of age, and closed reduction occasionally can be successful in children 18 months of age. Open reduction can be performed through an anterior, anteromedial, or medial approach; the choice depends on the experience of the surgeon and the particular dislocation.

The anterior approach requires more anatomical dissection but provides greater versatility because the pathological condition in the anterior and lateral aspects is easily reached and pelvic osteotomy can be performed through this approach if necessary.

The anteromedial approach described by Weinstein and Ponseti actually is an anterior approach to the hip through an anteromedial incision. The hip is approached in the interval between the pectineus muscle and the femoral neurovascular bundle. Weinstein and Ponseti recommended this approach for children up to the age of 24 months. Access to the lateral structures for dissection or osteotomy is not possible with this approach.

The medial (Ludloff) approach, although it is simpler and

involves less dissection, places the medial circumflex vessels at a higher risk and has been reported to be associated with a higher incidence of avascular necrosis. Mergen et al. and Castillo and Sherman reported avascular rates of 9.7% and 15%, respectively, with the use of the medial approach. Mergen et al. recommended this approach in infants between 7 and 18 months of age, and Castillo and Sherman recommended it only in those between 5 and 14 months of age.

◆ Anterior Approach

TECHNIQUE 27-3 *(Beaty, after Somerville)*

Make an anterior bikini incision from the middle of the iliac crest to a point midway between the anterosuperior iliac spine and the midline of the pelvis. The anterosuperior iliac crest should be at the midpoint of the incision, which can be placed 1 cm below the iliac crest (Fig. 27-12, *A*). Carry sharp dissection through the subcutaneous tissue to the deep fascia. Identify and enter the interval between the sartorius and tensor fasciae latae muscles, taking care to protect the lateral femoral cutaneous nerve by retracting it with a Penrose drain during the entire procedure. The presence of inguinal lymph nodes in the most medial dissection indicates the proximity of the neurovascular bundle. Detach the iliac apophysis from the ilium, beginning at the anterosuperior iliac spine and extending 4 cm posteriorly along the ilium. Subperiosteally dissect the tensor fasciae latae laterally to expose the ilium and the full extent of the anterolateral capsule.

Identify the origin of the sartorius muscle at the anterosuperior iliac crest, divide it, and allow it to retract distally. Next, dissect the tensor fasciae latae origin to the anteroinferior iliac spine. Place a retractor along the medial aspect of the anteroinferior spine onto the superior pubic ramus. Identify the psoas tendon in its groove on the superior pubic ramus and perform a recession tenotomy to facilitate placement of a right angle retractor in the groove on the superior pubic ramus normally occupied by the iliopsoas tendon. This retractor will protect the psoas muscle and neurovascular bundle anteriorly and assist in medial exposure. Identify the origins of both the direct and oblique heads of the rectus femoris muscle and perform a tenotomy approximately 1 cm distal to the anteroinferior iliac spine (Fig. 27-12, *B*). Tag the distal segment and allow the tendon to retract distally.

Identify the capsule of the hip joint anteriorly, medially, and laterally. A large amount of redundant capsule may be present laterally in the region of a false acetabulum. Make a T-shaped incision from the most medial aspect of the capsule to the most lateral and continue the incision along the anterior border of the femoral head and neck (Fig. 27-12, *C*). For more exposure, use Kocher clamps to retract the capsule. Identify the femoral head and the ligamentum teres; detach the ligamentum teres from the

continued

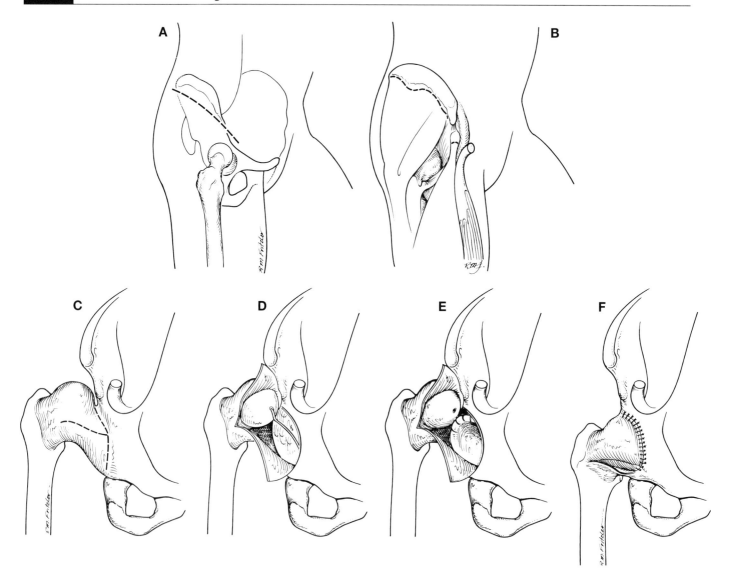

Fig. 27-12   Somerville technique of anterior open reduction in congenital dislocation of hip. **A,** Bikini incision. **B,** Division of sartorius and rectus femoris tendons and iliac epiphysis. **C,** T-shaped incision of capsule. **D,** Capsulotomy of hip and use of ligamentum teres to find true acetabulum. **E,** Radial incisions in acetabular labrum and removal of all pulvinar from depth of true acetabulum. **F,** Reduction and capsulorrhaphy after excision of redundant capsule.

Continued

femoral head and place on it a Kocher clamp. Trace the ligamentum teres to the true acetabulum and excise with a rongeur or sharp dissection any pulvinar in the true acetabulum (Fig. 27-12, *D*). Gently expose the bony articular surface of the acetabulum with its circumferential cartilage.

If a hypertrophied labrum is present, make several radial, T-shaped incisions laterally and superiorly to make enlargement of the true acetabulum easier (Fig. 27-12, *E*). Expose the acetabulum laterally, superiorly, medially, and inferiorly to the level of the deep transverse acetabular ligament, which should be divided to enlarge the most inferior aspect

of the acetabulum. Enlarge the entrance to the acetabulum with sequential incisions in the labrum or by excision of the fat from the innermost aspect of the acetabulum until the entrance is large enough to allow reduction of the femoral head without difficulty. After reducing the femoral head into the acetabulum, move the hip through a complete range of motion (including flexion, extension, adduction, and abduction), to determine the "safe zone" of reduction.

If the reduction is concentric and stable, reduce the femoral head and close the capsule, suturing the lateral flap of the T-shaped incision as far medially as possible to eliminate any redundant capsule in the region of the false

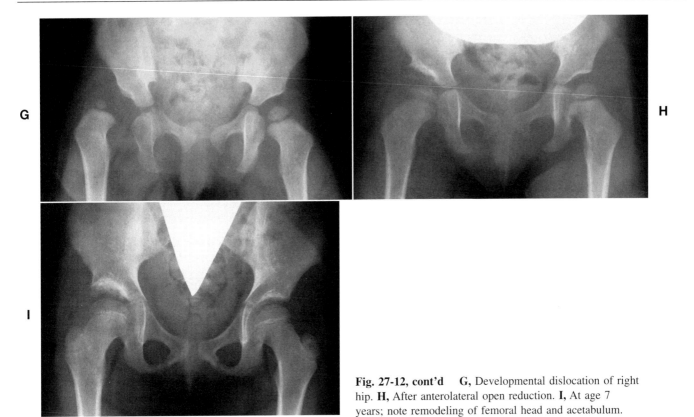

Fig. 27-12, cont'd   G, Developmental dislocation of right hip. **H,** After anterolateral open reduction. **I,** At age 7 years; note remodeling of femoral head and acetabulum.

acetabulum (Fig. 27-12, *F*). An adequate capsulorrhaphy will significantly improve stability of the hip. Place sutures in the tips of the T and along the superior border of the acetabulum. When capsulorrhaphy is completed, suture the rectus femoris tendon to its origin and the iliac apophysis to the fascia of the tensor fasciae latae along the iliac crest. Close the superficial fascial layers, the subcutaneous tissues, and the skin. Apply a double spica cast with the hips in 90 to 100 degrees of flexion and 40 to 55 degrees of abduction (Fig. 27-11, *G* to *I*).

AFTERTREATMENT. Roentgenograms or CT scans can be used to confirm reduction of the femoral head into the acetabulum. The spica cast is removed at 10 to 12 weeks. Sequential roentgenograms are used to assess development of the femoral head and acetabulum; these are obtained on a regular basis until the child reaches skeletal maturity.

◆ Anteromedial Approach

TECHNIQUE 27-4 *(Weinstein and Ponseti)*
With the patient supine, prepare and drape the affected extremity and hemipelvis free to allow full motion of the hip and knee. With the hip flexed to 70 degrees and in

unforced abduction, identify the neurovascular bundle and the superior and inferior borders of the adductor longus muscle. Make an incision from the inferior border of the adductor longus to just inferior to the femoral neurovascular bundle in the groin crease. Incise the skin and subcutaneous tissues down to the deep fascia, and incise the fascia over the adductor longus in the direction of the muscle fibers. Isolate the adductor longus, section it at its origin, and allow it to retract.

Follow the anterior branch of the obturator nerve proximally to its entrance into the thigh under the pectineus muscle. Gently retract superiorly the neurovascular bundle. Keep the anterior branch of the obturator nerve in sight, open the sheath overlying the pectineus muscle, and identify its superior and inferior borders. Identify and bluntly dissect the interval between the pectineus muscle and the femoral neurovascular bundle. Isolate the iliopsoas tendon in the inferior aspect of the wound, section it sharply, and allow it to retract.

With gentle retraction of the neurovascular bundle superiorly and the pectineus muscle inferiorly, isolate the hip joint capsule by blunt dissection. Make a small incision in the anteromedial capsule parallel to the anterior acetabular margin. Grasp the ligamentum teres with a Graham hook and bring it into the wound. Extend the capsular incision along the ligamentum teres to its insertion

continued

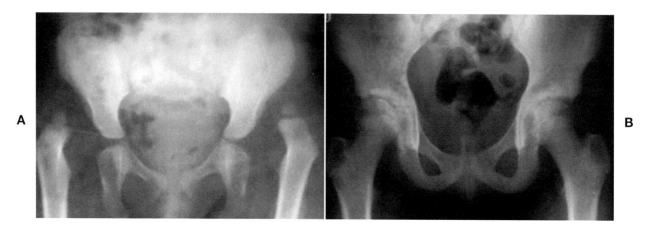

Fig. 27-13   Anteromedial open reduction. **A,** Bilateral congenital dislocation of hip in 32-month-old girl. **B,** At age 12 years, normal development of femoral head and acetabulum bilaterally. (Courtesy Stuart Weinstein, MD.)

on the femoral head. Rotate the leg to bring this attachment into view. If the ligamentum teres is hypertrophied or elongated, excise it to make reduction easier. Grasp the stump of the ligamentum teres with a Kocher clamp, and identify the interval between the ligament and the anteroinferomedial aspect of the joint capsule; mark this interval with a pair of scissors. Retract the pectineus muscle and sharply incise the anteromedial margin of the capsule.

Section the ligamentum teres at its base along with the transverse acetabular ligament to open up the "horseshoe" of the acetabulum and increase its diameter. Remove all pulvinar with a pituitary rongeur. Next, reduce the femoral head into the acetabulum and move the hip through a range of motion to test the stability of the reduction. Irrigate the wound copiously, leave the joint capsule open, and approximate the deep fascia with running absorbable sutures. Close the subcutaneous tissues and skin with absorbable sutures. Apply a spica cast with the hip in a position of maximal stability in flexion and mild abduction.

AFTERTREATMENT. The cast is worn for 10 to 12 weeks. If roentgenograms show satisfactory position of the hip 4 to 6 weeks after surgery, the portion of the cast below the knee is removed to allow knee motion and some hip rotation. After removal of the total cast, an abduction brace is worn full-time for 4 to 8 weeks; then it is worn only at night and during naps for 1 to 2 years, until normal acetabular development is evident (Fig. 27-13).

◆ *Medial Approach*

TECHNIQUE 27-5 *(Ludloff)*

Make a transverse incision centered at the anterior margin of the adductor longus, approximately 1 cm distal and parallel

to the inguinal ligament (Fig. 27-14). Open the fascia along the superior border of the adductor longus. Isolate this muscle, divide it close to its insertion on the pelvis, and retract it distally to expose the adductor brevis muscle in the inferior part of the wound and the pectineus muscle in the superior part of the wound. Identify the branches of the anterior obturator nerve on the surface of the adductor brevis muscle and with blunt dissection follow this nerve beneath the pectineus muscle. Free the posterior border of the pectineus muscle proximally to its insertion on the pelvis. Place a retractor beneath the pectineus muscle and retract it superiorly. Identify by palpation the lesser trochanter and the iliopsoas tendon. Open the fascial layer surrounding the tendon, pull the tendon into the wound with a right-angle clamp, and sharply divide it. With blunt dissection clear the pericapsular fat from the capsule. Dissect free the small branch of the medial circumflex artery that crosses the capsule inferiorly and preserve it. Incise the capsule in the direction of the femoral neck. Identify the transverse acetabular ligament and section it. If needed for reduction, perform additional release of the capsule. Reduce the hip in 90 to 100 degrees of flexion and 40 to 60 degrees of abduction. When the optimal position is determined, close the deep fascia and skin in routine fashion and apply a double spica cast. Obtain a CT scan after cast application to confirm reduction of the femoral head.

AFTERTREATMENT. Aftertreatment is similar to that after closed reduction (p. 1087) and varies according to the age of the child. Generally, 8 to 12 weeks of cast immobilization is sufficient.

Evaluation of Open Reduction. Zadeh, Catterall, Hashemi-Nejad, and Perry reported their results in 82 children (95 hips) in whom a test of stability after open reduction was

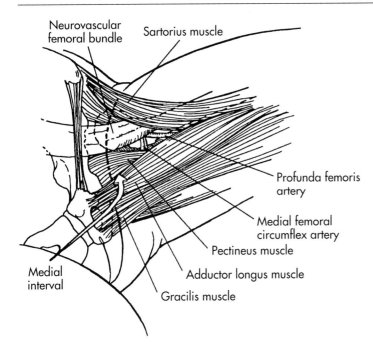

Fig. 27-14   Incision for medial (Ludloff) approach and open reduction.

used to determine the need for a concomitant osteotomy. Their criteria were as follows:

1. Hip stable in neutral position—no osteotomy
2. Hip stable in flexion and abduction—innominate osteotomy
3. Hip stable in internal rotation and abduction—proximal femoral derotational varus osteotomy
4. "Double-diameter" acetabulum with anterolateral deficiency—Pemberton-type osteotomy

Using these guidelines, they obtained satisfactory outcomes in 86% of patients; 7% required secondary procedures for persistent dysplasia.

Smith et al. suggested that the appearance of the acetabular teardrop figure after reduction of the hip in DDH may be the earliest roentgenographic sign that a stable, concentric reduction of the hip has been accomplished. Although their sample size was small (25 normal hips), Smith et al. found that 60% had a teardrop by age 12 months and all had a teardrop by age 18 months. Only 1 of 47 dislocated hips had a visible teardrop figure before reduction of the hip. All 38 hips that were stable after initial reduction and had a good roentgenographic result developed a teardrop within an average of 6.75 months after reduction. Hips that required further intervention to obtain stability did not develop a teardrop until a mean of 12.75 months, and the configuration of the teardrop usually was abnormal. The presence of a teardrop at 6 months after reduction predicted a satisfactory outcome in 93% of hips.

Special Problems

Teratological Dislocations. A teratological dislocation of the hip is one that occurs sometime before birth, resulting in significant anatomical distortion and resistance to treatment. It often occurs with other conditions such as arthrogry-posis, Larsen syndrome, myelomeningocele, and diastrophic dwarfism.

The anatomical changes in teratological dislocations are much more advanced than those in a typical congenital hip dislocation in a child of the same age. The acetabulum is small, with an oblique or flattened roof, the ligamentum teres is thickened, and the femoral head is of variable size and may be flattened on the medial side (Fig. 27-15). The hip joint is stiff and irreducible, and roentgenograms show superolateral displacement.

Most authors agree that closed reduction is not effective and that open reduction is necessary, but indications for treatment are not clear. Most agree that unilateral dislocations should be treated more aggressively than bilateral dislocations. Gruel et al. listed the ambulatory potential of the patient as the most important consideration in deciding whether to treat bilateral dislocations. The difficulty of successfully treating teratological dislocations is reflected in the results of Gruel et al. who found that of the 27 hips in their series, 44% had poor results and 70% had complications. Avascular necrosis occurred in 48% of hips, redislocation in 19%, and subluxation in 22%. Anterior open reduction and femoral shortening produced the best results with the fewest complications, whereas the worst results and most complications occurred in those hips treated by closed reduction.

Although multiple procedures may be required, good results can be obtained and a stable hip can be achieved in properly selected patients. Szöke et al. reported 80% good results in 25 hips of 16 patients with amyoplasia-type arthrogryposis after open reduction through a medial approach. They recommended this technique for children 3 to 6 months old and combined it with surgical correction of congenital contractures of the knee

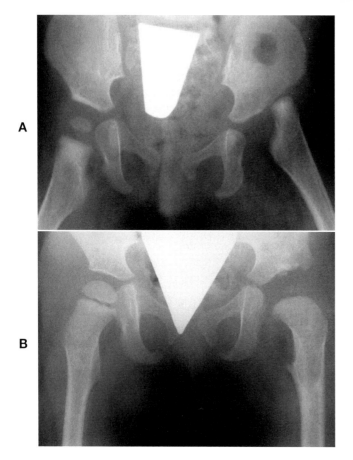

Fig. 27-15   **A,** Teratological dislocation of left hip in 18-month-old girl. **B,** Appearance at 3 years of age after primary femoral shortening, anterior open reduction, and innominate osteotomy.

and foot. In older children, primary femoral shortening and anterior open reduction, with or without pelvic osteotomy, is preferred.

Avascular Necrosis. The most serious complication associated with treatment of congenital dysplasia of the hip in early infancy is the development of avascular necrosis. Lehman et al., in their meta-analysis, estimated the rates of avascular necrosis to be 2.5/1000 in infants referred for treatment before 6 months of age and 109/1000 in those referred after 6 months of age.

Potential sequelae of avascular necrosis include femoral head deformity, acetabular dysplasia, lateral subluxation of the femoral head, relative overgrowth of the greater trochanter, and limb-length inequalities; osteoarthritis is a common late complication. Bucholz and Ogden, as well as Kalamchi and MacEwen, proposed classification systems based on morphological changes in the capital femoral epiphysis, the physis, and the proximal femoral metaphysis (Fig. 27-16). These classifications are useful in determining proper treatment and prognosis for a particular patient; however, the proper classification may not be identifiable on roentgenograms until the child is 4 to 6 years of age.

Treatment should be directed toward the clinical problems associated with each roentgenographic classification group. Many patients will not require any treatment during adolescence and young adulthood. In a few, femoral head deformity and acetabular dysplasia predisposing the hip joint to incongruity and persistent subluxation can be treated with either femoral osteotomy or appropriate pelvic osteotomy, or both.

Children with avascular necrosis after treatment of congenital dislocation of the hip should be followed to maturity with serial orthoroentgenograms. Bar-On, Huo, and DeLuca reported that of 25 patients with avascular necrosis of the femoral head complicating DDH, those treated early (1 to 3 years after the ischemic insult; average age, 2.7 years) with innominate osteotomy had significantly better results than those treated later (5 to 10 years after the ischemic insult) and those without pelvic osteotomy. Patients treated early also had less pain and fewer gait disturbances and required fewer additional procedures for limb-length inequality or greater trochanteric overgrowth. Bar-On et al. suggested that early innominate osteotomy induced spherical remodeling of the femoral head, with a resultant congruous hip joint, while with later osteotomy the femoral head was already deformed, with little potential for remodeling. Significant limb-length inequality can be corrected by appropriate techniques, usually a well-timed epiphysiodesis. Symptomatic overgrowth of the greater trochanter can be treated in older patients with greater trochanteric advancement, which will increase the abductor muscle resting length and increase the abductor lever arm (Fig. 27-17).

◆ *Trochanteric Advancement*

TECHNIQUE 27-6 *(Lloyd-Roberts and Swann)*

Approach the trochanter through a long lateral incision. Place a Gigli saw deep to the gluteus medius and minimus muscles and divide the trochanter at its base. Next, mobilize the gluteus muscles anteriorly and posteriorly as they are dissected off the joint capsule and strip them for a short distance from the ilium above. Displace the detached trochanter with its attached muscles distally to the lateral cortex of the femur while the hip is abducted. Bevel the femoral cortex to help reduce tension and improve placement of the trochanter. Secure the trochanter to the femur with screws and suture the femoral periosteum and vastus lateralis muscle. The top of the greater trochanter now should be positioned at the level of the center of the femoral head on anteroposterior roentgenogram. The trochanter usually requires advancement anteriorly as well as distally.

AFTERTREATMENT. The hip is protected by a spica cast in abduction for 3 to 6 weeks. A physical therapy program is begun for rehabilitation of the hip abductor musculature.

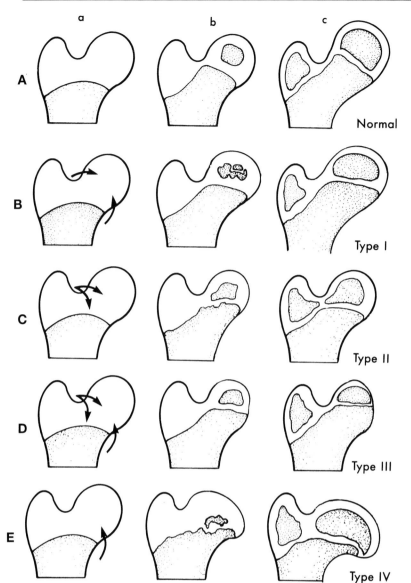

Fig. 27-16   Bucholz and Ogden classification of avascular necrosis of femoral head in congenital dislocation of hip. **A,** Normal femoral head at 2 months, 1 year, and 9 years of age. **B,** Type 1: *a*, sites of temporary vascular occlusion; *b*, irregular ossification in secondary center; *c*, normal epiphyseal contour, slight decrease in height of capital femoral ossification center. **C,** Type II: *a*, probable primary site of vascular occlusion; *b*, metaphyseal and epiphyseal irregularities; *c*, premature fusion of lateral metaphysis and epiphysis. **D,** Type III: *a*, sites of temporary vascular occlusion; *b*, impaired longitudinal growth of capital femoral epiphysis; *c*, irregularly shaped femoral head. **E,** Type IV: *a*, sites of temporary vascular occlusion; *b*, impaired longitudinal and latitudinal growth; *c*, premature epiphyseal closure. (Redrawn from Bucholz RW, Ogden JA: In *The hip*, St Louis, 1978, Mosby.)

Toddler (18 to 36 Months of Age)

Because of widespread screening of newborns, it is becoming less common for congenital dysplasia of the hip to go undetected beyond the age of 1 year. The older child with this condition has a wide perineum, shortened lower extremity, and hyperlordosis of the lower spine as a result of femoropelvic instability. For these children with well-established hip dysplasia, open reduction with femoral or pelvic osteotomy, or both, often is required. Persistent dysplasia can be corrected by a redirectional proximal femoral osteotomy in very young children. If the primary dysplasia is acetabular, pelvic redirectional osteotomy alone is more appropriate. Many older children, however, require both femoral and pelvic osteotomies if significant deformity is present on both sides of the joint.

Femoral Osteotomy in Dysplasia of Hip. Surgeons who recommend femoral osteotomies advise an operation on the pelvic side of the joint only after (1) the femoral head has been concentrically seated in the dysplastic acetabulum by such an osteotomy, (2) the joint has failed to develop satisfactorily, and (3) the growth potential of the acetabulum no longer exists. Opinions differ widely as to the age at which the acetabulum loses its ability to develop satisfactorily over a femoral head concentrically located; Kasser, Bowen, and MacEwen reported consistently good results in patients younger than 4 years old at the time of femoral osteotomy. Remodeling of the acetabulum occurred through the age of 8 years, but 4 of 13 hips in patients between the ages of 4 and 8 years showed persistent dysplasia despite the operation. The results were less predictable as the patients approached the age of 8 years. No benefit was derived from femoral osteotomy alone in 10 of 11 hips in patients older than 8 years of age. Femoral osteotomy is most frequently indicated with primary femoral shortening, but the technique is included here for completeness.

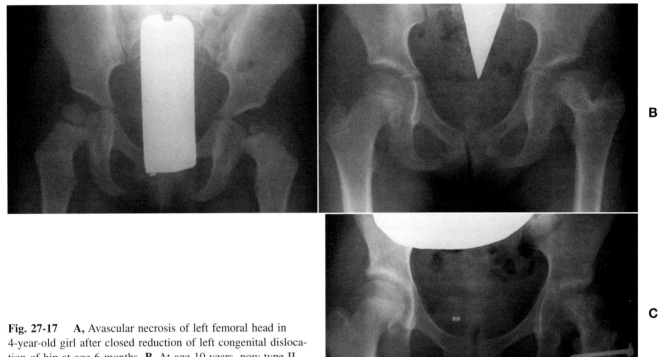

Fig. 27-17   A, Avascular necrosis of left femoral head in 4-year-old girl after closed reduction of left congenital dislocation of hip at age 6 months. **B,** At age 10 years, now type II avascular necrosis with premature lateral epiphyseal arrest and relative trochanteric overgrowth. **C,** At age 13 years, after transfer of trochanter distally and anteriorly.

◆ **Varus Derotational Osteotomy of the Femur in Hip Dysplasia, with Pediatric Hip Screw Fixation**

TECHNIQUE 27-7

Place the patient supine on a radiolucent operating table. Image intensification in the anteroposterior projection is desirable. Prepare and drape the affected extremity, leaving the unaffected leg draped free to allow intraoperative roentgenograms or imaging.

Make a lateral incision from the greater trochanter distally 8 to 12 cm, incise the iliotibial band, and reflect the vastus lateralis muscle to expose the lateral aspect of the femur. Make a transverse line in the femoral cortex with an osteotome to mark the level of the osteotomy at the level of the lesser trochanter or slightly distal. Correct positioning of the osteotomy can be verified with image intensification. Next, make a longitudinal orientation line on the anterior femoral cortex to determine correct rotation.

Drill a hole just distal to the greater trochanter and check its placement with the image intensifier. Place an appropriate guide pin of the proper length in the femoral neck with the aid of an adjustable angle guide (see Fig. 33-117, *A*).

Check the placement of the guide pin with image intensification. Once the guide pin is placed, use a per-cutaneous direct measuring gauge to determine the lag screw length. Set the adjustable positive stop on the combination reamer for the lag screw length determined by a percutaneous direct measuring gauge. Place the reamer over the guide pin and ream until the positive stop reaches the lateral cortex (see Fig. 33-117, *C*). It is prudent to periodically check the fluoroscopic image during reaming to ensure that the guide pin is not inadvertently advancing proximally into the epiphysis. Next, set the adjustable positive stop on the lag screw tap to the same length that was reamed. Tap until the positive stop reaches the lateral cortex. Then screw the appropriate intermediate compression screw over the guide pin (see Fig. 33-117, *D* and *E*).

Take the plate chosen during preoperative planning and insert its barrel over the barrel guide and onto the back of the lag screw. The plate angle will ultimately determine the final hip angle. Remove the barrel guide and insert a compressing screw to prevent the plate from disengaging during the reduction maneuver. Use the slotted screwdriver for the pediatric compressing screw or the hex screwdriver for the intermediate compressing screw. If the plate obscures the osteotomy site, loosen the screw and rotate the side plate.

Next, make the osteotomy cut at the transverse line on the cortex in a transverse or oblique direction, depending on the correction desired. If rotational, in addition to angular, correction is desired, complete the osteotomy through the medial cortex. Using the longitudinal mark in the femoral cortex as a guide, rotate the femur as needed to correct femoral anteversion (usually 15 to 30 degrees). Because the deformity is more rotational than angulatory, evaluate the position of the femur with roentgenograms or image intensification before continuing with varus correction. To achieve varus angulation, remove an appropriate wedge of bone from the medial cortex to effect a neck-shaft angle of 120 to 135 degrees.

To achieve compression, insert a drill or tap guide into the distal portion of the most distal compression slot. Drill through the medial cortex. If less compression is required, follow the same steps detailed above in the distal portion of either the second or third distal slots for up to 2.5 mm of compression.

Select the appropriate length bone screw and insert it using the hex screwdriver. Use the self-holding sleeve to keep the screw from disengaging from the screwdriver (see Fig. 33-117, *F*). Finally, in the most proximal slot, the intermediate combination drill/tap guide can be angled proximally so that the drill and ultimately the bone screw will cross the osteotomy line. Positioning the proximal bone screw in this way can provide additional stability at the osteotomy site. Insert screws into any remaining screw holes.

The lag screw can be inserted farther to provide more compression. To insert the lag screw for approximately 5 mm of compression, stop when the lateral cortex is midway between the two depth calibrations (see Fig. 33-117, *G*). To insert the lag screw for approximately 10 mm of compression, stop when the second depth calibration meets the lateral cortex (see Fig. 33-117, *H*).

Confirm the position of the fixation device and the proximal and distal fragments with an anteroposterior roentgenogram or image intensification. Irrigate the wound and close it in layers, inserting a suction drain if needed. Apply a one and one half spica cast.

AFTERTREATMENT. The spica cast is worn for 8 to 12 weeks, until union of the osteotomy occurs. The internal fixation can be removed at 12 to 24 months if desired.

Juvenile or Child (3 to 8 Years of Age)

The management of untreated congenital dislocation of the hip in a child over 3 years of age is difficult. By this age adaptive shortening of the periarticular structures and structural alterations in both the femoral head and the acetabulum have occurred. Dislocated hips in this age group require open reduction. Preoperative skeletal traction should not be used. Schoenecker and Strecker reported a 54% incidence of

avascular necrosis and a 31% incidence of redislocation after the use of skeletal traction in patients older than 3 years. Open reduction combined with femoral shortening resulted in no avascular necrosis and an 8% incidence of redislocation. Coleman reported an 8% incidence of avascular necrosis in his series of femoral shortening. Although femoral shortening aids in the reduction and decreases the potential for complications, it is technically demanding, as is treatment of the dislocated hip, in this older age group.

◆ Primary Femoral Shortening

Since the early 1990s the combination of primary open reduction and femoral shortening, with or without pelvic osteotomy, has been an accepted method of treatment of congenital hip dislocation in older children. This approach avoids expensive in-hospital traction, obtains predictable reduction, and results in a low rate of avascular necrosis.

Klisíc and Jankovic reported the use of combined procedures in both unilateral and bilateral dislocations, combining open reduction and femoral shortening with acetabular procedures as indicated (Fig. 27-18).

In a report of his experience with this technique in the treatment of congenital hip dislocation in older children, Wenger recommended primary femoral shortening, anterior open reduction, and capsulorrhaphy, with or without pelvic osteotomy as indicated, in children 3 years of age or older. He also emphasized the importance of correcting soft tissue deformity, as well as bony deformity, to prevent redislocation. Certain circumstances, such as teratological hip dislocation or a failed traction program, may make the procedure appropriate for younger children. A completely dislocated hip in an older child becomes fixed in a position superior to the true acetabulum. The degree of this superior migration ranges from severe subluxation (inferior head still adjacent to labrum), to dislocation with formation of a false acetabulum just superior to the true acetabulum, to severe dislocation with the femoral head high in the abductor musculature without formation of a false acetabulum. The extent of proximal migration determines the degree of deformation of the capsule and the extent of soft tissue reconstruction required to correct the deformity.

The capsular abnormality in the congenitally dislocated hip must be recognized and corrected to achieve successful open reduction. The methods for bony correction are well defined, perhaps because the techniques can be clearly illustrated and documented roentgenographically, but the soft tissue abnormalities and methods for their correction are not well described. As a result, a hip that appears reduced immediately after surgery may subluxate or redislocate with weight-bearing even though the bony procedure appears roentgenographically faultless.

The dislocation of the hip leads to adaptive enlargement of the hip capsule, with the capsule becoming nearly twice the normal size in the completely dislocated hip. The ligamentum teres hypertrophies and often becomes a partial weight-bearing structure. In older children this ligament occasionally avulses from the femoral head, retracting and reattaching to the inferior

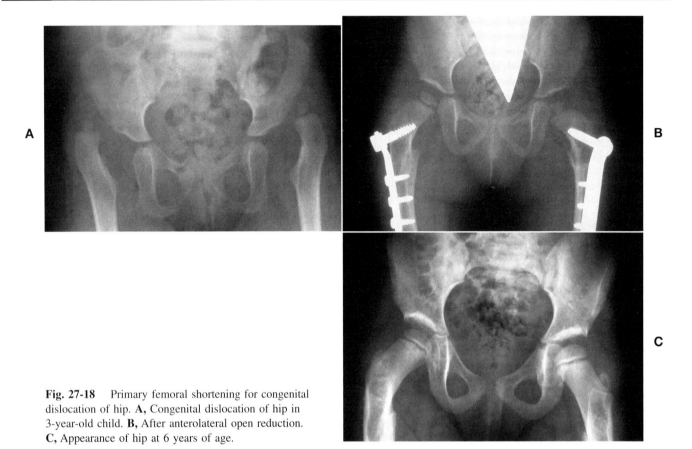

Fig. 27-18   Primary femoral shortening for congenital dislocation of hip. **A,** Congenital dislocation of hip in 3-year-old child. **B,** After anterolateral open reduction. **C,** Appearance of hip at 6 years of age.

capsule and forming a mass of tissue that may impede reduction. The fibrocartilaginous labrum is flattened superolaterally, with the attached hypertrophied capsule protruding into the overlying abductor muscle mass, which adheres to the displaced capsule. If the capsule is not separated adequately from the adherent overlying muscles, reduction is difficult and the chance of redislocation is increased.

In a high, severely dislocated hip the abductor muscles have contracted, and occasionally, despite prior traction or femoral shortening, these contracted muscles and fascia make it difficult to pull the proximal femur distal enough to fully reduce the femoral head (Fig. 27-19). In rare instances this requires release of the piriformis insertion or release of the anterior-most gluteus minimus fibers, or both, to allow adequate distal movement of the femoral head after femoral shortening. The middle and inferior portions of the capsule predictably are constricted by the overlying psoas tendon. The transverse acetabular ligament, crossing the base of the horseshoe-shaped true acetabulum, is contracted and thickened.

The following description of the technique for primary femoral shortening is a modification of the techniques described both by Klisíc and by Wenger and includes anterior open reduction and varus derotational osteotomy. These techniques are described on p. 1089 and p. 1096, respectively, and should be reviewed carefully before primary femoral shortening is performed (Fig. 27-20).

TECHNIQUE 27-8

Place the patient supine on the operating table with a small radiolucent pad beneath the affected hip. Prepare and drape the extremity in the usual manner to allow exposure of the pelvis and femur. Two incisions are made, an anterior ilioinguinal incision and a straight lateral incision, as described both for anterior open reduction (p. 1089) and for femoral osteotomy (p. 1096).

Through the anterior ilioinguinal incision, perform anterior open reduction as described (p. 1089), continuing the dissection to the point where capsulorrhaphy normally would be performed. Next, attend to the femoral shortening. Make a straight lateral incision from the tip of the greater trochanter to the distal third of the femoral shaft. Expose the shaft by dissection through the tensor fascia lata muscle, iliotibial band, and vastus lateralis muscle. Make a transverse mark on the femoral shaft at the level of the lesser trochanter to indicate the osteotomy site and make a longitudinal mark on the anterior border of the proximal shaft to orient derotation of the femur. Insert a lag screw into the femoral neck in the usual manner.

Estimate the amount of shortening that will be necessary from preoperative roentgenograms, measuring from the most proximal aspect of the femoral head to the triradiate cartilage. The amount of shortening generally required

continued

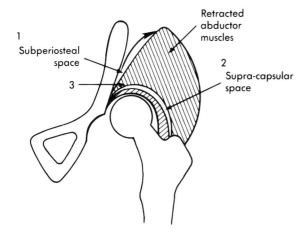

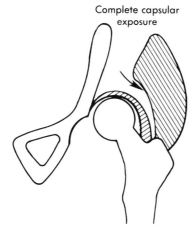

Fig. 27-19   Complete capsular exposure occasionally required in severe, high dislocation of hip. (Redrawn from Wenger DR: *Instr Course Lect* 38:343, 1989.)

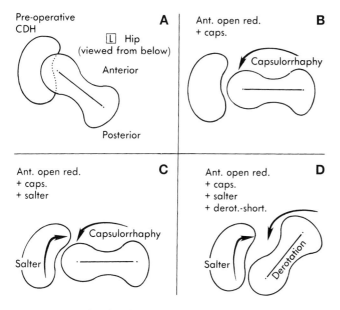

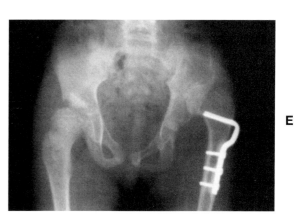

Fig. 27-20   **A,** Anteverted femur and acetabulum in untreated congenital dislocation of hip. **B,** Redirection of femoral neck by snug anterior capsulorrhaphy. **C,** Capsulorrhaphy and Salter innominate osteotomy. **D,** Capsulorrhaphy, Salter innominate osteotomy, and full femoral derotation. Combined in excess, this sequence can produce posterior dislocation. **E,** Open reduction, primary femoral shortening, derotation osteotomy, and Salter osteotomy produced fixed posterior hip dislocation in this 5-year-old girl. (**A** to **D** redrawn from Wenger DR: *Instr Course Lect* 38:343, 1989.)

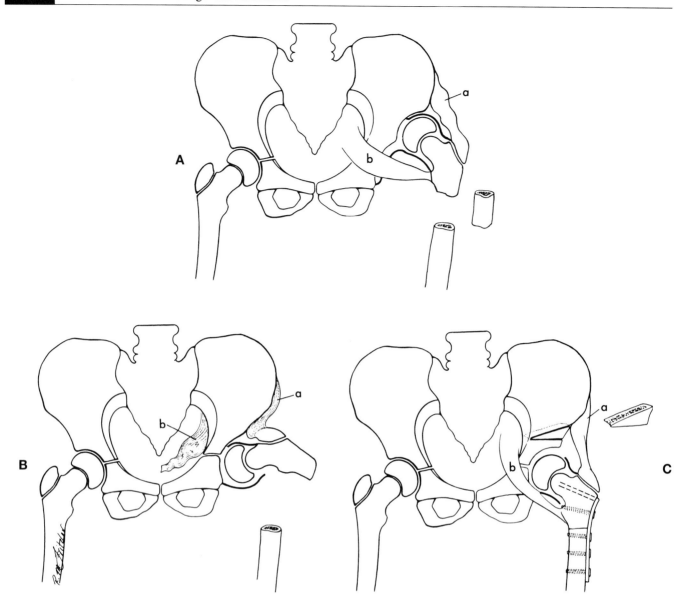

Fig. 27-21 Technique for open reduction, primary femoral shortening, and Salter osteotomy. **A,** Femoral head is dislocated. Gluteal muscles (*a*) are retracted and slightly shortened. Iliopsoas muscle (*b*) is intact. Capsule is interposed between femoral head and ilium. Segment of femur is resected. **B,** Proximal femur is abducted, iliopsoas tendon (*b*) is divided. Capsule is incised on inferior surface parallel to femoral neck. **C,** Operation is complete. Gluteal muscles (*a*) are tight. Iliopsoas muscle (*b*) is reattached. Salter osteotomy is completed with graft in place. Femoral fragments are fixed with pediatric hip screw.

varies from 1 to 3 cm. Perform an osteotomy of the femur slightly distal to the lag screw in the femoral neck. Make a second osteotomy at the appropriate distance distal to the first. Angle this osteotomy to allow varus and derotation of the femur as necessary. Remove the measured segment of the femoral shaft (Fig. 27-21).

Carefully incise subperiosteally the iliopsoas attachment to the lesser trochanter and the capsule attached to the medial femoral neck, avoiding the medial circumflex artery.

Gently reduce the femoral head into the acetabulum, using the lag screw in the femoral neck as a lever. Derotation of the proximal fragment of approximately 15 to 45 degrees usually is required. Next, appose the two segments of the femur and attach a side plate to the screw in the femoral neck and fix it to the distal femoral shaft. Use roentgenograms or image intensification to evaluate the femoral shortening and reduction of the femoral head.

At this point a Salter or Pemberton osteotomy, if

indicated to correct acetabular dysplasia, can be performed. A thorough and meticulous capsulorrhaphy should be performed as previously described. The most lateral flap of the capsule should be transposed medially to eliminate the redundant capsule of the false acetabulum (Fig. 27-22).

Irrigate both wounds and close them in the usual manner. Suction drains can be inserted if necessary. Apply a spica cast with the extremity in neutral rotation and slight flexion and abduction.

AFTERTREATMENT. The drains are removed 24 to 48 hours after surgery. The spica cast is removed at 8 to 12 weeks. Sequential roentgenograms are obtained to evaluate development of the femoral head and acetabulum. Although uncommon, limb-length discrepancy should be evaluated annually by clinical evaluation and, if necessary, scanograms.

Pelvic Osteotomy. Operations on the pelvis, alone or combined with open reduction, are useful in congenital dysplasia or dislocation of the hip to ensure or to increase stability of the joint. Those operations most often used are (1) osteotomy of the innominate bone (Salter), (2) acetabuloplasty (Pemberton), (3) osteotomies that free the acetabulum (Steel triple innominate osteotomy or "dial" acetabular osteotomy), (4) shelf operation (Staheli), and (5) innominate osteotomy with medial displacement of the acetabulum (Chiari). In an older child one of these operations can be combined with femoral osteotomy to correct femoral and acetabular abnormalities.

Osteotomy of the innominate bone, an operation devised by Salter, is useful only when any subluxation or dislocation has been reduced or can be reduced by open reduction at the time of osteotomy in a child 18 months to 6 years of age. The entire acetabulum together with the pubis and ischium is rotated as a unit, the symphysis pubis acting as a hinge. The osteotomy is held open anterolaterally by a wedge of bone, and thus the roof of the acetabulum is shifted more anteriorly and laterally. The osteotomy is contraindicated in patients with nonconcentric hips or severe dysplasia.

Acetabuloplasty is also useful only when any subluxation or dislocation has been reduced or can be reduced by open reduction at the time of operation in children at least 18 months old. In acetabuloplasty the inclination of the acetabular roof is decreased by an osteotomy of the ilium made superior to the acetabulum. Pemberton described a *pericapsular osteotomy of the ilium* in which the osteotomy is made through the full thickness of the bone from just superior to the anteroinferior iliac spine anteriorly to the triradiate cartilage posteriorly; the triradiate cartilage acts as a hinge on which the acetabular roof is rotated anteriorly and laterally. This procedure decreases the volume of the acetabulum and produces joint incongruity that requires remodeling.

Osteotomies that free the acetabulum have been devised by Steel and by Eppright. These operations free part of the

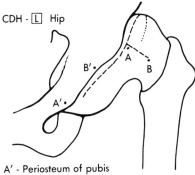

CDH - [L] Hip

A' - Periosteum of pubis
B' - Ant. inferior iliac spine

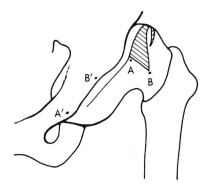

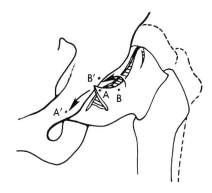

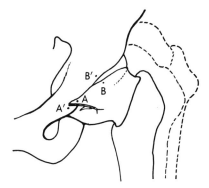

Fig. 27-22 Technique of capsulorrhaphy during open reduction of congenital dislocation of hip. (Redrawn from Wenger DR: *Instr Course Lect* 38:343, 1989.)

▼ **Table 27-1**   Recommended Osteotomies for Congenital Dislocation of the Hip

Osteotomy	Age	Indications
Salter innominate osteotomy	18 mo–6 yr	Congruous hip reduction; <10-15 degrees correction of acetabular index required
Pemberton acetabuloplasty	18 mo–10 yr	>10-15 degrees correction of acetabular index required; small femoral head, large acetabulum
Dial or Steel osteotomy	Skeletal maturity	Residual acetabular dysplasia; symptoms; congruous joint
Shelf procedure or Chiari osteotomy	Adolescent—skeletal maturity	Incongruous joint; symptoms; other osteotomy not possible

pelvis, creating a movable segment of bone that includes the acetabulum. They are indicated in adolescents and skeletally mature adults with residual dysplasia and subluxation in whom remodeling of the acetabulum can no longer be anticipated. These operations are useful because they place articular cartilage over the femoral head. On the other hand, the shelf operation and the operation of Chiari interpose capsular fibrous tissue between the femoral head and the reconstructed acetabulum.

In the triple innominate osteotomy (Steel), the ischium, the superior pubic ramus, and the ilium superior to the acetabulum are all divided, and the acetabulum is repositioned and stabilized by a bone graft and metal pins. In the pericapsular dial osteotomy of the acetabulum (Eppright), the entire acetabulum superiorly, posteriorly, inferiorly, and anteriorly is freed by osteotomy and as a single segment of bone is redirected to appropriately cover the femoral head.

The *shelf* procedure (Staheli) is useful for subluxations and dislocations that have been reduced and in which no other osteotomy will establish a congruous joint with apposition of the articular cartilage of the acetabulum to the femoral head. In a classic shelf operation the acetabular roof is extended laterally, posteriorly, or anteriorly, either by a graft or by turning distally over the femoral head the acetabular roof and part of the lateral cortex of the ilium superior to it.

Innominate osteotomy with medial displacement of the acetabulum, an operation devised by Chiari for patients over 4 years old, is a modified shelf operation that places the femoral head beneath a surface of bone and joint capsule and corrects the pathological lateral displacement of the femur. An osteotomy is made at the level of the acetabulum, and the femur and the acetabulum are displaced medially. The inferior surface of the proximal fragment forms a roof over the femoral head.

General recommendations for these osteotomies are summarized in Table 27-1.

◆ *Salter Innominate Osteotomy*

During open reduction of congenital dislocations of the hip, Salter observed that the entire acetabulum faces more anterolaterally than normal. Thus, when the hip is extended the femoral head is insufficiently "covered" anteriorly, and when it is adducted there is insufficient coverage superiorly. Salter's osteotomy of the innominate bone redirects the entire acetabulum so that its roof "covers" the femoral head both

anteriorly and superiorly. If indicated to correct acetabular dysplasia, any dislocation or subluxation must be reduced concentrically before this operation is performed; if not, then open reduction is carried out at the time of osteotomy. During the operation any contractures of the adductor or iliopsoas muscles are released by tenotomy, and in dislocations when the capsule is elongated, a capsulorrhaphy is carried out. Salter recommended his osteotomy in the primary treatment of congenital dislocation of the hip in children between the ages of 18 months and 6 years and in the primary treatment of congenital subluxation as late as early adulthood. He also recommended it in the secondary treatment of any residual or recurrent dislocation or subluxation after other methods of treatment within the age limits described (Fig. 27-23).

The following prerequisites are necessary for the success of this operation:

1. The femoral head must be positioned opposite the level of the acetabulum. This may require a period of traction before surgery or primary femoral shortening.
2. Contractures of the iliopsoas and adductor muscles must be released. This is indicated in subluxations and dislocations. Open reduction is performed for hip dislocation but usually is unnecessary for hip subluxation.
3. The femoral head must be reduced into the depth of the true acetabulum completely and concentrically. This generally requires careful open reduction and excision of any soft tissue, exclusive of the labrum, from the acetabulum.
4. The joint must be reasonably congruous.
5. The range of motion of the hip must be good, especially in abduction, internal rotation, and flexion.

In a cadaver study, Birnbaum et al. identified several structures that are at risk of injury during a Salter innominate osteotomy.

1. The lateral femoral cutaneous nerve may be injured during an anterior approach. Ensuring that the skin including the lateral femoral cutaneous nerve is pulled anteriorly will avoid this.
2. The nutrient vessels to the tensor fasciae latae muscle can be injured if retraction is too prolonged.
3. The sciatic nerve can be crushed or irritated by an inadequate subperiosteal approach during the pull on the Hohmann retractor.
4. An inadequate subperiosteal application of the medial Hohmann retractor can damage the obturator nerve.

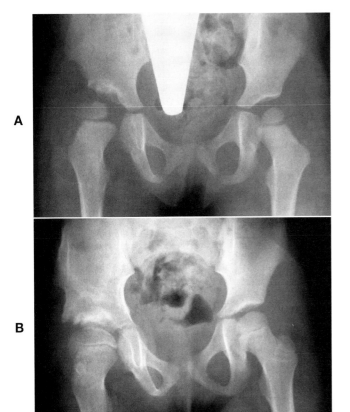

Fig. 27-23   Salter osteotomy for congenital dislocation of hip. **A,** Residual acetabular dysplasia and subluxation of right hip in 4-year-old girl in whom open reduction had been performed at age of 9 months. **B,** One year after repeat open reduction and Salter innominate osteotomy.

5. Too prolonged retraction of the iliopsoas muscle can cause compression of the femoral nerve.

They emphasized that, because of the narrow spatial connection between the anatomical pathways and the osteotomy area, strict subperiosteal dissection and careful use of retractors are essential to prevent nerve and vessel injuries.

TECHNIQUE 27-9 *(Including Open Reduction—Salter)*

Place the patient supine on the operating table with the thorax on the affected side elevated by a radiolucent sandbag. Drape the trunk on the affected side to the midline anteriorly and posteriorly and to the lower rib cage superiorly. Drape the lower extremity so that it can be moved freely during the operation. Next, release the adductor muscles by subcutaneous or open tenotomy. Make a skin incision beginning just inferior to the middle of the iliac crest, extending anteriorly to just inferior to the anterosuperior iliac spine and continuing to about the middle of the inguinal ligament. Decrease bleeding by applying pressure with sponges to the wound edges.

Bluntly dissect between the tensor fascia lata muscle laterally and the sartorius and rectus femoris medially and

expose the anterosuperior iliac spine. Next, dissect the rectus femoris from the underlying joint capsule and release its reflected head. Make a deep incision separating the iliac apophysis along the crest from the posterior end of the skin incision to the anterosuperior iliac spine anteriorly and then turning distally to the anteroinferior iliac spine.

Reflect the lateral part of the iliac apophysis and the periosteum from the lateral surface of the iliac crest in a continuous sheet inferiorly to the superior edge of the acetabulum and posteriorly to the greater sciatic notch. Free any adhesions of the joint capsule from the lateral surface of the ilium and from any false acetabulum. Expose the capsule anteriorly and laterally by dissecting bluntly the interval between it and the abductor muscles.

Next, pack the dissected spaces with large sponges to control bleeding and to increase the interval between the reflected periosteum and the sciatic notch. If concentric reduction of the femoral head into the acetabulum is impossible, open the capsule superiorly and anteriorly, parallel with and about 1 cm distal to the rim of the acetabulum.

Excise the ligamentum teres if it is hypertrophied. Next, gently reduce the femoral head into the acetabulum. Never excise the limbus. Incise the distal flap of capsule at right angles to the first incision, thus creating a T-shaped incision, and resect the inferolateral triangular flap so created. Test the stability of the joint; if the head becomes displaced superiorly from the acetabulum when the hip is adducted or anteriorly when it is extended or externally rotated, then osteotomy of the innominate bone is performed.

Next, allow the hip to redislocate and then strip the medial half of the iliac apophysis from the anterior half of the iliac crest and strip the periosteum from the medial surface of the ilium posteriorly and inferiorly to expose the entire medial aspect of the bone to the sciatic notch. Pack the surfaces thus exposed with sponges, again to control the loss of blood and to enlarge the interval between the periosteum and the bone. Next, expose the tendinous part of the iliopsoas muscle at the level of the pelvic brim. With scissors separate the tendinous part from the muscular part and divide the former while protecting the muscle. Pass a curved forceps subperiosteally medial to the ilium into the sciatic notch and with it grasp one end of a Gigli saw. Then gently retract the curved forceps to pass the Gigli saw into the sciatic notch.

Retract the tissues medially and laterally from the ilium and divide the bone with the saw in a straight line from the sciatic notch to the anteroinferior spine. Remove a full-thickness graft from the anterior part of the iliac crest (Fig. 27-24, *A*) and trim it to the shape of a wedge. Make the base of the wedge about as wide as the distance between the anterosuperior and anteroinferior iliac spines. With towel clips grasp each fragment of the osteotomized ilium. Next, insert a curved elevator into the sciatic notch and, by levering it anteriorly and by exerting traction on the towel

continued

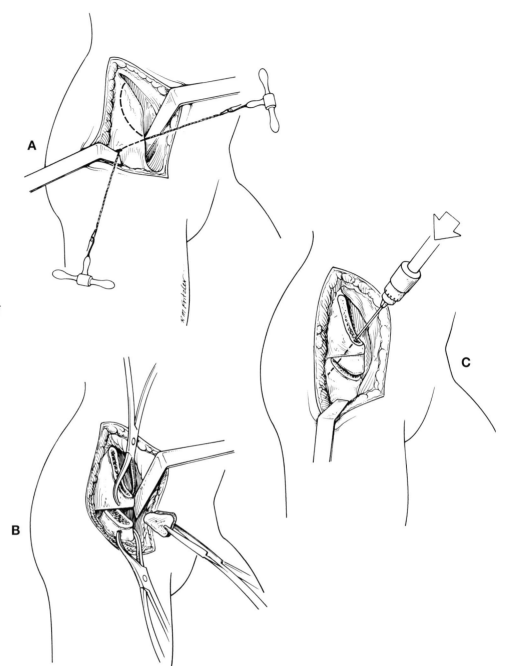

Fig. 27-24 Salter technique of osteotomy of innominate bone, including open reduction (see text). (Redrawn from Salter RB: *J Bone Joint Surg* 43B:518, 1961.)

clip that grasps the inferior fragment, shift this fragment anteriorly, inferiorly, and laterally to open the osteotomy anterolaterally. Be sure that the osteotomy remains closed posteriorly (Fig. 27-24, *B*). Placing the limb in a figure-four position makes displacement of the distal fragment easier.

Do not apply traction in a cephalad direction on the proximal fragment because this may dislocate the sacroiliac joint.

Next, insert the bone graft into the osteotomy and release the traction on the inferior fragment. Drill a strong

Kirschner wire through the remaining superior part of the ilium, through the graft, and into the inferior fragment (Fig. 27-24, *C*). Be sure that the Kirschner wire does not enter the acetabulum but that it does traverse all three fragments. Next, drill a second Kirschner wire parallel with the first, using the same precautions.

Reduce the femoral head again into the acetabulum and reevaluate its stability. Reduction should now be stable with the hip either in adduction or in slight external rotation. While closing the wound have an assistant hold the knee

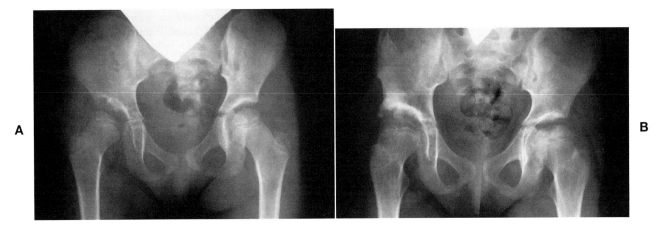

Fig. 27-25 Pemberton acetabuloplasty. **A,** Symptomatic residual acetabular dysplasia in 8-year-old girl after treatment of congenital dislocation of right hip. **B,** After Pemberton acetabuloplasty.

flexed and the hip slightly abducted, flexed, and internally rotated. Next, obliterate any residual pocket of capsule by performing a capsulorrhaphy.

Move the distal half of the lateral flap of capsule medially beyond the anteroinferior iliac spine. This brings the capsular edges together and increases the stability of reduction by keeping the hip internally rotated. Repair the capsule with interrupted sutures. Suture the sartorius and rectus femoris tendons to their origins. Suture together over the iliac crest the two halves of the iliac apophysis. Cut the Kirschner wires so that their anterior ends lie within the subcutaneous fat. Next, close the skin with a continuous subcuticular suture. With the hip held in the same position as during closure, apply a single spica cast.

AFTERTREATMENT. At 8 to 12 weeks the spica cast is removed, and with the patient under general or local anesthesia the Kirschner wires also are removed. The position of the osteotomy and of the hip is checked by roentgenograms.

◆ Pemberton Acetabuloplasty

The term *acetabuloplasty* designates operations that redirect the inclination of the acetabular roof by an osteotomy of the ilium superior to the acetabulum followed by levering of the roof inferiorly.

Pemberton devised an acetabuloplasty that he called *pericapsular osteotomy of the ilium* in which an osteotomy is made through the full thickness of the ilium, using the triradiate cartilage as the hinge about which the acetabular roof is rotated anteriorly and laterally. After a review of 115 hips in 91 patients followed for at least 2 years after surgery, Pemberton recommended this procedure for any dysplastic hip in patients between the age of 1 year and the age when the triradiate cartilage becomes too inflexible to serve as a hinge (about 12 years of age in girls and 14 years in boys), provided that any

subluxation or dislocation has been reduced or can be reduced at the time of osteotomy (Fig. 27-25).

Coleman, in a review of pericapsular and innominate osteotomies, noted that one advantage of the former operation is that internal fixation is not required, and thus a second, but minor, operation is avoided. Furthermore, a greater degree of correction can be achieved with less rotation of the acetabulum in the pericapsular osteotomy because the fulcrum, the triradiate cartilage, is nearer the site of desired correction. According to Coleman, however, Pemberton's operation is technically more difficult to perform. In addition, it alters the configuration and capacity of the acetabulum and can result in an incongruous relationship between it and the femoral head; consequently some remodeling of the acetabulum is required.

TECHNIQUE 27-10 *(Pemberton)*

Place the patient supine with a small radiolucent sandbag beneath the affected hip and expose the hip through an anterior iliofemoral approach. Make the superior part of the incision distal to and parallel with the iliac crest and extend it from the anterosuperior spine anteriorly to the middle of the crest posteriorly. Extend the distal part of the incision from the anterosuperior spine inferiorly for 5 cm parallel with the inguinal crease. Beginning at the crest, strip the gluteus and the tensor fascia lata muscles subperiosteally from the anterior third of the ilium distally to the joint capsule and posteriorly until the greater sciatic notch is exposed. Next, with a sharp elevator separate the iliac apophysis with its attached abdominal muscles from the anterior third of the iliac crest and then strip the muscles subperiosteally from the medial aspect of the ilium until the sciatic notch is again exposed. At this point open the capsule of the hip and remove any soft tissue that restricts reduction. Reduce the hip under direct vision and be sure that it is well seated; then redislocate it until the osteotomy has been made and propped open with a graft.

Next, insert two flat retractors subperiosteally into the

continued

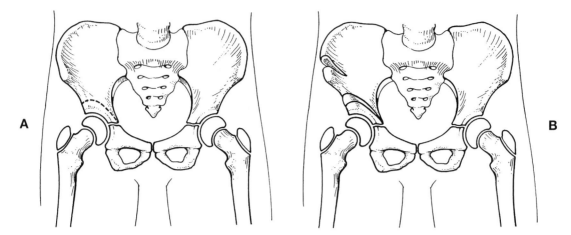

Fig. 27-26   Pemberton pericapsular osteotomy. **A,** Line of osteotomy beginning slightly superior to anteroinferior iliac spine and curving into triradiate cartilage. **B,** Completed osteotomy with acetabular roof in corrected position and wedge of bone impacted into open osteotomy site.

sciatic notch, one along the medial surface of the ilium and one along the lateral surface to keep the anterior third of the ilium exposed both medially and laterally. With a narrow curved osteotome cut through the lateral cortex of the ilium as follows. First, start slightly superior to the anteroinferior iliac spine and curve the osteotomy posteriorly about 1 cm proximal to and parallel with the joint capsule until the osteotome is seen to be well anterior to the retractor resting in the sciatic notch. Image intensification aids in confirming correct placement of the osteotomy.

From this point when driven farther, the blade of the osteotome disappears from sight, and it is therefore important to direct its tip sufficiently inferiorly so that it does not enter the sciatic notch but instead enters the ilioischial rim of the triradiate cartilage at its midpoint. After directing the osteotome properly, drive it 1.5 cm farther to complete the osteotomy of the lateral cortex of the ilium. With the same osteotome make a corresponding cut in the medial cortex of the ilium, starting anteriorly at the same point just superior to the anteroinferior iliac spine. Direct this cut posteriorly parallel with that in the lateral cortex until it reaches the triradiate cartilage (Fig. 27-26, *A*).

The direction in which the acetabular roof becomes displaced after the osteotomy is controlled by varying the position of the posterior part of the osteotomy of the medial cortex. The more anterior this part of the osteotomy, the less the acetabular roof rotates anteriorly; conversely, the more posterior this part of the osteotomy, the more the acetabular roof rotates anteriorly. After completing the osteotomy of the two cortices, insert a wide curved osteotome into the anterior part of the osteotomy and lever the distal fragment distally until the anterior edges of the two fragments are at least 2 to 3 cm apart.

The acetabular roof should be turned inferiorly far enough to result in an estimated acetabular index of 0 degrees on roentgenogram. Next, cut a narrow groove in the anteroposterior direction in each raw surface of the ilium. Resect a wedge of bone from the anterior part of the ilium, including the anterosuperior spine; then with a lamina spreader separate the osteotomy fragments and place the wedge of bone in the grooves made in the surfaces of the ilium; drive the wedge into place and firmly impact it. The acetabular roof should then remain fixed in the corrected position (Fig. 27-27, *B*). Hold the correction with a Kirschner wire, if necessary. If the hip has remained dislocated during the osteotomy, reduce it at this time. Perform a meticulous capsulorrhaphy for additional soft tissue stability. Suture the iliac apophysis over the remaining ilium and close the wound.

AFTERTREATMENT. With the hip in neutral position (or in slight abduction and internal rotation, if this has been found the most favorable position for closure of the wound), a spica cast is applied from the nipple line to the toes on the affected side and to above the knee on the opposite side. At 8 to 12 weeks the cast is removed, and the osteotomy is checked by roentgenograms.

◆ *Steel Osteotomy*

The Pemberton pericapsular osteotomy is limited by the mobility of the triradiate cartilage, and hinging on this cartilage can cause premature physeal closure. Although the Salter innominate osteotomy can be used in older patients, its results depend on the mobility of the symphysis pubis, and the amount of femoral head coverage is limited. Other, more complex osteotomies, such as those of Steel and Eppright, can provide more correction and improve femoral head coverage.

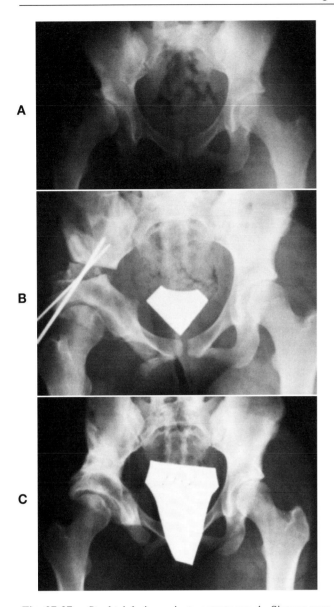

Fig. 27-27   Steel triple innominate osteotomy. **A,** Sixteen-year-old girl with painful right hip, subluxation, and acetabular dysplasia. **B,** After Steel osteotomy. **C,** One year after surgery. (Courtesy Randal Betz, MD, and Howard Steel, MD.)

In the *triple innominate osteotomy* developed by Steel, the ischium, the superior pubic ramus, and the ilium superior to the acetabulum are all divided, and the acetabulum is repositioned and stabilized by a bone graft and pins. The objective of this procedure is to establish a stable hip in anatomical position for dislocation or subluxation of the hip in older children when this is impossible by any one of the other osteotomies (Fig. 27-27). For the operation to be successful the articular surfaces of the joint must be congruous or become so once the acetabulum has been redirected so that a functional, painless range of motion will be achieved and a Trendelenburg gait will be absent. Steel reviewed 45 patients in whom 52 of his operations had been

performed. The results were satisfactory in 40 hips and unsatisfactory in 12. The unsatisfactory hips were painful and easily fatigued; in two the Trendelenburg test was positive, and in one significant motion had been lost.

Before surgery skeletal traction must be used until the femoral head is brought distally to the level of the acetabulum or femoral shortening must be performed; if necessary, any contracted muscles about the hip are released surgically.

Using three-dimensional CT scanning, Frick, Kim, and Wenger identified excessive (more than 10 degrees) external rotation of the acetabulum after triple innominate osteotomy in five hips, which included two with pubic osteotomy nonunions, two with ischial nonunions, and one with marked external rotation of the leg. They cautioned that the surgical technique for triple innominate osteotomy should be designed to avoid excessive external rotation of the acetabular fragment, which can result in (1) excessive external rotation of the lower limb, (2) decreased posterior coverage, (3) increased gaps at the pubic and ischial osteotomy sites with resultant higher rates of nonunion, and (4) lateralization of the joint center. Their technique modifications include avoidance of the "figure-of-four" maneuver to mobilize the acetabulum (they believe this promotes external rotation of the acetabulum); strict attention to the intraoperative landmarks of the proximal ilium and anterior inferior iliac spine, keeping the anterior inferior iliac spine in line with the plane of the proximal ilium to prevent external rotation; and use of a temporary Schanz screw in the acetabular segment to serve as a handle to guide the acetabulum into the correct position. Careful evaluation of the transverse plane acetabular position before and after provisional fixation is recommended to aid in preventing rotational malunions.

TECHNIQUE 27-11 *(Steel)*

Place the patient supine on the operating table and flex the hip and knee 90 degrees. Keep the hip in neutral abduction, adduction, and rotation. First drape the posterior aspect of the proximal thigh and the buttock, leaving the ischial tuberosity exposed. Make a transverse incision perpendicular to the long axis of the femoral shaft 1 cm proximal to the gluteal crease. Retract the gluteus maximus muscle laterally and expose the hamstring muscles at their ischial origin. By sharp dissection free the biceps femoris, the most superficial muscle in the area, from the ischium and expose the interval between the semimembranosus and the semitendinosus muscles. The sciatic nerve lies far enough laterally not to be endangered. Next, insert a curved hemostat in the interval between the origins of the semimembranosus and the semitendinosus deep to the ischium and into the obturator foramen. Elevate the origins of the obturator internus and externus and bring the tip of the hemostat out at the inferior margin of the ischial ramus. Be sure the hemostat remains in contact with the bone during its passage deep to the ramus. Next, with an osteotome directed posterolaterally and 45 degrees from the perpendicular, divide completely the ischial ramus. Allow the origin of the

continued

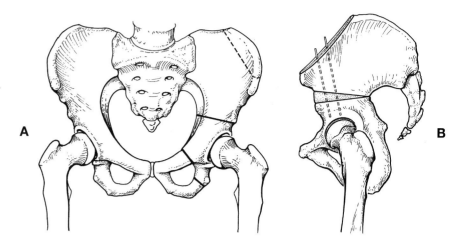

Fig. 27-28 Steel triple innominate osteotomy. **A,** Osteotomies to be performed in iliac wing and superior and inferior pubic rami. Note wedge of bone to be taken as graft from most superior portion of ilium. **B,** Lateral view showing graft in place and fixation with two Kirschner wires.

biceps femoris to fall into place. Next, suture the gluteus maximus to the deep fascia and close the skin.

Change gowns, gloves, and instruments and begin in the iliopubic area the second stage of the operation. As an alternative, the superior and inferior pubic rami can be dissected and divided through a medial adductor approach. If a posterior incision was chosen, however, proceed with a full skin preparation medially to the midline and superiorly to the costal margin and drape the extremity free. Through an anterior iliofemoral approach reflect the iliac and gluteal muscles from the wing of the ilium. Detach the sartorius and the lateral attachments of the inguinal ligament from the anterosuperior iliac spine and reflect them medially. Next, reflect the iliacus and psoas muscles subperiosteally from the inner surface of the pelvis; this protects the femoral neurovascular bundle. Next, divide the tendinous part of the origin of the iliopsoas and expose the pectineal tubercle. Detach the pectineus muscle subperiosteally from the superior pubic ramus and expose the bone 1 cm medial to the pubic tubercle. Pass a curved hemostat superior to the superior pubic ramus into the obturator foramen near the bone. With this hemostat penetrate the obturator fascia so that the tip of the hemostat is brought out inferior to the ramus. If the bone is especially thick, pass a second hemostat inferior to the ramus and direct it superiorly to contact the first one. Next, direct an osteotome posteromedially and 15 degrees from the perpendicular and perform an osteotomy of the pubic ramus.

The obturator artery, vein, and nerve are protected by the hemostat. Using the technique as described by Salter for innominate osteotomy, divide the ilium with a Gigli saw. When this osteotomy has been completed, free the periosteum and fascia from the medial wall of the pelvis to free the acetabular segment (Fig. 27-28). If the femoral head is subluxated or dislocated, open the capsule at this time and remove any tissue obstructing reduction. Reduce the femoral head as near as possible to the center of the triradiate cartilage and close the capsule.

Next, with a towel clip grasp the anteroinferior iliac spine and rotate the acetabular segment in the desired direction, usually anteriorly and laterally, until the femoral head is covered. In an older child, use a lamina spreader to open the osteotomy because the sacroiliac joint usually is more stable in this age group and is not likely to be subluxated. With the acetabular fragment in proper position, stabilize it with a triangular bone graft removed from the superior rim of the ilium. Transfix the graft with two pins that penetrate the inner wall of the ilium. Next, allow the pectineus and iliopsoas muscles to fall into place. Reattach the sartorius and the lateral end of the inguinal ligament to the anterosuperior iliac spine and close the wound in layers.

AFTERTREATMENT. A spica cast is applied with the hip in 20 degrees of abduction, 5 degrees of flexion, and neutral rotation. At 8 to 10 weeks the cast and pins are removed, and active and passive motion of the hip are started. All three osteotomies usually unite by 12 weeks after surgery, at which time progressive weight-bearing on crutches is started.

◆ **Dega Osteotomy**
In 1969 Dega described a transiliac osteotomy for the treatment of residual acetabular dysplasia secondary to congenital hip dysplasia or dislocation. This incomplete transiliac osteotomy involves osteotomy of the anterior and middle portions of the inner cortex of the ilium, leaving an intact hinge posteriorly consisting of the intact posteromedial iliac cortex and sciatic notch. The original technique and modifications and the results of the procedure have been described almost exclusively in the German and Polish literature. In 1996 Reichel and Hein reported 70 modified Dega acetabuloplasties done simultaneously with intertrochanteric osteotomies in 51 patients with developmental dysplasia. At long-term follow-up (average, 15 years), functional results were good or very good in 80%, fair in 11%, and poor in 9%. The rate of avascular necrosis was 5.7%. More recently, Grudziak and Ward reported their results

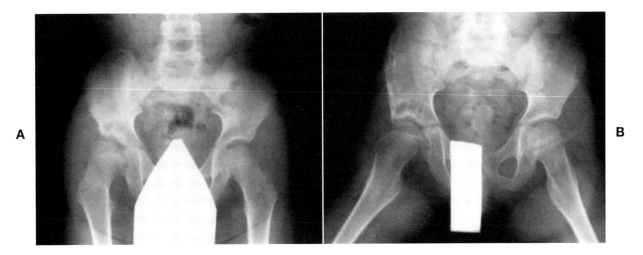

Fig. 27-29   Before (**A**) and after (**B**) Dega transiliac osteotomy.

with the Dega osteotomy for congenital hip dysplasia in 24 hips and presented a description of the technique. In their series 20 hips had concomitant femoral osteotomies and 13 had anterior open reductions of the hip in addition to the Dega osteotomy. Patients ranged in age from 23 months to 15 years and 10 months (average age, 5 years and 10 months). At an average follow-up of 55 months (range, 28 to 91 months), all patients had unlimited physical activity and no limp, and the average acetabular index was decreased from 33 degrees preoperatively to 12 degrees at follow-up. Grudziak and Ward suggested that the Dega osteotomy can both reorient and reshape the acetabulum; their roentgenographic results showed changes in the obturator foramen, the acetabular index, and the center-edge angle in most patients. Because of the variable hinge location, the Dega osteotomy can be done with either an open or closed triradiate cartilage, although Grudziak and Ward recommended that it be done before closure of the triradiate cartilage. They emphasized that this osteotomy is but one component of the comprehensive, complicated surgery required to treated severe congenital dysplasia of the hip in children of walking age. It must be accompanied by a satisfactory open reduction and an appropriate correction of proximal femoral deformity when needed (Fig. 27-29).

TECHNIQUE 27-12 *(Grudziak and Ward)*

Position the patient supine with the involved hip tilted up approximately 30 to 40 degrees by a bump placed at the midlumbar level. Make an extended anterolateral incision starting 1 cm inferior and posterior to the anterosuperior iliac spine and extending distally over the proximal part of the femur, centered over the greater trochanter (Fig. 27-30, *A*). Develop the interval between the tensor fasciae latae muscle posteriorly and the sartorius muscle anteriorly and release the sartorius from its origin on the anterosuperior iliac spine. Sharply reflect the abductor muscles off of the lateral wall of the ilium just distal to the

iliac apophysis but do not split the apophysis itself. Completely separate the abductor muscles and periosteum from the ilium and the hip capsule back to the sciatic notch, which is fully exposed, and insert an adult-size blunt Hohmann retractor into the notch. Do not dissect either the muscles or the periosteum off of the inner wall of the ilium. Separate the reflected head of the rectus femoris muscle from the hip capsule and incise it. Detach the tendon of the straight head of the rectus femoris muscle from the anteroinferior iliac spine only when necessary for proper exposure of the capsule. Isolate the tendinous portion of the iliopsoas muscle from the capsule and transect it either over the anteromedial aspect of the capsule just distal to the pelvic brim or more distally near its insertion. If required, reduce the hip and perform a femoral osteotomy with shortening and rotation to correct excessive anteversion.

Split the vastus lateralis fascia and muscle to expose the proximal part of the femur. If valgus correction was planned preoperatively, use a 90-degree AO infant blade-plate for fixation and reduce the true neck-shaft angle to 110 to 120 degrees. If shortening and rotation without valgus correction was planned, use a straight one-third tubular AO plate. Insert two small Kirschner wires into the femur, one above the osteotomy plane and the other below the level of the desired shortening, to aid in determining the amount of anteversion correction. Make the femoral osteotomy in the subtrochanteric or intertrochanteric region and allow the fragments to overlap as the femoral head is reduced deeply into the acetabulum. Shorten the femur equivalent to the amount of overlap. Use a bone clamp to obtain preliminary fixation of the straight plate or 90-degree blade plate. Flex the hip to 90 degrees and loosen the clamp so that enough external rotation of the distal fragment is added to make internal and external rotation of the hip symmetrical. Observation of the guide wires at this point reveals an estimated anteversion

continued

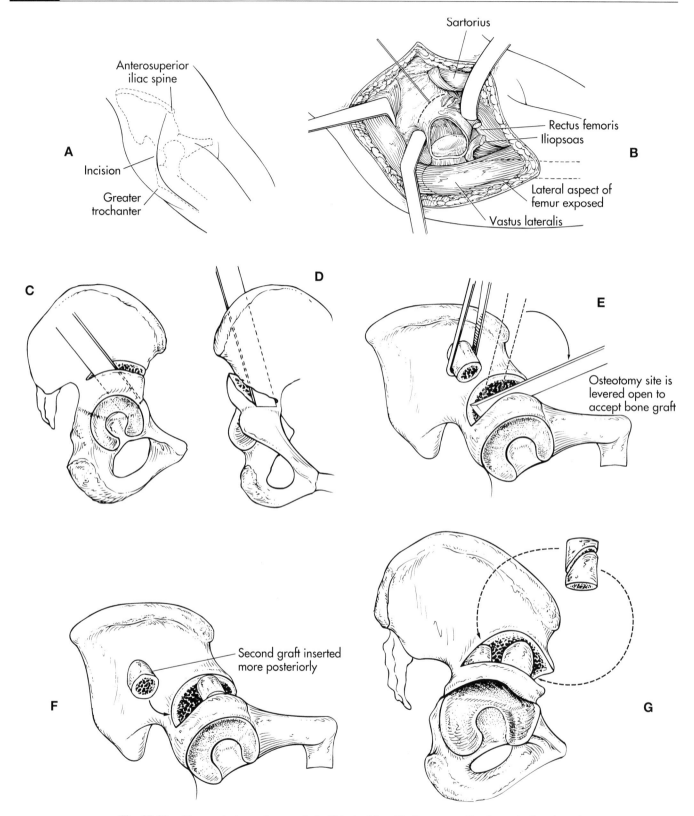

Fig. 27-30   Dega osteotomy (see text). **A,** Skin incision. **B,** Osteotomy line is marked on lateral cortex of ilium; guide wire is inserted to exit just above horizontal limb of triradiate cartilage. **C,** Osteotome penetrates inner cortex. **D,** View from inner side of pelvis shows intact posteromedial cortical hinge; the length of the intact inner cortex depends on the amount of anterior and lateral coverage desired. **E,** Osteotomy is levered open with osteotome or small laminar spreader. **F,** Two grafts large enough to keep osteotomy open at premeasured height are inserted. **G,** Larger graft is inserted anteriorly; posterior graft should be smaller to avoid loosening the anterior graft. (From Grudziak JS, Ward WT: *J Bone Joint Surg* 83A:845, 2001.)

correction ranging from 10 to 40 degrees. At this point, the femoral head will rest deeply in the still steep acetabulum and have a diminished tendency to dislocate with the leg in neutral position.

Next, make the Dega osteotomy to decrease acetabular dysplasia and to enhance containment of the femoral head. Mark the orientation of the osteotomy on the lateral cortex of the ilium (Fig. 27-30, B). The direction of the osteotomy is curvilinear when viewed from the lateral cortex, starting just above the anteroinferior iliac spine, curving gently cephalad and posteriorly to reach a point superior to the midpoint of the acetabulum, and then continuing posteriorly to end approximately 1 to 1.5 cm in front of the sciatic notch. The most cephalad extent of the osteotomy is in the middle of the acetabulum, at a point on the ilium determined by the steepness of the acetabulum. Very steep acetabular inclinations require a correspondingly higher midpoint. Insert a guide wire under fluoroscopic control at the most cephalad point of the curvilinear marking line, directing it caudally and medially to ensure that the osteotomy will exit at the appropriate level just above the horizontal limb of the triradiate cartilage. Use a straight 0.25- or 0.5-inch osteotome to make the bone cut, which extends obliquely medially and inferiorly, paralleling the guide wire to exit through the inner cortex just above the iliopubic and ilioischial limbs of the triradiate cartilage (Fig. 27-30, C), leaving the posterior one third of the inner cortex intact (Fig. 27-30, D). If predominantly anterior coverage is desired, cut the medial (inner) cortex over the anterior and middle portion, leaving only the posterior sciatic notch hinge intact. If more lateral coverage is desired, leave more of the medial cortex intact, resulting in a posteromedial hinge based on the posteromedial inner cortex and the entire sciatic notch. Generally, approximately one quarter to one third of the inner pelvic cortex is left intact posteriorly. With experience, the osteotomy cut might be done safely without fluoroscopic guidance, as in Dega's original description; however, we prefer to use fluoroscopy.

Use a 0.5-inch osteotome to gently lever open the osteotomy site either anteriorly or laterally in a controlled manner (Fig. 27-30, E). A small laminar spreader also is useful for this maneuver. Quite often, while the osteotomy site is being opened, the osteotomy cut on the outer cortex of the ilium propagates toward the sciatic notch as a greenstick fracture. However, since the posterior portion of the inner cortex is still intact, the outer cortical greenstick fracture does not weaken the recoil and stability at the osteotomy site.

Keep the osteotomy site open by inserting two correctly sized bone grafts (Fig. 27-30, F and G). Fashion the grafts from a bicortical segment of iliac crest bone or, alternatively, if femoral shortening has been done, use the segment of the femur that was removed. If there is a substantial gap at the osteotomy site, an autogenous femoral or iliac crest graft may not be sufficient. Under these circumstances, the height of the graft can be increased by using freeze-dried fibular allograft cut into trapezoidal sections. The correct graft height is determined by simply noting the opening of the osteotomy gap created by the laminar spreader or the levering osteotome. In congenital dysplasia, acetabular deficiency is most pronounced anteriorly, mandating placement of the larger graft more anteriorly. Wedge a smaller graft more posteriorly, just in front of the intact sciatic notch. Take care to ensure that both grafts are of an appropriate height and that the amount of correction of the dysplastic acetabulum provides enough coverage of the femoral head.

Once the grafts have been inserted, they are stable because of the inherent recoil at the osteotomy site produced by the intact sciatic notch. Metallic internal fixation is not necessary. Variations in the graft size and placement, extent of the outer and inner cortical cuts, and thickness of the acetabular fragment make it possible to both reorient and reshape the acetabulum. The more posterior the extent of the outer cortical cut, and the greater the amount of the inner cortex left intact, the more lateral the tilt of the acetabulum. A more cephalad starting point and a steeper osteotomy angle produce more lateral coverage. A more extensive cut through the inner cortex allows for more anterior coverage of the hip. Finally, the closer the osteotomy is to the acetabulum, the thinner and more pliable will be the acetabular fragment, theoretically allowing for more reshaping and less redirection to occur. These three-dimensional changes in the osteotomy are admittedly difficult to quantify, as is the true anatomical nature of a dysplastic hip. However, an experienced orthopaedic surgeon who is familiar with the spectrum of dysplastic hip pathology and who applies the principles described above should be able to perform an osteotomy that is precisely suited to the unique pathology of a given dysplastic hip. Once the osteotomy is done, satisfactory femoral head coverage can be appreciated and the hip should be stable during flexion and rotation.

After closure, apply a one and one half spica cast with the hip is neutral extension, approximately 20 degrees of internal rotation and 20 to 30 degrees of abduction.

AFTERTREATMENT. The cast is worn for 8 to 12 weeks, depending on the healing of the osteotomy site. After the cast is removed, progressive walking and range of motion are begun, but no formal physical therapy is prescribed.

Ganz (Bernese) Periacetabular Osteotomy. Ganz et al. developed a triplanar periacetabular osteotomy for adolescents and adults with dysplastic hips that require correction of congruency and containment to the femoral head. If significant degenerative changes involving the weight-bearing surface of the femoral head are present, a proximal femoral osteotomy can be added to provide uninvolved acetabular and proximal

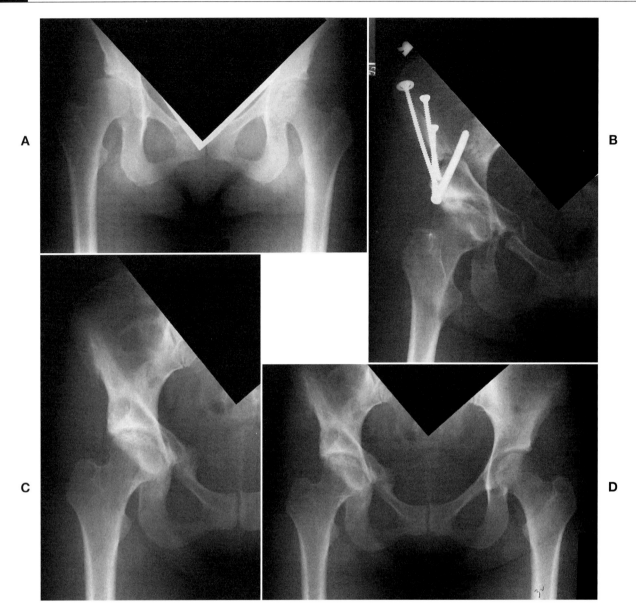

Fig. 27-31   A, Standing anteroposterior roentgenogram of 28-year-old woman with dysplastic right hip (lateral CE angle of 6 degrees). **B,** After Ganz osteotomy, lateral CE angle is 30 degrees, obliquity of weight-bearing zone of acetabulum has been eliminated, and femoral head is more medial in acetabulum. **C** and **D,** At 15 months after surgery, hardware has been removed, osteotomies are healed, cartilage space is widened, and weight-bearing portion of acetabulum is almost normal. (Courtesy Michael B. Millis, MD.)

femoral weight-bearing surfaces (Fig. 27-31). The reported advantages of periacetabular osteotomy include (1) only one approach is used; (2) a large amount of correction can be obtained in all directions, including the medial and lateral planes; (3) blood supply to the acetabulum is preserved; (4) the posterior column of the hemipelvis remains mechanically intact, allowing immediate crutch walking with minimal internal fixation; (5) the shape of the true pelvis is unaltered, permitting a normal child delivery; and (6) it can be combined with trochanteric osteotomy if needed. The technique for Ganz periacetabular osteotomy is described in Chapter 25.

◆ *Shelf Operations*

Shelf procedures have commonly been performed to enlarge the volume of the acetabulum; however, pelvic redirectional and displacement osteotomies have largely replaced this type of operation. The redirectional osteotomies are inappropriate in hips in which the femoral head and acetabulum are misshapen but still congruent, since redirection can cause incongruity.

Staheli described a slotted acetabular augmentation procedure to create a congruous acetabular extension in which the size and position of the augmentation can be easily controlled. A deficient acetabulum that cannot be corrected by redirec-

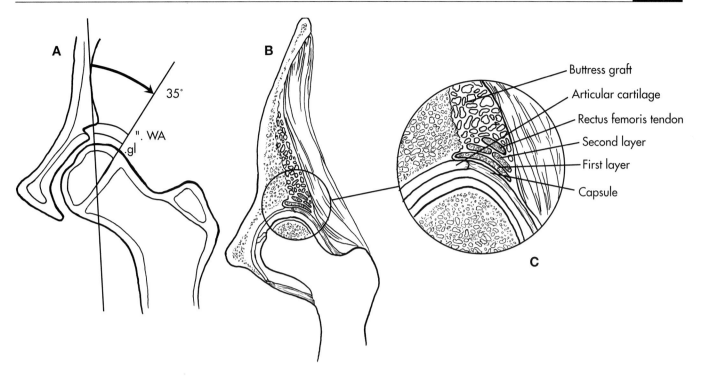

Fig. 27-32 Slotted acetabular augmentation of Staheli. **A,** Width of augmentation, *WA*, is determined preoperatively from standing anteroposterior roentgenogram of pelvis. CE angle and 35-degree angle are drawn. Graft length, *gl*, is sum of *WA* and slot depth. **B,** Objective of procedure is to provide congruous extension of acetabulum. **C,** Details of extension. (From Staheli LT: *J Pediatr Orthop* 1:321, 1981.)

tional pelvic osteotomy is the primary indication for this operation. Contraindications include dysplastic hips with spherical congruity suitable for redirectional osteotomy, hips requiring concurrent open reduction that must have supplementary stability, and patients unsuited for spica cast immobilization.

TECHNIQUE 27-13 *(Staheli)*

Before surgery the CE angle of Wiberg is determined from anteroposterior standing pelvic roentgenograms, and a normal CE angle (about 35 degrees) is drawn on the film. The additional width necessary to extend the existing acetabulum to achieve the normal angle is measured (Fig. 27-32). This determines the width of the augmentation; this measurement added to the depth of the slot gives the total graft length. If the patient is small or easily moved, the procedure is done on a standard operating table with the affected side elevated 15 degrees on a pad. For heavier patients, a fracture table is used and the involved limb is draped free.

Make a straight "bikini" skin incision 1 cm below and parallel to the iliac crest. Expose the hip joint through a standard iliofemoral approach. Divide the tendon of the reflected head of the rectus femoris muscle anteriorly and displace it posteriorly. If the capsule is abnormally thick (more than 6 to 7 mm), thin it by "filleting" with a scalpel.

The placement of the acetabular slot is the most critical part of the procedure; the slot must be created *exactly at the acetabular margin.* Determine the position of the slot by placing a probe into the joint to palpate the position of the acetabulum. Next, place a drill in the selected site and make an anteroposterior roentgenogram to verify correct position. The floor of the slot should be acetabular articular cartilage and little bone; the end and roof of the slot should be cancellous bone. The slot should be 1 cm deep.

Make the slot by drilling a series of holes with a 5/32-inch (4.5 mm) bit and join them with a narrow rongeur. Determine the length of the slot intraoperatively by the need for coverage. If excessive femoral anteversion is present, extend the slot anteriorly. If the acetabulum is deficient posteriorly, extend the slot in that direction.

Take thin strips of cortical and cancellous bone from the lateral surface of the ilium; cut these as long as possible. Extend the shallow decortication inferiorly from the iliac crest to the superior margin of the slot to ensure rapid fusion of the graft to the ilium. Do not remove the inner table of the ilium because this may change the contour of the pelvis.

Measure the depth of the slot and add this to the width of the augmentation as determined preoperatively. Select thin

continued

strips (1 mm) of cancellous bone and cut them into rectangles about 1 cm wide and of the appropriate length. Assemble these rectangular pieces on a moist sponge, cutting enough to provide a single layer the length of the augmentation. Apply the first layer radially from the slot with the concave side down to provide a congruous extension.

Select longer cancellous strips for the second layer and cut them to the length of the extension. Place these at right angles to the first layer and parallel to the acetabulum. They may be a little thicker (2 mm), especially the most lateral strip, to provide a well-defined lateral margin of the extension. Both layers must be of appropriate width and length. The augmentation should not extend too far anteriorly to avoid blocking hip flexion.

Secure these two layers of cancellous grafts by bringing the reflected head of the rectus femoris forward over the grafts and suturing it in its original position. A capsular flap can be substituted if this tendon is not available. Cut the remaining grafts into small pieces and pack them above but not beyond the initial layer. They are held in place by the reattached abductor muscles. Confirm the position and width of the graft by roentgenograms. After closure, apply a single hip spica cast with the hip in 15 degrees of abduction, 20 degrees of flexion, and neutral rotation (Fig. 27-33).

AFTERTREATMENT. The cast is removed after 6 weeks, and crutch walking is permitted with partial weight-bearing on the affected side until the graft is incorporated, usually at 3 to 4 months.

◆ Chiari Osteotomy

This is a capsular interposition arthroplasty and should be considered only in those instances when other reconstructions are impossible, that is, when the femoral head cannot be centered adequately in the acetabulum or in painfully subluxated hips with early signs of osteoarthritis. This procedure deepens the deficient acetabulum by medial displacement of the distal pelvic fragment and improves superolateral femoral coverage.

The Chiari procedure is an operation that places the femoral head beneath a surface of cancellous bone with the capacity for regeneration and corrects the lateral pathological displacement of the femur. An osteotomy of the pelvis is performed at the superior margin of the acetabulum, and the pelvis inferior to the osteotomy along with the femur is displaced medially (Fig. 27-34). The superior fragment of the osteotomy then becomes a shelf, and the capsule is interposed between it and the femoral head. After using this operation on more than 600 patients, 400 of whom have been observed for more than 2 years, Chiari recommended the operation in the following situations: (1) for congenital subluxations in patients 4 to 6 years old or older, including adults (including subluxations that

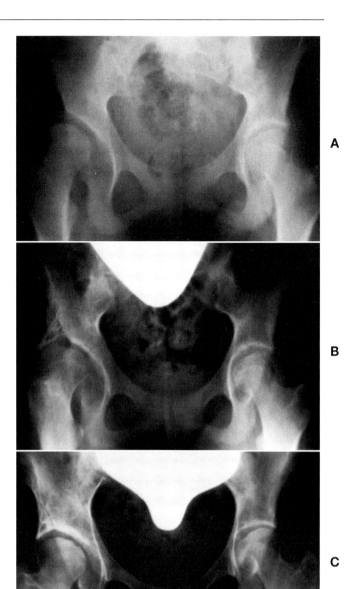

Fig. 27-33   Staheli slotted acetabular augmentation. **A,** Fourteen-year-old girl with painful right acetabular dysplasia. **B,** Four months after operation. **C,** One year after operation, excellent graft incorporation. (Courtesy Lynn Staheli, MD.)

persist after conservative treatment of dislocations and those previously not treated), (2) for untreated congenital dislocations in patients over 4 years old, soon after open or closed reduction, (3) for dysplastic hips with osteoarthritis, (4) for paralytic dislocations caused by muscular weakness or spasticity, and (5) for coxa magna after Perthes disease or avascular necrosis after treatment of congenital dysplasia. These indications are broader than those usually accepted by most pediatric orthopaedists. For children younger than about 10 years of age the osteotomy is not recommended in

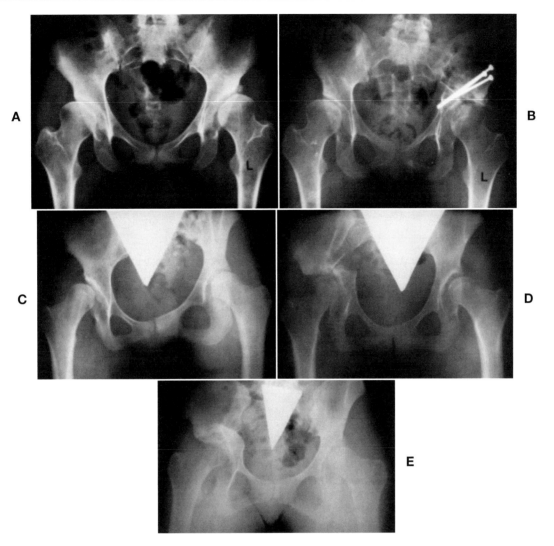

Fig. 27-34   Chiari osteotomy. **A,** Young adult with painful, bilateral acetabular dysplasia, greater on left than on right. **B,** After Chiari osteotomy of left hip. Note optional internal fixation and medial bone grafting. **C,** Bilateral acetabular dysplasia in 12-year-old girl. **D,** After surgery, right hip is completely displaced. **E,** One year after Chiari osteotomy. (**A** and **B** courtesy Randal Betz, MD.)

subluxations or in dislocations that can be reduced either surgically or conservatively and in which osteotomy of the innominate bone, acetabuloplasty, or osteotomies that free the acetabulum would result in a competent acetabulum. Some surgeons recommend the operation for patients in the second and later decades who have symptomatic early subluxation of the hip with acetabular dysplasia too severe to be treated by other pelvic osteotomies; for them innominate osteotomy with medial displacement is preferred to a shelf operation. Nakata et al. reported 96% excellent or good results in 96 hips after modified Chiari (dome) osteotomies done in 87 patients (average age, 29 years) with pain and disability because of osteoarthritis secondary to hip dysplasia. At an average follow-up of 13 years, only 4 of the hips had required total hip arthroplasty. The procedure also has been used in older children with underlying neuromuscular disorders and acetabular dysplasia.

Chiari's operation is a capsular arthroplasty because the capsule is interposed between the newly formed acetabular roof and the femoral head. Because the biomechanics of the hip are improved by displacing the hip nearer the midline, a Trendelenburg limp often is eliminated.

TECHNIQUE 27-14 *(Chiari)*

Place the patient supine on a fracture table with the feet fastened to the traction plate. Slightly abduct and externally rotate the affected hip. Make an anterolateral "bikini" incision about 10 cm long. Develop the interval between the tensor fascia lata and the sartorius muscles and laterally retract the former. Next, incise the iliac apophysis in line with the iliac crest. With a periosteal elevator detach the lateral half of the apophysis along with the tensor fascia lata muscle and the anterior part of the gluteus medius muscle.

continued

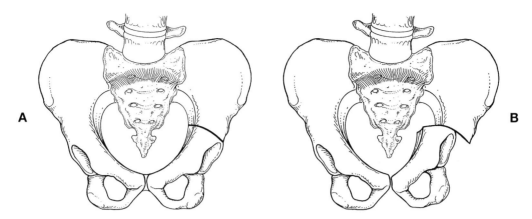

Fig. 27-35 Chiari medial displacement osteotomy. **A,** Line of osteotomy extending from immediately superior to lip of acetabulum into sciatic notch. Osteotomy can be curved to facilitate femoral head coverage. **B,** Completed osteotomy with medial displacement of distal fragment for interpositional capsular arthroplasty.

Dissect these muscles subperiosteally and retract them posteriorly. Insert a periosteal elevator between the capsule of the hip and the gluteus minimus. Dissect subperiosteally posteriorly to the point where the pelvis curves inferiorly. Next, with a curved periosteal elevator dissect subperiosteally farther posteriorly until the sciatic notch is reached. Replace this elevator with a flexible metal ribbon retractor 3 cm wide. This completes the dissection posteriorly. Next, return anteriorly to the medial aspect of the ilium. With a periosteal elevator strip the iliacus muscle and the underlying periosteum posteriorly to the sciatic notch.

Once the sciatic notch is reached, replace the elevator with a flexible metal ribbon retractor that touches and overlaps the ribbon retractor already in the notch. With curved scissors separate the rectus muscle and its reflected head from the capsule of the hip joint. Divide the reflected head. The osteotomy should be made with a Hohmann retractor precisely between the insertion of the capsule and the reflected head of the rectus, following the capsular insertion in a curved line and ending distal to the anteroinferior iliac spine anteriorly and in the sciatic notch posteriorly. Do not open or damage the capsule of the joint. After the line of the osteotomy has been determined, start the osteotomy with a straight, narrow osteotome, opening the lateral table of the ilium along this line.

At the beginning determine the exact position of the osteotome by image intensification or by roentgenograms. Direct the osteotomy superiorly approximately 20 degrees toward the inner table of the ilium (Fig. 27-35, *A*). Change the position of the osteotome as necessary to make the osteotomy curved superiorly. Do not direct the osteotomy more than 20 degrees superiorly because it might then enter the sacroiliac joint.

When the osteotomy has been completed, displace the hip medially by releasing the traction on the extremity and by forcing the limb into abduction. The distal fragment then displaces medially, hinging at the symphysis pubis (Fig. 27-35, *B*). If, however, the adductor muscles are extremely relaxed, it may be necessary to manipulate the head manually or to displace the distal fragment with an instrument. Be sure the distal fragment is displaced far enough medially (if necessary, 100% of the width of the ilium) so that the proximal fragment completely covers the femoral head. Internal fixation can be inserted to secure and maintain adequate displacement.

After the displacement has been completed, decrease the abduction of the limb to about 30 degrees. If the capsule is loose, perform a capsulorrhaphy. Next, check the position of the hip and the osteotomy by image intensification or by roentgenograms. Replace and suture the iliac apophysis and close the wound. Apply a spica cast with the hip in 20 to 30 degrees of abduction, neutral rotation, and neutral extension.

AFTERTREATMENT. In children and adults the cast is removed at 6 to 8 weeks, and active and passive exercises of the hip are started. Partial weight-bearing on crutches is allowed and progressed as tolerated.

Adolescent and Young Adult (Older Than 8 to 10 Years of Age)

In children older than 8 to 10 years of age or in young adults in whom the femoral head cannot be repositioned distally to the level of the acetabulum, only palliative salvaging operations are possible. Rarely a femoral shortening combined with a pelvic osteotomy could be considered, but the chances of creating a hip to last a lifetime are minimal. Reduction of a unilateral

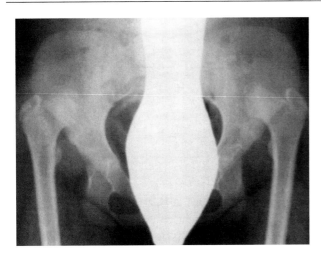

Fig. 27-36 Bilateral untreated congenital dislocation of hip in 12-year-old girl.

dislocation should be strongly considered, even in children 6 to 8 years of age. After some years degenerative arthritic changes develop in the hip joint. When these changes cause enough pain or limitation of motion to require additional surgery, a reconstructive operation such as a total hip arthroplasty may be indicated at the appropriate age. Aksoy and Musdal reported alleviation of pain and improvement in gait at an average 7-year follow-up after subtrochanteric valgus extension osteotomies in 35 patients (average age, 22 years) with unilateral or bilateral neglected congenital hip dislocations. The mean Harris Hip Score improved from 49 preoperatively to 72 postoperatively. Arthrodesis is now rarely indicated for old unreduced dislocations and is contraindicated for bilateral dislocations. In bilateral dislocations in this age group the hips should be left unreduced (Fig. 27-36), and total hip arthroplasties may be carried out during adulthood. Interestingly, degenerative joint disease is more likely to develop in early adulthood in a dislocated hip with a false acetabulum in the wing of the ilium than in a dislocated hip without formation of a false acetabulum. Patients with reduced femoral heads but painful acetabular dysplasia can be treated with an appropriate pelvic osteotomy (see Table 27-1).

Congenital and Developmental Coxa Vara

The term *congenital coxa vara* has been applied to two types of coxa vara seen in infancy and childhood. The first type is present at birth, is rare, and is associated with other congenital anomalies such as proximal femoral focal deficiency or anomalies in other parts of the body such as cleidocranial dysostosis. The second type, usually not discovered until the child is walking, is more common than the first and is associated with no other abnormality except possibly a congenitally short femur.

Coxa vara, often bilateral, is characterized by a progressive

decrease in the angle between the femoral neck and shaft, a progressive shortening of the limb, and the presence of a defect in the medial part of the neck. Microscopically, the tissue in this defect consists of cartilage that, because the columnar arrangement of its cells is irregular and ossification within it is atypical, resembles an abnormal physis. The adjacent metaphyseal bone is osteoporotic, its trabeculae being atrophic, and occasionally it contains large groups of cartilage cells. When walking is begun, the forces that the femoral neck must withstand are of course increased, and because the neck is weak, varus deformity gradually develops.

As the patient becomes older and heavier, the deformity increases until the greater trochanter eventually lies superior to the femoral head; furthermore, pseudarthrosis of the femoral neck may develop. In adults the trochanter may come to lie several inches superior to the head, and if pseudarthrosis is present, the head may be widely separated from the neck. After the age of 8 years the likelihood of obtaining a hip that will function normally rapidly diminishes.

The treatment of choice for correction of developmental coxa vara is subtrochanteric osteotomy to place the femoral neck and head in an appropriate valgus position with the shaft of the femur. Surgery can be delayed until the child is 4 or 5 years old to make internal fixation easier. Beals suggested that surgical treatment is indicated when coxa vara deformity is progressive, painful, unilateral, or associated with leg-length discrepancy. Surgery also is indicated when the neck-shaft angle is 110 degrees or less. The subtrochanteric osteotomy is fixed internally with either a blade-plate or screw-plate combination (Fig. 27-37). Although biomechanically this may provide enough rigid internal fixation to eliminate the need for postoperative immobilization, a spica cast can be worn until union is complete.

Regardless of the method of osteotomy, the deformity can recur, so children should be examined periodically after surgery until their growth is complete. Carroll, Coleman, and Stevens found that deformity recurred in 50% of 26 patients who had valgus osteotomies for coxa vara. Etiology, age at the time of surgery, type of osteotomy, and type of implant had no bearing on recurrence, but 95% of patients in whom Hilgenreiner's epiphyseal angle was corrected to less than 38 degrees had no recurrence of varus. The head-shaft angle was not reliable in determining adequacy of correction: two thirds of patients with correction to more than 135 degrees had recurrences and one third of those with correction to less than 135 degrees had satisfactory results. In addition, a significant number of children with coxa vara have associated femoral hypoplasia and limb-length discrepancy, which ultimately may require limb equalization.

◆ Valgus Osteotomy for Developmental Coxa Vara

TECHNIQUE 27-15

Perform an adductor tenotomy through a small medial incision. Expose the greater trochanter and proximal shaft of the femur through an 8- to 10-cm lateral, longitudinal

continued

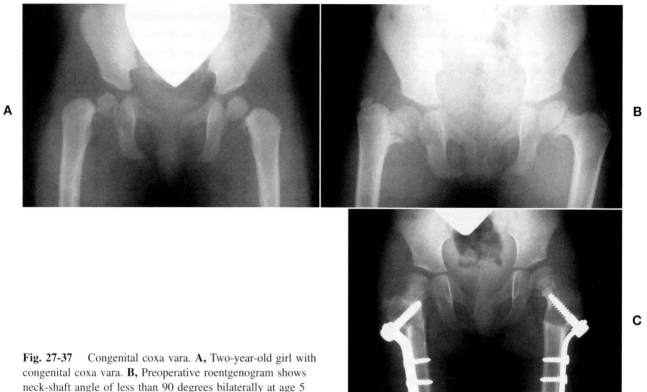

Fig. 27-37 Congenital coxa vara. **A,** Two-year-old girl with congenital coxa vara. **B,** Preoperative roentgenogram shows neck-shaft angle of less than 90 degrees bilaterally at age 5 years. **C,** After bilateral subtrochanteric osteotomies and internal fixation with pediatric hip screw.

incision. If a screw and side plate device is used for internal fixation, insert the screw in the midline of the femoral neck as determined by image intensification or both anteroposterior and lateral roentgenograms. Insert the screw as close as possible to the trochanteric apophysis without entering it. If possible, center the screw in the femoral neck distal to the abnormal physis. If this is technically impossible, center the screw in the femoral head. Next, make a transverse osteotomy slightly distal to the screw at about the level of the lesser trochanter. If necessary, take a small lateral wedge of bone to correct the neck-shaft angle to approximately 135 to 150 degrees. Next, fix the side plate to the femoral shaft in the usual manner. Irrigate the wound and close it in layers, inserting irrigation-suction drainage if desired. Apply a one and one half spica cast.

AFTERTREATMENT. The cast is removed at 8 to 12 weeks, when roentgenographic union of the osteotomy has occurred. Regular follow-up includes the assessment of possible recurrence of the deformity and the development of progressive limb-length discrepancy that requires additional treatment.

Exstrophy of Bladder

Exstrophy of the bladder occurs as a result of a congenital failure of fusion of the tissues of the midline of the pelvis. The

major anomaly is a maldevelopment of the lower part of the abdominal wall and the anterior wall of the bladder, so the anterior surface of the posterior wall of the bladder is exposed to the exterior. Hernias and other defects of the anterior abdominal wall also may be present more proximally. However, as noted by O'Phelan, the orthopaedic surgeon becomes involved in treatment because of the diastasis of the symphysis pubis, the lateral flare of the innominate bones, and the resultant lateral displacement and external rotation of the acetabula that, if left uncorrected, would result in a wide-based, waddling, externally rotated gait. Other orthopaedic anomalies may be present along with exstrophy of the bladder, including congenital dislocation or dysplasia of the hip and myelomeningocele.

ANTERIOR ILIAC OSTEOTOMIES AND APPROXIMATION OF SYMPHYSIS PUBIS

Because most of the urological structures are present or bifid, reconstruction is possible. However, unless the symphysis pubis is approximated, urological reconstruction is followed by complications such as the formation of fistulae or recurrences. These complications seem to be caused by tension placed on the soft tissues during closure, and this tension can be relieved by repair of the symphysis pubis. O'Phelan described the results of bilateral posterior iliac osteotomies and approximation of the symphysis (Fig. 27-38). More recently, Sponseller, Gearhart, and Jeffs recommended bilateral anterior iliac osteotomies, with internal or external fixation, citing advan-

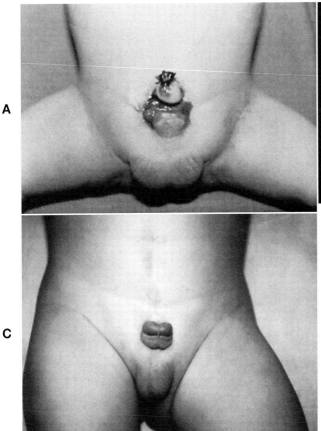
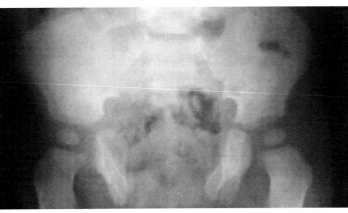

Fig. 27-38   A, Congenital exstrophy of bladder in newborn boy. **B,** Note pubic diastasis on roentgenogram at 1 year of age. **C,** After bilateral posterior iliac osteotomies and anterior reconstruction.

tages of increased mobility of the pubis and increased correction and avoidance of turning of the patient while under anesthesia for repeat preparation. Postoperative traction was not necessary in most of their patients. They reported no dehiscence, nonunions, or infections, and all older patients had normal gaits 4 months after surgery.

In a report of 25 patients with bladder exstrophy, Kasat and Borwankar identified 11 important factors in obtaining a successful primary closure: (1) proper patient selection, (2) a staged approach, (3) anterior approximation of the pubic bones with placement of the bladder and urethra in the true pelvis, (4) posterior bilateral iliac osteotomies when indicated, (5) double-layered closure of the bladder, (6) 2 weeks of proper ureteric catheter drainage, (7) prevention of infection, (8) prolonged and proper postoperative immobilization, (9) prompt treatment of bladder prolapse, (10) prevention of abdominal distention postoperatively, and (11) ruling out bladder outlet obstruction before removing the bladder catheter.

The three steps are performed as one operative procedure—first the anterior iliac osteotomies, then repair of the anterior structures by a urological surgeon, and finally repair of the symphysis pubis. A heavy, nonabsorbable suture can be substituted for wire fixation. Although described for treatment of older children or children with recurrent deformities, we prefer this technique for both early initial treatment and for older children (Fig. 27-39).

◆ Bilateral Anterior Iliac Osteotomies

TECHNIQUE 27-16 *(Sponseller, Gearhart, and Jeffs)*

Place the patient supine on the operating table and circumferentially prepare and drape the entire body below the umbilicus. Elevate the sacrum on folded towels. Make an anterior iliofemoral approach to the pelvis, similar to that used for a Salter osteotomy; both sides can be exposed simultaneously. Widely expose the medial iliac cortex and carefully elevate the periosteum posteriorly around the sciatic notch, using curved elevators and gauze sponges. With a Gigli saw, perform Salter innominate osteotomies. If the saw is difficult to pass, it can be threaded through on a leader of umbilical tape. In children younger than 6 months of age, use an oscillating saw because the force applied to the Gigli saw can cause preferential separation of the triradiate cartilage. Make the osteotomies from 5 mm above the anteroinferior iliac spine to the most cranial portion of the sciatic notch to leave a sizable inferior segment for internal fixation. Rotate the freed ischiopubic segments 30 to 45 degrees to bring the pubic rami together.

In children older than 6 months of age, a small external fixator, such as that used in the upper extremity, can be used with 2-mm pins for fixation. Increase the pin size to 4 mm

continued

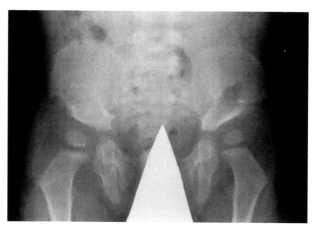

Fig. 27-39 **A,** Technique for reconstruction in exstrophy of bladder (see text). **B,** Postoperative roentgenogram after bilateral anterior Salter innominate osteotomies. (**A** redrawn from Sponseller PD, Gearhart JP, Jeffs RD: *J Urol* 146:137, 1991.)

for children between 4 and 10 years of age and to 5 mm for those older than 10 or 11 years old. Insert two pins in each iliac wing and two in each distal fragment. Predrilling may be necessary to prevent splitting of the bone in small infants. Place one distal fragment pin from the anteroinferior iliac spine to the notch, parallel and 5 to 10 mm inferior to the osteotomy, making sure the pin engages the deep posterior cortex of the notch. Insert another threaded pin just below this pin but externally angled 30 degrees. Close the wounds.

Have the urological surgeon prepare the operative field and identify the abnormal bladder and urethral structures. Use a single suture of 2-0 nylon in a horizontal mattress stitch to suture the pubic bones; tie it anterior to the neourethra and bladder neck while an assistant rotates the greater trochanters medially. Place heavy sutures of polyglactin in the rectus fascia just superficial to the pubic closure. After the pelvic ring is closed anteriorly, apply the external fixator. Again, good subperiosteal exposure is mandatory to ensure accurate pin placement away from the hip and triradiate cartilage.

The procedure can be modified to exclude external fixation by fixing both osteotomies with Kirschner wires and applying a spica cast to be worn for 8 to 12 weeks.

AFTERTREATMENT. Light Buck traction or a spica cast can be used for 1 to 2 weeks to maintain comfort and bed rest. This is mandatory in children younger than 1 year of age because they have relatively less cortical bone for fixation, but older children can be discharged from the hospital earlier if good external fixation is obtained. External fixation is continued for 4 weeks in children younger than 2 years of age and for 6 weeks in older children. Gradual resumption of activities is then allowed. No formal physical therapy program is necessary, but a walker is helpful during the first week of ambulation in older children.

References

CONGENITAL AND DEVELOPMENTAL DYSPLASIA OF HIP

Aksoy MC, Musdal Y: Subtrochanteric valgus-extension osteotomy for neglected congenital dislocation of the hip in young adults, *Acta Orthop Belg* 66:181, 2000.

Ando M, Gotoh E: Significance of inguinal folds for diagnosis of congenital dislocation of the hip in infants aged three to four months, *J Pediatr Orthop* 10:331, 1990.

Barlow TG: Early diagnosis and treatment of congenital dislocation of the hip, *J Bone Joint Surg* 44B:292, 1962.

Bar-On E, Huo MH, DeLuca PA: Early innominate osteotomy as a treatment for avascular necrosis complicating developmental hip dysplasia, *J Pediatr Orthop* B6:138, 1997.

Bar-On E, Myere S, Harari G, Porat S: Ultrasonography of the hip in developmental hip dysplasia, *J Bone Joint Surg* 80B:321, 1998.

Beoree NK, Clarke NM: Ultrasound imaging and secondary screening for congenital dislocation of the hip, *J Bone Joint Surg* 76B:525, 1994.

Berman L, Catterall A, Meire HB: Ultrasound of the hip: a review of the applications of a new technique, *Br J Radiol* 59:13, 1986.

Betz RR, Kumar J, Palmer CT, MacEwen GD: Chiari pelvic osteotomy in children and young adults, *J Bone Joint Surg* 70A:182, 1988.

Bialik V, Bialik BM, Blazer S, et al: Developmental dysplasia of the hip: a new approach to incidence, *Pediatrics* 103:93, 1999.

Birnbaum K, Pastor A, Prescher A, Heller KD: Complications of Chiari and Salter osteotomies: a cadaver study, *Surg Radiol Anat* 22:225, 2000.

Bos CF, Bloem JL, Obermann WR, et al: Magnetic resonance imaging in congenital dislocation of the hip, *J Bone Joint Surg* 70B:174, 1988.

Bowen J, Kassar J: *The pelvic harness*, Wilmington, Del, Dupont Institute (pamphlet).

Brien EW, Randolph DA Jr, Zahiri CA: Radiographic analysis to determine the treatment outcome in developmental dysplasia of the hip, *Am J Orthop* 29:773, 2000.

Brougham DI, Broughton NS, Cole WG, et al: Avascular necrosis following closed reduction of congenital dislocation of the hip: review of influencing factors and long-term follow-up, *J Bone Joint Surg* 72B:557, 1990.

Broughton NS, Brougham DI, Cole WG, Menelaus MB: Reliability of radiological measurements in the assessment of the child's hip, *J Bone Joint Surg* 71B:6, 1989.

Bucholz RW, Ogden JA: Patterns of ischemic necrosis of the proximal femur in nonoperatively treated congenital hip disease. In *The hip: Proceedings of the Sixth Open Scientific Meeting of the Hip Society*, St Louis, 1978, Mosby.

Campbell P, Tralow SD: Lateral tethering of the proximal femoral physis complicating the treatment of congenital hip dysplasia, *J Pediatr Orthop* 10:6, 1990.

Castelein RM, Korte J: Limited hip abduction in the infant, *J Pediatr Orthop* 21:668, 2001.

Castelein RM, Sauter AJM: Ultrasound screening for congenital dysplasia of the hip in newborns: its value, *J Pediatr Orthop* 8:666, 1988.

Castillo R, Sherman FC: Medial adductor open reduction for congenital dislocation of the hip, *J Pediatr Orthop* 10:335, 1990.

Chiari K: *Pelvic osteotomy as shelf operation*, Wien (Hofburg), 1963, Neuvième Congrès Internationale de Chirurgie Orthopédique.

Chiari K: Medial displacement osteotomy of the pelvis, *Clin Orthop* 98:55, 1974.

Chuinard EG: Femoral osteotomy in the treatment of congenital dysplasia of the hip, *Orthop Clin North Am* 3:157, 1972.

Coleman SS: The incomplete pericapsular (Pemberton) and innominate (Salter) osteotomies: a complete analysis, *Clin Orthop* 98:116, 1974.

Coleman SS: Treatment of congenital dislocation of the hip in the older child. In Ahstrom JP, ed: *Current practice in orthopaedic surgery*, vol 6, St Louis, 1975, Mosby.

Coleman SS: *Congenital dysplasia and dislocation of the hip*, St Louis, 1978, Mosby.

Coleman SS: Classics in orthopaedics: diagnosis and treatment of congenital hip dislocation. Paper presented at the Sixth Annual Meeting of the Mid-America Orthopaedic Association, Tucson, March 16, 1988.

Coleman SS, MacEwen GD: Congenital dislocation of the hip in infancy, *Instr Course Lect* 21:155, 1972.

Colton CL: Chiari osteotomy for acetabular dysplasia in young subjects, *J Bone Joint Surg* 54B:578, 1972.

Dega W: Selection of surgical methods in the treatment of congenital dislocation of the hip in children, *Chir Narzadow Ruchu Ortop Pol* 34:357, 1969.

Dega W, Króol J, Polakowski L: Surgical treatment of congenital dislocation of the hip in children: a one-stage procedure, *J Bone Joint Surg* 41A:920, 1959.

Edelson JG, Hirsch M, Weinberg H, et al: Congenital dislocation of the hip and computerized axial tomography, *J Bone Joint Surg* 66B:472, 1984.

Eppright RH: Dial osteotomy of the acetabulum, *J Bone Joint Surg* 58A:283, 1976.

Exner GU: Ultrasound screening for hip dysplasia in neonates, *J Pediatr Orthop* 8:656, 1988.

Eyre-Brook AL, Jones DA, Harris FC: Pemberton's acetabuloplasty for congenital dislocation or subluxation of the hip, *J Bone Joint Surg* 60B:18, 1978.

Ferguson AB Jr: Primary open reduction of congenital dislocation of the hip using a median adductor approach, *J Bone Joint Surg* 55A:671, 1973.

Fish DN, Herzenberg JE, Hensinger RN: Current practice in use of prereduction traction for congenital dislocation of the hip, *J Pediatr Orthop* 11:149, 1991.

Fletcher RR, Johnson CE II: Greater trochanteric advancement for the treatment of coxa brevis associated with congenital dislocation of the hip, *Orthopedics* 8:519, 1985.

Fong HC, Lu W, Li YH, Leong JC: Chiari osteotomy and shelf augmentation in the treatment of hip dysplasia, *J Pediatr Orthop* 20:740, 2000.

Frank GR, Michael HR: Treatment of congenital dislocation of the hip: results obtained with the Pemberton and Salter osteotomies, *South Med J* 60:975, 1967.

Frick SL, Kim SS, Wenger DR: Pre- and postoperative three-dimensional computed tomography analysis of triple innominate osteotomy for hip dysplasia, *J Pediatr Orthop* 20:116, 2000.

Gage JR, Winter RB: Avascular necrosis of the capital femoral epiphysis as a complication of closed reduction of congenital dislocation of the hip: a critical review of twenty years' experience at Gillette Children's Hospital, *J Bone Joint Surg* 54A:373, 1972.

Galeazzi R: Uber die Torsion des verrenkten oberen Femurendes und ihre Beseitigung, *Verhandl d Deutsch Gesellsch F Orthop Chir*, 1910, p 334.

Galpin RD, Roach JW, Wenger DR, et al: One-stage treatment of congenital dislocation of the hip, including femoral shortening, *J Bone Joint Surg* 71A:734, 1989.

Ganz R, Klaue K, Vinh TS, Mast JW: A new periacetabular osteotomy for the treatment of hip dysplasias, *Clin Orthop* 232:26, 1988.

Gravey M, Donoghue VB, Gorman WA, et al: Radiographic screening at four months of infants at risk for congenital hip dislocation, *J Bone Joint Surg* 74B:704, 1992.

Graf R: *Sonographie der Sauglinshufte Bucherei des Orthopaden*, Stuttgart, 1985, Ferdinand Enke Verlag.

Gregosiewicz A, Wósko I: Risk factors of avascular necrosis in the treatment of congenital dislocation of the hip, *J Pediatr Orthop* 8:17, 1988.

Grill F, Bensahel H, Canadell J, et al: The Pavlik harness in the treatment of congenital dislocating hip: report on a multicenter study of the European Paediatric Orthopaedic Society, *J Pediatr Orthop* 8:1, 1988.

Grudziak JS, Ward WT: Dega osteotomy for the treatment of congenital dysplasia of the hip, *J Bone Joint Surg* 83A:845, 2001.

Gruel CR, Birch JG, Roach JW, et al: Teratologic dislocation of the hip, *J Pediatr Orthop* 6:693, 1986.

Guille JT, Forlin E, Kumar SJ, et al: Triple osteotomy of the innominate bone in treatment of developmental dysplasia of the hip, *J Pediatr Orthop* 12:718, 1992.

Guille JT, Pizzutillo PD, MacEwen GD: Developmental dysplasia of the hip from birth to six months, *J Am Acad Orthop Surg* 8:232, 2000.

Hansson G, Jacobsen S: Ultrasonography screening for developmental dysplasia of the hip joint, *Acta Paediatr* 86:913, 1997.

Hangen DH, Kasser JR, Emans JB, et al: The Pavlik harness and developmental dysplasia of the hip: has ultrasound changed treatment patterns? *J Pediatr Orthop* 15:729, 1995.

Harris NH, Lloyd-Roberts GC, Gallien R: Acetabular development in congenital dislocation of the hip: with special reference to the indications for acetabuloplasty and pelvic or femoral realignment osteotomy, *J Bone Joint Surg* 57B:46, 1975.

Haynes RJ: Developmental dysplasia of the hip: etiology, pathogenesis, and examination and physical findings in the newborn, *Instr Course Lect* 50:535, 2001.

Henard DC, Calandruccio RA: Experimental production of roentgenographic and histological changes in the capital femoral epiphysis following abduction, extension and internal rotation of the hip, *J Bone Joint Surg* 52A:601, 1970 (abstract).

Hilgenreiner H: Zur Fruhdiagnose und Fruhbehandlung der angeborenen Huftgelenkverrenkung, *Med Clin* 21:1385, 1925.

Hoffman DV, Simmons EH, Barrington TW: The results of the Chiari osteotomy, *Clin Orthop* 98:162, 1974.

Ilfeld FW, Westin GW, Makin M, Paterson DC: Postnatal development dislocation of the hip. Poster exhibit, presented at the annual meeting of the American Academy of Orthopaedic Surgeons, Las Vegas, Feb 1989.

Inoue T, Naito M, Nomiyama H: Treatment of developmental dysplasia of the hip with the Pavlik harness: factors for predicting unsuccessful reduction, *J Pediatr Orthop B* 10:186, 2001.

Jones DA: Sub-capital coxa valga after varus osteotomy for congenital dislocation of the hip: a report of six cases with a minimum follow-up of nine years, *J Bone Joint Surg* 59B:152, 1977.

Jones GT, Schoenecker PL, Dias LS: Developmental hip dysplasia potentiated by inappropriate use of the Pavlik harness, *J Pediatr Orthop* 12:722, 1992.

Kahle WK, Anderson MB, Alpert J, et al: The value of preliminary traction in the treatment of congenital dislocation of the hip, *J Bone Joint Surg* 72A:1026, 1990.

Kalamchi A, MacEwen GD: Avascular necrosis following treatment of congenital dislocation of the hip, *J Bone Joint Surg* 62A:876, 1980.

Kalamchi A, MacFarlane R III: The Pavlik harness: results in patients over three months of age, *J Pediatr Orthop* 2:3, 1982.

Kasser JR, Bowen JR, MacEwen GD: Varus derotation osteotomy in the treatment of persistent dysplasia in congenital dislocation of the hip, *J Bone Joint Surg* 67A:195, 1985.

Kawaguchi AT, Otsuka NY, Delgado ED, et al: Magnetic resonance arthrography in children with developmental hip dysplasia, *Clin Orthop* 374:234, 2000.

Kay RM, Jaki KA, Skaggs DL: The effect of femoral rotation on the projected femoral neck-shaft angle, *J Pediatr Orthop* 20:736, 2000.

Kerry RM, Simonds GW: Long-term results of late nonoperative reduction of developmental dysplasia of the hip, *J Bone Joint Surg* 80B:78, 1998.

Kim HW, Morcuende JA, Dolan LA, Weinstein SL: Acetabular development in developmental dysplasia of the hip complicated by lateral growth disturbance of the capital femoral epiphysis, *J Bone Joint Surg* 82A:1692, 2000.

Klisíc P, Jankovic L: Combined procedure of open reduction and shortening of the femur in treatment of congenital dislocation of the hips in older children, *Clin Orthop* 119:60, 1976.

Klisíc P, Jankovic L, Basara V: Long-term results of combined operative reduction of the hip in older children, *J Pediatr Orthop* 8:532, 1988.

Krämer J, Schleberger R, Steffen R: Closed reduction by two-phase skin traction and functional splinting in mitigated abduction for treatment of congenital dislocation of the hip, *Clin Orthop* 258:27, 1990.

Kruczynski J: Avascular necrosis after nonoperative treatment of developmental hip dislocation: prognosis in 36 patients followed 17-26 years, *Acta Orthop Scand* 66:239, 1995.

Kumar SJ: Hip spica application for the treatment of congenital dislocation of the hip, *J Pediatr Orthop* 1:97, 1981.

Lang P, Gernant HK, Chagetz N, et al: Three-dimensional CT and MR imaging in congenital dislocation of the hip: clinical and technical considerations, *J Comput Assist Tomogr* 12:459, 1988.

Lehmann HP, Hinton R, Morello P, Santoli J: Developmental dysplasia of the hip practice guideline: technical report. Committee on Quality Improvement and Subcommittee on Developmental Dysplasia of the Hip, *Pediatrics* 105:E57, 2000.

Lerman JA, Emans JB, Millis MB, et al: Early failure of Pavlik harness treatment for developmental hip dysplasia: clinical and ultrasound predictors, *J Pediatr Orthop* 21:348, 2001.

Lin CJ, Lin YT, Lai KA: Intraoperative instability for developmental dysplasia of the hip in children 12 to 18 months of age as a guide to Salter osteotomy, *J Pediatr Orthop* 20:575, 2000.

Lloyd-Roberts GC, Swann M: Pitfalls in the management of congenital dislocation of the hip, *J Bone Joint Surg* 48B:666, 1966.

Ludloff K: Zur blutigen Eihrenkung der Angeborenen Huftluxation, *Z Orthop Chir* 22:272, 1908.

Luhmann SJ, Schoenecker PL, Anderson AM, Bassett GS: The prognostic importance of the ossific nucleus in the treatment of congenital dysplasia of the hip, *J Bone Joint Surg* 80A:1719, 1998.

MacEwen GD, Ramsey PL: The hip. In Lovell WW, Winter RB, eds: *Pediatric orthopaedics*, ed 1, Philadelphia, 1978, JB Lippincott.

Malvitz TA, Weinstein SL: Closed reduction for congenital dysplasia of the hip: functional and radiographic results after an average of thirty years, *J Bone Joint Surg* 76A:1777, 1994.

Mandel DM, Loder RT, Hensinger RN: The predictive value of computed tomography in the treatment of developmental dysplasia of the hip, *J Pediatr Orthop* 18:794, 1998.

Mankey MG, Arntz GT, Staheli LT: Open reduction through a medial approach for congenital dislocation of the hip, *J Bone Joint Surg* 75A:1334, 1993.

Mau H, Dorr WM, Henkel L, Lutsche J: Open reduction of congenital dislocation of the hip by Ludloff's method, *J Bone Joint Surg* 53A:1281, 1971.

McKay DW: A comparison of the innominate and the pericapsular osteotomy in the treatment of congenital dislocation of the hip, *Clin Orthop* 98:124, 1974.

McNally EG, Tasker A, Benson MK: MRI after operative reduction for developmental dysplasia of the hip, *J Bone Joint Surg* 79B:724, 1997.

Mergen E, Adyaman S, Omeroglu H, et al: Medial approach open reduction for congenital dislocation of the hip using the Ferguson procedure: a review of 31 hips, *Arch Orthop Trauma Surg* 110:169, 1991.

Mitchell GP: Arthrography in congenital displacement of the hip, *J Bone Joint Surg* 45B:88, 1963.

Mitchell GP: Chiari medial displacement osteotomy, *Clin Orthop* 98:146, 1974.

Moen C, Lindsey RW: Computerized tomography with routine arthrography in early evaluation of congenital hip dysplasia, *Orthop Rev* 15:71, 1986.

Mosley CF: Developmental hip dysplasia and dislocation: management of the older child, *Instr Course Lect* 50:547, 2001.

Mubarak SJ, Leach J, Wenger DR: Management of congenital dislocation of the hip in the infant, *Contemp Orthop* 15:29, 1987.

Murray KA, Crim JR: Radiographic imaging for treatment and follow-up of developmental dysplasia of the hip, *Semin Ultrasound CT MR* 22:306, 2001.

Nakata K, Masuhara K, Sugano N, et al: Dome (modified Chiari) pelvic osteotomy: 10- to 18-year follow-up study, *Clin Orthop* 389:102, 2001.

O'Hara JN, Bernard AA, Dwyer N: Early results of medial approach open reduction in congenital dislocation of the hip: use before walking age, *J Pediatr Orthop* 8:288, 1988.

Omeroglu H, Koparal S: The role of clinical examination and risk factors in the diagnosis and developmental dysplasia of the hip: a prospective study in 188 referred young infants, *Arch Orthop Trauma Surg* 121:7, 2001.

Ortolani M: Congenital hip dysplasia in the light of early and very early diagnosis, *Clin Orthop* 119:6, 1976.

Pavlik A: Functional treatment with a harness as a principle for the conservative treatment of congenital hip dislocations in infants, *Z Orthop* 89:341, 1957.

Pavlik A: Stirrups as an aid in the treatment of congenital dysplasias of the hip in children, *J Orthop Pediatr* 9:157, 1989 (translated by V Bialik, ND Reis).

Pemberton PA: Pericapsular osteotomy of the ilium for treatment of congenital subluxation and dislocation of the hip, *J Bone Joint Surg* 47A:65, 1965.

Pemberton PA: Pericapsular osteotomy of the ilium for treatment of congenitally dislocated hips, *Clin Orthop* 98:41, 1974.

Pérez A, Noguera JG: Experience with innominate osteotomy (Salter) and medial displacement osteotomy (Chiari) in the treatment of acetabular dysplasia: preliminary report of 82 operations, *Clin Orthop* 98:133, 1974.

Perkins G: Signs by which to diagnose congenital dislocation of the hip, *Lancet* 1:648, 1928.

Peterson HA, Klassen RA, McLeod RA, Hoffman AD: The use of computerized tomography in dislocation of the hip and femoral anteversion in children, *J Bone Joint Surg* 63B:198, 1981.

Race C, Herring JA: Congenital dislocation of the hip: evaluation of closed reduction, *J Pediatr Orthop* 3:166, 1983.

Ramsey PL, Lasser S, MacEwen GD: Congenital dislocation of the hip: use of the Pavlik harness in the child during the first six months of life, *J Bone Joint Surg* 58A:1000, 1976.

Reichel H, Hein W: Dega acetabuloplasty combined with intertrochanteric osteotomies: long-term results, *Clin Orthop* 323:234, 1996.

Ring PA: The treatment of unreduced congenital dislocation of the hip in adults, *J Bone Joint Surg* 41B:299, 1959.

Rosen A, Gamble JG, Vallier H, et al: Analysis of radiographic measurements as prognostic indicators of treatment success in patients with developmental dysplasia of the hip, *J Pediatr Orthop* B 8:118, 1999.

Roth A, Gibson DA, Hall JE: The experience of five orthopedic surgeons with innominate osteotomy in the treatment of congenital dislocation and subluxation of the hip, *Clin Orthop* 98:178, 1974.

Saies Ad, Foster BK, Lesquesne GW: The value of a new ultrasound stress test in assessment and treatment of clinically detected hip instability, *J Pediatr Orthop* 8:436, 1988.

Salter RB: Innominate osteotomy in the treatment of congenital dislocation and subluxation of the hip, *J Bone Joint Surg* 43B:518, 1961.

Salter RB: Role of innominate osteotomy in the treatment of congenital dislocation and subluxation of the hip in the older child, *J Bone Joint Surg* 48A:1413, 1966.

Salter RB: Specific guidelines in the application of the principle of innominate osteotomy, *Orthop Clin North Am* 3:149, 1972.

Salter RB, Dubos JP: The first fifteen years' personal experience with innominate osteotomy in the treatment of congenital dislocation and subluxation of the hip, *Clin Orthop* 98:72, 1974.

Salter RB, Hansson G, Thompson GH: Innominate osteotomy in the management of residual congenital subluxation of the hip in young adults, *Clin Orthop* 182:53, 1984.

Salvati EA, Wilson PD: Treatment of irreducible hip subluxation by Chiari's iliac osteotomy: a report of results in 19 cases, *Clin Orthop* 98:151, 1974.

Sanfridson J, Redlund-Johnell I, Uden A: Why is congenital dislocation of the hip still missed? Analysis of 96,891 infants screened in Malm 1956-1987, *Acta Orthop Scand* 62:87, 1991.

Schoenecker PL, Anderson DJ, Capelli AM: The acetabular response to proximal femoral varus rotational osteotomy: results after failure of post-reduction abduction splinting in patients who had congenital dislocation of the hip, *J Bone Joint Surg* 77A:990, 1995.

Schoenecker PL, Dollard PA, Sheridan JJ, et al: Closed reduction of developmental dislocation of the hip in children older than 18 months, *J Pediatr Orthop* 15:763, 1995.

Schoenecker PL, Strecker WB: Congenital dislocation of the hip in children: comparison of the effects of femoral shortening and of skeletal traction in treatment, *J Bone Joint Surg* 66A:21, 1984.

Schwartz DR: Acetabular development after reduction of congenital dislocation of the hip: a follow-up study of fifty hips, *J Bone Joint Surg* 47A:705, 1965.

Severin E: Congenital dislocation of the hip: development of the joint after closed reduction, *J Bone Joint Surg* 32A:507, 1950.

Shih CH, Shih HN: One-stage combined operation of congenital dislocation of the hips in older children, *J Pediatr Orthop* 8:535, 1988.

Skaggs DL, DuBois B, Kay RM, et al: A simplified valgus osteotomy of the proximal femur in children, *J Pediatr Orthop* B 9:114, 2000.

Smith JT, Matan A, Coleman SS, et al: The predictive value of the development of the acetabular teardrop figure in developmental dysplasia of the hip, *J Pediatr Orthop* 17:165, 1997.

Somerville EW: Development of congenital dislocation of the hip, *J Bone Joint Surg* 35B:568, 1953.

Somerville EW: Open reduction in congenital dislocation of hip, *J Bone Joint Surg* 35B:363, 1953.

Somerville EW: Results of treatment of 100 congenitally dislocated hips, *J Bone Joint Surg* 49B:258, 1967.

Somerville EW: A long-term follow-up of congenital dislocation of the hip, *J Bone Joint Surg* 60B:25, 1978.

Somerville EW, Scott JC: The direct approach to congenital dislocation of the hip, *J Bone Joint Surg* 39B:623, 1957.

Staheli LT: Technique: slotted acetabular augmentation, *J Pediatr Orthop* 1:321, 1981.

Staheli LT, Chew DE: Slotted acetabular augmentation in childhood and adolescence, *J Pediatr Orthop* 12:569, 1992.

Steel HH: Triple osteotomy of the innominate bone, *J Bone Joint Surg* 55A:343, 1973.

Sutherland DH, Greenfield R: Double innominate osteotomy, *J Bone Joint Surg* 59A:1082, 1977.

Suzuki S, Yamamuro T: Avascular necrosis in patients treated with the Pavlik harness for congenital dislocation of the hip, *J Bone Joint Surg* 72A:1048, 1990.

Szöke N, Kühll L, Heinrichs J: Ultrasound examination in the diagnosis of congenital hip dysplasia of newborns, *J Pediatr Orthop* 8:12, 1988.

Szöke G, Staheli LT, Jaffe K, Hall JG: Medial approach open reduction of hip dislocation in amyoplasia-type arthrogryposis, *J Pediatr Orthop* 16:127, 1996.

Taylor GR, Clarke NM: Monitoring the treatment of developmental dysplasia of the hip with the Pavlik harness: the role of ultrasound, *J Bone Joint Surg* 79B:719, 1997.

Thomas IH, Dunin AJ, Cole WG, et al: Avascular necrosis after open reduction for congenital dislocation of the hip: analysis of causative factors and natural history, *J Pediatr Orthop* 9:525, 1989.

Tien YC, Su JY, Lin CT, Lin SY: Ultrasonographic study of the coexistence of muscular torticollis and dysplasia of the hip, *J Pediatr Orthop* 21:343, 2001.

Toby EB, Koman LA, Bechtold RE, Nicastro JN: Postoperative computed tomographic evaluation of congenital hip dislocation, *J Pediatr Orthop* 7:667, 1987.

Tredwell SJ: Economic evaluation of neonatal screening for congenital dislocation of the hip, *J Pediatr Orthop* 10:327, 1990.

Trevor D, Johns DL, Fixsen JA: Acetabuloplasty in the treatment of congenital dislocation of the hip, *J Bone Joint Surg* 57B:167, 1975.

Tucci JJ, Kumar SJ, Guille JT et al: Late acetabular dysplasia following early successful Pavlik harness treatment of congenital dislocation of the hip, *J Pediatr Orthop* 11:501, 1991.

Utterback TD, MacEwen GD: Comparison of pelvic osteotomies for the surgical correction of the congenital hip, *Clin Orthop* 98:104, 1974.

Vengust R, Antolic V, Srakar F: Salter osteotomy for treatment of acetabular dysplasia in developmental dysplasia of the hip in patients under 10 years, *J Pediatr Orthop B* 10:30, 2001.

Viere R, Birch JG, Herring JA, et al: Use of the Pavlik harness in the treatment of CDH: an analysis of failures of treatment, *J Bone Joint Surg* 72A:238, 1990.

Wagner H: Osteotomies for congenital hip dislocation. In The Hip Society: *Proceedings of the fourth open scientific meeting of The Hip Society*, St Louis, 1976, Mosby.

Wagner H: Femoral osteotomies for congenital hip dislocation. In Weil VH, ed: *Progress in orthopaedic surgery*, vol 2, Berlin, 1978, Springer-Verlag.

Walsh JJ, Morrissy RT: Torticollis and hip dislocation, *J Pediatr Orthop* 18:219, 1998.

Waters P, Kurica K, Hall J, Micheli LJ: Salter innominate osteotomies in congenital dislocation of the hip, *J Pediatr Orthop* 8:650, 1988.

Weinstein SL, Ponseti IV: Congenital dislocation of the hip: open reduction through a medial approach, *J Bone Joint Surg* 61A:119, 1979.

Wenger DR: Congenital hip dislocation: techniques for primary open reduction including femoral shortening, *Instr Course Lect* 38:343, 1989.

Wenger DR, Lee CD, Kolman B: Derotational femoral shortening for developmental dislocation of the hip: special indications and results in the child younger than 2 years, *J Pediatr Orthop* 15:768, 1995.

Westin GW, Ilfeld FW, Makin M, Paterson D: Developmental hip dislocation, *Contemp Orthop* 16:17, 1988.

Willis RB: Developmental dysplasia of the hip: assessment and treatment before walking age, *Instr Course Lect* 50:541, 2001.

Wynne-Davies R: Acetabular dysplasia and familial joint laxity: two etiological factors in congenital dislocation of the hip: a review of 589 patients and their families, *J Bone Joint Surg* 52B:704, 1970.

Yoshitaka T, Mitani S, Aoki K, et al: Long-term follow-up of congenital subluxation of the hip, *J Pediatr Orthop* 21:474, 2001.

Zadeh HG, Catterall A, Hashemi-Jejad A, Perry RE: Test of stability as an aid to decide the need for osteotomy in association with open reduction in developmental dysplasia of the hip, *J Bone Joint Surg* 82B:17, 2000.

CONGENITAL AND DEVELOPMENTAL COXA VARA

Amstutz HC, Wilson PD Jr: Dysgenesis of the proximal femur (coxa vara) and its surgical management, *J Bone Joint Surg* 44A:1, 1962.

Beals RK: Coxa vara in childhood: evaluation and management, *J Am Acad Orthop Surg* 6:98, 1998.

Carroll K, Coleman S, Stevens PM: Coxa vara: surgical outcomes of valgus osteotomies, *J Pediatr Orthop* 17:220, 1997.

Fisher RL, Waskowitz WJ: Familial developmental coxa vara, *Clin Orthop* 86:2, 1972.

Kalamchi A, Cowell HR, Kim KI: Congenital deficiency of the femur, *J Pediatr Orthop* 4:285, 1984.

Kim HT, Chambers HG, Mubarak SJ, Wenger DR: Congenital coxa vara: computed tomographic analysis of femoral retroversion and the triangular metaphyseal fragment, *J Pediatr Orthop* 20:551, 2000.

Ogden JA, Lee KE, Rudicel SA, et al: Proximal femoral epiphysiolysis in the neonate, *J Pediatr Orthop* 4:285, 1984.

Pappas AM: Congenital abnormalities of the femur and related lower-extremity malformations: classification and treatment, *J Pediatr Orthop* 3:45, 1983.

Richie MF, Johnston CE II: Management of developmental coxa vara in cleidocranial dysostosis, *Orthopedics* 12:1001, 1989.

Weinstein JN, Kuo KN, Millar EA: Congenital coxa vara: a retrospective review, *J Pediatr Orthop* 4:70, 1984.

EXSTROPHY OF BLADDER

Aadlen RJ, O'Phelan EH, Chisholm TC, et al: Exstrophy of the bladder: long-term results of bilateral posterior iliac osteotomies and two-stage anatomic repair, *Clin Orthop* 151:193, 1980.

Cracciolo A III, Hall CB: Bilateral iliac osteotomy: the first stage in repair of exstrophy of the bladder, *Clin Orthop* 68:156, 1970.

Furnas DW, Haq MA, Somers G: One-stage reconstruction for exstrophy of the bladder in girls, *Plast Reconstr Surg* 56:61, 1975.

Greene WB, Dias LS, Lindseth RE, et al: Musculoskeletal problems in association with cloacal exstrophy, *J Bone Joint Surg* 73A:551, 1991.

Grotte G, Sevastikoglou JA: A modified technique for pelvic reconstruction in the treatment of exstrophy of the bladder, *Acta Orthop Scand* 37:197, 1966.

Gugenheim JJ, Gonzales ET Jr, Roth DR, Montagnino BA: Bilateral posterior pelvic resection osteotomies in patients with exstrophy of the bladder, *Clin Orthop* 364:70, 1999.

Jani MM, Sponseller PD, Gearhart JP, et al: The hip in adults with classic bladder exstrophy: a biomechanical analysis, *J Pediatr Orthop* 20:296, 2000.

Kantor R, Salai M, Ganel A: Orthopaedic long-term aspects of bladder exstrophy, *Clin Orthop* 335:240, 1997.

Kasat LS, Borwankar SS: Factors responsible for successful primary closure in bladder exstrophy, *Pediatr Surg Int* 16:194, 2000.

Loder RT, Dayioglu MM: Association of congenital vertebral malformations with bladder and cloacal exstrophy, *J Pediatr Orthop* 10:389, 1990.

O' Phelan EH: Iliac osteotomy in exstrophy of the bladder, *J Bone Joint Surg* 45A:1409, 1963.

Sponseller PD, Gearhart JP, Jeffs RD: Anterior innominate osteotomies for failure or late closure of bladder exstrophy, *J Urol* 146:137, 1991.

Yazici M, Kandermi U, Atilla B, Eryilmaz M: Rotational profile of lower extremities in bladder exstrophy patients with unapproximated pelvis: a clinical and radiologic study in children older than 7 years, *J Pediatr Orthop* 19:531, 1999.

Yazici M, Sozubir S, Kilicoglu G, et al: Three-dimensional anatomy of the pelvis in bladder exstrophy: description of bone pathology by using three-dimensional computed tomography and its clinical relevance, *J Pediatr Orthop* 18:132, 1998.

Congenital Anomalies of Trunk and Upper Extremity

James H. Beaty

Congenital elevation of the scapula, congenital torticollis, and congenital pseudarthrosis of the clavicle, radius, and ulna are discussed in this chapter. Congenital anomalies of the hand and certain others of the forearm are discussed in Chapter 76. Congenital conditions of the spine are discussed in Chapters 37, 38, and 41.

Congenital Elevation of Scapula (Sprengel Deformity)

In Sprengel deformity, the scapula lies more superiorly than it should in relation to the thoracic cage and usually is hypoplastic and misshapen. Other congenital anomalies may be present such as cervical ribs, malformations of ribs, and anomalies of the cervical vertebrae (Klippel-Feil syndrome); rarely one or more scapular muscles are partly or completely absent. Impairment never is severe unless the deformity is severe. If the deformity is mild, the scapula is only slightly elevated and is a bit smaller than normal, and its motion is only mildly limited; however, if the deformity is severe, the scapula is very small and can be so elevated that it almost touches the occiput. The patient's head often is deviated toward the affected side. In about one third of patients an extra ossicle, the omovertebral bone, is present; this is a rhomboidal plaque of cartilage and bone lying in a strong fascial sheath that extends from the superior angle of the scapula to the spinous process, lamina, or transverse process of one or more lower cervical vertebrae. Sometimes a well-developed joint is found between the omovertebral bone and the scapula; sometimes it is attached to the scapula by fibrous tissue only; rarely it forms a solid osseous ridge between the spinous processes and the scapula. In

a morphometric analysis using three-dimensional computed tomography (3D-CT), Cho et al. found that most of the affected scapulae in 15 patients with Sprengel deformity had a characteristic shape, with a decrease in the height-to-width ratio, and were larger than the contralateral scapulae. An inverse relationship was found between scapular rotation and superior displacement; and no significant difference was found in glenoid version. They suggested that the point of tethering of the omovertebral connection may determine the shape, rotation, and superior displacement of the scapula and that 3D-CT can be helpful in delineating the deformity and planning scapuloplasty.

If deformity and impairment are mild, no treatment is indicated; if they are more severe, surgery may be indicated, depending on the age of the patient and the severity of any associated deformities. The results of surgery occasionally are disappointing because the deformity is never simply elevation of the scapula; it is always complicated by malformations and contractures of the soft tissue structures of the region.

An operation to bring the scapula inferiorly to near its normal position can be attempted after the child is about 3 years old. However, the earlier surgery is performed after 3 years of age, the better the results, because the operation becomes more difficult as the child grows. In older children an attempt to bring the scapula inferiorly to its normal level can injure the brachial plexus.

Numerous operations have been described to correct Sprengel deformity. Two surgical techniques are commonly used. Green described surgical release of muscles from the scapula along with excision of the supraspinatus portion of the scapula and any omovertebral bone. The scapula is then moved inferiorly to a more normal position and the muscles are reattached. Leibovic, Ehrlich, and Zaleske modified the Green procedure by suturing the scapula into a pocket in the latissimus dorsi after rotating the scapula and moving it caudad to a more normal position. Bellemans and Lamourex also described a modification of the Green procedure in which the serratus anterior muscle was not dissected, and mobilization was begun immediately postoperatively. They reported an average abduction gain of 77 degrees using this technique in seven children. Woodward described transfer of the origin of the trapezius muscle to a more inferior position on the spinous processes. Greitemann, Rondhuis, and Karbowski prefer the Woodward procedure for patients with impaired function; for those with only cosmetic problems, resection of part of the superior angle of the scapula is preferred. They believe better results are obtained with the Woodward procedure because (1) the muscles are incised farther from the scapula, which lowers the risk of formation of a scar-keloid that may fix the scapula in poor position; (2) a larger mobilization is possible; and (3) the postoperative scar is not so thick as with Green's procedure. Borges et al. added excision of the prominent superomedial border of the scapula to the Woodward procedure for treatment of Sprengel deformity in 15 patients. At long-term follow-up (average 8 years), total shoulder abduction had improved an average of 35 degrees, and 13 of the 15 patients were satisfied with the results of their surgery. We generally prefer the Woodard procedure, and it is described here (Fig. 28-1).

In an effort to improve function of the shoulder, as well as the cosmetic appearance, Mears developed a procedure that includes partial resection of the scapula, removal of any omovertebral communication, and release of the long head of the triceps from the scapula. In the eight patients in whom this technique was used, average flexion improved from 100 degrees to 175 degrees and abduction improved from 90 degrees to 150 degrees. In two patients, hypertrophic scars formed at the curvilinear incision; this problem was eliminated by the use of a transverse incision in subsequent patients. Mears observed that a contracture of the long head of the triceps seems to represent a significant inhibition to full abduction in patients with Sprengel deformity and that release of this contracture allows increased abduction. Early postoperative active and active-assisted motion exercises of the shoulder are used to improve function.

Brachial plexus palsy is the most severe complication of surgery for Sprengel deformity. The scapula in this deformity is

Fig. 28-1   **A,** Sprengel deformity in 5-year-old boy *(left side).* **B,** Posteroanterior roentgenogram shows congenital elevation of left scapula. **C,** Posteroanterior roentgenogram after Woodward procedure.

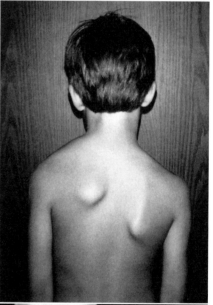

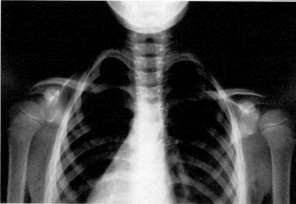

hypoplastic compared with the normal scapula. During surgery attention should be directed to placing the spine of the scapula at the same level as that on the opposite side, rather than aligning exactly the inferior angle of the scapulae. To avoid brachial plexus palsy, several authors recommended morselization of the clavicle on the ipsilateral side as a first step in the operative treatment of Sprengel deformity. This is not a routine part of surgical treatment but is recommended in severe deformity or in children who show signs of brachial plexus palsy after surgical correction. Greiteman et al., however, routinely perform an osteotomy of the clavicle to prevent this complication.

◆ WOODWARD OPERATION FOR CONGENITAL ELEVATION OF SCAPULA

TECHNIQUE 28-1

Place the patient prone on the operating table and prepare and drape both shoulders so that the involved shoulder girdle and the arm can be manipulated and the uninvolved scapula can be inspected in its normal position. Make a midline incision from the spinous process of the first cervical vertebra distally to that of the ninth thoracic vertebra (Fig. 28-2, A). Undermine the skin and subcutaneous tissues laterally to the medial border of the scapula. Next, identify the lateral border of the trapezius in the distal end of the incision and by blunt dissection separate it from the underlying latissimus dorsi muscle. By sharp dissection free the fascial sheath of origin of the trapezius from the spinous processes. Identify the origins of the rhomboideus major and minor muscles and by sharp dissection free them from the spinous processes. Next, free the rhomboids and the superior part of the trapezius from the muscles of the chest wall anterior to them. Retract the freed sheet of muscles laterally to expose any omovertebral bone or fibrous bands attached to the superior angle of the scapula. By extraperiosteal dissection excise any omovertebral bone, or if the bone is absent, excise any fibrous band or contracted levator scapulae; avoid injuring the spinal accessory nerve, the nerves to the rhomboids, and the transverse cervical artery. If the supraspinous part of the scapula is deformed, resect it along with its periosteum; this releases the levator scapulae (if not already excised), allowing the shoulder girdle to move more freely (Fig. 28-2, B). Divide transversely the remaining narrow attachment of the trapezius at the level of the fourth cervical vertebra. Displace the scapula along with the attached sheet of muscles distally until its spine lies at the same level as that of the opposite scapula (Fig. 28-2, C). While holding the scapula in this position, reattach the aponeuroses of the trapezius and rhomboids to the spinous processes at a more inferior level. In the distal part of the incision create a fold in the origin of the trapezius and either excise the excess tissue or incise the fold and overlap and suture in place the resultant free edges (Fig. 28-2, D).

AFTERTREATMENT. A Velpeau bandage is applied and is worn for about 2 weeks. Active and passive range-of-motion exercises are begun.

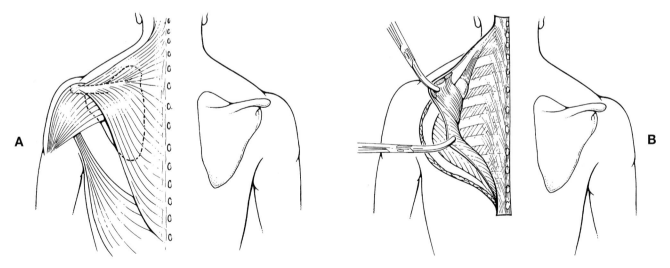

Fig. 28-2 Woodward operation for congenital elevation of scapula. **A,** Elevation of scapula, extensive origin of trapezius, and skin incision are shown. **B,** Skin has been incised in midline. Origins of trapezius and of rhomboideus major and minor have been freed from spinous processes, and these muscles have been retracted laterally. Levator scapulae, any omovertebral bone, and any deformed superior angle of scapula are to be excised. *Continued*

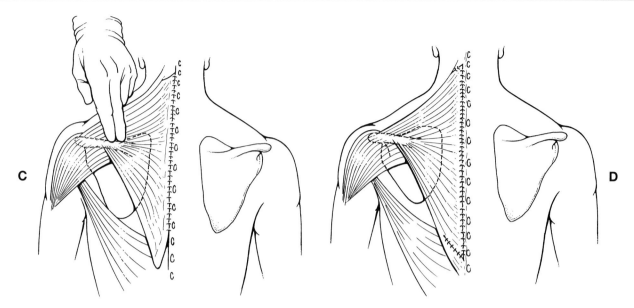

Fig. 28-2, cont'd   C, Remaining narrow attachment of trapezius superiorly has been divided at level of C4. Scapula and attached sheet of muscles have been displaced inferiorly, and aponeuroses of trapezius and rhomboids have been reattached to spinous processes at more inferior level. Thus a redundant fold of trapezius aponeurosis is formed inferiorly. **D,** Fold of trapezius aponeurosis has been incised, and resultant free edges have been overlapped and sutured in place. Free superior edge of trapezius has also been sutured. (Modified from Woodward JW: *J Bone Joint Surg* 43A:219, 1961.)

◆ MORSELIZATION OF CLAVICLE

TECHNIQUE 28-2
Make a straight incision over the clavicle extending from 1.5 cm lateral to the sternoclavicular joint to 1.5 cm medial to the acromioclavicular joint. Expose the clavicle subperiosteally. Next, divide the bone 2 cm from each end, remove it, and cut it into small pieces (morselize). Replace the pieces in the periosteal tube and close the tube with interrupted sutures. Close the subcutaneous tissues and skin in a routine manner.

Congenital Muscular Torticollis

Congenital muscular torticollis (CMT) is caused by fibromatosis within the sternocleidomastoid muscle. A mass either is palpable at birth or becomes so, usually during the first 2 weeks. It is more common on the right side than on the left side. It may involve the muscle diffusely, but more often it is localized near the clavicular attachment of the muscle. The mass attains maximal size within 1 or 2 months and then may remain the same size or become smaller; usually it diminishes and disappears within a year. If it fails to disappear, the muscle becomes permanently fibrotic and contracted and causes torticollis that is also permanent unless treated (Fig. 28-3).

Although CMT has been recognized for centuries, its cause remains unclear. Clinical studies have shown that infants with

CMT are more often the product of a difficult delivery and also have an increased incidence of associated musculoskeletal disorders, such as metatarsus adductus, developmental dysplasia of the hip, and talipes equinovarus. There is a reported incidence of congenital dislocation of the hip or dysplasia of the acetabulum ranging from 7% to 20% in children with CMT. Walsh and Morrissy examined 70 patients with CMT and found an 8% rate of hip disease. Careful screening and, if necessary, roentgenographic examination are indicated.

Various hypotheses of the cause of CMT include malposition of the fetus in utero, birth trauma, infection, and vascular injury. Davids, Wenger, and Mubarak found that MRI scans of 10 infants with CMT showed signals in the sternocleidomastoid muscle similar to those observed in the forearm and leg after compartment syndrome. Further investigation included cadaver dissections and injection studies, which defined the sternocleidomastoid muscle compartment; pressure measurements of three patients with CMT, which confirmed the presence of this compartment in vivo; and clinical review of 48 children with CMT, which showed a relation between birth position and the side affected by contracture. These findings led the authors to postulate that CMT may represent the sequela of an intrauterine or perinatal compartment syndrome (Fig. 28-4).

When CMT is seen in early infancy, it is impossible to tell whether the mass causing it will disappear spontaneously. Lin and Chou reported that ultrasonography can be useful in predicting which infants would require surgical treatment. In their study of 197 infants and children with CMT, all 27 patients in whom fibrotic change was limited to only the lower

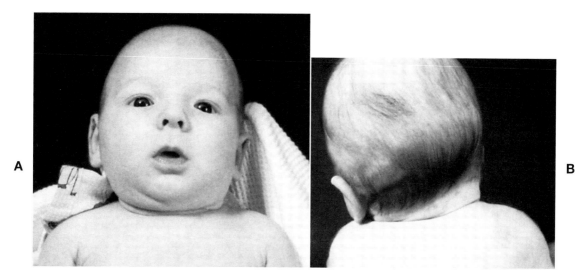

Fig. 28-3 Congenital torticollis *(left)* in 3-month-old girl. **A,** Anterior view. **B,** Posterior view. Note ear moving toward shoulder and chin, away from shoulder on affected left side.

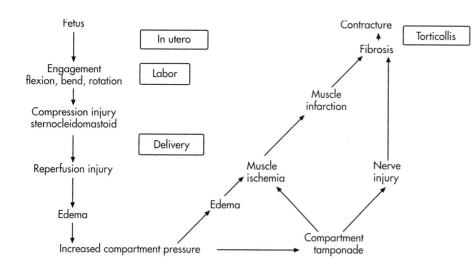

Fig. 28-4 Pathophysiology of congenital muscular torticollis (CMT) proposed by Davids, Wenger, and Mubarak, who suggested that CMT may represent the sequela of intrauterine or perinatal compartment syndrome. (From Davids JR, Wenger DR, Mubarak SJ: *J Pediatr Orthop* 13: 141, 1993.)

third of the SCM muscle recovered without surgery and only 6 (6%) of 93 patients with fibrotic changes limited to the middle and lower third or middle third required surgery, while 26 (35%) of 75 patients with whole muscle involvement required surgical release.

Only conservative treatment is indicated during infancy. The parents should be instructed to stretch the sternocleidomastoid muscle by manipulating the child's head manually. Excising the lesion during early infancy is unjustified; surgery should be delayed until evolution of the fibromatosis is complete, and then, if necessary, the muscle can be released at one or both ends. Coventry and Harris, in a study of 35 infants with CMT seen at the Mayo Clinic, found that conservative treatment at home by the family produced excellent results in 30; the other 5 needed surgical release of the muscle. Coventry and Harris believe that if the muscle is still contracted after the age of 1 year it should be released, but they also believe that surgery at

any age up to 12 years would produce as good a result as operation earlier because asymmetry of the face and skull could still correct itself during the remaining period of growth.

Canale, Griffin, and Hubbard evaluated 57 patients with CMT who were treated between 1941 and 1977 at the Campbell Clinic. They found that CMT did not resolve spontaneously if it persisted beyond the age of 1 year. Children who were treated during the first year of life had better results than those treated later, and an exercise program was more likely to be successful if the restriction of motion was less than 30 degrees and there was no facial asymmetry or the facial asymmetry was noted only by the examiner. Nonoperative therapy after the age of 1 year was rarely successful. Regardless of the type of treatment, established facial asymmetry and limitation of motion of more than 30 degrees at the beginning of treatment usually precluded a good result.

In a prospective study of 821 consecutive patients with

CMT, Cheng et al. divided the patients into three clinical groups: (1) sternomastoid tumor group (those with a clinically palpable sternomastoid tumor), (2) muscular groups (those with clinical thickening and tightness of the sternocleidomastoid muscle), and (3) postural torticollis (those with postural head tilt and clinical features of torticollis but without tightness or tumor of the sternocleidomastoid muscle). Analysis of their results demonstrated that the clinical group (sternomastoid tumor), an older age at presentation, difficulties with the birth, involvement of the right side, and rotation deformity of more than 15 degrees were all significantly associated with longer duration of treatment. The clinical group (sternomastoid tumor), age at presentation, more severe rotation deformity, and duration of treatment were all predictors of final score. Subsequent surgical treatment was required in 8% of patients in the sternomastoid tumor group, 3% of those in the muscular torticollis group, and none of those in the postural torticollis group. Controlled manual stretching was effective in about 95% of patients who were first seen before the age of 1 year.

Any permanent torticollis slowly becomes worse during growth. The head becomes inclined toward the affected side and the face toward the opposite side. If the deformity is severe, the ipsilateral shoulder becomes elevated, and the frontooccipital diameter of the skull may become less than normal. Such severe deformity could and should be prevented by surgery during early childhood. Surgery performed before the age of 6 to 8 years may allow remodeling of any facial asymmetry and plagiocephaly. Unfortunately many patients are first seen only after the deformities have become fixed and the remaining growth potential is insufficient to correct them (Fig. 28-5). Cheng and Tang, however, reported 81.8% excellent or good results in patients who were 10 years or older at the time of surgery and suggested that surgery can be beneficial in these older children.

Several operations have been devised to release the sternocleidomastoid muscle at the clavicle. Unipolar release of the muscle distally is appropriate for mild deformity. Bipolar release proximally and distally may be indicated for moderate and severe torticollis. Endoscopic release of the sternocleidomastoid muscle has been described, with suggested advantages of precise division of the muscle fibers, preservation of the neurovascular structures, and an inconspicuous scar; we have no experience with this technique and no large series have been reported.

◆ UNIPOLAR RELEASE

Ling, in a review of 103 patients treated for torticollis, found that open tenotomy of the sternocleidomastoid muscle could be followed by tethering of the scar to the deep structures, reattachment of the clavicular head or the sternal head of the sternocleidomastoid muscle, loss of contour of the muscle, failure to correct the tilt of the head, or failure of facial asymmetry to correct. Because tethering of the scar to the deep structures is common before the age of 1 year, he recommended

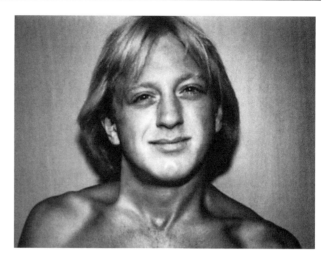

Fig. 28-5 Untreated torticollis *(right)* in 19-year-old man; note limited rotation and plagiocephaly.

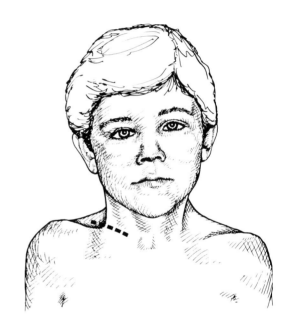

Fig. 28-6 Unipolar release for torticollis. Note line of skin incision.

that the operation be delayed until the child is between the ages of 1 and 4 years.

TECHNIQUE 28-3

Make an incision 5 cm long just superior to and parallel to the medial end of the clavicle (Fig. 28-6) and deepen it to the tendons of the sternal and clavicular attachments of the sternocleidomastoid muscle. Incise the tendon sheath longitudinally and pass a hemostat or other blunt instrument posterior to the tendons. Next, by traction on the hemostat

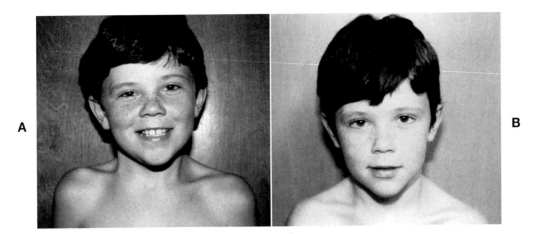

Fig. 28-7   Seven-year-old boy with right congenital muscular torticollis. **A,** Before unipolar supraclavicular release. **B,** After unipolar release; note scar superior to clavicle in transverse line of skin crease.

draw the tendons outside the wound and then superior and inferior to the hemostat; clamp them and resect 2.5 cm of their inferior ends. If contracted, divide the platysma muscle and adjacent fascia. Next, with the child's head turned toward the affected side and the chin depressed, explore the wound digitally for any remaining bands of contracted muscle or fascia, and if any are found, divide them under direct vision until the deformity can, if possible, be overcorrected. If after this procedure overcorrection is not possible, make a small transverse incision inferior to the mastoid process and carefully divide the muscle near the bone. Take care to avoid damaging the spinal accessory nerve. Close the wound or wounds and apply a bulky dressing that holds the head in the overcorrected position.

AFTERTREATMENT. At 1 week physical therapy, including manual stretching of the neck to maintain the overcorrected position, is begun. Manual stretching should be continued three times daily for 3 to 6 months; the use of plaster casts or braces usually is unnecessary (Fig. 28-7).

◆ BIPOLAR RELEASE

Surgical correction in children with severe deformity or after failed operation usually requires a bipolar release of the sternocleidomastoid muscle. Wirth et al. recommended bipolar release between the ages of 3 and 5 years in all patients who do not respond to nonoperative treatment. Chen and Ko reported excellent or good results in 10 of 18 patients ranging in age from 6 to 22 years (average age, 11 years) who were treated with bipolar (16) or distal (2) releases. All but 2 patients had improvement of facial asymmetry, and all but 1 had satisfactory

neck range of motion. They recommended bipolar release as the treatment of choice for CMT in patients older than 6 years of age. Ferkel et al. described a modified bipolar release and Z-plasty of the muscle for use in these circumstances.

TECHNIQUE 28-4 *(Ferkel et al.)*

Make a short transverse proximal incision behind the ear (Fig. 28-8, *A*) and divide the sternocleidomastoid muscle insertion transversely just distal to the tip of the mastoid process. With this limited incision the spinal accessory nerve is avoided, although the possibility that the nerve may take an anomalous route should be considered. Next, make a distal incision 4 to 5 cm long in line with the cervical skin creases, a fingerbreadth proximal to the medial end of the clavicle and the sternal notch. Divide the subcutaneous tissue and platysma muscle, exposing the clavicular and sternal attachments of the sternocleidomastoid muscle. Carefully avoid the anterior and external jugular veins and the carotid vessels and sheath during the dissection. Next, cut the clavicular portion of the muscle transversely and perform a Z-plasty on the sternal attachment so as to preserve the normal V-contour of the sternocleidomastoid muscle in the neckline (Fig. 28-8, *B* and *C*). Obtain the desired degree of correction by manipulating the head and neck during the release. Occasionally, release of additional contracted bands of fascia or muscle is necessary before closure. Close both wounds with subcuticular sutures.

AFTERTREATMENT. Physical therapy, consisting of stretching, muscle strengthening, and active range-of-motion exercises, is instituted in the early postoperative period. Head-halter traction or a cervical collar also can be used during the first 6 to 12 weeks after surgery (Fig. 28-9).

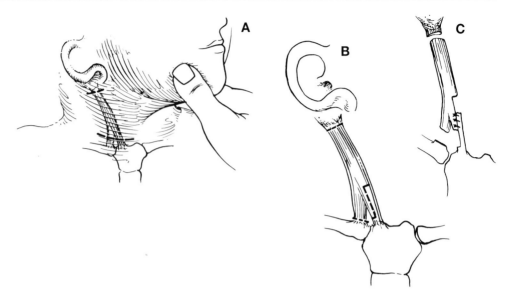

Fig. 28-8 Bipolar Z-plasty operation for torticollis. **A,** Skin incisions. **B,** Clavicular and mastoid attachments of sterno-cleidomastoid muscle are cut, and Z-plasty is performed on sternal origin. **C,** Completed operation; note preservation of medial portion of sternal attachment. (Redrawn from Ferkel RD, Westin GW, Dawson EG, Oppenheim WL: *J Bone Joint Surg* 65A:894, 1983.)

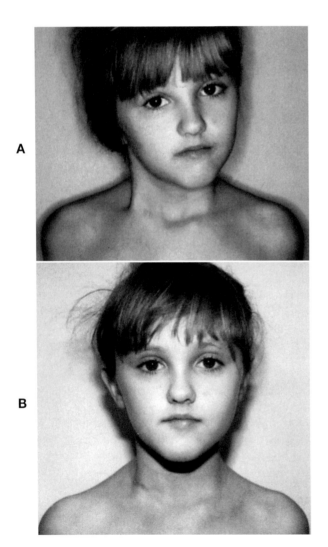

Fig. 28-9 Bipolar release for congenital torticollis. **A,** Severe congenital torticollis *(right)* in 8-year-old girl. **B,** After bipolar release.

Congenital Pseudarthrosis of Clavicle

Congenital pseudarthrosis of the clavicle is a rare anomaly. Several theories concerning its cause have been proposed. One is that since the clavicle develops in two separate masses by medial and lateral ossification centers, pseudarthrosis could be explained by failure of ossification of the precartilaginous bridge that would normally connect the two ossification centers. Another theory is that the lesion may be caused by direct pressure from the subclavian artery on the immature clavicle on the right. Congenital pseudarthrosis of the clavicle occurs almost invariably on the right side; bilateral involvement occurs in approximately 10% of patients. In a series of 60 unilateral lesions, 59 were on the right, and in the one patient with a pseudarthrosis on the left, dextrocardia was found. Pseudarthrosis of the clavicle is present at birth and usually is in the middle third of the clavicle (Fig. 28-10). The differential diagnoses include cleidocranial dysostosis and the rare nonunion after clavicular fracture.

Congenital pseudarthrosis of the clavicle may require treatment, not because of pain or hypermobility of the shoulder girdle, but usually because of an unacceptable appearance or occasionally because of pain in adolescent patients. Sales de Gauzy et al. described thoracic outlet syndrome in an adolescent with congenital pseudarthrosis of the clavicle. Hyperabduction of the arm caused compression of the subclavian artery by the medial end of the lateral clavicular fragment. After resection of the pseudarthrosis, iliac bone grafting, and plate fixation, the patient was pain free with total functional recovery. These authors suggested that, although congenital pseudarthrosis of the clavicle is asymptomatic in childhood, surgical treatment can restore normal morphology and prevent functional or vascular problems in adolescence and adulthood.

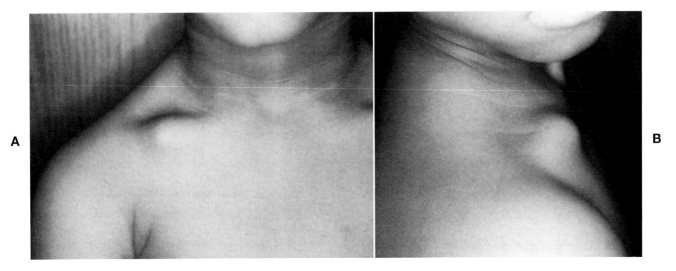

Fig. 28-10   Congenital pseudarthrosis of clavicle. **A,** Subcutaneous prominence in middle third of right clavicle in 4-year-old child. **B,** Lateral view.

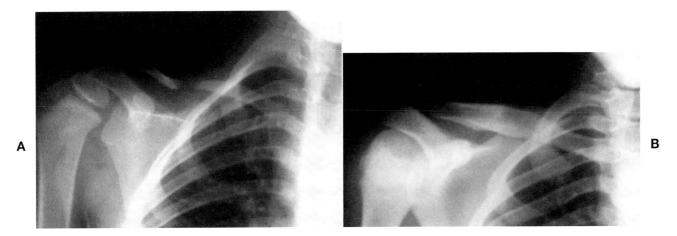

Fig. 28-11   **A,** Congenital pseudarthrosis of right clavicle before plating and bone grafting. **B,** At 7 years of age after plate removal.

Spontaneous union is unknown, and consequently any desired union requires open reduction and bone grafting. Most surgeons agree that the ideal time for grafting is between the ages of 3 and 5 years. Although it can be carried out at any age, the older the patient is, the more difficult is the grafting. Simple resection of the prominent ends of the bone has resulted in pain, prominence of the ends during movements of the shoulder, and asymmetry of the shoulder girdles. Grogan et al., however, reported the treatment of eight children with resection of fibrous pseudarthroses and sclerotic bone ends, careful dissection and preservation of the periosteal sleeve to maintain continuity, and approximation of bone ends, without bone grafting or internal fixation. All had bridging ossification by 6 to 8 weeks after surgery, and all were solidly healed by 14 weeks after surgery. Six of their eight patients were younger than 3 years of age at the time of surgery, but the two older children (5 and 6 years of age) also healed without internal

fixation. Grogan et al. suggested that early resection probably does not require the extensive grafting and internal fixation that are recommended for older children. Lorento Molto et al. also recommended early surgical treatment, citing good results in five children who were treated at ages ranging from 18 months to 4 years. The procedure in these children included excision of the pseudarthrosis, bone grafting, and fixation with an intramedullary Kirschner wire. Union was obtained in all patients within 6 weeks and all were satisfied with the cosmetic appearance.

Union is easier to obtain in congenital pseudarthrosis of the clavicle than in that of the tibia. Almost any type of bone grafting suitable for traumatic nonunion of the clavicle has been satisfactory in pseudarthrosis, but open reduction and internal fixation with plate and screws and autogenous iliac bone grafting have produced the best results, especially in older children (Fig. 28-11).

◆ OPEN REDUCTION AND ILIAC BONE GRAFTING

TECHNIQUE 28-5

Make a transverse 3-inch (7.5 cm) incision centered over the body of the clavicle, approximately a fingerbreadth above the superior border of the bone. Carry sharp dissection through the subcutaneous tissue to expose the clavicle, both medially and laterally and in the central third in the area of the pseudarthrosis. Expose the bone subperiosteally, taking care to protect the underlying neurovascular structures. Debride the site of the pseudarthrosis of all fibrous and cartilaginous tissue down to normal bone both medially and laterally. Bend a four-hole plate (either semitubular, dynamic compression, or acetabular reconstruction) to fit the contours of the bone. Next, fix the plate to the clavicle in the usual manner. Obtain autogenous iliac grafts and place them on the superior, inferior, and posterior aspects of the pseudarthrosis. Close the wound in layers and the skin with subcuticular sutures.

AFTERTREATMENT. A collar and cuff sling is worn for 2 to 3 weeks. The plate can be removed at 12 to 24 months or when roentgenographic union occurs.

Congenital Dislocation of Radial Head

Congenital dislocation of the radial head is rare but should be suspected when the head has been dislocated for a long time, there is no evidence that the ulna has been fractured, and the radial head appears abnormally small and misshapen. The roentgenographic findings are fairly characteristic. The radial shaft is abnormally long, and the ulna usually is abnormally bowed. The radial head is dislocated, frequently posteriorly but sometimes anteriorly; is rounded, showing little if any depression for articulation with the capitellum; and usually is smaller than normal; occasionally there is an area of ossification in the tissues about it. The capitellum also may be small, and the radial notch of the ulna that should articulate with the radial head may be small or absent (Fig. 28-12). Although bilaterality has been listed in older studies as a criterion for diagnosis of congenital dislocation of the radial head, more recent reports have confirmed the existence of unilateral dislocations.

Congenital dislocation of the radial head may be familial, especially on the paternal side, and may be associated with chondroosteodystrophy.

A congenitally dislocated radial head is irreducible either manually or surgically because of adaptive changes in the soft tissues and the absence of normal surfaces for articulation with the ulna and humerus. Consequently, open reduction of the dislocation and reconstruction of the annular ligament in childhood are inadvisable. Any impairment of function usually is caused by restriction of rotation of the forearm, and in children physical therapy to improve this motion is the only treatment indicated. If pain persists into adulthood, the radial head and neck can be excised. Any resection of the radial head should be postponed until growth is complete, but even then it may not improve motion because of the contractures of the soft tissues. Campbell, Waters, and Emans, however, reported good results after radial head excision in six patients (eight elbows) ranging in age from 10 to 15.5 years. Contrary to previously published data, excision of the radial head resulted in an increased range of motion and a decrease in elbow pain in all eight elbows.

Congenital Pseudarthrosis of Radius

Congenital pseudarthrosis of the radius is extremely rare. In patients with neurofibromatosis, the pseudarthrosis develops

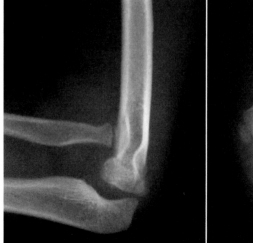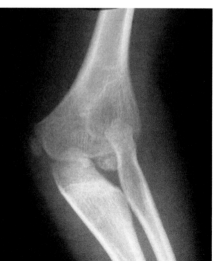

Fig. 28-12 Congenital dislocation of radial head. **A,** Lateral view. **B,** Anteroposterior view.

from a cyst in the radius, and patients usually have skin manifestations of neurofibromatosis or a strong family history of the disease.

In each instance reported, pseudarthrosis of the radius occurred in the distal third of the bone, and the distal fragment was quite short. Because the lesion is near the distal radial physis, the ends of the bone are attenuated and the ulna is relatively long. The treatment of choice is dual-onlay bone grafting as recommended by Boyd for congenital pseudarthrosis of the tibia (Chapter 26). This operation restores length, provides a viselike grip on the osteoporotic distal fragment, increases the size of the distal end of the proximal fragment, and usually results in satisfactory union (Fig. 28-13). Kameyama and Ogawa reported good results after complete resection of the involved radius, with the surrounding periosteum and soft tissue, and free vascularized fibular transfer. They suggested that the operation be delayed until skeletal maturity and that the arm be supported with a forearm brace until surgery is performed. In their review of the English literature Witoonchart et al. found that free vascular fibular grafting obtained the best union rate among the reported procedures: it was successful in 18 of 19 ulnar or radial pseudarthroses reported. Both Allieu et al. and Cheng et al. recommended free vascularized fibular grafting early, before the radial head is dislocated. Although the procedures in their patients were done at relatively young ages (20 months, 30 months, 5 years), Witoonchart et al. pointed out the difficulty of obtaining stable internal fixation in very young patients, in whom plate and screw fixation risks damage to the vascular supply of the periosteum around the fibular graft. They suggested that unstable fixation with only intramedullary and crossed Kirschner wires might have been the cause of a delayed

union in one of their patients. Vascular fibular grafting is described in Chapter 60.

Congenital Pseudarthrosis of Ulna

Congenital pseudarthrosis of the ulna in neurofibromatosis also is extremely rare. In their review of the English literature, Witoonchart et al. identified 29 patients with ulnar pseudarthrosis, 17 with radial pseudarthrosis, and 14 with pseudarthrosis of both bones. Of these 60, only 16 (27%) had no signs or family history of neurofibromatosis. The ulnar pseudarthrosis produces angulation of the radius, shortening of the forearm, and dislocation of the radial head (Fig. 28-14).

Various treatment methods have been described for congenital ulnar pseudarthrosis, including nonvascularized bone grafting with and without internal fixation, creation of a one-bone forearm, free vascularized fibular grafting, and the Ilizarov compression-distraction technique. Bone grafting of congenital pseudarthrosis of the ulna usually has failed, but because significant bowing of the radius develops in very young children, early surgery is indicated. If the pseudarthrosis has developed through a cystic lesion, early curettage of the cyst, internal fixation of the bone, and bone grafting usually are successful. In established pseudarthrosis with tapering of the ends of the bone, the distal ulna should be excised early to relieve its tethering effect on the radius; then the forearm is fitted with a suitable brace. If the radial head dislocates, it should be excised and a synostosis (one-bone forearm) produced between the radius and ulna (see Fig. 28-13). Osteotomy of the distal radius to correct bowing also may be indicated. Use of the Ilizarov device has been reported in

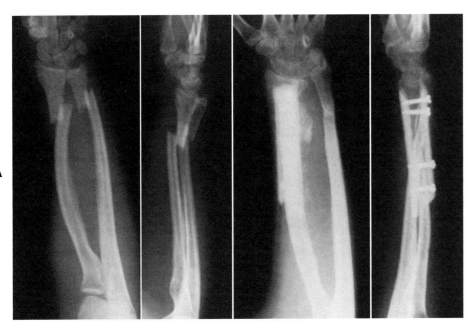

A   **B**

Fig. 28-13 Congenital pseudarthrosis of radius. **A,** Closed fractures of radius and ulna in child with manifestations of neurofibromatosis. **B,** Union of radius after dual onlay bone grafting.

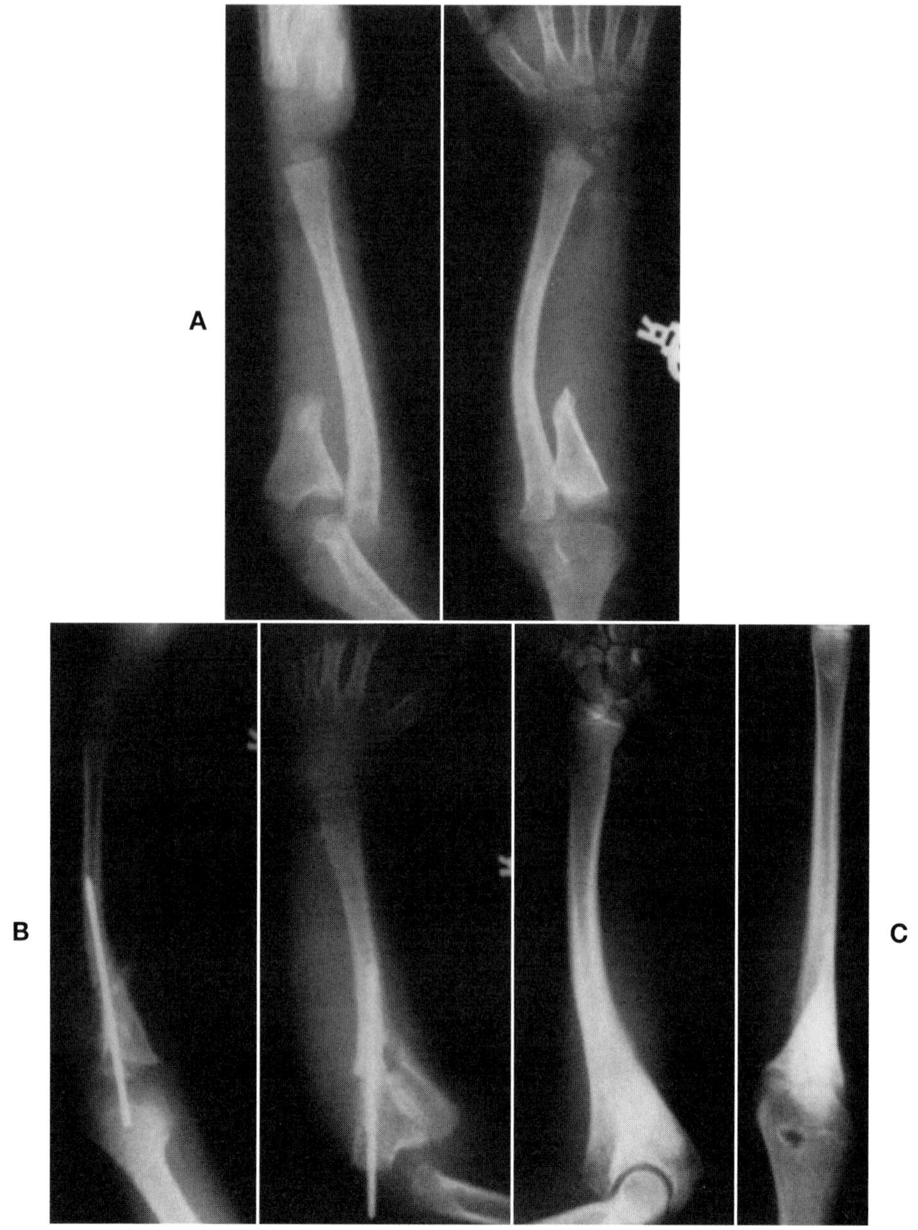

Fig. 28-14   Congenital pseudarthrosis of ulna with dislocation of radial head. **A,** Before surgery. **B,** After excision of radial head, creation of synostosis between proximal radius and ulna, and fixation with medullary nail. **C,** Final appearance of one-bone forearm.

patients with small pseudarthrosis "gaps" and bony fragments of acceptable quality.

◆ Congenital Radioulnar Synostosis

Congenital radioulnar synostosis usually involves the proximal ends of the radius and ulna, most often fixing the forearm in pronation. It is more often bilateral than unilateral. Familial predisposition is frequent, and the deformity seems to be transmitted on the paternal side of the family. Wilkie noted two types. In the first type the medullary canals of the radius and ulna are joined. The proximal end of the radius is malformed and is fused to the ulna for several centimeters (Fig. 28-15). The radius is longer and larger than the ulna, and its shaft

arches anteriorly more than normally. In the second type the radius is fairly normal, but its proximal end is dislocated either anteriorly or posteriorly and is fused to the proximal ulnar shaft; the fusion is neither as extensive nor as intimate as in the first type. Wilkie stated that the second type often is unilateral and that sometimes another deformity, such as a supernumerary thumb, absence of the thumb, or syndactylism, also is present.

Congenital radioulnar synostosis is difficult to treat. The fascial tissues are short and their fibers are abnormally directed, the interosseous membrane is narrow, and the supinator muscles may be abnormal or absent. The anomalies in the forearm may be so widespread that sometimes no rotation is possible, even after the radius and ulna have been separated and the interosseous membrane has been split throughout its length. Simply excising the fused part of the radius never improves

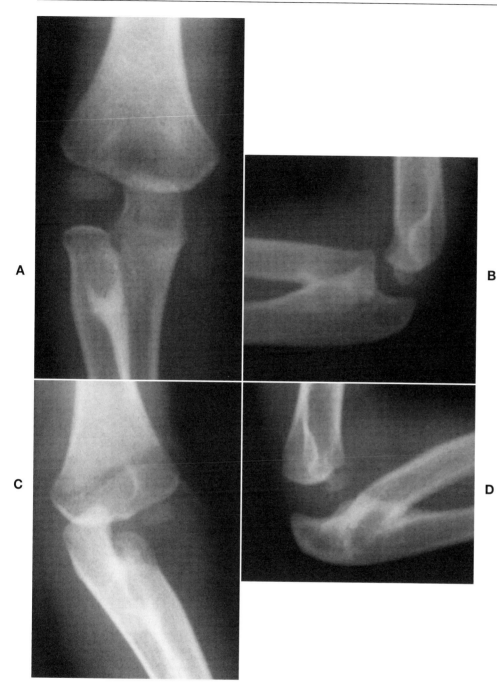

Fig. 28-15 Congenital radioulnar synostosis. **A** and **B,** First type: proximal radius and ulna are fused for 3 cm and radius is enlarged. **C** and **D,** Second type: radius is dislocated posteriorly and laterally.

function. It is inadvisable to perform any operation with the hope of obtaining pronation and supination. Fortunately, most patients are not disabled enough to justify an extensive operation. Any disabling pronation or supination deformity should be corrected by osteotomy; motion of the shoulder, especially when the elbow is extended, compensates well for the deformity in most children. Osteotomy occasionally is indicated in children with bilateral hyperpronation. One forearm can be positioned in neutral rotation to assist in hygiene. Seitz, Gordon, and Konsens reported the use of a small external fixation device after derotational osteotomy in a 2-year-old

child with congenital radioulnar synostosis. They cited as advantages to this technique precise rotational correction, adequate stabilization, and avoidance of cast immobilization.

Lin et al. described a two-stage technique for correction of severe forearm rotational deformities, including congenital radioulnar synostosis. Percutaneous drill-assisted osteotomies of both the radius and ulna are performed and are followed 10 days later by manipulation of the forearm into the desired functional position. No internal or external fixation is used; long-arm cast immobilization is used for 6 to 8 weeks. They reported functional improvement in 25 of 26 forearms,

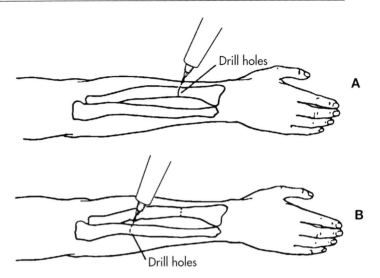

Fig. 28-16   Correction of congenital radioulnar synostosis with percutaneous drill-assisted osteotomies of radius (**A**) and ulna (**B**). Ten days later forearm is manipulated to more functional position. (From Lin HH, Strecker WB, Manske PR, et al: *J Pediatr Orthop* 15:53, 1995.)

including all 12 forearms with congenital radioulnar synostosis. Although the range of motion was not significantly changed, the arc of motion was in a more functional hand position.

TECHNIQUE 28-6 *(Lin et al.)*

Under tourniquet control, make a 1- to 2-cm incision over the dorsolateral ridge of the distal third of the radius (Fig. 28-16, *A*). Expose the bone subperiosteally and mark the osteotomy site with several fine drill holes that penetrate both cortices. Make a second small incision over the subcutaneous aspect of the proximal third of the ulna and similarly expose and drill this bone (Fig. 28-16, *B*). Use a sharp osteotome to complete the division of the radius and then the ulna. At this point, make no attempt to change the position of the arm. Deflate the tourniquet and obtain adequate hemostasis. Irrigate the wounds and close them with subcuticular sutures. Place a long arm cast over sterile dressings.

Ten days later, remove the cast with the patient under general anesthesia and supinate or pronate the forearm into the desired position. Obtain anteroposterior and lateral roentgenograms to confirm bony apposition and alignment. Generally, affected dominant extremities should be placed in 20 to 30 degrees of pronation and nondominant extremities in 20 degrees of supination. Check pulses carefully after manipulation and monitor the extremity closely to detect signs of compartment syndrome. Apply a long arm cast, which is worn for 6 to 8 weeks to allow complete healing of the osteotomies.

Kanaya and Ibaraki described a technique for mobilization of congenital radioulnar synostosis with use of a free vascularized fascio-fat graft to prevent recurrent ankylosis. The graft was obtained from the lateral aspect of the ipsilateral arm and reported minimal donor site morbidity and no difficulty with closure. The seven patients in whom this procedure was

done all had marked improvements in supination and pronation; at an almost 4-year average follow-up none had recurrent ankylosis or loss of the flap. The authors found that adding a radial osteotomy to the procedure prevented dislocation of the radial head and increased the arc of motion (83 degrees in those with osteotomy compared with 40 degrees in those without osteotomy). We have no experience with this technique.

References

CONGENITAL ELEVATION OF SCAPULA

Bellemans M, Lamoureux J: Results of surgical treatment of Sprengel deformity by a modified Green's procedure, *J Pediatr Orthop* 8:194, 1999.

Borges JLP, Shah A, Tores BC, Bowen JR: Modified Woodward procedure for Sprengel deformity of the shoulder: long-term results, *J Pediatr Orthop* 16:508, 1996.

Cho TJ, Choi IH, Chung CY, Hwang JK: The Sprengel deformity: morphometric analysis using 3D-CT and its clinical relevance, *J Bone Joint Surg* 82B:7121, 2000.

Chung SMK, Farahvar H: Surgery of the clavicle in Sprengel's deformity, *Clin Orthop* 116:138, 1976.

Chung SMK, Nissenbaum MM: Congenital and developmental defects of the shoulder, *Orthop Clin North Am* 6:381, 1975.

Galpin RD, Birch JG: Congenital elevation of the scapula (Sprengel's deformity), *Orthopedics* 10:965, 1987.

Green WT: The surgical correction of congenital elevation of the scapula (Sprengel's deformity), *J Bone Joint Surg* 39A:1439, 1957.

Green WT: Sprengel's deformity: congenital elevation of the scapula, *Instr Course Lect* 21:55, 1972.

Greitemann B, Rondhuis JJ, Karbowski A: Treatment of congenital elevation of the scapula: 10- (1-18) year follow-up of 37 cases of Sprengel's deformity, *Acta Orthop Scand* 64:365, 1993.

Halley DK, Eyring EJ: Congenital elevation of the scapula in a family, *Clin Orthop* 97:31, 1973.

Leibovic SJ, Ehrlich MG, Zaleske DJ: Sprengel deformity, *J Bone Joint Surg* 72A:192, 1990.

Mears DC: Partial resection of the scapula and a release of the long head of the triceps for the management of Sprengel's deformity, *J Pediatr Orthop* 21:242, 2001.

Orrell KG, Bell DF: Structural abnormality of the clavicle associated with Sprengel's deformity: a case report, *Clin Orthop* 258:157, 1990.

Robinson RA, Braun RM, Mack P, Zadek R: The surgical importance of the clavicular component of Sprengel's deformity, *J Bone Joint Surg* 49A:481, 1967 (abstract).

Woodward JW: Congenital elevation of the scapula: correction by release and transplantation of muscle origins: a preliminary report, *J Bone Joint Surg* 43A:219, 1961.

CONGENITAL MUSCULAR TORTICOLLIS

Brougham DI, Cole WG, Dickens DRV, Menelaus MB: Torticollis due to a combination of sternomastoid contracture and congenital vertebral anomalies, *J Bone Joint Surg* 71B:404, 1989.

Burstein FD, Cohen SR: Endoscopic surgical treatment for congenital muscular torticollis, *Plast Reconstr Surg* 101:40, 1998.

Canale ST, Griffin DW, Hubbard CN: Congenital muscular torticollis: a long-term follow-up, *J Bone Joint Surg* 64A:810, 1982.

Chen CE, Ko JY: Surgical treatment of muscular torticollis for patients above 6 years of age, *Arch Orthop Trauma Surg* 120:149, 2000.

Cheng JC, Tang SP: Outcome of surgical treatment of congenital muscular torticollis, *Clin Orthop* 362:190, 1999.

Cheng JC, Tang SP, Chen TM: Sternocleidomastoid pseudotumor and congenital muscular torticollis in infants: a prospective study of 510 cases, *J Pediatr* 134:712, 1999.

Cheng JC, Tang SP, Chen TM, et al: The clinical presentation and outcome of treatment of congenital muscular torticollis in infants: a study of 1086 cases, *J Pediatr Surg* 35:1091, 2000.

Cheng JCY, Wong MWN, Tang SP, et al: Clinical determinants of the outcome of manual stretching in the treatment of congenital muscular torticollis in infants: a prospective study of eight hundred and twenty-one cases, *J Bone Joint Surg* 83A:679, 2001.

Coventry MB, Harris L: Congenital muscular torticollis in infancy: some observations regarding treatment, *J Bone Joint Surg* 41A:815, 1959.

Davids JR, Wenger DR, Mubarak SJ: Congenital muscular torticollis: sequela of intrauterine or perinatal compartment syndrome, *J Pediatr Orthop* 13:141, 1993.

Demirbilek S, Atayurt HF: Congenital muscular torticollis and sternomastoid tumor: results of nonoperative treatment, *J Pediatr Surg* 34:549, 1999.

Ferkel RD, Westin GW, Dawson EG, Oppenheim WL: Muscular torticollis: a modified surgical approach, *J Bone Joint Surg* 65A: 894, 1983.

Hummer CD Jr, MacEwen GD: The coexistence of torticollis and congenital dysplasia of the hip, *J Bone Joint Surg* 54A:1255, 1972.

Lin JN, Chou ML: Ultrasonographic study of the sternocleidomastoid muscle in the management of congenital muscular torticollis, *J Pediatr Surg* 32:1648, 1997.

Ling CM: The influence of age on the results of open sternomastoid tenotomy in muscular torticollis, *Clin Orthop* 116:142, 1976.

Walsh JJ, Morrissy RT: Torticollis and hip dislocation, *J Pediatr Orthop* 18:219, 1998.

Wei JL, Schwartz KM, Weaver AL, Orvidas LJ: Pseudotumor of infancy and congenital muscular torticollis: 170 cases, *Laryngoscope* 111:688, 2001.

Wirth CJ, Hagena FW, Wuelker N, et al: Biterminal tenotomy for the treatment of congenital muscular torticollis: long-term results, *J Bone Joint Surg* 74A:417, 1992.

CONGENITAL PSEUDARTHROSES OF CLAVICLE, RADIUS, AND ULNA

Ali MS, Hooper G: Congenital pseudarthrosis of the ulna due to neurofibromatosis, *J Bone Joint Surg* 64B:600, 1982.

Allieu Y, Meyer zu Reckendorf G, Chammas M, Gomis R: Congenital pseudarthrosis of both forearm bones: long-term results of two cases managed by free vascularized fibular graft, *J Hand Surg* 24A:604, 1999.

Baldwin DM, Weiner DS: Congenital bowing and intraosseous neurofibroma of the ulna: a case report, *J Bone Joint Surg* 56A:803, 1974.

Bargar WL, Marcus RE, Ittleman FP: Late thoracic outlet syndrome secondary to pseudarthrosis of the clavicle, *J Trauma* 24:857, 1984.

Bayne LG: Congenital pseudarthrosis of the forearm, *Hand Clin* 1:457, 1985.

Bell DF: Congenital forearm pseudarthrosis: report of six cases and review of the literature, *J Pediatr Orthop* 9:438, 1989.

Boyd HB: Congenital pseudarthrosis: treatment by dual bone grafts, *J Bone Joint Surg* 23:497, 1941.

Boyd HB, Fox KW: Congenital pseudarthrosis: follow-up study after massive bone-grafting, *J Bone Joint Surg* 30A:274, 1948.

Brooks S: Bilateral congenital pseudarthrosis of the clavicles: case report and review of the literature, *Br J Clin Pract* 38:432, 1984.

Burge P, Benson M: Bilateral congenital pseudarthrosis of the olecranon, *J Bone Joint Surg* 69:460, 1987.

Cheng JCY, Hung LK, Bundoc RC: Congenital pseudarthrosis of the ulna, *J Hand Surg* 19B:238, 1994.

Fabry G, Lammens J, Van Melkebeek J, et al: Treatment of congenital pseudarthrosis with the Ilizarov technique, *J Pediatr Orthop* 8:67, 1988.

Gibson DA, Carroll N: Congenital pseudarthrosis of the clavicle, *J Bone Joint Surg* 52B:629, 1970.

Greenberg LA, Schwartz A: Congenital pseudarthrosis of the distal radius, *South Med J* 68:1053, 1975.

Grogan DP, Love SM, Guidera KJ, et al: Operative treatment of congenital pseudarthrosis of the clavicle, *J Pediatr Orthop* 11:176, 1991.

Herman S: Congenital bilateral pseudarthrosis of the clavicles, *Clin Orthop* 91:162, 1973.

Herring JA, Roach JW: Congenital pseudarthrosis of the radius (clinical conference), *J Pediatr Orthop* 5:367, 1985.

Kameyama O, Ogawa R: Pseudarthrosis of the radius associated with neurofibromatosis: report of a case and review of the literature, *J Pediatr Orthop* 10:128, 1990.

Lee KS, Lee SH, Ha KH, Lee SJ: Congenital pseudarthrosis of the ulna treated by free vascularized fibular graft: a case report, *Hand Surg* 5:61, 2000.

Lloyd-Roberts GC, Apley AG, Owen R: Reflections upon the aetiology of congenital pseudarthrosis of the clavicle: with a note on cranio-cleido dysostosis, *J Bone Joint Surg* 57B:24, 1975.

Masterson E, Earley MJ, Stephens MM: Congenital pseudarthrosis of the ulna treated by free vascularized fibular graft: a case report and review of methods of treatment, *J Hand Surg* 18B:285, 1993.

Mathoulin C, Gilbert A, Azze R: Congenital pseudarthrosis of the forearm: treatment of six cases with vascularized fibular graft and review of the literature, *Microsurgery* 14:252, 1993.

Lorente Molto FJ, Bonete Lluch DJ, Garrido IM: Congenital pseudarthrosis of the clavicle: a proposal for early surgical treatment, *J Pediatr Orthop* 21:689, 2001.

Ostrowski DM: Congenital pseudarthrosis of the forearm, *J Hand Surg* 14A:318, 1989 (letter).

Ostrowski DM, Eilert RE, Waldstein G: Congenital pseudarthrosis of the ulna: a report of two cases and a review of the literature, *J Pediatr Orthop* 5:463, 1985.

Ramelli GP, Slongo T, Tschappeler H, Weis J: Congenital pseudarthrosis of the ulnar and radius in two cases of neurofibromatosis type 1, *Pediatr Surg Int* 17:239, 2001.

Richin PF, Kranik A, Van Herpe L, Suffecool SL: Congenital pseudarthrosis of both bones of the forearm: a case report, *J Bone Joint Surg* 58A:1032, 1976.

Sales de Gauzy J, Baunin C, Puget C, et al: Congenital pseudarthrosis of the clavicle and thoracic outlet syndrome in adolescence, *J Pediatr Orthop* 8:299, 1999.

Schnall SB, King JD, Marrero G: Congenital pseudarthrosis of the clavicle: a review of the literature and surgical results of six cases, *J Pediatr Orthop* 8:318, 1988.

Schoenecker PL, Johnson GE, Howard B, et al: Congenital pseudarthrosis, *Orthop Rev* 21:885, 1992.

Sellers DS, Sowa DT, Moore JR, Weiland AJ: Congenital pseudarthrosis of the forearm, *J Hand Surg* 13A:89, 1988.

Sprague BL, Brown GA: Congenital pseudarthrosis of the radius, *J Bone Joint Surg* 56A:191, 1974.

Witoonchart K, Uerpairojkit C, Leechavengvongs S, Thuvasethakul P: Congenital pseudarthrosis of the forearm treated by free vascularized fibular graft: a report of three cases and a review of the literature, *J Hand Surg* 24A:1045, 1999.

Yougne D, Arford C: Congenital pseudarthrosis of the forearm and fibula: a case report, *Clin Orthop* 265, 1991.

Zaman M: Pseudoarthrosis of the radius associated with neurofibromatosis: a case report, *J Bone Joint Surg* 59A:977, 1977.

CONGENITAL DISLOCATION OF RADIAL HEAD

Agnew DK, Davis RJ: Congenital unilateral dislocation of the radial head, *J Pediatr Orthop* 13:526, 1993.

Bell S, Morrey B, Bianco A: Chronic posterior subluxation and dislocation of the radial head, *J Bone Joint Surg* 73A:392, 1991.

Campbell CC, Waters PM, Emans JB: Excision of the radial head for congenital dislocation, *J Bone Joint Surg* 74A:726, 1992.

Exarhou EI, Antoniou NK: Congenital dislocation of the head of the radius, *Acta Orthop Scand* 41:551, 1970.

Gattey PH, Wedge JH: Unilateral posterior dislocation of the radial head in identical twins, *J Pediatr Orthop* 6:220, 1986.

Gleason TF, Goldstein WM: Traumatic recurrent posterior dislocation of the radial head: a case report, *Clin Orthop* 184:186, 1984.

Keats S: Congenital bilateral dislocation of the head of the radius in a seven-year-old child, *Orthop Rev* 3:33, 1974.

Lancaster S, Horowitz M: Lateral idiopathic subluxation of the radial head: case report, *Clin Orthop* 214:170, 1987.

Luke DL, Schoenecker PL, Gilula LA: Imaging rounds 100: congenital dislocation of the radial head, *Orthop Rev* 18:911, 1989.

Menio GJ, Wenner SM: Radial head dislocations in children with below-elbow deficiencies, *J Hand Surg* 17A:891, 1992.

Miura T: Congenital dislocation of the radial head, *J Bone Joint Surg* 72B:477, 1990.

Mizuno K, Usui Y, Kohyama K, et al: Familial congenital unilateral anterior dislocation of the radial head: differentiation from traumatic dislocation by means of arthrography: a case report, *J Bone Joint Surg* 73A:1086, 1991.

Woo CC: Traumatic radial head subluxation in young children: a case report and literature review, *J Manipulative Physiol Ther* 10:191, 1987.

CONGENITAL RADIOULNAR SYNOSTOSIS

Bauer M, Jonsson K: Congenital radioulnar synostosis: radiological characteristics and hand function—case reports, *Scand J Plast Reconstr Surg Hand Surg* 22:251, 1988.

Dal Monte A, Andrisano A, Bungaro P, Mignani G: Congenital proximal radio-ulnar synostosis: clinical and anatomical features, *Ital J Orthop Traumatol* 13:201, 1987.

Dal Monte A, Andrisano A, Mignani G, Bungaro P: A critical review of the surgical treatment of congenital proximal radio-ulnar synostosis, *Ital J Orthop Traumatol* 13:181, 1987.

Griffet J, Berard J, Michel CR, et al: Les synostoses congenitales radio-cubitales superieures: a propos de 43 cas, *Int Orthop* 10:265, 1986.

Hankin FM, Smith PA, Kling TF Jr, Louis DS: Ulnar nerve palsy following rotational osteotomy of congenital radioulnar synostosis, *J Pediatr Orthop* 7:103, 1987.

Hansen OH, Andersen NO: Congenital radioulnar synostosis: report of 37 cases, *Acta Orthop Scand* 41:225, 1970.

Kanaya F, Ibaraki K: Mobilization of a congenital proximal radioulnar synostosis with use of a free vascularized fascio-fat graft, *J Bone Joint Surg* 80A:1186, 1998.

Lin HH, Strecker WB, Manske PR, et al: A surgical technique of radioulnar osteoclasis to correct severe forearm rotation deformities, *J Pediatr Orthop* 15:53, 1995.

Okrent DH, McFadden JC: Radiologic case study: congenital radio ulnar synostosis, *Orthopedics* 9:1452, 1986.

Seitz WH Jr, Gordon TL, Konsens RM: Congenital radioulnar synostosis: a new technique for derotational osteotomy, *Orthop Rev* 19:192, 1990.

Simmons BP, Southmayd WW, Riseborough EJ: Congenital radioulnar synostosis, *J Hand Surg* 8A:829, 1983.

Wilkie DPD: Congenital radio-ulnar synostosis, *Br J Surg* 1:366, 1913-1914.

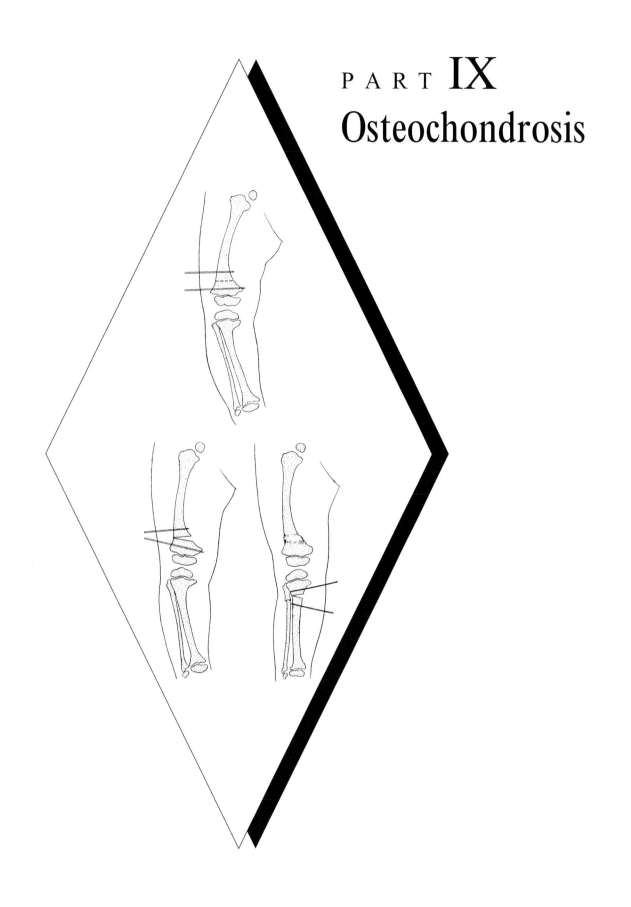

PART IX
Osteochondrosis

CHAPTER

29

Osteochondrosis or Epiphysitis and Other Miscellaneous Affections

S. Terry Canale

Osteochondrosis or Epiphysitis

The terms *osteochondrosis* and *epiphysitis* designate disorders of actively growing epiphyses. The disorder may be localized to a single epiphysis or occasionally may involve two or more epiphyses simultaneously or successively. The cause generally is unknown, but evidence indicates a lack of vascularity that may be the result of trauma, infection, or congenital malformation.

In some epiphyses osteochondrosis is distinctive enough to be easily recognized as a distinct clinical entity. On the other hand, osteochondrosis of some intraarticular epiphyses may closely resemble other diseases and requires careful diagnostic study. For example, multiple epiphyseal dysplasia may closely resemble Perthes disease of the hip. Roentgenograms of the ankle should be examined for the lateral narrowing or wedging of the distal tibial epiphysis that is characteristic of multiple epiphyseal dysplasia. In Perthes disease the bone age usually lags 1 to 2 years behind the chronological age, whereas the bone age usually is normal in multiple epiphyseal dysplasia.

After histologically studying excised specimens, Cohen and Wilkinson, Thompson and Dickinson, Rapp and Lazerte, and others concluded that Osgood-Schlatter disease is traumatic in origin but not associated with loss of vascularity and therefore should not be grouped with the osteochondroses.

Only those disorders of the epiphyses that sometimes require surgical treatment are discussed.

TRACTION EPIPHYSITIS OF FIFTH METATARSAL BASE (ISELIN DISEASE)

Iselin, in the German literature in 1912, described a traction epiphysitis of the base of the fifth metatarsal occurring in young adolescents at the time of appearance of the proximal epiphysis of the fifth metatarsal. This secondary center of ossification is a small, shell-shaped fleck of bone oriented slightly obliquely with respect to the metatarsal shaft and located on the lateral plantar aspect of the tuberosity (Fig. 29-1). Anatomical studies have shown that this bone is located within the cartilaginous flare onto which the peroneus brevis inserts. It is not usually visible on anteroposterior or lateral roentgenograms but can be seen on the oblique view. Hoerr et al. found this epiphysis visible on 198 of 200 oblique roentgenograms of children in their study. It appears in females at about age 10 years and in

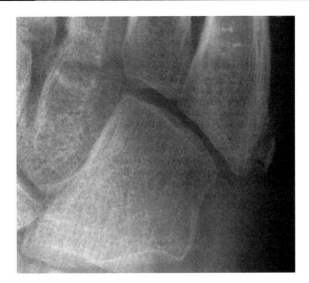

Fig. 29-1   Ossification of epiphysis on fifth metatarsal shaft.

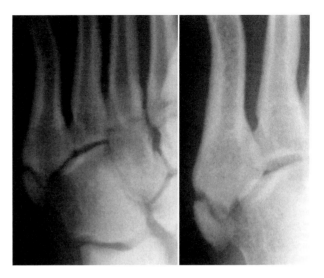

Fig. 29-3   Nonunion of fifth metatarsal as result of Iselin disease.

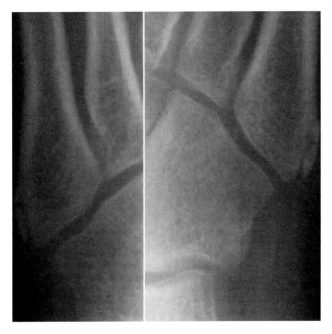

Fig. 29-2   Enlargement and fragmentation of epiphysis (Iselin disease).

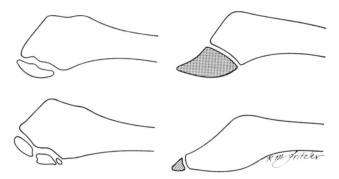

Fig. 29-4   Os vesalianum, as shown here, must be distinguished from Iselin disease.

males at about the age of 12 years; fusion occurs about 2 years later.

Iselin disease causes tenderness over a prominent proximal fifth metatarsal. Weight-bearing produces pain over the lateral aspect of the foot. Participation in sports requiring running, jumping, and cutting, causing inversion stresses on the forefoot, is a common factor. The affected area over the tuberosity is larger on the involved side, with soft tissue edema and local erythema. The area is tender to palpation at the insertion of the peroneus brevis, and resisted eversion and extreme plantar flexion and dorsiflexion of the foot elicit pain. Oblique

roentgenograms show enlargement and often fragmentation of the epiphysis (Fig. 29-2) and widening of the cartilaginous-osseous junction. Technetium 99 bone scanning shows increased uptake over the epiphysis. Nonunion of the fifth metatarsal (Fig. 29-3) has been reported in several adults as a result of Iselin disease and failure of fusion of the epiphysis.

The united epiphysis should not be mistaken for a fracture, nor should a fracture be mistaken for the epiphysis. Os vesalianum, a sesamoid in the peroneus brevis (Fig. 29-4), and traction epiphysitis with widening of the epiphysis must also be distinguished from Iselin disease.

According to Lehman et al., treatment is aimed at prevention of recurrent symptoms. For acute symptoms, initial treatment should decrease the stress reaction and acute inflammation caused by overpull of the peroneus brevis tendon. For mild symptoms, limitation of sports activity, application of ice, and administration of nonsteroidal antiinflammatory medication usually are sufficient. For severe symptoms, cast immobilization may be required. Internal fixation of the epiphysis is not indicated.

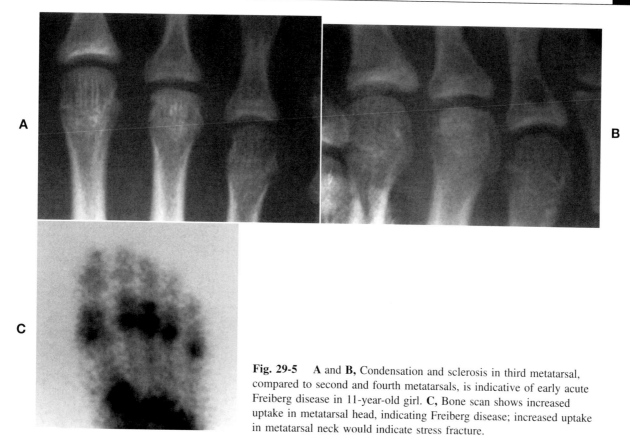

Fig. 29-5 **A** and **B,** Condensation and sclerosis in third metatarsal, compared to second and fourth metatarsals, is indicative of early acute Freiberg disease in 11-year-old girl. **C,** Bone scan shows increased uptake in metatarsal head, indicating Freiberg disease; increased uptake in metatarsal neck would indicate stress fracture.

OSTEOCHONDROSIS OF METATARSAL HEAD (FREIBERG INFRACTION)

Freiberg infraction usually occurs in the head of the second metatarsal but also has been seen in the third (Fig. 29-5) and, by Campbell and others, in the fourth and fifth metatarsals. Surgery is not recommended during the acute stage, which may persist for 6 months to 2 years. It may be indicated later because of pain, deformity, and disability. Occasionally a loose body is present (Fig. 29-6), and simply removing it may relieve the symptoms. Other procedures used include scraping the sclerotic area and replacing it with cancellous bone (Smillie procedure), total joint arthroplasty, and dorsal wedge osteotomy as described by Gauthier and Elbaz (Fig. 29-7). The surgical treatment of this disorder is discussed fully in Chapter 80.

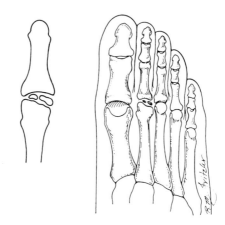

Fig. 29-6 Freiberg infarction of second metatarsal with two loose bodies.

OSTEOCHONDROSIS OF NAVICULAR (KÖHLER DISEASE)

Osteochondrosis of the tarsal navicular was originally described by Köhler in 1908. Karp noted that ossification centers of the navicular appear between the ages of 1.5 and 2 years in females and between 2.5 and 3 years in males. He found abnormalities of ossification, varying from minor irregularities in the size and shape of the navicular to gross changes indistinguishable from osteochondrosis. These abnormal ossi-fying nuclei were more common in late-appearing ossification centers of the navicular. Waugh described the blood supply to the navicular, noting numerous penetrating vessels in both children and adults. The development of the ossific nucleus was most frequently associated with a single artery, but the incorporation of other penetrating vessels as part of the vascular supply was variable; occasionally a single vessel was the sole supply until the age of 4 to 6 years. He postulated that delayed ossification might be the earliest event in the changes

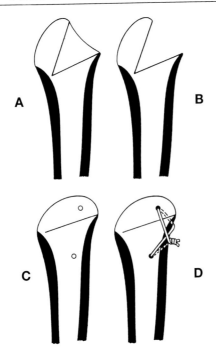

Fig. 29-7 Osteotomy for Freiberg infraction. **A,** Outline of bony wedge to be resected. **B,** Osteotomy of bony wedge. **C,** Closure of osteotomy. **D,** Fixation of osteotomy with wire. (Redrawn from Gauthier G, Elbaz R: *Clin Orthop* 142:93, 1979.)

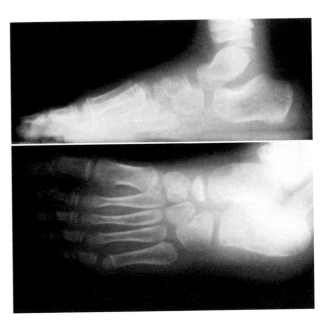

Fig. 29-8 Lateral and oblique roentgenograms show smaller and more sclerotic navicular characteristic of Köhler disease.

leading to irregular ossification and suggested that the lateness of ossification of the navicular subjects it to more pressure than the bony structures can withstand. Abnormal ossification may be a response of the unprotected, growing nucleus to normal stresses of weight-bearing. If osseous vessels are compressed as they pass through the junction between cartilage and bone, ischemia results and leads to reactive hyperemia and pain. Cowell and Williams, in a review of 21 patients with Köhler disease, found the diagnosis to be a clinical one requiring the presence of pain and tenderness in the area of the tarsal navicular associated with roentgenographic changes of sclerosis and diminished size of the bone (Fig. 29-8). They emphasized that the appearance of multiple ossification centers without an increase in density should not be confused with Köhler disease and that roentgenographic findings similar to Köhler disease in an asymptomatic foot should be considered an irregularity of ossification.

Cowell and Williams reported that patients treated with cast immobilization had quicker resolution of symptoms than those treated without casting. This is a self-limiting condition and operative treatment is rarely indicated.

Pain and disability occasionally develop after osteochondrosis when the navicular becomes distorted and sclerotic, the head of the talus becomes flattened, the articular surfaces of the two bones become fibrillated, and osteophytes form along the margin of the articular surfaces. Surgery is indicated when disabling symptoms persist. Arthrodesis is the only operation of value, and the calcaneocuboid joint is included because most of its function is lost when the talonavicular joint is fused. The midtarsal joints (talonavicular and calcaneocuboid) can be arthrodesed by a technique similar to that used for deformities in poliomyelitis (Chapter 31). The results of this operation usually are excellent; most patients become free of symptoms but may notice loss of lateral movements of the foot. When symptoms arise from the naviculocuneiform joints also, these joints should be included in the fusion. Here arthrodesis is difficult to secure; metallic internal fixation and inlay grafts of autogenous cancellous bone are helpful.

OSTEOCHONDRITIS OF ANKLE

Osteochondritis of the ankle in adults is discussed in Chapter 42. The natural history of this lesion in children with open physes appears to be similar to that of osteochondrosis of the knee in that with immobilization the lesion will heal in most children. Bauer et al., in a long-term (20 years or more) follow-up study of 30 children with osteochondritis of the ankle, found that only one patient developed severe arthritis. Only minor roentgenographic changes occurred in the rest of the patients, in contrast to osteochondritis of the knee, in which osteoarthritis is frequent. Two of the lesions in their series were located on the joint surfaces of the distal tibia, a site previously unreported. Bauer et al. noted that the lesions in children are indistinguishable from those in adults; however, because the lesions in children heal, there may be some variance in ossification of the talus (Fig. 29-9). Regardless of the cause, the initial treatment should be nonoperative.

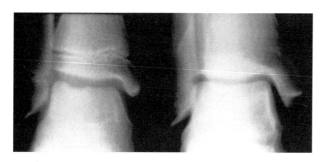

Fig. 29-9 *Left,* Osteochondritis dissecans in child with open distal tibial physes. *Right,* Three years later physes closed, patient was asymptomatic, and osteochondritis dissecans lesion was no longer present.

EPIPHYSITIS OF TIBIAL TUBEROSITY (OSGOOD-SCHLATTER DISEASE)

Surgery rarely is indicated for Osgood-Schlatter disease; the disorder usually becomes asymptomatic without treatment or with simple conservative measures such as the restriction of activities or cast immobilization for 3 to 6 weeks. Krause, Williams, and Catterall, in a review of the natural history of untreated Osgood-Schlatter disease in 69 knees in 50 patients, found that 76% of patients believed they had no limitation of activity, although only 60 could kneel without discomfort. Two distinct groups were identified: (1) those who before treatment had roentgenographic fragmentation and who had either separated ossicles or abnormally ossified tuberosities at follow-up and (2) those who before treatment had soft tissue swelling without roentgenographic fragmentation and who were asymptomatic at follow-up. In a prospective study of 17 patients with Osgood-Schlatter disease and 12 adolescents without anterior knee pain, Aparicio et al. noted a strong association between Osgood-Schlatter disease and patella alta. The increase in patellar height may require an increase in the force by the quadriceps to achieve full extension, which could be responsible for the apophyseal lesion. However, it can be argued that the patella alta is the result of chronic avulsion of the bony tuberosity. Robertsen et al. noted on histologic examination a pseudarthrosis covered with cartilage and no sign of inflammation. They suggested that persistent symptoms of Osgood-Schlatter disease for more than 2 years warrant exploration. Krause et al. concluded that symptoms of Osgood-Schlatter disease resolve spontaneously in most patients and that those who continue to have symptoms are likely to have distorted tibial tuberosities associated with fragmentation of the apophysis on initial roentgenograms. Lynch and Walsh described premature fusion of the anterior part of the upper tibial physis in two patients with Osgood-Schlatter disease who were treated nonoperatively, and they recommended screening for this rare complication.

Surgery may be considered if symptoms are persistent and severely disabling. However, Trial noted that after tibial sequestrectomy (removal of the fragments) results were no better than after conservative treatment. Bosworth recom-

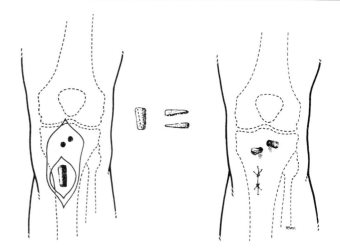

Fig. 29-10 Bosworth technique for insertion of bone pegs for Osgood-Schlatter disease (see text). (Redrawn from Bosworth DM: *J Bone Joint Surg* 16:829, 1934.)

mended inserting bone pegs into the tibial tuberosity; this procedure is simple and almost always relieves the symptoms. However, Thomson and Ferciot, as well as Flowers and Bhadreshwar, pointed out that an unsightly prominence remains after this operation. They recommended excision of the bony prominence through a longitudinal incision in the patellar tendon; longitudinal growth of the tibia was not disturbed after 41 operations in Thomson's series, 11 in Ferciot's series, and 42 in Flower and Bhadreshwar's series. Both Ogden and Roberts reported complications of Osgood-Schlatter disease whether treated surgically or not, including subluxations of the patella, patella alta, nonunion of the bony fragment to the tibia, and premature fusion of the anterior part of the epiphysis with resulting genu recurvatum. Because of the possibility of genu recurvatum, Høgh and Lund recommended delaying surgery until the apophysis has fused. We have removed only the ossicle with satisfactory results and believe the entire tuberosity should be excised only if it is significantly enlarged and the apophysis is closed.

◆ Insertion of Bone Pegs

TECHNIQUE 29-1 *(Bosworth)*

Make a longitudinal midline incision 7.5 cm long beginning at the distal third of the patellar tendon and continuing distally over the tibial tuberosity and tibial shaft (Fig. 29-10). Incise the periosteum longitudinally distal to the tuberosity. With an electric saw cut two matchstick pegs 4 cm long from the tibia; make the base of each peg larger than its tip. Then drill two holes through the tibial tuberosity—one near but not in contact with the proximal tibial physis and slanting proximally and laterally and the other also distal to the physis and slanting proximally and medially. Insert the pegs into these holes and resect their projecting ends.

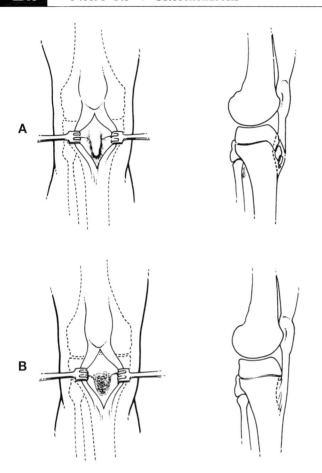

Fig. 29-11   Ferciot and Thomson excision of ununited tibial tuberosity. **A,** Tibial tuberosity has been exposed. **B,** Bony prominence has been excised. (Redrawn from Ferciot CF: *Clin Orthop* 5:204, 1955.)

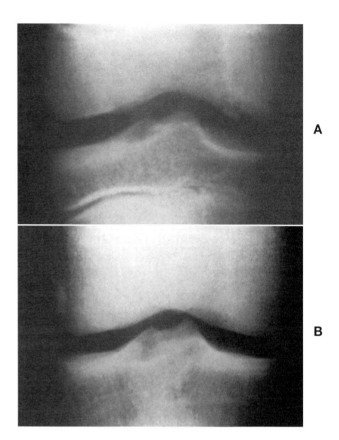

Fig. 29-12   **A,** Osteochondritis dissecans of medial femoral condyle in child with open physis. **B,** Four years later, physis is closed and lesion has healed.

AFTERTREATMENT. A cast is applied from groin to toes and is worn for 2 weeks. A cylinder walking cast is then worn for 4 more weeks.

◆ Excision of Ununited Tibial Tuberosity

TECHNIQUE 29-2 *(Ferciot; Thomson)*
Make a longitudinal incision centered over the tibial tuberosity. Expose the patellar tendon and incise it longitudinally (Fig. 29-11). Elevate the tendon laterally and medially and excise any loose fragments of bone and enough tibial cortex, cartilage, and cancellous bone to remove any bony prominence completely. Do not disturb the peripheral and distal margins of the insertion of the patellar tendon. Close the wound.

AFTERTREATMENT. A cylinder walking cast is applied and worn for 2 to 3 weeks. Exercises are then begun.

OSTEOCHONDRITIS DISSECANS OF KNEE

Osteochondritis dissecans of the knee in children with open physes usually heals when treated with cast immobilization. This treatment is preferable to excising the fragment early in life and creating a crater (Fig. 29-12). Hefti et al. in a multicenter study in 12 European countries studied 509 affected knees in 311 patients. Results were better in young patients than in adult patients. However, in the adolescent group, 22% of patients had abnormal knees at follow-up. The classic medial femoral condyle localization had a better prognosis than an unusual one. Patients with no effusion, a lesion less than 20 mm, and no gross detachment had significantly better results after conservative treatment than those who had undergone operation. If signs of detachment were present, the results were better after operative than after conservative treatment. Bradley and Dandy reported arthroscopic drilling of osteochondritis dissecans lesions in 11 children (11 knees) who had no signs of clinical or roentgenographic improvement after 6 months of conservative treatment. Relief of pain was noted within days of the operation, and roentgenographic healing occurred within 12

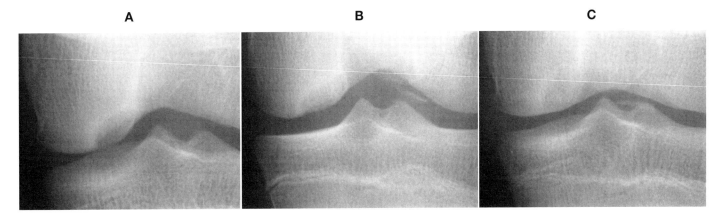

Fig. 29-13   A, Osteochondritis dissecans of medial femoral condyle treated with knee immobilizer in 13-year-old child with physis still open. **B,** At 3-month follow-up defect appears to be healing; possible osteochondral loose body noted. **C,** At 5-month follow-up patient is asymptomatic with healed lesion on roentgenogram and a loose body that is asymptomatic.

months in 9 of the 11 knees. Anderson et al. were able to repeat these findings with antegrade drilling in 20 knees of children in 1997. However, no such pain relief or healing was accomplished after surgery in four adults. Bradley and Dandy and Anderson et al. concluded that arthroscopic drilling of the lesion can be done before skeletal maturity in children who do not improve after prolonged conservative treatment. Nonoperative treatment always should be considered in patients with open physes (Fig. 29-13); however, specific indications for operative treatment of osteochondritis dissecans in children are prolonged pain without evidence of healing during a 6-month period, an unhealed lesion in which symptoms persist after physeal closure, a sclerotic lesion in the crater, and a troublesome loose body (Fig. 29-14). In skeletally mature individuals surgery is necessary to evaluate the lesion and implement treatment. DeSmet et al. noted that MRI is a highly sensitive method for detection of unstable osteochondritis dissecans. The presence of an underlying high-signal-intensity line, cystic area, or a focal articular defect indicates instability and may help in preoperative planning. Whether the lesion is drilled, excised, curetted, replaced and pinned, or bone grafted depends on the size, stability, and weight-bearing nature of the lesion, which can be determined only at surgery.

Osteochondritis dissecans of the knee in children should not be confused with anomalous ossification centers, as described by Smillie. Because these ossification centers may be present in both condyles and in both knees, comparison roentgenograms of the affected and unaffected knees are advised (Fig. 29-15). MRI findings appear to be different for anomalous ossification centers and osteochondritis dissecans. Newata et al. used MRI to examine posterolateral anomalous ossification centers of the knee and found the same signal intensity as the adjacent subchondral bone, which as noted above is quite different from osteochondritis dissecans lesions. Mitsuoka et al. suggested

that a discoid meniscus may cause osteochondritis dissecans during growth. Surgical procedures and techniques including the use and complications of Herbert screws, poly-L-lactic acid pins, and osteochondral grafts (mosaicplasty) are discussed in Chapter 43.

OSTEOCHONDRITIS DISSECANS OF PATELLA

Osteochondritis dissecans of the patella is a rare entity that affects the subchondral bone and articular surface and the cartilage overlying the surface of the patella. It may appear as an elliptical fragment within a crater. Rarely does it occur bilaterally, and it is frequently painful and quite debilitating. Boys between the ages of 10 and 15 are most commonly affected.

Osteochondritis dissecans of the patella should be differentiated from a dorsal defect of the patella so that surgical treatment will not be carried out on an asymptomatic defect (Table 29-1). The differences between the two are subtle but present. Unlike osteochondritis dissecans of the patella (Fig. 29-16, *A*), a dorsal defect is a simple, asymptomatic, subchondral defect in the superolateral portion of the patella that does not involve the articular cartilage and usually is an incidental finding on roentgenogram (Fig. 29-17, *A* and *B*). A sclerotic border occasionally is present, and 20% to 40% of the time it occurs bilaterally. Safran et al. stated that an MRI definitively shows that the dorsal defect does not involve the articular surface as compared with the osteochondritis dissecans (Figs. 29-16, *C* and *D*, and 29-17, *C* and *D*). A bone scan can also help differentiate between the two. In osteochondritis dissecans of the patella the bone scan is exceptionally "hot" in comparison to dorsal defects in which the bone scan is "cold" (Fig. 29-16, *B*).

Treatment of osteochondritis dissecans of the patella, especially in young children whose physes are still open, is

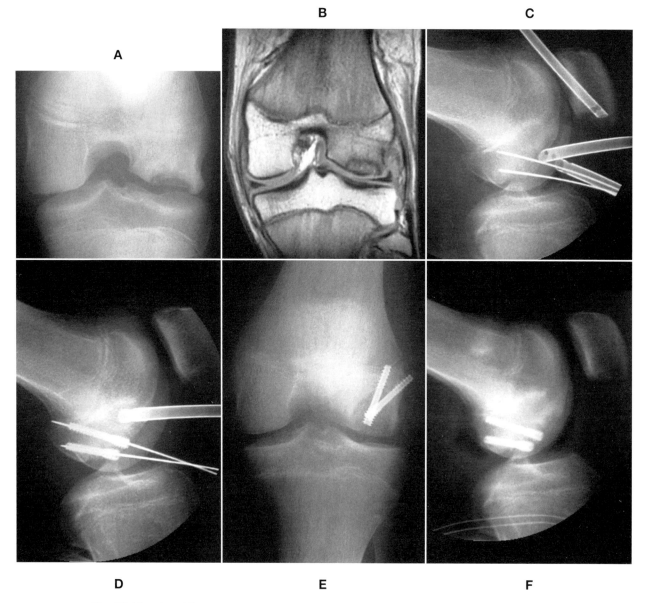

Fig. 29-14 **A** and **B,** Large osteochondritis dissecans defect on lateral femoral condyle seen on roentgenogram and magnetic resonance imaging. Chondroblastoma was ruled out in this patient with physes still open. **C** and **D,** After 9 months of unsuccessful conservative treatment, arthroscopy and Herbert screw fixation were performed. At the time of arthroscopy lesion was hinged but attached. Procedure requires use of image intensifier for correct guide pin placement and to avoid physis with Herbert screws. **E** and **F,** Postoperative anteroposterior and lateral roentgenograms with Herbert screws in acceptable position.

nonoperative if at all possible. Several of our patients have had a painful patella after excision of the fragment. Restriction of activities and immobilization for a period of time are recommended to avoid surgical excision. If conservative treatment fails, the lesion can be drilled, and if it is loose but still in the crater, the lesion can be internally fixed with a small diameter Herbert screw. We have had little luck with poly-L-lactic acid pins in this area. If a defect and an old loose body are present, the loose body should be removed and the crater debrided and drilled. If the loose body appears to have viable subchondral bone, the crater should be freshened and the loose body placed within the crater and internally fixed.

OSTEOCHONDROSIS OF CAPITELLUM (OSTEOCHONDRITIS DISSECANS)

Little Leaguer's elbow is a term that has been used loosely to describe changes in the elbow secondary to baseball pitching and usually limited to the capitellum, radial head, or medial epicondyle. We have seen both osteochondrosis and osteochondritis dissecans of the capitellum. The cause of both is

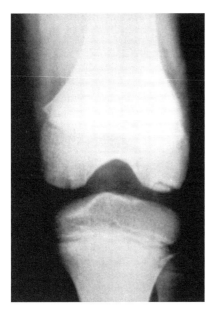

Fig. 29-15　Bilateral (medial and lateral) anomalous ossification centers in posterior aspects of femoral condyles (not osteochondritis dissecans).

Table 29-1　Differentiation of Osteochondritis Dissecans of Patella from Dorsal Defect of Patella

Osteochondritis Dissecans of Patella	Dorsal Defect of Patella
Usually symptomatic	Usually asymptomatic
Separation of chondral or osteochondral fragment from subchondral bone	Incidental finding on roentgenogram
Involves articular cartilage	Does not involve articular cartilage
	Round subchondral defect in superolateral portion of patella
	Occasionally sclerotic border
Rarely bilateral	20% to 40% bilateral occurrence
Bone scan hot	Bone scan cold

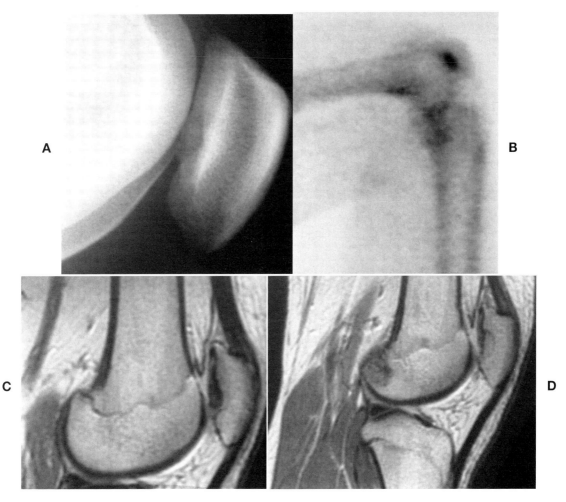

Fig. 29-16　Osteochondritis dissecans of patella. **A,** Lateral roentgenogram. **B,** Bone scan. **C** and **D,** MRI revealing osteocartilaginous fragment including articular cartilage within crater.

somewhat obscure and is not limited to throwing a baseball. Furthermore, a relationship may or may not exist between osteochondrosis and osteochondritis dissecans of the capitellum (Fig. 29-18). Woodward and Bianco, as well as Tullos and King, recommended excision of loose fragments only. Woodward and Bianco reported 42 patients with osteochondritis dissecans of the capitellum in whom some form of surgery was used in 38 elbows. Results were no better after drilling, curetting, or trimming the crater than after simple removal of the loose body. For several years after removal the range of motion increased, and eventually function of the elbow returned to normal. Bauer et al. reported 31 patients with osteochondrosis of the capitellum who were followed up for more than 20 years. Twenty-three patients were treated operatively. Impaired motion and pain with effort were the most common complaints, regardless of the type of treatment. Roentgenographic signs of degenerative joint disease were present in more than half of the elbows with reduction in range of motion. The diameter of the radial head was increased in comparison to the contralateral elbow in two thirds of the patients. If a loose body is not present, nonsurgical treatment usually is satisfactory especially if the lesion appears stable.

At follow-up, Ruch et al. noted a triangular avulsed fragment off the lateral capsule in patients with less than satisfactory surgical results. Takahara et al. examined 15

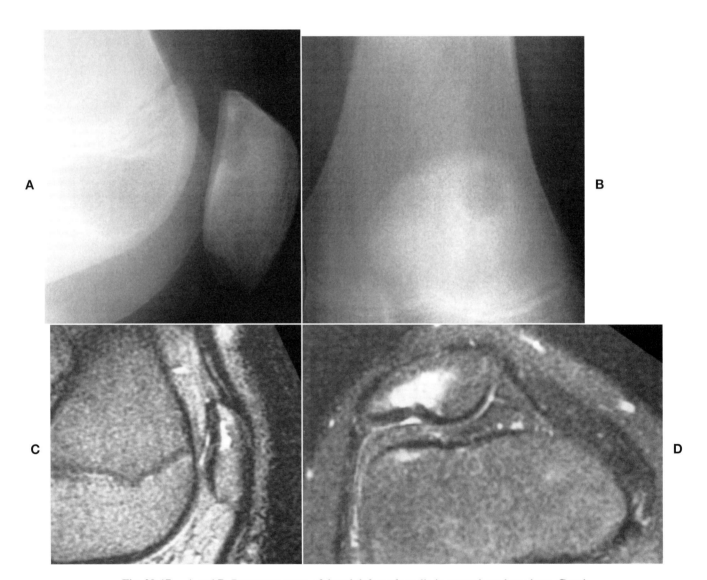

Fig. 29-17 **A** and **B,** Roentgenograms of dorsal defect of patella in superolateral quadrant. **C** and **D,** Magnetic resonance imaging revealing dorsal defect of patella with cystic defect noted but not involving the articular cartilage.

patients with osteochondritis dissecans of the elbow. At long-term follow-up, roentgenograms of those treated conservatively showed that three lesions had healed and nine had not. Their results suggest that osteochondritis dissecans of the capitellum has only a slight tendency to heal and that instability can cause failure of the lesion to heal. Furthermore, they described the long-term outcome of osteochondritis dissecans of the humeral capitellum in 53 patients. The average age of the patients at the time of treatment was 16.6 years (range, 10 to 34). The average follow-up was 12.6 years. Approximately 50% of patients, whether treated conservatively or with surgical removal of the fragment, had residual elbow symptoms that interfered with their activities of daily living, and they had poor results. Long-term poor results were associated with treatment of advanced lesions, osteochondritis, and large osteochondral defects. Klekamp et al. noted that instability of the radial head developed in a posterolateral direction in seven patients (two complete dislocations) at follow-up. Kuwahata and Inoue reported poor results after conservative treatment or simple excision but had satisfactory results after internal fixation with Herbert screws for large but stable lesions.

Arthroscopy (Chapter 49) and especially an elbow arthrogram or MRI may be indicated when a loose body is suspected but not seen on plain roentgenograms.

LEGG-CALVÉ-PERTHES DISEASE

The cause of Legg-Calvé-Perthes disease is unknown but has provoked considerable controversy. According to some authors an inherited thrombophilia appears to be present. Glueck et al. reported a resistance to activated protein C in 23 of 64 children with Perthes, which is many times greater than normal. They believe that this promotes thrombotic venous occlusion in the femoral vein causing bone death in the femoral head and ultimately leading to Legg-Calvé-Perthes disease. However, Arruda et al. and Gallistl et al. did not find an inherited hypercoagulability nor a deficiency in protein C activity, and they do not believe that inherited thrombophilia is associated with the avascular necrosis of Legg-Calvé-Perthes disease. Kealey et al. and Sievent et al. also concluded that coagulation deformities did not appear to be etiological factors in Legg-Calvé-Perthes disease.

Differentiating an irritable hip with transient synovitis from the acute symptoms of Legg-Calvé-Perthes disease can be difficult. In a report of two groups of patients—160 with irritable hip episodes and 120 with Legg-Calvé-Perthes disease—Erken and Katz described some distinguishing characteristics. Irritable hip syndrome occurs only twice as frequently in boys as in girls, whereas Legg-Calvé-Perthes disease occurs three times more frequently in boys than in girls. The average age of patients with irritable hips is 3 years, and the average age of those with Legg-Calvé-Perthes disease is 7 years. Children with irritable hips have an average duration of

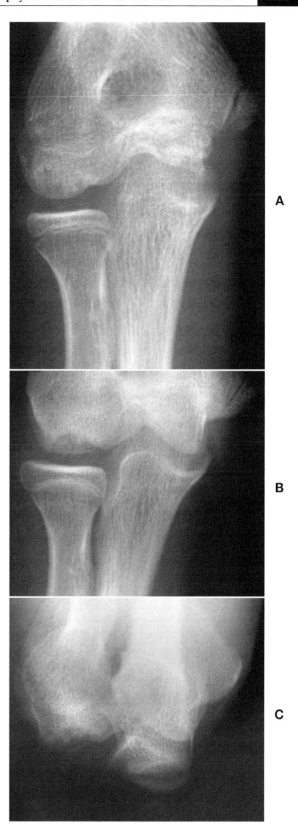

Fig. 29-18 **A,** Osteochondrosis of capitellum. Anteroposterior (**B**) and Jones (**C**) views 1 year later show evidence of some consolidation, but osteochondritis dissecans appears to be forming.

symptoms of 6 days, whereas those with Legg-Calvé-Perthes disease have symptoms present for an average of 6 weeks.

Using ultrasound evaluation, Futami et al. believed they were able to differentiate between transient synovitis with capsular distension caused by synovial effusion and Legg-Calvé-Perthes disease with thickening of the synovial membrane. Eggl et al. noted in nine patients capsular distention persisting longer than 6 weeks associated with the onset of Legg-Calvé-Perthes disease. Keenan and Clegg compared recurrent irritable hip syndrome with Perthes and found that only those with more than 2 years' delay in their bone age were in the early phases of Perthes disease at initial examination when the original hip roentgenograms were normal. A plain wrist roentgenogram was found to be a useful screening tool to determine who should have early repeat investigations such as roentgenograms or MRI.

Usually plain roentgenographic changes are delayed 6 weeks or more from the clinical onset of Legg-Calvé-Perthes. Bone scintigraphy and MRI can establish the diagnosis much earlier.

Once the diagnosis is established, the primary aim of treatment of Legg-Calvé-Perthes disease is containment of the femoral head within the acetabulum. If this is achieved, the femoral head can reform in a concentric manner by what Salter has termed "biological plasticity."

Lloyd-Roberts et al. classified patients with this disease into groups according to the amount of involvement of the capital femoral epiphysis: group I, partial head or less than half head involvement; groups II and III, more than half head involvement and sequestrum formation; and group IV, involvement of the entire epiphysis. Furthermore, they noted certain roentgenographic signs described as "head at risk" correlated positively with poor results, especially in patients in groups II, III, and IV. These head-at-risk signs include (1) lateral subluxation of the femoral head from the acetabulum, (2) speckled calcification lateral to the capital epiphysis, (3) diffuse metaphyseal reaction (metaphyseal cysts), (4) a horizontal physis, and (5) Gage sign, a radiolucent V-shaped defect in the lateral epiphysis and adjacent metaphysis. They recommended containment by femoral varus derotational osteotomy for older children in groups II, III, and IV with head-at-risk signs. Contraindications include an already malformed femoral head and delay of treatment of more than 8 months from onset of symptoms. Surgery is not recommended for any group I children or any child without the head-at-risk signs.

Salter and Thompson advocated determining the extent of involvement by describing the extent of a subchondral fracture in the superolateral portion of the femoral head. If the extent of the fracture (line) is less than 50% of the superior dome of the femoral head, the involvement is considered type A, and good results can be expected. If the extent of the fracture is more than 50% of the dome, the involvement is considered type B, and fair or poor results can be expected (Fig. 29-19). According to Salter and Thompson, this subchondral fracture and its entire extent can be observed roentgenographically earlier and more

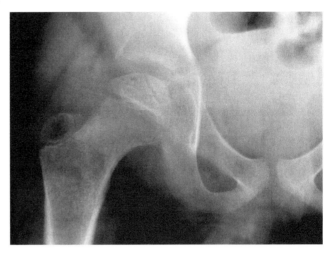

Fig. 29-19 Type B subchondral fracture involving more than 50% of femoral head.

readily than trying to determine the Catterall classification (8.1 months average). Furthermore, according to these authors, if the femoral head is graded as type B, then probably an operation such as an innominate osteotomy should be carried out. After statistical analysis of 116 hips affected with Perthes disease, Mukherjee and Fabry concluded that Salter and Thompson's classification is simple and accurate and can be applied early in the course of the disease to determine management. Song et al. reported that the extent of the subchondral fracture line, when present, is more accurate in predicting the extent of necrosis than is the extent of necrosis seen on MRI, which they believe does not have a consistent correlation. In our experience, however, subchondral fractures are present early in the course of the disease in only a third of patients, and although this classification is a reliable indicator in the group with fractures, it has little to offer in early treatment decisions for the other two thirds of patients.

Herring et al. described a classification based on the height of the lateral pillar: group A, no involvement of the lateral pillar; group B, at least 50% of lateral pillar height maintained; and group C, less than 50% of lateral pillar height maintained (Fig. 29-20). A statistically significant correlation was found between the final outcome (Stulberg classification) and the loss of pillar height. Patients in group A had uniformly good outcomes; those in group B who were younger than 9 years of age at onset had good outcomes, but those older than 9 years of age had less favorable results; those in group C had the worst results, with most having aspherical femoral heads, regardless of age at onset. Reproducibility of this classification system was confirmed by 78% of members of the Perthes study group who used it. Herring et al. noted that the advantages of this classification are (1) it can be easily applied during the active stages of the disease, and (2) the high correlation between the lateral pillar height and the amount of femoral head flattening at skeletal maturity allows accurate prediction of the natural history and treatment methods. Ritterbusch et al. compared the predictive value of the lateral pillar classification with the

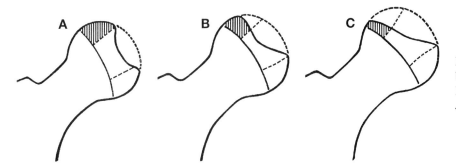

Fig. 29-20 Lateral pillar classification based on height of lateral pillar. (From Herring JA, Neustadt JB, Williams JJ, et al: *J Pediatr Orthop* 12:143, 1992.)

Catterall classification in 71 hips followed to skeletal maturity They concluded that the lateral pillar classification was a better predictor of Stulberg outcome than was the Catterall classification. Interobserver reliability of the lateral pillar classification also was better than that of the Catterall classification. Ippolito et al. found the Herring classification to be a reliable prognostic indicator at long-term follow-up in 49 patients.

We have in the past used a bone scan to try to determine early how much of the femoral head is involved. We compare the uptake (decreased) to that of the contralateral hip, similar to the method of Danigelis et al. and others. We do not make an absolute quantitative determination but rather compare general percentages. If the uptake is decreased less than 50% as compared with the opposite femoral head early in the course of the disease, then we consider the disease a Catterall group I or II and treat it appropriately. If the uptake is decreased more than 50%, we consider the disease a Catterall group III or IV, Salter type B, or lateral pillar type C, requiring a more aggressive treatment program.

In a study of 24 hips with Legg-Calvé-Perthes disease, Henderson et al. reported that MRI better delineated the extent and location of involvement than plain roentgenograms. They also noted that MRI is more accurate than roentgenograms in determining femoral head sphericity in some phases of the disease process. Furthermore, according to Uno, MRI appears to be superior to bone scintigraphy for depicting the extent of involvement in the early or evolutionary stage of Legg-Calvé-Perthes disease. Hosokawa et al. reported that MRI grading in early stages Legg-Calvé-Perthes disease predicted the ultimate outcome in a small group of patients. However, plain roentgenograms are considerably less costly and should be used for following the disease process. Song et al., using MRI, noted that the widened medial joint space on roentgenograms was filled with (1) overgrown cartilage in the initial stage, (2) both overgrown cartilage and widened true medial joint space at the fragmentation stage, and (3) widened true medial joint space at the healing stage. During the healing stage, widening of the medial joint space decreased or normalized because of ossification of overgrown cartilage despite the existence of lateral subluxation due to coxa magna. These authors concluded that widening of the medial joint space may be an indication of lateral subluxation of the original femoral head only at the fragmentation stage in Perthes disease.

Concerning bilaterality and gender, reports in the literature indicate that (1) patients with bilateral Perthes disease have more severe involvement than those with unilateral disease, because most have a Catterall III or IV or a Herring B or C classification, and 48% rate as a Stulberg 4 or 5 at skeletal maturity; and (2) boys and girls who have the same Catterall classification or lateral pillar classification at the time of initial evaluation can be expected to have similar outcomes according to the classification system of Stulberg et al.

Kelly and I at this clinic reviewed 80 children who had unilateral Perthes disease. The average follow-up was 22.4 years. Sixty-four of the eighty hips (84%) had good results; nine (11%) had fair results, that is, unsatisfactory roentgenographic appearance but normal clinical examination without symptoms; and seven (9%) had poor results, with both unsatisfactory roentgenographic appearance and significant symptoms. The conclusions from this series follow.

1. Most patients can be treated by noncontainment methods and obtain good results (84%).
2. Satisfactory clinical results frequently can be obtained at long-term follow-up despite an unsatisfactory roentgenographic appearance (9 hips).
3. The Catterall classification is a valid indicator of results but is not applicable as a therapeutic guide for an average of 8.1 months after onset.
4. Head-at-risk signs added little to the Catterall classification as a prognostic indicator or therapeutic guide.
5. All of the fair and poor results were in patients with Catterall III or IV involvement and onset of the disease at age 6 or later. (A Catterall III or IV classification is equivalent to Herring groups B and C.)

In the past some have used the classification system of Stulberg et al. as a basis for treatment during the active phase of Legg-Calvé-Perthes disease because it is a predictor of long-term outcome. However, Neyt et al. challenged the intrarater and interrater reliability and questioned the validity of treatment decisions, outcomes, and studies based on the Stulberg classification.

Roberts and Yngve and Bellyei and Mike reported that in younger children, instead of the femoral head remodeling, the acetabulum conforms and remodels to the shape of the femoral head, and therefore, to avoid a "hinged abduction," the femoral head must be placed in wide abduction to prevent subluxation.

Reinker found that hinge abduction occurred early in the course of Legg-Calvé-Perthes, frequently about an unossified portion of the femoral head, making detection difficult. Failure of movement of the lateral corner of the epiphysis under the edge of the acetabulum on an internally rotated and abducted roentgenogram is evidence of hinge abduction. Confirmation is easily obtained by arthrography. Both clinical and roentgenographic outcomes were worse in patients with unrelieved hinge abduction. Relief of hinging frequently can be accomplished by traction, and containment can then be maintained by appropriate surgery.

Fulford et al. compared the results of treatment with bed rest and skin traction followed by either a weight-relieving caliper (ischial weight-bearing brace) or by a proximal femoral varus osteotomy. The outcomes were similar in both groups (20% to 25% poor results) and could be predicted best by the arthrographic shape of the femoral head at presentation. They attributed the similarity in results to the common factor in the treatment protocols: the period of bed rest and traction with the hips in abduction until hip irritability decreased. In the past we have used the Scottish Rite brace, popularized by Purvis and others, because of the ability to place the legs in abduction and slight flexion. We now realize that this brace does not appear to offer any advantages over other methods of management, including no treatment, as noted by Meeham et al. and others. Furthermore, Harrison and Bassett noted that pulse electromagnetic frequency made no discernible difference in the outcome of Perthes. This raises the question of whether any treatment method produces better results than those obtained with no treatment. If observation alone is used, a vigorous physical therapy program, including active and active-assisted range-of-motion and muscle stretching exercises to the hip and knee, is recommended. We routinely place patients at bed rest with 3 pounds of skin traction until the synovitis subsides. Our current treatment protocol consists of explaining the natural history and length of time of the disease (24 to 36 months for the synovitis to resolve). A daily home physical therapy program to try to maintain a normal hip range of motion is instituted as noted above. Because Snyder has described poor results in younger children (ages 4 and 5), we are committed to treatment of children age 4 years and older. However, children ages 2 and 3 years who have Perthes disease can be observed and do not need aggressive treatment.

Loss of motion at any time indicates significant change in prognosis. If loss of motion is significant and subluxation laterally is occurring, then we, as well as Richards and Coleman, recommend closed reduction with the patient under general anesthesia and percutaneous adductor longus tenotomy, followed by an ambulatory abduction cast (Petrie) for 6 weeks or more. Kiepurska reported good results in 92 of 334 hips treated in ''broomstick'' casts and believes this method obtains better results than treatment by orthosis or femoral osteotomy.

We rarely recommend surgery for Perthes disease because of the complications possible after major hip surgery, whether it be a varus derotational osteotomy or an innominate osteotomy. It is easy to ''oversell'' an operation for Perthes

disease to the parents of a 6-year-old who have to face the possibility of brace wear for 12 to 18 months. To convince them that an operation and the wearing of a spica cast for 3 months is preferable to brace wear for 12 to 18 months is easy. Evans et al. compared a group of patients over the age of 6 years treated with abduction bracing to a group treated with varus derotational osteotomy and found treatment results were equal. However, if surgery is contemplated, then all the complications of major hip surgery should be explained to the parents before the procedure.

If surgery is indicated during the active phase of the disease, which procedure is best is controversial. Salter, Canale et al., Coleman et al., Paterson et al., and Maxted and Jackson achieved containment by a pelvic osteotomy above the hip joint (Fig. 29-21). Axer, Craig et al., Somerville, Lloyd-Roberts et al. and McElwain et al. stated that containment is best obtained by varus derotational osteotomy of the femur. All noted that an arthrogram or MRI before surgery is mandatory, first to determine if any flattening of the femoral head is present that would contraindicate an osteotomy of any type, and second to determine how much subluxation is present and how much surgical containment is necessary. Moberg et al. in a retrospective study of the surgical management of Legg-Calvé-Perthes disease described 16 femoral osteotomies and 18 innominate osteotomies. Their average follow-up was 7 years. The clinical results were the same for the two groups, and all patients were asymptomatic in the affected hips during daily activity. The roentgenographic results also were the same for the two groups with regard to measurements of the sphericity of the femoral head. Coverage of the femoral head by the acetabulum was better in the innominate osteotomy group. Crutcher and Staheli described a combined osteotomy (Salter pelvic osteotomy and varus femoral osteotomy) as a salvage procedure for severe Legg-Calvé-Perthes disease. The theoretical advantage of this combined procedure is that maximal femoral head containment can be achieved while avoiding the complications of either procedure alone, such as limb shortening, extreme neck-shaft varus angulation, and associated abductor weakness. All 14 patients reported by Crutcher and Staheli had severe involvement with poor prognoses, and initial nonoperative treatment was ineffective or poorly tolerated by the patients. Willett et al. recommend lateral shelf acetabuloplasty for older children who are not candidates for femoral osteotomies because of insufficient remodeling capacity and the likelihood that shortening of the femur will cause a persistent limp. Twenty of their patients who had poor prognoses were treated with acetabuloplasty (shelf procedure) and had better early results than 14 children who received no treatment.

Indications for reconstructive surgery in Perthes disease are (1) hinge abduction, for which valgus subtrochanteric osteotomy is indicated, (2) a malformed femoral head in late group III or residual group IV, for which Garceau's cheilectomy can be used, (3) a coxa magna, for which a shelf augmentation will provide coverage, (4) a large malformed femoral head with subluxation laterally, for which Chiari's pelvic osteotomy may

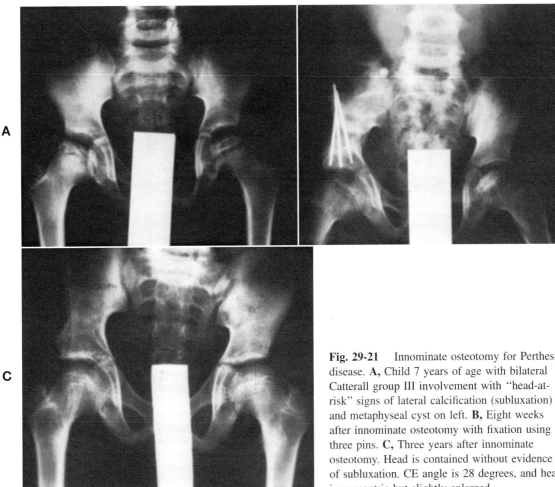

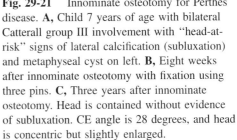

Fig. 29-21   Innominate osteotomy for Perthes disease. **A,** Child 7 years of age with bilateral Catterall group III involvement with "head-at-risk" signs of lateral calcification (subluxation) and metaphyseal cyst on left. **B,** Eight weeks after innominate osteotomy with fixation using three pins. **C,** Three years after innominate osteotomy. Head is contained without evidence of subluxation. CE angle is 28 degrees, and head is concentric but slightly enlarged.

be considered, and (5) capital femoral physeal arrest, for which trochanteric advancement or arrest can be performed.

An Ilizarov external fixator across the pelvis and hip has been used to reduce the femoral head to avoid hinge abduction and persistent subluxation. Kocaoglu et al. described 11 hips with category III or IV with signs of poor prognosis, or a Herring B or C at follow-up. Containment was sustained in only 4 of 11 hips. Because of the complications and low rate of success, they did not recommend the routine use of the Ilizarov technique.

◆ **Innominate Osteotomy**

The advantages of innominate osteotomy by either Salter's method or the Elizabethtown method (Fig. 29-22) include anterolateral coverage of the femoral head, lengthening of the extremity (possibly shortened by the avascular process), and avoidance of a second operation for plate removal. The disadvantages of innominate osteotomy include the inability sometimes to obtain proper containment of the femoral head, especially in older children, an increase in acetabular and hip joint pressure that may cause further avascular changes in the femoral head, and an increase in leg length on the operated side

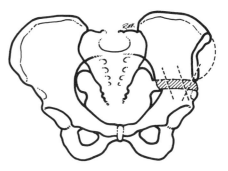

Fig. 29-22   Innominate osteotomy using quadrangular graft (see text). (From Canale ST, d'Anca AF, Cotler JM, Snedden HE: *J Bone Joint Surg* 54A:25, 1972.)

as compared with the normal side that may cause a relative adduction of the hip and uncover the femoral head.

In surgically treated patients older than 6 years of age with total head involvement and subluxation, Cotler and Wolfgang reported no further vascular compromise of the femoral head as indicated by avascular necrosis or chondrolysis. A faster healing rate (progression from one stage of the disease to the next in a shorter period) was not found after osteotomy; rather a change from one stage to the next was determined earlier, probably by the more frequent roentgenograms of hips that had been operated on.

Innominate osteotomy as described by Salter is included in the discussion of congenital deformities (see Chapter 26). It should be remembered that Salter's procedure includes iliopsoas release.

TECHNIQUE 29-3 *(Canale et al.)*

Through a Smith-Petersen approach to the hip (p. 58), release the sartorius, tensor fasciae latae, and rectus femoris and expose the anteroinferior iliac spine. Release the psoas tendon from its insertion and dissect subperiosteally on the inner and outer walls of the ilium down to the sciatic notch. Using retractors in the sciatic notch, with a right-angle clamp pass a Gigli saw through the notch. With the saw, carefully cut horizontally and anteriorly through the ilium as close as possible to the capsular attachment of the acetabulum. Maximally flex the knee and then flex and abduct the hip to open the osteotomy. Use a towel clip to pull the distal fragment of the osteotomy anteriorly and laterally. Take a full-thickness quadrilateral graft approximately 2 × 3 cm from the wing of the ilium according to the size of the space produced by opening the osteotomy (see Fig. 29-22). Predrill or precut the outline of the graft on the surfaces of the ilium to prevent fracture of the inner and outer cortices. Shape the quadrilateral graft carefully to fit the space produced and impact it into the osteotomy site. Use one or more threaded pins for fixation and leave the ends subcutaneous so that they can be removed later with local or general anesthesia.

Use the center edge angle of Wiberg (see Chapter 26) in the weight-bearing position at this time to assess by roentgenography the coverage and containment of the femoral head.

AFTERTREATMENT. The patient is immobilized for 10 to 12 weeks in a spica cast before the pins are removed. Range-of-motion exercises and full weight-bearing ambulation are then started, and roentgenographic evaluation is repeated.

◆ Lateral Shelf Procedure

TECHNIQUE 29-4 *(Willett et al.)*

Make a curved incision below the iliac crest, passing 1.5 cm below the anterosuperior iliac spine to avoid the lateral cutaneous nerve of the thigh. Strip the glutei subperiosteally from the outer table of the ilium to the level of insertion of the joint capsule. Mobilize and divide the reflected head of the rectus femoris. Create a trough in the bone immediately above the insertion of the capsule (Fig. 29-23, *A*). Raise a bony flap 3 cm wide × 3.5 cm long superiorly from the outer cortex of the ilium. Cut strips of cancellous graft from the ilium above the flap and insert them into the trough so that they form a canopy on the superior surface of the hip joint

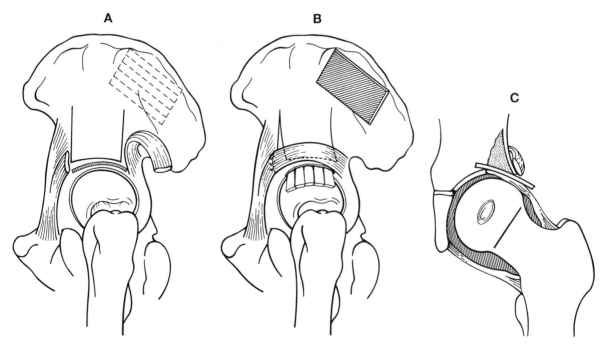

Fig. 29-23   Operative technique for lateral shelf acetabuloplasty (see text). (Redrawn from Bentley G, Greer RB: *Rob and Smith's operative surgery,* ed 4, London, 1991, Chapman & Hall.)

(Fig. 29-23, *B*). Pack the web-shaped space between the flap and the graft canopy with cancellous bone graft (Fig. 29-23, *C*). Repair the reflected head of rectus femoris over the created shelf. Close the wound in the usual manner and apply a spica cast.

AFTERTREATMENT. The spica cast is worn for 8 weeks. Protective weight-bearing in a single spica cast is continued for 6 additional weeks.

Varus Derotational Osteotomy

This procedure has been advocated by Axer, Craig et al., Somerville, and Lloyd-Roberts et al. The advantages of a varus derotational osteotomy of the proximal femur include the ability to obtain maximum coverage of the femoral head, especially in an older child, and the ability to correct excessive femoral anteversion with the same osteotomy (Fig. 29-24). Clancy and Steel performed incomplete intertrochanteric osteotomies on 53 patients with Perthes disease and compared the "healing" time roentgenographically with 36 patients who had nonoperative treatment. They concluded that intertrochanteric osteotomy did not alter the rate of healing of the disease. Lee et al. used serial scintigraphy to study the changes in blood flow in the femoral head after subtrochanteric femoral osteotomy in 25 patients with Legg-Calvé-Perthes disease and found that local blood flow did not increase significantly after osteotomy. The disadvantages of a varus derotational osteotomy include excessive varus angulation that may not correct with growth (especially in an older child), further shortening of an already shortened extremity, the possibility of a gluteus lurch produced by decreasing the length of the lever arm of the gluteal musculature, the possibility of nonunion of the osteotomy, and the requirement of a second operation to remove the internal fixation. As noted by Sponseller et al.,

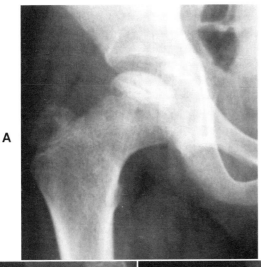

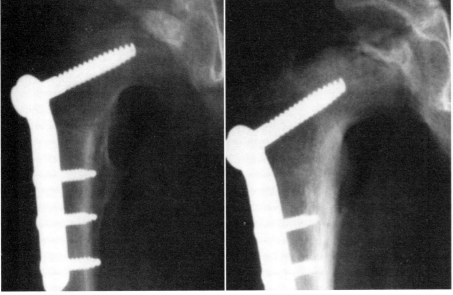

Fig. 29-24   A, Perthes disease in 7-year-old child with Catterall group III involvement. **B,** Immediately after varus osteotomy there is mild lateral subluxation. **C,** Eighteen months after operation, there is some remodeling of varus position and femoral head is better centered than immediately after surgery.

premature closure of the capital femoral physis may cause further varus deformity. Coates et al. reviewed the results of femoral osteotomy in 48 hips in children at skeletal maturity and noted that 29% had shortening and 25% had positive Trendelenburg signs; 58% obtained good results. When compared with the results of conservative treatment in 61 hips reported by Ippolito et al., the results of femoral osteotomy were better in all age groups except in children younger than 5 years of age.

A varus derotational osteotomy is the procedure of choice when containment of the femoral head is necessary but cannot be achieved with a brace for psychosocial or other reasons, when the child is from 8 to 10 years old and without leg length inequality, when on the arthrogram a majority of the femoral head is uncovered and the angle of Wiberg is decreased, and when there is a significant amount of femoral anteversion. Axer performs a subtrochanteric osteotomy early in the course of Perthes disease and uses the following plan.

An anteroposterior roentgenogram of the pelvis is taken with the lower extremities in internal rotation and parallel to each other (no abduction). If satisfactory containment of the femoral head is noted, derotational osteotomy alone is carried out. The degree of derotation is roughly estimated from the amount of internal rotation of the extremity, but further adjustments are made during the operation.

When internal rotation is seriously limited and remains so preoperatively after a 4-week period of bed rest with traction, varus osteotomy is carried out with the addition of extension that is produced by a slight backward tilt of the proximal fragment.

When internal rotation is sufficient, abduction of the extremity will bring about the desired containment of the femoral head. The degree of abduction is expressed by the angle formed by the shaft of the femur and a vertical line parallel to the midline of the pelvis. This angle represents the desired angle of the osteotomy (see technique). Since derotational osteotomy alone may result in lengthening of the extremity from stimulation of growth, a varus angle of 5 degrees to 10 degrees may be added.

Reliable information on acetabular containment of the femoral head, the size of the head, the flattening of the epiphysis, and the width of the medial joint space can be obtained from preoperative arthrography or MRI. The osteo-cartilaginous head of the femur should be covered adequately by the acetabular roof as the femur is abducted and the flattened segment of the femoral head is rotated into the depths of the acetabular fossa. Weiner et al. reviewed the results of femoral osteotomies in 79 hips and concluded that the amount of varus angulation should position the femoral head barely beneath the lateral rim of the acetabulum, avoiding excessive varus of less than 105 degrees. They also recommended performing a greater trochanteric epiphysiodesis at the time of femoral osteotomy to ensure remodeling of the neck-shaft angle and to prevent further varus deformity if the capital femoral physis is prematurely closed. Kitakoji et al. noted that in some patients after femoral varus osteotomy for Legg-Calvé-Perthes disease

additional operative techniques, such as a trochanteric epiphysiodesis, should be performed to prevent trochanteric prominence and medial displacement of the distal fragment that can lead to genu valgum. Furthermore, Matan et al. reported two groups of patients who had femoral varus osteotomies. One group also a trochanteric arrest (epiphysiodesis). At follow-up those with trochanteric arrest had a greater articulotrochanteric distance (ATD) (see Chapter 26), better range of motion, and less abductor weakness.

We use a varus (medial closing wedge) osteotomy fixed with an adolescent pediatric hip screw (Fig. 29-25).

◆ Varus Derotational Osteotomy with Adolescent Pediatric Hip Screw

TECHNIQUE 29-5 *(Stricker)*

Place the patient supine on the operating table with a roentgen cassette holder beneath the patient. Image intensification, positioned in the anteroposterior projection, is desirable. Prepare and drape the affected extremity, leaving it free to allow for intraoperative roentgenograms or imaging. Make a lateral incision from the greater trochanter distally 8 to 12 cm and reflect the vastus lateralis to expose the lateral aspect of the femur. Identify the femoral insertion of the gluteus maximus and make a transverse line in the femoral cortex with an osteotome to mark the level of the osteotomy at the level of the lesser trochanter or slightly distal (Fig. 29-25, *A*). Correct positioning of the osteotomy site can be verified with image intensification.

Once the lateral portion of the trochanter and the proximal lateral femur have been exposed, place a guide pin outside the capsule, anterior to the neck. Using the fluoroscopic image, determine the direction of the neck. Set the adjustable angle guide to 120 degrees, and position it against the lateral cortex. Attach the guide to the shaft with the plate clamp. Insert the guide pin through the cannulated portion of the adjustable angle guide and into the femoral neck (Fig. 29-25, *B*). Predrilling the lateral cortex with the twist drill can aid in placing the guide pin. Take care to ensure that the guide pin is placed in the center of the femoral neck within 5 mm of the proximal femoral physis without violating it or the trochanteric apophysis (Fig. 29-25, inset *1*). Verify guide pin placement in the anteroposterior and lateral views on the image.

Once the guide pin is placed within 5 mm of the physis, use the percutaneous direct measuring gauge to determine the lag screw length (Fig. 29-25, inset *2*).

Set the adjustable positive stop on the combination reamer to the lag screw length determined by the percutaneous direct measuring gauge. Place the reamer over the guide pin and ream until the positive stop reaches the lateral cortex (Fig. 29-25, *D*). Take care not to violate the physis. It is prudent to check the fluoroscopic image periodically during reaming to ensure that the guide pin is

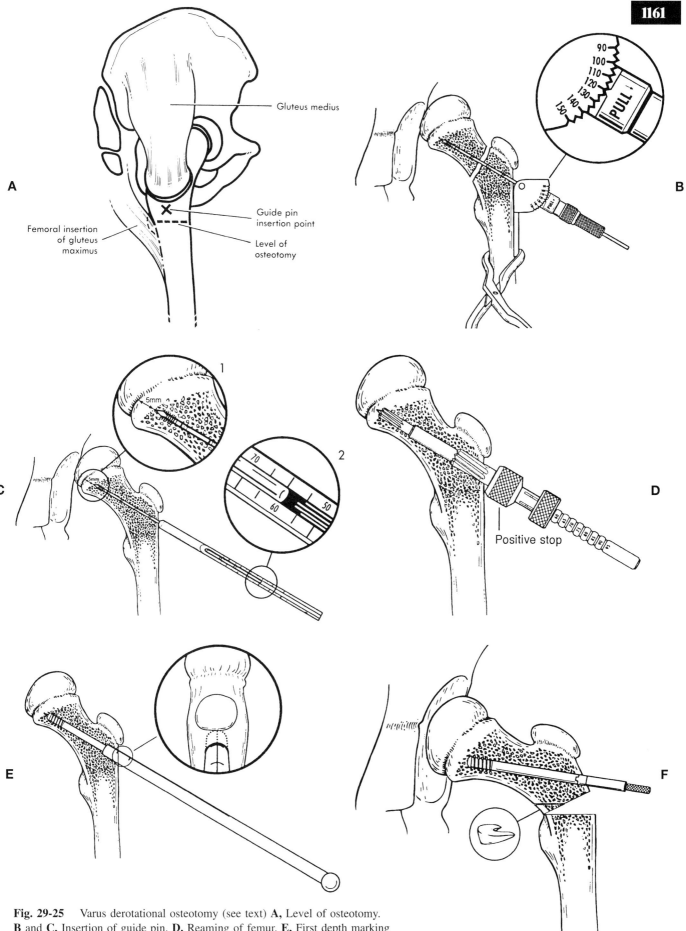

Fig. 29-25 Varus derotational osteotomy (see text) **A,** Level of osteotomy.
B and **C,** Insertion of guide pin. **D,** Reaming of femur. **E,** First depth marking
flush with lateral cortex. **F,** Removal of wedge to customize fit. *Continued*

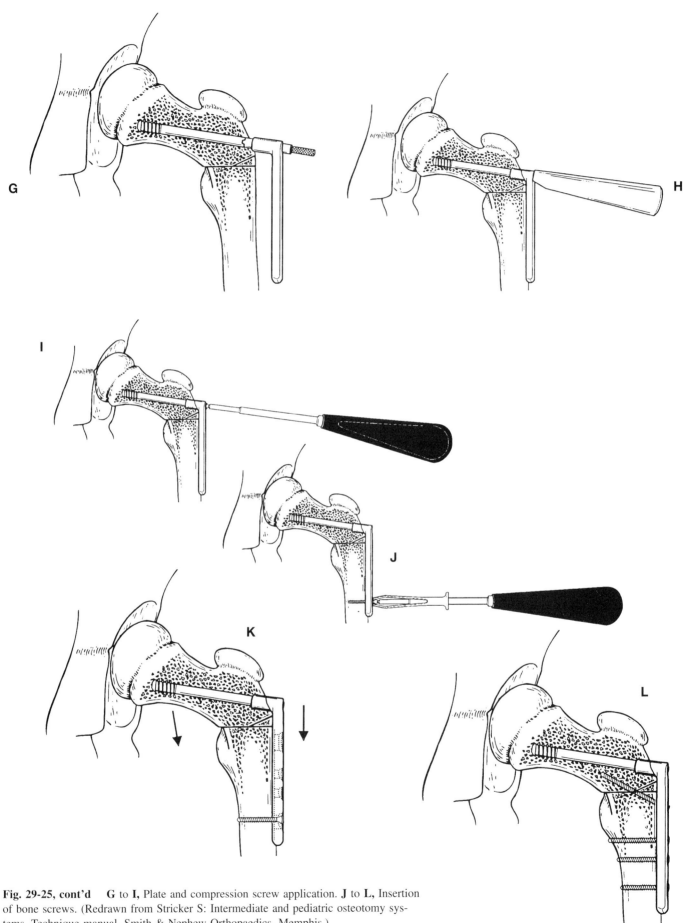

Fig. 29-25, cont'd **G** to **I,** Plate and compression screw application. **J** to **L,** Insertion of bone screws. (Redrawn from Stricker S: Intermediate and pediatric osteotomy systems. Technique manual, Smith & Nephew Orthopaedics, Memphis.)

not inadvertently advancing into the femoral epiphysis. Next, set the adjustable positive stop on the lag screw tap to the same length that was reamed. Tap until the positive stop reaches the lateral cortex. Insert the selected lag screw into the distal end of the insertion/removal wrench. Place it over the guide pin and into the reamed or tapped hole.

The lag screw is at the proper depth when (1) the insertion or removal wrench's first depth marking is flush with the lateral cortex (Fig. 29-25, E) and (2) the handle of the insertion or removal wrench is perpendicular to the shaft of the femur, with the longitudinal key line facing proximally. This positioning ensures that the plate barrel and lag screw shaft are properly keyed for rotational stability (Fig. 29-25, F). Remove the guide pin once the lag screw is at the appropriate length.

With the lag screw in place, perform the osteotomy (20-degree transverse osteotomy is illustrated). Make the cut as proximal as possible, just below the lag screw entry point, because the proximal metaphyseal bone usually heals better than the cortical subtrochanteric bone. In addition, the correction of the proximal femoral deformity is best accomplished close to the deformity, that is, as close to the femoral head as possible.

Insert the barrel guide into the back of the implanted lag screw to help position the proximal femur. The desired correction can be accomplished by tilting the head into valgus or, in this case, varus, removing wedges to customize the fit if needed (Fig. 29-25, G). Iliopsoas tenotomy or recession also may facilitate positioning of the osteotomy.

Take the plate chosen during preoperative planning (100 degrees × 76 mm × 4 holes in this case) and insert its barrel over the barrel guide and onto the back of the lag screw (Fig. 29-25, H). If necessary, insert the cannulated plate tamper over the barrel guide and tap it several times to fully seat the plate (Fig. 29-25, I).

Remove the barrel guide and insert a compressing screw to prevent the plate from disengaging during the reduction maneuver. Use the slotted screwdriver for the pediatric compressing screw or the hex screwdriver for the intermediate compressing screw (Fig. 29-25, J).

Reduce the osteotomy and secure the plate to the femur using the plate clamp. Check rotational position of the lower extremity in extension.

A range of 2.5 to 6.5 mm of femoral shaft compression is possible with the use of an intermediate osteotomy hip screw. To achieve up to 6.5 mm of compression, insert the drill guide end of the intermediate combination drill or tap guide into the distal portion of the most distal compression slot. Drill through to the medial cortex using the twist drill.

If less compression is required, follow the same steps detailed above in the distal portion of the either the second or third distal slots for up to 2.5 mm of compression. If no compression is needed, follow the same steps listed above, except begin by placing the intermediate combination

drill/tap guide in the proximal portion of the slot instead of the distal portion used for compression.

Next, insert the tap guide end of the intermediate combination drill or tap guide into the slot and insert the bone screw tap.

Insert the depth gauge through the slot and into the drilled or tapped hole. Make sure that the nose of the guide is fully inserted into the plate's slot. Insert the needle of the depth gauge and hook it on the medial cortex. Read the bone screw length measurement directly off of the depth gauge.

Select the appropriate length bone screw and insert it using the hex screwdriver. Use the self-holding sleeve to keep the screw from disengaging from the screwdriver.

In cases in which compression is being applied, the bone screw abuts the inclined distal aspect of the slot as it is being seated, forcing the plate and the attached proximal fragment slightly distally until resisted by compression of the osteotomy (Fig. 29-25, K). Follow the same steps for the remaining two slots.

Finally, in the most proximal slot, the intermediate combination drill or tap guide can be angled proximally so that the drill, and ultimately the bone screw, will cross the osteotomy line. Positioning the proximal bone screw in this way can provide additional stability at the osteotomy site (Fig. 29-25, L).

Irrigate the wound and close in layers, inserting a suction drain if needed. Apply a one and one-half spica cast.

AFTERTREATMENT. The spica cast is worn for 8 to 12 weeks, until union is effected. The internal fixation can be removed 12 to 24 months after the osteotomy if desired.

◆ ◆ ◆

Axer described a lateral opening wedge osteotomy for children 5 years of age and younger in which a prebent plate is used to hold the cortices apart laterally the measured amount. The defect laterally fills in rapidly in young children, but the open wedge may result in delayed or nonunion in children over 5 years of age. Since few children younger than 5 years are operated on in the United States, indications for this procedure are rare. His reversed wedge modification uses the removal of a wedge one half the calculated height based medially and its reversal for insertion laterally before fixation with the prebent plate. This method produces approximately the same amount of shortening as the opening wedge but not as much as complete removal and closure of the full height of the wedge medially.

◆ Lateral Opening Wedge Osteotomy

TECHNIQUE 29-6 *(Axer)*

With the patient supine on the operating table, drape the lower limb free for manipulation. Make a straight lateral incision beginning at the level of the middle of the greater

continued

Table 29-2   Table for Calculating Height of Base of Wedge To Be Removed for Varus Osteotomy*

Desired Angulatory Change (Degrees)	Femoral Shaft Width at Osteotomy Site (mm)												
	10	12.5	15	17.5	20	22.5	25	27.5	30	32.5	35	37.5	40
10	1.5	2.0	2.5	3.0	3.5	4.0	4.5	5.0	5.5	6.0	6.5	7.0	7.5
15	2.0	3.0	4.0	4.5	5.0	6.0	6.5	7.5	8.0	9.0	10.0	10.5	11.5
20	3.0	4.0	5.0	6.0	7.0	8.0	9.0	10.0	11.0	12.0	13.0	14.0	15.0
25	4.5	5.0	6.5	7.5	9.0	10.0	11.5	12.5	14.0	15.0	16.0	17.5	18.5
30	5.5	6.5	8.0	10.0	11.5	12.5	14.0	15.5	17.0	18.5	20.0	22.0	23.0
35	6.5	8.0	10.0	12.0	13.5	14.0	17.0	18.3	21.0	22.0	24.0	26.0	27.5
40	8.0	10.0	12.5	14.5	16.5	18.5	20.0	23.0	25.0	27.0	29.0	31.5	33.5

*Credited to Orkan and Roth. Data from Axer A: Personal communication, 1978.
The height of the base of the wedge in millimeters is read at the junction of the horizontal axis (desired degrees of angulatory change) and the vertical axis (width of the femoral shaft at the osteotomy site).

trochanter and continue it distally 10 to 13 cm. Expose subperiosteally the proximal part of the femur up to the origin of the vastus lateralis muscle. Apply a self-retaining bone clamp vertically on the femoral shaft as distally as possible while the lower extremity is held in full internal rotation. This clamp serves as an efficient retractor and enables the surgeon to control the distal fragment after osteotomy. Choose two Sherman bone plates of identical size so that half the length of the plate reaches from the base of the trochanter to the osteotomy site. Prebend one plate in the middle to the desired osteotomy angle and hold the other against the lateral aspect of the femur so that its proximal end reaches to the base of the greater trochanter. Make a transverse mark on the femoral shaft at the level of future osteotomy, corresponding with the midpart of the plate. Insert two long 7/64 inch (2.8 mm) drill points through the two proximal plate holes and through both femoral cortices and leave them there. Remove the plate and measure with calipers the width of the femoral shaft at the level of the subtrochanteric osteotomy. Read the length of the base of the wedge to be opened from the table credited by Axer to Orkan and Roth (Table 29-2). Then select either an opening wedge or reversed wedge technique for the osteotomy as indicated.

Opening Wedge Technique. While the extremity is held in internal rotation, divide the bone with an oscillating saw at the previously marked level. Hold the proximal fragment in slightly less than full internal rotation and in abduction with the help of the protruding long drill points. Bring the medial cortices of the distal and proximal fragments together after rotating the distal fragment externally until the patella points straight forward. Slip the prebent bone plate over the drill points and fix it to the proximal and distal fragments of the femoral shaft with two self-retaining bone clamps. Pay attention to the contact of the medial cortices and to an accurate fit of the plate to the outer surface of the bone so that the required varus angle is

established. Carefully attempt to internally rotate the extremity; a few degrees of rotation should be possible. Check the position of the patella to be sure that there is not too much external rotation of the foot at the midposition of the joint. Insert screws of proper length into the distal fragment and then into the proximal fragment, replacing the long drill points.

Reversed Wedge Technique. After calculating from the table the height of the base of the wedge to be removed, hold the extremity in internal rotation at the hip and mark a wedge half this height over the anterior surface of the femur with the base medially. Remove this wedge with an oscillating saw, rotate the distal fragment externally to the desired degree, turn the bone wedge 180 degrees, and insert it in the osteotomy with its base lateral or reversed. Since its base now is lateral, the varus angle obtained equals the angle that would be obtained with complete removal of a full-height bone wedge medially. Fix the bone fragments with the prebent plate as previously described with all cortices in contact. When the reversed bone wedge is not stable enough, fix it to the distal or proximal fragment with small Kirschner wires.

AFTERTREATMENT. A double spica plaster cast is applied and removed after 6 to 8 weeks or when union is confirmed by roentgenography. The child is encouraged to walk, in water initially if increased joint stiffness is noted. No restrictions are imposed on the child except for follow-up every 3 months in the first year.

Reconstructive Surgery in Perthes Disease

Valgus Extension Osteotomy. One residual of Legg-Calvé-Perthes disease is a malformed femoral head with resulting hinge abduction. Hinge abduction of the hip is an abnormal movement that occurs when the deformed femoral head fails to slide within the acetabulum. A trench is formed laterally,

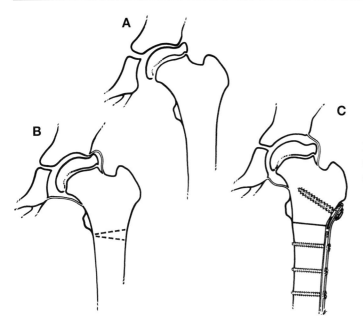

Fig. 29-26   Valgus osteotomy to reduce hinge abduction and increase flexion of hip; osteotomy is fixed with pediatric screw and side plate.

adjacent to a large uncovered portion of the deformed head anterolaterally. With the aid of image intensification, Snow et al. recognized late anterior impingement of the femoral head in four patients with Legg-Calvé-Perthes disease, all of whom had late-onset pain triggered by internal rotation. Three of the four were found to have articular surface damage and osteochondral projections at the area of anterior impingement. Arthroscopic debridement and proximal femoral osteotomies relieved symptoms in all four patients. We use a valgus extension osteotomy, as described by Catterall, fixed with a pediatric screw and side plate (Fig. 29-26) to relieve this obstruction.

Valgus Flexion Internal Rotation Osteotomy. Kim and Wenger, using three-dimensional CT scans in Legg-Calvé-Perthes, noted "functional retroversion" rather than femoral anteversion. As a result they recommended a valgus flexion internal rotation femoral osteotomy plus a simultaneous acetabuloplasty in patients with severe femoral head deformity. The combined procedure (1) corrects the functional coxa vara and hinge abduction (valgus osteotomy), (2) establishes a more normal articulation between the posteromedial portion of the true femoral head and the acetabulum while moving the anterolateral protruding portion of the femoral head away from the anterolateral acetabular margin (valgus-flexion osteotomy), (3) corrects external rotation deformity of the distal limb (internal rotation osteotomy), and (4) improves joint congruity and anterolateral femoral head coverage in hips with associated acetabular dysplasia.

◆ Cheilectomy

Occasionally, as a late residual of Perthes disease, a child will be left with a malformed femoral head, usually either a large mushroom shape (coxa plana) or a lateral protuberance of the head outside the acetabulum. For this lateral protuberance on the head, when the hip is painful and has a lack of abduction or a clicking sensation on abduction, Garceau recommended a cheilectomy for its removal (Fig. 29-27). When the head is mushroom-shaped, as in coxa plana, and subluxating from the acetabulum and when the hip is painful, coverage can be achieved by a Chiari osteotomy.

Preoperative evaluation for cheilectomy, as described by Sage and Clark at this clinic, includes determination as to whether the protuberance is anterior or posterior. In our experience it is usually anterior and lateral, and for this reason we usually use a lateral approach (p. 61).

TECHNIQUE 29-7 *(Sage and Clark)*

With the patient supine and the involved hip on a sandbag, begin an incision laterally approximately 5 cm proximal to the greater trochanter and carry it distally for 7.5 to 10 cm. Locate the interval between the gluteus medius and tensor fasciae latae muscles and carry the dissection proximally to expose the inferior branch of the superior gluteal nerve. Retract this nerve carefully because it innervates the tensor fasciae latae muscle. Complete the separation of the interval and expose the hip capsule. Open the capsule longitudinally along the anterosuperior surface of the femoral neck. Since the protuberance almost always lies laterally, it can then be seen either anteriorly or posteriorly. When it is more posterior, detach a small portion of the fibers of the gluteus medius tendon from the trochanter for exposure. Excise the entire protuberance with a sharp osteotome. Direct the osteotome away from the lateral edge of the proximal femoral physis to avoid its excision. Slipping of the capital femoral epiphysis has followed cheilectomy and may be related to excision of the lateral portion of the physis and the

continued

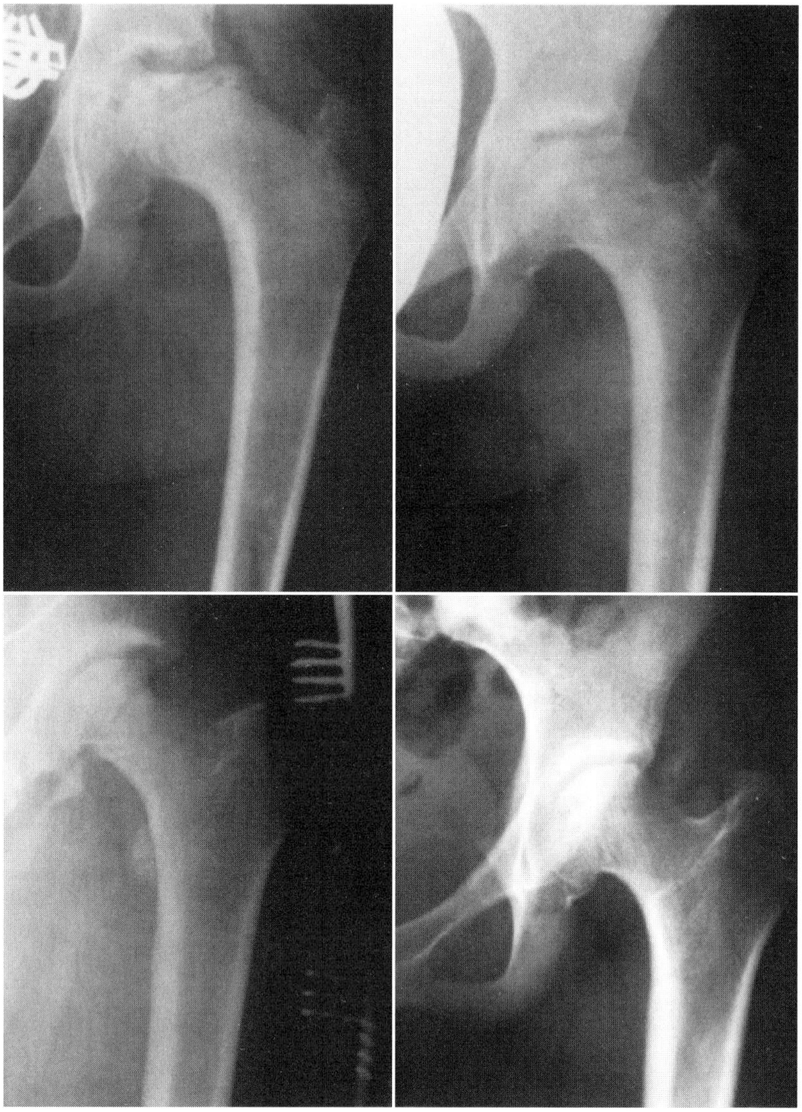

Fig. 29-27 Cheilectomy for Perthes disease. **A,** Roentgenogram of left hip of 7-year-old boy with Perthes disease who had been treated without containment and developed lateral subluxation of femoral head (late group III). **B,** Same patient in residual stage with coxa plana and lateral protuberance of femoral head outside acetabulum, which caused pain and limited abduction of hip. **C,** Roentgenogram made during surgery for cheilectomy. Large protruding area of bone has been excised. **D,** At follow-up several years later pain is relieved and motion, including abduction, is increased. Area of myositis ossificans or calcification is apparent in superior capsule of hip joint.

adjacent cortex of the neck. Check the range of motion, especially abduction, to be sure that a sufficient cheilectomy has been performed.

AFTERTREATMENT. The extremity is placed in balanced suspension, and over the next 2 to 3 weeks range-of-motion exercises, especially hip abduction, are carried out.

Shelf Procedure. If the hip is congruous, a Staheli or Catterall shelf augmentation procedure (Chapter 27) is performed for coxa magna and lack of acetabular coverage for the femoral head.

Chiari Osteotomy. The pelvic osteotomy described by Chiari (Fig. 29-28) has been used by us as a salvage procedure to accomplish coverage of a large flattened femoral head in an older child when the femoral head is subluxating and painful

(Fig. 29-29). It is described in detail in Chapter 27. Bennett et al. reported good results after 18 Chiari osteotomies performed for painful subluxation of hips after Legg-Calvé-Perthes disease. They believe that the clinical success of the procedure resulted from improved femoral head coverage and stability and decreased eccentricity.

◆ Trochanteric Advancement

Although trochanteric overgrowth can be caused by a number of conditions, including osteomyelitis, fracture, or congenital dysplasia, it occurs in Legg-Calvé-Perthes disease when the disease causes premature closure of the capital femoral physis. Whatever the mechanism, the result is the same: arrest of longitudinal growth of the femoral neck with continuation of growth of the greater trochanter (Fig. 29-30). According to Wagner, the functional consequences are always the same: elevation (overgrowth) of the trochanter decreases tension and

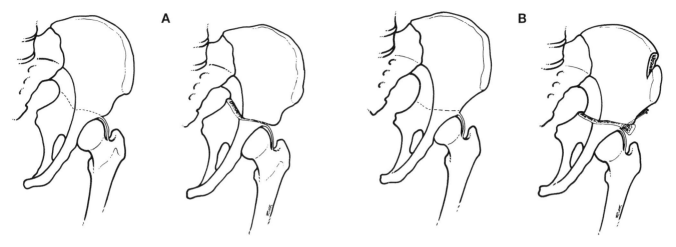

Fig. 29-28   **A,** Ideal Chiari osteotomy with 15-degree up-slope to obtain coverage in mild hip dysplasia. **B,** Chiari osteotomy with supplemental graft and shelf for severely dysplastic hip. (Redrawn from Graham S, Westin GW, Dawson E, Opppenheim WLl: *Clin Orthop* 208:249, 1986.)

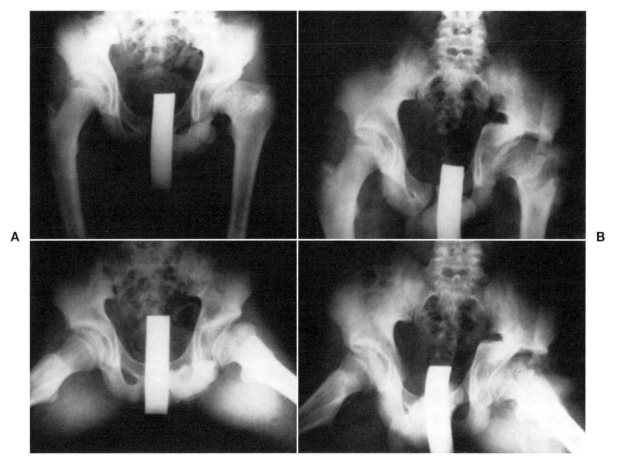

Fig. 29-29   Chiari osteotomy for residual Perthes disease. **A,** Anteroposterior and lateral roentgenograms showing residual Perthes disease (coxa plana) and subluxation in hip on right. **B,** Eight months after Chiari osteotomy with good coverage of femoral head.

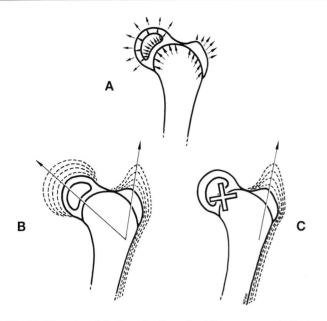

Fig. 29-30 **A** and **B,** Growth of proximal femur; arrows indicate site and direction of growth. **C,** If growth potential is impaired, longitudinal growth is arrested but greater trochanter continues to grow. (Redrawn from Wagner H, Holder J. In Schatzker J, ed: *Intertrochanteric osteotomy,* Berlin, 1984, Springer-Verlag.)

mechanical efficiency of the pelvic and trochanteric muscles; shortening of the femoral neck moves the greater trochanter closer to the center of rotation of the hip, decreasing the lever arm and mechanical advantage of the muscles and impairing muscular stabilization of the hip; the line of pull of the muscles becomes more vertical, increasing the pressure forces concentrated over a diminished area of hip joint surface; and impingement of the trochanter on the rim of the acetabular roof during abduction limits range of motion. Macnicol and Makris described a ''gear-stick'' sign of trochanteric impingement that is useful in the preoperative evaluation. This sign is based on the observation that hip abduction is limited by impingement of the greater trochanter on the ilium when the hip is extended, but full abduction is possible when the hip is fully flexed. The ''gear-stick'' sign is especially useful for differentiating between trochanteric impingement and other causes of limited abduction. Transfer of the greater trochanter distally restores normal tension to the trochanteric muscles and improves mechanical efficiency, puts a more horizontal pull on the pelvic and trochanteric muscle action to distribute forces over the hip joint more uniformly, and increases the length of the femoral neck to increase abduction and decrease acetabular impingement.

Premature closure of the proximal femoral physis often occurs after Perthes disease and may limit abduction and produce gluteal insufficiency. Lloyd-Roberts et al. described trochanteric advancement and the results obtained with the procedure in the late treatment of Perthes disease. The operation was performed in nine hips with premature proximal femoral physeal closure and the result was satisfactory in all.

According to Lloyd-Roberts et al. the procedure improves gluteal efficiency and increases the range of abduction, which was limited by impingement of the trochanter on the ilium. Doudoulakis reported the results of trochanteric advancement in 30 hips with premature arrest of the femoral physis from various causes. Twenty-seven had one or more operations before trochanteric advancement. All trochanters fused without complications after trochanteric advancement. Twenty-four hips that had positive Trendelenburg signs before surgery had negative signs after surgery, and hip abduction increased in 28 of the 30 hips. Alternative methods of treatment include abduction valgus osteotomy of the femur and trochanteric epiphysiodesis.

TECHNIQUE 29-8 *(Wagner)*

With the patient supine, approach the hip through a lateral incision. Incise the fascia lata longitudinally and release the vastus lateralis from the greater trochanter. Retract the gluteus medius muscle posteriorly and insert a Kirschner wire superiorly, parallel to the femoral neck and greater trochanteric physis and pointing toward the trochanteric fossa (Fig. 29-31, *A*). Confirm the placement of the guide wire by image intensification. Internally rotating the hip slightly will aid placement of the wire and allow better imaging. Make the osteotomy parallel to the Kirschner wire with a low-speed oscillating saw, completing it proximally with a flat osteotome (Fig. 29-31, *B*). Pry open the osteotomy until the medial cortex fractures (Fig. 29-31, *C* and *D*). Mobilize the greater trochanter first cephalad and with dissecting scissors remove any adhesions, joint capsule, and soft tissue flush with the medial surface of the trochanter, taking care to spare the blood vessels in the trochanteric fossa (Fig. 29-31, *E*). Once the greater trochanter is freed, transfer it distally and laterally. If excessive anteversion is present, it also can be transferred anteriorly. Using an osteotome, freshen the lateral femoral cortex to which the trochanter is to be attached. Place the trochanter against the lateral femoral cortex and check the position with image intensification. According to Wagner, the tip of the greater trochanter should be level with the center of the femoral head, and the distance between them should be 2 to 2.5 times the radius of the femoral head. When proper position is confirmed, fix the greater trochanter with two screws inserted in a cephalolateral to caudad direction (Fig. 29-31, *F*). These screws, with washers, should compress an area of bony contact between the trochanter and femur. Bury the screw heads by retracting all soft tissue to prevent soft tissue necrosis and local mechanical irritation from occurring postoperatively. Wagner uses a supplemental strong tension band suture that he believes helps absorb tensile forces from the pelvic and trochanteric muscles and prevents trochanteric avulsion; we have not found this suture to be necessary. No postoperative immobilization is required if the patient is compliant and the fixation is secure.

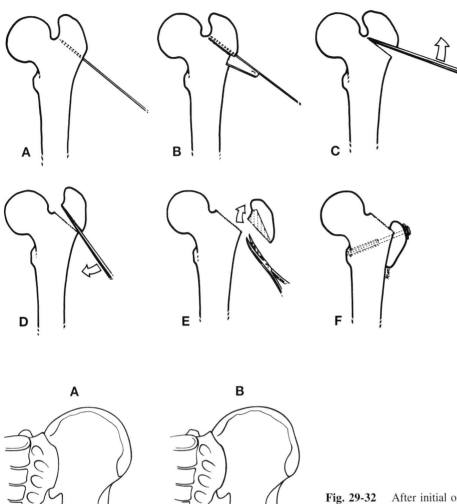

Fig. 29-31 Trochanteric advancement for trochanteric overgrowth (see text). (Redrawn from Wagner H, Holder J. In Schatzker J, ed: *Intertrochanteric osteotomy*, Berlin, 1984, Springer-Verlag.)

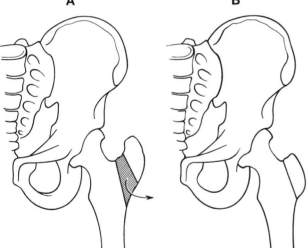

Fig. 29-32 After initial osteotomy of the greater trochanter, trapezoidal wedge of bone is removed. (Redrawn from Macnicol MF, Makris D: *J Bone Joint Surg* 73B:838, 1991.)

AFTERTREATMENT. Ambulation on crutches is begun at 7 days, but active exercises of the pelvic and trochanteric muscles are not permitted until 3 weeks. Sitting upright and flexing the hip also should be avoided because overpull of the gluteus medius muscle may cause loss of fixation.

TECHNIQUE 29-9 *(Macnicol)*

Approach the greater trochanter through a straight lateral incision under lateral image intensification. With a power saw, divide the base of the trochanter in line with the upper border of the femoral neck. Mobilize the trochanteric fragment and the gluteal muscles from their distal soft tissue attachment. Remove a thin wedge of bone from the posterolateral femoral cortex (Fig. 29-32) to provide a cancellous bone bed for the transferred trochanter and to ensure that the trochanter does not project too far laterally. Any undue prominence will cause friction of the fascia lata and produce discomfort and bursitis. Fix the trochanter with two compression screws to prevent rotation of the fragment and to allow early partial weight-bearing.

AFTERTREATMENT. A spica cast is not used, but patients walk with crutches by the end of the first postoperative week.

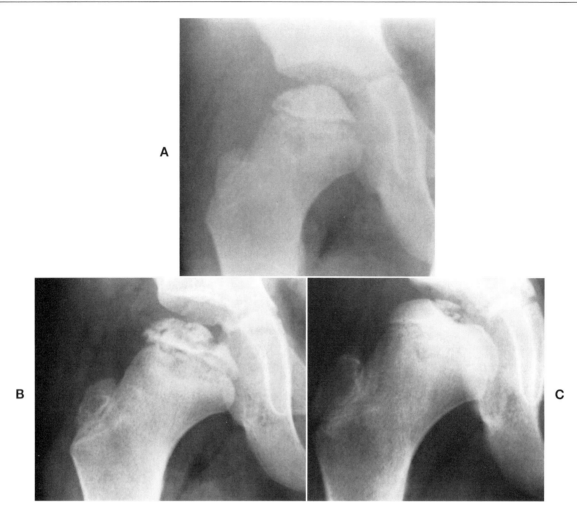

Fig. 29-33   Osteochondritis dissecans of hip. **A,** Onset of Perthes disease in 6-year-old patient. **B,** Fourteen months later, fragmentation and reossification stage. **C,** Persistent defect 5 years after onset.   *Continued*

Exercises to promote movement are gradually introduced, but upright sitting, abduction, flexion, and internal rotation are not forced.

◆ **Greater Trochanteric Epiphysiodesis**

TECHNIQUE 29-10
Approach the physis of the greater trochanter through a lateral incision and determine its location and orientation by inserting a Keith needle. If necessary, use roentgenograms to confirm its position. Use a small drill bit to outline the four corners of a rectangle that spans the lateral portion of the greater trochanteric epiphysis. Remove this lateral rectangle of cortical bone with osteotomies. Curet the physis, reverse the rectangle of bone, and replace it in its bed. Internal fixation is not necessary.

AFTERTREATMENT. Postoperative cast immobilization is not required unless curettage has been so vigorous that the physis of the greater trochanter has been excessively disrupted. Weight bearing is progressed as tolerated.

OSTEOCHONDRITIS DISSECANS OF HIP

Osteochondritis dissecans of the hip occurs most frequently after Perthes disease; it rarely occurs as an isolated entity. Rowe et al. reported osteochondritis dissecans in 7 of 363 (2%) hips with Legg-Calvé-Perthes disease. They noted a higher incidence in hips with worse prognoses. In children loose bodies secondary to Perthes disease, to the avascular necrosis of sickle cell disease, and to multiple epiphyseal dysplasia have to be ruled out before this diagnosis can be established. In adults idiopathic avascular necrosis, Gaucher disease, and occult trauma, such as a torn acetabular labrum, have to be considered in the differential diagnosis. Kamhi and MacEwen described seven children with Perthes disease who ultimately had "osteochondritis dissecans" of the hip. No treatment was necessary for most of these patients (Fig. 29-33). In the seven patients reported by Rowe et al., six did not require surgery, and the lesions healed in three.

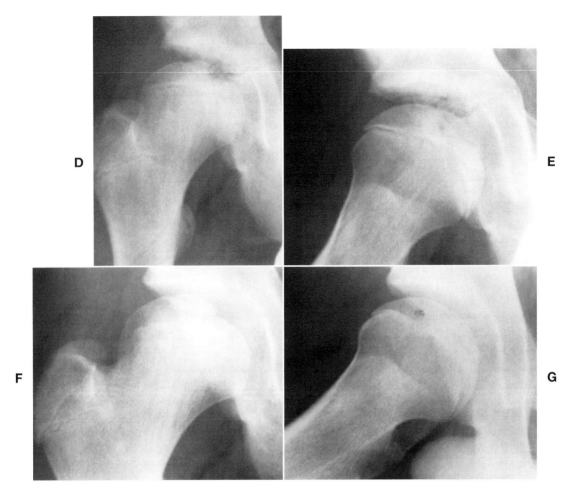

Fig. 29-33, cont'd   D, Osteochondritic lesion at 7 years with some evidence of healing. **E,** Lateral roentgenograms during same period show osteochondritic lesion. Note air arthrogram with smooth cartilage surface. **F,** At 8 years with osteochondritis; defect is healing. **G,** Lateral roentgenogram at same time shows no evidence of defect.

Guilleminet and Barbier described this lesion in the head of the femur not associated with any other affection in eight patients. It characteristically differs from its counterpart in the knee in that it almost always involves the weight-bearing portion of the hip, it almost always remains intact within its crater, and a loose body is only rarely found. However, because it involves a weight-bearing surface, late osteoarthritis frequently occurs. In children, the treatment by these authors and by Flashman and Ghormley was to restrict activity and occasionally brace the hip in the hope that healing and revascularization would occur. Kahmi and MacEwen, and others, described satisfactory results in children who had no treatment. They noted that operative treatment required dislocation of the hip joint with the risk of further vascular damage to the femoral head. In an asymptomatic child with osteochondritis dissecans of the hip, restriction of activity and prolonged observation are indicated to allow healing and revascularization.

Operative treatment is indicated for severe lesions with disabling symptoms. The choice of operative procedure depends on the extent and location of the lesion, the age and activity expectations of the patient, and the presence of degenerative joint changes. Flashman and Ghormley reported that, in their small series of adults, excision of the fragment was as successful as arthroplasty. They drilled the lesion to promote revascularization and recommended packing larger craters with cancellous bone to retain the articular surface contour. Removal of the loose fragment with curettage of the bed to bleeding bone produced good results in two patients reported by Hallel and Salvati. Lindholm and Osterman reported good results with internal fixation of the fragment with cortical bone pegs. Wood et al. reported 17 patients who had osteochondritis dissecans of the hip. In 5 of the 10 patients in whom surgery was performed it was necessary to dislocate the hip. No morbidity was noted as a result of the temporary surgical dislocation. Bowen et al. reported arthroscopic removal of the loose osteocartilaginous fragment in four patients, all of whom were asymptomatic or had improvement of symptoms approximately 1 year after the procedure. None of the procedures mentioned is recommended if severe osteoarthritic changes are present, and a procedure to redirect the femoral head (such as valgus extension osteotomy) is preferred.

In addition to removal of an osteochondritis lesion, arthroscopy of the hip may be indicated for synovial biopsy, removal of loose bodies, removal of debris and inspection of the labrum after fracture-dislocation, and partial or total synovectomy. Arthroscopy of the hip is not a simple procedure and should not be undertaken lightly. If the lesion is not anterior or anterolateral, it is difficult to see, and longitudinal traction should be used to increase the visibility of posterior or posterolateral lesions. A fracture table and image intensification are helpful in judging the correct amount of distraction and joint penetration. Anterior portals, as described by Bowen et al., are most often used, but the lateral portals, as described by Glick et al., may be necessary for more posteriorly located lesions. Arthroscopy of the hip is described in Chapter 48.

Hemophilia

Elective surgery for patients with either classic hemophilia (factor VIII deficiency), or hemophilia A and Christmas disease (factor IX deficiency), or hemophilia B has become possible and reasonable with the availability of factor VIII and factor IX concentrates. Previously only lifesaving surgery was performed, and mortality was high. Wound hematomas with massive sloughs and infection were common. However, only by expert management and strict control of the clotting mechanism can catastrophic complications be minimized, and therefore surgery in patients with hemophilia must not be undertaken casually. Weight-relieving calipers, wedging casts, and spring-loaded braces, such as the Dynasplint, can be used along with physical therapy to protect joints or to stretch soft tissue contractures. These measures may be as important as hematological management in avoiding surgery.

Finally, the current popularity of home therapy for hemophilic patients with self-administration of factor VIII or IX as soon as periarticular stiffness and pain occur may result in a lower incidence of degenerative arthritis and thus in fewer indications for major reconstructive procedures. Nilsson et al. have noted that factor given prophylactically from age 1 or 2 through adolescence, preventing the factor VIII concentration from falling below 1, appears to prevent hemophilic arthropathy, and only minor joint defects have been noted. The National Hemophiliac Foundation recommends the above; however, it should be pointed out that prophylactic factor given daily has to be given intravenously through a "central" line, which increases the possibility of contamination and infection. Recently, three changes have been noted regarding surgery in hemophiliacs: (1) decrease in the need for surgery, (2) increase in the age of the surgical patient, and (3) a change in types of operations performed.

The indications for surgery include the following:

1. Chronic, progressive hypertrophic synovial enlargement from repeated hemarthrosis that cannot be controlled by adequate factor replacement; preferably synovectomy is performed before the cartilage becomes thin and thus at least some of the articular cartilage is preserved. Timely synovectomy also may decrease the incidence of hemorrhage into the joint. This can be done by intraarticular radioisotope injection, arthroscopically, or open.

2. Severe soft tissue contractures that have not responded to nonoperative measures; for example, knee flexion contracture that is so severe that serial casting or a turn-buckle casting technique causes subluxation of the knee joint; supracondylar osteotomy of the femur has been beneficial in this instance, provided 70 to 80 degrees of knee motion remains and the contracture is not so severe that correction would result in excessive traction on the neurovascular bundle in the popliteal space. For correction of a knee flexion contracture of less than 45 degrees after conservative measures have failed, Rodriguez-Merchan et al. reported good results with hamstring release and posterior transverse capsulotomy. Correction by osteotomy of a contracture of more than 50 to 60 degrees probably should be done in stages and preferably after physeal closure.

3. A bony deformity severe enough to require osteotomy.

4. An expanding hematoma (pseudotumor) that continues to enlarge despite adequate factor replacement and possibly radiation therapy.

5. Useless or chronically infected extremities (amputation).

6. Severe arthritic changes with incapacitating pain and hemorrhage (total joint arthroplasty) (Fig. 29-34).

Post and Telfer and McCollough et al. reported small series of patients with hemophilia who had successful elective surgery. Successful surgery in hemophilia depends on a close working relationship between the orthopaedist and an experi-

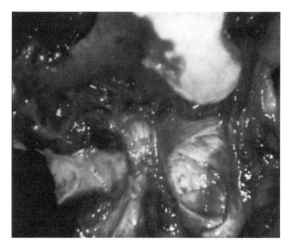

Fig. 29-34 Damaged knee joint with hemophilia (factor VIII deficiency). *Upper right,* Marked destruction and erosion of articular surface of femoral condyle. *Center,* Anterior cruciate ligament and intercondylar notch. Tibial plateaus are grossly eroded and articular surfaces and menisci destroyed by invasion of synovium.

enced hematologist. All hematological aspects of the patient's care must be the responsibility of the hematologist.

The hemorrhagic disorder must be accurately diagnosed before surgery is contemplated. Correct replacement of coagulation factors cannot be undertaken without precise identification and quantitation of the missing factor. Adequate reserve supplies of concentrate must be available in advance, and the supporting laboratory must be able to perform unlimited assays for the factor. It is also essential to determine within a few days of the operation whether the patient has developed an inhibitor against his deficient factor, since the inhibitor hinders hematological therapy and may eliminate the possibility of elective or semielective surgery. In addition, a factor assay should be obtained at the time of surgery. The hematocrit should be measured for several days after surgery, especially in blood groups A, B, and AB, since a Coombs-positive hemolytic anemia may develop. Preoperatively the patient's HIV and hepatitis status should be known. In patients with HIV or hepatitis, the extent of involvement should be investigated. T lymphocyte counts and other parameters should be known to determine the ability to heal and the potential for infection.

Post and Telfer emphasized meticulous surgical technique and detailed preoperative evaluation in this surgery. They recommended (1) as many procedures at one surgical session as the patient can tolerate; this reduces the times that the patient is at risk of bleeding complications and hepatitis and also reduces the high cost of the concentrate and the possibility of inducing an inhibitor; (2) meticulous aseptic technique and pneumatic tourniquets whenever possible; (3) tight, careful wound closure to avoid dead space; (4) avoidance of electrocautery because of the tendency of the coagulated areas to slough after surgery; (5) wound suction in deep wounds for a minimum of 24 hours; (6) no aspirin or other medications postoperatively that inhibit platelet function; and (7) as far as possible no intramuscular injections postoperatively for pain relief.

Post and Telfer and McCollough et al. reported that when coagulation is controlled with hematological therapy, wound slough or infection usually does not occur. Relief of pain and a substantial decrease in recurrent bleeding into joints usually result.

TOTAL JOINT ARTHROPLASTY

McCollough et al. found that synovectomy or total knee arthroplasty (Chapter 6) commonly was cost effective in that the cost of hematological maintenance (concentrate) was markedly lower after surgery. Total knee arthroplasty should be considered only if degenerative arthritis is advanced and range of motion is adequate, since the arthroplasty is unlikely to increase motion. Careful examination of the quadriceps mechanism and correction of any flexion contracture of more than 30 degrees are recommended before surgery. We also suspect that late complications similar to those seen in rheumatoid arthritis will develop because of disuse osteopenia (Fig. 29-35). Since most candidates for total knee arthroplasty in hemophilic arthropathy are relatively young, all other means of relieving the symptoms should be attempted first. Most often, both knees are involved and bilateral arthroplasties are indicated, although arthrodesis of one knee and total knee arthroplasty of the other is a reasonable alternative to bilateral arthroplasty, *provided* motion in the knee selected for arthroplasty is 80 to 90 degrees preoperatively.

Total hip arthroplasty (Chapter 7) is an appropriate operation for disabling hemophilic hip arthropathy. Nelson et al. described the results of 39 total hip arthroplasties in 38 patients with hemophilic arthropathy. Although a number of

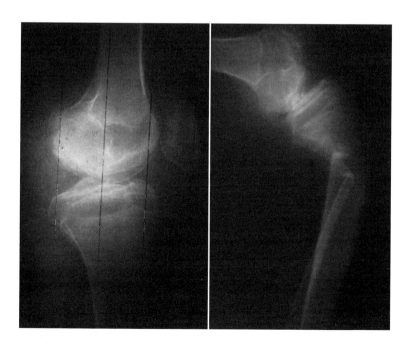

Fig. 29-35 Late complications of hemophilic arthropathy. Note osteopenia and resulting fractures due to manipulation.

total hip revisions were necessary, they noted that not only were some of these arthroplasties done in young patients, but the results may have been influenced by HIV.

SYNOVECTOMY

Although synovectomy of joints can decrease pain and the number of bleeding episodes in patients with hemophilia, it does not appear to alter the course of joint destruction. We performed 16 synovectomies of the knee in 14 children, adolescents, and young adults with hemophilia. Pain was eliminated or decreased in all patients, and the number of bleeding episodes dramatically decreased in all patients at 3-year follow-up. Some knee motion was lost in 5 patients. At long-term follow-up (average, 9 years) of 9 of these patients (11 knees), decreases in pain and frequency of bleeding episodes were sustained, but arthropathy had progressed in all 11 knees and 8 knees had lost motion compared to short-term follow-up. A disturbing finding in this group of patients was that, at long-term follow-up, all 9 were either HIV-positive or had developed AIDS.

Triantafyllou et al. described the results of open and arthroscopic synovectomies of the knee in patients with "classic" hemophilia, focusing on the number of bleeding episodes, the ranges of motion, and roentgenographic progression of hemophilic arthropathy. They noted that in both groups hemarthrosis was significantly reduced. In the open synovectomy group, knee range of motion decreased or remained unchanged in 75% and minimally increased in 25%, whereas in the arthroscopic group an increase of 80% and a decrease of 20% in range of motion were noted. In the open synovectomy group, 62% of knees required manipulation to improve range of motion, but in the arthroscopic group no manipulations were required. Hemophilic arthropathy progressed roentgenographically in most knees in both groups. The arthroscopic group required on the average longer operative time but required shorter hospitalization and less factor replacement. Both techniques reduced hemarthrosis; however, the arthroscopic procedure appeared to have less morbidity. Both Eickhoff et al. and Wiedel noted that, although arthroscopic synovectomy was a low-risk procedure and effective in reducing recurrent hemarthrosis and maintaining range of motion, deterioration of the joint continued, albeit at a slower rate.

The elbow is a frequent site (second only to the knee) of repeated hemorrhage followed by enlargement of the radial head and degenerative arthritis of the radiocapitellar and ulnar-trochlear articulations. We have been pleased with the relief of pain resulting from synovectomy of the elbow joint and excision of the radial head. Improvement in flexion and extension of the elbow cannot be expected, but increased forearm rotation frequently results.

Synovectomy also has proved beneficial for hemophilic arthropathy of the ankle. Greene described the results of open synovectomy of the ankle after failure of conservative treatment in five young patients with hemophilia who continued to have recurrent hemarthroses and hypertrophic synovitis characterized by boggy swelling of the ankle joint. At follow-up, the episodes of hemarthrosis requiring transfusion decreased significantly, and ankle range of motion increased in all of his patients. Greene recommended open synovectomy over arthroscopic synovectomy (see Chapter 48) because removal of the posterior synovial tissue from the crypts of the malleoli is difficult and may injure the articular cartilage even with the use of the posterolateral portal and distraction of the joint with an external fixator. Furthermore, rehabilitation of the ankle was relatively easy, even in the younger children in his series. However, Patti and Mayo believe that arthroscopic ankle synovectomy for recurrent hemarthrosis due to hemophilia is a viable alternative to open ankle synovectomy. Ankle, knee and elbow arthroscopic synovectomy are described in Chapters 48 and 49, respectively.

Radionuclide synovectomy, or synoviorthesis (destruction of synovial tissue by intraarticular injection of a radioactive agent), has produced encouraging results. The procedure has very little morbidity and can be done on an outpatient basis in the radiology department. The isotope appears to shrink the outer layer of synovium, decreasing pain, bleeding, and the recurrence rate. Repeat injections can be given to reduce the recurrence rate and the bleeds. Although Gilbert and Radomisli suggested that arthroscopic or open synovectomy is the treatment of choice in the hemophiliac population, they recommended radioactive synovectomy for patients with inhibitors to the clotting factor, advanced HIV, advanced hepatitis, or multiple joint involvement.

Siegel et al. reported improved range of motion and decreased frequency of hemorrhage in nearly 80% of adult patients treated with synoviorthesis of the elbow or knee using P-32 chromic phosphate. They recommend that synoviorthesis be done early, before the synovium enlarges. Erken described the use of radionuclides for the treatment of 58 joints in 35 patients who had hemophilic arthropathy. The patients were injected with 2 to 5 mCi of yttrium-90 silicate under local anesthesia. A preinjection arthrogram ensured correct placement of the needle. Immobilization of the joint was recommended for 3 days before surgery. After radionuclide injection, 47 joints were pain free and 13 remained free of hemorrhage. With this technique the hemorrhagic frequency decreased from four per month to two per year. The benefits of the procedure far outweighed the radiation risk. Although roentgenographic appearance of the joints showed little change, no worsening was noted. Five complications occurred—three needle track necroses from extravasation of the radiocolloid and two severely painful joints immediately after injection—as did one massive hemorrhagic episode. Erken recommended this form of treatment for hemophilic patients who fail to respond to intensive physical therapy and hematological therapy and for those who have inhibitors. He noted no ill effects, such as physeal closure, after radionuclide injection for hemophilic arthropathy in children and adolescents.

Rivard, Girard, and Belanger reported 92 synoviortheses in 48 patients who had chronic hemophilic synovitis. Colloidal P-32 chromic phosphate was injected intraarticularly, 1.0 mCi for knees and 0.5 mCi for other joints. The frequency and the amount of bleeding decreased in most of their patients. Range of motion improved or remained stable in 50% of the patients but continued to decrease in the other 50%. Roentgenographic scores worsened progressively despite the decreased frequency of hemarthrosis. Their patients were generally satisfied with the results.

In our experience, short-term results of radionuclide synovectomy of the ankle in children and adults have been encouraging because the nuclide appears to be able to penetrate posteriorly; however, the recurrence rate (need for a second synoviorthesis) seems to be higher than for open or arthroscopic synovectomy. Rodriguez-Merchan et al. evaluated synoviorthesis of the elbow and knees and noted that if two or three consecutive synviortheses within 3- to 6-month intervals

have been ineffective, or the roentgenographic score is more than two points (according to classification of the Orthopaedic Advisory Committee of the World Federation of Hemophilia), operative synovectomy is indicated.

ARTHRODESIS

Arthrodesis of the ankle (Chapter 3), shoulder (Chapter 4), and knee (Chapter 3) has been satisfactory in small series of patients with hemophilia. The use of internal fixation rather than external fixators that require transcutaneous pins is recommended to reduce bleeding and infection around the pins (Fig. 29-36). Fixed flexion contractures can be corrected by removing appropriate bone wedges at the time of arthrodesis. Gamble et al. recommended compression arthrodesis of the

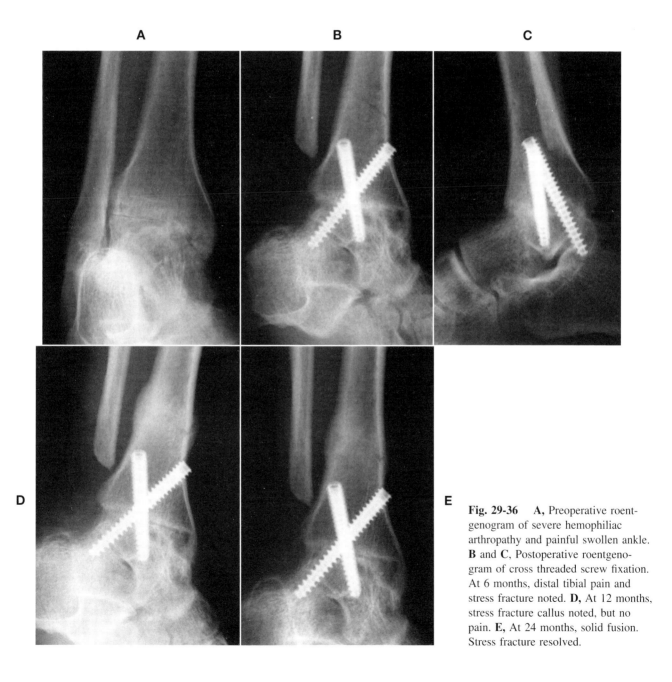

Fig. 29-36 **A,** Preoperative roentgenogram of severe hemophiliac arthropathy and painful swollen ankle. **B** and **C,** Postoperative roentgenogram of cross threaded screw fixation. At 6 months, distal tibial pain and stress fracture noted. **D,** At 12 months, stress fracture callus noted, but no pain. **E,** At 24 months, solid fusion. Stress fracture resolved.

ankle to alleviate pain, reduce bleeding episodes, and decrease equinus deformity in adults with established arthropathy and joint destruction. Despite the dismal prognosis, they also recommended early orthopaedic intervention for young children in whom bleeds are difficult to control because of lack of compliance. In their study of ankle arthropathy, they noted that some patients had severe problems before the age of 10 years and over half had problems before the age of 19 years. During the second decade of life, hemarthrosis occurred more often in the ankle than in the knee. Recurrent bleeding into the ankle joint, chronic synovitis, and overgrowth of the medial portion of the distal tibial physis were associated with an early onset of arthropathy in younger children, and usually osteonecrosis of the talus with collapse and flattening of the talar dome was evident.

OSTEOTOMY

For hemophilic patients with symptomatic bony deformities, osteotomies may be necessary. In patients with symptomatic genu varum deformities, proximal valgus closing wedge osteotomies may be performed (Chapter 26). Merchan and Galindo described 14 hemophilic patients with symptomatic genu varum who were treated with proximal valgus closing wedge osteotomies. They preferred to excise the tibiofibular syndesmosis rather than perform a fibular osteotomy. They noted that proximal tibial osteotomy is an effective and reliable treatment method.

COMPLICATIONS OF HEMOPHILIA

A rare, yet disabling and frequently life-threatening complication, iliac hemophilic pseudotumor, occurs in 1% to 2% of patients with factor VIII deficiency. Castañeda et al. noted two types of pseudotumors: one occurs primarily in the femur or pelvis in adults and has an exceptionally poor prognosis, and one occurs more distally in the extremities in children and has a better prognosis. They recommended factor replacement, immobilization, close observation, and avoidance of cyst aspiration. Operative resection for the adult-type pseudotumor may be life threatening, and amputation should be considered. Iwata et al. described the results of two patients who had large pseudotumors of the ilium removed. One patient had a favorable postoperative course, but the second patient, who had complete resection of the pseudotumor, died of postoperative bleeding and sepsis. Preoperative consideration of the tumor size and degree of infiltration is of utmost importance in operative management. Early excision eliminates the possibility of endogenous infection. Partial resection of huge tumors that leave the lateral wall intact for compression and recovery of function may be preferable to excision of the entire wall, leaving a huge dead space that allows massive hematoma and sepsis. Several studies have shown early promising results using radiation for pseudotumors that are inaccessible or not appropriate for resection.

In addition to involvement of various joints, nerve lesions also are common in patients with hemophilia. Katz et al. described 81 such peripheral nerve lesions. The femoral nerve was the most commonly involved, followed by the median nerve and the ulnar nerve. In 49% of the lesions, the nerves had full motor and sensory recovery after significant bleeds. In 34% a residual sensory deficit (normal motor) was present, and in 16% both persistent motor and sensory deficits were present. Patients who had inhibitors to factor VIII were significantly less likely to recover full motor or sensory function than those who did not have antibodies, and time to full motor recovery in these patients was significantly longer.

Hemophilia-related acquired immunodeficiency syndrome (AIDS) was first reported in the United States in 1981. Current estimates of the percentage of hemophilic patients with HIV antibodies range from 30% to 90%. Stehr-Green et al. reported that in the United States the median length of survival after diagnosis is 11.7 months in hemophiliacs with transfusion-associated AIDS. Before 1985 it was estimated that 90% of patients seen in hemophiliac clinics were HIV-positive, and a large percentage of patients also had laboratory evidence of hepatitis. The Centers for Disease Control and Prevention (CDC) estimated that 9000 or 45% of the hemophiliac population contracted AIDS and that 1900 patients actually died as the result of AIDS. The screening for the presence of HIV in blood and blood products for transfusion since 1985 and the development of monoclonal antibodies to factor VIII and of synthetically derived blood products have markedly decreased the rate of transmission; however, HIV cannot be identified in the "window" period by tests currently used to screen blood donors. Because of this increased risk of HIV infection in hemophilic patients, orthopaedic surgeons treating these patients should observe not only the universal precautions recommended by the CDC, but also the recommendations of the AAOS Task Force on AIDS and Orthopaedic Surgery published in 1989.

◆ SYNOVECTOMY OF KNEE

TECHNIQUE 29-11

Inflate a pneumatic tourniquet about the thigh. Through a medial parapatellar incision (p. 36), remove as much synovium from the knee capsule as possible. Removal of all synovium from the lateral gutter is extremely difficult, and considerable hemorrhage usually occurs in this area. Next remove synovium from the medial joint space, including over and around the medial meniscus and collateral ligament. Then remove synovium from the intercondylar notch and anterior cruciate ligament, and finally from the lateral joint space. Release the tourniquet and obtain meticulous hemostasis with electrocautery; this may require more time than the removal of the synovium. Tightly close the capsule and soft tissues in layers to obliterate any dead space; insert a closed suction drainage tube. If the medial capsule is redundant, oversew it to prevent recurrent dislocation of the patella.

AFTERTREATMENT. The knee is immobilized for 24 hours, and then motion is begun with the aid of the physical therapist and a continuous passive motion machine, if available. The drain is removed at 48 hours under adequate clotting factor replacement. Physical therapy is continued for 6 weeks; the continuous passive motion machine can be used at home.

ARTHROSCOPIC SYNOVECTOMY

Arthroscopic synovectomy is described in Chapter 48.

◆ SYNOVIORTHESIS FOR TREATMENT OF HEMOPHILIC ARTHROPATHY

TECHNIQUE 29-12
Replacement therapy for hemostasis at the time of the synoviorthesis is the same as that used for minor operations. For patients in whom an inhibitor is present, synoviorthesis is sometimes done without preparation for hemostasis. Using aseptic technique, anesthetize the skin with 2% procaine (without epinephrine) with a 23 gauge needle. Note free flow of procaine indicating the introduction of the needle into the intraarticular space. Withdraw synovial fluid when possible. Inject 2 to 5 ml of contrast medium and with roentgenography make sure there is no obvious leak from the synovial space. Inject colloidal P-32 chromic phosphate (Phosphocol P^{32}) intraarticularly. Use 1.0 mCi for knees and 0.5 mCi for other joints. Flush the needle with 2% lidocaine and remove. Apply a sterile plastic bandage and an appropriate immobilizer.

AFTERTREATMENT. The patient can bear weight immediately, but activity should be decreased for 48 hours.

◆ OPEN ANKLE SYNOVECTOMY

Transfusion of the missing clotting factor (factor VIII and IX) is based on the previously described protocol. Approximately 2 hours before the operation, the patient is given a transfusion to raise the level of the deficient clotting factor to close to 100%. Open synovectomy of the ankle is done through anteromedial, anterolateral, and posterior incisions.

TECHNIQUE 29-13 (Greene)
Place a sandbag underneath the lateral buttock to facilitate positioning of the ankle for the anterior portion of the synovectomy. Make an anteromedial incision 3 cm long just medial to the anterior tibialis tendon. Retract the anterior tibialis tendon laterally and retract the branches of the saphenous vein medially. Make a longitudinal incision in the joint capsule. Preserve the capsule even though it is stretched and attenuated by the underlying hypertrophic synovial tissue, since its presence may facilitate postoperative rehabilitation. Free the joint capsule from the adherent synovial tissue by sharp dissection. Remove all visible synovial tissue. Use small pituitary rongeurs to remove folds of synovial tissue that extend into the crypts between the talus and the medial malleolus. Make a 3 cm long anterolateral incision centered just lateral to the peroneus tertius tendon and retract this tendon medially. Open the joint capsule longitudinally and excise the synovial tissue in the same manner described for the anteromedial incision. Resect the folds of synovial tissue interposed between the talus and the lateral malleolus. Remove the sandbag beneath the ipsilateral buttock and place it beneath the contralateral buttock before making the posterior incision. Make a posterior incision approximately twice as long as the anterior incision and center it between the medial malleolus and the Achilles tendon. Open the sheath of the posterior tibialis tendon so that it can be retracted adequately. Dissect the other posterior tendons and the neurovascular structures away from the posterior portion of the capsule of the ankle joint. Place a retractor lateral to the flexor hallucis muscle and medial to the posterior tibialis tendon, permitting retraction of the soft tissue structures located posterior to the ankle joint. This provides full exposure of the posterior portion of the capsule. Incise the capsule horizontally from the medial malleolus to the distal end of the fibula. Dissect the insertion of synovial tissue on the talus and the distal end of the tibia. Use pituitary rongeurs to remove any residual folds of synovial tissue lying in the crypts of the malleoli. If the synovium cannot be removed from the capsule, or the capsule appears intimately involved, removal of large sections of the capsule may be necessary. According to Greene, postoperative rehabilitation may be impeded by extensive scar reaction in the posterior capsule. Once the synovectomy has been completed, deflate the pneumatic tourniquet and secure hemarthrosis meticulously. Repair the anterior portion of the capsule, but leave the posterior portion open and place a drain. Close the wounds in a standard fashion and immobilize the ankle joint in a neutral position with a bulky dressing augmented by a plaster-of-Paris splint.

AFTERTREATMENT. Patients who have a factor VIII deficiency should receive continuous transfusion therapy, and patients with factor IX deficiency should be given a bolus of factor IX every 12 hours. Transfusion should be continued throughout the duration of the hospital stay (7 to 10 days). After discharge, transfusion is given three times a week for 4 weeks. This regimen keeps the deficient clotting factor level sufficiently elevated to minimize the risk of a spontaneous hemarthrosis during the immediate postoperative period while the soft tissue reaction is resolving. The drain is removed on the first postoperative day, and active range-of-motion exercises with the aid of hydrotherapy are begun on the second postoperative day. Initially, weight-bearing is not permitted, and the ankle is intermittently splinted in a neutral position until range of motion of the ankle from neutral dorsiflexion to 25 degrees of plantar flexion is obtained. Discharge from the hospital is determined by the hematologist and the surgeon. Walking with crutches with touch-down weight-bearing is continued for approximately 5 weeks after discharge from the hospital.

Rickets, Osteomalacia, and Renal Osteodystrophy

Rickets is the bony manifestation of altered vitamin D, calcium, and phosphorous metabolism in a child; osteomalacia is the adult form. There are multiple causes of rickets and osteomalacia, and the various metabolic defects in rickets, osteomalacia, and renal osteodystrophy were reviewed by Mankin. Regardless of the cause of the abnormal metabolism, children with rickets have similar long bone and trunk deformities.

Because vitamin D deficiency has become less common in this country, rickets and osteomalacia are not often considered as differential diagnoses in patients who have extremity pain or deformity. However, the orthopaedist should remain familiar with the roentgenographic and laboratory findings that accompany these diseases. According to Mankin, the orthopaedist's responsibilities include establishing a diagnosis and treating osseous complications, such as fractures, slipped capital femoral epiphysis, and bowing of the extremities. When treating patients with rickets, osteomalacia, and renal dystrophy, the orthopaedist must always be concerned about the effect treatment may have on impaired calcium homeostasis.

In very young children with deformity, treatment of the metabolic defect supplemented by corrective splinting or bracing may correct the deformity (Fig. 29-37).

Evans et al. reported 10 patients with primary hypophosphatemic rickets who underwent 33 surgical procedures (19 on the femur and 14 on the tibia). Interestingly, 27 of the 33 procedures were for major long bone deformities and associated complications of surgery in three patients who were undiagnosed in early childhood. In seven patients who had early treatment (before 5 years of age) with inorganic phosphate and vitamin D, only six surgical procedures were performed, all but one of which were relatively simple tibial osteotomies at the proximal metaphysis to correct varus deformity. In prepubertal children or adolescents, medical management and bracing usually will not correct an established deformity. Ferris et al. reported 19 patients with hypophosphatemic rickets, including teenagers and young adults with knee problems. He found that diaphyseal osteotomies were best done over an intramedullary nail. Metaphyseal osteotomies were most successful using a blade plate at or close to maturity. Joint problems developed in patients in their early teens, with

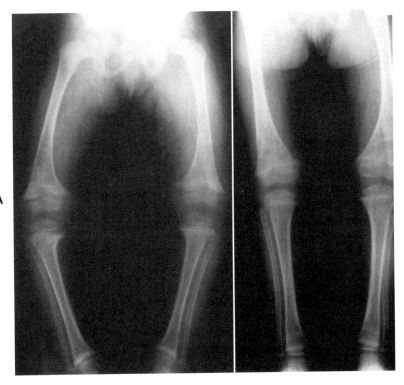

Fig. 29-37 Vitamin D–deficient rickets.
A, Standing roentgenogram of young child with nutritional rickets from vitamin D deficiency.
B, Same child 18 months later after treatment with vitamin D and braces.

osteochondritis lesions occurring in the knee, and late degenerative changes were noted in those in their twenties, with shedding of the articular cartilage. The older patients in this series developed incapacitating stiffness and immobility from calcification of the ligaments. Early osteotomy was recommended to ensure that the joints would be in a position of function if they became stiff.

Before surgery, management of the metabolic defect with vitamin D, phosphorus, and calcium or other appropriate measures should be carried out for several months. If the disease is not controlled metabolically, the deformity probably will recur after corrective osteotomy. However, large-dose vitamin D treatment should be discontinued for at least 3 weeks before surgery because otherwise hypercalcemia is likely to occur with immobilization.

If a water-soluble preparation of vitamin D, such as dihydrotachysterol, is used instead of cholecalciferol that is stored in the liver, the period without medication before surgery can be shortened. In addition, in hypophosphatemic vitamin D–resistant rickets, if the disease is controlled by using inorganic phosphate plus 50,000 units or less of vitamin D per day, symptoms of hypocalcemia during the immediate postoperative period are less likely to occur, even if the preoperative vitamin D medication is not discontinued. Evans et al. reported four procedures done for deformities secondary to vitamin D–resistant rickets, in which the vitamin D preparation was not discontinued before surgery. All patients were taking less than 50,000 units of vitamin D per day, and no symptoms of hypercalcemia developed. However, we still recommend stopping the administration of vitamin D 3 weeks before surgery because hypercalcemia can cause severe symptoms of anorexia, nausea, vomiting, weight loss, confusion, and even seizures. Mobilization of the patient as quickly as possible after surgery to allow early resumption of medical treatment will prevent delayed mineralization of the healing osteotomy and avoid recurrence of deformity with continued growth.

When deformity is severe in older children and there has been no previous medical treatment, after complete diagnostic studies are made, and if the patient does not have azotemic osteodystrophy, it may be better to proceed with the surgery with the patient in a less than homeostatic but compensated metabolic condition rather than to load the patient preoperatively with high doses of vitamin D, calcium, and phosphorus and run the risk of hypercalcemia and extraosseous calcification, especially in the kidney.

With azotemic osteodystrophy, expert preoperative and postoperative medical management is essential and ideally is done by a special team trained in the treatment of chronic renal failure. According to Cattell et al. and others, correction of anemia, adequate hydration, uremia control, and electrolyte balance are required for safe administration of anesthesia. Peritoneal dialysis or hemodialysis may be required before surgery. Cattell et al. and others noted that if attention is given to detail, children with azotemic osteodystrophy can successfully undergo orthopaedic surgery. Their requisites for surgery are a reasonable life expectancy, an intelligent and motivated

patient and parents, demonstrated improvement of bone lesions on medical management, deformities that can be corrected with one or two orthopaedic procedures, and the likelihood that the surgery will significantly reduce the patient's disability. Surgery for children with renal osteodystrophy and knee deformities is feasible, but Oppenheim et al. advised careful surgical planning and preoperative metabolic stabilization. They noted that patients who required repeated osteotomy appeared to have poor metabolic control during the initial surgery, which they measured by an increased alkaline phosphatase. Kanel and Price suggested using an external fixator to obtain precise correction of the deformities without interruption of medical management. Patients with resistant hypertension usually have short life expectancies and should not be considered as surgical candidates. In addition, when parathyroid autonomy is present and not controlled by parathyroidectomy and medical treatment, surgery is not indicated.

Sheridan et al. noted after a follow-up of over 40 years that lower extremity deformities were permanent. They suggested that corrective osteotomies for angulated lower extremities were protective in regard to degenerative arthritis of the knee.

The deformities that require surgical correction most often are genu varum and genu valgum. In genu varum usually the femur, tibia, and fibula are all deformed, often the latter two more severely; there is not only lateral bowing but also internal torsion. An osteotomy of the tibia and the fibula near the apex of the most severe bowing usually is required. Sometimes osteotomy of the femur also is necessary (Fig. 29-38). Osteotomies can be done bilaterally at one operation.

In genu valgum most of the bowing usually is in the femur, and a severe deformity in older children and in adults can be corrected by supracondylar osteotomy of the femur. The goal of both tibial and femoral osteotomies should be correction of deformity and alignment so that the plane of each knee joint is perfectly horizontal with the patient standing.

The techniques of osteotomy are described in the discussion of angular and torsional deformities (Chapter 26).

Tibia Vara (Blount Disease)

Erlacher is credited with the first description of tibia vara and internal tibial torsion (1922), but it was Blount's article in 1937 that prompted recognition of this disorder. Blount described tibia vara as "an osteochondrosis similar to coxa plana and Madelung's deformity but located at the medial side of the proximal tibial epiphysis." However, currently, tibia vara is considered an acquired disease of the proximal tibial metaphysis, rather than an epiphyseal dysplasia or osteochondrosis. The exact cause is unknown, but enchondral ossification appears to be altered. Suggested causative factors include infection, trauma, avascular necrosis, and a latent form of rickets, although none of these has been proved. A combination of hereditary and developmental factors is the most likely cause. Weight-bearing must be necessary for its development, since it

A   B   C

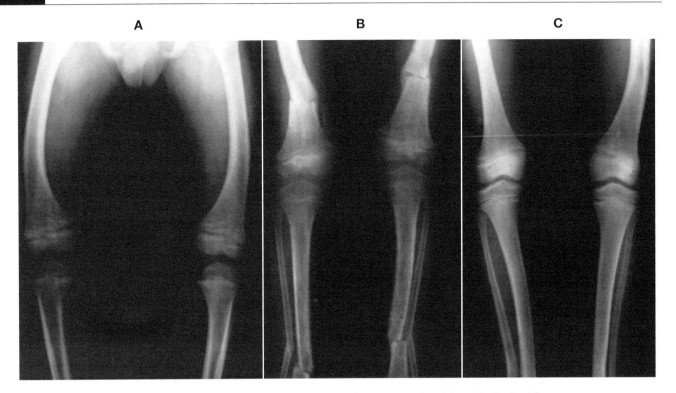

Fig. 29-38 Vitamin D–resistant rickets. **A,** Child before treatment has deformities in distal femurs. Tibias are not shown in this film. **B,** Three months after valgus osteotomies of distal femurs and tibias using pins incorporated in plaster above and below osteotomy sites. **C,** Two years after osteotomies; vitamin D–resistant rickets is well controlled with large doses of vitamin D, calcium, and phosphorus. There has been no recurrence of deformities.

does not occur in nonambulatory patients, and the relationship of early walking and obesity to Blount disease has been clearly documented.

Although the exact cause of tibia vara remains controversial, the clinical and roentgenographic findings are consistent. The abnormality is characterized by varus and internal torsion of the tibia and genu recurvatum. Blount distinguished, according to age at onset, two types of tibia vara: infantile, which begins before 8 years of age, and adolescent, which begins after 8 years of age but before skeletal maturity. The infantile form is difficult to differentiate from physiological bowing common in this age group, especially before the age of 2 years. Infantile tibia vara is bilateral and symmetrical in approximately 60% of affected children; physiological bowing is almost always bilateral. In Blount disease the varus deformity increases progressively, while physiological bowing tends to resolve with growth.

Although not nearly as common as the infantile form, adolescent Blount disease has been divided into two types: (1) an adolescent form occurring between the ages of 8 and 13 years caused by partial closure of the physis after trauma or infection and (2) "late-onset" tibia vara that occurs in obese children, especially black children, between the ages of 8 and 13, without a distinct cause. Thompson et al. noted that the histological changes that occur in patients with late-onset tibia

vara are markedly similar to those that occur in patients with infantile tibia vara or with slipped capital femoral epiphysis, suggesting a common cause for these conditions. They concluded that asymmetrical compressive shear forces across the proximal tibial physis promote disruption and cause compression and deviation of normal intercondylar ossification. Loder et al. reported 15 children with late-onset tibia vara, most of whom were obese black males. Fewer than half of the children had bilateral involvement. The average age of onset was 11 years, and all the children had histories of gradually progressive genu varum deformities. Most had knee pain, and the average preoperative tibiofemoral angle was 14 degrees.

In tibia vara, characteristically the medial half of the epiphysis as seen on roentgenograms is short, thin, and wedged; the physis is irregular in contour and slopes medially. The proximal metaphysis forms a projection medially that is often palpable, but this projection is not diagnostic of tibia vara. However, according to Smith medial metaphyseal fragmentation *is* pathognomonic for the development of a progressive tibia vara. The angular deformity occurs just distal to the projection.

Langenskiöld noted progression of epiphyseal changes and the deformity through six stages with growth and development (Fig. 29-39). At stage VI the medial portion of the epiphysis fuses at a 90-degree downward angle.

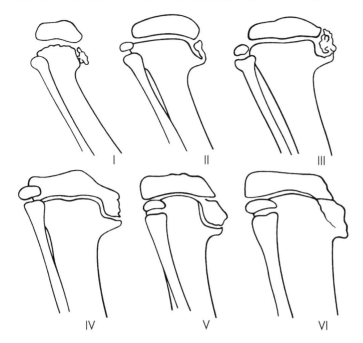

Fig. 29-39 Diagram of roentgenographic changes seen in infantile type of tibia vara and their development with increasing age. (From Langenskiöld A, Riska EB: *J Bone Joint Surg* 46A:1405, 1964.)

Vankka and Salenius described the normal progression of the tibiofemoral angle from pronounced varus before the age of 1 year to valgus between the ages of 1.5 and 3 years. Several authors have suggested that deviation from normal tibiofemoral angle development is indicative of Blount disease. Levine and Drennan reported that the metaphyseal-diaphyseal angle is an early indicator of Blount disease. In their study, most children with metaphyseal-diaphyseal angles of 11 degrees or more developed Blount disease, whereas children with angles of less than 11 degrees had physiological bowing that resolved with growth. This measurement is not an absolute prognosticator of Blount disease, but a metaphyseal-diaphyseal angle of more than 11 degrees warrants close observation (Fig. 29-40). Because of rotation, Drennan's angle is believed by some not to be reliable. Iwasawa et al. use MRI to predict late resolution of tibial bowing in Blount disease. O'Neill and MacEwen, in a roentgenographic study of 39 knees in bowlegged children younger than 30 months, found a poorer prognosis when the fibula was longer than the tibia and when proximal tibial angulation was more severe than distal femoral angulation. Although other angles of the femur and tibia at the knee can be determined (Fig. 29-41), once the deformity is present most authors agree that the mechanical axis of the limb, as it relates to the tibiofemoral angle on roentgenograms, should be the most functional measurement of the amount of deformity present (Fig. 29-42).

Kline et al. described femoral varus as a significant deformity of late-onset Blount disease. They demonstrated an average deformity of 10 degrees of femoral varus more than the calculated ideal femoral-tibial joint angle. This represented between 34% and 76% of the genu varum deformity of the affected limbs. They recommended that calculations be made on standing long-film roentgenograms to determine the amount of excessive femoral varus and that this should be corrected by

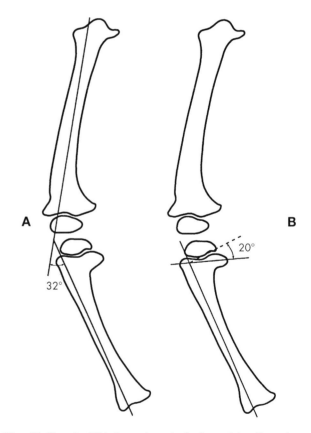

Fig. 29-40 **A,** Tibiofemoral angle is formed by lines drawn along longitudinal axes of tibia and femur. **B,** Metaphyseal-diaphyseal angle is formed by line drawn perpendicular to longitudinal axis of tibia and line drawn through two beaks of metaphysis to determine transverse axis of tibial metaphysis. (Redrawn from Levine AM, Drennan JC: *J Bone Joint Surg* 64A:1158, 1982.)

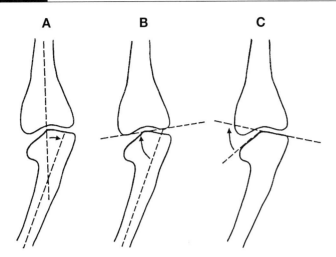

Fig. 29-41 **A,** Angle formed by femoral shaft and tibial shaft. **B,** Angle formed by femoral condyle and tibial shaft. **C,** Depression of the medial plateau of the tibia. (From Schoenecker PL, Johnston R, Rich MM, Capelli AM: *J Bone Joint Surg* 74A:351, 1992.)

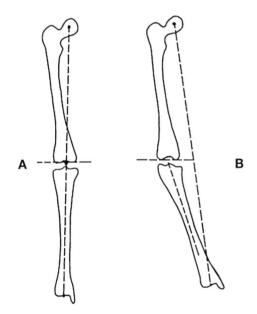

Fig. 29-42 Mechanical axis of limb as it relates to angle formed by femoral condyle and tibial shaft. **A,** Normal alignment. Angle formed by femoral condyle and tibial shaft is approximately 90 degrees. **B,** Tibia vara. Angle formed by femoral condyle and tibial shaft is less than 90 degrees. (From Schoenecker PL, Johnston R, Rich MM, Capelli AM: *J Bone Joint Surg* 74A:351, 1992.)

femoral osteotomy at the time of tibial osteotomy to avoid a subsequent compensatory deformity.

Siffert and Katz noted at arthrotomy in severe deformities a hypertrophied medial meniscus and a posteromedial depression of the articular surface of the tibia. At full extension the knee is stable, but as flexion of the knee progresses the medial condyle of the femur sinks into the depression posteromedially and relaxation of the tibial collateral ligament becomes obvious. Dalinka et al. also demonstrated with arthrography

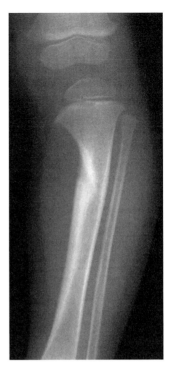

Fig. 29-43 Fibrocartilaginous dysplasia in proximal tibia with resultant varus deformity simulating "bowlegs" of Blount disease.

hypertrophy of the medial meniscus and the unossified cartilage of the medial tibial plateau.

Focal fibrocartilaginous dysplasia has been reported as a cause of tibia vara in a few patients. Bell described the characteristic roentgenographic appearance and unilateral nature of this lesion of the proximal medial metaphysis. Later reports suggest that this generally is a self-limiting condition that corrects spontaneously (Fig. 29-43) and that severe progression should be documented before valgus osteotomy is done. The proximal tibial physis has the potential to correct the deformity in the adjacent metaphysis, depending on the age of the patient and the severity of the deformity. Osteotomy is indicated only for significant deformity in an older child when spontaneous correction can no longer be expected.

The treatment of Blount disease depends on the age of the child and the severity of the varus deformity. Generally, observation or a trial of bracing is indicated for children between the ages of 2 and 5 years, but progressive deformity usually requires osteotomy. Raney et al., Richards et al., and Zionts and Shean all have recently reported that bracing at a young age (3 to 5 years) appears to have a favorable influence on the natural history of unilateral stage I or II Blount disease.

Recurrence of the deformity is not as frequent after osteotomy at an early age as after osteotomy when the child is older. Ferriter and Shapiro reported a recurrence rate of 76% in children undergoing osteotomy at 5 years of age or older, compared with a 31% recurrence rate in those in whom osteotomy was done at a younger age. Loder et al. and Johnston found that 88% of children younger than 4 years of age were successfully treated with one osteotomy, but only 32% of

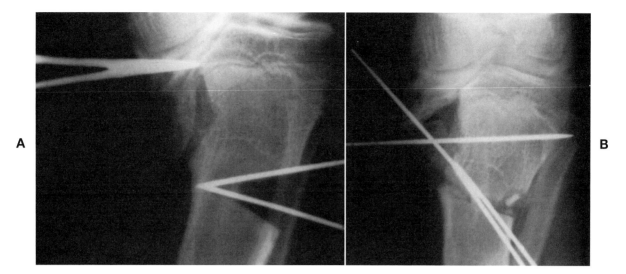

Fig. 29-44 Severe Blount disease. **A,** Closing wedge metaphyseal osteotomy. **B,** Epiphyseal elevation.

children older than 4 years of age had satisfactory results after a single osteotomy. Beaty et al. reported that early osteotomy (2 to 4 years of age) produced the best results, with only 1 of their 10 patients having recurrence of the deformity. Conversely, of 12 patients in whom osteotomy was done after the age of 5 years, 10 (83%) had recurrence of the deformity necessitating repeated osteotomy. They recommended valgus osteotomies of both the proximal tibia and fibula with mild overcorrection in young children.

Rab described a proximal tibial osteotomy for Blount disease in which a single-plane oblique cut allows simultaneous correction of varus and internal rotation and permits postoperative cast wedging if necessary to obtain appropriate position. More recently, Laurencin et al., in an effort to avoid neurovascular and physeal complications, described an oblique incomplete closing wedge osteotomy fixed with a lateral tension plate. Greene also described a chevron osteotomy in which opening and closing wedges can be made so that the limb length deformity present in moderate to severe tibia vara will not be increased. He prefers a crescent-shaped osteotomy, using a one half lateral closing wedge and using the graft medially in an opening wedge to maintain length. Internal fixation of the graft often is necessary.

One cause of recurrence of the deformity after osteotomy is a physeal bar. Greene listed the following criteria for deciding if tomographic studies should be done preoperatively to determine if a bony bar is present: (1) age of more than 5 years, (2) medial physeal slope of 50 to 70 degrees, (3) Langenskiöld grade IV roentgenographic changes, (4) body weight greater than the 95th percentile, and (5) black females who meet the previous criteria. Bony bridge resection should be considered in children with remaining growth potential and can be done in conjunction with tibial osteotomy if angulation is significant.

In children older than 9 years with more severe involvement, osteotomy alone, with bony bar resection, or with epiphysiodesis of the lateral tibial and the fibular physes may be

indicated. Medial physeal bar resection alone has been reported effective when premature closure of the physis is evident, but significant angular deformity will not be corrected by bar resection alone. Lateral tibial epiphysiodesis can be done, with or without osteotomy, after the age of 9 years but before skeletal maturity. For patients who do not have a bony bar but who are at risk for recurrence of the deformity, Greene modifies the tibial osteotomy by increasing the valgus alignment of the osteotomy, stapling the lateral aspect of the tibial physis, or epiphysiodesing the lateral tibial physis and the proximal fibular physis. In unilateral involvement, epiphysiodesis of the uninvolved leg may be indicated to correct leg length discrepancy.

For older patients in whom bracing and tibial osteotomy have failed to prevent progressive deformity, and when the risk of abnormal spontaneous medial epiphysiodesis is great, as evidenced by severe disorderly enchondral ossification, Ingram, Siffert, and others have suggested an intraepiphyseal osteotomy to correct severe joint instability and a valgus metaphyseal osteotomy to correct the varus angulation.

Gregosiewicz et al. reported satisfactory results after 13 double-elevating osteotomies (intraepiphyseal and metaphyseal). An essential element of this procedure is reconstruction of the horizontal level of the medial tibial plateau. They recommended this method for considerable depression of the medial femoral condyle within the defect of the tibial epiphyseal bone and when there is the possibility of a bony bridge between the metaphysis and epiphysis of the medial tibia.

Schoenecker et al. reported elevation of the medial tibial plateau in seven patients between the ages of 10 and 13 years who had severe varus deformities (Langenskiöld grades V and VI). The average varus deformity before surgery was 25 degrees. In addition to elevation of the depressed medial tibial plateau, they also performed metaphyseal valgus osteotomy to correct alignment of the tibia (Fig. 29-44).

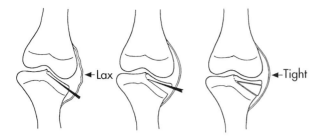

Fig. 29-45 Hemicondylar osteotomy. (From Zayer M: *Acta Orthop Scand* 63:350, 1992.)

Zayer described a hemicondylar tibial osteotomy through the epiphysis, but not through the physis, into the intercondylar notch (Fig. 29-45). His patients were older children with severe sloping of the medial tibial plateau and excessive ligamentous laxity. This method corrects the medial slope of the tibial epiphysis while avoiding the physis.

Because obesity, unequal limb lengths, and femoral deformity often are present in patients with Blount disease, Bell, as well as Coogan et al. recommended the Ilizarov technique as ideally suited for correction of deformity, as well as lengthening if needed, in adolescent patients. This technique allows adjustment of limb alignment postoperatively, if necessary, to obtain a perfect mechanical axis. Fixation of the

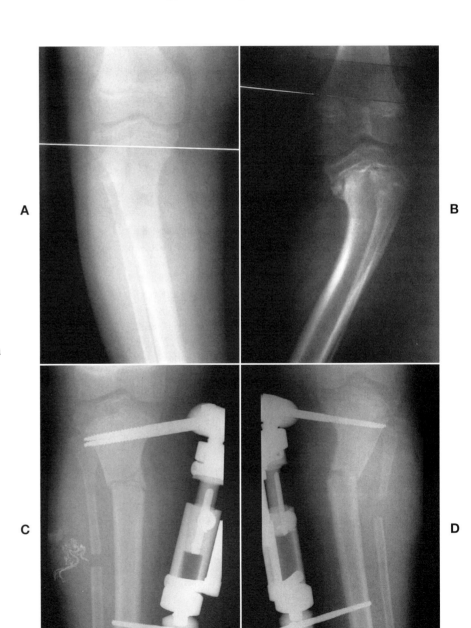

Fig. 29-46 **A** and **B,** Anteroposterior roentgenograms of severe bilateral tibia vara in obese adolescent. **C** and **D,** Roentgenograms of unilateral frame external fixators after metaphyseal osteotomies.

tibia is achieved through four proximal and four distal wires that are affixed to rings and then tensioned. Half-pin modifications also can be used. Bell reported no nerve palsies or compartment syndromes in 14 limbs treated with this technique. Also, external fixation to achieve stability after osteotomy and immediate correction appears to be an excellent method of treating an extremely obese patient for whom unilateral and especially bilateral casting is impractical. Price et al., Stanitski et al., and Gaudinez and Adar used a uniplanar external fixator especially for isolated frontal one-plane deformities with satisfactory results. The advantages appear to be ease of application, adjustability, early weight-bearing, the ability to lengthen the extremity, and avoiding a second operation to remove the hardware (Fig. 29-46).

◆ METAPHYSEAL OSTEOTOMY

The oblique osteotomy described by Rab begins at a point distal to the tibial tubercle, proximal to the posterior tibial metaphysis, and just distal to the physis and is done through a cosmetic transverse incision. Fasciotomy and fibular osteotomy are done through a separate incision. Because rigid internal fixation is not used, postoperative adjustments through cast wedging are possible.

Correction is obtained by rotating around the face of the oblique osteotomy and can be described best by considering the individual cuts in their anatomical planes (Fig. 29-47). Correction of a purely rotational deformity requires an osteotomy in the transverse plane, while purely varus or valgus correction requires osteotomy in the frontal (coronal) plane. An oblique osteotomy, directed from anterior-distal to posterior-proximal, splits the difference between the transverse and frontal planes. Rotation with its two faces in contact corrects varus and internal rotation. Osteotomy cuts that are more

vertical (frontal) correct more varus than internal rotation. More horizontal (transverse) cuts do the opposite. According to Rab, patients with Blount disease have almost equal amounts of varus and internal rotation, and in practice a 45-degree upward osteotomy provides adequate correction in most patients. He reports simultaneous correction of varus deformity up to 44 degrees and internal rotation up to 30 degrees. Figure 29-48 provides a quick estimate of the osteotomy angle when different degrees of external rotation and valgus correction are required. A mathematical model of the osteotomy rotations is shown in Fig. 29-49.

TECHNIQUE 29-14 *(Rab)*

Prepare and drape the patient in the usual manner and apply and inflate a tourniquet. Make a transverse incision at the

continued

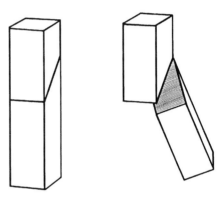

Fig. 29-47 Principle of oblique osteotomy. Rotation about face of cut produces both valgus and external rotation. (Redrawn from Rab GT: *J Pediatr Orthop* 8:715, 1988.)

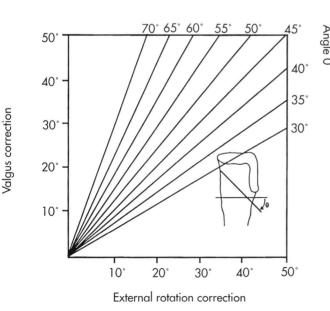

Osteotomy

Fig. 29-48 Nomogram for calculation of angle of oblique osteotomy. Desired valgus correction is found on vertical axis, and desired rotational correction is found on horizontal axis; intersection indicates osteotomy angle from horizontal as shown (inset). (Redrawn from Rab GT: *J Pediatr Orthop* 8:715, 1988.)

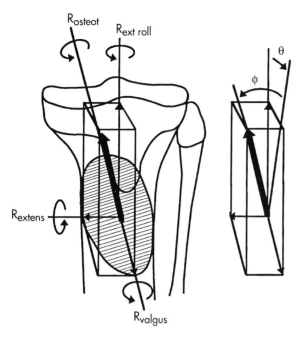

Fig. 29-49 Mathematic description of osteotomy rotations. Vectors represent rotation in frontal, transverse, and sagittal planes, and R_{osteot} is actual rotation about face of osteotomy cut. Vectors describing rotation are normal to (at right angles to) plane of osteotomy cut. (Redrawn from Rab GT: *J Pediatr Orthop* 8:715, 1988).

lower pole of the tibial tubercle (Fig. 29-50, *A*). Make a Y-shaped incision in the periosteum and dissect periosteally (including the pes anserinus insertion medially) until malleable or Blount retractors can be placed behind the tibia (Fig. 29-50, *B*). Elongate the periosteal incision distally, if necessary, to obtain subperiosteal protection posteriorly. Place a small Steinmann pin at a 45-degree angle 1 cm distal to the tibial tubercle and advance it under image intensifier control until it passes just into the posterior cortex (Fig. 29-50, *C*). Make sure the pin is distal to the physis at the posterior cortex on the image intensifier view. Measure the pin length and use a marking pen or steri-strip to mark the same length on the osteotomes and sagittal saw blades (Fig. 29-50, *D*). This serves as a reminder of the saw depth and can indicate if a lateral image intensifier exposure is appropriate. With the saw and osteotome, carefully make the osteotomy cut immediately distal to the Steinmann pin, checking frequently with image intensification (Fig. 29-50, *E*). As the cut nears completion, it may be helpful to make some of the cut from the anteromedial side of the tibia where subperiosteal exposure is better. Make a second small incision over the midfibula and excise a 1 to 2 cm subperiosteal segment of the fibula. Move the tibial osteotomy back and forth to free some of the posterior periosteum from the fragments. Drill a hole in the anteroposterior direction across the osteotomy cut lateral to the tibial tubercle. Rotate the osteotomy on its face by external rotation and valgus rotation (in Blount disease),

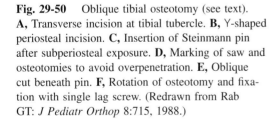

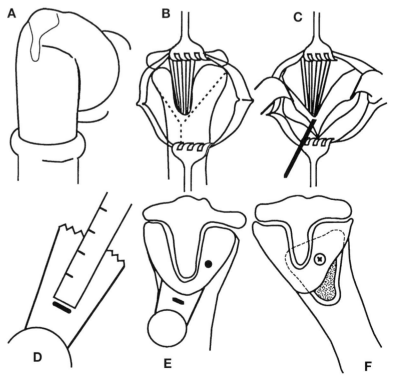

Fig. 29-50 Oblique tibial osteotomy (see text). **A,** Transverse incision at tibial tubercle. **B,** Y-shaped periosteal incision. **C,** Insertion of Steinmann pin after subperiosteal exposure. **D,** Marking of saw and osteotomies to avoid overpenetration. **E,** Oblique cut beneath pin. **F,** Rotation of osteotomy and fixation with single lag screw. (Redrawn from Rab GT: *J Pediatr Orthop* 8:715, 1988.)

overcorrecting if necessary. Through the drill hole secure the osteotomy with a single 3.5 mm cortical or cancellous lag screw overdrilled anteriorly (Fig. 29-50, *F*). Do not overtighten this screw. Perform a subcutaneous fasciotomy between the two incisions and release the tourniquet. Check for return of pulses, especially in the dorsalis pedis artery. Obtain hemostasis and close the wound over suction drains with fine absorbable subcutaneous and subcuticular sutures. Check both extremities for correct clinical alignment, which is very important at this stage. The single screw is loose enough to allow adjustment of the osteotomy position by cast wedging if necessary. Apply a long leg, bent-knee cast.

AFTERTREATMENT. The cast is changed at 4 weeks, and weight-bearing is allowed as tolerated if callus is visible on roentgenogram. The cast is worn for 8 weeks or until union is evident roentgenographically.

◆ CHEVRON OSTEOTOMY

Greene prefers an opening-closing chevron osteotomy that is a modification of the dome osteotomy and has the advantage of providing greater stability and minimal changes in leg length. Theoretical disadvantages are a slightly longer period of cast immobilization, which may be necessary to incorporate the wedge segment, and loss of correction caused by loss of fixation.

TECHNIQUE 29-15 *(Greene)*

Before surgery, make a paper template that outlines the desired lateral wedge. Place the patient supine on the operating table with a sandbag under the ipsilateral hip to improve exposure of the fibula. Prepare the leg from the toes to the proximal thigh. Preparing the foot allows more accurate evaluation of the tibial torsion and allows evaluation of the dorsalis pedis and posterior tibial pulses when the tourniquet is deflated. Begin the procedure with the fibular osteotomy. Expose the middle third of the fibula through the interval between the lateral and posterior compartments. Sharply incise the periosteum of the fibula and carefully elevate the periosteum circumferentially to prevent injury to the adjacent peroneal vessels. Remove a 1 cm segment of the fibula with a reciprocating saw. Cut the fibula obliquely, from superolateral to inferomedial direction. This allows the distal portion of the fibula to slide past the proximal fragment as the leg is brought from a varus to a valgus position.

For the tibial osteotomy, make a hockey-stick incision 4 to 5 cm distal to the tibial tubercle staying medial and lateral to the anterior spine of the tibia. Extend the incision to the tibial tubercle and curve it laterally toward the Gerdy tubercle. Sharply incise the periosteum immediately adjacent to the anterior compartment muscles. Incise the

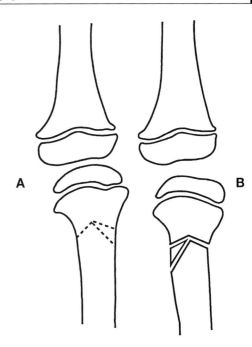

Fig. 29-51 Opening-closing chevron osteotomy. **A,** Osteotomy cuts. **B,** Lateral wedge is inserted medially. (From Greene WB: *J Bone Joint Surg* 75A:130, 1993.)

periosteum transversely just distal to the tibial tubercle and elevate it circumferentially so that curved retractors can be placed to protect the posterior soft tissues. Because of its triangular shape more care is required at the posterolateral and posteromedial edges of the tibia to ensure that dissection remains subperiosteal. Outline the osseous cuts on the anterior surface of the tibia with an osteotome or cautery (Fig. 29-51). The apex of the osteotomy should be just distal to the tibial tubercle. Drill a hole from anterior to posterior at this point to minimize the risk of extending the osteotomy beyond the desired location. Complete the osteotomy with an oscillating saw and remove the lateral wedge. Swing the distal tibia into the desired position of valgus and external rotation. Insert the lateral wedge medially in a position that will maintain the correction. Depending on the age of the child, the degree of obesity, and the stability of the osteotomy, a single pin or two crossed pins may be used for fixation if necessary. Use either smooth or threaded pins and predrill the diaphysis to make pin insertion easier and more accurate. Any pin used for fixation should cross the osteotomy and exit through the proximal cortex without crossing the physis. Release the tourniquet and check the circulation in the foot. If circulation is satisfactory and correction is adequate on roentgenograms, bury the ends of the pins beneath the skin to prevent pin track infection and skin ulceration. Perform subcutaneous fasciotomy in the anterolateral compartment. Close the fibular and tibial incisions, leaving the fascia open, and close the skin with

continued

subcuticular sutures. Apply a long leg, bent-knee cast with the knee flexed 45 degrees and the ankle in the neutral position.

AFTERTREATMENT. No weight-bearing is allowed for the first 4 weeks after surgery. The cast is changed at 4 weeks, and if healing is satisfactory on roentgenograms, the pins are removed and weight-bearing begun. Usually 8 to 10 weeks of immobilization are necessary, depending on the age of the child. The osteotomy must be protected long enough to minimize the risk of fracture that accompanies a quick resumption of vigorous play activity.

◆ EPIPHYSEAL AND METAPHYSEAL OSTEOTOMY

TECHNIQUE 29-16 *(Ingram, Canale, Beaty)*

Determine preoperatively the amount of wedge to be removed from the epiphyseal and metaphyseal areas (see Fig. 29-44) and whether a graft will be taken from the fibula or tibia. Prepare and drape the patient in the usual manner and apply and inflate a tourniquet. Expose the proximal tibia through a longitudinal incision approximately 10 cm long at the lateral border of the bone in the area of the physis. Carry the dissection through the soft tissue to expose the physis (Fig. 29-52). Continue subperiosteal exposure distally and place reverse retractors in the metaphyseal area of the bone into the area of the tibial collateral ligament attachment on the tibia. Make a short incision in the proximal third of the lateral compartment and carry soft tissue dissection down to the fibula, taking care to avoid the peroneal nerve. Remove a segment of the fibula approximately 1.5 cm long. If a graft is to be used beneath the tibial plateau, a longer segment of fibula may be required. Fasciotomy can be done through this incision or through the tibial incision. With an osteotome and mallet, make an osteotomy through the physis, resecting any bony bar (Fig. 29-52, *B*). Complete the osteotomy from the periphery to the center of the knee anteriorly to posteriorly, taking care to avoid vessels and nerves posteriorly. Place an elevator in the osteotomy site and gently pry open and elevate the medial tibial plateau until it is as nearly parallel as possible to the lateral tibial plateau (Fig. 29-52, *C*). If there is any offset of the osteotomy in the middle of the joint, arthrotomy can be done to inspect the joint; the abundant soft tissue and cartilage in the area of the tibial eminence act as a hinge, preventing any offset. Now cut the appropriate closing lateral wedge in the metaphysis and insert two parallel Steinmann pins. Place the wedge of bone (or bone graft from the fibula) beneath the elevated tibial plateau (Fig. 29-52, *D*); apply compression if desired (Fig. 29-52, *E*). Insert crossed Steinmann pins through the epiphysis and proximal tibial graft. Close the wound and

apply a long leg, bent-knee cast incorporating the pins in the plaster (Fig. 29-52, *F*) or in an external fixator apparatus.

AFTERTREATMENT. The pins in the osteotomy site are removed at 6 weeks, and those in the medial plateau are removed at 12 weeks. Cast immobilization is discontinued at 12 weeks, and range-of-motion exercises are begun.

◆ INTRAEPIPHYSEAL OSTEOTOMY

TECHNIQUE 29-17 *(Siffert; Støren)*

With the knee in extension, begin a medial longitudinal incision at the medial femoral epicondyle, extend it distally and anteriorly, and end it 2 cm medial and distal to the tibial tuberosity. (Siffert prefers a transverse incision along the medial joint line, curved distally to the tibial tuberosity.) Be careful to preserve the infrapatellar branch of the saphenous nerve at the inferior aspect of the wound. Open the knee joint through a capsular incision anterior to the tibial collateral ligament. The medial meniscus may be found hypertrophied; we try to preserve it. The capsular incision will allow inspection of the articular surface of the tibia as the osteotomy is made. With a scalpel, make a circumferential incision through the epiphyseal cartilage down to the primary ossification center of the proximal tibial epiphysis, extending from the posteromedial corner of the tibia to the anteromedial corner; make the incision midway between the articular surface and the prominent vascular ring of vessels penetrating the epiphysis just proximal to the physis. Then, using a ¾ inch (18 mm), gently curved osteotome, make an osteotomy through the medial aspect of the primary ossification center of the epiphysis. Because of the abnormal slope of the medial tibial plateau, the osteotomy parallels the articular surface medially and should reach the subchondral bone in the intercondylar area adjacent to the anterior cruciate ligament (Fig. 29-53). Gently elevate this segment, bringing the medial tibial plateau congruent with the medial femoral condyle and level with the lateral tibial plateau. Siffert states this should correct the genu recurvatum that is frequently present. Insert small cortical grafts from the medial proximal tibia (or bank bone) into the opened osteotomy. Since the articular depression is usually more posterior than anterior, grafts of different sizes and shapes are needed to maintain articular congruity and contact throughout a normal range of motion. It is important that the grafts be placed only in the opened wedge of the epiphyseal bone and not in the cartilage medially.

A medially based opening wedge osteotomy of the proximal tibia also may be required to correct varus of the tibia. Of course, a proximal fibular osteotomy is needed, and through the lateral incision required for the fibular osteotomy, we recommend a subcutaneous fasciotomy,

continued

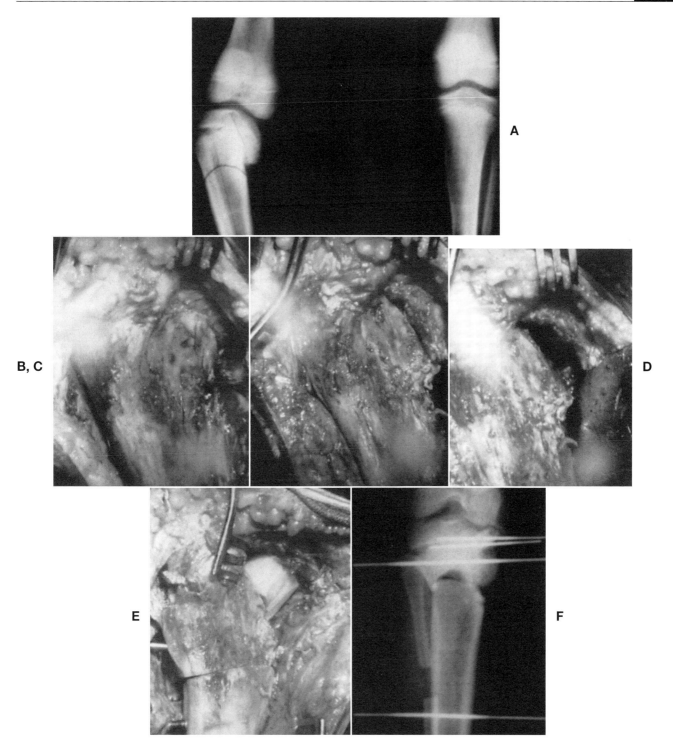

Fig. 29-52 Epiphyseal and metaphyseal osteotomy for tibia vara. **A,** Severe Blount disease with physis slipped 90 degrees. **B,** Exposure of physis. **C,** Osteotomy. **D,** Elevation of medial tibial plateau. **E,** Placement of bone graft under compression. **F,** Cast incorporating pins in plaster.

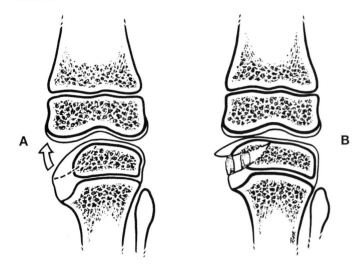

Fig. 29-53 Correction of intraarticular component of Blount disease by osteotomy of epiphysis. **A,** Incision made into epiphyseal cartilage at its midportion medially. Curved osteotomy directed laterally and proximally to subchondral intercondylar region paralleling articular surface. **B,** Osteotomized tibial condyle elevated on its intercondylar cartilage hinge to position of congruity with femur, and bone struts placed into gap to maintain contact in all planes of motion as well as to tighten medial ligament. (From Siffert RS: *J Ped Orthop* 2:81, 1982.)

taking care to protect the superficial peroneal nerve as it penetrates the deep investing fascia of the lower leg to become subcutaneous. We also insert a smooth Steinmann pin proximal and distal to the osteotomy of the proximal tibia, and with these incorporated in a long leg cast, the position of the osteotomy is maintained without a graft. A cortical graft can also be used in an opening wedge and is held with crossed Steinmann pins. The technique of osteotomy of the proximal tibia is described in the discussion of angular and torsional deformities (see Chapter 26).

A lateral epiphysiodesis can be done with any of the osteotomies by extending the subperiosteal dissection proximally to expose the physis. A curet or dental burr can be used to excise the cartilaginous physis. The technique for epiphysiodesis is described in Chapter 25.

NEUROVASCULAR COMPLICATIONS OF HIGH TIBIAL OSTEOTOMY

Neurovascular complications after an osteotomy for genu varum result most commonly from vascular occlusion or peroneal nerve palsy. Steel et al. have shown by arteriogram that at osteotomy, stretching of the anterior tibial artery occurs at the interosseous membrane with varus correction (as for genu valgum) and compression of the artery occurs with valgus correction (as for genu varum). Others have noted both a palsy

of the peroneal nerve and an anterior compartment syndrome. Regardless of the cause, early recognition is mandatory. Immediate diagnosis with return of the extremity to the preoperative position of deformity is beneficial regardless of the cause, especially since the causative factors may not be clearly evident in each patient. Sensory loss on the dorsum of the foot and loss of active dorsiflexion of the foot without pain usually are caused by paralysis of the common peroneal nerve. Decrease in dorsiflexion and severe pain on plantar flexion of the toes are the most common clinical signs of occlusion of the artery or of an anterior compartment syndrome (see Chapter 46).

Matsen and Staheli outlined appropriate treatment for each as follows:

1. For traction on the peroneal nerve (more common with varus correction), remove the cast and return the leg to the preoperative position. Then remove all pressure on the peroneal nerve and loosen all dressings from the thigh to the toes and observe closely.

2. For anterior compartment syndrome, remove the cast and return the leg to the preoperative position. Loosen all dressings from the thigh to the toes. If improvement does not occur immediately, then fasciotomy without delay is mandatory.

3. For anterior tibial artery occlusion remove the cast and return the leg to the preoperative position. Loosen all dressings from the thigh to the toes and observe closely. If immediate improvement is not evident, consider arteriography followed by appropriate surgery.

Congenital Affections

Most affections of bone seemingly of congenital origin may respond favorably to surgery. In Chapter 20 the surgical treatment of enchondromatosis (Ollier disease) and of hereditary multiple exostoses is described.

OSTEOGENESIS IMPERFECTA

Osteogenesis imperfecta is a disease apparently of the mesodermal tissues with abnormal or deficient collagen that has been demonstrated in bone, skin, sclerae, and dentine. The so-called diagnostic triad of blue sclerae, dentinogenesis imperfecta, and generalized osteoporosis in a patient with multiple fractures or bowing of the long bones usually is used clinically. There is no specific laboratory test for this disease. Multiple wormian bones around the base of the skull are a major finding only in the congenital type of osteogenesis imperfecta. Osteogenesis imperfecta congenita is characterized at birth by multiple fractures, bowing of the long bones, short extremities, and generalized osteoporosis. In addition, all of the patients with the congenital type in the series of Falvo et al. had dentinogenesis imperfecta and 92 had blue sclerae. In the classification suggested by Falvo et al., osteogenesis imperfecta tarda type 1 is differentiated from tarda type 2 by the presence of bowing of the long bones in type 1. The patients in the tarda type 2 classification without bowing apparently have a milder form of the disease. Fractures may be present at birth in both the tarda types of the disease even though very rarely in tarda type 2. *Only two characteristics are present in all patients with osteogenesis imperfecta: fractures and generalized osteoporosis.* In the series of 90 patients reported by Falvo et al., a few patients in each of the three diagnostic categories had white sclerae and 84 of the entire group had blue sclerae.

Daly et al. surveyed developmental milestones and walking ability in 59 children with osteogenesis imperfecta and related each to the Sillence and Shapiro classifications. They found that independent sitting by the age of 10 months was a predictor of walking as the main means of mobility, with 75% attaining this. Of the patients who did not achieve sitting by 10 months, walking became the main means of mobility in only 18%.

Orthopaedic surgery is most involved with the bowing of the long bones in osteogenesis imperfecta tarda type 1 in which progressively increasing deformities may cause deterioration in activity of these children from walkers to sitters and from braceable to unbraceable. Healing of fractures and osteotomies usually is quite satisfactory even though the healed bone may be no stronger than the original. Hyperplastic callus occasionally is seen after fractures and osteotomies. Because of frequently frail and disabling bone and joint deformities and fractures that preclude ambulation, Gerber et al. described a comprehensive rehabilitation program with long leg bracing that results in a high level of functional activity with an acceptable level of risk of fracture in children with osteogenesis imperfecta. Ring et al. used the Ilizarov method of lengthening to correct deformities of the lower extremity in six patients who had type I osteogenesis imperfecta. The average angular correction was 23 degrees. The seven limb segments gained an average of 6.6 cm. One of the six had a nonunion, and eighteen major complications occurred in six patients. Conversely, Papagelopoulos and Morrey reported favorable results with total hip (five) and total knee (three) arthroplasties for severe joint malalignment in patients with osteogenesis imperfecta. Patients should be examined for scoliosis before surgical procedures are undertaken. Widmann et al. noted that thoracic scoliosis of more than 60 degrees has severe adverse effects on pulmonary function in patients with osteogenesis imperfecta. This finding may partly explain the increased pulmonary morbidity in adult patients with osteogenesis imperfecta and scoliosis compared with that in the general population.

Multiple Osteotomies, Realignment, and Medullary Nail Fixation

The most successful surgical method of treating the deformities of osteogenesis imperfecta is based on the work of Sofield and Millar, who used a method of multiple osteotomies, realignment of fragments, and medullary nail fixation for long bones. This operation and its modifications are now widely used when surgical treatment of fresh fractures is indicated, as well as for correction of bowing and as prophylaxis to allow a child more activity without repeated fractures. Sofield and

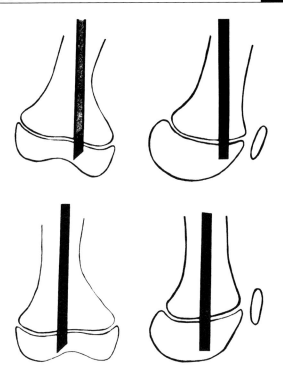

Fig. 29-54 Medullary rod positioning in osteotomies for osteogenesis imperfecta. *Above,* Incomplete reduction with poor position of rod. Rod is not centrally placed and is anterior in epiphysis. Physis is still tilted on both projections. *Below,* Complete reduction of end fragments and good central positioning of medullary rod. (From Tiley F, Albright JA: *J Bone Joint Surg* 55A:701, 1973.)

Millar reported no disturbances in growth when the smooth medullary nail penetrated the physis. Almost routinely the bone grows beyond the end of the nail, usually distally, since the bones of the lower extremities are the ones most commonly treated surgically. The bone extending beyond the end of the medullary nail tends to angulate, and the nail itself tends to cut out and allow deformity and a tendency to fracture at the end of the nail. Tiley and Albright recommended routine central placement of the rod across the physis to add length to the rod and postpone the problem of the rod becoming too short. The important points of treatment included adequate reduction of the ends of the long bones, proper placement of the rod in the metaphysis and epiphysis (Fig. 29-54), use of a hook on the femoral rods to prevent migration, use of a rod of adequate length, and incorporation of corrective forces in postoperative casts and braces.

Ryöppy et al. described 14 young children with severe osteogenesis imperfecta who were treated with closed or semiclosed intramedullary stabilization with nonexpandable rods and nails. In infants with a severe form of osteogenesis imperfecta, the operative technique was modified significantly from those presented earlier in the literature. Early intramedullary stabilization even soon after birth seemed justified in selected patients with severe osteogenesis imperfecta. Possibilities for motor development were improved, and later insertion of telescoping rods was easier. They performed the closed technique by osteoclasis and the semiclosed technique with limited open operation at the site of maximal angulation and subsequent limited osteotomy. They preferred this to open fragmentation because it is relatively easy, saves time, operative trauma is less, morbidity is lower, and several bones can be stabilized in one session. A possible solution to the rapid growing away from the nails appeared to be early stabilization with simple nonexpandable implants and, around the age of 4 years, insertion of telescoping nails. Ryöppy et al. believed that if an early, aggressive program of bone stabilization had been instituted in some of their older children who never learned to walk or who had lost their walking ability, these children would have gained years of active life.

Bailey and Dubow used a telescoping medullary rod with a small flange at its distal and proximal ends that are thus fixed within the bony epiphysis or cortex of the bone. With growth the rod elongates and allows the entire length of the long bone to remain reinforced for several years by the same internal support. Marafioti and Westin reported satisfactory experience with these rods, and of the several types of medullary rods that we have used in patients with this disease, these telescoping rods have produced the best results. Of the 153 multiple osteotomy and medullary nailing procedures reported by Marafioti and Westin, 47 used the telescoping rod and 105 used other standard types of medullary nails or pins. The incidence of reoperation was decreased 3½ times by the telescoping rod. Nicholas and James used intramedullary expandable rods for treatment of lower extremity deformities. All patients were in braces postoperatively. Nine patients who were previously nonambulatory were able to walk after surgery. Despite the high rate of complications, expandable nails corrected angular deformities, decreased the number of fractures, and allowed most previously nonambulatory children to walk.

Porat et al. evaluated operative intervention in 20 patients with osteogenesis imperfecta. Both nonelongating and elongating rods were used for fractures and angular deformities. Postoperatively, gait capacity improved in eight patients, regressed in three, and remained unchanged in nine. No preoperative ambulatory child regressed to a nonambulatory status. The complication rate was 72% for the Bailey-Dubow rod and 50% for the nonelongating rod, although the percentage of patients requiring reoperation was similar for both types of nails. There were no differences in the longevity of the two nails.

Gamble et al. described the complications of intramedullary rods in osteogenesis imperfecta and compared Bailey-Dubow rods with nonelongating rods. They concluded that intramedullary rods in patients with osteogenesis imperfecta are safe and have low operative morbidity. The complication rate was 69% for Bailey-Dubow rods and 55% for nonelongating rods. The most common complication for both groups was migration. The reoperation rate was higher for patients with nonelongating rods (29%) than for those with Bailey-Dubow rods (19%) (Fig. 29-55). The replacement rate was also higher for

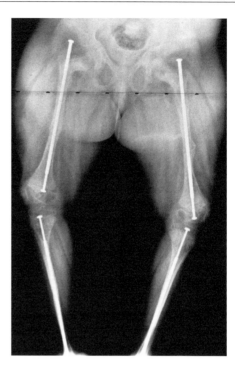

Fig. 29-55   Multiple osteotomies of femur and tibia and insertion of Bailey-Dubow elongating intramedullary rods in patient with osteogenesis imperfecta. (Courtesy Jay Cummings, MD.)

nonelongating rods. Thirty-four percent of the Bailey-Dubow complications involved the "T piece" and were potentially avoidable. They, as well as Janus et al., recommended the following: avoid loosening of the T junction of the obturator portion by either scoring the T piece before its insertion into the sleeve or stoutly crimping the sleeve after insertion of the T piece; place the T below the subchondral bone or below the periosteal-perichondral surface but not so deep that it migrates into the medullary canal; and after insertion, turn the T piece 90 degrees in the direction of insertion to help prevent backout. They concluded that, although the complications, reoperations, replacements, and number of migrations are not statistically different between the Bailey-Dubow group and the nonelongating group, the Bailey-Dubow group had fewer problems.

For the tibia, to allow use of the longest possible medullary rod, Williams reported a technique in which an extension is screwed onto the distal end of the rod and is pushed through the distal tibia and out the sole of the foot. After the fragments of the tibia are realigned, the nail is then reinserted in a retrograde fashion until the distal end lies just proximal to the surface of the ankle joint. The extension is then unscrewed, leaving the rod extending only into the distal tibial epiphysis.

Wilkinson et al. treated 74 bones in the lower limb in 28 children with the Sheffield Expanding IM rod system. This system was developed to avoid previous problems with other expanding systems. They found no evidence of epiphyseal damage after the procedure, and complication rates requiring rod exchange have been low (7%).

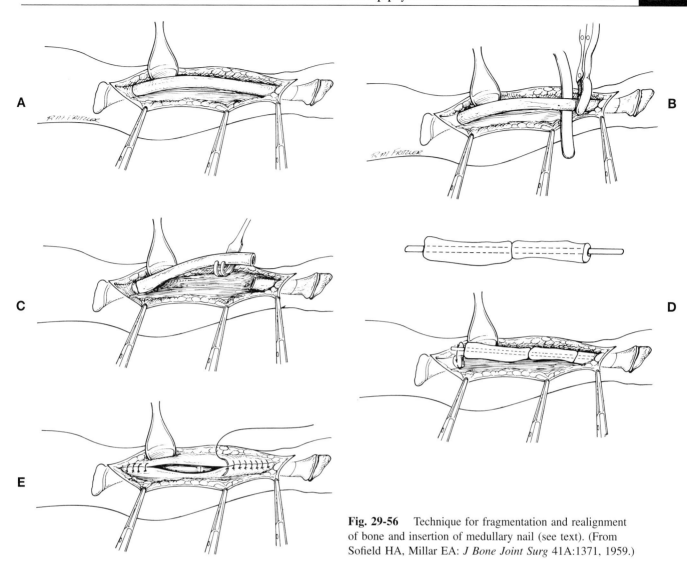

Fig. 29-56   Technique for fragmentation and realignment of bone and insertion of medullary nail (see text). (From Sofield HA, Millar EA: *J Bone Joint Surg* 41A:1371, 1959.)

◆ Osteotomy and Medullary Nailing

TECHNIQUE 29-18 *(Sofield and Millar)*

Expose the entire shaft of the bone subperiosteally, make an osteotomy through the proximal and the distal metaphyses, and carefully remove the shaft from the wound (Fig. 29-56). Study the shaft to determine how many times it must be osteotomized so that its segments can be threaded onto a straight medullary nail. Perform osteotomies, commonly three or four to correct the alignment, and skillfully shift and rotate the fragments end-to-end as necessary to align them on the straight nail. When the cortex of the bone is extremely thin, add homogeneous grafts. After the nail has been inserted, its distal end should lie in the medullary canal near the distal physis, and its proximal end should lie in the canal near the proximal physis, as in the tibia, or should project proximal to the proximal end of the bone, as in the femur, the ulna, or the humerus. (The techniques of

medullary nailing are described in Chapter 51.) This original Sofield technique is now modified routinely by us to extend the medullary nails into the bony epiphysis to the subchondral bone plate. Suture the periosteum over the bone and close the wound in a routine manner.

AFTERTREATMENT. The extremity is immobilized in a cast, and the immobilization is continued until the osteotomies have healed.

◆ Osteotomy and Medullary Nailing with Telescoping Rod

The internal fixation device used in this procedure consists of a hollow tube or sleeve with a solid rod that telescopes inside. For the femur it is used with one end anchored within the distal portion of the distal femoral epiphysis immediately adjacent to the knee joint and the proximal end in the superior portion of

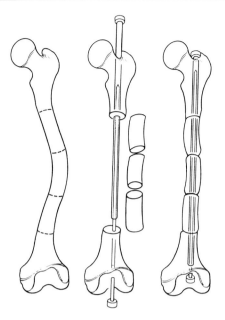

Fig. 29-57 Elongating medullary rods in treatment of osteogenesis imperfecta. *Left,* Multiple osteotomies are performed. *Center,* Proximal and distal joints are entered, and each half of rod is inserted. *Right,* Fragments are threaded onto rod that is telescoped together and T pieces on each end are gently rotated and sunk beneath articular surface. Both sleeve and rod (obturator) should be longer than illustrated, and each should be almost as long as bone. (From Marafioti RL, Westin GW: *J Bone Joint Surg* 59A:467, 1977.)

the neck at its junction with the greater trochanter. In the tibia each end is in a bony epiphysis adjacent to a joint.

TECHNIQUE 29-19 *(Bailey and Dubow)*
(Fig. 29-57)

Approach the femur subperiosteally as with the Sofield technique. Expose the intercondylar notch of the femur through a parapatellar incision, and for the tibia use a similar incision proximally and a transverse medial incision through the deltoid ligament distally to displace the talus and enter the ankle joint. The approach to the proximal part of the femur may require only a small incision placed directly over the end of the tubular sleeve as it is drilled proximally through the medullary canal and out the superior aspect of the neck just medial to the base of the greater trochanter. After osteotomies have been made in the metaphyses of the involved bone, make the multiple osteotomies as with the Sofield technique so that the segments can be lined up with insertion of the rod. The rod when collapsed should reach from the proximal to the distal end of the entire bone less 2 cm to allow a margin for error and for impaction of the shaft segments after the surgery. Fit the tubular sleeve with the special detachable drill point and drill through the medullary canal of one metaphysis, through the bony epiphysis, and into the joint, and then repeat this at the opposite end of the

bone. After drilling the medullary canal of all the fragments with the same drill point attached to the tubular sleeve, replace the drill point with the T-shaped flange that screws on the end of the tubular sleeve. At the other end of the bone insert the obturator rod across the joint through the articular cartilage and into the canal that was drilled in the metaphysis. Thread the fragments of the shaft on the sleeve portion of the rod and then place the other metaphysis in position with the obturator up inside the tubular sleeve. Manually kink with compression the T-shaped flange so that it will not loosen. Countersink the T-shaped end of the obturator through the articular cartilage and into the bony portion of the distal epiphysis. The sleeve end of the rod is then similarly impacted either into the joint cartilage of the proximal tibia or at the proximal end of the femur against the base of the trochanter. After roentgenograms are taken, close the periosteum around the fragments and close the remainder of the operative wounds.

AFTERTREATMENT. The patient is immobilized in a hip spica (femur) or long leg cast (tibia) cast until the osteotomies have healed.

Osteotomy and Medullary Nailing with Russell-Taylor Nail.
In an older child in whom disturbance of the physis will not cause a significant growth problem, a small-diameter medullary nail can be used, with or without proximal or distal locking. The Russell-Taylor Delta nail is available in an 8 mm diameter, and we have used this successfully in several older children with osteogenesis imperfecta. The guide wire is passed, in a closed manner, proximally to the point of angulation (Fig. 29-58, *A*). Through a small incision, an osteotomy is made at this site where the guide wire is impeded (Fig. 29-58, *B*). Then the medullary nail is inserted in a closed manner and locked both proximally and distally. The nail should extend as far distally as possible to prevent fracture distal to it. The technique for insertion of an interlocking medullary rod is described in Chapter 51.

DWARFISM (SHORT STATURE)

Dwarfism with disproportionate shortness of either the trunk or extremities has many different causes and is commonly difficult to classify. Goldberg noted, however, that certain orthopaedic problems are common to many of these patients. In an extensive review Kopits reported that the main areas of concern to orthopaedic surgeons are atlantoaxial instability, hip dysplasia, and malalignment of the lower extremities.

Cervical myelopathy and anomalies of the cervical spine are especially common in dwarfs with a disproportionately short trunk and are rare in achondroplasia. Dwarfs with a short trunk may exhibit a rudimentary or absent odontoid process with ligamentous laxity and resultant atlantoaxial instability.

Kopits described the first symptoms of myelopathy as a

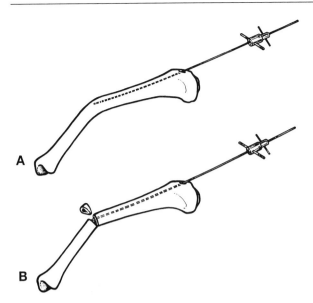

Fig. 29-58 Osteotomy and medullary nailing with Russell-Taylor nail (see text). **A,** Guide wire passed to point of angulation. **B,** Osteotomy. (Redrawn from Russell TA, Taylor JC, LaVelle DG: Russell-Taylor interlocking intramedullary nails, technique manual, 1985, Memphis, Richards Manufacturing.)

decrease in physical endurance and an early fatigue without neurological deficit. Neurological signs may develop later. Cord compression occurs because of bony displacement, ligamentous instability, and hypertrophy of the posterior longitudinal ligament. Often the spinal cord shifts laterally within the canal and accounts for the unilateral neurological signs and symptoms. Cord compression can also occur at the foramen magnum (achondroplastic dwarfs) or secondary to severe cervical kyphosis from ligamentous laxity. The diagnosis of atlantoaxial instability can be made from lateral flexion and extension roentgenographic views or with cineradiography. Kopits recommended cervical fusion only when (1) there are obvious clinical signs of compression myelopathy or (2) there is obliteration of the subarachnoid space around the cord in either flexion or extension as seen on gas myelography. Atlantoaxial instability demonstrated on roentgenograms or cineradiography is not in itself an indication for surgery, and prophylactic bracing is not indicated.

Kyphosis or scoliosis occurs commonly in short-trunk dwarfs, but with the exception of diastrophic dwarfs the scoliosis usually is mild and does not require surgery. Severe scoliosis is common in diastrophic dwarfs, and surgical correction and fusion seem to be the only reasonably effective treatment. With profound hypotonia, ligamentous laxity, and a collapsing spine, fusion may be necessary for stability while sitting.

Ligamentous laxity can cause kyphosis in achondroplasia. Severe progressive kyphoscoliosis with a posteriorly displaced vertebral body occasionally occurs in achondroplasia and in a variety of dwarfs. For neurological deficit, anterior decompres-

sion and fusion are best and are followed by posterior fusion when the deformity is greater than 60 degrees.

In the *lumbar spine,* profound lordosis, bulging intervertebral discs, and a narrowed spinal canal are characteristic of achondroplasia. Therefore by the third decade of life many of these patients complain of low back pain, have nerve root signs, and occasionally have a cauda equina syndrome and claudication. Laminectomy, cord and nerve root decompression, disc excision, and spinal fusion may ultimately be needed to relieve symptoms in some of these patients.

The *hip joint* in many dwarfing syndromes is spared as compared with the remainder of the lower extremity. Multiple epiphyseal dysplasia and spondyloepiphyseal dysplasia involve the epiphysis and may cause severe, early crippling arthritis. Hip fusion usually is not indicated in dwarfs for three reasons: (1) with extremely short stature, mobility is critical for activities of daily living such as dressing and stepping up stairs; (2) hip fusion may increase low back pain that already may be present from lumbar lordosis; and (3) hip fusion would further shorten a patient of already short stature. We have performed total hip arthroplasty in dwarfs with severe arthritis. Careful planning is necessary because nonstandard size femoral and acetabular components almost always are necessary. Bilateral dislocation of the hips is commonly seen in Morquio syndrome and usually is not vigorously treated (Fig. 29-59).

Two other conditions, *coxa vara* and *coxa valga,* occur in a substantial percentage of dwarfs. Coxa valga is commonly seen with Morquio syndrome and coxa vara with spondyloepiphyseal dysplasia (Fig. 29-60). Goldberg pointed out that varus and valgus osteotomies of the hips of patients with bone dysplasias should be done only rarely and after much study because of probable instability. Intertrochanteric osteotomies for severe coxa valga should be reserved for proven hip instability resulting from the valgus deformity, and for severe coxa vara they should be reserved for a waddling gait and cartilaginous defects. Varus and valgus osteotomies of the hip are described in Chapters 27 and 31.

A substantial percentage of dwarfs have either *genu varum* or *genu valgum.* In general, dwarfs with disproportionately short trunks have genu valgum, whereas those with disproportionately short extremities have genu varum. Angulation may be the result of ligamentous laxity, bowing of the proximal tibia and distal femur, or, as is characteristic of achondroplastic dwarfs, bowing of the distal tibia.

The deformity usually is progressive with an ultimate length discrepancy between the fibula and the tibia. Foot placement is in a forced varus or valgus position depending on the direction of angulation at the knees. Osteotomy at or near the site of the deformity is our preferred treatment. Bailey noted that in operating on recurrent genu valgum the surgeon should be prepared to release the lateral structures such as the iliotibial band and tighten the medial structures by reefing the vastus medialis. We have tried to control the deformity in young children with ambulatory "knock-knee" or "bowleg" braces. These braces are heavy and cumbersome and may actually promote ligamentous laxity, but in several patients we have

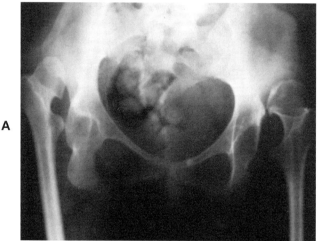

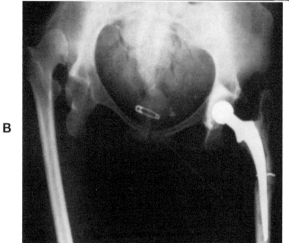

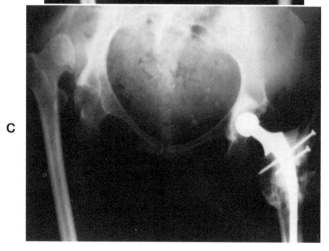

Fig. 29-59 **A,** Adult patient with Morquio disease with bilateral dislocated hips. Hip on right was painful and disabling. **B,** After total hip arthroplasty using custom-designed femoral component with small stem. Despite this, femoral shaft proximally was fractured during insertion. **C,** After revision of total hip arthroplasty with second custom-designed long stem femoral component and anchoring screws in methylmethacrylate. Result was satisfactory.

been able to stop the progression or improve the deformity (Fig. 29-61), and at a later age have performed an osteotomy without recurrence of the angulation. Kopits did not find braces to be satisfactory treatment.

Because of the disproportionate length of the extremities, especially the lower, limb lengthening has been attempted by several methods. Formerly, the most often used method in the United States has been that popularized by Wagner, which combines osteotomy with slow distraction (see Chapter 25). More recently, the Ilizarov and DeBastiani techniques have been reported to achieve greater lengthening with fewer complications. The frequency of complications and the lengthy immobilization period associated with limb lengthening by any method, however, have caused some authors to discourage its use, especially in dwarfs. Aldegheri reported 160 tibial lengthenings done for short stature using an Orthofix (Orthofix S.R.L.; Bussolengo, Verona, Italy) external fixator. The average gain in length was 7.8 cm ± 2.28 cm or 33%. Forty-six patients (29%) had complications. They pointed out that it is necessary to be aware of potential complications as well as the need for additional procedures to avoid predictable problems. These procedures include percutaneous tenotomy of the tendo calcaneus and fixation of the distal segment of the fibula to the tibia to maintain the integrity of the tibiofibular articulation and the alignment of the foot. Price noted that in many patients the amount of lengthening possible is not enough to achieve even the lowest percentile of normal height or to significantly decrease the difficulties in daily living. Others believe that any gain in height is beneficial both physically and psychologically. Limb lengthening should be attempted only in informed, cooperative patients committed to the lengthy procedure and with realistic expectations of the result.

Traumatic Physeal Arrest from Bridge of Bone

Physeal arrest after fracture in young children can produce significant limb shortening and angulatory deformity. Angulation osteotomies, epiphysiodesis of the involved epiphysis, and epiphysiodesis of the contralateral epiphysis are worthwhile and time-honored procedures to reduce angular deformity and limb length discrepancy.

Both Bright and Langenskiöld described resection of small, localized bony bridges (following fracture across a physis) that produced angular deformity or limb length discrepancy. They recommended this procedure for a young child with a significant deformity caused by a bony bridge across less than one half of the physis of a bone that is peripheral and accessible. Tomograms, CT scan, and MRI are helpful in determining the extent of the bony bridge.

After resection Langenskiöld filled the space with fat, and Bright with Silastic 382. Whereas the physis apparently does not regenerate in the area where the bony bridge was resected, the remaining normal physeal cartilage cells surrounding this

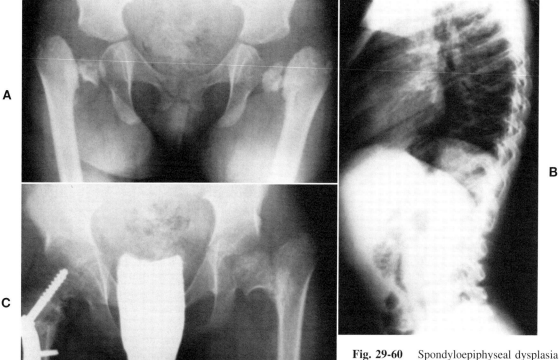

Fig. 29-60 Spondyloepiphyseal dysplasia. **A,** Severe bilateral coxa vara deformity. **B,** Platyspondyly in same patient. **C,** After valgus osteotomy of hip on left using Coventry lag screw. Cartilaginous defect is now more horizontal and under compression rather than shear.

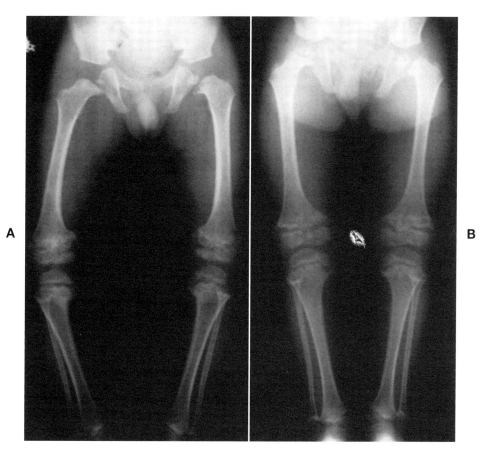

Fig. 29-61 Multiple epiphyseal dysplasia. **A,** Boy 4 years of age with weight-bearing roentgenogram showing delayed ossification of capital femoral epiphyses, coxa vara, and femoral and tibial bowing. **B,** One year after treatment in ambulatory bowleg braces. Femoral and tibial bowing is markedly improved.

area can produce bone in a more linear and orderly fashion than before. In a rabbit model, Lee et al. compared the results of interposition with physeal grafts, free fat, and Silastic after epiphysiodesis for correction of partial growth arrest. Clinical, roentgenographic, and histological studies showed physeal grafts (from the iliac crest) to be superior to Silastic in correcting angular deformity and contributing to the longitudinal growth of the tibia after resection of a large, peripherally situated bony bridge. Interposition of fat produced the worst results. We have resected a bony bridge in conjunction with an angulation osteotomy and used fat or silicone to fill the resected area.

Depending on the location of the physis and the amount of the deformity, we agree with MacEwen (personal communication) that bony bridge resection will not usually correct a significant angular deformity but that the resection may decrease the number of osteotomies necessary during the growth of a young child by decreasing the rate of recurrence of the angular deformity.

Ingram at this clinic described a technique for osteotomy at the level of the bony bridge adjacent and parallel to the physis. With this technique the bridge does not necessarily have to be peripheral. When the osteotomy is opened, the white, sclerotic bridge of bone can easily be differentiated from the normal cancellous metaphyseal bone with or without a magnifying optical loupe or microscope. The bridge is then resected with a dental burr, leaving only the normal physis and cancellous bone of the epiphysis and the metaphysis. A free graft of fat or a piece of silicone is then placed in the defect and the osteotomy is secured after insertion of a wedge of bone to correct deformity.

◆ BONY BRIDGE RESECTION

TECHNIQUE 29-20 (Langenskiöld)

Before the operation, exact localization and estimation of the size of the bony bridge by MRI, CT scans, and tomography in at least two planes are essential (Fig. 29-62, *A* and *B*). More than half of the physis should be normal, and the bony bridge should be peripheral, causing a progressive angular deformity or progressive discrepancy of leg length or both.

Expose the periphery of the physis by a suitable approach near the bony bridge. Use a tourniquet for a bloodless field for localization of the cartilaginous plate, which may be thin when close to the bridge. Use of a microscope or binocular loupe makes the procedure easier. Define the most peripheral part of the bony bridge and remove the overlying periosteum. Remove the bony bridge until the normal periphery of the physis is reached on both sides of the bridge and until the cartilaginous plate can be seen around the whole cavity. It is essential that no part of the bridge be left and that normal physeal cartilage not be removed unnecessarily. Release the tourniquet, and while hemostasis is

occurring secure a piece of fat from the subcutaneous tissue, preferably from the gluteal fold, to fill the cavity. Following cessation of bleeding, fill the cavity with the autogenous fat. When the resected cavity is irregular, divide the fat transplant into several pieces to ensure complete filling. To keep the autogenous fat in place, suture ligament, muscle, or subcutaneous tissue over the defect. Close the wound in layers without drainage.

◆ BONY BRIDGE RESECTION AND ANGULATION OSTEOTOMY

TECHNIQUE 29-21 (Ingram)

Accompanying a bony bridge there is usually not only angular deformity but also shortening, and an opening wedge osteotomy usually is indicated to gain length. Perform the osteotomy on the same side of the bone as the bony bridge causing the angular deformity (Fig. 29-62, *A* and *B*). Expose the metaphyseal area of the bone without damaging the periphery of the physis on the side of the bone where the bridge is located. After subperiosteal exposure place a guide pin in the metaphysis parallel to the physis and just adjacent to it, using either roentgenographic control or image intensifier fluoroscopy. The guide pin should penetrate or lie just adjacent to the bony bridge (Fig. 29-62, *C*). Perform an osteotomy at the level of the guide pin and open the osteotomy site wide with a laminar spreader. Using a small dental burr resect completely the white sclerotic bony bridge, using an operating microscope or a magnifying loupe for improved vision (Fig. 29-62, *D*). Carry the resection through the physis, making sure that all of the bony bridge is resected and that normal physeal cartilage appears on all sides of the cavity. This can be facilitated with the use of a dental mirror. After adequate resection obtain hemostasis and fill the area with autogenous fat obtained from the subcutaneous tissue at the incision or with a silicone implant. By inserting a wedge of autogenous bone into the osteotomy correct the angular deformity appropriately and secure the osteotomy with smooth pins (Fig. 29-62, *E*). Close the wound in layers and apply a sterile dressing and a plaster splint.

AFTERTREATMENT. Weight-bearing and activities should be limited until the osteotomy has completely healed and the pins are removed.

◆ PERIPHERAL AND LINEAR PHYSEAL BAR RESECTION

Peripheral and linear bars are more easily approached and identified than are central bars. The normal perichondral ring at the perimeter of the healthy physis is replaced by periosteum

Fig. 29-62 Traumatic epiphyseal arrest from bridge of bone. **A** and **B,** Anteroposterior roentgenograms and tomogram of lesion resulting from trauma to medial aspect of distal tibial epiphysis. **C** to **E,** Steps in operative technique of Ingram for excision of bony bar and wedge osteotomy of distal tibia (see text). **F,** Roentgenogram showing correction of deformity and defect at bony bridge site. (**C** to **F** from Canale ST, Harper MC: *AAOS Instr Course Lect* 30:85, 1981.)

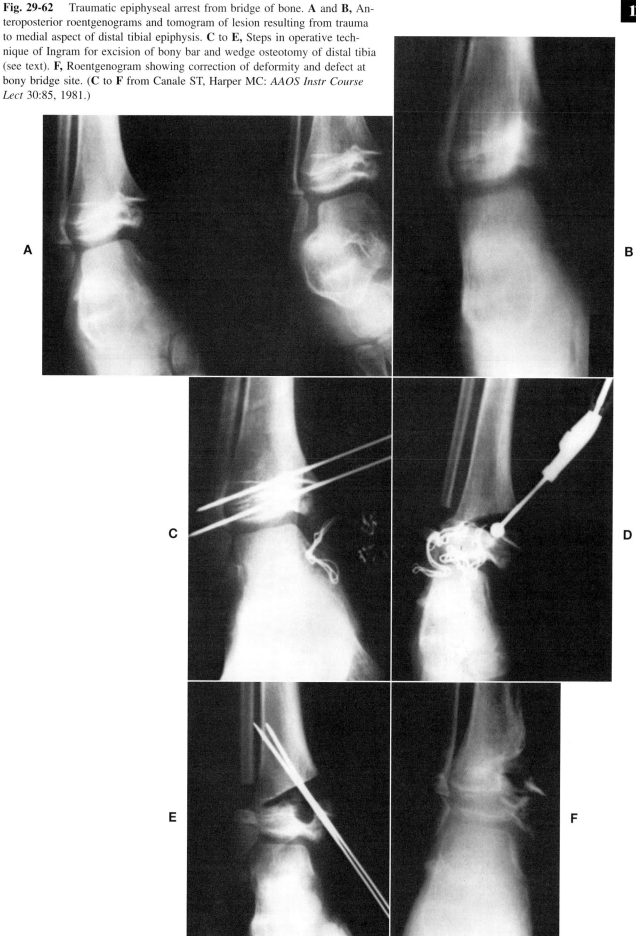

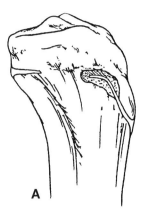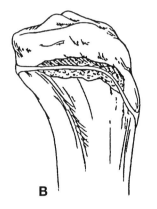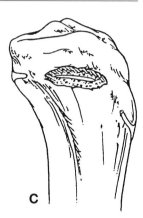

Fig. 29-63 Peripheral bar resection (see text). **A,** Fluoroscopy ensures that resection remains at level of physis. **B,** Resection continues until physis is visible throughout depth of cavity. **C,** Alternative method for exposure is periosteal stripping with fluoroscopic guidance. (Redrawn from Birch JG: *Op Tech Orthop* 3:166, 1993.)

over the bar and is easily stripped. According to Birch, Herring, and Wenger, peripheral bar resection involves scooping out the bar but leaving the residual healthy physis intact. This requires knowing where the bar meets the physis at the perimeter of the bone and the depth that the bar reaches into the physis.

TECHNIQUE 29-22 *(Birch et al.)*

Carefully expose the peripheral junction of the bar and the healthy perichondral ring at one, or preferably both, edges of the bar. This junction serves as an excellent starting point for removing the bar. Use fluoroscopy to ensure that the resection remains at the level of the physis and does not drift into the metaphysis or epiphysis (Fig. 29-63, *A*). Continue resection until the physis is visible from each edge of healthy perichondrium and throughout the depth of the cavity (Fig. 29-63, *B*). As an alternative, identify the bar with periosteal stripping and fluoroscopic guidance and develop a cavity directed toward the physis until it is identified (Fig. 29-63, *C*). Extend this cavity peripherally until healthy perichondrium is identified at either end of the bar. Fill the defect with autogenous fat from the area or from a small incision in the buttocks or groin.

◆ CENTRAL PHYSEAL BAR RESECTION

Central bars can be approached from the metaphyseal marrow cavity either through a metaphyseal cortical window or an osteotomy.

TECHNIQUE 29-23 *(Peterson)*

For bars extending completely across the physis, evaluate tomographic maps to determine surgical approach and ensure complete removal (Fig. 29-64). Approach centrally located bars (Fig. 29-65, *A*) through the metaphysis or epiphysis. Because the bar is not readily accessible through the transepiphyseal approach and because it usually requires traversing the joint, the transmetaphyseal approach is preferable, although it requires removal of a window of cortical bone and some cancellous metaphyseal bone to

Fig. 29-64 **A** to **C,** Elongated bar extending from anterior to posterior surfaces. Although all three have same appearance on anteroposterior view *(above)*, they have different contours on the transverse sections *(below)* (see text). (Redrawn from Peterson HA: *J Pediatr Orthop* 4:246, 1984.)

reach the bony bar (Fig. 29-65, *B*). After removal of the entire bar with a high-speed burr, inspect the normal physis with a small dental mirror (Fig. 29-65, *C*). The sides of the cavity should be flat and smooth (Fig. 29-66). Place metal markers, such as surgical clips, in the metaphysis and epiphysis to aid in accurate measurement of subsequent growth of the involved physis. Place these markers in cancellous bone, not in contact with the cavity, and in the same longitudinal plane proximally and distally to the defect. In a large cavity that is gravity dependent, pour liquid Cranioplast into the defect. If the cavity is not gravity dependent, place the Cranioplast in a syringe and push it into the defect through a short polyethylene tube (Fig. 29-67, *A*) or allow the Cranioplast to partially set and push it like putty into the defect. Allow as little Cranioplast as possible to remain in the metaphysis. After the

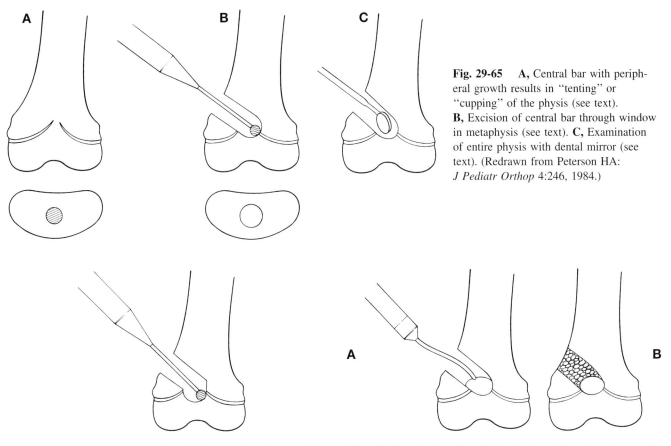

Fig. 29-65   **A,** Central bar with peripheral growth results in "tenting" or "cupping" of the physis (see text). **B,** Excision of central bar through window in metaphysis (see text). **C,** Examination of entire physis with dental mirror (see text). (Redrawn from Peterson HA: *J Pediatr Orthop* 4:246, 1984.)

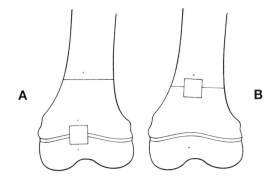

Fig. 29-66   Smoothing metaphyseal bone surface (see text). (Redrawn from Peterson HA: *J Pediatr Orthop* 4:246, 1984.)

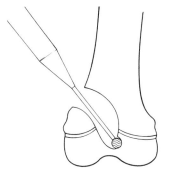

Fig. 29-67   **A,** Insertion of Cranioplast with syringe (see text). **B,** Bone graft filling remainder of defect (see text). (Redrawn from Peterson HA: *J Pediatr Orthop* 4:246, 1984.)

Fig. 29-68   **A,** Plug growing away from proximal marker and growth arrest line (see text). **B,** Plug remaining with metaphysis as epiphysis grows (see text). (Redrawn from Peterson HA: *J Pediatr Orthop* 4:2465, 1984.)

Fig. 29-69   Undermining of epiphysis (see text). (Redrawn from Peterson HA: *J Pediatr Orthop* 4:246, 1984.)

Cranioplast has set, fill the remainder of the metaphyseal cavity with cancellous bone (Fig. 29-67, *B*). The contour of the cavity also is important. Bar formation is less likely when the interposition material remains in the epiphysis (Fig. 29-68, *A*) than when the epiphysis grows away from it (Fig. 29-68, *B*). Methods of keeping the plug in the epiphysis include drilling holes in the cavity (undermining) (Fig. 29-69) and enlarging the cavity (Fig. 29-70).

AFTERTREATMENT. Joint motion is begun immediately. If osteotomy has not been done, no cast or other immobilization is necessary. Weight-bearing is encouraged on the day of

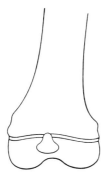

Fig. 29-70   "Collar button" contour of plug to act as anchor (see text). (Redrawn from Peterson HA: *J Pediatr Orthop* 4:246, 1984.)

surgery or as soon as comfort permits. Follow-up with scanograms continues until maturity.

References

OSTEOCHONDROSIS AND EPIPHYSITIS

Axer A: Personal communication, 1978.

Brighton CT: Clinical problems in epiphyseal plate growth and development. In American Academy of Orthopaedic Surgeons: *Instructional course lectures*, vol 23, St Louis, 1974, Mosby.

Cahill BR: Current concepts review. Osteochondritis dissecans, *J Bone Joint Surg* 79:471, 1997.

Chuinard EG, Logan ND: Varus-producing and derotational subtrochanteric osteotomy in the treatment of congenital dislocation of the hip, *J Bone Joint Surg* 45A:1397, 1963.

Duri ZA, Aichroth PM, Wilkins R, Jones J: Patellar tendonitis and anterior knee pain, *Am J Knee Surg* 12:99:1999.

Eaton GO: Long-term results of treatment in coxa plana: a follow-up study of eighty-eight patients, *J Bone Joint Surg* 49A:1031, 1967.

Ferciot C: Surgical management of anterior tibial epiphysis, *Clin Orthop* 5:204, 1955.

Ferguson AB, Gingrich RM: The normal and abnormal calcaneal apophysis and tarsal navicular, *Clin Orthop* 10:87, 1957.

Ferguson AB, Howorth MB: Coxa plana and related conditions at the hip, *J Bone Joint Surg* 16:781, 1934.

Hefti F, Buguiristain J, Krause R, et al: Osteochondritis dissecans: a multicenter study of the European Pediatric Orthopaedic Society, *J Pediatr Orthop B* 8:231, 1999.

Hoerr NL, Pyle SI, Francis CC: *Radiographic atlas of skeletal development of the foot and ankle*, Springfield, Ill, 1962, Charles C Thomas.

Iselin H: Wachstumsbeschwerden zur Zeit der Knochernen Entwicklung der Tuberosital metatarsi quint, *Deutsch Zeit Chir* 117:529, 1912.

Lehman RC, Gregg JR, Torg E: Iselin's disease, *Am J Sports Med* 14:494, 1986.

Lloyd-Roberts GC, Wetherill MH, Fraser M: Trochanteric advancement for premature arrest of the capital femoral epiphysis, *J Bone Joint Surg* 67B:20, 1985.

MacEwen GD, Ramsey PL: The hip. In Lovell WW, Winter RB, eds: *Pediatric orthopedics*, Philadelphia, 1978, JB Lippincott.

Miura H, Nagamine R, Urabe K, et al: Complications associated with Poly-L-lactic acid pins used for treating osteochondritis dissecans of the knee, *Arthroscopy* 15:1, 1999.

Nowinski RJ, Mehlman CT: Hyphenated history: Osgood-Schlatter disease, *Am J Orthop* 27:584, 1998.

Ogden JA: *Skeletal injury in the child*, Philadelphia, 1982, Lea & Febiger.

Peck DM: Apophyseal injuries in the young athlete, *Am Family Phys* 51:1891, 1995.

Richards BS, Coleman SS: Subluxation of the femoral head in coxa plana, *J Bone Joint Surg* 69A:1312, 1987.

Roberts JM: Fractures and dislocations of the knee. In Rockwood CA Jr, Wilkins KE, King RE, eds: *Fractures in children*, Philadelphia, 1984, JB Lippincott.

Yashar A, Loder RT, Hensinger, RN: Determination of skeletal age in children with Osgood-Schlatter disease by using radiographs of the knee, *J Pediatr Orthop* 15:298, 1995.

FREIBERG DISEASE, OSTEOCHONDROSIS OF ANKLE, KNEE, AND ELBOW, AND OSGOOD-SCHLATTER DISEASE

Anderson AF, Richards DB, Pagnani MJ, Hovis WD: Antegrade drilling for osteochondritis dissecans of the knee, *Arthroscopy* 13:319, 1997.

Aparicio G, Abril JC, Calvo E, Alvarez L: Radiologic study of patellar height in Osgood-Schlatter disease, *J Pediatr Orthop* 17:63, 1997.

Bauer M, Johnsson K, Josefsson PO, Lindén B: Osteochondritis dissecans of the elbow: a long-term follow-up study, *Clin Orthop* 284:156, 1992.

Bauer M, Johnsson K, Lindén B: Osteochondritis dissecans of the ankle: a 20-year follow-up study, *J Bone Joint Surg* 69B:93, 1987.

Baumgarten TE, Andrews JR, Satterwhite YE: The arthroscopic classification and treatment of osteochondritis dissecans of the capitellum, *Am J Sports Med* 26:520, 1998.

Berlet GC, Mascia A, Miniaci A: Treatment of unstable osteochondritis dissecans lesions of the knee using autogenous osteochondral grafts (mosaicplasty), *Arthroscopy* 15:312, 1999.

Binek R, Levinsohn EM, Bersani F, Rubenstein H: Freiberg disease complicating unrelated trauma, *Orthopedics* 11:753, 1988.

Bosworth DM: Autogenous bone pegging for epiphysitis of the tibial tubercle, *J Bone Joint Surg* 16:829, 1934.

Bradley J, Dandy DJ: Results of drilling osteochondritis dissecans before skeletal maturity, *J Bone Joint Surg* 71B:641, 1989.

Campbell WC: Infraction of the head of the second and third metatarsal bones: report of cases, *Am J Orthop Surg* 15:721, 1917.

Cohen B, Wilkinson RW: The Osgood-Schlatter lesion: a radiological and histological study, *Am J Surg* 95:731, 1958.

Cowell HR, Williams GA: Köhler's disease of the tarsal navicular, *Clin Orthop* 158:53, 1981.

De Inocencio J: Musculoskeletal pain in primary pediatric care: analysis of 1000 consecutive general pediatric clinic visits, *Pediatrics* 102:1, 1998.

Dervin GF, Keene GCR, Chissell HR: Biodegradable rods in adult osteochondritis dissecans of the knee, *Clin Orthop* 356:213, 1998.

DeSmet AA, Fisher DR, Graf BK, Lange RH: Osteochondritis dissecans of the knee: value of MR imaging in determining lesion stability and the presence of articular cartilage defects, *Am J Roentgenol* 155:549, 1990.

DeSmet AA, Ilahi OA, Graf BK: Reassessment of the MR criteria for stability of osteochondritis dissecans in the knee and ankle, *Skeletal Radiol* 25:159, 1996.

DeSmet AA, Ilahi OA, Graft BK: Untreated osteochondritis dissecans of the femoral condyles: prediction of patient outcome using radiographic and MR findings, *Skeletal Radiol* 26:463, 1997.

Ferciot CF: Surgical management of anterior tibial epiphysis, *Clin Orthop* 5:204, 1944.

Flowers MJ, Bhadreshwar DR: Tibial tuberosity excision for symptomatic Osgood-Schlatter disease, *J Pediatr Orthop* 15:292, 1995.

Freiberg AH: Infraction of the second metatarsal bone: a typical injury, *Surg Gynecol Obstet* 19:191, 1914.

Gauthier G, Elbaz R: Freiberg's infraction: a subchondral bone fatigue fracture: a new surgical treatment, *Clin Orthop* 142:93, 1979.

Green WT, Banks HH: Osteochondritis dissecans in children, *J Bone Joint Surg* 35A:26, 1953.

Helal B, Gibb P: Freiberg's disease: a suggested pattern of management, *Foot Ankle* 8:94, 1987.

Higashiyama I, Kumai T, Takakura Y, and Tamail S: Follow-up study of MRI for osteochondral lesion of the talus, *Foot Ankle* 21:127, 2000.

Higuera J, Laguna R, Peral M, et al: Osteochondritis dissecans of the talus during childhood and adolescence, *J Pediatr Orthop* 18:328, 1998.

Høgh J, Lund B: The sequelae of Osgood-Schlatter's disease in adults, *Int Orthop* 12:213, 1988.

Holmes SW Jr, Clancy WG Jr: Clinical classification of patellofemoral pain and dysfunction, *J Orthop Sports Phys Ther* 28:299, 1998.

Jakob RP, Miniaci A: A compression pinning system for osteochondritis dissecans of the knee, *Acta Orthop Scand* 60:319, 1989.

Janarv PM, Hesser U, Hirsch G: Osteochondral lesions in the radiocapitellar joint in the skeletally immature: radiographic, MRI, and arthroscopic findings in 13 consecutive cases, *J Pediatr Orthop* 17:311, 1997.

Judd DB, Kim DH, Hrutkay JM: Transient osteoporosis of the talus, *Foot Ankle Int* 21:134, 2000.

Kaeding CC, Whitehead R: Musculoskeletal injuries in adolescents, *Prim Care* 25:211, 1998.

Karp MG: Köhler's disease of the tarsal scaphoid: an end-result study, *J Bone Joint Surg* 19:84, 1937.

Klekamp J, Green NE, Mencio GA: Osteochondritis dissecans as a cause of development dislocation of the radial head, *Clin Orthop* 338:36, 1997.

Köhler A: Über eine häufige bisher anscheinend'-unbekannte Erkrankung einzelner kindlicher Knochen, *Münch Med Wochenschr* 45:1923, 1908.

Köhler A: Typical disease of the second metatarsophalangeal joint, *Am J Roentgenol* 10:705, 1923.

Krause BL, Williams JPR, Catterall A: Natural history of Osgood-Schlatter disease, *J Pediatr Orthop* 10:65, 1990.

Kumai T, Takakura Y, Higashiyama I, Tamai S: Arthroscopic drilling for the treatment of osteochondral lesions of the talus, *J Bone Joint Surg* 81A:1229, 1999.

Kuwahata Y, Inoue G: Osteochondritis dissecans of the elbow managed by Herbert screw fixation, *Orthopedics* 21:449, 1998.

Lynch MC, Walsh HPJ: Tibial recurvatum as a complication of Osgood-Schlatter's disease: report of two cases, *J Pediatr Orthop* 11:543, 1991.

Mandell GA, Harcke HT: Scintigraphic manifestations of infraction of the second metatarsal (Freiberg's disease), *J Nucl Med* 28:249, 1987.

Matsusue Y, Nakamur T, Suzuki S, Iwasaki R: Biodegradable pin fixation of osteochondral fragments of the knee, *Clin Orthop* 322:166, 1996.

McCarroll JR, Shelbourne KD, Patel DV: Anterior cruciate ligament reconstruction in athletes with an ossicle associated with Osgood-Schlatter's disease, *Arthroscopy* 12:556, 1996.

Mitsuoka T, Shino K, Hamada M, Horibe S: Osteochondritis dissecans of the lateral femoral condyle of the knee joint, *Arthroscopy* 15:20, 1999.

Miura H, Nagamine R, Urabe K, Matsuda S, et al: Complications associated with poly-L-lactic acid pins used for treating osteochondritis dissecans of the knee, *Arthroscopy* 15:1, 1999.

Newata K, Tewshima R, Morio Y, Hagino H: Anomalies of ossification in the posterolateral femoral condyle: assessment by MRI, *Pediatr Radiol* 29:781, 1999.

Ogden JA: *Skeletal injury in the child,* ed 2, Philadelphia, 1990, WB Saunders.

Ogilvie-Harris DJ, Sarrosa EA: Arthroscopic treatment after previous failed open surgery for osteochondritis dissecans of the talus, *Arthroscopy* 15:809, 1999.

Ogilvie-Harris DJ, Sarrosa EA: Arthroscopic treatment of osteochondritis dissecans of the talus, *Arthroscopy* 15:805, 1999.

Oka Y, Ohta K, Fukuda H: Bone-peg grafting for osteochondritis dissecans of the elbow, *Int Orthop* 23:53, 1999.

Paletta GA Jr, Bednarz PA, Stanitski CL, et al: The prognostic value of quantitative bone scan in knee osteochondritis dissecans: a preliminary experience, *Am J Sports Med* 26:7:1998.

Peterson RK, Savoie FH, Field LD: Osteochondritis dissecans of the elbow, *Instr Course Lect* 48:393, 1999.

Rapp IH, Lazerte G: Clinical pathological correlation in Osgood-Schlatter's disease, *South Med J* 51:909, 1958.

Roberts JM: Fractures and separations of the knee. In Rockwood CA Jr, Wilkins KE, King RE, eds: *Fractures in children,* ed 3, Philadelphia, 1991, JB Lippincott.

Robertsen K, Krsitensen O, Sommer J: Pseudoarthrosis between a patellar tendon ossicle and the tibial tuberosity in Osgood-Schlatter's disease, *Scand J Med Sci Sports* 6:57, 1996.

Ruch DS, Cory JW, Poehling GG: The arthroscopic management of osteochondritis dissecans of the adolescent elbow, *Arthroscopy* 14:797, 1998.

Safran MR, McDonough P, Seeger L, et al: Dorsal defect of the patella, *J Pediatr Orthop* 14:603, 1994.

Schenck RC, Goodnight JM: Current concepts review. Osteochondritis dissecans, *J Bone Joint Surg* 78A:439, 1996.

Slawski DP: High tibial osteotomy in the treatment of adult osteochondritis dissecans, *Clin Orthop* 341:155, 1997.

Smillie IS: Freiberg's infraction (Köhler's second disease), *J Bone Joint Surg* 39B:580, 1957.

Sueyoshi Y, Shimozaki E, Matsumoto T, and Tomita K: Two cases of dorsal defect of the patella with arthroscopically visible cartilage surface perforations, *Arthroscopy* 9:164, 1993.

Takahara M, Ogino T, Fukushima S, et al: Nonoperative treatment of osteochondritis dissecans of the humeral capitellum, *Am J Sports Med* 27:728, 1999.

Takahara M, Ogino T, Sasaki I, et al: Long-term outcome of osteochondritis dissecans of the humeral capitellum, *Clin Orthop* 363:108, 1999.

Taranow WS, Bisignani GA, Towers JD, Conti SF: Retrograde drilling of osteochondral lesions of the medial talar dome, *Foot Ankle Int* 20:474, 1999.

Thomee R, Augustsson J, Karlsson J: Patellofemoral pain syndrome: a review of current issues, *Sports Med* 28:245, 1999.

Thompson MS, Dickinson PH: Osgood-Schlatter's disease in the army, *Int Surg* 23:170, 1955.

Thomson JEM: Operative treatment of osteochondritis of the tibial tubercle, *J Bone Joint Surg* 38A:142, 1956.

Tol JL, Struijs PAA, Bossuyt PMM, et al: Treatment strategies in osteochondral defects of the talar dome: a systematic review, *Foot Ankle* 21:120, 2000.

Trial IA: Tibial sequestrectomy in the management of Osgood-Schlatter disease, *J Pediatr Orthop* 8:554, 1988.

Tullos JS, King JW: Lesions of the pitching arm in adolescents, *JAMA* 220:264, 1972.

Tuompo P, Arvela V, Partio EK, Rokkanen P: Osteochondritis dissecans of the knee fixed with biodegradable self-reinforced polyglycolide and polylactide rods in 24 patients, *Int Orthop* 21:355, 1997.

Victoroff BM, Marcus RE, Deutsch A: Arthroscopic bone peg fixation in the treatment of osteochondritis dissecans in the knee, *Arthroscopy* 12:506, 1996.

Waugh W: The ossification and vascularization of the tarsal navicular and their relation to Köhler's disease, *J Bone Joint Surg* 40B:765, 1958.

Wood JB, Klassen RA, Peterson HA: Osteochondritis dissecans of the femoral head in children and adolescents: a report of 17 cases, *J Pediatr Orthop* 15:313, 1995.

Woodward AH, Bianco AJ Jr: Osteochondritis dissecans of the elbow, *Clin Orthop* 110:35, 1975.

Yashar A, Loder RT, Hensinger RN: Determination of skeletal age in children with Osgood-Schlatter disease by using radiographs of the knee, *J Pediatr Orthop* 15:298, 1995.

Yoshida S, Ikata T, Takai H, et al: Osteochondritis dissecans of the femoral condyle in the growth stage, *Clin Orthop* 346:162, 1998.

Young MC, Fornasier VL, Cameron HU: Osteochondral disruption of the second metatarsal: a variant of Freiberg's infraction? *Foot Ankle Int* 8:103, 1987.

Zimbler S, Menkow S: Genu recurvatum: a possible complication after Osgood-Schlatter's disease, *J Bone Joint Surg* 66A:1129, 1984.

PERTHES DISEASE

Arruda VR, Belangero WD, Ozelo MC, et al: Inherited risk factors for thrombophilia among children with Legg-Calvé-Perthes disease, *J Pediatr Orthop* 19:84, 1999.

Axer A: Subtrochanteric osteotomy in the treatment of Perthes' disease, *J Bone Joint Surg* 47B:489, 1965.

Bellyei A, Mike G: Acetabular development in Legg-Calvé-Perthes disease, *Orthopedics* 11:407, 1988.

Bennett JT, Mazurek RG, Cash JD: Chiari's osteotomy in the treatment of Perthes' disease, *J Bone Joint Surg* 73B: 225, 1991.

Bowen JR, Kumar VP, Joyce JJ, Bowen JC: Osteochondritis dissecans following Perthes disease: arthroscopic-operative treatment, *Clin Orthop* 209:49, 1986.

Bowen JR, Schreiber FC, Foster BK, et al: Premature femoral neck physeal closure in Perthes' disease, *Clin Orthop* 171:24, 1982.

Cahuzac JPH, Onimus M, Trottmann F, et al: Chiari pelvic osteotomy in Perthes disease, *J Pediatr Orthop* 10:163, 1990.

Canale ST, d'Anca AF, Cotler JM, Snedden HE: Use of innominate osteotomy in Legg-Calvé-Perthes disease, *J Bone Joint Surg* 54A:25, 1972.

Canario AT, Williams L, Weintroub S, et al: A controlled study of the results of femoral osteotomy in severe Perthes disease, *J Bone Joint Surg* 62B:438, 1980.

Catterall A: The natural history of Perthes' disease, *J Bone Joint Surg* 53B:37, 1971.

Chiari K: Podiumdiskussion über die Beckenosteotomie, *Verh Dtsch Orthop Traum* 17:209, 1969.

Clancy M, Steel HH: The effect of an incomplete intertrochanteric osteotomy on Legg-Calvé-Perthes disease, *J Bone Joint Surg* 67A: 213, 1985.

Coates CJ, Paterson JMH, Woods KR, et al: Femoral osteotomy in Perthes' disease: results at maturity, *J Bone Joint Surg* 72B:581, 1990.

Coleman CR, Slager AF, Smith W: The effect of environmental influences on acetabular development, *Surg Forum* 9:775, 1958.

Cotler JM: Surgery in Legg-Calvé-Perthes syndrome. In American Academy of Orthopedic Surgeons: *Instructional course lectures*, vol 25, St Louis, 1976, Mosby.

Cotler JM, Wolfgang G: Femoral head containment following innominate osteotomy for coxa plana: a radiologic evaluation, *Orthop Rev* 5:27, 1976.

Craig WA, Pinder RC, Kramer WG: A review of one hundred hips operated on for Legg-Calvé-Perthes syndrome, *J Bone Joint Surg* 51A:814, 1969 (abstract).

Crutcher JP, Staheli LT: Combined osteotomy as a salvage procedure for severe Legg-Calvé-Perthes disease, *J Pediatr Orthop* 12:151, 1992.

Danigelis JA, Fisher RL, Ozonoff MB, Sziklas JJ: ^{99m}Tc-polyphosphate bone imaging in Legg-Perthes disease, *Radiology* 115:407, 1975.

Dorrell JH, Catterall A: The torn acetabular labrum, *J Bone Joint Surg* 68B:400, 1986.

Doudoulakis JK: Trochanteric advancement for premature arrest of the femoral-head growth plate: 6-year review of 30 hips, *Acta Orthop Scand* 62:92, 1991.

Eggl H, Drekonja T, Kaiser B, Dorn U: Ultrasonography in the diagnosis of transient synovitis of the hip and Legg-Calvé-Perthes disease, *J Pediatr Orthop B* 8:177, 1999.

Elsig JP, Exner GU, von Schulthess GK, Weitzel M: Case report: false-negative magnetic resonance imaging in early stage of Legg-Calvé-Perthes disease, *J Pediatr Orthop* 9:231, 1989.

Erken EHW, Katz K: Irritable hip and Perthes' disease, *J Pediatr Orthop* 10:322, 1990.

Evans IK, Deluca PA, Gage JR: A comparative study of ambulation-abduction bracing and varus derotation osteotomy in the treatment of severe Legg-Calvé-Perthes disease in children over 6 years of age, *J Pediatr Orthop* 8:676, 1988.

Farsetti P, Tudisco C, Caterini R, et al: The Herring lateral pillar classification for prognosis in Perthes disease: late results in 49 patients treated conservatively, *J Bone Joint Surg* 77B:739, 1995.

Fisher RL, Roderique JW, Brown DC, et al: The relationship of isotopic bone imaging findings to prognosis in Legg-Perthes disease, *Clin Orthop* 150:23, 1980.

Flashman FL, Ghormley RK: Osteochondritis dissecans of the head of the femur, *West J Surg* 57:221, 1949.

Fulford GE, Lunn PG, Macnicol MF: A prospective study of nonoperative and operative management for Perthes' disease, *J Pediatr Orthop* 13:281, 1993.

Futami T, Kasahara Y, Suzuki S, et al: Ultrasonography in transient synovitis and early Perthes' disease, *J Bone Joint Surg* 73B:635, 1991.

Gallistl S, Reitinger T, Linhart W, Muntean W: The role of inherited thrombotic disorders in the etiology of Legg-Calvé-Perthes disease, *J Pediatr Orthop* 19:82, 1999.

Garceau GJ: Surgical treatment of coxa plana, *J Bone Joint Surg* 46B:779, 1964.

Glick JM, Thompson TG, Gordon RB, et al: Hip arthroscopy by the lateral approach, *Arthroscopy* 3:4, 1987.

Glueck CJ, Brandt G, Gruppo R, et al: Resistance to activated protein C and Legg-Perthes disease, *Clin Orthop* 338:139, 1997.

Glueck CJ, Crawford A, Roy D, et al: Association of antithrombotic factor deficiencies and hypofibrinolysis with Legg-Perthes disease, *J Bone Joint Surg* 78A:3, 1996.

Gu Y, Da Paz Junior AC: Can an enlarged acetabulum cover the femoral head well in Legg-Calvé-Perthes disease? *J Pediatr Orthop B* 8:173, 1999.

Guille JT, Lipton GE, Szoke G, et al: Legg-Calvé-Perthes disease in girls: a comparison of the results with those seen in boys, *J Bone Joint Surg* 80A:1256, 1998.

Guilleminet M, Barbier JM: Osteochondritis dissecans of the hip, *J Bone Joint Surg* 22:327, 1940.

Hallel T, Salvati E: Osteochondritis dissecans following Legg-Calvé-Perthes disease, *J Bone Joint Surg* 58A:708, 1976.

Harrison MH, Bassett CA: Three results of a double-blind trial of pulsed electromagnetic frequency in the treatment of Perthes' disease, *J Pediatr Orthop* 17:264, 1997.

Harry JD, Gross RH: A quantitative method for evaluating results of treating Legg-Perthes syndrome, *J Pediatr Orthop* 7:671, 1987.

Hayek S, Kenet G, Lubetsky A, et al: Does thrombophilia play an aetiological role in Legg-Calvé-Perthes disease? *J Bone Joint Surg* 81B:686, 1999.

Henderson RC, Renner JB, Sturdivant MC, Greene WB: Evaluation of magnetic resonance imaging in Legg-Perthes disease: a prospective, blinded study, *J Pediatr Orthop* 10:289, 1990.

Herring JA: Management of Perthes' disease, *J Pediatr Orthop* 16:1, 1996.

Herring JA, Hotchkiss BL: Instructional case: Legg-Perthes disease versus multiple epiphyseal dysplasia, *J Pediatr Orthop* 7:341, 1987.

Herring JA, Neustadt JB, Williams JJ, et al: The lateral pillar classification of Legg-Calvé-Perthes disease, *J Pediatr Orthop* 12:143, 1992.

Herring JA, Williams JJ, Neustadt JN, Early JS: Evolution of femoral head deformity during the healing phase of Legg-Calvé-Perthes disease, *J Pediatr Orthop* 13:41, 1993.

Hoikka V, Poussa M, Yrjönen T, Österman K: Intertrochanteric varus osteotomy for Perthes' disease: radiographic changes after 2- to 16-year follow-up of 126 hips, *Acta Orthop Scand* 62:549, 1991.

Hosokawa M, Kim WC, Kubo T, et al: Preliminary report on usefulness of magnetic resonance imaging for outcome prediction in early-stage Legg-Calvé-Perthes disease, *J Pediatr Orthop B* 8:161, 1999.

Ippolito E, Tudisco C, Farsetti P: The long-term prognosis of unilateral Perthes' disease, *J Bone Joint Surg* 69B:243, 1987.

Ismail AM, Macnicol MF: Prognosis in Perthes' disease: a comparison of radiological predictors, *J Bone Joint Surg* 80B:310, 1998.

Joseph B, Srinivas G, Thomas R: Management of Perthes disease o late onset in southern India: the evaluation of a surgical method, *J Bone Joint Surg* 78B:625, 1996.

Kahle WK, Coleman SS: The value of the acetabular teardrop figure in assessing pediatric hip disorders, *J Pediatr Orthop* 12:586, 1992.

Kamegaya M, Shinada Y, Moriya H, et al: Acetabular remodeling in Perthes' disease after primary healing, *J Pediatr Orthop* 12:308, 1992.

Kamhi E, MacEwen GD: Osteochondritis dissecans in Legg-Calvé-Perthes disease, *J Bone Joint Surg* 57A:506, 1975.

Kealey WD, Mayne EE, McDonald W, et al: The role of coagulation abnormalities in the development of Perthes' disease, *J Bone Joint Surg* 82B:744, 2000.

Keenan WN, Clegg J: Perthes' disease after "irritable hip:" delayed bone shows the hip is a "marked man," *J Pediatr Orthop* 16:20, 1996.

Kelly FB Jr, Canale ST, Jones RR: Legg-Calvé-Perthes disease: long-term evaluation of non-containment treatment, *J Bone Joint Surg* 62A:400, 1980.

Kiepurska A: Late results of treatment of Perthes' disease by a functional method, *Clin Orthop* 272:76, 1991.

Kim HT, Wenger DR: "Functional retroversion" of the femoral head in Legg-Calvé-Perthes disease and epiphyseal dysplasia: analysis of head-neck deformity and its effect on limb position using three-dimensional computed tomography, *J Pediatr Orthop* 17:240, 1997.

Kim HT, Wenger DR: Surgical correction of "functional retroversion" and "functional coxa vara" in late Legg-Calvé-Perthes disease and epiphyseal dysplasia: correction of deformity defined by new imaging modalities, *J Pediatr Orthop* 17:247, 1997.

Kitakoji T, Hattori T, Iwata H: Femoral varus osteotomy in Legg-Calvé-Perthes disease: points at operation to prevent residual problems, *J Pediatr Orthop* 19:76, 1999.

Kocaoglu M, Kilicoglu OI, Goksan SB, Cakmak M: Ilizarov fixator for treatment of Legg-Calvé-Perthes disease, *J Pediatr Orthop B* 8:276, 1999.

Kruse RW, Guille JT, Bowen JR: Shelf arthroplasty in patients who have had Legg-Perthes disease, *J Bone Joint Surg* 64A:1338, 1991.

Lack W, Feldner-Busztin H, Ritschl P, Ramach, W: The results of surgical treatment for Perthes' disease, *J Pediatr Orthop* 9:197, 1989.

Landin LA, Danielsson LG, Wattsgard C: Transient synovitis of the hip: its incidence, epidemiology and relation to Perthes' disease, *J Bone Joint Surg* 69B:238, 1987.

Lee DY, Seong SC, Choi IH, et al: Changes of blood flow of the femoral head after subtrochanteric osteotomy in Legg-Perthes' disease: a serial scintigraphic study, *J Pediatr Orthop* 12:731, 1992.

Leitch JM, Paterson DC, Foster BK: Growth disturbance in Legg-Calvé-Perthes disease and the consequences of surgical treatment, *Clin Orthop* 262:178, 1991.

Lindholm TS, Osterman K: Internal fixation of the fragments of osteochondritis dissecans in the hip using bone transplants, *J Bone Joint Surg* 62B:43, 1980.

Lloyd-Roberts GC, Catterall A, Salamon PB: A controlled study of the indications for and the results of femoral osteotomy in Perthes disease, *J Bone Joint Surg* 58B:31, 1976.

Loder RT, Farley FA, Hensinger RN: Physeal slope in Perthes disease, *J Bone Joint Surg* 77B:736, 1995.

Macnicol MF, Makris D: Distal transfer of the greater trochanter, *J Bone Joint Surg* 73B:838, 1991.

Martinez AG, Weinstein SL: Recurrent Legg-Calvé-Perthes disease: case report and review of the literature, *J Bone Joint Surg* 73A:1081, 1991.

Martinez AG, Weinstein SL, Dietz FR: The weight-bearing abduction brace for the treatment of Legg-Perthes' disease, *J Bone Joint Surg* 74A:12, 1992.

Matan AJ, Stevens PM, Smith JT, Santora SD: Combination trochanteric arrest and intertrochanteric osteotomy for Perthes' disease, *J Pediatr Orthop* 16:10, 1996.

Maxted MJ, Jackson RK: Innominate osteotomy in Perthes' disease: a radiological survey of results, *J Bone Joint Surg* 67B:399, 1985.

Mazda K, Pennecot GF, Zeller R, Taussig G: Perthes' disease after the age of twelve years: role of the remaining growth, *J Bone Joint Surg* 81B:696, 1999.

McElwain JP, Regan BF, Dowling F, Fogarty E: Derotation varus osteotomy in Perthes disease, *J Pediatr Orthop* 5:195, 1985.

Meeham PL, Angel D, Nelson JM: The Scottish Rite abduction orthosis for the treatment of Legg-Perthes disease: a radiographic analysis, *J Bone Joint Surg* 74A:2, 1992.

Meiss L: Prognosis in Perthes' disease, *J Bone Joint Surg* 81B:180, 1999.

Moberg A, Hansson G, Kaniklides C: Results after femoral and innominate osteotomy in Legg-Calvé-Perthes disease, *Clin Orthop* 334:257, 1997.

Mose K: *Legg-Calvé-Perthes disease*, Copenhagen, 1964, Universitetsforlaget i Aarhus.

Muirhead-Allwood W, Catterall A: Treatment of Perthes' disease, the results of a trial management, *J Bone Joint Surg* 64B:285, 1982.

Mukherjee A, Fabry G: Evaluation of the prognostic indices in Legg-Calvé-Perthes disease: statistical analysis of 116 hips, *J Pediatr Orthop* 10:153, 1990.

Neyt JG, Weinstein SL, Spratt KF, et al: Stulberg classification system for evaluation of Legg-Calvé-Perthes disease: intrarater and interrater reliability, *J Bone Joint Surg* 81A:1209, 1999.

Paterson DC, Leitch JM, Foster BK: Results of innominate osteotomy in the treatment of Legg-Calvé-Perthes disease, *Clin Orthop* 266:96, 1991.

Petrie JG, Bitenc I: The abduction weight-bearing treatment in Legg-Calvé-Perthes disease, *J Bone Joint Surg* 49A:1483, 1967 (abstract).

Pinto MR, Peterson HA, Berquist TH: Magnetic resonance imaging in early diagnosis of Legg-Calvé-Perthes disease, *J Pediatr Orthop* 9:19, 1989.

Price CT, Day DD, Flynn JC: Behavioral sequelae of bracing versus surgery for Legg-Calvé-Perthes disease, *J Pediatr Orthop* 8:285, 1988.

Purvis JM, Dimon JH III, Meehan PL, et al: Preliminary experience with the Scottish Rite Hospital abduction orthosis for Legg-Perthes disease, *Clin Orthop* 150:49, 1980.

Quain S, Catterall A: Hinge abduction of the hip: diagnosis and treatment, *J Bone Joint Surg* 68B:61, 1986.

Ratliff AHC: Perthes' disease—a study of sixteen patients followed up for forty years. In Proceedings and Reports of Universities, Colleges, Councils, and Associations, *J Bone Joint Surg* 59B:248, 1977 (abstract).

Reinker KA: Early diagnosis and treatment of hinge abduction in Legg-Perthes disease, *J Pediatr Orthop* 16:3, 1996.

Richards BS, Coleman S: Subluxation of the femoral head in coxa plana, *J Bone Joint Surg* 69A:1312, 1987.

Ritterbusch JF, Shantharam SS, Gelinas C: Comparison of lateral pillar classification and Catterall classification of Legg-Calvé-Perthes disease, *J Pediatr Orthop* 13:200, 1993.

Roberts JM, Yngve DA: Acetabular hypertrophy in Legg-Calvé-Perthes disease, *J Pediatr Orthop* 5:416, 1985.

Robinson HJ, Putter H, Sigmond MB, et al: Innominate osteotomy in Perthes disease, *J Pediatr Orthop* 8:426, 1988.

Rowe SM, Kim HS, Yoon TR: Osteochondritis dissecans in Perthes' disease: report of 7 cases, *Acta Orthop Scand* 60:545, 1989.

Salter RB: Experimental and clinical aspects of Perthes' disease, *J Bone Joint Surg* 48B:393, 1966 (abstract).

Salter RB, Thompson GH: Legg-Calvé-Perthes disease: the prognostic significance of the subchondral fracture and a two-group classification of the femoral head involvement, *J Bone Joint Surg* 66A:479, 1984.

Serlo W, Heikkinen E, Puranen J: Preoperative Russell traction in Legg-Calvé-Perthes disease, *J Pediatr Orthop* 7:288, 1987.

Sirvent N, Fisher F, el Hayek T, et al: Absence of congenital prethrombotic disorders in children with Legg-Perthes disease, *J Pediatr Orthop B* 9:24, 2000.

Snow SW, Keret D, Scarangella S, Bowen JR: Anterior impingement of the femoral head: a late phenomenon of Legg-Calvé-Perthes' disease, *J Pediatr Orthop* 13:286, 1993.

Snyder CR: Legg-Perthes disease in the young hip: does it necessarily do well? *J Bone Joint Surg* 57A:751, 1975.

Somerville EW: Perthes disease of the hip, *J Bone Joint Surg* 53B:639, 1971.

Song HR, Lee SH, Na JB, et al: Comparison of MRI with subchondral fracture in the evaluation of extent of epiphyseal necrosis in the early stage of Legg-Calvé-Perthes disease, *J Pediatr Orthop* 19:70, 1999.

Song HR, Lee SH, Na JB, et al: Relationship between lateral subluxation and widening of medial joint space in Legg-Calvé-Perthes disease, *J Pediatr Orthop* 18:637, 1998.

Sponseller PD, Desai SS, Millis MB: Comparison of femoral and innominate osteotomies for the treatment of Legg-Calvé-Perthes disease, *J Bone Joint Surg* 70A:1131, 1988.

Steel HH, Clancy M: The effect of an incomplete intertrochanteric osteotomy on Legg-Calvé-Perthes' disease, *J Bone Joint Surg* 67A: 213, 1985.

Stricker S: Intermediate and pediatric osteotomy systems. Surgical Technique Manual, Smith & Nephew Orthopaedics, Memphis, Tennessee.

Stulberg SD, Cooperman DR, Wallensten R: The natural history of Legg-Calvé-Perthes disease, *J Bone Joint Surg* 63A:1095, 1981.

Suzuki S, Awaya G, Okada Y, et al: Examination by ultrasound of Legg-Calvé-Perthes disease, *Clin Orthop* 220:130, 1987.

Terjesen T, Østhus P: Ultrasound in the diagnosis and follow-up of transient synovitis of the hip, *J Pediatr Orthop* 11:608, 1991.

Thomas DP, Morgan G, Tayton K: Perthes' disease and the relevance of thrombophilia, *J Bone Joint Surg* 81B:691, 1999.

Thompson GH, Salter RB: Legg-Calvé-Perthes disease: current concepts and controversies, *Orthop Clin North Am* 18:617, 1987.

Thompson GH, Westin GW: Legg-Calvé-Perthes disease: results of discontinuing treatment in the early ossification phase, *Clin Orthop* 139:70, 1979.

Uno A, Hattori T, Noritake K, Suda H: Legg-Calvé-Perthes disease in the evolutionary period: comparison of magnetic resonance imaging with bone scintigraphy, *J Pediatr Orthop* 15:362, 1995.

Van den Bogaert G, de Rosa E, Moens P, et al: Bilateral Legg-Calvé-Perthes disease: different from unilateral disease? *J Pediatr Orthop B* 8:165, 1999.

Wagner H: Trochanteric advancement in the intertrochanteric osteotomy. In Schatzker J, ed: *The intertrochanteric osteotomy*, Berlin, 1984, Springer-Verlag.

Wang L, Bowen JR, Puniak MA, et al: An evaluation of various methods of treatment for Legg-Calvé-Perthes disease, *Clin Orthop* 314:225, 1995.

Weiner SD, Weiner DS, Riley PM: Pitfalls in treatment of Legg-Calvé-Perthes disease using proximal femoral varus osteotomy, *J Pediatr Orthop* 11:20, 1991.

Willett K, Hudson I, Catterall A: Lateral shelf acetabuloplasty: an operation for older children with Perthes' disease, *J Pediatr Orthop* 12:563, 1992.

HEMOPHILIA

American Academy of Orthopaedic Surgeons Task Force on AIDS and Orthopaedic Surgery: Recommendations for the prevention of human immunodeficiency virus (HIV) transmission in the practice of orthopaedic surgery, Park Ridge, Ill, 1989, The Academy.

Arnold WD, Hilgartner MW: Hemophilic arthropathy: current concepts of pathogenesis and management, *J Bone Joint Surg* 59A:287, 1977.

Aronstam AA, Wassef M, Hamad Z, Aston DL: The identification of high-risk elbow hemorrhages in adolescents with severe hemophilia, *Am J Pediatr* 98:776, 1981.

Battistella LR: Maintenance of musculoskeletal function in people with haemophilia, *Haemophilia* 4 (suppl 2):26, 1998.

Boardman KP, English P: Fractures and dislocations in hemophilia, *Clin Orthop* 148:221, 1980.

Buchanan GR, Holtkamp CA: Prolonged bleeding time in children and young adults with hemophilia, *Pediatrics* 66:951, 1980.

Canale ST, Dugdale M, Howard BC: Synovectomy of the knee in young patients with hemophilia, *South Med J* 81:1480, 1988.

Castañeda VL, Parmley RT, Bozzini M, Feldmeier JJ: Radiotherapy of pseudotumors of bone in hemophiliacs with circulating inhibitors to factor VIII, *Am J Hematol* 36:55, 1991.

Chen YF: Roentgen irradiation for chronic hemorrhage from an ulcer in a hemophiliac, *J Bone Joint Surg* 54A:1783, 1972.

Day AJ: Orthopedic management of hemophilia. In American Academy of Orthopaedic Surgeons: *Instructional course lectures*, vol 20, St Louis, 1971, Mosby.

Dugdale M: Personal communication, 1978.

Eickhoff HH, Koch W, Raderschadt G, Brackmann HH: Arthroscopy for chronic hemophilic synovitis of the knee, *Clin Orthop* 343:58, 1997.

Erken EHW: Radiocolloids in the management of hemophilic arthropathy in children and adolescents, *Clin Orthop* 264:129, 1991.

Feil E, Bentley G, Rizza CR: Fracture management in patients with haemophilia, *J Bone Joint Surg* 56B:643, 1974.

Floman Y, Niska M: Case report: dislocation of the hip joint complicating repeated hemarthrosis in hemophilia, *J Pediatr Orthop* 3:99, 1983.

Gamba G, Grignani G, Ascari E: Synoviorthesis versus synovectomy in the treatment of recurrent haemophilic haemarthrosis: long-term evaluation, *Thromb Haemost* 45:127, 1981.

Gamble JG, Bellah J, Rinsky LA, et al: Arthropathy of the ankle in hemophilia, *J Bone Joint Surg* 73A:1008, 1994.

Gilbert MS, Radomisli TE: Therapeutic options in the management of hemophilic synovitis, *Clin Orthop* 343:88, 1997.

Greene WB: Synovectomy of the ankle for hemophilic arthropathy, *J Bone Joint Surg* 76A:812, 1994.

Greene WB, Strickler EM: A modified isokinetic strengthening program for patients with severe hemophilia, *Dev Med Child Neurol* 25:189, 1983.

Hilgartner MW, Arnold WD: Hemophilic pseudotumor treated with replacement therapy and radiation: report of a case, *J Bone Joint Surg* 57A:1145, 1975.

Hofmann A, Wyatt R, Bybee B: Case report: septic arthritis of the knee in a 12-year-old hemophiliac, *J Pediatr Orthop* 4:498, 1984.

Hutchinson RJ, Penner JA, Hensinger RN: Anti-inhibitor coagulant complex (autoplex) in hemophilia inhibitor patients undergoing synovectomy, *Pediatrics* 71:631, 1983.

Iwata H, Oishi Y, Itoh A, et al: Surgical excision of hemophilic pseudotumor of the ilium, *Clin Orthop* 284:234, 1992.

Katz SG, Nelson IW, Atkins RM, et al: Peripheral nerve lesions in hemophilia, *J Bone Joint Surg* 73A:1016, 1991.

Keeley K, Buchanan G: Acute infraction of long bones in children with sickle cell anemia, *Pediatrics* 101:170, 1982.

Klein HG, Alter HJ: Blood transfusion and AIDS. *Information on AIDS for the practicing physician*, vol 2, Chicago, 1987, American Medical Association.

Koren A, Garty I, Katzuni E: Bone infraction in children with sickle cell disease: early diagnosis and differentiation from osteomyelitis, *Eur J Pediatr* 142:93, 1984.

LeBalc'h T, Ebelin M, Laurian Y, et al: Synovectomy of the elbow in young hemophilic patients, *J Bone Joint Surg* 69A:264, 1987.

Limbird TJ, Dennis SC: The treatment of hemophilic arthropathy by arthroscopic synovectomy, *Orthop Trans* 10:617, 1986 (abstract).

Lofqvist T, Nilsson IM, Petersson C: Orthopaedic surgery in hemophilia: 20 years' experience in Sweden, *Clin Orthop* 332:232, 1996.

Mackay SR: Orthopedic aspects of hemophilia. In American Academy of Orthopaedic Surgeons: *Instructional course lectures*, vol 22, St Louis, 1973, Mosby.

McCollough NC, Enis JE, Lovitt J, et al: Synovectomy or total replacement of the knee in hemophilia, *J Bone Joint Surg* 61A:69, 1979.

McCollough NC, Lovitt J, Enis JE, et al: Knee surgery in hemophiliacs, *Orthop Rev* 6:99, 1977.

Merchan ECR, Galindo E: Proximal tibial valgus osteotomy for hemophilic arthropathy of the knee, *Orthop Rev* 21:204, 1992.

Miller EH, Flessa HC, Glueck HI: The management of deep soft tissue bleeding and hemarthrosis in hemophilia, *Clin Orthop* 82:92, 1972.

Montane I, McCollough NC III, Lia EC: Synovectomy of the knee for hemophilic arthropathy, *J Bone Joint Surg* 68A:210, 1986.

Naveh Y, Berant M, Bialik V: Case report: vitamin K deficiency presenting with hemarthrosis, *J Pediatr Orthop* 4:630, 1984.

Nelson IW, Sivamurugan S, Lathem PD, et al: Total hip arthroplasty for hemophilic arthropathy, *Clin Orthop* 276:210, 1992.

Nicol RO, Menelau, MB: Synovectomy of the knee in hemophilia, *J Pediatr Orthop* 6:330, 1986.

Nilsson IM, Berntorp E, Löfqvist T, Pettersson H: Twenty-five years' experience of prophylactic treatment in severe haemophilia A and B, *J Intern Med* 232:25, 1992.

Pappo AS, Buchanan GR, Johnson A: Septic arthritis in children with hemophilia, *Am J Dis Child* 143:1226, 1989.

Patti JE, Mayo WE: Arthroscopic synovectomy for recurrent hemarthrosis of the ankle in hemophilia, *Arthroscopy* 12:652, 1996.

Pirich C, Pilger A, Schwameis E, et al: Radiation synovectomy using 165Dy ferric-hydroxide and oxidative DNA damage in patients with different types of arthritis, *J Nucl Med* 41:250, 2000.

Pootrakul P, Hungsprenges S, Fucharoen S, et al: Relation between erythropoiesis and bone metabolism in thalassemia, *N Engl J Med* 304:1470, 1981.

Post M, Telfer MC: Surgery in hemophilic patients, *J Bone Joint Surg* 57A:1136, 1975.

Post M, Watts G, Telfer M: Synovectomy in hemophilic arthropathy: a retrospective review of 17 cases, *Clin Orthop* 202:139, 1986.

Rivard GE: Synovectomy with radioactive colloids in hemophiliacs, *Prog Clin Biol Res* 324:215, 1990.

Rivard GE, Girard M, Belanger R, et al: Synoviorthesis with colloidal 32P chromic phosphate for the treatment of hemophilic arthropathy, *J Bone Joint Surg* 76A:481, 1994.

Rivard GE, Girard M, Cliche CL, et al: Synoviorthesis in patients with hemophilia and inhibitors, *Can Med Assoc J* 127:41, 1982.

Rodriguez-Merchan EC, Magallon M, Galindo E, Lopez-Cabarcos C: Hamstring release for fixed knee flexion contracture in hemophilia, *Clin Orthop* 343:63, 1997.

Rodriguez-Merchan EC, Magallon M, Galindo E, Lopez-Cabarcos C: Hemophilic synovitis of the knee and elbow, *Clin Orthop* 343:47, 1997.

Rosenthal RL, Graham JJ, Selirio E: Excision of pseudotumor with repair by bone graft of pathological fracture of femur in hemophilia, *J Bone Joint Surg* 55A:827, 1973.

Siegel HJ, Luck JV Jr, Siegel ME, et al: Hemarthrosis and synovitis associated with hemophilia: clinical use of P32 chromic phosphate synoviorthesis for treatment, *Radiology* 190:257, 1994.

Small M, Steven MM, Freeman PA, et al: Total knee arthroplasty in hemophilic arthritis, *J Bone Joint Surg* 65B:163, 1983.

Soreff J, Blomback M: Arthropathy in children with severe hemophilia A, *Acta Paediatr Scand* 69:667, 1980.

Speer DP: Early pathogenesis of hemophilic arthropathy: evolution of the subchondral cyst, *Clin Orthop* 185:250, 1984.

Staas WE Jr, Ditunno JF Jr, Gartland JJ, Shapiro SS: Lower extremity amputation in hemophilia: case report and review of surgical principles, *J Bone Joint Surg* 54A:1514, 1972.

Stehr-Green JK, Holman RC, Mahoney MA: Survival analysis of hemophilia-associated AIDS cases in the US, *Am J Public Health* 79:832, 1989.

Stehr-Green JK, Holman RC, Jason JM, et al: Hemophilia-associated AIDS in the United States, 1981 to September 1987, *Am J Public Health* 78:4, 1988.

Storti E, Traldi A, Tosatti E, et al: Synovectomy: a new approach to haemophilic arthropathy, *Acta Haematol* 41:193, 1969.

Triantafyllou SJ, Hanks GA, Handal JA, Greer RB: Open and arthroscopic synovectomy in hemophilic arthropathy of the knee, *Clin Orthop* 283:196, 1992.

Vas W, Cockshott WP, Martin RF, et al: Myositis ossificans in hemophilia, *Skeletal Radiol* 7:27, 1981.

Wiedel JD: Arthroscopic synovectomy for chronic hemophilic synovitis of the knee, *Arthroscopy* 1:205, 1985.

Wiedel JD: Arthroscopic synovectomy of the knee in hemophilia. 10- to 15-year follow-up, *Clin Orthop* 328:46, 1996.

RICKETS, OSTEOMALACIA, AND RENAL OSTEODYSTROPHY

Barrett IR, Papadimitriou DG: Skeletal disorders in children with renal failure, *J Pediatr Orthop* 16:264, 1996.

Callenbach JC, Sheehan MB, Abramson SJ, Hall RT: Etiologic factors in rickets of very low-birth-weight infants, *J Pediatr* 98:800, 1981.

Cattell HS, Levin S, Kopits S, Lyne ED: Reconstructive surgery in children with azotemic osteodystrophy, *J Bone Joint Surg* 53A:216, 1971.

Curtis JA, Kooh SW, Fraser D, Greenberg ML: Nutritional rickets in vegetarian children, *Can Med Assoc J* 128:150, 1983.

Doppelt SH: Vitamin D, rickets, and osteomalacia, *Orthop Clin North Am* 15:671, 1984.

Elmstedt E: Incidence of skeletal complications in renal graft recipients: effect of changes in pharmacotherapy, *Acta Orthop Scand* 53:853, 1982.

Evans GA, Arulanantham K, Gage JR: Primary hypophosphatemic rickets: effect of oral phosphate and vitamin D on growth and surgical treatment, *J Bone Joint Surg* 62A:1130, 1980.

Ferris B, Walker C, Jackson A, et al: The orthopedic management of hypophosphatemic rickets, *J Pediatr Orthop* 11:367, 1991.

Gefter W, Epstein DM, Anday EK, Dalinka MK: Rickets presenting as multiple fractures in premature infants on hyperalimentation, *Radiology* 142:371, 1982.

Greer FR, Searcy JE, Levin RS, et al: Bone mineral content and serum 25-hydroxy-vitamin D concentration in breast-fed infants with and without supplemental vitamin D, *J Pediatr* 98:696, 1981.

Herman MJ, Gulthuis DB: Incidental diagnosis of nutritional rickets after clavicle fracture, *Orthopedics* 22:254, 1999.

Holda ME, Ryan JR: Hepatobiliary rickets, *J Pediatr Orthop* 2:285, 1982.

Kanel JS, Price CT: Unilateral external fixation for corrective osteotomies in patients with hypophosphatemic rickets, *J Pediatr Orthop* 15:232, 1995.

Kanis JA: Vitamin D metabolism and its clinical application, *J Bone Joint Surg* 64B:542, 1982.

Klein KL, Maxwell MH: Renal osteodystrophy, *Orthop Clin North Am* 15:687, 1984.

Loder RT, Hensinger RN: Slipped capital femoral epiphysis associated with renal failure osteodystrophy, *J Pediatr Orthop* 17:205, 1997.

Loeffler R, Sherman F: The effect of treatment on growth and deformity in hypophosphatemic vitamin D–resistant rickets, *Clin Orthop* 162:4, 1982.

Lovinger RD: Rickets (grand round series), *Pediatrics* 66:365, 1980.

Mankin HJ: Rickets, osteomalacia, and renal osteodystrophy. 1, *J Bone Joint Surg* 56A:101, 1974.

Mankin HJ: Rickets, osteomalacia, and renal osteodystrophy. 2, *J Bone Joint Surg* 56A:352, 1974.

Mankin HJ: Metabolic bone disease, *J Bone Joint Surg* 76A:760, 1994.

Marie P, Pettifor J, Ross F, Glorieux F: Histological osteomalacia due to dietary calcium deficiency in children, *N Engl J Med* 307:584, 1982.

Masel J, Tudehope D, Cartwright D: Osteopenia and rickets in the extremely low birth weight infant—a survey of the incidence and a radiological classification, *Aust Radiol* 26:83, 1982.

Mason RS, Rohl PG, Lissner D, Posen S: Vitamin D metabolism in hypophosphatemic rickets, *Am J Dis Child* 136:909, 1982.

Nicol RO, Williams PF, Hill DJ: Transient osteopaenia of the hip in children, *J Pediatr Orthop* 4:590, 1984.

Oppenheim WL, Fischer SR, Salusky IB: Surgical correction of angular deformity of the knee in children with renal osteodystrophy, *J Pediatr Orthop* 17:41, 1997.

Opshaug O, Maurseth K, Howlid H: Vitamin D metabolism in hypophosphatasia, *Acta Pediatr Scand* 71:517, 1982.

Paterson CR: Case report: vitamin D deficiency rickets simulating child abuse, *J Pediatr Orthop* 1:423, 1981.

Rosenthal RE, Johnson HK, Richie RE: Massive skeletal trauma in renal transplant patients, *South Med J* 69:1582, 1976.

Scriver CR, Reade T, Halal F, et al: Autosomal hypophosphatemic bone disease responds to 1,25-(OH)$_2$D$_3$, *Arch Dis Child* 56:203, 1981.

Sheridan RN, Chiroff RT, Friedman EM: Operative and nonoperative treatment of rachitic lower extremity deformities: a long-term study with 46-year average follow-up, *Clin Orthop* 116:66, 1976.

Smith R: Idiopathic osteoporosis in the young, *J Bone Joint Surg* 62B:427, 1980.

Toomey F, Hoag R, Batton D, Vain N: Rickets associated with cholestasis and parenteral nutrition in premature infants, *Radiology* 142:85, 1982.

Touloukian RJ, Gertner JM: Vitamin D deficiency rickets as a late complication of the short gut syndrome during infancy, *J Pediatr Surg* 16:230, 1981.

TIBIA VARA

Beaty JH, Coscia MF, Holt M: Blount's disease. Paper presented at the Fifth Annual Meeting of the Southern Orthopedic Association, Edinburgh, Aug 4, 1988.

Beck CL, Burke SW, Roberts JM, Johnston CE III: Physeal bridge resection in infantile Blount disease, *J Pediatr Orthop* 7:161, 1987.

Bell DF: Treatment of adolescent Blount's disease using the Ilizarov technique, *Op Tech Orthop* 3:149, 1993.

Blount WP: Tibia vara: osteochondrosis deformans tibiae, *J Bone Joint Surg* 19:1, 1937.

Blount WP: Tibia vara: osteochondritis deformans tibia. In Adams JP, ed: *Current practice in orthopedic surgery*, vol 3, St Louis, 1966, Mosby.

Bradway JK, Klassen RA, Peterson HA: Blount disease: a review of the English literature, *J Pediatr Orthop* 7:471, 1987.

Bright RW: Operative correction of partial epiphyseal plate closure by osseous-bridge resection and silicone-rubber implant, *J Bone Joint Surg* 56A:655, 1974.

Canale ST, Harper MC: Biotrigonometric analysis and practical applications of osteotomies of tibia in children. In American Academy of Orthopaedic Surgeons: *Instructional course lectures*, vol 30, St Louis, 1981, Mosby.

Carter JR, Leeson MC, Thompson GH, et al: Late-onset tibia vara: a histopathologic analysis: a comparative evaluation with infantile tibia vara and slipped capital femoral epiphysis, *J Pediatr Orthop* 8:187, 1988.

Coogan PG, Fox JA, Fitch RD: Treatment of adolescent Blount disease with the circular external fixation device and distraction osteogenesis, *J Pediatr Orthop* 16:450, 1996.

Cook SD, Lavernia CJ, Burke SW, et al: A biomechanical analysis of the etiology of tibia vara, *J Pediatr Orthop* 3:449, 1983.

Dalinka MK, Coren G, Hensinger R, Irani RN: Arthrography in Blount's disease, *Radiology* 113:161, 1974.

Deitz WH, Gross WL, Kirkpatrick JA: Blount disease (tibia vara): another skeletal disorder associated with childhood obesity, *J Pediatr* 101:735, 1982.

De Palblos J, Azcarate J, Barrios C: Progressive opening-wedge osteotomy for angular long-bone deformities in adolescents, *J Bone Joint Surg* 77B:387, 1995.

Eggert P, Viemann M: Physiological bowlegs or infantile Blount's disease: Some new aspects on an old problem, *Pediatr Radiol* 26:349, 1996.

Erlacher P: Deformierended prozesse der Epiphysengegend bei Kindern, *Arch Orthop Unfallchir* 20:81, 1922.

Ferriter P, Shapiro F: Infantile tibia vara: factors affecting outcome following proximal tibial osteotomy, *J Pediatr Orthop* 7:1, 1987.

Fletcher R, D'Ambrosia R: Coxa vara in achondroplasia treated by valgus osteotomy, *Orthopedics* 6:1024, 1983.

Foreman KA, Robertson WW Jr: Radiographic measurement of infantile tibia vara, *J Pediatr Orthop* 5:452, 1985.

Gaudinez R, Adar U: Use of the Orthofix T-Garche fixator in the late-onset tibia vara, *J Pediatr Orthop* 16:455, 1996.

Golding JS, McNeil-Smith JD: Observations on the etiology of tibia vara, *J Bone Joint Surg* 45B:320, 1963.

Greene WB: Infantile tibia vara, *J Bone Joint Surg* 75A:130, 1993.

Greene WB: Genu varum and genu valgum in children: differential diagnosis and guidelines for evaluation, *Compr Ther* 22:22, 1996.

Gregosiewicz A, Wosko I, Kandzierski G, Drabik Z: Double-elevating osteotomy of tibiae in the treatment of severe cases of Blount's disease, *J Pediatr Orthop* 9:178, 1989.

Henderson RC, Kemp GJ Jr, Greene WB: Adolescent tibia vara: alternatives for operative treatment, *J Bone Joint Surg* 74A:342, 1992.

Herring JA, Ehrlich MG: Instructional case: valgus knee deformity—etiology and treatment, *J Pediatr Orthop* 3:527, 1983.

Herring JA, Wenger DR: Blount disease, *J Pediatr Orthop* 7:601, 1987.

Hoffman A, Jones RE, Herring JA: Blount's disease after skeletal maturity, *J Bone Joint Surg* 64A:1004, 1982.

Ingram AJ: Paralytic disorders. In Crenshaw AH, ed: *Campbell's Operative Orthopaedics*, ed 7, vol 4, St Louis, 1987, Mosby.

Iwasawa T, Inaba Y, Nishimura G, et al: MR findings of bowlegs in toddlers, *Pediatr Radiol* 29:826, 1999.

Johnston CE II: Late-onset tibia vara (adolescent's Blount's disease), *Orthopedics* 7:734, 1984.

Kariya Y, Taniguchi K, Yagisawa H, Ooi Y: Case report: focal fibrocartilaginous dysplasia: consideration of healing process, *J Pediatr Orthop* 11:545, 1991.

Kline SC, Bostrum M, Griffin PP: Femoral varus: an important component in late-onset Blount's disease, *J Pediatr Orthop* 12:197, 1992.

Kling TF Jr: Angular deformities of the lower limbs in children, *Orthop Clin North Am* 18:513, 1987.

Langenskiöld A: Tibia vara (osteochondrosis deformans tibiae), *Acta Chir Scand* 103:1, 1952.

Langenskiöld A: An operation for partial closure of an epiphyseal plate in children and its experimental basis, *J Bone Joint Surg* 57B:325, 1975.

Langenskiöld A: Tibia vara: osteochondrosis deformans tibiae (Blount's disease), *Clin Orthop* 158:77, 1981.

Langenskiöld A: Tibia vara: a critical review, *Clin Orthop* 246:195, 1989.

Langenskiöld A, Riska EB: Tibia vara (osteochondrosis deformans tibiae): a survey of seventy-one cases, *J Bone Joint Surg* 46A:1405, 1964.

Laurencin CT, Ferriter PJ, Millis MB: Oblique proximal tibial osteotomy for the correction of tibia vara in the young, *Clin Orthop* 327:218, 1996.

Levine A, Drennan J: Physiological bowing and tibia vara: the metaphyseal-diaphyseal angle in measurement of bowleg deformities, *J Bone Joint Surg* 64A:1158, 1982.

Lichtblau PO, Waxman BA: Blount's disease: a review of the literature and description of a new surgical procedure, *Contemp Orthop* 3:526, 1981.

Loder RT, Johnston CE II: Infantile tibia vara, *J Pediatr Orthop* 7:639, 1987.

Loder RT, Schaffer JJ, Bardenstein MB: Late-onset tibia vara, *J Pediatr Orthop* 11:162, 1991.

Matsen FA III, Staheli LT: Neurovascular complications following tibial osteotomy in children: a case report, *Clin Orthop* 110:210, 1975.

Meade WC, Schoenecker PL, Pierron RL, Capelli A: Blount's disease—a retrospective review and recommendations, *Orthop Trans* 6:372, 1982.

Medbo I: Tibia vara (osteochondrosis deformans tibiae or Blount's disease): treatment and follow-up examination, *Acta Orthop Scand* 34:323, 1964.

Mitchell EI, Chung SMK, Das MM, Gregg JR: A new radiographic grading system for Blount's disease evaluating the epiphyseal-metaphyseal angle, *Orthop Rev* 9:27, 1980.

Monticelli G, Spinelli R: A new method of treating the advanced stages of tibia vara (Blount's disease), *Ital J Orthop Traumatol* 10:295, 1984.

Mycoskie P: Complications of osteotomies about the knee in children, *Orthopedics* 4:1005, 1981.

Olney BW, Cole WG, Menelaus MB: Three additional cases of focal fibrocartilaginous dysplasia causing tibia vara, *J Pediatr Orthop* 10:405, 1990.

O'Neill DA, MacEwen GD: Early roentgenographic evaluation of bowlegged children, *J Pediatr Orthop* 2:547, 1982.

Oppenheim WL, Shayestehfar S, Salusky IB: Tibial physeal changes in renal osteodystrophy: lateral Blount's disease, *J Pediatr Orthop* 12:774, 1992.

Price CT, Scott DS, Greenberg DA: Dynamic axial external fixation in the surgical treatment of tibia vara, *J Pediatr Orthop* 15:263, 1995.

Rab GT: Oblique tibial osteotomy for Blount's disease (tibia vara), *J Pediatr Orthop* 8:715, 1988.

Raney EM, Topoleski TA, Yaghoubian R, et al: Orthotic treatment of infantile tibia vara, *J Pediatr Orthop* 18:670, 1998.

Richards BS, Katz DE, Sims JB: Effectiveness of brace treatment in early infantile Blount's disease, *J Pediatr Orthop* 18:374, 1998.

Salenius P, Vankka E: The development of the tibiofemoral angle in children, *J Bone Joint Surg* 57A:259, 1975.

Sasaki T, Yagi T, Monji J, et al: Transepiphyseal plate osteotomy for severe tibia vara in children: follow-up study of four cases, *J Pediatr Orthop* 6:61, 1986.

Schoenecker PL, Johnston R, Rich MM, Capelli AM: Elevation of the medial plateau of the tibia in the treatment of Blount disease, *J Bone Joint Surg* 74A:351, 1992.

Schoenecker PL, Meade WC, Pierron RL, et al: Blount's disease: a retrospective review and recommendations for treatment, *J Pediatr Orthop* 5:181, 1985.

Siffert RS: Intraepiphyseal osteotomy for progressive tibia vara: case report and rationale of management, *J Pediatr Orthop* 2:81, 1982.

Siffert RS, Katz JF: The intraarticular deformity in osteochondrosis deformans tibiae, *J Bone Joint Surg* 52A:800, 1970.

Smith CF: Current concepts review: tibia vara (Blount's disease), *J Bone Joint Surg* 64A:630, 1982.

Stanitski DF, Dahl M, Louie K, Grayhack J: Management of late-onset tibia vara in the obese patient by using circular external fixation, *J Pediatr Orthop* 17:691, 1997.

Stanitski DF, Srivastava P, Stanitski CL: Correction of proximal tibial deformities in adolescents with T-Garches external fixator, *J Pediatr Orthop* 18:512, 1998.

Steel HH, Sandrow RE, Sullivan PD: Complications of tibial osteotomy in children for genu varum or valgum: evidence that neurological changes are due to ischemia, *J Bone Joint Surg* 53A:1629, 1971.

Støren H: Operative elevation of the medial tibial joint surface in Blount's disease, *Acta Orthop Scand* 40:788, 1970.

Tachdjian MO: *Pediatric orthopedics*, Philadelphia, 1972, WB Saunders.

Thompson GH, Carter JR: Late-onset tibia vara (Blount's disease): current concepts, *Clin Orthop* 255:24, 1990.

Thompson GH, Carter JR, Smith CW: Late-onset tibia vara: a comparative analysis, *J Pediatr Orthop* 4:185, 1984

Volk AG, Kling TF Jr, Dias L, DeRosa GP: Blount's disease: follow-up to maturity, *Orthop Trans* 13:246, 1989.

Vankka E, Salenius P: Spontaneous correction of severe tibiofemoral deformity in growing children, *Acta Orthop Scand* 53:567, 1982.

Wenger DR, Mickelson M, Maynard JA: The evolution and histopathology of adolescent tibia vara, *J Pediatr Orthop* 4:78, 1984.

Zayer M: Hemicondylar tibial osteotomy in Blount's disease: a report of two cases, *Acta Orthop Scand* 63:350, 1992.

Zayer M: Tibia vara in focal fibrocartilaginous dysplasia: a report of two cases, *Acta Orthop Scand* 63:353, 1992.

Zionts LE, Shean CJ: Brace treatment of early infantile tibia vara, *J Pediatr Orthop* 18:102, 1998.

OSTEOGENESIS IMPERFECTA

Albright JA: Management overview of osteogenesis imperfecta, *Clin Orthop* 159:80, 1981.

Albright JA: Systemic treatment of osteogenesis imperfecta, *Clin Orthop* 159:88, 1981.

Bailey RW: Further clinical experience with the extensible nail, *Clin Orthop* 159:171, 1981.

Bailey RW, Dubow HI: Experimental and clinical studies of longitudinal bone growth: utilizing a new method of internal fixation crossing the epiphyseal plate, *J Bone Joint Surg* 47A:1669, 1965.

Bailey RW, Dubow HI: Evolution of the concept of an extensible nail accommodating to normal longitudinal bone growth: clinical considerations and implications, *Clin Orthop* 159:157, 1981.

Bauze RJ, Smith R, Francis MJO: A new look at osteogenesis imperfecta: a clinical, radiological, and biochemical study of forty-two patients, *J Bone Joint Surg* 57B:2, 1975.

Beighton P, Spranger J, Versveld G: Skeletal complications in osteogenesis imperfecta: a review of 153 South African patients, *S Afr Med J* 64:565, 1983.

Benson DR, Newman DC: The spine and surgical treatment in osteogenesis imperfecta, *Clin Orthop* 159:147, 1981.

Bergstrom L: Fragile bones and fragile ears, *Clin Orthop* 159:58, 1981.

Bleck EE: Nonoperative treatment of osteogenesis imperfecta: orthotic and mobility management, *Clin Orthop* 159:111, 1981.

Brown DM: Biomechanical abnormalities in osteogenesis imperfecta, *Clin Orthop* 159:75, 1981.

Bullough PG, Davidson DD, Lorenzo JC: The morbid anatomy of the skeleton in osteogenesis imperfecta, *Clin Orthop* 159:42, 1981.

Cozen L: Use of rods outside long bones for osteogenesis imperfecta: report of a case with a 16-year follow-up, *Orthop Rev* 10:129, 1981.

Cristofaro RL, Hoek KJ, Bonnett CA, Brown JC: Operative treatment of spine deformity in osteogenesis imperfecta, *Clin Orthop* 139:40, 1979.

Daly K, Wisbeach A, Sanpera I Jr, Fixsen JA: The prognosis for walking in osteogenesis imperfecta, *J Bone Joint Surg* 78B:477, 1996.

DeBastiani G, Aldegheri R, Renzi Brivio L, Trivella G: Limb lengthening by distraction of the epiphyseal plate: a comparison of two techniques in the rabbit, *J Bone Joint Surg* 68B:545, 1986.

DeBastiani G, Aldegheri R, Renzi Brivio L, Trivella G: Chondrodiastasis—controlled symmetrical distraction of the epiphyseal plate: limb lengthening in children, *J Bone Joint Surg* 68B:550, 1986.

DeBastiani G, Aldegheri R, Renzi Brivio L, Trivella G: Limb lengthening by callus distraction (callotasis), *J Pediatr Orthop* 7:129, 1987.

Eyre DR: Concepts in collagen biochemistry: evidence that collagenopathies underlie osteogenesis imperfecta, *Clin Orthop* 159: 97, 1981.

Falvo KA, Root L, Bullough PG: Osteogenesis imperfecta: clinical evaluation and management, *J Bone Joint Surg* 56A:783, 1974.

Gamble JG, Strudwick J, Rinsky LA, Bleck EE: Complications of intramedullary rods in osteogenesis imperfecta: Bailey-Dubow rods versus nonelongating rods, *J Pediatr Orthop* 8:645, 1988.

Gargan MF, Wisbeach A, Fixsen JA: Humeral rodding in osteogenesis imperfecta, *J Pediatr Orthop* 16:719, 1996.

Gerber LH, Binder H, Weintrob J, et al: Rehabilitation of children and infants with osteogenesis imperfecta: a program for ambulation, *Clin Orthop* 251:254, 1990.

Gertner JM, Root L: Osteogenesis imperfecta, *Orthop Clin North Am* 21:151, 1990.

Goldman AB, Davidson D, Pavlov H, Bullough PG: "Popcorn" calcifications: a prognostic sign in osteogenesis imperfecta, *Radiology* 136:351, 1980.

Ilizarov G: The principles of the Ilizarov method, *Bull Hosp Jt Dis* 48:1, 1988.

Janus GJ, Vanpaemel LA, Engelbert RH, Pruijs HE: Complications of the Bailey-Dubow elongating nail in osteogenesis imperfecta: 34 children with 110 nails, *J Pediatr Orthop* B 8:203, 1999.

King JD, Bobechko WP: Osteogenesis imperfecta: an orthopedic description and surgical review, *J Bone Joint Surg* 53B:72, 1971.

Laidlaw AT, Loder RT, Hensinger RN: Telescoping intramedullary rodding with Bailey-Dubow nails for recurrent pathologic fractures in children without osteogenesis imperfecta, *J Pediatr Orthop* 18:4, 1998.

Levin LS: The dentition in the osteogenesis imperfecta syndromes, *Clin Orthop* 159:64, 1981.

Libman RH: Anesthetic considerations for the patient with osteogenesis imperfecta, *Clin Orthop* 159:123, 1981.

Lubs HA, Travers H: Genetic counseling in osteogenesis imperfecta, *Clin Orthop* 159:36, 1981.

Luhmann SJ, Sheridan JJ, Capelli AM, Schoenecker PL: Management of lower extremity deformities in osteogenesis imperfecta with extensible intramedullary rod technique: a 20-year experience, *J Pediatr Orthop* 18:88, 1998.

Marafioti RL, Westin GW: Elongating intramedullary rods in the treatment of osteogenesis imperfecta, *J Bone Joint Surg* 59A:467, 1977.

Middleton RWD: Closed intramedullary rodding for osteogenesis imperfecta, *J Bone Joint Surg* 66B:652, 1984.

Millar EA: Observations on the surgical management of osteogenesis imperfecta, *Clin Orthop* 159:154, 1981.

Moorefield WG Jr, Miller GR: Aftermath of osteogenesis imperfecta: the disease in adulthood, *J Bone Joint Surg* 62A:113, 1980.

Morel R, Houghton GR: Pneumatic trouser splints in the treatment of severe osteogenesis imperfecta, *Acta Orthop Scand* 53:547, 1982.

Murray D, Young BH: Osteogenesis imperfecta treated by fixation with intramedullary rod, *South Med J* 53:1142, 1960.

Nicholas RW, James P: Telescoping intramedullary stabilization of the lower extremities for severe OI, *J Pediatr Orthop* 10:219, 1990.

Nielsen HE, Pedersen U, Hansen HH, Elbrønd O: Serum calcitonin and bone mineral content in patients with osteogenesis imperfecta, *Acta Orthop Scand* 50:639, 1979.

Niemann KMW: Surgical treatment of the tibia in osteogenesis imperfecta, *Clin Orthop* 159:134, 1981.

Papagelopoulos PJ, Morrey BF: Hip and knee replacement in osteogenesis imperfecta, *J Bone Joint Surg* 75A:572, 1993.

Paterson CR, McAllion S, Miller R: Osteogenesis imperfecta with dominant inheritance and normal sclerae, *J Bone Joint Surg* 65B:35, 1983.

Peterson LRA: Little people. In Morrey BF, ed: *Joint replacement arthroplasty*, New York, 1991, Churchill Livingstone.

Porat S, Heller E, Seidman DS, et al: Functional results of operations in OI: elongating and nonelongating rods, *J Pediatr Orthop* 11:200, 1991.

Ring D, Jupiter JB, Labropoulos PK, et al: Treatment of deformity of the lower limb in adults who have osteogenesis imperfecta, *J Bone Joint Surg* 78A:220, 1996.

Rodriguez RP, Bailey RW: Internal fixation of the femur in patients with osteogenesis imperfecta, *Clin Orthop* 159:126, 1981.

Root L: Upper limb surgery in osteogenesis imperfecta, *Clin Orthop* 159:141, 1981.

Russell TA, Taylor JC, LaVelle DG: Russell-Taylor interlocking intramedullary nails, Memphis, 1985, Richards Manufacturing.

Ryöppy S, Alberty A, Kaitila I: Early semiclosed intramedullary stabilization in osteogenesis imperfecta, *J Pediatr Orthop* 7:139, 1987.

Shapiro F: Consequences of an osteogenesis imperfecta diagnosis for survival and ambulation. *J Pediatr Orthop* 5:456, 1985.

Sillence D: Osteogenesis imperfecta: an expanding panorama of variants, *Clin Orthop* 159:11, 1981.

Sillence DO, Senn A, Danks DM: Genetic heterogeneity in osteogenesis imperfecta. *J Med Genet* 16:101, 1979.

Sofield HA, Millar EA: Fragmentation, realignment, and intramedullary rod fixation of deformities of the long bones in children: a 10-year appraisal, *J Bone Joint Surg* 41A:1371, 1959.

Tiley F, Albright JA: Osteogenesis imperfecta: treatment by multiple osteotomy and intramedullary rod insertion, *J Bone Joint Surg* 55A:701, 1973.

Villanueva AR, Frost HM: Bone formation in human osteogenesis imperfecta, measured by tetracycline bone labeling, *Acta Orthop Scand* 41:531, 1970.

Weil UH: Osteogenesis imperfecta: historical background, *Clin Orthop* 159:6, 1981.

Werner P, Metz L, Dubowski F: Nursing care of an osteogenesis imperfecta infant and child, *Clin Orthop* 159:108, 1981.

Widmann RF, Bitan FD, Laplaza FJ, et al: Spinal deformity, pulmonary compromise, and quality of life in osteogenesis imperfecta, *Spine* 15:1673, 1999.

Wilkinson JM, Scott BW, Clarke AM, Bell MJ: Surgical stabilisation of the lower limb in osteogenesis imperfecta using the Sheffield Telescopic Intramedullary Rod System, *J Bone Joint Surg* 80B:999, 1998.

Williams PF: Fragmentation and rodding in osteogenesis imperfecta, *J Bone Joint Surg* 47B:23, 1965.

Williams PF, Cole WHJ, Bailey RW, et al: Current aspects of the surgical treatment of osteogenesis imperfecta, *Clin Orthop* 96:288, 1973.

Wynne-Davies R, Gormley J: Clinical and genetic patterns in osteogenesis imperfecta, *Clin Orthop* 159:26, 1981.

Zionts LE, Ebramzadeh E, Stott NS: Complications in the use of the Bailey-Dubow extensible nail, *Clin Orthop* 348:186, 1998.

Ziv I, Rang M, Hoffman HJ: Paraplegia in osteogenesis imperfecta: a case report, *J Bone Joint Surg* 65B:184, 1983.

DWARFISM

Abe M, Shirai H, Okamoto M, Onomura T: Lengthening of the forearm by callus distraction, *J Hand Surg* 21B:151, 1996.

Aldegheri R: Distraction osteogenesis for lengthening of the tibia in patients who have limb-length discrepancy or short stature, *J Bone Joint Surg* 81A:624, 1999.

Bailey JA II: Orthopedic aspects of achondroplasia, *J Bone Joint Surg* 52A:1285, 1970.

Beals RK: Orthopedic aspects of the XO (Turner's) syndrome, *Clin Orthop* 97:19, 1973.

Beighton P, Craig J: Atlanto-axial subluxation in the Morquio syndrome: report of a case, *J Bone Joint Surg* 55B:478, 1973.

Borden SA, Kaplan FS, Fallon MD, et al: Metatrophic dwarfism, *J Bone Joint Surg* 69A:174, 1987.

De Bastiani G, Aldegheri R, Renzi-Brivio L, Trivella G: Limb lengthening by callus distraction (callotasis), *J Pediatr Orthop* 7:129, 1987.

Ganel A, Horoszowski H, Kamhin M, et al: Leg lengthening in achondroplastic children, *Clin Orthop* 144:194, 1979.

Goldberg MJ: Orthopedic aspects of bone dysplasias, *Orthop Clin North Am* 7:445, 1976.

Hollister DW, Lachman RS: Diastrophic dwarfism, *Clin Orthop* 114:61, 1976.

Ilizarov GA: The tension-stress effect on the genesis and growth of tissues. II. The influence of rate and frequency of distraction, *Clin Orthop* 239:263, 1989.

Kopits SE: Orthopedic complications of dwarfism, *Clin Orthop* 114: 153, 1976.

McKusick VA: *Heritable disorders of connective tissue*, ed 4, St Louis, 1972, Mosby.

Noonan KJ, Leyes M, Forriol F, Canadell J: Distraction osteogenesis of the lower extremity with use of monolateral external fixation: a study of 261 femoral and tibiae, *J Bone Joint Surg* 80A:793, 1998.

Paley D: Current techniques of limb lengthening, *J Pediatr Orthop* 8:73, 1988.

Polo A, Aldegheri R, Zambito A, et al: Lower-limb lengthening in short stature: an electrophysiological and clinical assessment of peripheral nerve function, *J Bone Joint Surg* 79B:1014, 1997.

Price CT: Metaphyseal and physeal lengthening, *AAOS Instr Course Lect* 38:331, 1989.

Scott CI Jr: Achondroplastic and hypochondroplastic dwarfism, *Clin Orthop* 114:18, 1976.

Simon D, Touati G, Prieur AM et al: Growth hormone treatment of short stature and metabolic dysfunction in juvenile chronic arthritis, *Acta Paediatr Suppl* 88:100, 1999.

Spranger JW, Langer LO Jr: Spondyloepiphyseal dysplasia congenita, *Radiology* 94:313, 1970.

Wagner H: Operative lengthening of the femur, *Clin Orthop* 136:125, 1978.

TRAUMATIC EPIPHYSEAL ARREST FROM BRIDGE OF BONE

Alford BA, Oshman DG, Sussman MD: Radiographic appearances following surgical correction of the partially fused epiphyseal plate, *Skeletal Radiol* 15:146, 1986.

Barash ES, Siffert ES: The potential for growth of experimentally produced hemiepiphysis, *J Bone Joint Surg* 48A:1548, 1966.

Birch JG, Herring JA, Wenger DR: Surgical anatomy of selected physes, *J Pediatr Orthop* 4:224, 1984.

Bright RW: Operative correction of partial epiphyseal plate closure by osseous bridge resection and silicone-rubber implant: an experimental study in dogs, *J Bone Joint Surg* 56A:655, 1974.

Canadell J, DePablos J: Breaking bony bridges by physeal distraction: a new approach, *Int Orthop* 9:223, 1985.

Carlson WO, Wenger DR: A mapping method to prepare for surgical excision of partial physeal arrest, *J Pediatr Orthop* 4:232, 1984.

Craig JG, Cramer KE, Cody DD, et al: Premature partial closure and other deformities of the growth plate: MR imaging and three-dimensional modeling, *Radiology* 210:835, 1999.

Friendenberg ZB: Reaction of the epiphysis to partial surgical resection, *J Bone Joint Surg* 39A:332, 1957.

Jowman-Giles R, Trochei M, Yeaters K, et al: Partial growth plate closure: apex view of bone scan, *J Pediatr Orthop* 5:109, 1985.

Klassen RA, Peterson HA: Excision of physeal bars: the Mayo Clinic experience, *Orthop Trans* 6:65, 1982 (abstract).

Langenskiöld A: Partial closure of epiphyseal plate: principles of treatment, *Int Orthop* 2:95, 1978.

Langenskiöld A: Surgical treatment of partial closure of the growth plate, *J Pediatr Orthop* 1:3, 1981.

Langenskiöld A, Videman T, Nevalainen T: The fate of fat transplants in operations for partial closure of the growth plate, *J Bone Joint Surg* 68B:234, 1986.

Lee EH, Gao GX, Bose K: Management of partial growth arrest: physis, fat, or Silastic? *J Pediatr Orthop* 13:368, 1993.

Lennox DW, Goldner RD, Sussman MD: Cartilage as an interposition material to prevent transphyseal bone bridge formation: an experimental model, *J Pediatr Orthop* 3:207, 1983.

Odgen JA: Current concepts review: the evaluation and treatment of partial physeal arrest, *J Bone Joint Surg* 69A:1297, 1987.

Odgen JA: *Skeletal injury in the child*, ed 2, Philadelphia, 1989, Lea & Febiger.

Osterman K: Operative elimination of partial epiphyseal closure: an experimental study, *Acta Orthop Scand* (suppl)147:1, 1972.

Peterson HA: Operative correction of post-fracture arrest of the epiphyseal plate: case report with 10-year follow-up, *J Bone Joint Surg* 62A:1018, 1980

Peterson HA: Partial growth arrest and its treatment, *J Pediatr Orthop* 4:246, 1984.

Peterson HA, Burkhart SS: Compression injury of the epiphyseal growth plate: fact or fiction? *J Pediatr Orthop* 1:377, 1981.

Porat S, Nyska M, Nyska A, Fields S: Assessment of bony bridge by computed tomography: experimental model in the rabbit and clinical application. *J Pediatr Orthop* 7:155, 1987.

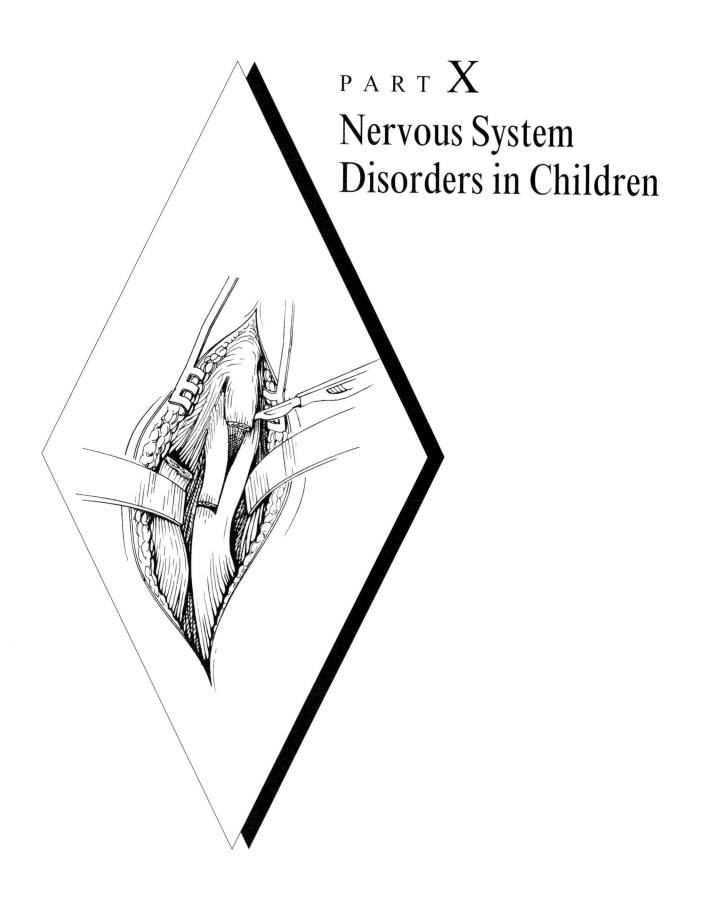

PART X
Nervous System Disorders in Children

CHAPTER

30 Cerebral Palsy

William C. Warner, Jr.

This chapter discusses cerebral palsy that occurs prenatally and perinatally, acquired cerebral palsy in children, and the treatment of adult patients recovering from cerebrovascular accident, or stroke.

Cerebral palsy is defined as a disorder of movement and posture caused by a nonprogressive defect or lesion in an immature brain. In the neurological literature, cerebral palsy is referred to as a "static encephalopathy." An immature brain attempts to heal itself but falls short, and the result is a fixed anatomical deficit that can lead to progressive deformity in a growing child or young adult from constant imbalance of muscle forces. At this time neurological injury cannot be reversed, and the role of orthopaedic surgeons in the treatment of children and adults with cerebral palsy is to improve function

and prevent the development of deformities by prescribing braces and by reestablishing the balance of muscle forces through soft tissue releases, transfers, or bony reconstructions. Although lesions that occur in the upper cervical cord just below the decussation of the pyramids do not technically fit the definition, they can be treated like cerebral palsy.

Children with cerebral palsy make up the largest group of pediatric patients with neuromuscular disorders in the United States. The occurrence of cerebral palsy in various countries and localities ranges from 0.6 to 5.9 patients per 1000 live births, varying according to the amount and type of prenatal care, the socioeconomic conditions of the parents, the environment, and the type of obstetrical and pediatric care the mother and child receive. In the United States the occurrence is approximately 2 per 1000 live births; there are approximately 25,000 new patients with cerebral palsy each year and approximately 400,000 children afflicted with cerebral palsy at any given time.

Neonatal intensive care units are saving more children of lower gestational age and lower birth weight than previously, resulting in a greater proportion of prematurely born infants who subsequently develop cerebral palsy. Infants with a birth weight of less than 1500 grams are more likely to have cerebral palsy, with a prevalence of 60 per 1000 compared with an overall prevalence of 3 per 1000 infants with normal birth weight. Although there is an increased prevalence of cerebral palsy in infants with a very low birth weight, the majority of these infants do not have cerebral palsy.

Cerebral palsy can be divided into six physiological types: spastic, athetoid, ataxic, hypotonic, rigid, and mixed. Spastic cerebral palsy is the most common type, occurring in about 70% to 80% of patients with cerebral palsy. Athetoid cerebral palsy is the next most common type, accounting for about 10% to 15% of cases. Athetoid cerebral palsy is further subdivided into five groups, each characterized by a type of abnormal posture movement: tension athetosis, dystonia, choreiform, ballismus, and rigidity.

Fewer than 5% of patients with cerebral palsy have the primary ataxia type. The mixed type has been found to account for an increasing number of patients, probably more than 10%, as we become better in detecting the various clinical types of abnormal movement and posture. As the immature brain develops, the clinical manifestations of the type of movement or posture disorder change.

The lesions in the brain that cause abnormality in movement or posture occur primarily in the following four areas: the cerebral cortex (spasticity), the midbrain or base of the brain (athetosis), the cerebellum (ataxia), and widespread brain involvement (mixed). Locating the causative lesion in the brain is easier now than in the past. Cerebral blood flow studies, computed tomography (CT), neuroultrasonography, and magnetic resonance imaging (MRI) can pinpoint the exact geographical location of the brain insult and at times define the type as well. Even with these methods of imaging the central nervous system, functional outcomes cannot be reliably predicted on the basis of neuroimaging studies performed during infancy. Therefore the development of a child who has had a central nervous system insult should be followed, and the child should be treated as indicated to maximize functional potential.

Etiology

The lesion responsible for cerebral palsy may have its origin in the prenatal, natal, or postnatal period. The prenatal period lasts from conception until the onset of labor, the natal period from the onset of labor until the actual time of delivery, and the postnatal period from the time of delivery until brain maturation at 2½ to 3 years, when a large part of myelinization has occurred. Some investigators have defined the perinatal period as the interval extending from the onset of labor to the seventh day after birth, when stability with the outside environment has been achieved.

Many lesions that cause cerebral palsy occur in the perinatal period, but increasing evidence shows that prenatal causes occur more often than suspected. Most reports show that at least 30% to 40% of cases of cerebral palsy can be related to prenatal causes. Nelson and Elleberg found that maternal mental retardation, birth weight below 2001 g, and fetal malformation were among the leading predictors.

PRENATAL CAUSES

Several prenatal causes have been implicated in the development of cerebral palsy, including maternal and pregnancy-specific problems.

Intrauterine and TORCH (*to*xoplasmosis, *r*ubella, *c*ytomegalovirus, and *h*erpes) infections may lead to cerebral palsy, which can be severe in some cases, especially if the infections occurred in the mother during the first and second trimesters of pregnancy. Children who were exposed to rubella in the first or second trimester usually have other congenital anomalies as well, including cataracts, congenital heart defects, deafness, and mental retardation. Infants born to mothers with metabolic disturbances, such as diabetes mellitus and thyroid abnormalities, or resultant toxemia, are at higher risk for cerebral palsy, as are infants born to mothers with mental retardation or epilepsy.

Anoxia, another cause of cerebral palsy, results in the prenatal period from various causes, including a ruptured placenta, placental infarction, maternal pneumonia, or cardiorespiratory disease. However, the incidence has been significantly reduced by fetal monitoring and improved obstetrical care. Erythroblastosis fetalis, which is caused by the destruction of fetal red blood cells by maternal antibodies with subsequent damage to the central nervous system, was formerly a common prenatal cause of cerebral palsy. However, the use of RhoGAM injection has made erythroblastosis fetalis rare in developed countries.

Chemical or alcohol dependency in a mother during pregnancy has been shown to increase the incidence of cerebral palsy. Children born to mothers addicted to "crack" cocaine during pregnancy, although not grossly spastic, may develop a mild but persistent hypotonicity. These children frequently are referred to early intervention programs and require persistent physical therapy to prevent the development of contractures; in some cases they require bracing and surgery.

Another cause of cerebral palsy in the prenatal period is a congenital brain defect. Children with a brain malformation, such as an absence of the corpus callosum, show unusual and mixed patterns of cerebral palsy.

NATAL CAUSES

Natal causes for cerebral palsy are trauma or asphyxia occurring during labor. Oxytocin augmentation, cord prolapse, and breech presentation have been associated with increased

Table 30-1	Grading System for Intraventricular Hemorrhage	
Grade	**Pathology**
I	Bleeding confined to germinal matrix
II	Bleeding extends into ventricles
III	Bleeding is complicated by dilatation of ventricles
IV	Bleeding extends into substance of brain

From Pellegrino L, Dormans JP: Definitions, etiology, and epidemiology of cerebral palsy. In Pellegrino L, Dormans JP, eds: *Caring for children with cerebral palsy,* Baltimore, 1998, Paul Brookes.

risk of cerebral palsy but only if accompanied by low Apgar scores. Current medical evidence, however, indicates that labor and delivery events account for a relatively small portion of patients with cerebral palsy. Nelson reported that asphyxia alone accounted for less than 10% of patients with cerebral palsy and that most patients with cerebral palsy had no signs of asphyxia in the perinatal period.

Prematurity is the most common natal cause of cerebral palsy. Low birth weight (less than 2268 g) and cerebral palsy have been known to be causally related. The blood vessels in a premature infant are fragile and subject to rupture, which can lead to periventricular hemorrhages. Periventricular hemorrhages are graded from I to IV according to severity (Table 30-1). Grades III and IV are associated with an increased risk for neurological sequelae, including hydrocephalus, mental retardation, and cerebral palsy. Approximately 10% of cerebral palsy patients weigh less than 1500 g at birth. In this low birth weight group, the risk of having cerebral palsy is 60 in 1000 compared with 3 in 1000 in infants weighing more than 2400 g or appropriate-for-gestational age. Even with the increased risk of cerebral palsy in premature infants, prematurity cannot solely be blamed for most of the cases, since 60% to 65% of afflicted children are born at full term.

POSTNATAL CAUSES

Encephalitis and meningitis can lead to a permanent brain injury, resulting in cerebral palsy. During the acute and postacute stages of encephalitis, motor deficit may progress with increasing involvement. After the acute stage, scarring ensues in the brain. The neurological lesion ultimately becomes stable, as does the motor deficit, unless infection recurs. Traumatic head injuries, caused by motor vehicle accidents and child abuse, account for a significant number of cases of cerebral palsy that develop in the postnatal period. Cerebral palsy resulting from trauma or associated hemorrhage usually is spastic. Patients with neurological disorders arising from trauma tend to improve with time, often for a year or more after the injury. In a study of children who suffered brain trauma, Brink and Hoffer related the prognosis for recovery directly to the level and length of unconsciousness after the initial insult. Deep coma for longer than 1 week results in a poor prognosis for any significant recovery.

Asphyxia from near-drowning or from being trapped in an enclosed space may result in disorders of movement that are often choreiform or severely rigid. Toddlers and teenage boys are the two largest groups that suffer brain injury from near-drowning accidents. Anoxic encephalopathy from near-drowning creates a hypertonic pattern seen with extreme rigidity, making it difficult to develop a seating system for these patients.

Surgery in patients injured through anoxic encephalopathy should be approached with caution because a simple release or correction of one deformity can lead to a rapid reversal of deformity from profound hypertonicity of the muscles.

Removal of brain tumors can result in a motor deficit, but after the immediate postoperative period, any remaining motor injury can be expected to be nonprogressive in patients with no residual disease. However, patients who have received aggressive chemotherapy and radiation therapy not only may develop static motor patterns as a result of the disease and surgery, but also may show progressive deterioration as a result of nervous system necrosis from radiation or chemotherapy. Patients who have been treated for brain tumors usually have unusual patterns of motor deficits and require individualized treatment.

The incidence of postnatal cerebral palsy arising from toxins, such as lead, had declined but is still seen as a cause for cerebral palsy.

Clinical Types

Most patients with cerebral palsy are found to have recognizable patterns of movement disorders, depending on what area of the brain is involved. This has allowed classification of cerebral palsy based on the neuropathic type of motor dysfunction. However, the common patterns of movement disorders that characterize cerebral palsy may not manifest until a child is 12 to 18 months of age. Often the child will be hypotonic and physically and developmentally delayed during the first year of life. Sometimes the only physical sign of cerebral palsy during the first year of life may be persistent infantile reflexes.

The most common clinical type of cerebral palsy is spasticity resulting from an injury to the pyramidal tracts in the immature brain. Spasticity is a state of increased tension in the muscles when they are passively lengthened, and it is caused by an exaggeration of the normal muscle stretch reflex. Spasticity is velocity dependent in that the faster the stretch is initiated, the greater the response to it. An exaggerated stretch reflex is pathognomonic of spasticity. In an exaggerated stretch reflex, resistance is felt as a sudden passive movement of the muscle, followed by relaxation of the muscle. This tightening and relaxation may become cyclical, with a fast passive stretch of the muscle resulting in clonus. Although patients with spasticity initially may be hypotonic, not all patients with hypotonia have spasticity. Most orthopaedic surgical procedures are designed for patients with spasticity.

The second most common clinical type of cerebral palsy is athetosis. Athetosis is a type of dyskinesia (abnormal movement caused by an extrapyramidal brain lesion). The movement disorder is one of continuous motion, and hypotonia may or may not be present. Joint contractures are not common in this type of cerebral palsy. Tendon lengthening in children with athetosis often is unpredictable, and can result create an opposite deformity that is more difficult to treat. Athetotic cerebral palsy can be subdivided into the following five patterns.

Tension athetosis. This condition results from deposition of bilirubin in the infant's basal ganglia. In the past this was more commonly the result of erythroblastosis fetalis, which was almost completely eradicated in developed countries over the past several generations; however, this condition is being seen again. Patients with tension athetosis are hypertonic but not hyperreflexive. There are no signs of clonus or other signs of spasticity; the tension in these muscles can literally be "shaken out." Associated problems in patients with tension athetosis include deafness and absence of an upward gaze.

Dystonic athetosis. These patients are in a continuous, tortuous, slow, twisting type of motion. All extremities, as well as the neck and trunk, tend to be involved.

Choreiform athetosis. More common than dystonic athetosis, this pattern is characterized by continual movement of the patient's wrist, fingers, ankles, toes, and tongue.

Dramatic ballismus athetosis. This type is characterized by trunk flailing that persists throughout the wakened state. These patients can injure themselves or their caregivers by this continuous dramatic movement of the trunk and proximal extremities.

Rigid athetosis. Patients with this type are the most hypertonic of all patients with cerebral palsy, yet there are no signs of spasticity and no evidence of clonus or hyperreflexia. These patients have extreme muscle stiffness, which may be of the "lead pipe" or "cogwheel" variety. When these patients undergo tendon release or neurectomy, the orthopaedic surgeon must use extreme caution so as not to create a fixed reversal of the deformity by overweakening an agonist and allowing the muscles' antagonists to drive the patient's rigidity in the opposite direction.

Ataxic cerebral palsy is uncommon and is probably the most misdiagnosed pattern or clinical type. It is a disturbance of coordinated movement and is usually the result of cerebellar dysfunction. Children with this disorder frequently are misdiagnosed as having spastic quadriplegia. Ataxia must be distinguished from spastic quadriplegia because tendon-lengthening procedures may result in a less functional gait that requires greater energy expenditure in the ataxic patient. Children with primary ataxia can improve over time, and although they may walk late, they often develop a near-normal gait and are able to function in an essentially normal manner.

Infants with hypotonic cerebral palsy are characterized by having low muscle tone and normal or increased deep tendon reflexes. Often hypotonia will last for 2 to 3 years and is most often a stage through which an infant passes before developing

overt spasticity or ataxia. The brain lesion initially may be masked by lack of myelination of the neural pathways.

The final clinical type of cerebral palsy is mixed cerebral palsy. Children with mixed cerebral palsy have both pyramidal and extrapyramidal motor control abnormalities. Patients with mixed cerebral palsy can have variable amounts of spasticity, athetosis, or ataxia.

GEOGRAPHICAL (ANATOMICAL) CLASSIFICATION

The geographical location, or the anatomical region of the body involved with the movement disorder, should be identified. Most of the time these geographical classifications refer to patients with spasticity; however, other clinical types, such as athetosis, may involve specific geographical locations rather than overall involvement.

Monoplegia

With monoplegia, only one extremity, either upper or lower, is affected. This is an extremely uncommon type of paresis and usually is seen after meningitis. Often the patient will have hemiplegia but the involvement of the ipsilateral upper or lower extremity is so mild that the patient will be classified as having monoplegia.

Hemiplegia

In hemiplegia, both extremities on the same side are affected and the upper extremity typically is more affected than the lower one. This motor pattern results from bleeding in the middle cerebral artery involving the central portion of one hemisphere. Because the sensory strip as well as the motor strip is involved, patients with spastic hemiplegia are found to have sensory disorders in the involved limbs. These sensory disorders do not necessarily involve pain or an elevated temperature, but rather may involve fine sensation. Absence of fine sensation in the upper extremity is predictive of a poor result if extensive upper extremity surgery is contemplated. Associated disorders in patients with hemiplegia include seizures and leg-length discrepancy of 1 to 2 cm shortening on the involved lower extremity.

Paraplegia

Much of the older literature on cerebral palsy lists spastic paraplegia as cerebral palsy prematurity. This is incorrect because these children actually have diplegia with the upper extremities involved, although not as severely as the lower extremities. In true spastic paraplegia, the patient's upper extremity gross and fine motor controls are completely normal. True spastic paraplegia is very rare, and if seen, a family history should be obtained to make sure there are no other causes, such as familial spastic paraplegia. Also, examination of the spine, including an MRI, is indicated to help determine whether the cerebral palsy has either a neoplastic cause or a mechanical cause, such as a diastematomyelia. These two diagnoses are not considered forms of cerebral palsy.

Diplegia

Spastic diplegia cerebral palsy is more often seen in premature infants, although not all premature infants develop spastic diplegia. Spastic diplegia results from a loss of blood flow in the region of the periventricular areas. Both lower extremities are always involved to a greater extent than the upper extremities. Physical examination of a child with spastic diplegia readily demonstrates gross and fine motor abnormalities in the upper limbs, although they may not be as prominent as in the lower extremities. Intelligence is usually normal.

Triplegia

Spastic triplegia cerebral palsy probably does not exist. In most patients the physical examination usually will reveal a pattern of three overly affected extremities and one minimally affected extremity. These patients can be very difficult to treat surgically because of the lack of symmetry between the upper extremities and the lower extremities and the difficulty in maintaining overall muscle balance.

Quadriplegia

In quadriplegia all four extremities are involved equally. Typically, the patient has neck and trunk control.

Double Hemiplegia

This type of geographical pattern is seen in patients who have sustained intraventricular bleeding in the middle cerebral artery in both hemispheres of the brain. Once again, the upper extremities are more involved than the lower extremities, and the treatment-associated problems are similar to those for patients with hemiplegia.

Total Body Involvement

In patients with total body involvement, all extremities are involved, as are the trunk and neck muscles. Frequently these patients require total care and cannot assist at all in the activities of daily living. They usually have problems with drooling, dysarthria, and dysphagia. These patients usually require specialized seating systems for care.

ASSOCIATED HANDICAPPING CONDITIONS

Almost all patients with a motor or postural deficit have some other impairment or disability. Many children with cerebral palsy have associated impairments or disabilities that have a greater effect on their ultimate prognosis.

Approximately 40% of all children with cerebral palsy have some abnormality of vision or oculomotor control, and at least 7% have a severe visual deficit. Commonly encountered visual impairments are myopia, amblyopia, strabismus, visual field defects, and cortical blindness. Because of the high incidence of visual problems associated with cerebral palsy, a visual screening examination should be part of the treatment protocol.

Hearing loss has been reported to occur in 10% to 25% of cerebral palsy patients. Seizures occur in about 30%, and are most often seen with patients who have hemiplegia and quadriplegia with mental retardation or in postnatally acquired syndromes.

Bulbar involvement can occur with drooling, difficulty swallowing, and speech impairment. Gastrointestinal problems, such as constipation, fecal impaction, impaired swallowing, esophageal reflux and hiatal hernia, often are seen in the more severely involved. Some of these impairments can lead to aspiration pneumonia and profound feeding problems resulting in malnutrition. Gastroesophageal reflux can sometimes be managed medically but often a surgical fundoplication is needed. Correction of associated malnutrition is best done by enteral feeding augmentation, but if this is not adequate or feasible then a gastrostomy or jejunostomy may be needed to correct the child's malnutrition. Bone mineral density has been reported to be decreased in children with spastic cerebral palsy. The two most important factors related to the decrease in bone mineral density were ambulatory status and nutritional status.

Emotional problems add to these handicapping conditions. The attitudes of the parents, the siblings, the community, and the treatment team are all important. The child's self-image plays an important role, especially during adolescence, when he is unable to keep up with his peers. As young adulthood is reached, concerns about employment, self-care, sexual gratification, marriage, and childbearing all cause anxiety and may lead to emotional instability.

Hoffer states that "the two most crucial abilities for any human being are the ability to think and the ability to communicate." Communication is important if one has cognitive ability. Communication aids often lead to the discovery of a normal cognitive ability in a child thought to be mentally retarded. In the absence of speech, some alternative for communication must be found so that cognitive abilities can function. As orthopaedic surgeons, we often place too much emphasis on the ability to walk and to do so in a more normal manner rather than on the habilitation of the child as a whole.

Treatment

Cerebral palsy is a nonprogressive neurological lesion. The brain lesion that causes the deficit in voluntary muscle control and posture, balance abnormalities, and disorders in tone remains constant. Even though the brain lesion is constant the natural history of cerebral palsy is not static. Growth and maturation of the child will often result in changing musculoskeletal problems.

The aim of management in cerebral palsy is to increase the patient's abilities as much as possible and minimize his impairments or disabilities. Attempts should be made to increase the patient's emotional maturity, physical independence, cognitive abilities, and speech or communication and to create a socioeconomic independence, as well as to create or improve his sense of self-worth. These may be idealistic goals, but can be tempered with a realistic appraisal of the patient's assorted abilities.

Adults with cerebral palsy rate the following, in order of

preference, for improving their quality of life: (1) education and communication, (2) activities of daily living, (3) mobility, and (4) ambulation. The focus of orthopaedic treatment has usually been on ambulation, with little attention to the other categories.

The goals of treatment may vary depending on the physiological and anatomic type of cerebral palsy and the amount of neurological involvement. Treatment goals should be individualized and be consistent with the expected benefits. For a patient with severe spastic quadriplegia, improving nursing care, hygiene, and sitting balance in a wheelchair should be the primary objective. In a patient with less severe spastic hemiplegia, the treatment goals may be to improve gait and make ambulation more energy efficient.

Numerous tests have been devised to predict and measure improvement in patients with cerebral palsy. A number of proven tests that measure these normal milestones are available, and we use them to compare a handicapped child's achievements with those of normal children. Some of the tests currently in use are the Gesell Developmental Scales, the Bayley Scales of Infant Development, the Denver Developmental Screening Test, and the Milani-Comparetti Motor Development Test.

Primitive reflex patterns of motor activity that are outgrown as the normal nervous system matures are demonstrated in children with cerebral palsy for longer periods of time after birth, and some remain permanently. Some cerebrocortical reactions needed for standing and walking in a normal child may develop fully, late, or not at all in a child with cerebral palsy. Other reflex patterns, on which integrated and skillful function of the motor system seems to be built, may be delayed or may never appear. In a child with cerebral palsy, these and other patterns of primitive motor activity should be sought and used to determine the patient's neurological age. By comparing this age with the child's chronological age, a neurological quotient can be established that may influence treatment and the prognosis for improvement. The continued presence of primitive reflex patterns can contribute to the development of deformities.

Johnson, Zuck, and Wingate; and Ingram, Withers, and Speltz developed tests that measure the rate at which motor and social skills are acquired by patients with cerebral palsy. By regular and repeated testing, they were able to assess the extent of the handicap, determine whether it was being influenced by the treatment program, and make tentative predictions concerning the future development of the patient. Ingram, Withers, and Speltz found that when the motor quotient (motor age times 100, divided by the chronological age) was 15 or lower, independent walking was unlikely, but when it was 25 or higher, walking could be expected. Using a test of motor performance similar to that described by Ingram, Withers, and Speltz, Beals studied 93 spastic paraplegic or diplegic patients followed to the age of 7 years or older. In an attempt to determine the severity of the handicap in a given patient, he developed a "severity index," which is a statement of the motor age in months at the chronological age of 3 years. Using this index, Beals attempted to predict the ultimate motor perfor-

mance of the individual patient and thus to establish realistic goals in treatment.

Paine observed that the presence of tonic neck reflexes usually is incompatible with independent standing balance and with the ability to make the alternating movements of the lower extremities necessary for walking. In his experience, if a child learns to sit alone before the age of 2 years, usually he will learn to walk independently. If a child learns to sit alone between the ages of 2 and 4 years, the likelihood of his learning to stand and walk independently is about 50%. If a child has not learned to sit alone before the age of 4 years, rarely will he learn to stand or walk without support. Finally, if a child has not learned to walk before the age of 8 years and if he does not have severe contractures that would otherwise prevent walking, it is unlikely he will ever learn to walk. Molnar and Gordon found that in children younger than 2 years of age independent sitting was not a good predictor for walking ability, but that after age 4 years the inability to sit predicted nonambulation.

Bleck studied the incidence and persistence of certain pathological reflexes in children with cerebral palsy and developed prognostic signs based on the presence or absence of infantile reflexes. A favorable sign in the prognosis for walking is sitting by the age of 2 years. One point was assigned to each automatic reflex definitely present that should not be so at 1 year of age, and one point was given for each automatic reflex normally present by 1 year but absent. A score of 2 or higher indicated a poor prognosis for walking, a score of 1 resulted in a guarded prognosis, and a score of 0 resulted in a good prognosis. In Bleck's experience, children with spastic hemiplegia usually walked by 21 months; most children with cerebral palsy usually walk by 7 years of age.

Poor prognostic signs for walking are (1) an imposable asymmetrical tonic neck reflex (Fig. 30-1, A); (2) a persistent Moro reflex (Fig. 30-1, B) (a loud noise or a sudden jerk of the table causes the upper limbs to extend away from the side of the body and then to come together in an embracing pattern); (3) a strong extensor thrust on vertical suspension (Fig. 30-1, C) (when the child is held upright by the armpits, the lower extremities stiffen out straight); (4) a persistent neck-righting reflex (Fig. 30-1, D) (when the head is turned, the shoulder, trunk, pelvis, and lower limbs follow the turned head); and (5) absence of the normal parachute reaction (Fig. 30-1, E) after 11 months (when the child is lifted horizontally by the waist and suddenly lowered to the table, normally the arms and hands extend to the table as though to protect from the fall).

Bleck also has analyzed pathological reflexes in children 1 to 8 years old. The reflexes recorded in the study were the symmetrical tonic neck reflex (Fig. 30-1, F), neck-righting reflex, foot placement reflex (Fig. 30-1, G), asymmetrical tonic neck reflex, Moro reflex, parachute reflex, and positive supporting reaction. Figure 30-2 shows the incidence of these various reflexes, on a scale of 0 to 8, in children with cerebral palsy who have not walked by age 8 years. The supporting reaction reflex is positive in practically all children who do not walk, the parachute reflex is absent in seven eighths of them, and the Moro and asymmetrical tonic reflexes are present in

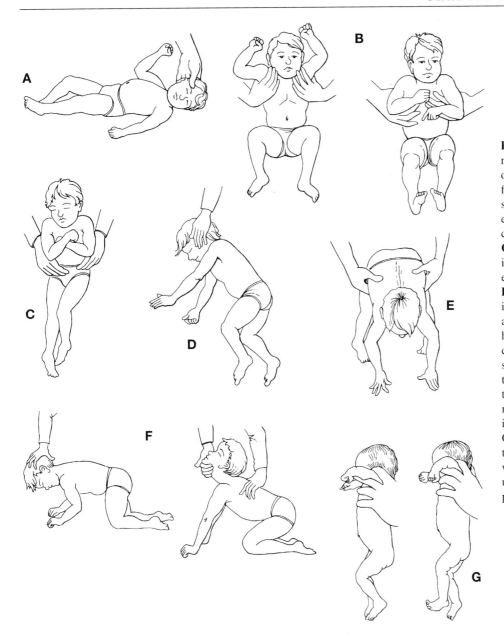

Fig. 30-1 **A,** Asymmetrical tonic neck reflex: as head is turned to one side, contralateral arm and knee flex. **B,** Moro reflex: as neck is suddenly extended, upper limbs extend away from body and then come together in embracing pattern. **C,** Extensor thrust reflex: as child is held upright by armpits, lower extremities stiffen out straight. **D,** Neck-righting reflex: as head is turned, shoulders, trunk, pelvis, and lower extremities follow turned head. **E,** Parachute reaction: as child is suspended at waist and suddenly lowered forward toward table, arms and hands extend to table in protective manner. **F,** Symmetrical tonic neck reflex: as neck is flexed, arms flex and legs extend. Opposite occurs as neck is extended. **G,** Foot placement reaction: when top of foot is stroked by underside of flat surface, child places foot on surface.

three fourths of these children. The persistence of these infantile automatisms indicates extensive, severe brain damage and a poor prognosis for ambulation, self-help, and the performance of activities of daily living.

GAIT ANALYSIS

Gait analysis has become a useful tool in the evaluation and treatment of patients with cerebral palsy. Evaluation should consist of a detailed physical examination, including documentation of range of motion of the hips, knees, and ankles. Visual assessment of the patient's gait should be done with attention to hips, knees, and ankles. Videotapes of the patient's gait may assist in this evaluation. Three-dimensional gait analyses give accurate and objective records of the gait. Joint movements (kinematics) are measured by tracking markers placed on the

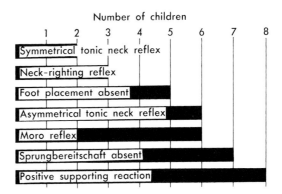

Fig. 30-2 Incidence of pathological reflexes in children with cerebral palsy who have not walked by 8 years of age (see text). (Courtesy EE Bleck, MD; from Goldner JL: *Instr Course Lect* 20:20, 1971.)

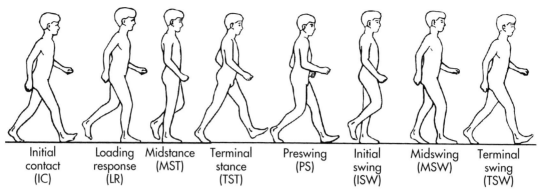

| Initial contact (IC) | Loading response (LR) | Midstance (MST) | Terminal stance (TST) | Preswing (PS) | Initial swing (ISW) | Midswing (MSW) | Terminal swing (TSW) |

Fig. 30-3   Gait cycle. Position of limbs at each phase represents general instantaneous position, because each joint is moving continually through each phase. (From Gage JR, DeLuca PA, Renshaw TS: *Instr Course Lect* 45:491, 1996.)

lower limbs with strategically placed cameras. Data from these recordings is used to construct a computer model of the patient's gait. Moments around each joint during the gait cycle can be calculated using a force plate embedded in the floor. Surface electrodes over major muscle groups can be used to detect muscle activity during specific segments of the gait cycle. With gait analysis, the individual components of the gait cycle can be investigated for pathology (Fig. 30-3). This is an extremely useful tool in the decision-making process in the treatment of cerebral palsy. Because of the expense, it is not readily available in all orthopaedic centers, therefore its role in routine clinical practice is still uncertain. Hughes et al. questioned the efficacy of gait analysis in deciding on treatment. He argued that these tests focus on the mechanical rather than functional outcome and that test results and subsequent surgical procedures depended on the subjective interpretation of gait laboratory analysts. Deluca et al. evaluated treatment recommendations after clinical examinations and videotapes of gait and compared them with treatment recommendations in the same patients after gait analysis. The initial surgical recommendations were changed in 52% of these patients after the gait analysis data were analyzed. The findings from gait analysis lead to 21 new procedures and the cancellation of 27 others. One of the most important advantages of gait analysis is the objective documentation of preoperative and postoperative function and the outcome of specific treatments (operative and nonoperative) for cerebral palsy.

INDICATIONS FOR SURGERY

Surgery is most often indicated in patients with spastic cerebral palsy and less often in those with dyskinesia. The chief role of surgery is to help correct local physical defects that interfere with the patient's rehabilitation, but it also can help to correct defects that interfere with nursing care.

The nonsurgical treatment of patients with cerebral palsy has been overemphasized in recent years, and thus the help that surgery can offer often has been overlooked. Statistical reports support the thesis that well-performed surgical procedures done on properly selected patients yield good results, provided that treatment after surgery is carefully managed. Surgery that is properly timed for specific indications may decrease the need for physical therapy and orthotic treatment.

During the course of conservative treatment, surgery often is necessary because progress has become arrested or because a new deformity or some other complication has developed. Usually surgery is only part of the total management of a patient with cerebral palsy. The indications and the proper time for surgery should be decided by the group of medical attendants responsible for the care of the specific patient. Much of the success of the operation depends on the care after surgery. Physical therapy and a bracing program may be needed to maintain the improvement gained from surgery.

Surgery is indicated less often for athetosis. Spastic paralysis affects individual muscles, but athetosis is characterized by the placing of parts in distorted positions by any muscles capable of doing so. Consequently, if athetoid muscles or groups of muscles responsible for a given distorted position are transferred or otherwise operated on, the athetosis may shift to other muscles of similar function to produce the same distorted position or a similar one; for example, the finger flexors may become affected after athetoid wrist flexors have been transferred to the dorsum of the wrist. Fortunately, when athetosis has been so shifted, the distorting muscles are usually weaker and are thus less harmful functionally and cosmetically; consequently, surgery is occasionally indicated, even though the athetosis may be expected to shift. Surgery also may be indicated for postural contractures, such as equinus deformities of the ankles and flexion contractures of the knees and hips, that result from prolonged sitting or lying in poor position. Surgery rarely will help a patient with athetosis to walk, but contractures may require release for better posture, as an aid in wheelchair transfer, and occasionally to stabilize a joint.

In cases involving rigidity, the brain is so severely damaged that surgery is rarely indicated except to correct major deformities, which may be caused by soft tissue contractures or bony abnormalities.

OPERATIONS USEFUL IN CEREBRAL PALSY

Surgery may be useful in cerebral palsy to (1) correct deformity, whether static, dynamic, or both; (2) balance muscle power; or (3) stabilize uncontrollable joints.

Static deformities are corrected chiefly by lengthening tendons and by capsulotomies, fasciotomies, and osteotomies, such as of the tarsal bones for varus or valgus deformity or of the tibia, femur, or forearm bones for angular or rotary deformity. Dynamic deformities are corrected, at least partially, by lengthening musculotendinous units (which also weakens the units) or by tenotomy of tendons such as the tibialis posterior, psoas, hamstring, hip adductor, and soleus muscles, or by tenotomy or myotomy of some muscles of the forearm and hand.

Balancing the muscle power acting on a joint is difficult in cerebral palsy. Some of the obstacles to satisfactory function after tendon transfers in patients with this affliction are (1) the impairment in voluntary control of muscles, (2) the slowness of voluntary movements, (3) the lowered threshold to stretch reflexes, (4) the frequency of associated sensory deficits, (5) the frequency with which antagonistic muscle groups exhibit synchronous activity without regard to the function being undertaken (dysphasic activity), (6) the fact that voluntary contraction of a spastic muscle begins simultaneously throughout the muscle, in contrast to a normal muscle, in which different parts contract at different times, and (7) the fact that coordinated and skillful use of a muscle, already difficult enough for the patient with cerebral palsy to learn when the muscle is in its normal location and serving its normal function, is even more difficult to learn when the function of the muscle has been changed or even reversed after surgery. For these and other reasons, most tendon transfers in cerebral palsy lack the highly coordinated function of most tendon transfers seen in poliomyelitis or peripheral nerve injury. Often their chief functions are to remove a dynamic but deforming force and to serve as a motorized tenodesis.

Rerouting a muscle to alter its function has limited popularity. Once a spastic muscle is transferred, it still retains its spasticity. The muscle may be weakened, but it is still spastic. For example, if the spastic tibialis posterior muscle is rerouted anteriorly through the interosseous membrane to the dorsum of the foot, it is changed from a spastic invertor and plantar flexor to a spastic dorsiflexor. The phasic activity of the muscle can be sorted out for decision making by kinetic electromyography.

Neurectomy of some of the motor branches of nerves to a particular muscle is based on the idea that by resecting some of the branches that innervate a spastic muscle, its strength may be diminished so that its power equals that of its antagonist; in practice, however, muscle balance is rarely if ever attained. To minimize errors in indications for neurectomy, Barnett has temporarily paralyzed the branches considered for neurectomy by exposing and crushing them. While the branches are regenerating, the effects of the contemplated neurectomy can be accurately evaluated, and if the desired results have been obtained, neurectomy is indicated. To obtain a more transient paralysis, the branches considered for neurectomy may be infiltrated with procaine; the immediate effects of such a paralysis are apparent, but the permanent effects and the patient's ability to learn new patterns of motor activity usually cannot be evaluated in such a short time. Often joint stabilization may be required and usually has predictable results.

TREATMENT AFTER SURGERY

Surgery in children with cerebral palsy is done to improve the deformity and function. To achieve the best results, surgical plans should include provisions for postoperative rehabilitation, which for the most part is directed by a physical therapist. Postoperative rehabilitation also may consist of splinting and bracing to maintain correction of a deformity obtained at the time of surgery. A particular brace or orthosis is described by the initials of the joints that it stabilizes. For example, an orthosis that stabilizes the ankle and foot is called an *ankle-foot orthosis (AFO);* one that also stabilizes the knee is called a *knee-ankle-foot orthosis (KAFO);* if the hip is included in the orthosis, it is known as an *HKAFO.* Lightweight plastic orthoses are more often used but in certain instances metal braces may still be used. The importance of a postoperative rehabilitation program should not be underestimated in achieving success of any surgical intervention for cerebral palsy.

MANAGEMENT OF SPASTICITY

Because cerebral palsy is the result of a central nervous system lesion, numerous operations on the central nervous system have been tried to modify this condition. These include operations on the spinal cord itself (such as longitudinal myelotomy), stereotactic surgery on the brain (such as cortex ablation), and procedures on the deep cerebellar nuclei or the thalamus for extrapyramidal lesions where motion disorders originate. Electrical stimulators have been implanted on the cerebellum or over the dorsal spinal cord, and some have advocated transcutaneous electric stimulators. The efficacy of these stimulators is uncertain.

Injections of various substances into muscles and around nerves may be used to weaken a muscle and improve the balance of forces across a joint to assess whether this will improve function. This usually is only temporary but may be of value to allow a stretching and strengthening physical therapy program. Short-acting local anesthetic agents injected into the vicinity of a specific nerve will inhibit the function of the innervated muscle. This allows the physician to observe the effect on a specific deformity from loss of the muscle's function. Injections of 45% alcohol will inhibit nerve transmission for approximately 6 weeks. These injections are painful and require general anesthesia. Phenol may be used to destroy the nerve fibers and will have a permanent effect.

Botulinum toxin was introduced in the early 1990s as a

treatment for spasticity in children with cerebral palsy. Botulinum toxin is a neurotoxin produced by *Clostridia* bacteria. This protein polypeptide chain irreversibly binds to the cholinergic terminal in the neuromuscular junction and inhibits the release of acetylcholine that is necessary for muscle contraction. The toxin will diffuse readily after injection into the muscle belly. The effect is seen 12 to 72 hours after injection and its effect will last 3 to 6 months. Recovery of tone results from the sprouting of new nerve terminals after injection. This technique has been useful in very young patients in whom there is a need to delay surgical intervention. Injections also may improve dynamic deformities to allow easier brace wear and improvement in physical therapy protocols. Until there is further experience with Botulinum toxin the effect on long-term functional outcomes remains uncertain.

Baclofen is an agonist of the neuroinhibitor gamma-aminobutyric acid that interferes with the release of excitatory transmitters that cause spasticity. It penetrates the blood-brain barrier poorly, restricting the effectiveness of the oral medicine. Continuous infusion of baclofen into the spinal canal has demonstrated efficacy in controlling spasticity. A programmable pump is implanted subcutaneously into the lateral abdominal wall and is attached to a catheter that tunnels under the skin and is connected to an intrathecal catheter (Fig. 30-4). The dose of a continuous infusion of baclofen is titrated to the desired clinical effect. The pump must be refilled with baclofen through a subcutaneous port about every 3 months. Studies on the use of baclofen pumps in children with cerebral palsy have reported improvement in the ability to perform activities of daily living and improvement in muscle tone, joint range of motion, and upper extremity function. Even with the decrease in spasticity, orthopaedic procedures may still be needed. Complications seen with the use of a baclofen pump are catheter-related problems, infection, cerebral spinal fluid leaks, and equipment failure.

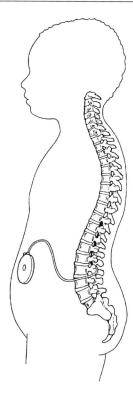

Fig. 30-4 Continuous intrathecal baclofen infusion. Baclofen is injected through skin to reservoir, which is located within surgically placed pump beneath skin of abdomen. The pump, which is about the size of a hockey puck, is programmable using a device placed against the skin and over the pump. Medication is continuously infused through catheter that tunnels under the skin and is inserted directly into spinal canal; baclofen mixes with spinal fluid, directly affecting spinal cord and decreasing spasticity. (From Reid S, Pellegrino L, Albinson-Scull S, Dormans JP: The management of spasticity. In Pellegrino L, Dormans JP, eds: *Caring for children with cerebral palsy,* Baltimore 1998, Paul Brookes.)

NEUROSURGICAL INTERVENTION

Selective dorsal rhizotomy is a method for reducing spasticity by sectioning a portion of the sensory nerve roots of the lumbosacral plexus. Altering the control exhibited by the anterior horn cells in the spinal cord reduces spasticity. The normal inhibitory influences of the gamma efferent system are deficient in cerebral palsy. Also, the ability to coordinate movement as mediated by the extrafusal fibers from the alpha motor neurons is abnormal. Selective posterior rhizotomy attempts to limit the stimulatory input from the muscle spindles in the lower limb that arrive by the afferent fibers in the dorsal roots. This is accomplished by using electromyographic readings to help identify which nerve rootlets are carrying abnormal information back to the alpha motor neurons, thus contributing to the increased hyperactivity of the stretch response and ultimately causing increased spasticity. The ideal candidate for selective dorsal root rhizotomy is a young child 3 to 8 years of age with spastic diplegia, voluntary motor control, reasonable intelligence and motivation, no fixed contractures, good trunk control, and severe or pure spasticity. Preterm or low-birth-weight patients are better candidates than full-term children because full-term children tend to have rigidity plus spasticity instead of pure spasticity. In the early postoperative period, the patient is weaker than before surgery and requires intensive physical therapy. Results thus far show lasting reduction in spasticity with increased hip, knee, and ankle range of motion. Increases in stride length and walking speed also have been reported.

Some of the complications seen after selective dorsal rhizotomy are significant and include muscle weakness, progressive hip subluxation or dysplasia, spondylolysis, spondylolisthesis, and increased lumbar lordosis. Patients with preexisting lumbar lordosis of more than 60 degrees on a sitting lateral roentgenogram are at risk for the development of postoperative lumbar hyperlordosis. Although selective dorsal root rhizotomy is effective in decreasing spasticity, it is estimated that up to 65% of these patients require additional orthopaedic procedures.

◆ Selective Posterior Rhizotomy

TECHNIQUE 30-1 *(As Described in General Terms by Oppenheim)*

The operation is performed with the patient prone and under general anesthesia. Through a limited midline laminectomy extending from L2 to L5, identify the L4 through S2 nerve roots. Intradurally, the posterior and anterior nerve roots are then separated and subdivided into 5 to 10 rootlets, which are analyzed by electrical stimulation and monitoring of their responses with EMG. The lower extremities must remain accessible at all times in order to observe the EMG and the muscles themselves for any sustained muscle contraction or spread of contractions to neighboring muscles. If the patient is a typical diplegic, this usually involves the testing of 45 to 50 nerve rootlets, and approximately 25% to 50% of them are transected after treatment.

AFTERTREATMENT. Postoperatively, some dysesthesias may be present, usually for 7 to 10 days, but they usually are transient, and seldom is any dysesthesia permanent. Transient weakness (at times profound) is a known sequel to this procedure. The patient is allowed to sit as soon as the wound has healed enough for the defect in the dura to seal. Functional improvement is expected in 6 to 12 months.

Gait studies have shown improvement in joint motion, stride length, and walking speed after surgery. Selective posterior rhizotomy reduces spasticity; it does not relieve or eliminate contractures. Its effect in preventing deformity in the bones and soft tissues can be determined only by long-term follow-up studies.

Foot

In cerebral palsy, spasticity can cause one or more of the following deformities of the foot: (1) equinus, (2) valgus, (3) varus, (4) talipes calcaneus, (5) adduction of the forefoot and hallux valgus with bunion formation, and (6) clawing of the toes.

EQUINUS DEFORMITY

Equinus deformity in spastic cerebral palsy can be treated by nonsurgical or surgical methods. Conservative treatment often is sufficient, but sometimes the deformity is so severe that surgery is indicated. In a young child the deformity often can be corrected conservatively by stretching the triceps surae both

manually and by using a brace. Inhibitive casts that are supposed to obliterate the plantar reflex are actually excellent holding casts that allow the stretched gastrocsoleus complex to lengthen. Cottalorda et al. and Brouwer et al. have both reported good results in controlling equinus deformity in children with spastic cerebral palsy. These most often are useful in children 3 years of age or younger. Once the desired amount of correction is obtained by serial casting, this position can be maintained with an ankle-foot orthosis. Tardieu and Tardieu have shown that stretching the soleus muscle 6 hours a day prevents contractures from developing. Unless a brace or orthosis is worn at night until skeletal maturity, the deformity usually recurs. The deformity tends to recur during growth because the tibia grows in length faster than the triceps surae, making the muscle group act like a bowstring. That the foot usually rests in an equinus position at night also is a factor.

Surgical Correction of Equinus Deformity

Surgery is indicated in equinus deformity when conservative treatment fails or when the deformity is so severe that conservative treatment would be ineffective. Because the equinus deformity tends to recur until growth is complete, the patient must be monitored until skeletal maturity.

◆ Open Lengthening of Tendo Calcaneus

Based on his observation that the tendo calcaneus rotates about 90 degrees on its longitudinal axis between insertion and origin, White in 1943 described his method of lengthening the tendo calcaneus. The rotation of the tendon fibers is from medial to lateral when viewed from the posterior aspect.

TECHNIQUE 30-2 *(White)*

Use a posteromedial incision to expose the tendo calcaneus from its insertion onto the calcaneus proximally for 10 cm. Near its insertion onto the calcaneus, divide the anterior two thirds of the tendon. Apply a moderate force in dorsiflexion to the foot and then divide the medial two thirds of the tendon 5 to 8 cm proximal to the site of the distal division. Forcefully dorsiflex the foot to lengthen the tendon (it slides on itself). Suturing the tendon usually is unnecessary, but it may be done when its continuity is doubtful. This method provides a smooth posterior surface of the tendon inferiorly, where little subcutaneous fat is present between it and the skin. Close the tendon sheath and skin and apply a long leg cast with the knee extended and the ankle in neutral dorsiflexion.

When heel varus accompanies the equinus, the two incisions may be altered to give a lateral insertion of the tendo calcaneus into the bone (Fig. 30-5).

AFTERTREATMENT. The patient is allowed to bear weight in the long leg cast the day after surgery. The cast is left in place with the knee in full extension for 3 weeks, and then a short leg cast is worn for an additional 3 weeks. This cast is then

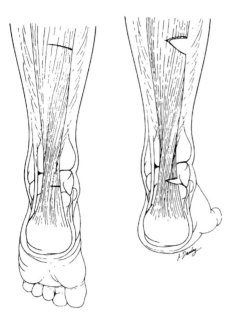
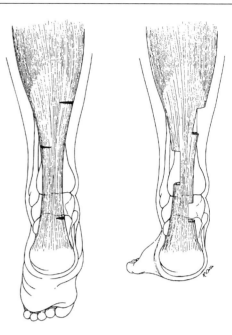

Fig. 30-5   Modification of White technique to effect more lateral insertion of tendo calcaneus onto calcaneus. Distal cut in tendon is made through its medial half, and proximal cut is made through posteromedial half of tendon. (Redrawn from Tachdjian MO: *Pediatric orthopaedics,* Philadelphia, 1972, WB Saunders.)

Fig. 30-6   Incisions for percutaneous tendo calcaneus lengthening. Cut ends slide on themselves with forceful dorsiflexion of foot. (Redrawn from Hsu JD, Hsu CL. In Jahss MH, ed: *Disorders of the foot,* Philadelphia, 1982, WB Saunders.)

removed and an AFO is fitted with the ankle in neutral dorsiflexion (right angle) for night use until longitudinal bone growth is complete. (See also the aftertreatment for Technique 30-3.) A short leg cast can be used initially, but the patient must be encouraged to straighten the knee, because flexion of the knee relaxes the gastrocnemius muscle.

TECHNIQUE 30-3 *(Hauser)*

Expose the tendon through a posteromedial incision. Incise two thirds of the tendon transversely at a level 8 to 12 cm proximal to its insertion by inserting a tenotome transversely into the tendon so that its flat surface faces anteroposteriorly and so that two thirds of the tendon is posterior to the blade. Turn the tenotome blade posteriorly and cut through the tendon to its posterior surface. Then incise the tendon 1.2 cm proximal to its insertion on the calcaneus as follows. Insert a curved tenotome anterior to the medial two thirds of the tendon and draw it posteromedially to partially divide the tendon at this point. Dorsiflex the foot, and the tendon will slide on itself and lengthen. It is beneficial to incise the plantaris tendon as it lies alongside the medial aspect of the tendo calcaneus. An effort should be made to repair the defects in the tendon sheath after the tendon has been lengthened to prevent the skin from adhering to the tendon by scar.

AFTERTREATMENT. A cast is applied from midthigh to toes with the knee in full extension and the ankle in neutral

dorsiflexion, making certain that the skin along the incision does not blanch when the foot is in neutral dorsiflexion. If it does blanch, it may slough in the postoperative period and cause scarring. If the skin blanches in these circumstances, allow the foot to fall into a little equinus before applying the cast. The foot can be brought up to neutral dorsiflexion at the first cast change. The long leg cast is removed at 6 weeks, and an AFO is used as a brace and as a night splint for as long as necessary to prevent recurrence of the equinus. Often a short leg cast may be used instead of a long leg cast.

Often a daytime orthosis will not be needed after lengthening because the dorsiflexor strength is then adequate to overcome the equinus thrust of the spastic triceps surae.

◆ Percutaneous Lengthening of Tendo Calcaneus

Moreau and Lake found that when performed on an outpatient basis, the technique was quick, inexpensive, and free of complications; 97% of their patients showed improvement in gait in a series of 90 legs so treated.

TECHNIQUE 30-4

With the patient prone and the leg prepared from a level above the knee to include the toes, extend the knee and dorsiflex the ankle to tense the tendo calcaneus so that it is subcutaneous, easily outlined, and away from the neurovascular structures anteriorly. Make three partial tenotomies in the tendo calcaneus (Fig. 30-6). Make the first medial, just

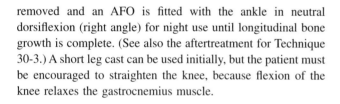

at the insertion of the tendon onto the calcaneus; cut through one half of the width of the tendon. Make the second tenotomy proximally and medially, just below the musculotendinous junction. Make the third laterally through half the width of the tendon midway between the two medial cuts. Dorsiflex the ankle to the desired angle. The incisions do not require closure, only a sterile dressing and a long leg cast with the knee in extension. The two incisions are on the medial side if the heel is in varus, as it usually is. If the heel is in valgus, two incisions are placed laterally and one medially in between.

AFTERTREATMENT. The aftertreatment is the same as that described for Technique 30-2.

◆ Semiopen Sliding Tenotomy of Tendo Calcaneus

The small incisions used for this procedure cause little scarring, which reduces postoperative morbidity and is preferred from a cosmetic standpoint. If equinus recurs, no extensive scarring is present in the skin and subcutaneous tissues or in the tendon itself.

TECHNIQUE 30-5

With the patient prone and the leg prepared from above the knee to include the toes, extend the knee fully and dorsiflex the ankle to tense the tendo calcaneus subcutaneously. Make two longitudinal incisions, each 2 cm long, centered over the tendo calcaneus, one at the level of its insertion onto the calcaneus and the other just below the musculotendinous junction. Deepen the lower incision down to the tendon and incise the tendon sheath. Cut the lateral half of the tendon just above its insertion (Fig. 30-7, *A*). Deepen the proximal incision down to the tendon sheath and incise it. Under direct view tenotomize the tendon of the plantaris and the posteromedial half of the tendo calcaneus.

Dorsiflex the ankle, and the cut portions of the tendon will slide on themselves to the desired length (Fig. 30-7, *B*). Close the incision with absorbable subcuticular sutures. Because the skin incisions are made vertically, they do not tend to open as the skin is tensed by dorsiflexing the ankle. Apply a sterile dressing and a long leg cast.

AFTERTREATMENT. The aftertreatment is the same as that described for Technique 30-3.

◆ ◆ ◆

Open lengthening is required in recurrent equinus because the normal rotation of the tendon fibers is no longer present and a sliding tenotomy cannot be done easily.

Posterior capsulotomy of the ankle may be needed in a patient with severe equinus deformity, especially if it is of long-standing duration. The posterior ankle capsule will be

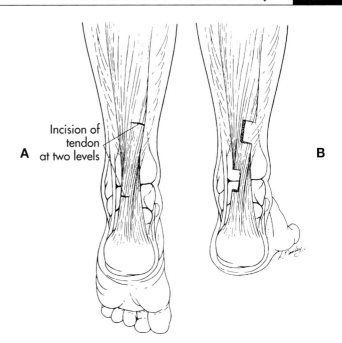

Fig. 30-7 Semiopen sliding lengthening of tendo calcaneus. **A,** Incision of tendon at two levels. **B,** Sliding lengthening by passive dorsiflexion of foot.

contracted, and in such instances posterior capsulotomy of the talotibial joint may be necessary to allow adequate ankle dorsiflexion.

◆ Lengthening of Gastrocnemius Muscle

The rest of this section discusses the type of deformity described by Silfverskiöld, in which the gastrocnemius muscle is the chief cause of equinus.

Strayer described an operation in which the aponeurotic tendon of the gastrocnemius is divided transversely near its junction with that of the soleus, the foot is dorsiflexed to the neutral position, and the retracted proximal part of the tendon is sutured to the underlying soleus. He concluded that the operation is helpful because it alters the proprioceptive impulses received from the extremity, and these impulses in turn modify the stretch reflexes. He reviewed his results in 23 patients and rated them as good or excellent in 16. The operation described by Strayer is similar in principle to that of Vulpius in which the aponeurotic tendon of the gastrocnemius is divided and its distal part is allowed to retract distally but is not sutured to the soleus.

Baker reported performing a procedure similar to the Silfverskiöld operation but without partial neurectomy of the tibial nerve. According to Calandriello, Scaglietti also has used a technique similar to that of Silfverskiöld. Olney, Williams, and Menelaus reviewed 219 aponeurotic lengthenings of the gastrocnemius in 156 patients. The rate of recurrence of deformity was high (48%). Recurrence was especially likely in children under 5 years of age.

Silver and Simon reported their experience with that operation of Silfverskiöld that combines transplantation of the heads of origin of the gastrocnemius with neurectomy of some branches of the tibial nerve. They had performed it 110 times, and only 5 times did the equinus deformity recur. According to them, these failures were each the result of weakness of the dorsiflexor muscles of the foot that was not properly evaluated before surgery.

Bassett and Baker reported their experiences with the three basic operations used to treat equinus deformity: neurectomy of branches of the tibial nerve, distal transplantation of the heads of origin of the gastrocnemius (gastrocnemius recession), and lengthening of the aponeurotic tendon of the gastrocnemius. Of 85 extremities treated by neurectomy, the deformity recurred in 26%; of 62 treated by gastrocnemius recession, it recurred in 16%; and of 447 treated by lengthening the aponeurotic tendon of the gastrocnemius using Baker's "tongue-in-groove" modification of the Vulpius operation, it recurred in only 4%. According to Bassett and Baker, when the deformity recurred, usually it had been incompletely corrected or care after surgery had been inadequate.

Craig and van Vuren used metal markers and roentgenograms made before, during, and after lengthening of the tendo calcaneus to demonstrate that the gastrocnemius cannot be sufficiently released by division of this tendon alone. In their opinion, to ensure relaxation of the gastrocnemius muscle, the operation of choice is a combination of gastrocnemius recession by the method of Strayer and lengthening of the tendo calcaneus to correct any deformity that may be caused by the shortened soleus. They reported 100 limbs treated by this method and followed for an average of 6 years after surgery; equinus deformity recurred in 9%, and a calcaneus deformity developed in 3%, resulting in insufficient push-off during walking. Their criterion for recurrence was inability to actively dorsiflex the foot above the neutral position with the knee extended.

This combined operation was developed because, in the opinion of Craig and van Vuren, the flat tendon and muscle belly of the gastrocnemius muscle are invariably adherent to the underlying soleus and therefore can retract only as far as the belly of the soleus retracts. Because the origin of the soleus extends halfway down the tibia and fibula, this muscle cannot retract farther proximally than the middle of the leg; proximal to this point the spastic gastrocnemius still exerts its pull on the underlying structures. To substantiate this opinion, the researchers attached a metal marker to the tendon of the gastrocnemius proximal to the soleus aponeurosis. The foot was then passively forced into maximal dorsiflexion with the knee extended, and a roentgenogram was made. Then the tendo calcaneus was lengthened, the foot was again forced into dorsiflexion with the knee extended, and a second roentgenogram was made, revealing that the marker had not moved much proximally as a result of the tendon lengthening. A gastrocnemius recession by the method of Strayer was performed, and only then did the marker move proximally to any marked degree on passive dorsiflexion of the foot with the knee

extended. According to Craig and van Vuren, reduction of spasm in the gastrocnemius is especially indicated when some of the equinus deformity is caused by a persistence of the positive support reflex or by the hyperactive stretch reflex.

For equinus deformity in spasticity in which the chief cause is contracture of or increased electrical activity within the gastrocnemius alone, one of the techniques described here (or a modification of one) is recommended; the choice of technique depends on the preference of the surgeon and on the findings in the specific patient. Considering the electromyographic findings before and after surgery by Perry et al. that tendon lengthening diminishes electrical activity within a muscle unit, partial neurectomy usually is not needed after lengthening of the gastrocnemius muscle.

TECHNIQUE 30-6 *(Silfverskiöld; Silver and Simon)*

With the patient under general anesthesia, place him prone on the operating table and apply a pneumatic tourniquet. Make a transverse incision in the popliteal fossa parallel with the skin creases, beginning at a point 1 cm lateral to the biceps femoris tendon and ending at a point 1 cm medial to the semitendinosus tendon. Deepen the incision transversely through the deep fascia and expose the two heads of origin of the gastrocnemius muscle. If a neurectomy is to be done, identify the tibial nerve and isolate its motor branches to the heads of origin of the gastrocnemius; one or two branches emerge from each side of the nerve and course obliquely distalward to the medial or lateral head. Pinch these branches gently to identify them. Then resect a small segment from enough of these branches to interrupt half or more of this innervation (Fig. 30-8, *A*); take great care to avoid injuring the popliteal vein, which lies immediately deep to the tibial nerve.

Now, use a curved clamp to elevate each head of the gastrocnemius muscle and free it from the posterior aspect of the femoral condyle by dividing it transversely near its attachment to the bone (Fig. 30-8, *B* and *C*); take care to avoid injuring the peroneal nerve, which courses near the lateral head. Then, by dissecting bluntly with a gauze sponge, elevate the two heads of the muscle until they are free to a level distal to the knee joint (Fig. 30-8, *D*). Close the wound routinely.

AFTERTREATMENT. A long leg cast is applied with the ankle dorsiflexed 10 degrees and the knee fully extended. A window is cut from the cast over the apex of the heel to prevent pressure sores. After 6 weeks the cast is removed, and rehabilitation is begun. Often, a well-padded short leg cast can be used for postoperative immobilization.

TECHNIQUE 30-7 *(Vulpius, Compere)*

Make a posterior longitudinal incision 7.5 cm long over the middle of the calf. Identify the medial sural cutaneous nerve

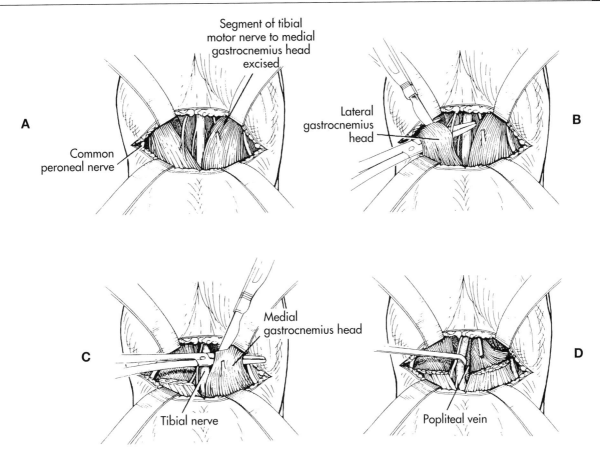

Fig. 30-8 Technique of Silfverskiöld as described by Silver and Simon. **A,** Segment has been resected from nerve to medial head of gastrocnemius. **B,** Lateral head of gastrocnemius is isolated, leaving its nerve intact. **C,** Medial head of gastrocnemius is isolated and divided. **D,** Both heads have been divided and have retracted distally. (Redrawn from Silver CM, Simon SD: *J Bone Joint Surg* 41A:1021, 1959.)

and retract it. Then expose the aponeurotic tendon of the gastrocnemius and make an inverted V-shaped incision through it (Fig. 30-9). Force the ankle into slight dorsiflexion and thus separate the segments of the tendon. If the aponeurosis of the soleus is also contracted, divide it but do not disturb the soleus muscle itself.

Baker modified the Vulpius technique by lengthening the aponeurotic tendon of the gastrocnemius in a "tongue-in-groove" fashion (Fig. 30-10).

AFTERTREATMENT. Postoperative care is similar to that used for the Silfverskiöld procedure.

TECHNIQUE 30-8 *(Strayer)*

With the patient prone and with a tourniquet inflated, make a posterior longitudinal incision 10 to 15 cm long over the middle of the calf (Fig. 30-11). Identify and retract the medial sural cutaneous nerve. Deepen the incision through the fascia to expose the gastrocnemius muscle; by blunt dissection separate this muscle from the underlying soleus distally to where its aponeurotic tendon joins that of the soleus to form the tendo calcaneus. Insert a probe or clamp deep to the gastrocnemius and sever its tendon. Then dorsiflex the foot; a gap 2 to 2.5 cm wide will appear between the segments of severed tendon. Then dissect the two muscle bellies from their medial and lateral attachments to the deep fascia proximally into the popliteal fossa and pass a finger from side to side beneath the muscle to completely separate the gastrocnemius from the soleus. This allows the gastrocnemius to retract farther proximally. Then suture the proximal part of the aponeurotic tendon to the underlying soleus with fine interrupted sutures at a level at least 2.5 cm more proximal than its original attachment. Close the wound with subcuticular catgut sutures so that the sutures need not be removed.

AFTERTREATMENT. Postoperative care is similar to that used for Silfverskiöld procedure or tendo calcaneus lengthening.

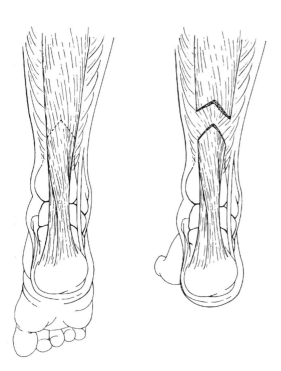

Fig. 30-9   Lengthening of gastrocnemius by Vulpius technique. (Courtesy EL Compere, MD, and WT Schnute, MD.)

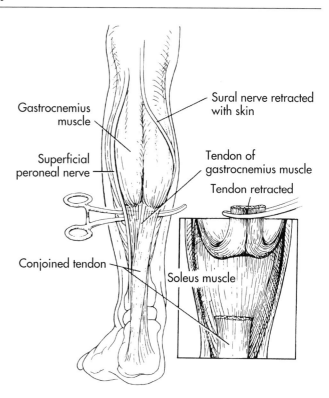

Fig. 30-11   Lengthening of gastrocnemius by Strayer technique (see text). (Redrawn from Strayer LM Jr: *J Bone Joint Surg* 32A:671, 1950.)

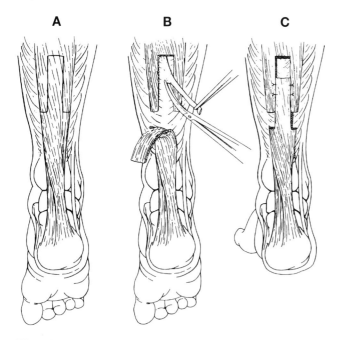

Fig. 30-10   Baker technique of aponeurotic lengthening of gastrocnemius muscle. **A,** Inverted-U incision is made through aponeurosis. **B,** Central aponeurosis of soleus is dissected free. **C,** After ankle is dorsiflexed, sliding end of tendon is sutured distally.

Muscle Transfer to Achieve Dorsiflexion. Ono et al. described an operation to achieve dorsiflexion of the foot. In this operation the flexor hallucis longus and flexor digitorum longus are transferred to the dorsum of the foot after tendo calcaneus lengthening. They believe this procedure is indicated in treating (1) recurrent equinus deformity and (2) poor voluntary control of the ankle dorsiflexors and failure to achieve dorsiflexion actively by tilting the body backward when in a standing position. They were able to achieve a heel-to-toe gait in two thirds of the 31 patients treated with the operation.

In an excellent review of the management of ankle and foot deformities in cerebral palsy, Fulford reported using a medial transfer of a gastrocnemius muscle belly, transferring it anteriorly on the tibia for dynamic equinus when plantar flexor power is excessive and dorsiflexor power is weak. As the first stage, he releases the medial head of the gastrocnemius from the femur through a transverse popliteal incision and then 6 weeks later opens the medial side of the incision and extends it distally along the medial side of the calf to the calcaneus. After the distal part of the medial belly of the gastrocnemius is freed by blunt dissection and its tendon is freed from the tendo calcaneus by sharp dissection, the entire muscle is passed subcutaneously around the medial side of the leg and the tendon is inserted just lateral to the midline on the dorsum of the foot. He advises crushing the nerve to the medial head of the gastrocnemius to prevent the muscle from contracting for about 6 weeks.

◆ **Anterior Transfer of Long Toe Flexors for Spastic Equinus and Equinovarus**

TECHNIQUE 30-9 *(Hiroshima et al.)*

Make a 10-cm incision over the back of the leg and lengthen the tendo calcaneus. Retract the triceps surae laterally and identify the flexor hallucis longus and flexor digitorum longus muscles. Dissect both muscles proximally to the junction of the middle and distal thirds of the leg and distally to the ankle. Make a second incision medially over the tuberosity of the navicular, reflect the abductor hallucis plantarward, and identify the extensor digitorum longus and the flexor hallucis longus at their crossing point. Divide the flexor digitorum longus here and retract it proximally through the first incision. Then free the flexor hallucis longus at the base of the hallux through a third incision on the plantar side of the first metatarsophalangeal joint and retract it also proximally through the initial incision. Then pass both tendons anteriorly through a large window in the interosseous space between the tibia and fibula, from posterior to anterior, and anchor both tendons in the base of the fourth metatarsal by forming a loop passing through the metatarsal.

AFTERTREATMENT. The leg is immobilized in a long leg cast with the knee flexed and the foot in the overcorrected position. Quadriceps-strengthening exercises are started the day after surgery. The cast is removed at 6 weeks, and exercises are begun to mobilize the foot and ankle. A short leg brace with a Klenzak ankle is used for standing and walking for the next 3 months. The foot is splinted at night to hold it in the corrected position.

◆ **Neurectomy of Branches of Tibial Nerve**

Occasionally neurectomy of branches of the tibial nerve to the gastrocnemius or soleus, or both, or advancement of the insertion of the tendo calcaneus may correct equinus deformity caused only by spasm of one or both muscles, but neurectomy alone is unsuccessful when the triceps surae is contracted.

Troublesome clonus on weight-bearing, however, usually can be reduced by neurectomy, as in Phelps' method, which is described here. Before surgery the surgeon should determine which muscle, the gastrocnemius or the soleus, is the cause of clonus; when clonus is caused chiefly by the gastrocnemius, it disappears or diminishes when the knee is flexed because the muscle takes origin proximal to the knee and flexion relaxes it; when clonus is caused chiefly by the soleus, changes in the position of the knee do not affect it because the soleus takes origin distal to the knee. Even when clonus is severe, lengthening of the tendo calcaneus at the time of neurectomy is inadvisable because after neurectomy the lengthening might be unnecessary. Usually resecting only one or two branches of the tibial nerve is sufficient to relieve clonus.

When the equinus deformity persisted after release of the patellar retinacula and transfer of the hamstring tendons to the femoral condyles, Eggers carried out neurectomy of the branches of the tibial nerve to the soleus alone. Lengthening the tendo calcaneus was then rarely necessary. Tolo and Sponseller reported 14 children who had this procedure and 11 in whom it had been combined with a tendo calcaneus lengthening. They used it in persistent clonus that interfered with walking. The deformity was not overcorrected in any of the children, and 12 of the 15 had no return of clonus. This neurectomy is described in the second technique here.

TECHNIQUE 30-10 *(Phelps)*

Make a transverse incision 7.5 cm long over the distal part of the popliteal fossa; this incision follows the flexion creases of the skin and is preferable to a longitudinal one because the scar does not tend to hypertrophy. Divide the fascia to expose the tibial nerve, which lies superficial to the vessels. Do not disturb the first branch of the nerve; it is purely sensory. The next two branches, one emerging from the medial side and the other from the lateral side of the nerve, course to the medial and lateral heads of the gastrocnemius muscle and are easily found and identified (Fig. 30-12). They enter the muscle close to the origin of its heads; the branch to the medial head divides into three twigs just before it disappears into the muscle, and the branch to the lateral head divides into two. Just distal to where these two branches emerge, a single branch emerges from the posterior surface of the tibial nerve and divides into two twigs, one to each head of the soleus muscle; farther distally, another branch that enters the medial head of the soleus emerges from the tibial nerve deep to the soleus. Stimulate each branch either by an electric current or by gently pressing it with a smooth forceps. While the branches are being stimulated, an assistant gently dorsiflexes the foot; thus the branch or branches chiefly responsible for the clonus or spasticity can be identified. Then decide which branches should be sacrificed, divide them where they emerge from the trunk, and avulse them from the muscle by winding each separately around a clamp.

When the decision has been made before surgery to resect only branches to the gastrocnemius, identifying branches to other muscles is unnecessary. Occasionally, however, when spasticity of the long toe flexors is disabling, branches of the tibial nerve to these muscles should be identified and resected.

AFTERTREATMENT. If only neurectomy has been carried out, a pressure dressing is usually sufficient immobilization. Exercises to reeducate the dorsiflexors are begun promptly after surgery, and walking is allowed as soon as the wound has healed.

TECHNIQUE 30-11 *(Eggers)*

With the patient prone, begin the incision at a point just posterior to the neck of the fibula and continue it distally

continued

Fig. 30-12   Exposure of tibial nerve and its branches for neurectomy. Most proximal and superficial branch to emerge is cutaneous one; next are medial and lateral branches to heads of gastrocnemius and soleus. Branch to tibialis posterior emerges at more distal level as nerve disappears beneath soleus. (Curved longitudinal skin incision that does not cross flexion crease at right angle, or transverse one, is preferred to incision shown here.)

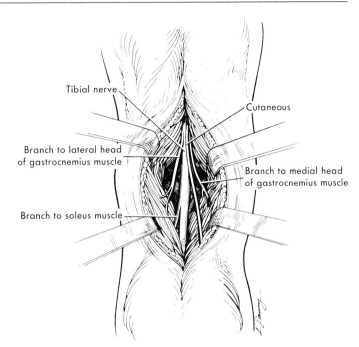

about 10 cm. Identify and protect the peroneal nerve. Locate and develop the interval between the gastrocnemius and soleus muscles; now retract the gastrocnemius posteriorly to expose the posterior surface of the soleus muscle in the floor of the wound. A triangular mass of fat is seen proximally and medially; in it courses the main branch to the soleus muscle, usually accompanied by a small vein. Trace the nerve into the soleus, where it usually terminates in two branches. After the nerve has been identified by stimulation, resect a segment from each of these two branches.

AFTERTREATMENT. The aftertreatment is the same as that described for Technique 30-10.

◆ **Anterior Advancement of Tendo Calcaneus**

Anterior advancement of the tendo calcaneus from the posterior tuberosity to the dorsum of the calcaneus immediately posterior to the subtalar joint will shorten the lever arm and weaken the triceps surae. This anterior advancement will decrease the resistance to ankle dorsiflexion by about 48%. Murphy described this technique.

TECHNIQUE 30-12 *(Murphy)*

With the patient prone and the foot under tourniquet control, make a posteromedial incision about 1 cm medial to the tendo calcaneus, beginning at the os calcis and extending it proximally for a length of 7.5 to 10 cm. Divide the subcutaneous tissue and tendon sheath in one plane in line with the skin incision (Fig. 30-13, *A*). Identify the tendo calcaneus and isolate by sharp and blunt dissection to its insertion. Detach it from the calcaneal tuberosity as far distally as possible to preserve length. Take care to avoid injury to the calcaneal apophysis (Fig. 30-13, *B*).

Place a Bunnell pull-out wire suture on the distal end of the tendo calcaneus. Mobilize the flexor hallucis longus tendon and retract medially. Expose the upper surface of the calcaneus. Drill a 0.6-cm hole from the superior part of the calcaneus immediately posterior to the subtalar joint to exit on the plantar aspect of the non-weight-bearing area of the calcaneus. Enlarge the hole with a curet if necessary (Fig. 30-13, *C*).

Pass the pull-out wire and tendo calcaneus through the drill hole and tie over a sterile, thick felt pad and a button on the plantar aspect of the foot with the ankle in 15 degrees of plantar flexion. The heel cord must be routed anterior to the flexor hallucis longus, otherwise the tendo calcaneus will reattach itself to its original insertion (Fig. 30-13, *D*).

Release the tourniquet, and after complete hemostasis, close the wound. Apply an above-knee cast with the ankle joint in 15 degrees of plantar flexion and the knee in 10 degrees of flexion.

AFTERTREATMENT. The cast and the pull-out wire are removed in 4 to 6 weeks. Physical therapy is begun to restore ankle motion and strength of the anterior tibial and triceps surae muscles.

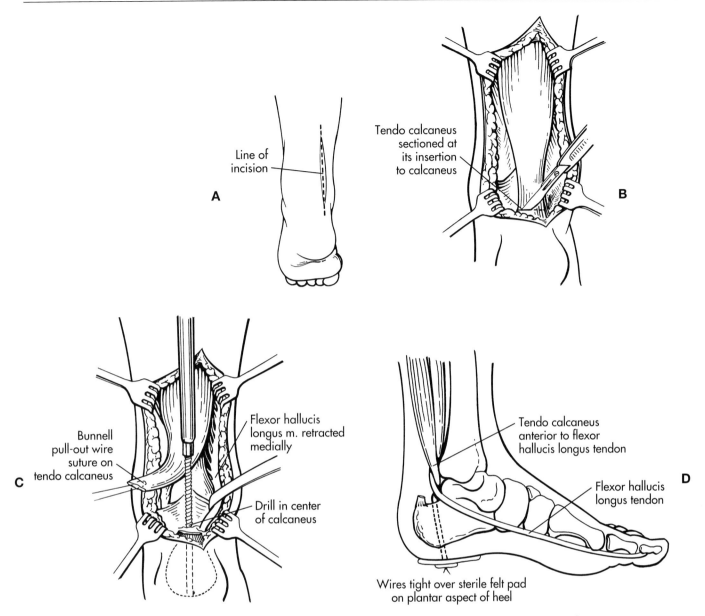

Fig. 30-13   Anterior advancement of tendo calcaneus. See text. (Redrawn from Tachdjian MO: *Pediatric orthopedics*, ed 2, Philadelphia, 1990, WB Saunders.)

VARUS OR VALGUS DEFORMITY

In cerebral palsy, varus or valgus deformity is most often accompanied by equinus, either of the forefoot or the hindfoot. Both neurological and biomechanical forces can cause these deformities. The position of the extremity above the ankle has a direct and indirect influence on the position of the foot; for example, in a diplegic patient with internally rotated and adducted hips and flexed knees external tibial torsion can develop that causes the foot to assume a valgus position. If the gastrocsoleus is spastic, there will be equinovalgus, that is, an equinus heel with the foot abducted or in valgus at the midtarsal joint. A patient with hemiplegia usually has an internally rotated thigh, but the knee usually comes into extension in the stance phase of gait, causing the foot to be internally rotated and to assume a varus posture. Neurological deformities usually are caused by retained primitive reflex patterns, inappropriate phasic activity of muscles during the gait cycle, absence of voluntary control of muscle activity, mass reflexes to stimuli of any type (labyrinthine, visual, auditory, or sensory), and an imbalance of agonist versus antagonist muscle activity.

In a study of 230 children, Bennett et al. found that in hemiplegia the foot deformity was equinus or equinovarus, and in diplegia or quadriplegia the foot deformity was valgus in 64% and varus in 36%.

Initially the deformity is dynamic, and it can be corrected and often controlled by some physiotherapeutic or orthotic means. If left uncorrected, however, an uncontrolled dynamic deformity will become fixed in the muscles, tendons, ligaments, and joint capsules and in the growing child will lead to bony deformities. Dynamic, static, and bony deformities require different approaches for proper treatment. The aim of treatment for dynamic deformities is to balance the muscles by lengthening or transferring a muscle-tendon complex. Static deformities also require muscle-tendon lengthening or transferring, but they also may require ligamentous or capsular releases about the joint. Bony deformities require realignment of the bones by osteotomy or arthrodesis. Dynamic muscle balance must be established once the bones have been realigned, otherwise the deformity will recur or the foot will remain poorly functional.

Varus deformity is more easily corrected surgically and is more functionally disabling in walking and standing. Valgus deformity is more difficult to correct surgically and is less functionally disabling. Consequently, surgery is done more often and more successfully for varus deformities than for valgus deformities.

Surgery is indicated to improve function when standing and walking, to aid in fitting the patient with shoes, to correct deformity when an orthosis will not hold it corrected, and to allow the extremity to be used without the impairment of an orthosis. When an orthosis is holding the deformity corrected and when other deformities in the same extremity require the continued use of an orthosis, then surgical correction is not indicated.

Varus Deformity

Varus deformity is most often accompanied by equinus. One must be sure that varus is not secondary to internal femoral or tibial torsion. Root has observed that when a child with a varus foot stands on his toes, the varus is accentuated by an overactive tibialis posterior muscle. Dynamic gait studies may show that the tibialis posterior tendon is active in the swing phase or it may be active continuously. In any event, in true varus or equinovarus of the foot, the tibialis posterior tendon usually is the offending structure. The other invertor muscles and weakness of the evertor muscles, whether actual or relative, may contribute to the deformity. Triceps surae spasticity or contracture adds considerably to the functional varus impairment. Hyperactivity of the anterior tibialis in combination or, rarely, alone can cause hindfoot varus. Operations on the invertor muscles of the foot include lengthening the tibialis posterior tendon, rerouting it from behind to in front of the medial malleolus, transferring its insertion through the interosseous membrane into the dorsum of the foot, and transferring part of it behind the tibia into the peroneus brevis. All of these tend to weaken its invertor action. Split transfer of the anterior tibialis is described in Technique 30-17.

Hoffer, Reiswig, Garrett, and Perry studied ambulatory electromyograms in patients with spastic varus hindfoot deformities and found inappropriate hyperactivity of the tibialis anterior tendon in some. For the patients with abnormal electromyograms, they devised a new procedure to correct

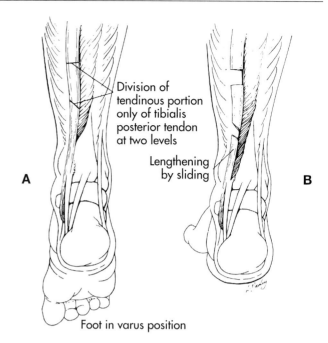

Fig. 30-14   Sliding lengthening of tibialis posterior tendon. **A,** Position of cuts in tendon. **B,** Lengthening by sliding.

deformity called the *split tibialis anterior tendon transfer.* It has been used extensively in adults with cerebrovascular accidents, and the results of 21 procedures performed in children with spastic cerebral palsy have been reported. In 15 feet fixed deformities required lengthening of the tendo calcaneus, lengthening of the tibialis posterior tendon, or release of the medial hindfoot. In six feet the deformity was dynamic, flexible, and correctable, and in these the split tibialis anterior transfer was performed as an isolated procedure. In only one instance was the procedure unsuccessful. In the remainder the split tendons worked with equal force in their spastic pattern as noted before surgery. In all of these patients, electromyograms before surgery revealed the tibialis anterior to be overactive and nonphasic; after surgery the gait electromyograms were often slightly modified but not dramatically so. When the gait electromyogram before surgery shows the tibialis anterior tendon to be neither overactive nor nonphasic, but there is phase reversal in the tibialis posterior muscle, transfer of the tibialis posterior is recommended.

Lengthening of Tibialis Posterior Tendon. The tibialis posterior tendon can be lengthened by a Z-plasty procedure, a step-cut procedure, or a sliding lengthening at its musculotendinous junction (Fig. 30-14, *A* and *B*). If the tendon is lengthened by a step-cut or Z-plasty procedure, it may bind down behind the medial malleolus in its tendon sheath and, with growth, act as a tether and cause the deformity to recur. In recurrent deformity, a previously lengthened tendon is less suitable for transfer because it is scarred and may be attenuated. Majestro, Ruda, and Frost described a modified lengthening of this tendon at its musculotendinous junction that is a more desirable procedure. If the deformity recurs, the tendon is more easily transferred because it will not have developed any intratendinous scarring. Majestro et al. reported only a 6% recurrence rate after this procedure. Intratendinous lengthening of the tibialis posterior tendon can be combined with an open tendo calcaneus lengthening through the same incision.

◆ *Z-Plasty Lengthening of Tibialis Posterior Tendon*

TECHNIQUE 30-13

Incise the skin longitudinally just above and posterior to the medial malleolus for a distance of 8 cm. By sharp dissection, divide the subcutaneous fat directly behind the medial border of the tibia down to the tendon sheath of the tibialis posterior tendon. Incise the tendon sheath directly over the tendon for 6 to 8 cm. Incise the tendon in its middle at the lower end of the incision and cut the lateral one half of the tendon; then incise the tendon in a proximal direction in line with its fibers for about 6 cm. At this proximal level, incise the tendon transversely medially to sever the medial one half of the tendon. Place the foot in the neutral position with regard to varus and neutral dorsiflexion. While holding the foot corrected, overlap the ends of the tendon and suture them together with nonabsorbable sutures. Repair the incision in the tendon sheath with small absorbable sutures. Close the subcutaneous tissue and skin with absorbable sutures and apply a short leg cast with the foot in the neutral or a slightly overcorrected position.

AFTERTREATMENT. Protected weight-bearing is allowed for 3 weeks, and then full weight-bearing in a short leg cast is allowed for an additional 3 weeks. When the cast is removed at 6 weeks, the foot is placed in an AFO to hold it in the corrected position. Daytime use of the AFO can be discontinued at 3 months. Protection of the foot in the corrected position with the AFO at night should be continued until skeletal growth of the limb is complete.

◆ *Step-Cut Lengthening of Tibialis Posterior Tendon*

TECHNIQUE 30-14

Expose the tendon sheath as described above but do not incise it over its length. Just above the medial malleolus, incise the lateral one half of the tendon sheath and the tendon. Move 6 to 8 cm proximally from this level and incise the medial one half of the tendon sheath and tendon. Dorsiflex the foot to the neutral position and forcibly correct the hindfoot and midfoot varus. The incised tendon should slide on itself within the sheath. Do not close the tendon sheath or suture the tendon. Close the subcutaneous tissues and skin in a routine fashion. Hold the foot and ankle in the corrected or a slightly overcorrected position and apply a short leg cast.

AFTERTREATMENT. The aftertreatment is the same as that described for Technique 30-13.

◆ **Intramuscular Lengthening of Tibialis Posterior Tendon**

TECHNIQUE 30-15 *(Majestro, Ruda, and Frost)*

With the patient supine and the pneumatic tourniquet inflated, make a longitudinal incision 3 cm long over the posteromedial corner of the tibia centered at the junction of the middle and distal thirds of the leg. Incise the deep fascia at this corner of the bone, identify the flexor digitorum longus, and retract it posteriorly. Now identify the musculotendinous junction of the tibialis posterior by placing a hemostat beneath it and by observing its action when inverting the foot without flexing the toes. Next, pass a curved hemostat beneath the tendinous part of the tibialis posterior, isolate this part from the muscle fibers that envelop it, and divide the tendon fibers completely, leaving the muscle fibers intact and allowing the tendon ends to retract freely within the muscle. Close the wound and apply a soft dressing.

AFTERTREATMENT. No cast is applied, and walking is allowed the day of surgery. The use of orthoses after surgery is not recommended until the final effect of the operation on motor balance of the foot during walking and running has been determined, usually at 2 months.

Rerouting Insertion of Tibialis Posterior Tendon Anterior to Medial Malleolus. Baker and Hill noted that when a spastic tibialis posterior muscle causes varus and internal rotational deformities of the foot, rerouting its tendon anterior to the medial malleolus improves alignment immediately. This was true in 34 feet in which the operation was used.

Bisla, Louis, and Albano reported anterior rerouting of the tibialis posterior tendon, as described by Baker and Hill, in 21 feet of 16 patients with cerebral palsy. In 5 the involvement was mild, in 10 moderate, and in 1 severe. On clinical evaluation after surgery, 4 were improved and in 14 there was no significant change. Varus or equinus deformity was not completely corrected in a single patient, and in 3 the equinovarus deformity increased significantly, requiring additional surgery. Examination both clinically and by electromyograms revealed neither voluntary nor involuntary action in the rerouted tendon.

A tendon so rerouted still acts as an invertor, although it is somewhat weakened. In our experience, anterior rerouting has not corrected the dynamic imbalance, and we no longer use the procedure.

Rerouting Insertion of Tibialis Posterior Tendon to Dorsum of Foot Through Interosseous Membrane. This operation has proved to be useful because it allows the tibialis posterior tendon to assist in dorsiflexion and removes a dynamic invertor and plantar flexor force. Bisla et al., Williams, Gritzka et al., and Root have all reported 80% or more excellent or good results after this procedure. On the other hand, Turner and Cooper found only 21% of their results were excellent or good, and in 71% of their patients the result was poor. Root stated that failures of this operation are caused by the following four factors: (1) unrecognized fixed varus deformity that cannot be corrected by a tendon transfer alone, and thus the varus deformity persists, (2) simultaneous tendo calcaneus lengthening, which can lead to a calcaneus deformity, (3) transplanting of the tendon too far laterally, which may lead to excessive valgus, and (4) insecure insertion of the tendon into the bone, which allows it to detach. Although originally we were enthusiastic about this procedure, 13 of 20 feet so treated have subsequently required a triple arthrodesis to correct heel and midfoot valgus. For this reason, we prefer one of the tendon-splitting transfer procedures to correct dynamic varus of the hindfoot or midfoot.

Split Tendon Transfers for Varus Deformity. In 1977 Kaufer reported treating varus deformities of the foot by split tendon transfer. The procedure was performed 30 times, 20 cases involving adults with deformities that arose after a stroke or central nervous system trauma and 10 cases involving patients with spastic cerebral palsy with varus deformities.

Any significant fixed deformity should be corrected before or during the transfer procedure. The split transfer functions reliably as a control mechanism only if the strongest deforming muscle is selected. The strongest deforming muscle usually is apparent in a varus deformity. When the tibialis posterior muscle is the principal deforming force, its tendon is prominent subcutaneously through the distal part of its course and, in addition to the adduction of the forefoot and varus of the heel, the metatarsals are in plantar flexion. When the tibialis anterior muscle is at fault, in addition to the varus deformity of the heel, adduction of the forefoot, and prominence of the tibialis anterior tendon in the subcutaneous tissues, the forefoot is supinated more and the metatarsals are in less plantar flexion.

If the tibialis posterior is the deforming structure, the plantar half of its tendon is detached from its insertion, is split proximally to the musculotendinous junction, is rerouted posterior to the tibia, and is then sutured to the peroneus brevis tendon. The tension is adjusted so that the foot rests in a neutral position when it dangles. If the tibialis anterior muscle is the major deforming force, its tendon is split to the musculotendinous junction and the lateral half is rerouted to the lateral border of the foot and is then sutured to the tendon of the peroneus brevis or is fixed in the cuboid. Again, the tension should be sufficient to allow the foot to rest in a neutral position when it dangles.

Of the first 30 feet in which this procedure was done by Kaufer, the postural deformity was corrected in 29. In one foot the deformity partially persisted, presumably as a result of failure of the tendon suture. In no instance did the deformity reverse, and all patients have been free of braces since surgery. Furthermore, the deformity has not tended to recur after an average of more than 5 years.

In 1985 Kling, Kaufer, and Hensinger reported excellent or good results in 34 of 37 patients with cerebral palsy who had undergone this operation, 26 of whom had reached skeletal maturity. In no instance did a calcaneus deformity result. Green, Griffin, and Shiavi have likewise reported good results. In our experience it has been a worthwhile procedure when combined with a tendo calcaneus lengthening.

◆ **Split Transfer of Tibialis Posterior Tendon**

TECHNIQUE 30-16 *(Kaufer)*

Begin a curvilinear incision at the tuberosity of the navicular and extend it inferiorly and posteriorly to the medial malleolus and then proximally to the posterior midline over the tendo calcaneus. Deepen the incision through the skin and subcutaneous tissue, and expose the tibialis posterior tendon sheath and the neurovascular bundle. Completely excise the tendon sheath over the tibialis posterior tendon except for a band 1 cm wide at the tip of the medial malleolus. Split the tibialis posterior tendon longitudinally into dorsal and plantar halves by a stab wound through it just distal to the medial malleolus. Introduce hemostats and split the tendon into two halves in the direction of its fibers proximally to the musculotendinous junction and distally to the tuberosity of the navicular. Continue the split beyond the tuberosity by sharp dissection, identify that part of the tendon that extends into the sole of the foot, divide this part, and withdraw it into the proximal part of the wound. Next carry out any necessary lengthening of the tendo calcaneus through the same incision. By blunt dissection separate the flexor tendons of the toes and the neurovascular bundle from the posterior aspect of the tibia and retract them posteriorly (Fig. 30-15). Retract farther laterally so that the fascia forming the peroneal muscle compartment can be seen in the depths of the wound. Excise a large window from this fascia and reposition the foot for access to its lateral side. Now make an incision from the tip of the lateral malleolus to the base of the fifth metatarsal and expose the peroneal tendons. Identify the peroneus brevis tendon and pass a tendon carrier proximally within its sheath posterior to the lateral malleolus. Reposition the foot, identify the tendon carrier within the peroneal muscle compartment, and bring it out through the window in the peroneal fascia and into the medial incision. Insert the freed half of the tibialis posterior tendon into the carrier, draw it through the peroneal muscle compartment and through the peroneal tendon sheath posterior to the lateral malleolus, and bring it out through the lateral incision next to the peroneus brevis tendon. Now close the medial wound. Place the foot in the corrected position with the forefoot abducted and pronated and suture the freed half of the tendon to the peroneus brevis tendon near its insertion and under tension so that the foot dangles in a neutral position (Fig. 30-15, *C* and *D*). Close the wound and apply a long leg plaster cast, holding the foot in the corrected position.

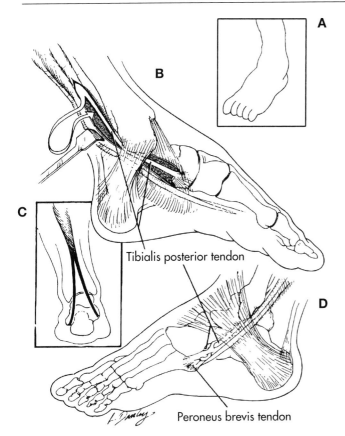

Fig. 30-15 Kaufer split transfer of tibialis posterior tendon for varus deformity. **A,** Foot is in varus position. **B,** Tibialis posterior tendon has been split, one half is freed distally, and flexor tendons of toes and neurovascular bundle are retracted posteriorly. **C** and **D,** Freed half of tendon is passed from medial to lateral behind tibia and sutured to peroneus brevis tendon near its insertion. (Courtesy H Kaufer, MD.)

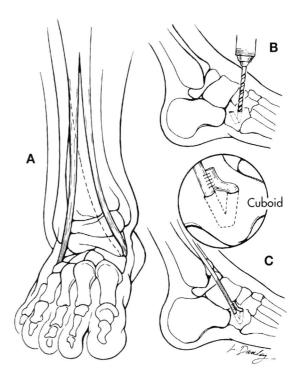

Fig. 30-16 Technique of Hoffer et al. of split transfer of tibialis anterior tendon for varus deformity. **A,** After transfer. **B,** Two holes are drilled in cuboid at converging angles to create tunnel in bone. **C,** One half of tibialis anterior tendon is passed through tunnel and sutured. Route of lateral one half of tibialis anterior tendon is shown. Transfer is completed. (Redrawn from Hoffer MM, Reiswig JA, Garrett AM, Perry J: *Orthop Clin North Am* 5:31, 1974.)

AFTERTREATMENT. At 2 months the cast is removed and a short leg walking cast is applied and worn for 2 more months. Then all external support is discontinued.

◆ Split Transfer of Tibialis Anterior Tendon

Hoffer et al. use this procedure when tibialis anterior hyperactivity causes a varus hindfoot and when the deformity is dynamic and correctable. Gait analysis by electromyography will confirm the hyperactivity of the tibialis anterior muscle in such patients. Barnes and Herring reported good results after split anterior tibial tendon transfer combined with an intramuscular lengthening of the posterior tibial tendon for varus deformity in patients with cerebral palsy. Hui et al. reported that for split tendon transfer, insertion onto the fourth metatarsal axis was the most effective route that produced maximal dorsiflexion with minimal supination and pronation. For a whole tendon transfer, the ideal site of insertion was along the third metatarsal axis.

This procedure is most appropriate when there is varus in the swing phase of gait with a clinically apparent functioning tibialis anterior muscle-tendon unit. If equinus is also present, lengthening of the tendo calcaneus and the tibialis posterior tendon may be necessary.

TECHNIQUE 30-17 *(Hoffer et al.)*

With the patient supine and a tourniquet inflated, make the first longitudinal incision on the dorsomedial aspect of the foot over the first cuneiform. Identify the tibialis anterior tendon at its insertion, split it, and insert an umbilical tape. Then make a second longitudinal incision over the anterolateral aspect of the ankle, identify the tibialis anterior tendon, and draw the umbilical tape into this second incision, splitting the tendon further. Then release the lateral half of the tendon distally, tag it, and bring it into the second incision. Now make a third short longitudinal incision over the dorsum of the cuboid. Pass the lateral half of the tendon subcutaneously into the third incision. Using a 7/64-inch (2.73-mm) drill bit, make two holes in the cuboid at converging angles (Fig. 30-16, *B*). Then use a small curet to join the depths of the holes, making a tunnel. Take care to

continued

preserve a roof of bone. Pass the slip of tendon through the tunnel and suture it on itself with the ankle in slight dorsiflexion (Fig. 30-16, *C*).

In children in whom the cuboid is too small to accept the split tendon through the drill holes, suturing the split anterior tibialis tendon to the peroneus brevis near its insertion on the fifth metatarsal has been found to give excellent results, and we now routinely use this anchor site instead of the cuboid tunnel. Before entering the tendon, the hindfoot is examined to make sure the tendo calcaneus is not excessively tight, which would place excessive stress on the split tendon transfer. In these situations a small gastrocnemius recession is performed through a separate posteromedial incision to help balance the hindfoot and ankle before the split tibialis anterior tendon is sutured to the peroneus brevis.

AFTERTREATMENT. A long leg cast is applied, and after 2 weeks weight-bearing in the cast is permitted. At 6 weeks the cast is discarded, and a weight-bearing orthosis is applied. A splint is used at night. At 6 months bracing is discontinued if possible.

Anterior Transfer of Tibialis Posterior Tendon. This technique is described in Chapter 31.

◆ Transfer of Extensor Hallucis Longus and Tibialis Anterior Tendons

Ono et al. advised the transfer of the flexor hallucis longus and flexor digitorum communis tendon to the dorsum of the foot for spastic equinovarus.

For equinovarus deformity of the foot, Tohen, Carmona, and Barrera transferred the extensor hallucis longus and tibialis anterior tendons to the dorsum of the foot at either its center or lateral side. In 14 feet in which the deformity could be manually reduced, the tendons were transferred to the proximal end of the second metatarsal, and in six in which the deformity could not be so reduced, they were transferred to the base of the fifth metatarsal. In addition to eliminating a dynamically deforming force, the newly created extensor responds to the abnormal Babinski reflex and to the triple flexion response as an active dorsiflexor of the ankle. In all feet the deformity was corrected and the transfer functioned actively after completion of an exercise program. In six feet the tendo calcaneus was lengthened at the time of tendon transfer, in three a triple arthrodesis was carried out at the time of transfer, and in one foot a triple arthrodesis and lengthening of the tendo calcaneus were performed and the tendons were transferred later.

TECHNIQUE 30-18 *(Tohen, Carmona, and Barrera)*

Make a longitudinal incision slightly curved laterally extending from the base of the first metatarsal proximally to the proximal phalanx of the great toe distally. Identify the

tibialis anterior and extensor hallucis longus tendons. Free the insertion of the tibialis anterior tendon, then divide the extensor hallucis longus tendon and suture its remaining distal end to the extensor hallucis brevis tendon. Next make a longitudinal incision 5 cm long proximal to the cruciate ligament of the ankle and lateral to the tibial crest. Through this incision locate the two tendons to be transferred and draw them into the wound. Then make three small incisions in the tibialis anterior tendon and weave the extensor hallucis longus tendon through them; sew the end of the tibialis anterior tendon to the extensor hallucis longus tendon while both are held under equal tension. Then pass this newly created conjoined tendon subcutaneously to the base of the second or fifth metatarsal (depending on the deformity as already mentioned) and anchor it subperiosteally or by the method of Cole (Fig. 1-8). Close the wound and apply a long leg cast.

AFTERTREATMENT. At 5 weeks the cast is removed. The muscles of the transfer are then reeducated by stimulating the sole of the foot so that they contract and by having the patient actively flex the hip while in a sitting position so that dorsiflexion of the foot is produced synergistically. At 6 or 7 weeks walking is resumed in a short leg brace that eliminates plantar flexion, and when the muscles of the transfer function well, the brace is discarded.

In any of these procedures, the flexor hallucis longus and the flexor digitorum communis may be so shortened as to require lengthening. These muscles will rarely prevent passive correction of the deformity, but they will draw the toes into marked plantar flexion once the hindfoot and forefoot have been corrected, making weight-bearing painful.

◆ Osteotomy of Calcaneus

Once the heel becomes fixed in varus, a corrective procedure on the bone is required, combined with a muscle-balancing soft tissue procedure. Osteotomy of the calcaneus as advocated by Dwyer will correct the varus of the heel and, unlike a triple arthrodesis, will not impair mobility in the subtalar or midtarsal joints.

Silver et al. reported a series of patients with cerebral palsy in whom an osteotomy of the calcaneus had been done for varus or valgus deformities of the foot. The operation is basically a modification of the Dwyer osteotomy (Fig. 30-17). It was performed on 27 feet in 20 children whose ages ranged from 2½ to 13 years and who had been observed for 2 to 5½ years after surgery. Twenty opening wedge osteotomies, which were held open by autoclaved homogenous tibial grafts, were done to correct valgus deformity; in 14 the result was excellent, in 4 a mild valgus deformity persisted, and in 2 a varus deformity was produced. Seven closing wedge osteotomies were done through a lateral approach to correct varus deformity, and the fragments

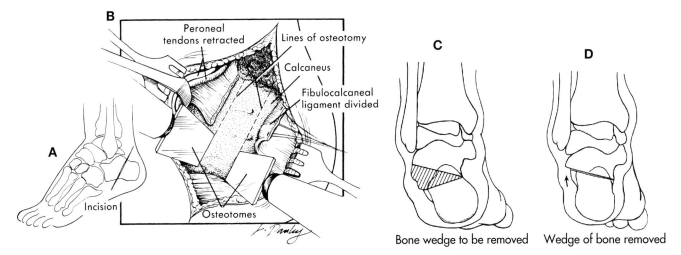

Fig. 30-17   Dwyer closing wedge osteotomy of calcaneus for varus heel. **A,** Lateral skin incision is made inferior and parallel to peroneal tendons. **B,** Wedge of bone is resected with its base laterally. **C,** Wedge of bone is tapered medially. **D,** Calcaneus is closed after bone has been removed, and varus deformity is corrected to slight valgus.

were fixed by staples; in 6 cases the result was excellent, and in 1 a valgus deformity was produced. In 11 of the 27 operations, procedures on the soft structures were carried out at the same time. Silver et al. recommended a minimum age of 3 years for this osteotomy, and they also recommended a triple arthrodesis in children 9 years old or older. In a later long-term study by Silver et al. of 100 patients, the effectiveness of this procedure was reaffirmed.

Opening wedge osteotomies of the calcaneus are not recommended. The skin laterally and medially along the bone is only slightly mobile, and opening wedges put tension on the suture line and tend to cause incisional skin sloughs. The medial calcaneal nerves also may be stretched by an opening wedge osteotomy made from the medial side, causing painful neuromas. For these reasons, a closing wedge resection osteotomy of the calcaneus is recommended. For varus deformities the incision is lateral and the base of the wedge of bone removed is lateral.

TECHNIQUE 30-19 *(Dwyer)*

Expose the lateral aspect of the foot through a curved incision parallel and about 1 cm posterior and inferior to the peroneus longus tendon (Fig. 30-17, *A*). Retract the superior wound edge until the tendon sheath of the peroneus longus is exposed. Strip the periosteum from the superior, lateral, and inferior surfaces of the calcaneus posterior to this tendon. Remove a wedge of bone from the calcaneus just inferior and posterior to the tendon and parallel with it (Fig. 30-17, *B*). Make the base of the wedge 8 to 12 mm wide as needed for correction of the deformity and taper the wedge medially to but not through the medial cortex of the calcaneus (Fig. 30-17, *C*). Manually break the medial cortex and close the gap in the bone. Bring the bony surfaces snugly together by pressing the foot into dorsiflexion against the pull of the tendo calcaneus (Fig. 30-17, *D*). Failure to

close the gap in the calcaneus indicates that a small piece of bone has been left behind at the apex of the wedge and should be removed. Now be certain that the varus deformity has been corrected and that the heel is in the neutral or a slightly varus position. Close the wound and apply a cast from the toes to the tibial tuberosity.

AFTERTREATMENT. Walking may be permitted as soon as soft tissue healing is secure. Cast immobilization is continued until the osteotomy is solid, usually no longer than 8 weeks.

Valgus Deformity

Hindfoot valgus deformity is more common in cerebral palsy than varus deformity, and it is more difficult to correct.

In cerebral palsy, valgus deformity can be caused by overpull of the peroneal and other evertor muscles and weakness, either relative or actual, of the invertor muscles. But Bassett and Baker and Keats and Kouten pointed out that the primary deforming factor in valgus deformity is most often contracture of the triceps surae. The contracted mechanism acts like a bowstring on the calcaneus and thus blocks normal dorsiflexion at the ankle joint. The desired dorsiflexion must then occur at the midtarsal joint, and as a part of this dorsiflexion the calcaneus usually rolls into eversion, removing the sustentaculum tali from its normal supporting position beneath the head of the talus. The forefoot abducts at the midtarsal joint, and the talus drops into a more medial and vertical position than normally. A standing lateral roentgenogram of the foot will indicate that the talus is in fact oriented vertically and standing on its head. The first step in correcting this deformity is to release the contracted triceps surae.

Initially, a valgus foot deformity should be treated conservatively with an orthosis or a shoe insert. If this approach is unsuccessful and the tendo calcaneus is tight, causing the foot to break in the midtarsal joint, tendo calcaneus lengthening and use of a shoe insert are indicated. Tight or spastic peroneus brevis and longus muscles may contribute to the deformity, and their tendons may require lengthening to correct the deformity.

Several operations have been suggested to alter the effect of the peroneal muscles on the valgus foot, but these have not gained much popularity. The peroneal tendons can be transferred to the midline dorsally, to the calcaneus, or to the tibialis posterior tendon. Perry and Hoffer have transferred the peroneus longus or peroneus brevis posteromedially into the tibialis posterior tendon if either or both are active during the stance phase only.

◆ Peroneus Brevis Elongation

TECHNIQUE 30-20 *(Fulford)*

Make an incision 3 cm long just proximal and posterior to the lateral malleolus. Enter the tendon sheath at the musculotendinous junction of the peroneus brevis muscle. Divide the peroneus brevis tendon transversely about 1 cm proximal to the lowest muscle fiber insertion on the tendon. Close the incision routinely.

AFTERTREATMENT. A short leg walking cast is applied and is molded to hold the foot in a varus position. Weight-bearing in the cast is allowed for approximately 6 weeks; the cast is then removed.

Extraarticular Arthrodesis of Subtalar Joint for Equinovalgus Deformity. Much has been written about the role of the Grice subtalar extraarticular arthrodesis for valgus deformity in cerebral palsy since Grice reported it in 1952. Keats and Kouten reported a series of 63 Grice operations for planovalgus deformity. To correct the equinus position of the talus and the lateral displacement of the calcaneus, they recommended opening the capsule of the talonavicular joint and, using a bone hook, reducing the head of the talus into its normal position over the sustentaculum tali before the bone grafts are locked in place. They also recommended homogenous bank bone for grafts, and in the 53 feet in which it was used, it caused no complications. The result was satisfactory in 61 feet in patients whose ages ranged from 2 to 8 years.

In 1974 Engstrom, Erikson, and Hjelmstedt studied the results of the Grice subtalar arthrodesis in 27 feet of patients with cerebral palsy. In 9 feet the grafts failed to unite, and in 6 they were either fully or partially absorbed. In 4 feet, abduction deformity of 15 to 30 degrees persisted, the foot was unstable, and weight-bearing was unsatisfactory. These researchers again emphasized the importance of correcting any existing deformity either before or during surgery, the use of strong autogenous bone for grafting, and the use of internal fixation to maintain the position until union has occurred.

Tohen et al. and others have reported their unsuccessful experience with the classic Grice procedure in a large number of patients. Despite this, the Grice subtalar extraarticular arthrodesis in most cases will stabilize a planovalgus foot deformity in cerebral palsy patients. It should be preceded or accompanied by operations that correct deformity of the soft structures and that attempt to balance muscle power. The bone grafts should be placed so that they lie at a right angle to the axis of motion of the subtalar joint and, as seen in a lateral roentgenogram of the foot, parallel to the weight-bearing axis of the leg, ankle, and foot. The dislocation of the head of the talus from the sustentaculum tali should be reduced before the grafts are inserted. Autogenous bone graft or bone bank bone can be used to obtain a fusion. The extremity should be immobilized until the fusion is solid. Jeray et al. reported good results with the use of a local bone graft technique for subtalar extraarticular arthrodesis.

Several modifications of the extraarticular subtalar fusion have appeared since Grice originally reported his procedure. Most are aimed at better retention of the calcaneus beneath the talus by some means, such as the use of a fibular graft or a perpendicular cancellous screw across the joint, because postoperative loss of position and nonunion have been among the complications. Other modifications include the use of other types of grafts and the donor areas from which they are obtained. A well-done extraarticular subtalar fusion has established itself as a useful procedure in the treatment of valgus foot deformities arising from cerebral palsy.

Baker and Hill described a different osteotomy of the calcaneus for correcting valgus deformities of the foot. It is a horizontal osteotomy made immediately beneath the posterior articular facet (Fig. 30-18). Its purpose is to correct the valgus inclination of this articular surface caused by prolonged weight-bearing with the foot in the deformed position. Forty-one such osteotomies were followed after surgery for an average of over 2 years. In 31 feet the osteotomy was the only operation performed on the bones; in 21 the result was satisfactory, in 2 a mild to moderate varus deformity was produced, and in 8 a mild valgus deformity persisted. In 10 feet the osteotomy was combined with the Grice extraarticular subtalar arthrodesis; in 5 the result was excellent, in 4 some valgus deformity persisted, and in 1 foot a varus deformity was produced.

The Grice-Green technique is described in Chapter 26.

◆ Modifications of Grice Extraarticular Subtalar Arthrodesis

TECHNIQUE 30-21 *(Dennyson and Fulford)*

Obliquely incise the skin in line with the skin creases over the sinus tarsi beginning anteriorly at the middle of the ankle and proceeding laterally to the peroneal tendons (Fig. 30-19, *A*). Incise and reflect as one flap the subcutaneous fat and the origins of the extensor brevis muscles. By sharp dissection excise the fat from the sinus tarsi down to bone proximally and distally. With a small gouge remove cortical bone from the apex of the sinus tarsi to expose cancellous bone on both the talar neck and the superior surface of the calcaneus. Do not remove the cortical bone from the outer part of the sinus tarsi where a transfixion screw is to pass.

Dorsally expose the small depression just behind the neck of the talus through a small separate skin incision and by blunt dissection between the neurovascular bundle and the tendons of the extensor digitorum longus. Hold the calcaneus in the corrected position and pass an awl from on top of the talus, through the talus, across the subtalar joint, and through the calcaneus. Direct the awl posteriorly, inferiorly, and slightly laterally so that it passes through cortical bone of the talus above and below and through cortical bone of the calcaneus above and inferolaterally. Use

the awl to determine the desired length of a screw needed for fixation and insert a screw in the hole. Remove chips of cancellous bone from the iliac crest and pack them into the sinus tarsi and against the bone that has been denuded on the talus and calcaneus (Fig. 30-19, *B*). Replace the extensor digitorum brevis and close the skin. Apply a short leg cast over padding. Mold it well around the heel and leave it in place for 6 to 8 weeks.

Barrasso, Wile, and Gage have modified this technique by using a Kirschner wire extending from the talus into the calcaneus as a guide for screw placement and as a holding device during screw insertion. They also do not decorticate the bone in the sinus tarsi until the screw has been placed across the subtalar joint.

Calcaneal Osteotomy. An effort has been made to preserve subtalar motion if possible by making an osteotomy of the calcaneus without removing a wedge of bone and translocating the inferior part of the calcaneus to a more medial position.

◆ Medial Displacement Sliding Osteotomy of Calcaneus

TECHNIQUE 30-22

Place the patient supine and apply a midthigh tourniquet. Expose the lateral surface of the calcaneus through an incision beginning near the lateral tuberosity of the tendo calcaneus attachment and extending distally and parallel to but inferior to the sural nerve. By blunt dissection expose the lateral surface of the calcaneus, reflecting the peroneal tendons and sural nerve superiorly. Using the plantar surface of the foot as a guide, place a Kirschner wire along the lateral side of the calcaneus and, with a roentgenogram of the foot, determine the appropriate placement of the osteotomy. It should not extend forward into the subtalar or calcaneocuboid joint. Make it transverse and parallel to the sole of the foot, beginning just posterior to the subtalar joint, and direct it plantarward toward the attachment of the plantar fascia to the calcaneus (Fig. 30-20, *A*). In making the osteotomy, protect the tendo calcaneus superiorly and the plantar muscles, vessels, and nerves inferiorly. Do not

continued

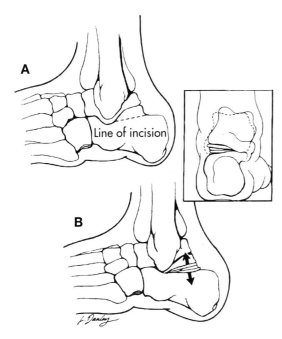

Fig. 30-18 Baker and Hill osteotomy of calcaneus to correct heel valgus. **A,** Broken line shows site of horizontal osteotomy made from lateral side; medial cortex is left intact to act as hinge. **B,** Osteotomy is opened enough laterally to place calcaneus in neutral position and is held open by homogenous bone grafts. (Redrawn from Baker LD, Hill LM: *J Bone Joint Surg* 46A:1, 1964.)

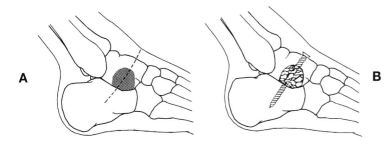

Fig. 30-19 Dennyson and Fulford technique of extra-articular subtalar arthrodesis using screw and cancellous bone chips. **A,** Skin incision and bone area curetted from lateral side of talus and calcaneus. **B,** Placement of iliac bone chips in side of talus and calcaneus after screw has been inserted across subtalar joint with heel in corrected position. (Redrawn from Dennyson WG, Fulford GE: *J Bone Joint Surg* 58B:507, 1976.)

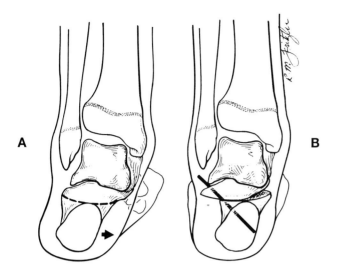

Fig. 30-20   Medial displacement of calcaneus for hindfoot valgus. **A,** Transverse osteotomy of calcaneus. **B,** Fixation with Kirschner wire after distal fragment has been shifted medially to place calcaneus in weight-bearing line of tibia.

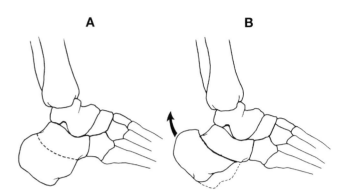

Fig. 30-21   Samilson technique of crescentic osteotomy of calcaneus. **A,** Line of osteotomy. **B,** Displacement of posterior fragment of calcaneus posterosuperiorly. (Redrawn from Samilson RL: Crescentic osteotomy of os calcis for calcaneocavus feet. In Bateman JE, ed: *Foot science,* Philadelphia, 1976, WB Saunders.)

penetrate the periosteum on the medial side of the bone. Once the osteotomy is complete, slide the inferior fragment medially to align the calcaneus with the tibia correctly. Insert a threaded Kirschner wire through the two fragments of calcaneus, downward and medially, for internal fixation (Fig. 30-20, *B*). Close the wound over suction drainage and apply a short leg cast.

AFTERTREATMENT. The cast is changed at 2 weeks, and the threaded Kirschner wire is removed. Another short leg cast is applied and is worn for 4 weeks.

Calcaneal Lengthening. Mosca reported a calcaneal lengthening osteotomy for the treatment of hindfoot valgus deformity, combined with tendo calcaneus lengthening. His technique is described in Chapter 79.

CALCANEUS DEFORMITY

Talipes calcaneus in spasticity usually is secondary to excessive or repeated lengthening of the tendo calcaneus either alone or in conjunction with neurectomy of branches of the tibial nerve. However, it also can develop as a primary deformity when the dorsiflexors of the foot are spastic and the triceps surae is weak. Surgical correction of talipes calcaneus in spasticity, whatever its cause, usually is unsatisfactory. If the dorsiflexors of the foot are spastic, the toe extensors can be partially denervated and the tibialis anterior tendon can be transferred to the tendo calcaneus, which is shortened at the same time. For calcaneo-cavus deformity caused by a spastic tibialis anterior muscle, Bleck advises stabilization of the subtalar joint by a Grice

procedure fixed with a screw and then transfer of the tibialis anterior tendon posteriorly into the calcaneus to strengthen plantar flexion (see Chapter 26). If this does not restore muscle balance, the peroneus longus and tibialis posterior tendons can both be inserted into the tendo calcaneus to further strengthen plantar flexion. The treatment of this condition in most instances is prevention by avoiding inappropriate lengthening or denervating procedures on the gastrocsoleus muscle group.

◆ Crescentic Osteotomy of Calcaneus

Occasionally talipes calcaneus is purely in the hindfoot and is accompanied by a cavus deformity in the midfoot. In such instances, Samilson has recommended a crescentic osteotomy of the calcaneus to lengthen the foot and elevate the base of the heel.

TECHNIQUE 30-23 *(Samilson)*

Inflate a midthigh tourniquet and incise the skin laterally over the calcaneus posterior to the subtalar joint and overlying the posterior tuberosity of the calcaneus. The peroneal tendons should lie anterior to the incision, and the incision should parallel them. Expose the lateral side of the calcaneus, protect the peroneal tendons, and then perform a plantar fasciotomy from the lateral surface of the foot. Make a crescentic osteotomy in the calcaneus with a motor saw using a curved blade or with a large curved osteotome (Fig. 30-21, *A*). Free the posterior tuberosity of the calcaneus and then shift it proximally and posteriorly in the line of the osteotomy to correct the calcaneocavus deformity (Fig. 30-21, *B*). Secure the fragments with a staple or a Kirschner wire and apply a short leg cast.

AFTERTREATMENT. The cast and staple or Kirschner wire are removed 6 weeks after surgery and full weight-bearing is allowed.

CAVUS DEFORMITY

Talipes cavus deformity is uncommon in cerebral palsy. It can occur as a hindfoot cavus in which the calcaneus is in a calcaneus position or as a forefoot cavus in which the apex of the angulation is at the midtarsal joints or distally. Hindfoot cavus is best treated by crescentic osteotomy of the calcaneus combined with plantar release as recommended by Samilson (see above). Forefoot cavus may respond to a plantar release and casting. In adolescents and adults, correction may require osteotomies as described in Chapter 32.

After skeletal maturity all residual deformities in the ankle, hindfoot, and midfoot can be corrected by a triple arthrodesis with appropriate wedge resections (see Chapter 31). Before undertaking a triple arthrodesis in a child with cerebral palsy, the surgeon always should obtain standing anteroposterior roentgenograms of the ankle. What often appears to be a valgus of the heel may in fact be valgus of the ankle mortise, which should be corrected by a supramalleolar osteotomy and realignment of the ankle rather than by creation of a secondary compensatory deformity in the subtalar joint (Fig. 30-22). Any external tibial torsion should be recognized before a triple arthrodesis is done because if the ankle joint is externally rotated, the foot will still appear to be in valgus and abduction after the triple arthrodesis.

◆ ADDUCTION DEFORMITY OF FOREFOOT

Bleck noted in 10 patients with spasticity an adduction deformity of the forefoot caused by spasticity of the abductor hallucis muscle that appeared after the triceps surae had been lengthened. The abductor hallucis becomes more active after this lengthening because a substitute pattern of muscle function develops. When the great toe is passively adducted at the metatarsophalangeal joint, the tight abductor hallucis tendon is palpable. To determine definitely that this muscle is the deforming one, it can be paralyzed by infiltrating it with procaine as a diagnostic procedure. An alternative method of making certain the abductor hallucis is the deforming force is to passively abduct the forefoot while holding the heel stable and the foot plantigrade and take a roentgenogram in the anteroposterior plane. If forefoot adduction can be passively corrected, Bleck recommends resecting a segment of the muscle and its tendon. Nine patients were observed for more than 2½ years after this operation was performed bilaterally; in 2 feet a hallux valgus deformity developed, but in the other 16 the adduction deformity did not increase, and the function and appearance of the feet were satisfactory.

TECHNIQUE 30-24 *(Bleck)*
Make a longitudinal incision 4 cm long over the medial aspect of the first metatarsal neck and curve it distally to the

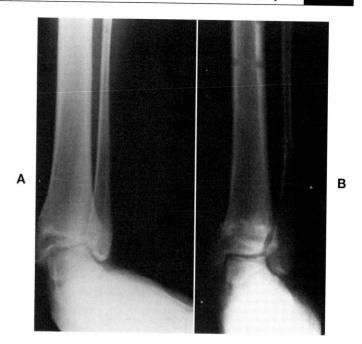

Fig. 30-22 A, Standing anteroposterior view of ankle demonstrating valgus deformity of ankle joint. **B,** Alignment of ankle achieved by supramalleolar osteotomy.

dorsomedial aspect of the proximal phalanx of the great toe. Expose and identify the abductor hallucis muscle and tendon and resect a segment of muscle and tendon 2.5 cm long. If the medial part of the capsule of the metatarsophalangeal joint is tight, do a partial capsulectomy. Close the wound, pad the medial border of the forefoot and great toe, and apply a boot cast molded to force the forefoot in abduction.

AFTERTREATMENT. At 6 weeks the cast is removed, and physical therapy is started.

◆ ◆ ◆

In an older child, forefoot adduction that cannot be corrected passively should be treated by osteotomies of the bases of all five metatarsals (see Chapter 26), metatarsal realignment, and internal fixation with Kirschner wires until union has occurred. Medial opening wedge midfoot osteotomy and grafting combined with a closing wedge midfoot osteotomy also has been used to correct this deformity.

Hallux Valgus

Hallux valgus deformity usually occurs secondary to equinovalgus in the foot, valgus in the heel, or external torsion of the tibia. As the foot pronates, the hallux is forced passively into abduction and hallux valgus results. The tendon of the extensor hallucis longus then subluxates into the space between the first and second metatarsals, and in this position it acts as an active adductor on the hallux. When the foot everts, the origin of the adductor hallucis arising from the peroneal tendon sheath is moved laterally and distally, thereby furthering its deforming influence on the hallux.

Correction of the equinovalgus, heel valgus, or external tibial torsion should precede any bunion procedure. If the hindfoot deformity is allowed to remain, recurrence of the hallux valgus is almost certain after any soft tissue procedure on the hallux, especially if arthrodesis of the metatarsophalangeal joint is not performed.

Root described a soft tissue procedure to correct hallux valgus after the foot has been balanced, which involves adductor hallucis release at the metatarsophalangeal joint and a lateral capsular release. The long toe extensor tendon is then isolated and passed through a subcutaneous tunnel along the medial side of the first metatarsophalangeal joint.

Correction of the hallux valgus may require fusion of the metatarsophalangeal joint by the McKeever method (see Chapter 78). In cerebral palsy patients the metatarsophalangeal fusion may give longer lasting and more predictable results.

Surgical procedures for hallux valgus are described in Chapter 78.

CLAWTOES

Clawtoe deformity is common in adolescents and adults with cerebral palsy. Although neurectomy of the lateral plantar nerve has been recommended for these deformities, we prefer to treat clawtoes by metatarsophalangeal joint capsulotomies and tenotomy of the long toe extensors to the lesser toes and proximal interphalangeal joint resections or fusions using Kirschner wire fixation until the bone and soft tissues are stable.

Surgical procedures for clawtoes are described in Chapter 38.

Knee and Hip Relationships

Deformities and disabilities of the knee in cerebral palsy are difficult to evaluate and treat. Pelvic, hip, knee, ankle, and foot deformities are interrelated. Muscle imbalance in the pelvis or the ankle and foot can cause deformities in the knee, and muscle imbalance in the knee can cause deformities in the pelvis, hip, or ankle. A number of muscles that cross the extensor and flexor sides of the hip and muscles that arise above the knee joint and that cause equinus or calcaneus deformities in the ankle also can cause deformities in the knee. These "two joint" muscles—the rectus femoris anteriorly, the gracilis, semitendinosus, and semimembranosus posteriorly (the medial hamstrings), and the biceps femoris (the lateral hamstrings)—all directly affect the position of the knee as well as the position of the hip. The gastrocnemius muscle originates above the knee joint and extends to the ankle joint, so it affects knee and ankle motion and position. A person who walks with his knees flexed does not necessarily have hamstrings that are tight or spastic. A person may walk with the knees in recurvatum, but this does

not mean that the quadriceps is overactive because this condition can be caused by an equinus contracture of the ankle or weakened hamstrings.

KNEE FLEXION DEFORMITY

Flexion, by far the most common knee deformity, can be caused by tight hamstring muscles, weak quadriceps muscle, or a combination of both. It can result from hip flexion deformities in which the hip flexors are spastic, the hip extensors are weak, or a combination of the two. It also can result from equinus of the ankles, or the so-called jump position, in which the hips are flexed, the knees are flexed, and the ankles are in equinus. It may be secondary to a weak triceps, in which the tendo calcaneus or another portion of the triceps surae has been overlengthened, or in which spastic ankle dorsiflexors overpull the ankles into calcaneus. If the ankles are in calcaneus, the knees must flex to get the forefeet on the ground.

To find the cause of knee flexion, the muscles must be assessed to determine whether the joint itself is contracted or whether the deformity is caused by spasticity. If possible, the strength of the muscles should be assessed, although this is difficult in a patient with cerebral palsy. It must be remembered that cerebral palsy is an upper motor neuron disorder caused by a lesion in the brain. The brain is geographically affected, and the body is regionally affected. Nerves to one specific muscle are not affected, but rather, nerves to a group of muscles are affected. If the hamstring muscles are spastic, then the quadriceps probably will be spastic too, perhaps to a lesser degree. The same is true for the gastrocnemius, the dorsiflexors of the foot, the flexors and extensors, and the abductors and adductors of the hip. It is not unusual to correct a knee flexion deformity by transferring or lengthening a hamstring and then have a spastic rectus femoris pull the knee into hyperextension because spasticity in the rectus femoris was not detected before the hamstring muscles were altered. An extended knee in the swing phase of gait tremendously hampers propulsion. If a person has flexed hips and extended knees, he may have difficulty even bending his knees enough to get up on a curbing or to climb steps. To effect this elevation, he must hike up his pelvis and abduct his hips.

The strength of the quadriceps muscle, whether it is under voluntary control and whether it has functional strength is best checked with the patient supine and his feet off the end of the table. Extend the hips and allow the knees to flex passively (Fig. 30-23, *A*) and then ask the patient to voluntarily extend his knees against resistance (Fig. 30-23, *B*). An opinion then can be formed as to the strength of the quadriceps. To determine if the rectus femoris muscle is spastic, turn the patient prone and do the prone rectus (Ely) test (Fig. 30-24). With the patient prone and the knees extended, flex the knees. If the rectus is spastic, the hips will flex and the buttocks will rise off the table when the rectus is thus stretched. It is best to do this test one side at a time to determine the relative spasticity in each rectus femoris.

The hamstring spasticity and contracture test is done with

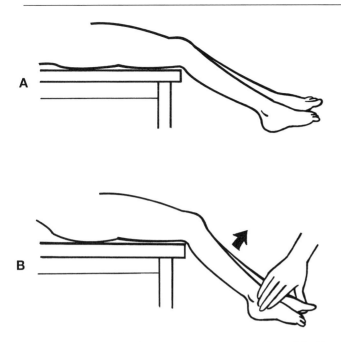

Fig. 30-23 Testing for quadriceps strength. **A,** With hips extended, knees are allowed to flex off end of table. **B,** Patient voluntarily extends knees from flexed position against resistance. (Redrawn from Evans EB: *Instr Course Lect* 20:42, 1971.)

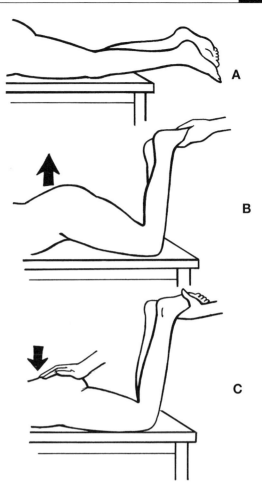

Fig. 30-24 Prone rectus test. **A,** Patient is prone, and knees are extended. **B,** Flexing knees causes buttocks to rise from table. **C,** Spasticity in rectus is overcome by downward pressure on buttocks. (Redrawn from Evans EB: *Instr Course Lect* 20:42, 1971.)

the patient prone and then supine (Fig. 30-25). With the patient prone, extend the hips as much as possible and exert gentle pressure on the calves. The angle that the femur and the tibia make after the spasticity has been overcome is the degree of absolute contracture of the soft tissues behind the knee. Next, place the patient supine to test hamstring spasticity. Stabilize the opposite knee in as much extension as possible and then raise the leg that is to be examined with the knee straight. If knee extension is limited as the hip is flexed, then either the medial or lateral hamstrings are tight. The patient also can be examined for medial hamstring spasticity in the prone position with the knees flexed and feet off the table. This relaxes the hamstrings proximally and allows the hip to be abducted if there is no contracture of the adductor muscles. Extend the knees. If extension is not possible unless the hip is adducted, the gracilis and medial hamstrings are tight. This also can be done with the patient supine and the hips and knees flexed (Fig. 30-26). To test for gastrocnemius contracture, the amount of equinus in the ankle is measured with the knee fully extended and then with the knee flexed (Fig. 30-27). If the ankle can be dorsiflexed more with the knee flexed than with it extended, there is gastrocnemius contracture or spasticity.

An absolute contracture of about 10 degrees is compatible with walking without flexing the hips and knees excessively. Contracture beyond 10 degrees should be corrected, usually by changing the strength of the hamstring muscles.

Weakened hamstrings are the major cause of recurvatum in the knees; thus only partial lengthening of the hamstring tendons is indicated in most instances. Selective lengthening of the gracilis and semitendinosus muscles with a Z-plasty

procedure and a recession of the semimembranosus are recommended. If the biceps femoris is determined to be tight, it is lengthened by incising its fascia.

◆ Fractional Lengthening of Hamstring Tendons
In 1942 Green and McDermott reported fractionally lengthening the hamstring tendons and other tendons about the knee in spastic flexion deformities. Some modification of their original operation is now used by most surgeons to modify spastic knee flexion when indicated.

Thometz, Simon, and Rosenthal reviewed the effectiveness of hamstring lengthening on 31 patients with cerebral palsy. All had preoperative and postoperative dynamic gait studies, including clinical evaluation, dynamic electromyographic patterns, velocity, cadence, stride length, and range and patterns of rotational motion of the knees, pelvis, hips, and ankle, especially the range of flexion and extension of the hips and ankles when the knees were in maximal extension. They concluded that overall, velocity, stride length, and cadence did

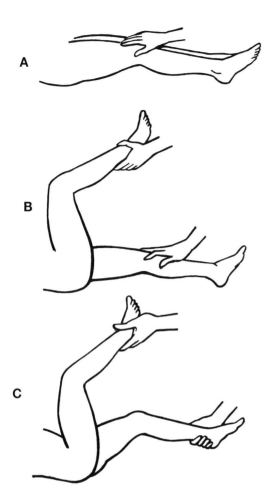

Fig. 30-25 Testing for hamstring spasticity and contracture. **A,** Patient is supine with hips extended. Pressure is exerted over knees, forcing them into extension. Flexion remaining in knees is absolute knee flexion contracture. **B,** Knee on side to be tested is flexed while opposite knee is stabilized in extension. **C,** Attempted flexion of hip results in more flexion of knee. (Redrawn from Evans EB: *Instr Course Lect* 20:42, 1971.)

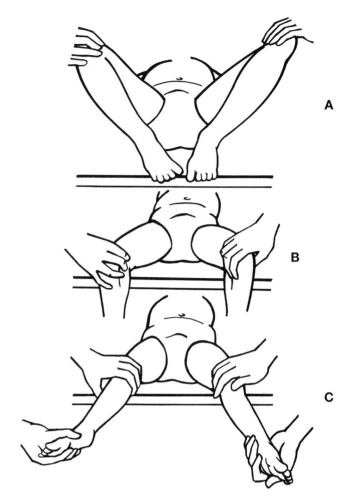

Fig. 30-26 Testing for adductor and medial hamstring tightness. **A,** Thighs abduct well with hips and knees flexed, indicating no adductor contracture. **B,** With hips extended and knees flexed, hips abduct well. **C,** With hips extended, bringing knees into extension causes thighs to adduct, indicating medial hamstring spasticity. (Redrawn from Evans EB: *Instr Course Lect* 20:42, 1971.)

not improve after hamstring lengthening, but knee extension in the stance phase improved markedly, although this was accompanied by a reduction in knee flexion in the swing phase. When the hamstrings and quadriceps were spastic, knee flexion during the swing phase of gait was markedly diminished.

TECHNIQUE 30-25 *(Tachdjian)*
Place the patient prone and inflate a midthigh tourniquet; then make a midline longitudinal incision beginning just above the popliteal crease and extend it 7 to 10 cm proximally (Fig. 30-28, *A*). Medial and lateral posterior incisions also can be used instead of a single midline incision. Divide the subcutaneous tissue and deep fascia in line with the skin incision. Protect the posterior femoral cutaneous nerve in the proximal part of the wound. Next,

identify the hamstring tendons by blunt dissection. Divide the tendon sheaths of each longitudinally and tag them with silk sutures. Expose the tendon of the biceps femoris laterally and isolate it from the peroneal nerve lying along its medial side. Pass a blunt instrument deep to the biceps tendon, incise its tendinous portion transversely at two levels 3 cm apart, and leave the muscle fibers intact (Fig. 30-28, *B*). The tendon lengthens over the muscle fibers as the hip is flexed and the knee is extended (Fig. 30-28, *C*). Next, isolate the semimembranosus tendon medially. Incise its tendon sheath and mark it as above. Divide its tendinous fibers on its deep side at two levels as in the biceps femoris (Fig. 30-28, *D*). Extend the knee and flex the hip, and the tendinous parts will slide on the muscle. Expose the

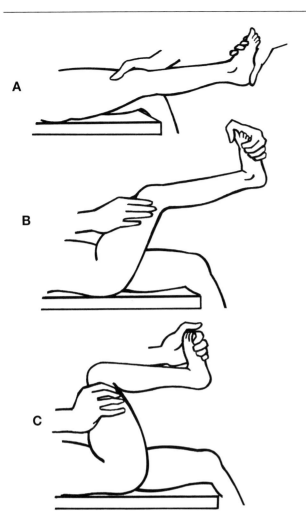

Fig. 30-27 Testing for gastrocnemius contracture and spasticity. **A,** With knee extended, equinus in ankle is noted. **B,** With knee flexed, ankle is easily dorsiflexed, indicating no soleus contracture. **C,** As knee is extended, ankle dorsiflexion is resisted by tight or spastic gastrocnemius muscles. (Redrawn from Evans EB: *Instr Course Lect* 20:42, 1971.)

semitendinosus tendon and divide the distal part of the tendon obliquely up to its muscle fibers. Incise the tendon transversely above and lengthen it in a similar manner or perform a Z-plasty procedure to lengthen the tendon (Fig. 30-28, *E*). Close all tendon sheaths meticulously but do not close the deep fascia (Fig. 30-28, *F*). After deflating the tourniquet, secure all bleeding points and close the subcutaneous tissues and skin. Apply a long leg cast with the knee in extension.

AFTERTREATMENT. Straight leg raising exercises are done 15 times a day while the cast is on to stretch the hamstring tendons. At 3 to 4 weeks, a new long leg cast is applied and bivalved so that active and passive exercises to alter knee

flexion and strengthen knee extension can be started. The patient is allowed to walk with crutches, and the cast is discontinued when a functional range of motion and muscle control of the knees are acquired.

◆ Distal Transfer of Rectus Femoris

Gage recommended distal transfer of the rectus femoris in the crouch gait in an effort to augment knee flexion while walking and to eliminate its extensor activity on the knee during the swing phase of gait. He noted that this operation has been effective in improving the swing phase of gait and foot clearance when appropriate prerequisites are observed: (1) any hamstring contracture must be corrected to allow full knee extension in midstance; (2) the foot must be plantigrade and stable in stance, which is accomplished either by surgery or with an orthosis; and (3) the foot progression line must be capable of producing a moment strong enough to maintain knee extension in midstance and terminal stance. He reported that malrotation of 10 degrees or less of the lower extremity can be corrected by appropriately transferring the distal insertion of the rectus femoris either medially for in-toeing or laterally for out-toeing. Inappropriate activity of the rectus femoris during preswing and swing must be demonstrated during gait analysis. Studies by Ounpuu et al. and Sutherland, Santi, and Abel have shown that transfer of the rectus femoris gives significantly better results in peak knee flexion during the swing phase of gait than simple release of the rectus femoris alone.

Rethlefsen et al. reported good results in 16 children after distal rectus femoris transfer. Significant improvement was seen in knee flexion and extension; however, stride length and gait velocity did not improve except in those patients who wore a postoperative orthosis. These authors noted that postoperative bracing may maximize surgical outcome in some patients.

TECHNIQUE 30-26 *(Gage)* (Fig. 30-29)

With the patient anesthetized and supine, make a longitudinal incision in the anterior thigh 5 to 6 cm proximal to the patella. Identify the rectus femoris proximally as it lies between the vastus lateralis and medialis. Separate the tendon of the rectus from the remainder of the quadriceps tendon but do not enter the knee joint. Dissect it free to approximately 3 cm proximal to the patella. Divide the tendon and separate it from the vastus intermedius, which it overlies. If the hamstrings are to be lengthened, transfer the distal end of the rectus femoris to the distal stump of the semitendinosus or to the gracilis muscle through an opening made in the medial intermuscular septum, or transfer it into the muscular part of the sartorius after an opening has been made in the medial intermuscular septum and the sartorius has been pulled through this opening into the anterior thigh distally. Pass the tendon through the sartorius and suture it onto itself. If the tendon is to be transferred laterally, pass it around the iliotibial band laterally and suture it back on itself.

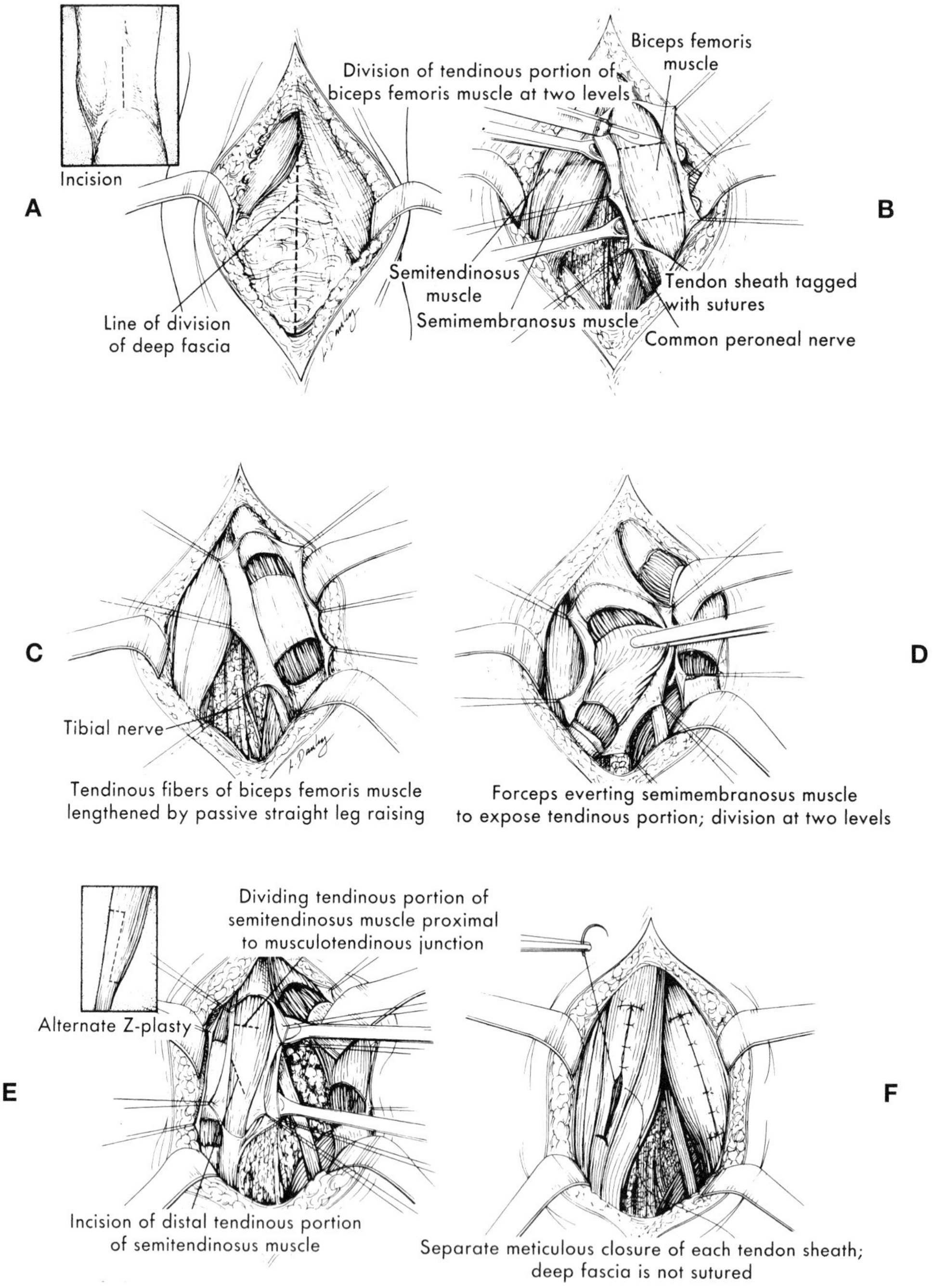

Fig. 30-28   Fractional lengthening of hamstrings. **A,** Skin incision and incision in deep fascia over back of knee. **B,** Incisions in tendon of biceps femoris in lateral compartment after its tendon sheath has been opened and retracted, with peroneal nerve protected medially. **C,** Tendon of biceps femoris lengthens as knee is extended and hip is flexed. **D,** Division of tendon of semimembranosus in similar fashion. **E,** Semitendinosus is lengthened by Z-plasty, as seen in inset, or by step-cuts in its tendon at multiple levels. **F,** Tendon sheaths of biceps femoris and semimembranosus are sutured before closure of wound. (Redrawn from Tachjdian MO: *Pediatric orthopaedics,* Philadelphia, 1972, WB Saunders.)

AFTERTREATMENT. Plaster immobilization is not necessary; instead, a foam-fabric knee immobilizer is used. The day after surgery the patient is allowed to sit in a reclining wheelchair and is gradually moved to the upright sitting position with the knee fully extended. Standing with support is allowed on the third day, and the knee immobilizer is removed for passive range-of-motion exercises for the knees. Walking without the knee immobilizer is started on the fourth or fifth day. At 4 weeks the physical therapist instructs the patient in vigorous exercises to strengthen the muscles while gait training continues. Gait will continue to improve until about 1 year after

surgery; then gait studies should be done to determine objectively the degree of improvement in gait and muscle balance.

◆ Lateral Transfer of Medial Hamstrings for Internal Rotational Deformity of Hip

Baker and Hill described an operation in which the semitendinosus tendon is transferred laterally to the anterior surface of the lateral femoral condyle for internal rotational deformity of the hip. They first used the procedure for an athetoid patient

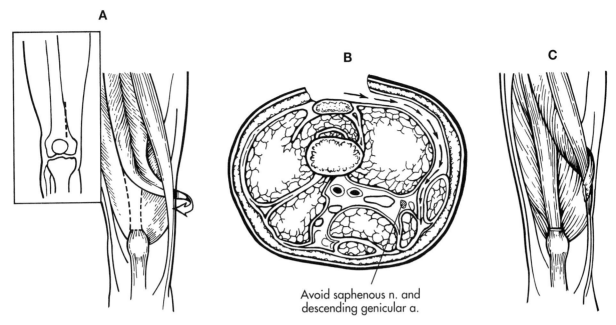

Fig. 30-29   Distal release or transfer of rectus femoris. **A,** Rectus femoris is separated from vastus medialis, vastus lateralis, and vastus intermedius. *Inset,* Longitudinal incision along medial side of distal third of rectus femoris. **B,** Rectus femoris may be transferred through medial intermuscular septum to sartorius if desired. **C,** Rectus femoris is sutured to sartorius.

with a dynamic deformity, but it also has proved useful when the tendon has been divided in the treatment of flexion deformity of the knee. The tendon is passed through a subcutaneous tunnel from the posteromedial aspect of the middle of the thigh to the anterior aspect of the lateral femoral condyle, where it is anchored opposite the superior pole of the patella.

Sutherland et al. used a technique of simultaneous electromyographic and photographic studies before and after surgery to record the timing of contraction of muscles, which coincided with the abnormal internal rotational movement at the hip. As a result of these studies, they transferred the semimembranosus and semitendinosus, as well as the gracilis if the adductors had not been previously released, to the lateral aspect of the femur and anchored them to the lateral intermuscular septum (Fig. 30-30).

TECHNIQUE 30-27 *(Sutherland et al.)*

With the patient prone, inflate a pneumatic tourniquet high on the thigh and make an S-shaped incision on the posterior aspect of the knee. Begin the incision proximally on the lateral aspect of the popliteal space over the biceps femoris tendon and extend it distally 7.5 cm, then medially across the popliteal space in the flexor crease, and then again distally for 5 cm over the insertion of the semitendinosus muscle (see Fig. 30-30, *A*). Mobilize the proximal flap. Pass a clamp beneath the semitendinosus and semimembranosus tendons and divide them near their insertions. If the adductors have not been previously released, identify the

gracilis tendon, free it proximally, and divide it near its insertion. Next gently mobilize the tibial and common peroneal nerves and develop the interval deep to the nerves but superficial to the femoral artery and vein and extend it down to the lateral intermuscular septum (Fig. 30-30, *B*). Incise the lateral intermuscular septum at its attachment to the periosteum of the femur just proximal to the lateral femoral condyle (Fig. 30-30, *C*). Gently tease the fibers of the vastus lateralis muscle away from the anterior surface of the intermuscular septum, pass the tendons through the incision in the septum, loop them around the septum, and suture them to themselves with interrupted nonabsorbable sutures (Fig. 30-30, *D*). Sometimes the semimembranosus alone is passed through the septum and the semitendinosus is sutured to it. The tendons must not be fixed under too much tension since Perry et al. have pointed out that this may cause inappropriate electrical activity in the transfer after surgery. Close the wound in layers and apply a long leg cast.

AFTERTREATMENT. At 4 weeks the cast is removed, and a walking cylinder cast is applied. At 6 weeks this cast is removed, and physical therapy is started.

RECURVATUM OF KNEE

Recurvatum may be primarily the result of quadriceps spasticity or quadriceps spasticity that is greater than any

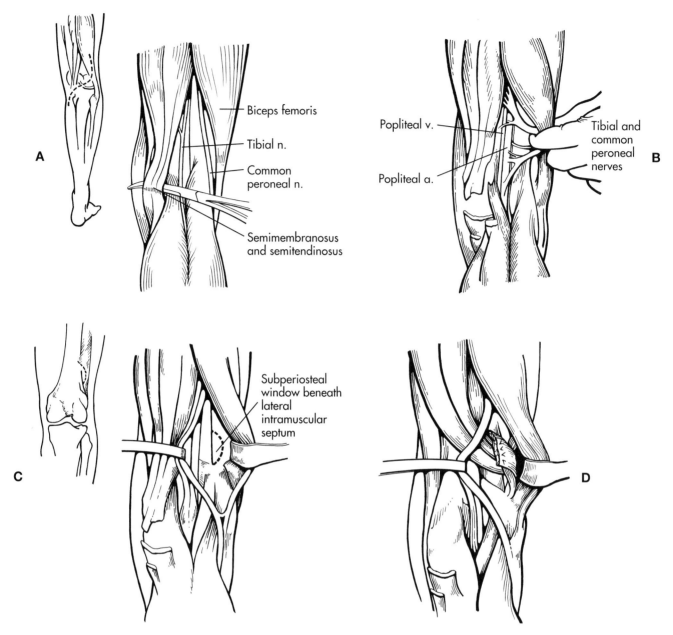

Fig. 30-30   Technique of Sutherland et al. for lateral transfer of medial hamstrings. **A,** *Inset,* Skin incision. Semitendinosus and semimembranosus tendons are divided. **B,** Tibial and common peroneal nerves are mobilized, and lateral intermuscular septum is exposed. **C,** Septum is incised at attachment to periosteum. **D,** Divided tendons are passed through incision in septum, looped around septum, and sutured to themselves. (Redrawn from Sutherland DH, Schottstaedt ER, Larsen LJ, et al: *J Bone Joint Surg* 51A:1070, 1969.)

spasticity of the hamstrings. It can be caused by hamstring weakness when the hamstrings have been lengthened too much or transferred, or by weakness of the gastrocnemius muscle when its proximal heads have been recessed. Recurvatum also may be secondary to equinus of the ankle; if a patient tries to put his foot on the ground with the ankle in equinus, the knee must go into recurvatum if the heel is to touch the surface.

The prone rectus (Ely) test is used to test for quadriceps spasticity. This test also can be done with the patient sitting. If

the rectus femoris is tight, it is lengthened at the hip or released at the knee, or its distal tendon is transferred posteriorly, either medially or laterally. Proximal lengthening of the rectus femoris can be done by the technique described by Sage.

To determine if recurvatum of the knee is secondary to equinus of the ankle, a short leg cast or ankle orthosis is applied with the ankle in neutral dorsiflexion. If the knee goes into recurvatum with the foot plantigrade, the recurvatum is secondary to either weakened hamstrings or a spastic quadriceps. If the ankle will not dorsiflex to neutral (right angle), the heel can be built up to compensate for the equinus. If the knee goes into recurvatum as this built-up heel touches the floor, equinus is not the cause of the recurvatum. If equinus is the cause, cast correction or surgery is indicated.

Recurvatum of the knee resulting from overlengthening or transfer of the hamstrings is difficult to treat. Even if the tendons can be replanted, the hamstrings will not regain normal strength because they will have been weakened by the previous surgery.

When activity in the rectus femoris is inappropriate, hamstring activity to achieve foot clearance can be augmented by a posterior transfer of the distal rectus. Root, Miller, and Kirz reviewed 20 patients in whom this operation had been done, along with hamstring releases, on 40 extremities for stiff-knee gait. At 1 year after surgery, knee flexion and extension during gait had improved and speed and cadence had increased.

Evans recommended that significant recurvatum of this nature be treated with bilateral long leg braces with a pelvic band. He recommended locking the knees at 20 degrees to prevent full extension and ankle stops at 5 degrees above a right angle. When hip control has been achieved, the pelvic band is removed but the long leg braces are retained for months or years until a satisfactory knee stance is achieved. He advised against flexion osteotomy for recurvatum.

◆ Recession of Rectus Femoris at the Hip

TECHNIQUE 30-28 *(Sage)*

Place the patient supine with a small elevation under the buttocks. Through the lower end of an iliofemoral approach (Technique 1-61), divide the fascia of the anterior thigh at the anterosuperior iliac spine, taking care not to injure the lateral femoral cutaneous nerve in this area. At the anterosuperior spine, separate the origin of the sartorius and the anterior border of the tensor fasciae latae. Retract the sartorius medially and the tensor fasciae latae laterally and elevate the latter muscle about 5 cm off the anterior edge of the outer iliac wing. Locate the straight head of the rectus femoris at its attachment to the anteroinferior iliac spine, lying between the medial border of the tensor fasciae latae and lateral to the iliacus (Fig. 30-31, *A*). Expose its straight head distally until the Y-bifurcation into the straight and reflected heads is found. By sharp and blunt dissection, clear the reflected head toward its origin proximally on the superior hip capsule. Free its attachment from the capsule and mark it with a suture. Follow the reflected head back to the Y-bifurcation and split it longitudinally along the course of its fibers distally toward the musculotendinous junction for at least 3 cm. Turn the scalpel anteriorly at this point and cut the attachment of the straight head from the remainder of the muscle and tendon, leaving it attached at the anteroinferior iliac spine (Fig. 30-31, *B*). Then extend the hip, flex

the knee, and suture the distal end of the straight head to the proximal end of the reflected head (Fig. 30-31, *C*). This effectively lengthens the tendon 5 cm but leaves it still attached to the anteroinferior iliac spine. Close the wound routinely.

KNEE VALGUS

Knee valgus usually is caused by a hip adduction deformity, which is coupled with internal rotation and flexion. Usually the valgus looks worse than it actually is because it is a combination of flexion and internal rotation that accentuates the appearance of valgus. Correction of the spastic hip adduction and internal rotational deformity is indicated. The hip adductors, the medial hamstrings, or the iliopsoas cause the deformity. The cause must be determined and corrected surgically, but in such patients the knee does not require surgery.

A tight iliotibial band also can cause knee valgus. This can be checked by positioning the patient on the contralateral side and having him flex the knee nearest the table up onto his abdomen. With the knee flexed, the hip being tested is flexed and abducted, moved from the position of flexion to extension, and then adducted. If the hip will not adduct without flexing, the iliotibial band is tight and can be palpated subcutaneously along the distal third of the thigh. The tight band should be resected by a Yount procedure (Chapter 31).

Severe valgus deformities of the ankle can cause structural knee valgus. It is rarely severe enough to warrant any surgery at the knee, but if it is, a supracondylar varus osteotomy can be performed. This deformity is more common in myelodysplasia than in cerebral palsy.

PATELLA ALTA

Patella alta causes chondromalacia. The patella rides above the femoral condyles, and the patellar tendon is lengthened (Fig. 30-32). This can be caused primarily by quadriceps spasticity or it can result from a marked knee flexion deformity of long duration. Plication of the patellar tendon is the procedure of choice for patella alta. Transplantation of the bony insertion of the patellar tendon distally is contraindicated because this condition usually occurs in growing children with open proximal tibial physes, and damage to the front of the physis can result in recurvatum of the knee. In severe flexion deformity of the knee with elongation of the patellar tendon, correction of the flexion deformity is all that is needed. Usually an operation on the patella is unnecessary because the quadriceps lag will disappear with time.

SUBLUXATION OR DISLOCATION OF PATELLA

Subluxation or dislocation of the patella can result from a valgus knee deformity. It also can be caused by flexion,

Fig. 30-31   Recession of origin of rectus femoris at hip. **A,** Y-bifurcate tendon of proximal end of rectus femoris is found between iliacus muscle and tensor fasciae latae after sartorius has been released and retracted. **B,** Straight head of rectus femoris is incised from its muscle as far distally as possible, leaving it attached to antero-inferior iliac spine above. Reflected head is then incised from hip capsule as far proximally as possible. **C,** Distal end of straight head is sutured to proximal end of reflected head, thus lengthening tendinous attachment proximally.

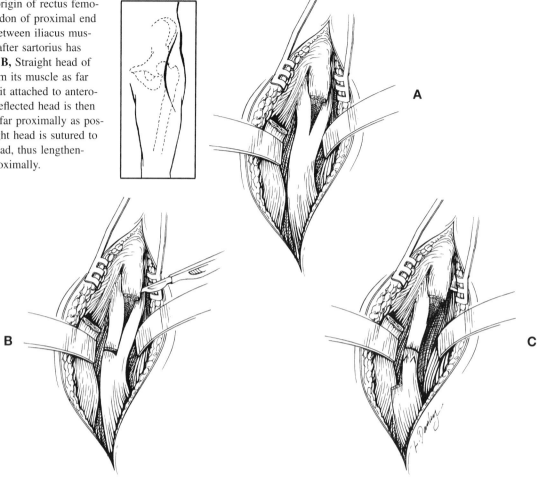

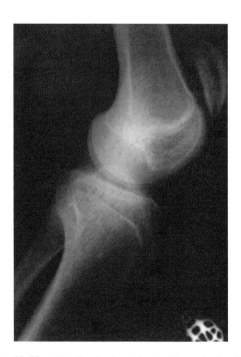

Fig. 30-32   Patella alta in patient with cerebral palsy.

adduction, and internal rotation contracture of the hip, which causes the quadriceps muscle to pull the patella laterally. If the patella becomes chronically dislocated, it should be reduced surgically because the knee cannot be adequately extended with a dislocated patella. Transferring the patellar tendon insertion (Chapter 45) by a soft tissue procedure is the preferred treatment. Lateral patellar retinacular release alone may suffice, but in chronic dislocation or subluxation it probably will not. Reefing the quadriceps tendon medially or transferring half of the patellar tendon medially into the upper tibia is the preferred method of alignment, along with releasing the patellar retinaculum (Chapter 45). If a valgus knee deformity is the cause of the patellar subluxation, a varus supracondylar osteotomy of the femur may be needed (Chapter 26).

Hip

Deformities of the hip in cerebral palsy are the second most common deformities encountered. They are caused by imbalance of muscle power, retained primitive reflexes, habitually faulty posture, absence of weight-bearing stimulation on bone, and growth. If the imbalance in muscle power is marked and if the faulty posture continues, adaptive changes develop in the soft tissues and bones. Anteversion of the femoral neck fails to correct spontaneously and even increases, and valgus deformity of the femoral neck caused by muscle imbalance and prolonged absence of weight-bearing gradually increases. The hip eventually may subluxate or dislocate. According to Baker, Dodelin, and Bassett, every patient with cerebral palsy who has appreciable involvement of the lower limbs should be considered to have abnormal hips until proved otherwise.

Sharrard stated that if hemiplegic spastic patients and other patients with nonspastic varieties of cerebral palsy are excluded, 92% of the remaining patients will show some degree of hip deformity, especially spastic, diplegic, triplegic, and quadriplegic patients.

In a study of the pathogenesis, incidence, and treatment of structural changes in 258 hips of 129 patients with cerebral palsy, Baker et al. found only 55 hips they considered entirely normal. There was valgus deformity of the femoral neck in 197, an increase in the obliquity of the acetabular roof in 160, subluxation in 42, and dislocation in 31; varus deformity of the neck was found in only 6. These researchers noted that valgus deformity of the neck was found by Banks in 179 of 180 hips of patients with cerebral palsy. They suggested that the strong overpull of the spastic muscles weakens and gradually overcomes the abductor muscles; this causes a decrease in stimulation and thus in growth of the greater trochanter and, in turn, a failure in development of the normal varus inclination of the femoral neck. They also proposed that if balanced muscle power about the hip can be established and normal alignment of the entire femur can be restored, later deformity of the hip can be prevented; precisely how and when these can be accomplished is the problem.

Therefore each patient should be examined both clinically and roentgenographically, and the examination should be repeated every 6 months to make sure the hips are not subluxating or dislocating or becoming dysplastic.

In discussing the early management of the hip in cerebral palsy, Scrutton stated that positional posturing has a strong influence on a tendency to subluxation, dislocation, and unwanted soft tissue contracture. He advocated early postural management for proper hip positioning and early soft tissue surgery to better balance the dynamic forces about the hip. Appropriate soft tissue surgery (such as releases) performed early are more effective. He agreed with Kalen and Bleck that the results of soft tissue surgery alone are better if done before the age of 5 years. He also agreed with Reimers that as soon as subluxation appears, an operation on the hip is indicated without allowing a further period of observation.

A roentgenographic method of recognizing and classifying subluxations and dislocations is important. The most practical method is based on the degree of migration of the femoral head from beneath the lateral border of the acetabulum. It was described by Beals in 1969, and Reimers labeled it the "migration percentage." It is measured by passing a line vertically from the lateral border of the acetabulum and then passing two vertical lines parallel to this original line, one along

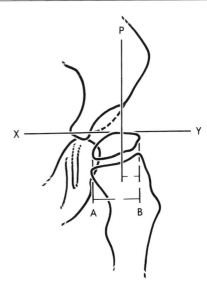

Fig. 30-33   Migration percentage: width of femoral head lateral to Perkins line divided by width of entire femoral head. (Redrawn from Reimers J, Poulsen S: *J Pediatr Orthop* 4:52, 1984.)

the lateral border of the femoral head epiphysis and the other along the medial border (Fig. 30-33). The width of the femoral head uncovered by the acetabulum is then divided by the width of the entire femoral head, and the result is multiplied by 100. The resulting figure is the migration percentage. Careful positioning for roentgenograms is necessary to produce accurate measurements. The patient should be supine, the patellae horizontal, and the hips together. Hips with a migration percentage of 0 are considered normal up to 4 years of age. Between 4 and 16 years of age migration should not exceed 5%. Reimers considered migration of more than 33% to denote subluxation and more than 100% to denote a dislocation. Others have considered a figure of 25% or less to signify a mild subluxation, from 26% to 50% a moderate subluxation, from 51% to 100% a severe subluxation, and more than 100% a dislocation.

It is important that the deformity of flexion and internal rotation be distinguished from adduction deformity, although they frequently coexist. Each can cause a scissors gait, but the treatment of each is different. The flexion–internal rotational deformity usually is caused by spastic internal rotators acting against weak external rotators; often spasticity of the tensor fasciae latae is a major cause. The habitually faulty postures in this deformity are assumed while sitting on the floor: the hips are flexed 90 degrees and fully rotated internally, the knees are flexed more than 90 degrees, and the legs and feet are externally rotated and positioned alongside the greater trochanters (the "reversed tailor position"). Often the child with cerebral palsy habitually sits in this position because it increases stability while sitting by broadening the base. This favors development of excessive internal torsion of the femur (anteversion of the femoral neck), external torsion of the tibia, and planovalgus deformity of the foot. This habit should be corrected as soon as possible. True adduction deformity is

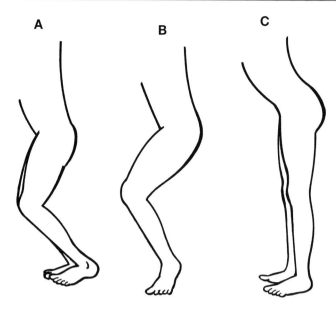

Fig. 30-34 Typical deformities of lower extremities and spine with flexed hip posture. **A,** Crouch posture. **B,** Jump posture. **C,** Extended lumbar spine with flexed hips and normal knees and ankles.

caused by spastic adductors acting against normal, less spastic, or weak abductors; the limbs are pulled together and do not rotate internally when forcibly separated by the examiner.

The relationships of flexion of the hip, with or without internal rotation, flexion of the knee, and dorsiflexion of the ankle, usually referred to as the "crouched position," have been discussed many times by Silfverskiöld, Bleck, Roosth, Samilson, Evans, Reimers, Sharrard, and others.

A patient with flexion deformities of the hips must flex the knees, overload the forefeet, and extend the lumbar spine to place the center of gravity over the weight-bearing surface. Likewise, a patient with fixed flexion deformities of the knees must flex the hips to place the center of gravity over the weight-bearing surface (Fig. 30-34, *A*). Furthermore, a patient with plantar flexion deformities of the ankles may flex the knees, hips, and lumbar spine for the same reason (Fig. 30-34, *B*). The decisions concerning whether the deformities are dynamic or fixed and which joint should be treated first and in what manner are controversial. For instance, if there are fixed plantar flexion deformities of the ankles and fixed flexion deformities of the hips and knees, and the deformities of the knees are corrected without correcting the deformities of the hips and ankles, genu recurvatum probably will develop, and because the posterior support of the hips has been decreased, increased flexion of the hips and increased lumbar lordosis also probably will develop. Therefore it is important to determine among the hip, knee, and ankle which joints are affected and the degree of any fixed deformities.

An isolated fixed deformity in any of the three joints that significantly interferes with the patient's activities can be corrected. If the fixed flexion deformity of the hip is from 15 to 30 degrees, most surgeons recommend intramuscular psoas tenotomy or psoas recession and resection of the rectus femoris.

If the deformity is more than 30 degrees, a more extensive anterior release is necessary, including the sartorius, tensor fasciae latae, and the anterior fibers of the gluteus medius and minimus. If significant flexion deformity of the knee persists after surgery, the hamstrings should be lengthened. If flexion contractures of the hip and knee and contracture of the tendo calcaneus coexist, then release of the contracted muscles beginning at the hip followed by release at the knee and ankle are indicated. One-stage, multilevel surgery to correct fixed contractures is recommended. This single-stage multilevel surgery is the preferred method instead of staged procedures performed at the hip, knee, and ankle.

The extent of surgery necessary to correct flexion deformity of the hip is also controversial. Bleck recommended recession of the psoas muscle and insertion of its tendon and the iliacus muscle fibers into the anterior capsule of the hip near the base of the femoral neck. He recommended this operation for children with flexion deformity of the hip of more than 15 degrees; the optimum age for surgery is from 7 to 9 years. The operation is also recommended in children with any one of the following three gait patterns: (1) flexed and internally rotated hips and flexed knees, (2) flexed and internally rotated hips and hyperextended knees, and (3) flexed and internally rotated hips and normal knees. Bleck performed additional surgery on these patients, depending on the analysis of the gait pattern and examination before surgery. In patients who walked with a scissors gait or had limited abduction of the hip to 15 degrees or less, adductor longus myotomy and neurectomy of the anterior branch of the obturator nerve were performed. In those who walked with hyperextended knees, the rectus femoris was released at its origin. In those who walked with flexed-knee gait patterns, the semitendinosus tendon was transferred to the medial femoral condyle and the semimembranosus was lengthened. Any contracture of the triceps surae was treated by lengthening the tendo calcaneus. The mean correction of the flexion deformity of the hip was 20 degrees; after surgery, passive internal rotation of the hip gradually decreased, and passive external rotation gradually increased. Subluxations of the hips in three nonambulatory patients were reduced.

According to Roosth, on the other hand, muscles that span two joints, namely the tensor fasciae latae, the rectus femoris, and the sartorius muscles, as well as the anterior fibers of the gluteus medius and minimus, cause flexion deformity of the hip, and release of these flexors of the hip at an early age without disturbing the psoas will eliminate the "crouch posture" and improve gait. At surgery he sequentially divided the different flexors of the hip and observed the flexion contracture after each muscle had been divided. When all of these muscles were sectioned, the deformity of the hip was relieved, but when all were not sectioned a flexion contracture of 15 degrees or less remained. Of 23 children with internal rotational deformity of the limbs before surgery, only one could not correct this deformity actively when examined after surgery.

Perry and Hoffer, Sutherland et al., Simon et al., Gage, and others have used kinetic electromyography and gait analysis to assess hip muscle dynamics and joint positions in patients with cerebral palsy. Hoffer used kinetic electromyography in patients who had flexed hip postures to differentiate between rectus femoris and iliopsoas hyperactivity. In the internally rotated, adducted gait, electromyograms have been used to differentiate between medial hamstring, gracilis, and adductor hyperactivity. Bleck used them in addition to determine the activity of the gluteus medius when considering whether to transfer them. He studied kinetic electromyograms about the hip in 25 patients with spastic hip muscle patterns. In all patients dysphasic activity was present in the adductors during the stance and swing phases of gait. In most patients the gluteus medius fired in phase, but its activity was prolonged. Kinetic electromyograms of 11 patients showed the iliacus to be phasic in five and dysphasic in six. He also studied the sartorius, rectus femoris, and the tensor fasciae latae—all hip flexors. The rectus was almost uniformly dysphasic. In hip extension deformity the hamstrings were found to be the offending muscles more often than the gluteus maximus. Gait analysis has come to play a major role in decision making concerning the dynamics of hip deformities.

The hip can become dislocated when its adductors, flexors, and internal rotators are spastic or rigid. The dislocation may be unilateral or bilateral, one hip may be dislocated and the opposite hip subluxated, or one hip may be dislocated and the opposite hip may present a combined abduction and external rotational deformity. The incidence of hip dislocation in cerebral palsy patients varies depending on the amount of neurological involvement but can range from 4% to 60%.

The goal in the treatment of the hip in a patient with cerebral palsy is prevention of progressive subluxation and dislocation. Early adductor releases have been effective in preventing further subluxation and dislocation in some patients. In other patients an adductor release and varus derotation osteotomy are needed. If there is significant acetabular dysplasia, an acetabuloplasty also should be performed.

ADDUCTION DEFORMITY

Adduction is the most common deformity of the hip in patients with cerebral palsy. It causes a scissoring gait and subluxation and dislocation of the hip. In a child with cerebral palsy, an adduction contracture of the hip is the earliest sign of impending subluxation.

In patients with early adduction contracture and early subluxation of the hip, an adductor longus tenotomy usually is sufficient to prevent further subluxation and dislocation of the hip. Adductor tenotomies usually are done bilaterally to prevent a windswept pelvis.

In more developed hips, tenotomy of the adductor longus may be required, as well as sectioning of all or part of the adductor brevis and gracilis. Surgery usually is required bilaterally. More extensive releases may be required on a more involved hip; a less involved hip may require a simple adductor tenotomy. In patients who are not ambulatory but who have marked adduction contractures that make hygiene activities difficult, extensive adductor tenotomies frequently are performed. Anterior obturator neurectomy can be done as well if

patients have a pure spastic pattern with no coexisting athetosis. Care must be taken not to perform an anterior obturator neurectomy in a patient with hypotonia as a result of athetoid cerebral palsy, especially in patients with rigid athetosis, because this can lead to an abduction external rotation deformity. Obturator neurectomy also should be used with caution in ambulatory cerebral palsy patients.

If the patient is noted to have a hip flexion contracture as well as an adduction contracture, iliopsoas release at the lesser trochanter or an iliopsoas recession at the pelvic brim may be performed. When releasing the iliopsoas at the lesser trochanter, care must be taken not to injure the medial circumflex femoral artery, resulting in a loss of vascularity to the femoral head. Likewise, an iliopsoas recession must be done with care so as not to confuse the femoral nerve with the tendon of the iliopsoas. Release of the iliopsoas at the lesser trochanter is recommended in nonambulatory patients, and a iliopsoas recession is recommended in ambulatory patients.

♦ Iliopsoas Recession

Bleck recommended iliopsoas recession when the hip internally rotates during walking and when passive external rotation of the hip is impossible if the joint is extended but is possible to 15 to 20 degrees if the joint is passively flexed to 90 degrees.

At the time of iliopsoas recession, other operations may be indicated, depending on the analysis of the gait pattern before surgery. If adductor spasm interferes with walking and if the hips cannot be passively abducted past 20 degrees, adductor tenotomy and neurectomy of the anterior branch of the obturator nerve may be indicated. If a child walks with the knees hyperextended, release or transfer of the rectus femoris at the hip or knee is indicated. If a child walks with the knees flexed and has not previously had surgery on the hamstrings, lengthening or transfer of the medial hamstrings may be indicated. If gait analysis shows prolongation of rectus femoris activity into the swing phase, a posterior transfer of the rectus femoris may be needed, with hamstring lengthening. If the foot is fixed in equinus deformity, lengthening of the tendo calcaneus or gastrocnemius is indicated.

TECHNIQUE 30-29 (Bleck)

Make an anterior iliofemoral incision beginning 1.5 cm distal to the anterosuperior iliac spine and coursing obliquely distally and medially for 10 to 15 cm, depending on the size of the patient (Fig. 30-35, A). Next, identify the sartorius muscle and retract it laterally. Then identify the femoral nerve and the medial and lateral borders of the iliacus muscle and separate the nerve from the muscle. The iliacus muscle fibers overlap the broad psoas tendon that hugs the anteromedial aspect of the capsule of the hip. Now divide the iliacus muscle transversely as far distally as possible and the psoas tendon at its attachment to the lesser trochanter (Fig. 30-35, B).

Transfer the psoas tendon superiorly and suture it to the anterior capsule of the hip joint near the base of the

continued

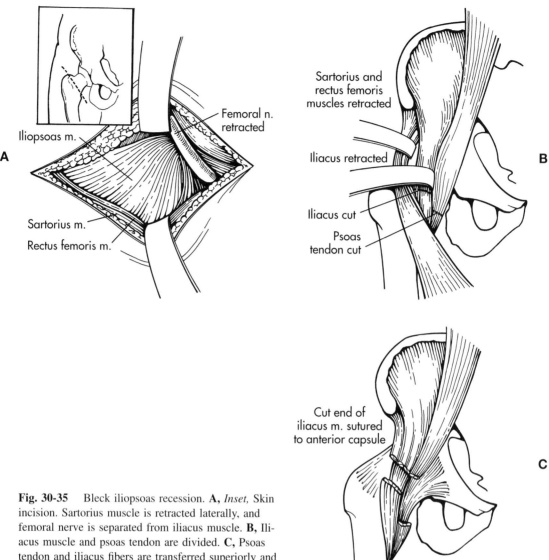

Fig. 30-35   Bleck iliopsoas recession. **A,** *Inset,* Skin incision. Sartorius muscle is retracted laterally, and femoral nerve is separated from iliacus muscle. **B,** Iliacus muscle and psoas tendon are divided. **C,** Psoas tendon and iliacus fibers are transferred superiorly and are sutured to anterior capsule. (Redrawn from Bleck EE: *J Bone Joint Surg* 53A:1468, 1971.)

femoral neck. Then suture the iliacus fibers to the capsule (Fig. 30-35, *C*).

AFTERTREATMENT. Immobilization in a cast is unnecessary. Bed rest, either prone or supine, is continued for 3 weeks.

◆ **Adductor Tenotomy and Anterior Obturator Neurectomy**

Adductor tenotomy is indicated for a patient with an adduction contracture, as indicated by a scissors gait, or for a child with early hip subluxation. An anterior obturator neurectomy can be added for patients who have a pure spastic pattern.

TECHNIQUE 30-30

Make a longitudinal 3-cm incision on the medial aspect of the thigh in line with the adductor longus muscle, or make a 3-cm transverse incision over the tendon of the adductor longus muscle. Dissect through the subcutaneous tissue and deep fascia. Separate the adductor longus muscle from the adductor brevis. Identify the anterior branch of the obturator nerve, coursing between the adductor longus and brevis muscles. Protect the branch of the anterior obturator nerve by retracting the adductor longus muscle away and cut the muscle transversely, using electrocautery to reduce bleeding. If the adduction contracture persists, examine the muscles to see if the primary source of the contracture is the

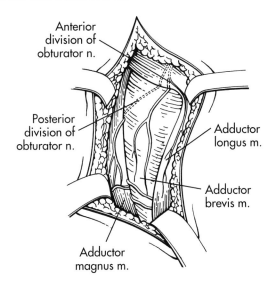

Fig. 30-36 Extrapelvic neurectomy of obturator nerve. Exposure of anterior and posterior divisions of obturator nerve; vessels on surfaces of adductor brevis and magnus muscles serve as guides. Note two branches of anterior division. If adductor spasm is mild, only anterior division is resected; if spasm is moderate or severe, both anterior and posterior divisions are resected.

gracilis or the adductor brevis. Use electrocautery to section parts or all of these muscles until the adduction contracture is relieved. The posterior branch of the obturator nerve is found beneath the adductor brevis muscle lying on the adductor magnus. If extensive release of the adductor brevis is indicated, identify and take care not to injure the posterior branch of the obturator nerve. After the adduction contracture has been relieved, if the patient is known to have a pure spastic pattern, perform an anterior obturator neurectomy if desired. Close the wound in layers (Fig. 30-36).

AFTERTREATMENT. Depending on the patient's mental status and the quality of the caregivers, bilateral leg casts and an abduction bar, a form-fitted abduction orthosis, or an abduction pillow may be worn until the patient is comfortable.

◆ Transfer of Adductor Origins to Ischium

Transferring the adductor origins to the ischium was first described by Nickel et al. for treating paralytic dislocation of the hip. It consists of transferring the origins of the adductor longus and gracilis posteriorly to the ischium and releasing the origins of the adductor brevis and anterior part of the adductor magnus.

Griffin, Wheelhouse, and Shiavi reported that patients treated by this operation walk with a narrower base, more security, less trunk shift, longer single support phase and stance, and more endurance than patients similarly involved but treated by adductor myotomy or obturator neurectomy or both.

Root and Spero reported the results of a 10-year study comparing adductor transfer (gracilis, adductor longus, and adductor brevis) to the ischium with adductor myotomy and anterior branch obturator neurectomy. They concluded that adductor transfers provided greater pelvic stability, reduced hip instability, and decreased hip flexion contracture more consistently than adductor myotomy and obturator neurectomy.

Reimers and Poulsen compared a similar group of patients using the two operations and found no significant difference in the results. For this reason, they abandoned the adductor transfer operation because it was technically more difficult and was more stressful to the child.

Scott et al. reported their results with adductor transfer and found pelvic obliquity and unilateral hip subluxation in a high percentage of patients who underwent adductor transfers. These complications led these authors to abandon this procedure.

The benefits of adductor transfer versus adductor myotomy are still controversial, but adductor transfer may be more beneficial in the ambulatory cerebral palsy patient. Beals, Thompson, and Beals reported 141 modified adductor transfers in 85 children with cerebral palsy. They found that the ambulatory status after surgery correlated with the severity of involvement. Four of 15 patients with a severity index of 10 or 11 and 6 of 8 of the patients with a severity index of ≥12 became independent walkers after surgery. Their intermediate and long-term results showed this procedure to be an effective method of achieving symmetric hip abduction in patients with cerebral palsy and abduction was maintained with a low incidence of recurrence.

TECHNIQUE 30-31 *(Couch, Derosa, and Throop)*

Place the patient in the lithotomy position with the buttocks resting at the end of the operating table. Position the legs in pelvic stirrups and, with 7.5 cm wide adhesive tape placed just proximal to the knees and attached to the uprights of the pelvic stirrup, hold the knees and thighs abducted as much as the contracted tissues permit. Carefully prepare the entire perineum, the buttocks, the lower abdomen, and the proximal thighs and drape the operative field, using paper draping from a gynecological pack. Sit between the patient's legs. Now begin an incision just superior to the tendon of the adductor longus and extend it posteriorly in a straight line to the ischial tuberosity, paralleling as closely as possible the borders of the inferior pubic ramus and the ischium. After the skin and subcutaneous tissues have been divided, use self-retaining retractors to increase the exposure. Identify the adductor longus tendon, tag it with a suture, and sever it from its origin on the pubic ramus with the cutting electrocautery. Next, also with the electrocautery, release the origins of the adductor brevis, gracilis, and anterior part of the adductor magnus next to the bone. End this dissection at the shiny fascia of the obturator externus. Now extend and

continued

slightly adduct the hip to allow the adductor longus tendon to reach the ischial tuberosity. Make an incision in the apophysis of the ischial tuberosity and push the adductor brevis, the adductor magnus, and the gracilis posteriorly toward the tuberosity, rolling them under the tendon of the adductor longus. Then free the adductor longus distally in the thigh, place it in a straight line, and secure it with several nonabsorbable sutures to the apophysis of the ischium. Now thoroughly irrigate the wound and close it. Place the child in long leg braces with a pelvic band.

AFTERTREATMENT. The child is kept in long leg braces with a pelvic band for 4 weeks. During the first 2 weeks the hip and knee locks are released occasionally for comfort and to allow the child to flex the hips about 45 degrees while eating. During the second week active and passive exercises of the hips and knees in the braces are begun. Four weeks after surgery the braces are discarded, and intensive physical therapy is started.

TECHNIQUE 30-32 *(Root)*

Incise the medial thigh 1 cm lateral and parallel to the groin crease, over the adductor longus, and carry the incision posteriorly for a distance of 6 cm. Dissect the fascia overlying the adductor longus to expose the insertion of the adductor longus and pectineus on the pubic ramus. Locate the interval between these muscles and identify and protect the branches of the obturator nerve. Using electrocautery, incise along the pubic ramus the origin of the gracilis, adductor longus, and adductor brevis. Strip the tendons from their insertion at the pubic ramus subperiosteally while preserving the thick fibrous periosteal origin of these muscles. Free the remainder of the adductor brevis muscular attachments by blunt dissection. With a clamp, grasp the freed periosteal attachments of the tendons and hold them alongside the ischial tuberosity while suturing them to the tuberosity with nonabsorbable sutures, the most distal part of insertion being on the anteroinferior aspect of the ischial tuberosity. Obtain meticulous hemostasis with the electrocautery. Close the wound in a standard manner and apply a double spica cast.

AFTERTREATMENT. The spica cast is left on for 3 weeks and then removed to begin mobilization exercises.

◆ Varus Derotational Osteotomy

With excessive anteversion and valgus deformity of the femur and a hip that is either subluxated or dislocated, a varus derotational osteotomy may be required in addition to soft tissue or pelvic corrective surgery to keep the hip reduced and stable. The corrective osteotomy usually can be made when any soft tissue correction is performed. It is best done at the level of the lesser trochanter through either a straight lateral or

posterior approach. In 1980 Root and Siegal reported 100 hips operated on through a posterior approach with the patient prone. The approach was relatively bloodless, and the image intensifier allowed easy viewing of the femur. Union occurred in 99% of patients. However, this approach cannot be used when an open reduction of the hip is anticipated.

TECHNIQUE 30-33 *(Root and Siegal)*

Place the patient prone on a table suitable for the image intensifier or anteroposterior roentgenograms. Drape the buttocks and lower extremities free in the sterile field. Make an incision 15 cm long over the greater trochanter beginning proximally in line with the fibers of the gluteus maximus and extending distally from the greater trochanter in line with the posterolateral border of the femur (Fig. 30-37, *A* and *B*). Deepen the incision through the fascia lata and gluteus maximus to expose the superior part of the posterior and posterolateral surfaces of the femur, including the greater trochanter. Using an electrocautery, detach the origin of the vastus lateralis from the proximal femur by a transverse cut at the base of the greater trochanter and a longitudinal cut along the linea aspera (Fig. 30-37, *C*). Reflect the vastus lateralis anteriorly from the lateral surface of the femur subperiosteally. At the level of the proximal edge of the lesser trochanter, use an electrocautery to cut proximally through the tendinous and muscular attachment of the quadratus femoris and reflect it from the back of the femur medially and distally. This allows palpation of the inferior surface of the neck of femur and identification of the lesser trochanter (Fig. 30-37, *D*). Isolate the iliopsoas tendon and free it from the lesser trochanter. The area of bone to be osteotomized is thus completely exposed. Perform an osteotomy at the level of the lesser trochanter (Fig. 30-37, *E*). Remove the wedge of bone calculated by preoperative measurements (Fig. 30-37, *F*) and place the neck-shaft angle at 100 to 110 degrees in patients younger than 8 years old. In older patients, the neck-shaft angle should be at 115 to 120 degrees.

Locate the proper level of the osteotomy cuts by using a guide wire in the neck of the femur for orientation (Fig. 30-37, *E*). It should be placed in the trochanter and upper femoral neck parallel with the intended proximal osteotomy cut. With the guide wire in proper position, insert an osteotome parallel with the guide wire and at the expected site of blade plate insertion into the subtrochanteric area of the femur. Verify the position of the osteotomy with the image intensifier or plain roentgenograms. Use the electrocautery to score a line in the bone posteriorly in line with the femoral shaft (vertically) as a later guide to rotational alignment (Fig. 30-37, *G*). Make the first osteotomy cut 1.5 to 2 cm below the level of the osteotome in the femoral neck and parallel to it, but not into the femoral neck. Make the second osteotomy cut distally at a right angle to the shaft of the femur and remove a medially based bone wedge of previously determined width to allow

continued

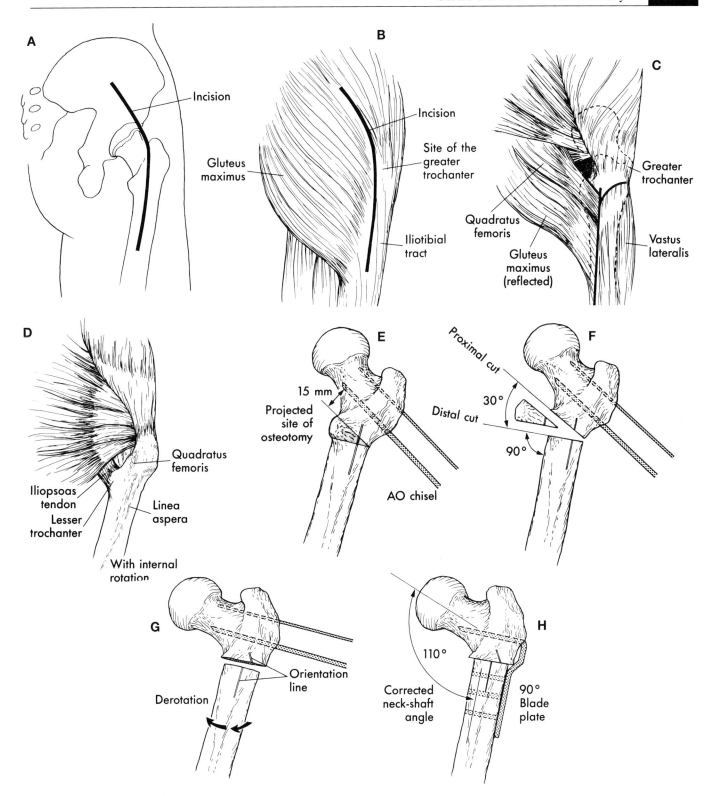

Fig. 30-37   Root and Siegal varus derotational osteotomy of hip. **A,** Skin incision. **B,** Incision through gluteus maximus and fascia lata (iliotibial tract). **C,** Greater trochanter, quadratus femoris, origin of vastus lateralis, tendinous attachment of gluteus maximus, and linea aspera are identified. **D,** Osteotomy site is exposed in area of lesser trochanter; psoas tendon can be released if necessary. **E,** Guide wire and chisel are inserted in parallel position. Shaded area represents wedge to be excised; scored line is for reference for later rotation. **F,** Location of osteotomy planes; proximal osteotomy is 15 mm distal to chisel. **G,** Rotation is accomplished by external rotation of femur. **H,** Osteotomy is fixed with AO plate and screws. (**A, C,** and **H** courtesy Leon Root, MD; **B** and **D** to **G** redrawn from Root L, Siegal T: *J Bone Joint Surg* 62A:571, 1980.)

the proper varus position of the neck of the femur. This wedge should include all or part of the lesser trochanter. The distal osteotomy should go to but not through the lateral cortex of the femur. Clamp the distal femur to the plate portion of the blade plate with a bone-holding forceps. This closes the open wedge–shaped space where the bone was removed. Check for proper positioning of the blade plate and the osteotomy with the image intensifier or roentgenograms. Release the bone clamp from the blade plate and derotate the femur to correct anteversion, using the previously scored longitudinal line on the posterior surface of the femur as a reference (Fig. 30-37, *H*). When corrective rotation has been made, again clamp the blade plate to the distal fragment for stability. Check for correction of anteversion by flexing the knee and rotating the hip. Approximately 15 to 20 degrees of internal rotation at the hip should be preserved. After proper rotation of the distal fragment has been determined, fix the blade plate to this fragment with screws and close the wound in a standard manner. Apply a hip spica cast.

A pediatric hip screw and side plate can be used effectively, as well as an angled blade plate. When performing a varus osteotomy using a screw and side plate configuration, it is advisable to perform a medial displacement osteotomy of the distal fragment. Screw and side plate configurations do not contain the offset found in angled blade plates; therefore, if a medial displacement osteotomy is not performed, lateralization of the femoral shaft after varus osteotomy results in tightening of the hip adductors— one of the main deforming forces of the hip. The technique can easily be incorporated at the time of osteotomy, as demonstrated in Fig. 30-38.

AFTERTREATMENT. The spica cast usually is removed 3 weeks after surgery but can be used longer if the fixation is questionable.

DISLOCATION

Dislocated or subluxated hips may become painful in many patients, and it cannot be predicted which will be painful and which will not. In a young child with a subluxation or dislocation, depending on the patient's medical condition, an aggressive approach usually should be taken to reduce a dislocation, relieve pain, improve perineal hygiene, improve balance when sitting and standing, and help prevent pelvic obliquity.

Drummond et al. noted that a dislocated hip usually is not disabling in a patient who is neurologically immature, extremely intellectually impaired, bedridden, and institutionalized. In 1974 they established the following four criteria for the open reduction of a dislocated hip: (1) the patient must be moderately mature neurologically and have moderate intelligence; (2) the patient should have walking ability or at least have sitting potential; (3) pelvic obliquity should have been corrected; and (4) the dislocation ideally should be unilateral.

In a 1979 study that included some of the same authors, Moreau et al. reviewed 88 hips in institutionalized adult patients with cerebral palsy (the average age was 26½ years); 41 of the 88 patients had unstable hips. In 24 patients the hips were dislocated, and in 9 they were subluxated. Pain was present in 11 of the patients who had dislocations. One third of the patients with hip subluxation or dislocation had problems with perineal care, and 14 of these had pelvic obliquity and scoliosis. Moreau et al. concluded that dislocation and subluxation should be prevented, but that surgery for a dislocated hip should be reserved for neurologically mature

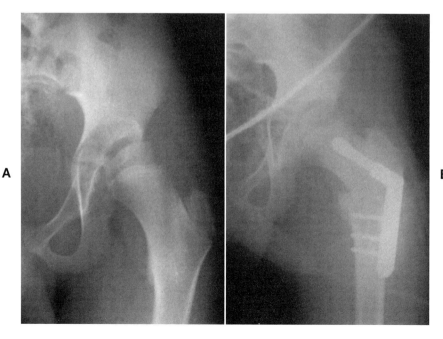

Fig. 30-38   Medial displacement osteotomy. Preoperative (**A**) and postoperative (**B**) roentgenograms.

patients and those with athetosis. They combined adductor release or varus derotational osteotomy of the femur with a femoral shortening, if needed, and open reduction of the hip, as well as iliopsoas muscle release. A Chiari osteotomy was performed 2 or 3 weeks later, and the hip was immobilized in a spica cast for 2 months.

Osterkamp, Cailloutte, and Hoffer reviewed a series of subluxated and dislocated hips that had been treated by a Chiari osteotomy after soft tissue surgery to better balance the muscles about the hip. They concluded that the Chiari osteotomy is useful in cerebral palsy. They found the osteotomy to be stable, and it prevented the hip from dislocating posteriorly. Lynne and Katcherian and others advocated a shelf procedure to augment the lateral acetabular coverage in residual dysplasia. They reported that a slotted acetabular augmentation graft (a shelf operation) can be combined with other soft tissue procedures, and provides good coverage posteriorly and superiorly.

Dietz and Knutson reported 23 patients with cerebral palsy who were treated with a Chiari pelvic osteotomy for hip subluxation or dislocation. The average follow-up exceeded 7 years. At final follow-up 79% of the hips were painless, and 88% tolerated unlimited sitting; 29% of the hips, however, had a migration index of 30% or higher. Resubluxation occurred largely in the first year after surgery. Flail hips had a greater migration index preoperatively and 1 year postoperatively. Seriously affected patients were treated without a concomitant femoral varus osteotomy.

Root et al. reported 31 patients with cerebral palsy who had surgical treatment for 35 severely subluxed or dislocated hips at a mean of 7 years after open reduction, pelvic osteotomy, primary femoral shortening and varus derotational osteotomy. At the latest follow-up examination, none of the hips was painful. In seven patients walking ability had improved, and patients confined to a wheelchair had better sitting balance. The authors concluded that a combined approach of proximal femoral and pelvic osteotomies provided coverage of the femoral head and reduced pain in the hip. They recommended the use of such an extensive approach in the treatment of severely involved hips.

McNerney et al. reported good results in 99 of 104 dysplastic hips treated with a one-stage correction that included soft tissue release, proximal femoral osteotomy, and acetabuloplasty.

◆ One-Stage Correction with San Diego Acetabuloplasty

TECHNIQUE 30-34 *(McNerney, Mubarak, Wenger)*

With the patient under anesthesia, approach the hip adductors through a transverse groin incision and lengthen them to obtain abduction of 60 degrees. Preserve the anterior branch of the obturator nerve. Lengthen the hamstrings (proximally in a nonwalking child and distally in a child with walking potential) to obtain a popliteal angle of 150 to 160 degrees. Release the iliopsoas at its insertion on the lesser trochanter through the interval between the neurovascular bundle and pectineus, taking care to avoid damage to the medial femoral circumflex artery. In a child with walking potential, perform the psoas tenotomy at the pelvic brim instead to preserve hip-flexor strength.

Approach the proximal femur laterally and perform a closing wedge femoral osteotomy. Secure the osteotomy with a 90-degree AO blade plate (Synthes, Inc., Paoli, Penn.). Shorten the femur as needed to reduce excessive soft tissue tension across the reduced hip. A final neck-shaft angle of 110 to 120 degrees and femoral anteversion of 10 to 20 degrees are desired, with the distal shaft medially translated according to the degree of varus performed (usually 1 cm). This is achieved by use of the AO blade plate with appropriate offset. Avoid creating excessive varus that will weaken the child's hip abductors and predispose the osteopenic bone to progressive varus, as well as hinder hip abduction.

Approach the acetabulum anteriorly. Split the iliac apophysis and expose the outer wall of the ilium subperiosteally to the sciatic notch posterior and to the anteroinferior iliac spine anteriorly. Expose the inner wall of the ilium subperiosteally over the anterior one third to allow later harvest of bone graft. Perform an open reduction with capsulorrhaphy at this time if the hip has a migration percentage of more than 70% or if the femoral head does not fully seat into the acetabulum.

Start the acetabuloplasty 1 cm above the lateral margin of the acetabulum, avoiding inadvertent extension into the acetabulum or damage to the lateral growth centers of the acetabulum. Make bicortical cuts over the anteroinferior iliac spine and posteriorly at the sciatic notch, using a retractor to protect the adjacent structures. Use of a large up-biting Kerrison rongeur helps establish the posterior bicortical cut in the sciatic notch. Make a unicortical cut through the outer table between these two points under image-intensification. Direct a straight or slightly curved osteotome toward the medial aspect of the triradiate cartilage to avoid fracturing into the hip joint.

The osteotomy should stop several millimeters away from the triradiate cartilage. To avoid physeal closure, never cross the triradiate cartilage with the osteotome. Rotate the acetabulum laterally and downward, hinging on the triradiate cartilage to correct the dysplasia and produce a horizontal sourcil (Fig. 30-39, *A*). Curet a small amount of cancellous bone from the osteotomy proximally to improve the stability of the subsequently placed bone grafts. Harvest the anterior crest of the ilium and fashion the trapezoidal segments of tricortical bone graft, with the base approximately the desired width of the hinged-open osteotomy (Fig. 30-39, *B*). Carefully impact three trapezoidal grafts in place. They should be quite stable and do not require internal fixation. Close the wound routinely and place the patient in a hip spica cast.

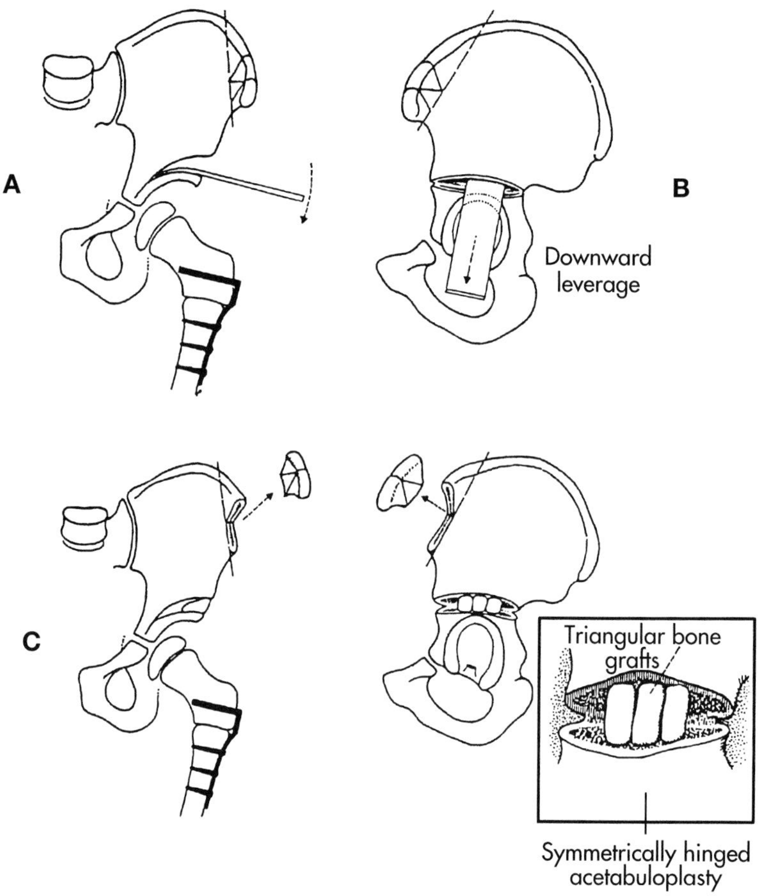

Fig. 30-39   Osteotomy stops several millimeters from triradiate cartilage and is then hinged open laterally to correct dysplasia. **A,** Tricortical segment of iliac wing is harvested for bone graft. **B,** Trapezoidal segments are fashioned to fit into osteotomy site. **C** and **D,** Three trapezoidal segments of tricortical bone graft are impacted into place to hold osteotomy site open. Elasticity of intact medial cortex holds bone grafts in place; therefore fixation is not required. (Redrawn from Mubarak, Valencia FG, Wenger DR: *J Bone Joint Surg* 74A:1347, 1992.)

AFTERTREATMENT. If the procedure is to be staged, a high spica cast is applied. Two to 4 weeks later, when the second stage is done, half of the cast can be removed for surgery on the contralateral hip while protecting the previously operated hip. The entire cast is replaced at the end of the second procedure. Patients should wear the spica cast for 4 to 6 weeks.

◆ **Slotted Acetabular Augmentation Graft**

TECHNIQUE 30-35 *(Lynne and Katcherian)*
With the patient supine and under general anesthesia, after appropriate soft tissues have been released, make a bikini incision inferior and parallel to the iliac crest. Deepen the incision to the iliac crest and separate the muscles and fascia from it extraperiosteally, thus exposing the origin of the reflected head of the rectus femoris and the joint capsule. Isolate the reflected head, divide it over the center of the femoral head, and reflect it anteriorly and posteriorly off the joint capsule (Fig. 30-40, *A*). Incise the joint capsule longitudinally through only half of its thickness and reflect the resulting flaps anteriorly and posteriorly (Fig. 30-40, *B*).

Insert a drill bit parallel to the femoral neck into the superior acetabular roof just deep to the articular cartilage (Fig. 30-40, *C*). Check the position of the drill bit by roentgenograms. Then, with drill holes, make a curved slot 1 cm deep in the superior acetabular rim parallel to the drill bit (Fig. 30-40, *D*). Remove a bone graft from the anterior ilium after marking its corners with four holes (Fig. 30-40, *E*). The graft should be approximately square and should be the width of the slot in the superior acetabular rim. Remove the outer table of the ilium between the four holes with an osteotome. Position the rectangular graft firmly in the slot superior to the acetabulum. Ensure a firm fit by modifying the graft or slot as needed. Close the two flaps in the capsule over the graft and suture the cut ends of the reflected head of the rectus femoris over the graft (Fig. 30-40, *F*). Curet cancellous bone from the iliac wing and place it between the graft and the ilium (Fig. 30-40, *G*). Close the wound routinely.

AFTERTREATMENT. A spica cast is applied and is worn for 6 weeks.

◆ ◆ ◆

In their review of 274 subluxated or dislocated hips in institutionalized patients, Samilson et al. found that the mean

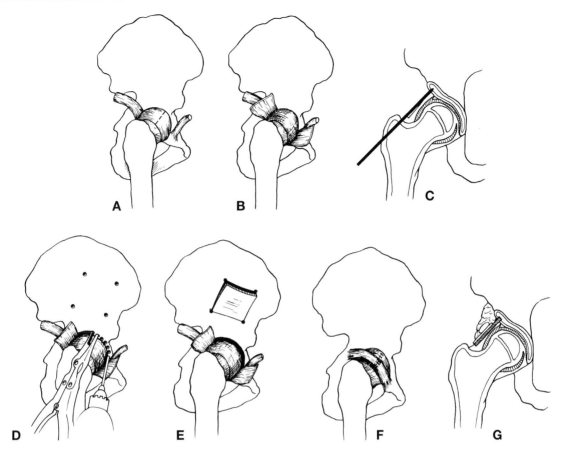

Fig. 30-40 Slotted acetabular augmentation (Lyne and Katcherian). **A,** Exposure of rectus femoris and joint capsule; capsule is incised through half of its thickness. **B,** Capsular flaps are reflected anteriorly and posteriorly. **C,** Drill bit is inserted in superior acetabular rim adjacent to capsule and just superior to acetabular articular cartilage. **D,** Curved slot is made in superior acetabular rim. **E,** Unicortical graft is harvested from outer table of ilium. **F,** Layers of capsule and reflected head of rectus are closed over graft. **G,** Cancellous graft from ilium is positioned over iliac graft. (Redrawn from Lyne ED, Katcherian DA: *J Pediatr Orthop* 8:278, 1988.)

age for dislocation was 7 years, and this has been the experience of others. They also found that pain from the dislocation was uncommon, occurring in only 6 patients, whereas perineal care was the primary indication for surgical treatment in 202 patients. They concluded that the proper treatment of subluxation was percutaneous adductor tenotomy (at times including the gracilis), open release of the iliopsoas and the rectus femoris, varus and derotational osteotomy of the femur to correct coxa valga and anteversion, and closed reduction of the hip.

Arthrodesis of the hip or total hip arthroplasty has been successful in a small number of skeletally mature patients with hip pain. Root recommended that the hip be arthrodesed in 45 degrees of flexion, 15 degrees of abduction, and neutral rotation. This procedure should be limited to the patient with total body involvement who has pain both when sitting and lying. Total hip arthroplasty usually is reserved for the adult ambulatory patient or the minimally involved patient with a painful subluxation or dislocation, although Gabos et al. reported good results in nonambulatory patients.

Modified Girdlestone procedures (see Chapter 17) and resection arthroplasties of the proximal femur with capsular interposition have been successful in the treatment of painful hip dislocations in cerebral palsy patients. Kalen and Gamble reviewed 18 hips in 15 patients who had proximal femoral resection arthroplasty at a mean age of 17.5 years with an average follow-up of 4.7 years. All patients were nonambulatory preoperatively, severely retarded, and totally dependent for all activities. In each patient nursing hygiene and care were made easier by the operation. Of the 10 patients with preoperative pain, 8 were improved by the procedure, and sitting and supine posture was improved in 8. Although some complications occurred, all nursing goals were achieved, and most patients were free of pain.

McCarthy et al. and Baxter and D'Astous reported good results from resection interposition arthroplasty of the proximal femur for dislocated hips in older children and adults. Their indications for this procedure, described by Castle and Schneider, were (1) an intolerance to sitting because of the nonfunctional position of the affected hip, (2) inability to provide proper perineal care, (3) decubitus ulceration, (4) severe pain during dressing or bathing, and (5) inability to walk. Heterotopic bone did form after surgery, but reoperation was rarely needed. Initially the hips were unstable, but instability diminished gradually with time.

◆ Resection Interposition Arthroplasty of Proximal Femur

TECHNIQUE 30-36 *(Castle and Schneider, as Modified by McCarthy et al.)*

After general anesthesia has been administered, place the patient supine with a sandbag elevating the affected hip. Make a straight lateral incision from 10 cm superior to the greater trochanter inferiorly along the proximal femur to inferior to the level of the lesser trochanter. Split the fascia of the tensor fasciae femoris and then extraperiosteally detach the insertions of the vastus lateralis and gluteus medius and minimus from the proximal femur. Detach the psoas tendon from the lesser trochanter and complete the exposure of the proximal femur extraperiosteally. Incise the periosteum circumferentially about the femur just distal to the insertion of the gluteus maximus or at the proposed level of femoral resection. Next, divide the short external rotators. Incise the capsule circumferentially and free it from the base of the femoral neck. Divide the ligamentum teres and remove the proximal femur (Fig. 30-41, *A*). Test the range of motion of the hip at this point and, if necessary for motion, tenotomize the proximal hamstrings through the same incision after identifying the sciatic nerve. If necessary, also release the adductors. Seal the acetabular cavity by oversewing the capsular edges. Cover the proximal end of the femur by attaching the vastus lateralis to the rectus femoris muscle. Next, interpose the gluteal muscles between the acetabulum and the proximal femur (Fig. 30-41, *B*). Secure meticulous hemostasis and close the wound over a suction drain.

AFTERTREATMENT. Skeletal traction is used for 3 to 6 weeks after surgery. A high level of vigilance must be maintained during these weeks to prevent the development of decubitus ulcers. Respiratory therapy, including cupping and postural drainage, should be performed once or twice daily. In patients in whom skeletal traction is discontinued after 3 weeks, skin traction is advised for an additional 3 weeks. If these patients are adults with profound cerebral palsy, they should be discharged to intermediate-care facilities where skin traction can be continued. The head of the bed is gradually elevated to prevent postural hypotension when the patient begins sitting.

As soon as soft tissue soreness subsides, gentle range of motion of the hip is performed daily. At first there may be some instability in the hip, but gradually, as the soft tissues stabilize, the hip becomes stable. Specialized seating should be arranged

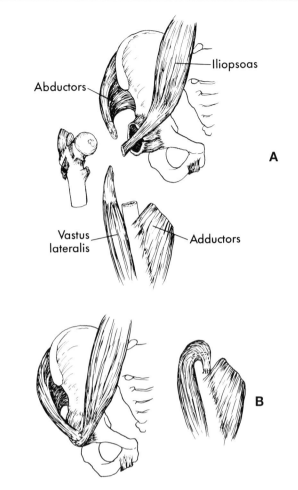

Fig. 30-41 Proximal femoral resection. **A,** Extraperiosteal approach, periosteal excision, and release of musculotendinous attachments. **B,** Interpositional arthroplasty: iliopsoas and abductors are sutured to hip capsule, and femoral stump is covered by vastus lateralis. (Redrawn from McCarthy RE, Simon S, Douglas B, et al: *J Bone Joint Surg* 70A:1011, 1988.)

as soon as possible to allow the patient the most comfort and to afford greater ease in patient care.

PELVIC OBLIQUITY, HIP DISLOCATION, AND SCOLIOSIS

The combination of pelvic obliquity, hip dislocation, and scoliosis is commonly seen in wheelchair-bound cerebral palsy patients. The scoliosis usually is a long C-shaped curve and may or may not be associated with pelvic obliquity and hip subluxation or dislocation. The best treatment for scoliosis associated with pelvic obliquity and hip subluxation or dislocation remains controversial.

Drummond et al. stated that pelvic obliquity in cerebral palsy was caused by a combination of scoliosis and contractures about the hip. In their review of 88 institutionalized adult patients, they found an incidence of hip dislocation that resulted in pelvic obliquity in 15% of patients. However, they concluded that a pelvic obliquity should be corrected before a paralytic hip deformity, for although the hip problem might be resolved surgically, a remaining pelvic obliquity would probably cause recurrence of the hip deformity. In their opinion, pelvic obliquity usually was caused by scoliosis.

Scoliosis is seen in about 7% of ambulatory patients with cerebral palsy and in 35% of those who are not ambulatory. Madigan and Wallace found that 64% of 272 patients with cerebral palsy who were institutionalized had scoliosis. The more common type of scoliosis is a long, gentle, C-shaped curve extending down into the pelvis, which with time becomes fixed, producing a fixed pelvic obliquity. A double S-curve occurs less commonly. Often a dislocated hip is also present. Drummond et al. reported that a thoracic lumbar spinal orthosis (TLSO) can control some curvatures and halt their progression for a time, but when use of such an orthosis was discontinued, the curvature in the spine recurred. They recommended corrective surgery and noted that often the fusion mass had to extend into the sacrum.

As Allen and Ferguson stated, an uncontrolled scoliosis can cause several problems. In the ambulatory patient, it can distort the trunk and make standing erect difficult or impossible. Hand support may be required to sit, meaning that the upper extremities cannot be used for other functions. Lying posture may be so distorted as to produce decubitus ulcers. Pelvic obliquity, produced by the scoliosis, can predispose the patient to hip dislocation, and cardiopulmonary function may be impaired.

Kalen, Conklin, and Sherman studied the effect of scoliosis on the cardiopulmonary state in a group of institutionalized and retarded patients with cerebral palsy. They compared a group of patients with scoliosis exceeding 20 degrees with another group with lesser degrees of scoliosis. They found no significant difference between the two groups in functional status, decubiti present, pulse, or oxygen saturation in the upright, dependent, and recumbent positions. They questioned whether correction of scoliosis in this type of patient is indicated in view of the serious complications that can occur with such major surgery.

Rinsky stated that in all patients with neuromuscular scoliosis the goals of treatment should be functionally oriented and related to loss of sitting balance, presence of pelvic obliquity, and presence of pain, rather than to the degree of the curve. According to him, a severe contracture in itself is not an indication for surgical correction of the scoliosis, but an inability to sit comfortably, uncontrolled by seating inserts in wheelchairs or with orthotics, does indicate a need for surgical correction and stabilization.

Cassidy et al. published a prospective care-burden study of 37 institutionalized patients with scoliosis and severe cerebral palsy to assess the effect of spinal stabilization on comfort, function, health, and ease of nursing care. Seventeen patients with a mean scoliosis of 37 degrees who had spinal fusion were compared with 20 patients with a mean scoliosis of 76 degrees who did not have fusion. No clinically significant differences

were noted in pain, the need for pulmonary medication or therapy, the presence of decubiti, patient function, or the time required for daily care. Subjectively, most health care workers believed that the patients who had undergone spinal fusion were more comfortable.

The treatment of paralytic scoliosis is discussed in Chapter 38.

When studying the relationship of scoliosis, pelvic obliquity, and dislocated hips, Lonstein and Beck reviewed 500 children treated by the Cerebral Palsy Spine Service at the Gillette Children's Hospital. They found no correlation between the frequency of dislocated hips, either bilateral or unilateral, and pelvic obliquity. All degrees of pelvic obliquity were found in children in whom both hips were dislocated. Furthermore, the frequency of hip dislocation on the same side as the elevated pelvis had no direct correlation with the degree of the pelvic obliquity. They also found that the convexity of a lumbar or thoracolumbar curve occurred on the side opposite the high side of the pelvis, but that in "windswept" hips there was no correlation between the direction of the windswept hips and the direction of the pelvic obliquity. Thus they concluded that hip dislocation and subluxation are the result of muscle imbalance about the hip and that pelvic obliquity and scoliosis are related to muscle imbalance of the trunk and independent of the position of the hips.

Upper Extremity

In cerebral palsy, upper extremity paralysis often is accompanied by sensory deficits, particularly in proprioception, stereognosis, barognosis, and light touch. There is seldom normal sensation in the hand of the paralyzed extremity. In many instances this sensory loss causes the patient to totally disregard the hand, and a direct relationship appears to exist between the use of the hand and its sensitivity or lack of it. When a patient uses an involved extremity to play, grasp, eat, or assist the opposite hand, it is functionally useful and can be improved by surgery. In an extremity that has been isolated from use by the patient, reconstructive surgery has seldom been of any benefit except to improve cosmesis and hand hygiene.

For a hand to function in grasp, release, pinch, and transfer activities, it must be able to reach the object to be handled. The hand may be so restrained by lack of motion at the shoulder and elbow that its maximal functional capacity cannot be achieved. If the hand is functional or can be made functional by surgical reconstruction, surgery on the shoulder, elbow, and forearm may be justified.

In spasticity the most common deformities are those of position: flexion of the fingers, flexion of the thumb with or without adduction, flexion of the wrist, pronation of the forearm, flexion of the elbow, and adduction and internal rotation of the shoulder.

The results of surgery on the upper extremity, in which the

goal is functional mobility, are poor compared with those of the lower extremity, in which the goal is painless stability.

Operations on the upper extremities are designed primarily to place the arm and forearm in a functional position and to enable the patient to extend the fingers and wrist while retaining active flexion of the fingers.

Not only the motor and sensory evaluation of the extremity, but also the patient's age and intellectual level should be considered when making a decision on surgery. More postoperative training is required after surgery of the upper extremities than with the lower extremities, and for this reason, age and cognition are of primary importance. Kinetic electromyographic evaluation is extremely useful when evaluating the upper extremity.

SHOULDER

Contracture of the shoulder or spasticity of the muscles that control it usually is not disabling enough to justify surgery. Deformity usually is one of adduction and internal rotation. When surgery is indicated, neurectomy of motor nerves to the involved muscles is impractical because the nerves are not easily accessible. For this reason, useful operations to correct the deformity are (1) the Fairbank operation as modified by Sever or procedures similar to those performed for obstetrical paralysis (Chapter 31) and (2) rotational osteotomy of the humerus done at the level of the deltoid tubercle (Chapter 31).

ELBOW

In an extremity in which the hand is functional or has been made so by surgery, an elbow flexion contracture inhibits its use by restricting the ability to reach forward. In a nonfunctional extremity, a flexion contracture at the elbow may cause skin breakdown in the antecubital fossa, which can be painful and result in poor skin hygiene. In such instances release of an elbow flexion contracture may be justified.

When a flexion contracture is released, attempts to gain full extension are avoided. The brachial artery and the median nerve have become shortened by the constant elbow flexion, and an effort to obtain full extension can result in neurovascular injury.

Mital reported the results of 50 anterior elbow releases in which there were no neurovascular complications and no recurrences of the deformity. Other operations that improve forearm supination and hand function by releasing the flexor-pronator muscle origins from the medial capsule result in a mild amount of elbow extension as well.

◆ Release of Elbow Flexion Contracture

Mital's indications for this operation are fixed elbow flexion contracture of 45 degrees or more or a functional flexion attitude of the elbow of 100 degrees (10 degrees above a right angle) that interferes with the ability to reach forward with a functional forearm and hand.

TECHNIQUE 30-37 *(Mital)*

With the patient supine and the arm fully draped, and with or without a tourniquet, approach the intercubital space through a gently curving, S-shaped incision over the flexor crease. If necessary, ligate the veins that cross the region transversely. Dissect the soft tissue and deep fascia to the muscle belly of the biceps proximally and then follow the muscle distally to its tendon and the lacertus fibrosis. Isolate the lacertus fibrosis and excise it (Fig. 30-42, *A*). Identify and protect the lateral antebrachial cutaneous nerve as it enters the area between the biceps and the brachialis laterally. Retract the nerve laterally, then flex the elbow partially and free the biceps tendon down to its insertion on the tuberosity of the proximal radius. Divide the biceps tendon for a Z-plasty lengthening (Fig. 30-42, *B*). The musculofascial surface of the brachialis muscle can then be seen under it. The radial nerve lies lateral to the brachialis muscle, and the brachial artery and median nerve lie medial to it. Identify and protect these structures. Extend the elbow maximally and circumferentially incise the aponeurotic tendinous fibers of the brachialis muscle at its distal end at one or two levels (Fig. 30-42, *C*). Then maximally extend the elbow and, if necessary, perform an anterior elbow capsulotomy. Allow the tourniquet to deflate and secure hemostasis. Then extend the elbow and repair the previously divided biceps tendon (Fig. 30-42, *D*). Ensure the integrity of the brachial artery and the median nerve. Close only the subcutaneous tissue and skin and immobilize the arm in a well-padded cast with the elbow maximally but not forcefully extended and the forearm fully supinated. Bivalve the cast and reapply it with straps at the operating table.

AFTERTREATMENT. The arm is elevated over the head for 48 hours, and finger motion is encouraged. The bivalved cast is loosened if any swelling occurs. At 4 days the dressing is changed, and at 5 days flexion-extension exercises out of the cast are begun. For 6 weeks after surgery the arm is replaced in the cast when the exercise period has been completed. Pronation-supination exercises are added to the routine 3 weeks after surgery. The bivalved cast is continued at night for 6 months. Maximal elbow motion usually is obtained 3 to 5 months after the operation.

FOREARM, WRIST, AND HAND

Deformities of the forearm, wrist, and hand are considered in Chapter 68 in the discussion of the hand in patients with cerebral palsy.

Adults with Cerebral Palsy

Through the pioneering efforts of many of the orthopaedists mentioned in this chapter, a generation of children with cerebral

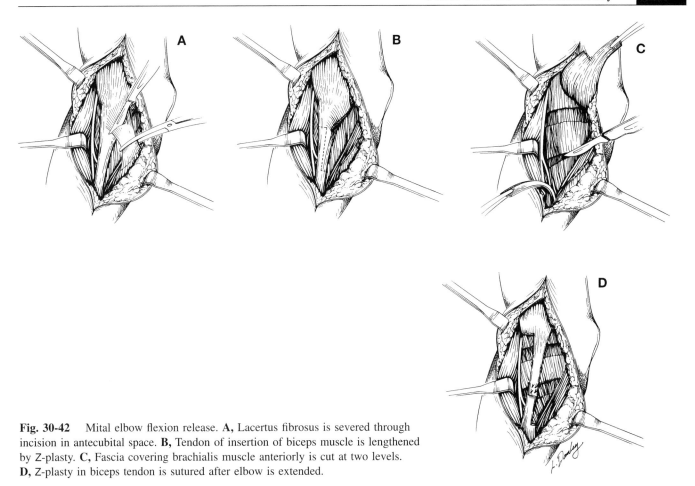

Fig. 30-42 Mital elbow flexion release. **A,** Lacertus fibrosus is severed through incision in antecubital space. **B,** Tendon of insertion of biceps muscle is lengthened by Z-plasty. **C,** Fascia covering brachialis muscle anteriorly is cut at two levels. **D,** Z-plasty in biceps tendon is sutured after elbow is extended.

palsy was taken from an existence of permanent gross contracture and total dependence in state hospitals to being cared for at home as part of a family. Many of these children were able to grow up in their family's community, attend school, and become a part of the workforce. After reaching adulthood these children no longer required orthopaedic surgical intervention and learned to live with the remaining neuromuscular disabilities. However, some of these individuals will return in their late thirties and early forties, when the compensatory mechanisms that they have relied on for so many years begin to fail. The precise number of adults with cerebral palsy is not known but has been estimated to be 400,000. These individuals often have knee instability, which arises from the development of recurvatum from ankle equinus and associated medial collateral ligament instability. Other common problems include degenerative hip disease, flat foot deformity, and scoliosis. Osteopenia also is frequently present in adults with cerebral palsy and may predispose them to fractures.

When treating an adult with cerebral palsy, it is important to first determine what is bothering the patient. The simple existence of a long-standing deformity does not necessitate surgical treatment. To design an effective treatment regimen, the orthopaedist must focus on the patient's needs and on the specific function recently lost. Currently, there are no long-term studies on the treatment of adults with cerebral palsy.

Hopefully, treatment recommendations can be made in the future.

Adult Stroke Patients

Much has been written about the orthopaedic evaluation and treatment of patients who have had cerebrovascular accidents, or strokes. Among those making significant contributions are Braun et al., Caldwell; Hoffer; McCollough; McKeever; Mooney; Perry and Nickel; and Roper, Waters, and Tracy.

LOWER EXTREMITY

Of patients who have had a stroke, 65% to 75% recover enough function in their lower extremities to permit them to walk. This is because the lower extremity does not depend as much on sensation for its function as does the upper extremity, and the activities necessary for walking are gross motor functions that are enhanced by primitive postural reflexes in the weight-bearing position. Most patients with residual hemiparesis require the use of an external support and a brace, at least initially, to become independently ambulatory.

Stroke orthotic positioning and range-of-motion exercises of the lower extremity begin in the early phases of recovery when prevention of contracture is the chief aim of treatment. This treatment extends through the period of motor recovery and gait training to the time when the neurological deficit becomes stationary and a definitive brace to aid in ambulation is required. In the early phase the paralysis is usually flaccid, and deformities result from poor positioning. Passive range-of-motion exercises help prevent undesirable patterning of movements, which often occurs in the recovery phase. Equinus deformity should be prevented by appropriate splinting, and frequently repeated range-of-motion exercises of all the joints of the extremity are indicated.

Preventing deformity of the lower extremities is greatly assisted by having the patient stand and walk as soon as his medical condition permits. Electrical stimulation of flaccid muscles in the postacute phase helps maintain strength, keeps joints mobilized, and as a sensorimotor educational tool may increase the awareness of the sensation of muscle contractions. All these help improve limb function after a stroke. In the immediate postacute phase this can be done by cutaneous stimulation, but later in the recovery phase electrodes can be placed directly on a motor nerve with stimulation controlled through an externally placed transmitter fired either manually or automatically by the positioning of the extremity.

Motor recovery usually occurs during the first 3 or 4 months, and the quality of gait can change considerably during this time. To become a functional ambulator, the patient must obtain adequate spontaneous improvement to allow voluntary control of the hip and knee. A brace for the ankle and foot usually is required, but any brace necessary to stabilize the knee is difficult to apply and manage and significantly interferes with walking. When maximal motor recovery has been obtained and the gait pattern has been stabilized, usually within 4 to 6 months, the patient should be fitted with a definitive brace. It must be the most functional, comfortable, and cosmetically acceptable one available that will control the gait defect.

Perry et al. contributed much to the understanding of the neurophysiology in both normal people and patients with stroke. They list seven neurological sources of motion. Two of these are sophisticated components of normal function (selected control and habitual control); five are forms of primitive control that normally are sublimated into a preparatory background but in the spastic patient are exposed as overt sources of motion (locomotor pattern, verticality, limb synergy, fast stretch, and slow stretch).

Selected control is the normal ability to move one joint independently of another, to contract an isolated muscle, or to select a desired combination of motions. How fast, strong, or continuous a motion is also can be controlled, and this is a cortical function. *Habitual control* is the normal automatic performance of a learned skill, such as walking, and probably arises from the basal ganglia. Primitive *locomotor patterns* are mass movements of flexion or extension. The patient can initiate or terminate the movements but cannot otherwise modify them. If the knee is extended, the ankle also is automatically plantar flexed and the hip is extended. The opposite movements occur in knee flexion. This voluntary

motion is preserved after a loss of cortical control and presumably is controlled by the midbrain. Control of *verticality* is a vestibular function and is an antigravity mechanism. When the body is erect, the extensor muscles have more tone than when it is supine, and standing creates a more intense stimulus than does sitting. In the upper extremity the flexor muscles respond in this manner. Primitive *limb synergy* is the result of a multisegmental spinal cord reflex, tying the action of the extensor muscles to the posture of the limb. Thus when the knee is extended, the tone of both the soleus and the gastrocnemius is greatly increased, making them much more sensitive to stretch than when the knee is flexed. Similarly, the tone in antagonistic muscles may be inhibited. It is this activity that confuses the results in the Silfverskiöld test used to differentiate contracture of the gastrocnemius from that of the soleus. The *fast stretch,* the stretch reflex characterized by the familiar clonic response, is caused by an intermittent burst of muscle activity. It is initiated by the velocity sensors in the muscle spindles. The *slow stretch* reflex is characterized by *rigidity,* a clinical term for continuous muscle reaction to stretch and often misinterpreted as joint contracture; however, when the patient is anesthetized and the muscles are relaxed, the deformity disappears. It is caused by the length-change sensors in the muscle spindles.

Primitive locomotor patterns and control of verticality, in addition to stretch reflex activity, are especially troublesome to the patient who is recovering from a stroke.

In addition to these motor problems, the stroke patient frequently has impaired sensation. Impaired proprioception is especially important, and this causes a delay or hesitancy in making a voluntary motor response. The duration of this delay indicates the time it takes to process the central nervous system signals, and if the delay is too great, walking is not a realistic goal.

Perry et al. also pointed out the importance of visual gait analysis and various standing tests, including double limb support, hemiparetic single limb stance, and hemiparetic limb flexion; the results of gait analysis and these various tests determine whether the patient can expect to walk and whether orthopaedic operations might be expected to reduce the handicap. Further information also is gained from kinesiologic electromyography, and some decisions for surgery cannot be made without this aid.

Surgery should be deferred until at least 6 months after the stroke. Most patients make rapid spontaneous recovery during the first 6 to 8 weeks. They then strengthen these gains and learn to live with their disability. Progress in control of the limb occurs, and this is a contribution that surgery cannot make. By 6 to 9 months after the stroke the patient will have obtained the maximal spontaneous improvement and must come to realize the permanence of the limitations. The results of surgery must be carefully and thoroughly explained to avoid unrealistic expectations after surgery. If nonoperative measures fail to control problems in hygiene or skin care, surgery is indicated. A surgical procedure is indicated if it is likely to improve function, such as making the patient brace free in ambulation or correcting severe deformity that makes an extremity braceable. Occasionally, surgery may improve cosmetic positioning in a grotesquely deformed extremity. Surgery most often is performed on the soft tissues, such as the muscle-tendon units, and rarely on the bony structures. Although improvement in a single deficit may be expected, restoration of normal function in the extremity is impossible.

Foot

Talipes equinovarus is the most common foot deformity in a stroke patient. Other deformities can occur, such as equinus without varus, varus of the forefoot, drop foot without spasticity in the triceps surae, occasionally planovalgus, and often in-curling of the toes.

Talipes Equinus. The goal of surgery is to correct talipes equinus in the midswing and midstance phases while preserving heel lift support in the terminal stance phase and accepting a flat-footed contact with the floor. The recommended operation is a closed subcutaneous triple hemisection of the tendo calcaneus. The distal cut is made medially proximal to the insertion of the tendon, the next is made 2.5 cm proximal to the first through the lateral half of the tendon, and the final one is made 2.5 cm proximal to the second through the medial half of the tendon. After surgery the foot is immobilized in a cast in a slightly equinus position so that walking does not stretch the tendon further. Walking in the cast is started immediately, and the cast is removed at 4 weeks.

Isolated contracture of the gastrocnemius muscle may be suspected when the plantar flexion deformity is mild and clonus in the soleus muscle is absent. It can be demonstrated by a nerve block and the traditional Silverskiöld test. In these patients gait electromyography shows prestance action in the gastrocnemius but not in the soleus.

◆ Talipes Equinovarus

Talipes equinovarus is commonly seen in stroke patients and can result from either dorsiflexor-evertor insufficiency or excess activity in their antagonists. The goal of surgery should be to render the patient free of bracing or to improve walking in a brace when proprioception is defective or the dorsiflexor muscles are inadequate. In the presence of moderate action of the tibialis anterior without assistance of the toe extensors, the equinus deformity is corrected by rebalancing the foot to eliminate the varus deformity. The tibialis anterior, the tibialis posterior, the soleus, the flexor hallucis longus, and the flexor digitorum longus, despite their swing phase and stance phase action, can be active well into the other phase and are often active continuously. Furthermore, they also can be inactive. Therefore varus deformity in either the swing or stance phase can be caused by any of these muscles. The tibialis posterior muscle-tendon unit rarely is a deforming force in the patient recovering from a stroke. Based on surgical experience and on the techniques of gait electromyography, Perry et al. recommend the following operation to correct equinovarus deformity. Three fourths of the tibialis anterior tendon is transferred

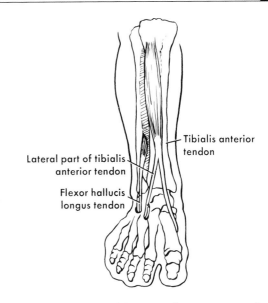

Fig. 30-43 Technique of Perry et al. to correct equinovarus deformity in stroke patients. Lateral three fourths of tibialis anterior tendon and flexor hallucis longus tendon are transferred to third cuneiform. Flexor digitorum longus is released (see text). (From Perry J, Waters RL: *Instr Course Lect* 24:40, 1975.)

laterally to the third cuneiform, the flexor hallucis longus tendon is transferred anteriorly to the same area, the flexor digitorum longus tendon is released, and the tibialis posterior tendon is not disturbed (Fig. 30-43).

TECHNIQUE 30-38 *(Perry et al.)*

Identify and expose the insertion of the tibialis anterior tendon. Separate and detach the lateral three fourths of the tendon from the medial one fourth. Bring the detached part out through an incision made just proximal to the ankle and route it subcutaneously to the dorsal surface of the third cuneiform. Here expose the cuneiform, drill converging holes into the bone, and use a curet to construct a tunnel. Loop the free part of the tendon through this tunnel to be anchored later. Then, in the arch of the foot, release the plantar flexors of the toes. Next, through a posterior incision identify the flexor hallucis longus tendon at its tunnel, detach it, and pass it anteriorly through a large window made in the interosseous membrane. Insert this tendon through the tunnel in the third cuneiform in the direction opposite to that of the tibialis anterior. Lengthen the tendo calcaneus as just described. With the ankle in neutral position and the foot slightly everted, sew the two tendons to themselves as loops and to each other. The flexor digitorum longus can be transferred instead of the flexor hallucis longus if the toe flexors are active in the swing phase of gait.

AFTERTREATMENT. Because the tendo calcaneus has been lengthened at the same time, a cast is applied with the foot in slight plantar flexion. At 6 weeks the cast is removed, and the foot is protected by a locked ankle brace for an additional 6 months. Because muscles in a hemiplegia patient pull with marked vigor or none at all, several months are necessary for the scar to mature enough not to yield under tension.

In 1976 Tracy reported satisfactory results from surgery in 32 of 35 adult hemiplegics with talipes equinovarus. He used an operation originally described by Mooney et al. consisting of triple hemisection of the tendo calcaneus, open Z-plasty lengthening and suturing of the tibialis posterior tendon just proximal to the medial malleolus, transfer of one half of the tibialis anterior tendon to the third cuneiform, and transverse division of the flexor digitorum brevis and flexor digitorum longus tendons at the base of each toe. All patients who could satisfactorily dorsiflex the foot after surgery had been able to contract the tibialis anterior selectively at will or had some activity in the muscle before surgery.

Varus. The tibialis anterior muscle usually is the deforming force in forefoot varus. A split tibialis anterior transfer (Technique 30-17) is the procedure of choice for this condition, although it does not correct a fixed hindfoot varus.

A short leg walking cast is worn for 6 weeks, and then an AFO is used when walking to protect the muscle transfer for 4 to 5 months more.

Planovalgus. If a pes planus preceded the stroke, in rare cases a planovalgus deformity may occur after the stroke. Spasticity of the triceps surae pulls the calcaneus laterally, and the peroneals may be hyperactive with no function occurring in the tibialis posterior tendon during stance.

If walking is impeded by pain, surgical correction is indicated. As in equinus deformity, the treatment involves lengthening of the tendo calcaneus and a triple-level hemitenotomy. The distal hemisection in the tendo calcaneus is performed in the lateral half of the tendon, however, to reduce the valgus placement or thrust of the tendon on the calcaneus.

If the peroneals are hyperactive during the stance phase, the peroneus brevis can be transferred medially into the tibialis posterior tendon to support the medial border of the foot, or the peroneus longus and brevis can be lengthened.

A triple arthrodesis ultimately may be required if an AFO does not control the deformity.

Toe Flexion. Toe flexion occurs at the metatarsophalangeal joint and is different from the clawtoe deformity seen in most neurological disorders in which extensors are hyperactive. Toe curling or toe flexion in the stroke patient occurs from overactivity of the long toe flexors. If all toes are involved, the flexor digitorum longus and the flexor hallucis longus can be tenotomized through a plantar incision along the medial border of the foot, reflecting the abductor hallucis plantarward and locating the tendons between the first and third layers of the plantar surface of the foot. An alternative is to tenotomize merely the toe flexors at the plantar surface of the metatarsophalangeal joints of all toes.

Knee

Flexion contractures of the knee, like other deformities in the stroke patient, are better prevented than treated. Although the hamstrings are important extensors of the hip, occasionally a patient with a flexion contracture of the knee and good power in the gluteus maximus and quadriceps muscles will benefit from release of the hamstrings or transfer of the medial hamstrings.

Deficient flexion of the knee during the swing phase, which produces a stiff-knee gait, usually is caused by increased electrical activity in the rectus femoris during the swing phase. Release of the rectus femoris from the patella by excision of its distal segment can result in 15 to 20 degrees of flexion of the knee during the swing phase.

Hip

The scissors gait caused by adductor spasticity is the only disability about the hip now treated surgically. To determine whether the adductors are necessary in flexion of the hip in a given patient, blocking of the obturator nerve, using a local anesthetic, is advisable. If the patient is unable to walk with the obturator nerve blocked, surgery will be of no benefit. On the other hand, if the gait is improved temporarily, neurectomy of the anterior branch of the obturator nerve is recommended. If the effect of the local anesthetic is prolonged, the nerve block can be repeated once or twice, and occasionally the results will be permanent.

Surgical release of a flexion contracture of the hip rarely is indicated in stroke patients because the decrease in the power of active flexion of the hip may make the patient unable to walk. When gait electromyography shows continuous activity in the flexors of the hip and in the medial hamstrings, releasing the iliopsoas, performing a tenotomy of the adductor longus, and transferring the medial hamstrings to the femur will sometimes allow the limb to assume an upright position.

UPPER EXTREMITY

The prognosis for recovering normal function in the upper extremity in stroke patients is poor, and approximately one third are left with a permanently functionless limb. The most important reason for this is that the patterns of neuromuscular activity in the normally functioning upper extremity are highly sophisticated and complex and are modified by multiple sophisticated sensory impulses. Permanent impairment in motor and sensory function in the upper extremity is incurable, and permanent impairment of function is to be expected. Thus rehabilitation of the arm and hand consists primarily of training the patient to accomplish the activities of daily living as a one-handed person. For patients who show sufficient neurological recovery, additional training for development of assistive function is indicated.

The orthopaedic surgeon may release contractures, weaken spastic muscles that cause imbalance and deformity, and transfer functioning muscle units to attempt to restore some balance in the extremity. These operations also can relieve persistent pain, which causes immobility and lack of participation in other areas of the rehabilitation program.

◆ Shoulder

Some stroke patients report pain localized precisely to the shoulder and specifically to the adductor and internal rotator groups of muscles. In others a hemicorporal type of diffuse discomfort is present and is untreatable by present methods. Patients with the first type of pain develop progressively decreasing ranges of motion in the joint despite intensive conservative treatment. They also have an exaggerated stretch reflex on rapid external rotation of the shoulder, abduction of less than 45 degrees, and internal rotation of less than 15 degrees. Surgery is recommended only for those patients who will have an exercise program available to them after surgery, for those who will participate in it fully, and for those who have a reasonable potential for rehabilitation. Braun et al. reviewed their initial experience with the operation described here and noted complete relief of pain and significant improvement in motion in 10 of the first 13 patients in whom it was used. Of 12 control patients with similar symptoms not treated by surgery, none had spontaneous resolution of the painful contracture of the joint.

TECHNIQUE 30-39 *(Braun et al.)*

Make an anterior deltopectoral approach to the shoulder. Identify the subscapularis tendon and cauterize the vascular bundle at its distal edge. Excise this tendon but preserve the anterior capsule of the shoulder joint. Palpate the tendon of the pectoralis major and with scissors passed distally along the humerus, cut its tendinous insertion.

AFTERTREATMENT. A sling is worn on the arm. A program of assisted range-of-motion exercises is begun within the first few days after surgery, and reciprocal pulley exercises are begun within the first 5 days. It is important to supervise the patient's participation in the exercises.

Elbow

Fixed flexion of the elbow seriously impairs function of the upper extremity. Anterior release in the antecubital fossa, however, is a major operation and can be followed by serious complications. Sometimes a fixed flexion deformity can be prevented by an open injection of phenol into the musculocutaneous nerve, carried out with minimal added dissection at the time the shoulder is released. This injection usually will allow the patient 6 months in which to develop adequate extensor muscles before motor power returns to the flexor muscles of the elbow supplied by this nerve.

Any necessary release is carried out through an S-shaped incision over the anterior aspect of the elbow. The neurovascular bundle is isolated and protected throughout the operation.

The biceps tendon is lengthened in a step-cut manner. The fascia over the brachialis muscle is divided and, if necessary, the brachialis itself is divided at its musculotendinous junction, the flexor-pronator origin is divided, the brachioradialis fascia is released, the capsule of the elbow joint is divided, the ulnar nerve is transplanted anteriorly, and the wound is closed over a drain. This operation is rarely used because the results are so uncertain.

PHENOL NERVE BLOCK

Braun et al. reported the results of injection of phenol into motor nerves in 24 adults and 10 children with spastic hemiplegia. The nerves were exposed surgically. That the correct nerve had been exposed was confirmed by a nerve stimulator, and the nerve was injected intraneurally with 3% to 5% phenol solution beneath the neural sheath and into the substance of the nerve. The volume of solution injected ranged from 2 to 5 ml within a 2-cm segment of the nerve. The injection was continued until electrical stimulation proximal to the site of injection revealed that the nerve had in fact been blocked. Such blocks in 18 patients initially resulted in improvement in 17, but review later revealed that 11 of these good results disappeared in 6 months. In two patients the deformity recurred in 1 year, and in only 2 patients did the good results last longer than 1 year. In these latter two some selective control of the antagonistic muscles was present before the injection. In four patients phenol block of the spastic flexor-pronator muscles was combined with transfer of the flexor carpi ulnaris tendon to the extensor carpi radialis brevis. Relaxation of the excessive flexor tone was seen during the 3 months required for strengthening of the transfer. These investigators concluded that open intraneural phenol nerve blocks can be expected to diminish muscle tone for about 6 months. During this time other treatment programs to prevent contractures or to strengthen and train weakened or transferred muscles can be carried out. A few patients showed prolonged benefits, and most of these had selective muscle control of their spastic muscles before the nerves were blocked.

In the stroke patient, phenol nerve blocks occasionally are indicated to change the paralysis from spastic to flaccid and thus make the extremity more responsive to corrective exercises, corrective posturing, or bracing. Phenol injections into nerves or motor end-plates is more often indicated in the patient who has experienced a head injury and in whom maximal recovery of function may not appear until 1½ to 3 years after injury.

FUNCTIONAL ELECTRICAL STIMULATION IN STROKE PATIENTS

Functional electrical stimulation (FES) is a product of modern electronic rehabilitation engineering whereby function is restored in paralyzed muscles by electrical stimulation. The aim is to have functional muscle control occur during stimulation, but occasionally a carryover occurs and the muscle comes under voluntary control even during periods without electrical stimulation. FES theoretically depends on one stimulation, such as heel lift, being transmitted through an antenna to an electrical implant, which then fires another signal to the nerve supply to the muscles, such as the peroneal nerve, to perform a function, such as dorsiflexion of the foot. The device needs to be small and cosmetically acceptable, and the activity of the stimulator should be partly under voluntary control otherwise too much stimulation may occur. FES is being used in the upper and lower extremities, around the foot and ankle to suppress spasticity, to correct scoliosis, for electrophrenic respiration, and in bladder control. There remains a need for external control of motor unit graduation, for synergistic activity in other muscles, and for some proprioceptive kinesthetic feedback.

References

GENERAL

Able MF, Damiano DL, Pannunzio M, Bush J: Muscle-tendon surgery in diplegic cerebral palsy: functional and mechanical changes, *J Pediatr Orthop* 19:366, 1999.

Allen MC: The appearance of selected primitive reflexes in a population of very low birthweight premature infants. Paper presented at the annual meeting of the American Academy of Cerebral Palsy and Developmental Medicine, Washington, DC, Oct 1984.

Allen MC, Capute AJ: Apgar score as predictor of outcome for premature infants, *Dev Med Child Neurol* 28 (suppl 53):18, 1986 (abstract).

Arvidsson J, Eksmyr R: Cerebral palsy and perinatal deaths in geographical defined populations with different perinatal services, *Dev Med Child Neurol* 26:709, 1984.

Astbury J, Orgill AA, Bajuk B, Yu VYH: Neurodevelopmental outcome, growth and health of extremely low-birthweight survivors: how soon can we tell? *Dev Med Child Neurol* 32:592, 1990.

Atkinson S, Stanley FJ: Spastic diplegia among children of low and normal birthweight, *Dev Med Child Neurol* 25:693, 1983.

Banks HH: Cerebral palsy. In Lovell WW, Winter RB, eds: *Pediatric orthopaedics,* ed 1, vol 1, Philadelphia, 1978, JB Lippincott.

Barnett HE: Orthopedic surgery in cerebral palsy, *JAMA* 150:1396, 1952.

Bayley N: *Bayley scales of mental and motor development,* New York, 1969, The Psychological Corp.

Beals RK: Spastic paraplegia and diplegia: an evaluation of non-surgical and surgical factors influencing the prognosis for ambulation, *J Bone Joint Surg* 48A:827, 1966.

Bennett FC, Chandler LS, Robinson NM, Sells CJ: Spastic diplegia in premature infants: etiological and diagnostic considerations, *Am J Dis Child* 135:732, 1981.

Bennett FC, Crowe T, Deitz J, TeKolste K: Childhood motor skills of premature infants. Paper presented at the annual meeting of the American Academy of Cerebral Palsy and Developmental Medicine, Washington, DC, Oct 1984.

Biasini FJ, Mindingall A: Developmental outcome of very low birthweight children, *Orthop Trans* 8:115, 1984.

Bleck EE: Cerebral palsy. In Bleck EE, Nagel DA, eds: *Physically handicapped children: a medical atlas for teachers,* New York, 1975, Grune & Stratton.

Bleck EE: Locomotor prognosis in cerebral palsy, *Dev Med Child Neurol* 17:18, 1975.

Bleck EE, ed: *Physically handicapped children: a medical atlas for teachers,* ed 2, New York, 1982, Grune & Stratton.

Bleck EE: *Orthopaedic management of cerebral palsy,* Philadelphia, 1979, WB Saunders.

Bleck EE: Where have all the CP children gone? The needs of adults, *Dev Med Child Neurol* 26:674, 1984.

Boscarino LF, Ounpuu S, Davis RB III, et al: Effects of selective dorsal rhizotomy on gait in children with cerebral palsy, *J Pediatr Orthop* 13:174, 1993.

Botte MJ, Nickel VL, Akeson WH: Spasticity and contracture: physiologic aspects of formation, *Clin Orthop* 233:7, 1988.

Bozynski ME, Nelson MN, Rosati-Skertich C, et al: Two-year longitudinal follow-up of premature infants weighing less than 1,200 grams at birth: sequelae of intracranial hemorrhage, *J Dev Behav Pediatr Trans* 5:346, 1984.

Brink JD, Hoffer MM: Rehabilitation of brain-injured children, *Orthop Clin North Am* 9:451, 1978.

Brown JK, Minns RA: Mechanisms of deformity in children with cerebral palsy, *Semin Orthop* 4:236, 1989.

Butler C: Effects of powered mobility on self-initiative behavior of very young, locomotor-disabled children. Paper presented at the annual meeting of the American Academy of Cerebral Palsy and Developmental Medicine, Washington, DC, 1984.

Campos da Paz A, Nomura AM, Braga LW, Burnett SM: Cerebral palsy: a retrospective study. Paper presented at the annual meeting of the Pediatric Orthopaedic Society, Vancouver, 1984.

Canadian Medical Protective Association and American Academy for Cerebral Palsy and Developmental Medicine: Perinatal asphyxia: its role in developmental deficits in children. Proceedings of a symposium held at Toronto, Oct 1988. Printed as a supplement to the Canadian Medical Association Journal, 1988.

Capute A, Palmer F: A pediatric overview of the spectrum of developmental disabilities, *J Dev Behav Pediatr* 1:66, 1980.

Capute AJ, Shapiro BK, Palmer FB: Spectrum of developmental disabilities, *Orthop Clin North Am* 12:3, 1981.

Carlson W, Carpenter B, Wenger D: Myoneural blocks for preoperative planning in cerebral palsy surgery. Paper presented at the annual meeting of the American Academy for Cerebral Palsy and Developmental Medicine, Chicago, 1983.

Carlson W, Carpenter B, Wenger D: Myoneural blocks for preoperative planning in cerebral palsy surgery, *Orthop Trans* 8:111, 1984 (abstract).

Cech D, Gallagher RJ: Infant motor assessment: Bayley scales of infant development as compared to the Chicago Infant Neuromotor Assessment. Paper presented at the annual meeting of the American Academy of Cerebral Palsy and Developmental Medicine, Washington, DC, Oct 1984.

Craig CL, Sosnoff F, Zimbler S: Seating in cerebral palsy: a possible advance. Paper presented at the annual meeting of the Pediatric Orthopaedic Society, Vancouver, 1984.

Dale A, Stanley FJ: An epidemiological study of cerebral palsy in Western Australia, 1956-1975. II. Spastic cerebral palsy and perinatal factors, *Dev Med Child Neurol* 22:13, 1980.

DeLuca PA, Davis III RB, Ounpuu S, et al: Alterations in surgical decision making in patients with cerebral palsy based on three-dimensional gait analysis, *J Pediatr Orthop* 17:608, 1997.

Denhoff E: Current status of infant stimulation or enrichment programs for children with developmental disabilities, *Pediatrics* 67:32, 1981.

Dennis SC, Green NE: Hereditary spastic paraplegia, *J Pediatr Orthop* 8:413, 1988.

Dierdorf SF, McNiece WL, Rao CC, et al: Effect of succinylcholine on plasma potassium in children with cerebral palsy, *Anesthesiology* 62:88, 1985.

Drennan JC: *Orthopaedic management of neuromuscular disorders,* Philadelphia, 1983, JB Lippincott.

Elliman AM, Bryan EM, Elliman AD, Palmer P, Dubowitz L: Denver developmental screening test and preterm infants, *Arch Dis Child* 60:20, 1985.

Evans P, Agassiz CDS, Pritchard FE, Nissen JJ: Symposium on cerebral palsy, *Proc R Soc Med* 44:82, 1951.

Evans P, Elliott M, Alberman E, Evans S: Prevalence and disabilities in 4 to 8 year olds with cerebral palsy, *Arch Dis Child* 60:940, 1985.

Fixsen JA: The role of orthopaedic surgery in cerebral palsy, *Semin Orthop* 4:215, 1989.

Florentino M: *A basis for sensorimotor development: normal and abnormal,* Springfield, Ill, 1981, Charles C Thomas.

Gage JR: Deformities of the knee and foot. Paper presented at American Academy for Cerebral Palsy and Developmental Medicine Symposium, Growing up with Cerebral Palsy, Wilmington, Del, April 1985.

Gage JR: Orthopaedic aspects of cerebral palsy. Paper presented at American Academy for Cerebral Palsy and Developmental Medicine Symposium, Growing up with Cerebral Palsy, Wilmington, Del, April 19-20, 1985.

Gage JR: *Gait analysis in cerebral palsy,* London, 1991, MacKeith.

Gage JR, DeLuca PA, Renshaw TS: Gait analysis: principles and applications with emphasis on its use in cerebral plasy, *Instr Course Lect* 46:491, 1996.

Gage JR, Fabian D, Hicks R, Tashman S: Pre- and postoperative gait analysis in patients with spastic diplegia: a preliminary report, *J Pediatr Orthop* 4:715, 1984.

Georgieff M, Hoffman-Williamson M, Spungen L, et al: Abnormal muscle tone as an indicator of later development in preterm infants, *Orthop Trans* 8:108, 1984 (abstract).

Gesell A, Amatruda CS: *Developmental diagnosis: normal and abnormal child development: clinical methods and pediatric applications,* ed 2, New York, 1947, Paul B Hoeber.

Gibbs FA, Gibbs EL, Perstein MA, Rich CL: Electroencephalographic and clinical aspects of cerebral palsy, *Pediatrics* 32:73, 1963.

Goldner JL: Cerebral palsy. I. General principles, *Instr Course Lect* 20:20, 1971.

Green WT, McDermott LJ: Operative treatment of cerebral palsy of spastic type, *JAMA* 118:434, 1942.

Gritzka TL, Aiona M, Pierce R: Intramuscular neurolysis as a diagnostic and therapeutic modality in cerebral palsy, *Dev Med Child Neurol* 29(55):22, 1987 (abstract).

Guralnick MJ, Heiser KE, Eaton AP, et al: Pediatricians' perceptions of the effectiveness of early intervention for at-risk and handicapped children, *J Dev Behav Pediatr* 9:12, 1988.

Hagberg B, Hagberg G, Olow I: Gains and hazards of intensive neonatal care: an analysis from Swedish cerebral palsy epidemiology, *Dev Med Child Neurol* 24:13, 1982.

Harris S: The school-aged child. Physical therapy: developmental vs. functional goals. Paper presented at American Academy for Cerebral Palsy and Developmental Medicine Symposium, Growing up with Cerebral Palsy, Wilmington, Del, April 1985.

Harris SR: Early predictors of spastic diplegia vs spastic hemiplegia, *Dev Med Child Neurol* 28(53):38, 1986 (abstract).

Harris SR, Tada WL: Providing developmental therapy services. In Garwood SG, Fewell RR: *Educating handicapped infants: issues in development and intervention,* Rockville, Md, 1983, Aspen Systems.

Henderson RC, Lin PP, Greene WB: Bone-mineral density in children and adolescents who have spastic cerebral palsy, *J Bone Joint Surg* 77A:1671, 1995.

Hensinger RN, Fraser B, Machello J, Taylor S: Head and neck control in the severely involved cerebral palsy patient. Paper presented at the annual meeting of the Pediatric Orthopaedic Society, Vancouver, 1984.

Herndon WA, Troup P, Yngve DA, Sullivan JA: Effects of neurodevelopmental treatment on movement patterns of children with cerebral palsy, *J Pediatr Orthop* 7:395, 1987.

Hoffer M, Brink J: Orthopedic management of acquired cerebral spasticity in childhood, *Clin Orthop* 110:224, 1975.

Hoffer MM: Basic considerations and classifications of cerebral palsy, *Instr Course Lect* 25:96, 1976.

Hoffer MM, Bullock M: The functional and social significance of orthopedic rehabilitation of mentally retarded patients with cerebral palsy, *Orthop Clin North Am* 12:185, 1981.

Hoffer MM, Knoebel RT, Roberts R: Contractures in cerebral palsy, *Clin Orthop* 219:70, 1987.

Hoffer MM, Koffman M: Cerebral palsy: the first three years, *Clin Orthop* 151:222, 1980.

Hoffer MM, Garrett A, Brink J, et al: The orthopaedic management of brain-injured children, *J Bone Joint Surg* 53A:567, 1971.

Hoffman-Williamson M et al: Comparable development progress in infants of birthweights less than 1000 grams and 1001-1500 grams, *Orthop Trans* 8:115, 1984 (abstract).

Holm VA: The causes of cerebral palsy: a contemporary perspective, *JAMA* 247:1473, 1982.

Hughes J Jacobs N: Normal human locomotion, *Prosthet Orthot Int* 3:4, 1979.

Ingram AJ, Withers E, Speltz E: Role of intensive physical and occupational therapy in the treatment of cerebral palsy: testing and results, *Arch Phys Med* 40:429, 1959.

Johnson DC, Damiano DL, Abel MF: The evolution of gait in childhood and adolescent cerebral palsy, *J Pediatr Orthop* 17:392, 1997.

Johnson MK: The use of motor age test in the evaluation of cerebral palsy patients. In American Academy of Orthopaedic Surgeons: *Instructional course lectures,* vol 9, Ann Arbor, Mich, 1952, JW Edwards.

Johnson MK, Zuck FN, Wingate K: The motor age test: measurement of motor handicaps in children with neuromuscular disorders such as cerebral palsy, *J Bone Joint Surg* 33A:698, 1951.

Kiely M, Lubin RA, Kiely JL: Descriptive epidemiology of cerebral palsy, *Pub Health Rev* 12:79, 1984.

Kling TF, Hensinger RN, Taylor SR: Transparent spinal orthosis for the neurologically handicapped child. Paper presented at the annual meeting of the American Academy for Cerebral Palsy and Developmental Medicine, Washington, DC, 1984.

Laborde JM, Solomonow M, Soboloff H: The effectiveness of surface electrical simulation in improving quadriceps strength and gait in young CP patients, *Dev Med Child Neurol* 28:26, 1986.

Lai KA, Kuo KN, Andriacchi TP: Relationship between dynamic deformities and joint moments in children with cerebral palsy, *J Pediatr Orthop* 8:690, 1988.

Lindsey RW, Drennan JC: Management of foot and knee deformities in the mentally retarded, *Orthop Clin North Am* 12:107, 1981.

Lipper EG, Voorhies T, Ross G, et al: Early neurological predictors of one-year outcome in birth-asphyxiated infants. Paper presented at the annual meeting of the American Academy of Cerebral Palsy and Developmental Medicine, Washington, DC, Oct 1984.

Lord J: Cerebral palsy: a clinical approach, *Arch Phys Med Rehabil* 65:542, 1984.

Mann R: Biomechanics in cerebral palsy, *Foot Ankle* 4:114, 1983.

Marquis PJ, Ruis NA, Lundy MS, Dillard RG: Primitive reflexes and early motor development in very low birth weight (VLBW) infants, *Orthop Trans* 8:108, 1984 (abstract).

Marty GR, Dias LS, Gaebler-Spira D: Selective posterior rhizotomy and soft-tissue procedures for the treatment of cerebral diplegia, *J Bone Joint Surg* 77A:713, 1995.

McKinlay IA: Therapy for cerebral palsy, *Semin Orthop* 4:220, 1989.

Milani-Comparetti A, Gidoni EA: Routine developmental examination in normal and retarded children, *Dev Med Child Neurol* 9:631, 1967.

Molnar GE, Gordon SV: Predictive value of clinical signs for early prognostication of motor function in cerebral palsy, *Arch Phys Med* 57:153, 1976.

Nelson MN, Bozynski MEA, Genaze D, et al: Comparative evaluation of motor development of 1,200 grams (or less) infants during the first postnatal year using the Bayley scales versus the Milani-Comparetti, *Orthop Trans* 8:108, 1984 (abstract).

Nelson KB, Ellenberg JH: Antecedents of cerebral palsy. Multivariate analysis of risk, *N Engl J Med* 10:315:81, 1986.

Nickel RE, Renken CA: The infant motor screen: a screening test for the early identification of infants with cerebral palsy, *Dev Med Child Neurol* 28(suppl 53):41, 1986 (abstract).

Norlin R, Odenrick P: Development of gait in spastic children with cerebral palsy, *J Pediatr Orthop* 6:674, 1986.

Norlin R, Tkaczuk H: One-session surgery for correction of lower extremity deformities in children with cerebral palsy, *J Pediatr Orthop* 5:208, 1985.

Nwaobi OM, Smith P: Effect of adaptive seating on pulmonary function of children with cerebral palsy, *Dev Med Child Neurol* 28(suppl 53):24, 1986.

Okawa A, Kajiura I, Hiroshima K: Physical therapeutic and surgical management in spastic diplegia: a Japanese experience, *Clin Orthop* 253:38, 1990.

O'Neill DL, Harris SR: Developing goals and objectives for handicapped children, *Phys Ther* 62:295, 1982.

O'Reilly DE, Walentynowicz JE: Etiological factors in cerebral palsy: an historical review, *Dev Med Child Neurol* 23:633, 1981.

Ough JL, Garland DE, Jordan C, Waters RL: Treatment of spastic joint contractures in mentally disabled adults, *Orthop Clin North Am* 12:143, 1981.

Paine RS: Cerebral palsy: symptoms and signs of diagnostic and prognostic significance. In Adams JP, ed: *Current practice in orthopaedic surgery,* vol 3, St Louis, 1966, Mosby.

Parmelee AH, Cohen SE: Neonatal follow-up services for infants at risk. In Harel S, Anastasiow NJ, eds: *The at-risk infant: psycho/socio/medical aspects,* Baltimore, 1985, Paul H Brookes.

Payne LZ, DeLuca PA: Heterotopic ossification after rhizotomy and femoral osteotomy, *J Pediatr Orthop* 13:733, 1993.

Pearson DT: Psychological needs of the handicapped. Paper presented at American Academy for Cerebral Palsy and Developmental Medicine Symposium, Growing up with Cerebral Palsy, Wilmington, Del, April 1985.

Pearson P, Williams CE: *Physical therapy services in the developmental disabilities,* Springfield, Ill, 1980, Charles C Thomas.

Pearson PH, Williams CE, eds: *Physical therapy services in the developmental disabilities,* Springfield, Ill, 1972, Charles C Thomas.

Pearson PH: The results of treatment: the horns of our dilemma, *Dev Med Child Neurol* 24:417, 1982.

Perry J, Simon S, Sutherland D: Gait analysis: an evaluation of measurement systems and their applications. Paper presented at the annual meeting of the American Academy for Cerebral Palsy and Developmental Medicine, Washington, DC, 1984.

Perry J, Hoffer MM, Antonelli D, et al: Electromyography before and after surgery for hip deformity in children with cerebral palsy: a comparison of clinical and electromyographic findings, *J Bone Joint Surg* 58A:201, 1976.

Pharoah POD: The epidemiology of cerebral palsy, *Semin Orthop* 4:205, 1989.

Phelps WM: Complications of orthopaedic surgery in the treatment of cerebral palsy, *Clin Orthop* 53:39, 1967.

Phelps WM: Treatment of paralytic disorders exclusive of poliomyelitis. In Bancroft FW, Marble JC: *Surgical treatment of the motor-skeletal system,* Philadelphia, 1951, JB Lippincott.

Piper MC, Silver KM: Resolution of neurological symptoms in the high-risk infant, *Dev Med Child Neurol* 28(suppl 53):14, 1986 (abstract).

Powell TG, Pharoah POD, Cooke RWI, et al: Cerebral palsy in low-birthweight infants. I. Spastic hemiplegia: associations with intrapartum stress, *Dev Med Child Neurol* 30:11, 1988.

Powell TG, Pharoah POD, Cooke RWI, et al: Cerebral palsy in low-birthweight infants. II. Spastic hemiplegia: associations with fetal immaturity, *Dev Med Child Neurol* 30:19, 1988.

Rang M, Douglas G, Bennet GC, Koreska J: Seating for children with cerebral palsy, *J Pediatr Orthop* 1:279, 1982.

Rang M, Silver R, de la Garza J: Cerebral palsy. In Lovell WW, Winter RB, eds: *Pediatric orthopaedics,* ed 2, vol 1, Philadelphia, 1986, JB Lippincott.

Reimers J: Static and dynamic problems in spastic cerebral palsy, *J Bone Joint Surg* 55B:822, 1973.

Roseberg LK, Blackman J, Sustik J: Assessment of motor dysfunction in infants: a computer-videodisc program, *Orthop Trans* 8:102, 1984 (abstract).

Rosenbaum PL: Early diagnosis of developmental delay. Paper presented at American Academy for Cerebral Palsy and Developmental Medicine Symposium, Growing up with Cerebral Palsy, Wilmington, Del, April 1985.

Samilson RL: Orthopaedic aspects of cerebral palsy, *Clin Dev Med* 52:183, 1975.

Samilson RL: *Orthopaedic aspects of cerebral palsy,* Philadelphia, 1975, JB Lippincott.

Samilson RL: Current concepts of surgical management of deformities of the lower extremities in cerebral palsy, *Clin Orthop* 158:99, 1981.

Samilson RL, Dillin L: Postural impositions on the foot and ankle from trunk, pelvis, hip, and knee in cerebral palsy, *Foot Ankle* 4:120, 1983.

Scrutton D, Gilbertson M: The physiotherapist's role in the treatment of cerebral palsy. In Samilson R, ed: *Orthopedic aspects of cerebral palsy,* Philadelphia, 1975, JB Lippincott.

Siegler EL, Beck LH: Stiffness: a pathophysiologic approach to diagnosis and treatment, *J Gen Intern Med* 4:533, 1989.

Tablan DJ: Clinical analysis of the brain-injured child: an analysis of 333 cases in the Philippines. In Samilson RL, ed: *Orthopedic aspects of cerebral palsy,* Philadelphia, 1975, JB Lippincott.

Tachdjian MO: Affections of brain and spinal cord. In Tachdjian MO: *Pediatric orthopaedics,* Philadelphia, 1972, JB Lippincott.

Tachdjian MO: The neuromuscular system. In Tachdjian MO: *Pediatric orthopaedics,* Philadelphia, 1972, WB Saunders.

Tachdjian MO, Minear WL: Sensory disturbances in the hands of children with cerebral palsy, *J Bone Joint Surg* 40A:85, 1958.

Taft LT: Intervention programs for infants with cerebral palsy: a clinician's view. In Brown CE, ed: *Infants at risk: assessment and intervention,* 1981, Johnson & Johnson Baby Products.

Tardieu G, Tardieu C: Cerebral palsy: mechanical evaluation and conservative correction of limb joint contractures, *Clin Orthop* 219:63, 1987.

Taylor S, Kling TF Jr: An improved system of orthotic management in neuromuscular disease. Paper presented at the annual meeting of the American Academy for Cerebral Palsy and Developmental Medicine, Chicago, 1983.

Taylor S, Kling TF Jr: An improved system of orthotic management in neuromuscular disease, *Orthop Trans* 8:105, 1984 (abstract).

Thompson G, Ragotzy S, Dixon C, et al: Treatment of spasticity via transcranial electrical stimulation in patients with cerebral palsy and severe mental retardation, *Dev Med Child Neurol* 28(suppl 53):36, 1986.

Thompson GH, Rubin IL, Bilenker RM, eds: *Comprehensive management of cerebral palsy,* New York, 1983, Grune & Stratton.

Vulpius O, Stoffel A: *Orthopädische Operationslehre,* ed 2, Stuttgart, 1920, Ferdinand Enke.

Watts HG: Editorial. Gait laboratory analysis for preoperative decision making in spastic cerebral palsy: is it all it's cracked up to be? *J Pediatr Orthop* 14:703, 1994.

Westin GW, Dye S: Conservative management of cerebral palsy in the growing child, *Foot Ankle* 4:160, 1983.

Williams SF, Ferguson-Pell M, Cochran GVB: Characterization and treatment patterns of 122 spastic diplegic patients. Paper presented at the annual meeting of the American Academy of Cerebral Palsy and Developmental Medicine, Washington, DC, Oct 1984.

Winters TF, Gage JR: Gait patterns in spastic hemiplegia secondary to cerebral palsy. Paper presented at the annual meeting of the American Academy for Cerebral Palsy and Developmental Medicine, Washington, DC, Oct 1984.

Wright T, Nicholson J: Physiotherapy for the spastic child: an evaluation, *Dev Med Child Neurol* 15:146, 1973.

Wright J, Rang M: The spastic mouse and the search for an animal model of spasticity in human beings, *Clin Orthop* 253:12, 1990.

Yale Clinic of Child Development: *The first five years of life: a guide to the study of the preschool child,* New York, 1940, Harper & Brothers.

Yngve DA, Chambers C: Vulpius and Z-lengthening, *J Pediatr Orthop* 16:759, 1996.

Young RR, Wiegner AW: Spasticity, *Clin Orthop* 219:50, 1987.

Zimbler S, Craig C, Harris J, et al: Orthotic management of severe scoliosis in spastic neuromuscular disease: results of treatment. Paper presented at the annual meeting of the American Academy for Cerebral Palsy and Developmental Medicine, Washington, DC, 1984.

NEUROSURGICAL TREATMENT

Albright AL, Barry MJ, Fasick MP, et al: Effects of continuous intrathecal baclofen infusion and selective posterior rhizotomy on upper extremity spasticity, *Pediatr Neurosurg* 23:82, 1995.

Albright AL, Cervi A, Singletary J: Intrathecal baclofen for spasticity in cerebral palsy, *JAMA* 265:1418, 1991.

Arens LJ, Peacock WJ, Peter J: Selective posterior rhizotomy: a long-term follow-up study, *Child Nerv Syst* 5:148, 1989.

Armstrong RW: Intrathecally administered baclofen for treatment of children with spasticity of cerebral origin, *J Neurosurg* 87:409, 1997.

Benedetti A, Colombo F, Alexandre A, Pellegri A: Posterior rhizotomies for spasticity in children affected by cerebral palsy, *J Neurosurg Sci* 26:179, 1982.

Berman B, Peacock WJ, Vaughan CL, Bridger RS: Assessment of patients with spastic cerebral palsy before and after rhizotomy, *Dev Med Child Neurol* 29(suppl 55):24, 1987 (abstract).

Cahan LD, Kundi MS, McPherson D, et al: Electrophysiologic studies in selective dorsal rhizotomy for spasticity in children with cerebral palsy, *Appl Neurophysiol* 50:459, 1987.

Cahan LD et al: Clinical, electrophysiologic and kinesiologic studies of selective dorsal rhizotomy, *J Pediatr Orthop* 9:487, 1989 (abstract).

Chicoine MR, Park TS, Kaufman BA: Selective dorsal rhizotomy and rates of orthopedic surgery in children with spastic cerebral palsy, *J Neurosurg* 86:34, 1997.

Chicoine MR, Park TS, Vogler GP, Kaufman BA: Predictors of ability to walk after selective dorsal rhizotomy in children with cerebral palsy, *Neurosurgery* 38:711, 1996.

Fasano VA, Broggi G, Zeme S: Intraoperative electrical stimulation for functional posterior rhizotomy, *Scand J Rehab Med Suppl* 17: 149, 1988.

Gerszten PC, Albright AL, Barry MJ: Effect on ambulation of continuous intrathecal baclofen infusion, *Pediatr Neurosurg* 27:40, 1997.

Gerszten PC, Albright AL, Johnstone GF: Intrathecal baclofen infusion and subsequent orthopedic surgery in patients with spastic cerebral palsy, *J Neurosurg* 88:1009, 1998.

Koman LA, Mooney JF, Smith BP, et al: Botulinum toxin type A neuromuscular blockade in the treatment of lower extremity spasticity in cerebral palsy: a randomized, double-blind, placebo-controlled trial, *J Pediatr Orthop* 20:108, 2000.

Kundi M, Cahan L, Starr A: Somatosensory evoked potentials in cerebral palsy after partial dorsal root rhizotomy, *Arch Neurol* 46:524, 1989.

Marty GR, Dias LS, Gaebler-Spira D: Selective posterior rhizotomy and soft-tissue procedures for the treatment of cerebral diplegia, *J Bone Joint Surg* 77A:713, 1995.

Mooney KLA, Leon WF: Botulinum toxin type A improved ankle function in children with cerebral palsy and dynamic equinus foot deformity, *J Pediatr Orthop* 20:108, 2000.

Neville BGR: Selective dorsal rhizotomy for spastic cerebral palsy, *Dev Med Child Neurol* 30:391, 1988.

Oppenheim WL: Selective posterior rhizotomy for spastic cerebral palsy: a review, *Clin Orthop* 253:20, 1990.

Oppenheim WL, Peacock WJ, Staudt LA, Gage JR: Selective posterior rhizotomy for cerebral palsy: issues and answers, Symposium held in San Francisco, Oct 1989.

Peacock WJ, Arens LJ: Selective posterior rhizotomy for the relief of spasticity in cerebral palsy, *S Afr Med J* 62:119, 1982.

Peacock WJ, Arens LJ, Berman B: Cerebral palsy spasticity: selective posterior rhizotomy, *Pediatr Neurosci* 13:61, 1987.

Peacock WJ, Staudt LA: Central and peripheral neurosurgical management of cerebral palsy, *Semin Orthop* 4:229, 1989.

Staudt LA, Peacock WJ: Selective posterior rhizotomy for treatment of spastic cerebral palsy, *Pediatr Phys Ther* 1:3, 1989.

Subramanian N, Vaughan CL, Peter JC, Arens LJ: Gait before and 10 years after rhizotomy in children with cerebral palsy spasticity, *J Neurosurg* 88:1014, 1998.

Vaughan CL, Berman B, Du Toit LL, Peacock WJ: Gait analysis of spastic children before and after selective posterior lumbar rhizotomy, *Dev Med Child Neurol* 29(suppl 55):25, 1987 (abstract).

Wright FV, Sheil EMH, Drake JH, et al: Evaluation of selective dorsal rhizotomy for the reduction of spasticity in cerebral palsy: a randomized controlled trial, *Dev Med Child Neurol* 40:239, 1998.

FOOT AND ANKLE

Adler N, Bleck EE, Rinsky LA: Gait electromyograms and surgical decisions for paralytic deformities of the foot, *Dev Med Child Neurol* 31:287, 1989.

Baker LD: A rational approach to the surgical needs of the cerebral palsy patient, *J Bone Joint Surg* 38A:313, 1956.

Baker LD: Triceps surae syndrome in cerebral palsy, *Arch Surg* 68:216, 1954.

Baker LD, Hill LM: Foot alignment in the cerebral palsy patient, *J Bone Joint Surg* 46A:1, 1964.

Banks HH: Equinus and cerebral palsy: its management, *Foot Ankle* 4:149, 1983.

Banks HH, Green WT: The correction of equinus deformity in cerebral palsy, *J Bone Joint Surg* 40A:1359, 1958.

Barnes MJ, Herring JA: Combined split anterior tibial-tendon transfer and intramuscular lengthening of the posterior tibial tendon. Results in patients who have a varus deformity of the foot due to spastic cerebral palsy, *J Bone Joint Surg* 73A:734, 1991.

Barrasso JA, Wile PB, Gage JR: Extraarticular subtalar arthrodesis with internal fixation, *J Pediatr Orthop* 4:555, 1984.

Bassett FH III, Baker LD: Equinus deformity in cerebral palsy. In Adams JP, ed: *Current practice in orthopaedic surgery,* vol 3, St Louis, 1966, Mosby.

Baumann JU, Zumstein M: Experience with a plastic ankle-foot orthosis for prevention of muscle contracture. Paper presented at the annual meeting of the American Academy for Cerebral Palsy and Developmental Medicine, Washington, DC, Oct 1984.

Bennett GC, Rang M, Jones D: Varus and valgus deformities of the foot in cerebral palsy, *Dev Med Child Neurol* 24:499, 1982.

Bisla RS, Louis HJ, Albano P: Transfer of tibialis posterior tendon in cerebral palsy, *J Bone Joint Surg* 58A:497, 1976.

Bleck EE: Forefoot problems in cerebral palsy: diagnosis and management, *Foot Ankle* 4:188, 1984.

Bleck EE, Rinsky LA: Decision making in surgical treatment of paralytic deformities of the foot with gait electromyograms, *Orthop Trans* 9:90, 1985.

Bleck EE: Spastic abductor hallucis, *Dev Med Child Neurol* 9:602, 1967.

Boss JA, Gugenheim JJ, Tullos HS: Dennyson-Fulford subtalar arthrodesis in fifty feet, *Orthop Trans* 8:63, 1984 (abstract).

Bowser BL, Dimitrijevic MM, Erdmann M, Solis IS: Effects of neuromuscular stimulation on passive ankle dorsiflexion in children with cerebral palsy: preliminary report, *Orthop Trans* 9:98, 1985.

Brouwer B, Davidson LK, Olney SJ: Serial casting in idiopathic toe-walkers and children with spastic cerebral palsy, *J Pediatr Orthop* 20:221, 2000.

Calandriello B: The detachment of gastrocnemius muscles in the treatment of spastic equinus foot, *Bull Hosp Jt Dis* 20:48, 1959.

Camacho FJ, Isunza A, Coutino B: Comparison of tendo-Achilles lengthening alone and combined with neuroectomy of the gastrocnemius muscle in the treatment of equinus deformity of the foot associated with clonus in children with cerebral palsy, *Orthopedics* 19:319, 1996.

Carpenter EB: Role of nerve blocks in the foot and ankle in cerebral palsy: therapeutic and diagnostic, *Foot Ankle* 4:164, 1983.

Cottalorda J, Gautheron V, Metton G, et al: Toe-walking in children younger than six years with cerebral palsy, *J Bone Joint Surg* 82B:541, 2000.

Craig JJ, van Vuren J: The importance of gastrocnemius recession in the correction of equinus deformity in cerebral palsy, *J Bone Joint Surg* 58B:84, 1976.

Dennyson WG, Fulford GE: Subtalar arthrodesis by cancellous grafts and metallic internal fixation, *J Bone Joint Surg* 58B:507, 1976.

Dias LS, Busch M, Tachdjian MO: Surgical treatment of severe hindfoot valgus by medial displacement osteotomy of the os calcis, *Orthop Trans* 11:35, 1987 (abstract).

Doute DA, Sponseller PD, Tolo VT, et al: Soleus neurectomy for dynamic ankle equinus in children with cerebral palsy, *Am J Orthop* 9:613, 1997.

Duncan WR, Mott DH: Foot reflexes and the use of the "inhibitive cast," *Foot Ankle* 4:45, 1983.

Eilert RE: Cavus foot in cerebral palsy, *Foot Ankle* 4:185, 1984.

Engstrom A, Erikson V, Hjelmstedt A: The results of extra-articular subtalar arthrodesis according to the Green-Grice method in cerebral palsy, *Acta Orthop Scand* 45:945, 1974.

Ford TB, Gaines RW: A systematic approach to the amount of Achilles tendon lengthening in cerebral palsy, *Dev Med Child Neurol* 28(suppl 53):7, 1986 (abstract).

Fulford GE: Surgical management of ankle and foot deformities in cerebral palsy, *Clin Orthop* 253:55, 1990.

Gaines RW, Ford TD: A systematic approach to the amount of Achilles tendon lengthening in cerebral palsy, *J Pediatr Orthop* 4:448, 1984.

Garbarino JL, Clancy M: A geometric method of calculating tendo Achilles lengthening, *J Pediatr Orthop* 5:573, 1985.

Graham HK, Fixsen JA: Lengthening of the calcaneal tendon in spastic hemiplegia by the White slide technique: a long-term review, *J Bone Joint Surg* 70B:472, 1988.

Green NE, Griffin PP, Shiavi R: Split posterior tibial-tendon transfer in cerebral palsy, *J Bone Joint Surg* 65A:748, 1983.

Green WT, Grice DS: The surgical correction of the paralytic foot. In American Academy of Orthopaedic Surgeons: *Instructional course lectures,* vol 9, Ann Arbor, Mich, 1952, JW Edwards.

Green WT, McDermott LJ: Operative treatment of cerebral palsy of the spastic type, *JAMA* 118:434, 1942.

Greene WB: Achilles tendon lengthening in cerebral palsy: comparison of inpatient versus ambulatory surgery, *J Pediatr Orthop* 7:256, 1987.

Grice DS: An extra-articular arthrodesis of the subastragalar joint for correction of paralytic flat feet in children, *J Bone Joint Surg* 34A:927, 1952.

Grice DS: Further experience with extra-articular arthrodesis of the subtalar joint, *J Bone Joint Surg* 36A:246, 1955.

Grice DS: The role of subtalar fusion in the treatment of valgus deformities of the feet, *Instr Course Lect* 16:127, 1959.

Gritzka TL, Staheli LT, Duncan WR: Posterior tibial tendon transfer through the interosseous membrane to correct equinovarus deformity in cerebral palsy: an initial experience, *Clin Orthop* 89:201, 1972.

Gross RH: A clinical study of the Batchelor subtalar arthrodesis, *J Bone Joint Surg* 58A:343, 1976.

Guttman G: Modification of the Grice-Green subtalar arthrodesis in children, *J Pediatr Orthop* 1:219, 1981.

Hauser ED: *Diseases of the foot,* Philadelphia, 1939, WB Saunders.

Hicks R, Durinick N, Gage JR: Differentiation of idiopathic toe-walking and cerebral palsy, *J Pediatr Orthop* 8:160, 1988.

Hiroshima K, Hamada S, Shimizu N, et al: Anterior transfer of the long toe flexors for the treatment of spastic equinovarus and equinus foot in cerebral palsy, *J Pediatr Orthop* 8:164, 1988.

Hoffer MM, Perry J: Pathodynamics of gait alterations in cerebral palsy and the significance of kinetic electromyography in evaluating foot and ankle problems, *Foot Ankle* 4:128, 1983.

Hoffer MM, Reiswig JA, Garrett AM, Perry J: The split anterior tibial tendon transfer in the treatment of spastic varus hindfoot of childhood, *Orthop Clin North Am* 5:31, 1974.

Hui JHP, Goh JCH, Lee EH: Biomechanical study of tibialis anterior tendon transfer, *Clin Orthop* 349:249, 1998.

Jahss MH: *Disorders of the foot,* Philadelphia, 1982, WB Saunders.

Jahss MH: Evaluation of the cavus foot for orthopedic treatment, *Clin Orthop* 181:52, 1983.

Javors JR, Klaaren HE: The Vulpius procedure for correction of equinus deformity in cerebral palsy, *J Pediatr Orthop* 7:191, 1987.

Jeray KJ, Rentz J, Ferguson RL: Local bone-graft technique for subtalar extraarticular arthrodesis in cerebral palsy, *J Pediatr Orthop* 18:75, 1998.

Kasser JR, MacEwen GD: Examination of the cerebral palsy patient with foot and ankle problems, *Foot Ankle* 4:135, 1983.

Kagaya H, Yamada S, Nagasawa T, et al: Split posterior tibial tendon transfer for varus deformity of the hindfoot, *Clin Orthop* 323:254, 1996.

Kaufer H: Split tendon transfers, *Orthop Trans* 1:191, 1977.

Keats S, Kouten J: Early surgical correction of the planovalgus foot in cerebral palsy: extra-articular arthrodesis of the subtalar joint, *Clin Orthop* 61:223, 1968.

Kennan MA, Creighton J, Garland DE, Moore TA: Surgical correction of spastic equinovarus deformity in the adult, *Orthop Trans* 8:195, 1984 (abstract).

King HA, Staheli LT: Torsional problems in cerebral palsy, *Foot Ankle* 4:180, 1984.

Kling TF Jr, Hensinger RN: The results of split posterior tibial tendon transfer in children with cerebral palsy, *Orthop Trans* 8:102, 1984 (abstract).

Kling TF Jr, Kaufer H, Hensinger RN: Split posterior tibial-tendon transfer in children with cerebral spastic paralysis and equinovarus deformity, *J Bone Joint Surg* 67A:186, 1985.

Koman LA, Mooney JF III, Goodman A, Nicastro JF: Management of valgus hindfoot deformity by medial displacement osteotomy. Paper presented at the annual meeting of the Pediatric Orthopaedic Society of North America, San Francisco, May 1990.

Majestro TC, Ruda R, Frost HM: Intramuscular lengthening of the posterior tibialis muscle, *Clin Orthop* 79:59, 1971.

Mann DC, Hoffer MM: Flat foot in spastic cerebral palsy, *Semin Orthop* 4:277, 1989.

McKeever DC: Arthrodesis of the first metatarsophalangeal joint for hallux valgus, hallux rigidus, and metatarsus primus varus, *J Bone Joint Surg* 34A:129, 1952.

Menelaus MB, Ross ERS: The management of curly and hammer toes by flexor tenotomy. Paper presented at the annual meeting of the Pediatric Orthopaedic Society, Vancouver, 1984.

Miller GM, Hsu JD, Hoffer MM, Rentfro R: Posterior tibial tendon transfer: a review of the literature and analysis of 74 procedures, *J Pediatr Orthop* 2:363, 1982.

Moreau MJ, Lake DM: Outpatient percutaneous heel cord lengthening in children, *J Pediatr Orthop* 7:253, 1987.

Mosca VS: Calcaneal lengthening for valgus deformity of the hindfoot, *J Bone Joint Surg* 77A:500, 1995.

Muburak SJ, Katz MM: Hereditary tendo-Achilles contractures. Paper presented at the annual meeting of the Pediatric Orthopaedic Society, Vancouver, 1984.

Ono K, Hiroshima K, Tada K, Inoue A: Anterior transfer of the toe flexors for equinovarus deformity of the foot, *Int Orthop* 4:255, 1980.

O'Reilly DE, Carter EE: Surgical treatment of equinus in cerebral palsy. Paper presented at the annual meeting of the American Academy for Cerebral Palsy and Developmental Medicine, Washington, DC, Oct 1984.

Perry J, Hoffer MM, Giovani P, et al: Gait analysis of the triceps surae in cerebral palsy: a preoperative and postoperative clinical and electromyographic study, *J Bone Joint Surg* 56A:511, 1974.

Pierrot AH, Murphy OB: Albert E. Klinkicht Award, 1972. Heel cord advancement. A new approach to the spastic equinus deformity, *Orthop Clin North Am* 5:117, 1974.

Phillips JE, Hooper G: A simple technique for arthrodesis of the first metatarsophalangeal joint, *J Bone Joint Surg* 68B:774, 1986.

Reimers J: Functional changes in the antagonists after lengthening the agonists in cerebral palsy. I. Triceps surae lengthening, *Clin Orthop* 253:30, 1990.

Root L: Varus and valgus foot in cerebral palsy and its management, *Foot Ankle* 4:174, 1984.

Root L, Miller SR, Kirz P: Posterior tibial-tendon transfer in patients with cerebral palsy, *J Bone Joint Surg* 69A:1133, 1987.

Rose SA, DeLuca PA, Davis RB III, et al: Kinematic and kinetic evaluation of the ankle after lengthening of the gastrocnemius fascia in children with cerebral palsy, *J Pediatr Orthop* 13:727, 1993.

Rosenthal RK: The use of orthotics in foot and ankle problems in cerebral palsy, *Foot Ankle* 4:195, 1984.

Sala DA, Grant AD, Kummer FJ: Equinus deformity in cerebral palsy: recurrence after tendo Achilles lengthening, *Dev Med Child Neurol* 39:45, 1997.

Samilson RL: Crescentic osteotomy of the os calcis for calcaneocavus feet. In Bateman JE, ed: *Foot science,* Philadelphia, 1976, WB Saunders.

Saraph V, Zwick EB, Uitz C, et al: The Baumann procedure for fixed contracture of the gastrosoleus in cerebral palsy, *J Bone Joint Surg* 82B:535, 2000.

Scott SM, Janes PC, Stevens PM: Grice subtalar arthrodesis followed to skeletal maturity, *J Pediatr Orthop* 8:176, 1988.

Segal LS, Mazur JM, Sienko SE, Mauterer M: Calcaneal gait in spastic diplegia after heel-cord lengthening: a preliminary study with gait analysis, *Dev Med Child Neurol* 29(suppl 55):5, 1987 (abstract).

Sharrard WJW, Bernstein S: Equinus deformity in cerebral palsy: a comparison between elongation of the tendo calcaneus and gastrocnemius recession, *J Bone Joint Surg* 54B:272, 1972.

Sharrard WJW, Smith TWD: Tenodesis of flexor hallucis longus for paralytic clawing of the hallux in childhood, *J Bone Joint Surg* 58B:224, 1976.

Silfverskiöld N: Reduction of the uncrossed two-joint muscles of the leg to one-joint muscles in spastic conditions, *Acta Chir Scand* 56:315, 1923-1924.

Silver CM, Simon SD: Gastrocnemius muscle recession (Silfverskiöld operation) for spastic equinus deformity in cerebral palsy, *J Bone Joint Surg* 41A:1021, 1959.

Silver CM, Simon SD, Litchman HM: Long term follow-up observations on calcaneal osteotomy, *Clin Orthop* 9:181, 1974.

Silver CM, Simon SD, Spindell E, et al: Calcaneal osteotomy for valgus and varus deformities of the foot in cerebral palsy: a preliminary report on twenty-seven operations, *J Bone Joint Surg* 49A:232, 1967.

Simon SR, Fernandez O, Rosenthal RK, Griffin P: The effect of heel cord lengthening and solid ankle foot orthosis on the gait of patients with cerebral palsy. Paper presented at the annual meeting of the American Academy for Cerebral Palsy and Developmental Medicine, Washington, DC, 1984.

Skinner SR, Lester DK: Dynamic EMG findings in valgus hindfoot deformity in spastic cerebral palsy, *Orthop Trans* 9:91, 1985 (abstract).

Stóffel A: The treatment of spastic contracture, *Am J Orthop Surg* 10:611, 1912-1913.

Strayer LM Jr: Gastrocnemius recession: five-year report of cases, *J Bone Joint Surg* 40A:1019, 1958.

Strayer LM Jr: Recession of the gastrocnemius: an operation to relieve spastic contracture of the calf muscles, *J Bone Joint Surg* 32A:671, 1950.

Strecker WB, Via MW, Oliver SK, Schoenecker PL: Heel cord advancement for treatment of equinus deformity in cerebral palsy, *J Pediatr Orthop* 10:105, 1990.

Sullivan JA, Schmidt FH, Gross RH: Comparison of percutaneous and open heel-cord techniques, *Dev Med Child Neurol* 29(suppl 55):4, 1987 (abstract).

Tohen ZA, Carmona PJ, Barrera JR: The utilization of abnormal reflexes in the treatment of spastic foot deformities: a preliminary report, *Clin Orthop* 47:77, 1966.

Tachdjian MO: *Pediatric orthopedics,* ed 2, Philadelphia, 1990, WB Saunders.

Tolo VT, Sponseller PD: Soleus neurectomy: an effective procedure in cerebral palsy, *Orthop Trans* 12:696, 1988 (abstract).

Townsend DR, Wells L, Lowenberg D: The Cincinnati incision for the split posterior tibial tendon transfer: a technical note, *J Pediatr Orthop* 10:667, 1990.

Trieshmann H, Millis M, Hall J, Watts H: Sliding calcaneal osteotomy for treatment of hindfoot deformity, *Orthop Trans* 4:305, 1980 (abstract).

Trumble T, Banta JV, Raycroft J, Curtis BH: Talectomy for equinovarus deformity in myelodysplasia. Paper presented at the annual meeting of the American Academy for Cerebral Palsy and Developmental Medicine, Washington, DC, Oct 1984.

Turner JW, Cooper RR: Anterior transfer of the tibialis posterior through the interosseous membrane, *Clin Orthop* 83:241, 1972.

Turner JW, Cooper RR: Posterior transposition of tibialis anterior through the interosseous membrane, *Clin Orthop* 79:71, 1971.

White JW: Torsion of the Achilles tendon: its surgical significance, *Arch Surg* 46:784, 1943.

Wilcox PG, Weiner DS: The Akron midtarsal dome osteotomy: preliminary review of a new surgical procedure for treatment of rigid pes cavus. Paper presented at the annual meeting of the American Academy for Cerebral Palsy and Developmental Medicine, Washington, DC, Oct 1984.

Williams PF, Menelaus MB: Triple arthrodesis by inlay grafting: a method suitable for the undeformed or valgus foot, *J Bone Joint Surg* 59B:333, 1977.

Williams PF: Restoration of muscle balance of the foot by transfer of the tibialis posterior, *J Bone Joint Surg* 58B:217, 1976.

Wills CA, Hoffer MM, Perry J: A comparison of foot-switch and EMG analysis of varus deformities of the feet of children with cerebral palsy, *Dev Med Child Neurol* 30:227, 1988.

Zimbler S, Craig C: Subtalar arthrodesis (Grice extra-articular type) for stabilization of the valgus foot in neuromuscular disease: long-term review, *Dev Med Child Neurol* 28(suppl 53):8, 1986 (abstract).

KNEE

Drummond DS, Rogala E, Templeton J, Cruess R: Proximal hamstring release for knee flexion and crouched posture in cerebral palsy, *J Bone Joint Surg* 56A:1598, 1974.

Eggers GWN: Surgical division of the patellar retinacula to improve extension of the knee joint in cerebral spastic paralysis, *J Bone Joint Surg* 32A:80, 1950.

Eggers GWN: Transplantation of hamstring tendons to femoral condyles in order to improve hip extension and to decrease knee flexion in cerebral spastic paralysis, *J Bone Joint Surg* 34A:827, 1952.

Evans EB: Cerebral palsy. III. Knee flexion deformity in cerebral palsy, *Instr Course Lect* 20:42, 1971.

Evans EB, Julian JD: Modifications of the hamstring transfer, *Dev Med Child Neurol* 8:539, 1966.

Evans EB: The status of surgery of the lower extremities in cerebral palsy, *Clin Orthop* 47:127, 1966.

Gage JR: Surgical treatment of knee dysfunction in cerebral palsy, *Clin Orthop* 253:45, 1990.

Gage JR: Deformities of the knee and foot. Paper presented at American Academy for Cerebral Palsy and Developmental Medicine Symposium, Growing up with Cerebral Palsy, Wilmington, Del, April 1985.

Gage JR, Perry J, Hicks R, et al: Rectus femoris transfer as a means of improving knee flexion in cerebral palsy, *Dev Med Child Neurol* 28(suppl 53):5, 1986 (abstract).

Grant AD, Small RD, Lehman WB: Correction of flexion deformity of the knee by supracondylar osteotomy, *Bull Hosp Jt Dis* 42:28, 1982.

Grogan DP, Lundy MS, Ogden JA: A method for early postoperative mobilization of the cerebral palsy patient using a removable abduction bar, *J Pediatr Orthop* 7:338, 1987.

Keenan MAE, Ure K, Smith CW, Jordan C: Hamstring release for knee flexion contracture in spastic adults, *Clin Orthop* 236:221, 1988.

Lloyd-Roberts GC, Jackson AM, Albert JS: Avulsion of the distal pole of the patella in cerebral palsy: a cause of deteriorating gait, *J Bone Joint Surg* 67B:252, 1985.

Mann RL, Root L: Long-term follow-up of distal hamstring releases in cerebral palsy, *Dev Med Child Neurol* 28(suppl 53):6, 1986 (abstract).

McCarroll HR: Surgical treatment of spastic paralysis, *Instr Course Lect* 6:134, 1949.

Olney BW, Williams PF, Menelaus MB: Treatment of spastic equinus by aponeurosis lengthening, *J Pediatr Orthop* 8:422, 1988.

Ounpuu S, Muik E, Davis RB III, et al: Rectus femoris surgery in children with cerebral palsy. I. The effect of rectus femoris transfer location on knee motion, *J Pediatr Orthop* 13:325, 1993.

Ounpuu S, Muik E, Davis RB III, et al: Rectus femoris surgery in children with cerebral palsy. II. A comparison between the effect of transfer and release of the distal rectus femoris on knee motion, *J Pediatr Orthop* 13:331, 1993.

Patrick JH: Techniques of psoas tenotomy and rectus femoris transfer: "new" operations for cerebral palsy diplegia—a description, *J Pediatr Orthop* 5B:242, 1996.

Perry J: Distal rectus femoris transfer, *Dev Med Child Neurol* 29:153, 1987.

Perry J, Hoffer MM, Antonelli D, et al: Electromyography before and after surgery for hip deformity in children with cerebral palsy, *J Bone Joint Surg* 58A:201, 1976.

Reimers J: Contracture of the hamstrings in spastic cerebral palsy: a study of three methods of operative correction, *J Bone Joint Surg* 56B:102, 1974.

Rethlefsen S, Tolo VT, Reynolds RA, Kay R: Outcome of hamstring lengthening and distal rectus femoris transfer surgery, *J Pediatr Orthop* 8B:75, 1999.

Root L, Angel D, Weiner L: Distal release or transfer of the rectus femoris muscle in cerebral palsy patients, *Orthop Trans* 12:561, 1988 (abstract).

Simon SR, Deutsch SD, Nuzzo RM, et al: Genu recurvatum in spastic cerebral palsy. Report on findings by gait analysis, *J Bone Joint Surg* 60:882, 1978.

Sullivan RC, Gehringer KM, Harris GF: A computer-assisted survey of results of medial hamstring surgery in children with cerebral palsy. Paper presented at the annual meeting of the American Academy for Cerebral Palsy and Developmental Medicine, Chicago, 1983.

Sutherland DH, Larsen LJ, Mann R: Rectus femoris release in selected patients with cerebral palsy: a preliminary report, *Dev Med Child Neurol* 17:26, 1975.

Sutherland DH, Santi M, Abel MF: Treatment of stiff-knee gait in cerebral palsy: a comparison by gait analysis of distal rectus femoris transfer versus proximal rectus release, *J Pediatr Orthop* 104:433, 1990.

Sutherland DH, Schottstaedt ER, Larsen LJ, et al: Clinical and electromyographic study of seven spastic children with internal rotation gait, *J Bone Joint Surg* 51A:1070, 1969.

Thometz J, Simon S, Rosenthal R: The effect on gait of lengthening of the medial hamstring in cerebral palsy, *J Bone Joint Surg* 71A: 345, 1989.

HIP

Abel MF, Blanco JS, Pavlovich L, Damiano DL: Asymmetric hip deformity and subluxation in cerebral palsy: an analysis of surgical treatment, *J Pediatr Orthop* 19:479, 1999.

Baciu CC: Translocation du muscle petit fessier dans la hanche spastique: a propos de onze cas, *Ann Chir* 38:435, 1984.

Baker LD, Dodelin R, Bassett FH III: Pathological changes in the hip in cerebral palsy: incidence, pathogenesis, and treatment—a preliminary report, *J Bone Joint Surg* 44A:1331, 1962.

Banks HH, Green WT: Adductor myotomy and obturator neurectomy for the correction of adduction contracture of the hip in cerebral palsy, *J Bone Joint Surg* 42A:111, 1960.

Baxter MP, D'Astous JL: Proximal femoral resection-interposition arthroplasty: salvage hip surgery for the severely disabled child with cerebral palsy, *J Pediatr Orthop* 6:681, 1986.

Beals RK: Developmental changes in the femur and acetabulum in spastic paraplegia and diplegia, *Dev Med Child Neurol* 11:303, 1969.

Beals TC, Thompson NE, Beals RK: Modified adductor muscle transfer in cerebral palsy, *J Pediatr Orthop* 18:522, 1998.

Black BE, Griffin PP: The cerebral palsied hip, *Clin Orthop* 338:42, 1997.

Bleck EE: Management of hip deformities in cerebral palsy. In Adams JP, ed: *Current practice in orthopaedic surgery,* vol 3, St Louis, 1966, Mosby.

Bleck EE: Cerebral palsy. IV. Hip deformities in cerebral palsy, *Instr Course Lect* 20:54, 1971.

Bleck EE: Postural and gait abnormalities caused by hip-flexion deformity in spastic cerebral palsy: treatment by iliopsoas recession, *J Bone Joint Surg* 53A:1468, 1971.

Bleck EE: The hip in cerebral palsy, *Orthop Clin North Am* 11:79, 1980.

Bos CFA, Rozing PM, Verbout AJ: Surgery for hip dislocation in cerebral palsy, *Acta Orthop Scand* 58:638, 1987.

Breed AL: The wind-swept hip in cerebral palsy, *Dev Med Child Neurol* 28(suppl 53):32, 1986 (abstract).

Breed AL, Kling TF Jr: Acetabular development in the spastic child with spastic quadriplegic cerebral palsy, *Dev Med Child Neurol* 28(suppl 53):30, 1986 (abstract).

Brunner R, Baumann JU: Long-term effects of intertrochanteric varus-derotation osteotomy on femur and acetabulum in spastic cerebral palsy: an 11- to 18-year follow-up study, *J Pediatr Orthop* 17:585, 1997.

Brunner R, Picard C, Robb J: Morphology of the acetabulum in hip dislocations caused by cerebral palsy, *J Pediatr Orthop* 6:207, 1997.

Brunner R, Robb JE: Inaccuracy of the migration percentage and center-edge angle in predicting femoral head displacement in cerebral palsy, *J Pediatr Orthop* 5:239, 1996.

Bunnell WP, Goncalves J: Varus derotational osteotomy of the hip in cerebral palsy. Paper presented at the annual meeting of the American Academy for Cerebral Palsy and Developmental Medicine, Washington, DC, Oct 1984.

Bunnell WP, Goncalves J: Varus derotational osteotomy of the hip in cerebral palsy, *J Pediatr Orthop* 5:375, 1985 (abstract).

Castle ME, Schneider C: Proximal femoral resection-interposition arthroplasty, *J Bone Joint Surg* 60A:1051, 1978.

Chiari K: Medial displacement osteotomy of the pelvis, *Clin Orthop* 98:55, 1974.

Cooke PH, Cole WG, Carey RPL: Dislocation of the hip in cerebral palsy: natural history and predictability, *J Bone Joint Surg* 71B:441, 1989.

Cornell MS, Hatrick C, Boyd R, Baird G, Spencer JD: The hip in children with cerebral palsy, *Clin Orthop* 340:165, 1997.

Cote PS, Drennan JC: The role of proximal femoral derotational osteotomy in pediatric acetabular dysplasia. Paper presented at the annual meeting of the American Academy of Orthopaedic Surgeons, Las Vegas, 1985.

Couch WH Jr, De Rosa GP, Throop FB: Thigh adductor transfer for spastic cerebral palsy, *Dev Med Child Neurol* 19:343, 1977.

Craig CL, Sosnoff F, Murray S, Zimbler S: Fixed-hip abduction contracture in the patient with cerebral palsy: a treatable and preventable deformity, *Dev Med Child Neurol* 28(suppl 53):33, 1986 (abstract).

Cristofaro RL, Blanco JS, Nelson JM: Hip reconstruction vs proximal femoral resection interposition arthroplasty in the treatment of spastic hip dislocation: a comparative study, *Orthop Trans* 12:578, 1988 (abstract).

Cristofaro RL, Taddonio RF, Gelb R: The effect of correction of spinal deformity and pelvic obliquity on hip stability in neuromuscular disease. Paper presented at the annual meeting of the American Academy for Cerebral Palsy and Developmental Medicine, Washington, DC, 1984.

DeLuca PA, Bueff HU: The fate of pelvic osteotomies in cerebral palsy, *Dev Med Child Neurol* 31(suppl 59):25, 1989 (abstract).

Dietz FR, Knutson LM: Chiari pelvic osteotomy in cerebral palsy, *J Pediatr Orthop* 15:372, 1995.

Drummond DS, Rogala EJ, Cruess R, Moreau M: The paralytic hip and pelvic obliquity in cerebral palsy and myelomeningocele, *Instr Course Lect* 28:7, 1979.

Evans EB, Julian JD: Modifications of the hamstring transfer, *Dev Med Child Neurol* 8:539, 1966.

Fulford GE, Brown JK: Position as a cause of deformity in children with cerebral palsy, *Dev Med Child Neurol* 18:305, 1976.

Gabos PG, Miller F, Galban MA, et al: Prosthetic interposition arthroplasty for the palliative treatment of end-stage spastic hip disease in nonambulatory patients with cerebral palsy, *J Pediatr Orthop* 19:796, 1999.

Gage JR: Gait analysis for decision making in cerebral palsy, *Bull Hosp Jt Dis* 43:147, 1983.

Gage JR, Perry J, Hicks RR, et al: Rectus femoris transfer to improve knee function of children with cerebral palsy, *Dev Med Child Neurol* 29:159, 1987.

Gamble JG, Rinsky LA, Bleck EE: Established hip dislocations in children with cerebral palsy, *Clin Orthop* 253:90, 1990.

Goldner JL: Hip adductor transfer compared with adductor tenotomy in cerebral palsy, *J Bone Joint Surg* 63A:1498, 1981 (letter).

Grant AD, Stongwater AM, Nelson J, Lehman WB: The femoral neck-metaphyseal angle, *Dev Med Child Neurol* 28(suppl 53):31, 1986.

Griffin PP, Wheelhouse WW, Shiavi R: Adductor transfer for adductor spasticity: clinical and electromyographic gait analysis, *Dev Med Child Neurol* 19:783, 1977.

Gross MS, Ibrahim K, Wehner J, Dvonch V: Combined surgical procedure for treatment of hip dislocation in cerebral palsy. Paper presented at the annual meeting of the American Academy for Cerebral Palsy and Developmental Medicine, Chicago, 1983.

Gross MS, Ibrahim K, Wehner J, Dvonch V: Combined surgical procedure for treatment of hip dislocation in cerebral palsy, *Orthop Trans* 8:113, 1984 (abstract).

Gurd AR: Surgical correction of myodesis of the hip in cerebral palsy. Paper presented at the annual meeting of the American Academy for Cerebral Palsy and Developmental Medicine, Chicago, 1983.

Gurd AR: Surgical correction of myodesis of the hip in cerebral palsy, *Orthop Trans* 8:112, 1984 (abstract).

Handelsman JE: The Chiari pelvic sliding osteotomy, *Orthop Clin North Am* 11:105, 1980.

Hiroshima K, Ono K: Correlation between muscle shortening and derangement of the hip joint in children with spastic cerebral palsy, *Clin Orthop* 144:186, 1979.

Hoffer MM, Prietto C, Koffman M: Supracondylar derotational osteotomy of the femur for internal rotation of the thigh in the cerebral palsied child, *J Bone Joint Surg* 63A:389, 1981.

Horstmann HM, Rosabal OG: Varus derotation osteotomy, *Orthop Trans* 8:113, 1984 (abstract).

Horstmann HM, Rosabal OG: Varus derotation osteotomy. Paper presented at the annual meeting of the American Academy for Cerebral Palsy and Developmental Medicine, Chicago, 1983.

Houkom JA, Roach JW, Wenger DR, et al: Treatment of acquired hip subluxation in cerebral palsy, *J Pediatr Orthop* 6:285, 1986.

Howard CB, McKibbin B, Williams LA, Mackie I: Factors affecting the incidence of hip dislocation in cerebral palsy, *J Bone Joint Surg* 67B:530, 1985.

Huang S, Eilert RE: Important radiographic signs for decision making in surgery of the hip in cerebral palsy. Paper presented at the annual meeting of the American Academy for Cerebral Palsy and Developmental Medicine, Washington, DC, Oct 1984.

Kaga CS, Huurman WW: Supracondylar derotation osteotomy of the femur for femoral anteversion, *Orthop Trans* 8:82, 1984 (abstract).

Kalen V, Bleck EE: Prevention of spastic paralytic subluxation and dislocation of the hip, *Orthop Trans* 8:112, 1984 (abstract).

Kalen V, Gamble JG: Resection arthroplasty of the hip in paralytic dislocations, *Orthop Trans* 8:113, 1984 (abstract).

Kalen V, Gamble JG: Resection arthroplasty of the hip in paralytic disorders, *Dev Med Child Neurol* 26:341, 1984.

Keats S: Combined adductor-gracilis tenotomy and selective obturator-nerve resection for the correction of adduction deformity of the hip in children with cerebral palsy, *J Bone Joint Surg* 39A:1087, 1957.

Kling TF Jr: Adductor release with and without obturator neurectomy in children with cerebral palsy, *Orthop Trans* 8:112, 1984 (abstract).

Kling TF Jr: Adductor release with and without obturator neurectomy in children with cerebral palsy. Paper presented at the annual meeting of the American Academy for Cerebral Palsy and Developmental Medicine, Chicago, 1983.

Koffman M: Proximal femoral resection or total hip replacement in severely disabled cerebral-spastic patients, *Orthop Clin North Am* 12:91, 1981.

Letts M, Shapiro L, Mulder K, Klassen O: The windblown hip syndrome in total body cerebral palsy, *J Pediatr Orthop* 4:55, 1984.

Lonstein JE, Beck K: Hip dislocation and subluxation in cerebral palsy. Paper presented at the annual meeting of the American Academy for Cerebral Palsy and Developmental Medicine, Chicago, 1983.

Lonstein JB, Beck K: Hip dislocation and subluxation in cerebral palsy. Paper presented at the annual meeting of the Pediatric Orthopaedic Society, Vancouver, 1984.

Lonstein JE, Beck K: Hip dislocation and subluxation in cerebral palsy. Paper presented at the annual meeting of the American Academy for Cerebral Palsy and Developmental Medicine, Washington, DC, Oct 1984.

Lonstein JE, Beck K: Hip dislocation and subluxation in cerebral palsy, *J Pediatr Orthop* 6:521, 1986.

Lundy DW, Ganey TM, Ogden JA, Guidera K: Pathologic morphology of the dislocated proximal femur in children with cerebral palsy, *J Pediatr Orthop* 18:528, 1998.

Lynne ED, Katcherian DA: Slotted acetabular augmentation in patients with neuromuscular disorders, *J Pediatr Orthop* 8:278, 1988.

Matsuo T, Hara H, Tada S: Selective lengthening of the psoas and rectus femoris and preservation of the iliacus for flexion deformity of the hip in cerebral palsy patients, *J Pediatr Orthop* 7:690, 1987.

Matsuo T, Tada S, Hajime T: Insufficiency of the hip adductor after anterior obturator neurectomy in 42 children with cerebral palsy, *J Pediatr Orthop* 6:686, 1986.

McCarthy RE, Simon S, Douglas B, et al: Proximal femoral resection to allow adults who have severe cerebral palsy to sit, *J Bone Joint Surg* 70A:1011, 1988.

McNerney NP, Mubarak SJ, Wenger DR: One-stage correction of the dysplastic hip in cerebral palsy with the San Diego acetabuloplasty: results and complications in 104 hips, *J Pediatr Orthop* 20:93, 2000.

Miller F, Dias RC, Dabney K, et al: Soft-tissue release for spastic hip subluxation in cerebral palsy, *J Pediatr Orthop* 17:571, 1997.

Moreau M, Cook PC, Ashton B: Adductor and psoas release for subluxation of the hip in children with spastic cerebral palsy, *J Pediatr Orthop* 15:672, 1995.

Moreau M, Drummond DS, Rogala E, et al: Natural history of the dislocated hip in spastic cerebral palsy, *Dev Med Child Neurol* 21:749, 1979.

Mubarak SJ, Mortensen W, Katz M: Combined pelvic (Dega) and femoral osteotomies in the treatment of paralytic hip dislocation, *J Pediatr Orthop* 7:493, 1987 (abstract).

Nickel VL, Perry J, Garrett A, Feiwell EN: Paralytic dislocation of the hip, *J Bone Joint Surg* 48A:1021, 1966.

Osterkamp J, Caillouette JT, Hoffer MM: Chiari osteotomy in cerebral palsy, *J Pediatr Orthop* 8:274, 1988.

Pemberton PA: Pericapsular osteotomy of the ilium in the treatment of congenital dislocation and subluxation of the hip, *J Bone Joint Surg* 47A:65, 1965.

Perry J: Distal rectus femoris transfer, *Dev Med Child Neurol* 29:153, 1987.

Perry J, Hoffer MM: Preoperative and postoperative dynamic electromyography as an aid in planning tendon transfers in children with cerebral palsy, *J Bone Joint Surg* 59A:531, 1977.

Perry J: Kinesiology of lower-extremity bracing, *Clin Orthop* 102:18, 1974.

Phelps WM: Prevention of acquired dislocation of the hip in cerebral palsy, *J Bone Joint Surg* 41A:440, 1959.

Pillard D, Benoit S, Taussig G: Résection élargie de l'éxtremitié supérieure du fémur chez l'enfant infirme moteur d'origine cérébrale (extensive excision of the upper end of the femur in cerebral palsy), *Rev Chir Orthop* 70:623, 1984.

Prichett JW: Treated and untreated unstable hips in severe cerebral palsy, *Dev Med Child Neurol* 32:3, 1990.

Ray RL, Ehrlich MG: Lateral hamstring transfer and gait improvement in the cerebral palsy patient, *J Bone Joint Surg* 61A:719, 1979.

Reimers J: The stability of the hip in children: a radiologic study of the results of muscle surgery in cerebral palsy, *Acta Orthop Scand Suppl* 184:1, 1980.

Reimers J: The stability of the hip in children, *Acta Orthop Scand Suppl* 184, 1980.

Reimers J, Poulsen S: Adductor transfer versus tenotomy for stability of the hip in spastic cerebral palsy, *J Pediatr Orthop* 4:52, 1984.

Roach JW, Herring JA, Norris EN: Treatment of acquired hip dysplasia in cerebral palsy. Paper presented at the annual meeting of the Pediatric Orthopaedic Society, Vancouver, 1984.

Roosth HP: Flexion deformity of the hip and knee in spastic cerebral palsy: treatment by early release of spastic hip-flexor muscles: technique and results in thirty-seven cases, *J Bone Joint Surg* 53A: 1489, 1971.

Root L: The hip in cerebral palsy. Paper presented at American Academy for Cerebral Palsy and Developmental Medicine Symposium, Growing up with Cerebral Palsy, Wilmington, Del, April 1985.

Root L, Bourman SN: Combined pelvic osteotomy with open reduction and femoral shortening for dislocated hips. Paper presented at the annual meeting of the American Academy for Cerebral Palsy and Developmental Medicine, Washington, DC, Oct 1984.

Root L, Laplaza FJ, Brourman SN, Angel DH: The severely unstable hip in cerebral palsy: treatment with open reduction, pelvic osteotomy, and femoral osteotomy with shortening, *J Bone Joint Surg* 77A:703, 1995.

Root L, Siegal T: Osteotomy of the hip in children: posterior approach, *J Bone Joint Surg* 62A:571, 1980.

Root L, Spero CR: Hip adductor transfer compared with adductor tenotomy in cerebral palsy, *J Bone Joint Surg* 63A:767, 1981.

Root L, Washington R: Pathological changes in the femoral head in cerebral palsy. Paper presented at the annual meeting of the American Academy for Cerebral Palsy and Developmental Medicine, Chicago, 1983.

Root L, Washington R: Pathological changes in the femoral head in cerebral palsy, *Orthop Trans* 8:111, 1984 (abstract).

Rosenthal RK: Soft tissue procedures about the hip in spastic cerebral palsy. Paper presented at the annual meeting of the American Academy for Cerebral Palsy and Developmental Medicine, Chicago, 1983.

Sage FP: Cerebral palsy. In Crenshaw AH, ed: *Campbell's operative orthopaedics*, St Louis, 1987, Mosby.

Salter RB: Innominate osteotomy in the treatment of congenital dislocation and subluxation of the hip, *J Bone Joint Surg* 43B:518, 1961.

Samilson RL: Orthopedic surgery of the hips and spine in retarded cerebral palsy patients, *Orthop Clin North Am* 12:83, 1981.

Samilson RL, Carson JJ, James P, Raney FL Jr: Results and complications of adductor tenotomy and obturator neurectomy in cerebral palsy, *Clin Orthop* 54:61, 1967.

Samilson RL, Trace P, Aamoth G, Green WM: Dislocation and subluxation of the hip in cerebral palsy: pathogenesis, natural history, and management, *J Bone Joint Surg* 54A:863, 1972.

Scott AC, Chambers C, Cain T: Adductor transfers in cerebral palsy: long-term results studied by gait analysis, *J Pediatr Orthop* 16:741, 1996.

Scrutton D: The early management of hips in cerebral palsy, *Dev Med Child Neurol* 31:108, 1989.

Seger BM, Dickson JH: Chiari osteotomy in the treatment of hip dysplasia: indications and long-term follow-up, *Orthop Trans* 8:62, 1984 (abstract).

Selva G, Miller F, Dabney KW: Anterior hip dislocation in children with cerebral palsy, *J Pediatr Orthop* 18:54, 1998.

Shapiro D, Craig CL, Shapiro J, Zimbler S: Management of the unstable hip of patients with cerebral palsy, *Dev Med Child Neurol* 28(suppl 53):32, 1986 (abstract).

Sharps CH, Clancy M, Steel HH: A long-term retrospective study of proximal hamstring release for hamstring contracture in cerebral palsy, *J Pediatr Orthop* 4:443, 1984.

Sharrard WJW: The hip in cerebral palsy. In Samilson RL: *Orthopaedic aspects of cerebral palsy*, Philadelphia, 1975, JB Lippincott.

Sharrard WJW, Allen JMH, Heaney SH, Prendiville GRG: Surgical prophylaxis of subluxation and dislocation of the hip in cerebral palsy, *J Bone Joint Surg* 57B:160, 1975.

Shea KG, Coleman SS, Carroll K, Van Boerum DH: Pemberton pericapsular osteotomy to treat a dysplastic hip in cerebral palsy, *J Bone Joint Surg* 79A:1342, 1997.

Silfverskiöld N: Reduction of the uncrossed two-joint muscles of the leg to one-joint muscles in spastic conditions, *Acta Chir Scand* 56:315, 1923-24.

Silver RL, Rang M, Chan J, de la Garza J: Adductor release in nonambulant children with cerebral palsy, *J Pediatr Orthop* 5:672, 1985.

Smith JT, Stevens PM: Combined adductor transfer, iliopsoas release, and proximal hamstring release in cerebral palsy, *J Pediatr Orthop* 9:1, 1989.

Song H-R, Carroll NC: Femoral varus derotation osteotomy with or without acetabuloplasty for unstable hips in cerebral palsy, *J Pediatr Orthop* 18:62, 1998.

Soutter R: A new operation for hip contractures in poliomyelitis, *Boston Med Surg J* 170:380, 1914.

Stasikelis PJ, Lee DD, Sullivan CM: Complications of osteotomies in severe cerebral palsy, *J Pediatr Orthop* 19:207, 1999.

Steel HH: Gluteus medius and minimus insertion advancement for correction of internal rotation gait in spastic cerebral palsy, *J Bone Joint Surg* 62A:919, 1980.

Stein GA, Hoffer MM, Koffman M: Long-term follow-up of proximal femoral varus derotation osteotomy for hip dislocations in cerebrospastic children. Paper presented at the annual meeting of the American Academy of Orthopaedic Surgeons, Las Vegas, 1985.

Stephenson CT, Griffith B, Donovan MM, Franklin T: The adductor transfer and iliopsoas release in the cerebral palsy hip, *Orthop Trans* 6:94, 1982 (abstract).

Sussman MD: Adductor and iliopsoas release: results after early mobilization. Paper presented at the annual meeting of the American Academy for Cerebral Palsy and Developmental Medicine, Chicago, 1983.

Sussman MD: Adductor and iliopsoas release: results after early mobilization, *Orthop Trans* 8:112, 1984 (abstract).

Sussman ME: Myositis ossification in young children following adductor and iliopsoas release. Paper presented at the annual meeting of the Pediatric Orthopaedic Society, Vancouver, 1984.

Sutherland DH: Gait analysis in cerebral palsy, *Dev Med Child Neurol* 20:807, 1978.

Sutherland DH, Olshen R, Cooper L, Woo SK: The development of mature gait, *J Bone Joint Surg* 62A:336, 1980.

Sutherland DH, Zilberfarb JL, Kaufman KR, et al: Psoas release at the pelvic brim in ambulatory patients with cerebral palsy: operative technique and functional outcome, *J Pediatr Orthop* 17:563, 1997.

Tachdjian MO, Minear WL: Hip dislocation in cerebral palsy, *J Bone Joint Surg* 38A:1358, 1956.

Terasawa K, Nakagomi T: Posterolateral transfer of internal rotators of the hips for correction of hip deformities in cerebral palsy: radiological assessment of results, *Dev Med Child Neurol* 29:5, 1987 (abstract).

Thompson GH et al: Chiari pelvic osteotomy: salvage for neuromuscular hip dysplasia and deformed femoral head, *J Pediatr Orthop* 8:115, 1988 (abstract).

Turker RJ, Lee R: Adductor tenotomies in children with quadriplegic cerebral palsy: longer term follow-up, *J Pediatr Orthop* 20:370, 2000.

Tylkowski CM, Price CT: Aponeurotic lengthening of the iliopsoas muscle for spastic hip-flexion deformities—assessment by gait analysis, *Dev Med Child Neurol* 28(suppl 53):4, 1986 (abstract).

Tylkowski CM, Rosenthal RK, Simon SR: Proximal femoral osteotomy in cerebral palsy, *Clin Orthop* 151:183, 1980.

Uematsu A, Bailey HL, Winter WGR, Brower TD: Results of posterior iliopsoas transfer for hip instability caused by cerebral palsy, *Clin Orthop* 126:183, 1977.

Vanden Brink KD, Beck KO, Comfort TH: Management of the hip in young children with severe cerebral palsy: a surgical dilemma. Paper presented at the annual meeting of the Pediatric Orthopaedic Society, Vancouver, 1984.

Vidal J et al: The success and limitations of adductor tenotomy in dysplasia of the hip in cerebral palsy, *Orthop Trans* 8:34, 1984 (abstract).

Weber M, Cabanela ME: Total hip arthroplasty in patients with cerebral palsy, *Orthopedics* 22:425, 1999.

Weinert C Jr, Ireland ML: Abduction osteotomy for the severely contracted hip in spastic quadriplegia: a new technique with rigid fixation using the compression hip screw system. Paper presented at the annual meeting of the American Academy for Cerebral Palsy and Developmental Medicine, Washington, DC, 1984.

Wenger DR, Carrell T: Chiari osteotomy and the migrating acetabulum: modifications to improve hip stability. Paper presented at the annual meeting of the Pediatric Orthopaedic Society, Vancouver, 1984.

Wheeler ME, Weinstein SL: Adductor tenotomy-obturator neurectomy, *J Pediatr Orthop* 4:48, 1984.

Widmann Rf, Do TT, Doyle SM, et al: Resection arthroplasty of the hip for patients with cerebral palsy: an outcome study, *J Pediatr Orthop* 19:805, 1999.

Yount IM: Hip fusion in the adolescent and young adult patient, *Orthop Trans* 12:578, 1988.

Zuckerman JD, Staheli LT, McLaughlin JF: Acetabular augmentation for progressive hip subluxation in cerebral palsy, *J Pediatr Orthop* 4:436, 1984.

SPINE

Akbarnia BA: Spinal deformity in patients with cerebral palsy. Paper presented at the annual meeting of the American Academy for Cerebral Palsy and Developmental Medicine, Chicago, 1983.

Akbarnia BA: Spinal deformity in patients with cerebral palsy, *Orthop Trans* 8:116, 1984 (abstract).

Allen BA Jr, Ferguson RL: L-rod instrumentation for scoliosis in cerebral palsy, *J Pediatr Orthop* 2:87, 1982.

Beck KO, Lonstein JE, Carlson JM: Functional evaluation of the sitting support orthosis for cerebral palsy, *Orthop Trans* 4:34, 1980 (abstract).

Bunnell WP: Spinal deformities in cerebral palsy. Paper presented at American Academy for Cerebral Palsy and Developmental Medicine Symposium, Growing up with Cerebral Palsy, Wilmington, Del, April 19-20, 1985.

Cassidy C, Craig CL, Perry A, et al: A reassessment of spinal stabilization in severe cerebral palsy, *J Pediatr Orthop* 14:731, 1994.

Charney EB, McMorrow M, Bruce DA, Sherk HH: Assessment of spinal deformities in children with myelomeningocele, *Orthop Trans* 8:116, 1984 (abstract).

Cristofaro RL, Taddonio RF, Gelb R: Stability in neuromuscular disease. Paper presented at the annual meeting of the American Academy for Cerebral Palsy and Developmental Medicine, Washington, DC, Oct 1984.

Fulford GE, Brown JK: Position as a cause of deformity in children with cerebral palsy, *Dev Med Child Neurol* 18:305, 1976.

Horstmann HM, Boyer B: Progression of scoliosis in cerebral palsy patients after skeletal maturity. Paper presented at the annual meeting of the American Academy for Cerebral Palsy and Developmental Medicine, Chicago, 1983.

Horstmann HM, Boyer B: Progression of scoliosis in cerebral palsy after skeletal maturity, *Orthop Trans* 8:116, 1984 (abstract).

Kalen V, Bleck EE, Rinsky LA: Preliminary results of Luque instrumentation in neuromuscular scoliosis. Paper presented at the annual meeting of the American Academy for Cerebral Palsy and Developmental Medicine, Washington, DC, 1984.

Kalen V, Conklin M, Sherman F: The effects of untreated scoliosis in severely involved cerebral palsy patients. Paper presented at the annual meeting of the Pediatric Orthopaedic Society of North America, San Francisco, May 1990.

Lonstein JE: Deformities of the spine in cerebral palsy, *Orthop Rev* 10:33, 1981.

Lonstein JE, Akbarnia BA: Operative treatment of spinal deformities in patients with cerebral palsy or mental retardation: an analysis of one hundred and seven cases, *J Bone Joint Surg* 65A:43, 1983.

Madigan RR, Wallace SL: Scoliosis in the institutionalized cerebral palsy population, *Spine* 6:583, 1981.

Mital MA, Belkin SC, Sullivan MA: An approach to head, neck and trunk stabilization and control in cerebral palsy by use of the Milwaukee brace, *Dev Med Child Neurol* 18:198, 1976.

Mubarak SJ, Kurz L, Schultz P, Park SM: Correlating scoliosis and pulmonary function in Duchenne muscular dystrophy, *Orthop Trans* 8:116, 1984 (abstract).

Rinsky LA: Surgery for spinal deformity in cerebral palsy, *Clin Orthop* 253:100, 1990.

Rinsky LA, Bleck E, Gamble J: The "growing" segmental spinal instrumentation technique in young children with progressive spinal deformity. Paper presented at the annual meeting of the American Academy for Cerebral Palsy and Developmental Medicine, Washington, DC, 1984.

Samilson RL: Orthopedic surgery of the hips and spine in retarded cerebral patients, *Orthop Clin North Am* 12:83, 1981.

Sharps CH, Bunnell WP: The natural history of scoliosis in cerebral palsy, *Dev Med Child Neurol* 28(suppl 53):19, 1986 (abstract).

Shufflebarger HL, Price CT, Riddick MF: L-rod instrumentation and spinal fusion: the Florida experience, *Orthop Trans* 8:43, 1984 (abstract).

Stanitski CL, Micheli LJ, Hall JE, Rosenthal RK: Surgical correction of spinal deformity in cerebral palsy, *Spine* 7:563, 1982.

Stegbauer SA, Lyne ED: Classification, natural history and etiology of scoliosis in the severely involved cerebral palsy patient, *Orthop Trans* 13:244, 1989 (abstract).

Thometz JG, Simons S, Griffin PP: Progression of scoliosis after skeletal maturity in institutionalized patients with cerebral palsy, *J Pediatr Orthop* 8:116, 1988 (abstract).

Thompson GH, Wilber RG, Shaffer JW, Nash CL: Segmental spinal instrumentation in spinal deformities, *Orthop Trans* 8:82, 1984 (abstract).

UPPER EXTREMITY

Craig CL, Ruby LK, Sosnoff F, Zimbler SZ: The upper extremity in Duchenne dystrophy: an unsolved problem. Paper presented at the annual meeting of the American Academy for Cerebral Palsy and Developmental Medicine, Washington, DC, 1984.

Hoffer MM, Perry J, Garcia M, Bullock D: Adduction contracture of the thumb in cerebral palsy: a preoperative electromyographic study, *J Bone Joint Surg* 65A:755, 1983.

House JH, Gwathmey FW, Fidler MO: A dynamic approach to the thumb-in-palm deformity in cerebral palsy: evaluation and results in fifty-six patients, *J Bone Joint Surg* 63A:216, 1981.

Manske PR: Extensor pollicis longus re-routing for treatment of spastic thumb in palm deformity, *Orthop Trans* 8:95, 1984 (abstract).

Mital MA: Flexion contractures and involuntary flexor bias in the upper extremities: its surgical management, *J Bone Joint Surg* 57A:1031, 1975 (abstract).

Mital MA: Lengthening of the elbow flexors in cerebral palsy, *J Bone Joint Surg* 61A:515, 1979.

Mital MA, Sakellarides HT: Surgery of the upper extremity in the retarded individual with spastic cerebral palsy, *Orthop Clin North Am* 12:127, 1981.

Mowery CA, Gelberman R, Roades CE: Upper extremity tendon transfers in cerebral palsy: an electromyographic and functional analysis. Paper presented at the annual meeting of the American Academy for Cerebral Palsy and Developmental Medicine, Washington, DC, 1984.

Mowery CA, Gelberman RH, Rhoades CE: Upper extremity tendon transfers in cerebral palsy: electromyographic and functional analysis, *J Pediatr Orthop* 5:69, 1985.

Patella V, Franchin B, Moretti B, Mori F: Arthrodesis of the wrist with mini-fixators in infantile cerebral palsy, *Ital J Orthop Traumatol* 10:75, 1984.

Patella V, Martucci G: Transposition of the pronator radii teres muscle to the radial extensors of the wrist in infantile cerebral paralysis: an improved operative technique, *Ital J Orthop Traumatol* 6:61, 1980.

Sakellarides HT: The management of the unbalanced wrist in cerebral palsy. Paper presented at the annual meeting of the American Academy for Cerebral Palsy and Developmental Medicine, Washington, DC, 1984.

Sakellarides HT, Mital MA, Lenzi WD: Treatment of pronation contractures of the forearm in cerebral palsy by changing the insertion of the pronator radii teres, *J Bone Joint Surg* 63A:645, 1981.

Sakellarides HT, Mital MA, Matza RA: The surgical treatment of the different types of "thumb-in-palm" deformities seen in cerebral palsy, *Orthop Trans* 4:9, 1980 (abstract).

Samilson RL, Morris JM: Surgical improvement of the cerebral-palsied upper limb: electromyographic studies and results of 128 operations, *J Bone Joint Surg* 46A:1203, 1964.

Skoff H, Woodbury DF: Current concepts review: management of the upper extremity in cerebral palsy, *J Bone Joint Surg* 67A:500, 1985.

Tachdjian MO: Affections of brain and spinal cord. In *Pediatric orthopaedics,* Philadelphia, 1972, WB Saunders.

Thometz JG, Tachdjian MO: Results of the flexor carpi ulnaris transfer in cerebral palsy. Paper presented at the annual meeting of the American Academy for Cerebral Palsy and Developmental Medicine, Washington, DC, 1984.

Zeitzew SL, Hoffer MM: Wrist arthrodesis in cerebral palsy, *Dev Med Child Neurol* 29(suppl 55):6, 1987 (abstract).

POSTNATAL CEREBRAL PALSY

Browne AO, McManus F: One-session surgery for bilateral correction of lower limb deformities in spastic diplegia, *J Pediatr Orthop* 7:259, 1987.

Dwyer FC: The treatment of relapsed club foot by the insertion of a wedge into the calcaneum, *J Bone Joint Surg* 45B:67, 1963.

Gage JR: Development disorders of gait. Paper presented at American Academy for Cerebral Palsy and Developmental Medicine Symposium: Growing up with cerebral palsy, Wilmington, Del, April 1985.

Green NE: The knee, ankle and foot in cerebral palsy. Paper presented at the annual meeting of the American Academy of Orthopaedic Surgeons, Las Vegas, 1985.

Hoffer MM, moderator: Symposium: management of cerebral palsy in the lower extremities, *Contemp Orthop* 16:79, 1988.

Jones ET, Knapp DR: Assessment and management of the lower extremity in cerebral palsy, *Orthop Clin North Am* 18:725, 1987.

Lindsey RW, Drennan JC: Management of foot and knee deformities in the mentally retarded, *Orthop Clin North Am* 12:107, 1981.

Norlin R, Tkaczuk H: One-session surgery for correction of lower extremity deformities in children with cerebral palsy, *J Pediatr Orthop* 5:208, 1985.

Perry J, Hoffer MM, Antonelli D, et al: Electromyography before and after surgery for hip deformity in children with cerebral palsy: a comparison of clinical and electromyographic findings, *J Bone Joint Surg* 58A:201, 1976.

Samilson RL: Current concepts of surgical management of deformities of the lower extremities in cerebral palsy, *Clin Orthop* 138:99, 1982.

Samilson RL, Dillin L: Postural impositions on the foot and ankle from trunk, pelvis, hip, and knee in cerebral palsy, *Foot Ankle* 4:120, 1983.

Tachdjian MO: Affections of brain and spinal cord. In Tachdjian MO: *Pediatric orthopaedics,* Philadelphia, 1972, WB Saunders.

Winters TF, Gage JR: Gait patterns in spastic hemiplegia secondary to cerebral palsy. Paper presented at the annual meeting of the Pediatric Orthopaedic Society, Vancouver, 1984.

ADULT STROKE PATIENT

Braun RM, Hoffer MM, Mooney V, et al: Phenol nerve block in the treatment of acquired spastic hemiplegia in the upper limb, *J Bone Joint Surg* 55A:580, 1973.

Braun RM, West F, Mooney V, et al: Surgical treatment of the painful shoulder contracture in the stroke patient, *J Bone Joint Surg* 53A:1307, 1971.

Caldwell C, Braun RM: Spasticity in the upper extremity, *Clin Orthop* 104:80, 1974.

Casey JM, Moore ML, Nickel VL: Spasticity: what to do when it becomes harmful, *J Musculoskel Med* Oct 1985, p 29.

Diamond M: Peripheral alcohol nerve blocks as an adjunct to the management of spasticity, *J Pediatr Orthop* 9:490, 1989 (abstract).

McCollough NC III: Orthopaedic evaluation and treatment of the stroke patient. I. Incidence and functional prognosis of hemiplegia, *Instr Course Lect* 24:21, 1975.

McCollough NC III: Orthopaedic evaluation and treatment of the stroke patient. II. Lower extremity management: orthotic management, *Instr Course Lect* 24:29, 1975.

McCollough NC III: Orthopaedic evaluation and treatment of the stroke patient. III. Upper extremity management: evaluation and management, *Instr Course Lect* 24:45, 1975.

McCollough NC III: Orthotic management in adult hemiplegia, *Clin Orthop* 131:38, 1978.

Mooney V, Perry J, Nickel VL: Surgical and non-surgical orthopaedic care of stroke, *J Bone Joint Surg* 49A:989, 1967.

Perry J: Orthopaedic evaluation and treatment of the stroke patient. I. Lower extremity management: examination—a neurologic basis for treatment, *Instr Course Lect* 24:26, 1975.

Perry J, Waters RL: Orthopaedic evaluation and treatment of the stroke patient. II. Lower extremity management: surgery, *Instr Course Lect* 24:26, 1975.

Perry J, Waters RL: Orthopaedic evaluation and treatment of the stroke patient. III. Upper extremity management: surgery, *Instr Course Lect* 24:45, 1975.

Perry J, Waters RL, Perrin T: Electromyographic analysis of equinovarus following stroke, *Clin Orthop* 131:47, 1978.

Perry J, Giovan P, Harris LJ, et al: The determinants of muscle action in the hemiparetic lower extremity (and their effect on the examination procedure), *Clin Orthop* 131:71, 1978.

Roper BA: The orthopedic management of the stroke patient, *Clin Orthop* 219:78, 1987.

Solomonow M: Restoration of movement by electrical stimulation: a contemporary view of the basic problems, *Orthopedics* 7:245, 1984.

Tracy HW: Operative treatment of the plantar-flexed inverted foot in adult hemiplegia, *J Bone Joint Surg* 58A:1142, 1976.

Waters RL: Stroke rehabilitation, *Clin Orthop* 131:2, 1978 (editorial comment).

Waters RL: Upper extremity surgery in stroke patients, *Clin Orthop* 131:30, 1978.

Waters RL, Perry J, Garland D: Surgical correction of gait abnormalities following stroke, *Clin Orthop* 131:54, 1978.

Waters RL, Frazier J, Garland DE, et al: Electromyographic gait analysis before and after operative treatment for hemiplegic equinus and equinovarus deformity, *J Bone Joint Surg* 64A:284, 1982.

Waters RL, Garland DE, Perry J, et al: Stiff-legged gait in hemiplegia: surgical correction, *J Bone Joint Surg* 61A:927, 1979.

31 Paralytic Disorders

William C. Warner, Jr.

POLIOMYELITIS

Acute anterior poliomyelitis is a viral infection localized in the anterior horn cells of the spinal cord and certain brainstem motor nuclei. One of three types of poliomyelitis viruses usually is the cause of infection, but other members of the enteroviral group can cause a condition clinically and pathologically indistinguishable from poliomyelitis. Initial invasion of the virus occurs through the gastrointestinal and respiratory tracts and spreads to the central nervous system through a hematogenous route.

Since the introduction and extensive use of the poliomyelitis vaccine, the incidence of acute anterior poliomyelitis in the Western world has dropped dramatically. Currently it most often affects children under the age of 5 years in developing tropical and subtropical countries and unimmunized persons in other temperate climates. Isolated outbreaks of poliomyelitis, however, have occurred in North America and Europe in the 1990s.

Administration of at least two and preferably three doses of the Sabin oral polio vaccine, containing all three types of attenuated virus, can prevent the disease. The use of the inactive poliovirus vaccine rather than the live attenuated virus vaccine still remains controversial. Live oral poliovirus vaccine (OPV) may immunize contacts who have not been vaccinated. However, Salk pointed out that live OPV places infants at special risk of paralysis from the live "spread virus." He also noted that licensed killed poliovirus vaccine provides as much protection as the live vaccine for vaccinated individuals and does not pose a risk to recipients or contacts. Outbreaks of paralytic poliomyelitis in the United States have been associated with the use of live poliovirus vaccine. The American Academy of Pediatrics recommends the expanded use of inactivated poliovirus vaccine (IPV) to eliminate vaccine-associated paralytic polio (VAPP). Only exclusive use of IPV can prevent vaccine-associated paralytic polio, but some experts believe that the optimal intestinal immunity induced by OPV is still needed to limit circulation of wild-type poliovirus if importation were to occur. The American Academy of Pediatrics has reported that each of three poliomyelitis vaccine schedules—IPV and OPV, IVP only, and OPV only—are all highly effective in protecting against poliomyelitis. Major factors in selecting the most appropriate immunization schedule are (1) the risk of VAPP, (2) the need for optimal intestinal immunity, (3) the cost of the vaccines, and (4) the parents' and provider's choice. When IVP is used, additional injections are necessary. Once additional combination vaccines are available, an IPV-only schedule should be feasible for all children in the United States. Oral poliovirus vaccine remains the vaccine of choice for global eradication in many parts of the world, specifically (1) in areas where wild-type poliovirus has either recently circulated or is currently circulating, (2) in most developing countries, where logistical issues and the higher cost of IPV prohibit its use, and (3) in places where inadequate sanitation necessitates an optimal mucosal barrier to wild-type poliovirus circulation.

Pathological Findings

Once the poliomyelitis virus invades the body through the oropharyngeal route, it multiplies in the alimentary tract lymph nodes and then spreads through the blood, acutely attacking the anterior horn ganglion cells of the spinal cord, especially in the lumbar and cervical enlargements. The incubation period ranges from 6 to 20 days. The anterior horn motor cells may be damaged directly by viral multiplication or toxic byproducts of the virus or indirectly by ischemia, edema, and hemorrhage in the glial tissues surrounding them. Destruction of the spinal cord occurs focally, and within 3 days wallerian degeneration is evident throughout the length of the individual nerve fiber. Macrophages and neutrophils surround and partially remove necrotic ganglion cells, and the inflammatory response gradually subsides. After 4 months, residual areas of gliosis and lymphocytic cells fill the area of destroyed motor cells in the spine. Reparative neuroglial cells proliferate. Continuous disease activity has been reported in spinal cord segments as long as 20 years after onset of the disease.

The number of individual muscles affected by the resultant flaccid paralysis and the severity of paralysis are variable; the clinical weakness is proportional to the number of lost motor units. According to Sharrard, weakness is clinically detectable only when more than 60% of the nerve cells supplying the muscle have been destroyed. Muscles innervated by the cervical and lumbar spinal segments are most often affected, and paralysis occurs twice as often in the lower extremity muscles as in upper extremity muscles. In the lower extremity, the most commonly affected muscles are the quadriceps, glutei, tibialis anterior, medial hamstrings, and hip flexors; in the upper extremity, the deltoid, triceps, and pectoralis major are most often affected.

The potential for recovery of muscle function depends on the recovery of damaged but not destroyed anterior horn cells. Most clinical recovery occurs during the first month after the acute illness and is almost complete within 6 months, although limited recovery may occur for about 2 years. According to Sharrard, a muscle paralyzed at 6 months remains paralyzed.

Clinical Course and Treatment

The course of poliomyelitis can be divided into three stages: acute, convalescent, and chronic. General guidelines for treatment are described here; specific indications and techniques for operative procedures are discussed in specific sections.

ACUTE STAGE

The acute stage generally lasts 7 to 10 days. Symptoms range from mild malaise to generalized encephalomyelitis with widespread paralysis. In younger children, systemic symptoms may include listlessness, sore throat, and a slight temperature elevation; these may resolve, but recurrent symptoms, including hyperesthesia or paresthesias in the extremities, severe headache, sore throat, vomiting, nuchal rigidity, back pain, and limitation of straight-leg raising, culminate in characteristically asymmetrical paralysis. In older children and adults, symptoms may include slight temperature elevation, marked flushing of the skin, and apprehension; muscular pain is common. Muscles are tender even to gentle palpation. Superficial reflexes usually are absent first, and deep tendon reflexes disappear when the muscle group is paralyzed. Differential diagnoses include Guillain-Barré syndrome and other forms of encephalomyelitis.

Treatment of poliomyelitis in the acute stage generally consists of bed rest, analgesics, hot packs, and anatomical positioning of the limbs to prevent flexion posturing and contractures. Padded foot boards, pillows, sandbags, or slings can help maintain position. Gentle, passive range-of-motion exercises of all joints should be carried out several times each day.

CONVALESCENT STAGE

The convalescent stage begins 2 days after the temperature returns to normal and continues for 2 years. Muscle power improves spontaneously during this stage, especially during the first 4 months and more gradually thereafter. Treatment during this stage is similar to that during the acute stage. Muscle strength should be assessed monthly for 6 months and then every 3 months. Physical therapy should emphasize muscle activity in normal patterns and development of maximal capability of individual muscles. Muscles with more than 80% return of strength recover spontaneously without specific therapy. According to Johnson, an individual muscle with less

than 30% of normal strength at 3 months should be considered permanently paralyzed.

Vigorous passive stretching exercises and wedging casts can be used for mild or moderate contractures. Surgical release of tight fascia and muscle aponeuroses and lengthening of tendons may be necessary for contractures persisting longer than 6 months. Orthoses should be used until no further recovery is anticipated.

CHRONIC STAGE

The chronic stage of poliomyelitis usually begins 24 months after the acute illness. It is during this time that the orthopaedist attempts to help the patient achieve maximal functional activity by management of the long-term consequences of muscle imbalance. The goals of treatment include correcting any significant muscle imbalances and preventing or correcting soft tissue or bony deformities. Static joint instability usually can be controlled indefinitely by orthoses. Dynamic joint instability eventually results in a fixed deformity that cannot be controlled with orthoses. Young children are more prone to develop bony deformity than are adults because of their growth potential. Soft tissue surgery, such as tendon transfers, should be done in young children before the development of any fixed bony changes; bony procedures for correcting a deformity usually can be delayed until skeletal growth is near completion.

Tendon Transfers

Tendon transfers are indicated when dynamic muscle imbalance results in a deformity that interferes with ambulation or function of the upper extremities. Surgery should be delayed until the maximal return of expected muscle strength in the involved muscle has been achieved. The objectives of a tendon transfer are (1) to provide active motor power to replace function of a paralyzed muscle or muscles, (2) to eliminate the deforming effect of a muscle when its antagonist is paralyzed, and (3) to improve stability by improving muscle balance.

Tendon transfer shifts a tendinous insertion from its normal attachment to another location so that its muscle can be substituted for a paralyzed muscle in the same region. In selecting a tendon for transfer, the factors that follow must be carefully considered:

1. The muscle to be transferred must be strong enough to accomplish what the paralyzed muscle did or to supplement the power of a partially paralyzed muscle. If the transferred muscle itself is weakened by paralysis, the expected action may be impossible or the muscle may function for a short time and then, because of overstretching, lose its power. A muscle to be transferred should have a rating of *good* or *better,* since a transferred muscle loses at least one grade in power after transfer.

2. For the transferred muscle to function efficiently, the freed end of the transferred tendon should be attached as close to the insertion of the paralyzed tendon as possible and should be routed in as direct a line as possible between the muscle's origin and its new insertion.

3. The transferred tendon should be retained in its own sheath or should be inserted into the sheath of another tendon; otherwise, it should be passed through tissues, such as subcutaneous fat, that will allow it to glide. Routing a tendon through tunnels in fascia or bone usually is not wise because scar tissue and adhesions will rapidly form.

4. The nerve and blood supply to the transferred muscle must not be impaired or traumatized in making the transfer.

5. The joint on which the muscle is to act must be in a satisfactory position; any contractures must be released before the tendon transfer. A transferred muscle cannot be expected to correct a fixed deformity.

6. The transferred tendon must be securely attached to bone under tension slightly greater than normal. If tension is insufficient, energy will be used in taking up slack in the musculotendinous unit rather than in producing the desired function.

7. Agonists are preferable to antagonists.

8. The tendon to be transferred should have, when possible, a range of excursion similar to the one it is reinforcing or replacing.

The anterior muscles of the leg are predominantly swing-phase muscles, and the posterior muscles, or flexors, are stance-phase muscles; in the thigh the quadriceps is characteristically a stance-phase muscle, and the hamstrings are swing-phase muscles. In general, phasic transfers retain their preoperative phasic activities; they also seem to regain their preoperative duration of contraction and electrical intensity. Many nonphasic muscle transfers retain their preoperative phasic activity and thus fail to assume the action of the muscles for which they are substituted. However, some nonphasic transfers are capable of phasic conversion. Some of the following factors seem to influence phasic conversion:

1. Often, a nonphasic muscle must be trained to assume the proper phase of the walking cycle after tendon transfer. Retraining of muscle function requires extensive physical therapy over several months.

2. Swing-phase transfers should not be mixed with stance-phase transfers. If these transfers are performed together, the nonphasic transferred muscle will have a high failure rate of phasic conversion.

3. Phasic conversion is not related to the amount of time that elapses between the onset of the disease and transfer of the muscle.

4. Bracing or splinting after surgery seems to have no effect on phasic conversion.

According to Mann, the ideal muscle for tendon transfer would have the same phasic activity as the paralyzed muscle, would be of about the same size in cross section and of equal strength, and could be placed in proper relationship to the axis of the joint to allow maximal mechanical effectiveness. Unfortunately, not all of these criteria can be met in every instance.

Paralytic deformities from muscle paralysis can be dynamic or static, and often both types are present. The extent to which the paralytic deformity is dynamic or static should be determined. A static deformity can be controlled with a brace in a growing child or with arthrodesis in an adult. In a growing child with dynamic deformity, recurrence is possible with arthrodesis alone; in a child with static deformity, however, recurrence after arthrodesis is rare. In a growing child with dynamic deformity, an appropriate tendon transfer with minimal external support redistributes muscle power, preventing permanent deformity until the patient is old enough for an arthrodesis.

Arthrodesis

A relaxed or flail joint is stabilized by partially or completely restricting its normal range of motion or by eliminating an abnormal motion. Although a properly constructed brace may work adequately to control a flail joint, a reconstructive operation that will not only eliminate the need for a brace but also improve function may be more effective. Arthrodesis is the most efficient method of permanent stabilization of a joint. Tenodeses that use flexor or extensor tendons to stabilize joints of the fingers (see Chapters 63 and 68) are notable exceptions, as are tenodeses of the peroneus longus or tendo calcaneus in paralytic calcaneus deformity; results are satisfactory here because the pull of gravity and body weight usually are not enough to overstretch the tendons.

Since the lower extremities are designed primarily to support the weight of the body, whether standing or walking, it is important that their joints be stable and their muscles have sufficient power. When the control of one or more joints of the foot and ankle is lost because of paralysis, stabilization may be required. In the upper extremity, on the other hand, reach, grasp, pinch, and release require more mobility than stability and more dexterity than power. Thus an operation to limit or obliterate motion in a joint of an upper extremity should be performed only after careful study of its advantages and disadvantages and of its general effect on the patient, especially in normal daily activity. Arthrodesis of the shoulder is useful for some patients but has certain disadvantages, cosmetic and functional, that must be weighed. Arthrodesis of the elbow is rarely indicated in poliomyelitis. Arthrodesis of the wrist, although useful for some patients, may increase the disability of other patients. For example, a patient who must use a wheelchair or crutches and has a wrist that is fused in the "optimal" position (for grasp and pinch) may be unable to lift himself from the chair or to manipulate crutches because he cannot shift his body weight to the palm of his hand with the wrist extended.

Foot and Ankle

Because the foot and ankle are the most dependent parts of the body and are subjected to significant amounts of stress, they are especially susceptible to deformity from paralysis. The most common deformities of the foot and ankle include clawtoes, cavovarus foot, dorsal bunion, talipes equinus, talipes equino-varus, talipes cavovarus, talipes equinovalgus, and talipes calcaneus. When the paralysis is of short duration, these dynamic deformities are not fixed and may be evident only on contraction of unopposed muscles or on weight-bearing; later, as a result of muscle imbalance, habitual posturing, growth, and abnormal weight-bearing alignment, a permanent deformity can occur from contracture of the soft tissues and from distortion of the normal contour of the bones.

Ambulation requires a stable plantigrade foot with even weight distribution between the heel and forefoot and no significant fixed deformity. Muscle transfer is performed to prevent the development of contractures, to balance the muscles responsible for dorsiflexion and plantar flexion and for inversion and eversion, and to reestablish as nearly normal a gait as possible. Arthrodesis to correct deformity or stabilize the joints usually should be delayed until about the age of 10 to 12 years to allow for adequate growth of the foot.

TENDON TRANSFERS

Tendon transfers about the foot and ankle after 10 years of age can be supplemented by arthrodesis to correct fixed deformities, to establish enough lateral stability for weight-bearing, and to compensate in part for the loss of function in the evertor and invertor muscles of the foot. When tendon transfers and arthrodesis are combined in the same operation, the arthrodesis should be performed first.

Transfer of a tendon usually is preferable to excision, not only to preserve function, but also to prevent further atrophy of the leg. When the paralysis is severe enough to require arthrodesis, there usually is some weakness of either the dorsiflexor or plantar flexor muscles. In this case the invertor or evertor muscles can be transferred to the midline of the foot either anteriorly or posteriorly into the calcaneus and tendo calcaneus. In the rare instance when a muscle function is discarded, 7 to 10 cm of its tendon should be excised to prevent scarring of the tendon ends by fibrous tissue.

After arthrodesis and tendon transfers, any deformities of the leg, such as excessive tibial torsion, genu varum, or genu valgum (bowlegs), should be corrected because otherwise they might cause recurrence of the foot deformity.

Paralysis of Specific Muscles

Isolated muscles may be paralyzed in patients with poliomyelitis, but more often combinations of muscles are affected. The specific muscle or muscles involved and the resulting muscle imbalance should be determined before treatment is started. Some of the more common deformities caused by muscle imbalance in the foot and ankle are described, according to the muscles involved. The exact pattern of muscle paralysis and the specific deformity that occurs must be carefully determined before any surgical intervention is undertaken.

Tibialis Anterior Muscle. Severe weakness or paralysis of the tibialis anterior muscle results in loss of dorsiflexion and inversion power and produces a slowly progressive deformity—equinus and cavus or varying degrees of plano-valgus—that is first evident in the swing phase of gait. The extensors of the long toe, which usually assist dorsiflexion, become overactive in an attempt to replace the paralyzed tibialis anterior muscle, causing hyperextension of the proximal phalanges and depression of the metatarsal heads. A cavovarus deformity occasionally results from unopposed activity of the peroneus longus combined with an active tibialis posterior muscle.

Passive stretching and serial casting can be tried before surgery to correct the equinus contracture. Posterior ankle capsulotomy and tendo calcaneus lengthening occasionally are required and are combined with anterior transfer of the peroneus longus to the base of the second metatarsal. The peroneus brevis is sutured to the stump of the peroneus longus to prevent a dorsal bunion. As an alternative, the extensor digitorum longus can be recessed to the dorsum of the midfoot to supply active dorsiflexion. Clawtoe deformity is managed by transfer of the long toe extensors into the metatarsal necks (see Chapter 83).

Plantar fasciotomy and release of intrinsic muscles may be necessary before tendon surgery for a fixed cavovarus deformity. In this situation the peroneus longus is transferred to the base of the second metatarsal, and the extensor hallucis longus is transferred to the neck of the first metatarsal. The clawtoe deformity frequently recurs because of reattachment of the extensor hallucis longus; this can be prevented by suturing its distal stump to the extensor hallucis brevis.

Tibialis Anterior and Posterior Muscles. If both the tibialis anterior and the tibialis posterior muscles are paralyzed, development of hindfoot and forefoot equinovalgus is more rapid and the deformity becomes fixed as the tendo calcaneus and peroneal muscles shorten. This deformity may be similar to congenital vertical talus on a standing lateral roentgenogram, but the apparent vertical talus is not confirmed when a plantar flexion lateral view is obtained. Serial casting is used before surgery to stretch the tight tendo calcaneus and avoid weakening the triceps surae. If the peroneal muscles are normal and both tibialis muscles are paralyzed, one of the peroneal muscles must be transferred. Because of its greater excursion, the peroneus longus is transferred to the base of the second metatarsal to replace the tibialis anterior and one of the long toe flexors replaces the tibialis posterior. The peroneus brevis is sutured to the distal stump of the peroneus longus tendon.

Tibialis Posterior Muscle. Isolated paralysis of the tibialis posterior muscle is rare but can result in hindfoot and forefoot eversion. Both the flexor hallucis longus and flexor digitorum longus have been used for tendon transfers in this situation. Through a posteromedial incision, the intrinsic plantar muscles are dissected sharply from their calcaneal origin, and one of the long toe flexors is exposed and divided. If the flexor digitorum longus is used, it is then dissected from its tendon sheath posterior and proximal to the medial malleolus, rerouted through the tibialis posterior sheath, and attached to the navicular. In rare cases, as an alternative, the extensor hallucis longus can be transferred posteriorly through the interosseous membrane and then through the tibialis posterior tunnel.

For children between the ages of 3 and 6 years, Axer recommended bringing the conjoined extensor digitorum longus and peroneus tertius tendons through a transverse tunnel in the talar neck and suturing the tendon back onto itself. For fixed equinus deformity, lengthening of the tendo calcaneus may be required before tendon transfer. For severe valgus he recommended transfer of the peroneus longus into the medial side of the talar neck and transfer of the peroneus brevis into the lateral side. Isolated transfer of the peroneus brevis should not be done because it can cause a forefoot inversion deformity. After surgery, cast immobilization is continued for 6 weeks, followed by 6 months of orthosis wear.

Tibialis Anterior, Toe Extensor, and Peroneal Muscles.
Progressively severe equinovarus deformity develops when the tibialis posterior and triceps surae are unopposed. The tibialis posterior increases forefoot equinus and cavus deformity by depressing the metatarsal head and shortening the medial arch of the foot. Further equinus and varus deformity results from contracture of the triceps surae, which acts as a fixed point toward which the plantar intrinsic muscles pull and increase forefoot adduction.

Stretching by serial casting may be attempted, but lengthening of the tendo calcaneus usually is required. Radical soft tissue release of the forefoot cavus deformity also may be necessary. Anterior transfer of the tibialis posterior to the base of the third metatarsal or middle cuneiform can be supplemented by anterior transfer of the long toe flexors. Arthrodesis usually is not required; the deformity can be controlled by physical therapy and orthoses. Watkins et al. obtained their best results with anterior transfer of the tibialis posterior in feet with varus deformities in which an overactive tibialis posterior was combined with good calf muscles and deficiencies in the dorsiflexors. Drennan described creation of a bony tunnel through either the base of the third metatarsal or the middle cuneiform and suture of the transfer to a button over a felt pad placed on the non-weight-bearing area of the plantar surface of the foot.

Peroneal Muscles.
Isolated paralysis of the peroneal muscles is rare in patients with poliomyelitis but can cause severe hindfoot varus deformity because of the unopposed activity of the tibialis posterior muscle. The calcaneus becomes inverted, the forefoot is adducted, and the varus deformity is increased by the action of the invertor muscles during gait. The unopposed tibialis anterior activity can cause a dorsal bunion (p. 1287). In this situation the tibialis anterior can be transferred laterally to the base of the second metatarsal; however, isolated transfer of the tibialis anterior can result in overactivity of the extensor hallucis longus, causing hyperextension of the hallux and development of a painful callus under the first metatarsal head. In children younger than 5 years of age, lengthening of the extensor hallucis longus tendon may be required. In children older than 5 years of age, the extensor hallucis longus should be transferred to the first metatarsal neck before the bony deformity becomes fixed.

Peroneal and Long Toe Extensor Muscles.
Paralysis of the peroneal muscles and long toe extensors causes a less severe equinovarus deformity that can be treated by transfer of the tibialis anterior to the base of the third metatarsal or the middle cuneiform.

Triceps Surae Muscles.
The triceps surae is a strong muscle group in the body, lifting the entire body weight with each step. Paralysis of the triceps surae, leaving the dorsiflexors unopposed, causes a rapidly progressive calcaneal deformity. Adequate tension of the tendo calcaneus is important to the normal function of the long toe flexors and extensors and to the intrinsic foot muscles. If the triceps surae is weak, the tibialis posterior, the peroneal muscles, and the long toe flexors cannot effectively plantar flex the hindfoot; however, they can depress the metatarsal heads and cause an equinus deformity. Shortening of the intrinsics and plantar fascia draws the metatarsal heads and the calcaneus together, much like a bowstring. The long axes of the tibia and the calcaneus coincide, negating any residual power in the triceps surae.

Keeping the foot in slight equinus during the acute stage of poliomyelitis helps prevent overstretching of the triceps surae, and the position is maintained in the convalescent stage. If the triceps surae is weak, early walking is discouraged. Serial standing roentgenograms should be obtained frequently, especially in children younger than 5 years of age, because of the rapid development of the deformity.

Surgical correction is indicated to prevent development of calcaneal deformity and to restore hindfoot plantar flexion. In the acute stage the only absolute indication for tendon transfer in children younger than 5 years of age is a progressive calcaneal deformity.

The combination of muscles transferred posteriorly depends on the residual strength of the triceps surae and the pattern of remaining muscle function. If the motor strength of the triceps surae is fair, posterior transfer of two or three muscles may be sufficient for normal gait. If the triceps surae is completely paralyzed, as many muscles as are available should be transferred. Plantar fasciotomy and intrinsic muscle release are required before tendon transfer in fixed forefoot cavus deformity.

The tibialis anterior can be transferred posteriorly as early as 18 months after the acute stage of poliomyelitis. This can be done as an isolated procedure if the lateral stabilizers are balanced and the strong toe extensors can be used for dorsiflexion. In more severe deformity, transfer of the toe extensors to the metatarsal heads and fusion of the interphalangeal joints may be required to prevent clawtoe deformity.

◆ *Posterior Transfer of Tibialis Anterior Tendon*

TECHNIQUE 31-1 *(Drennan)*
Take care to obtain maximal length of the tibialis anterior tendon, which may have shortened because of the calcaneal deformity the interosseous membrane. Split the insertion of

the tendo calcaneus longitudinally and develop osteoperiosteal flaps on the calcaneal tuberosity. Place the foot in maximal plantar flexion to ensure that the transfer is attached under appropriate tension. If necessary to obtain adequate plantar flexion, release other dorsal soft structures, including the ankle joint capsule, or lengthen the long toe extensors. If the attenuated tendo calcaneus requires shortening, use a Z-plasty technique, resecting redundant tendon from the proximal part. Attach the transferred tibialis anterior to the tuberosity of the calcaneus and to the distal stump of the tendo calcaneus, which has retained its normal attachment to the calcaneal tuberosity. Close the wound in normal fashion and apply a long leg cast with the foot in the plantar flexed position. The cast is worn for 5 weeks, and a brace is worn for an additional 4 months.

◆ ◆ ◆

If the invertors and evertors are balanced, a pure calcaneocavus deformity develops. Posterior transfer of only one set of these muscles causes instability and deformity. If the triceps surae strength is fair, transfer of the peroneus brevis and tibialis posterior to the heel is sufficient to control the calcaneus deformity and allow normal gait. Lateral imbalance requires transposition of the acting invertor or evertor to the heel. Both peroneals are transferred to the heel for calcaneovalgus deformity, and the tibialis posterior and flexor hallucis longus can be transferred for cavovarus deformity.

Westin and Defiore first recommended tenodesis of the tendo calcaneus to the fibula for paralytic calcaneovalgus deformity (Fig. 31-1). They used a T-shaped incision in the periosteum instead of a drill hole, with imbrication of the distal segment of the sectioned tendon below the periosteum. For mobile calcaneal deformities, Makin recommended transfer of the peroneus longus into a groove cut in the posterior

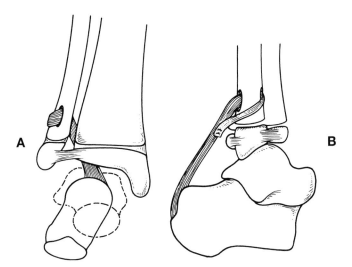

A   B

Fig. 31-1   Anterior (**A**) and lateral (**B**) views of tenodesis of tendo calcaneus to fibula.

calcaneus, without disturbance of the origin or insertion of the tendon. The tendon is freed proximal to the lateral malleolus and at the cuboid groove, and the foot is maximally plantar flexed, allowing the peroneus longus to displace posteriorly into the calcaneal groove, where it eventually unites with the bone. Extraarticular subtalar arthrodesis may be required as a second procedure.

In rare cases, if no invertors or evertors are present for transfer, the hamstrings can be used to replace the triceps surae. Prerequisites for this procedure include complete paralysis of the triceps surae, strong medial hamstrings or biceps femoris muscles, and strong ankle dorsiflexors and quadriceps muscles. The insertions of the semitendinosus and gracilis and occasionally the semimembranosus are mobilized, passed subcutaneously, and attached to the sagittally incised tendo calcaneus. A mattress suture at the proximal end of the tendo calcaneus prevents this incision from extending proximally. The tendons are sutured with the knee flexed to 25 degrees and the foot in plantar flexion.

Flail Foot.   When all muscles distal to the knee are paralyzed, equinus deformity results because of passive plantar flexion. The intrinsic muscles may retain some function, leading to forefoot equinus or cavoequinus deformity. Radical plantar release, sometimes combined with plantar neurectomy, usually controls this deformity. Midfoot wedge resection may be required for the forefoot equinus deformity in older patients.

◆ Dorsal Bunion

In this deformity the shaft of the first metatarsal is dorsiflexed and the great toe is plantar flexed; it usually results from muscle imbalance, although occasionally there may be other causes. In its early stages the deformity is not fixed but is present only on weight-bearing, especially walking; if the muscle imbalance is not corrected, however, the deformity will become fixed, although it remains more pronounced on weight-bearing (Fig. 31-2, *A*).

Usually only the metatarsophalangeal joint of the great toe is flexed, and on weight-bearing the first metatarsal head is displaced upward; thus the longitudinal axis of the metatarsal shaft can be horizontal, or its distal end can even be directed slightly upward. The first cuneiform also can be tilted upward. A small exostosis can form on the dorsum of the metatarsal head. When flexion of the great toe is severe enough, the metatarsophalangeal joint can subluxate and the dorsal part of the cartilage of the metatarsal head eventually can degenerate. The plantar part of the joint capsule and the flexor hallucis brevis muscle can become contracted.

Two types of muscle imbalance can cause a dorsal bunion: the most common dorsiflexes the first metatarsal, and the plantar flexion of the great toe is secondary; the less common plantar flexes the great toe, and dorsiflexion of the first metatarsal is secondary.

The most common imbalance is between the tibialis anterior and peroneus longus muscles; normally the tibialis anterior raises the first cuneiform and the base of the first metatarsal,

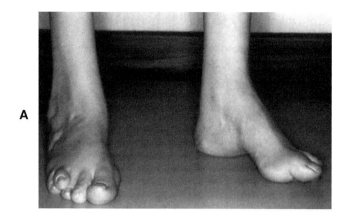

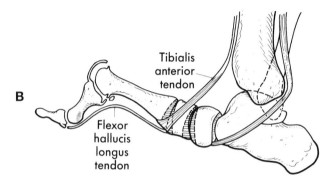

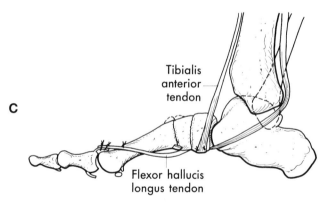

Fig. 31-2   **A,** Forefoot cavus deformity with mild dorsal bunion on left. **B,** Lapidus operation to correct dorsal bunion. *Shaded areas,* Bone to be resected and joints to be fused. **C,** Operation completed. Flexor hallucis longus has been converted to depressor of first metatarsal, and action of tibialis anterior as dorsiflexor of first metatarsal has been eliminated by transferring its insertion posteriorly. (Modified from Lapidus PW: *J Bone Joint Surg* 22:627, 1940.)

and the peroneus longus opposes this action. When the peroneus longus is weak or paralyzed or has been transferred elsewhere, the first metatarsal can be dorsiflexed by a strong tibialis anterior or by a muscle substituting for it. When the first metatarsal is dorsiflexed, the great toe becomes actively plantar flexed to establish a weight-bearing point for the medial side of the forefoot and to assist push-off in walking. Weakness of the dorsiflexor muscles of the great toe also may favor the development of this position of the toe. Lapidus and Hammond

observed that many dorsal bunions develop after ill-advised tendon transfers for residual poliomyelitis. In such patients the opposing actions of the peroneus longus and tibialis anterior muscles on the first metatarsal were considered in the transfers. Before any transfer of the peroneus longus tendon, the effect of its loss on the first metatarsal must be carefully considered. When the tibialis anterior is paralyzed and tendon transfer is feasible, the peroneus longus tendon or the tendons of the peroneus longus and peroneus brevis should be transferred to the third cuneiform rather than to the insertion of the tibialis anterior; as an alternative, Hammond suggested transferring the peroneus brevis tendon to the insertion of the tibialis anterior and leaving the peroneus longus tendon undisturbed. We believe that when the peroneus longus tendon is transferred, the proximal end of its distal segment should be securely fixed to bone at the level of division. When the triceps surae group is weak or paralyzed and the tibialis anterior and peroneus longus muscles are strong, the peroneus longus should not be transferred to the calcaneus unless the tibialis anterior is transferred to the midline of the foot. However, a dorsal bunion does not always follow ill-advised tendon transfers because the muscle imbalance may not be severe enough to cause it. When the deformity is progressive, surgery may simply consist of transferring the tibialis anterior (or the previously transferred peroneus longus) to the third cuneiform; correcting the deformity itself may then be unnecessary. But when the deformity is fixed, surgery must correct not only the muscle imbalance but also the deformity.

The second and less common muscle imbalance that can cause a dorsal bunion results from paralysis of all muscles controlling the foot except the triceps surae group, which may be of variable strength, and the long toe flexors, which are strong. These strong toe flexors help steady the foot in weight-bearing and sustain the push-off in walking. The flexor hallucis longus assumes a large share of this added function and with active use of the great toe may be almost constantly plantar flexed; the first metatarsal head is then displaced upward to accommodate it. A strong flexor hallucis brevis muscle also may help produce the deformity.

There are other, less common causes for the deformity. It can develop in conjunction with a hallux rigidus in which dorsiflexion of the first metatarsophalangeal joint is painful. The articular surfaces become irregular, and the plantar part of the joint capsule gradually contracts; proliferation of bone on the dorsum of the first metatarsal head often becomes pronounced and blocks dorsiflexion of the joint. When walking, the patient may then unconsciously supinate the foot and plantar flex the great toe to protect the weight-bearing pad of the great toe. A dorsal bunion also is sometimes seen in a severe congenital flatfoot with a rocker-bottom deformity.

TECHNIQUE 31-2 *(Lapidus)*

Make a longitudinal incision over the dorsomedial aspect of the first metatarsophalangeal joint to expose the dorsal part of the capsule. Outline a dorsal tongue-shaped flap of capsular tissue with its base attached to the proximal phalanx; open the joint by reflecting this flap distally. With an osteotome remove any abnormal bone from the dorsum of the metatarsal head. Now make a second longitudinal incision along the dorsomedial border of the forefoot and expose the first metatarsocuneiform joint and if necessary also the first naviculocuneiform joint. If the tibialis anterior is overactive, detach its tendon and transfer it to the second or third cuneiform on the dorsum of the foot or into the navicular. Thus the action of the tibialis anterior in dorsiflexion of the first metatarsal shaft is eliminated. Now remove a wedge of bone from the first metatarsocuneiform joint and if necessary also from the first naviculocuneiform joint (Fig. 31-2, *B*); the base of the wedge or wedges should be inferior, and their size will depend on the severity of the deformity. Lapidus pointed out that a metatarsus primus varus deformity, when present, can be corrected at the same time by following the principles of his bunion operation (Chapter 78). Now detach the flexor hallucis longus tendon from its insertion and pull it proximally into the incision over the forefoot. Drill an oblique tunnel in the shaft of the first metatarsal from its proximal plantar aspect to its distal dorsal aspect. Bring the end of the flexor hallucis longus tendon dorsally through this tunnel into the wound over the toe; this converts the flexor hallucis longus into a plantar flexor of the first metatarsal and eliminates its action in plantar flexing the great toe. Completely correct the flexion contracture of the great toe by subcutaneous plantar tenotomy and capsulotomy of the first metatarsophalangeal joint just proximal to the sesamoids.

Overlap the dorsal capsular flap to place the great toe in a few degrees of dorsiflexion; if there is hallux valgus, suture the flap with more tension on its medial side. Then anchor the distal end of the transferred flexor hallucis longus tendon into the capsular flap to passively reinforce the dorsal capsule. Also suture the tendon to the periosteum where it emerges from the metatarsal shaft (Fig. 31-2, *C*).

AFTERTREATMENT. A cast is applied from the toes to the knee with the foot in the correct position. After 2 weeks the cast is replaced by an unpadded walking cast that permits flexion of the great toe; weight-bearing gradually is resumed. At 8 to 10 weeks this cast is removed, an arch support is fitted in the shoe, and physical therapy is begun.

BONY PROCEDURES (OSTEOTOMY AND ARTHRODESIS)

The object of arthrodesis in patients with poliomyelitis is to reduce the number of joints the weakened or paralyzed muscles must control. The structural bony deformity must be corrected before a tendon transfer is performed. Stabilizing procedures for the foot and ankle are traditionally of five types: (1) calcaneal osteotomy, (2) extraarticular subtalar arthrodesis,

(3) triple arthrodesis, (4) ankle arthrodesis, and (5) bone blocks to limit motion at the ankle joint. These procedures can be performed singly or in combination with other procedures. The choice of operations depends on the age of the patient and the particular deformity that must be corrected.

Calcaneal Osteotomy
Calcaneal osteotomy (Chapter 26) can be performed for correction of hindfoot varus or valgus deformity in growing children. For cavovarus deformity, it can be combined with release of the intrinsic muscles and the plantar fascia, and for calcaneovarus deformity, with posterior displacement calcaneal osteotomy. Fixed valgus deformity may require medial displacement osteotomy in a plane parallel to the peroneal tendons.

Dillwyn-Evans Osteotomy
The Dillwyn-Evans osteotomy can be used for talipes calcaneovalgus deformity as an alternative to triple arthrodesis in children between the ages of 8 and 12 years. This osteotomy, the reverse of the original technique used in clubfeet, lengthens the calcaneus by a transverse osteotomy of the calcaneus and the insertion of a bone graft to open a wedge and lengthen the lateral border of the foot (Fig. 31-3).

◆ Subtalar Arthrodesis (Grice and Green; Dennyson and Fulford)
Paralytic equinovalgus deformity results from paralysis of the tibialis anterior and tibialis posterior and the unopposed action of the peroneals and triceps surae. The calcaneus is everted and displaced laterally and posteriorly. The sustentaculum tali no longer functions as the calcaneal buttress for the talar head, which shifts medially and into equinus. Hindfoot and forefoot equinovalgus deformities develop rapidly and, with growth, become fixed and require bony correction.

Grice and Green developed an extraarticular subtalar fusion to restore the height of the medial longitudinal arch in patients between the ages of 3 and 8 years. Ideally, this procedure is performed when the valgus deformity is localized to the subtalar joint and the calcaneus can be manipulated into its normal position beneath the talus. Careful clinical and roentgenographic examinations should determine whether the valgus deformity is located primarily in the subtalar joint or the ankle joint. If the forefoot is not mobile enough to be made plantigrade when the hindfoot is corrected, the procedure is contraindicated. The most common complications of the Grice and Green arthrodesis are varus deformity and increased ankle joint valgus because of overcorrection. Bone infection, pseudarthrosis, graft resorption, and degenerative arthritis of the metatarsal joints also have been reported.

Dennyson and Fulford described a technique for subtalar arthrodesis in which a screw is inserted across the subtalar joint for internal fixation and an iliac crest graft is placed in the sinus tarsi. Because the screw provides internal fixation, maintenance of the correct position is not dependent on the bone graft.

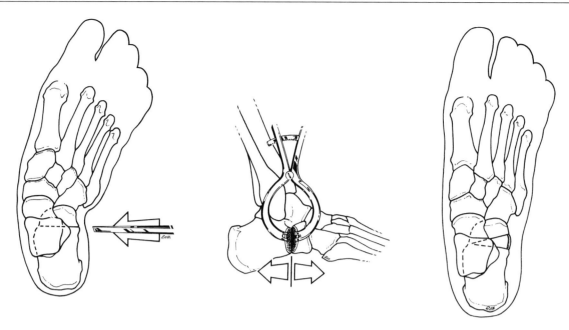

Fig. 31-3 Dillwyn-Evans procedure.

TECHNIQUE 31-3 *(Grice and Green)*

Make a short curvilinear incision on the lateral aspect of the foot directly over the subtalar joint. Carry the incision down through the soft tissues to expose the cruciate ligament overlying the joint. Split this ligament in the direction of its fibers and dissect the fatty and ligamentous tissues from the sinus tarsi. Dissect the short toe extensors from the calcaneus and reflect them distally. The relationship of the calcaneus to the talus now can be determined, and the mechanism of the deformity can be demonstrated. Place the foot in equinus and then invert it to position the calcaneus beneath the talus. A severe, long-standing deformity may require division of the posterior subtalar joint capsule or removal of a small piece of bone laterally from beneath the anterosuperior calcaneal articular surface. Insert an os-teotome or broad periosteal elevator into the sinus tarsi and block the subtalar joint to evaluate the stability of the graft and its proper size and position. Prepare the graft beds by removing a thin layer of cortical bone from the inferior surface of the talus and the superior surface of the calcaneus (Fig. 31-4).

Now make a linear incision over the anteromedial surface of the proximal tibial metaphysis, incise the periosteum, and take a block of bone large enough for two grafts (usually 3.5 to 4.5 cm long and 1.5 cm wide). As alternatives to tibial bone, take a short segment of the distal fibula or a circular segment of the iliac crest. Cut the grafts to fit the prepared beds. Use a rongeur to shape the grafts so that they can be countersunk into the cancellous bone to prevent lateral displacement. With the foot held in a slightly overcorrected position, place the grafts in the sinus tarsi. Evert the foot to lock the grafts in place. If a segment of the fibula or iliac crest is used, a smooth Kirschner wire can be used to hold the graft in place for 12 weeks. A screw can be inserted anteriorly from the talar neck into the calcaneus for rigid fixation. Apply a long leg cast with the knee flexed, the ankle in maximal dorsiflexion, and the foot in the corrected position.

AFTERTREATMENT. After 12 weeks of non-weight-bearing, the long leg cast is removed and a short leg walking cast is applied and worn for an additional 4 weeks.

TECHNIQUE 31-4 *(Dennyson and Fulford)*

Make an oblique incision in the line of the skin creases, centered over the sinus tarsi and extending from the middle of the front of the ankle proximally and laterally to the peroneal tendons (Fig. 31-5, *A*). Raise the origin of the extensor digitorum brevis, along with a pad of subcutaneous fat, proximally and reflect it distally to expose the sinus tarsi. Remove the fat from the sinus tarsi by sharp dissection close to the bone. With a narrow gouge, remove cortical bone from the apex of the sinus tarsi to expose cancellous bone on the undersurface of the talar neck and on the non-articular area in the upper calcaneal surface (Fig. 31-5, *B*). Do not remove cortical bone from the outer part of the sinus tarsi in the area through which the screw will pass. Expose the depression on the superior surface of the talar neck by blunt dissection between the tendon of the extensor

continued

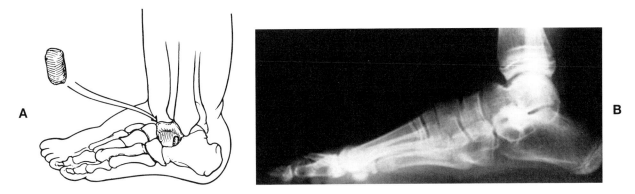

Fig. 31-4   Grice-Green subtalar fusion. Preparation of graft bed and placement of graft in lateral aspect of subtalar joint.

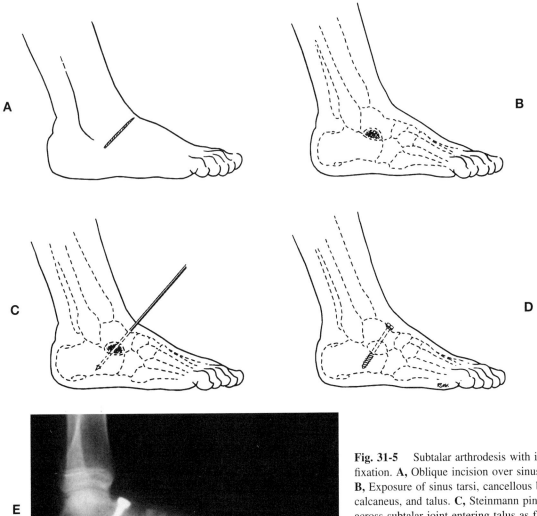

Fig. 31-5   Subtalar arthrodesis with internal fixation. **A,** Oblique incision over sinus tarsi. **B,** Exposure of sinus tarsi, cancellous bone of calcaneus, and talus. **C,** Steinmann pin is placed across subtalar joint entering talus as far distal as possible with foot held in corrected position. **D,** Screw is placed across subtalar joint from talar neck into calcaneus; sinus tarsi is filled with iliac crest bone graft. **E,** Roentgenogram of corrected foot with screw in place.

digitorum longus and the neurovascular bundle. Hold the calcaneus in its correct position and pass a bone awl from this depression, through the neck of the talus, and across the sinus tarsi to enter the upper surface of the calcaneus toward the lateral side until it pierces the cortex of the calcaneus at its inferolateral border (Fig. 31-5, *C*). The awl must pass through cortical bone on both the superior and inferior surfaces of the talar neck and on the superior and inferolateral surfaces of the calcaneus. Determine the length of the awl that is within the bones and insert a minifragment cancellous screw of the same length. Tighten the screw until its head is seated into the superior surface of the talus. Pack chips of cancellous bone from the iliac crest into the apex of the sinus tarsi (Fig. 31-5, *D*). Replace the extensor digitorum brevis and close the wound. Apply a long leg, non-weight-bearing cast.

AFTERTREATMENT. The long leg cast is removed at 6 to 8 weeks, and a short leg walking cast is applied and worn for an additional 4 to 6 weeks.

◆ Triple Arthrodesis

The most effective stabilizing procedure in the foot is triple arthrodesis: fusion of the subtalar, calcaneocuboid, and talonavicular joints. Triple arthrodesis limits motion of the foot and ankle to plantar flexion and dorsiflexion. It is indicated when most of the weakness and deformity are at the subtalar and midtarsal joints. Triple arthrodesis is performed (1) to obtain stable and static realignment of the foot, (2) to remove deforming forces, (3) to arrest progression of deformity, (4) to eliminate pain, (5) to eliminate the use of a short leg brace or to provide sufficient correction to allow fitting of a long leg brace to control the knee joint, and (6) to obtain a more normal-appearing foot. Generally, triple arthrodesis is reserved for severe deformity in children 12 years of age and older; occasionally it may be required in children 8 to 12 years of age with progressive, uncontrollable deformity.

The exact technique of triple arthrodesis depends on the type of deformity, and this should be determined before surgery. A paper tracing can be made from a lateral roentgenogram of the ankle, and the components of the subtalar joint are divided into three sections: the tibiotalar and calcaneal components and another comprising all the bones of the foot distal to the midtarsal joint. These are then reassembled with the foot in the corrected position so that the size and shape of the wedges to be removed can be measured accurately.

In talipes equinovalgus, the medial longitudinal arch of the foot is depressed, the talar head is enlarged and plantar flexed, and the forefoot is abducted. Raising the talar head and shifting the sustentaculum tali medially beneath the talar head and neck restores the arch. A medially based wedge consisting of a portion of the talar head and neck is excised (Fig. 31-6, *C*). When the hindfoot valgus deformity is corrected, the forefoot tends to supinate; this is controlled by midtarsal joint resection

with a medially based wedge. An additional medial incision may be required for resection of the talonavicular joint.

In talipes equinovarus, the enlarged talar head lies lateral to the midline axis of the foot and blocks dorsiflexion. A laterally based subtalar wedge, combined with midtarsal joint resection, places the talar head slightly medial to the midline axis of the foot (Fig. 31-6, *D*).

In talipes calcaneocavus, the arthrodesis should allow posterior displacement of the foot at the subtalar joint. After stripping of the plantar fascia, a wedge-shaped or cuneiform section of bone is removed to allow correction of the cavus deformity, and a wedge of bone is removed from the subtalar joint to correct the rotation of the calcaneus (Fig. 31-6, *D*).

The muscle balance of the foot and ankle determines how much the foot should be displaced posteriorly. Posterior displacement of the foot transfers its fulcrum (the ankle) anteriorly to a position near its center and lengthens its posterior lever arm; this is especially important when the triceps surae group is weak. If the foot is to be displaced as far posteriorly as possible, the procedure of Hoke or Dunn is used; the latter permits slightly more displacement than the former. When the ankle dorsiflexors and plantar flexors are equally strong, Ryerson's technique can be used.

TECHNIQUE 31-5

Make an oblique incision centered over the sinus tarsi in line with the skin creases on the lateral side of the foot, beginning dorsolaterally at the lateral border of the tendons of the long toe extensors at the level of the talonavicular joint (Fig. 31-6, *A*). Continue the incision posteriorly, angling plantarward and ending at the level of the peroneal tendons. Carefully protect the extensor and peroneal tendons and carry the incision sharply down through the sinus tarsi to the extensor digitorum brevis muscle. Reflect the origin of this muscle distally along with the fat in the sinus tarsi. Clean the remainder of the sinus tarsi of all tissue to expose the subtalar and calcaneocuboid joints and the lateral portion of the talonavicular joint.

Incise the capsules of the talonavicular, calcaneocuboid, and subtalar joints circumferentially to obtain as much mobility as possible. If this release allows the foot to be placed in a normal position, removal of large bony wedges is not required. If correction is impossible after soft tissue release, appropriate bony wedges are removed (Fig. 31-6, *C* and *D*).

Identify the anterior articular process of the calcaneus and excise it at the level of the floor of the sinus tarsi for better exposure of all joints. To make this osteotomy, use an osteotome placed parallel to the plantar surface of the foot; preserve the bone for grafting. Next, with an osteotome remove the articular surfaces of the calcaneocuboid joint to expose cancellous bone. Remove an equal amount from both bones unless wedge correction of a bony deformity is required (Fig. 31-6, *B*). Next, remove the distal portion of the head of the talus with ¼-inch and ½-inch straight and

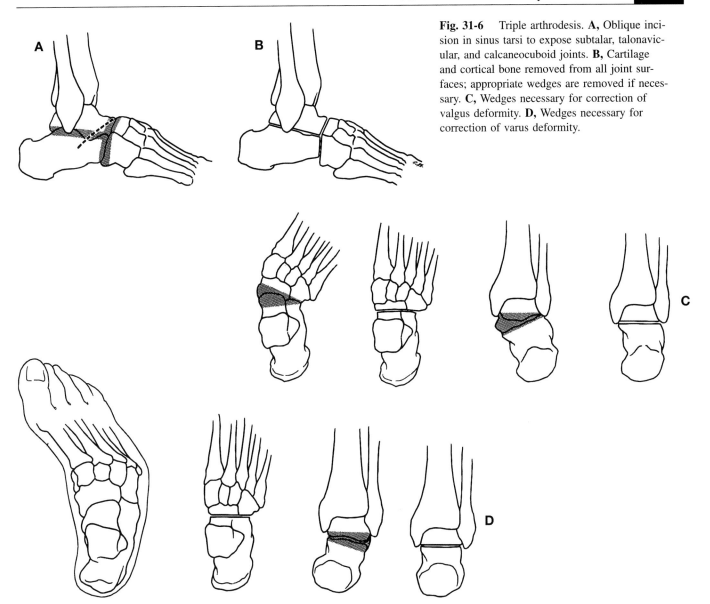

Fig. 31-6 Triple arthrodesis. **A,** Oblique incision in sinus tarsi to expose subtalar, talonavicular, and calcaneocuboid joints. **B,** Cartilage and cortical bone removed from all joint surfaces; appropriate wedges are removed if necessary. **C,** Wedges necessary for correction of valgus deformity. **D,** Wedges necessary for correction of varus deformity.

curved osteotomes. Remove only enough bone to expose the cancellous bone of the talar head unless a medial wedge is required to correct a fixed deformity. A small lamina spreader can be inserted for better exposure. A second medial incision may be necessary to expose the most medial portion of the talonavicular joint. Remove the proximal articular surface and subchondral bone of the navicular, and shape and roughen the surfaces for a snug fit with the talus. Excise the articular surfaces of the sustentaculum tali and the anterior facet of the subtalar joint.

Now approach the subtalar joint and completely remove its articular surfaces. For better exposure of the posterior portion, use the small lamina spreader to expose the subtalar joint. Remove appropriate wedges from this joint if necessary; otherwise, make the joint resections parallel to

the articular surfaces. Cut the removed bone into small pieces to be used for bone grafting. Place most of the bone graft around the talonavicular joint and in the depth of the sinus tarsi.

Correction is maintained with internal fixation, usually smooth Steinmann pins or Kirschner wires. Close the muscle pedicle of the extensor digitorum brevis over the sinus tarsi to reduce the dead space. Close the wound over a suction drain and apply a well-padded, short leg cast.

AFTERTREATMENT. Considerable bleeding from the drain and through the wound itself can be expected. The foot should be elevated to minimize swelling. The drain is removed at 24 to 48 hours. Walking with crutches or a walker, with touch-down weight-bearing on the operated foot, is allowed as tolerated. The cast and pins or wires are removed at 6 to 8 weeks, and a short leg walking cast is applied and worn until union is complete, usually 4 weeks more.

◆ Correction of Cavus Deformity

TECHNIQUE 31-6
Perform a medial radical plantar release to correct the contracted soft tissues bridging the longitudinal arch. Then forcibly correct the cavus deformity as much as possible. Now expose the calcaneocuboid, talonavicular, and subtalar joints through the incision described above. With an osteotome remove from the talonavicular and calcaneocuboid joints a wedge-shaped or cuneiform section of bone with its base anterior and large enough to correct the cavus deformity that remains after the plantar fascial stripping. Then dorsiflex the forefoot and appose the raw surfaces to see if the cavus is corrected; if so, expose the subtalar joint and remove from it a wedge of bone with its base posterior to correct the deformity or rotation of the calcaneus (Fig. 31-6, *D*). Be sure that all bone surfaces fit together well and that the foot is in satisfactory position before closing the wound.

AFTERTREATMENT. Correction usually is maintained with Steinmann pins or Kirschner wires. A cast is applied, and firm pressure is exerted on the sole of the foot while the plaster is setting to stretch the plantar structures as much as possible.

Miller and Irwin and Goldner and Irwin all advised postoperative manipulation of the foot. At 10 to 14 days the cast and sutures are removed, the foot is inspected, and roentgenograms are made. If the position is not satisfactory, the foot is manipulated with the patient under general anesthesia. A new cast, snug but properly padded, is then applied and is molded to the contour of the foot; this cast is removed at 12 weeks.

Complications of Triple Arthrodesis. The most common complication of triple arthrodesis is pseudarthrosis, especially of the talonavicular joint. The additional stress on the ankle joint caused by loss of mobility of the hindfoot can lead to the development of degenerative arthritis. Excessive resection of the talus can cause avascular necrosis, especially in adolescents; this usually is evident on roentgenograms 8 to 12 weeks after triple arthrodesis. Ligamentous laxity about the ankle joint may require ankle fusion. Muscle imbalance after hindfoot stabilization can lead to forefoot deformity; unopposed function of the tibialis anterior or peroneal muscles is the most common cause of this complication and should be corrected by tendon transfer. Residual deformity usually is caused by insufficient correction at surgery, inadequate immobilization, pseudarthrosis, or muscle imbalance.

Talectomy
Talectomy provides stability and posterior displacement of the foot and generally is recommended for children between the ages of 5 and 12 years when the deformity is not correctable by arthrodesis. Talectomy limits motion of the ankle joint, especially dorsiflexion, and creates a tibiotarsal ankylosis. Posterior displacement of the foot places the distal tibia over the center of the weight-bearing area, producing even weight distribution and good lateral stability. Appearance usually is satisfactory, pain is relieved, and special shoes or orthoses are not required.

The most common cause of failure of talectomy is muscle imbalance, usually the presence of a strong tibialis anterior or posterior muscle. Intrinsic muscle activity can cause contracture of the plantar fascia, resulting in a forefoot equinus deformity. In children younger than 5 years of age, recurrence of the deformity is frequent, and pain is common in those over 15 years of age, especially with inadequate excision of the entire talus. Tibiocalcaneal arthrodesis can be performed for failed talectomy and most commonly is indicated because of persistent pain. Carmack and Hallock recommended an anterior approach, leaving the foot in slight equinus. The technique of talectomy is described in Chapter 26.

◆ Lambrinudi Arthrodesis
The Lambrinudi arthrodesis is recommended for correction of isolated fixed equinus deformity in patients older than 10 years of age. Retained activity in the triceps surae, combined with inactive dorsiflexors and peroneals, causes the drop-foot deformity. The posterior talus abuts the undersurface of the tibia and the posterior ankle joint capsule contracts to create a fixed equinus deformity. In the Lambrinudi procedure a wedge of bone is removed from the plantar distal part of the talus so that the talus remains in complete equinus at the ankle joint while the remainder of the foot is repositioned to the desired degree of plantar flexion. Tendon resection or transfer may be necessary to prevent varus or valgus deformity if active muscle power remains. The Lambrinudi arthrodesis is not recommended for a flail foot or when hip or knee instability requires a brace. A good result depends on the strength of the dorsal ankle ligaments. If anterior subluxation of the talus is noted on a weight-bearing lateral roentgenogram, a two-stage pantalar arthrodesis is recommended.

Complications of the Lambrinudi arthrodesis include ankle instability, residual varus or valgus deformities caused by muscle imbalance, and pseudarthrosis of the talonavicular joint.

TECHNIQUE 31-7 *(Lambrinudi)*
With the foot and ankle in extreme plantar flexion, make a lateral roentgenogram and trace the film. Cut the tracing into three pieces along the outlines of the subtalar and midtarsal joints; from these pieces the exact amount of bone to be removed from the talus can be determined with accuracy before surgery. In the tracing the line representing the articulation of the talus with the tibia is left undisturbed, but that corresponding to its plantar and distal parts is to be cut so that when the navicular and the calcaneocuboid joint are

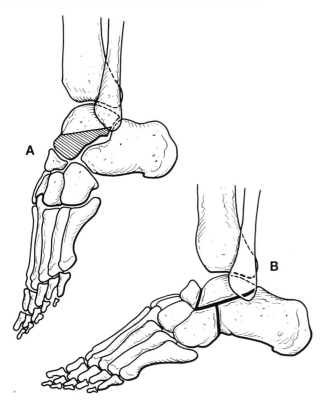

Fig. 31-7 Lambrinudi operation for talipes equinus. **A,** *Shaded area,* Part of talus to be resected. **B,** Sharp distal margin of remaining part of talus has been wedged into prepared trough in navicular, and raw osseous surfaces of talus, calcaneus, and cuboid have been apposed. (Redrawn from Hart VL: *J Bone Joint Surg* 22:937, 1940.)

later fitted to it the foot will be in 5 to 10 degrees of equinus relative to the tibia (Fig. 31-7) unless the extremity has shortened; more equinus may then be desirable.

Expose the sinus tarsi through a long lateral curved incision. Section the peroneal tendons by a Z-shaped cut, open the talonavicular and calcaneocuboid joints, and divide the interosseous and fibular collateral ligaments of the ankle to permit complete medial dislocation of the tarsus at the subtalar joint. With a small power saw (more accurate than a chisel or osteotome), remove the predetermined wedge of bone from the plantar and distal parts of the neck and body of the talus. Remove the cartilage and bone from the superior surface of the calcaneus to form a plane parallel with the longitudinal axis of the foot. Next make a V-shaped trough transversely in the inferior part of the proximal navicular and denude the calcaneocuboid joint of enough bone to correct any lateral deformity. Firmly wedge the sharp distal margin of the remaining part of the talus into the prepared trough in the navicular and appose the calcaneus and talus. Take care to place the distal margin of the talus well medially in the trough; otherwise, the position of the foot will not be satisfactory. The talus is now locked in the

ankle joint in complete equinus, and the foot cannot be further plantar flexed. Insert smooth Kirschner wires for fixation of the talonavicular and calcaneocuboid joints. Suture the peroneal tendons, close the wound in the routine manner, and apply a cast with the ankle in neutral or slight dorsiflexion.

AFTERTREATMENT. The cast and sutures are removed at 10 to 14 days, and the position of the foot is evaluated by roentgenograms. If the position is satisfactory, a short leg cast is applied, but weight-bearing is not allowed for another 6 weeks, after which a short leg walking cast is applied and is worn until fusion is complete, usually at 3 months.

Ankle Arthrodesis

Ankle fusion may be indicated for a flail foot or for recurrence of deformity after triple arthrodesis. Compression arthrodesis (Chapter 3) generally is recommended for older children and adolescents, and the Chuinard and Peterson fusion (Chapter 3) is recommended for skeletally immature patients because it does not disturb the distal tibial physis. Barr and Record recommended ankle arthrodesis for severe paralytic equinovarus deformities in adults when muscles suitable for transfer are not available; subcutaneous plantar fasciotomy and lengthening of the tendo calcaneus can be performed initially, followed by ankle arthrodesis.

Pantalar Arthrodesis

Pantalar arthrodesis is fusion of the tibiotalar, talonavicular, subtalar, and calcaneocuboid joints. For flail feet with paralyzed quadriceps, pantalar arthrodesis may be indicated to eliminate the need for long leg braces. Waugh, Wagner, and Stinchfield found a compensatory increase in forefoot motion that assisted in stance and gait in their patients with pantalar arthrodesis; the younger the patient, the more compensatory motion obtained. According to them, the ideal patient for this operation is one with a flail foot and ankle and normal muscles about the hip and knee. Absolute prerequisites for this procedure include a strong gluteus maximus to initiate toe-off during gait and a normally aligned knee with full extension or a few degrees of hyperextension.

The ankle should be fused in 5 to 10 degrees of equinus to produce the backward thrust on the knee joint necessary for stable weight-bearing. Excessive equinus position of the ankle results in pain and increased pressure under the metatarsal heads; acceptable plantar flexion should be confirmed with a lateral roentgenogram during surgery. Leibolt and King both recommended performing pantalar arthrodesis in two stages: the first in the foot and the second in the ankle, because it is difficult to achieve and maintain proper position of both the foot and ankle at the same time. However, in 116 pantalar arthrodeses, Waugh et al. found that results were the same regardless of whether the operation had been performed in one stage or two.

Complications of pantalar arthrodesis include pseudarthrosis, painful plantar callosities caused by unequal weight distribution, and excessive heel equinus, which causes increased pressure on the forefoot.

Posterior Bone Block

Campbell described a posterior bone block to eliminate ankle plantar flexion while retaining a functional range of dorsiflexion. He constructed a bony buttress on the posterior aspect of the talus and the superior surface of the calcaneus that impinged on the posterior lip of the distal tibia to prevent ankle plantar flexion. This technique rarely is indicated now, having been replaced by tendon transfer techniques and other arthrodesis procedures.

TENDON TRANSFER TECHNIQUES

Talipes Equinovarus

Talipes equinovarus caused by poliomyelitis is characterized by equinus deformity of the ankle, inversion of the heel, and, at the midtarsal joints, adduction and supination of the forefoot. When the deformity is of long duration, there also is a cavus deformity of the foot; clawing of the toes may develop secondary to substitution of motor patterns. In paralytic talipes equinovarus the peroneal muscles are paralyzed or severely weakened, but the tibialis posterior usually is normal; the tibialis anterior may be weakened or normal. The triceps surae is comparatively strong but becomes contracted by a combination of motor imbalance, growth, gravity, and posture. Treatment depends on the age of the patient, the forces causing the deformity, the severity of the deformity, and its rate of increase.

Anterior transfer of the tibialis posterior tendon removes a dynamic deforming force and aids active dorsiflexion of the foot (Fig. 31-8); however, transfer alone rarely restores active dorsiflexion. Rerouting of the tendon anterior to the medial malleolus diminishes its plantar flexion power and lengthens the tibialis posterior muscle; the deformity may not be corrected, however, because the muscle retains its varus pull. The entire tendon can be transferred through the interosseous membrane to the middle cuneiform or the tendon can be split, with the lateral half transferred to the cuboid.

◆ Anterior Transfer of Tibialis Posterior Tendon

TECHNIQUE 31-8 *(Barr)*

Make a skin incision on the medial side of the ankle beginning distally at the insertion of the tibialis posterior tendon and extending proximally over the tendon just posterior to the malleolus and from there proximally along the medial border of the tibia for 5 to 7.5 cm. Free the tendon from its insertion, preserving as much of its length as possible. Split its sheath and free it in a proximal direction

until the distal 5 cm of the muscle has been mobilized. Carefully preserve the nerves and vessels supplying the muscle. Make a second skin incision anteriorly; begin it distally at the level of the ankle joint and extend it proximally for 7.5 cm just lateral to the tibialis anterior tendon. Carry the dissection deep between the tendons of the tibialis anterior and the extensor hallucis longus, carefully preserving the dorsalis pedis artery; expose the interosseous membrane just proximal to the malleoli. Now cut a generous window in the interosseous membrane but avoid stripping the periosteum from the tibia or fibula. Then pass the tibialis posterior tendon through the window between the bones, taking care that it is not kinked, twisted, or constricted and that the vessels and nerves to the muscle are not damaged. Pass the tendon beneath the cruciate ligament, which can be divided if necessary to relieve pressure on the tendon. Expose the third cuneiform or the base of the third metatarsal through a transverse incision 2.5 cm long. Retract the extensor tendons, sharply incise the periosteum over the bone in a cruciate fashion, and fold back osteoperiosteal flaps. Now drill a hole through the bone in line with the tendon and large enough to receive it; anchor it in the bone with a pull-out wire. Be sure that the button on the plantar surface of the foot is well padded. Now suture the osteoperiosteal flaps to the tendon with two figure-eight silk sutures. Close the incision and apply a plaster cast to hold the foot in calcaneovalgus position.

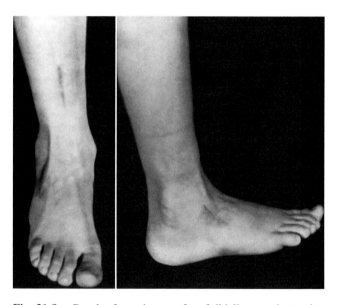

Fig. 31-8   Result of anterior transfer of tibialis posterior tendon through interosseous membrane. Foot is in mild valgus position, and result would have been better if transferred tendon had been anchored nearer midline of foot. Note small scar at normal insertion of tibialis posterior tendon and another over musculotendinous junction of tibialis posterior muscle and posterior to subcutaneous border of tibia.

Instead of the long medial incision used by Barr, we make a short longitudinal one to free the tibialis posterior tendon at its insertion and withdraw it through another incision 5 cm long at the musculotendinous junction just posterior to the subcutaneous border of the tibia (see Fig. 31-8). The tendon also can be anchored to bone by passing it through a hole drilled in the bone, looping it back, and suturing it to itself with nonabsorbable sutures.

AFTERTREATMENT. The cast is removed at 3 weeks, the wounds are inspected, the sutures are removed, and a short leg walking cast is applied with the foot in the neutral position and the ankle in slight dorsiflexion. Six weeks after surgery the cast is removed, and a program of rehabilitative exercises is started that is continued under supervision until a full range of active resisted function is obtained. The transfer is protected for 6 months by a double-bar foot-drop brace with an outside T-strap.

TECHNIQUE 31-9 *(Ober)*

Through a medial longitudinal incision 7.5 cm long, free the tibialis posterior tendon from its attachment to the navicular

(Fig. 31-9). Now make a second longitudinal medial incision 10 cm long centered over the musculotendinous junction of the tibialis posterior. Withdraw the tendon from the proximal wound and free the muscle belly well up on the tibia. Strip the periosteum obliquely on the medial surface of the tibia so that when the tendon is moved into the anterior tibial compartment only the belly of the muscle will come in contact with denuded bone. The tendon must not be in contact with the tibia. Make a third incision over the base of the third metatarsal, draw the tibialis posterior tendon from the second into the third incision, and anchor its distal end in the base of the third metatarsal.

AFTERTREATMENT. Aftertreatment is the same as for the Barr technique.

◆ Split Transfer of Tibialis Anterior Tendon

TECHNIQUE 31-10

Make a 2- to 3-cm longitudinal incision dorsomedially over the medial cuneiform (Fig. 31-10, *A*). Identify the tibialis

continued

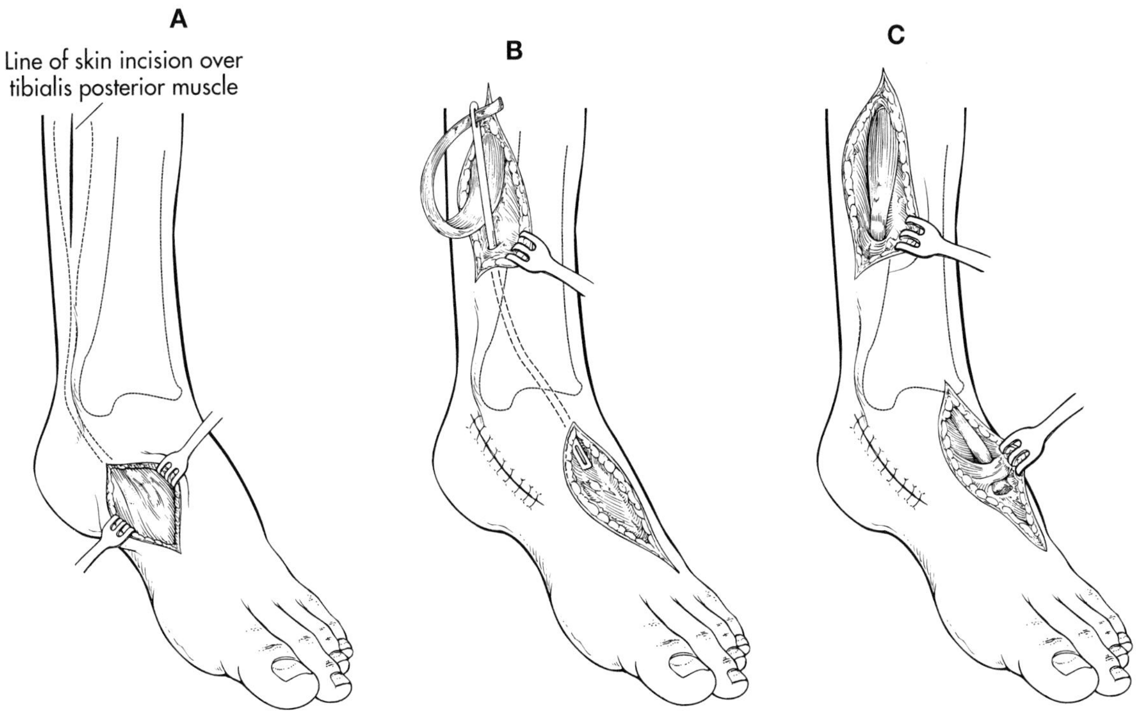

A
Line of skin incision over
tibialis posterior muscle

B

C

Fig. 31-9 Ober anterior transfer of tibialis posterior tendon. **A,** Insertion of tibialis posterior tendon has been exposed. Note line of skin incision over muscle. **B,** Tendon has been freed from its insertion, and muscle has been dissected from tibia. **C,** Tendon and muscle have been passed through anterior tibial compartment to dorsum of foot, and tendon has been anchored in third metatarsal. (Redrawn from Ober FR: *N Engl J Med* 209:52, 1933.)

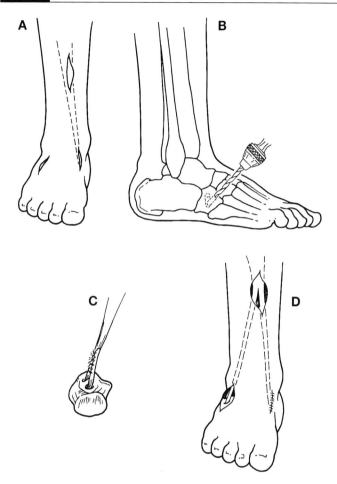

Fig. 31-10 Split transfer of tibialis anterior tendon. **A,** Three incisions: longitudinal over insertion of tibialis anterior tendon and longitudinally over distal leg and over cuboid. **B,** Two holes are drilled in cuboid. **C,** Split portion of tibialis anterior tendon is pulled into one hole and out the other and sutured to itself. **D,** New split portion of tendon in its redirected position. (Redrawn from Hoffer MM, Reiswig JA, Garrett AM, Perry J: *Orthop Clin North Am* 5:31, 1974.)

anterior tendon and split it longitudinally in the midportion. Detach the lateral half of the tendon from its insertion, preserving as much length as possible, and continue the split proximally to the extent of the incision. Make a second 2- to 3-cm incision anteriorly over the distal tibia, identify the tibialis anterior tendon sheath, and split it longitudinally. Continue the split in the tibialis anterior tendon proximally into this incision and up to the musculotendinous junction. Umbilical tape can be used to continue the split in the tendon. Place the tape into the split and bring its two ends into the proximal incision. Before the lateral half of the tendon is detached, continue the split to the musculotendinous junction by pulling on the tape. Once the split in the tendon is complete, detach the lateral half and bring it into the proximal wound.

Make a third 2- to 3-cm longitudinal incision over the cuboid on the dorsolateral aspect of the foot. Drill two holes in the cuboid, placing them as far away from each other as possible so that they meet well within the body of the cuboid (Fig. 31-10, *B*). Enlarge the holes with a curet if necessary but be certain to leave a bridge of bone between the two holes. Pass the split lateral portion of the tibialis anterior tendon distally through the subcutaneous tunnel from the proximal incision to the dorsolateral incision over the cuboid. Attach a nonabsorbable suture to the end of the tendon and pass it into one hole in the cuboid and out the other (Fig. 31-10, *C*). Hold the foot in dorsiflexion, pull the tendon tight, and suture the free end to the proximal portion of the tendon under moderate tension (Fig. 31-10, *D*).

As an alternative, drill a hole in the cuneiform through the plantar cortex, pass the tendon through this hole, and anchor it on the plantar aspect of the foot with a suture over felt and a button.

AFTERTREATMENT. A short leg cast is worn for 6 weeks. Hoffer et al. recommend the use of an ankle-foot orthosis for 6 months.

Split Transfer of Tibialis Posterior Tendon. This technique is used more often for patients with cerebral palsy and is described in Chapter 30.

Talipes Cavovarus

Paralytic talipes cavovarus can be caused by an imbalance of the extrinsic muscles or by persistent function of the short toe flexors and other intrinsic muscles when the foot is otherwise flail. Treatment of the cavus foot is discussed in Chapter 83.

Talipes Equinovalgus

Talipes equinovalgus usually develops when the tibialis anterior and posterior muscles are weak, the peroneus longus and peroneus brevis are strong, and the triceps surae is strong and contracted. The triceps surae pulls the foot into equinus and the peroneals into valgus position; when the extensor digitorum longus and the peroneus tertius muscles are also strong, they help to pull the foot into valgus position on walking. Structural changes in the bones and ligaments follow the muscle imbalance; eventually the plantar calcaneonavicular ligament becomes stretched and attenuated, the weight-bearing thrust shifts to the medial border of the foot, the forefoot abducts and pronates, and the head and neck of the talus become depressed and prominent on the medial side of the foot.

Treatment of this deformity in a skeletally immature foot is difficult. Subtalar arthrodesis and anterior transfer of the peroneus longus and brevis tendons usually will suffice until skeletal maturity is reached; if necessary, a triple arthrodesis can then be done. Failure to transfer the tendons is the usual cause of recurrence.

Paralysis of the tibialis anterior alone usually causes only a moderate valgus deformity that is more pronounced during dorsiflexion of the ankle and may disappear during plantar flexion. For this deformity, Fried and Hendel recommended transfer of the peroneus longus to the first cuneiform, transfer of the extensor digitorum longus, or the Jones procedure (Chapter 83). Paralysis of the tibialis posterior alone can cause a planovalgus deformity. Normally this muscle inverts the foot during plantar flexion, and when it is paralyzed, a valgus deformity develops. Since most of the functions of the foot are performed during plantar flexion, loss of the tibialis posterior is a severe impairment. Treatment of this deformity may involve transfer of the peroneus longus tendon, the flexor digitorum longus, the flexor hallucis longus, or the extensor hallucis longus. Paralysis of both the tibialis anterior and the tibialis posterior results in an extreme deformity similar to rocker-bottom flatfoot. For this deformity a transfer to replace the tibialis posterior is necessary, followed by another to replace the tibialis anterior if necessary. Extraarticular subtalar arthrodesis may be indicated for equinovalgus deformity in children 4 to 10 years of age. The equinus must be corrected by tendo calcaneus lengthening at surgery to allow the calcaneus to be brought far enough distally beneath the talus to correct the deformity. The technique of Grice and Green (Technique 31-3) or preferably of Dennyson and Fulford (Technique 31-4) can be used. Talipes equinovalgus in skeletally mature patients usually requires triple arthrodesis (Technique 31-5) and lengthening of the tendo calcaneus, followed in 4 to 6 weeks by appropriate tendon transfers.

◆ Peroneal Tendon Transfer

TECHNIQUE 31-11
Expose the tendons of the peroneus longus and peroneus brevis through an oblique incision paralleling the skin creases at a point midway between the distal tip of the lateral malleolus and the base of the fifth metatarsal. Divide the tendons as far distally as possible, securely suture the distal end of the peroneus longus to its sheath to prevent the development of a dorsal bunion, and free the tendons proximally to the posterior border of the lateral malleolus. (When they are to be transferred at the time of arthrodesis, they can be divided through a short extension of the routine incision, as shown in Fig. 31-6.) Make a second incision 5 cm long at the junction of the middle and distal thirds of the leg overlying the tendons. Gently withdraw the tendons from their sheaths, taking care not to disrupt the origin of the peroneus brevis muscle.

The new site of insertion of the peroneal tendons is determined by the severity of the deformity and the existing muscle power. When the extensor hallucis longus is functioning and is to be transferred to the neck of the first metatarsal, the peroneal tendons should be transferred to the lateral cuneiform; when no other functioning dorsiflexor is available, they should be transferred to the middle cuneiform anteriorly.

Expose the new site of insertion of the tendons through a short longitudinal incision. Retract the tendons of the extensor digitorum longus and make a cruciate or H-shaped cut in the periosteum of the recipient bone. Raise and fold back osteoperiosteal flaps and drill a hole in the bone large enough to receive the tendons. Then bring the tendons out beneath the cruciate crural ligament into this incision and anchor them side by side and under equal tension through a hole drilled in the bone, either by suturing them back on themselves or by securely fixing them to bone using a platform staple. As an alternative, drill a hole through the middle cuneiform and pull the tendons through the hole and then through a button on the plantar aspect of the foot.

When there is significant clawing of the great toe, the extensor hallucis longus tendon should be transferred to the neck of the first metatarsal, and the interphalangeal joint is fused (Jones procedure, Chapter 83). Residual clawing of the lateral four toes usually is of little or no significance after transfer of the peroneal and extensor hallucis longus tendons.

◆ Peroneus Longus, Flexor Digitorum Longus, or Flexor or Extensor Hallucis Longus Tendon Transfer

TECHNIQUE 31-12 *(Fried and Hendel)*
In this operation the tendon of the peroneus longus, flexor digitorum longus, flexor hallucis longus, or extensor hallucis longus can be transferred to replace a paralyzed tibialis posterior.

When the peroneus longus tendon is to be transferred, make a longitudinal incision 5 to 8 cm long laterally over the shaft of the fibula. After incising the fascia of the peroneal muscles, inspect them; if their color does not confirm their preoperative grading, the transfer will fail. Now make a second incision along the lateral border of the foot over the cuboid and the peroneus longus tendon. Free the tendon, divide it as far distally in the sole of the foot as possible, suture its distal end in its sheath, and withdraw the tendon through the first incision. By blunt dissection create a space between the triceps surae and the deep layer of leg muscles; from here make a wide tunnel posterior to the fibula and to the deep muscles and directed to a point proximal and posterior to the medial malleolus. Now make a small incision at this point and draw the peroneus longus tendon through the tunnel; it now emerges where the tibialis posterior tendon enters its sheath. Make a fourth incision 5 cm long over the middle of the medial side of the foot centered below the tuberosity of the navicular. Free and retract plantarward the anterior border of the abductor hallucis muscle and expose the tuberosity of the navicular and the insertion of the tibialis posterior tendon; proximal to the medial malleolus open the sheath of this tendon and into it introduce and advance a curved probe until it emerges

continued

with the tendon at the sole of the foot. Using the probe, pull the peroneus longus tendon through the same sheath, which is large enough to contain this second tendon. Now drill a narrow tunnel through the navicular, beginning on its plantar surface lateral to the tuberosity and emerging through its anterior surface. Pull the peroneus longus tendon through the tunnel in an anterior direction and anchor it with a Bunnell pull-out suture. Also suture it to the tibialis posterior tendon close to its insertion. Close the wounds and apply a short leg cast with the foot in slight equinus and varus position.

When the flexor digitorum longus tendon is to be transferred, make the incision near the medial malleolus as just described but extend it for about 7 cm. Free the three deep muscles and observe their color; if it is satisfactory, make the incision on the medial side of the foot as just described. Free and retract the short plantar muscles and expose the flexor digitorum longus tendon as it emerges from behind the medial malleolus. Free the tendon as far distally as possible, divide it, and withdraw it through the first incision; now pass it through the sheath of the tibialis posterior tendon and anchor it in the navicular as just described.

When the flexor hallucis longus tendon is to be transferred, use the same procedure as described for the flexor digitorum longus.

When the extensor hallucis longus tendon is to be transferred, cut it near the metatarsophalangeal joint of the great toe. Suture its distal end to the long extensor tendon of the second toe. Withdraw the proximal end through an anterolateral longitudinal incision over the distal part of the leg. Open the interosseous membrane widely, make the incision near the medial malleolus as previously described, and with a broad probe draw the tendon through the interosseous space and through the sheath of the tibialis posterior tendon to the insertion of that tendon. Then continue with the operation as described for transfer of the peroneus longus tendon.

AFTERTREATMENT. A short leg walking cast is applied. At 6 weeks the walking cast is removed, a splint is used at night, and muscle reeducation is started.

Talipes Calcaneus

Talipes calcaneus is a vicious, rapidly progressive paralytic deformity that results when the triceps surae is paralyzed and the other extrinsic foot muscles, especially those that dorsiflex the ankle, remain functional. Mild deformity in skeletally immature patients should be treated conservatively with braces or orthoses until the rate of progression of the deformity can be determined. For rapidly progressing deformities, especially in young children, Irwin recommended early tendon transfers. The goal of surgery in the skeletally immature foot is to stop progression of the deformity or to correct severe deformity

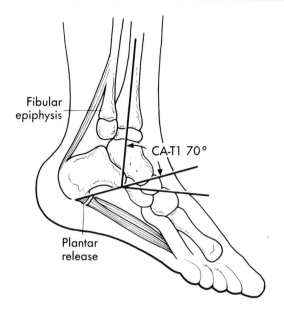

Fig. 31-11 Measurement of calcaneotibial angle (see text).

without damaging skeletal growth; arthrodesis may be necessary after skeletal maturity. If muscles of adequate power are available, tendons should be transferred early to improve function and avoid progressive deformity. If adequate muscles are not available, Westin recommended tenodesis of the tendo calcaneus to the fibula.

The calcaneotibial angle (Fig. 31-11) is formed by the intersection of the axis of the tibia with a line drawn along the plantar aspect of the calcaneus. Normally this angle measures between 70 and 80 degrees; in equinus deformity it is greater than 80 degrees, and in calcaneus deformity it is less than 70 degrees. In Westin's study of 66 patients, the average calcaneotibial angle before operation measured 55 degrees and at final follow-up was 76 degrees (Fig. 31-12). Westin also noted that when the tenodesis was fixed at 70 degrees or more at the time of surgery, the patient tended to develop a progressive equinus deformity with growth. Progressive equinus also was directly related to the patient's age at surgery: the younger the patient, the greater the calcaneotibial angle and the more likely the development of progressive equinus deformity with subsequent growth.

◆ **Tenodesis of Tendo Calcaneus**

TECHNIQUE 31-13 *(Westin)*

With the patient supine and tilted toward the nonoperative side, apply and inflate a pneumatic tourniquet. Make a posterolateral longitudinal incision just behind the posterior border of the fibula beginning 7 to 10 cm above the tip of the lateral malleolus and extending distally to the insertion of the tendo calcaneus on the calcaneus. Expose the tendon and section it transversely at the musculotendinous junction,

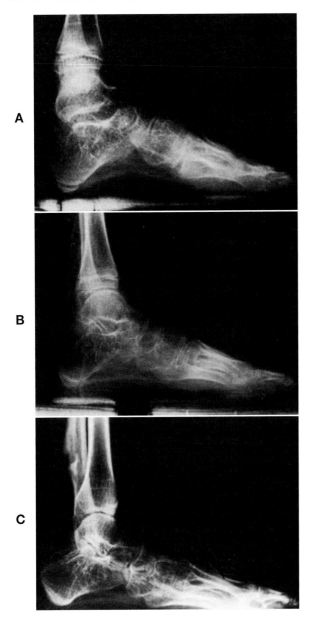

Fig. 31-12   Westin calcaneal tenodesis to fibula: preoperative **(A),** immediately after operation **(B),** and 3½ years after surgery **(C).** (Courtesy GW Westin, MD.)

usually 6 cm from its insertion. Stevens advised that the tendon be split eccentrically, leaving the lateral one fifth to prevent retraction. Transect the medial four fifths proximally. Expose the peroneus brevis and longus tendons, and if they are completely paralyzed or spastic, excise them. Expose the distal fibula, taking care not to damage the distal fibular physis. About 4 cm proximal to the distal physis, use a fine drill bit to make a transverse hole in an anteroposterior direction. Make the hole large enough for the tendo calcaneus to pass through it easily (Fig. 31-13, *A*). If the

tendon is too large, trim it longitudinally for about 2.5 cm. Bring the tendon through the hole and suture it to itself under enough tension to limit ankle dorsiflexion to 0 degrees (Fig. 31-13, *B*). Do not suture the tendon with the foot in too much equinus because of the possibility of causing a fixed equinus deformity.

In patients with active tibialis anterior tendons, simultaneous transfer of this tendon through the interosseous membrane to the calcaneus is indicated to avoid stretching of the tendo calcaneus after surgery (Fig. 31-13, *C*).

AFTERTREATMENT. Weight-bearing is allowed in a short leg cast with the ankle in 5 to 10 degrees of equinus. The cast is removed at 6 weeks, and an ankle-foot orthosis is fitted with the ankle in neutral position. Any residual cavus deformity is corrected by plantar release 3 to 6 months after tenodesis.

◆ ◆ ◆

In skeletally mature feet, initial surgery for talipes calcaneus consists of plantar fasciotomy and triple arthrodesis that corrects both the calcaneus and cavus deformities; the arthrodesis should displace the foot as far posteriorly as possible to lengthen its posterior lever arm (the calcaneus) and reduce the muscle power required to lift the heel. Six weeks after arthrodesis, the tendons of the peroneus longus and peroneus brevis and the tibialis posterior are transferred to the calcaneus, and when the extensor digitorum longus is functional, it can be transferred to a cuneiform, and the tibialis anterior also can then be transferred to the calcaneus.

◆ **Posterior Transfer of Peroneus Longus, Peroneus Brevis, and Tibialis Posterior Tendons**

TECHNIQUE 31-14
Expose the peroneus longus and peroneus brevis tendons through an oblique incision 2.5 cm long midway between the tip of the lateral malleolus and the base of the fifth metatarsal. Divide the tendons as far distally as possible and securely suture the distal end of the peroneus longus tendon to its sheath. Then bring the tendons out through a second incision overlying the peroneal sheath at the junction of the middle and distal thirds of the leg. If desired, suture the peroneus brevis at its musculotendinous junction to the peroneus longus tendon and discard the distal end of the peroneus brevis tendon. Expose the tibialis posterior tendon through a short incision over its insertion; free its distal end and gently bring it out through a second incision 2.5 cm long at its musculotendinous junction 5 cm proximal to the medial malleolus. Then reroute all three tendons subcutaneously to and out of a separate incision lateral and anterior to the insertion of the tendo calcaneus. Drill a hole in the superior surface of the posterior part of the calcaneus

continued

just lateral to the midline of the bone and enlarge it enough to receive the tendons; anchor the tendons in the hole with a large pull-out suture while holding the foot in equinus and the heel in the corrected position. An axial pin also can be inserted into the calcaneus and left in place for 6 weeks. With interrupted figure-eight sutures, transfix the tendons to the tendo calcaneus near its insertion; then close the wounds.

AFTERTREATMENT. The foot is immobilized in a long leg cast with the ankle in plantar flexion and the knee at 20 degrees. The pull-out sutures and cast (and axial pin, if used) are removed at 6 weeks, and physical therapy is started. Weight-bearing is not allowed until active plantar flexion is possible and dorsiflexion to the neutral position has been regained. The foot is protected for at least 6 more months by a reverse 90-degree ankle stop brace and an appropriate heel elevation.

◆ **Posterior Transfer of Tibialis Posterior, Peroneus Longus, and Flexor Hallucis Longus Tendons**

TECHNIQUE 31-15 *(Green and Grice)*
Place the patient prone for easier access to the heel. First, expose the tibialis posterior tendon through an oblique incision 3 or 4 cm long from just inferior to the medial malleolus to the plantar aspect of the talonavicular joint; open its sheath and divide it as close to bone as possible for maximal length. Then remove the peritenon from its distal 3 or 4 cm, scarify it, and insert a 1-0 or 2-0 braided silk suture into its distal end. When the flexor hallucis longus tendon also is to be transferred, expose it through this same incision where it lies posterior and lateral to the flexor digitorum longus tendon. At the proper level for the desired tendon length, place two braided silk sutures in the flexor hallucis longus tendon and divide it between them; suture the distal end of this tendon to the flexor digitorum longus tendon. Second, make a longitudinal medial incision, usually about 10 cm long, over the tibialis posterior muscle, extending distally from the junction of the middle and distal thirds of the leg. Open the medial compartment of the leg and identify the tibialis posterior and flexor hallucis longus muscle bellies. Using moist sponges, deliver the tendons of these two muscles into this wound. Third, make an incision parallel to the bottom of the foot from about a fingerbreadth distal to the lateral malleolus to the base of the fifth metatarsal. Expose the peroneus longus and peroneus brevis tendons throughout the length of the incision and divide that of the peroneus longus between sutures as far distally as possible in the sole of the foot and free its proximal end to behind the lateral malleolus. Then place a suture in the peroneus brevis tendon, detach it from its insertion on the fifth metatarsal, and suture it to the distal end of the

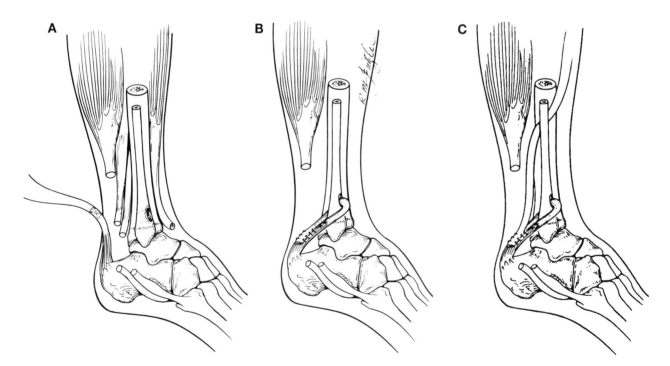

Fig. 31-13   Calcaneal tenodesis. **A,** After division of tendo calcaneus, tenotomy of peroneus brevis and longus, and detachment of tibialis anterior tendon from its insertion, transverse hole is made in fibula 2 cm proximal to epiphysis. **B,** Tendo calcaneus is passed through hole in fibula and sutured to itself. **C,** If necessary, tibialis anterior tendon can be passed through interosseous membrane and attached to calcaneus.

peroneus longus tendon. Fourth, make a lateral longitudinal incision over the posterior aspect of the fibula at the same level as the medial incision and deliver the peroneus longus tendon into it. Fifth, make a posterolateral transverse incision 6 cm long over the calcaneus in the part of the heel that neither strikes the ground nor presses against the shoe. Deepen the incision, reflect the skin flaps subcutaneously, and expose the tendo calcaneus and calcaneus. Beginning laterally, partially divide the tendo calcaneus at its insertion and reflect it medially, exposing the calcaneal apophysis. With a 9/64-inch (3.57-mm) drill bit, make a hole through the calcaneus beginning in the center of its apophysis and emerging through its plantar aspect near its lateral border. Enlarge the hole enough to receive the three tendons and ream its posterior end to make a shallow facet for their easier insertion.

Now, through the medial wound on the leg (the second incision), incise widely the intermuscular septum between the medial and posterior compartments; insert a tendon passer through the wound and along the anterior side of the tendo calcaneus to the transverse incision over the calcaneus. Thread the sutures in the ends of the tibialis posterior and flexor hallucis longus tendons through the tendon passer and deliver the tendons at the heel. Now, through the lateral wound on the leg (the fourth incision), open widely the intermuscular septum between the medial and posterior compartments in this area and pass the peroneus longus tendon to the heel. Pass all tendons through smooth tissues in a straight line from as far proximally as possible to avoid angulation. With a twisted wire probe bring the tendons through the hole in the calcaneus; suture them to the periosteum and ligamentous attachments where they emerge. When the dorsiflexors are weak, suture them under enough tension to hold the foot in 10 to 15 degrees of equinus, and when they are strong, in about 30 degrees of equinus. Also suture the tendons to the apophysis at the proximal end of the tunnel and to each other with 2-0 or 3-0 sutures. Replace the tendo calcaneus posterior to the transferred tendons and suture it in its original position. Close the wounds and apply a long leg cast with the foot in equinus.

AFTERTREATMENT. At 3 weeks the cast is bivalved, and exercises are started with the leg in the anterior half of the cast; the bivalved cast is reapplied between exercise periods. At first dorsiflexion exercises are not permitted, but later, guided reciprocal motion is allowed. The exercises are gradually increased, and at 6 weeks the patient is allowed to stand but not to bear full weight on the foot. The periods of partial weight-bearing on crutches are increased, depending on the effectiveness of the transfer, the cooperation of the patient, and his ability to control his motions. Usually at 6 to 8 weeks a single step is allowed, using crutches and an elevated heel; later more steps are allowed, using crutches and a plantar flexion spring brace with an elastic strap posteriorly. Crutches are continued for 6 to 12 months.

Knee

The disabilities caused by paralysis of the muscles acting across the knee joint include (1) flexion contracture of the knee, (2) quadriceps paralysis, (3) genu recurvatum, and (4) flail knee.

FLEXION CONTRACTURE OF KNEE

Flexion contracture of the knee can be caused by a contracture of the iliotibial band; contracture of this band can cause not only flexion contracture but also genu valgum and an external rotation deformity of the tibia on the femur. Flexion contracture also can be caused by paralysis of the quadriceps muscle when the hamstrings are normal or only partially paralyzed. When the biceps femoris is stronger than the medial hamstrings, there may again be genu valgum and an external rotation deformity of the tibia on the femur; often the tibia subluxates posteriorly on the femur.

Contractures of 15 to 20 degrees or less in young children can be treated with posterior hamstring lengthening and capsulotomy. More severe contractures usually require a supracondylar extension osteotomy of the femur (Fig. 31-14).

Flexion contractures of more than 70 degrees result in deformity of the articular surfaces of the knee. In a growing child with poliomyelitis, a decrease in pressure and a tendency toward posterior subluxation cause increased growth on the anterior surface of the proximal tibia and distal femur. The quadriceps expansion adheres to the femoral condyles and the collateral ligaments are unable to glide easily. Severe knee flexion contractures in growing children can be treated by division of the iliotibial band and hamstring tendons, combined with posterior capsulotomy. Skeletal traction after surgery is maintained through a pin in the distal tibia; a second pin in the proximal tibia pulls anteriorly to avoid posterior subluxation of the tibia. Long-term use of a long leg brace may be required to

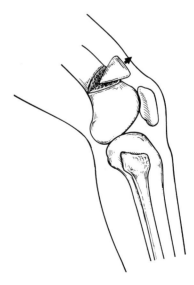

Fig. 31-14 Supracondylar extension osteotomy of femur for fixed knee flexion deformity in older child.

allow the joint to remodel. Supracondylar osteotomy may be required as a second-stage procedure in older patients near skeletal maturity.

QUADRICEPS PARALYSIS

Disability from paralysis of the quadriceps muscle is severe because the knee may be very unstable, especially if there is even a mild fixed flexion contracture. When there is slight recurvatum, the knee may be stable if the triceps surae is active.

Tendons usually are transferred about the knee joint to reinforce a weak or paralyzed quadriceps muscle; transfers are not necessary for paralysis of the hamstring muscles because in walking, gravity flexes the knee as the hip is flexed. Several muscles are available for transfer to the quadriceps tendon and patella: the biceps femoris, semitendinosus, sartorius, and tensor fasciae latae. When the power of certain other muscles is satisfactory, transfer of the biceps femoris has been the most successful. Transfer of one or more of the hamstring tendons is contraindicated unless one other flexor in the thigh and the triceps surae, which also acts as a knee flexor, are functioning. If a satisfactory result is to be expected after hamstring transfer, the power not only of the hamstrings but also of the hip flexors, the gluteus maximus, and the triceps surae must be fair or better; when the hip flexor muscles are less than fair, clearing the extremity from the floor may be difficult after surgery. Transfer of the tensor fasciae latae and sartorius muscles, although theoretically more satisfactory, is insufficient because these muscles are not strong enough to replace the quadriceps.

Ease in ascending or descending steps depends on the strength of the hip flexors and extensors. Strong hamstrings are necessary for active extension of the knee against gravity after the transfer; however, a weak medial hamstring can be transferred to serve as a checkrein on the patella to prevent it from dislocating laterally. A normal triceps surae is desirable because it aids in preventing genu recurvatum and remains as an active knee flexor after surgery; it may not, however, always prevent genu recurvatum, which can result from other factors. Recurvatum after hamstring transfers can be kept to a minimum if (1) strength in the triceps surae is fair or better, (2) the knee is not immobilized in hyperextension after surgery, (3) talipes equinus, when present, is corrected before weight-bearing is resumed, (4) postoperative bracing is used to prevent knee hyperextension, and (5) physical therapy is begun to promote active knee extension.

◆ Transfer of Biceps Femoris and Semitendinosus Tendons

TECHNIQUE 31-16
Make an incision along the anteromedial aspect of the knee to conform to the medial border of the quadriceps tendon, the patella, and the patellar tendon. Retract the lateral edge of the incision and expose the patella and the quadriceps tendon. Then incise longitudinally the lateral side of the thigh and leg from a point 7.5 cm distal to the head of the fibula to the junction of the proximal and middle thirds of the thigh. Isolate and retract the common peroneal nerve, which is near the medial side of the biceps tendon. With an osteotome, free the biceps tendon, along with a thin piece of bone, from the head of the fibula. Do not divide the fibular collateral ligament, which lies firmly adherent to the biceps tendon at its point of insertion. Free the tendon and its muscle belly proximally as far as the incision will permit; free the origin of the short head of the biceps proximally to where its nerve and blood supplies enter so that the new line of pull of the muscle may be as oblique as possible. Now create a subcutaneous tunnel from the first incision to the lateral thigh incision and make it wide enough for the transferred muscle belly to glide freely. To further increase the obliquity of pull of the transferred muscle, divide the iliotibial band, the fascia of the vastus lateralis, and the lateral intermuscular septum at a point distal to where the muscle will pass.

Beginning distally over the insertion of the medial hamstring tendons into the tibia, make a third incision longitudinally along the posteromedial aspect of the knee and extend it to the middle of the thigh. Locate the semitendinosus tendon; it inserts on the medial side of the tibia as far anteriorly as its crest and lies posterior to the tendon of the sartorius and distal to that of the gracilis. Divide the insertion of the semitendinosus tendon and free the muscle to the middle third of the thigh. Now reroute this muscle and tendon subcutaneously to emerge in the first incision over the knee.

Make an I-shaped incision through the fascia, quadriceps tendon, and periosteum over the anterior surface of the patella and strip these tissues medially and laterally. Next, with an 11/64-inch (4.36-mm) drill bit, make a hole transversely through the patella at the junction of its middle and proximal thirds; if necessary, enlarge the tunnel with a small curet. Then place the biceps tendon in line with and anterior to the quadriceps tendon, the patella, and the patellar tendon. Suture the biceps tendon to the patella with the knee in extension or hyperextension. When only the biceps tendon is transferred, close the soft tissues over the anterior aspect of the patella and the transferred tendon. With interrupted sutures fix the biceps tendon to the medial side of the quadriceps tendon. When the semitendinosus also is transferred, place it over the biceps and suture the two together with interrupted sutures; place additional sutures proximally and distally through the semitendinosus, quadriceps, and patellar tendons.

Crego and Fischer's technique differs from that just described. The insertion of the semitendinosus is detached from the tibia through an incision 2.5 cm long and is brought out through a posteromedial incision 7.5 cm long over its musculotendinous junction (Fig. 31-15). The enveloping

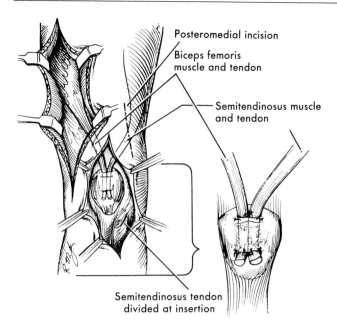

Posteromedial incision

Biceps femoris
muscle and tendon

Semitendinosus muscle
and tendon

Semitendinosus tendon
divided at insertion

Fig. 31-15 Transfer of semitendinosus and biceps femoris tendons to patella for quadriceps paralysis. (Modified from Schwartzmann JR, Crego CH Jr: *J Bone Joint Surg* 30A:541, 1948.)

fascia is incised to prevent acute angulation of the muscle, and the tendon is passed subcutaneously in a straight line to the patellar incision.

AFTERTREATMENT. With the knee in the neutral position, a long leg cast is applied. To prevent swelling, the extremity is elevated by raising the foot of the bed rather than by using pillows; otherwise, flexion of the hip may put too much tension on the transferred tendons.

At 3 weeks physical therapy and active and passive exercises are started. Knee flexion is gradually developed, and the hamstring muscles are reeducated. At 8 weeks weight-bearing is started, with the extremity supported by a controlled dial knee brace locked in extension. Knee motion is gradually allowed in the brace when the muscles of the transferred tendons are strong enough to extend the knee actively against considerable force. To prevent overstretching or strain of the muscles, a night splint is worn for at least 6 weeks and the brace for at least 12 weeks.

GENU RECURVATUM

In genu recurvatum the deformity is the opposite of that in a flexion contracture, and the knee is hyperextended. Mild genu recurvatum can cause some disability, but when the quadriceps is severely weakened or paralyzed, such a deformity is desirable because it stabilizes the knee in walking. However, severe genu recurvatum is significantly disabling.

Genu recurvatum from poliomyelitis is of two types: that

caused by structural articular and bony changes stemming from lack of power in the quadriceps, and that caused by relaxation of the soft tissues about the posterior aspect of the knee. In the first type the quadriceps lacks the power to lock the knee in extension; the hamstrings and triceps surae usually are normal. The pressures of weight-bearing and gravity cause changes in the tibial condyles and in the proximal third of the tibial shaft. The condyles become elongated posteriorly, their anterior margins are depressed compared with their posterior margins, and the angle of their articular surfaces to the long axis of the tibia, which is normally 90 degrees, becomes more acute. The proximal third of the tibial shaft usually bows posteriorly, and partial subluxation of the tibia may gradually occur. In the second type, both the hamstrings and the triceps surae muscles are weak. Hyperextension of the knee results from stretching of these muscles, often followed by stretching of the posterior capsular ligament.

The prognosis after correction of the first type of recurvatum is excellent: the skeletal deformity is corrected first, and then one or more hamstrings can be transferred to the patella. Irwin described an osteotomy of the proximal tibia to correct the first type of genu recurvatum caused by structural bone changes. Storen modified the Campbell osteotomy by immobilizing the fragments of the tibia with a Charnley clamp.

◆ Osteotomy of Tibia for Genu Recurvatum

TECHNIQUE 31-17 *(Irwin)*

Through a short longitudinal incision remove a section of the shaft of the fibula about 2.5 cm long from just distal to the neck. Pack the defect with chips from the sectioned piece of bone. Close the periosteum and overlying soft tissues. Through an anteromedial incision expose and, without entering the joint, osteotomize the proximal fourth of the tibia as follows. With a thin osteotome or a power saw, outline a tongue of bone but leave it attached to the anterior cortex of the distal fragment. Now, at a right angle to the longitudinal axis of the knee joint and parallel to its lateral plane, pass a Kirschner wire through the distal end of the proposed proximal fragment before the tibial shaft is divided. Then complete the osteotomy with a Gigli saw, an osteotome, or a power saw. Lift the proximal end of the distal fragment from its periosteal bed and remove from it a wedge of bone of predetermined size, its base being the posterior cortex. Replace the tongue in its recess in the proximal fragment and push the fragments firmly together. Suture the periosteum, which is quite thick in this area, firmly over the tongue; this is enough fixation to keep the fragments in position until a cast can be applied.

AFTERTREATMENT. The patient is placed on a fracture table, and the extremity is suspended to an overhead arm with traction through the Kirschner wire bow. The proximal fragment is hyperextended to its fullest extent by the weight of

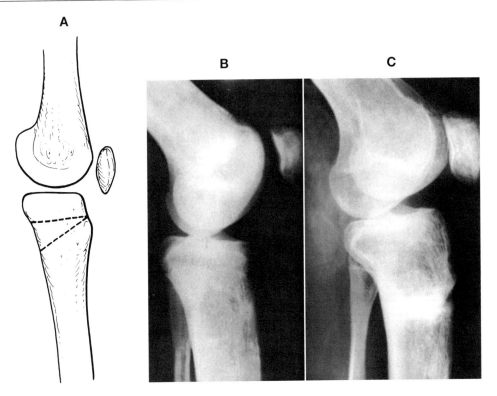

Fig. 31-16 Closing wedge osteotomy for genu recurvatum. **A,** Wedge of bone removed from tibia. **B,** Recurvatum secondary to anterior tilt of tibial plateau. **C,** Five months after operation.

the extremity and by pressure applied to the anterior surface of the distal thigh. With the extremity in this position, a long leg cast is applied. The position of the fragments and the general alignment of the extremity are checked by roentgenograms. When necessary, further changes in the position of the distal fragment are made by wedging the cast distal to the wire 10 to 14 days after surgery. The wire is removed at 6 weeks, and a new long leg cast is applied. At about 8 weeks the osteotomy usually is united, and the cast is removed. Full knee motion should be regained before any operation is done to correct the underlying cause of the recurvatum.

As an alternative, the osteotomy can be fixed with percutaneous Kirschner wires, an external fixator, or, in adults, rigid plate fixation.

Fig. 31-16 shows correction of genu recurvatum by the Campbell technique.

Soft Tissue Operations for Genu Recurvatum

Another type of genu recurvatum results from stretching of the posterior soft tissues. The prognosis is less certain after correction of this type of deformity; no muscles are available for transfer, the underlying cause cannot be corrected, and the deformity can recur. Perry, O'Brien, and Hodgson described an operation on the soft tissues, triple tenodesis of the knee, for correcting paralytic genu recurvatum. They pointed out that if the deformity is 30 degrees or less, prolonged bracing of the knee in flexion usually prevents an increase in deformity. However, when the deformity is severe, bracing is ineffective, the knee becomes unstable and weak, the gait is inefficient, and, in adults, pain is marked. Perry et al. listed the three following

principles that must be considered if operations on the soft tissues for genu recurvatum are to be successful.

1. The fibrous tissue mass used for tenodesis must be sufficient to withstand the stretching forces generated by walking; thus all available tendons must be used.
2. Healing tissues must be protected until they are fully mature. The operation should not be undertaken unless the surgeon is sure that the patient will conscientiously use a brace that limits extension to 15 degrees of flexion for 1 year.
3. The alignment and stability of the ankle must meet the basic requirements of gait. Any equinus deformity must be corrected to at least neutral. If the strength of the soleus is less than good on the standing test, this defect must be corrected by tendon transfer, tenodesis, or arthrodesis of the ankle in the neutral position.

◆ Triple Tenodesis for Genu Recurvatum

TECHNIQUE 31-18 *(Perry, O'Brien, and Hodgson)*

The operation consists of three parts: proximal advancement of the posterior capsule of the knee with the joint flexed 20 degrees, construction of a checkrein in the midline posteriorly using the tendons of the semitendinosus and gracilis, and creation of two diagonal straps posteriorly using the biceps tendon and the anterior half of the ilio-tibial band.

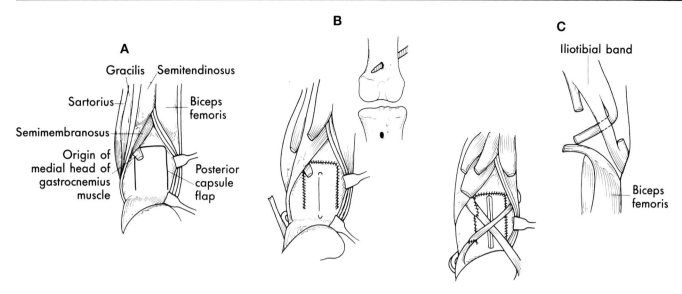

Fig. 31-17   Perry, O'Brien, and Hodgson operation for genu recurvatum. **A,** Origin of medial head of gastrocnemius has been released, leaving proximal strap. Broad flap of posterior capsule is released for future advancement. **B,** Semitendinosus and gracilis tendons are divided at musculotendinous junctions. Each is passed through tunnel in tibia, then across exterior of joint, and then through tunnel in femur. Flap of posterior capsule is advanced and sutured snugly with knee flexed 20 degrees. **C,** Cross straps are made with biceps femoris and iliotibial band (see text). (Redrawn from Perry J, O'Brien JP, Hodgson AR: *J Bone Joint Surg* 58A:978, 1976.)

Place the patient prone, apply a tourniquet high on the thigh, and place a large sandbag beneath the ankle to flex the knee about 20 degrees. Make an S-shaped incision beginning laterally parallel to and 1 cm anterior to the biceps tendon; extend it distally 4 cm to the transverse flexion crease of the knee; then carry it medially across the popliteal fossa; and finally extend it distally for 4 or 5 cm overlying or just medial to the semitendinosus tendon. Identify the sural nerve and retract it laterally. Then identify the tibial nerve and the popliteal artery and vein and protect them with a soft rubber tape. Next identify and free the peroneal nerve and protect it in a similar manner. Retract the neurovascular bundle laterally and identify the posterior part of the joint capsule. Detach the medial head of the gastrocnemius muscle in a step-cut fashion, preserving a long, strong proximal strap of the Z to be used in the tenodesis (Fig. 31-17, *A*). Next, use a knife to detach the joint capsule from its attachment to the femur just proximal to the condyles and the intercondylar notch. Detach the tendons of the gracilis and semitendinosus at their musculotendinous junctions and suture their proximal ends to the sartorius. Be sure to divide these tendons as far proximally as possible because all available length will be needed. Next, drill a hole in the tibia beginning at a point in the midline posteriorly inferior to the physis and emerging near the insertion of the pes anserinus; take care to avoid the physis. Next drill a hole in the femur beginning in the midline posteriorly proximal

to the femoral physis and emerging on the lateral aspect of the distal femur (Fig. 31-17, *B*). Draw the tendons of the gracilis and semitendinosus through the hole in the tibia, pass them posterior to the detached part of the capsule, and pull them through the hole in the femur to emerge on the lateral aspect of the distal femur; suture the tendons to the periosteum here under moderate tension with heavy nonabsorbable sutures with the knee flexed 20 degrees. Now advance the free edge of the joint capsule proximally on the femur until all slack has disappeared and suture it to the periosteum in its new position using nonabsorbable sutures. Detach the biceps tendon from its muscle, rotate it on its fibular insertion, and pass it across the posterior aspect of the joint deep to the neurovascular structures and anchor it to the femoral origin of the medial head of the gastrocnemius under moderate tension (Fig. 31-17, *C*). Next detach the anterior half of the iliotibial band from its insertion on the tibia, pass it deep to the intact part of the band, the biceps tendon, and the neurovascular structures, and suture it to the semimembranosus insertion on the tibia under moderate tension. If one of the tendons being used is of an active muscle, split that tendon and use only half of it in the tenodesis, leaving the other half attached at its insertion. Close the wound in layers and use suction drainage for 48 hours. Apply a well-padded cast from groin to toes with the knee flexed 30 degrees to prevent tension on the sutures.

AFTERTREATMENT. The cast is removed at 6 weeks, and a long leg brace that was fitted before surgery is applied. The brace is designed to limit extension of the knee to 15 degrees of flexion. Full weight-bearing is allowed in the brace, and at night a plaster shell is used to hold the knee flexed 15 degrees. Twelve months after surgery the patient is readmitted to the hospital, and the flexion contracture of the knee is corrected gradually to neutral by serial plaster casts; unprotected weight-bearing is then permitted. According to Perry, O'Brien, and Hodgson, it is extremely important that the soft tissues are completely healed before being subjected to excessive stretching caused by unprotected weight-bearing or by wedging plaster casts.

FLAIL KNEE

When the knee is unstable in all directions and muscle power sufficient to overcome this instability is not available for tendon transfer, either a long leg brace with a locking knee joint must be worn or the knee must be fused. Fusion of the knee in a good position not only permits a satisfactory gait but also improves it by eliminating the weight of the brace; on the other hand, fusion of the knee causes inconvenience while sitting. One option is to defer fusion until the patient is old enough to weigh its advantages and disadvantages before a final decision is made. For patients who are heavy laborers and would have trouble maintaining a brace, the advantages of being free of a brace outweigh the advantages of being able to sit with the knee flexed in a brace; in these patients, an arthrodesis is indicated. Others who sit much of the time may prefer to use a brace permanently. When both legs are badly paralyzed, one knee can be fused and the other stabilized with a brace.

Before an arthrodesis is performed, a cylinder cast can be applied on a trial basis, immobilizing the knee in the position in which it would be fused; this allows the patient to make an informed decision concerning the advantages and disadvantages of arthrodesis of the knee. The techniques of knee fusion are described in Chapter 3.

Tibia and Femur

Angular and torsional deformities of the tibia and femur are more often caused by conditions other than poliomyelitis, such as congenital abnormalities, metabolic disorders, or trauma, and the various osteotomies used for their treatment are discussed in Chapters 33 and 26.

Hip

Paralysis of the muscles about the hip can cause severe impairment. This may include flexion and abduction contractures of the hip, hip instability and limping caused by paralysis of the gluteus maximus and medius muscles, and paralytic hip dislocation.

FLEXION AND ABDUCTION CONTRACTURES OF HIP

An abduction contracture is the most common deformity associated with paralysis of the muscles about the hip; it usually occurs in conjunction with flexion and external rotation contractures of varying degrees. Less often a contracture of the hip may occur that consists of adduction with flexion and internal rotation. When contractures of the hip are severe and bilateral, locomotion is possible only as a quadruped; the upright position is possible after the contractures have been released.

Spasm of the hamstrings, the hip flexors, the tensor fasciae latae, and the hip abductors is common during the acute and convalescent stages of poliomyelitis. Straight-leg raising usually is limited. The patient assumes the frog position, with the knees and hips flexed and the extremities completely externally rotated. When this position is maintained for even a few weeks, secondary soft tissue contractures occur; thus a permanent deformity develops, especially when the gluteal muscles have been weakened. The deformity puts the gluteus maximus at a disadvantage and prevents its return to normal strength. If the faulty position is not corrected, growth of the contracted soft tissues will fail to keep pace with bone growth and the deformity will progressively increase. On the other hand, if positioning in bed is correct while muscle spasm is present and if the joints are carried through a full range of motion at regular intervals after the muscle spasm disappears, contractures can be prevented and soft tissues can be kept sufficiently long and elastic to meet normal functional demands.

The large expanse of the tensor fasciae latae must be recognized before the deforming possibilities of the iliotibial band can be appreciated. Proximally the fascia lata arises from the coccyx, the sacrum, the crest of the ilium, the inguinal ligament, and the pubic arch and invests the muscles of the thigh and buttock. Either the superficial or the deep layer is attached to most of the gluteus maximus muscle and to all of the tensor fasciae latae muscle. All the attachments of the fascia converge to form the iliotibial band on the lateral side of the thigh.

Contracture of the iliotibial band can contribute to the following deformities:

1. *Flexion, abduction, and external rotation contracture of the hip.* The iliotibial band lies lateral and anterior to the hip joint, and its contracture can cause flexion and abduction deformity. The hip is externally rotated for comfort and, if not corrected, the external rotators of the hip contract and contribute to a fixed deformity.
2. *Genu valgum and flexion contracture of the knee.* With growth, the contracted iliotibial band acts as a taut bowstring across the knee joint and gradually abducts and flexes the tibia.
3. *Limb length discrepancy.* Although the exact mechanism has not been clearly defined and may be related more to the loss of neurological and muscle function, a

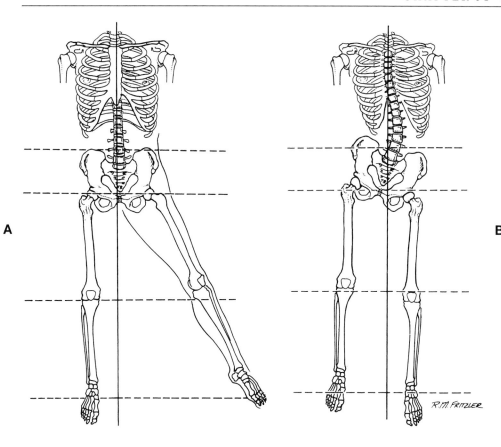

Fig. 31-18 **A,** In abduction contracture of hip, spine remains straight and pelvis level as long as hip is in abduction. **B,** When hip with abduction contracture is brought into weight-bearing position, pelvis must assume oblique position, causing scoliosis of lumbar spine. (Courtesy CE Irwin, MD.)

contracted iliotibial band on one side may be associated with considerable shortening of that extremity after years of growth.

4. *External tibial torsion, with or without knee joint subluxation.* Because of its lateral attachment distally, the iliotibial band gradually rotates the tibia and fibula externally on the femur; this rotation may be increased if the short head of the biceps is strong. When the deformity becomes extreme, the lateral tibial condyle subluxates on the lateral femoral condyle and the head of the fibula lies in the popliteal space.

5. *Secondary ankle and foot deformities.* With external torsion of the tibia, the axes of the ankle and knee joints are malaligned, causing structural changes that may require surgical correction.

6. *Pelvic obliquity.* When the iliotibial band is contracted and the patient is supine with the hip in abduction and flexion, the pelvis may remain at a right angle to the long axis of the spine (Fig. 31-18, *A*). When the patient stands, however, and the affected extremity is brought into the weight-bearing position (parallel to the vertical axis of the trunk), the pelvis assumes an oblique position: the iliac crest is low on the contracted side and high on the opposite side. The lateral thrust forces the pelvis toward the unaffected side. Further, the trunk muscles on the affected side lengthen, and those on the opposite side contract. An associated lumbar scoliosis can develop. If not corrected, the two contralateral contractures, that is,

the band on the affected side and the trunk muscles on the unaffected side, hold the pelvis in this oblique position until skeletal changes fix the deformity (Fig. 31-18, *B*).

7. *Increased lumbar lordosis.* Bilateral flexion contractures of the hip pull the proximal part of the pelvis anteriorly; for the trunk to assume an upright position, a compensatory increase in lumbar lordosis must develop.

A flexion and abduction contracture of the hip can be minimized or prevented in the early convalescent stage of poliomyelitis. The patient should be placed in bed with the hips in neutral rotation, slight abduction, and no flexion. All joints must be carried through a full range of passive motion several times daily; the hips must be stretched in extension, adduction, and internal rotation. To prevent rotation a bar similar to a Denis Browne splint is useful, especially when a knee roll is used to prevent a genu recurvatum deformity; the bar is clamped to the shoe soles to hold the feet in slight internal rotation. The contracture is carefully watched for in the acute and early convalescent stages; if found, it must be corrected before ambulation is allowed.

Irwin pointed out that secondary adaptive changes occur soon after the iliotibial band contracts and that the resulting deformity, regardless of its duration or of the patient's age, cannot be corrected by conservative measures; on the contrary, attempts at correction with traction will only increase the obliquity and hyperextension of the pelvis and cannot exert any helpful corrective force on the deformity.

Simple fasciotomies about the hip and knee may correct a

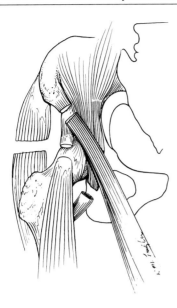

Fig. 31-19 Complete release of flexion-abduction–external rotation contracture of hip (see text).

minor contracture, but recurrence is common; they will not correct a severe contracture. For abduction and external rotation contractures, a complete release of the hip muscles (Ober-Yount procedure) is indicated. For severe deformities, complete release of all muscles from the iliac wing with transfer of the crest of the ilium (Campbell technique) is indicated.

◆ Complete Hip Release of Flexion, Abduction, and External Rotation Contracture

TECHNIQUE 31-19 *(Ober; Yount)*
With the patient in a lateral position, make a transverse incision medial and distal to the anterosuperior iliac spine, extending it laterally above the greater trochanter. Divide the iliopsoas tendon distally and excise 1 cm of it. Detach the sartorius from its origin in the anterosuperior iliac spine, detach the rectus from the anteroinferior iliac spine, and divide the tensor fasciae latae from its anterior border completely posteriorly (Fig. 31-19). Detach the gluteus medius and minimus and the short external rotators from their insertions on the trochanter. Retract the sciatic nerve posteriorly. Then open the hip capsule from anterior to posterior, parallel with the acetabular labrum. Close the wound over a suction drain and apply a hip spica cast with the hip in full extension, 10 degrees of abduction, and, if possible, internal rotation.

For the Yount procedure expose the fascia lata through a lateral longitudinal incision just proximal to the femoral condyle. Divide the iliotibial band and fascia lata posteriorly to the biceps tendon and anteriorly to the midline of the thigh at a level 2.5 cm proximal to the patella. At this level

excise a segment of the iliotibial band and lateral intermuscular septum 5 to 8 cm long. Before closing the wound, determine by palpation that all tight bands have been divided.

AFTERTREATMENT. The cast is removed at 2 weeks, and a long leg brace with a pelvic band is fitted with the hip in the same position.

◆ Complete Release of Muscles from Iliac Wing and Transfer of Crest of Ilium

TECHNIQUE 31-20 *(Campbell)*
Incise the skin along the anterior one half or two thirds of the iliac crest to the anterosuperior spine and then distally for 5 to 10 cm on the anterior surface of the thigh. Divide the superficial and deep fasciae to the crest of the ilium. Strip the origins of the tensor fasciae latae and gluteus medius and minimus muscles subperiosteally from the wing of the ilium down to the acetabulum (Fig. 31-20, *A*). Then free the proximal part of the sartorius from the tensor fasciae latae. With an osteotome resect the anterosuperior iliac spine along with the origin of the sartorius muscle and allow both to retract distally and posteriorly. Next denude the anterior border of the ilium down to the anteroinferior spine. Free subperiosteally the attachments of the abdominal muscles from the iliac crest (or resect a narrow strip of bone with the attachments). Strip the iliacus muscle subperiosteally from the inner table. Free the straight tendon of the rectus femoris muscle from the anteroinferior iliac spine and the reflected tendon from the anterior margin of the acetabulum or simply divide the conjoined tendon of the muscle. Releasing these contracted structures often will allow the hip to be hyperextended without increasing the lumbar lordosis; this is a most important point because in this situation correction may be more apparent than real. If the hip cannot be hyperextended, other contracted structures must be divided. If necessary, divide the capsule of the hip obliquely from proximally to distally and as a last resort free the iliopsoas muscle from the lesser trochanter by tenotomy.

After the deformity has been completely corrected, resect the redundant part of the denuded ilium with an osteotome (Fig. 31-20, *B*). Now suture the abdominal muscles to the edge of the gluteal muscles and tensor fasciae latae over the remaining rim of the ilium with interrupted sutures. Suture the superficial fascia on the medial side of the incision to the deep fascia on the lateral side to bring the skin incision 2.5 cm posterior to the rim of the ilium.

To preserve the iliac physis in a young child, modify the procedure as follows. Free the muscles subperiosteally from the lateral surface of the ilium. Detach the sartorius and rectus femoris as just described and, if necessary, release the

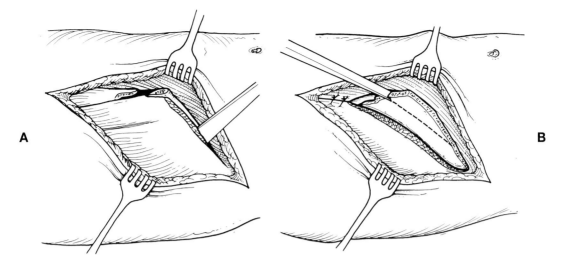

Fig. 31-20   Campbell transfer of crest of ilium for flexion contracture of hip. **A,** Origins of sartorius, tensor fasciae latae, and gluteus medius muscles are detached from ilium. **B,** Redundant part of ilium is resected.

capsule and iliopsoas muscle. Stripping the muscles from the medial surface of the ilium is unnecessary. Now with an osteotome remove a wedge of bone from the crest of the ilium distal to the physis from anterior to posterior; its apex should be as far posterior as the end of the incision and its base anterior and 2.5 cm or more in width, as necessary to correct the deformity. Then displace the crest of the ilium distally to contact the main part of the ilium and fix it in place with sutures through the soft tissues.

AFTERTREATMENT. When the deformity is mild, the hip is placed in hyperextension and about 10 degrees of abduction, and a spica cast is applied on the affected side and to above the knee on the opposite side. After 3 or 4 weeks the cast is removed, and the hip is mobilized. Support may be unnecessary during the day when the patient is on crutches; however, Buck extension or an appropriate splint should be used at night.

PARALYSIS OF GLUTEUS MAXIMUS AND MEDIUS MUSCLES

One of the most severe disabilities from poliomyelitis is caused by paralysis of the gluteus maximus muscle or the gluteus medius or both; the result is an unstable hip and an unsightly and fatiguing limp. During weight-bearing on the affected side when the gluteus medius alone is paralyzed, the trunk sways toward the affected side and the pelvis elevates on the opposite side (the "compensated" Trendelenburg gait). When the gluteus maximus alone is paralyzed, the body lurches backward. The strength of the gluteal muscles can be demonstrated by the Trendelenburg test: when a normal person bears weight on one extremity and flexes the other at the hip, the pelvis is

held on a horizontal plane and the gluteal folds are on the same level; when the gluteal muscles are impaired and weight is borne on the affected side, the level of the pelvis on the normal side will drop lower than that on the affected side; when the gluteal paralysis is severe, the test cannot be made because balance on the disabled extremity is impossible.

Because no apparatus will stabilize the pelvis when one or both of these muscles is paralyzed, function can be improved only by transferring muscular attachments to replace the gluteal muscles when feasible. These operations are only relatively successful. When the gluteal muscles are completely paralyzed, normal balance is never restored, and although the gluteal limp can be lessened, it remains; however, when the paralysis is only partial, the gait can be markedly improved.

◆ Transfer of External Oblique Muscle for Paralysis of Gluteus Medius Muscle

Anatomically the external oblique muscle is a good substitute for paralyzed abductors of the hip. Because its nerve supply is from a different spinal segment than that of the gluteus medius and minimus muscles, it is less likely to be paralyzed when these muscles are. Its aponeurosis is long and broad, its surfaces are well adapted for gliding movement, and after transfer its mechanical action on the greater trochanter is direct. Thomas, Thompson, and Straub described transfer of the external oblique muscle to the greater trochanter. Lindseth recommended posterolateral transfer of the fascia along with transfer of the adductor and external oblique muscles.

Transfer of the external oblique muscle has four advantages over transfer of the iliopsoas muscle: (1) the hip is not further weakened by elimination of the iliopsoas as a hip flexor; (2) muscle power is added to the hip by taking the muscle from the abdominal wall, where its absence is well tolerated; (3) the

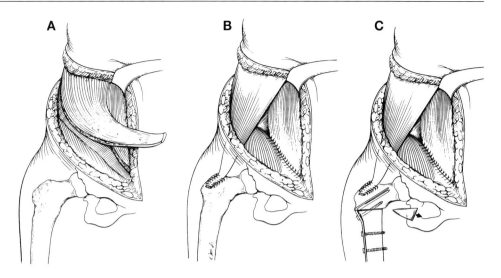

Fig. 31-21 External oblique transfer. **A,** With long oblique incision, muscle is freed distally. **B,** External oblique aponeurosis is attached to greater trochanter. **C,** Varus femoral osteotomy may be performed if necessary.

transfer functions synergistically, whereas iliopsoas transfer functions antagonistically; and (4) the ilium is not violated, allowing a pelvic osteotomy to be performed if necessary.

TECHNIQUE 31-21

With the patient supine and slightly tilted toward the nonoperative side, make an incision similar to that for the anterolateral approach to the hip (Chapter 1). Elevate the subcutaneous tissue from the external oblique aponeurosis all the way to the midline. Make an incision in the aponeurosis just at the level of the anterosuperior iliac spine, directed distally and medially, parallel to the inguinal ligament. At this point, direct the incision medially and proximally parallel to the linea alba. Carefully detach the external oblique muscle fibers from their insertion in the ilium, freeing the muscle from the underlying tissue by blunt dissection (Fig. 31-21, *A*). Now fold under and suture together the cut edges of the muscle and its aponeurosis to form a cone-shaped structure. Beginning at the pubis, repair the remaining aponeurosis of the muscle as far laterally as possible. Suture the remaining free edge of the aponeurosis to the underlying internal oblique muscle.

Perform adductor myotomy or adductor transfer to the ischium through a transverse incision beginning just anterior to the tendon of the adductor longus and extending down to the ischium. If the adductor transfer is performed, detach the tendons of the adductor longus, brevis, and anterior third of the magnus from the pubis and transfer them to the ischium with absorbable sutures.

Expose the greater trochanter through a separate lateral incision. The external oblique tendon aponeurosis can be inserted into the trochanter through either two holes, 1 cm in diameter and at right angles to each other, or through a posterolateral window hinged posteriorly. Make a large subcutaneous tunnel extending proximally from the original incision as far posterior as possible. Now pass the cone-

shaped strip of external oblique muscle distally through the tunnel, place the hip in 30 to 40 degrees of abduction, pass the tendon aponeurosis through the holes or window in the trochanter, and suture it firmly with nonabsorbable sutures or wire sutures (Fig. 31-21, *B*). If necessary, reattach the rectus anterior to the anteroinferior iliac crest and approximate and suture the iliac crest. Apply a hip spica cast with the hip in 25 to 30 degrees of abduction, extension, and internal rotation.

AFTERTREATMENT. At 6 weeks the cast is removed, and the child is admitted to the hospital for intensive physical therapy. A total body splint is fitted with the hip in 25 degrees of abduction and medial rotation.

◆ Posterior Transfer of Iliopsoas for Paralysis of Gluteus Medius and Maximus Muscles

Mustard devised an operation for weakness of the hip abductors in which the tendon of the iliopsoas muscle is transferred to the greater trochanter.

Sharrard modified Mustard's operation by transferring the iliopsoas tendon and the entire iliacus muscle posteriorly. This operation is more extensive than Mustard's but is superior to it when the gluteus maximus and gluteus medius are both paralyzed. Sharrard emphasized that open adductor tenotomy should always precede iliopsoas transfer.

TECHNIQUE 31-22 *(Sharrard)*

Place the patient on the operating table slightly tilted toward the nonoperative side. Through a transverse incision overlying the adductor longus, expose and divide the adductor muscles. Expose the lesser trochanter and detach it from the femur (Fig. 31-22, *A*). Then clear the psoas muscle as far proximally as possible. Make a second incision just below

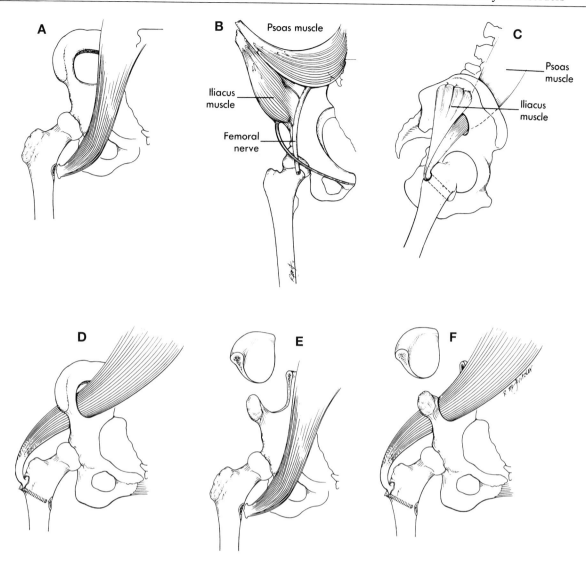

Fig. 31-22 Sharrard transfer of iliopsoas muscle. **A,** Iliopsoas tendon is released from lesser trochanter. **B,** Tendon and lesser trochanter are detached, iliacus and psoas muscles are elevated, origin of iliacus is freed, and hole is made in ilium. **C,** Iliopsoas tendon is passed from posterior to anterior through hole in greater trochanter. **D,** Iliopsoas muscle and lesser trochanter are secured to greater trochanter with screw. **E** and **F,** Modification of technique in which muscle and tendon are redirected laterally through notch in ilium and inserted into greater trochanter, as described by Weisinger et al. (**B** and **C** redrawn from Sharrard WJW: *J Bone Joint Surg* 46B:426, 1964.)

and parallel to the iliac crest. Detach the crest with the muscles of the abdominal wall and open the psoas muscle sheath. Locate the insertion of the muscle with a fingertip. Through the first incision, grasp the lesser trochanter with a Kocher forceps and pull it upward, within the psoas sheath and into the upper operative area (Fig. 31-22, *B*). Next expose the sartorius muscle and divide it in its proximal half. Allow the muscle to remain in the cartilaginous portion of the anterosuperior iliac spine, which is retracted medially. Identify the direct head on the rectus femoris muscle and divide it at its origin in the anteroinferior iliac spine. Identify

the reflected head of the rectus femoris muscle, dissect it free from the hip capsule, and elevate it posteriorly. If the hip is dislocated, open the capsule anteriorly and laterally, parallel to the labrum, excise the ligamentum teres, and remove any hypertrophic pulvinar. Reduce the hip joint.

Now make a hole through the iliac wing just lateral to the sacroiliac joint. Make an oval with its long axis longitudinal, its width slightly more than one third of that of the iliac wing, and its length 1½ times as long as its width. Then pass the iliopsoas tendon and the entire iliacus muscle through the hole (Fig. 31-22, *C*). Pass a finger from the gluteal region

continued

distally and posteriorly into the bursa deep to the gluteus maximus tendon and identify by touch the posterolateral aspect of the greater trochanter. By referring to this point expose the corresponding anterior aspect of the greater trochanter by dissecting through the fascia. Now with awls and burrs and from anteriorly to posteriorly make a hole through the greater trochanter until it is big enough to receive the tendon. Then, while the hip is held in abduction, extension, and neutral rotation, pass the end of the tendon through the buttock and from posteriorly to anteriorly through the tunnel in the greater trochanter (see Fig. 31-22, *C*). Secure the psoas and lesser trochanter to the greater trochanter with sutures or a screw (Fig. 31-22, *D*). Suture the origin of the iliacus muscle to the ilium inferior to the crest.

For severe coxa valga or anteversion that requires more than 20 to 30 degrees of abduction for stability, a varus derotation osteotomy with internal fixation can be performed before insertion and suturing of the iliopsoas tendon in the greater trochanter.

Wissinger, Turner, and Donaldson described a modification of the Sharrard transfer in which a "gutter," or notch, is cut into the posterolateral iliac crest rather than a window in the ilium. The muscle and its tendon can be redirected laterally through the notch and inserted into the greater trochanter (Fig. 31-22, *E* and *F*). This is technically simpler because the iliacus muscle is not transferred to the outside of the pelvis.

AFTERTREATMENT. The hip is immobilized for 6 weeks in an abduction spica cast.

PARALYTIC DISLOCATION OF HIP

If a child contracts poliomyelitis before the age of 2 years and the gluteal muscles become paralyzed but the flexors and adductors of the hip do not, the child may develop a paralytic dislocation of the hip before he is grown. That the combination of imbalance in muscle power, habitually faulty postures, and growth is important in producing deformity is illustrated nowhere better than in this situation. Generally, children with paralytic dislocation of the hip have normal strength of the flexors and adductors but paralysis of the gluteal muscles. Unless this muscle imbalance is corrected, dislocation is likely to recur regardless of other treatment. Dislocation also can develop because of fixed pelvic obliquity in which the contralateral hip is held in marked abduction, usually by a tight iliotibial band or a structural scoliosis. If the pelvic obliquity is not corrected, the hip gradually subluxates and eventually dislocates. Weakness of the abductor musculature retards the growth of the greater trochanteric apophysis. The proximal femoral capital epiphysis continues to grow away from the greater trochanter and increases the valgus deformity of the femoral neck; femoral anteversion also may be increased; and

the hip becomes mechanically unstable and gradually subluxates. The uneven pressure in the acetabulum causes an increased obliquity in the acetabular roof.

The goals of treatment of paralytic hip dislocations are reduction of the femoral head into the acetabulum and restoration of muscle balance. The bony deformity should be corrected before or at the time of any muscle-balancing procedures. Reduction of the hip in young children often can be achieved by simple abduction, sometimes aided by open adductor tenotomy and traction. Traction can be used to bring the femoral head opposite the acetabulum before closed reduction is attempted. If the hip cannot be reduced by traction, open reduction and adductor tenotomy may be required, in combination with primary femoral shortening, varus derotation osteotomy of the femur, and appropriate acetabular reconstructions (see Chapter 27). Hip arthrodesis rarely is indicated and should be used as the last alternative for treatment of a flail hip that requires stabilization or of an arthritic hip in a young adult that cannot be corrected with total hip arthroplasty. The Girdlestone procedure is the final option for failed correction of the dislocation.

Trunk

To understand the deformities and disabilities that may occur when the muscles of the trunk and hips are affected by poliomyelitis requires a knowledge of the normal actions and interactions of these muscles. Irwin described as follows the actions of the hip abductors and of the lateral trunk muscles during weight-bearing.

The different muscle groups, bone levers, and weight-bearing thrusts have a symmetrical and triangular relationship, as shown in Figs. 31-23 and 31-24. The line *BC* represents the abductor muscles of the hip; *AB*, the femoral head, neck, and trochanter, which provide a lever for the abductor muscles; *AC*, the weight-bearing thrust on the femoral head; *DF* and *CF*, the lateral trunk muscles; *CE*, the bone lever of the pelvis through which the trunk muscles act; and *FE*, the weight-bearing thrust through the midline of the pelvis from above. When the body is balanced, the triangles above and below the pelvis are symmetrical.

During normal walking the abductors of the hip on the weight-bearing side pull downward on the pelvis and the lateral trunk muscles on the opposite side pull upward; these two sets of muscles hold the pelvis at a right angle to the longitudinal axis of the trunk. The femoral head on the weight-bearing side serves as the fulcrum. The point of fixation of the trunk muscles (the ribs and spine) is less stable than that of the abductor muscles. Thus when *DF* elevates the pelvis, *CF* must provide counterfixation; *CF* in turn depends on the abductors of the hip, *BC*, for counterfixation. Thus with each step the femur on the weight-bearing side is the central point of action for this coordinated system of fixation and counterfixation. Each part of the system depends on the others for proper pelvic balance during walking.

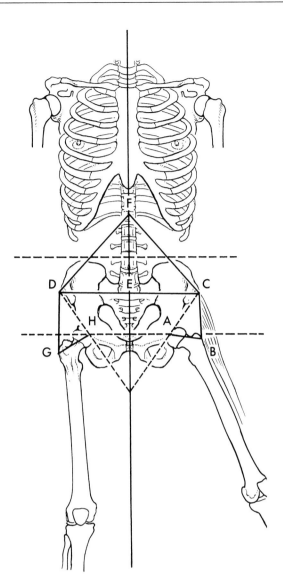

Fig. 31-23 Most true fixed pelvic obliquities are initiated by contractures below iliac crest (see text). (Redrawn from Irwin CE: *JAMA* 133:231, 1947.)

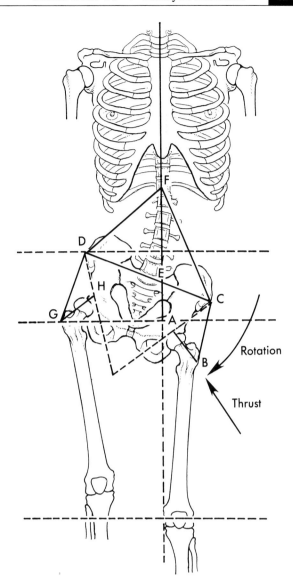

Fig. 31-24 Abnormal mechanical relationships are created when contracted hip is brought down into weight-bearing position (see text). (Redrawn from Irwin CE: *JAMA* 133:231, 1947.)

PELVIC OBLIQUITY

Irwin noted that when there is an abduction contracture of the hip, line *BC* is shortened; as the affected extremity is placed in the weight-bearing position, the femur, acting through the contracted abductor group, *BC*, depresses the pelvis on that side. During this motion the affected extremity and the pelvis act as a unit; the pelvis is displaced by the lateral thrust toward the opposite side, and thus the normal symmetry of the pelvis in relation to the weight-bearing thrust from above is altered. This thrust from above, *FE*, now closely approaches the affected hip, and the pelvis is tilted obliquely. The adducted position of the unaffected hip elongates the abductor muscles, *DG*, to about the same extent that the abductors on the affected side, *BC*, have been shortened, so even when the abductors,

DG, are normal, their contractility and efficiency are diminished. Moreover, the demand on these weakened muscles is increased by the increase in the length of line *DE*.

The trunk muscles also are affected by this asymmetry. The lateral trunk muscles, *CF*, become elongated, and their efficiency is impaired. The elongation of the abductors, *DG*, alters their interrelation with the lateral trunk muscles, *DF*, in providing a fixed point for contracture of the lateral trunk muscles, *CF*. The lateral trunk muscles, *CF*, normally elevate the pelvis on that side, but their position now prevents efficient function. Shortening of the lever, *EC*, places the trunk muscles, *CF*, at a further disadvantage. All these alterations in function and structure disrupt the mechanics of walking. When the contracted lateral trunk muscles, *DF*, and contracted hip abductors, *BC*, hold the pelvis in this position for long enough, its obliquity becomes fixed through adaptive changes in the spine.

When pelvic obliquity is associated with paralysis of the legs severe enough to require two long leg braces, walking is even more difficult. When the quadriceps is strong on the side of the abduction contracture (the apparently long extremity), the brace can be unlocked to allow knee flexion and walking is then possible, although with a marked limp. When the brace on the affected side cannot be unlocked and the heel on the opposite side (the apparently short extremity) is not elevated, the affected extremity must be widely abducted in walking; otherwise weight is borne only on the affected extremity, and the opposite one becomes almost useless.

Treatment

According to Irwin most pelvic obliquities arise from contractures distal to the iliac crest and few from unilateral weakness of the abdominal and lateral trunk muscles. Therefore when contractures are absent distal to the iliac crest, a pelvic obliquity should not be considered a true one but one secondary to scoliosis.

The early origin of a true pelvic obliquity from contracture of the iliotibial band has already been discussed (p. 1308). Before starting treatment, the degree of fixation of the lumbar scoliosis should be determined by roentgenograms. When the deformity is mild and the lumbar scoliosis is not fixed, the pelvic obliquity is corrected by treating the flexion and abduction contracture of the hip (p. 1310). When the pelvic obliquity is moderately severe and the lumbar scoliosis is fixed, the scoliosis is corrected first by instrumentation, as described in Chapter 38. After this treatment has been completed the contractures about the hip are released.

For adults with arthritic changes in the lumbar spine that make correction impossible, Irwin suggested that the weight borne on the adducted extremity (the apparently short one) be shifted nearer the midline by valgus osteotomy; a severe unilateral weakness of the gluteus medius also can be treated in this way. This procedure may enable a patient to walk who could not do so before. When the pelvic obliquity is extreme and the femoral head of the abducted extremity (the apparently long one) is almost within the center of gravity, varus osteotomy of the femur is indicated. The osteotomy usually is made at the level of the lesser trochanter, and the fragments are immobilized by appropriate internal fixation.

PARALYSIS OF MUSCLES OF ABDOMEN, BACK, SCAPULA, AND NECK

Severe disabilities can result from paralysis of the abdominal, back, scapular, and neck muscles. Imbalance in the trunk and shoulder muscles can produce a variety of deformities.

1. Weakness or paralysis of the rectus abdominis produces an anterior tilt of the pelvis and an increase in lumbar lordosis, both of which are exaggerated if the hip flexors are active.

2. Unilateral weakness of the quadratus lumborum produces a lateral deviation of the spine or a pelvic obliquity with secondary compensatory changes proximally. Unilateral weakness of the latissimus dorsi can produce a similar effect.

3. When the serratus anterior and pectoralis major are active, the rhomboids weak, and the shoulder drooping, the weight of the shoulder girdle is thrown anterior to the angle of the ribs and together with the pull of the active muscles tends to flatten them.

4. Contractures of unopposed muscles that pull diagonally or laterally, such as the transversalis, serratus anterior, and abdominal obliques, together with an unbalanced pull of the pectoralis major, latissimus dorsi, and quadratus lumborum, contribute to rotary and lateral deformities of the spine and ribs.

5. Paralysis of various muscles about the shoulder also can contribute to paralytic scoliosis in the cervical and upper thoracic spine, drooping and instability of the shoulder girdle, and deformity of the chest.

Muscle Transfers and Fascial Transplants for Paralysis of Scapular Muscles

Paralysis of the scapular muscles makes the scapula unstable and shoulder function inefficient; it may be indirectly responsible for high thoracic or cervicothoracic scoliosis. Numerous procedures to treat serratus anterior paralysis and trapezius and levator scapulae paralysis have been devised.

Serratus Anterior Paralysis. The following procedures were devised to treat this paralysis:

1. A fascial transplant to anchor the inferior angle of the scapula to the inferior border of the pectoralis major
2. Multiple fascial transplants extending from the vertebral border of the scapula to the fourth, fifth, sixth, and seventh thoracic spinous processes
3. Transfer of the teres major tendon from the humerus to the fifth and sixth ribs
4. Transfer of the coracoid insertion of the pectoralis minor muscle to the vertebral border of the scapula
5. Transfer of the coracoid insertion of the pectoralis minor to the inferior angle of the scapula
6. Transfer of pectoralis minor to distal third of scapula

Trapezius and Levator Scapulae Paralysis. The following procedures are used to treat this paralysis:

1. Fascial transplants extending from the spine of the scapula to the cervical muscles and to the first thoracic spinous process; also, anchoring of the inferior angle of the scapula to the adjacent paraspinal muscles for stability
2. Transplant of two fascial strips, one extending from the vertebral border of the scapula just proximal to its spine to the sixth cervical spinous process and the other from a point 6 cm distal to the first transplant to the third thoracic spinous process
3. A fascial transplant extending from the middle of the

vertebral border of the scapula to the spinous process of the second and third thoracic vertebrae and transfer of the insertion of the levator scapulae muscle lateralward on the spine of the scapula to a point adjacent to the acromion

Paralytic Scoliosis. The treatment of paralytic scoliosis is discussed in Chapter 38.

Shoulder

The disability caused by paralysis of the muscles about the shoulder can be diminished to some extent by tendon and muscle transfers or by arthrodesis of the joint; the pattern and severity of the paralysis determine which method is most appropriate. However, neither procedure is indicated unless the hand, forearm, and elbow have remained functional or have already been made so by reconstructive surgery.

Tendons and muscles are transferred to substitute for a paralyzed deltoid muscle or to reinforce a weak one. For these operations to be successful, power must be fair or better in the serratus anterior, the trapezius, and the short external rotators of the shoulder (for the trapezius transfer, power must be fair or better in the pectoralis major, the rhomboids, and the levator scapulae). When the short external rotators are below functional level, the latissimus dorsi or teres major can be transferred to the lateral aspect of the humerus to reinforce them (Harmon). When the supraspinatus is below functional level, Saha recommended transfer to the greater tuberosity of the levator scapulae, sternocleidomastoid, scalenus anterior, scalenus medius, or scalenus capitis; he preferred the levator scapulae. When the subscapularis is below functional level, he transferred to the lesser tuberosity either the pectoralis minor or the superior two digitations of the serratus anterior, or the latissimus dorsi or teres major posteriorly to a point exactly opposite the insertion of the subscapularis (here the action is backward although identical to that of the subscapularis after elevation above 90 degrees).

Arthrodesis of the shoulder may be indicated when the paralysis about the joint is extensive, provided that power in at least the serratus anterior and the trapezius is fair or better.

TENDON AND MUSCLE TRANSFERS FOR PARALYSIS OF DELTOID

Transfer of the insertion of the trapezius is the most satisfactory operation for complete paralysis of the deltoid. Bateman modified the Mayer technique by resecting a part of the spine of the scapula and including it in the transfer; this permits fixation of the transfer with screws after the muscle is pulled like a hood over the head of the humerus (Fig. 31-25). Saha also modified and improved the technique. The superior and middle trapezius is completely mobilized laterally from its origin, and thus the transfer is made 5 cm longer without endangering its nerve or blood supply; this added length greatly increases leverage of the transfer on the humerus. The entire insertion of the trapezius is freed by resecting the lateral clavicle, the acromion, and the adjoining part of the scapular spine; these are then anchored to the humerus by screws (Fig. 31-26).

Saha developed a functional classification of the muscles about the joint and recommended careful assessment of their strength before surgery. A summary of Saha's classification of the muscles of the shoulder follows.

1. *Prime movers:* the deltoid and clavicular head of the pectoralis major, which in lifting exert forces in three directions at the junction of the proximal and middle thirds of the humeral shaft axis.

2. *Steering group:* the subscapularis, the supraspinatus, and the infraspinatus. These muscles exert forces at the junction of the axes of the humeral head and neck and humeral shaft. As the arm is elevated the humeral head, by rolling and gliding movements, constantly changes its point of contact with the glenoid cavity. Although these muscles exert a little force in lifting the arm, their chief function is stabilizing the humeral head as it moves in the glenoid.

3. *Depressor group:* the pectoralis major (sternal head), latissimus dorsi, teres major, and teres minor. These muscles are intermediately located and exert their forces on the proximal fourth of the humeral shaft axis. During elevation they rotate the shaft, and in the last few degrees of this movement they depress the humeral head. They exert only minimal steering action on the head. Absence of their power would cause no apparent disability except that performance of the limb in lifting weights above the head would be diminished.

The classic methods of transferring a single muscle (or even several muscles to a common attachment) to restore abduction of the shoulder do not consider the functions of the steering muscles. When the steering muscles are paralyzed and a single muscle has been transferred to restore functions only of the deltoid, the arm cannot be elevated more than 90 degrees and scapulohumeral motion is significantly disturbed. Thus, for paralysis of the deltoid Saha transferred the entire insertion of the trapezius to the humerus to replace the anterior and middle parts of the muscle; however, he carefully evaluated the subscapularis, the supraspinatus, and the infraspinatus, and when any two are found paralyzed, he restored their functions also, because otherwise the effectiveness of the transferred trapezius as an elevator of the shoulder would be greatly reduced. As already mentioned, for paralysis of the subscapularis either the pectoralis minor or the superior two digitations of the serratus anterior can be transferred because either can be rerouted and anchored to the lesser tuberosity; or as an alternative procedure, the latissimus dorsi or the teres major can be transferred posteriorly to a point exactly opposite the lesser tuberosity. For paralysis of the supraspinatus the levator scapulae, sternocleidomastoid, scalenus anterior, scalenus medius, or scalenus capitis can be transferred to the greater tuberosity; of these the levator scapulae is the best because of

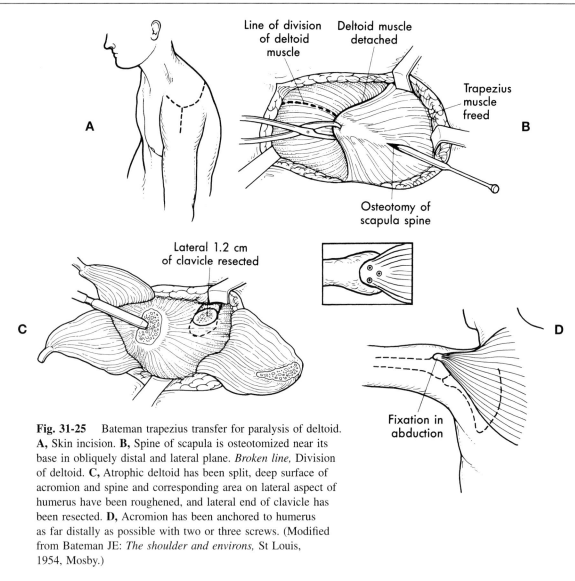

Fig. 31-25 Bateman trapezius transfer for paralysis of deltoid.
A, Skin incision. **B,** Spine of scapula is osteotomized near its
base in obliquely distal and lateral plane. *Broken line,* Division
of deltoid. **C,** Atrophic deltoid has been split, deep surface of
acromion and spine and corresponding area on lateral aspect of
humerus have been roughened, and lateral end of clavicle has
been resected. **D,** Acromion has been anchored to humerus
as far distally as possible with two or three screws. (Modified
from Bateman JE: *The shoulder and environs,* St Louis,
1954, Mosby.)

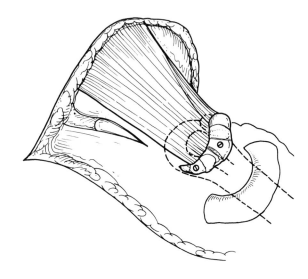

Fig. 31-26 Saha trapezius transfer for paralysis of deltoid. Entire insertion of trapezius along with attached lateral end of clavicle, acromioclavicular joint, and acromion and adjoining part of scapular spine have been
anchored to lateral aspect of humerus distal to tuberosities by two screws.
(Redrawn from Saha AK: *Acta Orthop Scand Suppl* 97:5 1967.)

the direction and length of its fibers. When suitable transfers are unavailable, the insertion of the trapezius can be anchored more anteriorly or posteriorly on the humerus to restore internal or external rotation.

Contractures of unopposed muscles about the shoulder rarely are severe enough to cause extreme disability; most can be corrected at the time of transfer or arthrodesis.

◆ Trapezius Transfer for Paralysis of Deltoid

TECHNIQUE 31-23 *(Bateman)*

With the patient prone, approach the shoulder through a T-shaped incision (see Fig. 31-25, *A*); extend the transverse part around the shoulder over the spine of the scapula and the acromion and end it just above the coracoid process; extend the longitudinal limb distally over the lateral aspect of the shoulder and upper arm for 6 cm. Mobilize the flaps, split the atrophic deltoid muscle, and expose the joint. Free of soft tissue the undersurface of the acromion and spine of the scapula. Now osteotomize the spine of the scapula near its base in an obliquely distal and lateral plane; thus, a broad cuff of the trapezius is freed, still attached to the spine and the acromion. Resect the lateral 2 cm of the clavicle, taking care to avoid damaging the coracoclavicular ligament. Roughen the deep surface of the acromion and spine, abduct the arm to 90 degrees, and at the appropriate level on the lateral aspect of the humerus, roughen a corresponding area. Now by firm traction bring the muscular cuff laterally over the humeral head and anchor the acromion to the humerus as far distally as possible with two or three screws (see Fig. 31-25, *D*). Immobilize the arm in a shoulder spica cast with the shoulder abducted to 90 degrees.

AFTERTREATMENT. Immobilization is continued for 8 weeks, but at 4 to 6 weeks the arm and shoulder part of the spica is bivalved to allow some movement. When the transplanted acromion has united with the humerus, the arm is placed on an abduction humeral splint and is gradually lowered to the side, and the muscle is reeducated by exercises.

TECHNIQUE 31-24 *(Saha)*

Make a saber-cut incision (see Fig. 31-26) convex medially; begin it anteriorly a little superior to the inferior margin of the anterior axillary fold at about its middle, extend it superiorly, then posteriorly, and finally inferiorly, and end it slightly inferior to the base of the scapular spine and 2.5 cm lateral to the vertebral border of the scapula. Mobilize the skin flaps and expose the trapezius medially to 2.5 cm medial to the vertebral border of the scapula; expose the acromion, the capsule of the acromioclavicular joint, the lateral third of the clavicle, and the entire origin of the paralyzed deltoid muscle. Next detach and reflect

laterally the origin of the deltoid and locate the anterior border of the trapezius. Identify the coronoid ligament and divide the clavicle just lateral to it. Then palpate the scapular notch, identify the acromion and the adjoining part of the scapular spine, and with a Gigli saw and beveling posteriorly, resect the spine. Now elevate the insertion of the trapezius along with the attached lateral end of the clavicle, the acromioclavicular joint, and the acromion and adjoining part of the scapular spine. Then free the trapezius from the superior border of the remaining part of the scapular spine medially to the base of the spine where the inferior fibers of the muscle glide over the triangular area of the scapula. Next free from the investing layer of deep cervical fascia the anterior border of the trapezius and raise the muscle from its bed for rerouting. Denude the inferior surfaces of the bones attached to the freed trapezius insertion; with forceps break these bones in several places but leave intact the periosteum on their superior surfaces. Denude also the area on the lateral aspect of the proximal humerus selected for attachment of the transfer. Then with the shoulder in neutral rotation and 45 degrees of abduction, anchor the transfer by two screws passed through fragments of bone and into the proximal humerus (see Fig. 31-26). When suitable transfers are unavailable to replace any paralyzed external or internal rotators, anchor the muscle a little more anteriorly or posteriorly. Transfers for paralysis of the subscapularis, supraspinatus, or infraspinatus are discussed later; when indicated, they should be performed at the time of trapezius transfer.

AFTERTREATMENT. A spica cast is applied with the shoulder abducted 45 degrees, neutrally rotated, and flexed in the plane of the scapula. At 10 days the sutures are removed, and roentgenograms are made to be sure that the humeral head has not become dislocated inferiorly. At 6 to 8 weeks the cast is removed, and active exercises are started.

◆ Transfer of Deltoid Origin for Partial Paralysis

TECHNIQUE 31-25 *(Harmon)*

Make a U-shaped incision 20 cm long extending from the middle third of the clavicle laterally and posteriorly around the shoulder just distal to the acromion to the middle of the spine of the scapula. Raise flaps of skin and subcutaneous tissue proximally and distally. Detach subperiosteally from its origin the active posterior part of the deltoid and free it distally from the deep structures for about one half its length, being careful not to injure the axillary nerve and its branches. Expose subperiosteally the lateral third of the clavicle, transfer the muscle flap anteriorly, and anchor it against the clavicle with interrupted nonabsorbable sutures through the adjacent soft tissues (Fig. 31-27).

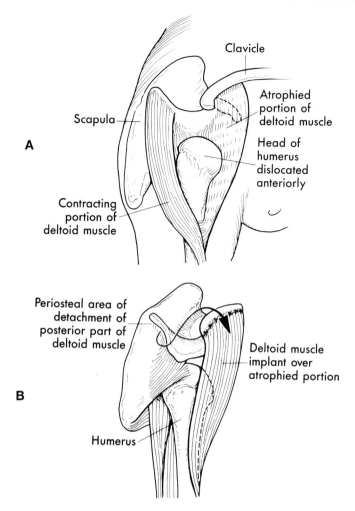

Fig. 31-27   Harmon transfer of origin of deltoid for partial paralysis. **A,** Posterior part of deltoid is functioning; middle and anterior parts are paralyzed. **B,** Transferred posterior part of deltoid is overlying atrophic anterior part. When transfer contracts, it prevents anterior dislocation of shoulder and exerts more direct abduction force than in its previous posterior location. (Redrawn from Harmon PH: *Surg Gynecol Obstet* 84:117, 1947.)

AFTERTREATMENT. A shoulder spica cast is applied, holding the arm abducted 75 degrees. At 3 weeks part of the cast is removed for massage and active exercise. At 6 weeks the entire cast is removed, and an abduction humeral splint is fitted to be worn for at least 4 months; supervised active exercises are continued during this time.

TENDON AND MUSCLE TRANSFERS FOR PARALYSIS OF SUBSCAPULARIS, SUPRASCAPULARIS, SUPRASPINATUS, OR INFRASPINATUS

Saha emphasized the importance of transfers for paralysis of the subscapularis, supraspinatus, or infraspinatus. According to him, when two of these three muscles are paralyzed, their functions must be restored by suitable transfers; this is just as necessary as the trapezius transfer for paralysis of the deltoid.

Without the function of these muscles or their substitutes, the effectiveness of the transferred trapezius in elevating the shoulder would be markedly reduced. Muscles suitable for transfer are those whose distal ends can be carried to the tuberosities of the humerus and whose general directions of pull correspond to those of the muscles they are to replace. The transfers should be rerouted close to the end of the axis of the humeral head and neck, or the desired functions will not be restored. The nerve and blood supply to any transferred muscle must, of course, be protected. Currently the most commonly performed transfers are transfer of the latissimus dorsi or teres major or both and posterior transfer of the pectoralis minor to the scapula. These transfers, when indicated, are carried out at the same time as the Saha trapezius transfer for paralysis of the deltoid. Consequently, in each instance the saber-cut incision will have been made, the lateral end of the clavicle and the acromion and adjoining part of the scapular spine will have been elevated, and the superior and middle trapezius will have been mobilized as already described.

◆ Transfer of Latissimus Dorsi or Teres Major or Both for Paralysis of Subscapularis or Infraspinatus

TECHNIQUE 31-26 *(Saha)*

Elevate the arm about 130 degrees. Then make an incision in the posterior axillary fold beginning in the upper arm about 6.5 cm inferior to the crease of the axilla and extending to the inferior angle of the scapula, crossing the crease in a zigzag manner. Expose and free the insertion of the latissimus dorsi and raise the muscle from its bed, taking care to preserve its nerve and blood supply. If the transfer is to be reinforced by the teres major, free and raise both muscles. Next fold the freed insertion on itself and close its margins by interrupted sutures; place in its end a strong mattress suture. Next, with a blunt instrument open the interval between the deltoid and long head of the triceps. Identify the tubercle at the inferior end of the greater tuberosity, carry the end of the transfer to this tubercle, and while holding the limb in neutral rotation, anchor the transfer there by interrupted sutures.

ARTHRODESIS

When paralysis about the shoulder is extensive, arthrodesis may be the procedure of choice, especially when there is a paralytic dislocation, the muscles of the forearm and hand are functional, and the serratus anterior and trapezius are strong. Motion of the scapula then compensates for lack of motion in the joint. Normal function of the forearm and hand is a prerequisite.

The position of the shoulder for arthrodesis is similar to that recommended for any shoulder fusion (Chapter 4). The angle of abduction should be determined on the basis of the clinical presentation of the arm's position in relation to the body. This angle traditionally is obtained by measuring the angle between the vertebral border of the scapula and the humerus; however, this frequently is difficult to determine on roentgenograms. Rowe and Leffert recommended that the position of the arm in shoulder arthrodesis be established with the arm at the side of the body, with enough clinically determined abduction of the arm from the side of the body to clear the axilla (15 to 20 degrees) and enough forward flexion (25 to 30 degrees) and internal rotation (40 to 50 degrees) to bring the hand to the midline of the body. An additional 10 degrees of abduction should be obtained in children with poliomyelitis when no internal fixation is used. When both shoulders must be fused, their positions should allow the patient to bring the hands together. A weak or flail shoulder should be fused in only slight abduction. Care must be taken to preserve the proximal humeral physis in skeletally immature patients. The techniques for shoulder arthrodesis are described in Chapter 4.

Elbow

Most operations for paralysis of the muscles acting across the elbow are designed to restore active flexion or extension of the joint. Operations to correct deformity or those to stabilize the joint, such as posterior bone block or arthrodesis, rarely are necessary.

MUSCLE AND TENDON TRANSFERS TO RESTORE ELBOW FLEXION

There are several methods of restoring active elbow flexion. Here, as elsewhere, the actual and the relative power of the remaining muscles must be accurately determined before a transfer procedure is chosen. Also, because the function of the hand is more important than flexion of the elbow, these operations should not be done when the muscles controlling the fingers are paralyzed unless their function has been or can be restored by tendon transfers. Several methods of restoring elbow flexion have been described: (1) flexorplasty (Steindler), (2) anterior transfer of the triceps tendon (Bunnell and Carroll), (3) transfer of part of the pectoralis major muscle (Clark), (4) transfer of the sternocleidomastoid muscle (Bunnell), (5) transfer of the pectoralis minor muscle (Spira), (6) transfer of the pectoralis major tendon (Brooks and Seddon), and (7) transfer of the latissimus dorsi muscle (Hovnanian).

◆ Flexorplasty

Flexorplasty consists of transferring the common origin of the pronator teres, the flexor carpi radialis, the palmaris longus, the flexor digitorum sublimis, and the flexor carpi ulnaris muscles from the medial epicondylar region of the humerus proximally about 5 cm. Its chief disadvantage is the frequent development of a pronation deformity of the forearm.

Flexorplasty is indicated when the biceps brachii and brachialis are paralyzed and the group of muscles arising from the medial epicondyle are fair or better in strength. The best results are obtained when the elbow flexors are only partially paralyzed and the finger and wrist flexors are normal. The

strength in active flexion and the range of motion of the elbow after surgery do not compare favorably with the normal, but the usefulness of the arm is nonetheless increased. When only the flexor digitorum sublimis is active, the elbow can be flexed only if the fingers are strongly flexed; this, of course, interferes with the function of the hand, and another method should be used to restore elbow flexion. According to Mayer and Green, unsuccessful results from this procedure usually are caused by overestimating the strength of the muscles to be transferred. A practical way to test them is to hold the patient's arm at a right angle to the body, rotate it to eliminate the influence of gravity, and then determine whether the muscles to be transferred can flex the elbow in this position; if not, this type of transfer will fail, and another should be used. In an attempt to minimize the loss of supination occurring after this procedure, Carroll and Gartland, Bunnell, and Mayer and Green modified the Steindler flexorplasty by moving the origin of the medial muscle mass not only proximally, as above, but also laterally onto the anterior surface of the humerus. Bunnell modified the technique by transferring the common muscle origin laterally on the humerus by means of a fascial transplant. This largely eliminates the action of the transferred muscle group in pronating the forearm.

TECHNIQUE 31-27 *(Bunnell)*

Make a curved longitudinal incision over the medial side of the elbow beginning 7.5 cm proximal to the medial epicondyle and extending distally posterior to the medial condyle and thence anteriorly on the volar surface of the forearm along the course of the pronator teres muscle. Locate the ulnar nerve posterior to the medial epicondyle and retract it posteriorly. Detach en bloc the common origin of the pronator teres, flexor carpi radialis, palmaris longus, flexor digitorum sublimis, and flexor carpi ulnaris from the medial epicondyle close to the periosteum. Free these muscles distally for 4 cm and prolong the common muscle origin with a free graft of fascia lata. Then advance this origin 5 cm up the lateral side rather than the medial side of the humerus (Fig. 31-28); this results in a moderate although not complete correction of the tendency of the transfer to pronate the forearm. Should a pronation deformity persist after this procedure, it can be corrected by transferring the tendon of the flexor carpi ulnaris around the ulnar margin of the forearm into the distal radius. Apply a cast with the elbow in acute flexion and the forearm midway between pronation and supination.

AFTERTREATMENT. At 2 weeks the cast is replaced by a splint that holds the arm in this same position for at least 6 weeks; physical therapy and active exercises are then started and are gradually increased to strengthen the transferred muscles.

◆ Anterior Transfer of Triceps

Anterior transfer of the triceps tendon can be done to regain active elbow flexion. One disadvantage of this transfer is that

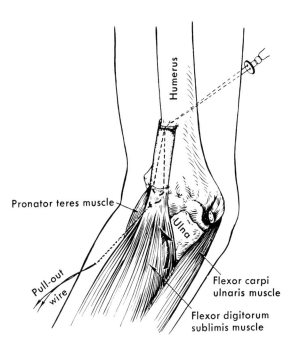

Fig. 31-28 Bunnell modification of Steindler flexorplasty. Common muscle origin is transferred laterally on humerus by means of fascial transplant. (Modified from Bunnell S: *J Bone Joint Surg* 33A:566, 1951.)

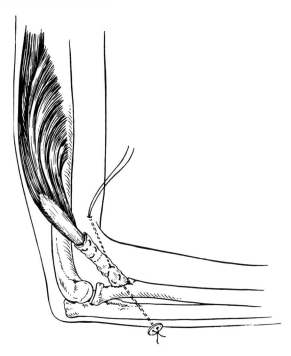

Fig. 31-29 Bunnell anterior transfer of triceps for paralysis of biceps. Triceps tendon prolonged by short graft of fascia or tendon, routed laterally, and inserted into tuberosity of radius by pull-out suture. (From Bunnell S: *J Bone Joint Surg* 33A:566, 1951.)

the triceps tendon will not reach the tuberosity of the radius; therefore a short graft of fascia or a tendon graft must be used to complete the transfer.

TECHNIQUE 31-28 *(Bunnell)*
Through a posterolateral incision expose the triceps tendon and divide it at its insertion. Dissect it from the posterior aspect of the distal fourth of the humerus and transfer it around the lateral aspect. Make an anterolateral curvilinear incision and retract the brachioradialis and pronator teres muscles to expose the tuberosity of the radius. Prolong the triceps tendon by a graft of fascia lata that is 4 cm long and wide enough to make a tube. Attach it to the roughened tuberosity of the radius with a steel pull-out suture passed to the dorsum of the forearm via a hole drilled through the tuberosity and the neck of the radius (Fig. 31-29). Flex the elbow, gently pull the suture taut to snug the tendon against the bone, and tie the suture over a padded button. Apply a cast with the elbow in acute flexion and the forearm midway between pronation and supination.

Carroll described a similar method of triceps transfer in which the tendon is passed superficial to the radial nerve and through a longitudinal slit in the biceps tendon and is sutured under tension with the elbow in flexion.

AFTERTREATMENT. At 2 weeks the cast is replaced by a splint that holds the arm in the same position for at least 6

weeks. The pull-out wire is removed at 4 weeks. Physical therapy and active exercises are begun at 6 weeks and are gradually increased.

◆ Transfer of Pectoralis Major Tendon
Brooks and Seddon described an operation to restore elbow flexion in which the entire pectoralis major muscle is used as the motor, and its tendon is prolonged distally by means of the long head of the biceps brachii. This transfer is contraindicated unless the biceps is completely paralyzed; they recommended it when flexorplasty is not applicable, when the distal part of the pectoralis major is weak but the proximal part is strong, or when both parts of the muscle are so weak that the entire muscle is needed for transfer. To avoid undesirable movements of the shoulder during elbow flexion after this procedure, muscular control of the shoulder and scapula must be good, or an arthrodesis of the shoulder should be performed.

TECHNIQUE 31-29 *(Brooks and Seddon)*
Make an incision from the distal end of the deltopectoral groove distally to the junction of the proximal and middle thirds of the arm. Detach the tendon of insertion of the pectoralis major as close to bone as possible and by blunt dissection mobilize the muscle from the chest wall proximally toward the clavicle (Fig. 31-30, *A*). Retract the deltoid laterally and superiorly and expose the tendon of

continued

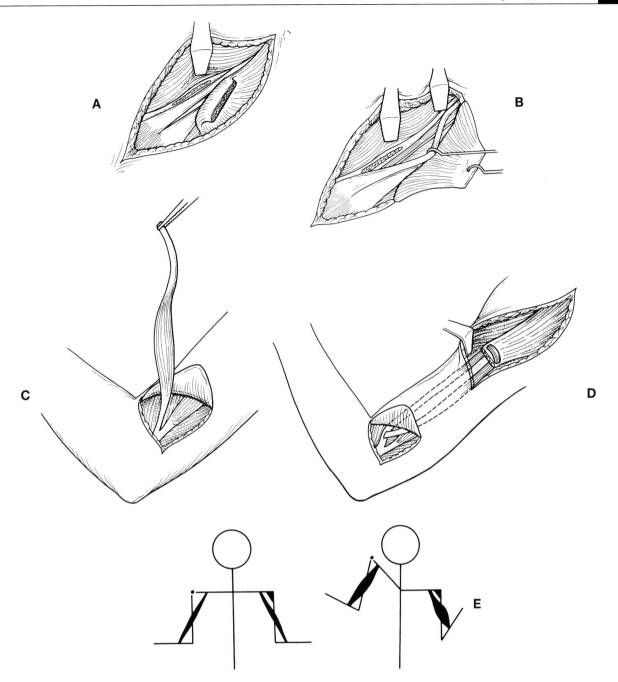

Fig. 31-30 Brooks-Seddon transfer of pectoralis major tendon for paralysis of elbow flexors. **A,** Insertion of pectoralis major is detached as close to bone as possible. **B,** Tendon of long head of biceps is exposed and divided at proximal end of bicipital groove. **C,** Tendon and muscle of long head of biceps are completely mobilized distally to tuberosity of radius by dividing all vessels and nerves that enter muscle proximal to elbow. **D,** Long head of biceps is passed through two slits in pectoralis major, is looped on itself so that its proximal tendon is brought into distal incision, and is sutured through slit in its distal tendon. **E,** To avoid undesirable movements of shoulder during elbow flexion after this transfer, muscular control of shoulder and scapula must be good, or shoulder must be fused. Left shoulder shown is flail; right has been fused. When transfer on left contracts, some of its force is wasted because of lack of control of shoulder, but on right, transfer moves only elbow. (Redrawn from Brooks DM, Seddon HJ: *J Bone Joint Surg* 41B:36, 1959.)

the long head of the biceps as it runs proximally into the shoulder joint; sever this tendon at the proximal end of the bicipital groove and withdraw it into the wound. By blunt and sharp dissection free the belly of the long head of the biceps from that of the short head and ligate and divide all vessels entering it. Now make an L-shaped incision at the elbow with its transverse limb in the flexor crease and its longitudinal limb extending proximally along the medial border of the biceps muscle. Now mobilize the long head of the biceps by dividing its remaining neurovascular bundles so that the tendon and muscle are completely freed distally to the tuberosity of the radius; withdraw the tendon and muscle through the distal incision (Fig. 31-30, *B* and *C*). (When the muscle belly is adherent to the overlying fascia, free it by sharp dissection.) Now replace the long head of the biceps in its original position and through the proximal incision pass its tendon and muscle belly through two slits in the tendon of the pectoralis major; loop the long head of the biceps on itself so that its proximal tendon is brought into the distal incision. Then, using silk, suture the end of the proximal tendon through a slit in the distal tendon (Fig. 31-30, *D*) and suture the tendon of the pectoralis major to the long head of the biceps at their junction. Close the incisions and apply a posterior plaster splint with the elbow in flexion.

AFTERTREATMENT. At 3 weeks the splint is removed, and muscle reeducation is started; care must be taken to extend the elbow gradually so that active flexion of more than 90 degrees is preserved. It may be 2 or 3 months before full extension is possible.

◆ Transfer of Latissimus Dorsi Muscle

Hovnanian described a method of restoring active elbow flexion by transferring the origin and belly of the latissimus dorsi to the arm and anchoring the origin near the radial tuberosity. This transfer is possible because the neurovascular bundle of the muscle is long and easily mobilized (Fig. 31-31, *A*); a similar transfer in which the origin is anchored to the olecranon to restore active extension also is possible.

TECHNIQUE 31-30 *(Hovnanian)*

Place the patient on his side with the affected extremity upward. Start the skin incision over the loin and extend it superiorly along the lateral border of the latissimus dorsi to the posterior axillary fold, distally along the medial aspect of the arm, and finally laterally to end in the antecubital fossa (Fig. 31-31, *B*). Carefully expose the dorsal and lateral aspects of the latissimus dorsi, leaving its investing fascia intact. Free the origin of the muscle by cutting across its musculofascial junction inferiorly and its muscle fibers superiorly. Then gradually free the muscle from the

underlying abdominal and flank muscles. Divide the four slips of the muscle that arise from the inferior four ribs and the few arising from the angle of the scapula. Carefully protect the neurovascular bundle that enters the superior third of the muscle. To prevent injury of the vessels to the latissimus dorsi, ligate their branches that anastomose with the lateral thoracic vessels. Identify and gently free the thoracodorsal nerve that supplies the muscle; its trunk is about 15 cm long and runs from the apex of the axilla along the deep surface of the muscle belly.

Next prepare a bed in the anteromedial aspect of the arm to receive the transfer. Carefully swing the transfer into this bed without twisting its vessels or nerve. To prevent kinking of the vessels, divide the intercostobrachial nerve and the lateral cutaneous branches of the third and fourth intercostal nerves; also free as necessary any fascial bands. Now suture the aponeurotic origin of the muscle to the biceps tendon and the periosteal tissues about the radial tuberosity, and the remaining origin to the sheaths of the forearm muscles and to the lacertus fibrosus (Fig. 31-31, *C*). Close the wound in layers and bandage the arm against the thorax with the elbow flexed and the forearm pronated.

AFTERTREATMENT. Exercises of the fingers are encouraged early. At 3 or 4 weeks the bandage is removed, and passive and active exercises of the elbow are started.

MUSCLE TRANSFERS FOR PARALYSIS OF TRICEPS

Weakness or paralysis of the triceps muscle usually is considered of little importance because gravity will extend the elbow passively in most positions that the arm assumes. However, a good triceps is essential to crutch walking or to shifting the body weight to the hands during such activities as moving from a bed to a wheelchair. A functioning triceps allows the patient to perform these activities by locking the elbow in extension. To place the hand on top of the head when the patient is erect, the triceps must be strong enough to extend the elbow against gravity; thrusting and pushing motions with the forearm also require a functional triceps. In other activities, strong active extension of the elbow is relatively unimportant in comparison with strong active flexion.

Posterior Deltoid Transfer (Moberg Procedure)

In 1975 Moberg described an operation to transfer the posterior third of the deltoid muscle to the triceps to restore active elbow extension in the quadriplegic patient. Patients with complete quadriplegia at the functioning level of C5 or C6 have active elbow flexion, shoulder flexion and abduction, and possibly wrist extension. Elbow extension is by gravity only, without triceps function (C7). Active extension is impossible. Ambulation is not a realistic goal in such patients. Rather, improved strength, mobility, and function were sought, as well as improved ability to reach overhead, to perform personal

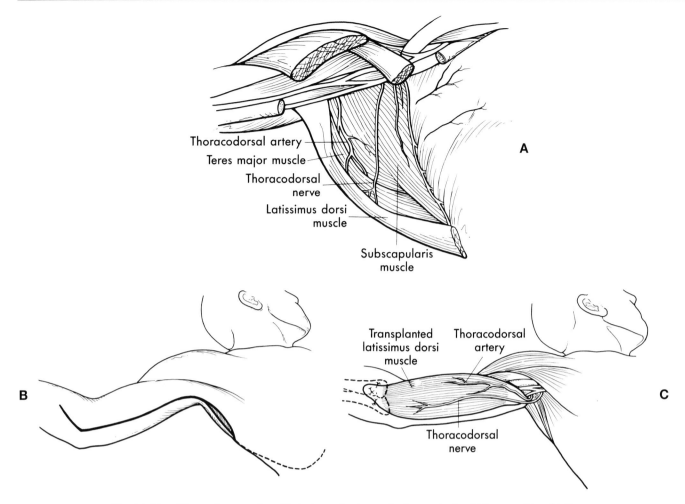

Fig. 31-31 Hovnanian transfer of latissimus dorsi muscle for paralysis of biceps and brachialis muscles. **A,** Normal anatomy of axilla; note that thoracodorsal nerve and artery are long and can be easily mobilized. **B,** Skin incision. **C,** Origin and belly of latissimus dorsi have been transferred to arm, and origin has been sutured to biceps tendon and to other structures distal to elbow joint. (Redrawn from Hovnanian AP: *Ann Surg* 143:493, 1956.)

hygiene and grooming, to relieve ischial pressure from the wheelchair, to achieve driving ability and wheelchair use, and to eat and control eating utensils.

Castro-Sierra and Lopez-Pita modified Moberg's procedure by the construction of tendinoperiosteal tongues proximally and distally instead of using the free tendon grafts from the foot. The posterior belly of the deltoid muscle is freed, along with the most distal insertion of the muscle and including a strip of periosteum 1 cm × 3 cm, continuous with the muscle and its insertion. Next a tongue of the triceps tendon 1.5- to 2-cm wide is developed by parallel incisions and including a continuous strip of periosteum similar to that above, if possible.

The length of the tendinoperiosteal tongues should be such that with the elbow extended and the arm adducted, their deep surfaces should appose when the triceps tendon is folded over 180 degrees. The angle of tendinous reflection is reinforced by a narrow sheet of Dacron wrapped around the grafts and sutured to the tongues and to itself.

Forearm

Operations on the forearm after poliomyelitis consist of tenotomy, fasciotomy, and osteotomy to correct deformities and tendon transfers to restore function.

PRONATION CONTRACTURE

Deformities of the forearm seldom are disabling enough in themselves to warrant surgery; the most common exception is a fixed pronation contracture from imbalance between the supinators and pronators. When the pronator teres is not strong enough to transfer to replace the paralyzed supinators, correcting the contracture alone is indicated, provided there is active flexion of the elbow. When the pronators of the forearm and the flexors of the wrist are active, however, function can be improved not only by correcting the pronation contracture, but also by transferring the flexor carpi ulnaris (Chapter 69).

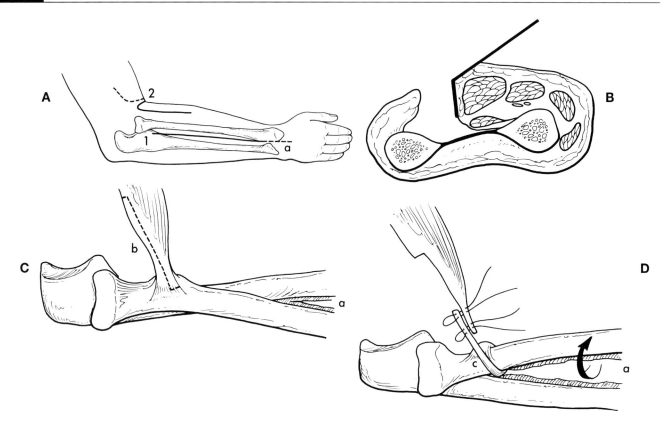

Fig. 31-32   Zancolli rerouting of biceps tendon for supination deformity of forearm. **A,** *1,* Dorsal skin incision is extended distally to *a* when distal radioulnar joint requires capsulotomy. *2,* Anterior incision to expose biceps tendon and radial head. **B,** Exposure of interosseous membrane by retracting dorsal muscles radially (see text). **C,** Broken line at *b* shows Z-plasty incision to be made in biceps tendon. Interosseous membrane has been divided at *a.* **D,** At *c,* biceps tendon has been divided by Z-plasty, distal segment has been rerouted around radial neck medially, and ends of tendon are being sutured together. Traction on tendon will now pronate forearm as indicated by arrow. (Redrawn from Zancolli EA: *J Bone Joint Surg* 49A:1275, 1967.)

Fixed supination deformity develops from muscle imbalance in which usually the pronators and finger flexors are weak and the biceps and wrist extensors are strong. The soft tissues, such as the interosseous membrane, contract, the bones become deformed, and eventually the radioulnar joints may dislocate. A fixed supination deformity combined with weak shoulder abduction markedly limits an otherwise functional hand. Recommended procedures for this deformity include rerouting of the biceps tendon (Zancolli) and manual osteoclasis of the middle thirds of the radius and ulna (Blount). The latter is recommended for children younger than 12 years of age with insufficient muscle power for tendon transfer.

◆ **Rerouting of Biceps Tendon for Supination Deformities of Forearm**

TECHNIQUE 31-31 *(Zancolli)*
If full passive pronation is already possible before surgery, omit the first part of the operation. Otherwise, make a longitudinal incision on the dorsum of the forearm over the

radial shaft (Fig. 31-32, *A, 1*). By blunt dissection expose the interosseous membrane and retract the dorsal muscles radialward to protect the posterior interosseous nerve (Fig. 31-32, *B*). Then divide the interosseous membrane throughout its length close to the ulna. If the dorsal ligaments of the distal radioulnar joint are contracted, extend the incision distally and perform a capsulotomy of this joint. If necessary, release the supinator muscle after identifying and protecting the posterior interosseous nerve in the proximal part of the incision. At this point in the operation full passive pronation of the forearm should be possible. Now make a second incision; begin it on the medial aspect of the arm proximal to the elbow and extend it distally to the flexion crease of the joint, then laterally across the joint in the crease, and then distally over the anterior aspect of the radial head (Fig. 31-32, *A, 2*). Identify and retract the median nerve and brachial artery. Divide the lacertus fibrosus and expose the insertion of the biceps tendon on the radial tuberosity. Now divide the biceps tendon by a long Z-plasty (Fig. 31-32, *C*). Then reroute the distal segment of the tendon around the radial neck medially, then posteriorly, and then laterally so that traction on it will pronate the forearm (Fig. 31-32, *D*). Then place the ends of the biceps tendon side-by-side and suture them together under tension that will maintain full pronation and yet allow extension of the elbow. If the radial head is subluxated or is dislocated, reduce it if possible and hold it in place by capsulorrhaphy of the radiohumeral joint; if the radial head cannot be reduced, excise it and transfer the proximal segment of the biceps tendon to the brachialis tendon. Close the incisions and apply a cast with the elbow flexed 90 degrees and the forearm moderately pronated.

AFTERTREATMENT. At about 3 weeks the cast and sutures are removed, and passive and active exercises are begun.

Wrist and Hand

The treatment of disabilities of the wrist and hand caused by paralysis is discussed in Chapter 68.

MYELOMENINGOCELE*
Epidemiology

Advances in medicine, surgery, and the allied health services have reduced the mortality rates in patients born with severe defects of the central nervous system. The challenge for orthopaedic surgeons is to assist these patients in attaining the best possible function within the limitations imposed on them by their physical handicap.

Myelomeningocele is the most common of the spectrum of conditions described as spina bifida. A myelomeningocele is a saclike structure containing cerebrospinal fluid and neural tissue (Fig. 31-33, *A*). The hernial protrusion of the spinal cord and its meninges through a defect in the vertebral canal results in variable neurological defects depending on the location and severity of the lesion.

The nervous system develops by the formation of a tubular structure (neurulation), and closure of this tube is completed by closure of the cranial and caudal neuropores at about days 24 to 26 of gestation. One theory about the cause of myelomeningocele is that the neural folds fail to fuse during this process. Another theory is that the defect occurs as a result of a rupture of a previously closed neural tube. Both theories have merit, but the exact embryological development is unknown.

The myelomeningocele is formed by the protrusion of dura

and arachnoid through the deficit in the vertebral arches. The spinal cord nerve roots are carried out into the fundus of the sac (Fig. 31-33, *B* and *C*). Other abnormalities of the spinal cord often occur with the myelomeningocele, including duplication of the cord, diastematomyelia, and severe vertebral bony anomalies such as defects in segmentation and failure of fusion of vertebral bodies, which cause congenital scoliosis, kyphosis, and kyphoscoliosis (see Chapters 38 and 41).

The incidence of myelomeningocele in the United States is 0.6 to 0.9 per 1000 births. The sibling recurrence is approximately 2% to 7%. Yates et al. showed an association between the susceptibility of offspring with neural tube defects and depressed red cell folate levels in the mother. They postulated that an inherent disorder of folate metabolism predisposes to neural tube defects. This theory was supported by Seller and Nevin, who reported a decreased incidence of neural tube defects in children whose mothers took periconceptional vitamins. The U.S. Food and Drug Administration (FDA) currently recommends that all women of childbearing age receive 0.4 mg folate before conception and during early pregnancy. The Centers for Disease Control and Prevention (CDC) recommend that women who are at high risk (i.e., those who have given birth to a prior affected child or who have a first-degree relative with a neural tube defect) receive 4 mg of folate per day. Prenatal diagnosis can be made by biochemical and enzyme evaluation, as well as by roentgenographic or ultrasound examination.

Associated Conditions

Most children with myelomeningocele will die if not treated; therefore most are treated with early closure of the defect and ventriculoperitoneal shunting. Myelomeningocele was believed to be nonprogressive, but studies have shown progressive neurological deterioration can occur, manifested by increasing levels of paralysis and decreasing upper extremity function. Hydrocephalus and associated hydrosyringomyelia, Arnold-Chiari malformation, and tethered cord syndrome have been associated with progressive neurological deterioration.

HYDROCEPHALUS

Of children with myelomeningocele, 80% to 90% have hydrocephalus that requires cerebrospinal shunting. The incidence is related to the neurological level of the lesion. Children who do not require shunting have a better prognosis for upper extremity function and trunk balance than those who require shunting. Even with improved designs, shunts can fail, resulting in neurological deterioration. Manifestations of shunt failure include signs of acute hydrocephaly, such as nausea, vomiting, and severe headaches. In older children the diagnosis may be more difficult, and shunt malfunction may be associated with increased irritability, decreased perceptual motor function, short attention span, intermittent headaches, increasing scoliosis, and increased level of paralysis.

---

*The author is indebted to Dr. Luciano Dias (Dias LS: Myelomeningocele. In Canale ST, Beaty JH, eds: *Operative pediatric orthopaedics,* St Louis, 1991, Mosby) for much of the information in this section.

Fig. 31-33 **A,** Infant with myelomeningocele. Lesion may be small extension (**B**) or large sessile protrusion (**C**).

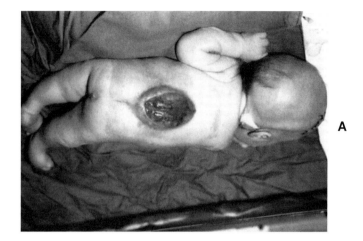

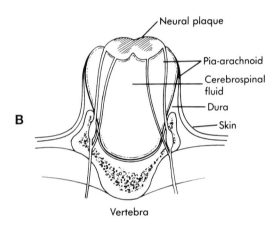

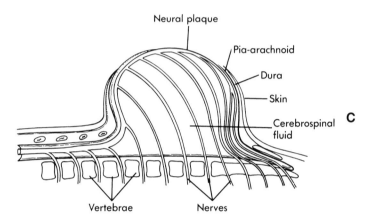

HYDROSYRINGOMYELIA

Hydrosyringomyelia is an accumulation of fluid in the enlarged central canal of the spinal cord. This usually is the result of hydrocephalus or an alteration in the normal cerebrospinal fluid dynamics. Hydrosyringomyelia can cause three problems in patients with myelomeningocele: (1) an increasing level of paralysis of the lower extremities, often associated with an increase in spasticity of the lower extremity, (2) progressive scoliosis, and (3) weakness in the hands and upper extremities. This condition can be diagnosed with magnetic resonance imaging; early treatment may reverse some of the neurological loss and scoliosis.

ARNOLD-CHIARI MALFORMATION

The Arnold-Chiari malformation (caudal displacement of the posterior lobe of the cerebellum) is a consistent finding in patients with myelomeningocele. The type II malformation is seen most often in children with myelomeningocele and is characterized by displacement of the medulla oblongata into the cervical neural canal through the foramen magnum. This malformation causes dysfunction of the lower cranial nerves, resulting in weakness or paralysis of vocal cords and difficulty in feeding, crying, and breathing. Sometimes these symptoms

are episodic, which makes diagnosis difficult. In childhood, symptoms may consist of nystagmus, stridor, difficulties in swallowing, and a depressed cough reflex. Spastic weakness of the upper extremities also may be present. Placement of a ventriculoperitoneal shunt to control hydrocephalus often resolves brainstem symptoms, and surgical decompression of the Arnold-Chiari malformation is not necessary. If brainstem compression symptoms remain after shunting, the posterior fossa and upper cervical spine will require surgical decompression.

TETHERED SPINAL CORD

Magnetic resonance imaging (MRI) shows signs of tethering of the spinal cord in most children with myelomeningocele, but only approximately 30% have clinical manifestations. Clinical signs are variable, but the most consistent are (1) loss of motor function, (2) development of spasticity in the lower extremities, primarily the medial hamstrings and ankle dorsiflexors and evertors, (3) development of scoliosis before the age of 6 years in the absence of congenital anomalies of the vertebral bodies, (4) back pain and increased lumbar lordosis in an older child, and (5) changes in urological function. MRI and, if necessary, computed tomography (CT), as well as myelographic evaluation, should be performed in any child suspected of having a

BOX 31-1 • Latex-Avoidance Protocol

Use of nonlatex gloves by surgical, anesthesia, and nursing personnel

Avoidance of any known latex product in the sterile field by the surgeon

Use of plastic anesthesia face mask for preoxygenation and positive-pressure ventilation

Use of nonlatex anesthetic reservoir bag for positive-pressure ventilation

Use of nonlatex tourniquet for intravenous catheter placement

Use of nonlatex blood pressure cuff/tubing, electrocardiogram leads, stethoscope

Use of nonlatex tape

Intravenous injection via stopcock rather than rubber injection port

From: Birmingham PK, Dsida RM, Grayhack JJ, et al: *J Pediatr Orthop* 16:799, 1996.

tethered cord syndrome. If clinical signs are documented, surgical treatment is indicated to prevent further deterioration of the motor function and to diminish the progress of spasticity and scoliosis. It is important to make an early diagnosis and start treatment because surgical release of the tethered cord rarely provides complete return of lost function.

LATEX HYPERSENSITIVITY

Latex hypersensitivity has been noted in children with myelomeningocele, with a reported incidence as high as 34%. The hypersensitivity is an immediate allergic reaction to latex exposure. It is recommended that all patients with myelomeningocele not be exposed to latex during surgery, including latex gloves and latex-containing accessories (catheters, adhesives, tourniquets, and anesthesia equipment) (Box 31-1). Dormans et al. recommended a pharmacological prophylaxis in addition to a latex-free environment (Table 31-1).

Classification

The most commonly used classification of myelomeningocele is based on the neurological level of the lesion (Fig. 31-34). Patients can be placed in one of three groups according to the level of the lesion and resultant muscle function.

Group I: thoracic or high lumbar level lesion, no quadriceps function. Community ambulation as adults in this group is rare unless trunk balance is excellent and upper extremity function is nearly normal.

Group II: low lumbar level lesion, functioning quadriceps and medial hamstring muscles, no gluteus medius function. Most children in this group require ankle-foot orthoses for support and crutches for trunk stability.

Group III: sacral level lesion, functioning quadriceps and gluteus medius muscles. Most children in this group can walk without external support and may or may not require ankle-foot orthoses.

Table 31-1 Prophylaxis for Latex Allergy

HIGH-RISK GROUP

A. Patient is admitted 24 hr before scheduled procedure

B. The following medications are administered IV before surgery and

For 72 hr postoperatively, administered every 6 hr (minimum, two doses)

	Dose	Max
Methylprednisolone	1 mg/kg	50 mg
Diphenhydramine	1 mg/kg	50 mg
Cimetidine	5 mg/kg	300 mg

C. Attempt to eliminate all latex-containing materials from the operating room environment.

MODERATE-RISK GROUP

A. Patient may be treated as outpatient

B. Oral medications are begun 24 hr before surgery (see below)

C. Medications are given every 6 hr for 24 hr before surgery with minimum of two doses

	Dose	Max
Prednisone	1 mg/kg	50 mg
Diphenhydramine	1 mg/kg	50 mg
Cimetidine	5 mg/kg	50 mg

D. Attempt to eliminate all latex-containing materials from the operating room environment

LOW-RISK GROUP

A. Patient may be treated as outpatient

B. Oral therapy is begun 12 hr before surgery

	Dose	Max
Prednisone	1 mg/kg	50 mg
Diphenhydramine	1 mg/kg	50 mg

C. The following are given 1 hr before surgery

	Dose	Max
Prednisone	1 mg/kg	50 mg
Diphenhydramine	1 mg/kg	50 mg

D. Attempt to eliminate all latex-containing materials from the operating room environment

From Dormans JP, Templeton J, Schriener MS, Delfico AJ: *J Pediatric Orthop* 17:622, 1997.

According to Asher and Olson, the difference in the ability to walk is significant between children with L4 level lesions and those with L3 level lesions. They stress that knee extensor power also is necessary for community ambulation. Children with L3 or L4 level lesions have the most to gain from orthopaedic treatment of musculoskeletal deformities.

Lindseth suggested that sensory level is a better way to define the level of paralysis, and this may better describe what is seen clinically. Muscles that can communicate with the brain through sensory feedback are functional, but muscles that cannot become flaccid or spastic, functioning only by reflex. A

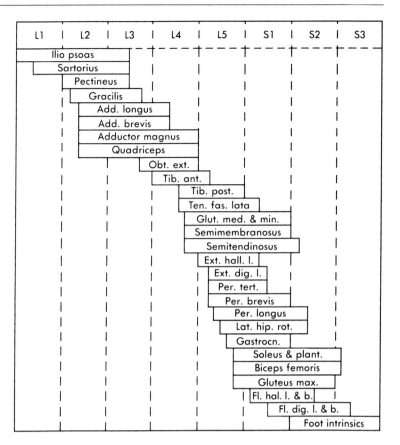

Fig. 31-34 Neurosegmental innervation of lower limb muscles. (From Sharrard WJW: *J Bone Joint Surg* 46B:427, 1964.)

sensory level classification also may be more reproducible between different observers.

Orthopaedic Evaluation

Orthopaedic evaluation of children with myelomeningocele should include the following:

1. Serial sensory and motor examinations to evaluate the neurological level of function. Absolute determination of the neurological level may not be possible before the child is 3 or 4 years old.
2. Sitting balance as an indication of central nervous system function. If one or two hands are required for support while sitting, the probability of ambulation is significantly decreased.
3. Upper extremity function, including decreased grip strength and atrophy of the thenar musculature (indications of hydromyelia).
4. Spinal curvature, as evaluated on yearly spinal roentgenograms, to detect development of scoliosis, kyphosis, and increased lumbar lordosis.
5. Range of motion, stability, and contractures of the hip.
6. Alignment, range of motion, contractures, and spasticity of the knee.
7. Rotational deformities, including external tibial torsion.
8. Ankle valgus deformity.
9. Other foot deformities, including congenital vertical talus or varus foot deformity.

Principles of Orthopaedic Management

Orthopaedic management should be tailored to meet specific goals during childhood, taking into account the expected function in adulthood. The goal of orthopaedic treatment is a stable posture. Ambulation is not the goal for every child. In spite of the best medical and surgical care, about 40% of children with myelomeningocele will not walk as adults. Quite often, however, the activities of daily living can be performed without lower extremity function. Surgery may be more detrimental than helpful, causing long-term disability. Before aggressive orthopaedic treatment is instituted, the lifetime prognosis for the patient should be considered. Only 30% of all patients with myelomeningocele are functionally independent, and only 30% of adults with myelomeningocele are employed full-time or part-time. Almost all patients with L2, or higher-level lesions are wheelchair users, and more than two thirds of those with lower level lesions (L3 to L5) use a wheelchair at least part of the time.

Most children achieve their maximal level of ambulation around the age of 4 years. If a child with myelomeningocele is not standing independently by the age of about 6 years, walking is unlikely. Prerequisites for walking include a spine balanced over the pelvis, absence of hip and knee contractures (or only mild contractures), and plantigrade, supple, braceable feet with the center of gravity centered over them. At least 80% of

Table 31-2 Foot Deformities in Patients with Myelomeningocele*

Level	Clubfoot	Calcaneovalgus Deformity	Vertical Talus	No Deformity
Thoracic	40	8	0	38
L1, L2	22	4	1	13
L3	24	21	9	
L4	50	4	0	14
L5	11	38	5	20
Sacral	19	4	0	41
Total	166	60	7	135

From Schafer ME, Dias LS: *Myelomeningocele: orthopaedic treatment,* Baltimore, 1983, Williams & Wilkins.
*In patients with asymmetrical paralysis, each foot was counted separately.

children with myelomeningocele have some impairment of their upper extremities; effective ambulation with low energy consumption and minimal bracing is possible in only about 50% of adult patients. Even though ambulation into adolescence and adulthood is unlikely, Mazur et al. have shown that children with high-level lesions benefit from walking during the first 10 years of life. Those who walk tend to be more mobile than children who never walk, and they have fewer fractures and skin pressure sores. If a child has functioning quadriceps and medial hamstring muscles, good sitting balance, and upper extremity function, all efforts should be made to achieve ambulation.

NONOPERATIVE MANAGEMENT

Orthotic treatment is aimed at obtaining effective mobility with minimal restriction. Bracing and splinting vary with the degree of motor deficit and trunk balance, and each child should be carefully evaluated by the orthopaedic surgeon, the orthotist, and the physical therapist. Children aged 12 to 18 months may benefit from the use of an A-frame for standing, and for children over 2 years of age, a parapodium supports the spine and allows a swing-to or swing-through gait with crutches or a walker. An ankle-foot orthosis (AFO) is used in children with low lumbar or sacral level lesions and fair quadriceps muscle function. The AFO should be rigid enough to provide ankle and foot stabilization and to maintain the ankle at 90 degrees. A knee-ankle-foot orthosis (KAFO) may be indicated for a child with a lumbar level lesion and weak quadriceps function to prevent abnormal valgus of the knee during the stance phase of gait. Children with high-level lesions often have excessive anterior pelvic tilt and lumbar lordosis and require a pelvic band, either as a conventional hip-knee-ankle-foot orthosis (HKAFO) or a reciprocating gait orthosis. The reciprocating gait orthosis also can be used in patients with upper lumbar lesions, allowing them to be upright and assisting them in attempts at ambulation. This brace provides the ability to walk in a reciprocal fashion by dynamically coupling the flexion of one hip to the simultaneous extension of the contralateral hip. For the reciprocating orthosis to be effective, the patient should have good upper extremity strength, trunk balance, and active hip flexion.

OPERATIVE MANAGEMENT

Orthopaedic deformities in children with myelomeningocele are caused by (1) muscle imbalance resulting from the neurological abnormality, (2) habitually assumed posture, and (3) associated congenital malformations. Surgical correction of deformities caused by any of these may be indicated. Most surgical procedures in patients with myelomeningocele are performed during the first 15 years of life. When surgical correction is indicated, the deformity should be completely and permanently corrected.

Menelaus listed several principles of orthopaedic management: multiple procedures should be done while the patient is under a single anesthetic; plaster immobilization, especially in recumbency, should be minimized because it fosters skeletal demineralization and secondary fractures; the orthopaedic treatment program must be integrated with the total treatment program; the absence of sensation, the increased likelihood of pathological fracture, and the increased danger of infection secondary to urinary tract problems must be constantly borne in mind; institutionalization must be kept at a minimum; and finally the sacrifices demanded of the family in terms of time, effort, expense, and separation must be minimized, lest these individual demands become collectively overwhelming.

Foot

Approximately 75% of children with myelomeningocele have foot deformities that can seriously limit function. These deformities can take many forms (Table 31-2), including clubfoot, acquired equinovarus, varus, metatarsus adductus, equinus, equinovalgus, congenital vertical talus, developmental vertical talus, calcaneus, calcaneovalgus, calcaneovarus, calcaneocavus, cavus, cavovarus, supination, pes planovalgus, and toe deformities.

The goal of orthopaedic treatment of foot deformities is a plantigrade, mobile, braceable foot. Muscle-balancing procedures that remove motors are more reliable than tendon transfer procedures. Bony deformities should be corrected by appropriate osteotomies that preserve joint motion; arthrodesis should be avoided if possible.

CLUBFOOT

Clubfoot is present at birth in approximately 30% of children with myelomeningocele. This deformity in myelomeningocele resembles that of arthrogryposis multiplex congenita and differs markedly from idiopathic clubfoot. It is characterized by severe rigidity, supination-varus deformity caused by the unopposed action of the tibialis anterior muscle, rotational malalignment of the calcaneus and talus, subluxation of the calcaneocuboid and talonavicular joints, and often a cavus component. Internal tibial torsion often is present. Recurrence of the deformity is frequent despite adequate surgical correction.

Surgery may be performed between the ages of 10 and 18 months. Radical posteromedial-lateral release through the Cincinnati incision (Chapter 26) is recommended. Tenotomies instead of tendon lengthening should be done to avoid any recurrence with growth. If the tibialis anterior tendon is active, simple tenotomy should be performed to prevent supination deformity. In older children, the imbalance between the medial and lateral columns of the foot may be so severe that it cannot be corrected by soft tissue release alone. Closing wedge osteotomy of the cuboid (Technique 26-8), lateral wedge resection of the distal calcaneus (Lichtblau procedure, Technique 26-13), or calcaneocuboid arthrodesis (Dillwyn-Evans procedure, see Fig. 31-3) may be required to shorten the lateral column. Talectomy (Technique 26-15) is indicated only as a salvage procedure for a severely deformed rigid clubfoot in an older child. The talus should be completely removed because any fragment left behind will resume its growth and cause recurrence of the deformity. Talectomy will correct the hindfoot deformity, but any adduction deformity should be corrected by shortening of the lateral column through the same incision. Severe forefoot deformities require midtarsal or metatarsal osteotomies (see Chapter 26).

VARUS DEFORMITY

Isolated varus deformity of the hindfoot is rare; it is more often associated with adduction deformity of the forefoot, cavus deformity, or supination deformity. Imbalance between the invertors and evertors should be carefully evaluated. For isolated, rigid hindfoot varus deformity, a closing wedge osteotomy is indicated. After removal of the lateral wedge (Fig. 31-35), the calcaneus should be translated laterally, if possible, to increase correction.

CAVOVARUS DEFORMITY

Cavovarus deformities occur mainly in children with sacral level lesions. The cavus is the primary deformity that causes the varus. The Coleman test (Fig. 32-19) helps to determine the rigidity of the varus deformity. For a supple deformity, radical plantar release (Technique 32-7) is indicated to correct the cavus deformity, without hindfoot bone surgery. If the varus deformity is rigid, in spite of plantar release with or without midtarsal osteotomy, a closing wedge osteotomy (Technique

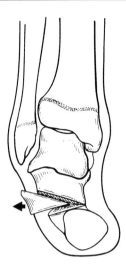

Fig. 31-35   Lateral closing wedge osteotomy of calcaneus for isolated varus deformity of hindfoot.

83-11) is indicated. Any muscle balance must be corrected either before the bony procedures or at the same time. Triple arthrodesis (Technique 31-5) rarely is indicated, although it can be used as a salvage procedure. Maynard et al. reported that foot rigidity, nonplantigrade position, and performance of an arthrodesis were risk factors for neuropathic foot ulcerations in patients with myelodysplasia.

SUPINATION DEFORMITY

Supination deformity of the forefoot occurs most frequently in children with L5 to S1 level lesions and is caused by the unopposed action of the tibialis anterior muscle when the peroneus brevis and peroneus longus are inactive. Adduction deformity also can be present. If the muscle imbalance is not corrected, the deformity becomes fixed. If the deformity is supple, simple tenotomy of the tibialis anterior tendon is adequate. If there is some gastrocsoleus activity and no spasticity, the tibialis anterior tendon can be transferred to the midfoot in line with the third metatarsal. Split tibialis anterior tendon transfer (Technique 31-10) occasionally can be used, with the lateral half of the tendon inserted in the cuboid. Osteotomy of the first cuneiform or the base of the first metatarsal may be required for residual bony deformity.

EQUINUS DEFORMITY

Equinus usually is an acquired deformity that can be prevented by bracing and splinting. It occurs more frequently in children with high lumbar or thoracic level lesions. For mild deformities, excision of about 2 cm of the tendo calcaneus through a transverse or vertical incision usually is sufficient. For more severe deformity, radical posterior release is required, including excision of all tendons and extensive capsulotomies of the ankle and subtalar joints. In rare cases, osteotomy or talectomy may be required for a symptomatic deformity.

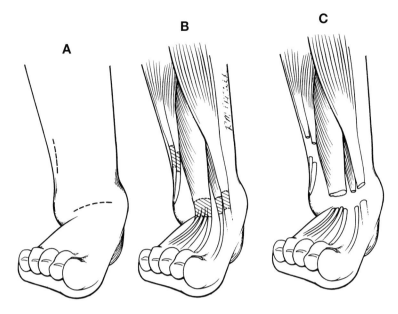

Fig. 31-36 Anterolateral release for calcaneus deformity (see text). **A,** Transverse and longitudinal incisions. **B** and **C,** Excision of portion of tendons and tendon sheaths.

CALCANEUS DEFORMITY

Approximately one third of children with myelomeningocele have calcaneus deformities, most frequently those with L5 to S1 level lesions. The most common form is a calcaneovalgus deformity caused by the active anterior leg muscles and inactive posterior muscles. Spasticity of the evertors and dorsiflexors may cause the deformity in children with high-level lesions. Untreated calcaneus deformity produces a bulky, prominent heel that is prone to pressure sores and makes shoe wear difficult. If the deformity is supple, as usually is the case, manipulation and splinting will bring the foot to a neutral position. Serial casting, followed by splinting, can be used for more rigid deformities. Muscle imbalance can be corrected early by simple tenotomy of all ankle dorsiflexors and tenotomy of the peroneus brevis and peroneus longus. After anterolateral release in some patients, spasticity develops in the gastrocsoleus muscle, causing an equinus deformity that requires tenotomy of the tendo calcaneus or posterior release. Posterior transfer of the anterior tibial tendon has been reported by Georgiadis and Aronson, Fraser and Hoffman, and Bliss and Menelaus to give good results even though a third to one half of the transfers have no active function; they recommended that this transfer be performed after 4 to 5 years of age. In older children with severe structural deformities, tendon transfers or tenotomies seldom achieve correction, and bony procedures are indicated.

◆ Anterolateral Release

TECHNIQUE 31-32

With the patient supine, apply and inflate a pneumatic tourniquet. Make a transverse incision about 2.5 cm long 2 to 3 cm above the ankle joint (Fig. 31-36, *A*). With sharp dissection, divide the superficial fascia to expose the tendons of the extensor hallucis longus, extensor digitorum communis, and tibialis anterior. Divide each tendon and excise at least 2 cm of each (Fig. 31-36, *B*). Locate the peroneus tertius tendon in the lateralmost part of the wound and divide it. Make a second longitudinal incision above the ankle joint lateral and posterior to the fibula (see Fig. 31-36, *A*). Identify and divide the peroneus brevis and longus tendons and excise a section of each (Fig. 31-36, *C*). Close the wounds and apply a short leg walking cast.

AFTERTREATMENT. The cast is worn for 10 days, and then an ankle-foot orthosis is fabricated for night wear.

◆ Transfer of Tibialis Anterior to Calcaneus

TECHNIQUE 31-33

With the patient supine, make an incision in the dorsal aspect of the foot at the level of the insertion of the tibialis anterior tendon at the base of the first metatarsal. Carefully detach the tendon from its insertion and free it as far proximally as possible. Make a second incision on the anterolateral aspect of the leg, just lateral to the tibial crest, about 3 to 5 cm above the ankle joint. Free the tendon as far distally as possible and bring it up into the proximal wound. Expose the interosseous membrane and make a wide opening in it. Make a third transverse incision posteriorly at the level of the insertion of the tendo calcaneus into the calcaneus. Using a tendon passer, bring the tibialis anterior tendon through the interosseous membrane, from anterior to posterior, down to the level of this incision. Drill a large hole in the calcaneus, starting posteriorly and medially and exiting laterally and plantarward. Pass a Bunnell suture

continued

through the tendon and use a Keith needle to draw the tendon through the hole. A button suture is not recommended because of pressure sores. Suture the tendon to the surrounding soft tissues to the level of its entrance into the calcaneus and to the tendo calcaneus. Close the wounds and apply a short leg cast.

HINDFOOT VALGUS

Valgus deformity at the ankle joint frequently exacerbates a hindfoot valgus deformity. Initially, this can be controlled with a well-fitted orthosis, but as the child becomes taller and heavier, control of the deformity is more difficult, pressure sores develop over the medial malleolus and the head of the talus, and surgical treatment is indicated. Clinical and roentgenographic measurements of the hindfoot valgus should be obtained; more than 10 mm of "lateral shift" of the calcaneus is significant. The Grice extraarticular arthrodesis (Technique 31-3) is the classic treatment for this problem, but frequently reported complications include resorption of the graft, nonunion, varus overcorrection, and residual valgus. Gallien, Morin, and Marquis reported successful subtalar arthrodesis in 61% of their patients; however, Ross and Lyne reported 80% unsatisfactory results with the procedure. Medial displacement osteotomy has been recommended for correction of hindfoot valgus so that arthrodesis of the subtalar joint can be avoided (see Chapter 3). The combination of hindfoot and ankle valgus should be considered; if the ankle deformity is more than 10 to 15 degrees, closing wedge osteotomy or hemiepiphysiodesis of the distal tibial epiphysis is recommended in addition to the calcaneal osteotomy.

VERTICAL TALUS

Vertical talus deformities occur in approximately 10% of children with myelomeningocele. The deformity is characterized by malalignment of the hindfoot and midfoot. The talus is almost vertical, the calcaneus is in equinus and valgus, the navicular is dislocated dorsally on the talus, and the cuboid may be subluxated dorsally in relation to the calcaneus. Two types of vertical talus, developmental and congenital, occur in children with myelomeningocele. Neither type can be corrected by conservative methods. In developmental vertical talus, the foot is more supple and the talonavicular dislocation can be reduced by plantar flexion of the foot. In congenital vertical talus, manipulation and serial casting may partially correct the soft tissue contractures in preparation for a complete posteromedial-lateral release (Chapter 26), which should be performed when the child is between 12 and 18 months old.

PES CAVUS DEFORMITY

Cavus deformity, alone or with clawing of the toes or varus of the hindfoot, occurs most often in children with sacral level lesions. It may cause painful callosities under the metatarsal heads and difficulty with shoe wear. As stressed by Paulos, Coleman, and Samuelson, plantar flexion of the first ray must be corrected for successful correction of the deformity. Although several procedures have been recommended for this deformity, few have been reported in patients with myelomeningocele. For an isolated cavus deformity with no hindfoot varus, radical plantar release is indicated. When varus deformity is present, medial subtalar release (Technique 26-13) is indicated. After surgery a short leg cast is applied, and 1 to 2 weeks later the deformity is gradually corrected by cast changes every week or every other week for 6 weeks. In older children with rigid cavus deformities, anterior first metatarsal closing wedge osteotomy (Technique 83-9) is indicated in addition to radical plantar release. For residual varus deformity, a Dwyer closing wedge osteotomy of the calcaneus (Technique 83-14) is recommended.

TOE DEFORMITIES

Clawtoe or hammer toe deformities occur more often in children with sacral level lesions and can cause problems with shoe and orthotic fitting. For clawtoe alone, simple tenotomy of the flexors at the level of the proximal phalanx usually is sufficient. The Jones procedure (tendon suspension, Technique 83-8) is indicated when clawing of the toes is associated with a cavus deformity. For clawing of the hallux, arthrodesis of the proximal interphalangeal joint (Technique 83-7) or tenodesis of the distal stump of the extensor pollicis longus to the extensor pollicis brevis is recommended. Alternatively, the Jones procedure can be performed on the hallux and the Hibbs transfer (Technique 83-10) on the other clawed toes.

Ankle

Progressive valgus deformity at the ankle or in combination with hindfoot valgus occurs most frequently in children with low lumbar level lesions. The strength of the gastrocsoleus muscle is diminished or absent, and excessive laxity of the tendo calcaneus allows marked passive ankle dorsiflexion. The medial malleolus is bulky, the head of the talus is shifted medially, and pressure ulcerations in these areas are common. The calcaneovalgus deformity usually appears early, but problems with orthotic fitting do not arise until the child is about 6 years old. Fibular shortening is common in children with L4, L5, or higher level lesions. In the paralytic limb, abnormal shortening of the fibula and lateral malleolus causes a valgus tilt of the talus, with subsequent valgus deformity at the ankle (Fig. 31-37). Shortening of the fibula alters the normal distribution of forces on the distal tibial articular surface and increases compression forces on the lateral portion of the tibial epiphysis, further inhibiting growth, whereas decreased compression on the medial portion of the tibial epiphysis accelerates growth. This imbalance causes the lateral wedging that produces a valgus inclination of the talus. The degree of lateral wedging of the tibial epiphysis correlates with the degree of fibular shortening.

To accurately evaluate valgus ankle deformity in children with myelomeningocele, three factors must be determined: (1) the degree of fibular shortening, (2) the degree of valgus tilt of the talus in the ankle mortise, and (3) the amount of "lateral

shift" of the calcaneus in relation to the weight-bearing axis of the tibia. Fibular shortening can be evaluated by measuring the distance between the distal fibular physis and the dome of the talus. In the normal ankle joint the distal fibular physis is 2 to 3 mm proximal to the dome of the talus in children up to 4 years of age (Fig. 31-38, *A*). Between the ages of 4 and 8 years, the physis is at the same level as the talar dome (Fig. 31-38, *B*), and in children older than 8 years of age, it is 2 to 3 mm distal to the talar dome (Fig. 31-38, *C*). Differences of more than 10 mm from these values are considered significant. The valgus tilt of the talus can be measured accurately on anteroposterior, weight-bearing roentgenograms. Malhotra classified ankle valgus into four stations based on the amount of ankle valgus and position of the fibular physis (Fig. 31-39). The lateral shift of the calcaneus is more difficult to determine. Stevens and Dias, Busch, and Tachdjian described roentgenographic techniques for evaluating ankle valgus and hindfoot alignment (Fig. 31-40, *A*). If the talar tilt exceeds 10 degrees, Stevens recommended tilting the roentgen tube appropriately to obtain a true lateral weight-bearing view of the foot. On this view, the weight-bearing axis of the tibia is drawn, and the distance from this line to the center of the calcaneus is measured. Dias et al. also used an anteroposterior weight-bearing view, directing the beam horizontally and preserving the coronal relationship in both dimensions. They positioned the foot in slight dorsiflexion

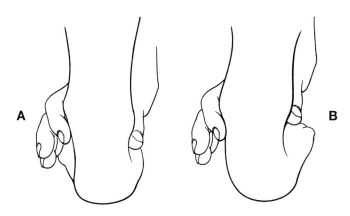

Fig. 31-37 **A,** Posterior view of right foot of normal child with correct alignment of malleoli and hindfoot. **B,** In child with myelomeningocele, medial malleolus is prominent and lateral malleolus is shortened, causing valgus deformity of ankle.

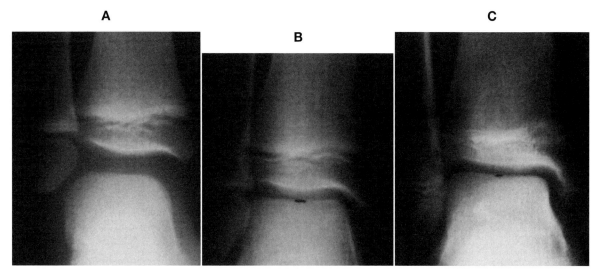

Fig. 31-38 Normal position of distal fibular physis. **A,** Proximal to dome of talus in children up to 4 years of age. **B,** Level with dome of talus in children between 4 and 8 years of age. **C,** Distal to dome of talus in children older than 8 years of age.

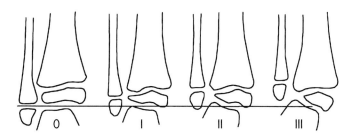

Fig. 31-39 Malhotra classification of ankle valgus. Station 0 is normal with fibular physis at level of plafond. Stations I to III correspond with progressive valgus as indicated by the proximal position of the fibular physis. (From Stevens PM, Bell RM: *J Pediatric Orthop* 17:9, 1997).

by placing a hard foam wedge under the plantar surface but not under the calcaneus and positioning the cassette behind the foot and ankle. The normal lateral shift of the calcaneus is from 5 to 10 mm (Fig. 31-40, *B*); if the center of the calcaneus is more than 10 mm lateral to the weight-bearing line, excessive valgus is present (Fig. 31-40, *C*). This technique is useful to determine before surgery if the valgus deformity is at the ankle or subtalar level.

Operative treatment is indicated when the ankle valgus deformity causes problems with orthotic fitting and cannot be relieved with orthoses. Tenodesis of the tendo calcaneus to the fibula (see Fig. 31-1) was described by Westin and Defiore for patients with poliomyelitis; Dias, and Stevens and Toomey have reported its use in patients with myelomeningocele. Tendo calcaneus tenodesis is indicated for valgus talar tilt between 10 and 25 degrees in patients between the ages of 6 and 10 years (see Fig. 31-9). Other procedures may be indicated for severe bony deformities, including hemiepiphysiodesis for mild deformity in children with remaining growth and supramalleolar derotation osteotomy for severe angular deformity. Medial sliding osteotomy of the calcaneus may be indicated if the valgus deformity is in the subtalar joint and calcaneus.

HEMIEPIPHYSIODESIS OF DISTAL TIBIAL EPIPHYSIS

Burkus, Moore, and Raycroft recommended hemiepiphysiodesis of the distal tibial epiphysis in young children with valgus deformities of less than 20 degrees and mild fibular shortening. Through a medial incision at the ankle, the medial aspect of the epiphysis is exposed, and epiphysiodesis is performed by either a percutaneous or an open method (Fig. 31-41). The growth arrest of the medial physis combined with continued growth of the lateral side gradually corrects the lateral wedging of the tibial epiphysis. If overcorrection occurs, the epiphysiodesis should be completed laterally. This procedure does not correct any rotational component of the deformity, and derotation osteotomy of the distal tibia and fibula may be required. Beals described a surface epiphysiodesis of the ankle to correct ankle valgus. He removed a strip of cortical bone 1 cm wide, 2 cm long, and 0.5 cm deep across the physis of the medial distal tibia. A piece of intact bone was then placed across the physis to obtain the surface epiphysiodesis.

Stevens and Belle and Davids et al. reported good results with screw epiphysiodesis for correction of ankle valgus. This technique involves placing a vertical 4.5-mm screw across the medial malleolar physis to retard growth. This allows gradual correction of ankle valgus. Davids et al. found a median rate of correction of 0.59 degrees per month. They also noted that, if the single screw was removed, growth resumed and deformity recurred at a rate of 0.60 degrees per month. Stevens and Belle recommended this procedure in children over the age of 6 years.

◆ Screw Epiphysiodesis

TECHNIQUE 31-34
Place the patient supine. Make a 3-mm stab wound over the medial malleolus. Use image intensification to properly position the incision. Insert a guide pin from the 4.5-mm

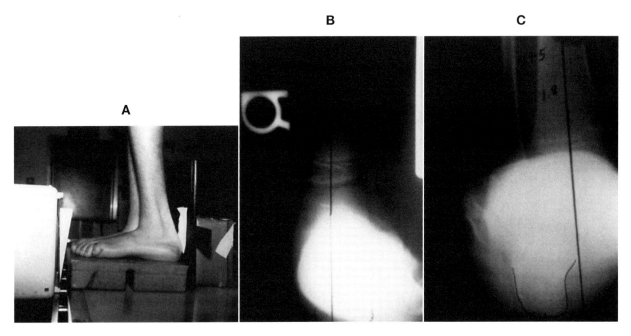

Fig. 31-40   Roentgenographic technique for evaluation of ankle valgus. **A,** Roentgenographic technique for weight-bearing view. **B,** Normal shift of calcaneus is 5 to 10 mm. **C,** Lateral shift of 15 to 18 mm indicates excessive valgus.

cannulated screw set into the medial malleolus and advance it proximally and medially across the distal tibial physis. Confirm the position of the guide pin by image intensification. The guide pin should be as vertical as possible in the medial one fourth of the medial distal tibial physis in the anteroposterior plane. In the sagittal plane the guide pin should cross the physis through its middle third. Place a tap over the guide pin and tap the bone across the physis. Insert a fully threaded, cannulated screw over the guide pin until it is completely seated.

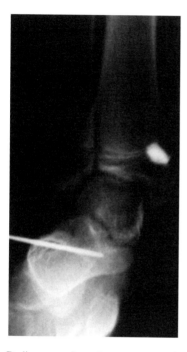

Fig. 31-41 Radiopaque dye shows extent of medial hemiepiphysiodesis of distal tibial epiphysis.

◆ SUPRAMALLEOLAR VARUS DEROTATION OSTEOTOMY

Supramalleolar osteotomy is recommended for children older than 10 years of age with low lumbar level lesions, severe fibular shortening (more than 10 to 20 mm), valgus tilt of more than 20 degrees, and external tibial torsion.

TECHNIQUE 31-35

With the patient supine, make an anterior longitudinal incision at the distal third of the leg. Expose the distal tibia and identify the epiphysis. Make a second incision over the distal third of the fibula and perform an oblique osteotomy beginning laterally and extending distally and medially, depending on the degree of valgus to be corrected. Make the medial-based wedge osteotomy as distal on the tibia as possible (Fig. 31-42, *A*). At the time of correction of the valgus, rotate the distal fragment internally to correct external tibial torsion. Use two Kirschner wires to temporarily hold the fragments in place and obtain roentgenograms to evaluate correction of the valgus deformity. The talus should be horizontal and the lateral malleolus lower than the medial malleolus. Staples or Kirschner wires or, in patients nearing skeletal maturity, a plate and screws (Fig. 31-42, *B*) can be used for internal fixation. Close the wounds and apply a long leg cast with the ankle and foot in neutral.

AFTERTREATMENT. Partial weight-bearing with crutches is allowed immediately. At 3 weeks the cast is changed to a below-knee cast, and full weight-bearing is allowed. The Kirschner wires can be removed at 8 to 12 weeks.

◆ ◆ ◆

Abraham et al. described a similar technique for supramalleolar osteotomy but used staples for fixation of the osteotomy site. They found that the best results were obtained when the tibiotalar axis was corrected to 5 degrees of varus (Fig. 31-43).

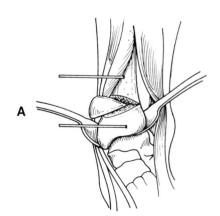
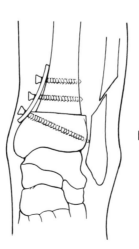

Fig. 31-42 Supramalleolar varus derotation osteotomy for severe ankle valgus deformity in adolescents. **A,** Removal of medial bone wedge from distal tibial metaphysis. **B,** Fixation of osteotomy with plate and screws.

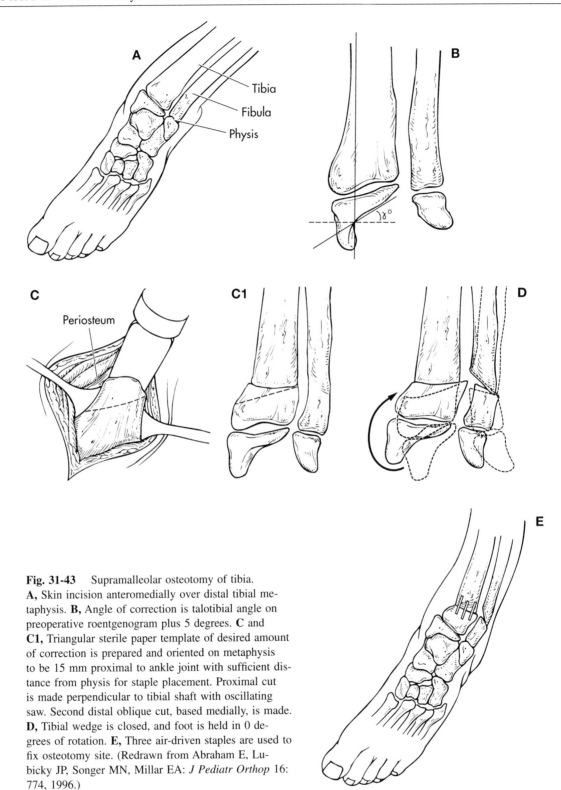

Fig. 31-43 Supramalleolar osteotomy of tibia.
A, Skin incision anteromedially over distal tibial metaphysis. **B,** Angle of correction is talotibial angle on preoperative roentgenogram plus 5 degrees. **C** and **C1,** Triangular sterile paper template of desired amount of correction is prepared and oriented on metaphysis to be 15 mm proximal to ankle joint with sufficient distance from physis for staple placement. Proximal cut is made perpendicular to tibial shaft with oscillating saw. Second distal oblique cut, based medially, is made. **D,** Tibial wedge is closed, and foot is held in 0 degrees of rotation. **E,** Three air-driven staples are used to fix osteotomy site. (Redrawn from Abraham E, Lubicky JP, Songer MN, Millar EA: *J Pediatr Orthop* 16: 774, 1996.)

Rotational deformities of the lower extremity can cause functional problems in patients with myelomeningocele. Toeing-out can result either from an external rotation deformity of the hip or from external tibial torsion. Toeing-in frequently occurs in patients with fourth or fifth lumbar level lesions because of an imbalance between the medial and lateral hamstrings. The hamstrings tend to remain active during the stance phase of gait, and when the biceps femoris is paralyzed, the muscle imbalance produces a toeing-in gait. Another cause for toeing-in is residual internal tibial torsion.

Rotation deformity of the hip and external and internal tibial torsion can be corrected by derotation osteotomies. Dias et al. corrected the dynamic toeing-in gait by transferring the semitendinosus laterally to the biceps tendon.

Knee

Deformities of the knee in patients with myelomeningocele are of four types: (1) flexion contracture, (2) extension contracture, (3) valgus deformity, and (4) varus deformity.

FLEXION CONTRACTURE

Flexion contractures are more common than extension contractures. About half of children with thoracic or lumbar level lesions have knee flexion contractures. Contractures of up to 20 degrees are common at birth, but most correct spontaneously. Knee flexion contractures may become fixed because of (1) the typical position assumed when supine: hips in abduction, flexion, and external rotation, knees in flexion, and feet in equinus; (2) gradual contracture of the hamstring and biceps muscles, with contracture of the posterior knee capsule from quadriceps weakness and prolonged sitting; (3) spasticity of the hamstrings that may occur with the tethered cord syndrome; and (4) paralysis of the gastrocsoleus and gluteus maximus muscles. Knee flexion contractures caused by positioning in children with high-level lesions often can be prevented by early splinting and a well-supervised home physical therapy program. In children with low lumbar lesions, the flexion deformity usually occurs later, after the age of 10 years, and orthoses do not prevent its gradual development. Radical flexor release usually is required for contractures of 15 to 30 degrees, especially in children who walk with below-knee orthoses. Supracondylar extension osteotomy of the femur (see Fig. 31-14) generally is required for contractures of more than 30 to 45 degrees in older children who are community ambulators and in whom radical flexor release was unsuccessful. If a hip flexion contracture is present, both hip and knee contractures should be corrected at the same time. No surgical treatment is indicated in older children who are not community ambulators if the contracture does not interfere with mobility.

◆ Radical Flexor Release

TECHNIQUE 31-36

Make a medial and a lateral vertical incision just above the flexor crease. In a child with a high-level lesion, identify and divide the medial hamstring tendons (semitendinosus, semimembranosus, gracilis, and sartorius). Resect part of each tendon (Fig. 31-44, *A*). Laterally, identify, divide, and resect the biceps tendon and the iliotibial band. In a child with a low lumbar-level lesion, intramuscularly lengthen the biceps and semimembranosus to preserve some flexor power. Next, free the origin of the gastrocnemius from

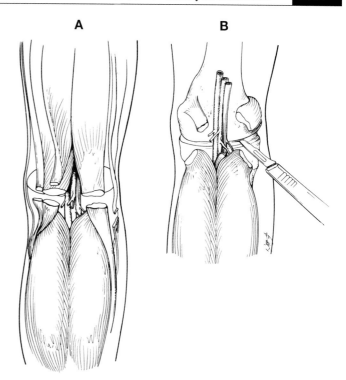

Fig. 31-44 Radical release of flexor tendons for flexion contracture of knee. **A,** All flexor tendons are divided, and about 3 cm of each is resected. **B,** Gastrocnemius origin from femoral condyle is divided and retracted; capsule is completely divided. If full extension is not obtained, posterior cruciate ligament is divided.

the medial and lateral condyles, exposing the posterior knee capsule, and perform an extensive capsulectomy (Fig. 31-44, *B*). If full extension is not obtained, divide the medial and lateral collateral ligaments and the posterior cruciate ligament. Close the wound over a suction drain and apply a long leg cast with the knee in full extension. If the flexion contracture is greater than 45 degrees, because of the possibility of vascular problems, the first cast should be applied with the knee in 20 to 30 degrees of flexion and gradually brought to full extension through serial cast changes.

AFTERTREATMENT. The cast is removed at 14 days, and a long leg splint is used at night. For children with low lumbar level lesions, intensive physical therapy for strengthening of the quadriceps mechanism is imperative after cast removal.

EXTENSION CONTRACTURE

Extension contractures usually are bilateral and are frequently associated with other congenital anomalies such as dislocation of the ipsilateral hip, external rotation contracture of the hip, equinovarus deformity of the foot, and occasionally valgus deformity of the knee. Knee extension contracture can seriously impair ambulation and make wheelchair sitting and transfer in and out of an automobile difficult. Serial casting, attempting to flex the knee to at least 90 degrees, is successful in most patients. If this does not correct the contracture, lengthening of the quadriceps mechanism is indicated. Several methods of lengthening have been described, including "anterior circumcision" (Dupré and Walker) in which all of the structures in front and at the side of the knee are divided by subcutaneous tenotomy, Z-plasty of the extensor mechanism combined with anterior capsulotomy (Parsch and Manner), and V-Y quadriceps lengthening (Curtis and Fisher).

VARUS OR VALGUS DEFORMITY

Varus or valgus deformity of the knee can be caused by malunion of a supracondylar fracture of the femur or proximal metaphyseal fracture of the tibia. Contracture of the iliotibial band also can cause a valgus deformity. For mild deformities, no treatment is indicated. If the iliotibial band is contracted, its distal portion should be divided 2.5 cm proximal to the patella (p. 1309). More severe deformities that interfere with bracing and mobility require either supracondylar or tibial osteotomy with internal fixation.

Hip

Deformities or instability of the hip in children with myelomeningocele can be caused by muscle imbalance, congenital dysplasia, or both. Nearly half the children with myelomeningocele have either hip subluxation or dislocation, and hip contractures can be more of a problem than the dislocation. Abduction or adduction contractures of the hip can cause infrapelvic obliquity, which can interfere with ambulation and bracing. Treatment of hip dislocations in these children differs significantly from that of congenital hip dislocation. Because of the different levels of paralysis and the combination of mixed and flaccid paralysis, treatment must be individualized.

FLEXION CONTRACTURE

Flexion deformity of the hip occurs most frequently in children with high lumbar or thoracic level lesions and is caused by the unopposed action of the hip flexors (iliopsoas, sartorius, and rectus), by long periods of lying supine or sitting, or by spasticity of the hip flexors. Hip flexion contractures must be distinguished from the physiological flexion position, and the amount of hip flexion should be determined by the Thomas test. Shurtleff et al. found that in the first 27 months of life, the deformity diminished except in patients with lesions at T12 or above. Because of this tendency to improve, hip flexion deformities rarely should be surgically treated before 24 months of age. Surgical release is indicated for contractures that interfere with bracing or walking but rarely is required for those of less than 20 degrees. Knee flexion contractures, which commonly occur with the hip contractures, should be corrected at the same time as the hip contracture.

Anterior hip release involves release of the sartorius, rectus femoris, iliopsoas, tensor fasciae latae muscles, the anterior hip capsule, and the iliopsoas tendon. This procedure should adequately correct flexion contractures of up to 60 degrees. If deformity remains after release, subtrochanteric extension osteotomy is indicated but should be postponed until the patient is near skeletal maturity to avoid recurrence of the deformity.

◆ Anterior Hip Release

TECHNIQUE 31-37

Make a "bikini" skin incision slightly distal and parallel to the iliac crest, extending it obliquely along the inguinal crease. Identify and protect the neurovascular bundle medially. Identify the iliopsoas tendon as far distally as possible and divide it transversely. Detach the sartorius muscle from its origin on the superior iliac crest. Identify the rectus insertion in the anteroinferior iliac crest and detach it. Laterally, identify the tensor fasciae latae muscle and, after carefully separating it from the fascia, divide the fascia transversely completely posterior to the anterior border of the gluteal muscles to expose the anterior hip capsule. If any residual flexion contracture remains, open the joint capsule transversely about 2 cm from the acetabular labrum. Place a suction drain in the wound, suture the subcutaneous tissue with interrupted sutures, and approximate the skin edges with subcuticular nylon sutures. Apply a hip spica cast with the hip in full extension, 10 degrees of abduction, and neutral rotation.

In children with low lumbar level lesions, this release greatly reduces hip flexor power and may impair mobility. A free tendon graft, using part of the tensor fasciae latae, can be used to reattach the sartorius to the anterosuperior iliac crest, and the rectus tendon can be sutured distal to the sartorius muscle in the hip capsule.

AFTERTREATMENT. Early weight-bearing for 2 to 3 hours a day is encouraged. The spica cast is removed at 4 to 6 weeks, and a total body splint is fitted with the hip in the same position.

FLEXION-ABDUCTION–EXTERNAL ROTATION CONTRACTURE

Flexion-abduction–external rotation contractures are common in children with thoracic level lesions and complete paralysis of the muscles of the lower extremity. Continuous external rotation of the hip in the supine position causes contractures of the posterior hip capsule and short external rotator muscles; this can be prevented by the use of night splints (total body splints) and range-of-motion exercises. Complete hip release (Technique 31-19) is indicated only when the deformity interferes with bracing. If both hips are contracted, as is often the case, both should be corrected at the same time.

EXTERNAL ROTATION CONTRACTURE

Isolated external rotation contracture of the hip occasionally occurs in children with low lumbar level lesions. Initially, bracing and physical therapy will help improve the external rotation contracture. If the external hip rotation persists after the child is 5 or 6 years old, a subtrochanteric medial rotation osteotomy (Chapter 30) is indicated.

ABDUCTION CONTRACTURE

Isolated unilateral abduction contracture is a common cause of pelvic obliquity, scoliosis, and difficulty in sitting and ambulation. It generally is caused by contracture of the tensor fasciae latae but may occur after iliopsoas transfer. It is common in children with high-level lesions and can be prevented by early splinting and physical therapy. Fascial release is indicated when the abduction contracture causes pelvic obliquity and scoliosis and interferes with function.

◆ Fascial Release

TECHNIQUE 31-38

Incise the skin along the anterior one half or two thirds of the iliac crest to the anterosuperior iliac spine. Divide all thigh fascial and tendinous structures around the anterolateral aspect of the hip; fascia lata, fascia over the gluteus medius and gluteus minimus, and tensor fasciae latae. Do not divide the muscle tissue, only the enveloping fascial structures. Fasciotomy of the fascia lata distally, as described by Yount (Technique 31-19), also may be required. Close the wound over a suction drain and apply a hip spica cast with the operated hip in neutral abduction and the opposite hip in 20 degrees of abduction, enough to permit perineal care.

AFTERTREATMENT. The cast is removed at 2 weeks, and a total body splint is fitted.

ADDUCTION CONTRACTURE

Adduction contractures are common with dislocation or subluxation of the hip in children with high-level lesions because of spasticity and contracture of the adductor muscles. Surgery is indicated when the contracture causes pelvic obliquity and interferes with sitting or walking. Adductor release may be combined with operative treatment of hip subluxation or dislocation.

◆ Adductor Release

TECHNIQUE 31-39

Make a transverse inguinal incision 2 to 3 cm long just distal to the inguinal crease over the adductor longus tendon. Open the superficial fascia to expose the adductor longus tendon.

Using electrocautery, divide the tendon close to its insertion on the pubic ramus. If necessary, divide the muscle fibers of the gracilis proximally and completely divide the adductor brevis muscle fibers, taking care to protect the anterior branch of the obturator nerve. At least 45 degrees of abduction should be possible. Close the wound over a suction drain and apply a spica cast with the hip in 25 to 30 degrees of abduction.

AFTERTREATMENT. The cast is removed at 2 weeks, and a total body splint is fitted with the hip in 25 degrees of abduction.

HIP SUBLUXATION AND DISLOCATION

More than half of children with myelomeningocele have hip subluxation or dislocation. Congenital, teratological, or paralytic dislocation may be present at birth. Congenital hip dislocation occurs in children with sacral level lesions without muscle imbalance. Treatment should follow standard conservative methods (Pavlik harness, traction and closed reduction, and spica cast immobilization). Teratological dislocations usually occur in children with high-level lesions. Initial roentgenograms show a dysplastic acetabulum, with the head of the femur displaced proximally; these dislocations should not be treated initially.

Paralytic subluxation or dislocation is the most common type, occurring in 50% to 70% of children with low-level (L3 or L4) lesions. Dislocation occurs most frequently during the first 3 years of life because of an imbalance between abduction and adduction forces. Dislocations in older children usually are caused by contractures or spasticity of the unopposed adductors and flexors associated with a tethered cord syndrome or hydromyelia.

Reduction of hip dislocations in children with myelomeningocele is controversial. Barden, Meyer, and Stelling found no correlation between the status of the hip and the ability to walk in children observed for 20 years. Feiwell, Sakai, and Blatt reported that reduction did not improve range of motion, did not reduce pain, and did not reduce the amount of bracing required. They stressed that maintaining a level pelvis and flexible hips was more important than reduction of the hip dislocation. The goal of treatment should be maximal function rather than roentgenographic reduction. Soft tissue release alone is indicated in patients without functional quadriceps muscles because only occasionally do they remain community ambulators as adults. Open reduction is appropriate only for those children with strong quadriceps muscles bilaterally, normal trunk balance, and normal upper extremity function. Bilateral or unilateral hip dislocation or subluxation in children with high-level lesions does not require extensive surgical treatment, but soft tissue contractures should be corrected. More aggressive treatment is indicated for children with low-level lumbar lesions who are likely to maintain their ambulatory potential.

In addition to open reduction of the femoral head into the acetabulum, muscle imbalance, contractures, bony deformities, and capsular laxity must be corrected. Lee and Carroll recommended iliopsoas transfer with adductor release, capsulorrhaphy, and acetabuloplasty in addition to open reduction. The Sharrard iliopsoas transfer through the posterolateral ilium (Technique 31-22) is most often used. Reported success rates of posterior iliopsoas transfer range from 20% to 95%. Roye et al. discouraged bilateral iliopsoas transfers because the resulting weakness of the hip flexors can impede ambulation. Thomas, Thompson, and Straub described a method of transferring the external oblique muscle to the greater trochanter (Technique 31-21). McKay recommended transfer in conjunction with femoral osteotomy. Lindseth recommended posterolateral transfer of the tensor fascia lata with transfer of the adductor and external oblique muscles.

◆ Transfer of Adductors, External Oblique, and Tensor Fasciae Latae

TECHNIQUE 31-40 *(Phillips and Lindseth)*

Place the patient supine. Expose the adductor muscles through a transverse incision beginning just anterior to the tendon of the adductor longus and extending posteriorly to the ischium. Incise the fascia longitudinally. Detach the tendons of the gracilis, adductor longus, and brevis and the anterior third of the magnus from the pubis. Carry the dissection posteriorly to the ischial tuberosity and suture the detached origins of the adductor muscles to the ischium with nonabsorbable sutures. Take care not to disrupt the anterior branch of the obturator nerve that supplies the adductor muscles.

Transfer the external abdominal oblique muscle to the gluteus medius tendon or preferably to the greater trochanter, as described by Thomas, Thompson, and Straub.

Make an oblique skin incision extending from the posterior third of the iliac crest to the anterosuperior iliac spine (Fig. 31-45, *A*). Curve the incision distally and posteriorly to the junction of the proximal and middle third of the femur. With sharp and blunt dissection, raise skin flaps to expose the fascia of the leg from the lateral border of the sartorius to the level of the greater trochanter. Expose the external oblique similarly from the iliac crest to the posterosuperior iliac spine and from its costal origin to the pubis (Fig. 31-45, *B*). Make two incisions approximately 1 cm apart in the aponeurosis of the external oblique parallel to the Poupart ligament and join them close to the pubis at the external ring. Extend the superior incision proximally along the medial border of the muscle belly until the costal margin is reached. Free the muscle from the underlying internal oblique by blunt dissection until the posterior aspect is reached in the Petit triangle. Elevate the muscle fibers from the iliac crest by cutting from posterior to anterior along the crest. Close the defect that remains in the

aponeurosis of the external oblique beginning at the pubis and extending as far laterally as possible. Fold the cut edges of the muscle and aponeurosis over and suture with a single suture at the muscle-tendinous junction. Weave a heavy, nonabsorbable suture through the aponeurosis in preparation for transfer (Fig. 31-45, *C*).

Attention is then directed to the tensor fasciae latae. Detach the origin of the tensor fasciae latae from the ilium. Separate the muscle along its anterior border from the sartorius down to its insertion into the iliotibial band. Divide the iliotibial band transversely to the posterior part of the thigh. Carry the incision in the iliotibial band proximally to the insertion of the oblique fibers of the tensor fasciae latae and the tendon of the gluteus maximus. Take care to preserve the superior gluteal nerve and arteries beneath the gluteus medius muscle approximately 1 cm distal and posterior to the anterosuperior spine (Fig. 31-45, *D*). Abduct the hip and fold the origin of the tensor fasciae latae back on itself to the limit allowed by the neurovascular bundle, then suture it to the ilium with nonabsorbable sutures so that its origin overlies the gluteus medius muscle. Do not attach the distal end to the gluteus maximus tendon until the end of the procedure.

The hip, proximal femur, and ilium are now easily accessible for indicated corrective procedures such as open reduction of the hip, capsular plication, proximal femoral osteotomy, and acetabular augmentation. The origins of the rectus femoris and the psoas tendon are not routinely divided, although they can be released at this time if there is a hip flexion contracture.

With the patient maximally relaxed or paralyzed, transfer the tendon of the external oblique to the greater trochanter. Drill a hole in the greater trochanter and pass the tendon of the external oblique from posterior to anterior and suture it back on itself. The muscle should reach the greater trochanter and should follow a straight line from the rib cage to the trochanter; if it does not, the borders of the muscle should be inspected to ensure that they are free from all attachments (Fig. 31-45, *D*). Weave the distal end of the tensor fasciae latae through the tendon of the gluteus maximus while the hip is abducted approximately 20 degrees.

AFTERTREATMENT. A hip spica cast is applied postoperatively with the hips in extension and abducted 20 degrees. The child is encouraged to stand in the cast to prevent osteopenia. The cast is removed 1 month after surgery, and physical therapy is started. The patient is returned to the braces used before the operation. Any modification in bracing is made as indicated on follow-up.

For severe acetabular dysplasia, a shelf procedure (Chapter 27) or Chiari pelvic osteotomy (Chapter 27) can be performed at the same time as the transfer. If more than 20 to 30 degrees of abduction is necessary to maintain concentric

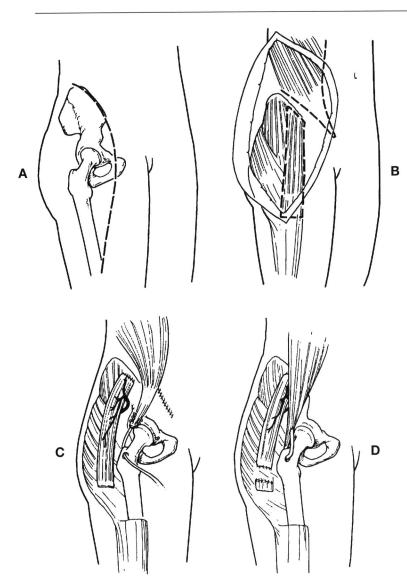

A

B

C

D

Fig. 31-45 Transfer of adductors, external oblique, and tensor fasciae latae. **A,** Skin incision. **B,** Skin flaps are elevated to expose fascia of leg and external oblique muscle. **C,** Cut edges of external oblique muscle and aponeurosis are folded over and sutured. Defect in aponeurosis is sutured. Origin of tensor fasciae latae on ilium is detached, with care being taken to preserve neurovascular bundle. Remainder of muscle is prepared for transfer. **D,** Tendon of external oblique is transferred to greater trochanter from posterior to anterior. Distal end of tensor fasciae latae is woven through tendon of gluteus maximus. (From Phillips DP, Lindseth RE: *J Pediatr Orthop* 12:712, 1992.)

reduction of the hip, a varus femoral osteotomy is indicated. Even with these procedures to correct acetabular dysplasia there is a high failure rate if muscle-balancing procedures are not included as part of the procedure.

◆ Proximal Femoral Resection and Interposition Arthroplasty

Severe joint stiffness is one of the most disabling results of hip surgery in patients with myelomeningocele. If the hip is stiff in extension, the child cannot sit; if it is stiff in flexion, the child cannot stand; if it is stiff "in between," the child can neither sit nor stand. Treatment of this complication rarely has been discussed. Resection of the femoral head and neck is not effective. Castle and Schneider reported proximal femoral resection and interposition arthroplasty in severely retarded, multiply handicapped children with dislocated hips and severe adduction contractures of the lower extremity.

TECHNIQUE 31-41 *(Baxter and D'Astous)*

Position the patient with a sandbag beneath the affected hip. Make a straight lateral approach beginning 10 cm proximal to the greater trochanter and extending down to the proximal femur. Split the fascia lata. Detach the vastus lateralis and gluteus maximus from their insertions and detach them from the greater trochanter. Identify the psoas tendon and detach its distal insertion on the lesser trochanter to expose extraperiosteally the proximal femur. Incise the periosteum circumferentially just distal to the gluteus maximus insertion and transect the bone at this level. Divide the short external rotators. Incise the capsule circumferentially at the level of the basal neck. Cut the ligamentous teres, remove the proximal femur, and test the range of motion of the hip. If necessary, perform a proximal hamstring tenotomy through the same incision after identifying the sciatic nerve.

continued

Adductor release also can be performed through a separate groin incision. Seal the acetabular cavity by oversewing the capsular edges. Cover the proximal end of the femur with the vastus lateralis and rectus femoris muscles. Interpose the gluteal muscles between the closed acetabulum and the covered end of the proximal femur to act as a further soft tissue cushion. Close the wound in layers over a suction drain.

AFTERTREATMENT. The operated lower extremity is placed in Russell traction in abduction until the soft tissues have healed, and then gentle range-of-motion exercises are begun.

PELVIC OBLIQUITY

Pelvic obliquity is common in patients with myelomeningocele. In addition to predisposing the hip to dislocation, it interferes with sitting, standing, and walking, and it can lead to ulceration under the prominent ischial tuberosity. Mayer described three types of pelvic obliquity: (1) infrapelvic, caused by contracture of the abductor and tensor fasciae latae muscles of one hip and contracture of the adductors of the opposite hip; (2) suprapelvic, caused by uncompensated scoliosis resulting from bony deformity of the lumbosacral spine or severe paralytic scoliosis; and (3) pelvic, caused by bony deformity of the sacrum and sacroiliac joint, such as partial sacral agenesis, causing asymmetry of the pelvis. Infrapelvic obliquity can be prevented by splinting, range-of-motion exercises, and positioning, but when hip contractures are well established, soft tissue release is required. Occasionally, more severe deformities require proximal femoral osteotomy. Suprapelvic obliquity can be corrected by control of the scoliosis by orthoses or spinal fusion. If severe scoliosis cannot be completely corrected, bony pelvic obliquity becomes fixed.

According to Lindseth, obliquity of 20 degrees is sufficient to interfere with walking and to produce ischial decubitus ulcerations; he recommended pelvic osteotomy in this instance. Before osteotomy, hip contractures should be released and the scoliosis should be corrected by spinal fusion. The degree of correction of pelvic obliquity is determined preoperatively from appropriate roentgenograms of the pelvis and spine (Fig. 31-46, *A*). The maximal correction obtainable with bilateral iliac osteotomies is 40 degrees.

◆ Pelvic Osteotomy

TECHNIQUE 31-42 *(Lindseth)*

The approach is similar to that described by O'Phelan for iliac osteotomy to correct exstrophy of the bladder (Chapter 27). With the child prone, make bilateral, inverted, L-shaped incisions beginning above the iliac crest, proceeding medially to the posterosuperior iliac spine, and

then curving downward along each side of the sacrum to the sciatic notch. Detach the iliac apophysis by splitting it longitudinally starting at the anterosuperior iliac spine and proceeding posteriorly (Fig. 31-46, *B*). Retract the paraspinal muscles, the quadratus lumborum muscle, and the iliac muscles medially along the inner half of the epiphysis and the inner periosteum of the ilium. After the sacral origin of the gluteus maximus has been detached from the sacrum, divide the outer periosteum of the ilium longitudinally just lateral to the posteromedial iliac border, extending from the posterosuperior iliac spine down to the sciatic notch. Strip the outer periosteum, along the gluteus muscles and the outer half of the epiphysis, from the outer table of the ilium, taking care to avoid damaging the superior and inferior gluteal vessels and nerves. Retract the soft tissues down to the sciatic notch and protect them by inserting malleable retractors. Next, make bilateral osteotomies approximately 2 cm lateral to each sacroiliac joint. The size of the wedge is determined by the amount of the correction desired and is limited to no more than one third of the iliac crest; the base of the wedge usually is about 2.5 cm long (Fig. 31-46, *C*).

After the wedge of bone has been removed, correct the deformity by pulling on the limb on the short side and pushing up on the limb on the long side (see Fig. 31-46, C). Usually this closes the osteotomy on the long side. If upper migration of the ilium onto the sacrum is severe, trim the excess iliac crest. Close the wedge osteotomy with two threaded pins or sutures through drill holes. Then use a spreader to open the osteotomy on the opposite (short) side sufficiently to receive the graft. Use two Kirschner wires to hold the graft in place (Fig. 31-46, *D*). Close the wound over suction-irrigation drains and apply a double full-hip spica cast.

AFTERTREATMENT. The cast is worn for 2 weeks. The Kirschner wires are removed when roentgenograms show sufficient healing of the osteotomy.

Spine

SCOLIOSIS

Paralytic spinal deformities have been reported in up to 90% of patients with myelomeningocele. Scoliosis is the most common deformity and usually is progressive. The incidence of scoliosis is related to the level of the bony defect and the level of paralysis. Moe et al. noted a 100% incidence of scoliosis with T12 lesions, 80% with L2 lesions, 70% with L3 lesions, 60% with L4 lesions, 25% with L5 lesions, and 5% with S1 lesions. The curves develop gradually until the child reaches the age of 10 years and may increase rapidly with the adolescent growth spurt. Raycroft and Curtis differentiated between developmen-

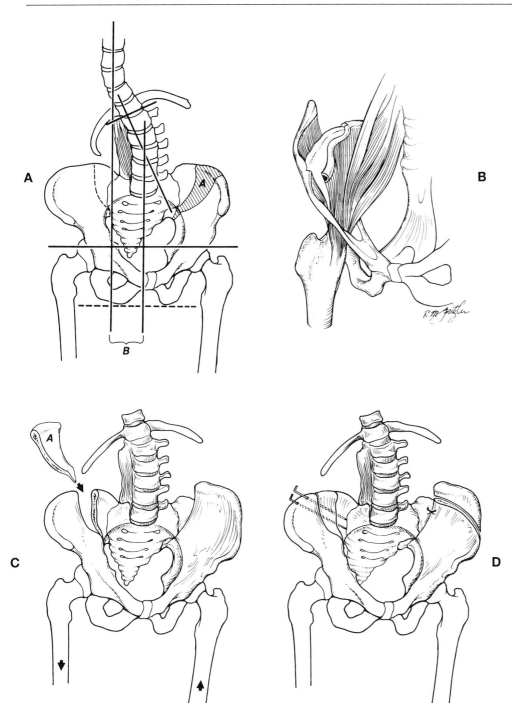

Fig. 31-46   Pelvic osteotomy for pelvic obliquity, as described by Lindseth. **A,** Preoperative determination of size of iliac wedge to be removed and transferred. **B,** Exposure of ilium. **C,** After bilateral osteotomies and removal of wedge from low side, deformity is corrected. **D,** Transferred iliac wedge is fixed with two Kirschner wires. (Redrawn from Lindseth RE: *J Bone Joint Surg* 60A:17, 1978.)

tal (no vertebral anomalies) and congenital (structural disorganization of the vertebral bodies) scoliosis in patients with myelomeningocele. The two types were almost evenly divided in their patients. Raycroft and Curtis suggested muscle imbalance and habitual posturing as causes of developmental scoliosis because 70% of patients also had dislocated hips and 83% had pelvic obliquity. Developmental curves occur later than congenital curves, are more flexible, and usually are in the lumbar area with compensatory curves above and below. Several authors have suggested that developmental scoliosis

can be caused in some patients by hydromyelia or a tethered cord syndrome, and an early onset of scoliosis (before the age of 6 years) frequently occurs in patients with these lesions.

Spinal roentgenograms should be obtained at least once each year, beginning when the child is 5 years old. If any scoliosis is detected, further evaluation is indicated. MRI should be performed to determine if hydromyelia or a tethered spinal cord is present. The use of a molded, bivalved, polypropylene body jacket (thoracic-lumbar-sacral orthosis) is recommended for daytime wear when the curve is greater than

30 degrees. Bracing slows curve progression and delays surgical intervention but does not halt the progress of most curves. Indications for spinal fusion include a progressive increase in angular deformity that cannot be controlled by bracing, unacceptable deformities, and progressive thoracic lordosis. Anterior spinal fusion, followed by posterior fusion, may be necessary for severe curves (Fig. 31-47). Contraindications to surgery include short life expectancy, uncontrollable hydrocephalus, failure to thrive, and marked mental retardation with no hope of independent function.

KYPHOSIS

The most severe spinal deformity in patients with myelomeningocele is congenital kyphosis; it occurs in approximately 10% of patients. The kyphosis usually is present at birth and may make sac closure difficult. The curve generally extends from the lower thoracic level to the sacral spine, with its apex in the midlumbar region. The deformity usually is progressive.

Congenital kyphosis is unresponsive to bracing and usually requires surgery for correction. The goal of treatment of the kyphosis is not to obtain a normal spine but to provide sitting balance without the use of the arms and hands for support. Other goals are to increase the lumbar height to allow room for abdominal contents and provide better mechanics for breathing and to prevent pressure sores by reducing the kyphotic prominence.

Surgical techniques for spinal fusion in scoliosis and correction of kyphosis are described in Chapter 38. Complications of spinal surgery in patients with myelomeningocele are significantly greater than in patients with idiopathic scoliosis. The most common complication is failure of fusion, reported to occur in as many as 40% of patients. Infection rates as high as 8% also have been reported.

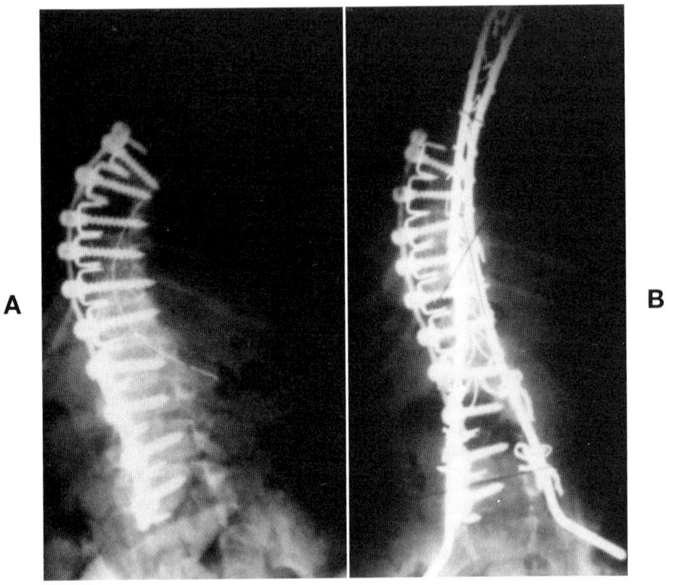

A **B**

Fig. 31-47 Correction of severe scoliosis with anterior fusion with Dwyer instrumentation (**A**) followed by posterior fusion with Luque rods (**B**).

ARTHROGRYPOSIS MULTIPLEX CONGENITA

Arthrogryposis multiplex congenita, or multiple congenital contractures, is a nonprogressive syndrome characterized by deformed, rigid joints. The involved muscles or muscle groups are atrophied or absent. The involved extremities appear cylindrical, fusiform, or cone shaped and have diminished skin creases and subcutaneous tissue. Contracture of the joint capsule and periarticular tissues is present. Dislocation of the joints is common, especially of the hip and knee. Sensation and intellect are normal (Fig. 31-48). The incidence of arthrogryposis is 1 in 3000 live births.

More than 150 specific entities can be associated with what has been known as arthrogryposis multiplex congenita; because it is no longer considered a discrete clinical entity, the term *multiple congenital contractures* is preferred. The deformities may result from neurogenic, myogenic, skeletal, or environmental factors. Most cases of arthrogryposis are neurogenic in origin. The neurogenic causes result from a congenital or acquired defect in the organization or number of anterior horn

Fig. 31-48 Newborn with arthrogryposis multiplex congenita. Note orthopaedic conditions: congenital dislocation of knees, teratological clubfeet, internal rotation contractures of shoulder, extension contractures of elbow, and flexion contractures of wrist.

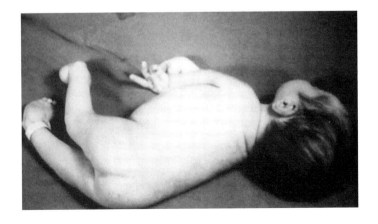

cells, roots, peripheral nerves, or motor end plates, producing muscular weakness and resultant joint immobility at critical stages of intrauterine development (Table 31-3). Myopathic multiple congenital contractures, which account for 10% or fewer of patients, appear to be transmitted as an autosomal recessive disorder. Genetic evaluation is recommended for patients with arthrogryposis. Limited intrauterine movement is common to all types of arthrogryposis. Histological analysis shows a small muscle mass with fibrosis and fat between the muscle fibers. Myopathic and neuropathic features often are found in the muscle. The periarticular soft tissue structures are fibrotic and create a fibrous ankylosis.

Clinical examination remains the best modality for establishing the diagnosis of arthrogryposis multiplex congenita. Neurological assessment, electromyography and nerve conduction studies, serum enzyme tests, and muscle biopsy can help to determine the underlying diagnosis. Roentgenographic examination will assess the integrity of the skeletal system, especially the presence or absence of dislocated hips or knees, scoliosis, and other skeletal anomalies. The most common lower extremity deformities are rigid clubfoot and fixed extension or

Table 31-3 Some Deformities in Patients with Arthrogryposis Multiplex Congenita

Pattern of Deformity	Level
UPPER LIMB	
Type I: adduction and/or medial rotation of shoulder, extension of elbow, pronation of forearm, flexion and ulnar deviation of wrist (in addition, two patients had weak intrinsic muscles of the hand, indicating T1 involvement)	C5, C6
Type II: adduction and/or medial rotation of shoulder, flexion deformity of elbow, flexion and ulnar deviation of wrist (in addition, two patients had weak intrinsic muscles, indicating T1 involvement)	Partial C5, C6, partial C7
LOWER LIMB	
Type III: flexion and adduction of hip (with dislocation in five limbs), extension of knee, equinovarus of foot (in addition, two patients had weak intrinsic muscles, indicating S3 involvement)	L4, L5, S1
Type IV: flexion of knee, equinovarus of foot	L3, L4, partial L5
Type V: flexion and abduction of hip, flexion of knee, equinovarus of foot	L3, L4, patchy S1-2
Type VI: flexion of hip, extension of knee with valgus, equinus of foot	L4, L5
Type VII: equinus of foot	L4
Type VIII: equinovarus of foot, weak intrinsic muscles of foot	L4, patchy L5, S3

From Brown LM, Robson MJ, Sharrard WJW: *J Bone Joint Surg* 62B:4, 1980.

flexion contractures of the knees. Major problems in the upper extremity usually are immobile, adducted, and internally rotated shoulders; elbow contractures; severe, fixed palmar flexion and ulnar deviated deformities of the wrist; and contractures of the metacarpophalangeal and interphalangeal joints. Involvement usually is bilateral but not always symmetrical. Scoliosis has been reported to occur in 10% to 30% of patients.

Treatment

Most children with arthrogryposis have a relatively good prognosis, therefore treatment should be focused on obtaining maximal function. Palmer et al. devised a program of passive stretching exercises for each contracted joint, to be followed by serial splinting with custom thermoplastic splints. Although they reported significant gains in extremity function and a reduction in the need for corrective surgery, most authors have reported that any improvement after physical therapy is transient at best and that recurrence of the deformity is likely. Drummond et al. outlined some principles of orthopaedic management of patients with multiple congenital contractures:

1. Muscle balance should be established if functioning muscles are available for transfer.
2. Recurrence of the deformity is the rule because the dense, inelastic soft tissues about the joints do not properly elongate with growth.
3. Tenotomies should be accompanied by capsulotomy and capsulectomy on the concave side of the joint, followed by prolonged plaster and then orthotic support to prevent or at least delay recurrence of the deformity.
4. Maximal safely obtainable correction should be achieved at the time of surgery. The use of wedging or corrective casts after surgery is of little additional benefit.
5. Osteotomies to correct deformity or transfer the range of motion to a more useful arc are beneficial but only at or near skeletal maturity; otherwise, the deformity will recur with growth.

These principles remain as guidelines for the treatment of arthrogryposis except that prolonged casting has been replaced with early motion and prolonged bracing.

LOWER EXTREMITY

The rigid foot deformity in multiple congenital contractures usually is a clubfoot or congenital vertical talus. The goal of treatment is conversion of the rigid deformed foot into a rigid plantigrade foot; a normal foot is not a realistic goal of treatment. If the valgus foot is plantigrade, treatment usually is not required. The most common foot deformity is clubfoot. Manipulation and serial casting of an arthrogrypotic clubfoot may lead to some correction, but surgery eventually is required in almost all patients, usually between the ages of 6 and 18 months. An extensive posteromedial and posterolateral release (Technique 26-10) is recommended. If the deformity recurs in

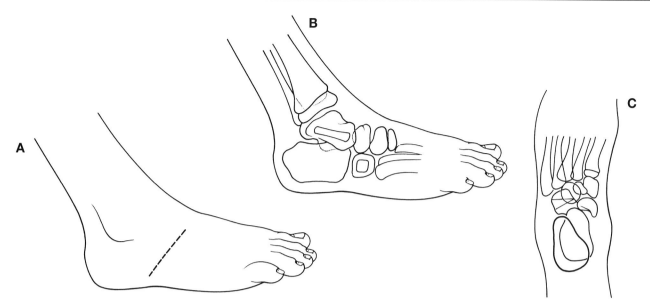

Fig. 31-49   Cancellectomy of talus and cuboid. **A,** Incision. **B,** Windows in talus and cuboid to expose cancellous bone. **C,** Closing wedge osteotomy in cuboid. (**A** redrawn from Gross RH: *Clin Orthop* 194:99, 1985; **B** and **C** redrawn from Spires TD et al: *J Pediatr Orthop* 4:706, 1984.)

a young child or is so severe it cannot be corrected by posteromedial soft tissue release, talectomy is indicated. Gross described a technique of cancellectomy of the talus and cuboid in which a window is created in the dorsal cortex of the cuboid and lateral cortex of the neck and body of the talus (Fig. 31-49). All cancellous bone is carefully curetted, and the deformity is corrected by manual manipulation. He credited Verebelyi with the original description of the technique, and he cited reports of Ogston and Kopits of its use in patients with myelomeningocele. Triple arthrodesis may be performed for rigid deformity in adolescents.

The most common knee deformity in multiple congenital contractures is a fixed flexion contracture. Initial treatment is by serial splinting or casting in progressive degrees of extension. Ambulation is possible with a residual knee flexion contracture of 15 degrees. If complete correction has not been obtained by 6 to 12 months of age, posterior medial and lateral hamstring lengthening and knee capsulotomies are indicated. Supracondylar extension osteotomy of the distal femur may be required to correct a contracture and allow use of orthoses. Extension osteotomies should be done when the patient is near skeletal maturity to decrease the risk of recurrent deformity with growth. If osteotomies are done before skeletal maturity DelBello and Watts found that the deformity recurred at a rate of 1 degree per month. Even with this tendency for recurrence about 50% correction was maintained. When soft tissue webbing is associated with knee flexion contracture, a circular-frame external fixator can be used to achieve gradual correction. Contracture of the quadriceps mechanism can cause hyperextension of the knee, which again is treated initially by serial casting. If the deformity does not respond to conservative

treatment by 6 to 12 months of age, surgical correction by quadricepsplasty (Technique 24-2) is recommended.

The hip is involved in approximately 80% of patients with multiple congenital contractures. In general, hip deformities should be treated by passive stretching exercises, beginning in infancy. If conservative measures fail, surgical correction of the hip deformity should be delayed until deformities of the feet and then the knees have been corrected. Traditional recommendations are that bilateral teratological hip dislocations should not be reduced because reduction may not improve function. Szöke et al. reported good results with early open reduction using a medial approach to the hip. This approach was used for unilateral and bilateral hip dislocations. The authors recommended surgery between 3 and 6 months of age. If surgical intervention is done between the ages of 12 and 36 months, a one-stage open reduction, primary femoral shortening, and possible pelvic osteotomy are recommended. Unilateral dislocation of the hip, whether flexible or rigid, should be reduced surgically and placed in a functional position to avoid potential pelvic obliquity and scoliosis.

UPPER EXTREMITY

Correction of upper extremity deformities should be delayed until ambulation has been achieved, usually until the age of 3 to 4 years. The goal of treatment of upper extremity deformities is to provide optimal function of the hand in the activities of daily living. Function may be adequate in spite of severe deformity, and surgical intervention has the risk of loss of function. Weakness and stiffness about the shoulder do not significantly impair function and usually require no treatment.

Proximal humeral rotation osteotomy (Technique 31-44) may be indicated for severe internal rotation deformity. Deformity of the elbow usually means severe limitation of either flexion or extension. The stiff flexed elbow is not a severe impairment, and surgery is not indicated. Fixed extension elbow deformity, especially if bilateral, is a severe functional impairment. Surgical options available for the fixed extended elbow are tricepsplasty, triceps transfer, flexorplasty, and pectoralis major transfer. Lengthening of the triceps mechanism and posterior capsulotomy are the most reliable and durable of available surgical procedures. Triceps transfer can be done to regain elbow flexion but over time a flexion contracture often occurs. Tricepsplasty on one elbow and triceps transfer on the opposite side allow basic activities of feeding and toileting, as well as apposition of the hands for bimanual activities. Steindler flexorplasty rarely is indicated in children with multiple congenital contractures because the wrist flexors usually are both inactive and contracted.

Wrist stabilization in the optimal functional position probably is the single most beneficial procedure in patients with multiple congenital contractures, but determination of the best position for function must be made carefully. Mild ulnar deviation and dorsiflexion between 5 and 20 degrees will prove to be the most satisfactory position. After skeletal maturity has been reached, wrist fusion can be performed by traditional methods when required. In younger children, Williams recommended sacrificing the carpal bones and radius and inserting a medullary nail through the third metacarpal, the carpals, and the radius. If the wrist and hand need to be repositioned, a procedure analogous to those for centralization for radial clubhand (Chapter 76) can be performed.

Scoliosis

Scoliosis has been reported to occur in 10% to 30% of patients with multiple congenital contractures, generally associated with neuromuscular weakness or pelvic obliquity. If the deformity is severe and progressive, early surgical intervention is warranted. The indications and techniques for treatment of scoliosis in patients with multiple congenital contractures are the same as those for patients with other neuromuscular disorders (Chapter 38).

BRACHIAL PLEXUS PALSY

Brachial plexus palsy may be seen after injury to the brachial plexus during birth. Reported incidences range from 0.1% to 0.4% of live births. Numerous risk factors have been identified, including large birth weight, breech presentation, shoulder dystocia, prolonged labor, and forceps delivery. The severity of the palsy depends on which roots of the brachial plexus have been injured and the extent of injury. Although the incidence of birth palsy has remained the same, the severity of birth palsies has diminished.

Brachial plexus palsy is classified according to the location of the injury of the brachial plexus. Seddon classified the injuries into three types and Sunderland into five. The most common types are upper plexus palsy (Erb-Duchenne), in which the supraspinatus and infraspinatus muscles are the most frequently paralyzed; whole plexus palsy ("mixed"), in which there is complete sensory and motor paralysis of the entire extremity because of severe injury in all roots of the brachial plexus; and lower plexus palsy (Klumpke), in which the muscles of the forearm and hand together with parts served by the cervical sympathetic chain are paralyzed after injury of the eighth cervical and first thoracic nerve roots. The injury to the brachial plexus can range from neurapraxia or axonotmesis to rupture of roots and avulsion from the spinal cord. Upper root level injuries (C5-C6) occur most frequently (approximately 90% of patients) and have the best prognosis; lower plexus and whole plexus injuries have the worst prognosis but are much less common. Geutjens found a higher incidence of avulsion of the upper roots in babies with brachial plexus palsy who were born breech. The babies with avulsions of the upper roots had a worse prognosis for recovery after exploration and microsurgical-grafting. Narakas proposed a more detailed classification based on the clinical course of children with brachial plexus palsies during the first 8 weeks after birth; his classification includes a prognosis for each type of injury (Table 31-4).

Clinical Features

The diagnosis usually is evident at birth. In upper root involvement, the arm is held in internal rotation and active abduction is limited. The elbow may be slightly flexed or in complete extension. The thumb is flexed, and occasionally the fingers will not extend. In complete paralysis, the entire arm and hand is flail. Pinching produces no reaction. Vasomotor impairment may be indicated by the relative paleness of the involved extremity. Roentgenograms of the shoulder may reveal fracture of the proximal humeral epiphysis or fracture of the clavicle. A clavicular fracture occurs in association with plexus palsy in 10% to 15% of patients. Pseudoparalysis from a clavicular or proximal humeral fracture should resolve within 10 to 21 days. If limited motion persists after 1 month of age most likely a concomitant brachial plexus palsy is present. A septic shoulder in an infant also can cause a pseudoparalysis, which can be differentiated from a brachial plexus palsy by evidence of systemic illness and resolution of the pseudoparalysis after the infection is treated.

Characteristic deformities usually develop promptly. The shoulder becomes flexed, internally rotated, and slightly abducted; active abduction of the joint decreases; and external rotation disappears (Fig. 31-50). The shoulder may become posteriorly subluxated and eventually dislocated, or the humeral head becomes flattened against the glenoid. Waters reported that the natural history of untreated brachial plexus birth palsy with residual weakness is progressive glenohumeral

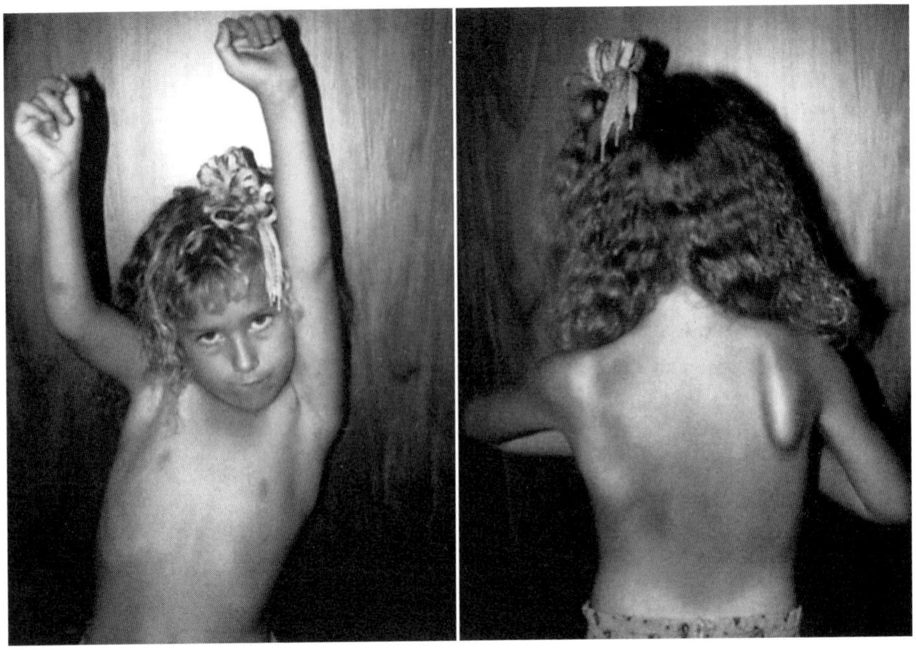

Fig. 31-50   Anterior (**A**) and posterior (**B**) views of child with brachial plexus palsy. Note winging of scapula.

Table 31-4   Classification and Prognosis in Obstetrical Palsy

	Clinical Picture	Recovery
Type I	C5-6	Complete or almost in 1-8 wk
Type II	C5-6	Elbow flexion: 1-4 wk
		Elbow extension: 1-8 wk
	C7	Limited shoulder: 6-30 wk
Type III	C5-6	Poor shoulder: 10-40 wk
		Elbow flexion: 16-40 wk
	C7	Elbow extension: 16-20 wk
		Wrist: 40-60 wk
	C8-T1 (no Horner sign)	Hand complete: 1-3 wk
Type IV	C5-7	Poor shoulder: 10-40 wk
		Elbow flexion: 16-40 wk
	C8	Elbow extension incomplete, poor: 20-60 wk or nil
	T1 (temporary Horner sign)	Wrist: 40-60 wk
		Hand complete: 20-60 wk
Type V	C5-7	Shoulder and elbow as above
	C7	
	C8	Wrist poor or only extension; poor flexion or none
	T1	
	C8-T1 (Horner sign usually present)	Very poor hand with no or weak flexors and extensors; no intrinsics

Modified from Narakas AO. In Bora FW Jr, ed: *The pediatric upper extremity: diagnosis and management,* Philadelphia, 1986, WB Saunders.

deformity from persistent muscle imbalance. Advanced glenoid changes were seen by the time the child was 2 years old. He classified the glenohumeral deformity into seven types based on CT and MRI findings (Table 31-5). Evaluation of the brachial plexus injury may include clinical evaluation, electrical diagnostic studies, myelography, CT, and MRI. Combined myelography, CT, and MRI are more reliable than myelography alone. Large diverticulae and meningoceles are indicative of root avulsions.

Treatment

Minimal injuries respond well to conservative treatment and, although recovery may require as long as 18 months, usually residual disability or deformity is slight. Most authors report significant recovery within the first 3 months, with slower recovery occurring within the next 6 to 12 months. Jackson, Hoffer, and Parrish reported that all their patients who

Table 31-5 Computed Tomography/Magnetic Resonance Imaging (CT/MRI) Classification of Glenohumeral Deformity in Chronic Brachial Plexus Birth Palsies

Type	CT/MRI Findings
I	Normal glenohumeral joint
II	Minimal glenoid hypoplasia (>5 degrees increased retroversion)
III	Posterior subluxation of the humeral head
IV	Development of a false glenoid
V	Posterior flattening of the humeral head
VI	Infantile dislocation
VII	Proximal humeral growth arrest

From Waters PM: The upper limb. In Morrissy RT, Weinstein SL, eds: *Lovell and Winter's pediatric orthopaedics,* Philadelphia, 2001, Lippincott Williams & Wilkins.

recovered fully did so within 1 year, and Greenwald, Schute, and Shiveley reported complete recovery in 92% of patients within 3 months. Gilbert and Tassin, and Millesi have suggested that if no evidence of deltoid or biceps recovery is seen by the age of 3 months, surgical exploration should be considered. The Toronto scale has been used to predict poor outcomes if microsurgical repair or grafting is not done. This scale consists of grading elbow flexion, elbow extension, wrist extension, finger extension, and thumb extension. These muscle groups are scored as 0 (no motion), 1 (motion present but limited), or 2 (normal motion) for a maximal score of 12. Michelow et al. found that a score of less than 3.5 predicted a poor long-term outcome without microsurgery.

The aim of treatment in the initial stages is prevention of contractures of muscles and joints. Gentle passive exercises are begun to maintain full range of passive motion of all joints of the upper extremity, especially full extension of the fingers, hand, and wrist, full pronation, and supination of the forearm, full extension of the elbow, and full abduction, extension, and external rotation of the shoulder. Splinting is discouraged by most authors, but Perry et al. recommended functional bracing to encourage early hand use. Microsurgical nerve repair or grafting has been reported to give satisfactory results in carefully selected patients. Kawabata et al., as well as others, used CT scanning and myelography, followed by electromyographic and nerve conduction velocity studies. If these studies show root avulsion from the spinal cord, they recommended no surgery. If the CT scan and myelogram are normal, they recommended exploration of the brachial plexus and repair of any injuries. Most authors recommend electromyography and CT myelography or MRI evaluation before surgical intervention. The timing of microsurgical intervention still is controversial and ranges from 1 to 6 months. The indications for microsurgical intervention are the absence of biceps recovery (usually by 3 months of age), a Toronto score of less than 3.5, and total plexopathy with Horner syndrome.

Surgery in unresolved brachial plexus palsy usually is directed toward improving shoulder function and joint contrac-

tures. Sever recommended anterior subscapularis release to correct mild to moderate internal rotation contracture. Hoffer recommended in addition an anterior release transfer of the latissimus dorsi and teres major to the rotator cuff to improve function. Wickstrom and others recommended external rotation osteotomy of the humerus for severe fixed rotation contracture.

Waters recommended that patients with grade I (normal), II (mild increase in glenoid retroversion), or mild grade III (slight posterior subluxation) glenohumeral deformities have an anterior musculotendinous lengthening of the pectoralis major and posterior latissimus dorsi and teres major transfer to the rotator cuff. Patients with advanced grade III, grade IV, or grade V glenohumeral deformities should have a humeral derotation osteotomy.

Elbow flexion and forearm supination deformities can occur with a Klumpke palsy (C8-T1) or a mixed brachial plexus lesion. Progressive deformities occur because of weak or absent triceps, pronator teres, and pronator quadratus muscles with an intact biceps muscle. This creates progressive elbow flexion and supination deformity from the unopposed biceps muscle. Radial head dislocation may occur, and the wrist and hand usually are held in extreme dorsiflexion because of the unopposed wrist dorsiflexors. The biceps tendon can be Z-lengthened and rerouted around the radius to convert it from a supinator to a pronator (see Technique 31-32); this improves elbow extension and forearm pronation.

◆ ANTERIOR SHOULDER RELEASE

TECHNIQUE 31-43 *(Fairbank, Sever)*

Make an incision on the anterior aspect of the shoulder in the deltopectoral groove distally from the tip of the coracoid process to a point distal to the tendinous insertion of the pectoralis major muscle; divide this tendon parallel to the humerus. Then retract the anterior margin of the deltoid laterally and the pectoralis major medially and expose the coracobrachialis muscle. With the shoulder externally rotated and abducted, trace the coracobrachialis superiorly to the coracoid process. If the coracoid is elongated, resect 0.5 to 1 cm of its tip together with the insertions of the coracobrachialis, the short head of the biceps, and the pectoralis minor muscles; this resection increases the range of motion of the shoulder in external rotation and abduction. Now locate the inferior edge of the subscapularis tendon at its insertion on the lesser tuberosity of the humerus, elevate it with a grooved director (Fig. 31-51), and divide it completely without incising the capsule. External rotation and abduction of the shoulder should then be almost normal. A curved prolongation of the acromion may interfere with abduction and with reduction of any mild posterior subluxation of the joint; in this event either resect this obstructing part or divide the acromion and elevate this part.

AFTERTREATMENT. An abduction splint that holds the shoulder in abduction and mild external rotation is applied and

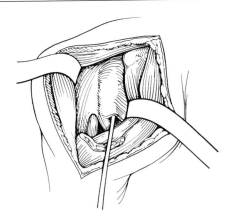

Fig. 31-51 Anterior shoulder release for internal rotation contracture in brachial plexus palsy.

is worn constantly for 2 weeks and intermittently for another 4 weeks. Active exercises are started early and are continued until maximal improvement has occurred.

◆ ROTATIONAL OSTEOTOMY OF HUMERUS

TECHNIQUE 31-44 *(Rogers)*

Approach the humerus anteriorly between the deltoid and pectoralis major muscles. With the arm abducted, perform an osteotomy 5 cm distal to the joint. Under direct vision externally rotate the distal fragment of the humerus 90 degrees; be sure the fragments are then apposed. Kirschner wire fixation can be used if needed. Close the wound.

AFTERTREATMENT. With the shoulder abducted 40 degrees, the elbow flexed 90 degrees, and the forearm supinated, a shoulder spica cast is applied and is worn for 8 to 12 weeks. Kirschner wires, if used, are removed at the time of cast removal.

◆ RELEASE OF INTERNAL ROTATION CONTRACTURE AND TRANSFER OF LATISSIMUS DORSI AND TERES MAJOR

When performed before the age of 6 years, the Sever-L'Episcopo procedure, as modified by Green, improves external rotation of the shoulder by releasing the internal rotation contracture and transferring the latissimus dorsi and teres major posteriorly to provide active external rotation.

TECHNIQUE 31-45 *(Sever-L'Episcopo, Green)*

Place a sandbag under the upper part of the chest for proper exposure. Prepare and drape in the usual manner. An adequate amount of whole blood should be available for transfusion. Make an anterior incision beginning over the coracoid process and extending distally along the deltopec-

toral groove for 12 cm (Fig. 31-52, *A*). Identify the cephalic vein and ligate or retract with a few fibers of the deltoid muscle. With blunt dissection, develop the interval between the pectoral and deltoid muscles. Expose the coracobrachialis, the short head of the biceps, the coracoid process, the insertion of the tendinous portion of the subscapularis, and the insertion of the pectoralis major. Detach the short head of the biceps and coracobrachialis from their origin on the coracoid process and reflect downward.

In the distal part of the wound, expose the insertion of the pectoralis major at its humeral attachment (Fig. 31-52, *B*). With a periosteal elevator, reflect the muscle fibers of the pectoralis major medially to expose the tendinous portion of its insertion. To perform Z-lengthening, divide the distal half of the tendinous insertion of the pectoralis major immediately on the humeral shaft (Fig. 31-52, *C*).

Divide the upper half of the tendinous portion of the pectoralis major as far medially as good aponeurotic tendinous material exists, usually 4 to 5 cm from its insertion (Fig. 31-52, *D*). Later, the distal tendon stump will be attached to the proximal tendon left inserted on the humerus, thus providing further length to the pectoralis major. The reattachment of the tendon more proximally permits a greater degree of shoulder abduction but still allows rotary function. Apply whip sutures to the tendon still attached to the shaft and to the portion of the tendon attached to the muscle. Expose the subscapularis muscle over the head of the humerus. Starting medially with a blunt instrument, separate the subscapularis and elevate it from the capsule. Do not open the shoulder capsule. With a knife, lengthen the subscapularis tendon by an oblique cut (Fig. 31-52, *E*). Starting medially, split the tendon into anterior and posterior halves, becoming more superficial laterally and completing the division at the insertion of the subscapularis into the humerus. Again, take care not to open the capsule. Once the subscapularis has been divided, the shoulder joint will abduct and externally rotate freely. If the coracoid process is elongated, hooked downward and laterally, and limits external rotation, it should be resected to its base. Likewise, if the acromion process is beaked downward and obstructs shoulder abduction, partially resect it.

Next, identify the insertions of the latissimus dorsi and teres major and expose by separating them from adjacent tissues both anteriorly and posteriorly. The attachment of the latissimus dorsi is superior and anterior to that of the teres major. Divide both tendons immediately on bone and suture each tendon with a whip stitch. Then, with the patient turned over on the side and with the patient's arm adducted across the chest, make a 7- to 8-cm incision over the deltoid-triceps interval (Fig. 31-52, *F*). Retract the deltoid muscle anteriorly and the long head of the triceps posteriorly. Be careful not to damage the radial and axillary nerves. Subperiosteally expose the lateral surface of the proximal

continued

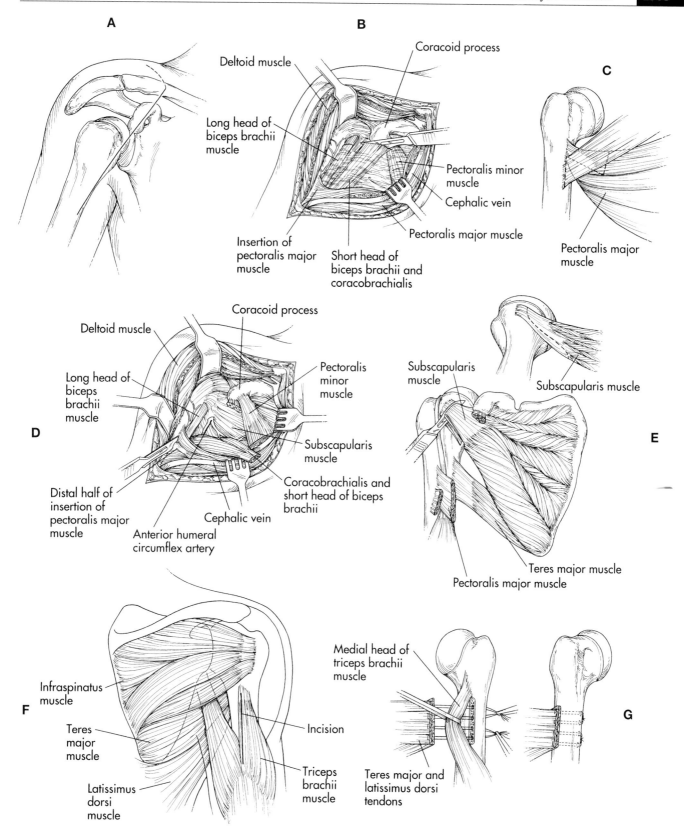

A

B

Coracoid process

Deltoid muscle

Long head of
biceps brachii
muscle

C

Pectoralis minor
muscle

Cephalic vein

Pectoralis major muscle

Insertion of
pectoralis major
muscle

Short head of
biceps brachii and
coracobrachialis

Pectoralis major
muscle

Coracoid process

Deltoid muscle

Long head of
biceps
brachii
muscle

Pectoralis
minor
muscle

Subscapularis
muscle

Subscapularis muscle

D

Subscapularis
muscle

E

Distal half of
insertion of
pectoralis major
muscle

Coracobrachialis and
short head of biceps
brachii

Cephalic vein

Anterior humeral
circumflex artery

Teres major muscle

Pectoralis major muscle

Infraspinatus
muscle

Medial head of
triceps brachii
muscle

F

Teres
major
muscle

Incision

G

Latissimus
dorsi
muscle

Triceps
brachii
muscle

Teres major and
latissimus dorsi
tendons

Fig. 31-52   Sever-L'Episcopo and Green procedure. **A,** Anterior incision. **B,** Exposure of insertion
of pectoralis major at humeral attachment. **C,** Incisions of tendinous insertion of pectoralis major for
Z-lengthening. **D,** Distal half of tendinous insertion of pectoralis major on shaft of humerus is
divided. **E,** Subscapularis is divided by oblique cut. **F,** Incision over deltoid-triceps interval. **G,** Teres
major and latissimus dorsi tendons are attached to cleft in lateral humerus.   *Continued*

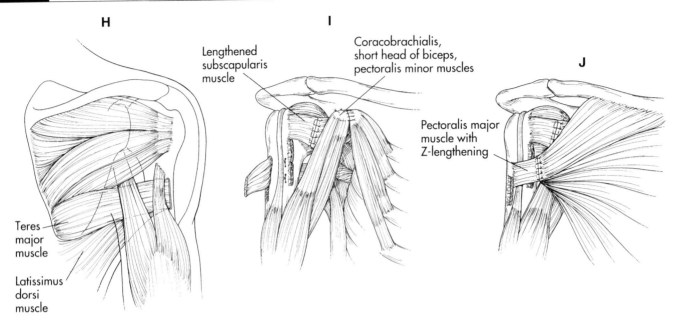

Fig. 31-52, cont'd   H, Back view showing reattachment of muscles. **I** and **J,** Front views showing reattachment of muscles. (Redrawn from Tachdjian MO, ed: *Pediatric orthopedics,* ed 2, Philadelphia, 1990, WB Saunders.)

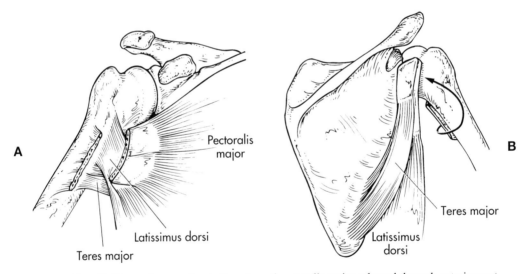

Fig. 31-53   **Hoffer tendon transfer. **A, Insertion of pectoralis major released through anterior part of incision. **B,** Combined insertions *(arrow)* of latissimus dorsi *(LAT)* and teres major *(TM)* released through posterior part of incision. Closed reduction is then performed, and tendons are sutured to rotator cuff. (Redrawn from: Hoffer MM: *J Bone Joint Surg* 80A:997, 1998.)

diaphysis of the humerus. Make a 5-cm longitudinal cleft using drills, an osteotome, and a curet.

Drill four holes from the depth of the cleft coming out on the medial surface of the humeral shaft at the site of the former insertion of the teres major and latissimus dorsi muscles. Identify the tendons of the latissimus dorsi and teres major in the anterior wound and deliver them into the posterior incision so that their line of pull is straight from

their origins to the proposed site of attachment on the lateral humerus. Draw the latissimus dorsi and teres major tendons into the slot in the humerus and tie securely into position with 1-0 silk sutures in the front (Fig. 31-52, *G* and *H*).

Suture the subscapularis tendon, which is lengthened "on the flat," at its divided ends to provide maximal lengthening. Suture the pectoralis major in a similar way. Reattach the coracobrachialis and short head of the biceps to the base of the coracoid process. If the coracobrachialis and short head of the biceps are short, lengthen them at their musculotendinous junction (Fig. 31-52, *I* and *J*). The lengthened muscles should be of sufficient length to permit complete external rotation in abduction without undue tension. Close the wound in the usual manner and immobilize the upper limb in a previously prepared, bivalved shoulder spica cast that holds the shoulder in 90 degrees of abduction, 90 degrees of external rotation, and 20 degrees of forward flexion. Position the elbow in 80 to 90 degrees of flexion. Place the forearm and hand in a functional neutral position.

AFTERTREATMENT. Exercises are begun 3 weeks after surgery to develop abduction and external rotation of the shoulder, as well as shoulder adduction and internal rotation. Particular emphasis is given to developing the function and strength of the transferred muscles. When the arm adducts satisfactorily, a sling is used during the day and the bivalved shoulder spica cast is worn at night. The night support is continued for 3 to 6 more months. Exercises are performed for many months or years to preserve functional range of motion of the shoulder and to maintain muscle control.

Hoffer reported transfer of the latissimus dorsi and the teres major to the rotator cuff, which has a stabilizing effect on the rotator cuff and increases glenohumeral abduction and external rotation (Fig. 31-53).

References

POLIOMYELITIS

Barr JS: The management of poliomyelitis: the late stage. In *Poliomyelitis, First International Poliomyelitis Congress,* Philadelphia, 1949, JB Lippincott.

Green WT, Grice DS: The management of chronic poliomyelitis, *Instr Course Lect* 9:85, 1952.

Huckstep RL: *Poliomyelitis: a guide for developing countries, including appliances and rehabilitation for the disabled,* Edinburgh, 1975, Churchill Livingstone.

Johnson EW Jr: Results of modern methods of treatment of poliomyelitis, *J Bone Joint Surg* 27:223, 1945.

Mayer L: Tendon transplantations on the lower extremity, *Instr Course Lect* 6:189, 1949.

Ober FR: Tendon transplantation in the lower extremity, *N Engl J Med* 209:52, 1933.

Salk D: Polio immunization policy in the United States: a new challenge for a new generation, *Am J Public Health* 78:296, 1988.

Seddon HJ: Reconstructive surgery of the upper extremity. In *Poliomyelitis, Second International Poliomyelitis Congress,* Philadelphia, 1952, JB Lippincott.

Steindler A: *Orthopedic operations: indications, technique, and end results,* Springfield, Ill, 1940, Charles C Thomas.

Vulpius O: Zur Kasuistik der Schnen transplantation, *Münch Med Wochenschr* 16, 1897.

FOOT AND ANKLE

Axer A: Into-talus transposition of tendons for correction of paralytic valgus foot after poliomyelitis in children, *J Bone Joint Surg* 42A: 1119, 1960.

Barr JS: Transference of posterior tibial tendon for paralytic talipes equinovarus. Personal communication, July and Oct 1954.

Barr JS, Record EE: Arthrodesis of the ankle for correction of foot deformity, *Surg Clin North Am* 27:1281, 1947.

Barr JS, Record EE: Arthrodesis of the ankle joint, *N Engl J Med* 248:53, 1953.

Beals RK: The treatment of ankle valgus by surface epiphysiodesis, *Clin Orthop* 266:162, 1991.

Bényi P: A modified Lambrinudi operation for drop foot, *J Bone Joint Surg* 42B:333, 1960.

Blount WP: Forward transference of posterior tibial tendon for paralytic talipes equinovarus. Personal communication, July 1954.

Brindley H Sr, Brindley H Jr: Extra-articular subtalar arthrodesis, *Orthop Trans* 6:188, 1982.

Brown A: A simple method of fusion of the subtalar joint in children, *J Bone Joint Surg* 50B:369, 1968.

Campbell WC: An operation for the correction of "drop-foot," *J Bone Joint Surg* 5:815, 1923.

Campbell WC: End results of operation for correction of drop-foot, *JAMA* 85:1927, 1925.

Carmack JC, Hallock H: Tibiotarsal arthrodesis after astragalectomy: a report of eight cases, *J Bone Joint Surg* 29:476, 1947.

Crego CH Jr, McCarroll HR: Recurrent deformities in stabilized paralytic feet: a report of 1100 consecutive stabilizations in poliomyelitis, *J Bone Joint Surg* 20:609, 1938.

Davids JR, Valadie AL, Ferguson RL, et al: Surgical management of ankle valgus in children: use of a transphyseal medial malleolar screw, *J Pediatr Orthop* 17:3, 1997.

Dennyson WG, Fulford GE: Subtalar arthrodesis by cancellous grafts and metallic internal fixation, *J Bone Joint Surg* 58B:507, 1976.

Dias LS, Busch M, Tachdjian MO: Surgical treatment of severe hindfoot valgus by medial displacement osteotomy of the os calcis, *Orthop Trans* 11:35, 1987.

Dillwyn-Evans D: Relapsed clubfoot, *J Bone Joint Surg* 43B:722, 1961.

Dunn N: Suggestions based on ten years' experience of arthrodesis of the tarsus in the treatment of deformities of the foot. In *Robert Jones' birthday volume,* London, 1928, Oxford University Press.

Dwyer FC: Osteotomy of the calcaneum for pes cavus, *J Bone Joint Surg* 41B:80, 1959.

Evans D: Relapsed club foot, *J Bone Joint Surg* 43B:722, 1961.

Evans D: Calcaneo-valgus deformity, *J Bone Joint Surg* 57B:270, 1975.

Evans EL: Astragalectomy. In *Robert Jones' birthday volume,* London, 1928, Oxford University Press.

Fried A, Hendel C: Paralytic valgus deformity of the ankle: replacement of the paralyzed tibialis posterior by the peronaeus longus, *J Bone Joint Surg* 39A:921, 1957.

Fried A, Moyseyev S: Paralytic valgus deformity of the foot: treatment by replacement of paralyzed tibialis posterior muscle: a long-term follow-up study, *J Bone Joint Surg* 52A:1674, 1970.

Goldner JL, Irwin CE: Paralytic deformities of the foot, *Instr Course Lect* 5:190, 1948.

Goldner JL, Irwin CE: Clawing of the great toe in paralytic equinovalgus: mechanism and treatment, *Duke Correspondence Club Letter,* July 7, 1949.

Green WT, Grice DS: The surgical correction of the paralytic foot, *Instr Course Lect* 10:343, 1953.

Green WT, Grice DS: The management of calcaneus deformity, *Instr Course Lect* 13:135, 1956.

Grice DS: An extra-articular arthrodesis of the subastragalar joint for correction of paralytic flat feet in children, *J Bone Joint Surg* 34A:927, 1952.

Grice DS: Further experience with extra-articular arthrodesis of the subtalar joint, *J Bone Joint Surg* 36A:246, 1955.

Grice DS: The role of subtalar fusion in the treatment of valgus deformities of the feet, *Instr Course Lect* 16:127, 1959.

Gross RH: A clinical study of the Batchelor subtalar arthrodesis, *J Bone Joint Surg* 58A:343, 1976.

Hammond G: Elevation of the first metatarsal bone with hallux equinus, *Surgery* 13:240, 1943.

Hart VL: Lambrinudi operation for drop-foot, *J Bone Joint Surg* 22:937, 1940.

Hibbs RA: An operation for "claw-foot," *JAMA* 73:1583, 1919.

Hoffer MM, Reiswig JA, Garrett AM, Perry J: The split anterior tibial tendon transfer in the treatment of spastic varus hindfoot of childhood, *Orthop Clin North Am* 5:31, 1974.

Hoke M: An operation for stabilizing paralytic feet, *J Orthop Surg* 3:494, 1921.

Hsu LCS, O'Brien JP, Yau ACMC, Hodgson AR: Valgus deformity of the ankle in children with fibular pseudarthrosis: results of treatment by bone-grafting of the fibula, *J Bone Joint Surg* 56A:503, 1974.

Hsu LCS, O'Brien JP, Yau ACMC, Hodgson AR: Batchelor's extra-articular subtalar arthrodesis, *J Bone Joint Surg* 58A:243, 1976.

Hsu LCS, Yau ACMC, O'Brien JP, Hodgson AR: Valgus deformity of the ankle resulting from fibular resection for a graft in subtalar fusion in children, *J Bone Joint Surg* 54A:585, 1972.

Irwin CE: The calcaneus foot, *South Med J* 44:191, 1951.

Irwin CE: Equinovalgus deformity in the immature foot: extra-articular subtalar arthrodesis, *Piedmont Orthopaedic Society Letter,* 1954.

Irwin CE: The calcaneus foot: a revision, *Instr Course Lect* 15:135, 1958.

Jones R: The soldier's foot and the treatment of common deformities of the foot. II. Claw-foot, *Br Med J* 1:749, 1916.

King BB: Ankle fusion for correction of paralytic drop foot and calcaneus deformities, *Arch Surg* 40:90, 1940.

Lahdenranta U, Pylkkänen P: Subtalar extra-articular fusion in the treatment of valgus and varus deformities in children: a review of 162 operations in 136 patients, *Acta Orthop Scand* 43:438, 1972.

Lambrinudi C: New operation on drop-foot, *Br J Surg* 15:193, 1927.

Lapidus PW: "Dorsal bunion": its mechanics and operative correction, *J Bone Joint Surg* 22:627, 1940.

Leibolt FL: Pantalar arthrodesis in poliomyelitis, *Surgery* 6:31, 1939.

Lipscomb PR, Sanchez JJ: Anterior transplantation of the posterior tibial tendon for persistent palsy of the common peroneal nerve, *J Bone Joint Surg* 43A:60, 1961.

MacKenzie IG: Lambrinudi's arthrodesis, *J Bone Joint Surg* 41B:738, 1959.

Mann RA: Tendon transfers and electromyography, *Clin Orthop* 85:64, 1972.

Miller OL: Surgical management of pes calcaneus, *J Bone Joint Surg* 18:169, 1936.

Ryerson EW: Arthrodesing operations on the feet, *J Bone Joint Surg* 5:453, 1923.

Sharrard WJ, Grosfield I: The management of deformity and paralysis of the foot in myelomeningocele, *J Bone Joint Surg* 50B:456, 1968.

Steindler A: Stripping of the os calcis, *J Orthop Surg* 2:8, 1920.

Steindler A: The treatment of the flail ankle: panastragaloid arthrodesis, *J Bone Joint Surg* 5:284, 1923.

Stevens PM, Belle RM: Screw epiphysiodesis for ankle valgus, *J Pediatr Orthop* 17:9, 1997.

Tachdjian MO: *Pediatric orthopaedics,* ed 2, Philadelphia, 1990, WB Saunders.

Thompson TC: Astragalectomy and the treatment of calcaneovalgus, *J Bone Joint Surg* 21:627, 1939.

Turner JW, Cooper RR: Posterior transposition of tibialis anterior through the interosseous membrane, *Clin Orthop* 79:71, 1971.

Turner JW, Cooper RR: Anterior transfer of the tibialis posterior through the interosseous membrane, *Clin Orthop* 83:241, 1972.

Watkins MB, Jones JB, Ryder CT Jr, Brown TH Jr: Transplantation of the posterior tibial tendon, *J Bone Joint Surg* 36A:1181, 1954.

Waugh TR, Wagner J, Stinchfield FE: An evaluation of pantalar arthrodesis: a follow-up study of one hundred and sixteen operations, *J Bone Joint Surg* 47A:1315, 1965.

Westin W: Tendo Achilles tenodesis to the fibula, update, personal communication, 1985.

KNEE

Asirvatham R, Rooney RJ, Watts H: Proximal tibial extension medial rotation osteotomy to correct knee flexion contracture and lateral rotation deformity of the tibia after polio, *J Pediatr Orthop* 11:646, 1991.

Conner AN: The treatment of flexion contractures of the knee in poliomyelitis, *J Bone Joint Surg* 52B:138, 1970.

Crego CH Jr, Fischer FJ: Transplantation of the biceps femoris for the relief of quadriceps femoris paralysis in residual poliomyelitis, *J Bone Joint Surg* 13:515, 1931.

Irwin CE: Genu recurvatum following poliomyelitis: controlled method of operative correction, *JAMA* 120:277, 1942.

Leong JC, Alade CO, Fang D: Supracondylar femoral osteotomy for knee flexion contracture resulting from poliomyelitis, *J Bone Joint Surg* 64B:198, 1982.

Mestikawy M, Zeier FG: Tendon transfers for poliomyelitis of the lower limb in Guinean children, *Clin Orthop* 75:188, 1971.

Ober FR: Tendon transplantation in the lower extremity, *N Engl J Med* 209:52, 1933.

Perry J, O'Brien JP, Hodgson AR: Triple tenodesis of the knee: a soft-tissue operation for the correction of paralytic genu recurvatum, *J Bone Joint Surg* 58A:978, 1976.

Schwartzmann JR, Crego CH Jr: Hamstring-tendon transplantation for the relief of quadriceps femoris paralysis in residual poliomyelitis: a follow-up study of 134 cases, *J Bone Joint Surg* 30A:541, 1948.

Storen G: Genu recurvatum: treatment by wedge osteotomy of tibia with use of compression, *Acta Chir Scand* 114:40, 1957.

Yount CC: An operation to improve function in quadriceps paralysis, *J Bone Joint Surg* 20:314, 1938.

HIP

Barr JS: Poliomyelitic hip deformity and the erector spinae transplant, *JAMA* 144:813, 1950.

Bjerkreim I: Secondary dysplasia and osteoarthrosis of the hip joint in functional and in fixed obliquity of the pelvis, *Acta Orthop Scand* 45:873, 1974.

Cabaud HE, Westin GW, Connelly S: Tendon transfers in the paralytic hip, *J Bone Joint Surg* 61A:1035, 1979.

Campbell WC: Transference of the crest of the ilium for flexion contracture of the hip, *South Med J* 166:235, 1912.

Eberle CF: Pelvic obliquity and the unstable hip after poliomyelitis, *J Bone Joint Surg* 64B:300, 1982.

Hammesfahr R, Topple S, Yoo K, et al: Abductor paralysis and the role of the external abdominal oblique transfer, *Orthopedics* 6:315, 1983.

Irwin CE: The iliotibial band, its role in producing deformity in poliomyelitis, *J Bone Joint Surg* 31A:141, 1949.

Johnson EW Jr: Contractures of the iliotibial band, *Surg Gynecol Obstet* 96:599, 1953.

Jones GB: Paralytic dislocation of the hip, *J Bone Joint Surg* 36B:375, 1954.

Jones GB: Paralytic dislocation of the hip, *J Bone Joint Surg* 44B:573, 1962.

Katz DE, Haideri N, Song K, Wyrick P: Comparative study of conventional hip-knee-ankle-foot orthosis versus reciprocating-gait orthosis for children with high-level paraparesis, *J Pediatr Orthop* 17:377, 1997.

Miller GR, Irwin CE: Paralytic dislocations of the hip, *Duke Correspondence Club Letter,* Sept 6, 1948.

Mustard WT: A follow-up study of iliopsoas transfer for hip instability, *J Bone Joint Surg* 41B:289, 1959.

Ober FR: An operation for relief of paralysis of the gluteus maximus muscle, *JAMA* 88:1063, 1927.

Parker B, Walker G: Posterior psoas transfer and hip instability in lumbar myelomeningocele, *J Bone Joint Surg* 57B:53, 1975.

Samilson RL, Tsou P, Aamoth G, Green WM: Dislocation and subluxation of the hip in cerebral palsy: pathogenesis, natural history and management, *J Bone Joint Surg* 54A:863, 1972.

Sharrard WJ: Posterior iliopsoas transplantation in the treatment of paralytic dislocation of the hip, *J Bone Joint Surg* 46B:426, 1964.

Thomas LI, Thompson TC, Straub LR: Transplantation of the external oblique muscle for abductor paralysis, *J Bone Joint Surg* 32A:207, 1950.

Yount CC: The role of the tensor fasciae femoris in certain deformities of the lower extremity, *J Bone Joint Surg* 8:171, 1926.

TRUNK

Axer A: Transposition of gluteus maximus, tensor fasciae latae and ilio-tibial band for paralysis of lateral abdominal muscles in children after poliomyelitis: a preliminary report, *J Bone Joint Surg* 40B:644, 1958.

Clark JMP, Axer A: A muscle-tendon transposition for paralysis of the lateral abdominal muscles in poliomyelitis, *J Bone Joint Surg* 38B:475, 1956.

Irwin CE: Subtrochanteric osteotomy in poliomyelitis, *JAMA* 133: 231, 1947.

Mayer L: The significance of the iliocostal fascial graft in the treatment of paralytic deformities of the trunk, *J Bone Joint Surg* 26:257, 1944.

Perry J, Nickel VL: Total cervical-spine fusion for neck paralysis, *J Bone Joint Surg* 41A:37, 1959.

Perry J, Nickel VL, Garrett AL: Capital fascial transplants adjunct to spine fusion in flaccid neck paralysis, *Clin Orthop* 24:128, 1962.

SHOULDER

Barr JS, Freiberg JA, Colonna PC, Pemberton PA: A survey of end results on stabilization of the paralytic shoulder: report of the research committee of the American Orthopaedic Association, *J Bone Joint Surg* 24:699, 1942.

Bateman JE: *The shoulder and environs,* St Louis, 1954, Mosby.

Harmon PH: Anterior transplantation of the posterior deltoid for shoulder palsy and dislocation in poliomyelitis, *Surg Gynecol Obstet* 84:117, 1947.

Harmon PH: Surgical reconstruction of the paralytic shoulder by multiple muscle transplantations, *J Bone Joint Surg* 32A:583, 1950.

Makin M: Early arthrodesis for a flail shoulder in young children, *J Bone Joint Surg* 59A:317, 1977.

Mayer L: The physiological method of tendon transplantation, *Surg Gynecol Obstet* 22:182, 1916.

Ober FR: An operation to relieve paralysis of the deltoid muscle, *JAMA* 99:2182, 1932.

Ober FR: Transplantation to improve the function of the shoulder joint and extensor function of the elbow joint, *Instr Course Lect* 2:274, 1944.

Rowe CR, Leffert RD: Advances in arthrodesis of the shoulder. In Rowe CR, ed: *The shoulder,* New York, 1988, Churchill Livingstone.

Saha AK: Surgery of the paralyzed and flail shoulder, *Acta Orthop Scand Suppl* 97:5 1967.

Steindler A: The reconstruction of upper extremity in spinal and cerebral paralysis, *Instr Course Lect* 6:120, 1949.

Steindler A: Reconstruction of the poliomyelitic upper extremity, *Bull Hosp Jt Dis* 15:21, 1954.

Vastamäki M: Pectoralis minor transfer in serratus anterior paralysis, *Acta Orthop Scand* 55:293, 1984.

ELBOW AND FOREARM

Ahmad I: Restoration of elbow flexion by a new operative technique, *Clin Orthop* 106:186, 1975.

Blount WP: Osteoclasis for supination deformities in children, *J Bone Joint Surg* 22:300, 1940.

Brooks DM, Seddon HJ: Pectoral transplantation for paralysis of the flexors of the elbow: a new technique, *J Bone Joint Surg* 41B:36, 1959.

Bunnell S: Restoring flexion to the paralytic elbow, *J Bone Joint Surg* 33A:566, 1951.

Carroll RE: Restoration of flexor power to the flail elbow by transplantation of the triceps tendon, *Surg Gynecol Obstet* 95:685, 1952.

Carroll RE, Gartland JJ: Flexorplasty of the elbow: an evaluation of a method, *J Bone Joint Surg* 35A:706, 1953.

Carroll RE, Hill NA: Triceps transfer to restore elbow flexion: a study of fifteen patients with paralytic lesions and arthrogryposis, *J Bone Joint Surg* 52A:239, 1970.

Castro-Sierra A, Lopez-Pita A: A new surgical technique to correct triceps paralysis, *Hand* 15:42, 1983.

Clark JMP: Reconstruction of biceps brachii by pectoral muscle transplantation, *Br J Surg* 34:180, 1946.

duToit GT, Levy SJ: Transposition of latissimus dorsi for paralysis of triceps brachii: report of a case, *J Bone Joint Surg* 49B:135, 1967.

Dutton RO, Dawson EB: Elbow flexorplasty: an analysis of long-term results, *J Bone Joint Surg* 63A:1064, 1981.

Green WT, Banks HH: Flexor carpi ulnaris transplant in cerebral palsy, *J Bone Joint Surg* 44A:1343, 1962.

Harmon PH: Muscle transplantation for triceps palsy: the technique of utilizing the latissimus dorsi, *J Bone Joint Surg* 31A:409, 1949.

Hovnanian AP: Latissimus dorsi transplantation for loss of flexion or extension at the elbow: a preliminary report on technic, *Ann Surg* 143:493, 1956.

Lindholm TS, Einola S: Flexorplasty of paralytic elbows: analysis of late functional results, *Acta Orthop Scand* 44:1, 1973.

Mayer L, Green W: Experiences with the Steindler flexorplasty at the elbow, *J Bone Joint Surg* 36A:775, 1954.

Moberg E: Surgical treatment for absent single hand grip and elbow extension in quadriplegia, *J Bone Joint Surg* 57A:196, 1975.

Ober FR, Barr JS: Brachioradialis muscle transposition for triceps weakness, *Surg Gynecol Obstet* 67:105, 1938.

Owings R, Wickstrom J, Perry J, Nickel VL: Biceps brachii rerouting in treatment of paralytic supination contracture of the forearm, *J Bone Joint Surg* 53A:137, 1971.

Raczka R, Braun R, Waters RL: Posterior deltoid-to-triceps transfer in quadriplegia, *Clin Orthop* 187:163, 1984.

Samii K: Transplantation of the clavicular head of the pectoralis major for paralysis of the elbow flexors, *Am Dig Foreign Orthop Lit* 61, 1970.

Seddon HJ: Transplantation of pectoralis major for paralysis of the flexors of the elbow, *Proc Royal Soc Med* 42:837, 1949.

Segal A, Seddon HJ, Brooks DM: Treatment of paralysis of the flexors of the elbow, *J Bone Joint Surg* 41B:44, 1959.

Spira E: Replacement of biceps brachii by pectoralis minor transplant: report of a case, *J Bone Joint Surg* 39B:126, 1957.

Steindler A: Muscle and tendon transplantation at the elbow, *Instr Course Lect* 2:276, 1944.

Zancolli EA: Paralytic supination contracture of the forearm, *J Bone Joint Surg* 49A:1275, 1967.

Zancolli E, Mitre H: Latissimus dorsi transfer to restore elbow flexion: an appraisal of eight cases, *J Bone Joint Surg* 55A:1265, 1973.

MYELOMENINGOCELE

Abraham E, Lubicky JP, Songer MN, Millar EA: Supramalleolar osteotomy for ankle valgus in myelomeningocele, *J Pediatr Orthop* 16:774, 1996.

Abraham E, Verinder DGR, Sharrard WJW: The treatment of flexion contracture of the knee in myelomeningocele, *J Bone Joint Surg* 59B:433, 1977.

Allen BL, Ferguson RL: The operative treatment of myelomeningocele spinal deformity, *Orthop Clin North Am* 10:845, 1979.

Altman R, Altman DA: Imaging of spinal dysraphism, *Am J Neurol Radiol* 8:533, 1987.

American Academy of Orthopaedic Surgeons: *Symposium on myelomeningocele,* St Louis, 1972, Mosby.

Aprin H, Kilfoyle RM: Extension contracture of the knees in patients with meningomyelocele, *Clin Orthop* 144:260, 1979.

Archibeck MJ, Smith JT, Carroll KL, et al: Surgical release of tethered spinal cord: survivorship analysis and orthopedic outcome, *J Pediatr Orthop* 17:773, 1997.

Asher M, Olson J: Factors affecting the ambulatory status of patients with spina bifida cystica, *J Bone Joint Surg* 65A:350, 1983.

Banta JV, Becker G: The natural history of scoliosis in myelomeningocele, *Orthop Trans* 10:18, 1986.

Banta JV, Park SM: Improvement in pulmonary function in patients having combined anterior and posterior spine fusion for myelomeningocele scoliosis, *Spine* 8:765, 1983.

Banta JV, Sutherland DH, Wyatt M: Anterior tibial transfer to the os calcis with Achilles tenodesis for calcaneal deformity in myelomeningocele, *J Pediatr Orthop* 1:125, 1981.

Barden GA, Meyer LC, Stelling FH III: Myelodysplastics: fate of those followed for 20 years or more, *J Bone Joint Surg* 57A:643, 1975.

Baxter MP, D'Astous JL: Proximal femoral resection interposition arthroplasty: salvage hip surgery for the severely disabled child with cerebral palsy, *J Pediatr Orthop* 6:681, 1986.

Bazih J, Gross RH: Hip surgery in the lumbar level myelomeningocele patient, *J Pediatr Orthop* 1:405, 1981.

Beaty JH, Canale ST: Orthopaedic aspects of myelomeningocele, *J Bone Joint Surg* 72A:626, 1990.

Benton LJ, Salvati EA, Root L: Reconstructive surgery in the myelomeningocele hip, *Clin Orthop* 110:261, 1975.

Birmingham PK, Dsida RM, Grayhack JJ, et al: Do latex precautions in children with myelodysplasia reduce intraoperative allergic reactions? *J Pediatr Orthop* 16:799, 1996.

Bliss HG, Menelaus MB: The results of transfer of the tibialis anterior to the heel in patients who have a myelomeningocele, *J Bone Joint Surg* 68A:1258, 1986.

Blount WP: Unequal leg length in children, *Surg Clin North Am* 38:1107, 1958.

Brinker MR, Rosenfeld SR, Feiwell E, et al: Myelomeningocele at the sacral level, *J Bone Joint Surg* 76A:1293, 1994.

Brock DJH, Sutcliffe RG: Alpha-fetoprotein in the antenatal diagnosis of anencephaly and spina bifida, *Lancet* 2:197, 1972.

Brocklehurst G, ed: *Spina bifida for the clinician,* Philadelphia, 1976, JB Lippincott.

Broughton NS, Brougham DI, Cole WG, Menelaus MB: Reliability of radiological measurements in the assessment of the child's hip, *J Bone Joint Surg* 71B:6, 1989.

Broughton NS, Graham G, Menelaus MB: The high incidence of foot deformity in patients with high-level spina bifida, *J Bone Joint Surg* 76B:548, 1994.

Broughton NS, Menelaus MB, Cole WG, Shurtleff DB: The natural history of hip deformity in myelomeningocele, *J Bone Joint Surg* 75B:760, 1993.

Bunch WH, Cass AS, Bensman AS, Long DM: *Modern management of myelomeningocele,* St Louis, 1972, Warren H Green.

Bunch WH, Hakala MW: Iliopsoas transfers in children with myelomeningocele, *J Bone Joint Surg* 66A:224, 1984.

Bunch WH, Scarff TB, Dvonch VM: Progressive loss in myelomeningocele patients, *Orthop Trans* 7:185, 1983.

Burkus JK, Moore DW, Raycroft JF: Valgus deformity of the ankle in myelodysplastic patients: correction by stapling of the medial part of the distal tibial physis, *J Bone Joint Surg* 65A:1157, 1983.

Canale G, Scarsi M, Mastragostino S: Hip deformity and dislocation in spina bifida, *Ital J Orthop Traumatol* 18:155, 1992.

Canale ST, Hammond NL III, Cotler JM, Snedden HE: Pelvic displacement osteotomy for chronic hip dislocation in myelodysplasia, *J Bone Joint Surg* 57A:177, 1975.

Carroll NC: The orthotic management of the spina bifida child, *Clin Orthop* 102:108, 1974.

Carroll NC: Assessment and management of the lower extremity in myelodysplasia, *Orthop Clin North Am* 18:709, 1987.

Carroll NC, Sharrard WJW: Long-term follow-up of posterior ilio psoas transplantation for paralytic dislocation of the hip, *J Bone Joint Surg* 54A:551, 1972.

Castle ME, Schneider C: Proximal femoral resection interposition arthroplasty, *J Bone Joint Surg* 60A:1051, 1978.

Charney EB, Melchionni JB, Smith DR: Community ambulation by children with myelomeningocele and high-level paralysis, *J Pediatr Orthop* 11:579, 1991.

Correll J, Gabler C: The effect of soft tissue release of the hips on walking in myelomeningocele, *J Pediatr Orthop* 9:148, 2000.

Crandall RC, Birkebak RC, Winter RB: The role of hip location and dislocation in the functional status of the myelodysplastic patient: a review of 100 patients, *Orthopedics* 12:675, 1988.

Crawford AH, Marxen JL, Osterfield DL: The Cincinnati incision: a comprehensive approach for surgical procedures of the foot and ankle in childhood, *J Bone Joint Surg* 64A:1355, 1982.

Cruess RL, Turner NS: Paralysis of hip abductor muscles in spina bifida: results of treatment by the Mustard procedure, *J Bone Joint Surg* 52A:1364, 1970.

Curtis BH: The hip in the myelomeningocele child, *Clin Orthop* 90:11, 1973.

Curtis BH, Fisher RL: Congenital hyperextension with anterior subluxation of the knee: surgical treatment and long-term observations, *J Bone Joint Surg* 51A:255, 1969.

Cyphers SM, Feiwell E: Review of the Girdlestone-Taylor procedure for clawtoes in myelodysplasia, *Foot Ankle* 8:229, 1988.

DeSouza LJ, Carroll N: Ambulation of the braced myelomeningocele patient, *J Bone Joint Surg* 58A:1112, 1976.

Dias L: Surgical management of knee contractures in myelomeningocele, *J Pediatr Orthop* 2:127, 1982.

Dias LS: Ankle valgus in children with myelomeningocele, *Dev Med Child Neurol* 20:627, 1981.

Dias LS: Valgus deformity of the ankle joint: pathogenesis of fibular shortening, *J Pediatr Orthop* 5:176, 1985.

Dias LS, Busch M, Tachdjian MO: Surgical treatment of severe hindfoot valgus by medial displacement osteotomy of the os calcis, *Orthop Trans* 11:35, 1987.

Dias LS, Hill JS: Evaluation of treatment of hip for subluxation in myelomeningocele by intertrochanteric varus derotation femoral osteotomy, *Orthop Clin North Am* 11:31, 1980.

Dias LS, Jasty MJ, Collins P: Rotational deformities of the lower limb in myelomeningocele: evaluation and treatment, *J Bone Joint Surg* 66A:215, 1984.

Dias LS, Stern LS: Talectomy in the treatment of resistant talipes equinovarus deformity in myelomeningocele and arthrogryposis, *J Pediatr Orthop* 7:39, 1987.

Donaldson WF: Hip problems in the child with myelomeningocele. In American Academy of Orthopedic Surgeons: *Symposium on myelomeningocele,* St Louis, 1972, Mosby.

Dormans JP, Templeton J, Schreinder MS, Delfico AJ: Intraoperative latex anaphylaxis in children: classification and prophylaxis of patients at risk, *J Pediatr Orthop* 17:622, 1997.

Douglas R, Larson PF, D'Ambrosia R, McCall RE: The LSU reciprocation—joint orthosis, *Orthopedics* 6:834, 1983.

Drennan JC: Orthotic management of the myelomeningocele spine, *Dev Med Child Neurol* 18:97, 1976.

Drennan JC, Sharrard WJW: The pathological anatomy of convex pes valgus, *J Bone Joint Surg* 53B:455, 1971.

Drennan JC, Banta JV, Bunch WH, Lindseth RE: Symposium: current concepts in the management of myelomeningocele, *Contemp Orthop* 19:63, 1989.

Drummond DF, Moreau M, Cruess RL: The results and complications of surgery for the paralytic hip and spine in myelomeningocele, *J Bone Joint Surg* 62B:49, 1980.

Duckworth T, Smith TWD: The treatment of paralytic convex pes valgus, *J Bone Joint Surg* 56B:305, 1974.

Dunteman RC, Vankoski SJ, Dias LS: Internal derotation osteotomy of the tibia: pre- and postoperative gait analysis in persons with high sacral myelomeningocele, *J Pediatr Orthop* 20:623, 2000.

Dupré P, Walker G: Knee problems associated with spina bifida, *Dev Med Child Neurol* 14(27):152, 1972.

Dwyer AF, Newton NC, Sherwood AA: An anterior approach to scoliosis: a preliminary report, *Clin Orthop* 62:192, 1969.

Evans D: Calcaneo-valgus deformity, *J Bone Joint Surg* 57B:270, 1975.

Feiwell E: Surgery of the hip in myelomeningocele as related to adult goals, *Clin Orthop* 148:87, 1980.

Feiwell E: Selection of appropriate treatment for patients with myelomeningocele, *Orthop Clin North Am* 12:101, 1981.

Feiwell E, Sakai D, Blatt T: The effect of hip reduction on function in patients with myelomeningocele: potential gains and hazards of surgical treatment, *J Bone Joint Surg* 60A:169, 1978.

Flandry F, Burke S, Roberts JM, et al: Functional ambulation in myelodysplasia: the effect of orthotic selection on physical and physiologic performance, *J Pediatr Orthop* 6:661, 1986.

Fraser RK, Hoffman EB: Calcaneus deformity in the ambulant patient with myelomeningocele, *J Bone Joint Surg* 73B:994, 1991.

Fraser RK, Hoffman EB, Sparks LT, Buccimazza SS: The unstable hip and mid-lumbar myelomeningocele, *J Bone Joint Surg* 74B: 143, 1992.

Fraser RK, Menelaus MB: The management of tibial torsion in patients with spina bifida, *J Bone Joint Surg* 75B:495, 1993.

Freehafer AA, Vessely JC, Mack RP: Iliopsoas muscle transfer in the treatment of myelomeningocele patients with paralytic hip deformities, *J Bone Joint Surg* 54A:1715, 1972.

Freeman JM: *Practical management of meningomyelocele,* Baltimore, 1974, University Park Press.

Gallien R, Morin F, Marquis F: Subtalar arthrodesis in children, *J Pediatr Orthop* 9:59, 1989.

Georgiadis GM, Aronson DD: Posterior transfer of the anterior tibial tendon in children who have a myelomeningocele, *J Bone Joint Surg* 72A:392, 1990.

Gross PM, Lyne D: The Grice procedures: indications and evaluation of long-term results, *Clin Orthop* 153:194, 1980.

Guidera KJ, Smith S, Raney E, et al: Use of the reciprocating gait orthosis in myelodysplasia, *J Pediatr Orthop* 13:341, 1993.

Hall JE, Poitras B: The management of kyphosis in patients with myelomeningocele, *Clin Orthop* 128:33, 1977.

Hall PV, Lindseth RE, Campbell RC, Kalsbeck JE: Myelodysplasia and developmental scoliosis: a manifestation of syringomyelia, *Spine* 1:48, 1976.

Harris MB, Banta JV: Cost of skin care in the myelomeningocele population, *J Pediatr Orthop* 10:355, 1990.

Hay MC, Walker G: Plantar pressures in healthy children and in children with myelomeningocele, *J Bone Joint Surg* 55B:828, 1973.

Hedemann JS, Gillespie R: Management of myelomeningocele kyphosis in the older child by kyphectomy and segmental spinal instrumentation, *Spine* 12:37, 1987.

Hoffer M, Feiwell E, Perry R, et al: Functional ambulation in patients with myelomeningocele, *J Bone Joint Surg* 55A:137, 1973.

Huff CW, Ramsey PL: Myelodysplasia: the influence of the quadriceps and hip abductor muscles on ambulatory function and stability of the hip, *J Bone Joint Surg* 60A:432, 1978.

Hull WJ, Moe JN, Winter RB: Spinal deformity in myelomeningocele: natural history, evaluation, and treatment, *J Bone Joint Surg* 56A:1767, 1974.

Jackson RD, Padgett TS, Donovan MM: Posterior iliopsoas transfer in myelodysplasia, *J Bone Joint Surg* 61A:40, 1979.

Jones R: Certain operative procedures in the paralysis of children, with special reference to poliomyelitis, *Br Med J* 2:1520, 1911.

Kumar SJ, Cowell HR, Townsend P: Physeal, metaphyseal, and diaphyseal injuries of the lower extremities in children with myelomeningocele, *J Pediatr Orthop* 4:25, 1984.

Lee EH, Carroll NC: Hip stability and ambulatory status in myelomeningocele, *J Pediatr Orthop* 5:522, 1985.

Letherman KD, Dickson RA: Congenital kyphosis in myelomeningocele: vertebral body resection and posterior spinal fusion, *Spine* 3:222, 1978.

Levitt RL, Canale ST, Gartland JJ: Surgical correction of foot deformity in the older patient with myelomeningocele, *Orthop Clin North Am* 5:19, 1974.

Lichtblau S: Medial and lateral release operation for clubfoot: preliminary report, *J Bone Joint Surg* 55A:1377, 1973.

Lim R, Dias L, Vankoski S, et al: Valgus knee stress in lumbosacral myelomeningocele: a gait-analysis evaluation, *J Pediatr Orthop* 18:428, 1998.

Lindseth RE: Treatment of the lower extremity in children paralyzed by meningocele (birth to 18 months), *Instr Course Lect* 25:76, 1976.

Lindseth RE: Posterior iliac osteotomy for fixed pelvic obliquity, *J Bone Joint Surg* 60A:17, 1978.

Lindseth RE, Seltzer L: Vertebral excision for kyphosis in children with myelomeningocele, *J Bone Joint Surg* 61A:699, 1979.

Lock TR, Aronson DD: Fractures in patients who have myelomeningocele, *J Bone Joint Surg* 71A:1153, 1989.

London JT, Nichols O: Paralytic dislocation of the hip in myelodysplasia: the role of the adductor transfer, *J Bone Joint Surg* 57A:501, 1975.

Lonstein JE, Bradford DS, Winter RB: *Moe's textbook of scoliosis and other spinal deformities,* ed 3, Philadelphia, 1994, WB Saunders.

Lorber J: Results of treatment of myelomeningocele: an analysis of 270 consecutive cases with criteria for selection for the future, *Arch Dis Child* 47:854, 1972.

Lorber J: Selective treatment of myelomeningocele: to treat or not to treat? *Pediatrics* 53:307, 1974.

Lorber J: Some paediatric aspects of myelomeningocele, *Acta Orthop Scand* 46:350, 1975.

Lorber J, Stewart CR, Ward AM: Alpha-fetoprotein in antenatal diagnosis of anencephaly and spina bifida, *Lancet* 1:1187, 1973.

Makin M: Tibio-fibular relationship in paralysed limbs, *J Bone Joint Surg* 47B:500, 1965.

Malhotra D, Puri R, Owen R: Valgus deformity of the ankle in children with spina bifida aperta, *J Bone Joint Surg* 66B:381, 1984.

Mannor DA, Weinstein SL, Dietz FR: Long-term follow-up of Chiari pelvic osteotomy in myelomeningocele, *J Pediatr Orthop* 16:769, 1996.

Marshall PD, Broughton NS, Menelaus MB, Graham HK: Surgical release of knee flexion contractures in myelomeningocele, *J Bone Joint Surg* 78B:912, 1996.

Mayer L: Further studies of fixed pelvic obliquity, *J Bone Joint Surg* 18:27, 1936.

Maynard MJ, Weiner LS, Burke SW: Neuropathic foot ulceration in patients with myelodysplasia, *J Pediatr Orthop* 12:786, 1992.

Mazur J, Menelaus MB, Dickens DRV, Doig WG: Efficacy of surgical management for scoliosis in myelomeningocele: correction of deformity and alteration of functional status, *J Pediatr Orthop* 6:568, 1986.

Mazur JM, Menelaus MB, Hudson I, Stillwell A: Hand function in patients with spina bifida cystica, *J Pediatr Orthop* 6:442, 1986.

Mazur JM, Stillwell A, Menelaus M: The significance of spasticity in the upper and lower limbs in myelomeningocele, *J Bone Joint Surg* 68B:213, 1986.

Mazur JM, Shurtleff D, Menelaus MB, et al: Orthopaedic management of high-level spina bifida: early walking compared with early use of a wheelchair, *J Bone Joint Surg* 71A:56, 1989.

McCall RE, Schmidt WT: Clinical experience with the reciprocal gait orthosis in myelodysplasia, *J Pediatr Orthop* 6:157, 1986.

McKay DW: McKay hip stabilization in myelomeningocele, *Orthop Trans* 1:87, 1977.

McLaughlin TP, Banta JV, Gahm NH, Raycroft JF: Intraspinal rhizotomy and distal cordectomy in patients with myelomeningocele, *J Bone Joint Surg* 68:88, 1986.

McMaster MJ: Anterior and posterior instrumentation and fusion of thoracolumbar scoliosis due to myelomeningocele, *J Bone Joint Surg* 69B:20, 1987.

McMaster MJ: The long-term results of kyphectomy and spinal stabilization in children with myelomeningocele, *Spine* 13:417, 1988.

Menelaus M: *The orthopaedic management of spina bifida cystica,* ed 2, Edinburgh, 1980, Churchill Livingstone.

Menelaus MB: Talectomy for equinovarus deformity in arthrogryposis and spina bifida, *J Bone Joint Surg* 53B:468, 1971.

Menelaus MB: Orthopaedic management of children with myelomeningocele: a plea for realistic goals, *Dev Med Child Neurol* 18:3, 1976.

Menelaus MB: Progress in the management of the paralytic hip in myelomeningocele, *Orthop Clin North Am* 11:17, 1980.

Menelaus MB, Broughton NS: Letter to the editor, *J Bone Joint Surg* 79A:1750, 1997.

Moe JH, Winter RB, Bradford DS, Lonstein JE: *Scoliosis and other spinal deformities,* Philadelphia, 1978, WB Saunders.

Molloy MK: The unstable paralytic hip: treatment by combined pelvic and femoral osteotomy and transiliac psoas transfer, *J Pediatr Orthop* 6:533, 1986.

Mustard WT: Iliopsoas transfer for weakness of the hip abductors, *J Bone Joint Surg* 34A:647, 1952.

Nicol RO, Menelaus MB: Correction of combined tibial torsion and valgus deformity of the foot, *J Bone Joint Surg* 65B:641, 1983.

Olney BW, Menelaus MB: Triple arthrodesis of the foot in spina bifida patients, *J Bone Joint Surg* 70B:234, 1988.

O'Phelan EH: Iliac osteotomy in exstrophy of the bladder, *J Bone Joint Surg* 45A:409, 1963.

Osebold WR, Mayfield JK, Winter RB, Moe JM: Surgical treatment of paralytic scoliosis associated with myelomeningocele, *J Bone Joint Surg* 64A:841, 1982.

Parker B, Walker G: Posterior psoas transfer and hip instability in lumbar myelomeningocele, *J Bone Joint Surg* 57B:53, 1975.

Parsch K, Manner G: Prevention and treatment of knee problems in children with spina bifida, *Dev Med Child Neurol* 18:114, 1976.

Paulos L, Coleman SS, Samuelson KM: Pes cavovarus, *J Bone Joint Surg* 62A:942, 1980.

Phillips DL, Field RE, Broughton NS, Menelaus MB: Reciprocating orthosis for children with myelomeningocele: a comparison of two types, *J Bone Joint Surg* 77B:110, 1995.

Phillips DP, Lindseth RE: Ambulation after transfer of adductors, external oblique, and tensor fasciae latae in myelomeningocele, *J Pediatr Orthop* 12:712, 1992.

Pierz K, Banta J, Thomson J, et al: The effect of tethered cord release on scoliosis in myelomeningocele, *J Pediatr Orthop* 20:362, 2000.

Piggott H: The natural history of scoliosis in myelodysplasia, *J Bone Joint Surg* 62B:54, 1980.

Olney BW, Menelaus MB: Triple arthrodesis of the foot in spina bifida patients, *J Bone Joint Surg* 70B:234, 1988.

Raycroft JF: Abduction splinting of the hip joints in myelodysplastic infants, *J Pediatr Orthop* 7:686, 1987.

Raycroft JF, Curtis BH: Spinal curvature in myelomeningocele. In American Academy of Orthopaedic Surgeons: *Symposium on myelomeningocele,* St Louis, 1972, Mosby.

Raycroft TF: Posterior iliopsoas transfer—long term results in patients treated at Newington Children's Hospital, *Orthop Trans* 11:454, 1987.

Roberts JA, Bennet GC, MacKenzie JR: Physeal widening in children with myelomeningocele, *J Bone Joint Surg* 71B:30, 1989.

Robinson JM, Hewson JE, Parker PM: The walking ability of fourteen- to seventeen-year-old teenagers with spina bifida: a physiotherapy study, *Z Kinderchir* 31:421, 1980.

Rose J, Gamble JG, Lee J, et al: The energy expenditure index: a method to quantitate and compare walking energy expenditures for children and adolescents, *J Pediatr Orthop* 11:571, 1991.

Rose GK, Sankarankutt M, Stallard J: A clinical review of the orthotic treatment of myelomeningocele patients, *J Bone Joint Surg* 65B:242, 1983.

Ross PM, Lyne D: The Grice procedure: indications and evaluation of long-term results, *Clin Orthop* 153:195, 1980.

Roy DR, Crawford AH: Idiopathic chondrolysis of hip: management by subtotal capsulectomy and aggressive rehabilitation, *J Pediatr Orthop* 8:203, 1988.

Roye DP Jr, Morden ML, Madsen N: Treatment of the hip in myelomeningocele: a review of 200 patients. Paper presented at the annual meeting of the Pediatric Orthopaedic Society of North America, Toronto, May 1987.

Rueda J, Carroll NC: Hip instability in patients with myelomeningocele, *J Bone Joint Surg* 54B:422, 1972.

Samuelsson L, Eklöf O: Scoliosis in myelomeningocele, *Acta Orthop Scand* 59:122, 1988.

Samuelsson L, Eklöf O: Hip instability in myelomeningocele: 158 patients followed for 15 years, *Acta Orthop Scand* 61:3, 1990.

Samuelsson L, Skoog M: Ambulation in patients with myelomeningocele: a multivariate statistical analysis, *J Pediatr Orthop* 8:569, 1988.

Sanda JPS, Skinner SR, Banto PS: Posterior transfer of tibialis anterior in low level myelodysplasia, *Dev Med Child Neurol* 26:100, 1984.

Schafer MF, Dias LS: *Myelomeningocele: orthopaedic treatment,* Baltimore, 1983, Williams & Wilkins.

Schopler SA, Menelaus MB: Significance of the strength of the quadriceps muscles in children with myelomeningocele, *J Pediatr Orthop* 7:507, 1987.

Schurtleff DB, Menelaus MB, Staheli LT, et al: Natural history of flexion deformity of the hip in myelodysplasia, *J Pediatr Orthop* 6:666, 1986.

Segal LS, Mann DC, Feiwell E, Hoffer MM: Equinovarus deformity in arthrogryposis and myelomeningocele: evaluation of primary talectomy, *Foot Ankle* 10:12, 1989.

Seller MJ, Nevin NC: Periconceptional vitamin supplementation and the prevention of neural tube defects in south-east England and Northern Ireland, *J Med Genet* 21:325, 1984.

Sharrard WJW: Posterior iliopsoas transplantation in the treatment of paralytic dislocation of the hip, *J Bone Joint Surg* 46B:426, 1964.

Sharrard WJW: Paralytic deformity in the lower limb, *J Bone Joint Surg* 49B:731, 1967.

Sharrard WJW: Spinal osteotomy for congenital kyphosis in myelomeningocele, *J Bone Joint Surg* 50B:466, 1968.

Sharrard WJW: Long-term follow-up of posterior iliopsoas transplantation in the treatment of paralytic dislocation of the hip, *J Bone Joint Surg* 52B:779, 1970.

Sharrard WJW: The orthopaedic surgery of spina bifida, *Clin Orthop* 92:195, 1973.

Sharrard WJW: The orthopaedic management of spina bifida, *Acta Orthop Scand* 46:356, 1975.

Sharrard WJW, Drennan JC: Osteotomy-excision of the spine for lumbar kyphosis in older children with myelomeningocele, *J Bone Joint Surg* 54B:50, 1972.

Sharrard WJW, Grosfield I: The management of deformity and paralysis of the foot in myelomeningocele, *J Bone Joint Surg* 50B:456, 1968.

Sharrard WJW, Webb J: Supra-malleolar wedge osteotomy of the tibia in children with myelomeningocele, *J Bone Joint Surg* 56B:458, 1974.

Sharrard WJW, Zachary RB, Lorber J: Survival and paralysis in open myelomeningocele with special reference to the time of repair of the spinal lesion, *Dev Med Child Neurol* 9:35, 1967.

Sharrard WJW, Zachary RB, Lorber J: The long-term evaluation of a trial of immediate and delayed closure of spina bifida cystica, *Clin Orthop* 50:197, 1967.

Sharrard WJW, Zachary RB, Lorber J, Bruce AM: A controlled trial of immediate and delayed closure of spina bifida cystica, *Arch Dis Child* 38:18, 1963.

Sherk HH, Amos MD: Talectomy in the treatment of the myelomeningocele patient, *Clin Orthop* 110:218, 1975.

Sherk HH, Marchinski LJ, Clancy M, Melchonni J: Ground reaction forces on the plantar surface of the foot after talectomy in the myelomeningocele, *J Pediatr Orthop* 9:269, 1989.

Sherk HH, Melchionne J, Smith R: The natural history of hip dislocation in ambulatory myelomeningoceles, *Z Kinderchir* 42:48, 1987.

Shurtleff DB, Goiney R, Gordon LH, Livermore N: Myelodysplasia: the natural history of kyphosis and scoliosis: a preliminary report, *Dev Med Child Neurol* 18(suppl 37):126, 1976.

Shurtleff DB, Menelaus MB, Staheli LT, et al: Natural history of flexion deformity of the hip in myelodysplasia, *J Pediatr Orthop* 6:666, 1986.

Smyth BT, Piggot J, Forsythe WI, Merrett JD: A controlled trial of immediate and delayed closure of myelomeningocele, *J Bone Joint Surg* 56B:297, 1974.

Stevens PM: Relative hypoplasia of fibula and associated ankle valgus, *J Pediatr Orthop* 7:605, 1987.

Stevens PM: Effect of ankle valgus on radiographic appearance of the hindfoot, *J Pediatr Orthop* 8:184, 1988.

Stevens PM, Toomey E: Fibular-Achilles tenodesis for paralytic ankle valgus, *J Pediatr Orthop* 8:169, 1988.

Stillwell A, Menelaus M: Walking ability in mature patients with spina bifida, *J Pediatr Orthop* 3:184, 1983.

Stillwell A, Menelaus M: Walking ability after transplantation of the iliopsoas, *J Bone Joint Surg* 66B:656, 1984.

Swank SM et al: Spina bifida: a review of 10 years' experience with 198 children. Paper presented at the American Academy of Cerebral Palsy and Developmental Medicine, Toronto, Oct 1987.

Taylor LJ: Excision of the proximal end of the femur for hip stiffness in myelomeningocele, *J Bone Joint Surg* 68B:75, 1986.

Thomas LI, Thompson TC, Straub LR: Transplantation of the external oblique muscle for abductor paralysis, *J Bone Joint Surg* 32A:207, 1950.

Thomsen M, Lang RD, Carstens C: Results of kyphectomy with the technique of Warner and Fackler in children with myelodysplasia, *J Pediatr Orthop* 9:143, 2000.

Tosi LL, Buck BD, Nason SS, McKay DW: Dislocation of the hip in myelomeningocele, *J Bone Joint Surg* 78A:664, 1996.

Trieshmann H, Millis M, Hall J, Watts H: Sliding calcaneal osteotomy for treatment of hindfoot deformity, *Orthop Trans* 4:305, 1980.

Trumble T, Banta JV, Raycroft JF, Curtis BH: Talectomy for equinovarus deformity in myelodysplasia, *J Bone Joint Surg* 67A:21, 1985.

Vogel LC, Schrader T, Lubicky JP: Latex allergy in children and adolescents with spinal cord injuries, *J Pediatr Orthop* 15:517, 1995.

Walker G: The early management of varus feet in myelomeningocele, *J Bone Joint Surg* 53B:462, 1971.

Weisl H, Fairclough JA, Jones DG: Stabilisation of the hip in myelomeningocele: comparison of posterior iliopsoas transfer and varus-rotation osteotomy, *J Bone Joint Surg* 70B:29, 1988.

Westin GW, Defiore RJ: Tenodesis of the tendo-Achilles to the fibula for a paralytic calcaneus deformity, *J Bone Joint Surg* 56A:1541, 1975.

Williams JJ, Graham GP, Dunne KB, Menelaus MB: Late knee problems in myelomeningocele, *J Pediatr Orthop* 13:701, 1993.

Winter RB, Carlson JM: Modern orthotics for spinal deformities, *Clin Orthop* 126:74, 1977.

Wissinger LA, Turner T, Donaldson WF: Posterior iliopsoas transfer: a treatment for some myelodysplastic hips, *Orthopedics* 3:865, 1980.

Wright JG, Menelaus MB, Broughton NS, Shurtleff D: Natural history of knee contractures in myelomeningocele, *J Pediatr Orthop* 11:725, 1991.

Wright JG, Menelaus MB, Broughton NS, Shurtleff D: Lower extremity alignment in children with spina bifida, *J Pediatr Orthop* 12:232, 1992.

Yates JR, Ferguson-Smith MA, Shenkin A, et al: Is disordered folate metabolism the basis for the genetic predisposition to neural tube defects? *Clin Genet* 31:279, 1987.

Yngve DA, Douglas R, Roberts JM: The reciprocating gait orthosis in myelomeningocele, *J Pediatr Orthop* 4:304, 1984.

Yngve DA, Douglas R, Roberts JM: The reciprocating gait orthosis in myelomeningocele, *J Pediatr Orthop* 4:304, 1984.

Yngve DA, Lindseth RE: Effectiveness of muscle transfers in myelomeningocele hips measured by radiographic indices, *J Pediatr Orthop* 2:121, 1982.

Yount CC: The role of the tensor fasciae femoris in certain deformities of the lower extremities, *J Bone Joint Surg* 8:171, 1926.

ARTHROGRYPOSIS MULTIPLEX CONGENITA

Akazawa H, Oda K, Mitani S, et al: Surgical management of hip dislocation in children with arthrogryposis multiplex congenita, *J Bone Joint Surg* 80B:636, 1998.

Atkins RM, Bell MJ, Sharrard WJ: Arthrogryposis: pectoralis major transfer for paralysis of elbow flexion in children, *J Bone Joint Surg* 67B:640, 1985.

Axt MW, Niethard FU, Döderlein L, Weber M: Principles of treatment of the upper extremity in arthrogryposis multiplex congenita type I, *J Pediatr Orthop* 6:179, 1986.

Banker BQ: Neuropathologic aspects of arthrogryposis multiplex congenita, *Clin Orthop* 194:30, 1985.

Bayne LG: Hand assessment and management in arthrogryposis multiplex congenita, *Clin Orthop* 194:68, 1985.

Brown LM, Robson MJ, Sharrard WJW: The pathophysiology of arthrogryposis multiplex congenita neurologica, *J Bone Joint Surg* 62B:291, 1980.

Carlson WO, Speck GJ, Vicari V, Wenger DR: Arthrogryposis multiplex congenita: a long-term follow-up study, *Clin Orthop* 194:115, 1985.

Cassis N, Capdevila R: Talectomy for clubfoot in arthrogryposis, *J Pediatr Orthop* 20:652, 2000.

DelBello DA, Watts HG: Distal femoral extension osteotomy for knee flexion contracture in patients with arthrogryposis, *J Pediatr Orthop* 16:122, 1996.

Diamond LS, Alegado R: Perinatal fractures in arthrogryposis multiplex congenita, *J Pediatr Orthop* 1:189, 1981.

Drummond DS, Cruess RL: The management of the foot and ankle in arthrogryposis multiplex congenita, *J Bone Joint Surg* 60B:96, 1978.

Drummond DS, Siller TN, Cruess RL: The management of arthrogryposis multiplex congenita, *Instr Course Lect* 23:79, 1974.

D'Souza H, Aroojis A, Chawara GS: Talectomy in arthrogryposis: analysis of results, *J Pediatr Orthop* 18:760, 1998.

Fairbank HAT: Birth palsy: subluxation of the shoulder-joint in infants and young children, *Lancet* 1:1217, 1913.

Fedrizzi E, Botteon G, Inverno M, et al: Neurogenic arthrogryposis multiplex congenita: clinical and MRI findings, *Pediatr Neurol* 9:343, 1993.

Friedlander HL, Westin GW, Wood WL Jr: Arthrogryposis multiplex congenita, *J Bone Joint Surg* 50A:89, 1968.

Green ADL, Fixsen JA, Lloyd-Roberts GC: Talectomy for arthrogryposis multiplex congenita, *J Bone Joint Surg* 66B:697, 1984.

Green WT, Tachdjian MO: Correction of residual deformities of the shoulder in obstetrical palsy, *J Bone Joint Surg* 45A:1544, 1963.

Gross RH: The role of the Verebelyi-Ogston procedure in the management of the arthrogrypotic foot, *Clin Orthop* 194:99, 1985.

Guidera KJ, Drennan JC: Foot and ankle deformities in arthrogryposis multiplex congenita, *Clin Orthop* 194:93, 1985.

Guidera KJ, Kortright L, Barber V, Ogden JA: Radiographic changes in arthrogrypotic knees, *Skel Radiol* 20:193, 1991.

Hahn G: Arthrogryposis: pediatric review and habilitative aspects, *Clin Orthop* 194:104, 1985.

Hall JG: Genetic aspects of arthrogryposis multiplex congenita, *Clin Orthop* 194:44, 1985.

Herron LD, Westin GW, Dawson EG: Scoliosis in arthrogryposis multiplex congenita, *J Bone Joint Surg* 60A:293, 1978.

Hoffer MM, Swank S, Eastman F, et al: Ambulation in severe arthrogryposis, *J Pediatr Orthop* 3:293, 1983.

Hsu LCS, Jaffray D, Leong JCY: Talectomy for clubfoot in arthrogryposis, *J Bone Joint Surg* 66B:694, 1984.

Huurman WW, Jacobsen ST: The hip in arthrogryposis multiplex congenita, *Clin Orthop* 194:81, 1985.

Kopits S: Orthopaedic management. In Freeman J, ed: *Practical management of meningomyelocele*, Baltimore, 1974, University Park Press.

L'Episcopo JB: Tendon transplantation in obstetrical paralysis, *Am J Surg* 25:122, 1934.

Letts M, Davidson D: The role of bilateral talectomy in the management of bilateral rigid clubfeet, *Am J Orthop* 28:106, 1999.

Mennen U: Early corrective surgery of the wrist and elbow in arthrogryposis multiplex congenita, *J Hand Surg* 18B:304, 1993.

Murray C, Fixsen JA: Management of knee deformity in classical arthrogryposis multiplex congenital (amyoplasia congenita), *J Pediatr Orthop* 6:186, 1997.

Ogston A: A new principle of curing club-foot in severe cases in children a few years old, *Br Med J* 1:1524, 1902.

Palmer PM, MacEwan GD, Bowen JR, Mathews PA: Passive motion for infants with arthrogryposis, *Clin Orthop* 194:54, 1985.

Sarwark JF, MacEwen GD, Scott CI: Amyoplasia: a common form of arthrogryposis, *J Bone Joint Surg* 72A:465, 1990.

Sever JW: The results of a new operation for obstetrical paralysis, *Am J Orthop Surg* 16:248, 1918.

Shapiro F, Specht L: The diagnosis and orthopaedic treatment of childhood spinal muscular atrophy, peripheral neuropathy, Friedreich ataxia, and arthrogryposis, *J Bone Joint Surg* 75A:1699, 1993.

Sodergard J, Ryöppy S: The knee in arthrogryposis multiplex congenita, *J Pediatr Orthop* 10:177, 1990.

Sodergard J, Ryöppy S: Foot deformities in arthrogryposis multiplex congenita, *J Pediatr Orthop* 14:768, 1994.

Solund K, Sonne-Holm S, Kjolbye JE: Talectomy for equinovarus deformity in arthrogryposis: a 13- (2-20) year review of 17 feet, *Acta Orthop Scand* 62:372, 1991.

Staheli LT, Chew DE, Elliott JS, et al: Management of hip dislocations in children with arthrogryposis, *J Pediatr Orthop* 7:681, 1987.

St Clair HS, Zimbler S: A plan of management and treatment results in the arthrogrypotic hip, *Clin Orthop* 194:74, 1985.

Swinyard CA, Bleck EE: The etiology of arthrogryposis (multiple congenital contracture), *Clin Orthop* 194:15, 1985.

Szöke G, Staheli LT, Jaffe K, et al: Medial-approach open reduction dislocation in amyoplasia-type arthrogryposis, *J Pediatr Orthop* 16:127, 1996.

Thomas B, Schopler S, Wood W, Oppenheim WL: The knee in arthrogryposis, *Clin Orthop* 194:87, 1985.

Thompson GH, Bilenker RM: Comprehensive management of arthrogryposis multiplex congenita, *Clin Orthop* 194:6, 1985.

Verebelyi L: Angeborner Klupfuss, dirch subperiostales evidement des talus geheilt, *Pester Med Chir Presse* 14:224, 1877.

Wenner SM, Saperia BS: Proximal row carpectomy in arthrogrypotic wrist deformity, *J Hand Surg* 12A:523, 1987.

Williams PF: The management of arthrogryposis, *Orthop Clin North Am* 6:967, 1978.

Williams PF: Management of upper limb problems in arthrogryposis, *Clin Orthop* 194:60, 1985.

Williams PF: Personal communication, 1985.

Wynne-Davies RW, Williams PF, O'Connor JBF: The 1960's epidemic of arthrogryposis multiplex congenita, *J Bone Joint Surg* 63B:76, 1981.

Yingsakmongkol W, Kumar SJ: Scoliosis in arthrogryposis multiplex congenital: results after nonsurgical and surgical treatment, *J Pediatr Orthop* 20:656, 2000.

BRACHIAL PLEXUS

Al Zahrani S: Modified rotational osteotomy of the humerus for Erb's palsy, *Int Orthop* 17:202, 1993.

Boome RS, Kaye JC: Obstetric traction injuries of the brachial plexus: natural history, indications for surgical repair and results, *J Bone Joint Surg* 70B:571, 1988.

Brown KLB: Review of obstetrical palsies: nonoperative treatment, *Clin Plast Surg* 11:181, 1984.

Bunnell S: Tendon transfers in the hand and forearm, *Instr Course Lect* 6:106, 1949.

Bunnell S: *Surgery of the hand*, ed 3, Philadelphia, 1956, JB Lippincott.

Buschmann WR, Sager G: Orthopaedic considerations in obstetric brachial plexus palsy, *Orthop Rev* 16:290, 1987.

Chung SMK, Nissenbaum MM: Obstetrical paralysis, *Orthop Clin North Am* 6:393, 1975.

Déjerine-Klumpke A: *Des polynévrites en général et des paralysies et atrophies saturnines en particulier: etude clinique et anatomo-pathologique*, Paris, 1889, Ancienne Librairie Germer Bailliére et Cie.

Episcopo JB: Tendon transplantation in obstetrical paralysis, *Am J Surg* 25:122, 1934.

Erb W: Ueber eine eigenthiumliche Localization von Lachmungen in Plexus Brachialis, *Verhandl Naturhist Med Verin* 1:130, 1874.

Geutjens G, Gilbert A, Helsen K: Obstetric brachial plexus palsy associated with breech delivery: a different pattern of injury, *J Bone Joint Surg* 78B:303, 1996.

Gilbert A, Razabone R, Amar-Khodja S: Indications and results of brachial plexus surgery in obstetrical palsy, *Orthop Clin North Am* 19:91, 1988.

Gilbert A, Tassin JL: Surgical repair of the brachial plexus in obstetric paralysis, *Chirurgie* 110:70, 1984.

Goddard NJ, Fixsen JA: Rotation osteotomy of the humerus for birth injuries of the brachial plexus, *J Bone Joint Surg* 66B:257, 1984.

Green WT, Tachdjian MO: Correction of residual deformity of the shoulder from obstetrical palsy, *J Bone Joint Surg* 45A:1544, 1963.

Greenwald AG, Schute PC, Shiveley JL: Brachial plexus birth palsy: a 10-year report on the incidence and prognosis, *J Pediatr Orthop* 4:689, 1984.

Hardy AE: Birth injuries of the brachial plexus: incidence and prognosis, *J Bone Joint Surg* 63B:98, 1981.

Hentz V, Meyer R: Brachial plexus microsurgery in children, *Microsurgery* 12:175, 1991.

Hoffer MM, Phipps GJ: Closed reduction and tendon transfer for treatment of dislocation of the glenohumeral joint secondary to brachial plexus birth palsy, *J Bone Joint Surg* 80A:997, 1998.

Hoffer MM, Wickenden R, Roper R: Brachial plexus birth palsies: results of tendon transfers to the rotator cuff, *J Bone Joint Surg* 60A:691, 1978.

Jackson ST, Hoffer MM, Parrish N: Brachial plexus palsy in the newborn, *J Bone Joint Surg* 70A:1217, 1988.

Jones SJ: Diagnostic value of peripheral and spinal somatosensory evoked potential in traction lesions of the brachial plexus, *Clin Plast Surg* 2:167, 1984.

Kawabata H, Masada K, Tsuyuguchi Y, et al: Early microsurgical reconstruction in birth palsy, *Clin Orthop* 215:233, 1987.

Kirkos JM, Papadopoulos IA: Late treatment of brachial plexus palsy secondary to birth injuries: rotational osteotomy of the proximal part of the humerus, *J Bone Joint Surg* 80A:1477, 1998.

Klumpke A: Paralysies radiculaires du plexus brachial; paralysies radiculaires inferieures; de la partipation des filets sympathiques oculopupillaires dan ces paralysies, *Rev Med* 5:739, 1885.

Leffert RD: Clinical diagnosis, testing, and electromyographic study in brachial plexus traction injuries, *Orthop Clin North Am* 237:24, 1988.

Meyer RD: Treatment of adult and obstetrical brachial plexus injuries, *Orthopedics* 9:899, 1986.

Michelow BJ, Clarke HM, Curtis CG, et al: The natural history of obstetrical brachial plexus palsy, *Plast Reconstr Surg* 93:675, 1994.

Millesi H: Surgical management of brachial plexus injuries, *J Hand Surg* 2:367, 1977.

Narakas A: Brachial plexus surgery, *Orthop Clin North Am* 12:303, 1981.

Narakas AO: Injuries to the brachial plexus. In Bora FW Jr, ed: *The pediatric upper extremity: diagnosis and management,* Philadelphia, 1986, WB Saunders.

Narakas A: The treatment of brachial plexus injuries, *Int Orthop* 9:29, 1985.

Pearl ML, Edgerton BW: Glenoid deformity secondary to brachial plexus birth palsy, *J Bone Joint Surg* 80A:659, 1998.

Perry J, Hsu J, Barber L, Hoffer M: Orthoses in patients with brachial plexus injuries, *Arch Phys Med Rehabil* 55:132, 1974.

Riordan DC: Tendon transplantation in median nerve and ulnar nerve paralysis, *J Bone Joint Surg* 35A:312, 1953.

Rogers MH: An operation for the correction of deformity due to obstetrical paralysis, *Boston Med Surg J* 174:163, 1916.

Seddon HJ: Brachial plexus injuries, *J Bone Joint Surg* 31B:3, 1949.

Sever JW: The results of a new operation for obstetrical paralysis, *Am J Orthop Surg* 16:248, 1918.

Sever JW: Obstetric paralysis, *JAMA* 85:1862, 1925.

Sever JW: Obstetrical paralysis, *Surg Gynecol Obstet* 44:547, 1927.

Solonen KA, Telaranta T, Ryöppy S: Early reconstruction of birth injuries of the brachial plexus, *J Pediatr Orthop* 1:367, 1981.

Sugioka H: Evoked potentials in the investigation of traumatic lesions of the peripheral nerve and the brachial plexus, *Clin Orthop* 184:85, 1984.

Sunderland S: *Nerves and nerve injuries,* ed 2, New York, 1978, Churchill Livingstone.

Tada K, Tsuyuguchi Y, Kawai H: Birth palsy: natural recovery course and combined root avulsion, *J Pediatr Orthop* 4:279, 1984.

Terzis JK, Liberson WT, Levine R: Obstetric brachial plexus palsy, *Hand Clin* 2:773, 1986.

Waters PM: Comparison of the natural history, the outcome of microsurgical repair, and the outcome of operative reconstruction in brachial plexus birth palsy, *J Bone Joint Surg* 81A:649, 1999.

Waters PM: The upper limb. In Morrissy RT, Weinstein SL, eds: *Lovell and Winter's Pediatric orthopaedics,* Philadelphia, 2001, Lippincott Williams & Wilkins.

Waters PM, Peljovich AE: Shoulder reconstruction in patients with chronic brachial plexus birth palsy, *Clin Orthop* 364:144, 1999.

Waters PM, Smith GR, Jaramillo D: Glenohumeral deformity secondary to brachial plexus birth palsy, *J Bone Joint Surg* 80A:668, 1998.

Wickstrom J: Birth injuries of the brachial plexus: treatment of defects in the shoulder, *Clin Orthop* 23:187, 1962.

Zancolli EA: Classification and management of the shoulder in birth palsy, *Orthop Clin North Am* 12:433, 1980.

CHAPTER

32 Neuromuscular Disorders

William C. Warner, Jr.

Neuromuscular disease in children includes conditions that affect the spinal cord, peripheral nerves, neuromuscular junctions, and muscles. Accurate diagnosis is essential because the procedures commonly used to treat deformities in patients with neuromuscular disease such as poliomyelitis or cerebral palsy may not be appropriate for hereditary neuromuscular conditions. The diagnosis is made on the basis of clinical history, detailed family history, physical examination, and laboratory testing (including serum enzyme studies, especially serum levels of creatinine phosphokinase and aldolase), electromyography, nerve conduction velocity studies, and nerve and muscle biopsies. Serum enzyme levels of creatinine phosphokinase generally are elevated, but the increase varies dramatically from levels of 50 to 100 times normal in patients with some dystrophic muscle conditions (such as Duchenne muscular dystrophy) to only slight increases (1 to 2 times normal) in some patients with congenital myopathy or spinal muscular atrophy.

Nerve or muscle biopsy, or both, is useful for precise diagnosis. The muscle to be biopsied must be involved but still functioning—usually the deltoid, vastus lateralis, or gastrocnemius muscles. The biopsy specimen should not be taken from the region of musculotendinous junctions because the normal fibrous tissue septa can be confused with the pathological fibrosis. Specimens should be about 10 mm long and 3 mm deep and should be fixed in glutaraldehyde, in preparation for electron microscopy. The specimen of muscle that is to be processed for light microscopy should be frozen in liquid nitrogen within a few minutes after removal. The specimen should not be placed into saline solution or formalin. For nerve biopsy, the sural nerve usually is chosen. This nerve can be accessed laterally between the tendo calcaneus and the lateral malleolus just proximal to the level of the tibiotalar joint. The entire width of the nerve should be taken for a length of 3 to 4 cm. Atraumatic technique is essential in either type of biopsy for meaningful results.

Tremendous advances have been made in the 1990s in the understanding of the genetic basis of neuromuscular disorders. Through advances in molecular biology, chromosome locations for various abnormal genes are being identified, characterized, and sequenced (Table 32-1). In certain diseases, such as Duchenne and Becker muscular dystrophy, not only have the genes been localized, cloned, and sequenced, but the biochemical basis for these diseases is now understood. The gene responsible for Duchenne and Becker muscular dystrophy is located in the xp21 region of the X chromosome. This region is responsible for the coding of the dystrophin protein. Dystrophin testing (dystrophin immunoblotting) can be used as a biochemical test for muscular dystrophy; it is also useful for the differentiation of Duchenne muscular dystrophy from Becker muscular dystrophy.

Orthopaedic treatment has been aimed at preventing the worsening of deformities and providing stability to the skeletal system to improve the quality of life for these children. Although a cure is possible with gene therapy, orthopaedic treatment is still necessary to improve the quality of life for

Table 32-1 Classification of Major Muscular Dystrophies

Disease	Locus	Protein
X-LINKED RECESSIVE		
Duchenne-Becker dystrophy	xp21	Dystrophin
Emery-Dreifuss dystrophy	xp28	Emerin
AUTOSOMAL DOMINANT (AD)		
Myotonic dystrophy	19q	Myotonin
Facioscapulohumeral dystrophy	4q	?
LGMD—1A	5q	?
LGMD—B	Other	?
AUTOSOMAL RECESSIVE (AR)		
LGMD—2A	15q	Calpain
LGMD—2B	2q	?
LGMD—2C	13q	γ-Sarcoglycan
LGMD—2D	17q	α-Sarcoglycan
LGMD—2E	4q	β-Sarcoglycan
LGMD—2F	5q	δ-Sarcoglycan
MISCELLANEOUS OTHER		
Congenital Dystrophies		
Congenital muscular (AR)	6q	Merosin
Fukuyama disease (AR)	9q13	?
Congenital Myopathies		
Central core disease (AD)	19q	Ryanodine receptor
	14q	Myosin
Nemaline rod disease (AD)	1q22	Tropomyosin
Myotubular myopathies	Xq26	?
Distal muscular dystrophy (AD)	14q	?
Oculopharyngeal dystrophy (AD)	14q	?

From Brown RH Jr, Phil D: *Annu Rev Med* 48:457, 1997.

most children no matter how severely impaired. Louis et al. reported 34 surgical procedures performed over a 12-year period to improve sitting posture, care, and comfort in a select population of individuals with severe multiple impairments. Significant improvement was found in most patients, and no patient was made worse. Bleck listed the priorities of patients with severe neuromuscular diseases: the ability to communicate with other people and the ability to perform many activities of daily living, mobility, and ambulation. The role of the orthopaedic surgeon in achieving these goals includes prescribing orthoses for lower extremity control to facilitate transfer to and from wheelchairs, preventing or correcting joint contractures, and maintaining appropriate standing and sitting postures. Treatment must be individualized for each patient. The choice and timing of the procedures depend on the particular disorder, the severity of involvement, the ambulatory status of the patient, and the experience of the physician. This chapter includes some of the common neuromuscular disorders in children that frequently require surgical intervention.

General Treatment Considerations

FRACTURES

Fractures are common in children with neuromuscular disease because of disuse osteoporosis and frequent falls. Larson and Henderson found a significant decrease in bone mineral density on DEXA scans in boys with Duchenne muscular dystrophy, with 44% sustaining fractures. Most fractures are nondisplaced metaphyseal fractures that heal rapidly. Minimally displaced metaphyseal fractures of the lower limbs should be splinted so that walking can be resumed quickly. If braces are being used, they can be enlarged to accommodate the fractured limb and allow progressive weight-bearing. Displaced diaphyseal fractures can be treated with cast-braces or, rarely, open reduction and internal fixation to allow walking during fracture healing. Medical treatment of disuse osteopenia can be of some benefit in decreasing the incidence of fractures in this patient population.

ORTHOSES

Spinal bracing usually is accomplished with a polypropylene plastic shell with a soft foam polyethylene lining, in the form of either an anterior and posterior (bivalved) total-contact orthosis or an anterior-opening thoracic-lumbar-sacral orthosis (TSLO) with lumbar lordotic contouring. Bracing helps with sitting balance and may slow but will not prevent the progression of spinal deformity. Knee-ankle-foot orthoses provide stability for patients with proximal muscle weakness. A pelvic band with hip and knee locks can be added if necessary. Ankle-foot orthoses help to position the ankle and foot in a plantigrade position in an effort to prevent progressive equinus and equinovarus deformities.

SEATING SYSTEMS

For most children with severe neuromuscular disease, walking is difficult and frustrating, and a wheelchair eventually may be needed. The chair—whether manual or electric—must be carefully contoured. A narrow chair with a firm seat increases pelvic support, and a firm back in slight extension supports the spine. Lateral spine supports built into the chair may help sitting balance but usually will not alter the progression of scoliosis. Specialized seating clinics can provide custom-fitted chairs with numerous options for daily use. These custom-fitted chairs will accommodate any spinal deformity and pelvic obliquity that are present.

Differentiation of Muscle Disease from Nerve Disease

In addition to the history, physical examination, and routine laboratory studies, special tests such as the electromyogram, muscle tissue biopsy, serum enzyme, and molecular and genetic studies help differentiate the two diseases.

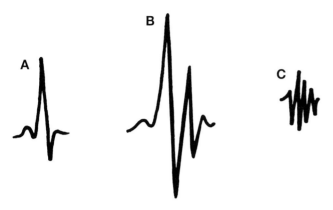

Fig. 32-1 Motor units seen in electromyography. **A,** Normal triphasic motor unit potential. **B,** Large polyphasic motor units as seen in neurogenic disorders such as spinal muscular atrophy, in which they also are reduced in number. **C,** Small polyphasic motor units as seen in muscular dystrophy. These usually are of normal number. (Courtesy Tulio E Bertorini, MD.)

ELECTROMYOGRAPHIC STUDIES

In an electromyogram of normal muscle, resting muscles usually are relatively electrosilent; on voluntary contraction of a normal muscle the electromyogram shows a characteristic frequency, duration, and amplitude action potential (Fig. 32-1). In a myopathy the electromyogram shows increased frequency, decreased amplitude, and decreased duration of the motor action potentials. In a neuropathy it shows decreased frequency and increased amplitude and duration of the action potentials. In a neuropathy nerve conduction velocities usually are slowed; in a myopathy the nerve conduction velocities usually are normal. Myotonic dystrophy is characterized by an increase in frequency, duration, and amplitude of the action potentials on needle electrode insertion, which gradually decreases over time. These action potentials when amplified create the "dive-bomber" sound that is almost universal in this disease.

MUSCLE TISSUE BIOPSY

Interpretation of the muscle tissue biopsy will differentiate not only myopathy from neuropathy, but also the various types of congenital dystrophy from one another. In addition to the usual hematoxylin and eosin stain, special stains and techniques, such as the Gomori modified trichrome stain, NDH-TR stain, and the alizarin red S stain, are helpful. Electron microscopy also is beneficial.

Histopathological study of muscle affected by myopathy shows an increased fibrosis in and between muscle spindles, with necrosis of the fibers (Fig. 32-2, *B*). Later, deposition of fat within the fibers occurs, accompanied by hyaline and granular degeneration of the fibers. The number of nuclei is increased with migration of some nuclei to the center of the fibers. Some small groups of inflammatory cells also may be seen, and in polymyositis inflammatory cells are markedly increased. Special histochemical stains that can demonstrate muscle fiber

type show a preponderance of type I fibers. In normal skeletal muscle the ratio of type I to type II fibers is 1:2 (Fig. 32-2, *A*). In some dystrophies other than the Duchenne type fiber splitting is apparent. Calcium accumulation in muscle fibers also has been demonstrated.

The microscopic picture in neuropathy is quite different (Fig. 32-2, *C*). There is little or no increase in fibrous tissue, and small, angular, atrophic fibers are present between groups of normal-sized muscle fibers. Special stains that demonstrate fiber type show that 80% of the fibers are type II.

An adequate biopsy must be obtained to make a correct diagnosis. An open muscle biopsy usually is performed, but in some cases a needle biopsy in small children has proved satisfactory. Muscles that are totally involved should not be used; biopsies of muscles suspected of early involvement are indicated. As an example, the muscle bellies of the gastrocnemius in a patient with Duchenne muscular dystrophy usually are involved early and are a poor site to obtain material for a biopsy, whereas the quadriceps (especially the vastus lateralis at midthigh) and rectus abdominis usually show early involvement without total replacement of the muscle spindles by fibrous tissue or fat. Biopsies of these muscles usually are the most reliable.

One must be careful when securing a biopsy specimen that the muscle is maintained at its normal length between clamps (Fig. 32-3) or sutures (Fig. 32-4) and that the biopsy specimen has not been violated by a needle electrode during an electromyogram or infiltrated with a local anesthetic before the biopsy. Biopsy needles should have a minimal core diameter of 3 mm.

A second sample of muscle tissue should be taken at the time of biopsy and sent for dystrophin analysis (dystrophin immunoblotting). Dystrophin is a muscle protein that has been found to be absent, decreased, or modified in certain types of dystrophy. The measurement and quantification of this protein combined with the clinical picture of certain types of muscular dystrophy have added significantly to the ability to diagnose various dystrophies.

Regional block anesthesia is preferred; a general anesthetic may be necessary but carries the known risk of anesthetic complications such as malignant hyperthermia.

◆ Open Muscle Biopsy

TECHNIQUE 32-1

Block the area regionally with 1% lidocaine and make a 1.5-cm incision through the skin and subcutaneous tissues. Carefully split the enveloping fascia to clearly expose the muscle bundles from which the biopsy specimen is to be taken. Using a special double clamp (Fig. 32-3) or silk sutures approximately 2 cm apart (Fig. 32-4), grasp the muscle and section around the outside of the arms of the clamp or sutures. Prevent bleeding within the muscle and take only small biopsy specimens. Take more than one specimen, since different stains need different preservative

continued

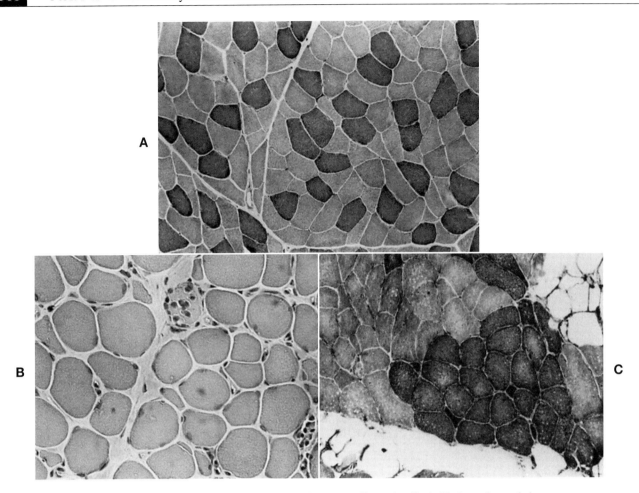

Fig. 32-2   **A,** Normal muscle biopsy (except for one small angular fiber). Notice polygonal shape of myofibrils, normal distribution of type I and type II fibers, and normal connective tissue of endomysium (NADH-TR stain, ×125). **B,** Muscular dystrophy. Fibers are more rounded, some fibers have internalized nuclei, and others are atrophic. One muscle fiber is necrotic and is undergoing phagocytosis. Connective tissue between fibers is increased (H&E stain, ×295). **C,** Chronic neurogenic atrophy (juvenile spinal muscular atrophy). Notice grouping of fibers of same type and some atrophic angular fibers. Fat is increased between muscle fascicles. (NADH-TR stain, ×125). (Courtesy Tulio E Bertorini, MD.)

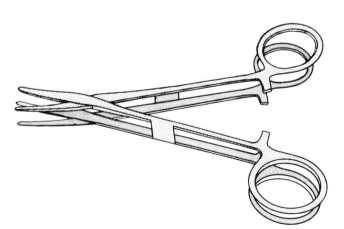

Fig. 32-3   Two hemostats bound together to preserve length when securing muscle biopsy. (From Cruess RL, Rennie WRJ: *Adult orthopaedics,* New York, 1984, Churchill Livingstone.)

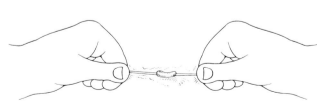

Fig. 32-4   Muscle length maintained by muscle biopsy done on outer side of previously placed sutures. (Redrawn from Curtis B: *Instr Course Lect* 19:78, 1970.)

techniques; for example, some histochemical changes are best demonstrated on fresh frozen sections that have had special staining. The pathologist should know in advance that a muscle biopsy is to be done so that special fixative techniques, such as freezing with liquid nitrogen, are readily available when the specimen is received.

◆ Percutaneous Muscle Biopsy

Mubarak, Chambers, and Wenger described percutaneous muscle biopsy in 379 patients. This procedure can be performed in an outpatient clinic with only local anesthesia.

TECHNIQUE 32-2 *(Mubarak, Chambers, Wenger)*

Prepare the biopsy site with iodophor paint. Place a fenestrated adhesive drape over the site. Infiltrate the skin and subcutaneous tissue with 5 to 8 ml of 1% lidocaine without epinephrine. When the quadriceps is being biopsied, also anesthetize the fascia. Check the Bergström biopsy needle to ensure a smooth sliding of the cutter within the trocar. Cut the K-50 tube at an angle and place it into the end of the cutting needle with the other end attached to a 10-ml syringe.

Use a no. 11 scalpel blade to make a small stab wound in the skin and fascia lata at about the midthigh level. Insert the Bergström needle into the muscle, preferably the rectus femoris, at an oblique angle. Pull the needle back about one half of its length and have an assistant apply suction with the 10-ml syringe. This allows muscle to be pulled into the cutting chamber. Cut by compressing the cutter into the trocar. Remove the Bergström apparatus from the thigh. Remove the muscle samples from the chamber with a fine needle and place on saline-soaked gauze in a petri dish. Through the same incision and track, reinsert the Bergström needle and repeat the procedure until five or six samples have been obtained. Close the small wound with ¼-inch Steri-Strips.

AFTERTREATMENT. Dressing sponges are applied and held in place with foam tape to serve as a compressive, but not constricting, bandage for 2 days. The Steri-Strips are left in place for 10 days; no perioperative antibiotics or narcotic analgesics are necessary.

SERUM ENZYME ASSAYS

Serum enzyme assays are extremely helpful, especially the level of serum creatine phosphokinase in the blood. Serum glutamic-oxaloacetic transaminase and serum glutamic-pyruvic transaminase levels are less specific; although elevated, they also are elevated in other conditions, such as myocardial infarction, myocardial myopathy, or liver disease, as is lactic dehydrogenase.

Creatine phosphokinase elevation is extremely important in the diagnosis in the early stages of Duchenne muscular dystrophy. It usually is not elevated in liver disease. It is elevated in myocardial infarction but not to the level seen in a patient with early muscular dystrophy. In affected newborns and children in the first year of life, the creatine phosphokinase level may be 200 to 300 times the normal level. The level may fall in the later stages of the disease, when the greater muscle mass has already deteriorated and there is less breakdown of muscle mass than in the earlier stages. This test is extremely beneficial in detecting the carrier state of Duchenne and Becker muscular dystrophies because creatine phosphokinase usually is elevated in the carrier female. A muscle provocation test also is beneficial in detecting the female carrier state, because creatine phosphokinase levels rise higher after strenuous exercise in carrier females than in noncarrier females.

Blood and urine chemistry studies are beneficial in making a diagnosis. Skeletal muscles produce creatinine in their metabolism of creatine. In dystrophic muscles, serum creatine is not used as much as usual, and creatinine is not produced in as great a quantity. This leads to excess creatine in the blood and thus in the urine. Urine creatine is excessive in dystrophic patients in the active stage of muscle breakdown. Any process that causes muscle breakdown, however, such as excessive exercise, diabetes mellitus, starvation in which carbohydrate intake is reduced, and also in the neuropathies, can cause an excess of creatine in the urine. In myotonic dystrophy, because of the reduced ability of the liver to produce creatine phosphate, blood creatine is decreased.

DNA mutation analysis (polymerase chain reaction or DNA blot analysis) can provide a definitive diagnosis of Duchenne or Becker muscular dystrophy. These tests also can help identify the carrier and may allow prenatal diagnosis in some cases. These DNA tests can be done from a small sample of blood or amniotic fluid.

Muscular Dystrophy

The muscular dystrophies are a group of hereditary disorders of skeletal muscle that produce progressive degeneration of skeletal muscle and associated weakness. The X-linked dystrophies are more common and include Duchenne muscular dystrophy, Becker muscular dystrophy, and Emery-Dreifuss muscular dystrophy. Limb-girdle muscular dystrophy and congenital muscular dystrophy are the two most common autosomal recessive muscular dystrophies. Facioscapulohumeral muscular dystrophy is inherited as an autosomal dominant trait (see Table 32-1).

DUCHENNE MUSCULAR DYSTROPHY

Duchenne muscular dystrophy, a sex-linked recessive inherited trait, occurs in males and in females with Turner syndrome; carriers are female. It is reported to occur in 1 in 3500 live births. There is a family history in 70% of patients, and the

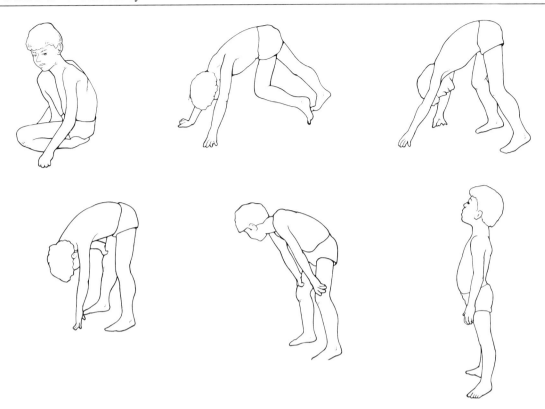

Fig. 32-5   Gower sign. Child must use his hands to rise from sitting position. (Redrawn from Siegel IM: *Clinical management of muscle disease,* London, 1977, William Heinemann.)

condition occurs as a spontaneous mutation in about 30% of patients.

Duchenne muscular dystrophy is the result of a mutation in the xp-21 region of the X chromosome, which encodes the 400 kilodalton in protein dystrophin. In patients with Duchenne muscular dystrophy, the total absence of this in transcellular protein results in progressive muscle degeneration and loss of function.

Children with Duchenne muscular dystrophy usually reach early motor milestones at appropriate times, but independent ambulation may be delayed and many are initially toe-walkers. Clinical features include large, firm calf muscles, the tendency to toe-walking, a widely based, lordotic stance, a waddling Trendelenburg gait, and a positive Gower test indicative of proximal muscle weakness (Fig. 32-5). The diagnosis usually is obvious by the time the child is 5 or 6 years old. Diagnosis is confirmed by a dramatically elevated level of creatinine phosphokinase (50 to 100 times normal) and DNA analysis of blood samples. Muscle biopsy demonstrates variations in fiber size in internal nuclei, split fibers, degenerating or regenerating fibers, and fibrofatty tissue deposition. Dystrophin testing of the muscle biopsy will confirm the type of muscular dystrophy (Fig. 32-6).

Physical Examination

The degree of muscular weakness depends on the age of the patient. Because the proximal musculature weakens before the distal muscles, examination of the lower extremities demonstrates an early weakness of gluteal muscle strength. The weakness in the proximal muscles of the lower extremity can be demonstrated by a decrease in the ability to rise from the floor without assistance of the upper extremities (Gower's sign). The calf pseudohypertrophy is caused by infiltration of the muscle by fat and fibrosis, giving the calves the feel of hard rubber (Fig. 32-7). The extrinsic muscles of the foot and ankle retain their strength longer than the proximal muscles of the hip and knee. The posterior tibial muscle retains its strength for the longest time. This pattern of weakness causes an equinovarus deformity of the foot. Weakness of the shoulder girdle musculature can be demonstrated by the Meryon sign, which is elicited by lifting the child with one arm encircling the child's chest. Most children contract the muscles about the shoulder to increase shoulder stability and facilitate lifting. In children with muscular dystrophy, however, the arms abduct because of the severe shoulder abductor muscle weakness until they eventually slide through the examiner's arms unless the chest is tightly encircled. Later in the disease process, the Thomas test demonstrates hip flexion contracture, and the Ober test demonstrates an abduction contracture of the hip.

Orthopaedic Treatment

The major goal of early treatment is to maintain functional ambulation as long as possible. Between the ages of 8 to 14 years (with a median of 10 years), children with Duchenne

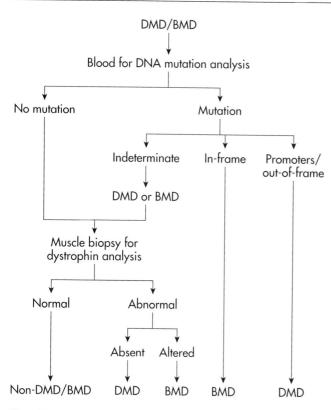

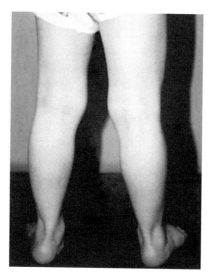

Fig. 32-7   Calf pseudohypertrophy in muscular dystrophy.

Fig. 32-6   Flow chart of process for molecular diagnostic evaluation of patients in whom diagnosis of Duchenne muscular dystrophy *(DMD)* or Becker muscular dystrophy *(BMD)* is suspected. (From Shapiro F, Specht L: *J Bone Joint Surg* 75A:439, 1993.)

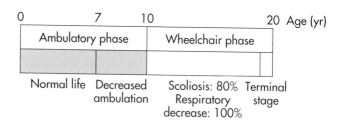

Fig. 32-8   Graph of natural course of Duchenne muscular dystrophy: age-related stages (From Rideau Y, Duport G, Delaubier A, et al: *Semin Neurol* 15:9, 1995.)

muscular dystrophy typically have a sensation of locking of the joints. Contractures of the lower extremity require early treatment to prolong the child's ability to ambulate, if even for 1 to 2 years, which is important to the child and the family and helps delay the inevitable progression of scoliosis. This requires prevention or retardation of the development of contractures of the lower extremity, which would eventually prohibit ambulation. It is easier to keep patients walking than to induce them to resume walking once they have stopped. When children with Duchenne muscular dystrophy stop walking, they also become more susceptible to the development of scoliosis and severe contractures of the lower extremities. Scoliosis develops in nearly all children with Duchenne muscular dystrophy, usually when they require aided mobility or shortly after becoming wheelchair bound.

If surgical correction of lower extremity contractures is debatable, three approaches have been used:

1. *Ambulatory approach.* The goal of surgery during the ambulatory period is to correct any contractures in the lower extremity while the patient is still ambulatory. Rideau recommends early aggressive surgery. His indications for surgery are: first appearance of contractures in lower extremities, a plateau in muscle strength, usually around 5 to 6 years of age, and difficulty

maintaining upright posture with the feet together. He believes surgery should be performed before deterioration of Gower's maneuver time or time to rise from the floor. Other surgeons recommend surgery later in the ambulatory phase, just before the cessation of ambulation.

2. *Rehabilitative approach.* Surgery is performed after the patient has lost the ability to walk but with the intention that walking will resume. Surgery during this stage usually only allows for minimal ambulation with braces.

3. *Palliative approach.* The palliative approach treats only contractures that interfere with shoe wear and comfortable positioning in a wheelchair.

Currently the most common approach is to correct contractures just before the patient has a significant decline in ambulation and before the patient has to use a wheelchair (ambulatory approach) (Fig. 32-8).

Mild equinus contractures of the feet can help force the knee into extension, which in turn helps prevent the knee buckling caused by severe weakness of the quadriceps. Stretching exercises and nightly bracing can be used to prevent the contractures from becoming severe. Flexion and abduction contractures of the hip, however, impede ambulation and should be minimized. Exercises to stretch the hip muscles and lower extremity braces worn at night to prevent the child's sleeping in a frog position are helpful initially. If surgery is indicated, the foot and hip contractures should be released simultaneously, usually through percutaneous incisions. Ambulation should be resumed immediately after surgery if possible. Polypropylene braces are preferred to long-term casting. Prolonged immobilization must be avoided to prevent or limit the progressive muscle weakness caused by disuse.

◆ Percutaneous Release of Hip Flexion and Abduction Contractures and Tendo Calcaneus Contracture

TECHNIQUE 32-3 *(Green)*

With the child supine on the operating table, prepare and drape both lower extremities from the iliac crests to the toes. First flex and then extend the hip to be released, holding the hip in adduction to place tension on the muscles to be released; keep the opposite hip in maximal flexion to flatten the lumbar spine. Insert a no. 15 knife blade percutaneously just medial and just distal to the anterosuperior iliac spine (Fig. 32-9). Release the sartorius muscle first, then the tensor fasciae femoris muscle. Push the knife laterally and subcutaneously—without cutting the skin—to release the tensor fasciae latae completely. Bring the knife to the original insertion point and push it deeper to release the rectus femoris completely. Take care to avoid the neurovascular structures of the anterior thigh. Next, approximately 3 to 4 cm proximal to the upper pole of the patella, percutaneously release the fascia lata laterally through a stab wound in its midportion. Push the knife almost to the femur to release the lateral intermuscular septum completely. Now perform a percutaneous release of the tendo calcaneus. Apply long leg casts with the feet in neutral position and with the heels well padded to prevent pressure ulcers.

AFTERTREATMENT. The patient is mobilized immediately after surgery. If tolerated, a few steps are allowed. Walker-assisted ambulation is begun as soon as possible, and once

transfer is achieved, the patient is placed on a regular bed and physical therapy is continued. The casts are bivalved, and bilateral polypropylene long leg orthoses are fitted as soon as possible. Patients are discharged from the hospital as soon as they can ambulate independently with a walker.

Rideau Technique. Rideau et al. described a similar technique but with an open procedure to release the hip flexor contractures and lateral thigh contractures. They also excised the iliotibial band and the lateral intermuscular septum (Fig. 32-10).

◆ Transfer of Posterior Tibialis Tendon to Dorsum of Foot

In patients with marked overpull of the posterior tibialis muscle, Greene found that transfer of the posterior tibialis tendon to the dorsum of the foot combined with other tenotomies or tendon lengthening gave better results than posterior tibial tendon lengthening alone. Although transfer of the posterior tibialis tendon is technically more demanding and has a higher perioperative complication rate, Greene noted that the patients retained the plantigrade posture of their feet, even after walking ceased. Despite the more extensive surgical procedure, early ambulation of the patients was not impeded.

TECHNIQUE 32-4 *(Greene)*

Place the patient supine; after placing a tourniquet make a 3-cm incision starting medially at the neck of the talus and extending to the navicular (Fig. 32-11, *A*). Open the sheath of the posterior tibial tendon from the distal extent of the flexor retinaculum to the navicular. Release the tendon from its bony insertions, preserving as much length as possible. Make a second incision 6 to 8 cm long vertically between the tendo calcaneus and the medial distal tibia. The tendo calcaneus can be lengthened through the same incision if necessary. Incise the posterior tibial tendon sheath and pull the distal portion of the tendon through the second operative wound. Make a third incision 6 cm long lateral to the

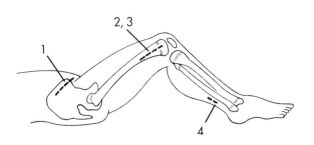

Fig. 32-9 Tenotomy sites for release of hip flexors *(1)*, tenor fasciae latae and fascia lata *(2 and 3)*, and tendo calcaneus *(4)*. (Redrawn from Siegel IM: *Clin Pediatr* 19:386, 1980.)

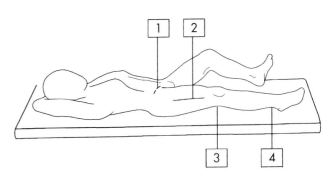

Fig. 32-10 Surgical sites for musculotendinous releases to bilaterally reduce contractures of the hip *(1)*, thigh *(2)*, knee *(3)*, and ankle *(4)*. (Redrawn from Rideau Y, Duport G, Delaubier A, et al: *Semin Neurol* 15:9, 1995.)

anterior crest of the tibia and extend it to the superior extensor retinaculum (Fig. 32-11, *B*). Incise the anterior compartment fascia and retract the tibialis anterior tendon laterally. Carefully incise the interosseous membrane on the lateral aspect of the tibia adjacent to its tibial insertion for a distance of 3 cm. Enlarge the opening by proximal and distal horizontal cuts, extending halfway across the interosseous membrane. Pass a curved clamp close to the tibia from the anterior compartment proximally into the second incision. Keep the curved clamp on the tibia to prevent injury to the peroneal vessels. After grasping the posterior tibialis tendon and pulling it into the third incision, inspect the tendon through the second incision to make sure that it has neither twisted on itself nor ensnared the flexor digitorum longus tendon. Make a fourth incision 3 cm long on the dorsum of the foot in the region of the middle cuneiform. Incise the periosteum of the middle cuneiform and expose the central portion of the bone. Drill a hole 5 to 8 mm to insert the tendon through the middle of the cuneiform. Pass a Kelly clamp subcutaneously from the third incision to the fourth incision distally to create a subcutaneous tract for the posterior tibialis tendon. Pull the tendon through the subcutaneous tract with a tendon passer. Holding on to the sutures tied to the end of the posterior tibialis tendon, pass the tendon into the hole in the middle cuneiform and pass the sutures through the dorsum of the foot with the aid of straight needles. Release the tourniquet. Inspect, irrigate, and close the wounds. After the wounds have been closed tie the suture over a felt pad and button on the plantar aspect on

the foot with the foot in a neutral position (Fig. 32-11, *C*). Apply a long leg cast with the knee extended and the ankle in neutral position.

AFTERTREATMENT. Standing and walking are allowed 24 to 48 hours after surgery. A long leg cast is worn for 4 to 6 weeks, and a knee-ankle-foot orthosis is worn permanently.

◆ Transfer of Posterior Tibialis Tendon to Dorsum of Base of Second Metatarsal

In a personal communication Mubarak described transfer of the posterior tibialis tendon to the dorsum of the base of the second metatarsal. Mubarak prefers this technique to that of Greene because more distal placement of the posterior tibialis tendon increases the lever arm in dorsiflexion of the ankle, and the technique allows easier plantar flexion and dorsiflexion balancing of the ankle at the time of surgery.

TECHNIQUE 32-5 *(Mubarak)* (Fig. 32-12)

With the patient supine and a tourniquet in place, make a 3-cm incision over the insertion of the posterior tibialis tendon on the navicular. Open the sheath of the posterior tibialis tendon from the anterior aspect of the medial malleolus to the navicular. Release the tendon from the bony insertions, preserving as much length as possible. Make a second incision in the posteromedial calf in the region of the myotendinous junction of the posterior tibialis tendon. A

continued

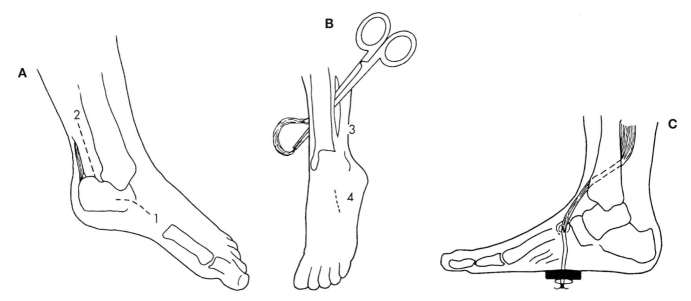

Fig. 32-11   Posterior tibialis tendon transfer. **A,** First and second incisions. **B,** Third and fourth incisions and clamp placement for pulling posterior tibialis tendon from posterior to anterior compartment of leg. **C,** Position of transplanted tendon and suture tied over felt pad and button on plantar aspect of foot. (From Greene WB: *Foot Ankle* 13:526, 1992.)

Fig. 32-12 **A,** Posterior tibialis tendon removed from insertion. Length can be effectively doubled by splitting at myotendinous junction to cut end. Secure midpoint at lengthened tendon with suture. **B,** Lengthened tendon is passed through hole in interosseous membrane (posterior to anterior) and subcutaneously across anterior aspect of ankle. **C,** Lengthened tendon is pulled subcutaneously across dorsum of midfoot, looped around base of second metatarsal, and sutured to itself with enough tension to hold ankle in neutral.

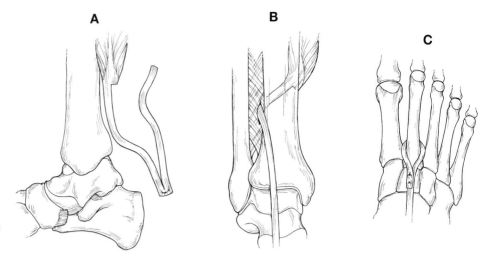

gastrocnemius recession can be performed through this incision if necessary, but excessive lengthening of the triceps surae complex should be avoided to prevent the development of a crouched gait postoperatively. Open the posterior tibial tendon sheath and pull the tendon through the sheath into the calf wound. At the myotendinous junction of the tibialis posterior, incise the tendon transversely halfway through its width. Extend this incision distally to within 0.5 cm of the cut insertion of the tibialis tendon. Secure the distal aspect of the tendon with a single suture to prevent the longitudinal cut from extending out to the end of the tendon. This procedure effectively doubles the length of the posterior tibialis tendon (Fig. 32-12, *A*). Make a third incision, 6 cm long lateral to the anterior crest of the tibia, extending it to the superior extensor retinaculum. Perform an anterior compartment fasciotomy and retract the tibialis anterior tendon laterally. Incise the interosseous membrane of the lateral aspect of the tibia for a distance of 3 cm. Take a Kelly clamp and place it through the anterior compartment wound across the interosseous membrane and into the deep posterior compartment. Grasp the end of the lengthened posterior tibialis tendon and bring it through the interosseous membrane into the anterior compartment of the calf (Fig. 32-12, *B*). Make another incision, 2 to 3 cm long, over the base of the second metatarsal. Dissect down to the base of the second metatarsal and subperiosteally dissect around the base of the second metatarsal circumferentially. Take the elongated tibialis posterior tendon and tunnel it subcutaneously into the incision over the dorsum of the second metatarsal. Loop the tendon around the base of the second metatarsal as a sling and tie it to itself with the appropriate tension on the ankle to hold it into a neutral plantar flexion and dorsiflexion (Fig. 32-12, *C*). Release the

tourniquet and inspect the tibial vessels to make sure that they are not being kinked by the transferred tendon. Irrigate the wounds and close them in a standard fashion.

AFTERTREATMENT. Aftertreatment is the same as for transfer of the posterior tibialis tendon to the dorsum of the foot (p. 1371).

◆ ◆ ◆

Equinus contractures can be corrected by a percutaneous tendo calcaneus lengthening or an open tendo calcaneus lengthening (see Chapter 30).

Although release of contractures usually allows another 2 to 3 years of ambulation, by the age of 12 to 13 years most children with Duchenne muscular dystrophy can no longer walk, and spinal deformity becomes the primary problem. Scoliosis affects almost all children with Duchenne muscular dystrophy, and the curve usually is progressive (Fig. 32-13). Scoliosis produces pelvic obliquity, which makes sitting increasingly difficult. Bracing and wheelchair spinal-support systems may slow progression of the curve somewhat, but spinal fusion ultimately is required for most patients.

Once a patient becomes nonambulatory the scoliosis almost invariably worsens and significant kyphosis develops. Many authors recommend spinal arthrodesis at the onset of scoliosis when the curve is only 10 to 20 degrees. Given the natural history of the condition, delaying surgery until the curve reaches 40 or 50 degrees has no advantage and can make surgery more complicated because of the worsening of cardiac and pulmonary function during the delay. Most authors recommend that the forced vital capacity of the lungs be 50% or more of normal to reduce pulmonary complications to an acceptable level. Cambridge and Drennan list forced

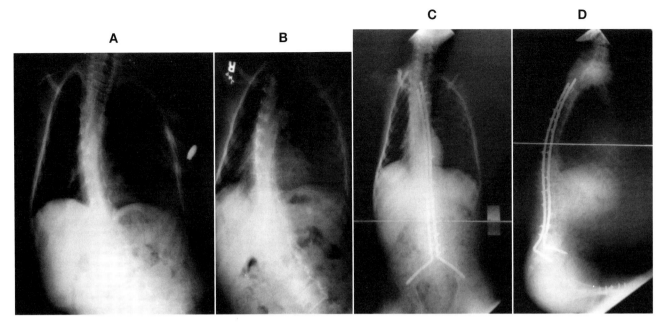

Fig. 32-13 **A** and **B,** Roentgenograms of patient with scoliosis. **C** and **D,** Postoperative roentgenograms after treatment with Luque-Galveston technique.

vital capacity of less than 35% as a relative contraindication to surgery and as evidence of significant cardiomyopathy. Surgery can still be done when vital capacity is less than 50%, but the risk of pulmonary and cardiac complications increases.

Posterior spinal fusion with segmental instrumentation is the operation of choice. The fusion of the entire thoracolumbar spine must extend to the proximal thoracic spine to prevent postoperative kyphosis above the fusion. Facet joint arthrodesis should be performed at every level, using autogenous or allograft bone graft as needed. Most authors have recommended that fusion extend to the pelvis, either with bone grafting alone or with extension of the rods into the ilium by the Galveston technique. Because of associated osteopenia of bone, the possibility of the rods cutting out of the pelvis is significant. Mubarak et al. reported satisfactory results with fusion to the fifth lumbar vertebra without extension of the fusion to the sacrum. Alman and Kim found that if the apex of the curve was below L1 and instrumentation and fusion were stopped short of the pelvis, progression of pelvic obliquity occurred. He recommended instrumentation and fusion to the pelvis if the apex of the curve was at or below L1.

OTHER VARIANTS OF MUSCULAR DYSTROPHY

Becker Muscular Dystrophy

Becker muscular dystrophy is a mild, slowly progressive form of sex-linked recessive muscular dystrophy that occurs in 1 in every 30,000 live male births. The affected gene in Becker muscular dystrophy is identical to that in Duchenne muscular dystrophy, but patients with Becker muscular dystrophy show some evidence of a functional intracellular dystrophin. The dystrophin in Becker muscular dystrophy, although present, is either altered in size or decreased in amount, or both. The severity of the disease is dependent on the amount of functional dystrophin in the muscles. Genetic studies and dystrophin testing now allow the clinician to better define severe forms of Becker muscular dystrophy. Serum creatine phosphokinase levels are highest before muscle weakness is clinically apparent and can be 10 to 20 times normal levels. Onset of symptoms usually occurs after the age of 7 years, and patients may live to their midforties or later. Cardiac involvement is much less frequent.

The orthopaedic treatment of Becker muscular dystrophy depends on the severity of the disease. In patients with large amounts of functional dystrophin, orthopaedic procedures frequently are not needed until after childhood, and in patients with more severe forms of the disease, treatment consideration is the same as for Duchenne muscular dystrophy. Contractures of the foot and overpull of the posterior tibialis muscle can be effectively treated with tendo calcaneus lengthening and posterior tibial tendon transfers with good long-term results. Patients rarely need soft tissue releases about the hip. Because scoliosis rarely occurs in patients with Becker muscular dystrophy, no definitive recommendations exist in the literature, and treatment must be individualized.

Emery-Dreifuss Muscular Dystrophy

Emery-Dreifuss muscular dystrophy is an X-linked recessive disorder, with the fully developed disease seen only in boys, although milder disease has been reported in girls. During the first few years of life, patients have muscle weakness, an awkward gait, and a tendency for toe-walking. The full syndrome, usually occurring in the second decade of life, is characterized by fixed equinus deformities of the ankles, flexion contractures of the elbows, extension contracture of the neck, and tightness of the lumbar paravertebral muscles. A significant factor in the diagnosis and treatment of Emery-Dreifuss muscular dystrophy is the presence of cardiac abnormalities, consisting of bradycardia and atrial ventricular conduction defects that can lead to complete heart block. It is important to recognize Emery-Dreifuss muscular dystrophy because of the cardiac abnormalities that initially are almost always asymptomatic but lead to a high incidence of sudden cardiac death, which may be averted by a cardiac pacemaker.

Orthopaedic treatment of Emery-Dreifuss muscular dystrophy involves release of the heel cord contractures, as well as other muscles about the foot. Successful results of release of elbow contractures have not been reported. Contractures about the neck and back should be treated conservatively with range of motion, although full range of motion should not be expected.

Limb-Girdle Dystrophy

Limb-girdle dystrophy is an autosomal recessive disorder, although an autosomal dominant pattern of inheritance has been reported in some families. The clinical characteristics are indistinguishable from those of Becker muscular dystrophy, but normal dystrophin is noted on laboratory examination. The disease may occur in the first to fourth decades of life; the later the onset, the more rapid the progression. Weakness may be in the muscles of either the shoulders or the pelvis (Fig. 32-14). Lower extremity weakness may involve the gluteus maximus, the iliopsoas, and the quadriceps. Upper extremity weakness may involve the trapezius, the serratus anterior, the rhomboids, the latissimus dorsi, and the pectoralis major. Some weakness may develop in the prime movers of the fingers and wrists as well. Surgery is seldom required in patients with limb-girdle dystrophy. Stabilization of the scapula to the ribs may be required for winging of the scapula, and in rare cases muscle transfers about the wrist may be needed.

Facioscapulohumeral Muscular Dystrophy

Facioscapulohumeral muscular dystrophy is an autosomal dominant condition with characteristic weakness of the facial and shoulder-girdle muscles (Fig. 32-15). The affected gene appears to be located on chromosome 4. Onset of the disease may be in early childhood, in which case the disease runs a rapid, progressive course, confining most children to a wheelchair by the age of 8 to 9 years; or onset may occur in patients from 15 to 35 years of age, in which case the disease progresses more slowly. The most striking clinical manifestation is facial weakness with an inability to whistle, purse the lips, wrinkle the brow, or blow out the cheeks. The greatest functional impairments are the inability to abduct and flex the arms at the

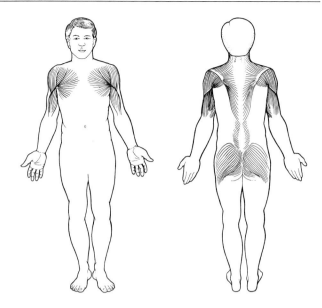

Fig. 32-14   Pattern of weakness in limb-girdle dystrophy. (Redrawn from Siegel IM: *Clinical management of muscle disease,* London, 1977, William Heinemann.)

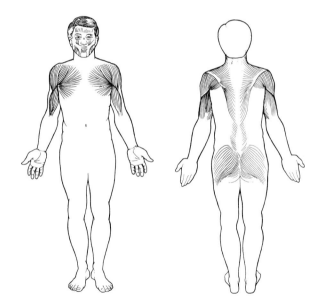

Fig. 32-15   Pattern of weakness in facioscapulohumeral dystrophy.

glenohumeral joints and winging of the scapula, both caused by progressive weakness of the muscles that fix the scapula to the thoracic wall, while the muscles that abduct the glenohumeral joint remain strong. As the disease progresses, weakness of the lower extremities, especially in the peroneal and the tibialis anterior muscles, results in a footdrop that requires the use of an ankle-foot orthosis. Sometimes a quadriceps muscle is involved, requiring expansion of the orthosis to a knee-ankle-foot orthosis. Scoliosis is rare, although extreme lumbar lordosis is common.

The inability to functionally flex and abduct the shoulder usually is treated by stabilization of the scapula, with scapulothoracic arthrodesis. Scapulothoracic fusion with strut grafts or with plates and screws as described by Letournel et al. provides a satisfactory fusion of the medial border of the scapula to the posterior thoracic ribs; however, it is associated with significant complications, including pneumothorax, pleural effusion, atelectasis, and pseudarthrosis. Jakab and Gledhill described a simplified technique for scapulocostal fusion in patients with facioscapulohumeral muscular dystrophy.

◆ Scapulothoracic Fusion

TECHNIQUE 32-6 *(Jakab and Gledhill)*
Place the patient prone and manually position the scapula at 15 to 20 degrees of external rotation. Make an oblique 12-inch incision over the medial border of the scapula and transect the trapezius muscle. Release the rhomboids and levator scapula from their scapular insertions and elevate the supraspinatus, infraspinatus, and subscapularis muscles subperiosteally for 2 cm from the medial border of the scapula. Excise a 2-cm strip of subscapularis muscles to allow approximation of the scapula to the thoracic wall. Usually ribs 3 through 7 are exposed subperiosteally for 2 cm. Pass double 16-gauge Luque wires subperiosteally under each rib. Use a sharp towel clip to make holes 1 cm from the medial ledge of the scapular points corresponding from the wired ribs (Fig. 32-16). Use a burr to decorticate the posterior surface of the exposed rib margins in the corresponding points along the anterior surface of the scapula. Place strips of cancellous allograft taken from the posterior iliac crest between the denuded ribs and scapula. Tighten the wires sequentially.

AFTERTREATMENT. A sling is worn for 3 to 4 days. Active abduction is possible 3 weeks after surgery without the need for physical therapy.

◆ ◆ ◆

Copeland et al. have described a similar fusion technique, but instead of using Luque wires, the scapula is stabilized to the fourth, fifth, and sixth ribs with screws. A shoulder spica is recommended for 1 month (Fig. 32-17).

Congenital Dystrophies
Congenital dystrophies include relatively rare conditions such as nemaline dystrophy, central core myopathy, myotubular myopathy, congenital fiber disproportion, and multicore and minicore disease. Congenital myopathies and congenital muscular dystrophies are defined by the histological appear-

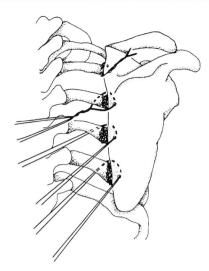

Fig. 32-16   Scapulocostal fusion (rib 7 also can be fused). (From Jakab E, Gledhill RB: *J Pediatr* 13:749, 1993.)

ance of the muscle biopsy rather than by specific clinical or molecular criteria. Electron microscopy may be needed to differentiate some of the types. Weakness and contractures at birth can cause hip dislocation, clubfeet, or other deformities. Respiratory weakness and difficulty with feeding and swallowing are common. The clinical appearance is one of dysmorphism, with kyphoscoliosis, chest deformities, a long face, and a high palate. Muscle tissue gradually is replaced with fibrous tissue, and contractures can become severe. Treatment is aimed at keeping the patient ambulatory and preventing contractures by exercises and orthotic splinting. Equinus and varus deformities of the feet may require releases if they interfere with ambulation. Congenital dislocation of the hip and clubfoot deformity are treated conventionally, but recurrence is frequent.

Myotonic Dystrophy
Myotonic dystrophy is characterized by an inability of the muscles to relax after contraction. It is progressive and usually is present at birth, although it may develop in childhood. Inheritance is most often autosomal dominant but may be autosomal recessive. In addition to the inability of the muscles to relax, muscle weakness causes the most functional impairment. Other defects include hyperostosis of the skull, frontal and temporal baldness, gonadal atrophy, dysphasia, dysarthria, electrocardiographic abnormalities, and mental retardation. The characteristic clinical appearance is a tent-shaped mouth, facial diplegia, and dull expression. About half of the children with myotonic dystrophy have clubfoot deformities, and hip dysplasia and scoliosis may exist. The hip dysplasia is treated conventionally but, because of capsular laxity, may not respond as readily as in other children. Serial casting can correct equinovarus deformity early on, but recurrence is likely and extensile release usually is required;

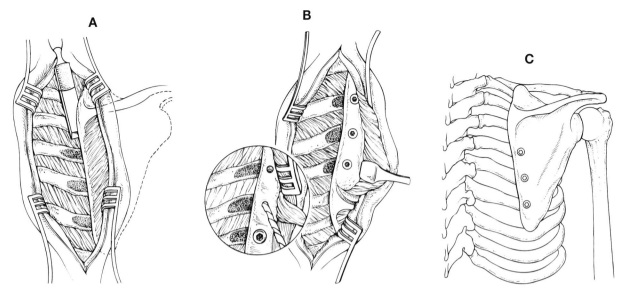

Fig. 32-17   Copeland technique. **A,** Decortication of ribs. **B** and **C,** Drilling and insertion of rib screws after application of cancellous bone graft. (Redrawn from Copeland SA, Levy O, Warner GC, Dodenhoff RM: *Clin Orthop* 368:80, 1999.)

triple arthrodesis may be required at skeletal maturity if recurrence is frequent despite extensile releases. In patients with marked clubfoot deformity, extensive posteromedial release may not be sufficient to correct the deformity, and a talectomy may be needed. An ankle-foot orthosis, which frequently is needed for weakness in dorsiflexion, usually can maintain postoperative correction. In some adolescent patients scoliosis develops and should be treated with the same principles as for the treatment of idiopathic scoliosis. The high incidence of cardiac abnormalities and decreased pulmonary function will increase the risk of surgery and may prohibit surgery in these patients.

Charcot-Marie-Tooth Disease (Peroneal Muscular Atrophy)

Charcot-Marie-Tooth disease is an inherited degenerative disorder of the central and peripheral nervous systems that causes muscle atrophy and loss of proprioception. It usually is an autosomal dominant trait but can be X-linked recessive or autosomal recessive. Muscle atrophy is steadily progressive in most patients with the autosomal dominant form; less often, the disease arrests completely or manifests intermittently. The recessive forms have an early onset (first or second decade) and are more rapidly progressive. Initial complaints usually are general weakness of the foot and an unsteady gait. Foot problems include pain under the metatarsal heads, claw toes, foot fatigue, and difficulty in wearing regular shoes. Distal loss of proprioception and spinal ataxia are common. Charcot-Marie-Tooth disease should be suspected in patients with claw toes, high arches, thin legs, poor balance, and an unsteady gait.

In addition to physical examination and family history, electromyograms, showing an increased amplitude in duration of response and slow nerve conduction velocity, typically confirm the diagnosis.

Advances in molecular biology have improved the ability to confirm the diagnosis of Charcot-Marie-Tooth disease and to differentiate between variants of the condition. A mutation of the connexin 32 gene has been found to be associated with the most common form of X-linked Charcot-Marie-Tooth disease (CMTX1). Type IA Charcot-Marie-Tooth disease (CMTIA), or hereditary neuropathy with liability to pressure palsies (HNPP), has been associated with a duplication or deletion of the peripheral myelin protein 22 gene (PMP22). This association has been found in 70% of patients with CMTIA. Southern blot analysis can now be performed in commercial laboratories to confirm the presence or absence of these genetic abnormalities. The use of molecular biology may allow orthopaedic surgeons to make more specific treatment recommendations for patients with the variants of Charcot-Marie-Tooth disease.

CAVOVARUS FOOT DEFORMITY

Charcot-Marie-Tooth disease is the most common neuromuscular cause of cavovarus foot deformity in children. This is a complex deformity of the forefoot and hindfoot. Surgery often is required to stabilize the foot. Although there is little question that the cavovarus deformity is caused by muscle imbalance, theories explaining which muscles are involved and how the imbalances produce the rigid cavovarus deformity do not completely account for the clinical deformity. The neuropathic cavovarus deformity of Charcot-Marie-Tooth disease has been suggested to be caused by a combination of intrinsic and extrinsic weakness, beginning with weakness of the intrinsic

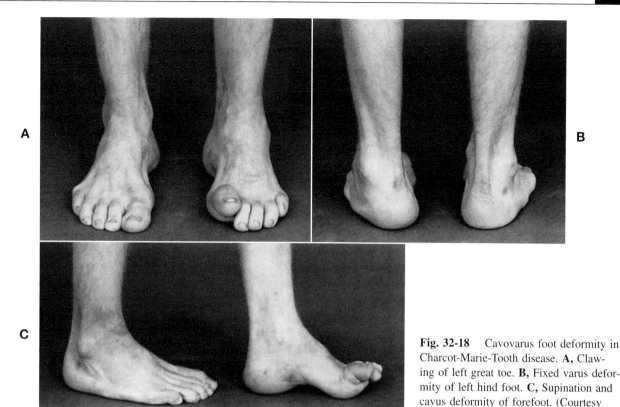

Fig. 32-18   Cavovarus foot deformity in Charcot-Marie-Tooth disease. **A,** Clawing of left great toe. **B,** Fixed varus deformity of left hind foot. **C,** Supination and cavus deformity of forefoot. (Courtesy Jay Cummings, MD.)

foot muscles and the tibialis anterior, with normal strength of the tibialis posterior and peroneus longus. The triceps surae also is weak and may be contracted. The forefoot is pulled into equinus relative to the hindfoot, and the first ray becomes plantarflexed. The long toe extensors attempt to assist the weak tibialis anterior in dorsiflexion but contribute to metatarsal plantar flexion, and the foot is pronated into a valgus position with mild adduction of the metatarsals. Initially the foot is supple and plantigrade with weight-bearing, but as the forefoot becomes more rigidly pronated, the hindfoot assumes a varus position. Weight-bearing becomes a "tripod" mechanism, with weight borne on the heel and the first and fifth metatarsal heads (Fig. 32-18).

Clinical and Roentgenographic Evaluation

Clinical evaluation of the cavovarus deformity includes determination of the rigidity of the hindfoot varus, usually with the block test of Coleman (Fig. 32-19), and assessment of individual muscle strength and overall balance. Careful examination of the peripheral and central nervous systems is required, including electromyography and nerve conduction velocity studies.

Standard anteroposterior, lateral, and oblique roentgenograms are the most useful methods for evaluating the child's foot; however, to determine any significant relationships between the bones, it is essential that the anteroposterior and lateral views be made with the foot in a weight-bearing or simulated weight-bearing position. Anteroposterior views

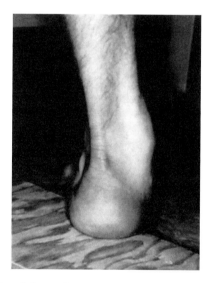

Fig. 32-19   Coleman block test shows flexible hindfoot. Heel placed on 1-inch block with plantarflexed forefoot on floor.

document the degree of forefoot adduction. The degree of cavus can be estimated on the lateral view by determining Meary's angle, the angle between the long axis of the first metatarsal and long axis of the talus; the normal angle is 0. Roentgenograms using the Coleman block test demonstrate the correction of the varus deformity if the hindfoot is flexible.

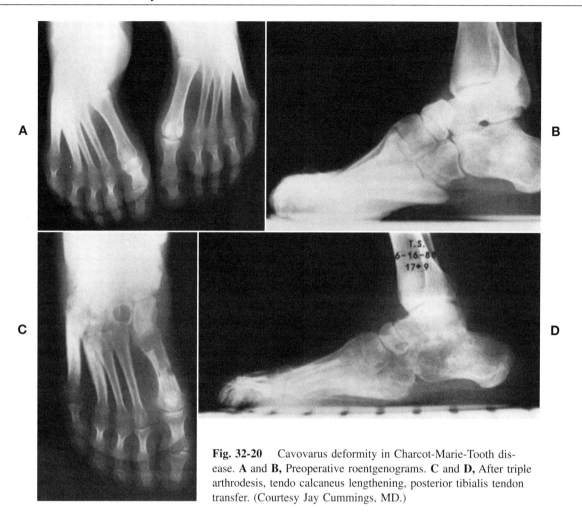

Fig. 32-20 Cavovarus deformity in Charcot-Marie-Tooth disease. **A** and **B,** Preoperative roentgenograms. **C** and **D,** After triple arthrodesis, tendo calcaneus lengthening, posterior tibialis tendon transfer. (Courtesy Jay Cummings, MD.)

Orthopaedic Treatment

Treatment is determined by the age of the patient and the cause and severity of the deformity. Nonoperative treatment of the cavovarus foot generally has been unsuccessful. Surgical procedures are of three types: soft tissue (plantar fascia release, tendon release or transfer), osteotomy (metatarsal, midfoot, calcaneal), and joint stabilizing (triple arthrodesis).

Experience in the treatment of foot deformities in Charcot-Marie-Tooth disease has demonstrated that early, aggressive treatment when the hindfoot is flexible and early soft tissue releases can delay the need for more extensive reconstructive procedures. Even in young patients with a fixed hindfoot deformity, limited soft tissue release, combined with a first metatarsal or calcaneal osteotomy, or both, can provide a satisfactory functional outcome without sacrificing the hindfoot and midfoot joint motion that is lost after triple arthrodesis. Because of early degenerative changes in the ankle, forefoot, and midfoot, triple arthrodesis should serve as a salvage procedure for patients in whom other procedures were unsuccessful or in patients with untreated fixed deformities (Fig. 32-20).

Children younger than 8 years of age with supple hindfeet usually respond to plantar releases and appropriate tendon transfers. Bradley and Coleman use a more extensive plantar medial release and osteotomy of the first metatarsal for rigid forefoot deformity. In children younger than 12 years of age with rigid hindfoot deformities, radical plantar-medial release, first metatarsal osteotomy, and a calcaneal osteotomy usually correct the deformity. In a fixed hindfoot with a prominent calcaneus, a Dwyer lateral closing wedge osteotomy may be preferred to shorten the heel (Technique 30-19). If the heel is not prominent, a sliding calcaneal osteotomy (Technique 30-22) gives satisfactory results.

Wukich and Bowen reported that only 14% of patients with Charcot-Marie-Tooth disease required triple arthrodesis (Chapter 79) and recommended soft tissue procedures and osteotomies in skeletally immature feet and those with less severe deformity. The Hoke arthrodesis or a modification of it is most often recommended. Appropriate wedge resections correct both the hindfoot varus and midfoot component of the cavus deformity; soft tissue release and muscle balancing are required for the forefoot deformity. In the most severe deformities, a Lambrinudi triple arthrodesis can produce a painless plantigrade foot. Wukich and Bowen recommend

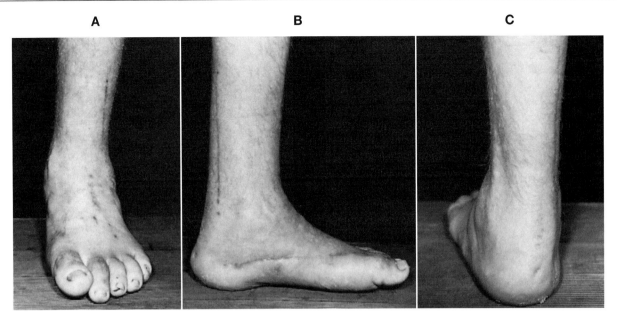

Fig. 32-21 Clinical appearance of foot in Fig. 32-20 after triple arthrodesis, tendo calcaneus lengthening, and posterior tibialis tendon transfer. **A,** Anterior view. **B,** Medial correction of cavus. **C,** Posterior correction of hindfoot varus. (Courtesy Jay Cummings, MD.)

restoring hindfoot stability with triple arthrodesis and transferring the posterior tibial tendon anteriorly to eliminate the need for a postoperative drop-foot brace. They reported good or excellent results in 88% of their patients treated with this method. McCluskey, Lovell, and Cummings recommended tendo calcaneus lengthening with triple arthrodesis after correction of the forefoot (Fig. 32-21).

Flexible clawtoe deformity usually is corrected without additional surgery when the midfoot deformity is corrected. For clawing in a young child without severe weakness of the anterior tibial muscle, the toe extensors can be transferred to the metatarsal necks with tenodesis of the interphalangeal joint of the great toe (Jones procedure). For adolescents or children with severe weakness of the anterior tibial muscle, all the long toe extensors can be transferred to the middle cuneiform with fusion of the interphalangeal joint (Hibbs procedure). For severe deformity, the posterior tibial tendon can be transferred anteriorly to the middle cuneiform instead of the long toe extensors (Technique 32-12).

Surgical procedures usually are staged. The initial procedure is a radical plantar or plantar-medial release, with a dorsal closing wedge osteotomy of the first metatarsal base if necessary. Tendo calcaneus lengthening should not be performed as part of the initial procedure because the force used to dorsiflex the forefoot would dorsiflex the calcaneus into an unacceptable position. If the hindfoot is flexible and a posterior release is not necessary, posterior tibial tendon transfer can be done as part of the initial procedure for severe anterior tibial weakness.

◆ Radical Plantar-Medial Release and Dorsal Closing Wedge Osteotomy

TECHNIQUE 32-7 *(Coleman)*

Make a curved incision over the medial aspect of the foot, extending anteriorly from the calcaneus to the base of the first metatarsal (Fig. 32-22, *A*). Identify the origin of the abductor hallucis and separate it from its bony and soft tissue attachments both proximally and distally, but leave it attached at its origin and insertion. Identify the posterior neurovascular bundle as it divides into medial and lateral branches and enters the intrinsic musculature of the foot. Identify the tendinous origin of the abductor at its attachment on the calcaneus between the medial and lateral plantar branches of the nerve and artery and sever it to free the origin of the abductor hallucis. Identify the long toe flexors as they course along the plantar aspect of the foot and section the retinaculum of the tendons. Sever the origins of the plantar aponeurosis, the abductor hallucis, and the short flexors from their attachments to the calcaneus (Fig. 32-22, *B*) and gently dissect this entire musculotendinous mass distally and extraperiosteally as far as the calcaneocuboid joint.

If the first metatarsal remains in plantar flexion after this release, make a dorsally based closing wedge osteotomy immediately distal to the physis, removing enough bone to correct the lateral talo–first metatarsal angle to 0. Fix the osteotomy with a smooth Steinmann pin or Kirschner wire.

continued

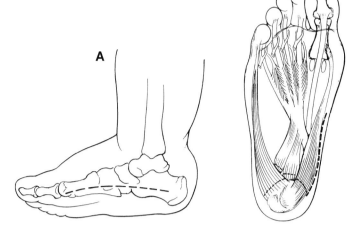

Fig. 32-22 Radical plantar-medial release and dorsal closing wedge osteotomy for cavovarus deformity. **A,** Incision. **B,** Release of musculotendinous mass. (Redrawn from Coleman SS: *Complex foot deformities in children,* Philadelphia, 1983, Lea & Febiger.)

Close the wound in routine fashion and apply a short leg cast with the foot in the corrected position.

AFTERTREATMENT. If there is excessive tension on the wound, the foot can be casted in slight plantar flexion. A new cast should be applied at 2 weeks with the foot in a fully corrected position. The pins and cast are removed at 6 to 8 weeks.

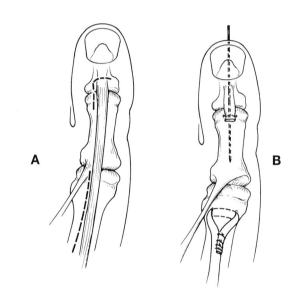

Fig. 32-23 Transfer of extensor hallucis longus tendon for claw toe deformity (Jones procedure). **A,** Incisions. **B,** Completed procedure.

◆ **Transfer of Extensor Hallucis Longus Tendon for Clawtoe Deformity**

TECHNIQUE 32-8 *(Jones)*
Expose the interphalangeal joint of the great toe through an L-shaped incision (Fig. 32-23). Retract the flap of skin and subcutaneous tissue medially and proximally and expose the tendon of the extensor hallucis longus. Cut the tendon transversely 1 cm proximal to the joint and expose the joint. Excise the cartilage, approximate the joint surfaces, and insert a 5/64-inch intramedullary Kirschner wire or screw for fixation. Clip the wire off just outside the skin. Now expose the neck of the first metatarsal through a 2.5-cm dorsomedial incision extending distally to the proximal extensor skin crease. Dissect free the extensor hallucis longus tendon but protect the short extensor tendon. Cleanly and carefully excise the sheath of the long extensor tendon throughout the length of the proximal incision. Beginning on the inferomedial aspect of the first metatarsal neck, drill a hole transverse to the long axis of the bone to emerge on the dorsolateral aspect of the neck. Now pass the tendon through the hole and suture it to itself with interrupted sutures. The same procedure can be performed on adjacent toes with clawing. Close the wounds and apply a short leg walking cast with the ankle in neutral position.

AFTERTREATMENT. Walking with crutches is allowed in 2 to 3 days. At 3 weeks the cast and skin sutures are removed and a short leg walking cast is applied. At 6 weeks the walking cast and Kirschner wire are removed, and active exercises are begun.

◆ **Transfer of Extensor Tendons to Middle Cuneiform**

TECHNIQUE 32-9 *(Hibbs)*
Make a curved incision 7.5 to 10 cm long on the dorsum of the foot lateral to the midline and expose the common extensor tendons (Fig. 32-24). Divide the tendons as far distally as feasible, draw their proximal ends through a tunnel in the third cuneiform, and fix them with a

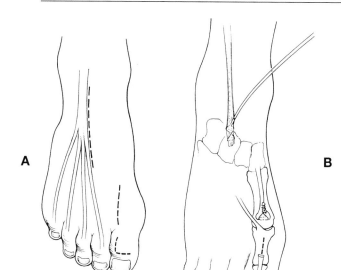

A

B

Fig. 32-24 Transfer of extensor tendons to middle cuneiform for claw toe deformity (Hibbs procedure). **A,** Incisions. **B,** Completed procedure combined with Jones procedure.

nonabsorbable suture. As an alternative, use a plantar button and felt with a Bunnell pull-out stitch. Close the wounds and apply a plaster boot cast with the foot in the corrected position.

AFTERTREATMENT. The cast and plantar button are removed at 6 weeks.

◆ ◆ ◆

In patients with advanced Charcot-Marie-Tooth disease, a triple arthrodesis may be necessary to establish a plantigrade foot; however, triple arthrodesis should not be routinely done in younger patients with less severe disease because degenerative changes of the ankle may result. In patients who have not had limited procedures during early adolescence but have major hindfoot, midfoot, and forefoot deformities, a triple arthrodesis may be the only treatment alternative. In severe deformity, a more extensive procedure, such as a Lambrinudi triple arthrodesis, can be performed. Techniques for triple arthrodesis are outlined in Chapter 31.

HIP DYSPLASIA

Acetabular dysplasia has been reported in patients with Charcot-Marie-Tooth disease. The treating physician should be aware of this association. If hip dysplasia is present, it should be corrected with pelvic and femoral osteotomies.

SPINAL DEFORMITIES

Scoliosis is uncommon in association with Charcot-Marie-Tooth disease, occurring in only approximately 10% of patients. The curve usually is mild to moderate and often does not require any treatment. In patients with Charcot-Marie-

Tooth disease, Hensinger and MacEwen reported associated kyphosis in half their patients with scoliosis. They reported that nonoperative treatment with a brace was well tolerated and successfully controlled the curve in many patients. Generally, spinal deformities in children with Charcot-Marie-Tooth disease can be managed by the same techniques used for idiopathic scoliosis.

CHARCOT-MARIE-TOOTH VARIANTS

Genetic analysis of patients with the autosomal dominant form of Charcot-Marie-Tooth disease demonstrates duplication of chromosome 17. A human peripheral myelin protein gene is contained within the duplication, and an abnormality in this gene encodes a myelin protein, which is the etiological basis for Charcot-Marie-Tooth disease.

Roussy-Lévy syndrome (hereditary areflexic dystaxia) is an autosomal dominant disease with the clinical characteristics of classic Charcot-Marie-Tooth disease plus a static tremor in the hands. The disease usually begins in infancy and is benign until adolescence. It is characterized by severe alterations in nerve conduction and sensory dysfunction.

Déjérine-Sottas syndrome (familial interstitial hypertrophic neuritis) usually is an autosomal recessive disease but may show an autosomal dominant inheritance with variable penetrance. The disease usually begins in infancy but may not appear until adolescence. Along with the classic pes cavus deformity, marked sensory loss occurs in all four extremities, and patients also may have clubfoot or kyphoscoliosis.

Refsum disease is an autosomal recessive disorder beginning in childhood or puberty in which the spinal fluid protein is increased. It is accompanied by retinitis pigmentosa and is characterized by a hypertrophic neuropathy with ataxia and areflexia. Distal sensory and motor loss occurs in the hands and feet. The course is unpredictable, with repeated reactivations and remissions, but the prognosis is poor.

Neuronal type Charcot-Marie-Tooth disease is an autosomal dominant disease with a usually late onset (middle age or later). The small muscles of the hands are not as weak as in other forms of the disease, but the ankle muscles and plantar muscles of the feet are much weaker and more atrophic.

Friedreich Ataxia

Friedreich ataxia is an autosomal recessive condition characterized by spinocerebellar degeneration. The prevalence of Friedreich ataxia is approximately 1 in 50,000. The abnormal gene is located on chromosome 9, but the definitive biochemical abnormality is not yet known. The variants and the wide phenotype in presentation suggests that the gene is affected through a variety of mutations. An ataxic gait usually is the presenting symptom, with onset routinely between 7 and 15 years of age. The diagnosis is suggested by the clinical triad of ataxia, areflexia, and a positive Babinski reflex. The disease is progressive, and almost all patients are wheelchair bound by the first or second decade of life. Patients typically demonstrate progressive dysarthria or weakness, decreased vibratory sense in the lower extremities, cardiomyopathy, pes cavus, and scoliosis. Knee jerk and ankle jerk reflexes are lost quite early. Patients usually die in the fourth or fifth decades of life as a result of progressive cardiomyopathy, pneumonia, and aspiration.

The primary concern of the orthopaedist is the correction of foot and spinal deformities. In patients with Friedreich ataxia, the plantar reflex sometimes is so great that when standing is attempted, the feet and toes immediately plantarflex and the tibialis posterior tendon pulls the forefoot into equinovarus. If general anesthesia is contraindicated because of myocardial involvement or other medical conditions, tenotomies of the tendo calcaneus, the tibialis posterior tendon at the ankle, and the toe flexors at the plantar side of the metatarsophalangeal joints can be done with the patient under local anesthesia. Surgery should be delayed in patients who are able to walk and who have deformities that are either supple or can be controlled in braces; however, the cavovarus deformities tend to worsen and become rigid. In patients with rigid cavovarus deformity, primary triple arthrodesis provides a solid base of support with a fixed plantigrade foot. Because most patients become wheelchair bound, later development of ankle and midfoot degenerative changes seldom is clinically significant. Tibialis posterior tenotomy lengthening or transfer should be combined with the triple arthrodesis. Bracing is routinely required after surgery.

Labelle et al., in a study of 56 patients with Friedreich ataxia and scoliosis, found that the curve patterns were similar to those of idiopathic scoliosis, many curves were not progressive, no relationship existed between muscle weakness and the curvature, and the onset of the scoliosis before puberty was the major factor in progression. However, as opposed to idiopathic scoliosis, kyphosis frequently was noted in patients with Freidreich ataxia. They recommended that curves of less than 40 degrees should be observed and curves of more than 60 degrees should be treated surgically; treatment of curves between 40 and 60 degrees is based primarily on the patient's age at onset of the disease, age at which the scoliosis was first recognized, and evidence of the curve's progression. Stabilization of the spine should be performed when the curve is greater than 40 to 50 degrees and the patient is no longer ambulatory. A single-stage posterior arthrodesis with segmental instrumentation is the treatment of choice (Chapter 38). The fusion should extend from the upper thoracic spine to the lower region of the lumbar spine.

Spinal Muscular Atrophy

Spinal muscular atrophy is an inherited degenerative disease of the anterior horn cells of the spinal cord that occurs in 1 in 20,000 births. It generally is transmitted by an autosomal recessive gene, but other hereditary patterns have been described. Hoffmann (1893) and Werdnig (1894) first described an infantile condition of generalized weakness that resulted in early death from respiratory failure, and in 1956 Kugelberg and Welander described a similar condition of juvenile onset that was less progressive in nature. In the acute infantile type (type I) severe generalized weakness manifests in patients younger than 6 months, and terminal respiratory failure occurs early. A chronic infantile type (type II) occurs during the middle of the first year and, after initial progression of weakness, may remain static for long periods. The juvenile type (type III) develops later, with gradual onset of weakness and a slowly progressive course. In patients with spinal muscular atrophy, blood creatine phosphokinase or aldolase is either normal or mildly elevated. Electromyography studies reveal muscle denervation. Nerve conduction velocities are normal. Genetic studies have demonstrated the defective gene to be located on chromosome 5. In 98% of patients with spinal muscular atrophy, deletions of either exon 7 or 8 have been identified in the survival motor neuron (SMN) gene. Advances in molecular biology have now made a test for this gene and its potential deletions commercially available. The three types of spinal muscular atrophy appear to result from different mutations of the same gene.

Clinical characteristics of spinal muscular atrophy include severe weakness and hypotonia, areflexia, fine tremor of the fingers, fasciculation of the tongue, and normal sensation. Proximal muscles are affected more than distal ones, and the lower extremities usually are weaker than the upper extremities. Evans, Drennan, and Russman proposed a functional classification to aid in planning long-term orthopaedic care: group I patients never develop the strength to sit independently and have poor head control; group II patients develop head control and can sit but are unable to walk; group III patients can pull themselves up and walk in a limited fashion, frequently with the use of orthoses; and group IV patients develop the ability to walk and run normally and to climb stairs before onset of the weakness.

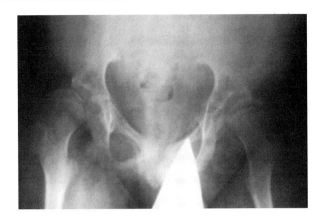

Fig. 32-25 Coxa valga deformity and subluxation in 12-year-old child with spinal muscular atrophy.

Orthopaedic treatment generally is required for hip and spine problems. Children with type I spinal muscular atrophy are markedly hypotonic and generally succumb to the disease early in life. In these patients, orthopaedic reconstruction is not warranted; however, patients with type I spinal muscular atrophy may develop fractures that heal quickly with appropriate splinting. Many children with infantile spinal muscular atrophy (Werdnig-Hoffmann disease) are never able to walk even with braces, but most patients with the juvenile form (Kugelberg-Welander disease) are able to walk for many years. Gentle passive range-of-motion exercises and positioning instructions can be beneficial initially. Surgical release of contractures rarely is required. Because of the absence of movement and weight-bearing, coxa valga deformity of the hip is frequent, and unilateral or bilateral hip subluxation may occur (Fig. 32-25). Since many of these children are sitters, a stable and comfortable sitting position is essential. In nonambulatory patients, proximal femoral varus derotational osteotomy (Technique 30-33) produces a more stable sitting base; this procedure is not indicated if the child is ambulatory. Valgus subtrochanteric osteotomy or distal transfer of the greater trochanter may be indicated for severe coxa vara deformity in ambulatory patients. Efforts should be made to maintain the reduction of the hips for good sitting balance and prevention of pain and pelvic obliquity, even if repeat procedures are necessary for recurrent coxa valga and hip subluxation.

Among children with spinal muscular atrophy who survive childhood, scoliosis becomes the greatest threat during adolescence. The prevalence of scoliosis is nearly 100% in children with type II spinal muscular atrophy and in children with type III muscular atrophy who become nonambulatory. It usually is progressive and severe and can limit daily function and cause cardiopulmonary problems. Bracing may be indicated during the growing years to slow curve progression, but spinal stabilization is ultimately required in almost all adolescent patients. Several authors have emphasized the importance of early surgery before the curve becomes severe and rigid. The treatment of choice is a long posterior fusion,

using segmental instrumentation. In some patients, these rods and the fusion are extended to the pelvis by means of the Galveston technique. Fusion generally should extend beyond that indicated for idiopathic scoliosis because curve progression above the level of the fusion is likely.

Intraoperative and postoperative complications are frequent in these patients, and thorough preoperative evaluation is mandatory. Hensinger and MacEwen and Piasecki et al. noted that the frequency of respiratory tract infections before surgery and the vital capacity of the lungs are good indicators of the patient's ability to tolerate surgery. Tracheostomy should be considered for any patient with frequent preoperative respiratory tract infections and a vital capacity of less than 35% of normal.

References

GENERAL
Allen BL Jr, Ferguson RL: The Galveston technique of pelvic fixation with L-rod instrumentation of the spine, *Spine* 9:388, 1984.

Bach JR: Letter to the editor, *J Bone Joint Surg* 77A:649, 1995.

Botte MJ, Keenan MAE, Abrams RA: Heterotopic ossification in neuromuscular disorders, *Orthopedics* 20:335, 1997.

Bleck EE: *Orthopaedic management of cerebral palsy,* Philadelphia, 1979, WB Saunders.

Brumsen C, Neveen A, Hamdy T, Papapoulos SE: Long-term effects of bisphosphonates on the growing skeleton, *Medicine* 76:266, 1997.

Clark MW: New developments in activity for young people with disabilities. Paper presented at Pediatric Orthopedic Society of North America, Boston, May 1986.

Crawford AH, Jucharzyk D, Roy DR, Bilbo J: Subtalar stabilization of the planovalgus foot by staple arthroereisis in young children who have neuromuscular problems, *J Bone Joint Surg* 72A:840, 1990.

DiLiberti JH, D'Agostino AN, Cole G: Needle muscle biopsy in infants and children, *J Pediatr* 103:566, 1983.

Drennan JC: *Orthopaedic management of neuromuscular disorders,* Philadelphia, 1983, JB Lippincott.

Drennan JC: Neuromuscular disorders. In Morrissy RT, ed: *Lovell and Winter's pediatric orthopaedics,* ed 3, vol 2, Philadelphia, 1990, JB Lippincott.

Gardner-Medwin D: Clinical features and classification of muscular dystrophies, *Br Med Bull* 36:109, 1980.

Glorieux FH, Bishop NJ, Plotkin H, et al: Cyclic administration of pamidronate in children with severe osteogenesis imperfecta, *N Engl J Med* 339:947, 1998.

Gower WR: Clinical lecture on pseudo-hypertrophic muscular paralysis, *Lancet* 2:1, 1879.

Green NE: The orthopaedic care of children with muscular dystrophy, *AAOS Instr Course Lect* 36:267, 1987.

Hageman G, Ippel EPF, Beemer FA, et al: The diagnostic management of newborns with congenital contractures: a nosologic study of 75 cases, *Am J Med Genet* 30:883, 1988.

Ingram AJ: Paralytic disorders. In Crenshaw AH, ed: *Campbell's operative orthopaedics,* ed 7, St Louis, 1987, Mosby.

Jablecki CK: Electromyography in infants and children, *J Child Neurol* 1:297, 1986.

Kim H, Wenger DR: Location of acetabular deficiency and associated hip dislocation in neuromuscular hip dysplasia: three-dimensional computed tomographic analysis, *J Pediatr Orthop* 17:143, 1997.

Koch SJ, Aergo DE, Bowser B: Outpatient rehabilitation for chronic neuromuscular diseases, *Am J Phys Med Rehabil* 65:245, 1986.

Kunkel LM: The Welcome lecture, 1988. Muscular dystrophy: a time of hope, *Proc R Soc Lond* 237:1, 1989.

Lonstein JE, Renshaw TS: Neuromuscular spine deformities, *Instr Course Lect* 36:285, 1987.

Louis DS, Hensinger RN, Fraser BA, et al: Surgical management of the severely multiply handicapped individual, *J Pediatr Orthop* 9:15, 1989.

Mubarak SJ, Chambers HG, Wenger DR: Percutaneous muscle biopsy in the diagnosis of neuromuscular disease, *J Pediatr Orthop* 12:191, 1992.

O'Neill DL, Harris SR: Developing goals and objectives for handicapped children, *Phys Ther* 62:295, 1982.

Rinsky LA, Gamble JG, Bleck EE: Segmental instrumentation without fusion in children with progressive scoliosis, *J Pediatr Orthop* 5:687, 1985.

Sage FP: Inheritable progressive neuromuscular diseases. In Crenshaw AH, ed: *Campbell's operative orthopaedics,* ed 7, St Louis, 1987, Mosby.

Sanchez AA, Rathjen KE, Mubarak SJ: Subtalar staple arthroereisis for planovalgus foot deformity in children with neuromuscular disease, *J Pediatr Orthop* 19:34, 1999.

Shapiro F, Bresnan MJ: Current concepts review: orthopaedic management of childhood neuromuscular disease. II. Diseases of muscle, *J Bone Joint Surg* 64A:1102, 1982.

Shapiro F, Specht L: Current concepts review: the diagnosis and orthopaedic treatment of childhood spinal muscular atrophy, peripheral neuropathy, Friedreich ataxia, and arthrogryposis, *J Bone Joint Surg* 75A:1699, 1993.

Shapiro F, Specht L: Current concepts review: the diagnosis and orthopaedic treatment of inherited muscular diseases of childhood, *J Bone Joint Surg* 75A:439, 1993.

Shaw NJ, White CP, Fraser WD, Rosenbloom L: Osteopenia in cerebral palsy, *Arch Dis Child* 71:235, 1994.

Siegel IM: *The clinical management of muscle disease: a practical manual of diagnosis and treatment,* London, 1977, William Heinemann.

Siegel IM: Diagnosis, management, and orthopaedic treatment of muscular dystrophy, *Instr Course Lect* 30:3, 1981.

Tachdjian MO: *Pediatric orthopedics,* ed 2, Philadelphia, 1990, WB Saunders.

Vedantam R, Capelli AM, Schoenecker PL: Subtalar arthroereisis for the correction of planovalgus foot in children with neuromuscular disorders, *J Pediatr Orthop* 18:294, 1998.

Yazici M, Ahser MA, Hardacker JW: The safety and efficacy of Isola-Galveston instrumentation and arthrodesis in the treatment of neuromuscular spinal deformities, *J Bone Joint Surg* 82A:524, 2000.

MUSCULAR DYSTROPHY—GENERAL

Bailey RO, Marzulo DC, Hans MB: Muscular dystrophy: infantile fascioscapulohumeral muscular dystrophy—new observations, *Acta Neurol Scand* 74:51, 1986.

Becker PE: Two new families of benign sex-linked recessive muscular dystrophy, *Rev Can Biol* 21:551, 1962.

Berman AT, Garbarino JL, Rosenberg H, et al: Muscle biopsy: proper surgical technique, *Clin Orthop* 198:240, 1985.

Bowen TR, Miller F, Mackenzie W: Comparison of oxygen consumption measurements in children with cerebral palsy to children with muscular dystrophy, *J Pediatr Orthop* 19:133, 1999.

Brown RH, Phil D: Dystrophy-associated proteins and the muscular dystrophies, *Annu Rev Med* 48:457, 1997.

Copeland SA, Levy O, Warner GC, Dodenhoff RM: The shoulder in patients with muscular dystrophy, *Clin Orthop* 368:80, 1999.

Gardner-Medwin D: Clinical features and classification of muscular dystrophies, *Br Med Bull* 36:109, 1980.

Green NE: The orthopaedic care of children with muscular dystrophy, *Instr Course Lect* 36:267, 1987.

Hsu JD, Hoffer MM: Posterior tibial tendon transfer anteriorly through the interosseous membrane, *Clin Orthop* 131:202, 1978.

Roy L, Gibson D: Pseudohypertrophic muscular dystrophy and its surgical management: review of 30 patients, *Can J Surg* 13:13, 1970.

Shapiro F, Bresnan MJ: Current concepts review: orthopaedic management of childhood neuromuscular disease. Part II. Diseases of muscle, *J Bone Joint Surg* 64A:1102, 1982.

Siegel IM: *The clinical management of muscle disease: a practical manual of diagnosis and treatment,* London, 1977, William Heinemann.

Siegel IM: Diagnosis, management, and orthopaedic treatment of muscular dystrophy. In American Academy of Orthopaedic Surgeons: *Instructional course lectures,* vol 30, St Louis, 1981, Mosby.

Spencer GE Jr: Orthopaedic considerations in the management of muscular dystrophy, *Curr Prac Orthop Surg* 5:279, 1973.

DUCHENNE MUSCULAR DYSTROPHY

Alman BA, Kim HKW: Pelvic obliquity after fusion of the spine in Duchenne muscular dystrophy, *J Bone Joint Surg* 81B:821, 1999.

Bleck EE: Mobility of patients with Duchenne muscular dystrophy (letter), *Dev Med Child Neurol* 21:823, 1979.

Bridwell KH, Baldus C, Iffrig TM, et al: Process measures and patient/parent evaluation of surgical management of spinal deformities in patients with progressive flaccid neuromuscular scoliosis (Duchenne's muscular dystrophy and spinal muscle atrophy), *Spine* 24:1300, 1999.

Brook PD, Kennedy JD, Stern LM, et al: Spinal fusion in Duchenne's muscular dystrophy, *J Pediatr Orthop* 16:324, 1996.

Brown JC: Muscular dystrophy, *Practitioner* 226:1031, 1982.

Brownell AKW, Paasuke RT, Elash A, et al: Malignant hyperthermia in Duchenne muscular dystrophy, *Anesthesiology* 58:180, 1983.

Cambridge W, Drennan JC: Scoliosis associated with Duchenne muscular dystrophy, *J Pediatr Orthop* 7:436, 1987.

Cooper RR: Skeletal muscle and muscle disorders. In Cruess RL, Rennie WRJ: *Adult orthopaedics,* vol 1, New York, 1984, Churchill Livingstone.

Crisp DE, Ziter FA, Bray PF: Diagnostic delay in Duchenne's muscular dystrophy, *JAMA* 247:478, 1982.

Douglas R, Larson PF, Ambrosia RD, et al: The LSU reciprocation-gait orthosis, *Orthopedics* 6:834, 1983.

Drennan JC, Bondurant M: Paralytic disorders. In American Academy of Orthopaedic Surgeons: *Atlas of orthotics,* ed 2, St Louis, 1985, Mosby.

Firth M, Gardner-Medwin D, Hoskin G, et al: Interviews with parents of boys suffering from Duchenne muscular dystrophy, *Dev Med Child Neurol* 25:466, 1983.

Fletcher R, Blennow G, Olsson AK et al: Malignant hyperthermia in a myopathic child: prolonged postoperative course requiring dantrolene, *Acta Anaesth Scand* 26:435, 1982.

Fowler WM Jr: Rehabilitation management of muscular dystrophy and related disorders. II. Comprehensive care, *Arch Phys Med Rehabil* 63:322, 1982.

Fowler WM Jr, Taylor M: Rehabilitation management of muscular dystrophy and related disorders. I. The role of exercise, *Arch Phys Med Rehabil* 63:319, 1982.

Galasko CSB, Delaney C, Morris P: Spinal stabilisation in Duchenne muscular dystrophy, *J Bone Joint Surg* 74B:210, 1992.

Gardner-Medwin D, Johnston HM: Severe muscular dystrophy in girls, *J Neurol Sci* 64:79, 1984.

Gibson DA, Koreska J, Robertson D, et al: The management of spinal deformity in Duchenne's muscular dystrophy, *Orthop Clin North Am* 9:437, 1978.

Goertzen M, Baltzer A, Voit T: Clinical results of early orthopaedic management in Duchenne muscular dystrophy, *Neuropediatrics* 26:257, 1995.

Granata C, Giannini S, Ballestrazzi L, Merlini L: Early surgery in Duchenne muscular dystrophy, *Neuromusc Disord* 4:87, 1994.

Green NE: The orthopaedic care of children with muscular dystrophy, *Instr Course Lect* 36:267, 1987.

Greene W: Transfer versus lengthening of the posterior tibial tendon in Duchenne's muscular dystrophy, *Foot Ankle* 13:526, 1992.

Hahn A, Bach JR, Delaubier A, Renardel-Irani A, et al: Clinical implications of maximal respiratory pressure determinations for individuals with Duchenne muscular dystropy, *Arch Phys Med Rehabil* 78:1:1997.

Hoffman EP, Kunkel LM: Dystrophin abnormalities in Duchenne/Becker muscular dystrophy, *Neuron* 2:1019, 1989.

Hoffman EP, Brown RH, Kunkel LM: Dystrophin: the protein product of Duchenne muscular dystrophy locus, *Cell* 51:919, 1987.

Hsu JD: Orthopedic approaches for the treatment of lower-extremity contractures in the Duchenne muscular dystrophy patient in the United States and Canada, *Semin Neurol* 15:6, 1995.

Hsu JD: The natural history of spine curvature progression in the nonambulatory Duchenne muscular dystrophy patient, *Spine* 8:771, 1983.

Hsu JD, Hsu CL: Motor unit disease. In Jahss MH, ed: *Disorders of the foot,* Philadelphia, 1982, WB Saunders.

Hsu JD, Lewis JE: Challenges in the care of the retarded child with Duchenne muscular dystrophy, *Orthop Clin North Am* 12:73, 1981.

Hsu JD, Hall VD, Swank S, et al: Control of spine curvature in the Duchenne muscular dystrophy (DMD) patient. In *Proceedings of the Scoliosis Research Society,* Denver, 1982, Scoliosis Research Society.

Kelfer HM, Singer WD, Reynolds RN: Malignant hyperthermia in a child with Duchenne muscular dystrophy, *Pediatrics* 71:118, 1983.

Kennedy JD, Staples AJ, Brook PD, et al: Effect of spinal surgery on lung function in Duchenne muscular dystrophy, *Thorax* 50:1173, 1995.

Kurz LT, Mubarak SJ, Schultz P, et al: Correlation of scoliosis and pulmonary function in Duchenne muscular dystrophy, *J Pediatr Orthop* 3:347, 1983.

Lane RJM, Robinow M, Roses AD: The genetic status of mothers of isolated cases of Duchenne muscular dystrophy, *J Med Genet* 20:1, 1983.

LaPrade RF, Rowe DE: The operative treatment of scoliosis in Duchenne muscular dystrophy, *Orthop Rev* 21:39, 1992.

Larson CM, Henderson RC: Bone mineral density and fractures in boys with Duchenne muscular dystrophy, *J Pediatr Orthop* 20:71, 2000.

Lutter LD, Carlson M, Winner RB, et al: Spine curvatures in progressive muscular dystrophy. Paper presented at the Annual Meeting of the Pediatric Orthopaedic Society, Vancouver, May 1984.

Manzur AY, Hyde SA, Rodillo E, et al: A randomized controlled trial of early surgery in Duchenne muscular dystrophy, *Neuromusc Disord* 2:379, 1992.

Marchesi D, Arlet V, Stricker U, Aebi M: Modification of the original Luque technique in the treatment of Duchenne's neuromuscular scoliosis, *J Pediatr Orthop* 17:743, 1997.

Marchildon MB: Malignant hyperthermia: current concepts, *Arch Surg* 117:349, 1982.

McDonald CM, Abresch RT, Carter GT, et al: Profiles of neuromuscular diseases. Duchenne muscular dystrophy, *Am J Phys Med Rehabil* 74 (suppl):S70, 1995.

Melkonian GJ, Cristofaro RL, Perry J, et al: Dynamic gait electromyography study in Duchenne muscular dystrophy (DMD) patients, *Foot Ankle* 1:78, 1980.

Mendell JR, Moxley RT, Griggs RC et al: Randomized, double-blind six-month trial of prednisone in Duchenne's muscular dystrophy, *N Engl J Med* 320:1592, 1989.

Miller RG, Chalmers AC, Dao H, et al: The effect of spine fusion on respiratory function in Duchenne muscular dystrophy, *Neurology* 41:38, 1991.

Miller F, Moseley CF, Koreska J: Spinal fusion in Duchenne muscular dystrophy, *Dev Med Child Neurol* 34:775, 1992.

Miller F, Moseley CF, Koreska J, Levison H: Pulmonary function and scoliosis in Duchenne dystrophy, *J Pediatr Orthop* 8:133, 1988.

Moser H: Duchenne muscular dystrophy: pathogenetic aspects and genetic prevention, *Hum Genet* 66:17, 1984.

Mubarak SJ et al: Correlating scoliosis and pulmonary function in Duchenne muscular dystrophy. Paper presented at the American Academy for Cerebral Palsy and Developmental Medicine Annual Meeting, Chicago, 1983.

Mubarak SJ, Morin WD, Leach J: Spinal fusion in Duchenne muscular dystrophy—fixation and fusion to the sacropelvis? *J Pediatr Orthop* 13:7562, 1993.

Ramirez N, Richards BS, Warren PD, Williams GR: Complications after posterior spinal fusion in Duchenne's muscular dystrophy, *J Pediatr Orthop* 17:109, 1997.

Renshaw TS: Treatment of Duchenne's muscular dystrophy, *JAMA* 248:922, 1982.

Rideau Y, Duport G, Delaubier A, et al: Early treatment to preserve quality of locomotion for children with Duchenne muscular dystrophy, *Semin Neurol* 15:9, 1995.

Rochelle J, Bowen JR, Ray S: Pediatric foot deformities in progressive neuromuscular disease, *Contemp Orthop* 8:41, 1984.

Seeger BR, Caudrey DJ, Little JD: Progression of equinus deformity in Duchenne muscular dystrophy, *Arch Phys Med Rehabil* 66:286, 1985.

Seeger BR, Sutherland AD, Clark MS: Orthotic management of scoliosis in Duchenne muscular dystrophy, *Arch Phys Med Rehabil* 65:83, 1984.

Shapiro F, Sethna N, Colan S, et al: Spinal fusion in Duchenne muscular dystrophy: a multidisciplinary approach, *Muscle Nerve* 15:604, 1992.

Siegel IM: Maintenance of ambulation in Duchenne muscular dystrophy: the role of the orthopedic surgeon, *Clin Pediatr* 19:383, 1980.

Smith AD, Koreska J, Moseley CF: Progression of scoliosis in Duchenne muscular dystrophy, *J Bone Joint Surg* 71A:1066, 1989.

Sussman MD: Advantage of early spinal stabilization and fusion in patients with Duchenne muscular dystrophy, *J Pediatr Orthop* 4:531, 1984.

Sutherland DH, Olshen R, Cooper L, et al: The pathomechanics of gait in Duchenne muscular dystrophy, *Dev Med Child Neurol* 23:3, 1981.

Swank SM, Brown JC, Perry RE: Spinal fusion in Duchenne's muscular dystrophy, *Spine* 7:484, 1982.

Vignos PJ, Wagner MB, Kaplan JS, et al: Predicting the success of reambulation in patients with Duchenne muscular dystrophy, *J Bone Joint Surg* 65A:719, 1983.

Vignos PJ, Wagner MB, Karlinchak B, Katirji B: Evaluation of a program for long-term treatment of Duchenne muscular dystrophy, *J Bone Joint Surg* 78A:1844, 1996.

Weimann RL, Gibson DA, Moseley CF, et al: Surgical stabilization of the spine in Duchenne muscular dystrophy, *Spine* 8:776, 1983.

Yasuma F, Sakai M: Scoliosis in Duchenne muscular dystrophy, *Respiration* 66:463, 1999.

BECKER MUSCULAR DYSTROPHY

Becker PE, Kiener F: Eine neue x-chromosomale Muskeldystrophie, *Arch Psychiatr Nervenkr* 193:427, 1955.

Emery AEH, Skinner R: Clinical studies in benign (Becker type) X-linked muscular dystrophy, *Clin Genet* 10:189, 1976.

Fowler WM Jr: Rehabilitation management of muscular dystrophy and related disorders. II. Comprehensive care, *Arch Phys Med Rehabil* 63:322, 1982.

Grimm T: Genetic counseling in Becker type X-linked muscular dystrophy. I. Theoretical considerations, *Am J Med Genet* 18:713, 1984.

Grimm T: Genetic counseling in Becker type X-linked muscular dystrophy. II. Practical considerations, *Am J Med Genet* 18:719, 1984.

Herrmann FH, Spiegler AWJ: Carrier detection in X-linked Becker muscular dystrophy by muscle provocation test (MPT), *J Neurol Sci* 62:141, 1983.

Khan RH, MacNicol MF: Bilateral patellar subluxation secondary to Becker muscular dystrophy: a case report, *J Bone Joint Surg* 64A: 777, 1982.

Kloster R: Benign X-linked muscular dystrophy (Becker type): a kindred with very slow rate of progression, *Acta Neurol Scand* 68:344, 1983.

McDonald CM, Abresch RT, Carter GT, et al: Profiles of neuromuscular diseases. Becker's muscular dystrophy, *Am J Phys Med Rehabil* 74 (suppl):S93, 1995.

LIMB-GIRDLE DYSTROPHY

Fowler WM Jr: Rehabilitation management of muscular dystrophy and related disorders. II. Comprehensive care, *Arch Phys Med Rehabil* 63:322, 1982.

Fowler WM Jr, Nayak NN: Slowly progressive proximal weakness: limb-girdle syndromes, *Arch Phys Med Rehabil* 64:527, 1983.

McDonald CM, Johnson ER, Abresch RT, et al: Profiles of neuromuscular diseases: limb-girdle syndromes, *Am J Phys Med Rehabil* 74(suppl): S117, 1995.

EMERY-DREIFUSS MUSCULAR DYSTROPHY

Morrison P, Jago RH: Emery-Dreifuss muscular dystrophy, *Anesthesia* 46:33, 1991.

Shapiro F, Specht L: Orthopedic deformities in Emery-Dreifuss muscular dystrophy, *J Pediatr Orthop* 11:336, 1991.

Zacharias AS, Wagener ME, Warren ST, Hopkins LC: Emery-Dreifuss muscular dystrophy, *Semin Neurol* 19:67, 1999.

FACIOSCAPULOHUMERAL DYSTROPHY

Fowler WM Jr: Rehabilitation management of muscular dystrophy, and related disorders. II. Comprehensive care, *Arch Phys Med Rehabil* 63:322, 1982.

Jakab E, Gledhill RB: Simplified technique for scapulocostal fusion in the facioscapulohumeral dystrophy, *J Pediatr Orthop* 13:749, 1993.

Kocialkowski A, Frostick SP, Wallace WA: One-stage bilateral thoracoscapular fusion using allografts, *Clin Orthop* 273:264, 1991.

Letournel E, Fardeau M, Lyltle JO, et al: Scapulothoracic arthrodesis for patients who have facioscapulohumeral muscular dystrophy, *J Bone Joint Surg* 72A:78, 1990.

McGarry J, Garg B, Silbert S: Death in childhood due to facioscapulohumeral dystrophy, *Acta Neurol Scand* 68:61, 1983.

Padberg G, Erikson AW, Volkers WS, et al: Linkage studies in autosomal dominant facioscapulohumeral muscular dystrophy, *J Neurol Sci* 65:261, 1984.

Shapiro F, Specht L, Korf BR: Locomotor problems in infantile facioscapulohumeral muscular dystrophy, *Acta Orthop Scand* 62:367, 1991.

CONGENITAL DYSTROPHY

Cornelio F, Di Donato S: Myopathies due to enzyme deficiencies, *J Neurol* 232:329, 1985.

Cunliffe M, Burrows FA: Anaesthetic implications of nemaline rod myopathy, *Can Anaesth Soc J* 32:543, 1985.

Eeg-Olofsson O, Henriksson KG, Thornell LE, et al: Early infant death in nemaline (rod) myopathy, *Brain Dev* 5:53, 1983.

Fowler WM Jr: Rehabilitation management of muscular dystrophy and related disorders. II. Comprehensive care, *Arch Phys Med Rehabil* 63:322, 1982.

Jones R, Kahn R, Hughes, S, et al: Congenital muscular dystrophy: the importance of early diagnosis and orthopaedic management in the long-term prognosis, *J Bone Joint Surg* 61B:13, 1979.

McMenamin JB, Becker LE, Murphy EG: Congenital muscular dystrophy: a clinicopathologic report of 24 cases, *J Pediatr* 100:692, 1982.

McMenamin JB, Becker LE, Murphy EG: Fukuyama-type congenital muscular dystrophy, *J Pediatr* 100:580, 1982.

MYOTONIC DYSTROPHY

Begin R, Bureau MA, Lupien L, et al: Pathogenesis of respiratory insufficiency in myotonic dystrophy: the mechanical factors, *Am Rev Respir Dis* 125:312, 1982.

Hawley RJ, Gottdiener JS, Gay JA, et al: Families with myotonic dystrophy with and without cardiac involvement, *Arch Intern Med* 143:2134, 1983.

Johnson ER, Abresch RT, Carter GT, et al: Profiles of neuromuscular diseases. Myotonic dystrophy, *Am J Phys Med Rehabil* 74(suppl):104, 1995.

O'Brien TA, Harper PS: Course, prognosis and complications of childhood-onset myotonic dystrophy, *Dev Med Child Neurol* 26:62, 1984.

Ray S, Bowen JR, Marks HG: Foot deformity in myotonic dystrophy, *Foot Ankle* 5:125, 1984.

CHARCOT-MARIE-TOOTH DISEASE

Aktas S, Sussman MD: The radiological analysis of pes cavus deformity in Charcot Marie Tooth disease, *J Pediatr Orthop* 9:137, 2000.

Alexander IJ, Johnson KA: Assessment and management of pes cavus in Charcot-Marie-Tooth disease, *Clin Orthop* 246:273, 1989.

Bradley GW, Coleman SS: Treatment of the calcaneocavus foot deformity, *J Bone Joint Surg* 63A:1159, 1981.

Charcot JM, Marie P: Sur une forme particuliere d'atrophie musculaire souvent familiale debutant par les pied et les jambes et atteignant plus tard les mains, *Rev Med* p 96, 1886.

Coleman SS: *Complex foot deformities in children,* Philadelphia, 1983, Lea & Febiger.

Coleman SS, Chestnut WJ: A simple test for hind foot flexibility in the cavovarus foot, *Clin Orthop* 123:60, 1977.

Daher YH, Lonstein JE, Winter RB, et al: Spinal deformities in patients with Charcot-Marie-Tooth disease: a review of 21 patients, *Clin Orthop* 202:219, 1986.

Dejerine J, Sottas J: Sur la neurite interstitielle hypertrophique et progressive de l'enfance, *CR Soc Biol* 45:63, 1893.

Fuller JE, DeLuca PA: Acetabular dysplasia and Charcot-Marie-Tooth disease in a family, *J Bone Joint Surg* 77A:1087, 1995.

Dwyer FC: The treatment of relapsed club foot by the insertion of a wedge into the calcaneum, *J Bone Joint Surg* 45B:67, 1963.

Gould N: Surgery in advanced Charcot-Marie-Tooth disease, *Foot Ankle* 4:267, 1984.

Hensinger RN, MacEwen GD: Spinal deformity associated with heritable neurologic conditions: spinal muscular atrophy, Friedreich's ataxia, familial dysautonomia, and Charcot-Marie-Tooth disease, *J Bone Joint Surg* 58A:13, 1978.

Hibbs RA: An operation for "claw-foot," *JAMA* 73:1583, 1919.

Jones R: The soldier's foot and the treatment of common deformities of the foot. II. Claw-foot, *Br Med J* 1:749, 1916.

Kirkpatrick JS, Goldner JL, Goldner RD: Revision arthrodesis for tibiotalar pseudarthrosis with fibular onlay-inlay graft and internal screw fixation, *Clin Orthop* 268:29, 1991.

Kumar SJ, Marks HG, Bowen JR, et al: Hip dysplasia associated with Charcot-Marie-Tooth disease in the older child and adolescent, *J Pediatr Orthop* 5:511, 1985.

Lorenzetti D, Pareyson D, Sghirlanzoni A, et al: A 1.5-Mb deletion in 17p11.2-p12 is frequently observed in Italian families with hereditary neuropathy with liability to pressure palsies, *Am J Hum Genet* 56:91, 1995.

Lupski JR, Chance PF, Garcia CA: Inherited primary peripheral neuropathies: molecular genetics and clinical implications of CMT1A and HNPP, *JAMA* 270:2326, 1993.

Lupski JR, de-Oca-Luna RM, Slaugenhaupt S, et al: DNA duplication associated with Charcot-Marie-Tooth disease type 1A, *Cell* 66:219, 1991.

Mann RA, Missirian J: Pathophysiology of Charcot-Marie-Tooth disease, *Clin Orthop* 234:221, 1988.

McCluskey WP, Lovell WW, Cummings RJ: The cavovarus foot deformity: etiology and management, *Clin Orthop* 247:27, 1989.

Medhat MA, Krantz H: Neuropathic ankle joint in Charcot-Marie-Tooth disease after triple arthrodesis of the foot, *Orthop Rev* 17:873, 1988.

Miller GM, Hsu JD, Hoffer MM, et al: Posterior tibial tendon transfer: a review of the literature and analysis of 74 procedures, *J Pediatr Orthop* 2:363, 1982.

Patel PI, Roa BB, Welcher AA, et al: The gene for the peripheral myelin protein PMP-22 is a candidate for Charcot-Marie-Tooth disease type 1A, *Nat Genet* 1:159, 1992.

Paulos L, Coleman SS, Samuelson KM: Pes cavovarus: review of a surgical approach using selective soft-tissue procedures, *J Bone Joint Surg* 62A:942, 1980.

Refsum S: Heredopathia atactica polyneuritiformis: a familial syndrome not hitherto described, *Acta Psych Neurol Suppl* 38:1, 1946.

Roa BB, Garcia CA, Suter U, et al: Charcot-Marie-Tooth disease type 1A: association with a spontaneous point mutation in the PMP22 gene, *N Engl J Med* 329:96, 1993.

Rochelle J, Bowen JR, Ray S: Pediatric foot deformities in progressive neuromuscular disease, *Contemp Orthop* 8:41, 1984.

Roussy G, Levy G: Sept case d'une maladie familiale particuliere: troubles de la marche, pieds, bots et areflexie tendineuse generalisee, avec accesoirement, *Rev Neurol* 54:427, 1926.

Sabir M, Lyttle D: Pathogenesis of Charcot-Marie-Tooth disease: gait analysis and electrophysiologic, genetic, histopathologic, and enzyme studies in a kinship, *Clin Orthop* 184:223, 1984.

Samilson RL, Dillin W: Cavus, cavovarus, and calcaneocavus: an update, *Clin Orthop* 177:125, 1983.

Sherman FC, Westin GW: Plantar release in the correction of deformities of the foot in childhood, *J Bone Joint Surg* 63A:1382, 1981.

Siffert RS, del Torto U: "Beak" triple arthrodesis for severe cavus deformity, *Clin Orthop* 181:64, 1983.

Steindler A: Stripping of the os calcis, *J Orthop Surg* 2:8, 1920.

Timmerman V, Nellis E, Van Hul W, et al: The peripheral myelin protein gene PMP-22 is contained within the Charcot-Marie-Tooth disease type 1A duplications, *Nat Genet* 1:171, 1992

Tooth HH: *The peroneal type of progressive muscular atrophy,* London, 1886, HK Lewis.

Valentijn LJ, Bolhuis PA, Zorn A, et al: The peripheral myelin gene PMP-22/GAS-3 is duplicated in Charcot-Marie-Tooth disease type IA, *Nat Genet* 1:166, 1992

Wetmore RS, Drennan JC: Long-term results of triple arthrodesis in Charcot-Marie-Tooth disease, *J Bone Joint Surg* 71A:417, 1989.

Wukich DK, Bowen JR: A long-term study of triple arthrodesis for correction of pes cavovarus in Charcot-Marie-Tooth disease, *J Pediatr Orthop* 9:433, 1989.

FRIEDREICH ATAXIA

Cady RB, Bobechko WP: Incidence, natural history, and treatment of scoliosis in Friedreich's ataxia, *J Pediatr Orthop* 4:673, 1984.

Hensinger RN, MacEwen GD: Spinal deformity associated with heritable neurologic conditions: spinal muscular atrophy, Friedreich's ataxia, familial dysautonomia, and Charcot-Marie-Tooth disease, *J Bone Joint Surg* 58A:13, 1978.

Labelle H, Thome S, Duhaime M et al: Natural history of scoliosis in Friedreich's ataxia, *J Bone Joint Surg* 68A:564, 1986.

Levitt RL, Canale ST, Cooke AJ, et al: The role of foot surgery in progressive neuromuscular disorders in children, *J Bone Joint Surg* 55A:1396, 1973.

Paulos L, Coleman SS, Samuelson KM: Pes cavovarus: review of a surgical approach using selective soft-tissue procedures, *J Bone Joint Surg* 62A:942, 1980.

Rochelle J, Bowen JR, Ray S: Pediatric foot deformities in progressive neuromuscular disease, *Contemp Orthop* 8:41, 1984.

Rothschild H, Shoji H, McCormick D: Heel deformity in hereditary spastic paraplegia, *Clin Orthop* 160:48, 1981.

Shapiro F, Bresnan MJ: Current concepts review: orthopaedic management of childhood neuromuscular disease. II. Peripheral neuropathies, Friedreich's ataxia, and arthrogryposis multiplex congenita, *J Bone Joint Surg* 64A:949, 1982.

Tynan MC, Klenerman L, Helliwell MA, et al: Investigation of muscle imbalance in the leg in symptomatic forefoot pes cavus: a multidisciplinary study, *Foot Ankle* 13:489, 1992.

SPINAL MUSCULAR ATROPHY

Aprin H, Bowen JR, MacEwen GD: Spine fusion in patients with spinal muscular atrophy, *J Bone Joint Surg* 64A:1179, 1982.

Bell DF, Moseley CF, Koreska J: Unit rod segmental spinal instrumentation in the management of patients with progressive neuromuscular spinal deformity, *Spine* 14:1301, 1989.

Daher YH, Lonstein JE, Winter RB, et al: Spinal surgery in spinal muscular atrophy, *J Pediatr Orthop* 5:391, 1985.

Drennan JC: Skeletal deformities in spinal muscular atrophy. In Abstracts of Association of Bone and Joint Surgeons, *Clin Orthop* 133:266, 1978.

Evans GA, Drennan JC, Russman BS: Functional classification and orthopaedic management of spinal muscular atrophy, *J Bone Joint Surg* 63B:516, 1981.

Ferguson RL, Allen BL: Segmental spinal instrumentation for routine scoliotic curve, *Contemp Orthop* 2:450, 1980.

Granata C, Merlini L, Magni E, et al: Spinal muscular atrophy: natural history and orthopaedic treatment of scoliosis, *Spine* 14:760, 1989.

Hahnen E, Forkert R, Marke C, et al: Molecular analysis of candidate genes on chromosome 5q13 in autosomal recessive spinal muscular atrophy: evidence of homozygous deletions of SMN gene in unaffected individuals, *Hum Mol Genet* 4:1927, 1995.

Hensinger RN, MacEwen GD: Spinal deformity associated with heritable neurological conditions: spinal muscular atrophy, Friedreich's ataxia, familial dysautonomia, and Charcot-Marie-Tooth disease, *J Bone Joint Surg* 58A:13, 1976.

Hoffmann J: Ueber chronische spinale Muskelatrophie im Kindersalter, auf familiarer Basis, *Dtsch Z Nervenheulkd* 3:427, 1893.

Hsu JD, Grollman T, Hoffer M, et al: The orthopaedic management of spinal muscular atrophy, *J Bone Joint Surg* 55B:663, 1973.

Kugelberg E, Welander L: Heredofamilial juvenile muscular atrophy simulating muscular dystrophy, *Arch Neurol Psychiatry* 75:500, 1956.

Lefebvre S, Burglen L, Reboullet S, et al: Identification and characterization of a spinal muscular atrophy–determining gene, *Cell* 80:155, 1995.

Merlini L, Granata C, Bonfiglioli S, et al: Scoliosis in spinal muscular atrophy: natural history and management, *Dev Med Child Neurol* 31:501, 1989.

Phillips DP, Roye DP, Farcy JPC, et al: Surgical treatment of scoliosis in a spinal muscular atrophy population, *Spine* 15:942, 1990.

Piasecki JO, Mahinpour S, Levine DB: Long-term follow-up of spinal fusion in spinal muscular atrophy, *Clin Orthop* 207:44, 1986.

Shapiro F, Bresnan MJ: Current concepts review: orthopaedic management of childhood neuromuscular disease. I. Spinal muscular atrophy, *J Bone Joint Surg* 64A:785, 1982.

van der Steege G, Grootscholten PM, van der Vlies P, et al: PCR-based DNA test to confirm clinical diagnosis of autosomal recessive spinal muscular atrophy, *Lancet* 345:985, 1995.

Werdnig G: Die frühinfantile progressive spinale Amyotrophie, *Arch Psychiatr Nervenkr* 26:706, 1894.

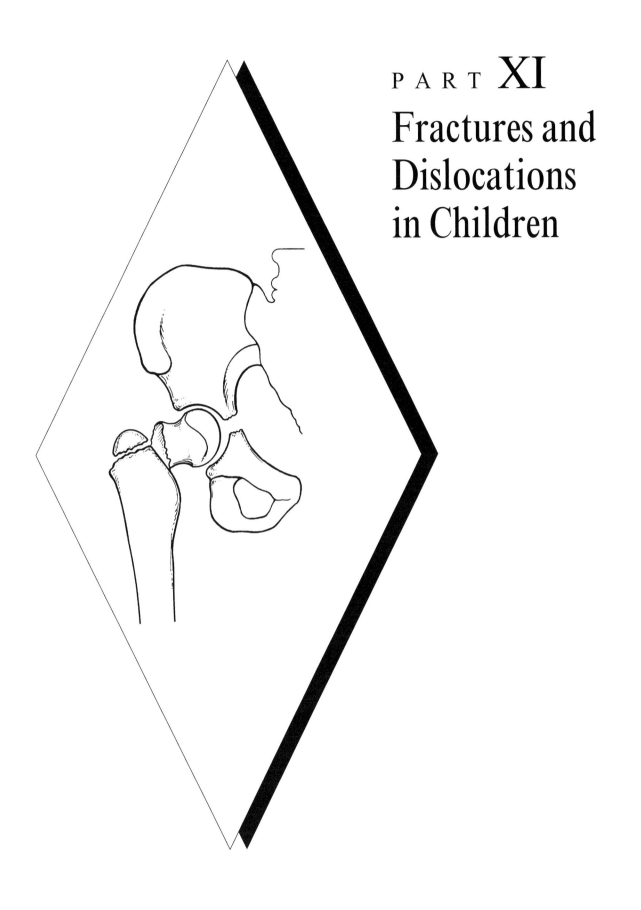

PART XI

Fractures and
Dislocations
in Children

33 Fractures and Dislocations in Children

S. Terry Canale

Fractures and soft tissue injuries in children are different from those in adults. According to Currey and Butler, children's bones are more malleable, allowing a plastic type of "bowing" injury. They also tend to be weaker and as a result can absorb more energy before breaking. The periosteum is thicker than in adults and usually remains intact on one side of the fracture, which helps stabilize any reduction, decreases the amount of displacement, and probably is a factor in the lower incidence of open fractures in children than in adults. Fractures adjacent to joints and angulated in their plane of motion in younger children will remodel; however, varus and valgus angulation and rotational malalignment may not correct so readily. Finally, the long bones of children have epiphyses and physes, the latter of which appear to be the weakest points in the child's skeleton. These weak links account for the significant difference between the location of fractures in children and adults. Furthermore, the epiphyses and physes are parts in which the normal anatomy should be preserved. Thus the dilemma: the physes, the weakest points in the bones and the sites of many children's fractures, are also the structures that must be preserved in as nearly normal condition as possible to avoid growth arrest and angular deformities.

This chapter discusses mainly those fractures in children that require operative treatment. Some fractures (those of the lateral humeral condyle, femoral neck, and distal tibial epiphysis) are described as "fractures of necessity," for which surgery is almost always necessary. Other fractures rarely if ever require open reduction and internal fixation. Although such treatment may result in a higher incidence of union, it should be remembered that closed fractures in children rarely result in nonunion. As Boyd noted, if nonunion does occur in a child, it is probably "open," pathological, or iatrogenic; if not, then the nonunion is much more refractory to treatment than a nonunion in an adult.

Growth of bone is determined by the age of the patient, and in a young child it will compensate for imperfection in apposition and to some extent for imperfect alignment and even shortening. This latter compensation is exemplified by fractures of the femur, which may stimulate overgrowth of the extremity. In very young children, fractures of the shafts of the humerus and femur usually heal and grow normally regardless of the alignment and position of the fragments. Historically, Blount established general rules concerning the prognosis of fractures of the shafts of long bones and the amount of spontaneous correction of any angular deformity to be expected. His rules are based on the age of the child, the location of the fracture, and the degree of angulation. Greater angulation is acceptable when the child is young and the deformity is near the end of the bone. Reduction must be almost perfect if the child is near maturity or if the fracture is near the middle of the bone. Spontaneous correction of an angular deformity is greatest when the angulation is in the plane of motion of a nearby hinged joint; for example, in fractures just proximal to the knee, elbow, or wrist, angulation with its apex toward the flexor aspect of the joint usually results in surprisingly little deformity. Flexion is limited somewhat, but the restriction of motion usually is not disabling. Hyperextension, if present, usually is insignificant. Function often returns to normal unless the fracture occurs near the end of the growth period. Angulation in any other direction probably will persist at least to some extent. Rotational deformities are permanent.

Karaharju et al. noted that compensatory physeal growth plays an important role in remodeling diaphyseal fractures in animals. Although varus or valgus angulation may correct spontaneously to some extent after fractures of long bones in children, an excessive amount of angulation cannot be expected to correct and will cause significant angular deformity. Such a deformity is not only cosmetically distasteful but also may affect function of the joints above and below it. For this reason every effort should be made to correct varus or valgus angulation at the time of fracture. The extremities tolerate valgus angulation of the long bones more readily than varus angulation, especially the lower extremities. In the humerus and, to some extent, in the femur, a mechanism at the shoulder and hip (ball and socket) joints appears to compensate to some degree for malrotation.

Physeal Injuries

The occurrence of certain fractures is related to the age of the child. In a review of 2650 long bone fractures in children up to 16 years of age, Mann and Rajmaira found that physeal injuries accounted for 30% of the fractures and occurred twice as often in the upper extremities as in the lower extremities. Girls with physeal fractures were an average of 1.5 years younger than boys with the same type of fracture in the same location. We, as well as others, have noted a rather consistent fracture pattern for each physis and adjacent joint. As an example, most lateral humeral condylar fractures occur between the ages of 3 and 7 years, with only one or two fracture patterns. Ankle fractures in children caused by an adduction force almost always are located across the distal tibial physis at the medial plafond and may occur in either young or older children. Conversely, almost all physeal fractures on the lateral side of the distal tibia occur in older children. They are Salter-Harris type III fractures and occur as the physis is closing in this area (Tillaux fracture).

Injuries that involve the physis and the epiphysis historically have caused cessation of growth and resultant angular deformities. These injuries have been classified by Weber et al., Poland, Ogden, and others, but the most commonly used classification is that of Salter and Harris, which is based on the roentgenographic appearance of the fracture (Fig. 33-1). This classification depicts the amount of involvement of the physis, the epiphysis, and the joint. The higher the classification, the more likely is physeal arrest or joint incongruity to occur. Type I fractures are epiphyseal separations through the physis only, with or without displacement. Stress roentgenograms are useful in determining whether this fracture is present. Type II fractures have a metaphyseal spike attached to the separated epiphysis (Thurston-Holland sign) with the separation also through the physis. Type III is a physeal separation with a fracture through the epiphysis into the joint with joint incongruity when the fracture is displaced. Type IV is a fracture through the metaphysis, through the physis, through the epiphysis, and into the joint, also with possible joint incongruity. Type V fracture, which can be diagnosed only in retrospect, is a compression fracture of the physis, producing permanent damage. Peterson questioned the validity of the Salter-Harris type V compression injury of the physis, noting, among other things, the uniform complete closure of the physis in injuries in which other fracture patterns not caused by compressive forces occur in the same extremity. He suggested that more investigation is necessary to determine why the physis uniformly closes prematurely. Rang modified the Salter and Harris classification, describing a "bruise" or contusion to the periphery of the physis. This seemingly minor injury can cause scarring, tethering, and arrest of the periphery of the physis, which may be the most crucial area regarding angular deformity.

Ogden devised a more complicated classification but one that fits almost every fracture pattern in every physis. His first five classes are basically the same as those of Salter and Harris, except for subclasses used for peculiar fracture patterns in special joints, such as the hip, and for certain traction epiphyses. His type VI fracture is similar to that described by Rang. The type VII fracture is an intraarticular osteochondral fracture. Types VIII and IX fractures are not epiphyseal or physeal fractures but appear to stimulate the physes and contribute to longitudinal bone growth.

Peterson described two previously unclassified physeal fractures. The first is a fracture completely across the metaphysis with a linear longitudinal extension to the physis (Fig. 33-2). The fracture usually does not extend along the physis. In the second fracture, a portion of the physis is missing. This is always an open fracture that requires open reduction and internal fixation and often requires late reconstructive surgery because of premature physeal closure.

Smith et al. noted that magnetic resonance imaging (MRI) scans taken within 10 days of fracture may change the Salter-Harris classification, especially in confusing fracture patterns that are difficult to interpret on roentgenograms. They noted that MRI performed early (between 3 and 17 weeks after fracture) can demonstrate transphyseal bridging or altered growth lines in physeal fractures before these become apparent on plain roentgenograms.

We routinely use the Salter-Harris classification and realize that any physeal injury may result in growth disturbance, although it is more common after Salter-Harris types III, IV, and V fractures. Most types I and II fractures can be treated by closed reduction. Types III and IV fractures often require open reduction and internal fixation to reposition the fragments anatomically and to fix them securely so that growth in the physis may continue and the joint will be congruous. An example is a type IV injury of the lateral humeral condyle, which, as mentioned previously, is a "fracture of necessity" and almost always requires open reduction and internal fixation. If not treated adequately, this fracture will not unite, causing joint incongruity and angular deformity. In type V fractures the cartilage cells of the physis are crushed and, regardless of the form of treatment, growth disturbance can occur. In fact, a type V fracture usually is diagnosed only in retrospect when a growth disturbance develops.

The indications for open reduction of physeal fractures are given in detail in the appropriate sections of this chapter. If a fracture involves a physis, the parents should be informed fully at the time of fracture concerning the possibility of growth disturbance.

Although the Salter-Harris classification has been an excellent one, some fractures do not behave as predicted, in that not all types I and II fractures do well after closed reduction and not all types III and IV fractures do not do well after open reduction. A type II distal femoral physeal fracture that is significantly displaced often results in growth arrest and angular deformity. A gentle closed anatomical reduction of this fracture is required to avoid crushing or otherwise injuring the germinal cells in the physis in the proximal fragment; even so, the physis may close prematurely. Although many authors indicate that nondisplaced types III and IV distal tibial fractures can be treated closed, Bright noted that nondisplaced fractures of these types that become displaced in the cast may develop a physeal bony bridge, and for this reason he recommended that almost all types III and IV fractures be treated by open reduction and internal fixation, regardless of the amount of displacement. In his series, smooth pins crossing the physis for fixation may have contributed to the formation of some bony bridges. Crossing the physis with any form of fixation should be avoided if possible (Fig. 33-3). In types III and IV fractures the pins should cross the epiphysis in the fractured areas, and in types II and IV they should cross the metaphysis rather than the physis, if at all possible. Böstman et al. described the use of biodegradable fixation (polyglycolic acid) across the physis for fixation of distal humeral physeal fractures. They obtained excellent temporary fixation without secondary displacement or signs of growth disturbance, except for severe displacement of one supracondylar fracture in which the polyglycolide pins broke. Because of their good results, and the fact that a second

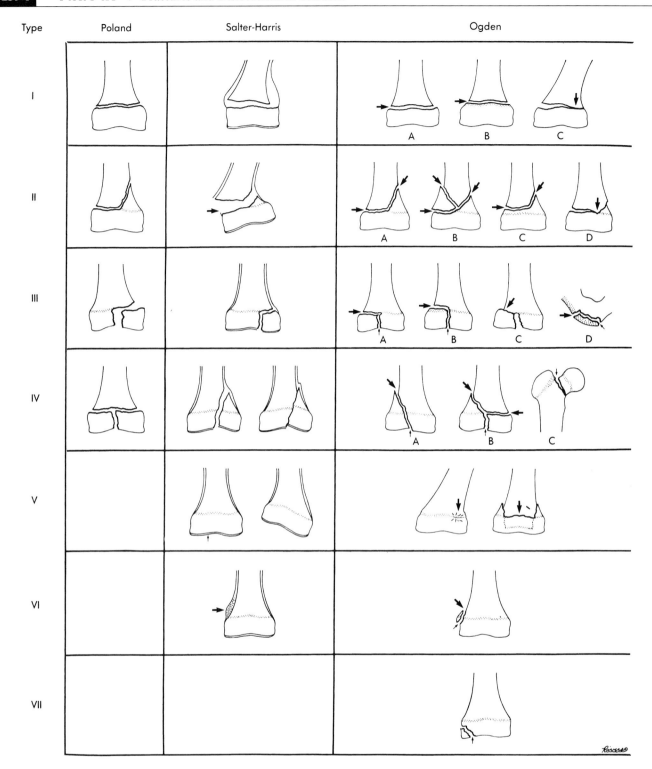

Fig. 33-1   Classification of physeal injuries by Poland, Salter and Harris, and Ogden. All three systems are similar, but from left to right are increasingly complex. Salter-Harris classification is a refinement of Poland's system, and Ogden's classification, which is all-inclusive, adds more subclasses to simpler systems.

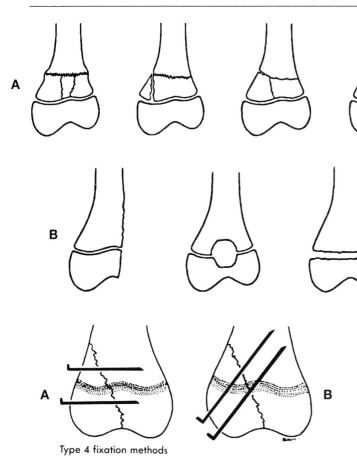

Fig. 33-2 A, Fractures of metaphysis with extension to physis. **B,** Fractures of physis with portion of physis missing. (From Peterson HA: *J Pediatr Orthop* 14:431, 1994.)

Type 4 fixation methods

Fig. 33-3 Fixation of physeal fracture. **A,** Correct placement of parallel smooth pins across epiphysis and metaphysis. **B,** Smooth pins should cross physis only if necessary to hold reduction. (From Ogden JA: *Skeletal injury in the child*, Philadelphia, 1982, Lea & Febiger.)

procedure for hardware removal is not required, they recommended biodegradable fixation for physeal fractures.

In older children osteotomy is indicated for a bony bridge or physeal bar with angular deformity (Chapter 29). In younger children, Langenskiöld and Bright both described a technique for bony bridge resection and the interposition of fat or some inert material for this complication. We have used successfully a combination of bony bar resection and osteotomy. Peterson stated that in general in younger children, if the angular deformity is less than 20 degrees, bony bridge resection alone can be used; however, if the deformity is greater than 20 degrees, then bony bridge resection plus osteotomy is indicated. Of course, these figures vary depending on which extremity and which angular deformity is present. In general, more angular deformity can be tolerated in the upper extremity than in the lower, more valgus deformity can be tolerated than varus deformity, and more flexion deformity can be tolerated than extension deformity. In the lower extremity more deformity can be tolerated proximally than distally (the same varus angle in the hip can be compensated for better than in the knee, and least well in the ankle).

If growth ceases symmetrically across the physis and shortening is significant in a younger child, epiphysiodesis of the opposite limb can be performed using several techniques (Chapter 26), including a percutaneous epiphysiodesis under control of an image intensifier. The techniques of femoral and tibial shortening or lengthening can be used for leg length inequality in an older child. For evaluation of the lower extremity, the Green-Anderson tables, as well as the Moseley straight line graph (Chapter 26), should be used with special attention to detail. In the upper extremity, length is not as important to function as in the lower extremity. Pritchett studied physeal activity in the upper extremity and found that growth occurs 1 or 2 years earlier in females than in males. Approximately 80% of the growth of the humerus occurs at the proximal physis; in the ulna and radius, approximately 85% occurs at the distal physes (Fig. 33-4).

Open Fractures

The classification and principles of treatment of open fractures in adults also apply in children. However, in a young child the history concerning the mechanism of the injury, the environment in which it occurred, and the last oral intake may not be as accurate or reliable as in an adult. Regardless of the classification of an open wound, where and how the accident took place are critical in treatment. If the history is questionable, an open fracture should be treated as if contaminated. We, as well as Roy and Crawford, have seen several "type I" puncture wounds (see Gustilo's classification, Chapter 50) in both-bone forearm fractures that became sealed over with a seroma, producing a perfect medium for *Bacillus clostridium* and gas gangrene, and resulting in above-elbow amputations. Fee et al. reported five patients with gas gangrene in both-bone forearm fractures, four of which were in children who fell from a height. The proximal fragment protruded and became contaminated by soil; the small wounds were

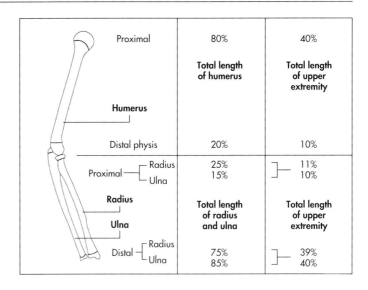

Fig. 33-4 Approximately 80% of growth of humerus occurs at proximal physis; in ulna and radius, approximately 85% occurs at distal physis.

minimally debrided and loosely closed. For this reason we have treated minor open wounds as major ones if the history is in any way questionable. It is important not to close the open wound. Some wounds in open fractures are being enlarged, irrigated, and debrided in a sterile operating suite in the emergency department, especially if general anesthesia is contraindicated. As a general rule, however, all open fractures should be irrigated and debrided thoroughly in the regular operating room with the patient under general or regional block anesthesia, and the patient should be admitted for observation and routine treatment with intravenous antibiotics.

Reports have indicated good results with external fixation of fractures in children, but all stress the necessity of avoiding the physis with the transfixing pins and using adequate incisions for pin insertion to prevent skin necrosis and infection. The report of results and complications after primary external fixation of 40 open lower extremity diaphyseal fractures in children by Golz et al. does not support the general assumption that Gustilo types II and III open diaphyseal fractures heal readily in children. Their patients under the age of 17 years had high incidences of delayed union and nonunion. The incidence of chronic infection was lower than that in adults with similar injuries. Frequent (every 36 to 48 hours) and vigorous debridement and irrigation of the open wound and adequate stabilization of the fracture seem to decrease the rates of nonunion and infection.

Rarely, after closed reduction of a fracture (without any skeletal traction pins or local anesthetic injection at the fracture) hematogenous osteomyelitis occurs at the fracture.

Pathological Fractures

As complications from anesthesia and infection decrease, more pathological fractures in children can be treated operatively, possibly decreasing morbidity and immobilization. Children with pathological fractures should not have to tolerate long periods of immobilization, which make their bones more osteoporotic. Open reduction and internal fixation frequently are beneficial, as in patients with osteogenesis imperfecta. Children who have large defects that require bone grafting likewise can benefit from surgery. Entities such as pseudarthrosis of the tibia from neurofibromatosis, fractures through cystic areas as in unicameral bone cysts, and multiple fractures of long bones in children with myelomeningocele or osteogenesis imperfecta may require open reduction and internal fixation. In children in whom conservative management may be impeded because of head injury or multiple trauma, some fractures may benefit from open reduction and internal fixation. Each of these entities and their resultant fractures are discussed in other chapters of this book.

Fractures at Birth and Fractures Caused by Child Abuse

Two groups of special fractures in children must be mentioned even though operative treatment usually is unnecessary. In the first group are fractures that are present at birth. These fractures occur most commonly in the clavicle, humerus, hip, and femur. They rarely require surgery but frequently are diagnosed as pseudopalsy, infection, or dislocation. Torode and Donnan described 12 children with obstetric paralysis and posterior dislocation of the humeral head. All 12 were treated with open reduction via an anterior approach. The age range at the time of surgery was from 7 months to 7 years. They believe that dislocation of the shoulder in association with obstetric paralysis is not rare, as previously believed, and once diagnosed, the dislocation can be treated satisfactorily by a single anterior open reduction of the shoulder.

The second group of special fractures are those caused by child abuse. The highest percentage of child abuse occurs between birth and 2 years of age. In any child under 2 years old

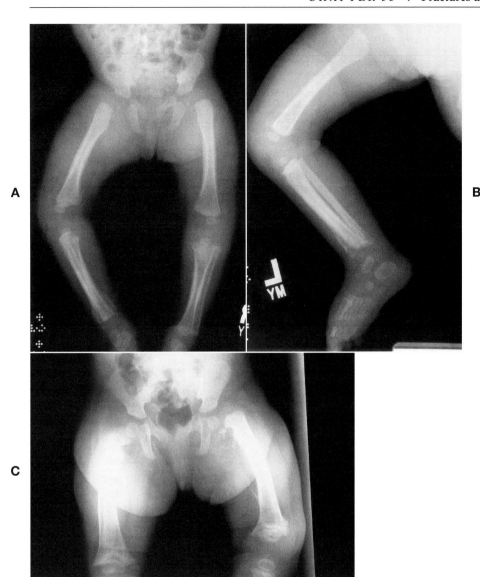

Fig. 33-5   **A** and **B,** Metaphyseal and epiphyseal changes in different stages of fracture healing of bones of knees and ankles, with apparent involvement of femur and hip **(C).**   *Continued*

with a significant fracture and a questionable history of its occurrence, child abuse should be suspected. To rule out this possibility, a bone scan or a skeletal survey generally is indicated. Multiple fractures in different stages of healing are almost always indicative of child abuse. Multiple areas of large ecchymoses in different stages of resolution (from black and blue to brown and green) also are pathognomonic of child abuse. Other, less common findings include skin burns, ocular changes, hematuria, and abdominal signs. Epiphyseal-metaphyseal ("corner") fractures are almost always pathognomonic of child abuse because the pulling and twisting forces necessary to produce these injuries rarely are accidental (Fig. 33-5). The most common sites of fractures caused by child abuse are the humerus, tibia, and femur. Every state requires physicians to report suspected child abuse. Definite knowledge or a specific diagnosis is not required. It is probably unfortunate that few fractures in this age group require open reduction and internal fixation. If they did, some abused children might actually benefit from surgery by being sheltered from those

abusing them. Regardless, the orthopaedic surgeon should protect the child who has a fracture caused by child abuse and should inform the parents of his legal responsibility to make a report.

General Principles of Operative Fracture Treatment in Children

Few children's fractures require open reduction and internal fixation. If open reduction is necessary, these general principles of operative treatment should be followed:

1. Do not think that all fractures in children will remodel completely and that adequate reduction is unnecessary.
2. Know the special surgical anatomy of the physes. Each physis, besides being undulated, also is unique in contour at each joint and is not just a flat plate.
3. If an open reduction is necessary, reposition the frag-

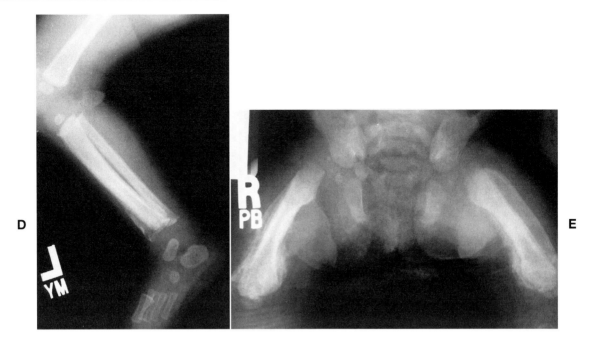

Fig. 33-5, cont'd   D and **E,** At follow-up, extensive changes are present in tibia, ankle, knees, femoral shaft, and hip.

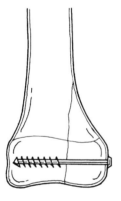

Fig. 33-6   Fixation of physeal fracture. If threaded pins or cancellous screws are used, they should cross epiphysis or metaphysis and not physis. (From Weber BG, Brunner C, Freuler F, eds: *Treatment of fractures in children and adolescents*, New York, 1980, Springer-Verlag.)

ments as anatomically as possible. This is especially important at the physis. The cartilaginous fragment should be in anatomical position; otherwise, the resulting offset will cause a bony bridge and joint incongruity.

  4. Use adequate fixation but not more than is necessary, keeping in mind the possibility of early mobilization in certain situations.
  5. Use fixation that can be removed readily.
  6. Use smooth rather than threaded pins.
  7. Try not to cross the physis, but rather parallel it in the epiphysis or pin the fracture spike in the metaphysis (Figs. 33-3 and 33-6).

  8. Avoid unnecessary drill holes that later may become iatrogenically created pathological fractures.
  9. Avoid pin penetration into joints.
  10. Use a plastic type of closure with absorbable suture.
  11. Immobilize the noncompliant child adequately.
  12. Watch for neurovascular insufficiency during convalescence.
  13. Warn the parents about early operative complications and late complications such as bony bridge formation, angular deformity, and avascular necrosis before they develop.

Hand and Wrist Fractures, Dislocations, and Fracture-Dislocations

The indications for operative treatment of closed fractures of the hand in adults are rare and are even rarer in children because an angulated bone in children tends to remodel. The exception to this is a fracture involving a physis, which requires anatomical reduction and thus occasionally operative treatment. The time of physiological closure of the physes should be noted in the phalanges and metacarpals because closure generally occurs earlier here than in other physes. Closure is earlier distally (phalanges) and later proximally (the distal radius), and once the physes have closed, a child's fracture can be treated as an adult's. Adequate reduction of phalangeal and metacarpal fractures should be obtained, even though some remodeling can be expected, and anatomical reduction of the

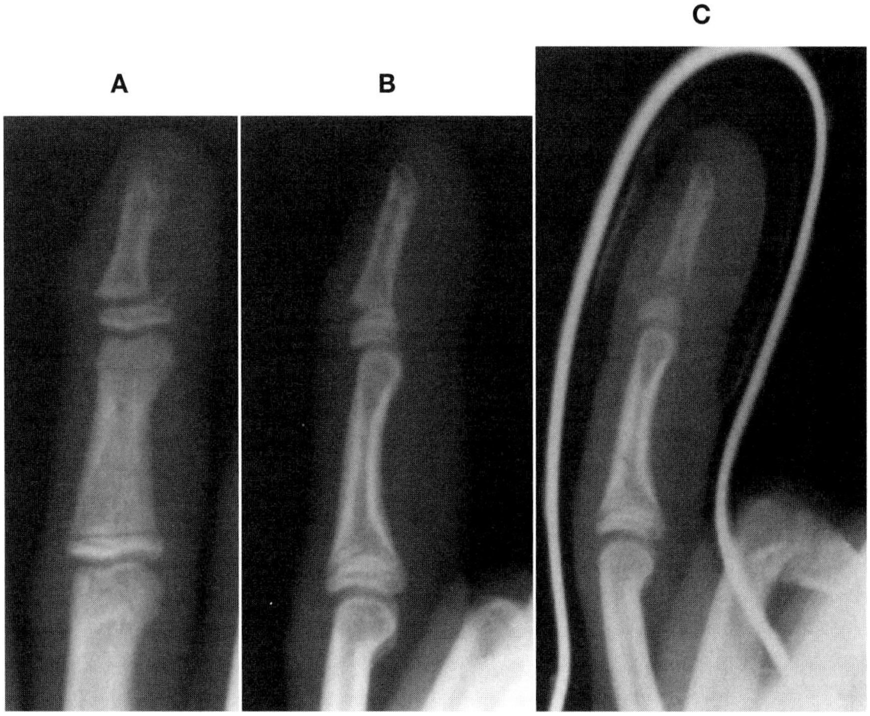

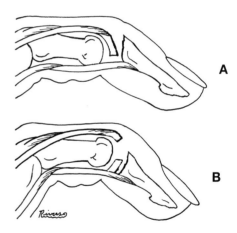

Fig. 33-7 Rare pediatric mallet finger. **A** and **B,** Salter-Harris type II fracture of distal phalanx. **C,** After closed reduction and application of hyperextension splint.

physes is necessary to prevent degenerative joint changes and angular deformity.

We reviewed 180 fractures or fracture-dislocations of the hand in children; 21 were physeal fractures, and only 4 required open reduction. Of these, one was an irreducible dorsal dislocation of a proximal interphalangeal joint that was 7 months old; one was a Salter-Harris type IV fracture; one was an open Salter-Harris type I fracture of the distal phalanx; and one involved multiple fractures and soft tissue injuries of the second, third, fourth, and fifth proximal phalanges.

PHALANGEAL FRACTURES

Phalangeal fractures probably are the most frequent hand fractures in children. Of 57 physeal phalangeal fractures in children, Crick et al. found 35 in the middle phalanx and 22 in the distal phalanx. Salter-Harris type III injuries were the most common (51%) and occurred primarily in older children (average age, 13 years); type II fractures were the second most common (37%), and type I fractures were relatively uncommon (12%).

Avulsion injuries of a distal phalanx and physis can produce a Salter-Harris type I or III fracture (Fig. 33-7). Adequate closed reduction of type I fractures will produce satisfactory results. Type III fractures of the distal phalanx produce a "mallet" finger. In a young child this usually requires only an accurate closed reduction, but if this cannot be obtained and held, open reduction and internal fixation are indicated (Fig. 33-8). Kirner congenital deformity should not be mistaken for a distal phalangeal fracture. Roentgenograms of the opposite hand also show the Kirner deformity. A large

Fig. 33-8 Two types of mallet equivalent physeal fractures in child. **A,** Salter-Harris type I fracture. **B,** Salter-Harris type III fracture. (Redrawn from Wood VE: *Orthop Clin North Am* 7:527, 1976.)

percentage of physeal separations occur in the middle and proximal phalanges, most commonly Salter-Harris type II. Type III fractures do occur, but types I and IV fractures are extremely rare in the phalanges (Fig. 33-9). Most type II fractures can be treated satisfactorily by closed methods. A type III fracture requires an anatomical reduction. If this cannot be obtained closed, then open reduction and internal fixation are necessary (Fig. 33-10).

Diaphyseal fractures also occur in the phalanges. Most distal and middle phalangeal fractures can be treated by closed reduction. Occasionally in older children, as in adults, the reduction cannot be maintained and internal fixation may be required, as reported by Greene and Anderson; Rang; Coonrad and Pohlman; and Campbell (Fig. 33-11). Stahl and Jupiter described tension band wiring in the treatment of Salter-Harris types III and IV avulsion fractures in the hand. With the placement of a small-gauge wire through the insertion of the ligament into the fracture fragment, accurate reduction and

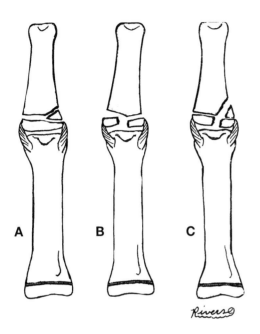

Fig. 33-9   Three types of physeal fractures of phalanges. **A,** Salter-Harris fracture type II. **B,** Type III fracture. **C,** Rare type IV fracture. (Redrawn from O'Brien ET: Fractures of the hand and wrist. In Rockwood CA Jr, Wilkins KE, King RE, eds: *Fractures in children*, Philadelphia, 1984, JB Lippincott.)

stability that allow early mobilization are achieved. This avoids the physis and many of the pitfalls and complications of other methods of internal fixation (Fig. 33-12).

Most phalangeal neck fractures also can be treated by closed methods; open reduction is required only if a severe angular deformity persists in an older child. Some degree of remodeling will occur in most younger children. Exceptions to this have been noted by Wood and by Dixon and Moon, who found that the volar plate can become interposed between the fracture fragments after rotation and angulation of the head fragment; this requires open reduction (Fig. 33-13). The technique for open reduction of this persistent deformity is described in Chapter 64.

Several types of intraarticular fractures of the phalanges can occur: condylar (Figs. 33-14 and 33-15, *A*), T-condylar (Fig. 33-15, *B*), or osteochondral (Fig. 33-15, *C*). Open reduction is indicated if the intraarticular component is displaced and is large enough to be fixed internally (see Chapter 64 for technique).

METACARPAL FRACTURES

Most fractures of the bases of the metacarpals in children can be treated by closed reduction and observation. Most metacarpal shaft fractures likewise do not require open reduction. Normal rotation should be confirmed by the ability to flex the fingers into the palm (Chapter 64). If troublesome malrotation persists, it will not remodel, and therefore open reduction and internal fixation are indicated. Green noted that for multiple metacarpal shaft fractures in children open reduction and internal fixation occasionally are indicated for stability, as in adults (Chapter 64). A significant intraarticular metacarpal head fracture also may require open reduction and internal fixation.

Fig. 33-10   Salter-Harris type III or IV fracture of proximal phalanx. **A,** Displacement of fracture. **B,** At time of open reduction and internal fixation with smooth pins across physis.

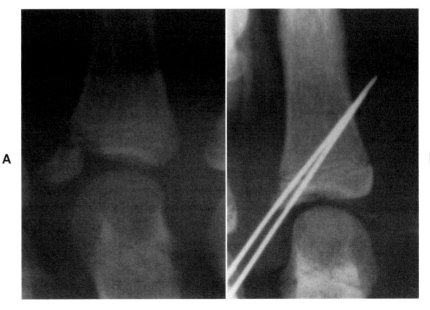

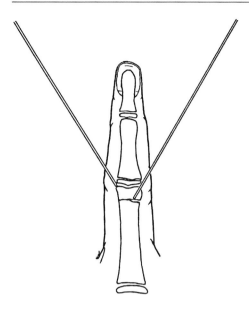

Fig. 33-11   In percutaneous fixation short distal fracture fragment is clinically lined up with middle phalanx by gentle hyperextension of PIP joint. Kirschner wire is aligned clinically with middle phalanx on lateral side and drilled into distal fragment. Second Kirschner wire is inserted on other side at 45-degree angle to proximal phalanx. With both Kirschner wires in distal fragment only, fracture is reduced with PIP joint in slight flexion and wires drilled across fracture to emerge at mid-phalanx.

A

Anteroposterior   Lateral

Hole

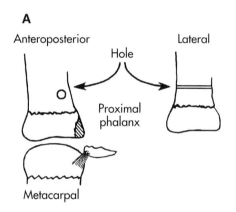

Proximal
phalanx

Metacarpal

B

Hole

Fig. 33-12   Figure-of-eight tension wire fixation. **A,** Displaced avulsed epiphyseal fracture with drill hole. **B,** Drill hole made vertically distal to physis. **C,** Wire passed through hole and through insertion of ligament on fragment in figure-of-eight fashion. **D,** Wire tightened. (Redrawn from Stahl S, Jupiter JB: *J Pediatr Orthop* 19:233, 1999.)

C   **D**

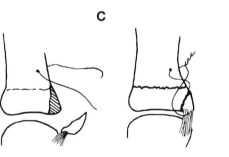

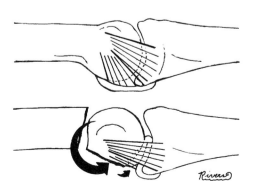

Fig. 33-13   Phalangeal neck fracture with interposition of volar plate. (Redrawn from Wood VE: *Orthop Clin North Am* 7:527, 1976.)

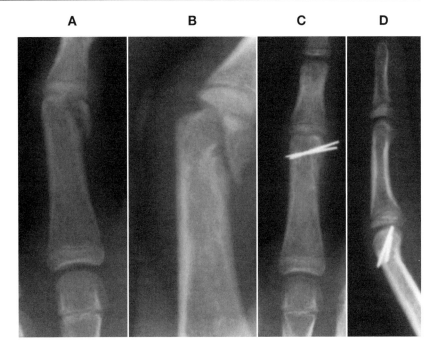

Fig. 33-14   **A** and **B,** Fracture with displacement. Condylar intraarticular fracture of proximal phalanx. **C** and **D,** After open reduction and internal fixation with transverse pins.

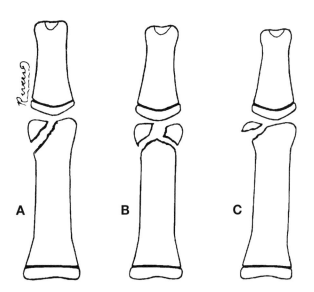

Fig. 33-15   Types of intraarticular condylar fractures. **A,** Single condyle. **B,** Both condyles. **C,** Osteochondral fracture. (Redrawn from O'Brien ET: Fractures of the hand and wrist region. In Rockwood CA Jr, Wilkins KE, King RE, eds: *Fractures in children,* Philadelphia, 1984, JB Lippincott.)

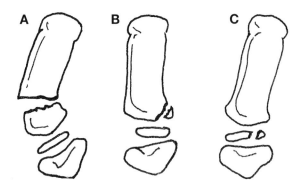

Fig. 33-16   Classification of thumb metacarpal fractures. **A,** Type A, metaphyseal fracture. **B,** Type B, Salter-Harris type II fracture. **C,** Type C, Salter-Harris type III fracture. (Redrawn from O'Brien ET: Fractures of the hand and wrist region. In Rockwood CA Jr, Wilkins KE, King RE, eds: *Fractures in children,* Philadelphia, 1984, JB Lippincott.)

Thumb Metacarpal Fractures

Most thumb metacarpal fractures occur at the base where the physis is located, rather than at the metacarpal head, as in the other metacarpals. However, as a rare variant, the thumb metacarpal may have a physis at both the proximal and distal ends. A fracture of the thumb metacarpal base does not require open reduction but is treated in an abduction thumb spica cast. The physeal fracture that occurs most often in this area is a Salter-Harris type II injury, and it can be treated by closed reduction without causing physeal arrest (Fig. 33-16, *A* and *B*). However, pediatric Bennett fracture does occur, which is a Salter-Harris type III fracture (Fig. 33-16, *C*). A Bennett fracture (equivalent to an adult's gamekeeper thumb) (Fig. 33-17) is intraarticular, and in a child it can result in a bony bridge if not treated properly. Closed reduction and percutaneous pin fixation or open reduction and internal fixation with smooth pins, as in an adult Bennett fracture, probably are indicated (Chapter 64). Occasionally, in an older child, a fracture of the base of the first metacarpal that does not involve the physis (Rolando fracture) can be satisfactorily reduced and pinned percutaneously with the aid of image intensification (Fig. 33-18). Regarding the use of image intensification, especially in hand surgery, the radiolucent

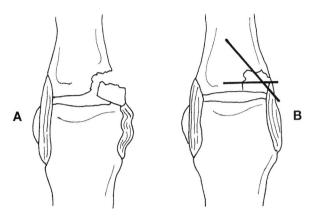

Fig. 33-17 Example of gamekeeper thumb. **A,** Type III physeal fracture. **B,** After open reduction and internal fixation with pins. (Redrawn from Wood VE: *Orthop Clin North Am* 7:527, 1976.)

surface plate of the C-arm should not be used as an operating table. Waseem and Kenny and Matthews reported the dangers of this practice. Penetration of the tube by drill bits and wires can result in electrocution of the surgeon and patient.

◆ Open Reduction and Internal Fixation of Physeal Fractures of Phalanges and Metacarpals

TECHNIQUE 33-1

Make a straight midlateral incision (Chapter 61) over the involved physis. After soft tissue dissection and retraction, mobilize the neurovascular structures and lateral bands. Now expose the physis, but take care not to damage it or the perichondral ring or periosteum overlying it. Carefully mobilize the fragments; clean out any small fragments or hematoma. With small hand surgery instruments, reduce the fracture anatomically. Make sure the reduction is satisfactory at both the physis and joint surface. Now with a power drill (low torque, high speed), transfix the fracture with two smooth parallel pins, preferably either in the metaphysis or epiphysis. Crossed pins and pins that cross the physis generally should be avoided, but sometimes small fracture fragments cannot be adequately transfixed and held otherwise. Cut off the pins beneath the skin but leave them long enough to be removed easily in the office as an outpatient. Close the soft tissues appropriately and apply a splint or cast.

AFTERTREATMENT. The pins are removed at 4 weeks, and a range-of-motion exercise program is started at that time or shortly thereafter. This program should be taught to the parents and the patient and should concentrate on active range of motion only. (Passive range-of-motion exercises in the child cause the child to withdraw or guard against any motion at all.) The parents should be warned of the possibility of growth arrest

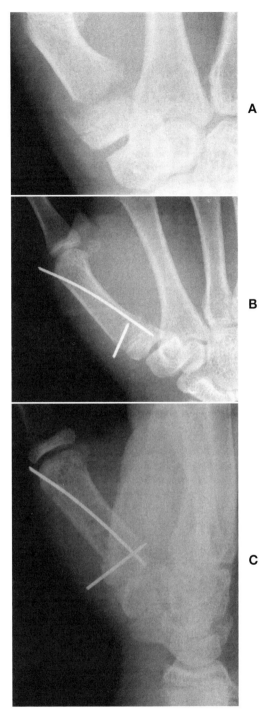

Fig. 33-18 **A,** Displaced fracture of base of thumb not involving physis (Rolando fracture) in older child. **B** and **C,** After closed reduction with aid of image intensification and fixation with smooth pins in acceptable position.

with subsequent angular deformity. The parents also should be warned, according to O'Brien, of the possibility of avascular necrosis of the phalangeal or metacarpal heads after fractures in this area, similar to that in Freiberg disease of the metatarsal heads.

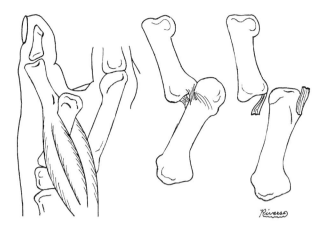

Fig. 33-19   Dislocation of metacarpophalangeal joint of thumb. (Redrawn from Wood VE: *Orthop Clin North Am* 7:527, 1976.)

DISLOCATIONS

Dislocations of the joints of the hand in children are even rarer than in adults, primarily because of the weakness of the physes, which separate instead of the adjacent joint's becoming dislocated. However, because of ligamentous laxity and the malleability of cartilage, dislocations do occur. Dislocations of the distal interphalangeal joint are extremely rare. More commonly, dislocations occur in the proximal interphalangeal joint, where the middle phalanx dislocates dorsally or laterally on the proximal phalanx. Fracture-dislocations are uncommon and open reduction and internal fixation are not indicated unless the dislocation is irreducible because of the interposition of soft tissue structures, such as the volar plate. Dislocations can occur at the metacarpophalangeal joint, especially of the thumb; this usually is a dorsal dislocation and generally can be reduced by closed methods. If the dislocation is complex and complete, as described by Farabeuf, McLaughlin, and Green and Terry, with the volar plate interposed and the metacarpal encircled by the heads of the flexor pollicis brevis muscle, then open reduction usually is necessary (Fig. 33-19). The thumb metacarpal head also can be caught in a tight sling formed by the flexor pollicis brevis and adductor pollicis, with the flexor pollicis longus displaced ulnarward; this also requires open reduction.

O'Brien described a gamekeeper thumb in children that results in ulnar instability of the thumb metacarpal, either from rupture of the ulnar collateral ligament or a Salter-Harris type I or III physeal fracture of the proximal phalanx. He recommended open reduction and internal fixation for type III physeal fractures; the operative technique for this fracture is the same as for other phalangeal physeal fractures. Repair of ruptures of the ulnar collateral ligament of the thumb is described in Chapter 64.

One of the more common dislocations is of the second metacarpophalangeal joint. Kaplan described the mechanism of this injury and noted that the metacarpal head is buttonholed through the palmar fascia with the flexor tendons on its ulnar

side and the lumbrical muscles on the radial side. The volar plate is torn and turned dorsally to become caught between the metacarpal head and the base of the proximal phalanx. Closed reduction of this dislocation almost always fails, and open reduction usually is indicated. Techniques for reduction of thumb and index metacarpophalangeal joint dislocations are described in Chapter 64.

Carpometacarpal and wrist dislocations are extremely rare in children, and their treatment is the same as in adults (Chapter 66).

OTHER FRACTURES AND FRACTURE-DISLOCATIONS

Injuries of the carpal bones generally are considered rare in children, but Nafie found that they constituted 3.9% (82 of 2102 fractures) of all fractures of the wrist in children and suggested that many of these injuries are overlooked. The scaphoid was involved in 71 patients, the triquetrum in 5, the trapezium in 3, the hamate in 2, and the trapezoid in 1. The scaphoid is the largest bone in the proximal row of the carpus, and ossification begins here between the ages of 5 and 6 years and is completed between the ages of 13 and 15 years. Before ossification the scaphoid is almost completely cartilaginous, accounting for the fewer scaphoid fractures in younger children. In Nafie's series, all patients with fracture of the scaphoid were at least 9 years old, and fractures of the waist of the scaphoid did not occur in any patient younger than 11 years old. Fractures of the other carpal bones also occurred at about the time of ossification: triquetrum, between the ages of 12 and 13 years; trapezium and trapezoid, between 13 and 14 years; and hamate, at 15 years. The correct diagnosis was made in 50% of patients before roentgenographic examination. The most common clinical signs of scaphoid fracture are dorsal swelling of the wrist, tenderness in the anatomical snuffbox and over the distal part of the radius, and painful dorsiflexion of the wrist or extension of the thumb. In 37% of patients the correct diagnosis was not made after initial roentgenograms were examined. All but one of the fractures were treated with thumb-abduction spica casting or splinting with good results. One scaphoid nonunion was discovered 18 months after injury when treatment was sought for a trivial wrist injury; union was obtained after autogenous cancellous bone grafting and Kirschner wire fixation.

Vahvanen and Westerlund in 1980 reviewed 108 fractures of the carpal scaphoid in children. All the fractures healed completely in a thumb spica cast. However, most of the fractures were avulsions of the distal third of the scaphoid. Some were waist fractures, and only a few were in the proximal pole. Fractures of the proximal pole, although rare, appear to heal uneventfully when treated by prolonged immobilization. Avulsion fractures in the distal third of the scaphoid are common in children and usually require only immobilization in an adequate plaster cast. Gamble and Simmons reported bilateral scaphoid fractures in a child.

A painful nonunion of the proximal scaphoid, which in

A   B   C

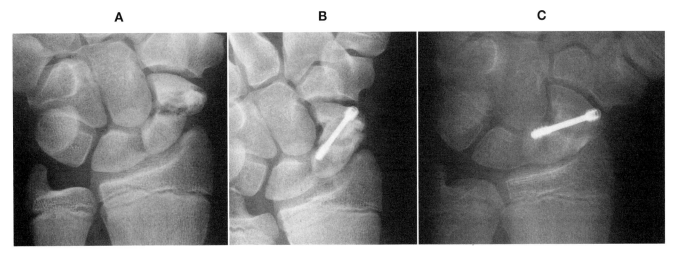

Fig. 33-20   A, Nonunion of waist of scaphoid in child with open physes of distal radius and ulna. **B,** After open reduction and internal fixation with Herbert compression screw. **C,** At 1 year, nonunion has healed.

children is extremely rare, should be treated surgically as in an adult if it limits the activities of daily living. A dorsal or volar approach can be used. Smooth pins should be considered for internal fixation in young children because this is a primary ossification center with potential growth remaining; otherwise, a compression screw can be used (Fig. 33-20). Mintzer and Waters described 13 pediatric scaphoid fracture nonunions in 12 children treated over an 18-year period; 4 were treated by using the Matti-Russe procedure (Chapter 66), and 9 were treated with Herbert screw fixation and iliac crest bone grafting. All fractures had clinical and radiographic union. They recommended the use of one Herbert screw because the length of time of postoperative immobilization in the Herbert screw group was significantly less than that in the Matti-Russe group.

Bipartite scaphoid has been described by Greene et al. and others. Some have speculated that bipartite scaphoid may be an ununited waist fracture that has taken on the characteristics of a bipartite bone.

Letts and Esser reported that fractures of the triquetrum in children often are subtle flake avulsion or impingement fractures that require good oblique roentgenograms for recognition. The incidence of these fractures probably is much higher than currently known because many are misdiagnosed as wrist sprains or type I physeal injuries of the distal radius and ulna. Three weeks of cast immobilization usually is sufficient treatment.

Forearm Fractures

Forearm fractures are extremely common in children. Most fractures at any level need not and should not be treated by open reduction and internal fixation. For closed reduction most authors agree that for distal fractures the arm should be placed in pronation; for fractures of the middle third, in neutral position; and for proximal fractures, in supination. King stated

that the radial bicipital tuberosity proximally and the radial styloid distally are best seen in maximal supination and he recommended that these two landmarks be properly aligned on the anteroposterior roentgenogram.

FRACTURES OF DISTAL THIRD OF FOREARM

Fractures of the distal third of the forearm are extremely common. Blount noted that approximately 75% of fractures of the forearm are in the distal third, and that these almost never require open reduction and internal fixation. Most are dorsally displaced and in the plane of motion of the joint, and they will remodel satisfactorily if remodeling potential remains. Besides single or both-bone fractures, physeal fractures of the distal radius and ulna occur. Salter-Harris types I and II fractures are common; types III and IV fractures are extremely rare. These physeal injuries usually do not require surgery. Open reduction and internal fixation have been described after closed reduction has failed for a reason such as the interposition of periosteum between the fragments. However, Lee et al. reported 10 children with premature closure of the distal radial physis after either physeal compression injuries (Salter-Harris type V fractures) or repeated forceful attempts at reduction. They noted that these injuries do not require repeated attempts at reduction if the initial reduction achieves apposition of more than 50%.

Zehntner et al. reported growth disturbance caused by partial closure of the distal radial physis after trauma (pseudo-Madelung deformity) and described an opening wedge osteotomy of the radius to correct the relationship between the radius and ulna (Fig. 33-21). Ulnar shortening can be performed for premature closure of the distal radial physis, as noted by Lee et al., and Irani et al., as well as O'Brien, described ulnar lengthening for proximal ulnar growth arrest. Distal ulnar growth arrest also can occur as noted by Nelson et al. Golz et al. reviewed 18 patients and 2 traumatic

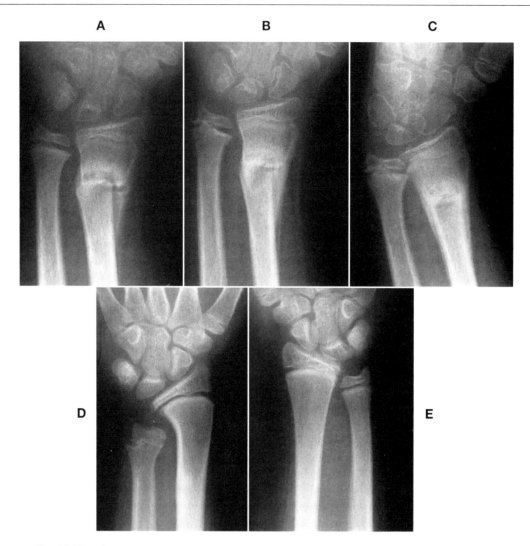

Fig. 33-21   **A,** Fracture of distal radius with what appears to be Salter-Harris type I fracture of distal ulna 2 weeks after injury. **B,** At 4 months, remodeling of radius is apparent; ulna appears normal. **C,** At 6 months, radius appears almost totally remodeled but with suggestion of bony bridge of ulnar physis. At 2 years, growth arrest and shortening of ulna are obvious secondary to Salter-Harris type I or V fracture. **D,** Ulnar deviation of the radius resulted from tethering of ulna (pseudo-Madelung deformity). Ulnar lengthening or shortening angulation osteotomy of radius may be necessary when child is older. **E,** Contralateral normal distal radius.

amputation specimens with injuries involving the distal ulnar physis and found that type I injuries were the most common fracture pattern. Premature physeal closure and ulnar shortening occurred in 55% of patients. Ray et al. described the treatment options, which included epiphysiodesis, ulnar lengthening, radial osteotomy, and the Sauve-Kapandji procedure (Technique 66-23). Other consequences of premature physeal closure included radial bowing, ulnar angulation of the distal radius, and ulnar translocation of the carpus.

Occasionally reduction is lost in a distal third greenstick fracture of the radius or of the radius and ulna, causing unacceptable volar angulation. Furthermore, a completely displaced, distal both-bone fracture of the radius and ulna can be difficult to reduce. However, either of these troublesome

fractures can almost always be treated by closed methods. Voto et al. reported 90 patients with reangulation and redisplacement after closed reduction of forearm fractures. Although remanipulation was performed between 1 and 2 weeks after injury in most patients, the authors found that nonphyseal fractures could be safely remanipulated up to 24 days after injury. They estimated that 7% of pediatric forearm fractures treated by closed reduction reangulate or displace and recommended remanipulation as a safe, effective method for obtaining and maintaining reduction.

Holmes and Louis noted in three children entrapment of the pronator quadratus that prevented closed reduction of distal radial fractures. They postulated that this probably occurs more frequently than reported in the literature when volar angulation and dorsal translation of the distal fragment are present. Open reduction was performed through a dorsal approach between the third and fourth dorsal compartments with ulnar retraction of the extensor pollicis longus and the common digital extensors, revealing the fracture and the interposed pronator quadratus.

Only rarely is surgical treatment required for severely displaced fragments with soft tissue interposition. Sometimes an open distal fracture that requires irrigation and debridement is inherently unstable, and some form of internal fixation may be necessary. Smooth Steinmann pins can be used across the physis through the radial styloid. A metal plate, however small, should not be used in this area because of the possibility of damaging the physis. If the fragments are in good alignment, internal fixation is unnecessary. Satisfactory remodeling of angular deformities usually occurs if the fracture is in the plane of motion of the wrist joint. Remodeling will not, however, correct rotational deformities. Furthermore, some loss of pronation and supination can occur because of loss of the interosseous space if varus or valgus angulation persists.

FRACTURES OF MIDDLE THIRD OF FOREARM

Fractures of the middle third of the forearm rarely require open reduction, especially in younger children in whom significant fracture remodeling can be expected. Vittas et al. emphasized the importance of the physis in fracture remodeling in children, noting that this importance decreases in late childhood and is less pronounced in the midshaft than in the distal forearm. Their study correlated with the experimental study by Karaharju, Ryöppy, and Makiner, who found that physeal growth plays an important role in the remodeling process of diaphyseal fractures in animals and that despite a lack of correction of fracture angulation, correction at the physis occurred as a secondary reaction to angulation. Price et al., in a study of 39 malunited diaphyseal both-bone forearm fractures, found that distal fractures had a better prognosis than more proximal fractures. In their patients, mild loss of forearm rotation was not disabling. They recommended closed reduction as the treatment of choice for skeletally immature patients with diaphyseal fractures of the radius and ulna, and noted that rotational alignment should be accurately restored, using the position of the radial tuberosity as a guide. Although anatomical alignment is ideal, Price et al. believe that 40 degrees of malrotation, 10 degrees of angulation, complete displacement, and loss of radial angle can be accepted rather than resorting to open reduction.

According to Weber et al., operative treatment is indicated for (1) an open fracture, (2) fracture in an older child (shortly before maturity), (3) malunion, (4) a fracture that is irreducible because of soft tissue interposition, or (5) multiple refractures occurring in a short period of time. We agree with Nielson and Simonsen that open reduction also is indicated in an older child when several attempts at closed reductions have failed. As King noted, in an older child when remodeling is not expected, open reduction and internal fixation are preferable to malunion and

loss of motion. Fuller and McCullough noted that, with gross malunion, correction of the deformity did not occur in girls after 8 years of age or in boys after 10 years of age. Although the complications of infection and scar formation may be more likely, open reduction with internal fixation is preferable to open reduction without internal fixation; the use of internal fixation avoids the complications of nonunion or recurrence of the malposition. Of the 177 fractures of the forearm in children in our series, only two had open reduction and internal fixation, and both were middle third fractures in older children with malreductions after several closed attempts; both had internal fixation with compression plates. Open reduction and internal fixation for both-bone fractures is described in Technique 54-20. The compression plate should not cross an open physis, even in an older child. Vainionpää et al. used small compression plates, one third tubular plates, and medullary Kirschner wires for fixation in 14 patients with severely displaced diaphyseal fractures of both bones of the forearm (Fig. 33-22). They recommended open reduction and internal fixation for all severely displaced fractures of the forearm.

Lascombes et al. obtained excellent results and full ranges of motion in 92% of 85 forearm fractures treated with elastic intramedullary nails. They recommend this fixation for displaced forearm fractures in children older than 10 years of age and in younger children when conservative treatment fails. Verstreken et al. reported good results with medullary nailing of completely displaced shaft fractures in six children. They recommended closed nailing through a distal approach to avoid extensive dissection and to allow motion of the extremity immediately after surgery, as Wyrsch et al. noted.

Flynn and Waters described intramedullary pin fixation of either the radius or ulna for both-bone fractures for which closed reduction has failed. Their rationale for treatment consisted of stabilizing only one bone while rotating the other into reduction. Their results were uniformly good, repeated anesthesia was avoided, and malreduction was prevented without using adult both-bone plating and hardware. As noted by Cullen et al., excellent results with the use of intramedullary pins can be expected, but complications related to surgical technique are common. Shoemaker et al. described nine complications in eight patients using intramedullary Kirschner wires. These included loss of reduction after wire removal, refracture, deep infection, pin-site infection, transient anterior interosseous nerve palsy, and a skin ulcer over a buried wire. They recommended stabilizing both the radius and ulna with an intramedullary Kirschner wire and burying wire under the skin for 3 months.

Compression plate fixation techniques can be used in older children as in adults, but the physis must be avoided. It must be remembered that open reduction may result in nonunion, infection, nerve injury, ischemic contracture, or radioulnar synostosis. Van der Reis et al. compared retrospectively 23 patients who were treated with plate and screw fixation and 18 who were treated with intramedullary nailing of unstable forearm fractures. Indications for operative treatment included open, irreducible, and unstable fractures. Excellent results were

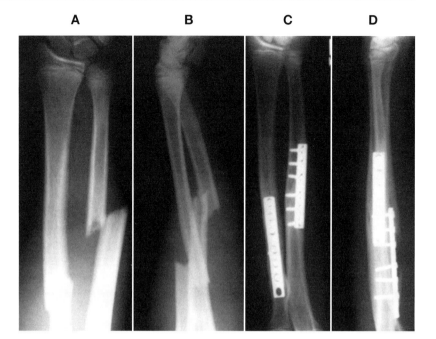

Fig. 33-22 **A** and **B,** Severely displaced both-bone forearm fractures. **C** and **D,** After open reduction and internal fixation with AO plates.

obtained in 78% of both groups. The functional results, rate of union, and rate of complications were statistically similar for both groups. However, intramedullary fixation allowed shorter operative time, minimal soft tissue dissection, ease of hardware removal, and early motion after nail removal and gave excellent cosmetic results.

◆ Closed Intramedullary Nailing

TECHNIQUE 33-2 *(Verstreken et al.)*
Place the child in the decubitus position with the affected arm on a lateral table. Apply a pneumatic tourniquet if open reduction is required, but do not inflate it. Make a 1-cm longitudinal incision on the lateral side of the distal metaphysis of the less displaced bone. With a brad awl, drill a hole in the bone 1 cm proximal to the metaphysis, first perpendicularly and then obliquely toward the elbow. Depending on the diameter of the bone, choose a titanium blunted pin of the appropriate size. The pins range in size from 15 to 25/10 mm, and the proximal ends are bent 30 degrees. Introduce the pin into the bone bent side first and push it, with a hammer if necessary, to the fracture site (Fig. 33-23). Reduce the fracture by external manipulation and fix the pin in the proximal metaphysis. Repeat the procedure for the other bone. Bend the outer tips of the pins and cut them 5 to 10 mm from the bone. Use one to two stitches to close the skin wounds.

AFTERTREATMENT. Immediate motion is allowed, and discharge from the hospital usually is allowed on the first or second day. Sports are avoided for 2 months. Pins are removed by simple extraction at 3 months.

King and Stanitski and Micheli reported ipsilateral both-bone fractures and supracondylar fracture of the humerus, and we have seen this injury. This has been described as a "floating elbow." The supracondylar fracture is reduced and pinned percutaneously to stabilize the elbow, and the forearm fracture is reduced by closed methods. Closed reduction and percutaneous pinning (reduction pinning) of a supracondylar fracture is described in Technique 33-13.

FRACTURES OF PROXIMAL THIRD OF FOREARM

Fractures of the proximal third of the forearm are rare. Because of the possibility of radial head dislocation proximally and radioulnar dissociation distally, roentgenograms of the elbow and wrist joints should always be obtained in any forearm fracture. Holdsworth and Sloan noted that only 7% of both-bone fractures were in the proximal third and did not recommend open reduction and internal fixation in children under 12 years of age. Walker and Rang found that proximal forearm fractures in young children may be unstable when the elbow is flexed but are stable when the elbow is extended. They treated 15 such fractures with immobilization in a long arm cast with the elbow extended. All patients had normal elbow movement at 2 weeks and full forearm rotation at follow-up. Although an extended-elbow cast is awkward, they believe it provides an acceptable alternative to internal fixation for some unstable fractures in young children. Because of poor results after nonoperative treatment in older children, surgical treat-

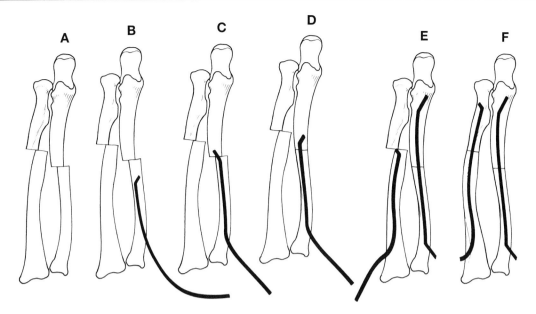

Fig. 33-23   Medullary nailing of both-bone fractures of forearm. **A,** Displaced both-bone fractures. **B,** Pin is introduced into least displaced bone, bent side first. **C,** Pin is advanced to fracture site. **D,** Fracture is reduced by external manipulation and pin is advanced into proximal metaphysis. **E,** Fracture of other bone is reduced and fixed in same manner. **F,** Both pins in place. (Redrawn from Verstreken L, Delronge G, Lamoureux J: *J Pediatr Orthop* 8:450, 1988.)

ment may be indicated. In proximal both-bone fractures, radioulnar synostosis may develop.

Cross-Union (Synostosis)

Cross-union is a rare complication of fractures of the forearm in children, but when both bones are united by a single callus, supination and pronation are impossible and the forearm will not be completely functional. Several factors have been suggested as contributing to the development of cross-union, including severe initial displacement, displacement after reduction, periosteal interposition, surgery, delayed surgery, remanipulation, excision of the radial head, and fractures at the same level in the radius and ulna (Fig. 33-24). Vince and Miller reported 10 cross-unions in children and classified them according to location: type 1, intraarticular in the distal third; type 2, nonarticular in the distal or middle third; and type 3, in the proximal third. Type 3 cross-unions were the most frequent and occurred after mild injury and nonoperative treatment, as well as after severe trauma; type 2 cross-unions consistently occurred after severe trauma; and there were no type 1 cross-unions. They concluded that the risk of cross-union is increased by surgical trauma to the soft tissues between the radius and ulna and that excision of the radial head alone was a greater risk factor than open reduction alone. Although their results after excision of the cross-union were not as good as in adults, they noted that delaying excision until the child is skeletally mature may preclude regaining full pronation and supination because of soft tissue contractures.

Plastic Deformation

Because of the plastic nature of children's bones, the long bones frequently bend or bow rather than break. Most plastic deformities in the radius and ulna occur in children between the ages of 2 and 15 years. In a review of reported plastic deformation of the forearm, Mabrey and Fitch found the ulna bowed in 83% of patients and the radius in 50%. In addition to the cosmetic deformity, bowing of one or both bones of the forearm may cause limitation of pronation and supination as the bowed bones encroach on the interosseous space. According to Borden, physiological remodeling in younger children eventually may permit full pronation and supination, but this is unlikely to occur in older children with uncorrected deformity. Untreated severe plastic deformation of the forearm may result in cosmetic deformity and loss of forearm rotation. Sanders and Heckman suggested reduction of any plastic deformity that prevents reduction of a concomitant fracture or dislocation. Angulation of less than 20 degrees in young children usually will remodel satisfactorily, but they suggested consideration of reduction in children older than 4 years or in any child with a deformity of more than 20 degrees, especially if it limits pronation and supination. Nimityongskul et al. reported four children with plastic deformation of the forearm and reviewed treatment recommendations in the literature. On the basis of the age of the patient and the severity of the deformity, they recommended, that (1) in children older than 10 years of age, deformities of 15 degrees or more should be manipulated and corrected; (2) in children between 6 and 10 years of age,

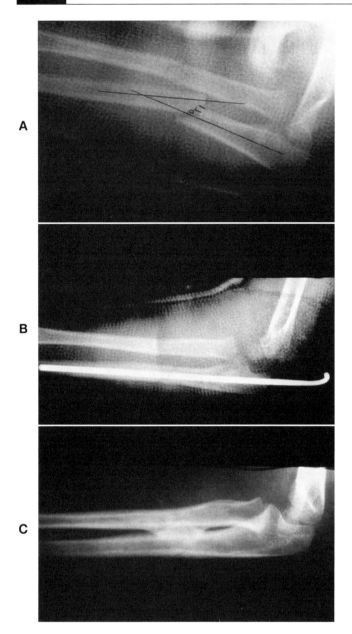

Fig. 33-24   A, Evidence of radial head dislocation after closed reduction and casting of both-bone fractures at junction of proximal and middle thirds of radius and ulna. **B,** After open reduction and internal fixation of ulna and closed reduction of radius and radial head. **C,** At follow-up, synostosis (cross union) between radius and ulna at fracture with decreased pronation and supination.

correction of deformities of 20 degrees of more should be attempted; and (3) in children 5 years of age and younger, no correction is necessary because remodeling most likely will restore correct anatomy and function. If reduction is attempted, parents should be warned that fracture of one or both bones may be necessary.

Sanders and Heckman described a method of closed reduction of plastic deformation of the forearm and reported an average correction of 85% of the angulation in eight patients.

Their technique consists of applying a transversely directed force both proximal and distal to the apex of the bow with the apex placed over a rolled towel. Usually this is performed with the patient under general anesthesia. Since the bowing may occur in more than one plane, sequential forces are applied to correct the deformity in both planes. Care is taken to avoid placing force over the physes. With the application of a force of 20 to 32 kg, the deformity gradually corrects over 2 to 3 minutes. If the other bone is fractured, it is then treated by the method that would have been chosen had plastic deformation not occurred. A long arm cast is applied with the elbow in 90 degrees of flexion and the forearm in full supination; the cast is worn from 6 to 8 weeks. Several important points must be remembered about this technique: (1) adequate anesthesia is essential, (2) the most deformed bone should be reduced first, (3) pressure is applied to the distal and proximal ends of the forearm adjacent but not directly over the physes, and (4) force must be applied gradually to prevent fracture. King modified the technique of Sanders and Heckman by using the surgeon's knee as a fulcrum and applying the corrective force for 5 to 8 minutes. He suggested that 85% of the deformity should be corrected before the cast is applied.

Monteggia and Galeazzi Fractures

A special fracture-dislocation of the forearm was described by Monteggia, and an analogous but reverse fracture-dislocation was described by Galeazzi. These seemingly benign fractures of the radius and ulna, with occult dislocation of the radial head proximally (Monteggia) or of the ulnar head distally (Galeazzi), can result in poor function if not diagnosed and treated properly.

Monteggia Fracture. In Monteggia fractures roentgenograms of the elbow are sometimes not made and even when they are, a subtle dislocation or subluxation of the radial head often is not recognized. The radial head should always point through the middle of the capitellum in any position, especially on the lateral roentgenogram. This can be confirmed by drawing on the roentgenogram a straight line through the radial head; in any position, this line should pass through the center of the capitellum. Four types of Monteggia fractures, as well as three "equivalent" types, have been described. The most common is a fracture of the proximal third of the ulna, anterior angulation of the fracture, and anterior dislocation of the radial head (Fig. 33-25, *A*). The second most common is fracture of the proximal ulna, posterior angulation of the fracture, and posterior dislocation of the radial head (Fig. 33-25, *B*). Lateral angulation of the proximal ulnar fracture may result in a rare third type with a lateral dislocation of the radial head (Fig. 33-25, *C*). In addition, Bado and Barquet and Caresani described a rare fourth type with a proximal both-bone fracture and anterior dislocation of the radial head (Fig. 33-25, *D*).

More recently, several authors have suggested that, although this classification may be related to the mechanism of injury, it has no relationship to the treatment or results of these injuries in children. Wiley and Galey proposed a three-part classification of the dislocation of the radial head associated with

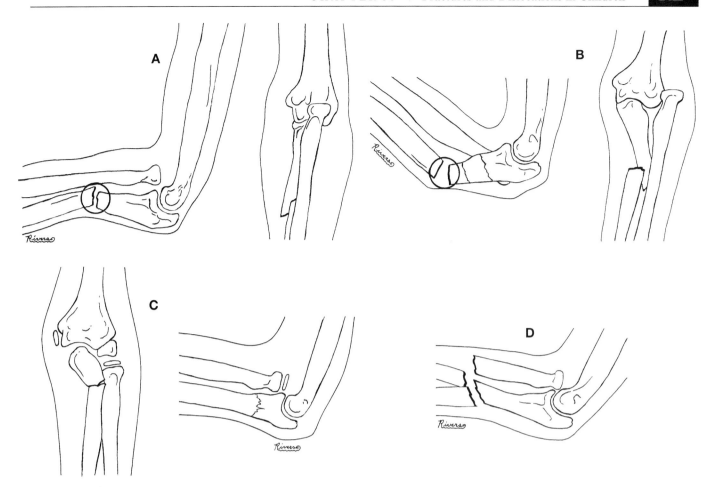

Fig. 33-25   Types of Monteggia fractures. **A,** Type I with anterior dislocation of radial head and anterior angulation of ulnar fracture. **B,** Type II with posterior dislocation of radial head and posterior angulation of ulnar fracture. **C,** Type III with lateral dislocation of radial head and lateral angulation of ulnar fracture. **D,** Rare type IV with fractures of radial and ulnar shafts and dislocation of radial head. (Redrawn from Bado JL: *Clin Orthop* 50:71, 1967).

fracture of the proximal ulna: type I, anterior; type II, posterior; and type III, lateral. Letts et al. suggested a more extensive classification system to include Monteggia equivalents in which there is bowing, or "greensticking," of the ulna (Fig. 33-26). Onley and Menelaus, on the other hand, found the Bado classification applicable to children's fractures in their series of 102 Monteggia lesions. In 197 Monteggia lesions reported in the literature (Reckling, Bruce et al., Letts et al., Wiley and Galey, and Onley and Menelaus), Bado type I lesions were by far the most common (59%), followed by type III lesions (26%); types II (5%) and IV (1%) were rare. Onley and Menelaus found a type I equivalent (ulnar fracture associated with radial neck fracture or separation of the proximal radial epiphysis) in 14 of their 102 patients. In their report of 46 dislocations of the radial head associated with olecranon fracture, Theodorou et al. found the dislocation to be lateral in 23 (58%), posterolateral in 13 (28%), anterolateral in 8 (17.4%), and anterior in 2 (4.3%); they found no posterior dislocations.

Most Monteggia fractures can be treated by closed methods. If the recommended maneuvers do not produce an adequate reduction, then interposition of the annular ligament or the capsule may be present, and an open reduction may be necessary.

Three Monteggia "equivalent" fractures have been described: (1) isolated radial head dislocation (p. 1415) (Fig. 33-27), (2) fracture of the proximal ulna with fracture of the radial neck, and (3) both-bone proximal third fractures with the radial fracture more proximal than the ulnar fracture. Proper alignment often cannot be obtained in Monteggia equivalents, and open reduction may be necessary. Monteggia equivalent lesions are extremely rare, but just as in Monteggia fractures, they must be handled expertly.

In Monteggia fractures if open reduction of the radial head is performed, internal fixation of the proximal ulna is carried out only in older children. Myositis or synostosis in this area is common, and stripping of the soft tissues including the periosteum should be minimal. In adolescents, the ulna should

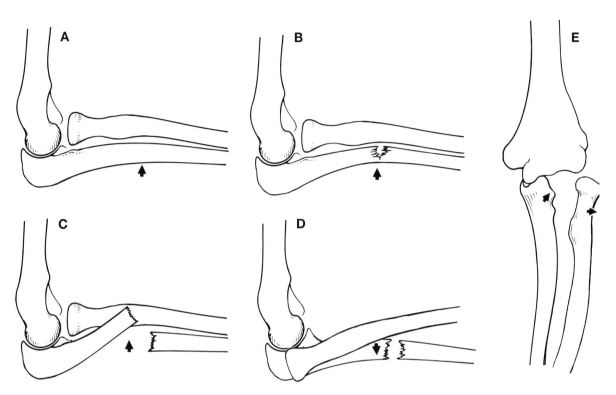

Fig. 33-26   Classification of pediatric Monteggia fracture-dislocations. **A,** Anterior bend. **B,** Anterior greenstick. **C,** Anterior complete. **D,** Posterior. **E,** Lateral. (Redrawn from Letts M, Locht R, Weins J: *J Bone Joint Surg* 67B:724, 1985.)

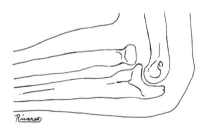

Fig. 33-27   Monteggia equivalent with isolated anterior dislocation of radial head. (Redrawn from Bado JL: *Clin Orthop* 50:71, 1967.)

be fixed with a plate or medullary nail at the time of reduction of the radial head. We routinely use the Boyd approach (see Technique 1-96). King recommended two separate incisions to avoid myositis or synostosis. Any material caught in the radiocapitellar articulation should be removed and the dislocation should be stabilized, preferably by repairing the annular ligament and flexing the elbow to 120 degrees. We have held the radiocapitellar articulation with a pin inserted across the radial head and neck and into the capitellum. Technically, this is an exacting procedure, and the results have not always been satisfactory. The dangers of the transcapitellar pin are well known; however, when necessary, a large, smooth pin as described by King can be used. The parents should be warned

of possible pin tract infection or breakage of the pin. Open reduction and internal fixation of acute Monteggia fractures are described in Chapter 54.

Posterior and anterior interosseous nerve lesions and proximal radioulnar synostosis have been described in Monteggia fractures and their equivalents. Historically, after Monteggia fractures with chronic persistent radial head dislocation or chronic untreated isolated radial head dislocations, the dislocation has been ignored until skeletal maturity. At that time, if necessary, the radial head is resected. Resection of the radial head in a child leads to angular deformity at both the elbow and the wrist. If the dislocation is symptomatic, it should be resected only at skeletal maturity. In 15 older children in whom the radial head was resected, Speed and Boyd noted only 3 in whom any abnormality developed at the distal radioulnar joint. In these, approximately 1 cm of radial shortening was seen at the level of the radial styloid. The distal ulna was somewhat prominent, and the hands were slightly deviated toward the radius. Speed and Boyd found that, although resecting the radial head may be theoretically objectionable, practically the procedure in older patients does not produce any significant consequences. Campbell et al. also reported that, contrary to published data, excision of the radial head for congenital dislocation in older children increased the range of motion and decreased elbow pain in their patients.

According to reports in the literature the radial head can be

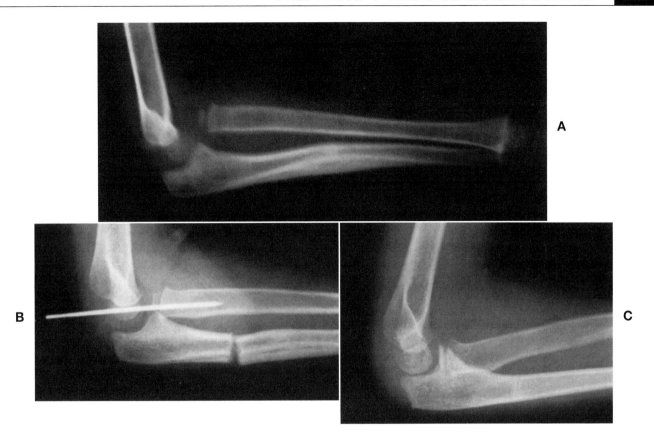

Fig. 33-28 Malunion of ulna and anterior dislocation of radial head. **A,** Before treatment. **B,** After Bell Tawse procedure using triceps fascia, insertion of transcapitellar pin, and extension osteotomy of ulna. **C,** At 3 years after surgery, showing maintenance of radial head reduction. Sclerosis of radial head is worrisome.

reduced satisfactorily as late as 6 months or even longer after traumatic dislocation. This generally requires osteotomy of the angulated ulna followed by open reduction of the radial head, reconstruction of the annular ligament with fascia or other soft tissue, and stabilization of the radial head in normal position against the capitellum. Bell Tawse, Lloyd-Roberts and Bucknill, and King have all described satisfactory results. We have treated eight children by this method with satisfactory results; one child in whom the osteotomy was not done had an unsatisfactory result. If the ulna has malunited, regardless of how little or how much remodeling has taken place, an osteotomy usually is necessary to "lengthen" the ulna and produce a stable radial head reduction. Boyd used a slip of fascia from the extensor aponeurosis to reconstruct the torn or attenuated annular ligament (see Technique 54-19). Bell Tawse used a central slip of the triceps fascia, and Lloyd-Roberts used the lateral aspect of the triceps fascia attached distally. Oblique pin fixation from the radial neck to the olecranon and proximal ulna can be used if the reduction is unstable, but this is technically difficult. If necessary, we reluctantly use a transcapitellar pin to hold the reduction in older children (Fig. 33-28) and a medullary pin or compression plate to fix the osteotomy of the ulna. In younger children, internal fixation of the ulna usually is unnecessary. This operation should not

be performed for congenital dislocation of the radial head. Congenital dislocations usually are posterior, in contrast to the usual anterior dislocation seen after trauma. Further, the congenitally dislocated radial head does not appear to be well formed as is a normal radial head that has been traumatically dislocated, and congenital dislocation is bilateral in at least 40% of the patients.

◆ Open Reduction of Old Monteggia Fracture in Children

TECHNIQUE 33-3 *(Speed and Boyd)*

Expose both the fracture of the ulna and the dislocation of the radial head through the Boyd approach (Technique 1-96). If the ulna has united in malposition, make an osteotomy through the area of union and fix it internally with either a compression plate or a medullary nail. Reposition the head of the radius anatomically after removing any portion of the annular ligament that may be caught in the radiohumeral articulation. If the annular ligament cannot be repaired adequately, free a strip of fascia, 1.3 cm wide and approximately 11.5 cm long, from the

continued

muscles of the forearm, leaving it attached to the proximal ulna (see Fig. 54-86). Pass the fascial strip between the radial notch of the ulna and the tuberosity of the radius and around the neck of the radius. Fasten it to itself with interrupted nonabsorbable sutures. If the proximal radius is still unstable, maintain reduction with an oblique pin from the radius to the proximal ulna or fix it with a large, smooth, transarticular Steinmann pin as described in the next technique. Irrigate the wound and close it in layers. Keep the forearm slightly supinated and apply a sterile dressing and a long arm cast.

AFTERTREATMENT. The parents should be warned about possible transcapitellar pin breakage and infection. The cast and pin are removed at 3 to 6 weeks, and range-of-motion exercises are begun.

TECHNIQUE 33-4 *(Bell Tawse; Lloyd-Roberts and Bucknill; King)*

Place the patient supine on the operating table; prepare and drape the arm in the usual fashion on a hand table. Make a longitudinal incision centered over the apex of the ulnar fracture and carry the soft tissue dissection down to the malaligned fracture. Perform an osteotomy at the apex of the fracture. If the malunion is angulated anteriorly, pull the proximal fragment into hyperextension. In a young child, overriding of the fragments is acceptable. Now make a Boyd approach. Carry the dissection down to the radial head, remove the capsule and interposed remnant of annular ligament that is blocking reduction of the radial head against the capitellum, and reduce the proximal radius. Free a central or lateral slip of the triceps fascia, as described by Bell Tawse, Lloyd-Roberts and Bucknill, and King. This slip should be 8 cm long × 1 cm wide and is left attached distally to the ulna adjacent to the radial neck. Pass the fascia from medial to lateral around the radial neck and through holes drilled in the ulna and suture it to itself (Fig. 33-29). Check the radial head reduction. Introduce a large, smooth, Steinmann pin through the capitellum, across the joint, and into the head and neck of the radius, as described by Lloyd-Roberts (Fig. 33-30). Bend its proximal end outside the skin. If internal fixation is necessary in older children, fix the ulna with a long medullary Steinmann pin or a compression plate. Apply a long arm cast with the elbow in 90 degrees of flexion and the forearm in mild supination.

AFTERTREATMENT. Aftertreatment is the same as for the Speed and Boyd technique.

Galeazzi Fracture-Dislocation.

Galeazzi fracture-dislocations, fracture of the radius with disruption of the distal radioulnar joint, are rare in children. Walsh et al. reported that fewer than 5% of all radial shaft fractures in children are

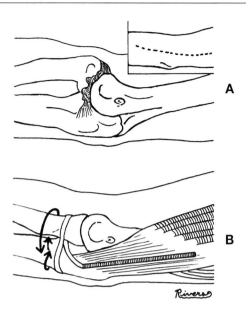

Fig. 33-29 Bell Tawse procedure. **A,** Pathological condition at radiohumeral joint. *Inset,* Skin incision. **B,** Use of fascial strip from triceps tendon to reconstruct annular ligament. (Redrawn after Bell Tawse AJ: *J Bone Joint Surg* 47B:718, 1965.)

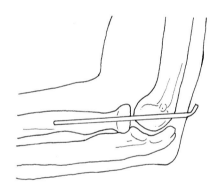

Fig. 33-30 Transcapitellar pin used after reduction of chronic dislocation of radial head. (Redrawn from Hurst LC, Dubrow EN: *J Pediatr Orthop* 3:227, 1983.)

associated with obvious disruption of the distal radioulnar joint. They divided 41 fracture-dislocations into two groups: fractures in the distal third of the radius (Fig. 33-31, *A*) and fractures at the junction of the middle and distal thirds (Fig. 33-31, *B*). These two groups were further classified as anterior or posterior dislocations. Most fractures within the distal third of the radius were associated with anterior dislocation of the ulnar head; conversely, most fractures at the junction of the distal and middle thirds were associated with posterior dislocations. Like Monteggia lesions, Galeazzi fracture-dislocations are often unrecognized. Walsh et al. reported that in 41% of their patients the injury to the distal radioulnar joint was not recognized initially.

Most of these injuries in children can be treated by closed reduction. Once the radius is restored to length and the angulation is corrected, the distal radioulnar joint will reduce

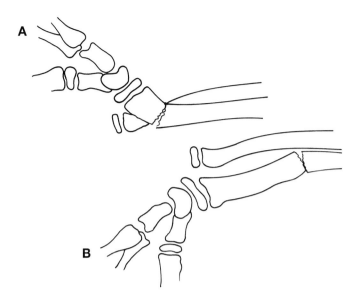

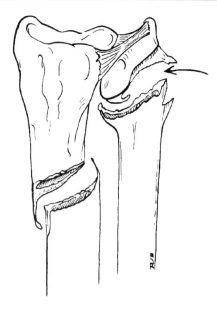

Fig. 33-31   **A,** Fracture-dislocation within distal third of forearm with posterior displacement of radius. **B,** Classic Galeazzi injury with radial fracture at junction of middle and distal thirds; distal radius is anteriorly displaced. (Redrawn from Walsh HPJ, McLaren CAN, Owen R: *J Bone Joint Surg* 69B:731, 1987.)

Fig. 33-32   Variant of Galeazzi fracture-dislocation. Interposed periosteum may block reduction. (From Landfried MJ, Stenclik M, Susi JG: *J Pediatr Orthop* 11:332, 1991.)

and become stable. Mikic reported good results after conservative treatment of 14 Galeazzi fractures in children, and Walsh et al. reported excellent or good results in 92% of fractures treated closed. The three poor results in the series of Walsh et al. were fractures of the distal third treated with below-elbow plaster casts. They recommended verifying relocation of the joint after reduction of the radial fracture and immobilization in an above-elbow cast with the forearm in supination. If closed reduction cannot be obtained, open reduction and internal fixation of the radius with a compression plate (Technique 54-20) are indicated, especially in older children.

Landfried et al. described a variant of the Galeazzi fracture-dislocation in children in which separation of the distal radioulnar joint occurred through a displaced Salter-Harris type II physeal fracture of the distal ulna (Fig. 33-32). In adults radioulnar dislocation cannot occur without disruption of the triangular fibrocartilage complex, but in children with open physes the distal ulnar physis can avulse before rupture of the complex. Closed reduction could not be obtained in any of their three patients with this injury, and at the time of open reduction and internal fixation, interposition of the periosteum blocked reduction.

Isolated Dislocations of Radial Head

Isolated dislocations of the radial head are rare. Dislocations usually occur in conjunction with fractures of the ulna; however, because of the plasticity of bone in children, an acute isolated anterior dislocation can occur, as well as an extremely rare lateral or posterior dislocation without fracture of the ulna.

The clinical diagnosis of radial head dislocation with or without ulnar fracture often is difficult. A delay in diagnosis from 1 week to 18 months has been noted by several authors to result in an increased number of children who required open treatment and who had less satisfactory results.

Lincoln and Mubarak, in a study of traumatic radial head dislocations with and without fracture of the ulna, challenged the existence of an "isolated" traumatic radial head dislocation. Using the "ulnar bow sign," they found injury to the ulna in five patients with isolated traumatic radial head dislocations. The ulnar bow sign is determined by drawing a straight line on the roentgenogram along the dorsal border of the ulna from the level of the olecranon to the distal ulnar metaphysis. The maximal perpendicular distance of this line from the ulnar shaft is measured and the location of maximal bowing along the ulnar shaft is recorded. Their results showed that the location of maximal ulnar bowing after radial head dislocation without ulnar fracture uniformly occurred near the mid ulna, at a mean distance of 45 mm ± 2% from the proximal end, and averaged 3.9 ± 0.4 mm. In a control group, however, maximal ulnar bowing was less than 1 mm from the straight line drawn along the dorsal ulnar border. They asserted that ulnar bowing of more than 1 mm may signify the presence of a serious injury to the forearm and may help alert the physician to an undetected radial head dislocation (Fig. 33-33). Lincoln and Mubarak suggested that the diagnosis of traumatic isolated radial head dislocation is probably a misnomer for an injury that is more accurately described as a minimal Monteggia fracture-dislocation.

Vesely reported 17 isolated dislocations of the radial head; 13 were anterior; 3 were lateral, and 1 was posterior. Only 4

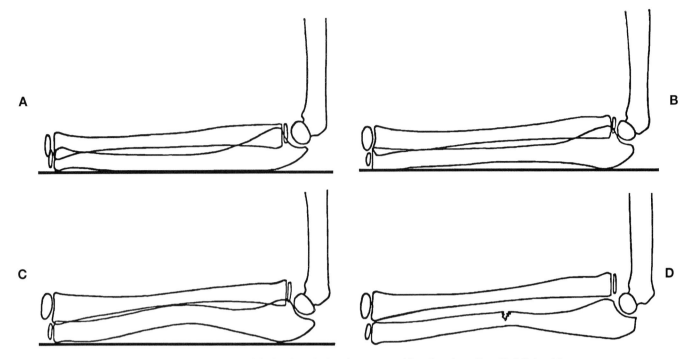

Fig. 33-33 **A,** Normal straight border of ulna demonstrated by ulnar bow line. **B,** Minimal bow. **C,** Anterior bend. **D,** Anterior greenstick. (From Lincoln TL, Mubarak SJ, *J Pediatr Orthop* 14:455, 1994.)

Fig. 33-34 Overcorrection with posterior convexity and elongation of ulna for anterior dislocation of radial head. (Redrawn from Hirayama T, Takemitsu Y, Yagihara K, Mikita A: *J Bone Joint Surg* 69B:639, 1987.)

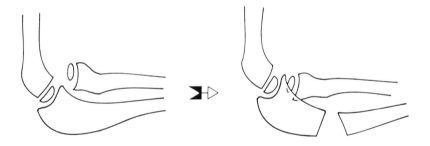

required open reduction. After closed manipulation of an anterior dislocation, the forearm should be held in supination with the elbow flexed to 90 degrees. Conversely, in a posterior dislocation the forearm should be held in a position of pronation with the elbow at 90 degrees. Open reduction is indicated only when the dislocation has persisted for over 3 weeks or when closed manipulation has not been successful. For open reduction we have used the Boyd approach, repairing the annular ligament and using a pin placed obliquely or a transcapitellar pin when necessary. Reduction should be maintained for 3 weeks or longer in an older child. The pin is then removed and the cast is worn for an additional 3 weeks. As noted by Vesely, complications of open reduction include redislocation and proximal radioulnar synostosis.

Hirayama et al. reported good results in nine chronic posttraumatic dislocations after osteotomy of the ulna with overcorrection of the angular deformity and elongation of the bone. They suggested that the interosseous membrane of the forearm is the most important structure in maintaining the corrected position of the radial head.

◆ OSTEOTOMY OF ULNA AND OVERCORRECTION OF ANGULAR DEFORMITY

TECHNIQUE 33-5 *(Hirayama et al.)*

After inflation of a pneumatic tourniquet on the upper arm, make a posterolateral skin incision extending from above the elbow to a point sufficient to expose the joint and the proximal third of the ulna. Then excise the scar tissue around the radiohumeral and proximal radioulnar joints. Perform a subperiosteal osteotomy of the ulna 5 cm below the olecranon. Distract the osteotomy by about 1 cm to lengthen the ulna and angulate it to produce overcorrection of the deformity. Correct anterior displacement of the radial head by posterior angulation of the ulna (Fig. 33-34) and lateral dislocation by medial angulation (Fig. 33-35). Hold the osteotomy with a metal plate bent to an angle of about 15 degrees. Be sure the repositioned radial head lies in the radial notch of the ulna to ensure proper spacing of the radiohumeral joint and to prevent excessive pressure on

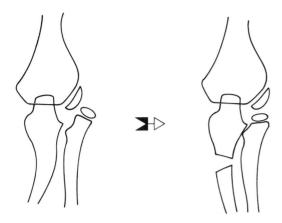

Fig. 33-35   Overcorrection with medial convexity and elongation of ulna for lateral dislocation of radial head. (Redrawn from Hirayama T, Takemitsu Y, Yagihara K, Mikita A: *J Bone Joint Surg* 69B:639, 1987.)

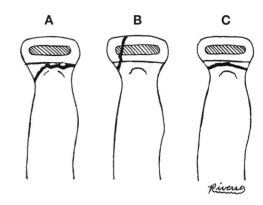

Fig. 33-36   Wilkins classification of radial neck fractures. **A,** Salter-Harris type II fracture. **B,** Salter-Harris type IV fracture. **C,** Salter-Harris type I fracture. (Redrawn from Wilkins KE: Fractures and dislocations of the elbow region. In Rockwood CA Jr, Wilkins KE, King RE, eds: *Fractures in children*, Philadelphia, 1984, JB Lippincott.)

the radial head. Before wound closure, test the stability of the repositioned head by flexion, extension, pronation, and supination. Approximate the anconeus muscle but do not repair the annular ligament. Apply a plaster splint with the elbow in 90 degrees of flexion and full supination.

AFTERTREATMENT. The cast is removed at 4 weeks, and active movements are begun.

Elbow Joint Fracture and Dislocations

RADIAL HEAD AND NECK FRACTURES

The ages of children with radial neck fractures usually fall between 4 and 14 years, primarily because ossification of the radial head usually does not begin before 5 years of age. The normal anatomical angulation of the radial neck in children has been erroneously diagnosed as a buckle fracture in this area. Most fractures in children are of the radial neck and not the radial head. Fractures of the epiphysis of the radial head are usually Salter-Harris type IV fractures. Most radial neck fractures occur through the metaphysis, but they can occur through the physis, with a metaphyseal spike of bone producing a characteristic Salter-Harris type II epiphyseal injury.

Numerous classifications of radial neck fractures have appeared, including those of Vostal, Newman, O'Brien, and Jeffery. Wilkins combined the classifications of Jeffery and Newman: type A, Salter-Harris types I and II injuries of the proximal radial epiphyses; type B, Salter-Harris type IV injuries of the proximal radial epiphyses; type C, fractures involving only the proximal radial metaphysis; type D,

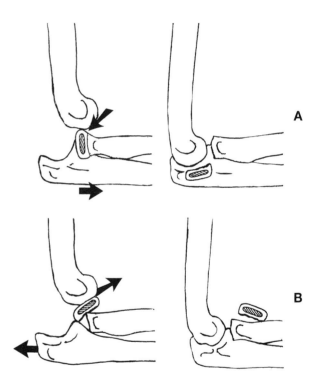

Fig. 33-37   **A,** Fracture occurring when elbow dislocation is reduced. **B,** Fractures occurring at time of elbow dislocation. (**A** from Jeffery CC: *J Bone Joint Surg* 32B:314, 1950; **B** from Newman JH: *Injury* 9:114, 1977.)

fractures occurring when a dislocated elbow is being reduced (Fig. 33-36); and type E, fractures occurring in conjunction with the elbow dislocation (Fig. 33-37). The fractures can be angulated, translocated (shifted), or totally displaced (Fig. 33-38). After dislocation of the elbow the proximal fragment can be loose in the joint, or it can be trapped, which prevents reduction (Fig. 33-39).

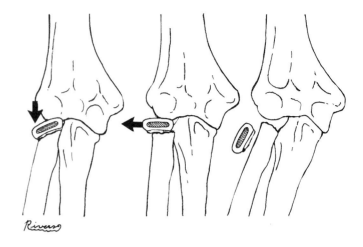

Fig. 33-38 Examples of angulation, translocation, and total displacement of radial neck fractures. (Redrawn from Wilkins KE. In Rockwood CA Jr, Wilkins KE, and King RE, eds: *Fractures in children*, Philadelphia, 1984, JB Lippincott.)

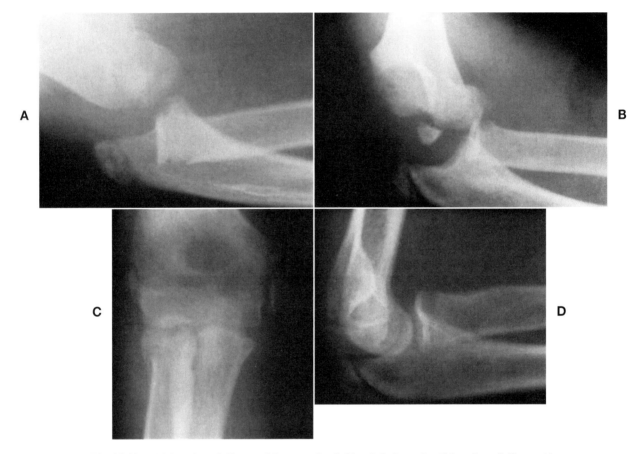

Fig. 33-39 Dislocation of elbow and fracture of radial head. **A,** Posterior dislocation of elbow with suggestion of osteochondral fragment from radial head fracture. **B,** Oblique roentgenogram showing loose fragments of radial head entrapped within joint. **C and D,** After open reduction and excision of loose fragment. Obvious ossification around both collateral ligaments and callus in area of radial head and neck are seen in **C.**

Between 30 and 45 degrees of residual angulation usually is accepted in closed treatment with satisfactory results. A significantly angulated radial head and neck fracture often can be reduced closed to an angle of less than 45 degrees. According to Tibone and Stoltz, results are not as good in older children with radial head and neck fractures or in children with other associated upper extremity injuries, usually on the medial aspect of the elbow. The best results are obtained if treatment is initiated early, and closed reduction to an acceptable position (30 to 45 degrees) is achieved. Steinberg et al. reported that severely displaced fractures had better results after open reduction, but moderately displaced fractures did just as well

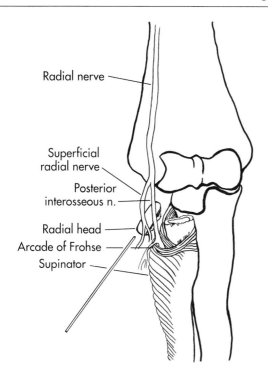

Fig. 33-40   Radial neck fracture in relation to arcade of Frohse. During percutaneous reduction, wire should be introduced on ulnar side of radius to avoid deep branch of radial nerve. (Redrawn from Bernstein SM, McKeever P, Bernstein L: *J Pediatr Orthop* 13:85, 1993.)

after closed treatment. From their data and review of the literature, they concluded that angulation of 30 degrees or less is compatible with a good result.

Pesudo et al. suggested using a percutaneous pin with the aid of an image intensifier to manipulate and reduce the angulation of the fracture fragments. Bernstein et al. reported satisfactory results in 15 patients using this technique (Fig. 33-40). Gonzalez-Herranz et al. treated 17 displaced radial neck fractures (O'Brien types II and III) in children between the ages of 6 and 16 years with closed intramedullary pinning according to the Metaizeau technique. This technique consists of inserting a curved steel Kirschner wire that is sharply bent at the last 1.5 cm through the distal radial metaphysis into the medullary canal. The wire is advanced until the point fixes in the epiphysis and then elevates and replaces it under the lateral condyle. The pin is turned around its long axis through 180 degrees, producing a medial shift of the radial head, thereby reducing it. Excellent results were observed in 94%. Overgrowth of the radial head was present in three patients without functional impairment. These authors recommend this closed method of treatment because it is simple, easy to perform, and has few complications.

If a satisfactory closed reduction cannot be obtained, then open reduction should be carried out for any angulation greater than 45 degrees. Surgery should be performed within 5 to 7 days of injury in an effort to prevent myositis ossificans of the elbow, which seems to occur more often after delayed surgical treatment. We routinely use a lateral incision (Technique 1-88)

and have found that internal fixation is necessary; sutures in the periosteum are not adequate internal fixation. One or more oblique pins can be inserted across the fracture fragments, although this is technically difficult. A large transcapitellar wire, which is technically easier to insert, also can be used; however, the parents should be warned of possible intraarticular breakage of the wire or infection. Merchan reported that in 36 children with transarticular internal fixation of radial head and neck fractures, the Kirschner wires bent in 4 and broke at the joint in 2. Fowles and Kassab reported 23 radial neck fractures; 15 with angulation of more than 60 degrees were treated by open reduction and internal fixation with transarticular Kirschner wires through the humerus and radius. Because the Kirschner wires broke at the joint in two patients, they recommended avoiding the humerus by inserting the wires obliquely. Their worst results were in children with other injuries of the same elbow treated by open reduction, but they attributed this to the severity of the injury rather than to the surgery itself. Contrary to our experience Wedge and Robertson noted that open reduction without internal fixation produced equally good results as open reduction with internal fixation. The complications after open reduction include loss of motion, premature physeal closure, nonunion of the radial neck, avascular necrosis of the radial head, radioulnar synostosis, and myositis ossificans, as well as possible injury to the posterior interosseous nerve. If no treatment is carried out and the angulation is greater than 45 degrees, pronation and supination may be limited significantly. If this is a problem after skeletal maturity, the radial head can be excised. Before skeletal maturity is reached, radial head resection may result in proximal radioulnar synostosis, cubitus valgus, and radial deviation of the hand.

◆ Closed and Open Reduction of Radial Neck Fractures

TECHNIQUE 33-6

Use a general anesthetic. Place the patient supine and apply straight longitudinal traction. Use the manipulative technique as described by Patterson. Have an assistant hold the arm proximally, with one hand placed medially against the distal humerus, and apply straight longitudinal distal traction. Then apply a varus force to the forearm and digital pressure directly over the tilted radial head to complete the reduction. Hold the forearm in 90 degrees of flexion and in pronation (Fig. 33-41).

If this manipulation reduction is unsuccessful, the technique described by Pesudo et al. and Bernstein et al. can be tried. Have the assistant hold the arm with the shoulder abducted to 90 degrees and the forearm held in supination. With the use of an image intensifier and in a sterile operating field, introduce a Kirschner wire through the skin on the radial side of the elbow down to the angulated and displaced radial head and neck. Bernstein et al. suggest introducing the

continued

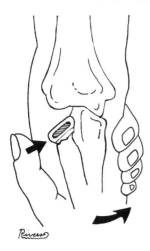

Fig. 33-41   Mechanism of reduction of radial neck fracture (see text). (Redrawn from Ogden JA: *Skeletal injury in the child*, Philadelphia, 1982, Lea & Febiger.)

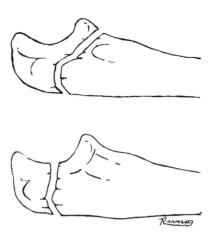

Fig. 33-42   Two types of olecranon physeal fractures. Regardless of type, if displacement is significant, open reduction and internal fixation are probably indicated. (Redrawn from Wilkins KE: Fractures and dislocations of the elbow region. In Rockwood CA Jr, Wilkins KE, King RE, eds: *Fractures in children*, Philadelphia, 1984, JB Lippincott.)

wire on the ulnar side of the radius to avoid the arcade of Frohse, which the deep branch of the radial nerve traverses (see Fig. 33-40). Disimpact and push the radial head into anatomical position with the Kirschner wire. Remove the wire and flex the elbow to 90 degrees. Apply a cast in the neutral position and leave it on for 4 to 6 weeks.

If these maneuvers are unsuccessful in reducing the fracture to less than 45 degrees of angulation, prepare for an open reduction. After preparing and draping the patient in the usual fashion, approach the dislocation through a Boyd approach (Technique 1-96). Remove any debris or torn annular ligament. Reduce the fracture gently. Secure the fixation with small Kirschner wires placed obliquely across fracture into the proximal radius. If this is impossible, then use a large transcapitellar pin across the joint and through the fracture site. If the annular ligament is torn, repair it. Close the incision in the standard fashion, holding the forearm in neutral rotation or in pronation and the elbow in 90 degrees of flexion, and apply a long arm cast.

AFTERTREATMENT. The pins are removed at approximately 3 to 6 weeks, but the cast is continued for 6 to 8 weeks because of the possibility of delayed union.

OLECRANON FRACTURES

Pure physeal fractures of the olecranon are extremely rare and are confusing because of the complexity of the secondary ossification centers of the proximal ulna. The epiphysis fuses to the metaphysis at about age 14. However, a sclerotic margin at the site of fusion may persist through adulthood and may be mistaken for a fracture. Two types of physeal fracture patterns were noted by Grantham and Kiernan and Wilkins (Fig. 33-42). The first type is purely physeal; the second type occurs in older

children and has a large metaphyseal fragment attached to the epiphysis. Papavasiliou et al. classified isolated fractures of the olecranon in children as intraarticular (group A) and extraarticular (group B). Included in the intraarticular fractures are simple crack fractures, fractures with minimal displacement, complete fractures of the olecranon involving the articular cartilage and with slight dorsal displacement of the proximal fragment, and grossly displaced fractures. A greenstick fracture is the only extraarticular fracture. They found that the fractures tended to be displaced in older children but not in young children, which they attributed to the thicker articular cartilage in younger children. Graves and Canale classified 44 olecranon fractures in children as those with less than 5 mm of displacement, those with more than 5 mm of displacement, and open fractures. Evans and Graham devised a classification and management algorithm that is extensive but complex and is in agreement with Schoenecker's. If displacement, especially intraarticular, is more than 3 to 4 mm, then open reduction and internal fixation are indicated (Box 33-1).

Regardless of the type of fracture, if significant displacement persists after attempts at closed reduction, open reduction and internal fixation with tension band wiring should be performed as in adult fractures (Technique 54-13). Matthews recommended open reduction and fixation for displacement of 4 mm or more, and Wilkins recommended palpation of the defect in the olecranon or flexion of the elbow to determine stability; if either suggests instability, he recommended open reduction and internal fixation with tension band wires secured over axial pins. Of the 15 isolated olecranon fractures in the series of Papavasiliou et al., 10 minimally displaced fractures were treated conservatively with excellent results, 4 grossly displaced fractures were treated operatively with some loss of extension, and 1 untreated fracture resulted in some loss of

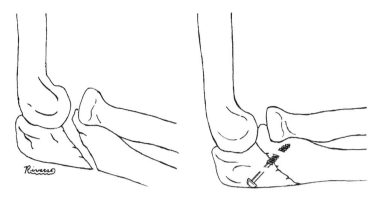

Fig. 33-43 Metaphyseal intraarticular olecranon fracture that is unstable and requires open reduction and internal fixation, here with oblique screw. (Redrawn from Wilkins KE: Fractures and dislocations of the elbow region. In Rockwood CA Jr, Wilkins KE, King RE, eds: *Fractures in children*, Philadelphia, 1984, JB Lippincott.)

> **BOX 33-1 • Classification of Olecranon Fractures in Children**
>
> A. Anatomic site
>   1. Epiphyseal (apophyseal)
>   a. Extraarticular, olecranon-tip fracture
>   b. Intraarticular
>   2. Physeal (Harris-Salter equivalents)
>   3. Metaphyseal
>   a. Juxtaphyseal
>   b. True metaphyseal
>   4. Combined olecranon-coronoid process injury
> B. Fracture configuration (angulation of the fracture line to the long axis of the ulna in degrees)
>   1. Transverse (<30 degrees)
>   2. Oblique (30-60 degrees)
>   3. Longitudinal (>60 degrees)
> C. Intraarticular displacement
>   1. <2 mm displacement
>   2. 2-4 mm displacement
>   3. >4 mm displacement
> D. Associated injuries (ipsilateral elbow and upper limb)
>   1. Radial head/neck fracture
>   2. Radial head dislocation/subluxation (Monteggia variant)
>   3. Lateral humeral condylar physeal injury
>   4. Medial humeral condylar physeal injury
>   5. Supracondylar humeral fracture
>   6. Distal radial/ulnar fracture

From Evans MC, Graham HK: *J Pediatric Orthop* 19:559, 1999.

extension and flexion. In the 44 olecranon fractures reviewed by Graves and Canale, fractures with less than 5 mm of displacement were treated with a posterior plaster splint or long arm cast until the fracture was not tender, then with a collar and cuff for 3 to 4 weeks; good results were obtained in 28 of 30 patients. Of 9 fractures with more than 5 mm of displacement treated with open reduction and tension band wiring, with or without axial fixation, or with interfragmentary screw fixation, 7 had satisfactory results. Two open fractures treated with surgical debridement and irrigation and internal fixation had good results. They noted no growth abnormalities of the olecranon apophysis, regardless of the type of fracture. The primary cause of unsatisfactory results in their patients was loss of motion in both flexion and extension.

Metaphyseal fractures occur from either flexion or extension injuries. The extension injuries usually are associated with a valgus component following a shearing injury pattern, as described by Wilkins and others. Regardless of type, if the fracture is stable after closed reduction, surgery rarely is necessary. However, if the reduction is unstable and the fracture is intraarticular, open reduction and internal fixation with axial pins, tension band wires, or oblique screws may be necessary (Figs. 33-43 and 33-44). Techniques for open reduction and internal fixation of olecranon fractures are described in Chapter 54.

FRACTURES OF CORONOID PROCESS

Regan and Morrey classified fractures of the coronoid process as type I, a small chip fracture; type II, a fracture involving less than 50% of the process; and type III, a fracture involving more than 50% of the process (Fig. 33-45). They recommended closed treatment for types I and II fractures and open reduction and internal fixation for type III fractures if possible.

ELBOW DISLOCATIONS
Acute Dislocations

Dislocation of the elbow in children is rare. Blount cited an incidence of 6% of all children's fractures and dislocations involving the elbow. Wilkins reviewed three large series of traumatic dislocations of the elbow in all age groups, those of Linscheid and Wheeler, of Neviaser and Wickstrom, and of Roberts, and noted that 29% of the dislocations occurred between the ages of 10 and 20 years and 18% occurred before the age of 10, with the youngest patient being 4 years old. Thus approximately half of all elbow dislocations occur in people younger than 20 years old.

Most pure dislocations are posterior, but they can occur anteriorly, medially, or laterally. Rare proximal radioulnar joint disruption (divergent dislocation) can occur either in the anteroposterior plane or the medial transverse plane. Regardless of the type, most elbow dislocations can be reduced closed. The primary indications for open reduction are the inability to obtain a closed reduction and an open dislocation. If an open reduction of a closed dislocation is necessary, it is probably

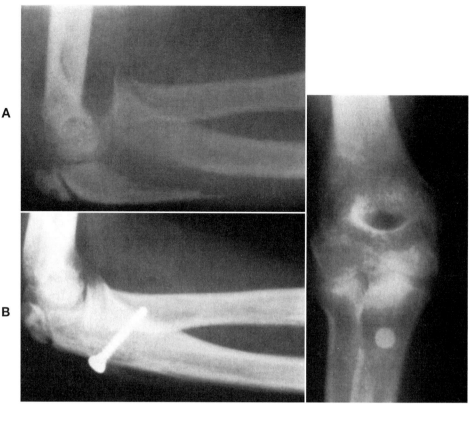

Fig. 33-44 Shearing intraarticular metaphyseal olecranon fracture, with displacement and instability. **A,** Before treatment. **B** and **C,** After open reduction and internal fixation with oblique cancellous screw.

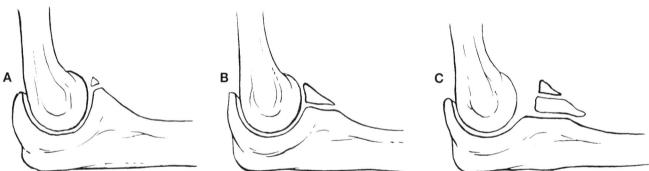

Fig. 33-45 Classification of coronoid fractures: **A,** Type I, small fragment avulsion. **B,** Type II, involvement of less than 50% of coronoid process. **C,** Type III, involvement of more than 50% of coronoid process. (From Regan W, Morrey BF: *Orthopedics* 15:845, 1992.)

because of a fracture, most commonly of the medial epicondyle or radial neck. Open dislocations usually have arterial injuries that also require surgery. Once the reduction is achieved, the dislocation usually is stable but the elbow should be immobilized for approximately 6 weeks. Wilkins noted a complication rate of 11% in the previously noted series. The complications included involvement of all three major nerves about the elbow. As noted by Hallet, the median nerve can become trapped and block reduction. Arterial injuries can occur, especially in open dislocations, as well as myositis ossificans, recurrent dislocations, osteochondral fractures, and a rare iatrogenic proximal radioulnar translocation after reduction.

Chronic Recurrent Elbow Dislocations

Recurrent dislocations, although rare, do occur, most often in adolescents. We have seen several patients with chronic recurrent dislocations that were worrisome because of a lack of understanding of the pathological condition. Four primary underlying causes of recurrent dislocation of the elbow have been suggested in the literature: (1) a shallow trochlear notch that allows easy dislocation of the olecranon from the trochlea; (2) capsular laxity of the elbow, either medial, lateral, or combined; (3) intraarticular fractures that cause instability of the olecranon in the trochlea, either medial or lateral; and (4) congenital laxity of the medial and lateral ligaments about the elbow. Often the cause consists of a combination of two or more of these conditions.

A thorough evaluation of the specific pathological condition is mandatory and should include (1) anteroposterior and lateral roentgenograms of both elbows for comparison, with special attention to any dysplasia of the distal humerus, particularly a shallow trochlear notch (any osseous loose bodies or articular fractures also can be noted); (2) varus and valgus stress roentgenograms of both elbows to determine any medial or lateral ligamentous instability; (3) arthrogram, which may be helpful in patients with a suspected intraarticular condylar fracture or loose body; and (4) fluoroscopic examination during surgery. Arthroscopy of the elbow also has been performed to evaluate elbow instability.

The surgical procedure should be selected to correct the specific condition. If plain roentgenograms reveal a shallow trochlear notch and stress roentgenograms and arthrograms are normal, transfer of the biceps or triceps tendon or both is appropriate. Reichenheim transferred the biceps tendon into the coracoid process of the ulna, suturing it to the periosteum on the anterior aspect of the coronoid process with two smooth wires. King modified Reichenheim's technique by passing the tendon through a drill hole in the coronoid to the subcutaneous border of the ulna, where it was sutured. Kapel formed a "cruciate" ligament by threading a strip of biceps tendon through a drill hole in the small partition of bone separating the coronoid and olecranon fossae and suturing it to the tip of the olecranon; a central slip of triceps tendon was pulled through the same hole and sutured to the coronoid process.

If stress roentgenograms reveal significant ligamentous laxity, capsular repair and imbrication are appropriate. For medial and lateral laxity, Osborne and Cotterill performed posterolateral repair by making transverse holes through the lateral condyle, placing sutures through the holes and the posterolateral part of the capsule, and fixing the capsule tightly to the bone; when needed, the medial aspect of the capsule was similarly repaired. For laxity isolated to the medial aspect, Schwab et al. advanced the medial collateral ligament and medial epicondyle posteriorly and fixed the epicondyle to the humerus with a screw. For isolated lateral laxity, Hassmann et al. removed the cortex of the lateral epicondylar area, made drill holes through the lateral epicondyle, and passed sutures through the holes and reattached the shortened capsuloligamentous structures.

If a roentgenogram or arthrogram reveals an intraarticular pathological condition, this must be evaluated at the time of capsular and ligamentous reconstruction. Medial or lateral arthrotomy, or both, may be required to remove loose bodies or to repair large osteochondral fractures.

Hassmann et al., Osborne and Cotterill, Symeonides et al., and Trias and Comeau believe that posterolateral instability is the most common posttraumatic lesion. Their procedures include soft tissue repair and reconstruction on the lateral side of the elbow, reinforcement of this area, and reattachment of the lateral collateral ligament. However, as noted by Herring and Sullivan, it is important to document the type of dislocation,

because a lateral reconstruction may cause only further dislocations if the dislocation is other than lateral. Other techniques of reconstruction for treatment of recurrent dislocations of the elbow are described in Chapter 45.

Old Unreduced Elbow Dislocations

Speed, at this clinic, noted that when dislocations of the elbow remained unreduced for 3 months or longer, a satisfactory functional result could still be obtained by an open reduction, and the results were better than after extensive arthroplasty procedures in immature patients. Fowles et al. reported 15 children with untreated posterior dislocations of the elbow; 3 had a satisfactory painless range of motion, whereas 12 had stiff elbows and were treated operatively between 3 weeks and 3 years after injury. Of these 12 patients, 11 had improved motion, but 1 had a rigid myositis ossificans. Fowles et al. recommended operative reduction as late as 3 years after injury, asserting that open reduction is always worth trying in a child. They recommended an interval of conservative treatment for those seen from 3 weeks to 2 months after dislocation. Initially, they used a lateral incision, but in their last nine patients they used the Speed technique and a posterior approach (Campbell) and found it superior for exposure and the ability to use the Speed V-Y muscle-plasty (Technique 58-15).

The technique used by Speed for persistent chronic (old) dislocations of the elbow in adults is described in Technique 58-15.

◆ Open Reduction of Untreated (Chronic) Posterior Dislocation of Elbow in Children

TECHNIQUE 33-7 *(Fowles et al.)*
Expose the elbow posteriorly through a Campbell posterolateral approach (Technique 1-85). Free subperiosteally all muscle attachments from the distal humerus, both anteriorly and posteriorly. Release the attachments of the joint capsule around the humeral condyles. Expose the joint circumferentially and detach the collateral ligaments from their proximal insertions. A fibrous ankylosis forms in most patients with the elbow in 30 to 60 degrees of flexion, and old articular fractures may be obscured by fibrous tissue within the joint. Release the thick, fibrotic, contracted capsule and resect portions as necessary. Remove all the fibrous tissue from the joint, taking care to protect the underlying cartilage. Excise scar tissue carefully because it is often difficult to distinguish firm white scar from normal articular cartilage. Also remove subperiosteal new bone when it is an obstacle to reduction of the dislocation. If the triceps is tight, preventing reduction or limiting flexion to about 30 degrees after reduction, lengthen the muscle using Speed's V-Y muscle-plasty (see Technique 58-15). Gently reduce the elbow. If the reduction is still difficult, release further the soft tissues proximally around the humerus and distally from the olecranon and the annular ligament until

continued

the elbow can be reduced without force. Do not reattach the ligaments to bone to avoid making the repair too tight. If the ulnar nerve is tight or was compressed preoperatively, then transpose it anteriorly. Check the stability of the reduction manually at 90 degrees of flexion. If the joint redislocates easily, insert one or two Kirschner wires through the olecranon and into the humerus with the elbow flexed to 70 degrees. Close the wound and apply a long arm cast with the forearm in neutral rotation.

AFTERTREATMENT. The cast and any Kirschner wires are removed at 2 to 3 weeks. Active mobilization of the elbow is started slowly and is encouraged.

DISTAL HUMERAL FRACTURES

Fractures of the distal humerus in children are most often supracondylar or involve a single condyle. Certain features are common to all condylar fractures. First, the roentgenograms may be misleading because (1) the fragment consists mainly of cartilage; (2) in an immature child the fragment seems smaller than it actually is; and (3) the displacement, although it is indeed pronounced, may not seem appreciable. Second, strong flexor and extensor muscle groups attached to the separated medial and lateral condyles, respectively, often rotate and displace the involved condyle by their pull. Even if closed reduction is possible, this rotational pull on the fragment frequently redisplaces the fragment after closed reduction. Third, although free access to the fracture is obtained at surgery, accurate fitting of the fracture surfaces and the physis may be difficult. Fourth, after reduction the need for some type of internal fixation is easily demonstrated if the attached muscles are placed under slight tension; the gentlest traction will displace the fragment. Fifth, after internal fixation, the smooth Kirschner wires usually should be removed at 4 to 6 weeks. Although in theory pins crossing the physis may cause growth disturbance, this is rare; here as elsewhere it is sometimes necessary for the pins to pass through the physis.

Boyd and Altenberg studied fractures of the elbow in children seen at this clinic: 713 fractures in patients 12 years of age or younger, distributed as indicated in Table 33-1. Supracondylar fractures occurred most often (about 65%); condylar fractures occurred in about 25% of the children.

Because the fragment consists mainly of cartilage, roentgenograms may be misleading; the fragment may appear smaller than its actual size and even significant displacement may not be appreciated.

Skaggs and Mirzayan noted in a prospective study that 76% of children with a posterior fat pad sign ultimately had a fracture. Of the 45 patients, 34 had a supracondylar fracture of the humerus; 9 (26%) had a fracture of the proximal part of the ulna; 4 (12%) had a fracture of the lateral condyle; and 3 (9%) had a fracture of the radial neck. Their results support the practice of treating children who have a history of trauma to the elbow and an elevated posterior fat pad but no other

▷ **Table 33-1** Elbow Fractures in Children

	No. Cases	Percentage
Supracondylar fractures	465	65.4
Condylar fractures		25.3
Lateral condyle	124	
Medial epicondyle	33	
Medial condyle	23	
Fractures of neck of radius	34	4.7
Monteggia fractures	16	2.2
Olecranon fractures	12	1.6
T-condylar fractures	6	0.8
Total	713	100.0

roentgenographic evidence of fracture as if they have a non-displaced fracture about the elbow.

Arthrography has been suggested as a means of determining injury patterns before complete ossification of the elbow. Hansen et al. concluded that arthrographic examination to outline the cartilaginous structures about the distal humerus may be the most satisfactory nonoperative means of establishing the correct diagnosis and providing proper treatment of elbow injuries in children. Yates and Sullivan found that after arthrogram the original diagnosis and treatment were altered in almost 20% of their patients. The injury pattern most often misdiagnosed was the lateral condylar fracture. They believe arthrography is especially useful in condylar fractures and periarticular fractures in which anatomical alignment cannot be determined from plain roentgenograms, but they note that the need for arthrography should be infrequent when proper roentgenograms, including comparison views of the opposite elbow, are obtained. Ultrasonography and MRI may make the "invasive" arthrogram unnecessary.

Failure to diagnose and treat fractures of the distal humerus adequately in children can result in severe complications:

1. *Nonunion:* This is most common after single condylar fractures.
2. *Malunion:* Disturbances in the carrying angle of the elbow may result from either nonunion or physeal growth disturbance. Cubitus varus deformity after supracondylar fractures most frequently results from malunion. Increase in carrying angle or cubitus valgus deformity is more common after lateral condylar fractures and results predominantly from nonunion.
3. *Physeal growth disturbances:* This is most often the result of a Salter-Harris type III or IV physeal injury and can lead to either cubitus varus or cubitus valgus.
4. *Avascular necrosis of the condyle:* This complication is relatively rare, but when it does occur it may cause a slowly progressive cubitus varus or valgus deformity.
5. *Acute neurocirculatory compromise:* Acute compromise of either the neural or circulatory status in the extremity is not uncommon after fractures about the elbow in children. Fortunately, most compromises are transient and lead to no permanent complications when adequate

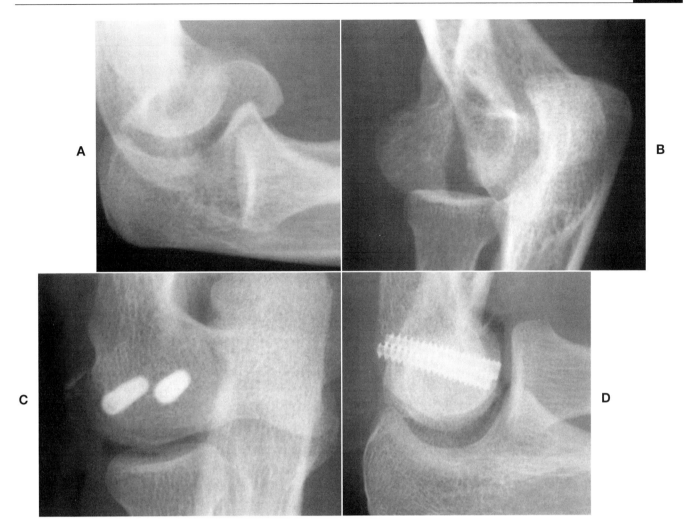

Fig. 33-46   **A** and **B,** Lateral and oblique roentgenograms revealing displaced capitellar fracture in 16-year-old. **C** and **D,** Anteroposterior and lateral roentgenograms after open reduction and internal fixation with Acuflex screws.

treatment is instituted immediately. The most serious of all vascular complications about the elbow is a Volkmann contracture (Chapter 71), which results in an ugly deformity that often renders the hand and forearm practically useless.

Oh et al. noted residual cubitus varus in 7 of 12 patients younger than the age of 3 years who had separation of the distal humeral epiphysis; 6 of the 7 had varying degrees of avascular necrosis. Although they recommended percutaneous fixation, they noted that avascular necrosis occurred in younger children regardless of the type of treatment.

Damage to nerves and impairment of circulation should be suspected in all fractures of the elbow in children. The surgeon is spared embarrassment by discovering such injuries before rather than after treatment; this is especially true for supracondylar fractures. If no examination is performed, a medicolegal dilemma can result when neurovascular function is recorded as being normal preoperatively and then becomes abnormal postoperatively. If the patient can bend the fingers with the metacarpophalangeal joints extended and can appose the thumb to the little finger, the three major nerve trunks are intact. The sensory distribution of these nerves also should be tested. When the circulation is impaired, the radial pulse is diminished or absent, the capillary circulation is sluggish, and swelling, cyanosis, and paresthesia or anesthesia of the hand and fingers occur. Testing of the nerves and vessels should be repeated after treatment. Close and frequent observation of the neurocirculatory status in the hand is important in aftertreatment, and any impairment requires immediate attention.

CAPITELLAR FRACTURES

Although fractures of the capitellum are rare, especially in children, they can significantly limit elbow motion and cause disability if they remain undiagnosed. Type I fractures of the capitellum consist of a large fragment of cancellous bone and possibly part of the trochlea; type II fractures usually are cartilaginous and may include a small fragment of subchondral bone; and type III are comminuted fractures (Fig. 33-46). Treatment has included closed reduction, open reduction and internal fixation, and excision of the fragment. Letts et al. reported excellent results in five of six children who had accurate open reduction and internal fixation of type I capitellar fractures. Internal fixation methods included Kirschner wires, Herbert screws, or cannulated screws. One patient required a reoperation to remove an exostosis block to flexion.

LATERAL CONDYLAR FRACTURES

Fractures of the lateral condyle of the humerus are quite common and occur at approximately the age of 6 years. In fact, they are the most common distal humeral epiphyseal fracture. They are more common than those of the medial epicondyle, the medial condyle, or the fracture-separation of the entire distal epiphysis. Milch described two basic types of lateral condylar fractures. In the type I fracture, the fracture line courses medially to the trochlea through and into the capitellar-trochlear groove. This type I fracture is rare; however, because of the location of the fracture line it is a true Salter-Harris type IV fracture but is frequently stable (Fig. 33-47). Roentgenograms usually reveal a small, wafer-shaped bony metaphyseal fragment, and stress roentgenograms are valuable in noting any motion at the fracture site, implying instability. In the type II fracture described by Milch, which is more common, the fracture line extends into the area of the

trochlea and produces inherent instability of the elbow because of the ability of the distal fragment and the forearm not only to angulate but to translate into a lateral position. It has been argued that this Milch type II fracture is in reality a Salter-Harris type II fracture rather than, as traditionally thought, a Salter-Harris type IV injury. Lateral condylar fractures also have been classified according to the amount of displacement: (1) undisplaced, (2) moderately displaced, and (3) completely displaced and rotated (Fig. 33-48). Roentgenographic classifications have been proposed by Badelon et al. and Finnbogason et al. Finnbogason et al. described roentgenographic criteria for determining fracture stability, which they used in planning the initial treatment (Fig. 33-49): type A, fracture through the lateral humeral condyle with minimal lateral gap—a stable fracture; type B, fracture through the lateral humeral condyle to the epiphyseal cartilage with a lateral gap—a fracture with undefinable risk; type C, fracture through the lateral humeral condyle with the fracture gap as wide laterally as medially—a fracture with high risk of later displacement.

Sometimes it is difficult to determine the amount of displacement, if any; when doubt exists, the fracture should be treated as displaced. We have seen what was believed to be a benign nondisplaced fracture that, 1 week after casting, became completely displaced and required open reduction and internal fixation. Speed and Boyd repeatedly noted that these fractures are notorious for complications, with the worst being that of nonunion with subsequent migration proximally of the nonunited fragment, an increase in the carrying angle (cubitus valgus), and tardy ulnar nerve palsy (Fig. 33-50). Speed, in reviewing his results, found them to be so unsatisfactory after closed treatment that open reduction and internal fixation were necessary; thus the term, "the fracture of necessity." Others believe that if the fracture is nondisplaced (Milch type I with inherent stability), only cast immobilization is necessary. However, if this treatment is used, close observation every 5 to 7 days is necessary. Further, good roentgenograms out of plaster should be made at each visit to determine the status of the fracture. This may require considerable time and effort, and open reduction and internal fixation may be preferable. As mentioned previously, if the fracture is displaced and rotated, open reduction and internal fixation always are required.

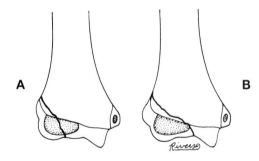

Fig. 33-47 Lateral humeral condylar fractures. **A,** Milch type I fracture, which is a Salter-Harris type IV epiphyseal fracture. **B,** Milch type II fracture, which is a Salter-Harris type II epiphyseal fracture. (Redrawn from Milch H: *J Trauma* 4:592, 1964.)

Fig. 33-48 Different stages of displacement of lateral condylar fracture: undisplaced, moderately displaced, and completely displaced and rotated. (Redrawn from Jakob R, Fowles JV, Rang M, Kassab MT: *J Bone Joint Surg* 57B:430, 1975.)

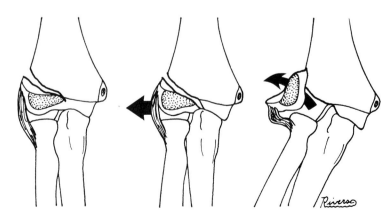

Beaty and Wood reviewed the results of treatment at this clinic, from 1944 through 1983 in 53 children who returned for long-term evaluation. Of these, 75% had open reduction and internal fixation and 25% had closed cast treatment. All 32 patients who were treated initially by open reduction and internal fixation achieved union; in this group, 2 patients developed avascular necrosis of the capitellum, and 4 had trochlear physeal arrest (Fig. 33-51). There were no deep infections. Of 14 patients initially treated by closed methods, nonunions developed in 4. Also 5 nonunions were seen at

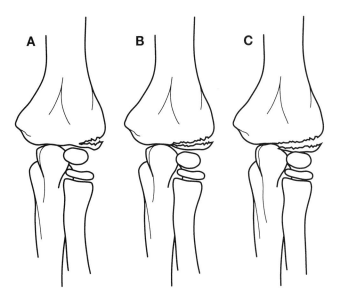

Fig. 33-49 **A,** Fracture through lateral humeral condyle with minimal lateral gap. **B,** Fracture through lateral humeral condyle to epiphyseal cartilage with lateral gap. **C,** Fracture through lateral humeral condyle with fracture gap as wide laterally as medially, a fracture with high risk of later displacement. (Redrawn from Finnbogason T, Karlsson G, Lindberg L, Mortensson W: *J Pediatr Orthop* 15:422, 1995.)

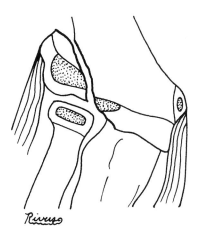

Fig. 33-50 Nonunion of lateral condyle with fragment migrating proximally, producing cubitus valgus deformity and possible tardy ulnar nerve palsy. (Redrawn from Ogden JA: *Skeletal injury in the child*, Philadelphia, 1982, Lea & Febiger.)

long-term follow-up; 1 had a failure of closed treatment as mentioned above, and 4 were unrecognized and untreated fractures. All had cubitus valgus deformity and weakness with loss of elbow motion and occasional pain; 3 had tardy ulnar nerve palsy.

From these results, it is obvious that open reduction and internal fixation are necessary for displaced fractures; the proper treatment of nondisplaced fractures is the problem. As noted in this series, some nondisplaced fractures will heal uneventfully. Beaty and Wood used varus and valgus stress roentgenograms to determine if the fracture was stable and had an intact cartilaginous hinge. If displacement occurs when the fracture is stressed, then the hinge probably is not intact and the fracture is unstable; therefore open reduction and internal fixation are indicated. Conversely, if no displacement occurs when the fracture is stressed, cast immobilization alone may be justified. Beaty and Wood recommended observing these patients extremely closely with serial casting and roentgenograms for 6 to 8 weeks.

Mintzer et al. reported 12 children who had lateral condylar fractures of the distal humerus with less than 2 mm of displacement. Intraoperative arthrograms of each elbow demonstrated no articular incongruity associated with minimal rotation of the distal fracture fragment. Closed reduction was performed, and these fractures were pinned percutaneously with the aid of image intensification, eliminating the need for open reduction and internal fixation. Their results were uniformly excellent. They recommended percutaneous pinning for lateral condylar fractures with less than 2 mm of displacement and congruent joint surfaces.

Kamegaya et al. studied 12 children who had minimally displaced lateral humeral condyle fractures. To determine the stability, they used MRI to study the distal humerus and elbow joint. Two types of fractures were identified: types I and II. In type I the fracture line coursed from the lateral metaphysis to the physis but not through it. In type II the line crossed the physis to enter the joint space. They concluded that MRI distinguishes the potentially unstable fracture (type II) from the stable, minimally displaced fracture (type I). They recommended percutaneous pin fixation for unstable, displaced fractures.

If open reduction is necessary, we use routinely a lateral approach, replacing the fragment without significant dissection and fixing it internally with pins or screws. Different authors have suggested various forms of fixation, including (1) suture fixation, which is inadequate; (2) smooth pin fixation, preferably with two pins, either through the epiphysis or through the metaphyseal spike; and (3) screw fixation, preferably through the metaphyseal area. However, Conner and Smith used a Glasgow screw through the physis and through the epiphysis and did not notice any growth disturbance (Fig. 33-52). Speed noted that screws could be put through the physis, and he had little difficulty with cubitus valgus resulting from premature closure in his patients.

Significant complications can develop from this injury, as mentioned previously; the worst of these probably is a

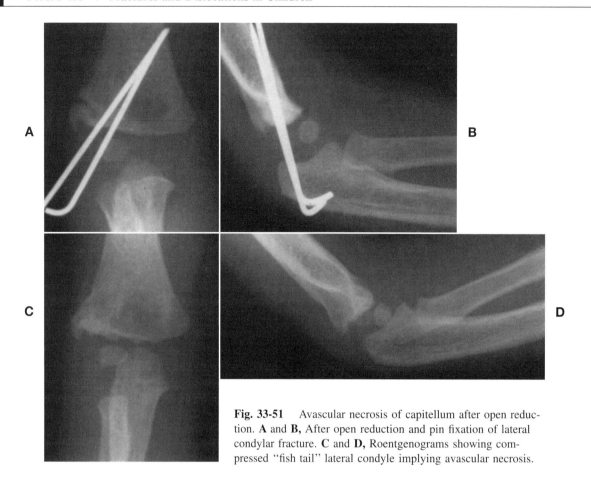

Fig. 33-51   Avascular necrosis of capitellum after open reduction. **A** and **B,** After open reduction and pin fixation of lateral condylar fracture. **C** and **D,** Roentgenograms showing compressed "fish tail" lateral condyle implying avascular necrosis.

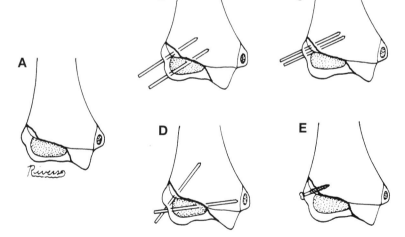

Fig. 33-52   Different methods of fixation of lateral condylar fractures. **A,** Fracture pattern. **B,** Parallel pins. **C,** Parallel pins through metaphysis only. **D,** Cross pin fixation. **E,** Cancellous screw fixation. (Redrawn from Wadsworth TG: *Clin Orthop* 85:127, 1972.)

nonunion with resultant cubitus valgus. Nonunion must be differentiated from delayed union. Flynn and Richards noted that immobilization of the fracture even with minimal displacement for at least 12 weeks often is necessary. Others have noted delay in union resulting from external immobilization or inadequate internal fixation. If union is not achieved at 12 weeks, Flynn and Richards suggested using a small wedge-shaped bone graft across the metaphyseal fragment with or without supplemental smooth pin fixation. Jeffery used bone grafting with supplemental screw fixation. Some believe that if

the elbow appears to be stable and is not painful, and all that is present is a lucent line with no motion of the fracture fragment on stress views, then observation and prolonged immobilization may be all that are necessary. However, if motion is present or a nonunion appears to be developing, then early operation as suggested by Flynn and Richards or Jeffery is indicated. Beaty and Wood described five condylar fractures treated late by surgery for delayed union, the latest treatment being 2 years after the fracture. All five fractures ultimately united. Internal fixation was used in each, but bone grafts were applied in only one. In late surgery for nonunion, (1) the surgeon should be experienced in children's elbow surgery, (2) the amount of displacement should be 1 cm or less, and (3) the nonunion should be compressed and not widely exposed at surgery.

◆ **Open Reduction and Internal Fixation**

TECHNIQUE 33-8

Expose the elbow through a Kocher lateral J approach (Fig. 1-108). Carry the dissection down to the lateral humeral condyle. Expose both posterior and anterior surfaces of the joint by separating the fibers of the common extensor muscle mass. Limit soft tissue detachment to only that necessary to expose the fragment, the fracture, and the joint. The displacement and the size of the fragment are always greater than is apparent on the roentgenograms, since much of the fragment is cartilaginous. The fragment usually is rotated as well as displaced. Irrigate the joint to remove blood clots and debris, reduce the articular surface accurately, and confirm the reduction by observing the articular surface, particularly at the trochlear ridge. Hold the position with a small tenaculum, bone holder, or towel clip. If a large metaphyseal fragment is present, insert two smooth Kirschner wires across it into the medial portion of the metaphysis; if necessary for secure fixation, insert the wires across the physis. If the epiphyseal portion is small, insert two smooth Kirschner wires across the condyle, across the physis, and into the humeral metaphysis. Direct the wires at an angle of 45 to 60 degrees; check the reduction and the position of the internal fixation by roentgenograms before closing the wound. Cut off the ends of the wires beneath the skin, but leave them long enough to allow easy removal (Fig. 33-53). Place the arm in a posterior plaster splint with the elbow flexed 90 degrees.

AFTERTREATMENT. Immobilization should continue for approximately 6 weeks. At the end of that time the pins can be removed if union is progressing. Gentle active motion of the elbow is then usually resumed intermittently out of the splint. The splint is not removed permanently until the roentgenograms show solid union. These fractures are notorious for late and delayed union (Flynn et al.), and some require immobilization with intermittent range-of-motion exercises for as long as 12 weeks.

◆ **Open Reduction and Internal Fixation with Bone Grafting for Nonunion or Delayed Union of Minimally Displaced Fractures**

Flynn described open reduction and internal fixation with bone grafting for early established nonunion of the lateral condyle. He noted that function will be satisfactory after surgery if the segment is in an acceptable position (Fig. 33-54, *A*) and the physis of the condylar fragment is open.

TECHNIQUE 33-9 *(Flynn et al.; Jeffery)*

Expose the fracture as described for open reduction. Limit soft tissue dissection to only that necessary to expose the fragment and the nonunion. Through the distal limb of the incision, expose the proximal ulna and take from it a "peg" bone graft 5 mm wide × 2.5 to 3 cm long, depending on the age of the child and the size of the lateral condylar fragment. Expose the fragment carefully but do not disturb the fibrous union. Do not attempt to freshen the fracture fragments. Identify the physis, either visually or roentgenographically, but do not disturb it. Drill a hole for the peg graft through the metaphyseal portion of the condylar fragment and into the metaphysis of the proximal fragment (Fig. 33-54, *B*), taking special care to avoid the physis. Insert the peg graft into the hole and impact it soundly across the fibrous union. If desired, use an iliac cancellous bone graft instead (Jeffery). Insert a heavy pin, cancellous screw, or cannulated screw adjacent to the graft. If the fragment is small, the fixation may, by necessity, have to cross the physis. Try to draw the condylar fragment firmly against the metaphysis. Penetration of the opposite cortex of the humerus may be necessary.

AFTERTREATMENT. The limb is immobilized in plaster with the elbow at 90 degrees of flexion and the forearm in neutral rotation for 12 weeks. The pin or screw can then be removed, and active exercises are begun.

ESTABLISHED NONUNION WITH CUBITUS VALGUS

Cubitus valgus appears to occur, not from premature closure of the capitellar physis, but from nonunion with proximal migration of the lateral condyle (Fig. 33-55). This occurs most often after displaced fractures. Wilkins pointed out that this nonunion may be similar to some nonunions in other areas of the skeleton such as in the carpal scaphoid. In that nonunion, if displacement of the proximal fragment is significant, the cartilaginous articular surface of the distal fragment comes in contact with the bony surface of the proximal fragment, and in such a situation union will not occur.

Masada et al. reported the results of 3 procedures in 30 elbows with old established nonunions of the lateral condyles: 9 had anterior transposition of the ulnar nerve, 4 had corrective osteotomy and anterior transposition of the ulnar nerve, and 17 had osteosynthesis of the nonunion combined with neurolysis and anterior transposition of the ulnar nerve, with or without corrective osteotomy of the humerus. Of the 30 patients, 15 had been apprehensive when using the elbow because of lateral instability or had pain in the elbow. Although the pain and apprehension disappeared in 13 of these 15 patients who were treated by osteosynthesis, the range of elbow motion decreased in all but 3. Masada et al. concluded that osteosynthesis is indicated for the treatment of nonunion of the lateral humeral condyle only if the patient has severe pain in the elbow or is

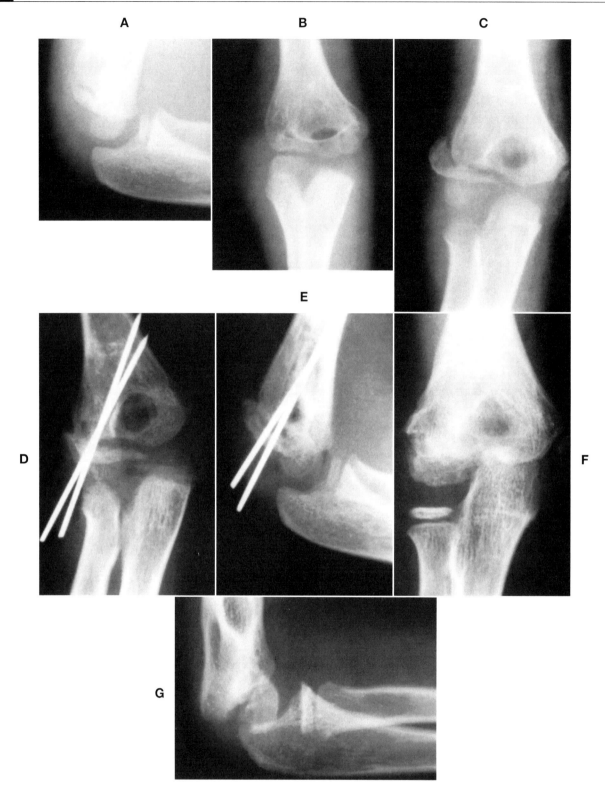

Fig. 33-53 **A** and **B,** Roentgenograms showing undisplaced lateral condylar fracture. Fracture was treated in long arm cast. **C,** "Jones view" at 3 weeks showing displacement. **D** and **E,** After open reduction and fixation with smooth wires. **F** and **G,** At 6 months wires have been removed and union is complete.

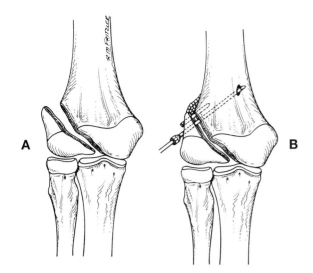

Fig. 33-54 **A,** Nonunion of lateral condyle with distal fragment in acceptable position for bone grafting and internal fixation. **B,** Transfixed, freshened, bone-grafted nonunion; physis of condylar fragment is not violated by pin or graft. (Redrawn from Flynn JC: *J Pediatr Orthop* 9:694, 1989.)

apprehensive about using the elbow because of lateral instability.

Milch devised two osteotomies for nonunion of the lateral condyle; with each, internal fixation and bone grafting are recommended. In Milch type I fractures (Salter-Harris type IV) there is little lateral displacement when the nonunion is seen relatively early. As a result, the cubitus valgus usually is not as marked. A closing wedge medial osteotomy as described by Speed or an opening wedge lateral osteotomy as described by Milch can be carried out in these nonunions (Fig. 33-56). We combine the osteotomy with an autogenous bone graft and smooth pin fixation to the epiphysis.

In Milch type II fractures there is significant lateral displacement of the fragment and some rotation. Consequently, a simple opening wedge lateral osteotomy results in an unacceptable medial prominence, as well as placing the distal humerus and forearm in unacceptable alignment (Fig. 33-57, *A* and *B*). Milch therefore recommended an opening wedge displacement osteotomy (Fig. 33-57, *C* and *D*).

If tardy ulnar nerve palsy has developed because of the nonunion and cubitus valgus, we correct the angular deformity and observe the palsy. If angular deformity is minimal and a tardy ulnar nerve palsy is present, an anterior transposition of the nerve is indicated (Chapter 59).

◆ Osteotomies for Established Cubitus Valgus Secondary to Nonunion or Growth Arrest

TECHNIQUE 33-10 *(Milch)*

Place the patient prone with the forearm supported on an arm board. Use a posterior muscle-splitting incision, exposing the lower end of the humerus, but do not open the elbow joint. Split the fibers of the triceps muscle, retract them, and identify the ulnar nerve. When indicated for treatment of tardy ulnar nerve palsy, detach the flexor group of muscles from the medial epicondyle and transplant the nerve anteriorly. Now reattach the flexor muscles. As a landmark, note the upper limit of the condylar fragment. Perform a simple transverse osteotomy at the level of the intersection of the forearm axis with the lateral cortex of the humerus (Fig. 33-57, *A* and *B*). For type II (Milch) cubitus valgus deformity, an extensive osteotomy is necessary. Notch the inferior surface of the proximal fragment to receive the apex of the superior surface of the distal fragment, which is moved laterally (Fig. 33-57, *C* and *D*). Adduct the distal fragment until the excessive angle of abduction (valgus) has been reduced to the normal carrying angle, controlling the amount of correction by roentgenograms made with the extremity and the fragments in extension. When correction is satisfactory, fix the fragments by inserting two smooth crossed Kirschner wires, carefully flex the elbow, and immobilize it in plaster at 90 degrees.

AFTERTREATMENT. The cast is left on for 6 to 12 weeks, depending on the age of the child and evidence of bony union. The wires are removed and motion is encouraged at that time.

MEDIAL EPICONDYLAR FRACTURES

Most fractures of the medial epicondylar epiphysis are acute avulsion injuries caused by overpull of the forearm flexor tendon; occasionally they are avulsed by the ulnar collateral ligament of the elbow, as described by Woods and Tullos and others. Most nondisplaced or minimally displaced fractures can be treated by closed methods. Significantly displaced fractures may require more extensive treatment. These fractures can occur in dislocation of the elbow, and the fragment may or may not become caught in the joint, preventing reduction of the dislocation. Indications for open reduction include (1) rotation and displacement of more than 1 cm because of the resulting weakness of the forearm flexors or cosmetic deformity (Fig. 33-58), (2) persistent entrapment of a fracture fragment in the joint after reduction of an elbow dislocation, (3) ulnar nerve dysfunction, and (4) valgus instability. Woods and Tullos recommended valgus stressing of the elbow to test stability. If the elbow is unstable after this fracture, especially in high-performance athletes who use their upper extremities, fixation of the collateral (anterior oblique) ligament and the fragment is indicated.

Most medial epicondylar fractures do not require surgery. The fracture is considered significantly displaced only if distal displacement is more than 1 cm or the fragment is caught within the joint. Hines et al. recommend operative treatment of these fractures displaced more than 2 mm and reported 96% good results with operative treatment, noting decreased motion only in patients in whom arthrotomy was required for removal

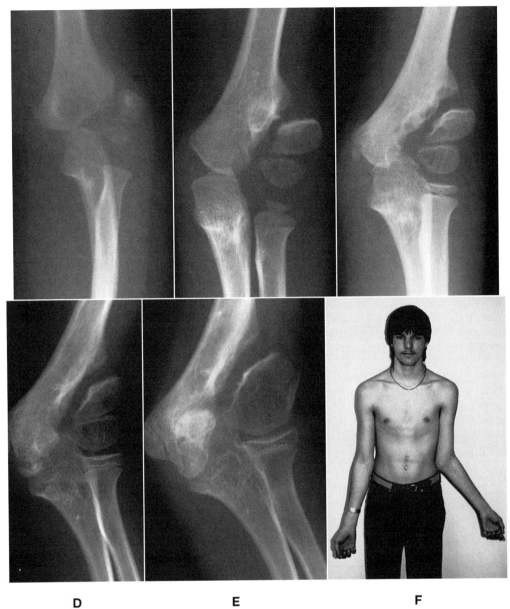

A B C

D E F

Fig. 33-55 **A,** Fracture of lateral humeral condyle in 5-year-old child. **B,** Established nonunion at 1 year after treatment by observation only. **C,** Capitellum and condyle appear to have migrated proximally at 3 years. **D,** At 5 years after injury, severe nonunion with prominent cubitus valgus. **E,** At age 16 years, patient has severe cubitus valgus and mild ulnar nerve symptoms. **F,** Clinical photograph at age 16 years shows cubitus valgus deformity.

Fig. 33-56 Correction of cubitus valgus by osteotomy. **A,** Cubitus valgus secondary to nonunion of lateral humeral condyle. **B,** Opening wedge osteotomy laterally to restore alignment. (Redrawn from Milch H: *Clin Orthop* 6:120, 1955.)

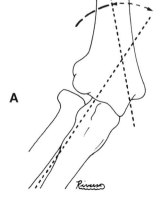

A

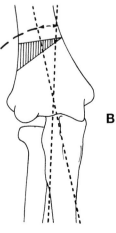

B

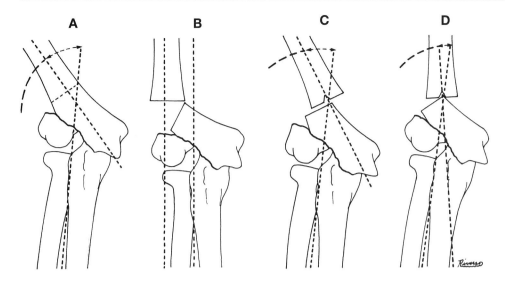

Fig. 33-57 **A** and **B,** Milch type II significantly displaced lateral condylar fracture, in which simple osteotomy would result in unacceptable alignment. **C** and **D,** Osteotomy with lateral displacement of distal humeral fragment, aligning arm satisfactorily with forearm. (Redrawn from Milch H: *Clin Orthop* 6:120, 1955.)

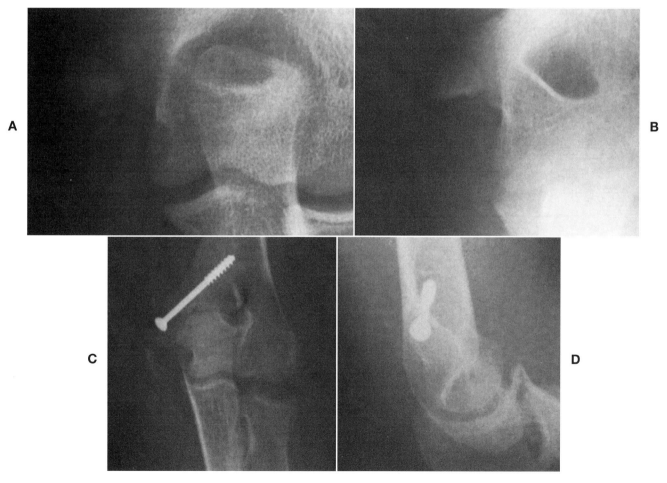

Fig. 33-58 **A,** Severely displaced fracture of medial epicondyle. **B,** Stress view shows more displacement and rotation. **C** and **D,** After open reduction and internal fixation with cancellous lag screw.

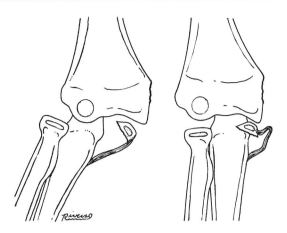

Fig. 33-59 Intraarticular displacement of medial epicondyle and entrapment within joint after reduction of dislocation of elbow. (Redrawn from Ogden JA: *Skeletal injury in the child*, Philadelphia, 1982, Lea & Febiger.)

of an entrapped fracture fragment and in one patient with inadequate pin fixation.

Ulnar nerve paresthesias can occur with this fracture; therefore the fragment should be reduced as accurately as possible. Early transposition of the ulnar nerve, however, does not appear to be justified. If the fragment is trapped in the joint, the elbow will almost always remain dislocated because of the large size of the fragment and its attachment to the flexor muscles (Fig. 33-59). If the fragment is small, it can be difficult to see on the anteroposterior roentgenogram after successful reduction of the dislocation. The fragment may be overlapped by the distal humeral epiphysis, or it may be confused with one of the ossification centers of the trochlea. Thus the diagnosis may be missed. The medial epicondyle should be identified and its location noted after every elbow dislocation. Comparison anteroposterior and lateral roentgenograms of the opposite elbow can be helpful. According to Patrick, if the epicondyle can be seen on the lateral roentgenogram, then it is caught within the joint. If the fragment remains caught within the joint, a closed reduction should be attempted with the forearm supinated and stressed in valgus with the patient under general anesthesia. Passive dorsiflexion of the fingers may help put traction on the epiphysis. If closed methods fail, then open reduction is required with removal of the fragment from the joint and either excision or reduction and internal fixation of the fragment (Fig. 33-60).

For an old dislocation with entrapment of the epicondyle within the joint, Patrick advised that the fragment be left alone rather than removed. Contrary to this, Fowles and Kassab reported six children with this complication after closed reduction of elbow dislocations. They were seen, on an average, 14 weeks after injury. The elbows were painful, and the average range of flexion was 22 degrees. Two of the children had ulnar nerve symptoms that disappeared after operation. The epicondyle in all six was removed from the joint and was either reattached to the humerus or excised and the muscle was reattached. Two children had an anterior transposition of the ulnar nerve. At follow-up, flexion was dramatically increased, and none of the children had pain.

◆ **Displaced or Entrapped Medial Epicondyle**

TECHNIQUE 33-11
Begin a medial incision 7.5 cm long just distal to the elbow and carry it proximally parallel to the medial surface of the humerus. If the fragment is entrapped within the elbow joint when the normal location of the medial epicondyle is exposed, only the raw surface of the condyle is seen; no loose fragment is visible. The ulnar nerve lies posteriorly. The medial capsule, the musculotendinous origin of the long flexor muscles, and the epicondyle are folded within the joint, covering the lower part of the coronoid fossa and process. With a small tenaculum, remove the epicondyle with its soft tissue attachments from within the joint. Now consider the fragment simply as a displaced epicondylar fracture. Replace the epicondyle accurately, and fix it with a screw or Kirschner wire. If the fracture is old or the fragment small and this is not possible, excise the fragment and suture the flexor muscles to the distal humeral metaphysis. Transfer the ulnar nerve anteriorly (Chapter 59) if necessary (Fowles and Kassab). Suture the tear in the capsule and forearm muscles, close the wound, and apply a posterior plaster splint with the elbow flexed 90 degrees.

AFTERTREATMENT. The splint is worn for 4 weeks. Then the arm is supported by a sling permitting active motion of the elbow but preventing forced dorsiflexion of the wrist or supination of the forearm. At 6 weeks the wire or screw is removed and normal activities are resumed gradually.

MEDIAL CONDYLAR FRACTURES

Fractures of the medial humeral condyle in adults and children are among the least common injuries of the elbow. Kilfoyle described three types: type I, a greenstick or impacted fracture; type II, a fracture through the humeral condyle into the joint with little or no displacement; and type III, an epiphyseal fracture that is intraarticular and involves the medial condyle with the fragment displaced and rotated (Fig. 33-61). Type III fractures account for only 25% of medial condylar fractures and occur most frequently in older children. Type I fractures are more common in younger children. Types I and undisplaced type II fractures can be treated by observation and posterior splinting; however, a nonunion of the medial condyle can occur, as well as the formation of a bony bridge (Fig. 33-62). Displacement of type II fractures can be difficult to determine; if displacement is suspected, open reduction and internal fixation are appropriate to avoid growth disturbance and nonunion. Type III fractures should be treated by open

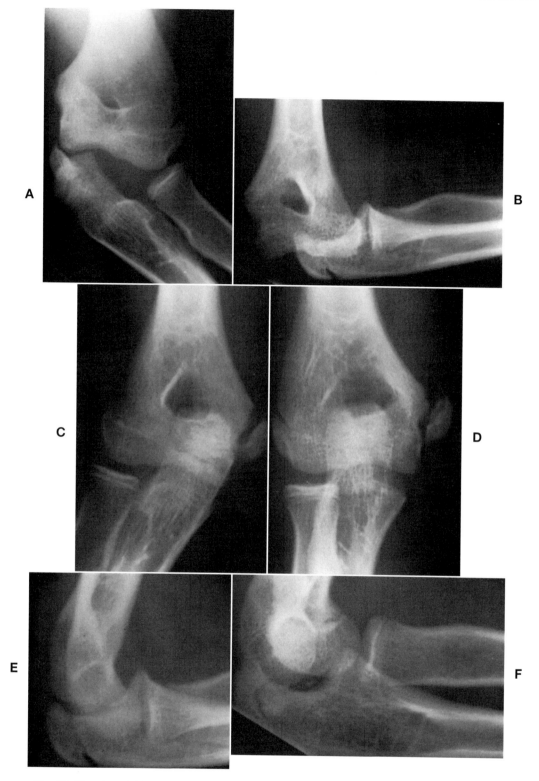

Fig. 33-60 **A** and **B,** Dislocation of elbow with displacement of medial epicondyle. **C** and **D,** Satisfactory closed reduction with medial epicondyle mildly displaced. **E,** Lateral view shows excellent reduction. **F,** Oblique view, however, reveals small fragment within joint.

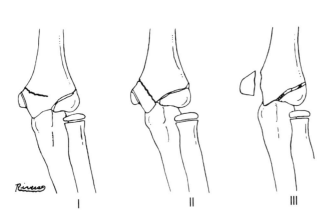

Fig. 33-61 Three types of medial condylar fractures described by Kilfoyle: type I, impacted; type II, epiphyseal and intraarticular; and type III, displacement of entire medial condyle. (Redrawn from Kilfoyle RM: *Clin Orthop* 41:43, 1965.)

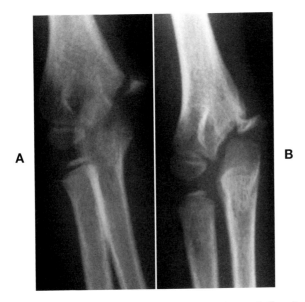

Fig. 33-62 **A,** This fracture of medial condyle was believed to be fracture of medial epicondyle. **B,** At 12 weeks after injury, nonunion of medial condyle is obvious.

reduction and internal fixation. Early diagnosis, accurate reduction, and internal fixation are essential to avoid growth disturbance, articular roughening, and functional disability, as in any Salter-Harris type III or IV fracture. Undiagnosed and untreated fractures may require supracondylar closing wedge valgus osteotomy to correct cubitus varus deformity and improve elbow range of motion. Papavasiliou et al. reported satisfactory results in 11 nondisplaced fractures treated non-operatively, 2 acutely displaced fractures treated with percutaneous pinning, and 2 untreated fractures (2 years after injury) treated with supracondylar closing wedge valgus osteotomy fixed with Kirschner wires.

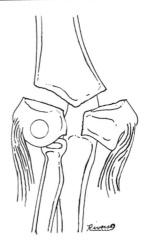

Fig. 33-63 T-condylar fracture of humerus. (Redrawn from Ogden JA: *Skeletal injury in the child,* Philadelphia, 1982, Lea & Febiger.)

◆ **Open Reduction and Internal Fixation**

TECHNIQUE 33-12

Begin a medial incision just distal to the fractured condyle and extend it proximally 7.5 cm parallel to the long axis of the humerus. Carry the dissection down to bone. Then isolate the ulnar nerve and retract it posteriorly. The capsule usually is ruptured widely and need not be incised for exposure of the fracture. Carefully examine the detached condyle and remove all loose particles of bone. The fragment is surprisingly large, and often a part of the capitellum is included. Gently reduce the fracture, and hold it with a towel clip without disturbing the soft tissue attachments of the fragment. Restore the normal contour of the articular surfaces. Insert two smooth Kirschner wires through the condylar fragment and into the humerus in a proximal and lateral direction. Two wires are necessary to prevent rotation of the fragment. Use smooth Kirschner wires rather than screws because they are less likely to injure the physis. Before closing the incision, verify the position of the wires and the fragment by roentgenograms. Cut off the wires beneath the skin, leaving them long enough to allow easy removal. Close the wound and apply a plaster splint with the elbow flexed 90 degrees.

AFTERTREATMENT. The aftertreatment is the same as that described for fracture of the lateral condyle (p. 1429).

◆ ◆ ◆

Other fractures of the distal humerus, such as lateral epicondylar fractures, usually do not require operative treatment. Conversely, the rare osteochondral fractures of the capitellum or trochlea in children may require arthrotomy or operative arthroscopy with either excision of the fragment or open reduction and internal fixation by pinning the intraarticular fragment. The rare displaced T-condylar fracture that causes

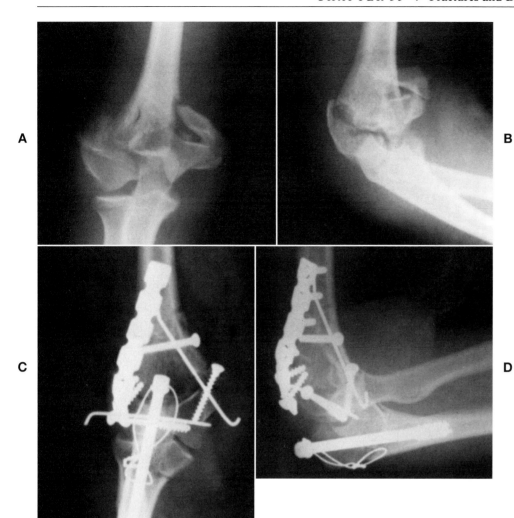

Fig. 33-64 **A** and **B,** Severely comminuted T-condylar fracture of elbow in 13-year-old child. **C** and **D,** After open reduction and internal fixation with transverse cancellous screws and contoured plate on shaft; olecranon osteotomy was performed for better exposure of intraarticular condylar fragments. Early motion was encouraged.

joint incongruity (Fig. 33-63) requires open reduction and internal fixation the same as does the T-condylar adult fracture. Jarvis and D'Astous reported satisfactory results using a posterior approach, splitting the triceps, and avoiding extensive dissection for fear of avascular necrosis of the trochlea. Kasser, Richards, and Millis evaluated nine complex humeral fractures treated by open reduction through a triceps-dividing approach, as described by Campbell (Technique 1-85). At 3.5-year follow-up, all patients had good results clinically and by Cybex testing. They recommended triceps division rather than olecranon osteotomy in children who require open reduction of complex distal humeral fractures. Occasionally osteotomy of the olecranon may be necessary for adequate exposure. Re et al., after reviewing 17 T-condylar fractures from the same institution as Kasser et al., recommended the posteromedial (Bryan-Morrey) approach (Technique 1-87) and the use of olecranon osteotomies because these results showed statistically significant better extension at follow-up than those obtained with the use of the triceps-splitting approach.

The condyles are secured to each other first, with screws or Kirschner wires, and are then fixed to the shaft with Kirschner wires or plates, depending on the age of the child (Fig. 33-64).

Postoperatively, the arm is immobilized for only 1 to 3 weeks before an active range-of-motion exercise program is begun. Older adolescents can be treated as adults, with open reduction, rigid internal fixation, and early range of motion. Technique for open reduction of T-condylar fractures is described in Chapter 54.

Peterson described a triplane fracture of the distal humeral epiphysis, and he believes this particular fracture pattern is the same as occurs in the ankle. Its treatment in the elbow should include anatomical reduction and maintenance of reduction. If this cannot be accomplished by closed methods, then open reduction and internal fixation should be carried out as in the T-condylar fracture.

SUPRACONDYLAR FRACTURES

Much attention has been paid to the problem of malreduction of supracondylar fractures of the humerus in children. In the past, cubitus varus or cubitus valgus frequently was thought to occur because of growth arrest of the distal humeral physis, rather than because of malreduction of the fracture. Wilkins, reviewing 4520 fractures in 31 major series, made several

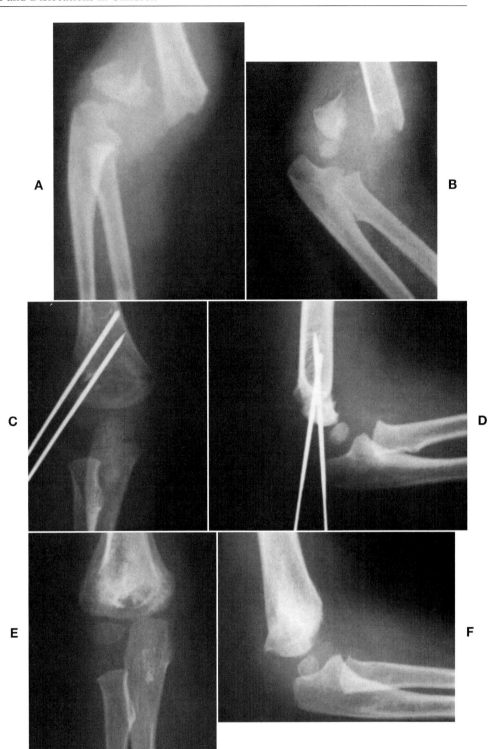

Fig. 33-65 Internal fixation of supracondylar fracture. **A** and **B,** Severely displaced type III supracondylar fracture. **C** and **D,** After closed reduction and percutaneous pinning. **E** and **F,** Good result soon after removal of pins.

pertinent observations: (1) 97.7% of the fractures were of the extension type, and only 2.2% were of the flexion type; (2) most occurred in males, especially between the ages of 5 and 8 years; and (3) a Volkmann ischemic contracture occurred in 0.5% of the fractures; the radial, median, and ulnar nerves were involved in that order of frequency.

Prevention of cubitus varus or cubitus valgus by obtaining

as anatomical a reduction as possible is necessary. No longer is it acceptable to hear "not bad for a supracondylar fracture." Dameron listed, depending on the type of fracture, four basic types of treatment: (1) side-arm skin traction, (2) overhead skeletal traction, (3) closed reduction and casting, with or without percutaneous pinning, and (4) open reduction and internal fixation. Gartland proposed a useful classification for supracondylar fractures: type I, undisplaced; type II, displaced with intact posterior cortex; and type III, displaced with no cortical contract. His classification also noted whether the fracture is displaced posteromedially or posterolaterally. Type I nondisplaced fractures can be satisfactorily treated closed with external fixation, such as a plaster cast. Type II fractures are displaced and are difficult to reduce and to hold reduced by external methods. Type III fractures are displaced posteromedially or posterolaterally with no cortical contact and the periosteum may be stripped; reduction is difficult, and maintaining reduction is almost impossible without some form of internal fixation (Fig. 33-65).

An occasional author has mentioned holding the reduction by extension of the elbow to get good roentgenograms and to avoid any cubitus varus or valgus. In fact, this appears to be the biggest problem in the treatment of these fractures: obtaining satisfactory roentgenograms to determine whether any cubitus varus or valgus is present. Technically, whether using the roentgenographic unit or an image intensifier, the machine should be moved into the anteroposterior and lateral positions rather than moving the child's elbow and losing the reduction. Various methods of overhead traction have been recommended, as well as side-arm traction. Better roentgenograms sometimes can be taken in these positions, although lengthy hospitalization is required. The three most common reasons for residual cubitus varus or valgus deformity are (1) the inability to interpret poor roentgenograms and thus acceptance of less than adequate reduction, (2) the inability to interpret good roentgenograms because of a lack of knowledge of the pathophysiology of the fracture, and (3) the loss of reduction. The lateral roentgenogram appears to be no problem. The Jones view in the anteroposterior plane should be taken properly with the elbow flexed maximally, the cassette underneath the elbow, and the tube at a 90-degree angle to the cassette. The Baumann angle, as well as any offset at the fracture site, tilting, or angulation, should be observed. An anterior spike on the lateral view usually implies rotation rather than posterior displacement. A crescent sign, described by Marion et al., implies tilt either medially or laterally (Fig. 33-66).

Attempts have been made to correlate various roentgenographic measurements with adequate fracture reduction. The Baumann angle (Fig. 33-67) is the most frequently cited method of assessing fracture reduction and has been reported to correlate well with the final carrying angle, not to change significantly from the time of initial reduction to final follow-up, and not to be obscured or invalidated by elbow flexion or pronation. The common formula is that a change of 5 degrees in the Baumann angle corresponds to a 2-degree change in the clinical carrying angle. Williamson et al. found that an average of 72 degrees (64 to 81 degrees) could be considered a normal Baumann angle and that as long as the angle did not exceed 81 degrees, cubitus varus would not occur. A template can be used to make measurement of this angle easier (Fig. 33-68). Dodge found, however, that orientation of the roentgen beam more than 20 degrees from perpendicular in the cephalad-caudad direction invalidates the measurement.

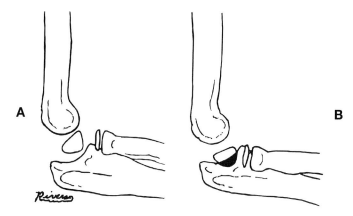

Fig. 33-66 Crescent sign. **A,** Normal lateral view of elbow. **B,** In varus deformity, part of ulna overlies distal humeral epiphyses, producing crescent sign. (Redrawn from Marion J, LaGrange J, Faysse R, Rigault P: *Rev Chir Orthop* 48:337, 1962.)

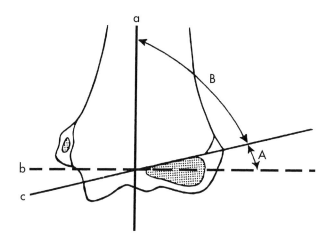

Fig. 33-67 Baumann angle. *a,* Midline diaphysis of humeral shaft. *b,* Line perpendicular to midline. *c,* Line through physis of lateral condyle. Angle *A* is original Baumann angle. Angle *B* is more commonly used currently.

Webb and Sherman found the Baumann angle to correlate with the carrying angle, but inaccuracy of measurement increased in young children and adolescents, so they recommended its use only in comparison with the normal elbow. Using CT, Mohammad et al. found Baumann's angle to be an inaccurate indicator of the carrying angle in the treatment of displaced supracondylar fractures.

Oppenheim et al. suggested that the humeral-ulnar-wrist angle is the most consistent and accurate method of approximating the true carrying angle. Webb and Sherman also found its accuracy rate higher than the Baumann angle. O'Brien et al., in an unpublished study, reported that the metaphyseal-diaphyseal angle (Fig. 33-69) was more accurate than the Baumann angle in determining the adequacy of reduction. Biyani et al. described a measurement of the medial epicondylar epiphyseal angle to determine the accuracy of

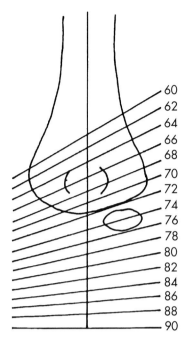

Fig. 33-68   Measurement of Baumann angle with overlay grid of angles. (Redrawn from Williamson DM, Coates CJ, Miller RK, et al: *J Pediatr Orthop* 12:636, 1992.)

reduction of supracondylar fractures, but our results with this measurement have been so variable that we no longer use it.

In this fracture, cubitus valgus causes little problem, primarily because the carrying angle is 5 to 7 degrees of physiological valgus, and anything more than this is an accentuation of the normal. Conversely, cubitus varus produces a distasteful cosmetic deformity but only rarely any limitation of motion. Many authors have demonstrated that pure posterior displacement causes little deformity and that pure horizontal rotation will likewise cause little deformity because rotation is adequately compensated for at the shoulder joint. Coronal tilting can occur with opening of the lateral aspect of the fracture site, causing angulation into a varus position, or with impaction of the medial side of the fracture site, again resulting in cubitus varus (Fig. 33-70). As noted by Wilkins and others, horizontal rotation predisposes to coronal tilting, and a combination of horizontal rotation, coronal tilting, and posterior displacement can result in a three-dimensional deformity of cubitus varus (Fig. 33-71). The crescent sign and the fishtail sign anteriorly both imply angulation and rotation. When they are seen on the lateral view, the anterior or Jones view should be studied closely for loss of the Baumann angle, coronal tilting secondary to lateral displacement, or medial impaction at the

Fig. 33-69   Metaphyseal-diaphyseal angle. On anteroposterior roentgenogram, transverse line is drawn through metaphysis at widest point, longitudinal line is drawn through axis of diaphysis; angle is measured between lateral portion of metaphyseal line and proximal portion of diaphyseal line. **A,** Normal angle is 90 degrees. **B,** Angle greater than 90 degrees indicates varus angulation. **C,** Angle less than 90 degrees indicates valgus angulation. (Courtesy RE Eilert, MD.)

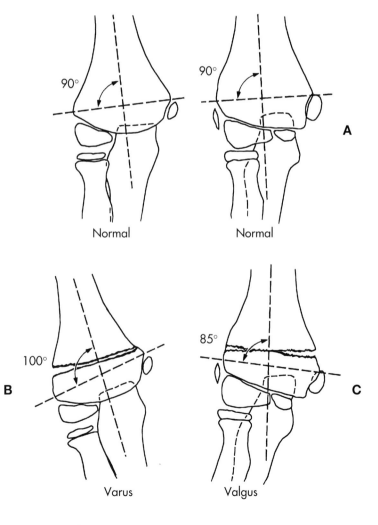

fracture site. By a mechanism that is not completely understood, varus tilting is reduced by pronation of the forearm that closes the fracture laterally (Fig. 33-72). Whether external immobilization or pin fixation is used, the forearm should be placed in the pronated position to decrease the varus tilt and resultant cubitus varus.

Closed reduction with splint or cast immobilization has traditionally been recommended for displaced supracondylar fractures, but loss of reduction and the necessity of repeated manipulations have been frequently reported to cause elbow stiffness and physeal damage. Pirone et al. reported that closed reduction and casting of displaced fractures resulted in a lower percentage of good results and higher percentages of early and late complications compared with skeletal traction, percutaneous pinning, and open reduction; they recommended cast treatment only for undisplaced fractures. Criteria for closed reduction are easy reduction, stable fracture, minimal swelling, and no vascular compromise. Several authors have described reduction of the fracture in extension and maintenance of the reduction through the use of the triceps bridge by holding the elbow in flexion if the pulse and vasculature tolerate this.

However, Mapes and Hennrikus, using Doppler ultrasonography, concluded that in displaced extension supracondylar fractures, vascular safety is enhanced by extending the elbow and supinating the forearm. An occasional author has reported holding the reduction by extension of the elbow. Bosanquet and Middleton reported good results with skin traction in full extension. They attributed the lack of cubitus varus or valgus deformity to good roentgenographic techniques. Skeletal traction using either an olecranon pin or screw applied with either side-arm or overhead positioning also has been widely recommended because of the advantages of increased mobility, decreased pain and swelling, and improved alignment. Ippolito et al. reported good results at long-term follow-up in 81% of nondisplaced and 78% of displaced fractures treated conservatively. Their treatment regimen included overhead skeletal traction for 2 to 10 days until reduction of the overriding fragments was obtained, further reduction of the fracture with the patient under general anesthesia, and application of a long plaster cast, including the traction bow, with the elbow in 90 degrees of flexion and the forearm pronated. The overhead traction position was maintained for another 2 to 3 days, after

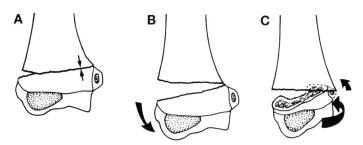

Fig. 33-70 Mechanism of coronal tilting. **A,** Impaction of fracture medially. **B,** Tilting of fragment medially. **C,** Horizontal rotation. (Redrawn from Marion J, LaGrange J, Faysse R, Rigault P: *Rev Chir Orthop* 48:337, 1962.)

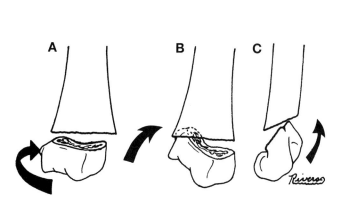

Fig. 33-71 Three static components that combine to produce cubitus varus. **A,** Horizontal rotation. **B,** Coronal tilting. **C,** Anterior angulation. (Redrawn from Wilkins KE: Fractures and dislocations of the elbow region. In Rockwood CA Jr, Wilkins KE, King RE, eds: *Fractures in children*, Philadelphia, 1984, JB Lippincott.)

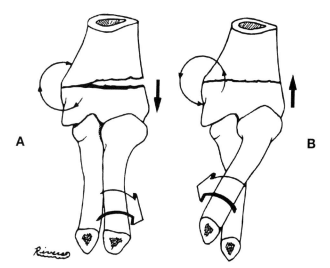

Fig. 33-72 Reduction of lateral tilt by pronation of forearm. **A,** Supination opening fracture laterally. **B,** Pronation closing fracture laterally. (Redrawn from Abraham E, Powers T, Witt P, Ray RD: *Clin Orthop* 171:309, 1982.)

which the long plaster cast was connected to a shoulder spica cast. After 2 weeks, the traction bow was removed through a window in the cast. The use of a cast averaged 4.5 weeks. The incidence of cubitus varus was 7.5% and of cubitus valgus 5.6%, both of which occurred most frequently after displaced fractures. Spontaneous correction of the deformity occurred with growth in 3 patients with cubitus varus and in 13 with cubitus valgus. Kramhøft et al. reported excellent or good results in 60 severely displaced supracondylar fractures after closed reduction and vertical skeletal traction with a screw in the olecranon. Eight fractures lost reduction and required reduction with the patients under general anesthesia. The length of hospitalization (average, 2.6 weeks) was cited as the major disadvantage of the method, which they believed was offset by the reduction in serious complications. Worlock and Colton reported the use of overhead olecranon traction through an olecranon screw and traction clip in 27 severely displaced supracondylar fractures; 22 (81%) had excellent results, and 5 had good results. Two had mild cubitus varus deformities. Worlock and Colton recommend this method as technically easy to perform and without significant complications. Pirone et al. obtained equally good results in displaced fractures with overhead traction through an olecranon screw as with percutaneous pinning, and they recommend traction for the grossly swollen elbow in which the osseous landmarks are obscured and reduction is difficult or impossible. Most displaced Gartland type II and reducible type III fractures are treated by percutaneous pinning.

Closed Reduction and Percutaneous Pinning

As noted by Dameron, closed reduction is difficult not only to achieve, but also to maintain because of the thinness of bone of the distal humerus between the coronoid and olecranon, where most supracondylar fractures occur. For this reason, many authors have described percutaneous pinning techniques, and these techniques have become the treatment of choice for most supracondylar fractures. Swenson, Casiano, and Flynn et al. used two crossed pins. Arino et al. recommended two lateral pins, and Foster and Paterson used two lateral "divergent" pins (Fig. 33-73), whereas Fowles and Kassab used one lateral oblique pin and a second vertical pin through the olecranon. Haddad et al. used two pins laterally and one medially. Herzenberg et al., in animal studies, found that medial and lateral pin fixation provides more stability than lateral pinning alone. Wilkins recommended placing the initial pin medially so that it will aid in the reduction.

Graves and Beaty reported good results in 61 of 64 (95%) type III supracondylar fractures treated with closed reduction and percutaneous pinning. Of the three fractures with unsatisfactory results, two had been fixed in a varus position with medial and lateral pins and one fixed in good alignment with two lateral pins had lost fixation and position postoperatively. They recommended medial and lateral pinning for added stability, but noted that if bony landmarks cannot be palpated because of edema or if injury to the ulnar nerve with a medial pin is of concern, then lateral pinning alone may be preferred.

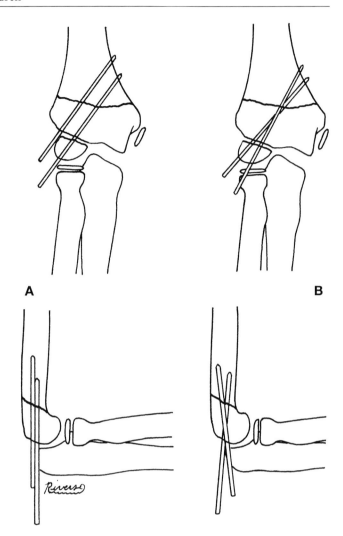

Fig. 33-73   Pinning of supracondylar fracture. **A,** Two lateral pins are inserted parallel, crossing fracture site and opposite medial cortex. **B,** Divergent pins crossing same structures. (Redrawn from Arino VL, Lluch EE, Ramirez AM, et al: *J Bone Joint Surg* 59A:914, 1977.)

Transient and permanent ulnar nerve damage are rare in all reports. Royce et al. reported neurological complications in 4 of 143 children (2.7%) after Kirschner wire fixation of supracondylar fractures. Late ulnar neurapraxia occurred in 2 patients, and in the other 2 patients nerve injuries (one ulnar and one radial) were caused by insertion of the Kirschner wires. Lyons et al. described ulnar nerve palsies after closed or open reduction and percutaneous pinning for supracondylar fractures in 17 patients who had normal neurologic examinations preoperatively. Only 4 had the medial pins removed, and 2 others had explorations, which showed no interruption of the nerve. Although all patients had complete return of function eventually, many did not have complete return of function until after 4 months. They concluded that nerve palsies occurring after percutaneous pinning of the supracondylar fracture usually resolve spontaneously.

Because of these complications, Royce et al. recommended two lateral wires for fixation if the fracture is stable after closed reduction. For comminuted or unstable fractures, medial and lateral pins are used. To prevent nerve injury when a medial pin is used, they recommended using a small incision over the medial epicondyle and placing a drill guide on the bone, through which the wire is inserted. The pins should be angulated superiorly approximately 40 degrees and posteriorly 10 degrees. The pins must continue into the opposite cortex to provide solid fixation. Smooth pins are preferred. Some authors have advised placing the patient prone with the elbow flexed rather than supine. We routinely use the supine position; however, we have tried the prone position, and it does provide easier accessibility for pin placement, but orientation of the fragments with the patient prone is difficult even when the image intensifier is being used.

Percutaneous fixation after closed reduction has the advantage of providing excellent stability of the supracondylar fracture in any position of the elbow (Fig. 33-74). However, the ultimate result will be only as good as the initial reduction and does not depend on the placement of the pins. If the fracture is not satisfactorily reduced and is held in an unsatisfactory position with pins, the outcome will be unsatisfactory, just as if no pin fixation were used. Aronson and Prager evaluated the quality of reduction by measuring the Baumann angle after reduction; they accepted the reduction if the Baumann angle of the fractured extremity was within 4 degrees of that of the normal extremity. Although as many as 21% of the fractures treated in this manner have a small degree of residual cubitus varus, this is primarily because a poor position was accepted at the time of pinning.

The flexion type of fracture occurs in only 2% to 3% of all supracondylar fractures, according to Wilkins. In displaced flexion fractures Fowles and Kassab noted that ulnar nerve lesions are common, the reduction is more difficult, the results are worse than in extension fractures, and these anteriorly displaced fractures should be considered for accurate reduction and percutaneous pinning.

◆ **Closed Reduction and Percutaneous Pinning of Supracondylar Fracture**

TECHNIQUE 33-13
Place the patient prone or supine on a fracture table. Prepare and drape the elbow. Then outline the posterior triangle of the elbow joint—the medial and lateral epicondyles and the olecranon. Reduce the fracture by applying longitudinal traction, extending the fracture, and manipulating with the thumbs to correct lateral tilt, medial impaction, or posterior displacement. Flex the elbow to neutral. Crisscross two smooth Steinmann pins through the condyles and metaphysis, one to exit above the medial epicondyle and one to exit above the lateral epicondyle. Angle the medial pin 40 degrees from the axis of the humeral shaft and direct it

10 degrees posteriorly, carefully avoiding the ulnar nerve. After engagement of the shaft, use an image intensifier to make sure the pin engages the opposite lateral cortex proximally. Repeat the procedure for the lateral pin. For the most rigid biomechanical construct, the pins should cross in the middle of the humerus several centimeters proximal to and not at the fracture site. Cut the pins off either outside or beneath the skin and bend their ends so that they will not migrate proximally but can be retrieved easily in the office. Check and note the radial pulse.

AFTERTREATMENT. A long arm posterior plaster splint is worn for 3 weeks. Ulnar, radial, and median nerve function should be checked after anesthesia. The pins are removed at 3 weeks, and another posterior splint is applied. At 4 weeks intermittent active range-of-motion exercises are started at home; they should be taught by the physical therapist to the child and the parent, explaining that the child is to carry out his own active range-of-motion program. Passive motion or forceful manipulative motion must be avoided in children because they will decrease the range of motion and frighten the child.

TECHNIQUE 33-14 (Modified by Thometz, and Aronson and Prager)
Position the patient supine and use image intensification to determine the direction of displacement and the status of the soft tissues of the injured extremity. Supinate and pronate the forearm to tighten the lateral and medial soft tissue hinges, respectively; flex and extend the elbow to tighten the posterior and anterior hinges, respectively. For the rare flexion supracondylar fracture with anterior displacement of the distal fragment, extend the elbow to obtain satisfactory closed reduction.

For the more common extension type of supracondylar fracture, with countertraction on the humerus, apply traction to the forearm and examine the fracture with image intensification. Pronate or supinate the forearm to rotate the distal fragment into correct rotational alignment with the proximal fragment. Translate the distal fragment in a similar manner to correct medial or lateral displacement. While maintaining traction and precise forearm rotation, gently flex the elbow. Place gentle pressure on the olecranon as the elbow is flexed to correct posterior displacement of the distal fragment. Now maximally flex the elbow and pronate the forearm to lock the posterior and medial soft tissue hinges. Confirm the anteroposterior reduction with image intensification, aiming the beam through the forearm and rotating the humerus from medial to lateral. Confirm lateral reduction by externally rotating the shoulder to obtain a lateral view of the elbow.

Maintain reduction while performing closed percutaneous pinning with image intensification to verify that the two

continued

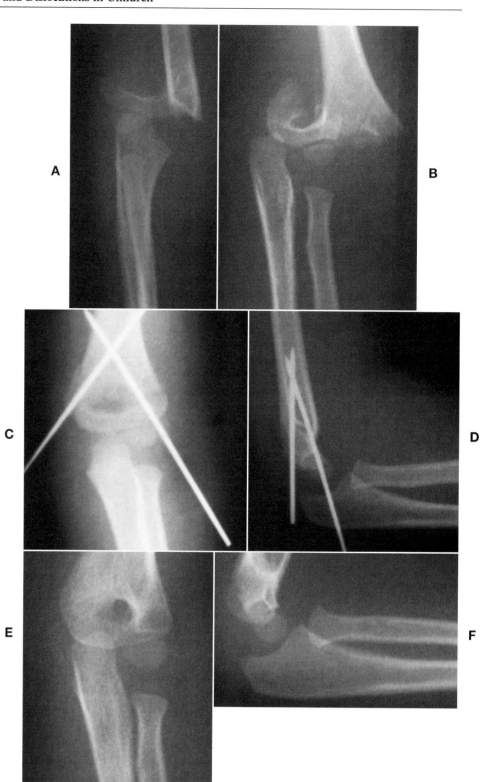

Fig. 33-74   Closed reduction and percutaneous pinning of supracondylar fracture. **A** and **B,** Severely displaced type III supracondylar fracture. **C** and **D,** After closed reduction and percutaneous pinning. Smooth pins crossed and caught opposite cortex. **E** and **F,** At 2 years normal architecture including alignment.

lateral pins engage both fracture fragments (Fig. 33-75). After the pins are inserted, extend the elbow as far as possible without bending the pins. Compare the carrying angle with that of the normal extremity and obtain true anteroposterior roentgenograms of both forearms to judge the quality of reduction. Carefully position the arm with the medial and lateral epicondyles parallel to the cassette. Direct the roentgen beam to obtain a true anteroposterior view of the distal humerus. Use the Baumann angle to further evaluate the quality of reduction (p. 1439).

AFTERTREATMENT. Aftertreatment is the same as for fixation with crossed pins (p. 1443).

◆ Open Reduction and Internal Fixation

Open reduction and internal fixation of supracondylar fractures are indicated when closed reduction is unsatisfactory. In a type III displaced fracture with no cortical contact and completely detached periosteum, and with the fracture fragment "puckering" or even penetrating the skin (open fracture), a satisfactory closed reduction may not be possible. If, after one or two attempts at closed reduction with the child under general anesthesia, the fragments cannot be reduced and held by percutaneous pinning, open reduction and internal fixation are indicated.

According to Rasool and Naidoo manipulation should be avoided in displaced type III posterolateral supracondylar fractures with neurovascular deficit if clinical evidence indicates that the fracture fragment has buttonholed through the brachialis muscle, since the neurovascular bundle may be trapped in the fracture site. If the elbow is so severely swollen that a closed reduction cannot be maintained, then olecranon traction can be used for several days, followed by closed or, if necessary, open reduction. Other indications for open reduction include open fractures that require irrigation and debridement and fractures complicated by vascular injury. Possible complications of open reduction include infection, vascular injury, myositis ossificans, excessive callus formation with residual stiffness, and decreased range of motion.

If open reduction and internal fixation are to be carried out, they should be performed after the swelling has decreased but not later than 5 days after injury, since the possibility of myositis ossificans apparently increases after that time. We prefer a lateral approach; others have used posterior, medial, anterolateral, and antecubital approaches. Kekomäki et al., using an antecubital approach, as well as Danielsson and Pettersson, using a medial approach, described good results using open reduction and internal fixation of severely displaced fractures that could not be reduced or had significant vascular embarrassment. They also recommended fasciotomy at the same time. Gruber and Hudson treated 31 difficult fractures with open reduction and internal fixation and obtained satisfactory results even in the most severe fractures.

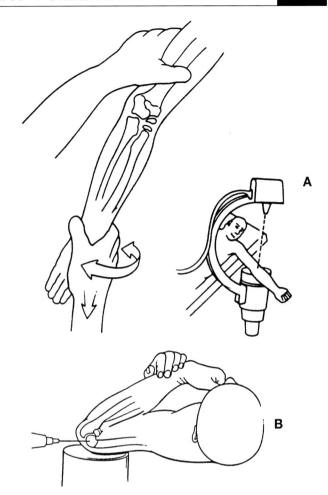

Fig. 33-75 **A,** Rotational deformity and displacement evaluated with image intensification; anatomical correction of these deformities must be obtained before elbow is fixed. **B,** Accurate position of pins ensured by image intensification during procedure. (Redrawn from Aronson DD, Prager BI: *Clin Orthop* 219:174, 1987.)

TECHNIQUE 33-15

Prepare and drape the arm in the usual fashion with the patient supine. Make a curved incision over the lateral humeral condyle, beginning about 2 cm distal to the olecranon and carrying it proximally for about 6 cm above the condyle. Dissect the soft tissue, including the anconeus and common extensor origins, and retract these anteriorly and posteriorly respectively. Make sure the radial nerve is retracted posteriorly. A large hematoma may require evacuation before the fracture can be seen. Observe the supracondylar fragment, and note its alignment with the proximal fragment. Use a small curet to remove any hematoma at the fracture site. Note any interdigitations on the ends of the bone and by matching them, reduce the fracture. Use two crossed Steinmann pins in a manner similar to that described for percutaneous pinning. Image

continued

intensification simplifies pin placement, as does a power drill. Cut the pins off outside the skin for easy removal later. Close the incision in layers.

AFTERTREATMENT. A posterior plaster splint is applied, and the radial pulse and neurological function are checked after anesthesia. The pins are removed at 3 to 4 weeks, and an active, not passive, range-of-motion program is started.

Early Complications

Neurological compromise—usually a neurapraxia—is reported to occur in 3% to 22% of patients with supracondylar fractures. Any of the peripheral nerves—median, anterior interosseous, radial, or ulnar—may be damaged, and mixed nerve lesions have been reported. Complete return of nerve function is usual, although this may require several months. Some authors recommend surgical exploration if nerve function has not returned within 6 to 8 weeks of reduction, whereas others recommend allowing a minimum of 2 months for resolution. Continued nerve palsies after fracture may indicate nerve entrapment in the fracture callus. Culp et al. reported 18 neural injuries in children with supracondylar humeral fractures, 9 of which resolved spontaneously an average of 2.5 months after injury. The remaining 9 lesions were explored at an average of 7.5 months after injury. Neurolysis was performed on 8, and 1 completely lacerated nerve required grafting. They concluded that observation should be the initial approach, but if clinical or electromyographic evidence of neural function is not present at 5 months after injury, exploration and neurolysis are indicated. If the nerve is in continuity, the prognosis after neurolysis is excellent. Amillo and Mora reported 25 neural injuries at the elbow joint in children. Findings at surgery revealed discontinuity of the affected nerve trunk in 8 patients; 17 had a constrictive lesion with the nerve trunk in continuity. The surgical technique in 8 involved repair by interfascicular grafting and epineural suture, and 17 by neurolysis. Excellent results were found in nearly 80% of the continuous lesions treated by neurolysis. In discontinuous lesions, 66% had excellent results with grafting.

Injury to the brachial artery occurs in as many as 10% of patients with supracondylar fractures. Often the problem is corrected once the fracture has been reduced and circulation has returned to normal. Most authors recommend close observation of vascular status after reduction; if circulation does not return to normal (with the elbow flexed to less than 45 degrees) within about 5 minutes, consultation with a vascular surgeon is recommended and surgical exploration of the brachial artery may be necessary. Besides the clinical indications of capillary refill and pulse, Doppler measurements or a pulse oximeter have been recommended for evaluating circulation after reduction. Vasli reported the use of Doppler waveform analysis in which the equipment is connected to a spectrum analyzer, producing a picture of the velocity

waveform that can be compared with the normal extremity and easily interpreted. An arteriogram usually is not recommended unless entrapment or severing of the artery is suspected. Sabharwal et al. used a combination of segmental pressure monitoring, color-flow duplex scanning, and magnetic resonance angiography (MRA) in evaluating patency of the brachial artery and collateral circulation across the elbow.

Shaw et al. reported rapid reduction with Kirschner wire stabilization without arteriogram in 17 children with signs of vascular impairment after supracondylar humeral fractures. In three patients in whom satisfactory blood supply to the hand was not present after reduction, brachial artery exploration was performed. They reported no vascular complications at follow-up. Because of these findings, Shaw et al. concluded that arteriography is not indicated before reduction of supracondylar fractures. Garbuz et al. reported 22 children with a supracondylar fracture and an absent radial pulse. They concluded that the initial treatment for children who have displaced supracondylar fractures with an absent radial pulse should be closed reduction, Kirschner wire fixation, and immobilization in less than 90 degrees of flexion. Children with a well-perfused hand but an absent radial pulse after satisfactory closed reduction do not necessarily require routine exploration of the brachial artery. Garbuz et al., as well as Rang, did not recommend open reduction even if the distal pulse is absent after reduction; they noted that the pulse usually returns within a week or two after reduction, often quite suddenly. Unusually severe ischemic pain after reduction is an indication of vascular problems. Disappearance of the radial pulse with attempts at fracture reduction (not in an acutely flexed position) implies interposition of the artery in the fracture site and requires surgical exploration.

Compartment syndrome is an uncommon but serious complication of supracondylar fractures. Compartment syndromes occur as the result of hypoxic damage caused by interruption of the circulation to the muscles. Any evidence of compartment syndrome requires vascular consultation, compartment pressure measurements, and possibly fasciotomy. Fasciotomy is recommended in the presence of clinical signs of compartment syndrome, such as undue pain and a palpable firmness in the forearm. Wilkins pointed out that the morbidity caused by fasciotomy is minimal, while that caused by an untreated compartment syndrome is much greater. The general indications for fasciotomy are (1) clinical signs such as demonstrable motor or sensory loss, (2) compartment pressures above 35 mm Hg (slit or wick catheter technique) or above 40 mm Hg (needle technique), and (3) interrupted arterial circulation to the extremity for more than 4 hours. A number of techniques have been advocated for fasciotomy of the forearm, but the standard Henry approach (Fig. 33-76), as recommended by Eaton and Green and Gelberman et al., is most often used.

Late Complications

Cubitus varus is the most common angular deformity that results from supracondylar fractures in children. Cubitus valgus, although mentioned in the literature as causing tardy

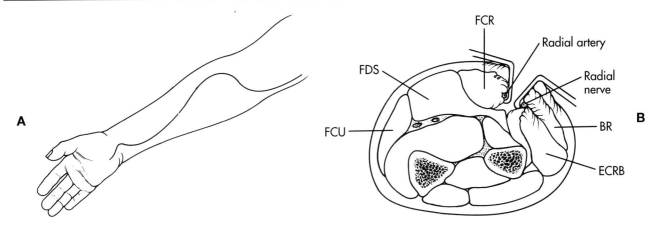

Fig. 33-76   **A,** Henry approach to volar aspect of forearm. **B,** Henry approach to superficial and deep compartments of forearm. *FCR,* Flexor carpi radialis; *BR,* brachioradialis; *ECRB,* extensor carpi radialis brevis; *FCU,* flexor carpi ulnaris; *FDS,* flexor digitorum superficialis. (Redrawn from Rorabeck CH: *Instr Course Lect* 32:102, 1983.)

ulnar nerve palsy, rarely occurs and is more often caused by nonunion of lateral condylar fractures.

Several causes for cubitus varus have been suggested. Medial displacement and rotation of the distal fragment have been blamed most often, but Smith proved in his experimental studies that varus tilting of the distal fragment was the most important cause of change in the carrying angle. He also showed that rotation of the distal fragment does not cause cubitus varus but is the single most important factor leading to medial tilt. LaBelle et al. found varus tilting of the distal fragment to be the cause of deformity in all of their patients with cubitus varus after supracondylar fracture. Growth disturbance in the distal humerus, especially overgrowth of the lateral condyle, can occur. Kasser noted that osteonecrosis and delayed growth of the trochlea, with relative overgrowth of the normal lateral side of the distal humeral epiphysis, is a rare cause of progressive cubitus varus deformity after supracondylar fracture. This progressive growth abnormality cannot be prevented by stabilization of the distal fragment.

Davids et al. described lateral condylar fractures after malunited supracondylar fractures of the humerus with subsequent cubitus varus deformity. They postulated that torsional moment and shear force generated across the capitellar physis by a fall are increased with varus malalignment. Thus they suggested that posttraumatic cubitus varus may predispose a child to subsequent lateral condylar fracture and that this deformity should be viewed as more than just a cosmetic problem.

Beals noted that the normal carrying angle increases from childhood to adulthood. For this reason an increase in valgus is not as cosmetically noticeable as a complete reversal to a varus position.

Rotational malalignment may occur but is not a significant deformity. Malrotation of the distal humerus is compensated for to a large degree by the shoulder joint. As a result the rotational component in cubitus varus deformities is of little consequence, and all that is necessary for correction of the cubitus varus

deformity is a lateral closing wedge osteotomy. However, occasionally a hyperextension deformity requires the addition of a flexion component.

Three basic types of osteotomies have been described: a medial opening wedge osteotomy with a bone graft, an oblique osteotomy with derotation, and a lateral closing wedge osteotomy. King and Secor described the medial opening wedge osteotomy. The disadvantages of this osteotomy are that it gains length, which is not a problem in the upper extremity, and it creates a certain amount of inherent instability. Lengthening the medial aspect of the humerus also can stretch and damage the ulnar nerve unless it is transposed anteriorly. An oblique osteotomy can be beneficial, but the derotation described is probably not necessary for the reasons given earlier. Amspacher and Messenbaugh reported good results with an oblique osteotomy fixed with cortical screws, but this procedure attempts to correct a two-plane deformity with one osteotomy and requires rotation to correct the varus deformity. Uchida et al. described a three-dimensional osteotomy for correction of cubitus varus deformity, in which medial and posterior tilt and rotation of the distal fragment can be corrected if necessary (Fig. 33-77).

In our experience and that of others, a lateral closing wedge osteotomy is the easiest, safest, and inherently the most stable osteotomy. The primary difference in the types of lateral closing wedge osteotomies are the methods of fixation that include the use of two screws and a wire attached between them, plate fixation, compression fixation, crossed Kirschner wires, and staples; some have used no fixation. In the literature Kirschner wire fixation is the most prevalent method of holding the osteotomy. We also have frequently used this method. However, loosening of the fixation with recurrent deformity has been noted, as well as pin track infections, osteomyelitis, skin slough, nerve palsy, and rarely aneurysm of the brachial artery. Roach and Hernandez reported their results of corrective osteotomy for cubitus varus deformity and noted that unstable internal fixation allowed the osteotomy fragments to slip into a

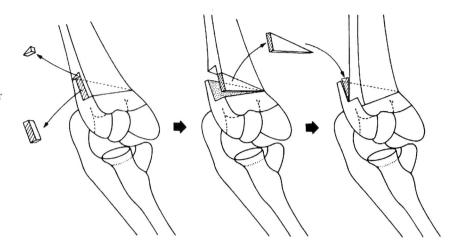

Fig. 33-77   Three-dimensional osteotomy for correction of cubitus varus deformity. Medial and posterior tilt are corrected. After osteotomy, distal fragment is compacted with proximal fragment by adding external rotation by wedge of humeral cortex. Bone graft is added if necessary. (From Uchida Y, Ogata K, Sugioka Y: *J Pediatr Orthop* 11:327, 1991).

varus position in a number of patients. They attributed this to nonrigid internal fixation and recommended a two-hole lateral plate and a percutaneous medial pin to increase stability.

Voss et al. described a uniplanar supracondylar closing wedge humeral osteotomy with preset Kirschner wires for correction of posttraumatic cubitus varus deformity in 36 patients. They described their technique as being simple with good correction and minimal complications.

French used two parallel screws that are attached by a single figure-eight wire that is tightened for fixation. Bellemore et al. reported their results using a modified French technique in 27 children with cubitus varus after supracondylar fractures. Their primary indication was unacceptable cosmetic deformity. They compared three sets of children who had a closing wedge osteotomy: (1) those with external fixation alone, such as a plaster cast, (2) those with Kirschner wire fixation, and (3) those with a modified French technique. Their results as to loss of fixation, correction of deformity, and complications were superior using the modified French technique, and they concluded that this method is safe and satisfactory (Fig. 33-78).

DeRosa and Graziano reported good and excellent results in 10 of 11 patients with a step-cut osteotomy technique fixed with a single cortical screw. The one patient with a poor result had persistent varus caused by unrecognized fracture of the cortical spike, which caused loss of fixation. They reported no ulnar or radial nerve injuries, infections, nonunions, or hypertrophic scars, and all patients retained preoperative ranges of motion. They concluded that this osteotomy with single-screw fixation is a safe procedure that can correct multiple planes of deformity, but they emphasized the importance of careful preoperative planning and special attention to surgical detail.

◆ **Lateral Closing Wedge Osteotomy**

TECHNIQUE 33-16 *(Voss et al.)*
After standard preparation and draping and inflation of the tourniquet, approach the elbow through a lateral incision. With fluoroscopic guidance, insert two Kirschner wires into the lateral condyle before osteotomy and advance them just distal to the planned distal cut (Fig. 33-79, *A*). Be prepared to advance these proximally after the closing wedge osteotomy has been made. Make a closing wedge osteotomy laterally, leaving the medial cortex intact (Fig. 33-79, *A* and *B*). Weaken the medial cortex using drill holes and a rongeur. Apply a forceful valgus stress to complete the osteotomy with the forearm in pronation and the elbow flexed. Close the osteotomy and advance the Kirschner wires from the lateral condyle into the medial cortex of the proximal fragment (Fig. 33-79, *B*). Leave the wires buried under the skin. A third wire can be used if necessary for stability. Close the wound in layers and splint the arm in 90 degrees of flexion and full pronation.

AFTERTREATMENT. The wires are removed at approximately 6 to 8 weeks after surgery, and a range-of-motion program is started.

TECHNIQUE 33-17 *(French)*
Expose the distal humerus through a posterior longitudinal incision and split the triceps muscle and aponeurosis. Detach the lateral half of the triceps from its insertion and reflect it proximally; the posterior surface and lateral border of the humerus are now visible, and the ulnar nerve can be exposed. Insert two drill points to act as guides in making the osteotomy and check their position by roentgenograms. Before the bone is divided, insert one screw above and one screw below the drill points and parallel with them, but insert the distal screw in the anterior part of the distal fragment and the proximal screw in the posterior part of the proximal fragment (Fig. 33-80). Using a reciprocating motor saw, excise the wedge of bone from between the drill points; divide the bone but leave the periosteum intact medially to act as a hinge. Approximate the cut surfaces and correct the rotation deformity by rotating the distal fragment externally until the distal screw is directly distal to the

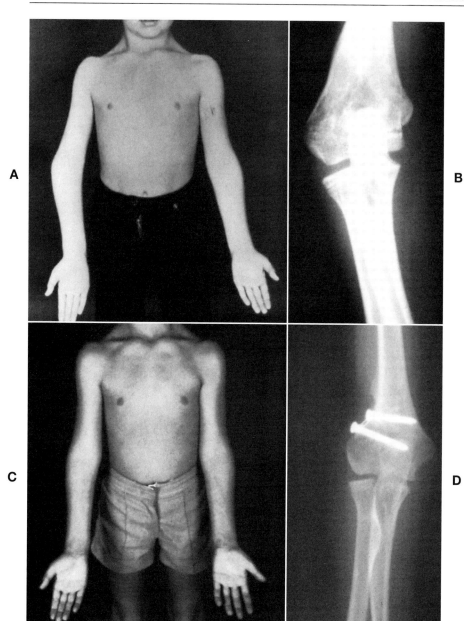

Fig. 33-78 **A** and **B,** Clinical photograph and roentgenogram of moderate cubitus varus secondary to supracondylar fracture. **C** and **D,** Clinical photograph and roentgenogram after French technique of supracondylar osteotomy. (From Bellemore MC, Barrett IR, Middleton RWD: *J Bone Joint Surg* 66B:566, 1984.)

proximal screw. Maintain this position by tightening a wire loop around the heads of the two screws. Close the wound. With this type of fixation the danger of damaging the physis is minimized.

AFTERTREATMENT. Aftertreatment is the same as for the modified French technique described next.

TECHNIQUE 33-18 (French, Modified by Bellemore et al.)

Make a posterolateral incision and split the triceps. Detach the triceps from its insertion and reflect it proximally. Lift the middle two thirds of the muscle from the humerus subperiosteally, taking care to protect the neurovascular bundle. Outline a laterally based wedge on the bone, ending just short of the medial cortex. Place one screw in the lateral cortex proximally, above the proposed osteotomy, and another distally, below the proposed osteotomy, at an angle approximating that of the wedge to be resected. Then resect the wedge with an oscillating saw, leaving its apex intact at the medial cortex. Extend the elbow and close the wedge by fracturing the medial cortex, carefully retaining a periosteal hinge. Place the forearm in supination and evaluate the carrying angle. If it is satisfactory, tighten a wire loop around the heads of the screws to firmly appose the cut surfaces. If necessary, correct any rotational deformity at this time by offsetting the distal screw. Then derotate the

continued

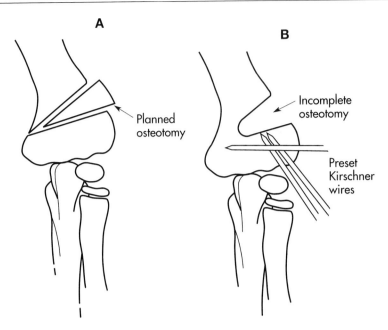

Fig. 33-79   **A,** Wedge to be removed from affected arm is determined on preoperative roentgenogram. **B,** Preset Kirschner wires and incomplete osteotomy. (Redrawn from Voss FR, Kasser JR, Trepman E, et al: *J Pediatr Orthop* 14:474, 1994.)

distal fragment, correct for rotational deformity, and align it with the superior screw. Tighten the wires around the screw heads.

AFTERTREATMENT. The elbow is flexed 90 degrees with the forearm in neutral rotation in a posterior plastic splint for 3 weeks. An active mobilization program is started at that time.

◆ **Oblique Osteotomy with Derotation**

TECHNIQUE 33-19 *(Amspacher and Messenbaugh)*

With the patient prone and a pneumatic tourniquet in place, expose the elbow posteriorly through a longitudinal incision that fashions a tongue of triceps fascia and divides the triceps muscle in line with its fibers (Technique 1-85). Expose subperiosteally the supracondylar part of the humerus, taking care to protect the radial and ulnar nerves in the periphery of the wound. Use an oscillating saw to make an oblique osteotomy about 3.8 cm proximal to the distal end of the humerus, directing it from posteriorly above to anteriorly below; complete it anteriorly with an osteotome. Then tilt and rotate the distal fragment until the internal rotation and cubitus varus have been corrected. With the fragments in proper position, fix them with a screw inserted across the middle of the osteotomy.

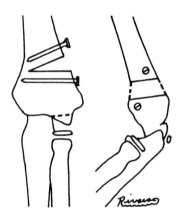

Fig. 33-80   French closing wedge osteotomy using screw and wire fixation. (Redrawn from French PR: *Lancet* 2:439, 1959.)

AFTERTREATMENT. The arm is immobilized in a long arm splint or cast until union is solid at 4 to 6 weeks.

◆ **Step-Cut Osteotomy**

TECHNIQUE 33-20 *(Derosa and Graziano)*

With the patient prone and a tourniquet inflated, make a posterior approach to the distal humerus (Technique 1-85) and reflect the triceps tendon, taking care to protect both the ulnar and radial nerves. Using a template constructed preoperatively, make a lateral closing wedge osteotomy in the metaphyseal region superior to the olecranon fossa. Place the apex of the template (angle to be corrected) medially with the superior margin perpendicular to the humeral shaft. Join the inferior margin to the superior margin to outline the osteotomy (Fig. 33-81, *A*). Remove the osteotomy wedge, leaving a lateral spike of bone on the distal fragment. Some trimming of the lateral part of the proximal fragment may be necessary for close approximation of the osteotomy. Temporarily fix the osteotomy with crossed Kirschner wires and examine the arm for any remaining deformity. If necessary, correct rotational malalignment and hyperextension deformity. Next, insert a cortical screw as a lag screw through the lateral spike into the proximal fragment and remove the Kirschner wires (Fig. 33-81, *B*). Close the wound in a routine manner and apply a long arm cast with the elbow in slight flexion and the forearm in full supination.

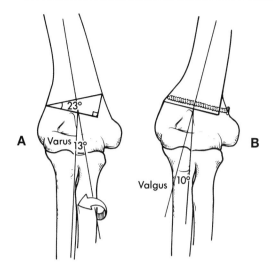

Fig. 33-81 **A,** Osteotomy designed to correct cubitus varus deformity of 13 degrees. Distal fragment can be rotated to correct additional deformity. **B,** After wedge removal and closure, screw is used for fixation. (Redrawn from De Rosa GP, Graziano GP: *Clin Orthop* 236:160, 1988.)

AFTERTREATMENT. The cast is removed at 4 weeks, and active range-of-motion exercises are begun. A posterior shell is used for protection between exercise periods until union is obtained.

SEPARATION OF ENTIRE DISTAL HUMERAL EPIPHYSIS

In younger children the entire distal humeral epiphysis may separate from the humerus in the same area in which supracondylar fractures occur in older children. Although this area is thicker in younger children, it is weaker because it is epiphyseal cartilage (Fig. 33-82). DeLee et al. classified these separations into three groups based on the age of the child and the degree of ossification of the lateral condylar epiphysis. Group A fractures are seen in infants before the secondary ossification center of the lateral condyle appears. These usually are Salter-Harris type I physeal injuries. Because of the lack of ossification of the epiphysis, they can be mistaken for elbow dislocations. According to Barrett et al. and others, these fractures can occur as a birth injury or in newborns, but more important, they can be caused in this age group by child abuse. Group B fractures occur between the ages of 1 and 3 years, when the ossification center of the lateral condylar epiphysis is definitely present, and may be Salter-Harris type I or II fracture. Group C fractures occur in older children and produce a large metaphyseal fragment, displaced most commonly laterally but possibly medially or posteriorly. Groups A and B fractures are almost always displaced medially or posteromedially.

Although separation of the entire epiphysis is rare, it must be differentiated from a dislocation of the elbow in newborns and from a lateral condylar fracture, which usually is a Salter-Harris type IV epiphyseal separation, in older children (Fig. 33-83). This complete separation usually is a Salter-Harris type II fracture and does not necessarily require open reduction and internal fixation, in contrast to most lateral condylar

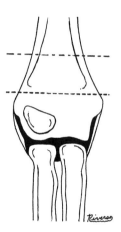

Fig. 33-82 Horizontal lines indicate proximal area where supracondylar fracture occurs and distal area where physeal fracture-separation occurs in wider part of distal humerus in younger age group. (Redrawn from Mizuno K, Hirohata K, Kashiwagi D: *J Bone Joint Surg* 61A:570, 1979.)

fractures. Roentgenographically, both the radial head and proximal ulna are displaced as a unit in relationship to the distal humerus in this epiphyseal fracture-separation (Fig. 33-84). If this relationship, usually posteromedial, is seen and stays equidistant, then the diagnosis of separation of the entire distal humeral epiphysis should be considered. In older children in whom the lateral epiphysis is ossified, a constant relationship is maintained between the visible epiphysis and the radial head.

Yates and Sullivan, Akbarnia et al., Hansen et al., and others noted that arthrography is more accurate than standard roentgenography in the diagnosis of some elbow injuries in young children. They emphasized that distal humeral injuries in

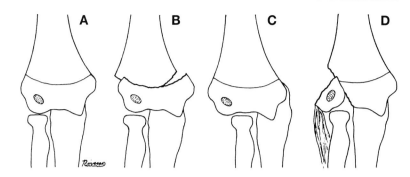

Fig. 33-83 Elbow injuries that may be confused clinically. **A,** Normal elbow before three centers of ossification appear. **B,** Separation of entire distal humeral epiphysis. **C,** Dislocation of elbow. **D,** Lateral condylar fracture. (Redrawn from Mizuno K, Hirohata K, Kashiwagi D: *J Bone Joint Surg* 61A: 570, 1979.)

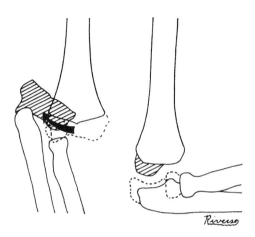

Fig. 33-84 Fracture-separation of entire distal humeral epiphysis displaced posteromedially. Note radial head and proximal ulna displacing as unit in relation to distal humerus. (Redrawn from Barrett WP, Almquist EA, Staheli LT: *J Pediatr Orthop* 4:618, 1984.)

young children can be extremely difficult to diagnose because the cartilaginous ossification centers may not be visible on the roentgenograms; this is especially true in young children in whom the ossific nucleus of the capitellum is not present. With arthrography, using either single- or double-contrast, they were able to confirm a diagnosis and alter treatment in a number of children. Some children thought to have condylar fractures actually had transverse epiphyseal fracture-separations (Salter-Harris type II fractures), and several thought to have intraarticular fractures actually had supracondylar fractures. Some children originally considered for surgery were thus treated nonoperatively after an accurate arthrographic diagnosis. Because they are noninvasive procedures, ultrasonography and MRI are being used to identify nonossified fracture fragments and to establish the diagnosis. This physeal separation injury is included here to emphasize that open reduction and internal fixation are not always necessary because the separation is a Salter-Harris type I or II fracture and will remodel, according to DeLee et al., because it is in the plane of flexion and extension of the elbow. Wilkins showed that most of these fractures remodel without residual deformity, and he stated that many open reductions with internal fixation occurred because these injuries were confused with supracondylar or lateral condylar fractures.

In a small child, a group A fracture usually can be reduced satisfactorily and immobilized in a posterior plaster splint. In an older child with a group C fracture, treatment recommendations include closed reduction with the patient under general anesthesia and cast immobilization. If the fracture is displaced medially, a pronated position probably should be used after reduction. After satisfactory reduction, a long arm cast or a posterior plaster splint should be applied if the separation is stable. If the fracture is unstable after satisfactory closed reduction, smooth pins can be used to stabilize the fracture, similar to the treatment for supracondylar fractures, to prevent the complications of malunion or nonunion (p. 1443). Holda, Manoli, and LaMont noted in seven patients that the separated fragment was almost always medially displaced, and five had mild cubitus varus. Because of this, they recommended treating these fractures aggressively, as with displaced supracondylar fractures, to prevent cubitus varus from a malunion. If a satisfactory reduction could not be obtained or maintained, open reduction and internal fixation with pins were carried out. Mizuno and associates, before the report of DeLee et al., reported six patients in whom open reduction and internal fixation were carried out, in some because of confusion over the diagnosis. They recommended an arthrogram to aid in diagnosis, as well as gentle closed reduction; if reduction was unsatisfactory, open reduction and internal fixation with smooth pins were carried out.

Because this is a Salter-Harris type I or II fracture with remodeling potential, open reduction and internal fixation are indicated only in those fractures with severe displacement that cannot be reduced and held by closed methods.

◆ Open Reduction and Internal Fixation

TECHNIQUE 33-21 *(Mizuno et al.)*
Approach the distal humerus through a long posterior longitudinal incision. Carry the soft tissue dissection down to the subperiosteal area and retract the ulnar nerve medially. Detach the triceps insertion with a cartilaginous piece of the olecranon and reflect it posteriorly and superiorly to expose the fracture. Clean away any debris including small hematomas and fracture fragments. Expose both fragments and gently reduce the epiphyseal separation.

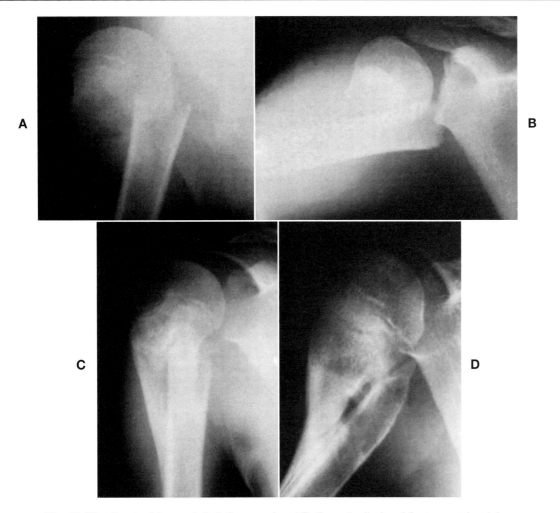

Fig. 33-85   Proximal humeral shaft fracture. **A** and **B,** Severely displaced fracture not involving physis. **C** and **D,** Good remodeling of fracture with satisfactory range of motion after poor reduction.

Insert crossed Kirschner wires through the lateral and medial humeral condyles as for a supracondylar fracture. Irrigate the wound copiously. Apply a posterior splint with the elbow at 90 degrees of flexion. Check the radial pulse.

AFTERTREATMENT. Aftertreatment is the same as for open reduction of supracondylar fractures (p. 1446).

Fractures of Shaft and Proximal End of Humerus

Fractures of the midshaft of the humerus in children always unite; if they are treated in a hanging arm cast, shortening, angulation, and rotary deformity are minimal, and open reduction is almost never indicated. Occasionally, in a fracture at the junction of the middle and distal thirds, the radial nerve is intact but its function disappears after reduction. This should alert the surgeon that the nerve is probably entrapped between the fracture fragments; exploration of the nerve and internal fixation of the fracture, even in children, are then indicated as in adults (Chapter 54).

Although the proximal shaft occasionally fractures (Fig. 33-85), fractures of the proximal humerus are usually physeal, most commonly Salter-Harris type II injuries. Salter-Harris type I fractures do occur but are more common in younger children, whereas types III and IV fractures are rare (Fig. 33-86). A severe fracture or physeal injury in a young child should cause suspicion of child abuse. Neer and Horowitz classified fractures involving the proximal humeral physis according to the amount of displacement. A grade I fracture is displaced less than 5 mm, whereas a grade IV fracture involves total displacement. Salter-Harris types I and II fractures of the proximal humerus rarely require operative treatment (Fig. 33-87). Larsen et al., in their report of 65 patients with proximal humeral metaphyseal or physeal fracture-separation, found that full remodeling occurred. They concluded that

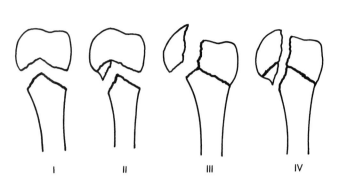

Fig. 33-86 Salter-Harris classification of proximal humeral physeal injuries. Types I and II are extremely common; types III and IV are extremely rare. (Redrawn from Dameron TB, Rockwood CA Jr: Fractures and dislocations of the shoulder. In Rockwood CA Jr, Wilkins KE, King RE, eds: *Fractures in children*, Philadelphia, 1984, JB Lippincott.)

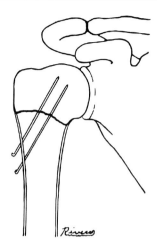

Fig. 33-88 Closed reduction and percutaneous pinning of proximal physeal separation. Two wires cross physis. (Redrawn from Megerl F: Fractures of the proximal humerus. In Weber BG, Brunner C, Freuler F, eds: *Treatment of fractures in children and adolescents*, New York, 1980, Springer-Verlag.)

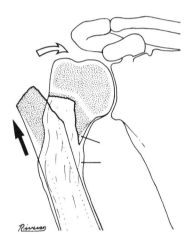

Fig. 33-87 Remodeling potential of proximal humeral physeal fracture because of periosteal sleeve. (Redrawn from Ogden JA: *Skeletal injury in the child*, Philadelphia, 1982, Lea & Febiger.)

nonoperative treatment is appropriate for proximal humeral fractures in children up to the age of 15 years, even when the fracture is extensively displaced. Dameron and Reibel noted 11 ways to treat displaced Salter-Harris types I and II fractures in this area; most are conservative, but percutaneous pinning and open reduction and internal fixation are included. If the fracture is severely displaced, a closed reduction may be necessary, followed by some form of traction or percutaneous pinning with the aid of an image intensifier. In our experience, open reduction is indicated if the distal fragment is buttonholed completely through the deltoid muscle, is impinging against the skin, and cannot be repositioned by closed methods. The open reduction should be done through a short deltoid-splitting approach, taking care not to damage the axillary nerve, or a

short deltopectoral approach. The shaft is reduced through the split deltoid muscle and the fracture is pinned percutaneously. Beringer et al. reported 48 patients with severely displaced proximal humeral epiphyseal fractures. Nine patients underwent open treatment, and three of the nine had complications severe enough for the authors to recommend avoiding operative intervention with few exceptions.

◆ CLOSED REDUCTION AND CASTING OR PERCUTANEOUS PINNING

TECHNIQUE 33-22 *(Sherk and Probst)*

With the patient supine, manipulate the distal fragment into slight external rotation, 90 degrees of flexion, and 70 degrees of abduction using image intensification. This will bring the fragments together satisfactorily. This maneuver should push the upper part of the shaft back through the rent in the deltoid muscle and anterior periosteum and correct the anterior angulation. Have an assistant support the proximal fragment to help achieve and maintain the reduction. Test for stability by bringing the distal fragment down out of flexion and abduction. If the reduction remains stable, apply a Velpeau dressing to be worn for 4 or 5 weeks until union is sufficient to permit gentle shoulder motion. If the fracture becomes redisplaced immediately after reduction, repeat the reduction maneuver and keep the arm supported in the salute position. Apply either a spica cast or skin traction in this position. As an alternative, drill one or two smooth Steinmann pins through the lateral shaft in a proximal direction into the humeral head to maintain the reduction. Cut the pins beneath the skin to be removed at 3 to 4 weeks (Fig. 33-88). Immobilize the arm in the neutral position.

◆ ◆ ◆

Open reduction also may be indicated for (1) the rare displaced Salter-Harris types III and IV fractures, (2) interposition of the biceps tendon in the fracture site, (3) fracture-dislocations, and (4) open fractures. Open reduction and internal fixation of Salter-Harris type III or type IV fractures, as well as biceps interposition and fracture-dislocations, are similar to the surgical procedures necessary for Neer type III or type IV fractures in adults (see Chapter 54).

Acromioclavicular Dislocations

Dameron and Reibel and Rockwood described five types of acromioclavicular injuries in children (Fig. 33-89). A type I injury is a contusion of the joint not sufficient to rupture the acromioclavicular or the coracoclavicular ligaments. A type II injury damages the acromioclavicular ligaments but not the coracoclavicular ligaments; a partial periosteal sleeve (tube) tear also occurs. In a type III injury, the acromioclavicular ligament is completely ruptured, but the coracoclavicular ligaments are intact inasmuch as they are still attached to the periosteum. The clavicle is unstable and is displaced superiorly through a rent in the periosteal tube (pseudodislocation). A type IV injury is identical to type III except that in addition to being displaced superiorly, the clavicle is also displaced posteriorly. The type V injury is severe; the acromioclavicular ligaments are disrupted, and, although the coracoclavicular ligaments are still attached to the periosteal sleeve, the clavicle is now unstable and its lateral end is buried in the trapezius and deltoid muscles or has pierced them and is located under the skin in the posterior aspect of the shoulder. In many types III, IV, and V dislocations, an unrecognized fracture of the distal end of the clavicle occurs, with the acromioclavicular and coracoclavicular ligaments remaining intact and attached to the empty periosteal tube or to the most distal fragment. This pseudodislocation was originally described by Katznelson et al. According to Curtis, Dameron and Reibel, and Rockwood, in children and adolescents up to age 15, types I, II, and III acromioclavicular separations, even with a fracture of the distal third of the clavicle, can be treated by nonoperative means. In patients older than 15, type III injuries may require more aggressive treatment. Open reduction and internal fixation should be considered for markedly displaced types IV and V fractures (Chapter 54). Falstie-Jensen and Mikkelsen believe that, because the incidence of complete rupture of the periosteum of the lateral part of the clavicle is unknown, it is possible to have instead a total rupture of the coracoclavicular ligaments, and they believe that the amount of periosteal damage can be determined only at surgery; therefore they recommended operative treatment for types IV and V lesions. According to them, although new bone will form from the periosteal envelope, the lateral end of the clavicle will become Y-shaped and will be unsightly and uncomfortable if the injury is not treated operatively.

In types IV and V acromioclavicular dislocations, it is

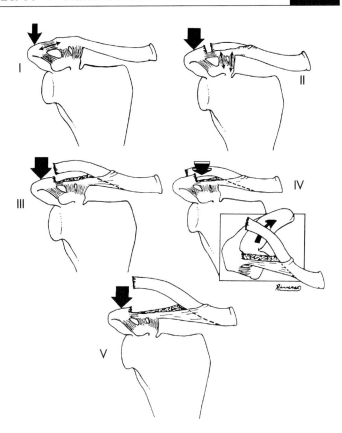

Fig. 33-89 Five types of acromioclavicular separation occurring in children (see text). Acromioclavicular and coracoclavicular ligaments are attached to periosteal tube even though distal end of clavicle is significantly displaced in types III, IV, and V. (Redrawn from Dameron TB, Rockwood CA Jr: Fractures and dislocations of the shoulder. In Rockwood CA Jr, Wilkins KE, King RE, eds: *Fractures in children*, Philadelphia, 1984, JB Lippincott.)

important to disengage the distal clavicle from the trapezius and deltoid muscles. If this is not successful by closed means, surgery is indicated to remove the clavicle from the muscles and replace it in the periosteal tube. The periosteal tube should be repaired and the deltoid-trapezius muscle fascia should be imbricated superiorly over the clavicle. If the repair is unstable, then internal fixation is required, as in adults, by either acromioclavicular or coracoclavicular fixation, as described in Chapter 54.

Fractures and Dislocations of Clavicle

Fractures of the clavicle can be classified into those occurring in the outer (distal), middle, and proximal (medial) thirds. Fractures of the distal or outer third of the clavicle heal satisfactorily without surgical treatment because the periosteal tube remains intact at the fracture site. The ligamentous attachments also remain intact. Remodeling of the fracture will

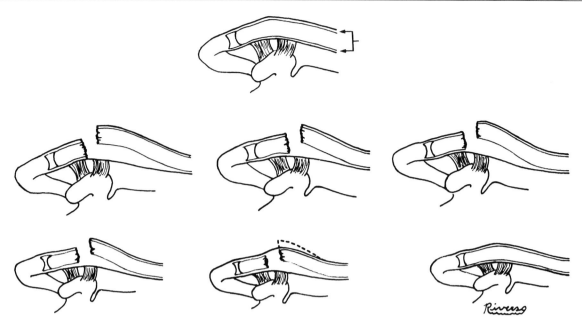

Fig. 33-90 Distal clavicle fracture with coracoclavicular and coracoacromial ligaments still intact or at least attached to periosteal tube. Fracture in child will remodel satisfactorily without surgery. (Redrawn from Rockwood CA Jr: Fractures and dislocations of the ends of the clavicle, scapula, and glenohumeral joint. In Rockwood CA Jr, Wilkins KE, King RE, eds: *Fractures in children*, Philadelphia, 1984, JB Lippincott.)

occur along the intact periosteal tube (Fig. 33-90). Some authors state that when the supportive coracoclavicular ligaments are disrupted, fractures of the distal clavicle in adults require surgery to reduce and align the fracture properly. Because of the periosteal tube, fracture of the distal clavicle in children is not analogous to that in adults, and surgery is not necessary.

Havranek reported 10 distal physeal clavicular injuries, 9 of which were treated conservatively either by closed reduction, figure-eight bandage, or Desault bandage. One fracture was treated with open reduction and internal fixation because of severe displacement of the central fragment and deformity of the shoulder. All fractures healed without functional impairment, but 7 of the 9 patients treated conservatively had visible deformity of the affected shoulder. He recommended open reduction for cosmesis if displacement of the central metaphyseal fragment results in shortening of the clavicle and deformity of the shoulder. Wilkes and Hoffer, on the other hand, reported 38 clavicular fractures in children with head injuries, all of which healed without immobilization and exhibited excellent remodeling. All patients recovered complete shoulder range of motion. Two lateral fractures resulted in "double" clavicles, one of which required surgery for removal of a tender bony prominence. If surgery is indicated in an older adolescent, the operative treatment is as in Technique 54-1.

Fractures of the midshaft of the clavicle rarely require surgical treatment. Open reduction usually is condemned because it appears to increase the incidences of delayed union and nonunion. If the fracture is tenting the skin, it can be reduced beneath the trapezius with a towel clip with the patient under either general or local anesthesia. Fractures of the clavicle in children should not be confused with congenital pseudarthrosis of the clavicle, as discussed in Chapter 28.

Besides debridement of an open fracture, the only indications for surgery in a midshaft clavicular fracture in a child are a vascular injury complicating the fracture, which should be treated as a vascular emergency, and an established nonunion caused by trauma (Fig. 33-91).

Fractures of the proximal or medial third of the clavicle are difficult to diagnose. The cephalic tilt view, shot at 45 degrees cephalad as recommended by Curtis, Dameron and Reibel, and Rockwood, is helpful in differentiating between a dislocation of the sternoclavicular joint, which rarely occurs in children, and a Salter-Harris type I or II fracture of the proximal clavicular physis, which is quite common. The medial physis of the clavicle usually does not fuse until ages 20 to 24 years, and most injuries that are thought to be anterior dislocations of the sternoclavicular joint in children and young adults are actually Salter-Harris types I and II fractures of the proximal clavicle (Fig. 33-92). A "knot" usually appears 2 weeks after injury at the medial end of the clavicle. These physeal fractures should be treated conservatively. Reduction is easy but cannot be maintained. Nevertheless, these fractures will remodel and leave only a small anterior prominence. Operative treatment is not justified, and Rockwood has described numerous complications of ill-advised operations on these benign injuries.

For possible true dislocations of the sternoclavicular joint we obtain a 45-degree cephalad tilt supine roentgenographic view, as described by Rockwood. In the absence of a proximal fracture or physeal separation, the entire clavicle, if dislocated

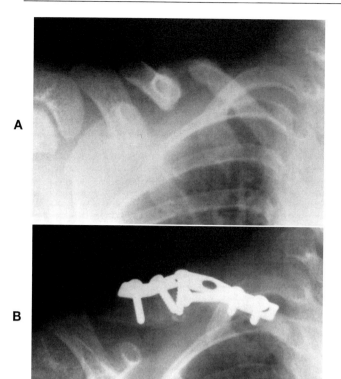

A

B

Fig. 33-91 **A,** Nonunion of clavicle *(right)* in 3-year-old child. Although traumatic fracture of the clavicle in a child of this age is rare, this was not considered congenital pseudarthrosis of clavicle, which also almost always occurs on right side, is present at young age, and produces "rounded" bone ends. **B,** At surgery, new callus was found around fracture fragments; open reduction and internal fixation with semitubular plate were performed, and union was obtained.

anteriorly, will be cephalad as compared with the contralateral uninvolved medial end of the clavicle. In a posterior dislocation, which is extremely rare, it will be caudad to the uninvolved contralateral medial end of the clavicle. The treatment of sternoclavicular dislocations is discussed in Chapter 57.

Spine Fractures and Dislocations

CERVICAL SPINE

Cervical spine fractures are not as common in children as in adults. They do occur in newborn infants from child abuse, in young children with congenital anomalies such as Down syndrome, and in older children from accidents such as occur in diving. The cervical region is more flexible in children than in adults. In fact, it is difficult to differentiate the normal from the abnormal on flexion and extension roentgenograms of the cervical spine of a child. Fielding came to several conclusions concerning the mobility between C1 and C2 on lateral roentgenograms in adults. Anterior displacement of the atlas of

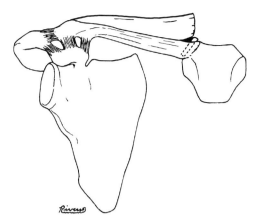

Fig. 33-92 Injury shown is Salter-Harris type I physeal separation of medial clavicle rather than dislocation of sternoclavicular joint. (Redrawn from Rockwood CA Jr: Fractures and dislocations of the ends of the clavicle, scapula, and glenohumeral joint. In Rockwood CA Jr, Wilkins KE, King RE, eds: *Fractures in children*, Philadelphia, 1984, JB Lippincott.)

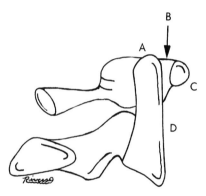

Fig. 33-93 Relationships of atlas and axis. *A,* Apical epiphysis. *B,* Space between odontoid and atlas anteriorly, which may be over 3 mm in children. *C,* Anterior arch of atlas. *D,* Basilar odontoid synchondrosis or cartilaginous plate, which may fuse between 7 and 10 years of age. (Redrawn from Cattell HS, Filtzer DL: *J Bone Joint Surg* 26A:1295, 1965.)

up to 3 mm is within the range of normal. When the distance between the odontoid process and the arch of C1 is between 3 and 5 mm, the transverse ligaments are ruptured. When the distance is greater than 10 to 12 mm, all the ligaments have failed. Cattell and Filtzer noted in their study that a minimum of 3 mm and even more of anterior displacement of the atlas in flexion was a normal variation in 14 asymptomatic children 1 to 7 years old (Fig. 33-93). This difference between adults and children probably is caused by mobility and ligamentous laxity. Pseudosubluxation of C2 on C3, originally noted by Bailey, has also been described by Cattell and Filtzer. They noted significant anterior displacement of C2 on C3 in flexion in young children without symptoms and noted that pseudosubluxation is a normal variant. This normal pseudosubluxation was noted primarily in children between the ages of 1 and 7 years but did occur in older children and also in the relationship of C3 to C4, but to a lesser degree. These examples are given because it is important to distinguish normal variants from acute fractures or fracture-dislocations.

Fielding outlined these and other normal roentgenographic variations that may be misinterpreted as acute injuries:

1. The apical ossification center of the odontoid, which may be confused with an acute fracture
2. Secondary ossification centers at the tips of the transverse and spinous processes, which may be confused with avulsion fractures
3. Incomplete ossification, especially of the odontoid process, with apparent superior subluxation of the anterior arch of C1
4. Persistence of the synchondrosis (physis) at the base of the odontoid
5. Anterior wedging in a vertebral body, which may be misinterpreted as a compression fracture or a subluxation
6. Hypermobility "pseudosubluxation," especially of C2 anterior to C3
7. Increase in the atlanto-dens interval of up to 4 mm
8. Absence of the ossification of the anterior arch of C1 in the first year of life, which suggests posterior displacement of C1 on the odontoid
9. Physiological variations in the width of the soft tissue swelling anterior to the cervical spine
10. Overlying anatomy, such as the ears, braided hair, teeth, or the hyoid bone
11. Horizontally placed facets in the normal child, which create the illusion of a pillar fracture
12. Congenital anomalies such as os odontoideum, spina bifida, and lack of segmentation
13. Less-than-normal lateral lordotic posture of the neck

Radionuclide bone scanning, tomography, CT scanning, and MRI may be helpful in distinguishing normal growth variants from traumatic injuries in the cervical spine.

Herzenberg et al. described modifications of the standard backboard for safer alignment of the spine during transport of young children with cervical spine injuries. In their study of 10 children younger than 7 years, they found that unstable injuries of the cervical spine had anterior angulation or translation or both, and that extension was the proper position for reduction in all 10. Because young children have a large head in comparison to the rest of the body, positioning on a standard backboard may force the neck into relative kyphosis. Herzenberg et al. recommended the use of a recess for the occiput to lower the head or a double mattress pad to raise the chest and prevent undesirable cervical flexion.

Atlantoaxial Fracture-Dislocations

Lesions in the area from the occiput to the atlas or C1 are extremely rare and are usually lethal. Henrys et al. noted a high incidence of cervical spine injuries occurring from C1 to C4 in children as compared with adult injuries, which are more prevalent from C3 to C7. Fielding reported four lesions occurring at the C1-2 interval in children: (1) ligamentous laxity related to inflammation or other local affliction, (2) rotary deformity, (3) traumatic ligamentous disruption, and (4) odontoid fracture.

Atlantoaxial displacement caused by inflammation, after an upper respiratory tract viral infection, tuberculosis, syphilis, poliomyelitis, juvenile rheumatoid arthritis, or ankylosing spondylitis, or in Down syndrome or eosinophilic granuloma, should not be confused with traumatic ligamentous disruption. A careful history and physical and roentgenographic examinations, including CT scans, should determine if a significant traumatic injury has occurred. With appropriate treatment of the inflammation or other affliction, and cervical traction in extension to stabilize the vertebrae, most atlantoaxial displacements do well. However, Marar and Balachandran reported nontraumatic atlantoaxial dislocations in 12 children, 3 of whom had posterior cervical spine fusion because of persistent symptoms and neurological signs from unreduced dislocations after 6 weeks of treatment with traction.

Lateral rotary displacement of the odontoid-axial area is relatively common and is one of the most common causes of traumatic torticollis. Bailey noted four different types of rotary displacement. Regardless of type, most rotary deformities require little more than head-halter traction, muscle relaxants, and bed rest. However, Fielding noted that some of these deformities may become fixed, especially if rotary displacement is significant. He recommended a C1 and C2 fusion for stability and to maintain correction when the following conditions are present: (1) persistent neurological involvement, (2) significant anterior rotary displacement, (3) failure to achieve or maintain correction if the deformity has been present for longer than 3 months, and (4) recurrence of the deformity after an adequate trial of conservative management, consisting of at least 6 weeks of immobilization.

Traumatic ligamentous disruption is difficult to diagnose in children because in flexion there may be 3 mm or more of anterior displacement of the atlas on the axis without significant trauma. Fielding suggested that if there is evidence of significant trauma and more than 5 mm of displacement, then a definite ligamentous rupture has occurred. If the rupture is acute, he recommended, and we agree, that reduction in extension by traction should be carried out; later a halo cast is used to hold the reduction for 8 to 12 weeks. Then flexion and extension roentgenograms should be obtained. According to Fielding, if the displacement and symptoms persist, fusion of C1 to C2 should be performed (Chapter 35).

Fractures of the Odontoid

Failure of ossification of the apical odontoid process or lack of synchondrotic fusion of the base of the odontoid should not be confused with a fracture (see Fig. 33-93). The synchondrosis (physis) of the base of the odontoid usually closes by age 7, but it can persist roentgenographically for 2 to 4 years longer. As a result, most fractures of the odontoid process in children occur around the age of 7 or earlier and almost invariably occur between the odontoid process and the body of the second

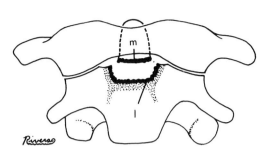

Fig. 33-94   Pattern of odontoid fractures. *m* marks level of usual adult fractures. *l* marks area of childhood fractures at synchondrosis. (Redrawn from Ogden JA: *Skeletal injury in the child*, Philadelphia, 1982, Lea & Febiger.)

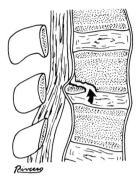

Fig. 33-95   Posterior physeal injury that can mimic ruptured disc. Avulsion of ring apophysis has produced displaced fragment that presses on nerve root. (Redrawn from Ogden JA: *Skeletal injury in the child*, Philadelphia, 1982, Lea & Febiger.)

cervical vertebra, at or near the synchondrosis (Fig. 33-94). Sherk, Nicholson, and Chung found that odontoid fractures in children younger than 7 years old that are treated promptly usually heal without sequelae. The fractures usually can be reduced by passive manipulation or recumbency on a divided mattress and head-halter traction in extension. Immobilization in the reduced position for 2 to 3 months in a neck brace or a halo cast or vest should result in healing. A halo cast should not be applied until the fracture is reduced. If the acute fracture cannot be reduced, then skeletal traction with tongs or even closed manipulative reduction with the patient under general anesthesia may be necessary. Traction should be used carefully because of the possibility of dangerous distraction. Sherk et al. and Gertzbein noted good results in these fractures in children, which contrasts sharply with the results and difficulties encountered in the same injury in adults, as noted by Anderson and D'Alonzo. Odent et al. reviewed 15 odontoid fractures in children younger than 6 years of age, 8 of whom had neurological involvement. Conservatively treated fractures fused without problems; however 3 patients whose initial management was operative had complications postoperatively.

Congenital anomalies such as an os odontoideum or a rudimentary odontoid may contribute to C1 to C2 instability, especially in adolescent athletes; these children should be watched closely for any evidence of instability. If symptoms justify it, the cervical spine should be fused as in adults (Chapter 37).

C3 to C7 Fractures and Dislocations

Fractures below C2 in young children are extremely rare and difficult to diagnose, since anterior wedging of an end plate often can be present, simulating an anterior compression fracture of a vertebral body. Furthermore, because of more horizontal facets and ligamentous laxity in a child, anterior displacement of the superior vertebra 3 mm or more can, as previously noted, simulate a dislocation (pseudodislocation). Eosinophilic granuloma and vertebral plana should not be mistaken for a traumatic fracture; these are pathological collapses that will heal uneventfully. A significant fracture or a

fracture-dislocation of the cervical spine may require stabilization as in adults (Chapter 35).

Fielding, as well as Anderson and D'Alonzo and Edmonson, noted that fusion of the cervical spine in children occurs more rapidly than in adults. The fusion mass in children develops more rapidly and profusely, and consequently it is prudent to explore only the area in which the fusion is indicated. Otherwise, extension of the fusion above or below the area of fracture or dislocation may result in a more extensive fusion than is necessary, with ultimately more stiffness of the neck. This is especially true in C1 to C2 arthrodesis, where a generous superior and inferior exposure will result in an occiput to C3 fusion, which is unnecessary.

THORACIC AND LUMBAR SPINE FRACTURES

Fractures in the thoracic and lumbar spine in children are rarer than fractures in the cervical spine. They do occur in newborn infants from child abuse, in older children from moving vehicular accidents, and in teenagers from sports and recreational activities. Eosinophilic granuloma, Gaucher disease, metastatic disease, osteogenesis imperfecta, idiopathic juvenile osteoporosis, and Scheuermann disease may all simulate acute traumatic compression fractures in children. Hensinger described an anterior wedge compression fracture simulating Scheuermann disease in the thoracolumbar and lumbar spines. He suggested that these are actually microfractures that may occur in adolescent weight lifters and especially in female gymnasts. Scheuermann disease in the thoracic spine, and traumatic spondylolysis and spondylolisthesis, are described elsewhere (Chapter 38).

Lowrey and others noted that a displaced fragment of a lumbar vertebral ring epiphysis in adolescents may simulate disc rupture (Fig. 33-95). The finding at surgery in each patient was a displaced bony fragment from the apophyseal ring, which was deficient posteriorly. Others have noted that an end plate physeal fracture and herniated disc material also can cause neurological sequelae. Regardless, an MRI is the diagnostic procedure of choice.

Kewalramani and Tori reviewed 97 children with spinal cord trauma, two thirds in the cervical area and one third in the thoracic and lumbar areas. Most had complete spinal cord lesions. Of the 35 injuries in the thoracic and lumbar areas, most fractures and dislocations complicated by cord injuries occurred from T1 to T12, with few lumbar lesions. Others have noted that, because of the elasticity of a child's spine and the cartilaginous nature of the vertebrae, forces are transmitted over many segments and multiple fractures may occur. Most thoracolumbar fractures with associated neurological loss are associated with vertebral body fractures; some have neural arch fractures and subluxation rather than dislocation. Hensinger noted that restoration of height of a compressed vertebra caused by fractures in children is partly the result of hypervascularity of the reparative response and stimulation of the physis. This probably accounts for the infrequent occurrence of kyphosis in children with multiple compression fractures. Hensinger pointed out that operative treatment in a young child is indicated only in the presence of significant neurological involvement, persistent frank dislocation, or a block on the myelogram. We also have noted that most anterior compression fractures in children heal without sequelae, and some height of the vertebra is gained after the fracture. This also occurs after multiple fractures, and little kyphotic residual should be expected. In compression fractures the type of treatment does not appear to affect the outcome, and several days to several weeks of bed rest usually is all that is necessary for symptoms to disappear completely. The more complex fractures, such as burst fractures with fragments protruding into the spinal canal, the rare "Chance" fracture, and the fracture-dislocation should be managed similarly to those in adults (Chapter 35).

Reid et al. and Rumball and Jarvis noted an association between pediatric Chance fractures caused by seat belt use and intraabdominal injuries, especially when the child has a "seat-belt" sign (abdominal contusion consisting of ecchymosis and bruising in a band that corresponds to the position of the seat belt across the abdomen). In the presence of a neurological deficit after a burst fracture-dislocation or Chance fracture, open reduction should be carried out and the fracture stabilized by internal fixation (Fig. 33-96).

Operative indications and techniques for fractures of the thoracic and lumbar spine in children are similar to those in adults (Chapter 35). Laminectomy is indicated only rarely, and then for progression of neurological deficit; otherwise, it should be avoided, as in adults.

The major complication of thoracic spine fractures in children is paraplegia. The sequelae of paraplegia have been outlined by Hensinger and others and include (1) increase in the number of long bone fractures, (2) paralytic hip dislocations, (3) decubitus ulcers, (4) flexion contractures, (5) genitourinary complications, and (6) progressive spinal deformity, including scoliosis, kyphosis, and lordosis. Age, type of injury, and amount of spasticity seem to be the most important factors in the development of significant spinal deformity, which can occur at all levels. The management of paralytic kyphoscoliosis is described in Chapter 38.

Pelvic Fractures

Fractures of the pelvis in children are unusual. Open reduction and internal fixation rarely are necessary for these fractures. Generally the long-term results of conservative treatment are satisfactory because of the remodeling potential of the pelvis in children. However, soft tissue injuries occurring in conjunction with pelvic fractures may be severe and require emergency treatment. Many pelvic fractures occur in children struck by moving vehicles. Associated injuries include skull, cervical, facial, and long bone fractures; subdural hematomas, cerebral contusions and concussions; lung contusions; hemothorax; hemopneumothorax; ruptured diaphragm; and lacerations of the spleen, liver, and kidney. Injuries that may be associated with and adjacent to pelvic fractures include damage to major blood vessels, retroperitoneal bleeding, rectal tears, and rupture or laceration of the urethra or bladder. Bond et al. noted that the location and number of pelvic fractures were strongly associated with the probability of abdominal injury: 1% for isolated pubic fractures, 15% for iliac or sacral fractures, and 60% for multiple fractures of the pelvic ring. Because of these other injuries, mortality in children is high, ranging from 9% to 18%. Rieger and Brug reviewed 54 major pelvic fractures and noted that 87% had associated pelvic or extrapelvic (soft tissue) injuries; 14.8% died. Most patients (70.4%) were treated conservatively. They believe the principles of management in children should not differ greatly from those in adults. Serious associated pelvic or extrapelvic injuries may pose more treatment problems than the actual pelvic fractures.

Torode and Zieg reported 11 deaths in 141 patients with pelvic fractures, and 40% of patients with type IV injuries (Fig. 33-97) required laparotomy because of other injuries. Frequently a child who has what roentgenographically appears to be a minor pelvic fracture also has suffered significant and possibly life-threatening soft tissue injuries about the pelvis.

The pelvis in children differs from that in adults in that (1) more malleability is present because of the nature of the bone itself, the increased elasticity of joints, and the ability of the cartilaginous structures to absorb energy; (2) the elasticity of the joints about the pelvis is greater, which may allow for significant displacement and result in fracture of only one area rather than the traditional double break in the pelvic ring seen in adults; (3) the cartilage at the apophyses is inherently weak as compared with bone, so avulsion fractures occur more frequently in children and adolescents than in adults; and (4) fractures into the triradiate cartilage can occur, causing growth arrest, which results in leg length inequality and faulty development of the acetabulum.

Numerous classification systems have been devised for pelvic fractures in children. Torode and Zieg proposed a four-part classification of pelvic fractures (see Fig. 33-97): type I, avulsion of the bony elements of the pelvis; type II, iliac wing fractures; type III, simple ring fractures, including those involving the pubic rami or disruptions of the pubic symphysis; and type IV, ring disruption fractures, which create an unstable segment of the pelvic ring, including bilateral pubic rami

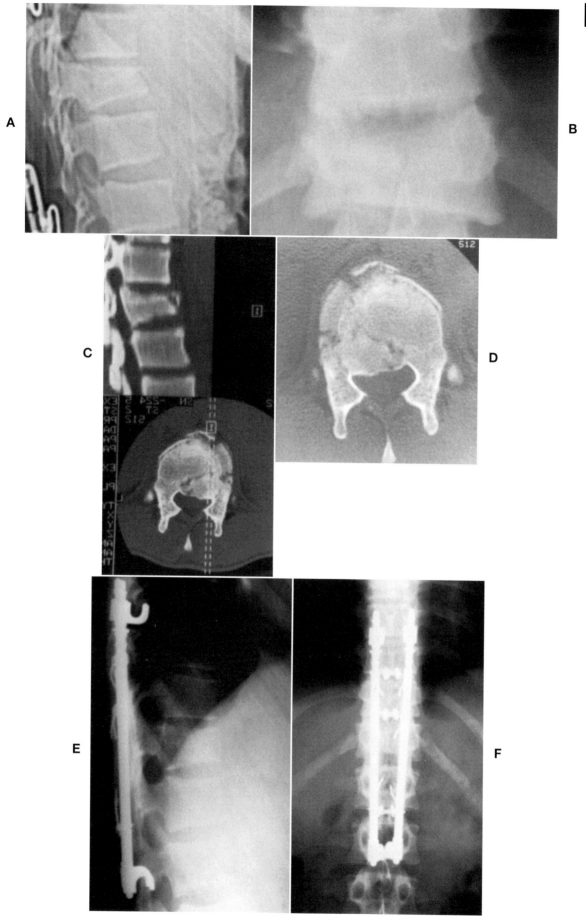

Fig. 33-96   A and B, Burst and compression fractures of T12 in 14-year-old child. C and D, CT scan shows over 50% compromise of canal. E and F, Restoration of vertebral height after reduction.

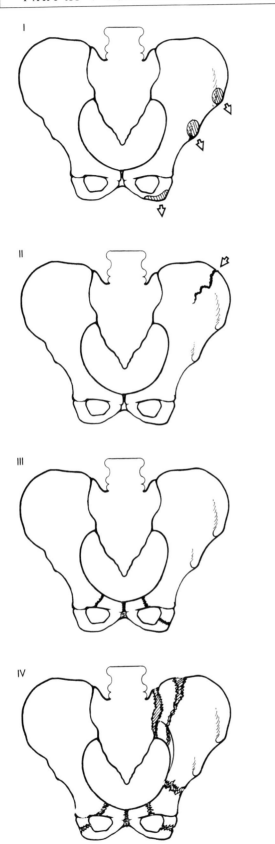

Fig. 33-97   Classification of pelvic fractures (see text). (Redrawn from Torode I, Zieg D: *J Pediatr Orthop* 5:76, 1985.)

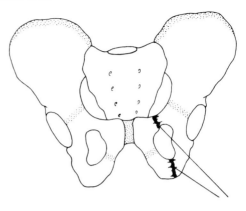

Fig. 33-98   Single break in pelvic ring, with two ipsilateral rami fractures. (Redrawn from Ogden JA: *Skeletal injury in the child*, Philadelphia, 1982, Lea & Febiger.)

(straddle) fractures (Fig. 33-98), fractures involving either the right or left pubic rami or the pubic symphysis and a fracture through the posterior elements or disruption of the sacroiliac joint, and fractures involving the anterior structures and acetabular portion of the pelvic ring. This classification does not include acetabular fractures. Quinby and Rang classified pelvic fractures into three categories: uncomplicated fractures, fractures with visceral injuries requiring surgical exploration, and fractures associated with immediate massive hemorrhage. Although this classification is useful concerning the patient's ultimate outcome, its emphasis is on associated soft tissue injuries rather than on the pelvic fracture itself. Moreno et al. described four types of "fracture geometry" based on roentgenographic appearance and used to identify patients at risk for severe hemorrhage. Classifications by Letournel, Judet, Pennal, Tile, Ogden, and the AO/ASIF group emphasize fracture stability. Young and Burgess classified pelvic fractures according to the direction of force: lateral compression, anteroposterior compression, vertical shear, and combined mechanisms. Key and Conwell's classification of pelvic fractures in adults is based on the number of breaks in the pelvic ring. Their system, which includes acetabular fractures, also is applicable in children (Fig. 33-99). We have evaluated 134 pelvic fractures in children; the percentages of the individual bones and types of fractures are given in Table 33-2. The Orthopaedic Trauma Association (OTA) devised a classification scheme that consists of three main types and numerous subtypes: A, lesion sparing (or with no displacement of) posterior arch; B, incomplete disruption of posterior arch, partially stable; C, complete disruption of posterior arch, unstable.

Comparison among studies using different systems is difficult, and the most useful information is whether a fracture is stable or unstable. Most pelvic fractures in children are stable.

AVULSION FRACTURES

Avulsion fractures occur most commonly in adolescent athletes; they occur in the anterosuperior and anteroinferior

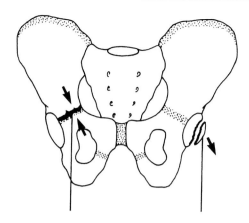

Fig. 33-99 Small acetabular rim fracture *(right)* and triradiate cartilage compression fracture *(left)*. (Redrawn from Ogden JA: *Skeletal injury in the child*, Philadelphia, 1982, Lea & Febiger.)

Table 33-2   Distribution of Pelvic Fractures in Children, Campbell Clinic Series (134 Patients)*

I—Individual Bones 66.5%				II—Single Break 11.9%			III—Double Break 11.9%			IV—Acetabulum 9.7%			
A	**B**	**C**	**D**	**A**	**B**	**C**	**A**	**B**	**C**	**A**	**B**	**C**	**D**
13.4%	33.6%	18%	1.5%	8.2%	3%	0.7%	3%	8.2%	0.7%	0.7%	6%	0	3%

COMPARISON WITH OTHER SERIES

	Dunn†	Peltier†	Reed†	Hall, Klassen, Ilstrup‡	Campbell Clinic‡
	(115 pts.)	(186 pts.)	(84 pts.)	(204 pts.)	(134 pts.)
I—Individual bones		10%	60.5%	24.5%	66.5%
II—Single break	70%	39%	2.5%	18.6%	11.9%
III—Double break	30%	27%	32.0%	31.9%	11.9%
IV—Acetabulum	Not included	24%	5%	7.8%	9.7%
				(17.2% acetabulum and	
				pelvis)	

From Rockwood CA Jr, Wilkins KD, King RE, editors: *Fractures in children,* ed 3, vol 3, Philadelphia, 1991, JB Lippincott.
*Classification of Key and Conwell.
†Adult series.
‡Children's series.

iliac spines and in the ischial tuberosity and are caused by overpull of the sartorius muscle, rectus femoris muscle, and hamstring muscles, respectively. Fernbach and Wilkinson reported 20 avulsion fractures of the apophyses of the pelvis and proximal femur, most of which occurred in male adolescents engaged in competitive sports; 6 of these fractures involved the ischial tuberosity, 5 the lesser femoral trochanter, 4 the anteroinferior iliac spine, 4 the anterosuperior iliac spine, and 1 the iliac crest apophysis (Fig. 33-100). Approximately 13% of injuries in our series were avulsion injuries. Operative treatment for these injuries is rarely if ever indicated. Results were as good in those treated conservatively as in those treated with open reduction and internal fixation of the fragments regardless of the amount of displacement. Rarely, excessive callus formation or myositis ossificans will occur after a displaced ischial tuberosity fracture. In two of our patients it was necessary to excise the fragment and the callus rather than reattach the fragment. Recurrence of some excessive callus or

myositis ossificans occurred, but these two patients have continued their athletic activity. Sundar and Carty described 32 avulsion fractures of the pelvis in adolescents (average age, 13.8 years) seen at an average 44-month follow-up; 10 patients had disability persisting into adulthood and limitation of sports activity, and 6 patients continued to have persistent symptoms. Although they advocated surgical exploration and removal of ununited fragments, Sundar and Carty cautioned that surgical treatment does not guarantee the return of the athlete to the same standard as before the injury. Any of these avulsion injuries, especially in the area of the ischium, can be confused with infection, myositis ossificans, and even Ewing sarcoma.

PELVIC FRACTURES

Three physical signs commonly associated with pelvic fractures were described by Milch: (1) Destot sign—a large superficial hematoma formation beneath the inguinal ligament or in the scrotum, (2) Roux sign—a decrease in the distance of the greater trochanter to the pubic spine on the affected side in lateral compression fractures, and (3) Earle sign—a bony prominence or large hematoma, as well as tenderness on rectal examination, indicating a significant pelvic fracture. Posterior

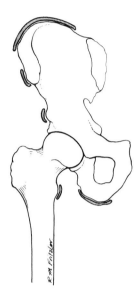

Fig. 33-100   Distribution of 20 avulsion fractures in children: iliac crest, 1; anterosuperior iliac spine, 4; anteroinferior iliac spine, 4; lesser trochanter, 5; ischium or ischial apophysis, 6. (Redrawn from Fernbach SK, Wilkinson RH: *Am J Roentgenol* 137:581, 1981.)

pressure on the iliac crest causes pain at the fracture site as the pelvic ring is opened, and compression of the pelvic ring at the iliac crest from lateral to medial causes pain and possibly crepitation. Downward pressure on the symphysis pubis and posteriorly on the sacroiliac joints causes pain and motion if a break in the pelvic ring is present. Pain in the inguinal area can be elicited by flexion and extension of the hips.

As already mentioned, most pelvic fractures in children can be treated closed, usually by a few days or weeks at bed rest. Any residual deformity usually is unimportant or remodels with growth. Nierenberg et al. reported good to excellent functional results despite roentgenographic evidence of pelvic deformities after conservative treatment of pelvic fractures in 20 children. They suggested that treatment guidelines for pelvic fractures are not the same for children as for adults, and they recommended that surgery, either external or internal fixation, be used only when conventional methods have been exhausted. Occasionally, a significant diastasis of the symphysis requires bed rest in a pelvic sling, followed by a spica cast in the reduced position. We also have used a pelvic external fixator to close the diastasis of the symphysis (Fig. 33-101). According to Mears and Fu, symphysis pubis and sacroiliac subluxations should be treated as aggressively in children as in adults because little or no remodeling occurs to compensate for joint subluxations or dislocations. The technique of external fixation of pelvic fractures is described in Chapter 53.

The Malgaigne fracture, a double vertical fracture in the pelvic ring or a fracture with a dislocation, renders the hemipelvis unstable, but fortunately it is less common in children than in adults. A CT scan may be helpful in

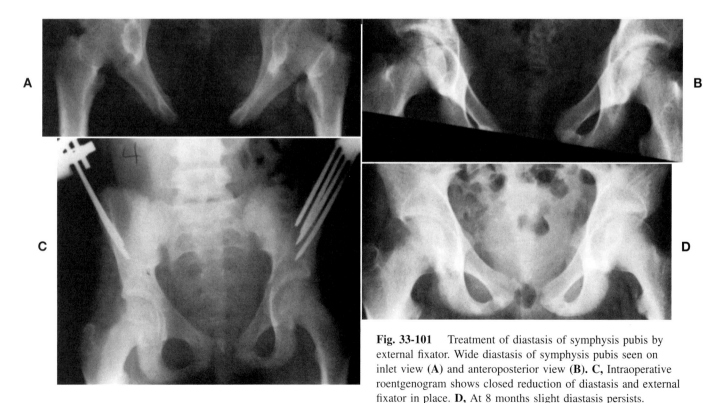

Fig. 33-101   Treatment of diastasis of symphysis pubis by external fixator. Wide diastasis of symphysis pubis seen on inlet view (**A**) and anteroposterior view (**B**). **C,** Intraoperative roentgenogram shows closed reduction of diastasis and external fixator in place. **D,** At 8 months slight diastasis persists.

determining the amount of joint displacement. Various methods of treatment for Malgaigne or severely comminuted fractures have been described. In the past, we have used a combination of skeletal traction and a pelvic sling. Occasionally a spica cast is applied incorporating the pelvic sling while the pelvic traction is still in place. We have on numerous occasions used an external fixator or a combination of open reduction and internal fixation for anterior and posterior instability.

ACETABULAR FRACTURES

Acetabular fracture-dislocations in children differ from those in adults because they can be caused by trivial trauma in children. Further, damage to the triradiate cartilage in the child may cause growth arrest and a shallow, dysplastic acetabulum (Fig. 33-102). A CT scan may help determine the extent of acetabular involvement and femoral head stability. The classification of acetabular fractures is based on the extent of acetabular involvement: (1) small fragments most often associated with dislocation of the hip (see Fig. 33-99), (2) linear fractures associated with pelvic fractures without displacement, (3) large linear fractures with hip joint instability, and (4) central fracture-dislocations.

Reduction of a hip dislocation may reveal a small chip fracture from the posterior margin of the acetabulum, but the hip usually is stable. Roentgenograms before reduction often reveal the occult fragment more readily than films taken after the reduction. Union almost always occurs. Occasionally, an osteochondral fragment may be caught within the hip joint after an apparently satisfactory reduction. Roentgenograms of the opposite hip should be taken for comparison to make sure that the reduction is congruous (see p. 1480, Traumatic Hip Dislocations). Stable linear fractures require only conservative treatment; a period of non-weight-bearing on crutches is all that is necessary. Linear fractures producing hip joint instability require skeletal traction and an accurate reduction. This injury usually occurs in older children, and treatment should be the same as for adults. In these patients, skeletal traction has been recommended for 6 to 12 weeks in adults to prevent superior displacement of the acetabular roof. However, depending on the skeletal age of the child, this lengthy period of traction may not be necessary, but it is better to continue traction longer than necessary rather than allow superior displacement of the fragment. Recently we have used open reduction to obtain a congruous reduction and avoid prolonged traction and bed rest.

Central fracture-dislocations in children should be reduced promptly because the triradiate cartilage may be involved. Gepstein et al. found that after surgically induced premature triradiate cartilage fusion in young rabbits, acetabular dysplasia occurred 5 weeks after operation in all animals and hip dislocation in 9 weeks in half. Heeg, Visser, and Oostvogel reported that of four patients with injuries of the triradiate cartilage, three had premature fusion of the cartilage and two of these developed acetabular deformity and hip subluxation. Because injury to the triradiate cartilage is easily missed on initial roentgenograms, they recommend that all patients with

pelvic trauma be followed clinically and roentgenographically for at least 1 year. Bucholz et al. noted two main patterns of growth plate disruption in nine patients with triradiate cartilage injuries: a Salter-Harris type I or II injury, which had a favorable prognosis for continued normal acetabular growth, and a Salter-Harris type V crushing injury, which had a

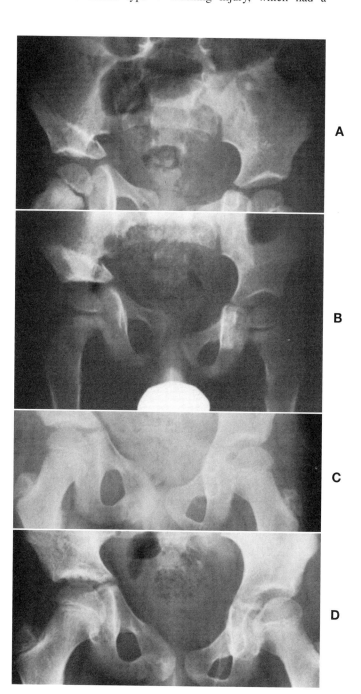

Fig. 33-102 Premature closure of triradiate cartilage. **A,** Fracture of right ilium is obvious. Fracture on left was not identified. **B,** At 4 months fracture on right again seen. At left, acetabulum shows increased sclerosis caused by ischial fracture into acetabulum. **C,** At 5 years premature closure of left triradiate cartilage. **D,** At 6 years premature closure of left triradiate cartilage and subluxation of femoral head caused by shallow acetabulum.

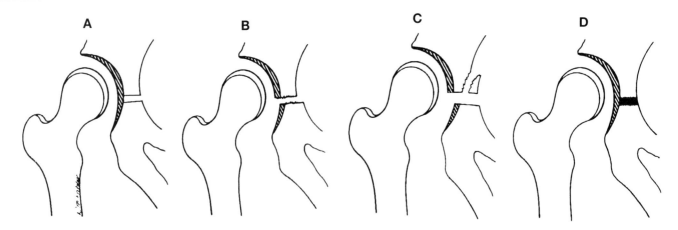

Fig. 33-103   Schematic representation of hemipelvis and types of injuries. **A,** Normal hemipelvis. **B,** Salter-Harris type I fracture. **C,** Salter-Harris type II fracture. **D,** Salter-Harris type V fracture. (From Scuderi G, Bronson MJ: *Clin Orthop* 217:179, 1987.)

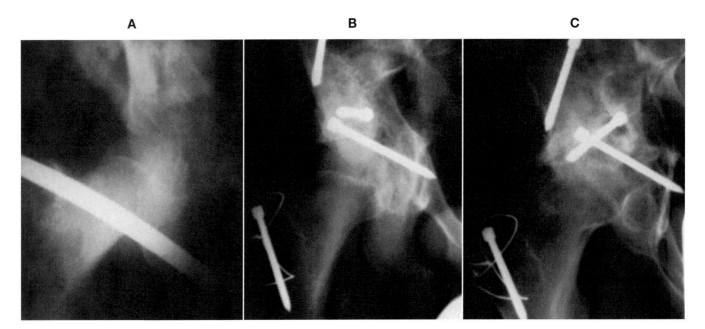

Fig. 33-104   **A,** Severe fracture-dislocation of hip. **B,** After open reduction and internal fixation of acetabulum. **C,** At long-term follow-up, severe ankylosis of hip caused by traumatic arthritis secondary to avascular necrosis or chondrolysis.

poor prognosis because of premature closure of the triradiate physes secondary to formation of a medial osseous bridge (Fig. 33-103). In both patterns the prognosis was dependent on the age of the patient at the time of injury. In younger children, especially those younger than 10 years, abnormal acetabular growth was frequent and resulted in a shallow acetabulum. By skeletal maturity, disparate growth increased the incongruity of the hip joint and led to progressive subluxation. They recommended acetabular reconstruction for correction of the gradual subluxation of the femoral head.

Longitudinal skeletal traction is necessary. If this is not adequate, then lateral traction should be added to ensure a satisfactory reduction. Occasionally, open reduction and inter-

nal fixation may be necessary as in adults (Chapter 53), although Heeg et al. found that operative reduction, required for unstable posterior fracture-dislocations and irreducible central fracture-dislocations, did not improve results in their patients, especially those with type V fractures (Fig. 33-104).

Hip Fractures in Children

Hip fractures include fractures of the head, neck, and intertrochanteric region of the femur. They differ from pelvic and acetabular fractures because, although they can occur in conjunction with a life-threatening injury, they more commonly produce late complications of avascular necrosis, coxa vara, nonunion, and premature physeal closure. The importance of operating on a child's hip is not easily understood or accepted by the parents. However, aggressive treatment of hip fractures in children is necessary to prevent these late complications.

Hip fractures probably make up less than 1% of all children's fractures, and most orthopaedic surgeons treat such fractures only a few times during their career. We have collected data on 86 fractures of the hip in children since 1922. In 1975 we reported the results of 61 of these fractures. The data given here will be from the 61 fractures previously reported, as well as examples from what we have learned and applied to 35 fractures treated later. In general, the child's hip differs from the adult's because the physis can contribute to a type I transepiphyseal separation in which the capital femoral epiphysis may stay within the acetabulum or may be dislocated. Further, the blood vessels to the femoral head are easily damaged, and a high incidence of avascular necrosis occurs in cervical and transepiphyseal fractures in children, even higher than in adults. Growth arrest in the physis can cause shortening of up to 15% of the total extremity. Varus or valgus angulation of the femoral neck also can occur from arrest of only one side of the physis. Hip fractures in children also differ from those in adults because a child can tolerate immobilization much more readily than an adult, and thus more choices for treatment are available, including traction, a spica cast, and bed rest, in addition to operative treatment. Internal fixation with threaded pins often is used in adult hip fractures and also can be used through the capital femoral physis in a child to secure firm fixation of the femoral neck. However, in an infant, this can cause premature physeal closure and significant leg length inequality (Fig. 33-105).

We have used the classification employed by Ingram and Bachynski in 1957 at this clinic (Fig. 33-106). This is the same classification proposed by Delbet and popularized by Colonna: type I, transepiphyseal separations with or without dislocation of the femoral head from the acetabulum; type II, transcervical fractures, displaced and nondisplaced; type III, cervicotrochanteric fractures, displaced and nondisplaced; and type IV, intertrochanteric fractures.

TYPE I, TRANSEPIPHYSEAL SEPARATIONS

The results of the transepiphyseal separations are the worst of any fractures in our series. All five patients with transepiphyseal separations had dislocation of the femoral head from the acetabulum, and all these children developed avascular necrosis. Closed reduction and fixation with pins through a short lateral incision should be performed in an older child if possible. However, open reduction was necessary in all but one of our patients. These transepiphyseal separations with dislocation often occur in young children in whom fixation with threaded screws or pins can cause premature physeal closure. The physis should be crossed only by smooth pins when internal fixation is necessary.

We have used specially made smooth pins, similar to

Knowles pins but without threads, to try to prevent premature physeal closure. However, smooth pins do not back out with collapse at the fracture site, as do the threaded pins. In fact, because of the sharp points, the smooth pins seem to migrate toward the acetabulum if any collapse occurs. If the femoral head is not dislocated from the acetabulum, closed reduction can be carried out, with the aid of image intensification, by longitudinal traction in abduction and internal rotation, and internal fixation through a percutaneous stab wound or a small lateral incision with Knowles pins, cannulated hip screws, or smooth pins can be done (Fig. 33-107). The number of pins needed depends on the size of the child; we have found that two Knowles pins usually are too few and five are too many. With the larger-diameter cannulated hip screw, two or even one may be sufficient. If the femoral head is dislocated and there is any doubt about whether it is dislocated anteriorly or posteriorly, a CT scan is helpful. If an open reduction is necessary and the head is dislocated anteriorly, a Watson-Jones approach anteriorly (Chapter 1) allows reduction and insertion of pins or screws under direct vision. If the head is dislocated posteriorly, a modified Gibson approach (Chapter 1) should be used.

Forlin et al. reported treatment of transepiphyseal fractures in five young children (8 to 26 months of age) with spica casting without closed or open reduction. Four of the five fractures healed with varus deformities, but in two children with open proximal femoral physes the deformities corrected with growth. These authors recommended spica casting without reduction in children younger than 2 years of age and later correction of coxa vara or limb length discrepancy by osteotomy if necessary.

In newborns an entity called *proximal femoral epiphysiolysis* occasionally occurs in which the physis separates probably at birth. If not considered, it may be confused with congenital dislocation or infection of the hip. An arthrogram is generally necessary to make the diagnosis early. At approximately 2 weeks after the separation, callus may be seen along the medial border of the femoral neck. Operative treatment with internal fixation is not needed for this separation. Clinical signs, such as pseudoparalysis of the lower extremity, and laboratory studies should aid in differentiating proximal femoral epiphysiolysis from infection. An arthrogram or MRI is necessary to differentiate the disorder from early congenital dislocation of the hip.

TYPE II, TRANSCERVICAL FRACTURES

Transcervical fractures occur more often than other hip fractures in children. Unfortunately, most of these are displaced, and the amount of displacement appears to be directly related to the development of avascular necrosis. The avascular necrosis rate for our entire series was 43%, and for the type II transcervical fractures it was 52%. We believe that the displacement is responsible for the vascular insufficiency and that the maximal amount of displacement probably occurs at the time of injury. However, Boitzy, as well as Rang, reported excellent results in 11 and 13 patients, respectively, none of

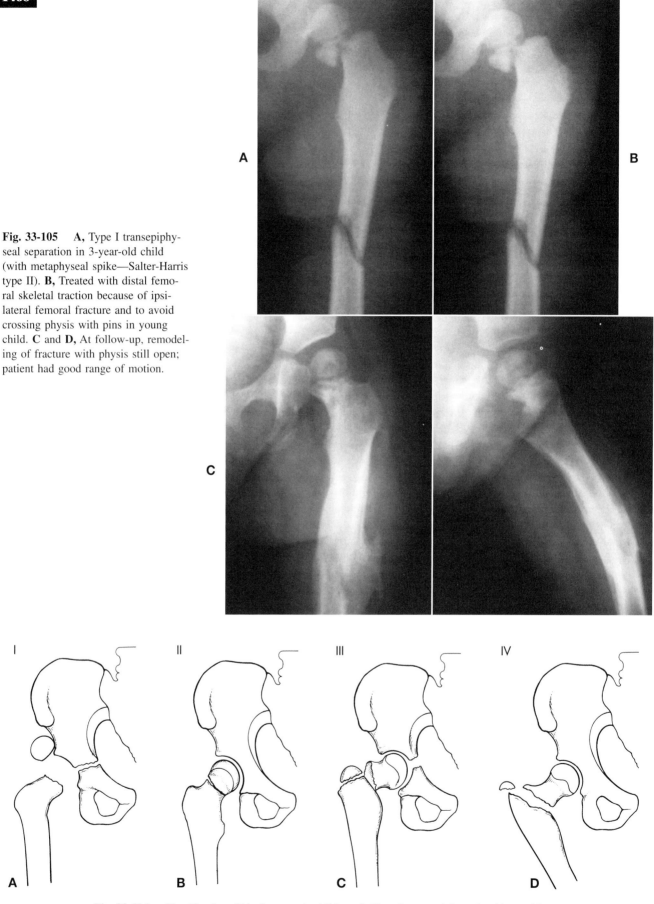

Fig. 33-105 **A,** Type I transepiphyseal separation in 3-year-old child (with metaphyseal spike—Salter-Harris type II). **B,** Treated with distal femoral skeletal traction because of ipsilateral femoral fracture and to avoid crossing physis with pins in young child. **C** and **D,** At follow-up, remodeling of fracture with physis still open; patient had good range of motion.

Fig. 33-106 Classification of hip fractures in children. **A,** Type I, transepiphyseal, with or without dislocation from acetabulum. **B,** Type II, transcervical. **C,** Type III, cervicotrochanteric (basicervical). **D,** Type IV, intertrochanteric.

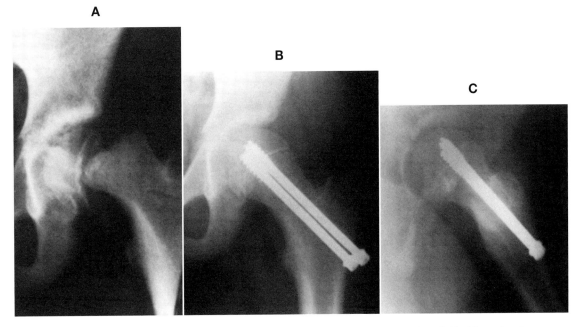

Fig. 33-107 Type I, transepiphyseal separation. **A,** Before treatment. **B** and **C,** After closed reduction and fixation with cannulated hip screws.

whom developed avascular necrosis. According to Boitzy, capsular distention and subsequent tamponade of the vessels may increase the incidence of avascular necrosis, and consequently evacuation of the hematoma early by either aspiration or capsular release and early internal fixation can decrease the rate of avascular necrosis (Fig. 33-108). Gerber et al. reviewed from seven Swiss (AO) hospitals 28 femoral neck fractures in children, which were treated as recommended by Weber et al. with early release of the distended capsule and internal fixation. Their experience, contrary to that of Weber et al., was that early open reduction and internal fixation still resulted in an incidence of avascular necrosis of 30%. The occurrence of avascular necrosis was related to the degree of initial fracture displacement and also to the location of the fracture. Type II transcervical fractures were at greater risk (50%) than type III fractures. They concluded that immediate open reduction and internal fixation did not prevent avascular necrosis after displaced types II and III fractures.

Internal fixation is recommended for all type II fractures because most are unstable. Almost invariably, both displaced and nondisplaced type II transcervical fractures "drift" into coxa vara if treated only by external fixation or by closed reduction and external fixation (spica cast). Nonunion also can occur if internal fixation is not used. The rate of coxa vara in our patients was extremely low with the use of internal fixation, as compared with Lam's series of patients in whom internal fixation was not uniformly used. Why the avascular necrosis rate was lower in Lam's series than in Ratliff's or ours is not understood. A gentle closed reduction, similar to that for adult femoral neck fractures, should be carried out with longitudinal traction, abduction, and internal rotation, followed by fixation with either Knowles pins or cannulated hip screws. Percutaneous pinning can be done with the use of an image intensifier.

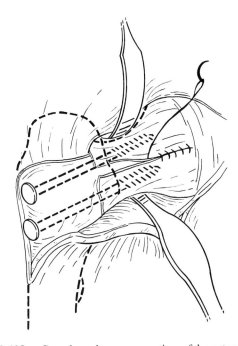

Fig. 33-108 Capsular release; evacuation of hematoma, open reduction and internal fixation with pins, and repair of capsule done as emergency. (Redrawn from Boitzy A: Fractures of the proximal femur. In Weber BG, Brunner C, Freuler F, eds: *Treatment of fractures in children and adolescents*, New York, 1980, Springer-Verlag.)

The head and neck of a child's femur are extremely hard, and the use of triflanged nails or other similar devices should be avoided for fear of distraction of the fracture and possible separation of the capital femoral epiphysis. In small children, two Knowles pins may suffice, although three can be used. We

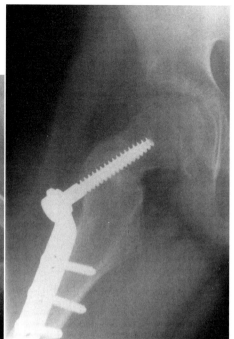

Fig. 33-109   **A,** Displaced type III (cervicotrochanteric) fracture. **B,** After fixation with cannulated screw and attached side plate for better fixation of unstable fracture.

A

B

routinely use two cannulated hip screws. Swiontkowski and Winquist recommend 4.5-mm AO cortical screws inserted short of the physis and overdrilled in the proximal fragment for a lag effect. Because of numerous problems with noncompliance, a spica cast with the hip abducted is used for 6 weeks.

TYPE III, CERVICOTROCHANTERIC FRACTURES

Type III fractures (cervicotrochanteric) are similar to those occurring at the base of the femoral neck in adults, although avascular necrosis after this fracture in children is more common than in adults. If the fracture is truly nondisplaced, then treatment in an abduction spica cast after a period of traction is recommended. If the fracture is displaced, closed reduction and internal fixation with Knowles pins or cannulated hip screws should be carried out. More recently, because of several nonunions, we have used a cannulated screw with a side plate for fixation of "low" cervicotrochanteric fractures in older children (Fig. 33-109). If whether the fracture has been displaced is questionable, then it should be treated as a displaced fracture. Several fractures in our series were thought to be nondisplaced and were treated in spica casts only to have them angulate into an unacceptable varus position.

TYPE IV, INTERTROCHANTERIC FRACTURES

In the Campbell Clinic series, type IV fractures (intertrochanteric) resulted in fewer complications than the other types. Because of the child's osteogenic potential in the trochanteric area, rapid union almost always occurs, usually within 6 to 8 weeks. Initially, we use skeletal traction to obtain an acceptable reduction. After the alignment appears to be stable, at 2 to 3 weeks depending on the age of the child, an abduction spica

cast is applied and is worn 6 to 10 weeks. Occasionally, when the fracture cannot be reduced with traction, closed manipulation can be used followed by an abduction spica cast. On other occasions internal fixation may be optimal treatment. The type of internal fixation used depends on the age of the child. Because the fracture is some distance from the physis, the internal fixation device should not cross it.

TREATMENT RECOMMENDATIONS

In summary, our treatment recommendations are as follows:
1. Type I, transepiphyseal separations without dislocations—gentle closed reduction and internal fixation; with dislocation—gentle closed reduction, then, if not successful, immediate open reduction and fixation with Knowles pins or cannulated hip screws
2. Type II, transcervical—closed reduction and internal fixation regardless of the amount of displacement
3. Type III, cervicotrochanteric fractures, if displaced—gentle closed reduction and internal fixation; if not displaced—abduction spica cast
4. Type IV, intertrochanteric fractures—skin or skeletal traction, abduction spica cast; internal fixation may be necessary if the fracture cannot be reduced and held in a spica cast or if traction followed by casting is not an option.

Several types of cannulated cancellous screws are available (Fig. 33-110). King noted that these screws are sometimes difficult to retrieve because their threads do not cut in reverse. The fixation device should be removed 7 to 12 months after fracture, when union is ensured, or at the first signs of avascular necrosis. We try to avoid penetrating the physis, especially in children younger than 9 years in whom the cannulated hip

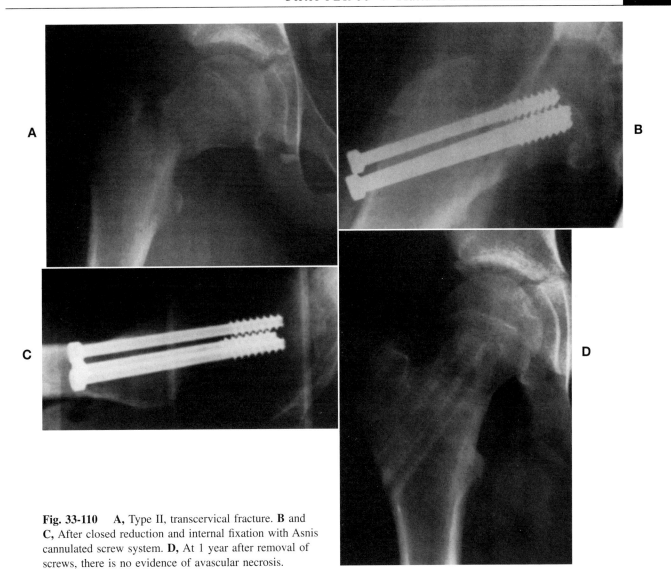

Fig. 33-110   **A,** Type II, transcervical fracture. **B** and **C,** After closed reduction and internal fixation with Asnis cannulated screw system. **D,** At 1 year after removal of screws, there is no evidence of avascular necrosis.

screws may give better purchase, but if it must be crossed, especially in younger children, then smooth pins are used.

The most serious complication of hip fractures in children is avascular necrosis, which occurred in 43% of our patients: type I, 100%; type II, 52%; type III, 27% and type IV, 14%. Two studies have confirmed the frequency of this complication after hip fractures in children. Forlin et al. reported that avascular necrosis developed in 14 of 16 children (87.5%) with displaced femoral neck fractures. Davison and Weinstein reported avascular necrosis in 9 (47%) of 19 children with hip fractures, 7 of whom required operative treatment.

Ratliff described three types of avascular necrosis: type I, whole head involvement; type II, partial head involvement; and type III, an area of avascular necrosis from the fracture line to the physis (Fig. 33-111). In several children under the age of 10 years, with type I or II avascular necrosis, removal of the Knowles pins followed by an "abduction containment" orthosis has produced acceptable results. We have arbitrarily "contained" the femoral head for 1 year (Fig. 33-112).

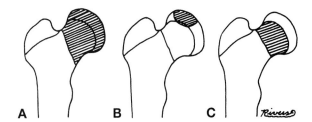

Fig. 33-111   Three types of avascular necrosis. **A,** Type I, total head involvement. **B,** Type II, segmental involvement. **C,** Type III involvement from fracture line to physis. (Redrawn from Ratliff AHC: *J Bone Joint Surg* 44B:528, 1962.)

Coxa vara occurred in our series less often than in other series, probably because of the routine use of internal fixation. In the children with coxa vara in our series, if the neck-shaft angle was more than 120 degrees in a young child, remodeling occurred to some degree, and even if it did not, it caused little disability. However, if the neck-shaft angle was between 100

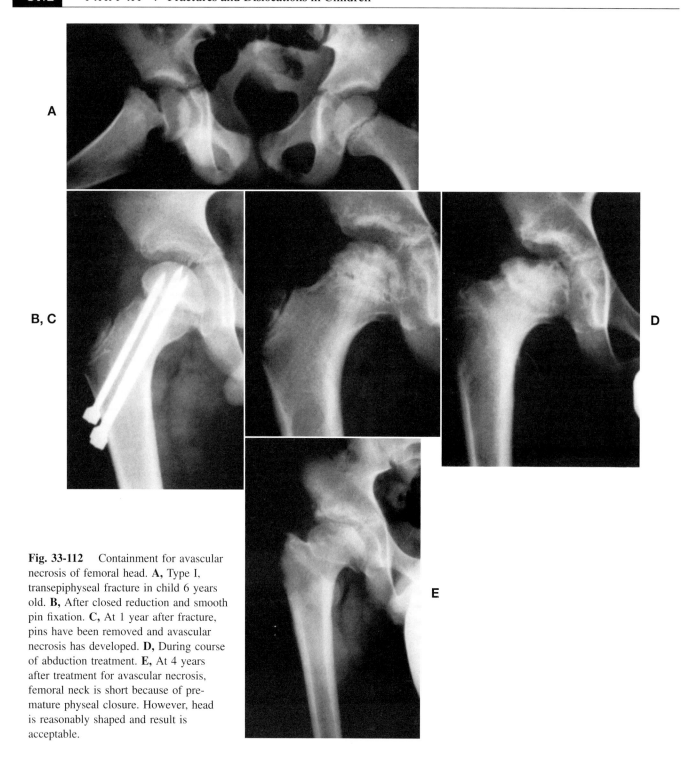

Fig. 33-112 Containment for avascular necrosis of femoral head. **A,** Type I, transepiphyseal fracture in child 6 years old. **B,** After closed reduction and smooth pin fixation. **C,** At 1 year after fracture, pins have been removed and avascular necrosis has developed. **D,** During course of abduction treatment. **E,** At 4 years after treatment for avascular necrosis, femoral neck is short because of premature physeal closure. However, head is reasonably shaped and result is acceptable.

and 110 degrees, the coxa vara deformity did not remodel but persisted. Significant coxa vara causes a shortened extremity and an abductor or gluteal lurch, as well as delayed degenerative joint changes. For these reasons we have routinely used a subtrochanteric valgus osteotomy for persistent coxa vara deformity and for nonunion (Fig. 33-113). A closing wedge osteotomy just distal to the greater trochanter, using a pediatric lag screw with a side plate for internal fixation, is

preferred. Although nonunion of the osteotomy is rare, we still apply a one and one half spica cast that is worn for 12 weeks.

The nonunion rate in our series was low, 6.5%. This we also attribute to the use of internal fixation. Operative treatment for nonunion should be undertaken as soon as possible. We have used a valgus subtrochanteric osteotomy, as recommended by Ratliff, to make the nonunion more horizontal and allow compressive vertical forces to aid in union. This osteotomy can

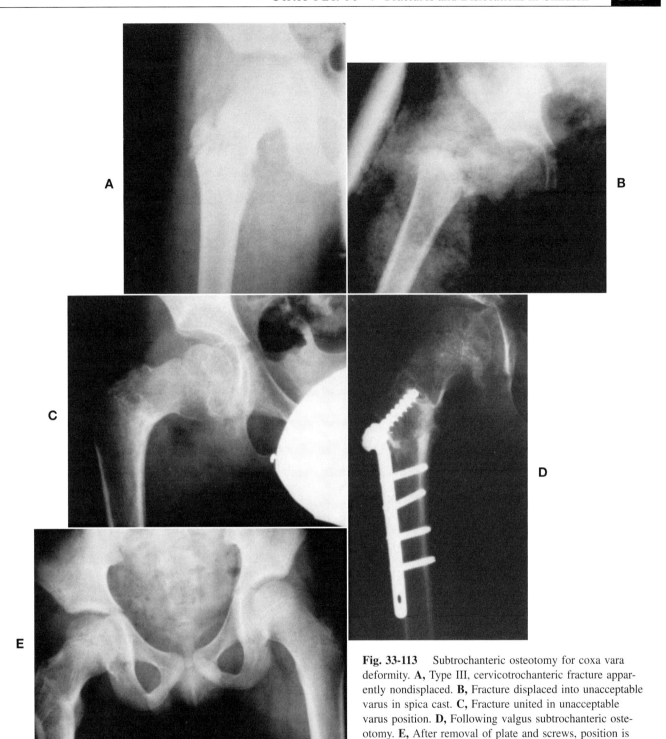

Fig. 33-113 Subtrochanteric osteotomy for coxa vara deformity. **A,** Type III, cervicotrochanteric fracture apparently nondisplaced. **B,** Fracture displaced into unacceptable varus in spica cast. **C,** Fracture united in unacceptable varus position. **D,** Following valgus subtrochanteric osteotomy. **E,** After removal of plate and screws, position is acceptable.

be augmented, if necessary, with bone grafts. Internal fixation is routinely employed across the nonunion site, and a spica cast is worn for 12 weeks (Fig. 33-114).

Premature physeal closure occurred in our series at a higher rate than in other series. Of the children with Knowles pins crossing the physis, 87% had premature physeal closure. Because the capital femoral physis contributes 15% of the growth of the entire lower extremity and normally closes earlier than most of the other lower extremity physes, shortening was less than 2 cm in most of the children involved. The discrepancy was more than 2 cm only in those children in whom avascular necrosis also developed. Nevertheless, we have tried to avoid penetrating the physis, especially in a young child. Leg length inequality should be determined with scanograms and carefully recorded. Epiphysiodesis in the opposite extremity can be done if necessary.

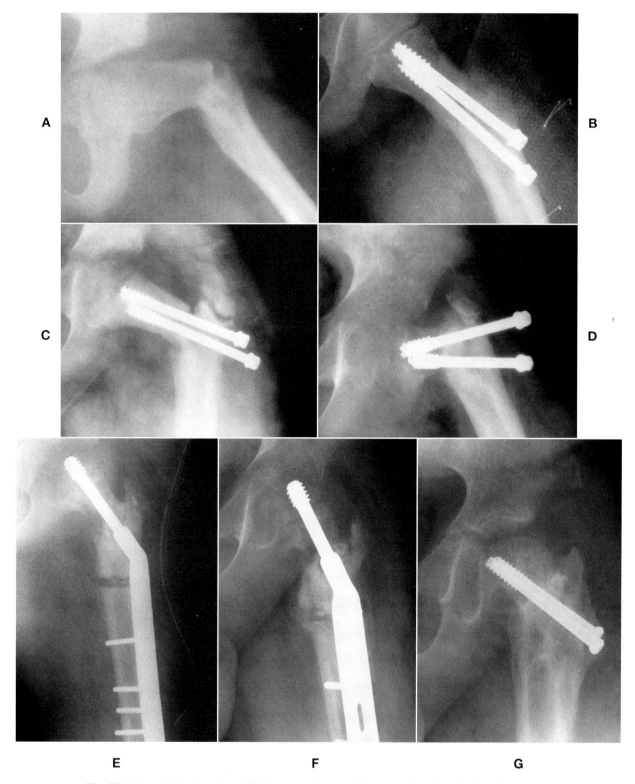

Fig. 33-114   **A,** Displaced type III (cervicotrochanteric) fracture. **B,** After closed reduction and internal fixation, fracture is in good alignment in spica cast. **C,** Early evidence of nonunion. **D,** Definite evidence of nonunion, with pins backing out and severe coxa vara deformity. **E** and **F,** After subtrochanteric valgus osteotomy and internal fixation with side plate and bone graft. **G,** Persistent nonunion required second bone grafting procedure and internal fixation with cannulated screws before union was obtained.

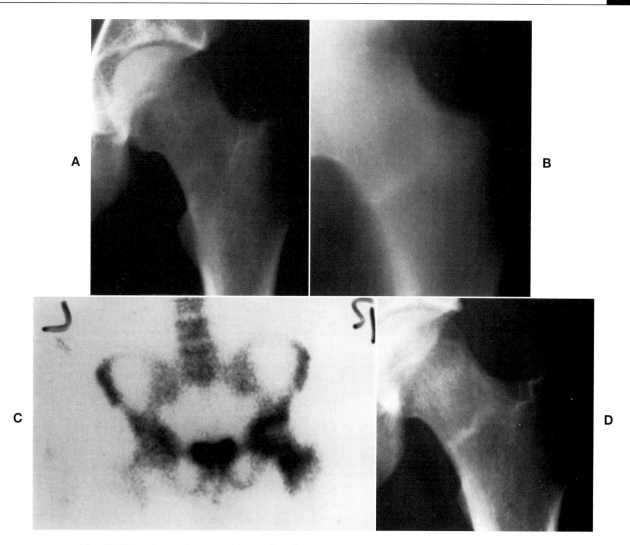

Fig. 33-115   Stress fracture of femoral neck. **A,** Roentgenogram showing possible faint inferior femoral neck fracture. **B,** Tomogram showing definite evidence of compression type of stress fracture in inferior femoral neck. **C,** Bone scan showing increased uptake in this area. **D,** Roentgenogram made 3 weeks later revealing callus formation in inferior neck at stress fracture.

Infection is uncommon after hip fractures in children. Of 86 patients in our two series, only 1 patient (1%) in the early group developed an infection after open reduction performed 2 months after a fracture-dislocation. Lam's and Ratliff's studies report similar low incidence of infection. Davison and Weinstein reported septic arthritis in 2 of their 19 patients, both of whom also had avascular necrosis.

Chondrolysis after hip fractures in children has been reported by Forlin et al. in 7 of 16 patients (44%), but this complication has not been found by other investigators. All 7 patients with chondrolysis also had avascular necrosis and all had poor results.

Stress fractures of the femoral neck, as noted by Wolfgang, can occur in children, especially in adolescents. Devas noted two types: (1) a transverse type in the superior portion of the femoral neck, which may become displaced and

cause severe morbidity, and (2) a compression stress fracture in the inferior portion of the femoral neck, which rarely becomes displaced, although mild varus deformity has occurred in young patients (Fig. 33-115). Internal fixation with a screw or pin is recommended for the transverse type, whereas the compression type may be treated by non-weight-bearing and limitation of the child's activity. St. Pierre et al. reported five femoral neck stress fractures in children and adolescents and recommended activity modification and rest as effective treatment measures; however, they warned that a stress fracture can progress to a complete fracture if proper treatment is not begun and the child is allowed to continue the same activity.

The technique for closed reduction and percutaneous pin or screw fixation is described in the section on slipped capital femoral epiphysis (p. 1485).

◆ Closed Reduction and Internal Fixation

TECHNIQUE 33-23

Place the child supine on a fracture table and attach the feet to the traction stirrups. Carry out a gentle closed reduction by applying longitudinal traction, abduction, and internal rotation. Check the reduction with anteroposterior and lateral roentgenograms or with an image intensifier. If reduction is satisfactory, prepare and drape the involved hip. With the use of an image intensifier, make a stab wound percutaneously or a 7-cm incision just distal to the greater trochanter and dissect through the fascia lata. Reflect the vastus lateralis anteriorly, exposing the proximal femoral shaft. Elevate the periosteum and place reverse retractors around the proximal femur to aid in exposure. With an image intensifier, determine the correct placement for a drill hole in the lateral shaft of the femur. With a power drill and a 9/64-inch drill bit, drill a hole in the lateral cortex. Through the hole drill a guide pin across the fracture site and proximally into the femoral neck. In young children it is important to avoid penetrating the physis, if possible. Verify the correct position of the guide pin with the image intensifier. Measure the exact length of the portion of the guide pin in the bone. Then drill a Knowles pin or a cannulated hip screw the same length as the measured length of the guide pin parallel to or over it across the fracture site. Remove the guide pin and place a second Knowles pin or cannulated screw parallel to the first through the guide pin hole. Use a minimum of two Knowles pins or one 6.0 cannulated screw. We generally use three Knowles pins or two 6.0 cannulated screws, depending on the size of the child and the femoral neck. Place the pins or screws parallel and in a "cluster" formation. Close the incision and apply a one and one half spica cast with the hip in the abducted position.

AFTERTREATMENT. The spica cast is worn for 6 weeks, and the patient progresses to weight-bearing on crutches during the next 6 weeks. The pins or screws should be removed at 1 year when the fracture has united or when there is evidence of avascular necrosis.

◆ Open Reduction and Internal Fixation

TECHNIQUE 33-24 *(Weber et al. and Boitzy)*

Place the patient supine and drape the limb so that it can be moved freely during the operation. Use a Watson-Jones approach to the hip joint (Technique 1-50). Incise the hip joint capsule longitudinally and evacuate and flush out the hematoma, which usually is under pressure. Reduce the fracture with a periosteal elevator. This can be made easier by appropriate traction and internal rotation of the extremity.

Temporarily stabilize the fracture with Kirschner wires and check the reduction in the region of the calcar. Then fix the fracture permanently with cancellous screws fitted with washers. The screw threads should be in the proximal fragment only and not across the physis of the femoral head. Confirm the reduction roentgenographically and close the hip capsule.

An anterior approach, such as the Watson-Jones, can be used for displaced type II and type III fractures, and for type I transepiphyseal separations when the femoral head is dislocated from the acetabulum anteriorly. If the femoral head is dislocated posteriorly, a modified Gibson approach (Technique 1-55) is used. The femoral head may be devoid of all blood supply. However, it should be replaced in the acetabulum, making sure there are no cartilaginous or osseous fragments in the joint, and then fixed to the femoral neck with Knowles pins or cancellous screws.

AFTERTREATMENT. A below-knee cast with a transverse bar is applied with the leg in 10 to 15 degrees of internal rotation. At 2 weeks the cast is removed and the patient begins active mobilization without weight-bearing. A Thomas weight-relieving caliper is worn for 8 to 10 months, and the pins are removed at 12 months.

◆ Valgus Subtrochanteric Osteotomy for Acquired Coxa Vara or Nonunion

TECHNIQUE 33-25

Place the patient on a fracture table with an image intensifier or roentgenographic equipment in place to obtain antero-posterior and lateral roentgenograms. Prepare and drape the hip in the usual fashion. If bone grafts are to be used, prepare and drape the iliac crest also. Make a straight lateral longitudinal incision beginning at the greater trochanter and extending distally for 8 to 10 cm. Carry the dissection down to the lateral aspect of the femur. Elevate the periosteum and insert reverse retractors around the femur subperiosteally to expose the lateral aspect of the bone.

Determine preoperatively the amount of valgus necessary to align the hip properly by comparing roentgenograms with those of the contralateral hip. We have used trigonometric functions to evaluate the effect of proximal femoral osteotomy. If either a varus or valgus osteotomy is performed in the subtrochanteric or trochanteric area, the length of the femoral head and neck fragment does not change; only the angles and the leg length change (Fig. 33-116). The amount of change in leg length can be computed by determining the change in the two angles. Thus the change in leg length or (Δh) is equal to the length of the point from the middle of the osteotomy site to the

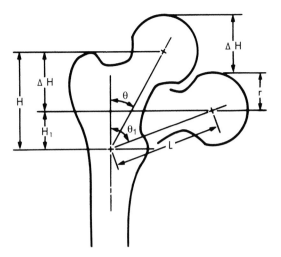

Fig. 33-116 Illustration of constant head-neck length, *L,* change in angles θ to θ₁, and ultimately the change in height ΔH. Formula is used to determine change in height; ΔH is equal to *L*(cos θ₁ – cos θ). (From Harper MD, Canale ST, Cobb RM: *J Pediatr Orthop* 3:431, 1983.)

middle of the femoral head *(L)* times the cosine of one angle minus the cosine of the new angle:

$$\Delta h = L \, (\cos \theta_1 - \cos \theta)$$

Therefore, going from a varus position to a valgus position increases the leg length, or Δh, and conversely, going from a valgus position to a varus position decreases the leg length, or Δh.

Because of the difficulty of using sine and cosine tables, Table 33-3 is included. The original angle (L) is given for head-neck segments of 2, 3, and 4 cm. The estimated increase or decrease in leg length or (Δh) is given for the "desired angle" obtained by a varus or valgus osteotomy.

Once the angle of correction is determined, the appropriate laterally based closing wedge osteotomy can be determined. First determine the diameter of the bone by drilling a guide pin transversely through the femur. Determine the correct size of the wedge by using a template, tangent tables (W = tangent of the angle × the diameter), or the formula W = .02 × diameter × angle. Outline the appropriate closing wedge osteotomy in the subtrochanteric area.

After preparation of the osteotomy site, attention should be turned to placement of an intermediate hip compression screw. Drill a hole just distal to the greater trochanter and check its placement with the image intensifier. Place an appropriate guide pin of the proper length in the femoral neck with the aid of an adjustable angle guide (Fig. 33-117, *A*). If the child is young, avoid crossing the physis if possible. If the nonunion is proximal, crossing

the physis may be necessary to gain union. It should be remembered that the proximal femoral physis contributes 30% to the growth of the femur and only 15% to the entire lower extremity (Fig. 33-117, *B*). Many times it is preferable to obtain union of the femoral neck and worry about minor to moderate leg length inequality afterward. Check the placement of the guide pin with image intensification. Once the guide pin is placed, use a percutaneous direct measuring gauge to determine the lag screw length. Set the adjustable positive stop on the combination reamer for the lag screw length determined by a percutaneous direct measuring gauge. Place the reamer over the guide pin and ream until the positive stop reaches the lateral cortex (Fig. 33-117, *C*). It is prudent to check the fluoroscopic image periodically during reaming to ensure that the guide pin is not inadvertently advancing proximally into the epiphysis. Next, set the adjustable positive stop on the lag screw tap to the same length that was reamed. Tap until the positive stop reaches the lateral cortex. Then screw the appropriate intermediate compression screw over the guide pin (Fig. 33-117, *D* and *E*).

Take the plate chosen during preoperative planning and insert its barrel over the barrel guide and onto the back of the lag screw. The plate angle ultimately determines the final hip angle. Remove the barrel guide and insert a compressing screw to prevent the plate from disengaging during the reduction maneuver. Use the slotted screwdriver for the pediatric compressing screw or the hex screwdriver for the intermediate compressing screw. If the plate obscures the osteotomy site, loosen the screw and rotate the side plate. Make the appropriate angled osteotomy using a power saw. Remove the wedge and align the two fragments. Reduce the osteotomy and secure the plate to the femur using the plate clamp. Check rotational position of the lower extremity in extension.

To achieve compression, insert a drill or tap guide into the distal portion of the most distal compression slot. Drill through the medial cortex. If less compression is required, follow the same steps detailed above in the distal portion of either the second or third distal slots for up to 2.5 mm of compression.

Select the appropriate length bone screw and insert it using the hex screwdriver. Use the self-holding sleeve to keep the screw from disengaging from the screwdriver (Fig. 33-117, *F*). Finally, in the most proximal slot, the intermediate combination drill/tap guide can be angled proximally so that the drill, and, ultimately, the bone screw will cross the osteotomy line. Positioning the proximal bone screw in this way can provide additional stability at the osteotomy site. Insert screws into any remaining screw holes.

The lag screw can be inserted farther to afford compression across the nonunion. To insert the lag screw

continued

Table 33-3 Estimates of Leg Length Change for a Variety of Angulation Changes

L, Original Angle (Degrees)	Desired Angle (Degrees)								
	90	100	110	120	130	135	140	150	160
2 cm									
90	0	0.3	0.6	1.0	1.3	1.4	1.5	1.7	1.9
100	−0.3	0	0.3	0.7	0.9	1.1	1.2	1.4	1.5
110	−0.6	−0.3	0	0.3	0.6	0.7	0.9	1.0	1.2
120	−1.0	−0.7	−0.3	0	0.3	0.4	0.5	0.7	0.9
130	−1.3	−0.9	−0.6	−0.3	0	0.1	0.2	0.4	0.6
135	−1.4	−1.1	−0.7	−0.4	−0.1	0	0.1	0.3	0.5
140	−1.5	−1.2	−0.9	−0.5	−0.2	−0.1	0	0.2	0.3
150	−1.7	−1.4	−1.0	−0.7	−0.4	−0.3	−0.2	0	0.1
160	−1.9	−1.5	−1.2	−0.9	−0.6	−0.5	−0.3	−0.1	0
3 cm									
90	0	0.5	1.0	1.5	1.9	2.1	2.3	2.6	2.8
100	−0.5	0	0.5	1.0	1.4	1.6	1.8	2.1	2.3
110	−1.0	−0.5	0	0.5	0.9	1.1	1.3	1.6	1.8
120	−1.5	−1.0	−0.5	0	0.4	0.6	0.8	1.1	1.3
130	−1.9	−1.4	−0.9	−0.4	0	0.2	0.4	0.7	0.9
135	−2.1	−1.6	−1.1	−0.6	−0.2	0	0.2	0.5	0.7
140	−2.3	−1.8	−1.3	−0.8	−0.4	−0.2	0	0.3	0.5
150	−2.6	−2.1	−1.6	−1.1	−0.7	−0.5	−0.3	0	0.2
160	−2.8	−2.3	−1.8	−1.3	−0.9	−0.7	−0.5	−0.2	0
4 cm									
90	0	0.7	1.4	2.0	2.6	2.8	3.1	3.5	3.8
100	−0.7	0	0.7	1.3	1.9	2.1	2.4	2.8	3.1
110	−1.4	−0.7	0	0.6	1.2	1.5	1.7	2.1	2.4
120	−2.0	−1.3	−0.6	0	0.6	0.8	1.1	1.5	1.8
130	−2.6	−1.9	−1.2	−0.6	0	0.3	0.5	0.9	1.2
135	−2.8	−2.1	−1.5	−0.8	−0.3	0	0.2	0.6	0.9
140	−3.1	−2.4	−1.7	−1.1	−0.5	−0.2	0	0.4	0.7
150	−3.5	−2.8	−2.1	−1.5	−0.9	−0.6	−0.4	0	0.3
160	−3.8	−3.1	−2.4	−1.8	−1.2	−0.9	−0.7	−0.3	0
5 cm									
90	0	0.9	1.7	2.5	3.2	3.5	3.8	4.3	4.7
100	−0.9	0	0.8	1.6	2.3	2.7	3.0	3.5	3.8
110	−1.7	−0.8	0.8	1.5	1.8	2.2	2.6	3.0	
120	−2.5	−1.6	−0.8	0	0.7	1.0	1.3	1.8	2.2
130	−3.2	−2.3	−1.5	−0.7	0	0.3	0.6	1.1	1.5
135	−3.5	−2.7	−1.8	−1.0	−0.3	0	0.3	0.8	1.2
140	−3.8	−3.0	−2.2	−1.3	−0.6	−0.3	0	0.5	0.9
150	−4.3	−3.5	−2.6	−1.8	−1.1	−0.8	−0.5	0	0.4
160	−4.7	−3.8	−3.0	−2.2	−1.5	−1.2	−0.9	−0.4	0
6 cm									
90	0	1.0	2.1	3.0	3.9	4.2	4.6	5.2	5.6
100	−1.0	0	1.0	2.0	2.8	3.2	3.6	4.2	4.6
110	−2.1	−1.0	0	0.9	1.8	2.2	2.5	3.1	3.6
120	−3.0	−2.0	−0.9	0	0.9	1.2	1.6	2.2	2.6
130	−3.9	−2.8	−1.8	−0.9	0	0.4	0.7	1.3	1.8
135	−4.2	−3.2	−2.2	−1.2	−0.4	0	0.4	1.0	1.4
140	−4.6	−3.6	−2.5	−1.6	−0.7	−0.4	0	0.6	1.0
150	−5.2	−4.2	−3.1	−2.2	−1.3	−1.0	−0.6	0	0.4
160	−5.6	−4.6	−3.6	−2.6	−1.8	−1.4	−1.0	−0.4	0

From Harper MC, Canale ST, Cobb RM: *J Pediatr Orthop* 3:431-434, 1983.
Left-hand column is different angles, with L (the length of the neck to the center of the head) being 2 cm, 3 cm, 4 cm, 5 cm, and 6 cm, going from the original angle in the left-hand column to the desired angle in leg right-hand column, and the change in Δh, or height (in centimeters).

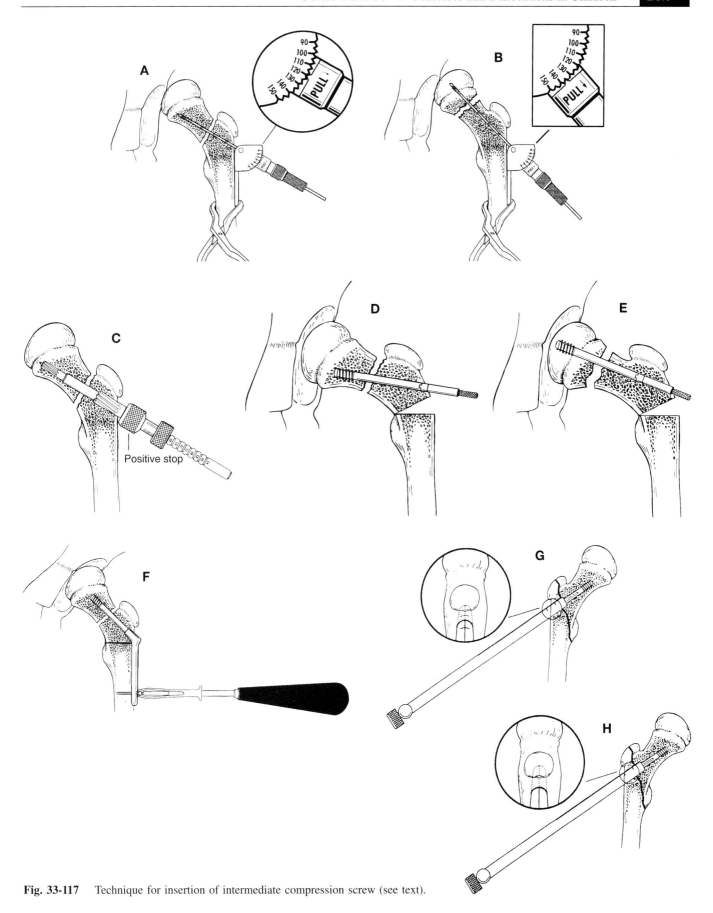

Fig. 33-117 Technique for insertion of intermediate compression screw (see text).

for approximately 5 mm of compression, stop when the lateral cortex is midway between the two depth calibrations (Fig. 33-117, *G*). To insert the lag screw for approximately 10 mm of compression, stop when the second depth calibration meets the lateral cortex (Fig. 33-117, *H*).

Close the wound in layers. Insert a suction drainage tube and apply a one and one half spica cast with the hip in 30 to 40 degrees of abduction.

For fixation of a nonunion the intermediate compression hip screw should cross the nonunion site. The nonunion appears to heal better if it is made more horizontal by placing the hip in a valgus position at the subtrochanteric osteotomy site. The fibrous tissue need not be removed from the nonunion. A cancellous or cortical bone graft placed across the nonunion site may be helpful in older children. The graft is inserted by drilling a hole the size of the graft up through the femoral neck adjacent and parallel to the fixation device. Care should be taken not to loosen the device. A cortical graft from the tibia or fibula can be used, but we prefer cancellous bone from the iliac crest. We have not used a bone graft routinely in this procedure. In younger children with good internal fixation, making the nonunion more horizontal has been all that is necessary. A smaller version of the compression hip screw is available for infants. Blount described an osteotomy similar to this for adult nonunions (Chapter 56).

AFTERTREATMENT. The spica cast should be worn for approximately 12 weeks, depending on the age of the child. Then the cast is removed, and touch-down weight-bearing on crutches is begun.

Traumatic Hip Dislocations in Children

Traumatic hip dislocations in children are more common than hip fractures, although they are also rare. Trivial injury may cause a hip dislocation in young children primarily because their immature cartilage is pliable and their ligaments are lax. MacFarlane noted that half the hip dislocations in children occurred between the ages of 12 and 15 years, but Gartland and Brenner found an equal age distribution in 248 patients. Libri et al. and Hamilton and Broughton reported that their 22 patients fell into two distinct groups: those between 2 and 5 years of age (8 patients) and those between 11 and 15 years of age (14 patients). As in adults, posterior dislocations are more common than anterior ones. Factors that influence the ultimate result after dislocations of the hip are (1) the severity of the injury, (2) the interval between injury and reduction, (3) the type of treatment, (4) the period of non-weight-bearing, (5) whether recurrent dislocation develops, (6) whether

avascular necrosis develops, and (7) whether reduction was incomplete because of the interposition of an object in the joint.

We reviewed our results in 30 children with traumatic hip dislocations and found that the more severe the injury, the worse the results. Hips left unreduced for more than 24 hours had poor results, and avascular necrosis of the femoral head developed more frequently than in those reduced promptly. However, the interval between injury and reduction, a critical factor in dislocations in adults, seems less important in children. Gartland and Brenner, Petrini and Grassi, and Libri et al. found little correlation between time to reduction and final result. Closed reduction, when successful, produced better results than open reduction. However, open reduction may be necessary for more severe injuries. Contrary to previous reports, the period of non-weight-bearing did not influence the development of avascular necrosis of the femoral head.

Recurrent dislocation also is more common in children than in adults because of cartilaginous pliability and ligamentous laxity. In fact, Rang noted a higher incidence of recurrent dislocation in children with hyperlaxity syndromes, especially Down syndrome. He recommended posterior plication of the capsule and a bony procedure, such as an innominate or varus osteotomy.

Avascular necrosis of the femoral head does occur after simple dislocation of the hip in an estimated 10% to 26% of adults and 8% to 10% of children (Fig. 33-118). Delays in reduction and the severity of the injury probably influence the development of avascular necrosis.

Complete reduction may be prevented by interposition of the capsule, labrum, other soft tissue, or an osteocartilaginous fragment. Roentgenograms of both hips should be made after closed reduction to compare the width of the joint spaces. If the involved joint space is wider and the Shenton line is broken, an incongruous reduction should be suspected (Fig. 33-119). An attempt to disengage the interposed object may be made by moving the hip through a full range of motion with the child under general anesthesia. The femoral head should not be completely redislocated during this maneuver. If this is not successful, a CT scan frequently reveals the entrapped object (Fig. 33-120). Altenberg described an inverted labrum causing severe traumatic arthritis of the hip at an early age, and for this reason we recommend open reduction and removal of the offending material. For posterior dislocations a posterior approach, such as a modified Gibson (Technique 1-55) or Moore (Technique 1-57) approach, should be used. For anterior dislocations an anterior approach, such as the Smith-Petersen (Technique 1-47), is used. If the direction of dislocation cannot be determined, a posterior approach is used because this is the more common direction of dislocation. At open reduction, the hip should be redislocated and the acetabulum checked for loose bony fragments or an inverted limbus or other soft tissue. Reduction should be confirmed roentgenographically in the operating room, ensuring that the width of the joint space has returned to normal. The technique for open reduction of an incongruous closed reduction is the same as for irreducible hip dislocation and is described in Chapter 52.

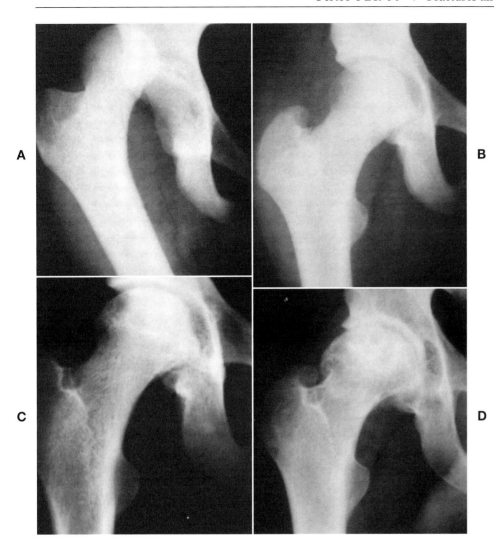

A

B

C

D

Fig. 33-118 Avascular necrosis of femoral head after hip dislocation. **A,** Traumatic dislocation in older child. **B,** After satisfactory closed reduction. **C,** At 1 year after reduction, suggestion of early avascular necrosis. **D,** At 8 years after reduction, cystic appearance of avascular necrosis.

Occasionally, an ipsilateral femoral fracture occurs at the time of hip dislocation. The treatment of this combination of injuries is described in Chapter 52.

Slipped Capital Femoral Epiphysis

A type I transepiphyseal fracture-separation and a slipped capital femoral epiphysis (SCFE) are both epiphyseal separations, but controversy over their natural histories and pathogenesis separates the two disorders. Type I transepiphyseal separations generally are caused by high-energy trauma, whereas SCFE can occur insidiously and minor trauma can cause acute separation or a chronic slip. Type I transepiphyseal separations are most common in younger children, whereas SCFE occurs in a distinct older age group (between the ages of 10 and 16 years); 78% of patients with SCFE are adolescents in the rapid growth phase. SCFE occurs more frequently in obese children and is almost twice as common in males as in females. It occurs approximately twice as often in black

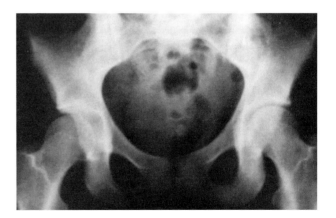

Fig. 33-119 Incongruous reduction of hip. Roentgenogram of both hips after what was thought to be successful closed reduction of traumatic dislocation of right hip in adolescent. However, reduction is incongruous, as shown by break in Shenton line and increase in width of joint space.

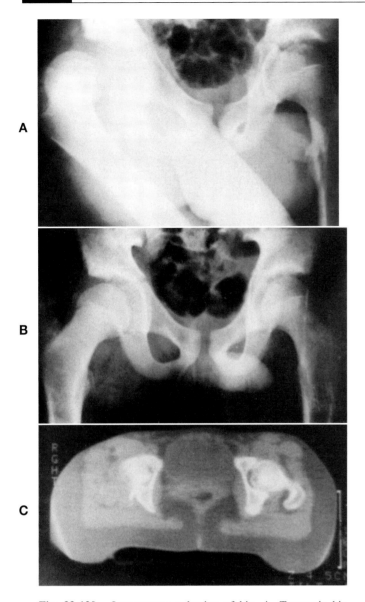

Fig. 33-120 Incongruous reduction of hip. **A,** Traumatic hip dislocation in adolescent. **B,** After two attempts at closed reduction, joint space is still too wide and Shenton line is broken. **C,** CT scan shows osteocartilaginous fragment in acetabulum impeding reduction; open reduction was necessary.

children as in white children. The left hip is affected twice as often as the right, and bilateral involvement is reported to occur in from 25% to 40% of children. When bilateral slips occur, the second slip usually occurs within 12 to 18 months of the initial slip.

Several etiological factors have been suggested for SCFE, including local trauma, mechanical factors (especially obesity), inflammatory conditions, endocrine disorders (such as hypothyroidism, hypopituitarism, and chronic renal disease), and genetic factors. Loder, Wittenberg, and DeSilva found that of 85 children with endocrine disorders and SCFE, 40% had hypothyroidism and 25% had growth hormone deficiencies.

Futami et al. arthroscopically examined the hip joints of five children before treatment of SCFE. They found erosion of the anterosuperior articular cartilage, damage to the posterolateral acetabular labrum, and cartilaginous erosion and a transverse cleft on the anterior surface of the femoral head. They believe that these findings support the hypothesis that all pathomechanisms of SCFE are traumatic. Although shear forces generally are cited as causative factors, Aronson and Tursky suggested that torsional forces also play a role in SCFE. Of 15 acute slips in their study, torsion was the primary force in 6, and in all 15 internal rotation or torsion was necessary for reduction. The true cause of SCFE probably is multifactorial: a physis that is weakened by some underlying condition fails when it is subjected to more than normal stress, resulting in slipping of the proximal femoral epiphysis.

The clinical symptoms and roentgenographic signs of SCFE vary according to the type of slip but usually include pain in the groin, medial thigh, or knee and limitation of hip motion, especially internal rotation. SCFE should be suspected in patients between the ages of 10 and 16 who complain of vague knee pain, which may be referred pain from the hip. Matava et al. noted that patients with SCFE who had distal thigh or knee pain or both as their chief complaint were more likely to receive a misdiagnosis or delay in diagnosis and undergo unnecessary or uninformative roentgenographic evaluations.

Patients with chronic slips may have mild or moderate shortening of the affected extremity and the leg may be in fixed external rotation.

The diagnosis of SCFE usually is apparent from anteroposterior roentgenograms, but special views may be helpful. A cross-table, or true, lateral view can help determine the extent of posterior displacement of the epiphysis, and a "frog-leg" lateral view best shows subtle slipping. The frog-leg lateral view should be avoided, however, in patients with acute slips for fear of causing further slipping of the epiphysis. CT scanning may help confirm the diagnosis in patients with early, mild slipping that is not apparent on roentgenograms. The use of ultrasonography and MRI for diagnosis and evaluation of SCFE has been reported, but neither seems to add useful information to that obtained from plain roentgenograms.

SCFE has traditionally been classified according to the duration of symptoms and the severity of the slip. Acute slips are those with a sudden onset of usually severe symptoms that have been present for less than 2 weeks. Roentgenograms show the epiphyseal displacement with no evidence of bone healing or remodeling. Chronic slips are characterized by gradual onset and symptoms of more than 2 weeks' duration. Some bony healing and remodeling along the posterior and medial femoral neck usually are visible on roentgenograms. Acute-on-chronic slips are those with symptoms lasting longer than 1 month and a recent sudden exacerbation of pain after a relatively trivial injury. Preslip is an essentially roentgenographic finding of irregularity, widening, and indistinctness of the physis. On anteroposterior roentgenograms, the normal femoral head-shaft angle is 145 degrees; on the lateral view it is 170 degrees or more. Mild slipping (grade I) exists when the neck is displaced

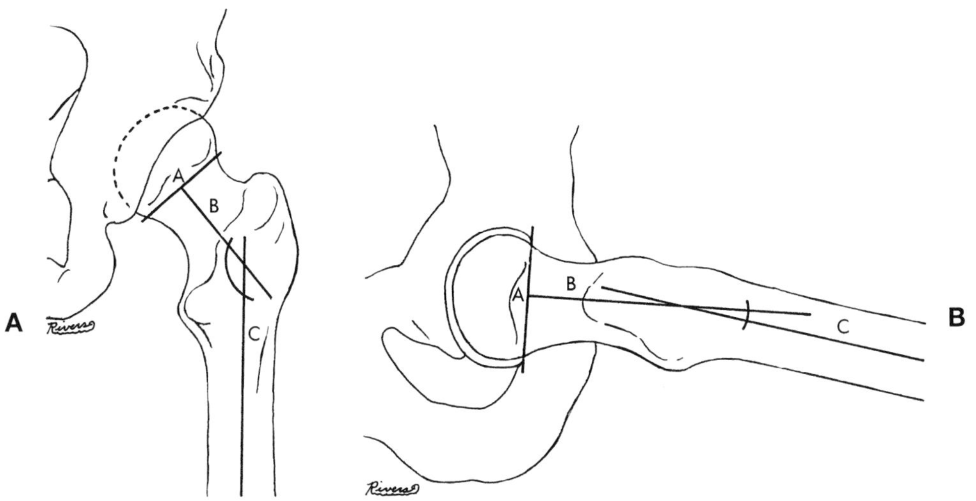

Fig. 33-121 Measurement of head-shaft angle on anteroposterior and lateral roentgenograms. Line *A* connects peripheral portions of physis. Line *B* is perpendicular to line *A*, and line *C* is in long axis of femoral shaft. Intersection of lines *B* and *C* forms head-shaft angle in both views. (Redrawn from Rao JP, Francis AM, Siwek CW: *J Bone Joint Surg* 66A:1169, 1984.)

less than one third of the diameter of the femoral head or when the head-shaft angle deviates from normal by 30 degrees or less on either projection (Fig. 33-121). In moderate slipping (grade II), the neck is displaced between one third and one half of the diameter of the femoral head, or the head-shaft angle deviates between 30 and 60 degrees from normal on either view. Severe slipping (grade III) is characterized by neck displacement of more than half the diameter of the head, or deviation of the head-shaft angle of more than 60 degrees. In most large series of SCFE, 60% to 90% of slips are classified as chronic, and over half are classified as mild slips. Ingram et al. in 1982 reported 329 slips treated at this clinic between 1935 and 1973. Of these, 11% were acute, 60% were chronic, 23% were acute-on-chronic, and 6% were preslips. Mild slipping was present in 51%, moderate slipping in 22%, and severe slipping in 17%.

Loder et al. described a simple two-part classification of SCFE based on the stability of the physis. They classify a slip as unstable if severe pain prevents walking, even with crutches, regardless of the duration of symptoms. With a stable slip, walking is possible, with or without crutches. In their report of 55 slips (38 acute, 17 acute-on-chronic), 30 were unstable, and 25 were stable. Fourteen slips were mild, 16 moderate, and 25 severe. Satisfactory results were obtained in 96% of stable slips, compared to 47% of unstable slips. Kallio et al. used sonography to classify 26 slips as acute (joint effusion), chronic (remodeling but no joint effusion), or acute-on-chronic (both effusion and remodeling). Acute and acute-on-chronic slips were considered unstable, and chronic slips were considered stable.

TREATMENT

The ideal treatment of SCFE should prevent additional slipping of the epiphysis and stimulate early physeal closure, while avoiding the complications of avascular necrosis, chondrolysis, and osteoarthritis. Stabilization of the slip and closure of the physis are relatively easy to obtain by a variety of methods;

however, prevention of complications has proved more difficult.

Nonoperative treatment by traction and spica cast immobilization has been reported to prevent further slipping in 82% to 97% of patients and to result in premature physeal closure in as many as 82%; however, complications have been frequently reported after this treatment method and include recurrent slipping after cast removal (18%), chondrolysis (from 19% to 76%), avascular necrosis of the femoral head (7%), skin ulcers (16%), and psychosocial complications. Ordenberg et al. confirmed the inadequacy of closed reduction and casting in their study of 72 patients 25 to 72 years after treatment. Most patients had pain and limited hip function, and 35% had required surgery for osteoarthritis as adults, compared with an untreated group in which only 2 of 49 (4%) required subsequent operation.

Davidson et al., in a comparison of 63 slips treated with casting to 369 slips treated with pin fixation, found that the prevalence of avascular necrosis was lower after cast treatment (1.6%) than after pinning (3%), but chondrolysis was much more frequent after cast treatment (14.3%) than after pinning (1.9%). Meier et al. also reported a high prevalence of chondrolysis after cast treatment (53%). Betz et al., however, reported chondrolysis in only 5 of 37 hips (13.5%) and no avascular necrosis. They recommended at least 12 weeks of immobilization and suggested cast treatment as an alternative to pin fixation.

Methods of operative treatment of SCFE have included percutaneous and open in situ pinning, open reduction and internal fixation, epiphysiodesis, osteotomy, and reconstruction by arthroplasty, arthrodesis, or cheilectomy. Each technique has its proponents and opponents, and the choice of treatment must be individualized for each child, depending on age, type of slip, and severity of displacement.

In Situ Pin or Screw Fixation

Percutaneous in situ pinning is currently the most often used treatment for mild, moderate, and some severe acute or chronic

SCFE. Open in situ pinning may be indicated for more severe acute or acute-on-chronic slipping. In the past, Knowles pins, threaded Steinmann pins, hip compression screws, and cannulated screw systems all have been used successfully for fixation. Although earlier reports indicated that two or three pins were necessary for stability and the results of multiple pinning generally have been satisfactory, reports now recommend the use of a single, larger-diameter central pin or screw because single pin insertion is technically simpler than insertion of multiple pins.

The development of pediatric cannulated screws for insertion over guide wires has made fixation of SCFE easier and more accurate. These screws have reverse-cutting flutes that make removal easier, and they usually are self-tapping. Whether pins or cannulated hip screws are used, they should not be removed for at least 12 months or until the physis closes.

Kibiloski et al. performed a biomechanical analysis of single- versus double-screw fixation of SCFE in bovine specimens. The specimens were subjected to physiological shear loads across the epiphysis (100 cycles at 1.1 Hz; 400 N for slow walking, and 900 N for fast walking). These authors noted no significant difference in creep in those with two screws and those with one and thus recommended single screw fixation.

O'Beirne et al. reported single-pin fixation of 18 slipped epiphyses (8 acute and 10 chronic; 15 mild, 2 moderate, and 1 severe) and prophylactic pinning of 15 contralateral hips. All patients had satisfactory clinical results, with no slip progression, no pin breakage, and no late reslips. Aronson and Loder also reported the use of single cannulated screw fixation in 97 slips in which chondrolysis developed in 3. Blanco et al. compared multiple-pin to single-pin fixation in 114 hips and found that complications occurred in only 4.6% of hips with single pins, whereas 36% of those with multiple pins had complications. Laplaza and Burke noted evidence of the epiphysis "growing off" the pins in 18% of the hips treated with threaded Steinmann and Knowles pins. No hips with cannulated screws continued to "grow" after surgery.

Carney et al. reported long-term follow-up (41 years) of 155 hips treated for SCFE with various techniques. They concluded that, regardless of the severity of the slip, in situ pinning provided the best long-term function and delay of degenerative arthritis with a low risk of complications.

Although for many years we obtained satisfactory results with multiple Knowles pinning of SCFE, we now prefer the single-pin technique. We have used percutaneous single cannulated screw fixation in over 500 hips and have found that morbidity is less and pin placement is more accurate because it is not limited by a lateral incision. We generally use two screws for acute (unstable) slips and one for chronic slips (stable), although Goodman et al. suggested that single screw fixation is adequate for treating uncomplicated acute and acute-on-chronic SCFE.

Persistent pin penetration has been the most serious disadvantage of in situ pinning. Adverse effects attributed to unrecognized pin penetration include joint sepsis, localized acetabular erosion, synovitis, postoperative hip pain, chon-

drolysis, and late degenerative osteoarthritis. The incidence of pin penetration has been reported to range from 14% to 60%.

Walters and Simon were among the first to recognize this complication, and they noted that, because the femoral head is spherical in a three-dimensional plane, two-plane roentgenograms may not reveal penetration of pins or screws into the hip joint. The pins should be placed in the femoral neck and into the center of the head in the "safe" zone to avoid pin penetration. Various techniques have been recommended to lower the risk of pin penetration. Volz and Martin, Walters and Simon, Rooks and Schmitt, Cowell, and Orr et al., among others, described complex mathematical formulas for determining accurate pin placement, as well as roentgenographic techniques and templates. Lehman et al. (1984) and Shaw recommended the use of a cannulated hip screw with injection of radiopaque dye to detect pin penetration. More recently, based on roentgenographic measurements and a mathematical formula, Rooks et al., as a practical clinical guide, recommended that the pin tip be advanced to 8 mm or one third of the femoral head radius from subchondral bone, whichever projection is the closest. This places the actual tip 7 to 18 mm from the subchondral bone, leaving a safe margin. Bassett reported the use of endoscopy for direct visual confirmation of cannulated screw placement in 12 patients.

The incidence of pin penetration also has been decreased by the use of a single screw or pin rather than multiple pins. Aronson and Carlson reported excellent results in 54 of 58 hips in which a single cannulated screw was used for in situ pinning of SCFE; avascular necrosis developed in 1 hip, and chondrolysis did not develop in any. One subtrochanteric fracture occurred after pinning, and in 2 hips the degree of slippage of the capital femoral epiphysis increased. They suggested placing the screw in the center of the femoral head to decrease the prevalence of screw penetration (Fig. 33-122).

Several authors, including Menche and Lehman, Rab and Simon, and Moseley, have emphasized the use of a rotating fluoroscopic beam to detect penetration. This is the method we prefer. We view the hip while rotating the image intensifier through an arc from the anteroposterior to the lateral position; the hip also can be moved into the frog-leg position during this rotation. This maneuver is helpful but not totally foolproof; it can give false negative results because the image intensifier does not revolve a complete 360 degrees.

As Morrissy emphasized, in situ pinning is a roentgenographic technique, and good quality roentgenograms or image intensification must be available for successful pinning. He noted two common errors: passing the pin obliquely toward the anterior surface rather than the center of the femoral head and passing the pin out the posterior neck and into the head. His solution was to select the starting point of the fixation device on the basis of the position of the femoral head, starting the device on the femoral neck so that when it leaves the neck, it enters the femoral head perpendicular to the physeal surface and in its center. He contended that this starting point is on the anterior rather than lateral aspect of the femoral neck, and the farther the femoral head has slipped posteriorly, the more anterior this starting position must be.

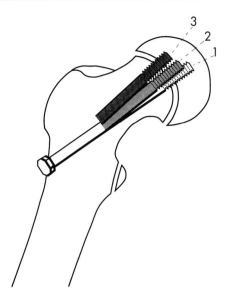

Fig. 33-122 Screw positions in proximal femur. Position *1*, central axis of screw is located over center line of femoral head or within distance equal to one half diameter of screw (ideal position). Position *2*, distance between axis of screw and center line of femoral head is between one half and one screw diameter. Position *3*, axis of screw is more than one screw diameter from center line. Position is given as two numbers: first for position of screw on anteroposterior roentgenogram and second for position as seen on lateral view. Ideal position is 1. (From Aronson DD, Carlson WE: *J Bone Joint Surg* 74A:810, 1992.)

We have used a fluoroscopic technique based on geometric axioms in more than 100 children to determine preoperatively the appropriate site to allow the guide wire for the cannulated screw system to be placed through a minimal incision or a simple stab (puncture) wound. The geometric principles concern the intersection of skin planes with the line of correct insertion of the screw. There are some limitations in exactness of this technique because the skin lines and their intersection are made on mobile soft tissue and the guide wires are flexible. Also, the guide wire or pin may "walk" along the cortical bone to an unacceptable position. Thus the starting point and alignment must be confirmed fluoroscopically before advancing the wire. This technique simply aids in localizing and minimizing the skin incision and helps determine the approximate angle of the guide wire and pin, but it does not prevent technical errors of pin placement.

◆ **Determining Entry Point for Cannulated Screw Fixation of Slipped Epiphysis**

TECHNIQUE 33-26 *(Canale et al.)*

Place the patient supine so that anteroposterior and lateral fluoroscopic views can be obtained without repositioning the patient or the extremity; a fracture table can be used. The entire proximal femoral epiphysis and hip joint space should be clearly visible on both views. Prepare and drape the extremity to allow free access to the entire anterior surface of the thigh and as far medially as the pubis in the inguinal area. A fluoroscopic C-arm is used for an anteroposterior and an exact lateral image. On the lateral view the femoral neck should be parallel to the femoral shaft.

Place a guide wire on the anterior aspect of the thigh (Fig. 33-123, *A*) so that the anteroposterior image shows it in the desired varus-valgus position (Fig. 33-123, *B*) and mark the position of the guide wire on the anterior surface of the thigh with a marking pen. Then place the guide along the lateral aspect of the thigh (Fig. 33-123, *C*) so that it is in the correct anteroposterior position on fluoroscopic image (Fig. 33-123, *D*) and mark the position of the wire on the skin. In (SCFE) the epiphysis is displaced posteriorly relative to the femoral neck and this lateral guide wire angles from anterior to posterior and appears on fluoroscopic image to enter at the anterior femoral neck. The two skin lines should intersect on the anterolateral aspect of the thigh (Fig. 33-123, *E*). The greater the degree of the slip (the more posterior the epiphysis), the more anterior the intersection (Fig. 33-123, *F*).

Now place a guide wire, drill, or pin through either a small lateral incision or a simple stab (puncture) wound (Fig. 33-123, *G*) at the intersection of the two skin lines. Monitor proper alignment, position, and depth of insertion in the proximal femoral epiphysis on anteroposterior and lateral fluoroscopic images. Insert internal fixation in the routine manner.

TECHNIQUE 33-27 *(Morrissy)*

Place the patient on the fracture table with the affected leg abducted 10 to 15 degrees and internally rotated as far as possible without force. This brings the femoral neck as close as possible to parallel to the floor to assist in obtaining true anterior and lateral image views. Position the image intensifier between the legs so that anteroposterior and lateral views can be obtained by moving the tube around the arc of the machine (Fig. 33-124). After standard preparation and draping and under image control, insert a Kirschner wire percutaneously through the anterolateral area of the thigh down to the femoral neck (Fig. 33-125), adjusting the guide wire on the anteroposterior projection to determine the axis of the femoral neck. Obtain a lateral view to determine the amount of posterior inclination necessary. When the starting point on the femoral neck and amount of posterior inclination have been estimated, insert the guide assembly through a small puncture wound. Advance the guide assembly to the physis and confirm placement in the central axis of the femoral head by image intensification. If the position is correct, advance the guide assembly across the plate. (If positioning is incorrect, insert a second guide assembly using the first to determine what correction in the starting point or angulation is necessary.) When the proper

continued

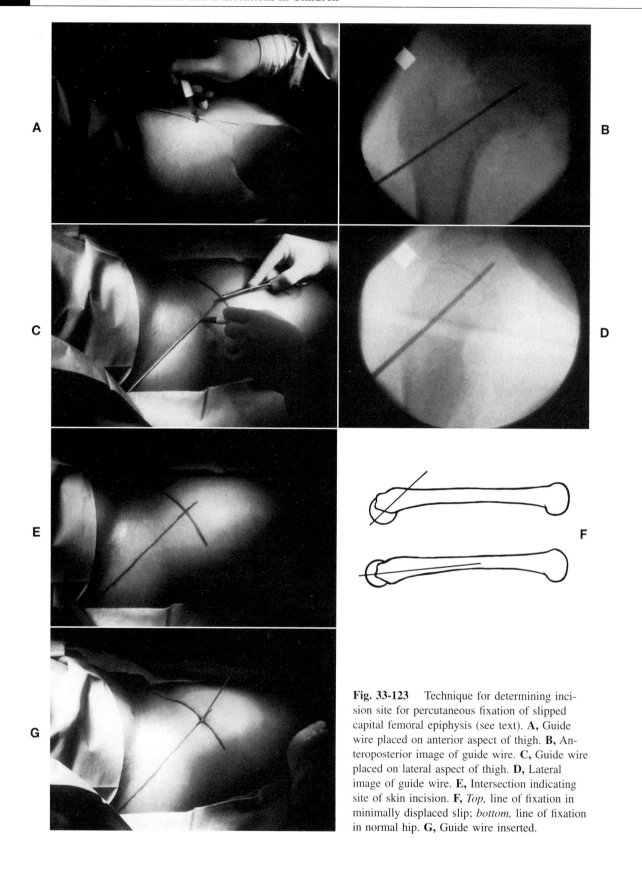

Fig. 33-123   Technique for determining incision site for percutaneous fixation of slipped capital femoral epiphysis (see text). **A,** Guide wire placed on anterior aspect of thigh. **B,** Anteroposterior image of guide wire. **C,** Guide wire placed on lateral aspect of thigh. **D,** Lateral image of guide wire. **E,** Intersection indicating site of skin incision. **F,** *Top,* line of fixation in minimally displaced slip; *bottom,* line of fixation in normal hip. **G,** Guide wire inserted.

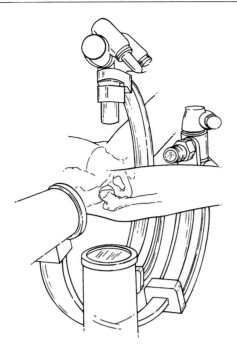

Fig. 33-124 Percutaneous in situ fixation of slipped capital femoral epiphysis. Positioning of image intensifier to allow rotation necessary to obtain lateral and anteroposterior views. (From Morrissy RT: *J Pediatr Orthop* 10:347, 1990.)

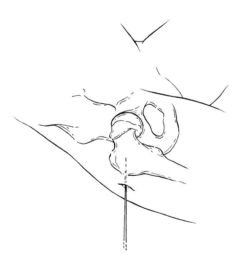

Fig. 33-125 Kirschner wire passed percutaneously to estimated starting point on femur.

depth is reached (at least 0.5 cm from subchondral bone), remove the cannula and leave the guide wire in the bone. Determine the correct screw length by passing a guide wire of identical length along the one in the bone and measuring the difference. Advance the correct length screw over the guide pin and then remove the pin. Remove the leg from the traction device and move it in multiple directions, using both anteroposterior and lateral views to confirm that the

screw does not penetrate the joint. Close the stab wound with a single subcuticular suture.

If two screws are deemed necessary for an acute slip, the first screw should lie in the central axis of the femoral head and the second below it, avoiding the superolateral quadrant. The second screw should stop at least 8 mm from the subchondral bone.

AFTERTREATMENT. Range-of-motion exercises are begun the day after surgery. Most patients begin walking with a three-point partial weight-bearing crutch gait on the first day after surgery and are discharged the same day. Crutches are used until all signs of synovitis are gone and motion is free and painless (usually 1 week). All rigorous sports and other activities are forbidden until the physes have closed. The screws are removed after physeal closure has been demonstrated roentgenographically. The easiest method of removal is to pass a guide wire into the cannula of the screw under image control to allow the screwdriver to be guided into the head of the screw over the guide wire.

TECHNIQUE 33-28 *(Asnis)*

Place the patient supine on a fracture table. Reduce the fracture or, rarely, the slipped capital femoral epiphysis only if necessary and confirm the reduction and position by two-plane roentgenograms or image intensification. Make an 8-cm lateral incision, starting at the prominence of the greater trochanter and extending distally. Split the fascia lata and vastus lateralis in line with the incision and retract their edges. Select a point 3 to 4 cm below the greater trochanter, midway between the anterior and posterior femoral cortices. Then at this point drive a two-part guide pin assembly into the lateral femoral neck and direct it across the fracture site, or the physis in a slipped capital femoral epiphysis, and into the femoral head. Confirm the position of the pin assembly with roentgenograms or an image intensifier. If the position is not acceptable, estimate the angle between this pin and another necessary for correction and insert another guide pin assembly. Place an adjustable pin guide system (Fig. 33-126) over the malaligned guide pin assembly and, using the estimated angle, insert another guide pin assembly in the proper location. Release both friction locks, and remove the malaligned guide pin assembly.

Next, use the fixed pin guide, which contains a grid of different-sized triangles. Select the desired triangle depending on the size of the femoral neck (Fig. 33-127). Drive two more guide pin assemblies into the femoral head with the aid of the fixed pin guide. Check the length and position of the guide pin assemblies with roentgenograms or the image intensifier. Place the tips of the guide pin assemblies 7 to 10 mm from the subchondral bone. Then tap the inner pin of each guide pin assembly gently with a mallet until its lateral end is flush with the lateral end of the outer component.

continued

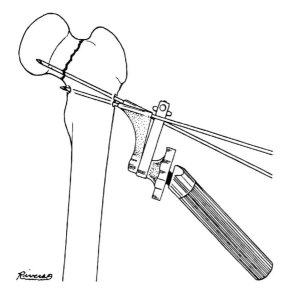

Fig. 33-126 Adjustable pin guide system for use over mal-aligned pin assembly by placing second guide pin in proper location in femoral head and neck. (Redrawn from Asnis SE: *The Asnis guided screw system technique manual*, Rutherford, NJ, 1984, Courtesy Howmedica.)

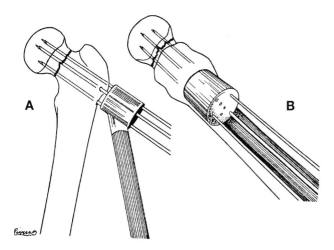

Fig. 33-127 Placement of two or more guide pin assemblies into femoral head and neck with aid of fixed pin guide. **A,** Anteroposterior view. **B,** Lateral view. (Redrawn from Asnis SE: *The Asnis guided screw system technique manual*, Rutherford, NJ, 1984, Courtesy Howmedica.)

Remove each outer component with the power driver, leaving the inner guide pin in place. For each guide pin determine the screw length by holding the depth gauge against the femoral cortex along the pin and reading off the depth of penetration of the pin. Tap the outer femoral cortex at each guide pin with a cannulated tap placed over the pin. Now insert a cannulated screw over each guide pin, and tighten each with the cannulated screwdriver (Fig. 33-128).

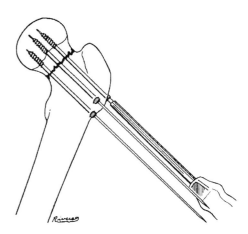

Fig. 33-128 Insertion of cannulated screw with screwdriver and removal of guide pins. (Redrawn from Asnis SE: *The Asnis guided screw system technique manual*, Rutherford, NJ, 1984, Courtesy Howmedica.)

Check the placement of the screws by image intensification, and if a screw is not of ideal length remove it over the guide pin and replace it with one of appropriate length. Now remove the guide pins and close the wound.

AFTERTREATMENT. A spica cast generally is unnecessary unless any large drill holes are not filled with screws, thereby acting as "stress risers." The patient should be non-weight-bearing on crutches for 4 to 6 weeks.

Lehman et al. described another cannulated hip screw that is inserted over a guide pin for hip fractures in children and for slipped capital femoral epiphyses.

TECHNIQUE 33-29 *(Lyden; Lehman et al.)*

Place the patient supine and drape the affected hip in the usual manner. Reduce the fracture or, rarely, the slipped capital femoral epiphysis, if required, and verify the position roentgenographically. Then with a standard lateral approach, open the skin, fascia, and muscle down to the lateral femur. Make a hole in the lateral cortex of the femur with a 4.8-mm (3/16-inch) diameter "trocar pointed" Steinmann pin. This cortical aperture should be 40 to 50 mm below the crest of the greater trochanter (or opposite the middle of the lesser trochanter) to allow pin placement at 135 degrees (Fig. 33-129, *A*). Next, introduce a 2.4-mm (3/32-inch) smooth guide pin across the fracture or across the slipped physis in an acceptable position and depth in the femoral

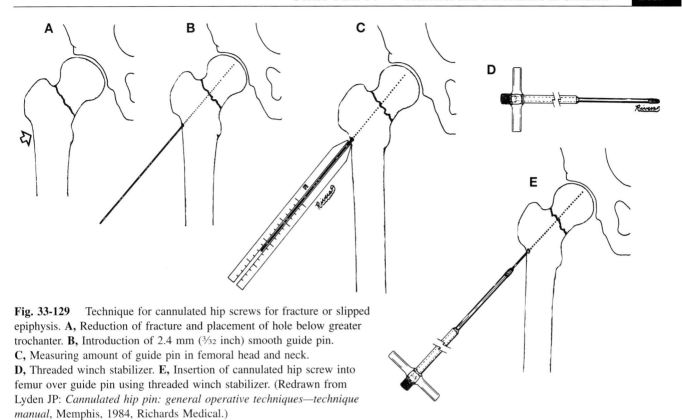

Fig. 33-129 Technique for cannulated hip screws for fracture or slipped epiphysis. **A,** Reduction of fracture and placement of hole below greater trochanter. **B,** Introduction of 2.4 mm (³⁄₃₂ inch) smooth guide pin. **C,** Measuring amount of guide pin in femoral head and neck. **D,** Threaded winch stabilizer. **E,** Insertion of cannulated hip screw into femur over guide pin using threaded winch stabilizer. (Redrawn from Lyden JP: *Cannulated hip pin: general operative techniques—technique manual*, Memphis, 1984, Richards Medical.)

head. The tip should engage subchondral bone (Fig. 33-129, *B*). If the pin is poorly positioned, withdraw and reinsert it into the femoral neck and central in the head. If more than one screw is used, the second and third screws should parallel the first, with their threads not touching. A triangular configuration is preferred. Use a measuring gauge to determine the length of the cannulated screw required (Fig. 33-129, *C*) or merely hold a second guide wire along the initial one to measure the length. Then connect the winch to the cannulated screw of appropriate length by means of a threaded winch stabilizer (Fig. 33-129, *D*). Place the screw over the guide pin and insert it into the femur (Fig. 33-129, *E*). The flutes of the cannulated screw will cut through the cancellous bone until the beveled shoulders seat on the lateral cortex. If self-tapping of the bone is difficult, especially in the femoral head, an appropriate reamer and tap should be used first. After the first screw is satisfactorily positioned, insert additional screws with or without the use of an alignment guide (Fig. 33-130). The number of screws chosen depends on the stability of the fracture or "slip," the quality of bone, and the adequacy of pin placement. Subsequent screws can be inserted with the initial guide wire protruding distally to act as an insertion guide. The second screw may go in freehand by using a 4.8-mm

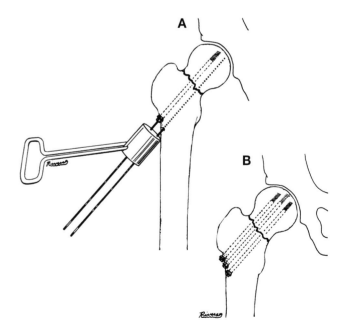

Fig. 33-130 **A,** Insertion of guide pins through alignment guide. **B,** Three cannulated screws have been inserted. (Redrawn from Lyden JP: *Cannulated hip pin: general operative techniques—technique manual*, Memphis, 1984, Richards Medical.)

continued

Steinmann pin and the alignment guide and then the cannulated screw. Alternatively, if the correct length of the subsequent screw is assured, follow the initial screw with a 4.8-mm Steinmann pin to create a femoral hole and then insert the subsequent cannulated screws directly without the intermediate guide alignment.

Lehman modified this technique somewhat for slipped capital femoral epiphyses. If self-tapping of the cannulated bone is difficult, use a reamer over the guide wire first; then use a tap before inserting the screws of appropriate size. Because the reamer or tap may advance the guide wire across the femoral head into the hip joint, remove the guide wire as the reamer or tap reaches the epiphysis. If the guide wire is not removed at this point, roentgenographic control is absolutely necessary during the advancement of the reamer or tap to be certain that the guide wire does not advance through the femoral head.

AFTERTREATMENT. The aftertreatment is similar to that described for the Asnis technique.

Prophylactic Pinning of Contralateral Slips

Bilateral involvement has been reported in 21% to 80% of patients with SCFE. Symptomatic slipping of the contralateral slip after unilateral slipping has been estimated to occur in 12.5% of patients before skeletal maturity, and asymptomatic slipping of the contralateral hip in as many as 40%. In the series of Ingram et al. bilateral slips occurred in 32% of children; however, only 16% of the second slipped epiphyses occurred after treatment of the original slipped epiphysis. Loder, Aronson, and Greenfield reported 82 bilateral slips in 224 children (37%); half were diagnosed simultaneously and half sequentially. Compared with the children in whom bilateral slips were diagnosed simultaneously, children in whom the slips were diagnosed sequentially had a shorter duration of symptoms before diagnosis of the first slip, were younger at the time of diagnosis of the first slip, and tended to be more obese. In 88%, the second slip was diagnosed within 18 months of the first slip. They, as well as Steel and Betz et al., recommended frequent follow-up examinations for the first 2 years after diagnosis of a unilateral slip, especially in girls 12 years old or younger and in boys 14 years old or younger.

Because of the relative infrequency of a symptomatic contralateral slip and the frequency of complications such as chondrolysis after pinning, prophylactic pinning of the contralateral hip usually is not performed. This has been further emphasized by Johnson and Hernandez, who analyzed their results of prophylactic pinning and noted that it was indicated only in rare instances, such as in high-risk, noncompliant patients or patients with epiphysiolysis from irradiation therapy or renal failure. Kumm et al. performed prophylactic dynamic screw fixation of 34 unaffected hips using a single cannulated screw and dynamic screw fixation, respectively, with no complications. Their study supports the prophylactic treatment of the asymptomatic hip.

Closed Reduction

Manipulative reduction has been reported for acute (unstable) and acute-on-chronic slips with moderate and severe displacement by Fairbank, Aadalen et al., and Griffith, among others. Boyer et al., however, reported that slips treated without reduction, even moderate and severe slips, had better results when pinned in situ than after manipulative reduction. Carney et al. reported the development of avascular necrosis in 12 of 39 (31%) hips in which reduction was attempted and in only 6 of 116 (5%) hips in which no reduction was attempted. Although an association of avascular necrosis with manipulative reduction has been suggested, the development of avascular necrosis may be related to the severity of the slip rather than to the manipulative reduction, provided that only a very gentle reduction is performed. It probably is best, however, to manipulate only severe, acute (unstable) slips that may be technically difficult or impossible to pin in situ. We occasionally perform a gentle reduction only if gradual reduction has failed and the position of the epiphysis is unacceptable. This is performed with the patient on a fracture table, and internal rotation alone usually is sufficient to obtain adequate reduction. An acute separation in a previously normal hip usually can be reduced easily; no attempt should be made to reduce it by forceful manipulation. Because of the risk of avascular necrosis, we no longer use the Boyd technique of closed reduction. Casey et al. suggested that a gradual reduction by skin traction and internal rotation over 3 to 4 days is less traumatic to the epiphysis than manipulative reduction (Fig. 33-131). None of their 16 patients treated by this method developed avascular necrosis, whereas avascular necrosis developed in 5 of 36 treated with manipulative reduction.

The closed reduction should be checked roentgenographically or with image intensification, and the epiphysis should be fixed with a cannulated hip screw (p. 1485).

Open Reduction

Because of the possibility that biomechanical disturbances caused by the tilt of the epiphysis will cause early degenerative joint changes, open reduction, limited osteotomy, and internal fixation, if necessary, have been recommended if a severe acute or chronic slip cannot be reduced closed. Avascular necrosis has been reported after open reduction, and Compere in 1950 noted the importance of protecting the posterior retinacular vessels during open reduction. Dunn emphasized the need to shorten the femoral neck to prevent tension on the posterior vessels when the epiphysis is reduced, making the procedure a closing wedge osteotomy rather than a simple open reduction. Szypryt et al. compared the results of Dunn's open reduction with the more conservative Heyman-Herndon epiphysiodesis and concluded that, whereas the Heyman-Herndon procedure gave consistently good results for moderate slips, Dunn's procedure gave better results for severe slips. They recommended a realignment procedure for slips of more than 50%.

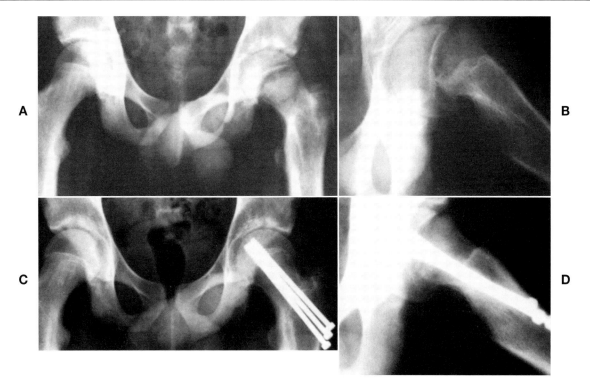

Fig. 33-131 **A** and **B,** Acute slipped capital femoral epiphysis with moderate displacement. **C** and **D,** After in situ pinning with cannulated cancellous hip screws.

Broughton et al. reported open reduction of severe slips in 115 patients with an average follow-up of almost 13 years. In 70 patients with chronic slips and open physes, avascular necrosis occurred in 2 (2.8%), chondrolysis in 5 (7%), and both in 1; however, in 38 patients with acute-on-chronic slips, avascular necrosis occurred in 6 (16%), chondrolysis in 1, and both in 3. Of 7 patients with partially fused physes, only 1 had a satisfactory result, leading these authors to conclude that open reduction should not be performed in hips with a partially fused physis. Aronson and Tursky reported successful open reduction of nine acute slips, with no avascular necrosis or chondrolysis, and they suggested that restoration of functional motion may decrease the risk of osteoarthritis.

Bone Peg Epiphysiodesis

Bone peg epiphysiodesis was originally described by Ferguson and Howorth in 1931, and its popularity has increased because of reported complications after pin or screw penetration into the joint. Weiner et al. reported their results of 185 bone peg epiphysiodeses over a 30-year period. Of 26 acute slips, avascular necrosis developed in only 2, and chondrolysis developed in only 1. Of 159 chronic slips, 4 had further slipping, caused by acute trauma in 2, graft absorption in 1, and malplacement of the graft in 1. Avascular necrosis developed in only one hip, and chondrolysis developed in none. These authors cited as advantages of bone peg epiphysiodesis rapid physeal closure and low incidences of complications, especially chondrolysis. Roberts (personal communication), as well as Bloom and Crawford, also reported that the long-term results

were better after bone peg epiphysiodesis than after in situ pinning of moderate or severe slips but recommended in situ pinning for mild acute or chronic slips. Zahrawi et al., in their report of 105 hips treated for mostly mild slips, concluded that in situ pinning is more predictable, has fewer complications, and produces better long-term results than bone peg epiphysiodesis. Ward and Wood reported physeal fusion in 12 of 17 open bone graft epiphysiodeses. Eight grafts either resorbed, moved, or fractured postoperatively, leading them to conclude that graft insufficiency is common in single bone grafts and causes an increase in severity of slip and failure of physeal fusion. Other disadvantages of open bone peg epiphysiodesis include longer operating time, increased blood loss, longer hospitalization, and longer rehabilitation. After bone peg epiphysiodesis of acute slips, spica cast immobilization may be necessary for 6 weeks or more to prevent further slipping. Because of postoperative complications, including avascular necrosis, chondrolysis, infection, thigh hypesthesias, and heterotopic ossification, and the need for lengthy immobilization, as well as economic concerns, Roy and Crawford no longer recommend bone peg epiphysiodesis for stable (chronic) slips.

Although the procedure traditionally has been performed through an anterior iliofemoral approach, Weiner et al. described an anterolateral approach that simplifies the technique. In a report of 32 epiphysiodeses performed with the anterolateral approach, they cited advantages of reduced operating time, less blood loss, avoidance of damage to the lateral femoral cutaneous nerve, and improved wound healing.

Fig. 33-132 **A,** Anterior approach to hip and H-shaped capsular incision. **B,** Use of hollow mill to create tunnel across physis as seen in anteroposterior and lateral views. **C,** Sandwiched iliac bone grafts are driven across physis. (Redrawn from Weiner DS, Weiner S, Melby A, Hoyt WA Jr: *J Pediatr Orthop* 4:145, 1984.)

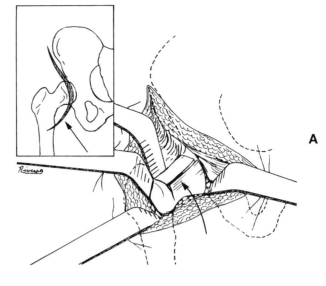

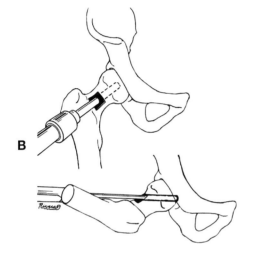

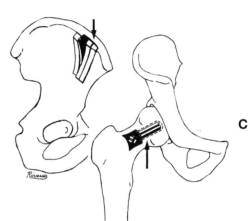

◆ **Bone Peg Epiphysiodesis Through Anterolateral Approach**

TECHNIQUE 33-30 *(Weiner et al.)*

Make a midlateral incision beginning 4 to 5 inches (10 to 12 cm) below the level of the greater trochanter in the lateral midline of the upper portion of the thigh, proceeding proximally to the greater trochanter and then angling obliquely to the anterosuperior iliac spine (Fig. 33-132, *A*, inset). Split the tensor fasciae femoris proximally to the level of the anterosuperior iliac spine. Retract the tensor anteriorly and posteriorly to expose the underlying anterior portion of the gluteal musculature. Retract posteriorly the most anterior fibers of the gluteus medius to expose the joint capsule. Make an H-shaped incision in the capsule and place large cobra retractors around the femoral neck (Fig. 33-132, *A*). If a bony prominence ("hump") on the anterolateral metaphyseal region resulting from the slipping is severe enough to act as an impediment to motion, remove

it with an osteotome. Fashion a square or rectangular window in the anterior surface of the femoral neck. Then insert a large, hollow "mill" through the window and drill it across the physis into the epiphysis under image intensifier control. Remove a cylindrical core, consisting of metaphyseal bone, physis, and a portion of the epiphyseal bone, thereby guaranteeing passage of the mill across the physis and into the epiphysis (Fig. 33-132, *B*). Enlarge the cylindrical tunnel with a curet and remove more of the physis. Remove sections of corticocancellous bone from the outer layer of the ilium. Sandwich them together and drive this composite bone peg across the physis into the epiphysis (Fig. 33-132, *C*).

AFTERTREATMENT. In acute slips when the femoral head is mobile, a spica cast should be applied with the femoral head in the reduced position with the graft in place. The cast is worn for 6 weeks, and then touch-down weight-bearing is allowed. In chronic slips, after bed rest for 48 to 96 hours, the patient ambulates on crutches. Weight-bearing can be started at approximately 10 weeks.

◆ ◆ ◆

In an effort to simplify bone peg epiphysiodesis, Schmidt et al. developed a percutaneous, fluoroscopically guided technique using cortical allograft inserted through a hole drilled in the lateral femoral cortex, passed through the femoral neck and across the physis. Much of this procedure is similar to that for percutaneous pin fixation (p. 1485), except that, rather than a cannulated screw, a 10-mm reamer is inserted over the guide pin and the reamed tunnel is filled with a cortical strut allograft. The authors reported that this makes operative time and morbidity not significantly different from single-screw fixation. They reported 35 excellent, 1 good, and 2 fair results in mild and moderate slips with this technique, although 6 patients (16%) had major postoperative complications, including avascular necrosis, chondrolysis, femoral neck and intertrochanteric fractures, and progressive coxa vara deformities.

Osteotomy

Because moderately or severely displaced chronic slips produce permanent irregularities in the femoral head and acetabulum, some form of realignment procedure often is indicated to restore the normal relationship of the femoral head and neck and possibly delay the onset of degenerative joint disease. Carney et al., however, reported that in a long-term follow-up patients with osteotomies had worse scores on the Iowa hip rating with each passing decade than did patients without hip realignment procedures. They recommended in situ fixation regardless of the severity of the slip. Crawford's indications for osteotomy were problems with gait, sitting, or cosmetic appearance after 1 year; he recommended this delay in realignment after stabilization because of the capacity of the capital femoral epiphysis to remodel. Kallio et al., after serial sonographic examination of 26 slips with pin fixation, concluded that metaphyseal resorption continued at the rate of 2 mm every 3 weeks until the physeal "step-off" was smooth in the anterior aspect of the femoral neck. They recommended sonography as an accurate method for evaluating and classifying the remodeling after fixation of SCFE. Strong et al. noted remodeling of the femoral neck and epiphysis after internal fixation across the physis in 55 hips. Of 71 mild slips, only 1 (5%) remodeled, 5 of 23 moderate slips (22%) remodeled, and all 11 severe slips (100%) remodeled. Their findings support the use of internal fixation and a delay of 2 years after pinning before consideration of realignment of femoral neck osteotomies.

Osteotomy also may be indicated for malunion of a chronic slip in poor position; malunited slipped epiphysis differs from a chronic slip only in that in the former the physis has fused and further slipping will not occur.

There are two basic types of osteotomy: closing wedge osteotomy through the femoral neck, usually near the physis to correct the deformity, and compensatory osteotomy through the

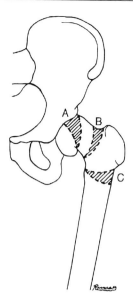

Fig. 33-133 Osteotomies for slipped capital femoral epiphysis. *A,* Through neck near epiphysis. *B,* Through base of neck. *C,* Through trochanteric region. (Redrawn from Crawford AH: *Instr Course Lect* 33:327, 1984.)

trochanteric region to produce a deformity in the opposite direction (Fig. 33-133). The advantage of osteotomy through the femoral neck is that the deformity itself is corrected, but incidences of avascular necrosis ranging from 2% to 100% and of chondrolysis from 3% to 37% have been associated with this procedure. For this reason, we rarely make an osteotomy in the femoral neck. For completeness, four femoral neck osteotomies are described: (1) the technique of Fish, (2) the technique of Dunn just distal to the slip, (3) the base of the neck technique of Kramer et al., and (4) the technique of Abraham et al.

Compensatory osteotomies in the trochanteric region, as well as partial cheilectomy, to reduce deformity also are described (pp. 1495 to 1500).

◆ Cuneiform Osteotomy of Femoral Neck (Fish)

Although some of our worst results followed osteotomy of the femoral neck, reduction by a cuneiform osteotomy made just distal to the physis and internal fixation may be necessary for a severe chronic or acute-on-chronic slip. The reported incidences of avascular necrosis and chondrolysis after this procedure have been exceptionally high. However, Fish reported long-term follow-up (average of 13 years, 4 months) of 61 patients (66 hips) with displacement severe enough (more than 30 degrees) to require correction by cuneiform osteotomy of the femoral neck just distal to the physis. Results were excellent in 55 hips, good in 6, fair in 2, and poor in 3. Avascular necrosis developed in 3 hips (4.5%), chondrolysis in 2 (3%), and osteoarthritis in 6 (9%). Pin penetration was noted in all hips with osteoarthritis. Nishiyama et al. followed 15 patients (18 hips) who had subcapital wedge osteotomy for severe slips. Only 1 patient had a poor result; he developed both

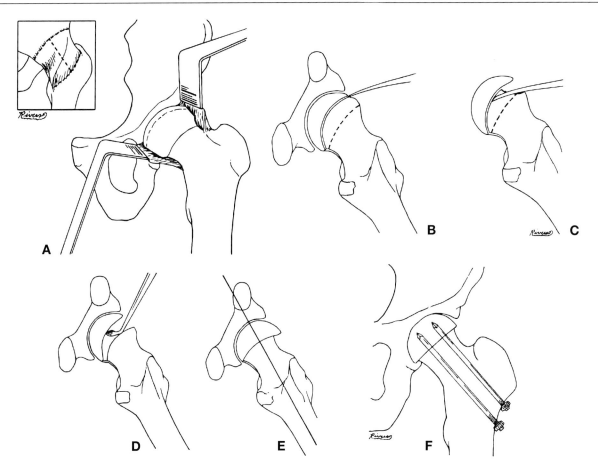

Fig. 33-134   Fish technique for cuneiform osteotomy of femoral neck. Femoral head and neck are exposed. **A,** *Inset,* Joint capsule is incised longitudinally, and then transverse incision is made at each end of longitudinal incision so that physis can be identified. **B,** Osteotomy is made distal to physis. **C,** Wedge of bone is removed in small pieces with osteotome and mallet. **D,** More bone is removed with small curet or curved osteotome. **E,** Anatomical alignment is obtained. After wedge is removed, diameter of femoral head is often greater than that of femoral neck. **F,** Epiphysis is fixed to femoral neck with three or four pins. (Redrawn from Fish JB: *J Bone Joint Surg* 66A:1153, 1984.)

avascular necrosis and chondrolysis. Both Fish and Nishiyama et al. believe this is the only operation that restores an accurate anatomical relationship between the head and neck of the femur. Fish recommended it for moderate and severe slips of 30 degrees or more, and Nishiyama et al. recommended it for severe slips of more than 60 degrees. DeRosa et al. reported 19 good, 4 fair, and 4 poor results after cuneiform osteotomy in 23 patients with 27 severe slips; avascular necrosis occurred in 15%. They recommend this procedure only for severe slips in patients with open physes.

TECHNIQUE 33-31 *(Fish)*

Place the patient supine on a standard operating table with a radiolucent roll beneath the involved side of the pelvis to elevate it. Drape the limb free to allow manipulation of the hip during the osteotomy and for roentgenographic determination of the position of the femoral head and the pins used for internal rotation (gentle manipulation under anesthesia is done only for patients with an acute slip). Make an anterolateral approach to the hip (Technique 1-49) and carry the dissection between the tensor fasciae latae and gluteus medius to the anterior aspect of the capsule of the hip joint. Generously expose the capsule proximal to the rim of the acetabulum. Open the capsule longitudinally and then make transverse incisions at each end of the longitudinal incision to expose the femoral neck (Fig. 33-134, *A*). Carefully retract the capsule with either appropriate clamps or Meyerding retractors. Identify the capital femoral epiphysis, which usually is barely visible at the rim of the acetabulum. The projecting portion of the neck should be obvious. Locate the physis with the aid of a Keith needle or small, sharp, curved osteotome. Determine the size of the wedge to be removed by noting the degree of slip and the position of the epiphysis. Remove enough bone to allow effortless anatomical reduction of the head and neck. Make the base of the wedge anteriorly and superiorly for correct positioning of the epiphysis. Generally, a wider wedge superiorly is necessary in a more severe slip. Shape the wedge of the bone to be removed so that the curved contour of the epiphysis will match the corresponding curved cancellous surface of the femoral neck. After determining the size of the wedge, remove the bone gently in small pieces with an osteotome and mallet (Fig. 33-134, *B* and *C*). Approach the posterior aspect of the neck with caution to avoid vascular damage. This area can be cleared with a small curet or a hand-held curved osteotome (Fig. 33-134, *D* and *E*). After removing sufficient bone, reduce the epiphysis by flexion, abduction, and internal rotation of the limb. If insufficient bone has been removed and the reduction is forceful, too much tension may be placed on the posterior periosteum, capsule, and vessels. After reduction, fix the epiphysis to the neck with three or four pins. Use pins that are 6 inches (15.2 cm) long and threaded on one half of their lengths, with a knurled nut on the threads. Do not allow the pins to penetrate the articular cartilage of the epiphysis, but do penetrate the epiphysis deeply enough to obtain firm fixation. Use anteroposterior and frog-leg lateral roentgenograms to determine the position of the pins. Screw down the knurled nuts to the femoral cortex and cut the pins next to the nuts (Fig. 33-134, *F*).

AFTERTREATMENT. The patient should be free in bed, with the involved limb supported on pillows. When comfortable, he is allowed out of bed, using crutches with only touch-down weight-bearing on the involved limb. Full weight-bearing is permitted after roentgenograms show the osteotomy to be completely healed, at approximately 5 months. Then the pins are removed, and full activity is allowed 2 months later.

◆ Cuneiform Osteotomy of Femoral Neck (Dunn)

Dunn described an osteotomy for severe chronic slips in children with open physes; he emphasized that this procedure should not be done if the physis is closed. He bases his technique on two well-known facts: (1) the slip of the femoral head strips the periosteum from the back of the femoral neck and a beak of new bone is laid down beneath it (Fig. 33-135, *A*), and (2) the main retinacular blood supply runs up the back of the femoral neck; a lateral approach allows stripping of the periosteum and its contained vessels under direct vision (Fig. 33-135, *B*) to avoid damaging the blood supply to the femoral head.

TECHNIQUE 33-32 *(Dunn)*

Through a lateral approach (Chapter 1), make an incision in the periosteum and elevate the posterior vascular covering of the femoral neck (Fig. 33-135, *C*). Make two osteotomy cuts, one in the long axis of the neck to remove the bony

beak and the second at right angles to the neck to shorten it by 3 to 4 mm (Fig. 33-135, *D*). Appose the surfaces of the osteotomy and insert three threaded pins up the femoral neck to its cut surface. Reduce the deformity and confirm position on roentgenograms. In the lateral view the head should appear to sit squarely on the neck (Fig. 33-135, *E*), but in the anteroposterior view the head should be tilted into about 20 degrees of valgus (Fig. 33-135, *F*). When reduction is satisfactory, drive the pins into the femoral head. Close the wound in the usual manner.

AFTERTREATMENT. For a reliable, mature child, if internal fixation is secure, putting the extremity in balanced suspension for early motion is preferred. Otherwise, a cast is applied from the nipple line to the toes on the affected side, holding the extremity in neutral rotation and moderate abduction, and to above the knee on the opposite side. The cast is removed at about 4 weeks, and active and passive motions are begun and gradually increased. About 2 weeks later walking is allowed with crutches, bearing the weight of the affected extremity on the floor but without bearing weight through the hip. At 3 to 4 months after surgery, partial weight-bearing is permitted. Full weight-bearing is not allowed until roentgenograms show union of the osteotomy.

◆ Compensatory Basilar Osteotomy of Femoral Neck

Kramer et al. described a compensatory osteotomy of the base of the femoral neck that corrects the varus and retroversion components of moderate or severe chronic SCFE. They suggested that it is safer than an osteotomy made near or at the physis because the line of the osteotomy is distal to the major blood supply in the posterior retinaculum. Threaded pins are used for fixation of the osteotomy and the epiphysis. Not only is the anatomical relationship of the proximal femur restored, but also further slipping is prevented.

TECHNIQUE 33-33 *(Kramer et al.)*

Determine preoperatively the size of wedge to be removed by measuring the degree of the slip. Determine on anteroposterior roentgenograms the head and neck angle. Use paper tracings of the anteroposterior and lateral roentgenograms and cut with scissors the wedge on the tracing paper to determine the amount of bone to be removed and the results to be obtained.

Approach the hip laterally. Begin the skin incision 2 cm distal and lateral to the anterosuperior iliac spine and curve it distally and posteriorly over the greater trochanter and then distally along the lateral surface of the femoral shaft to a point 10 cm distal to the base of the trochanter. Incise longitudinally the fascia lata. Develop the interval between the gluteus medius and tensor fasciae latae. Carry the dissection proximally to the inferior branch of the superior

continued

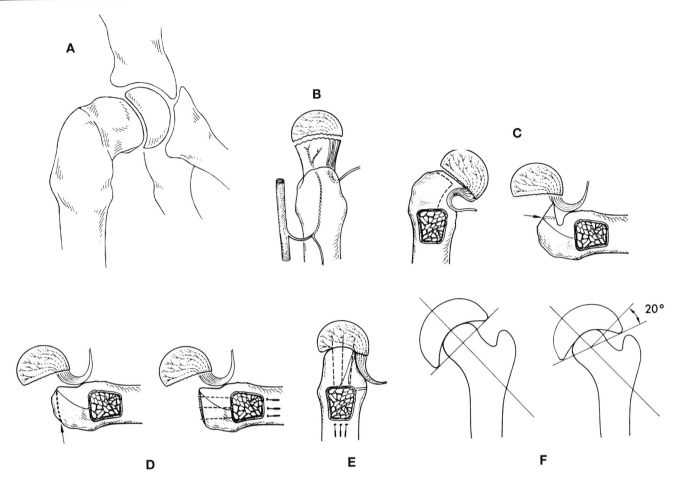

Fig. 33-135 **A,** Diagram showing beak of new bone. **B,** Normal hip exposed from lateral side showing vascular synovium on back of neck and avascular anterior surface. **C,** Incision in synovium and head detached, preserving blood supply and exposing beak of new bone (*arrow* indicates first cut). **D,** Beak has been removed (*arrow* indicates second cut), and threaded pins are inserted into shortened neck. **E,** Head square on neck in lateral view; deformity is reduced and pinned, and blood supply is intact. **F,** *Left,* Head is square on neck. This is incorrect. *Right,* Head should be tilted to give valgus alignment of about 20 degrees. (From Dunn DM: *The hip: Proceedings of the Third Open Scientific Meeting of the Hip Society,* St Louis, 1975, Mosby.)

gluteal nerve, which innervates the latter muscle. Incise the capsule of the hip joint longitudinally along the anterosuperior surface of the femoral neck. Release widely the capsular attachment along the anterior intertrochanteric line. Reflect distally the vastus lateralis to expose the base of the greater trochanter and the proximal part of the femoral shaft. With the capsule of the hip joint open, identify the junction between the articular cartilage of the femoral head and the callus and the junction of the callus with the normal cortex of the femoral neck. Compare the distance between these two junctions with the calculations made from the paper cutouts of the roentgenograms. The widest part of the wedge will be in line with the widest part of the slip, in the anterior and superior aspects of the neck (Fig. 33-136, *A* and *B*). Make the more distal osteotomy cut first, perpendicular to

the femoral neck and following the anterior intertrochanteric line from proximal to distal. Extend this osteotomy cut to the posterior cortex but leave this cortex intact. Make the second osteotomy cut with the blade of the osteotome directed obliquely so that its cutting edge stays distal to the posterior retinacular blood supply. The capsule with the blood supply reaches to the intertrochanteric line anteriorly, but posteriorly the lateral third of the neck is extracapsular. Therefore, according to Kramer et al., an osteotomy made through the region of the anterior intertrochanteric line lies distal to the posterior retinacular vessels. Drill one or two 5-mm threaded Steinmann pins into the femoral neck proximally to ensure that the proximal portion of the femur is kept under control before completing the osteotomy (Fig. 33-136, *A* and *B*). Complete the osteotomy,

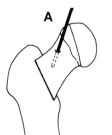 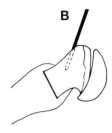 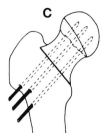 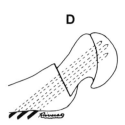

Fig. 33-136   **A** and **B,** Widest part of wedge (at base of neck) is in line with widest part of slip, correcting both varus and retroversion components, and Steinmann pin is inserted into femoral neck to control proximal fragment. If wedge is too wide anteriorly, retroversion will be overly corrected. Most common mistake is to make wedge too narrow superiorly, resulting in incomplete correction of varus. **C** and **D,** Osteotomy is closed and 5-mm threaded Steinmann pins are inserted from outer cortex of femoral shaft through femoral neck, across osteotomy site, and into head. Pins fix osteotomy, and since they cross physis, they prevent any further slip. (Redrawn by H Mohagheg, MD; from Kramer WG, Craig WA, Noel S: *J Bone Joint Surg* 58A:796, 1976.)

taking care that the osteotome does not fully penetrate the posterior cortex. Insert several 5-mm threaded Steinmann pins from the outer cortex of the femoral shaft through the femoral neck. Complete the osteotomy by greensticking the posterior cortex and removing the wedge of bone. Advance the threaded Steinmann pins across the osteotomy site and the physis to prevent further slipping (Fig. 33-136, *C* and *D*). Close the capsule of the hip with interrupted sutures. Clip off the pins close to the femoral shaft. Close the wound in layers. If epiphysiodesis of the greater trochanter is necessary, do it at this time.

AFTERTREATMENT. Bed rest is prescribed for 2 to 3 weeks, followed by non-weight-bearing. Partial weight-bearing is allowed depending on the stability of the osteotomy and the weight of the patient. The threaded Steinmann pins should be removed only after the physis has fused.

◆ **Extracapsular Base-of-Neck Osteotomy**

Abraham et al. reported good or excellent results in 32 of 36 hips (89%) after extracapsular base-of-neck osteotomies; avascular necrosis did not occur in any patient. They recommended this osteotomy as safe and effective in preventing further slipping and improving hip range of motion in patients with severe chronic slips; however, it does not affect limb length discrepancy. They noted that with severe slips the amount of correction of varus and posterior tilt of the femoral head is limited and complete restoration of a normal head-shaft angle may not be possible or necessary. Removal of a wedge larger than 20 mm compromises femoral neck length and may greatly increase femoral anteversion. Also, pinning across the osteotomy site becomes more difficult when correction of more than 55 degrees of varus or valgus is attempted. These same restrictions also are applicable to intracapsular base-of-neck

osteotomies and to the Southwick procedure (trochanteric osteotomy).

TECHNIQUE 33-34 *(Abraham et al.)*

Before surgery, the head-shaft angle is determined on lateral roentgenograms by measuring the angle formed by the epiphyseal line and the femoral shaft in the affected limb (Fig. 33-137) and comparing it to the contralateral side (or to 145 degrees). The head-shaft angle for posterior tilt or retroversion is determined on a frog-leg view and compared with the contralateral side (or to 10 degrees). The differences between the abnormal and normal angles are used to determine the size of the wedges removed during osteotomy.

Secure the anesthetized patient on a fracture table and maximally internally rotate the involved limb by gently moving the foot plate. Widely abduct the contralateral leg to make placement of fluoroscopic equipment easier. Obtain permanent anteroposterior and "shoot-through" lateral roentgenograms to confirm the chronicity of the slip and to better outline the femoral head. Prepare and drape the hip and patellar areas appropriately. Make a standard anterolateral approach and place a Charnley retractor deep to the iliotibial band. Locate the anterior joint tissue or intertrochanteric line between the gluteus medius and the vastus lateralis muscles. With a periosteal elevator, carefully elevate the anterior iliofemoral ligament. Place a narrow-tipped Hohmann retractor around the femoral neck superiorly and deep to the ischiofemoral ligament. Place another retractor deep to the iliofemoral ligament proximal to the lesser trochanter.

Delineate a triangle on the anterior surface of the femoral neck to indicate the two-plane wedge osteotomy. Locate the proximal cut by placing a 3-cm-long Kirschner wire on the anterior surface of the femur from the lesser to the greater trochanter at the base of the neck along the edge of

continued

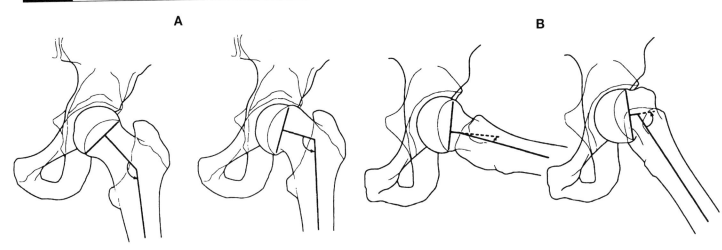

Fig. 33-137   Extracapsular base-of-neck osteotomy: measurement of head-shaft angles on roentgenogram. **A,** Normal anteroposterior angle compared with slipped capital femoral epiphysis. **B,** Normal lateral angle compared with slipped capital femoral epiphysis. (From Abraham E, Garst J, Barmada R: *J Pediatr Orthop* 13:294, 1993.)

the capsule (Fig. 33-138, *A*). Confirm this position by fluoroscopy. Use a wide osteotome to mark the bone along the wire. Externally rotate the leg and drill a second Kirschner wire in the anteroposterior plane just distal to the guide wire (Fig. 33-138, *B*). Place this wire vertical to the anterior surface of the femoral neck. Rotate the limb internally and obtain a lateral fluoroscopic view to confirm correct wire placement.

Begin the second distal osteotomy line from the lesser trochanter to the growth plate of the greater trochanter. The angle at which this line is made from the first osteotomy line depends on the amount of correction needed. Usually, a 15-mm-wide wedge, measured superiorly, to the baseline of the triangle is needed. Make the osteotomy cuts with a saw, converging them posteriorly to make a single osteotomy along the posterior cortex. Completely remove the wedge of bone, especially superiorly, for maximal correction (Fig. 33-138, *C*). While maintaining traction to prevent proximal migration of the femur, internally rotate the leg until the wedge closes completely. Abducting the leg also helps to close the osteotomy. When the patella can be internally rotated 15 degrees, adequate correction has been achieved. Remove additional bone from the metaphyseal side if necessary, but remove a maximum of 20 mm in the bony wedge. Fix the osteotomy with three or four cannulated screws (Fig. 33-138, *D*). Use the first guide wire to temporarily hold the osteotomy in the desired position. Use only one screw to span the physis of the femoral head, avoiding the superolateral quadrant. Check alignment and screw placement on permanent roentgenograms before closing the wound. Usually the iliofemoral ligament and capsule are not reattached, but if they are excessively elevated from the bone, suture or staple them back to the

anterior femur to preserve anterior joint stability. Close the wound in routine fashion and apply a sterile dressing.

AFTERTREATMENT. Partial weight-bearing with crutches is allowed for 6 to 8 weeks, and then full weight-bearing is allowed. Weight-bearing as tolerated is permitted after bilateral osteotomies.

Intertrochanteric Osteotomy. When a capital femoral epiphysis has chronically slipped and has united in a poor position, a trochanteric osteotomy to produce an opposite deformity may be indicated. Although our rate of chondrolysis has been nearly the same after trochanteric osteotomy as after closing wedge osteotomy of the femoral neck, the rate of avascular necrosis has been sufficiently lower to justify its use. If a trochanteric osteotomy is used for a chronic slip, the physis will still be open, and it should be fixed with pins or screws either before or at the time of osteotomy. This is imperative if a hip compression screw is to be used for fixation because further displacement of the femoral epiphysis can occur during screw insertion.

To correct a deformity consisting mainly of coxa vara but with some external rotation and hyperextension, a closing wedge trochanteric osteotomy is sufficient. The base of the wedge removed laterally should be wide enough to correct the coxa vara. The deformity also can be corrected by an opening wedge osteotomy based medially and wide enough to correct the coxa vara.

Correcting a deformity consisting of coxa vara, hyperextension, and moderate or severe external rotation is more difficult. This triple deformity may be corrected by a ball-and-socket osteotomy made at the level of the lesser trochanter following the guidelines of a biplane wedge osteotomy as origi-

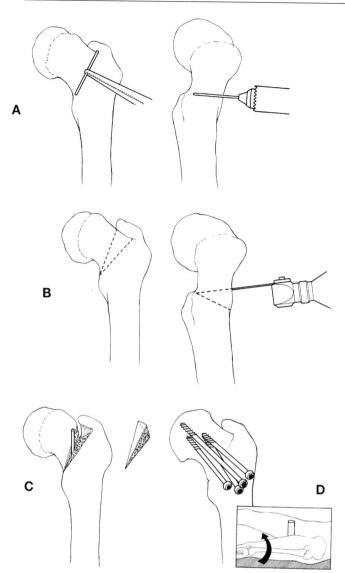

Fig. 33-138   Extracapsular base-of-neck osteotomy (see text). **A,** Determination of proximal osteotomy cut. **B,** Osteotomy cuts. **C,** Removal of bony wedge. **D,** Fixation with cannulated screws. (Redrawn from Abraham E, Garst J, Barmada R: *J Pediatr Orthop* 13:294, 1993.)

nally described by Southwick and made at the same level (Fig. 33-139). A ball-and-socket osteotomy in which the proximal fragment is concave and the distal fragment is convex can be made at the level of the lesser trochanter. It permits correction of the three components of the deformity: hyperextension, coxa vara, and external rotation. With careful planning a compression hip screw with side plate or a blade plate can be bent to the proper angle before surgery and used for fixation. The biplane osteotomy, which corrects varus and hyperextension, also dynamically corrects the third deformity, external rotation. This operation is better technically than the ball-and-socket osteotomy but is more difficult to perform, and we have had difficulty procuring both right and left plates at different angles.

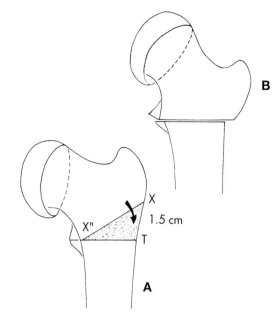

Fig. 33-139   **A,** After transverse line has been scribed on anterior and lateral surfaces of bone at level of lesser trochanter, junction of lateral and anterior surface is identified and marked as orientation mark (*X-T*). Usual size of wedge to be removed is indicated 1.5 cm along anterolateral orientation mark. **B,** Position as seen in postoperative anteroposterior roentgenogram. (Redrawn from Clark CR, Southwick WO, Ogden JA: *Instr Course Lect* 29:90, 1980.)

◆ *Ball-and-Socket Trochanteric Osteotomy*

TECHNIQUE 33-35
Plan carefully before surgery. Make tracings of anteroposterior and lateral roentgenograms and measure them accurately to determine exactly the severity of the deformity. With paper cutouts determine the position in which the fragments should be fixed.

Through a lateral approach (Chapter 1) expose the trochanteric region and the proximal 7.5 to 10 cm of the femoral shaft. Insert a guide pin transversely through the femur at the level of the lesser trochanter and verify its position by roentgenograms. Now with an osteotome make reference marks on the trochanter and the proximal shaft to be used in determining how much to rotate, flex, and abduct the distal fragment at the time of internal fixation. At the level of the lesser trochanter outline on the bone an osteotomy convex proximally. Along this outline make multiple holes in the cortices with a drill and complete the osteotomy with an osteotome directed proximally. Now the distal fragment is convex and the proximal fragment is concave. Next abduct, flex, and internally rotate the distal fragment appropriately as determined before surgery and fix the fragments with a blade plate or compression hip screw as in a trochanteric fracture.

AFTERTREATMENT. Whether a spica cast is applied depends on the firmness of fixation. Usually a cast is unnecessary. The care after surgery usually is about the same as that outlined for basilar osteotomy of the femoral neck (p. 1498).

Cheilectomy

When a prominence on the anterosuperior aspect of the femoral neck blocks internal rotation or abduction by impinging against the acetabulum, it is resected, as described by Heyman in 1949 and by Herndon in 1972.

Simple resection of the prominence removes the obstruction and improves motion. This procedure was first described by Whitman in 1909 according to Heyman. When the coxa vara and external rotational deformity are not severe, this operation alone may be sufficient. When the deformity is severe, resection of the prominence is combined with trochanteric osteotomy. The procedure is similar to that of cheilectomy as described by Garceau for femoral head deformity caused by Perthes disease. Herndon recommended removing the prominence and, if the epiphysis is still open, carrying out a capital femoral epiphysiodesis. Removal of the entire prominence may involve the removal of considerably more bone than was anticipated from examination of roentgenograms before surgery. Care should be taken to preserve the integrity of the neck of the femur and the physis, since fractures of the neck of the femur and further acute slipping of the epiphysis may occur when too much is excised. Intraarticular epiphysiodesis using bone from the crest of the ilium was recommended by Herndon.

COMPLICATIONS OF SLIPPED CAPITAL FEMORAL EPIPHYSIS

Avascular Necrosis

Avascular necrosis has been reported to occur in 10% to 15% of patients with SCFE, although more recent reports of in situ pinning with cannulated screws generally report lower incidences (0% to 5%). Avascular necrosis is rare in untreated patients and probably results from interruption of the retrograde blood supply by the original injury and appears more common in unstable (acute) slips, by forceful repetitive manipulations, by open reduction, or by osteotomy of the femoral neck. Ingram et al. found avascular necrosis more common with moderate and severe displacement and after femoral neck osteotomy (33%), open reduction and pinning (27%), and closed reduction with Knowles pinning (27%). It was less common with mild displacement and after in situ fixation (1.5%) and trochanteric osteotomy (10%). Of 22 patients in the series who had no surgical treatment, chondrolysis developed in 5 and avascular necrosis developed in 2. However, 2 of these patients had a manipulative reduction and a spica cast.

Although tamponade of the blood supply to the proximal femoral epiphysis as a result of acute hemorrhage within the capsule of the hip has been suggested as a cause of avascular necrosis, no evidence has indicated that immediate aspiration of the hip joint is effective in preventing avascular necrosis. Superolateral placement of pins also has been associated with the development of avascular necrosis, or at least with exacerbation of the process.

Both Herman et al. and Loder et al. suggested that instability may be the best predictor of avascular necrosis after acute slips. In the series of Loder et al., avascular necrosis occurred in 9 (47%) of 19 acute, unstable slips and in 3 of 9 such slips in the series of Herman et al.

We identified 36 patients in whom avascular necrosis developed after treatment of SCFE. Of 22 patients (24 hips) who were evaluated at an average of 31 years after treatment, 9 have undergone reconstructive surgery—4 during adolescence and 5 during adulthood. The remaining 13 patients (15 hips) have had no further operations, but all show degenerative changes on current roentgenograms. The natural history appears to be that of gradual degenerative changes for which reconstructive surgery most often can be delayed until adulthood.

Treatment guidelines for avascular necrosis after SCFE are essentially the same as for treatment of avascular necrosis after hip fracture (p. 1471).

Chondrolysis

The diagnosis of chondrolysis requires a joint space less than 3 mm wide (normal, 4 to 6 mm) and a decreased range of motion of the hip joint. Of the 79 patients in whom chondrolysis developed in the series of Ingram et al, it was present in 12 at first examination. It occurred more often in blacks and in females than in whites and males. However, in their review of 44 hips in black children treated for SCFE, Spero et al. reported a 6.8% incidence of chondrolysis and a 4.5% incidence of avascular necrosis, which are not significantly different from the incidences of these complications in white children. Obesity, which was more common in black children than in white children, did correlate with the frequency of bilateral disease (52%). These findings were similar to those of Kennedy and Weiner, who concluded that black children with SCFE do not have poorer outcomes than white children. Aronson and Loder also reported chondrolysis in only 3 of 97 black children in whom a single cannulated screw was used for fixation.

Pin penetration into the joint has been the most frequently cited cause of chondrolysis. Walters and Simon reported a high incidence of chondrolysis after pin penetration into the joint, but Bennet et al., using computer techniques, noted that, although pin penetration frequently occurs, it does not substantially influence the development of chondrolysis. Sternlicht et al. used a rabbit model to study the role of pin protrusion in the etiology of chondrolysis. They found that after pin protrusion the loss of proteoglycans in the articular cartilage averaged approximately 30% and matched the increase in neutral protease activity. This would seem to account for the loss of height that occurs with chondrolysis, but in their study the joint space did not narrow; rather, it increased. This suggests that some other factor is necessary to produce chondrolysis, such as a slip or an immune response.

In the series of Ingram et al., the incidence of chondrolysis

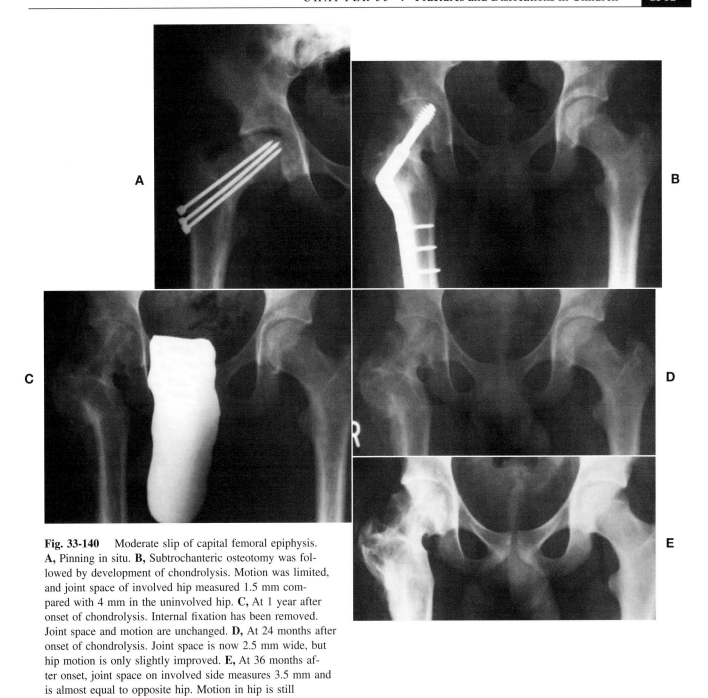

Fig. 33-140   Moderate slip of capital femoral epiphysis. **A,** Pinning in situ. **B,** Subtrochanteric osteotomy was followed by development of chondrolysis. Motion was limited, and joint space of involved hip measured 1.5 mm compared with 4 mm in the uninvolved hip. **C,** At 1 year after onset of chondrolysis. Internal fixation has been removed. Joint space and motion are unchanged. **D,** At 24 months after onset of chondrolysis. Joint space is now 2.5 mm wide, but hip motion is only slightly improved. **E,** At 36 months after onset, joint space on involved side measures 3.5 mm and is almost equal to opposite hip. Motion in hip is still decreased.

was lower in acute slips (11%) than in chronic or acute-on-chronic slips (31%). Chondrolysis occurred after trochanteric osteotomy (59%), open reduction (55%), and femoral neck osteotomy (37%), but it occurred also after closed reduction and in situ fixation (13%). When pins protruded through the femoral head into the joint postoperatively, 51% developed chondrolysis. Chondrolysis was present before any treatment in 12% of the patients and thus cannot be considered as a complication exclusively of surgical treatment (Fig. 33-140). When chondrolysis appeared, it usually was diagnosed within the first 6 to 9 months of observation and almost always within

the first year. The joint space was rapidly lost, usually reaching its worst state within 6 to 9 months when severely limited hip motion usually became apparent. Subsequently the width of the joint space usually increased slowly and hip motion increased slightly. Most patients ultimately achieved a joint space 4 mm or more in width. Arthritic spurring of both the femoral head and the acetabulum had occurred by the time this point was reached. The time required for these changes to develop was long, varying from 18 months to 4 years after onset.

Mandell et al. reported that evidence of marked periarticular uptake and premature fusion of the greater trochanteric physis (as indicated by decreased activity) on bone scintigraphy are reliable indicators of chondrolysis. These changes preceded roentgenographic evidence of chondrolysis in five patients.

Although fibrous ankylosis of the hip joint often occurs after chondrolysis, spontaneous partial cartilage recovery has been reported. Vrettos and Hoffman reported partial reconstitution of the joint space (average, 2.6 mm) in 14 hips with chondrolysis after SCFE; 64% of patients had good functional results at an average 13-year follow-up. However, Carney et al. reported continued deterioration in hip function at an average follow-up of 41 years.

Bed rest, traction, salicylates, phenylbutazone, steroids, and physical therapy have not modified the course of chondrolysis. We have had some success with intraarticular cortisone injection and surgical manipulation, followed by a vigorous in-hospital exercise program. Crawford recommended subtotal circumferential capsulectomy, operative manipulation, and postoperative continued passive motion with bupivacaine analgesia for joints unresponsive to traction and physical therapy. If severe joint space narrowing persists with limitation of joint motion, arthrodesis or arthroplasty should be considered.

Femoral Neck Fracture

Femoral fractures have been infrequently reported as a complication of in situ fixation of SCFE, although subtrochanteric fractures have been reported by several authors. Cameron et al. reported five subtrochanteric fractures at an average of 2.5 months after 164 pinnings with a variety of devices. All were caused by significant trauma, usually a fall, all were transverse fractures, and all were related to a "low" entry point of the device through the lateral cortex. Schmidt and Gregg collected reports of 10 subtrochanteric fractures after fixation of SCFE with multiple pins. Five of the 10 fractures occurred through unused drill holes. Greenough et al. reported three subtrochanteric fractures in their series of 83 hips: one 13 days after surgery and two 26 and 29 days after nail removal. Of 308 hips fixed with multiple pins, Riley et al. reported one subtrochanteric fracture (0.3%) at a screw-bone interface. Of 58 hips with single screw fixation, Aronson and Carlson found one subtrochanteric fracture (1.7%) in an overweight patient who fell 7 months after screw removal; the fracture was not through an area of screw fixation. We have described four patients with subtrochanteric fractures through unused drill holes below screw fixation (Fig. 33-141). After trying various methods of treatment for the subtrochanteric fracture, we now recommend immediate open reduction of the fracture and internal fixation with a hip screw and a long sideplate while maintaining the reduction of SCFE.

Femoral neck fracture after in situ pinning of SCFE is even less common. Baynham et al. reported two such fractures at 2 and 6 months after surgery and suggested that thermal injury caused by reaming of the femoral neck before screw insertion was a causative factor. Koval et al. reported a suspected stress fracture of the femoral neck 7 months after pinning in a patient in whom no extraneous drill holes were made and no reaming

of the proximal end of the femur was done before insertion of the screw. None of these three femoral neck fractures was displaced and none occurred through a bone-screw interface. Koval et al. successfully treated the stress fracture with spica casting. Baynham et al. reported healing of one femoral neck fracture with weight relief alone; the other required a vascularized pedicle bone graft.

We have described and treated two patients with displaced femoral neck fractures after in situ fixation of SCFE. In both, treatment of the femoral neck fractures was difficult, and results were less than satisfactory. One fracture was anatomically reduced after removal of the original fixation; two cannulated screws and a Knowles pin were placed anteriorly in the femoral neck across the fracture. The other fracture was reduced by internally rotating the extremity through the fracture site; two cannulated screws were placed through the medullary canal of the femoral neck without penetrating the joint anteriorly. The rotation of the extremity through the fracture site acted much like a compensatory osteotomy, placing the hip more anterior relative to the femoral neck and allowing internal fixation to be placed more laterally. One patient developed avascular necrosis, which was not surprising given the high incidence of avascular necrosis after femoral neck fractures in children and the additional risk associated with a posteriorly displaced and already compromised femoral head secondary to SCFE, which has an overall avascular necrosis rate of 13%. The same patient also developed chondrolysis. The other patient had a less than satisfactory reduction and delayed union that required prolonged spica cast immobilization. It is possible that the inadvertent rotation through the fracture site resulted in an inadequate reduction that contributed to the development of nonunion.

As more reports are accumulated, femoral fractures after in situ fixation of SCFE may be found to be more frequent than currently appreciated. The likelihood of this complication can perhaps be decreased by avoiding drilling unnecessary holes in the bone during surgery and by avoiding overzealous reaming of the femoral neck. Because fractures can occur just distal to the pins through the femoral neck, pins probably should be removed after the physis has fused, at least 1 year after insertion. However, Crandall et al. reviewed their results after pin removal from 43 hips, including Knowles pins, Steinmann pins, Hagie pins, and cannulated steel pins. Bone overgrowth made pin extraction difficult in all types, and Steinmann and Knowles pins broke during removal. According to Lee et al., titanium devices caused a significant increase in problems with retrieval because of osteointegration (direct contact of bone with metal). Vresilovic et al. reported that cannulated steel pins with reverse cutting threads were easier to remove than Knowles, Steinmann, or Hagie pins and Vitallium screws. The authors of both these studies concluded that pin removal was not without costs and risks and that the question of whether a pin must be removed at the end of treatment remains unanswered. Because we have had so many complications after pin or screw removal, we currently are leaving pins and screws in place after treatment of SCFE.

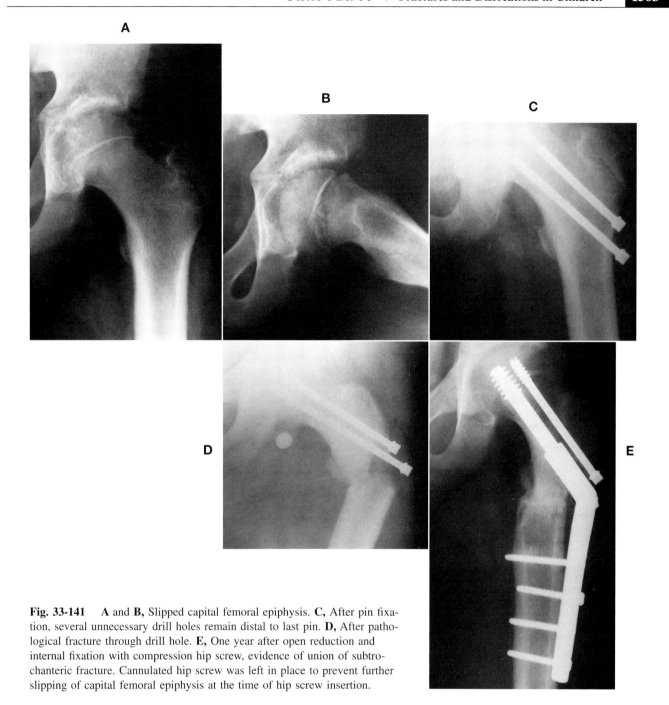

Fig. 33-141   **A** and **B,** Slipped capital femoral epiphysis. **C,** After pin fixation, several unnecessary drill holes remain distal to last pin. **D,** After pathological fracture through drill hole. **E,** One year after open reduction and internal fixation with compression hip screw, evidence of union of subtrochanteric fracture. Cannulated hip screw was left in place to prevent further slipping of capital femoral epiphysis at the time of hip screw insertion.

Continued Slipping

Continued slipping occurred in seven of our patients who refused treatment and in two treated by immobilization in spica casts. In two hips the epiphysis continued to slip because the Knowles pins were not placed far enough proximally or were removed before the physis had fused completely.

Femoral Fractures

Fractures of the femur usually are classified according to location as subtrochanteric; proximal, middle, and distal thirds

of the shaft; supracondylar, and distal femoral physeal. Fractures occur most commonly in the middle third. According to Hinton et al., the annual rate of femoral shaft fractures in children in Maryland between 1990 and 1996 was 19.15 per 100,000. With regard to age, the distribution was bimodal, with peaks at 2 and 17 years. Boys had higher rates of fracture than did girls at all ages, and blacks had higher rates than did whites. The primary mechanisms of fracture were age-dependent and included falls for children younger than 6 years old, motor vehicle–pedestrian accidents for those 6 to 9 years old, and motor vehicle accidents for teenagers. Firearm-related injuries accounted for 15% of the fractures among black adolescents.

Adverse socioeconomic conditions were significantly associated with higher rates of fracture.

Most femoral fractures in children are closed injuries and traditionally have been treated by closed methods. Management of pediatric femoral fractures as noted by Carey and Galpin has gradually evolved in the past decade toward operative approaches because of a desire for more rapid recovery and reintegration of the patients, with the recognition that prolonged immobilization can have negative effects even in children. Economic pressures also are factors in selecting operative treatment. External fixation, compression plating, and intramedullary nailing all have been advocated.

Besides the usual mechanisms of injury, femoral fractures can occur at birth, can be caused by child abuse, or can be pathological. Kasser noted that 30% of femoral fractures in children younger than 4 years of age are caused by child abuse. In children younger than 1 year of age, 70% of femoral fractures are abuse related. Abuse should be suspected if any of the following are present: (1) unreasonable history, (2) inappropriate delay in coming to the hospital, (3) previous history of abuse, (4) evidence of other fractures in various stages of healing, (5) multiple acute fractures, and (6) characteristic fracture patterns.

Quite often other serious injuries that require treatment also are present. If a child sustains enough trauma to fracture the largest bone in his body, he may have occult abdominal or other injuries. Examination of the ipsilateral knee is mandatory because of a 4% incidence of instability, as noted by Robertson et al.

FEMORAL SHAFT FRACTURES (OR DIAPHYSEAL FEMORAL FRACTURES)

In proximal shaft and subtrochanteric fractures, the proximal fragment usually is in a position of flexion, abduction, and external rotation because of the unopposed pull of the iliopsoas, abductor, and short external rotator muscles (Fig. 33-142). The adductors and extensors are intact in midshaft fractures, and the distal fragment usually is in satisfactory alignment except for some external rotation. In supracondylar fractures, the distal fragment is in a position of hyperextension because of the overpull of the gastrocnemius. The muscle imbalances are important when aligning the distal fragment to the proximal fragment in traction or a spica cast.

If alignment and length are maintained, mild malrotation usually corrects with growth. Strong et al. performed midshaft femoral osteotomies on 16 rabbits, internally rotated the limb, and applied external fixators until the osteotomies healed. They found that an average of 55% of rotational remodeling occurred spontaneously. The findings are similar to those of Schneider in canine studies. Both experimental studies support the clinical experience that few patients with mild malrotation of fractures of long bones have complaints as adults. Wallace and Hoffman reported an average 85% correction in 28 children who had angular deformities of 10 to 26 degrees after unilateral fractures of the middle third of the femoral shaft. Most of the correction

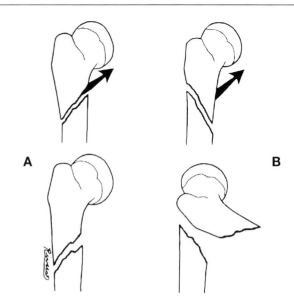

Fig. 33-142   Subtrochanteric fracture may be stable or unstable. **A,** If proximal spike of bone is posterior, often fracture is stable. **B,** Conversely, if proximal spike is anterior, often fracture is unstable and 90-90 traction is necessary. (Redrawn from Rang M: *Children's fractures,* Philadelphia, 1981, JB Lippincott.)

Table 33-4   General Treatment Guidelines in Children with Femoral Shaft Fractures

Age	Recommended Treatment
Birth to 6 years	Immediate spica casting
	Traction followed by spica casting
6 to 10 years	Traction followed by spica casting
	External fixation
	Fixation with flexible nonreamed intramedullary rods
11 years or older Children with multiple fractures or head injury	Locked intramedullary nailing

(74%) occurred at the physis; 26% occurred at the fracture. These authors concluded that in children younger than 13 years of age, malunion of as much as 25 degrees in any plane will remodel enough to give normal alignment of the joint surfaces.

Staheli defined the ideal treatment of femoral shaft fractures in children as one that controls alignment and length, does not compress or elevate the extremity excessively, is comfortable for the child and convenient for the family, and causes the least negative psychological impact possible. Determining the ideal treatment for each child depends on the age of the child, the location and type of fractures, the family environment, the knowledge and ability of the surgeon, and to a lesser degree financial considerations. Our general treatment recommendations (Table 33-4) are similar to those of Kasser.

Table 33-5   Cost of Treatment of Femoral Shaft Fractures

Series	Immediate (Early Spica)	Skeletal Traction Spica	IM Rod	External Fixation
Newton and Mubarak	$5494	$21,093	$21,359	
Clinkscales and Peterson	$5490	$16,273	$16,056	$16,394
Stans et al.	$5264	$15,980	$15,495	$14,478
Yandow et al.	$1867	$11,171		
Nork and Hoffinger		$22,396		$11,520
Coyte et al.	$5970			$ 7626
	(Canadian $)			(Canadian $)

The comparative economics of nonoperative and operative treatment have been evaluated by several authors. The charges or cost included both hospital and physician charges (orthopaedists, radiologists, and anesthesiologists). Table 33-5 gives the cost or charges in different series of patients. The differences seen in each series are not comparable because of many variables. However, on average, immediate or early spica casting (traction spica) cost less than prolonged traction with spica casting, intramedullary rods, or external fixation. Prolonged skeletal traction and spica casting, intramedullary rods, or external fixation were frequently the same in cost. The cost of reoperations for malrotation or removal of hardware was also similar for the three groups.

Immediate spica casting of femoral shaft fractures in children has been recommended by several authors, including Clement and Colton, Griffin et al., Irani et al., Neer and Cadman, Nork et al., and Staheli and Sheridan; best results with this method seem to be obtained in infants and young children. Illgen et al. reviewed 114 children who had early spica treatment and recommended it as treatment of choice in children younger than 6 years of age.

Hughes et al. reviewed 23 children treated with early spica casting to determine the effect of this treatment on family, school, and other support systems. They identified patient mobility as the most difficult problem, followed by toileting, hygiene, time off work for parents, and schooling. They suggested that spica cast treatment is easier for preschool children than for school-aged children, and they recommended counseling and careful planning before spica cast application.

The primary problems with immediate spica casting are shortening and angulation of the fracture in high-energy femoral shaft fractures. Pollak et al. reported shortening and angulation that required repeat reduction or other treatment in 12 (50%) of 23 closed, high-energy femoral shaft fractures in children younger than 10 years of age; only 2 (8%) of low-energy fractures required repeat closed reduction

Thompson et al. described early spica cast treatment in 100 children between the ages of 2 to 10 years for uncomplicated isolated closed femoral shaft fractures. Eighty-one (81%) of the children had an acceptable outcome, and 19 (19%) had an unacceptable outcome, with more than 25 mm of fracture fragment overlap after clinical healing. These authors described

a new clinical test, the telescope test, that had a sensitivity of 80% and a specificity of 85% for predicting outcome. The relative risk for failure of spica cast treatment with a positive telescope test was 20.4%. They recommended that children 2 to 10 years of age with uncomplicated femoral shaft fractures and a negative telescope test be treated appropriately in most cases with early application of a spica cast. Unfortunately, the test is difficult to administer without heavily sedating the child.

Czertak and Hennrikus recommended early spica casting in 90-90 position to avoid shortening and angulation. Twenty-three consecutive children younger than 6 years with a closed femoral shaft fracture stemming from low-energy trauma were treated with an early spica cast.

Stannard et al. used a Pavlik harness instead of a spica cast in 16 infants between birth and 18 months of age. They cited as advantages of using a Pavlik harness, ease of application without anesthesia, minimal hospitalization (less than 24 hours), easy reduction, ability to adjust the harness, minimal costs, and ease in diaper changing, nursing, and bonding. However, they advised careful consideration of parent reliability before choosing this method of treatment.

Aronson, Singer, and Higgins reported excellent results in 54 children with femoral fractures treated with 90-90 skeletal traction and spica casting. Their study showed that pins for skeletal traction should be placed parallel to the axis of the knee joint (Fig. 33-143) and that fractures in children older than 11 years should be reduced without overriding. The average time in traction of their patients was 24 days, and the hip-spica cast was worn an average of 58 days. In an effort to lower cost, Boman, Gardell, and Janarv recommended a home 90-90 skeletal traction program in preschool children. At long-term follow-up of 33 children treated with immediate spica casting or skeletal traction followed by spica casting, Hennrikus et al. found persistent deficits in strength of the quadriceps muscle as measured by Cybex II testing. The only etiological factor that correlated with this weakness was the amount of initial displacement of the fracture. Despite this weakness, no patient had clinical problems at follow-up.

Adolescents do not tolerate prolonged immobilization as well as younger children, and Humberger and Eyring reported high incidences of knee pain, angulation at the fracture, and difficulty in maintaining length when 90-90 traction

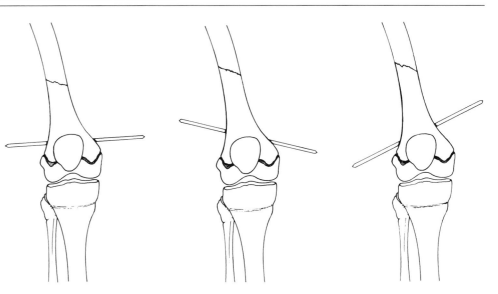

Fig. 33-143 Position of pin in traction is either horizontal (optimal) or oblique. Oblique pins are either "to varus" or "to valgus," reflecting resultant pull of traction bow. (Redrawn from Aronson DD, Singer RM, Higgins RF: *J Bone Joint Surg* 69A:1435, 1987.)

treatment was used in children older than 10 years. Kirby et al. and Ziv et al. also noted that prolonged traction and spica casting in adolescents frequently result in limb shortening and leg length discrepancy, malunion, pin track infection, loss of joint motion, and muscle atrophy.

At our institution, skeletal or skin traction is applied in children younger than 6 years of age, depending on the age of the child and the level of the fracture. Longitudinal traction or traction at a 45-degree angle with 4 to 10 pounds of weight is recommended. Overhead skin traction should not be used for femoral fractures in this age group because of the increased risk of neurovascular compromise. Neurovascular status and skin condition should be monitored carefully while the child is in traction. When length and alignment are achieved, a spica cast is applied. In children between the ages of 6 and 10 years, the age at which most femoral fractures occur, skeletal traction usually is appropriate, with the application of a spica cast after approximately 2 to 3 weeks of traction. Early, but not immediate, spica casting can be used for low-energy fractures with less than 2 to 3 cm of shortening. In older or larger children in whom skin traction may not be adequate, a 5/64-inch Steinmann pin can be inserted in the proximal tibia. If a tibial pin is used, it should be placed distal to the tibial tubercle and the proximal tibial physis to minimize the risk of growth disturbance and genu recurvatum deformity. A distal femoral traction pin rarely may be necessary for a distal supracondylar fractures because of skin problems or for 90-90 degree traction in a proximal femoral fracture with anterior displacement.

Peroneal nerve palsy is a rare complication of skin or skeletal traction and casting. Weiss et al. reported peroneal nerve palsies in 4 of 110 patients treated with 90-90 traction and casting, and two of our patients younger than 2 years of age developed peroneal nerve palsies after skin traction and spica casting. Spontaneous recovery occurs in most patients.

External fixation has been recommended for treatment of femoral shaft fractures in children. Evanoff, Strong, and

MacIntosh reported the use of external fixation until fracture consolidation in 25 femoral fractures and 21 tibial fractures in skeletally immature patients, most of whom had multiple fractures or head injuries. All fractures consolidated with the fixators in place, and most patients regained preoperative joint motion. Eighty-four percent of fractures lost no position in the fixator; the remaining 16% lost fewer than 5 degrees. These authors recommended external fixation of all femoral fractures in children between the ages of 3 and 13 years. Sola et al. recommended an auxiliary pin when using an Orthofix monolateral fixator to enhance stability and to avoid having to remanipulate the fracture after loss of reduction. Four of 22 femurs without an auxiliary pin went on to malunion. No femur with an auxiliary pin had malunion.

Blasier, Aronson, and Tursky used primary external fixation with early weight-bearing for 139 femoral fractures in children. The fixators were left in place an average of 11.4 weeks. Of those examined at 2-year follow-up, 15 of 18 had an average of 8.7 mm overgrowth, and 3 had an average shortening of 7.7 mm. Refracture rate was 1.4%, and although pin tract infection requiring antibiotic treatment developed in 6, osteomyelitis did not develop in any of the patients. These authors recommended external fixation using a monolateral fixator with four half-pins that are predrilled and hand screwed laterally into the bone as an alternative to casting for the treatment of isolated femoral fractures in children ages 4 to 12 years.

Probe et al. reported refractures after frame removal in two adolescent patients treated with external fixation. They suggested that refracture is a clinical expression of the detrimental effects of prolonged rigidity imposed by the external fixator. Skaggs et al. noted secondary fractures in 12% of their patients. Five fractures occurred at the original fracture site and one through a pin site. They noted a statistically significant association between the number of cortices demonstrating bridging callus (on both anteroposterior and lateral views) at the time of fixator removal and the rate of refracture.

A   B   C   D

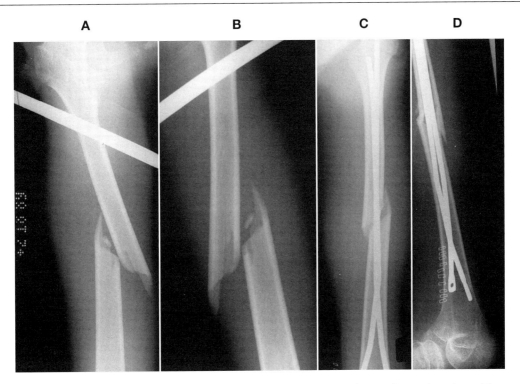

Fig. 33-144   **A** and **B,** Angulated femoral shaft fracture in 9-year-old, severely spastic patient with extreme flexion contracture. **C** and **D,** After percutaneous fixation with medullary Enders pins avoiding proximal and distal physes.

Fractures showing fewer than three cortices of bridging callus had a 33% refracture rate, whereas fractures with three or four cortices of bridging callus had a 4% rate of refracture.

Gregory, Pevny, and Teague in a retrospective study of 27 pediatric patients identified 8 major complications (30%) in 6 patients and 29 minor complications (107%) in 20 patients. The major complications included 2 refractures, 2 fractures through pin sites, 1 postimmobilization supracondylar femoral fracture, 1 persistent pin track infection requiring early pin removal, 1 malreduction, and 1 loss of reduction. Of the patients with minor complications, 14 had pin track infections requiring oral antibiotics, 5 refused to go to school with a fixator in place, 5 were dissatisfied with scar appearance, and 5 had clinically insignificant malunions. These authors recommended that if external fixation is chosen as the method of treatment for pediatric femoral fractures, careful attention must be paid to operative technique and postoperative treatment to minimize complications.

Occasionally, in a young child with polytrauma, open fracture, or severe head injury, a small fragment external fixator with 4-mm pins can be used. The technique of external fixation of fractures of the femur is described in Chapter 51.

Early good results using flexible (Ender) or elastic stable (Nancy) intramedullary rods have been reported by several European authors and by Heinrich et al., Fein et al., Kissel and Miller, and Mann et al. in the United States. Mann et al. successfully used Ender nailing in 16 patients with an average age of 12 years, 7 months (Fig. 33-144). Heinrich et al., in a

prospective study of 78 femoral fractures in 77 children aged 2¾ years to 18 years, noted at follow-up mild varus or valgus angulation (11%) and mild anterior or posterior malalignment (8%) after fixation with flexible intramedullary nails. However, 68 of the children had equal leg lengths at follow-up, and 8 had minimal rotational malalignment of an average 8 degrees. They reported that stabilization of selected pediatric diaphyseal fractures with flexible intramedullary nails obtained results comparable to nonoperative treatment but with less disruption of family life and shorter hospitalization. Ligier et al. reported the use of elastic stable intramedullary nails (ESIN) in 123 fractures of the femoral shaft in patients ranging from 5 to 16 years of age; all fractures united and no patient complained of disability or had gait abnormalities at follow-up. Most reports recommend this technique for children ages 6 to 10 years in whom traction or external fixation has not been selected as an option and in whom both the proximal and distal femoral physes need to be avoided. Bar On et al., in a prospective study comparing external fixation with flexible intramedullary nailing in children, noted that flexible intramedullary nailing had fewer complications, and the parents were more satisfied. They recommended the use of flexible intramedullary nailing for fractures of the femoral shaft that require surgery and reserve external fixation for open or severely comminuted fractures.

Rigid intramedullary fixation of femoral shaft fractures in adolescents has been reported to result in high rates of union with short hospital stays and brief periods of immobilization (Fig. 33-145). Kirby et al. reported excellent results with

A   B   C   D

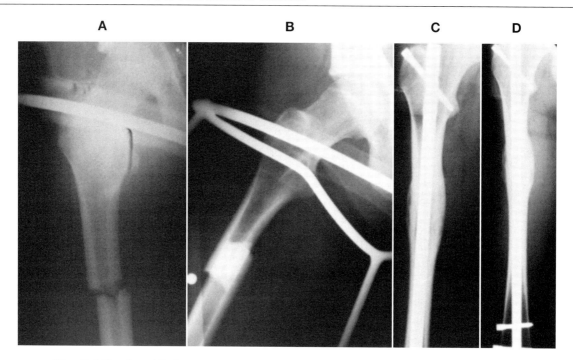

Fig. 33-145   **A** and **B,** Fracture of proximal third of femur in 14-year-old boy. **C** and **D,** After closed medullary nailing with proximal and distal interlocking screws.

Küntscher nailing of 13 fractures in patients with an average age of 12 years, 7 months. Reeves et al. compared the results of traction and subsequent casting with rigid fixation in a large series of adolescent femoral shaft fractures. The traction and casting group had a mean hospital stay of 26 days. The operative group had a mean hospital stay of 9 days and had fewer complications than the nonoperative group. They concluded that intramedullary rodding and shorter hospitalization have psychological, social, educational, and some economic advantages over conservative treatment.

Herndon et al. compared nonoperative treatment with intramedullary nailing in 45 femoral fractures and found the incidence of malunion was significantly decreased in the fractures treated operatively. They used Küntscher nails, Ender nails, Rush rods, and interlocking nails, and although they did not recommend one device over another, they used interlocking nails for comminuted fractures and Ender nails for younger patients. They now use closed intramedullary nailing for almost all femoral shaft fractures in patients older than 10 years. Buford et al. studied 60 adolescents (average age, 12 years) with femoral fractures treated with intramedullary nailing. MRI scans were obtained to evaluate subclinical avascular necrosis of the femoral head. All patients had open physes at the time of surgery. Implants were removed in 33 patients at an average of 10 months after nailing. Two patients had subclinical avascular necrosis as seen on MRI. In one, avascular necrosis developed in both femoral heads 1 year after nail removal. The second patient had asymptomatic marrow changes on MRI consistent with avascular necrosis with no femoral head collapse. These authors concluded that intramedullary nailing of pediatric

femoral fractures is a safe treatment option. Momberger et al. concurred with these findings. In a study of 50 femoral shaft fractures treated with reamed, interlocking, intramedullary nailing, no patient developed osseous necrosis of the femoral head or significant proximal deformity. Their surgical technique included a starting point on the medial greater trochanter avoiding the piriformis fossa. They used overreaming a guide pin under fluoroscopy rather than an awl. No attempt was made to spare the trochanteric apophysis from reaming. All nails, which averaged 9 mm, were statically locked. Despite intramedullary nailing through the greater trochanteric apophysis, articulotrochanteric distance measurements increased only 4.5 mm at their latest follow-up.

In a review of our results of intramedullary nailing of 31 femoral fractures in 30 adolescents ranging in age from 10 to 15 years (average, 12.3 years), we found that all 31 fractures united without evidence of trochanteric overgrowth or coxa valga deformity. Two patients had bony overgrowth of more than 2 cm (2.5 cm and 2.8 cm). Other complications included one superficial distal wound infection that resolved after intravenous antibiotic therapy, decreased sensation in the distribution of the deep peroneal nerve in one patient and in the distribution of the pudendal nerve in another; both neurological problems resolved spontaneously. Mild heterotopic ossification over the nail proximally was found in three patients. Asymptomatic segmental avascular necrosis developed in one patient and was not visible on roentgenograms until 15 months after fracture. The cause may have been the initial injury, an unrecognized hip injury, injury to the blood supply of the femoral head and neck during nail insertion, or dissection

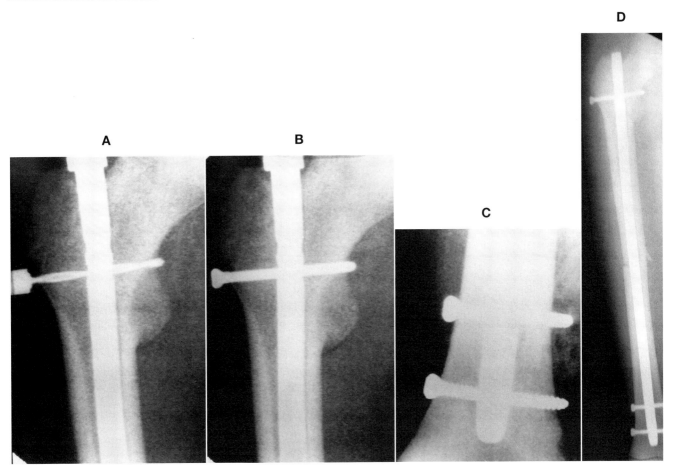

Fig. 33-146 Pediatric intramedullary nail. **A,** Drill bit across femur and nail. **B,** Screw in place. **C,** More distal holes for transverse fixation to avoid physis and produce better fixation more distally. **D,** Eight-mm pediatric nail in place.

during nail removal. All nails were removed at an average of 14 months after injury; no refractures or femoral neck fractures occurred after nail removal. Because of the few complications and high rate of union in our patients, we believe intramedullary nailing is a reasonable choice for the treatment of femoral shaft fractures in older adolescents (12 to 16 years of age) and in patients from 10 to 16 years of age with multiple trauma or head injuries.

The length and diameter of the intramedullary nail may somewhat limit the use of this technique, but the development of a smaller (8 to 9 mm diameter) pediatric nail expands its application. This pediatric nail also has a transverse proximal interlocking screw that avoids the greater trochanter and more-distal screw holes in the nail to avoid the physis (Fig. 33-146). Delta femoral nails (10 or 11 mm) or standard femoral nails (12 mm) also can be used in older adolescents with wider medullary canals.

The technique of locked intramedullary nailing of the femur is described in Chapter 51. To lower the risk of avascular necrosis, it is important to limit dissection to the tip of the greater trochanter, without extending to the capsule or the midportion of the femoral neck. Dissection should be limited to the lateral aspect of the greater trochanter and not into the piriformis fossa. This prevents dissection near the origin of the lateral ascending cervical artery, which is medial to the piriformis fossa. The proximal end of the nail should be left long (up to 1 cm) to make later removal easier. Nails can be removed 9 to 18 months after roentgenographic union to prevent bony overgrowth over the proximal tip of the nail.

◆ Flexible Intramedullary Rod Fixation

Most femoral shaft fractures in children can be stabilized using retrograde fixation. Three points of fixation, established around the fracture or the medullary canal, must be "stacked" with multiple nails at the fracture to prevent angulation. Usually, medial and lateral insertion sites are used, but a single insertion site, either medial or lateral, can be used in the distal femoral metaphysis. Two divergent C-configuration nails or one C- and one S-configuration nail (bent by the surgeon at a point approximately 5 cm distal to the eyelet) are routine; additional nails can be added if necessary. Special expertise is needed to stabilize subtrochanteric fractures and fractures of the distal third of the femur; antegrade insertion commonly is used for the latter.

TECHNIQUE 33-36 *(Heinrich et al.)*

Retrograde Fixation. Use longitudinal traction, preferably on a fracture table. Apply a sterile tourniquet to the leg at approximately 100 mg Hg above the systolic blood pressure. Identify the physis by fluoroscopy and mark its location on the skin. Make a 5- to 6-cm medial incision, extending proximally from a point 1.5 cm distal to the physis. Incise the soft tissue and fascia overlying the vastus medialis muscle and anteriorly reflect the muscle by blunt dissection, leaving the femoral periosteum intact. Through a similar lateral approach, cut the iliotibial band in line with its fibers. Reflect the vastus lateralis muscle anteriorly, leaving the periosteum intact on the lateral aspect of the distal femur. Use a 4-mm to 4.5-mm drill bit with a tissue protector to make a hole in the cortex on the medial and lateral distal femoral metaphysis at a point approximately 3 cm proximal to the physis. Tilt the drill in a cephalad direction to prepare a tract for the nail after the entry portal has been made. Lay one of the selected nails over the thigh and determine that it is of the appropriate length by fluoroscopy. The nail should extend from the level of the distal femoral physis to a point approximately 2 cm distal to the capital femoral physis and 1 cm distal to the greater trochanteric physis. At a point 1.5 cm from the blunt end, bend the tip of the nail approximately 25 degrees so that it will "bounce" off the cortical bone on the inside of the medullary canal. Rotate the nail through an arc of approximately 30 degrees while the tip is in contact with the opposite cortex to prevent it from becoming imbedded. After it bounces off the opposite cortex, drive the nail to the fracture with fluoroscopic guidance. Manipulate the thigh and pass the nail across the fracture. Insert a second rod into the medullary canal from the opposite side of the distal femur and drive it across the fracture and then drive both nails into their final positions. The eyelet of the nail should rest several millimeters proximal to the distal femoral physis. Bend the eyelet away from the bone (10 to 15 degrees) to make nail removal easier.

If an additional nail is needed on the same side as the first nail, make an entry portal anterior or posterior to the first portal. Drive another nail into place, taking care not to twist it around the first nail as it is rotated to the opposite cortex and passes across the fracture. Be careful to prevent distraction while the nails are driven into place. Release longitudinal traction after the nails cross the fracture and use manual compression if necessary to prevent distraction. Check fracture alignment and nail position by fluoroscopy. Release the tourniquet, obtain hemostasis, and close the wound in layers.

Antegrade Fixation. Make an approximately 5-cm longitudinal incision at the metaphyseal-diaphyseal junction just below the greater trochanter. Cut the subcutaneous tissue and the iliotibial band in line with the skin incision. Split the vastus lateralis muscle in line with its fibers to expose the lateral cortex of the proximal femur. Drill a 4- to 4.5-mm hole in the cortex at the metaphyseal-diaphyseal junction. Insert an S-configured nail into the medullary canal and drive it across the fracture. Drill a second 4- to 4.5-mm hole adjacent to the first, insert a C-configured nail into the medullary canal, and drive it across the fracture. Starting with the S-shaped nail, drive both nails into their final positions.

AFTERTREATMENT. Children with stable fractures and whose parents are compliant may be kept non-weight-bearing without external support for approximately 2 weeks, during which an exercise program for the hip and knee is begun. Weight-bearing is begun at 2 weeks after the fracture is stabilized. Children with comminuted fractures or noncompliant parents are immobilized in a long leg cast and pelvic band. The below-knee segment is removed at 1 week to allow knee motion. The remaining portion of the cast is removed 1 week later and weight-bearing is begun. Nails are removed after the fracture is united, usually at about 3 to 4 months for isolated femoral fractures.

◆ Nancy Nail (Stable Elastic Intramedullary Nail)

TECHNIQUE 33-37 *(Ligier et al.)*

Place the patient on an orthopaedic table and reduce the fracture partially by traction guided by fluoroscopy (Fig. 33-147, *A* and *B*). Use blunt-ended nails of quality steel (cold-hammered at 140°) or titanium. The nails should be 45 cm long with diameters of 3, 3.5, or 4 mm, depending on the child's weight and age. Prepare the nails preoperatively by angling them at 45 degrees about 2 cm from one end to facilitate penetration of the medullary canal and also bend them into an even curve over their entire length. With the help of a T-handle and by rotation movements of the wrist, introduce the nails through a longitudinal drill hole, 4- to 5-mm in diameter, made in the distal femoral metaphysis just above the physis. Use two nails, one lateral and one medial, to stabilize the fracture. Carefully push both up the medullary canal to the already-reduced fracture site. After touching the opposite internal cortex, the nails bend themselves in the direction of the long bone's axis. The nails should cross distal to the fracture site (normally 4 to 6 cm distal) (Fig. 33-147, *C*). Rotate the T-handle or manipulate the limb to direct the pins into the opposite fragment. If the first is impeded, try the second with the aid of an image intensifier. Make sure both nails are in the canal across the fracture site. When they pass the fracture level, release traction, pushing the nails farther and fixing their tips in the

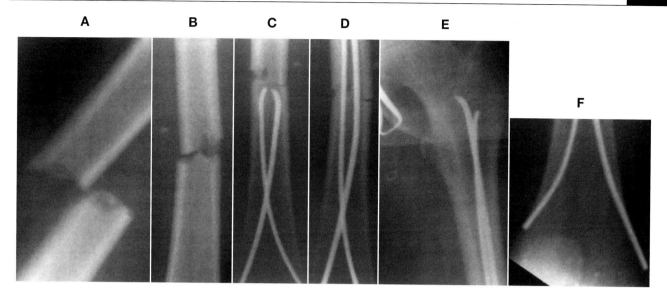

Fig. 33-147 Nancy nail technique. Roentgenograms of femoral fracture before **(A)** and after **(B)** reduction on fracture table. **C,** Both Nancy nails are placed (medial and lateral) to cross well below fracture site and stopped temporarily at fracture site for ease of passage. **D,** Both nails are driven past fracture site by manipulating distal fragment, hugging wall of intramedullary canal as necessary. **E,** Nails are then driven into greater trochanteric and cervical area. **F,** Distal portion of nails are left slightly protruding for ease of removal, but not too long to prevent knee motion.

spongy tissue of the metaphysis, without their passing through the physis (Fig. 33-147, *D*). Small distractions can be corrected by rotation of the pins. Avoid residual angulation by making sure that the nails are introduced at the same level so that they have identical curvatures (Fig. 33-147, *E*). Leave the distal portion of the nails slightly protruding for ease of removal (Fig. 33-147, *F*).

If the technique is performed correctly, the fracture is finally stabilized by two nails, each with three points of fixation. The fixation is elastic but sufficiently stable to allow automatic small position corrections by limited movements during the limb's loading.

AFTERTREATMENT. Postoperatively, the limb is rested on a pillow. A knee immobilizer may give more comfort. Mobilization using crutches without weight-bearing is allowed as soon as the fracture causes no pain. A spica cast can be used if rotation or angulation is evident after the procedure. At the beginning of the third week, partial weight-bearing is allowed. After the appearance of calcified external callus, full weight-bearing is allowed. Nails are removed at the beginning of the third postoperative month or whenever the surgeon is positive that healing has occurred. Antibiotics are not necessary after surgery unless infection or inflammation is present.

◆　◆　◆

Compression plating of femoral fractures in children and adolescents has been reported by Robertson et al., by Hansen, and by Ward et al. Hansen used AO compression plates for

fixation of 13 femoral shaft fractures in 12 children with an average age of 11 years. All fractures healed without angulation or rotation and with a mean overgrowth of 7 mm. All patients had unrestricted ranges of motion of the hip and knee. Ward et al. reported good fracture healing without leg length discrepancy after compression plating of femoral fractures in 25 children aged 6 to 16 years. They recommended compression plate fixation for patients with severe head injury or multiple trauma. Because of the possibility of plate failure, they used supplemental bone grafting in fractures with medial cortex comminution. Although rare, stress fracture may occur through the screw holes during the first few months after plate removal.

Complications

The most common complication after femoral shaft fractures in children is leg length discrepancy, usually resulting from "overgrowth" of the injured femur. The exact cause of this overgrowth is still not known, but it has been attributed to age, gender, fracture type, fracture level, handedness, and amount of overriding of the fracture fragments. Age seems to be the most constant factor, but fractures in the proximal third of the femur and oblique comminuted fractures also have been associated with relatively greater growth acceleration. According to Staheli, shortening is more likely in patients older than 10 years of age, and overgrowth is more likely in those between 2 and 10 years of age, especially if traction has been used.

Although some angular deformity occurs after femoral shaft fractures in children, it usually remodels with growth. The acceptable amount of angular deformity is controversial, but as a general guideline, angulation of more than 15 degrees in the coronal plane and 20 degrees in the sagittal plane is unacceptable. However, this varies according to the age of the child, and as much as 45 degrees of angulation in the sagittal plane may be acceptable in an infant. Genu recurvatum deformity of the proximal tibia has been reported after traction pin or wire placement through or near the anterior aspect of the proximal tibial physis, excessive traction, pin track infection, and prolonged cast immobilization. Occasionally a significant angular deformity requires corrective osteotomy, but this should be delayed at least a year unless function is impaired. Torsional deformities have been reported to occur in one third to two thirds of children with femoral shaft fractures; however, most of these are mild (less than 10 degrees) and asymptomatic and rarely require treatment.

Delayed union and nonunion of femoral shaft fractures are rare in children and occur most often after open fractures, fractures with segmental bone loss or soft tissue interposed between the fragments, and subtrochanteric fractures that have been poorly aligned in traction. Delayed union in a young child whose femoral fracture has been treated with casting probably should be treated by continuing cast immobilization until bridging callus forms. Rarely, bone grafting and internal fixation may be required for nonunion in an older child; an interlocking intramedullary nail usually is preferred for fixation in children older than 10 to 12 years of age.

FRACTURES OF DISTAL FEMORAL PHYSIS

Fractures of the distal femoral physis are not as common as physeal injuries elsewhere, accounting for only 7% of physeal injuries of the lower extremity. At this clinic, we see about seven or eight of these injuries each year. At the distal femur, Salter-Harris type II physeal fractures cause more severe physeal arrests than in other parts of the skeleton. Occult Salter-Harris type V compression fractures with premature closure of the physis also occur more frequently in this location.

Salter-Harris type I fractures of the distal femoral physis rarely need operative treatment. In past years many of these fractures were displaced anteriorly because they were caused by large "spoke wheels." Today these fractures are caused more often by motor vehicle accidents or by a varus or valgus force encountered in athletic activities, and many are

undisplaced (Fig. 33-148). Stress roentgenograms may be helpful in differentiating a tear of a collateral ligament from a type I epiphyseal separation. Salter-Harris type II fractures are most common and occur in older children. Displacement usually is in the coronal plane, although it can be in the anteroposterior plane. Physeal arrest is more frequent after this fracture than after type II fractures in other locations.

In an experimental study in rabbits, Mäkelä et al. found that destruction of as little as 7% of the cross-sectional area of the distal femoral physis caused permanent growth disturbance and shortening of the femur. According to Roberts, the portion of the physis beneath the metaphyseal fracture spike (Thurston-Holland sign) usually is spared. If the metaphyseal spike is medial, valgus deformity may occur because of lateral closure of the physis. If the spike is lateral, then varus angulation may follow.

Salter-Harris type III fractures rarely occur. The amount of displacement is important because joint incongruity results if anatomical alignment is not restored, and a bony bridge develops if the physis is not realigned exactly (Fig. 33-149, *A*). A Salter-Harris type IV fracture is even more uncommon. It likewise requires accurate reduction. The metaphyseal spike of bone that occurs with this type of fracture is worrisome because

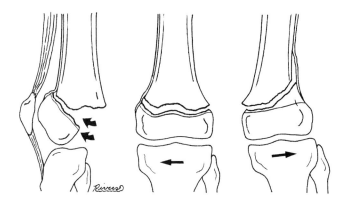

Fig. 33-148 Various angulations of distal femoral physeal fractures, including posterior angulation, varus angulation, and valgus angulation. (Redrawn from Ogden JA: *Skeletal injury in the child*, Philadelphia, 1982, Lea & Febiger.)

Fig. 33-149 **A,** Salter-Harris type III distal femoral physeal fracture that requires anatomical reduction. **B,** Various types of Salter-Harris III and IV fracture-separations, including unicondylar, bicondylar, and combination of types III and IV, which is triplane fracture. (Redrawn from Ogden JA: *Skeletal injury in the child*, Philadelphia, 1982, Lea & Febiger.)

A

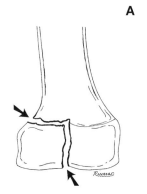

B

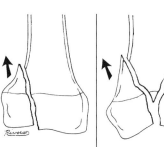
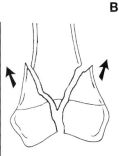
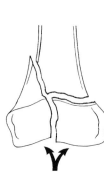

of the increased possibility of physeal arrest from bony bridge formation (Fig. 33-149, B).

Most type V fractures are either unrecognized or misdiagnosed as Salter-Harris type I fractures. When late premature physeal closure occurs, a retrospective diagnosis of a Salter-Harris type V compression injury is made. Hresko and Kasser reported physeal arrest in seven patients with "nonphyseal" fractures of the lower extremity in whom the physeal injury was not recognized until an average of 12 months after injury when gross angular deformities were present. Whether this is a true compression injury, with premature closure uniformly across the distal femoral physis, was questioned by Peterson and Burkhart, who speculated whether this uniform premature physeal closure could be caused by some other mechanism, such as prolonged immobilization or even some undiscovered mechanism.

Roberts and Rang, as well as others, have noted that an avulsion injury can occur at the edge of the physis, especially on the medial side. A small fragment, including a portion of the perichondrium and underlying bone, may be torn off the femur when the proximal attachment of a collateral ligament is avulsed. This uncommon injury, although assumed to be benign, can lead to localized premature physeal arrest. If physeal arrest from a bony bridge is located at the most peripheral edge of a physis, severe angular deformity can occur.

Surgery is often necessary in displaced types I and II and almost all types III and IV distal femoral physeal fractures. Displacement should be reduced by closed methods as perfectly as possible without excessive trauma to the physis. Repeated manipulations should be avoided. Stephens et al. postulated that repeated manipulations, especially of type II fractures, grind the distal portion of the proximal fragment of the metaphysis into the cartilage of the physis on the distal fragment and thus cause premature physeal closure.

Czitrom et al. concluded that the Salter-Harris classification is a good indicator of the mechanism of injury and the prognosis of distal femoral physeal injuries, noting that most types I and II fractures did well, with an average loss of length of 1 cm, which was of no clinical significance. They concluded that unsatisfactory results in type II physeal injuries were caused by inadequate reduction or associated injuries. Lombardo and Harvey, however, reported unsatisfactory results in type II fractures and concluded that the Salter-Harris classification is an unreliable indication of prognosis. Cassebaum and Patterson reported significant and measurable growth disturbance in 40% of the distal femoral physeal injuries and an alarmingly high incidence in Salter-Harris types I and II fractures.

Thomson et al. analyzed 30 consecutive fractures and concluded that the best results after displaced fractures were obtained with gentle anatomical reduction and internal fixation with pins. They noted that long leg cast immobilization without pin fixation is not adequate to maintain reduction, and they advised close follow-up of a fracture that has not been internally fixed. Also, patients should be made aware of the

potential for late complications related to physeal damage, especially in severely displaced fractures. Riseborough et al. suggested that the final results can be improved by anatomical reduction and more frequent use of internal fixation, not only in types III and IV fractures but also in type II fractures (Fig. 33-150).

Types I and II fractures usually are reduced with the patient under general anesthesia, and the reduction is maintained in a spica cast. These fractures are noted for redisplacement, especially if they are initially displaced anteriorly. Varus and valgus types I and II fractures can be treated, if watched closely, in a long leg cast. Closed reduction can be made easier by the use of a traction bow on a Kirschner wire in the proximal tibia. This wire can be incorporated into the cast to maintain the reduction. Reduction should be 90% by traction or distraction and only 10% by leverage or manipulation. Most types I and II physeal fractures do not require anatomical reduction because the fracture occurs through the zone of provisional calcification of the physis, leaving the cells responsible for growth with the ossified epiphysis, although Salter-Harris types I and II fractures in the distal femur may be an exception. If a less than anatomical reduction results but acceptable general alignment and position are obtained, then union and satisfactory growth and remodeling can be expected, especially in children younger than 10 years of age in whom as much as 20 degrees of posterior angulation will remodel. In older patients nearer skeletal maturity, only slight anteroposterior displacement and no more than 5 degrees of varus-valgus angulation are acceptable. According to Salter it is better to accept a less than anatomical reduction with the possibility of an osteotomy later than to use forceful or repeated manipulation. In older children a closed reduction can be carried out, but because of inherent instability, percutaneous cross wire fixation with the aid of image intensification may be necessary to maintain reduction (Fig. 33-151). The pins should cross the metaphysis to prevent rotation of the epiphysis. Rarely, a Salter-Harris I or II fracture cannot be satisfactorily reduced closed because of interposition of soft tissue, and open reduction and internal fixation then become necessary.

In adolescents, a large metaphyseal spike (Thurston-Holland fragment) can be fixed with two cannulated screws. Salter-Harris types III and IV fractures require anatomical reduction. If this cannot be achieved by closed methods, open reduction and internal fixation are indicated. The amount of displacement that is acceptable in type III fractures has not been determined conclusively, but most authors report 2 mm or less as acceptable for closed reduction. We believe that if the surgeon thinks realistically that the amount of displacement can be decreased by performing an open reduction, then this should be carried out. CT scans and tomograms are helpful. The problem with these sophisticated techniques is the interpretation and standardization of the amount of displacement that is acceptable with closed treatment. Generally, displacement will appear to be greater on CT scans and tomograms than on the plain roentgenograms, and how much displacement is acceptable has not been properly documented.

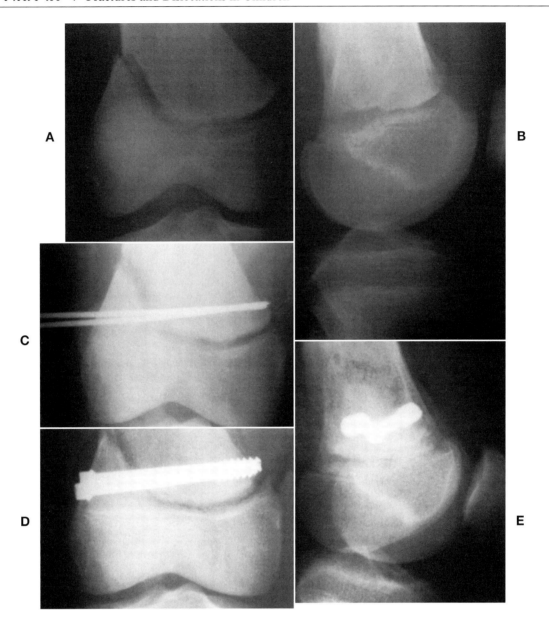

Fig. 33-150   **A** and **B,** Displaced Salter-Harris type II fracture of distal femoral physis could be reduced by closed means, but reduction could not be maintained. **C,** Guide wires hold fracture reduction before placement of cannulated screw. **D** and **E,** Fixation with cannulated screw.

◆ Closed or Open Reduction

TECHNIQUE 33-38

Carry out closed reduction for Salter-Harris types I and II fractures. If the reduction is satisfactory, apply a spica or long leg cast, depending on the direction of the original displacement. If reduction cannot be maintained, insert crossed, smooth 2.4-mm (3/32-inch) unthreaded Steinmann pins through the medial and lateral condyles and into the metaphysis (see Fig. 33-151). If a large metaphyseal spike (Salter-Harris II) is present after closed reduction, horizontal percutaneous pins or screws can be used as described below.

If the Salter-Harris I or II fracture cannot be reduced closed, then expose the epiphysis through a lateral longitudinal incision, as described in Chapter 51 for intercondylar fractures. Reduce the separation as gently and completely as possible by manual traction and minimal leverage. If the use of instruments is necessary, avoid injury to the physis. Remove any interposed soft tissue and gently maneuver the epiphysis into position. Once reduction is achieved, drill 2.4-mm unthreaded pins through the medial and lateral condyles so that they cross near the center of the physis and enter the metaphysis. Cut the pins off beneath the

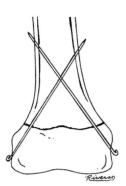

Fig. 33-151 Cross wire fixation with aid of image intensifier. Smooth pins should be used and should penetrate opposite cortex. (Redrawn from Weber BG, Brunner C, Freuler F, eds: *Treatment of fractures in children and adolescents*, New York, 1980, Springer-Verlag.)

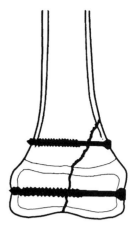

Fig. 33-152 Salter-Harris type IV fracture metaphyseal spike is secured transversely with cancellous screw. (Redrawn from Weber BG, Brunner C, Freuler F, eds: *Treatment of fractures in children and adolescents*, New York, 1980, Springer-Verlag.)

skin. If the pins are inserted as described and removed at 4 to 6 weeks, they are unlikely to cause any growth disturbance. If a type II or IV fracture has a large metaphyseal spike, then rather than using smooth crossed pins, drill two 2.4-mm threaded pins or a cancellous screw (Fig. 33-152) through the metaphysis of the spike into the proximal metaphyseal portion of the fracture. This should provide good stability and avoids crossing the physis. If the fragment is too small, then cross the physis with smooth crossed pins.

If the injury is a displaced Salter-Harris type III fracture, expose the displaced condyle through either an anteromedial or anterolateral incision, depending on which condyle is involved. An arthrotomy is necessary to ensure an anatomical reduction of the articular surface. Drill a large smooth pin, a Knowles pin, a cancellous screw, or a guide pin for cannulated cancellous screws into the displaced condyle to manipulate it. Gently and carefully reduce the displaced condyle into position with the pin or screw. Then insert the pin or screw transversely into the intact opposite condyle without crossing the physis. Confirm the reduction by roentgenograms. Threaded or cancellous screws can be used across the epiphysis, as long as they do not involve, penetrate, or cross the physis; however, smooth pins are preferable. These pins should be cut off beneath the skin for easy removal later.

Growth disturbance occurs frequently after type IV fractures if an anatomical reduction is not achieved and fixation is not secure. Arthrotomy usually is required to ensure anatomical reduction at the articular surface. Approach the fracture either anteromedially or anterolaterally, depending on which condyle is involved or on which side the metaphyseal spike is present. Reduce the articular

surface and the physis precisely with smooth pins, Knowles pins, or cancellous screws. Secure the fragment to the intact condyle, again with transverse fixation, without crossing the physis if possible. If, as in type II fractures, a large displaced metaphyseal spike is present, reduce the fracture anatomically with traction and secure the metaphyseal spike to the proximal metaphyseal fragment with threaded pins, screws, or cancellous bone screws (Fig. 33-153). If the metaphyseal spike is not large enough to ensure rigid fixation or if transverse fixation of the epiphysis cannot be secured, then smooth pins can be inserted across the physis.

AFTERTREATMENT. When the initial displacement is anterior, a long leg or single spica cast, depending on the stability, is applied with the knee in 45 degrees of flexion. These fractures are comparable to supracondylar fractures of the humerus in that the quadriceps and flexed knee are comparable to the triceps and flexed elbow in the maintenance of reduction. If the initial displacement is posterior, then the knee should be immobilized in extension. Union usually occurs at 4 to 6 weeks. The cast and any temporary pins can then be removed and an exercise program begun. Weight-bearing can be permitted at 8 to 10 weeks.

Complications. The immediate complications of closed or open reduction include vascular impairment, peroneal nerve palsy, and recurrent displacement and angulation. Late complications include joint stiffness and physeal arrest. All children with fractures of the distal femoral physis should be observed periodically until skeletal maturity. Epiphysiodesis of the contralateral extremity may be necessary because of premature physeal arrest with shortening or angulation or both. Angular deformity caused by bony bridge formation is common in distal femoral physeal fractures. Bony bridge resection and epiphysiodesis of the opposite extremity, as well as osteotomy, may be necessary to equalize leg lengths and correct angular deformity (Chapter 26).

Knee Fractures

PATELLAR FRACTURES

It is estimated that only 1% of all fractures occur in the patella and that only 1% of these occur in the immature skeleton, so fractures of the patella in children are extremely rare. They usually occur in older children. Some fractures, especially osteochondral and small peripheral fractures, as well as "sleeve-" type fractures, can be caused by acute dislocation of

the patella, which is common in children. In adolescents, "jumper's knee" and Sinding-Larsen-Johansson syndrome occur quite frequently. These are avulsion injuries of the proximal and distal poles of the patella and should be considered chronic repetitive ligamentous injuries. Bipartite patella should not be confused with a patellar fracture, although it can be misleading because bipartite patella occasionally is painful in adolescent athletes. However, in bipartite patella the edges of the defect usually are rounded, the condition is bilateral in approximately 50% of children, and it is almost always in the superolateral quadrant of the bone. Congenital absence of the patella or congenital hypoplasia may be seen in onycho-osteodysplasia or nail-patella syndrome and may be confusing. Fractures of the distal pole of the patella and even transverse fractures of the patella occur quite often in children with cerebral palsy and spasticity of the quadriceps muscle.

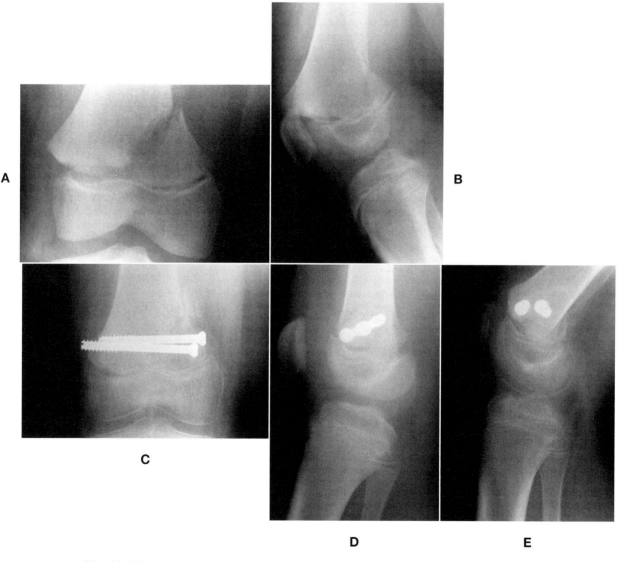

Fig. 33-153   **A** and **B,** Salter-Harris type II fracture of distal femoral physis with small metaphyseal spike. **C** and **D,** After closed reduction and percutaneous pinning. **E,** Two weeks after surgery, loss of reduction occurred because of inadequate fixation through metaphyseal spike only.

A sleeve-type of fracture of the distal pole of the patella has been described. Often only a fleck of bone is seen on the roentgenogram, giving a falsely benign appearance; however, a rather large, cartilaginous "sleeve" is attached to the patellar tendon which, if not replaced properly when healed and ossified, will be malaligned and will produce an abnormally elongated patella and patellar mechanism (Fig. 33-154). If this fracture occurs in conjunction with dislocation or subluxation of the patella, the elongation of the patellar mechanism makes the dislocation more unstable.

Patellar fractures should be classified according to location, type, and amount of displacement (Fig. 33-155). We (Maguire and Canale) reviewed 67 patellar fractures in 66 children at an average age of 12.4 years. Nineteen fractures were comminuted, 18 were transverse, 15 were chip fractures, 6 were vertical, and 2 were sleeve fractures; 7 fractures could not be classified from the available roentgenograms. The results of treatment were analyzed in 24 patients who were followed for more than 2 years (average follow-up, 9.5 years). Treatment followed guidelines generally accepted for patellar fractures in adults, but the large number of ipsilateral lower extremity fractures often dictated that treatment be determined according to the associated injury. Overall results were good in 13 patients, fair in 8, and poor in 3. Even though the numbers were too small for statistical analysis, some general trends were evident. We agree with other authors that restoration of the extensor mechanism is essential; results were less than optimal when this was not accomplished. Open reduction and internal fixation produced good results in our patients, and we found no growth disturbance after the use of cerclage wires. The number of patients treated in this manner is small, however, and their injuries occurred near skeletal maturity. The wires were removed after the fracture healed. Total patellectomy for displaced, comminuted fractures without ipsilateral tibial or femoral fractures was not associated with a poor result.

Because of the possibility of growth disturbance and because of frequent breakage of wires in children, we routinely remove wires, pins, and screws, preferably before they break. If the fracture occurs in conjunction with an acute or recurrent dislocation of the patella, a limited lateral release and medial reefing of the retinaculum may be indicated; we have had little experience with this. An osteochondral fracture of the patella or lateral femoral condyle should be suspected when acute patellar dislocation occurs.

We have seen one patient with an unrecognized sleeve fracture in conjunction with an acute dislocation of the patella (Fig. 33-156). On roentgenogram only a fleck of bone was noted at the distal pole of the patella; however, the patella was riding high, and a defect was present that should have been noticed clinically. The fracture was allowed to heal in a malaligned, elongated position, and when ossification occurred, the distal patella was malaligned. The child had no significant ligamentous laxity, but the deformed area on the inferior pole of the patella was painful. Approximately 18 months after injury, the inferior fracture fragment was excised because of pain. The pain was relieved, but recurrent dislocation of the patella was a problem; after the proximal tibial physis closed, the patellar mechanism distally was realigned. If the defect or the size of the fragment is uncertain, an MRI will reveal the extent of both the cartilage and bone fragment.

Because in a sleeve fracture a large cartilaginous fragment usually is attached to the fleck of bone, anatomical reduction,

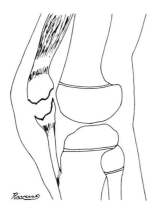

Fig. 33-154 Substantial sleeve of avulsed cartilage when seen on roentgenogram appears as only a "fleck" of bone and looks benign. (Redrawn from Houghton GR, Ackroyd CE: *J Bone Joint Surg* 61B:165, 1979.)

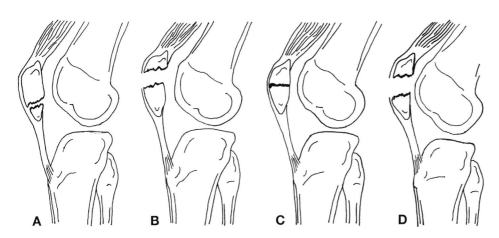

A **B** **C** **D**

Fig. 33-155 Types of patellar fracture. **A,** Inferior pole. **B,** Superior pole. **C,** Transverse undisplaced midsubstance. **D,** Transverse displaced midsubstance. (Redrawn from Ogden JA: *Skeletal injury in the child,* Philadelphia, 1982, Lea & Febiger.)

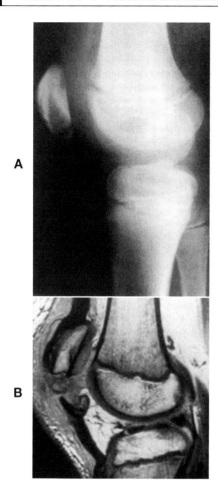

Fig. 33-156   A, Apparent minor inferior pole patellar fracture. **B,** MRI reveals extent of sleeve fracture.

either closed or open, is required. Malunion of the fracture may be painful and require excision of the distal fragment. If the sleeve fracture was caused by dislocation of the patella, healing in an elongated position may contribute to chronic recurrent dislocation.

The technique for open reduction and internal fixation of patellar fractures in children is the same as in adults (Chapter 43); however, because the sleeve fracture of the patella is peculiar to children, the technique of reduction and fixation is described here.

◆ Open Reduction and Internal Fixation of Sleeve Fracture

TECHNIQUE 33-39 *(Houghton and Ackroyd)*
Place the patient supine on the operating table and prepare the leg in the usual fashion; use a tourniquet. Approach the inferior pole of the patella through a 7-cm medial parapatellar incision, using only the distal portion. Expose the distal pole patellar fracture. Irrigate the fracture copiously with saline and with a small curet remove any

clots and loose cancellous bone. Reduce the fragment with a small bone holder. Observe the fracture fragments anteriorly and try to observe the reduction posteriorly on the articular surface. If this is not possible, use a gloved finger to feel for any angulation or offset on the articular surface. Then perform a tension band wiring with two Kirschner wires (Chapter 51). After reduction of the fracture, place two parallel longitudinal Steinmann pins across the fracture site. Leave them protruding approximately ¼ inch (0.5 cm) distally for easy removal. Then place a tension band wire from the superior to the inferior pole of the patella, crossing itself and incorporating the parallel pins (Fig. 33-157). Tighten the wire sufficiently but not enough to overly compress and angulate the fracture fragments. Close the wound in layers and apply an appropriate cast with the knee in mild flexion.

AFTERTREATMENT. At 3 to 4 weeks the cast is removed and range-of-motion exercises are started. The AO group recommends early motion in flexion after tension band wiring, which, according to the tension band principle, holds the reduction. However, this is unnecessary in a young child.

FRACTURES OF INTERCONDYLAR EMINENCE OF TIBIA

Tibial intercondylar eminence fractures have been classified into three types by Meyers and McKeever: type I, little or no displacement; type II, elevated anteriorly and proximally, with some displacement but with a cartilaginous hinge; and type III, complete displacement (Fig. 33-158). The goal of treatment is to reduce the fragment as well as possible, and this has been done traditionally by extending the knee. However, simply extending the knee may not reposition the fragment satisfactorily and it may heal with the anterior cruciate ligament relaxed.

An increasing number of reports have associated ligament injuries in children with fractures of the tibial intercondylar eminence. Several authors have reported varying amounts of ligamentous laxity after these fractures, regardless of treatment methods. Baxter and Wiley, in a study of 45 fractures, reported that 51% of patients had a positive anterior drawer test at follow-up and that all patients had a measurable loss of extension, ranging from 4 to 15 degrees; 64% of them were aware of the difference between their knees. Baxter and Wiley found that open reduction did not eliminate the cruciate ligament laxity or persistent loss of extension.

According to Grönkvist et al., younger children will compensate somewhat for any anterior instability as the skeleton grows, but in older children, some anterior instability will persist. They recommended operative repair, especially in older children, if satisfactory closed reduction cannot be obtained. According to Roberts and Lovell, the greatest complication of this fracture, if it remains displaced, is a lack of full extension of the knee rather than anterior instability. In

A   B   C

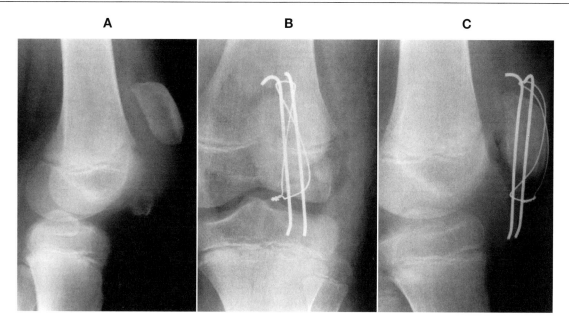

Fig. 33-157   **A,** Patellar "sleeve" fracture. **B** and **C,** After reduction and fixation with Kirschner wires and tension band wiring.

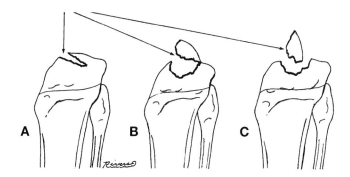

Fig. 33-158   Fractures of intercondylar eminence of tibia. **A,** Type I, avulsion fracture, nondisplaced. **B,** Type II, hinged fracture, displaced but posterior rim remains intact. **C,** Type III, completely displaced fracture. (Redrawn from Roberts JM: Fractures and dislocations of the knee. In Rockwood CA Jr, Wilkins KE, King RE, eds: *Fractures in children*, Philadelphia, 1984, JB Lippincott.)

their report of 50 patients with tibial eminence fractures, Willis et al. noted that although most children have objective evidence of anterior cruciate ligament laxity at long-term follow-up, few have subjective complaints. They found clinical signs of anterior instability in 64% of their patients and objective (KT-1000 arthrometer testing) evidence of laxity in 74%; however, only 10% of patients complained of pain and none complained of instability at follow-up. No correlation was found between long-term stability and method of treatment (open or closed). They concluded that most anterior tibial eminence fractures should be treated by closed reduction and immobilization in extension, with open reduction and internal fixation reserved for irreducible fractures, and that arthroscopy may be useful to ensure adequate reduction of the fragment. Willis et al. warned that the long-term prognosis of tibial

eminence fractures remains guarded because of persistent anterior cruciate ligament laxity.

Most authors agree that placement of the knee joint in full extension will reduce the fragment quite satisfactorily in types I and II fractures. Aspiration of the hemarthrosis from a tense knee joint also may be beneficial. Occasionally, in types II and III fractures, interposition (impingement) of a meniscus may prevent reduction. In these instances open reduction should be performed. Meyers and McKeever recommended open reduction of displaced types II and III fractures. For types I and II fractures, we aspirate any significant hemarthrosis and apply a cylinder or long leg cast with the knee in full extension. Type III fractures also are treated initially by aspiration and extension. If the reduction is successful, the leg is immobilized in a long leg cast. Otherwise, for types II and III fractures, open reduction and internal fixation are carried out (Fig. 33-159). We prefer a medial parapatellar incision to expose the tibial spine, anterior cruciate ligament, and anterior horns of both menisci to make sure they are not trapped beneath the fragment. We use a nonabsorbable suture or a wire passed through the distalmost portion of the anterior cruciate ligament and brought out distally through holes drilled in the proximal tibial epiphysis, avoiding the physis. This can be done arthroscopically with the use of an anterior cruciate ligament but is technically difficult. The arthroscopic technique is described in Chapter 48.

◆ Open Reduction and Internal Fixation

TECHNIQUE 33-40
Expose the knee through the distal portion of an anteromedial parapatellar incision (Technique 1-25). Open the capsule medially to expose the fracture fragments and the

continued

Fig. 33-159 **A,** Type III tibial eminence fracture that could not be reduced closed. **B,** Lateral roentgenograms after open reduction and fixation with nonabsorbable sutures. Entrapped meniscus that prevented closed reduction was found at time of surgery.

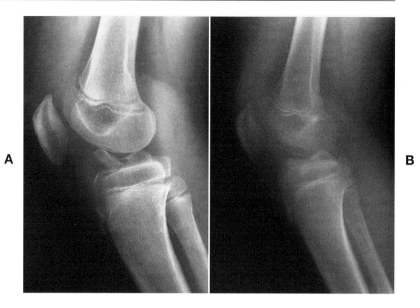

Fig. 33-160 Types of avulsion fracture of tibial tuberosity. **A,** Type I, through secondary ossification center. **B,** Type II, at junction of primary and secondary ossification centers. **C,** Type III, across primary ossification center (Salter-Harris type III) with physis near closing posteriorly. (Redrawn from Roberts JM: Fractures and dislocations of the knee. In Rockwood CA Jr, Wilkins KE, King RE, eds: *Fractures in children*, Philadelphia, 1984, JB Lippincott.)

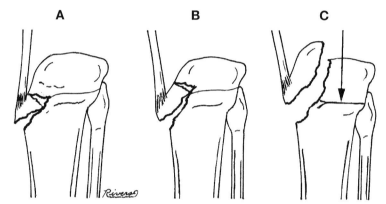

defect in the proximal tibia. Examine the medial meniscus and then with retraction examine the anterior horn of the lateral meniscus to make sure the menisci are not impeding the reduction. Place the knee in extension and reduce the fragment after any clots and cancellous bone have been removed from the defect. Drill two holes from distal to proximal through the tibial epiphysis. Take care to drill the holes proximal to the physis. The holes should enter the joint (1) just medial and lateral to the fracture fragments or (2) into the defect and into the fragment itself if it is large enough. Pass either a 19-gauge or 18-gauge wire, or a 1-0 nonabsorbable suture, through the distalmost portion of the anterior cruciate ligament just proximal to the fracture fragment. Now with suture carriers pass the ends of the suture through the drill holes and tie them on themselves after the reduction is satisfactory. Flex and extend the knee to make sure the reduction is stable. Irrigate and close the wound.

AFTERTREATMENT. A cast is applied with the knee in full extension. At 4 to 6 weeks, the cast is removed and range-of-motion exercises are started.

TIBIAL TUBEROSITY FRACTURES

Fractures of the tibial tuberosity usually occur in older children and were classified by Watson-Jones: type I, a small fragment that is displaced superiorly; type II, a larger fragment involving the secondary center of ossification and the proximal tibial physis, which is hinged upward; and type III, a fracture that passes proximally and posteriorly across the physis and proximal articular surface of the tibia (a Salter-Harris type III physeal fracture (Fig. 33-160). This classification is important because type III fractures in younger children, if not anatomically reduced and held, can result in bony bridge formation, causing anterior growth arrest and hyperextension deformity. However, as noted by Ogden et al., this complication is unlikely because these fractures usually occur in older adolescents (Fig. 33-161). Roberts pointed out that because of imprecise definition of this entity as compared with Osgood-Schlatter disease and Salter-Harris type III injuries of the proximal tibial physis, the results are quite confusing. He noted the differences between Osgood-Schlatter disease and traumatic avulsion of the tibial tuberosity. In Osgood-Schlatter disease the injury often is insidious with mild symptoms and partial disability; symptomatic and supportive treatment is all that is necessary, the prognosis is good, and only occasionally

A   B   C

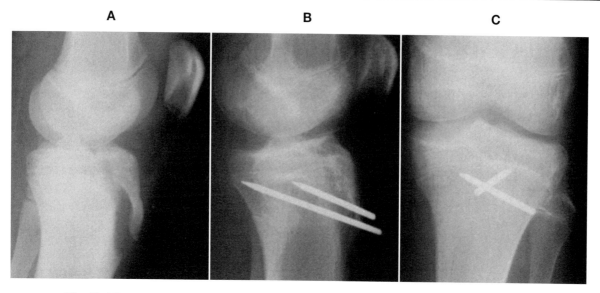

Fig. 33-161 Tibial tuberosity fracture. **A,** Watson-Jones type III fracture (Salter-Harris type III) extending into knee joint. **B** and **C,** After open reduction and internal fixation with smooth pins, avoiding physis.

are symptoms prolonged by an ununited ossicle. Conversely, in acute traumatic avulsions of the tibial tuberosity, pain and swelling occur immediately and standing or walking is impossible. Open reduction and internal fixation often are necessary and are followed by rapid healing and return to full activity.

Hand et al. recommended open reduction and internal fixation of types II and III fractures and noted that a large periosteal flap can prevent an adequate closed reduction. Ogden et al. recommended surgery for (1) significant displacement of one or more fragments of the tuberosity anteriorly and superiorly and (2) extension of the fracture through the proximal tibial epiphysis into the knee joint, with disruption of the joint surface (Salter-Harris type III). We treat most of these fractures closed, especially types I and II fractures. Reduction should be carried out with the knee in extension, followed by casting. If displacement of more than 0.5 cm persists, then open anatomical reduction is indicated. If closed methods are used, serial roentgenograms, especially in the lateral plane, must be made frequently to ensure that proximal displacement does not occur because of the quadriceps pull. A displaced Salter-Harris type III fracture should be treated by open reduction and internal fixation, as described for proximal tibial physeal fractures. For Watson-Jones types I and II avulsions of the tibial tuberosity, screw fixation can be used in a large fragment in older children. However, smooth wires or pins should be used if the fragment is smaller or comminuted in younger children. A large periosteal flap may be avulsed from the adjacent metaphysis medially, laterally, or distally and should be sutured in its original position at the time of repair. According to Ogden, this adds intrinsic stability to the reduction. It is hoped that with healing, fusion will occur across the traction apophysis only.

◆ Open Reduction and Internal Fixation

TECHNIQUE 33-41
Make an anteromedial incision 5 cm long adjacent to the tibial tuberosity and parallel to the patellar tendon. Carry the dissection laterally over the tibial tuberosity and the insertion of the patellar tendon. Expose the fracture and clean its base with a curet. Do not dissect completely free the attachments of the tibial tuberosity. Identify any large periosteal flap, which may be avulsed medially, laterally, bilaterally, or distally. If it is frayed, resect some of it. If not, retain it for stability. Reduce the fracture with the knee in full extension. Insert two small pins across the fracture. If the fragment is large and in an older child, a cancellous bone screw can be used quite satisfactorily; make sure the head of the screw is buried deeply enough not to cause chronic discomfort from contusions in the area. Check the reduction with roentgenograms. Suture any periosteal flap and close the wound in layers.

AFTERTREATMENT. A cylinder cast is applied with the knee in full extension. At 4 to 6 weeks the cast is removed, and if smooth pins have been used, they also are removed at that time.

OSTEOCHONDRAL FRACTURES

Osteochondral fractures of the knee occur primarily on the cartilaginous surfaces of the medial or lateral femoral condyle or the patella. They may be caused by direct forces applied against the femur or patella or by dislocation of the patella itself (Fig. 33-162). Nietosvaara et al. reported 72 acute patellar dislocations, 39 of which had associated osteochondral

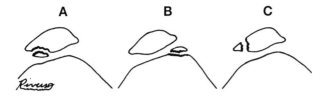

Fig. 33-162   Three locations of osteochondral fractures caused by dislocation of patella. **A,** Inferior surface of patella. **B,** Femoral condyle. **C,** Medial surface of patella. (Redrawn from Rang M: *Children's fractures,* Philadelphia, 1981, JB Lippincott.)

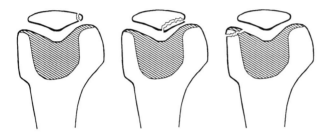

Fig. 33-163   Distribution of osteochondral fractures in 72 acute patellar dislocations. Medial marginal patellar avulsions, 15; intraarticular fractures, 15; inferomedial patellar facet, 7; lateral femoral condyle, 5; combined fracture, 3.

fractures; 50% of these fractures were capsular avulsions of the medial patellar margin, and 50% were loose intraarticular fragments detached from the patella or the lateral femoral condyles. The intraarticular fragments were found only after spontaneous relocation of the patella. The femoral fractures consistently involved the edge of the articular surface and the middle third of the condylar arc (Fig. 33-163). Usually a significant hemarthrosis follows the traumatic episode. If ligamentous instability is not present and the aspirate of the knee is sanguineous (hemarthrosis), then an osteochondral fracture should be suspected, even though quite often the fragment is not bony and cannot be seen on roentgenograms. Occasionally, just a faint density or fleck of subchondral bone can be identified. This small osseous fragment usually is part of an osteocartilaginous loose body that at surgery will be surprisingly large. Arthroscopy is indicated to locate, identify, and remove the loose body. The defect in the patella or femur also should be identified. All but exceptionally large fragments should be excised. A fragment, if it is recently displaced from an osseous crater, can be replaced in the crater and fixed internally, as for treatment of osteochondritis dissecans (Chapters 42 and 43).

FLOATING KNEE INJURIES

Although not actually an injury of the knee joint, "floating knee" describes the flail knee joint segment resulting from a fracture of the shafts or adjacent metaphyses of the ipsilateral femur and tibia. This is an uncommon injury in children, most often resulting from motor vehicle accidents, and usually is associated with major soft tissue damage, open fractures, and head injuries. Letts et al. proposed a five-part classification of these injuries (Fig. 33-164): type A, both femoral and tibial fractures are closed diaphyseal fractures; type B, one fracture is diaphyseal, one is metaphyseal, and both are closed; type C, one fracture is diaphyseal, the other is an epiphyseal displacement; type D, one fracture is open with major soft tissue injury; and type E, both fractures are open with major soft tissue injury. Their basic recommendation for treatment of these injuries is that at least one fracture (usually the tibial) must be rigidly fixed by open reduction and internal fixation. If mobilization of the child is essential, internal fixation of both fractures may be indicated. In older children, intramedullary nailing may be more appropriate than plate fixation. Open fractures with major soft tissue injury should be left open and stabilized with external fixation (Fig. 33-165). Bohn and Durbin described the results of ipsilateral fractures of the femur and tibia in children and adolescents with an average follow-up of 6.8 years. In children younger than 10 years of age, an average of 8.1 cm of femoral and tibial overgrowth occurred. Most children younger than 10 years were treated successfully with closed methods. In children older than 10 years who were treated with reduction and fixation (intramedullary rods, plates, external fixator) of the femoral fracture, a high complication rate was noted, as well as frequent concomitant injuries to the ligaments of the knee that resulted in long-term dysfunction of the extremity. At follow-up, over 50% had a poor result because of limb length discrepancy, angular deformity, or instability of the knee, particularly ligamentous instability.

Acute Dislocations of Knee

Acute dislocations of the knee and of the proximal tibiofibular joint are extremely rare in children. Those of the knee seldom require surgical treatment. Ogden reported a large series of subluxations and dislocations of the proximal tibiofibular joint. Most of these can be treated by closed reduction. The problem is in identifying the pathological condition and the subtle roentgenographic changes.

Tibial and Fibular Fractures

Fractures of the tibia and fibula require operative treatment only when they cannot be reduced, when they are open, or occasionally when they occur in the proximal or distal tibial physis. Otherwise, fractures of the tibia and fibula can be treated closed. One of the more worrisome fractures is the incomplete metaphyseal fracture of the proximal tibia. Fracture of the proximal tibial epiphysis also deserves special attention because of its proximity to the popliteal artery, which may be injured when the tibial shaft is posteriorly displaced (Fig. 33-166). Fractures of the distal tibial and fibular physes also are of special concern because, if not treated properly, varus and valgus angulation may occur in older children, and a

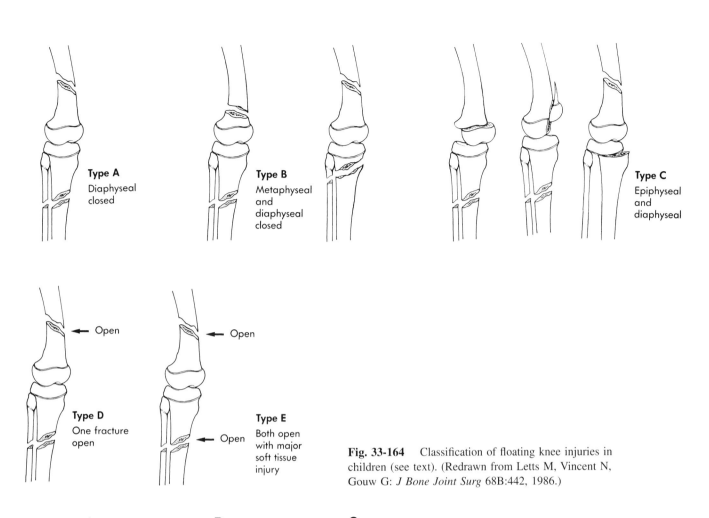

Type A
Diaphyseal
closed

Type B
Metaphyseal
and
diaphyseal
closed

Type C
Epiphyseal
and
diaphyseal

← Open

Type D
One fracture
open

← Open

Type E
Both open
with major
soft tissue
injury

← Open

Fig. 33-164   Classification of floating knee injuries in children (see text). (Redrawn from Letts M, Vincent N, Gouw G: *J Bone Joint Surg* 68B:442, 1986.)

A   **B**   **C**

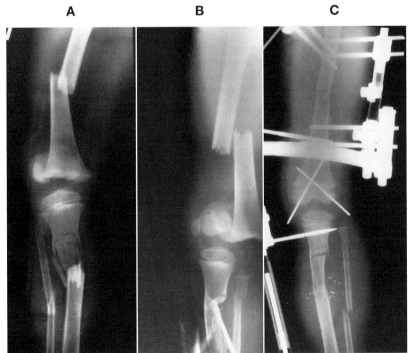

Fig. 33-165   **A** and **B,** Severe floating knee injury with midshaft fracture of femur, Salter-Harris type I fracture of distal femoral physis, and comminuted fracture of tibial shaft. **C,** After internal fixation of distal femoral physeal fracture with crossed pins and external fixation of fractures of femoral and tibial shafts.

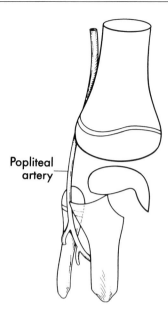

Fig. 33-166   Salter-Harris types I and II fractures with posterior displacement of tibial shaft may injure popliteal artery.

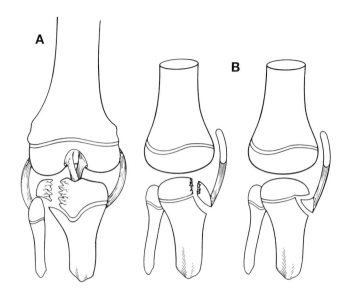

Fig. 33-167   Salter-Harris type III fracture of proximal tibia. **A,** Fracture analogous to tibial plateau fracture. **B,** Fracture through tibial tuberosity and across epiphysis into knee joint somewhat similar to avulsion of epiphysis of tibial tuberosity.

bony bridge may form causing angular deformity in younger children.

PROXIMAL TIBIAL PHYSEAL FRACTURES

In 1965 Aitken reported 14 children with proximal tibial physeal fractures and made two pertinent observations. First, fewer ligaments are attached to the proximal tibial physis than to the distal femoral physis. As a result, the distal femoral physis separates more often than the proximal tibial physis. In fact, at this clinic we see approximately seven or eight distal femoral physeal separations per year compared with one proximal tibial physeal separation per year. However, we have seen an increased number of the "tongue" type Salter-Harris type III fractures through the tibial physis and into the joint. The second observation of Aitken was that the proximal tibial shaft when displaced posteriorly comes in close proximity to the popliteal artery, which may be injured in Salter-Harris types I and II fractures (Fig. 33-166). Wozasek et al. reported that 4 of 30 patients (13%) with injuries of the proximal tibial physis, half of which were displaced, had peripheral ischemia.

Shelton and Canale reviewed 39 proximal tibial epiphyseal fractures treated at this clinic between 1951 and 1976. They occurred in older children (average age of 14.2 years). Of the fractures 23 were displaced and 16 were nondisplaced; 9 were type I fractures, 17 were type II, 10 were type III, and only 3 were type IV. Treatment was according to the Salter-Harris recommendations (p. 1393). Of the 9 type I fractures, 8 were treated satisfactorily by closed reduction. One had persistent posterior displacement and a transection of the popliteal artery with subsequent transmetatarsal amputation and equinus deformity of the foot.

Results were satisfactory in most of the type II fractures, even though one child subsequently had 2 inches (5 cm) of shortening. Most of these fractures could be reduced easily and held in a bent-knee cast. One required a fasciotomy and one an arthrotomy. One fracture was manipulated 8 weeks after injury because this fracture in an older child was allowed to heal in 40 degrees of angulation, which was considered unacceptable.

Of the 10 type III fractures, two different types occurred: one was basically a tibial plateau fracture (Fig. 33-167, *A*), and the other, a type III fracture starting at the physis of the tibial tuberosity and extending up into the joint and across the proximal tibial physis. These fractures are not considered avulsions of the tibial tuberosity but rather are fractures of the physis of the tibial tuberosity that extend as Salter-Harris type III fractures into the joint; they almost always require open reduction and internal fixation (Fig. 33-168). These are large tongue-type fractures that extend from the medial to lateral side of the knee, lifting the tibial tuberosity and the proximal tibial physis up anteriorly and superiorly. For each of the two types of type III fractures the exposure required is extensive and should be undertaken only after complete understanding of the anatomy. Fixation with cancellous screws or threaded or smooth pins is carried out for most of these fractures. In two patients the results were unsatisfactory because of joint incongruity and late traumatic arthritis.

The three type IV fractures were treated primarily as tibial plateau fractures. One had an incomplete reduction and developed traumatic arthritis. One had ligamentous instability, and stress roentgenograms helped in making the diagnosis (Fig. 33-169).

Stress roentgenograms also can help in the diagnosis of a nondisplaced type I fracture. Tomograms and CT scans can

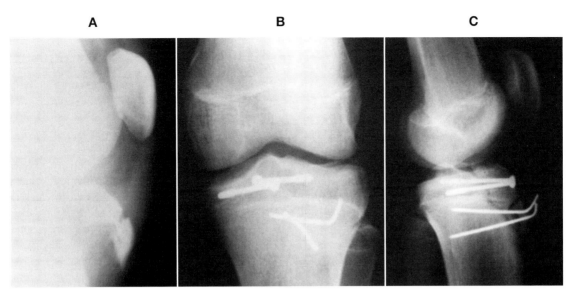

Fig. 33-168 **A,** Salter-Harris type III fracture of proximal tibial physis. **B** and **C,** After open reduction and internal fixation.

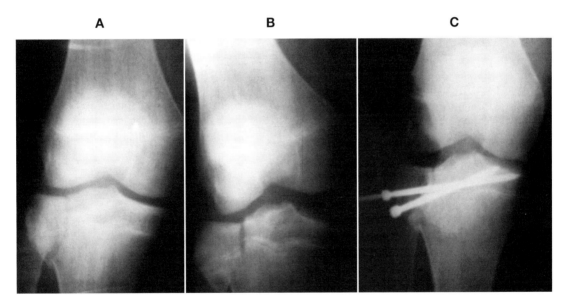

Fig. 33-169 Physeal fracture with major ligamentous injury. **A,** Nondisplaced Salter-Harris type IV fracture. **B,** Stress roentgenograms show fracture displacement and medial joint line opening, implying tibial collateral ligament injury. **C,** At time of open reduction and internal fixation.

help determine the amount of displacement. However, as mentioned previously in discussing injuries of the distal femoral physis, proper interpretation of these special, sophisticated, roentgenographic techniques is required to determine how much displacement is excessive and requires open reduction and internal fixation.

In our patients, complications included anterior compartment syndrome, transient and permanent peroneal nerve palsy, arterial thrombosis, angular deformity, and leg length inequality. Any suggestion of ischemic changes, a compartment

syndrome, or peroneal nerve palsy requires that immediate action be taken in the emergency department. Appropriate treatment for each is given in Chapter 46. Leg length inequality of more than 1 inch (2.5 cm) occurred in 2 of the 39 children. Two children had joint incongruity and angular deformity. These complications can be treated by epiphysiodesis, osteotomy, and bony bridge resection.

In summary this fracture is rare and usually occurs in maturing adolescents, especially those engaged in athletics. The roentgenograms often show little evidence of injury, but the CT scan and tomograms can reveal significant displacement. Thus the roentgenograms can give a false sense of security in an injury that can produce deformity and disability.

◆ Open Reduction and Internal Fixation

TECHNIQUE 33-42

Prepare the patient and drape the knee in the usual fashion. Inflate the tourniquet. Make a long medial or lateral parapatellar incision, depending on the location of the fracture. Carry the soft tissue dissection down to the fracture and expose the fracture widely. The Salter-Harris type III or IV injury frequently is a tongue-type fracture anteriorly with the entire tibial tuberosity elevated and hinged posteriorly. Dissect both medially and laterally into the joint until the physeal fracture is seen. It may be located in the midportion of the joint or even posteriorly. Elevate the entire physeal fragment. Wash out any debris and remove all soft tissues such as periosteum from the fracture so that the reduction is not impeded. Now reduce the fracture anatomically. This should be similar to closing a hinge, and if any soft tissue is entrapped, the hinge will not close completely when the knee is extended. After the reduction, observe for joint congruity and reduction of the fracture at its peripheral margins.

In a vertical fracture, insert transverse pins for fixation. Because the patient usually is an older child, threaded pins, screws, or cancellous bone screws can be used. In younger children use smooth pins transversely or horizontally. Irrigate the wound copiously with saline. Close the wound in the usual manner and apply a bent-knee cast.

AFTERTREATMENT. The cast remains in place for 4 to 6 weeks. At 2 weeks a window is made in it for removal of sutures and change of dressing. Gentle mobilization of the knee should be started between 4 and 6 weeks, depending on the age of the child.

PROXIMAL TIBIAL METAPHYSEAL FRACTURES

Displaced fractures of the proximal tibial metaphysis are of concern because of their proximity to the posterior tibial artery, as is true of fractures of the proximal tibial physis, and the possibility of damaging the vasculature of the leg. Fractures of the proximal tibial metaphysis, especially those that are nondisplaced, can, with or without an associated proximal fibular fracture, produce a valgus angular deformity. Roentgenograms reveal a benign "greenstick" nondisplaced fracture pattern in a child 3 to 8 years old. Frequently the fracture is treated in a straight or bent-knee cast and heals uneventfully with apparently satisfactory alignment. Later the tibia is noted to have a significant valgus angulation as compared with the opposite tibia. This excess valgus may not have been preventable, and for this reason, the parents should be told at

the beginning of treatment about the possibility of this complication.

At what point the valgus angulation occurs and why it occurs are still unknown; however, numerous explanations have been advanced and include the following:

1. Asymmetrical growth stimulation of the proximal tibial physis. Houghton and Rooker surgically lacerated the proximal tibial periosteum medially in animals and noted a resultant valgus angulation.
2. Asymmetrical growth stimulation of the medial proximal metaphysis from asymmetrical vascular response has been suggested by several authors, including Dias and Giegerich; Green; Herring and Moseley; Ogden; and Jordan et al.. They postulated that an unbalanced vascular healing response occurs after injury to the metaphysis, causing the medial side of the tibia to outgrow the lateral side. Zionts et al. reported that technetium bone scanning in one patient 5 months after injury demonstrated increased uptake at the proximal tibial physis with proportionally greater uptake on the medial side, suggesting a relative increase in vascularity and consequent overgrowth of the medial portion of the metaphysis. A study by Ogden et al. corroborated an overgrowth mechanism as the most likely cause of valgus deformity, and they concluded that the angulation is actually an accelerated physiological response that coincides with the age range in which children gradually shift from physiological genu varum to genu valgum.
3. The tibial physis is stimulated more or for a longer period than the fibular physis, which may or may not have been fractured. This would cause a tethering effect, with the tibia overgrowing more medially than the fibula laterally, pulling the extremity into a valgus position. This theory has been supported by Taylor and by Jackson and Cozen.
4. Rang suggested that the valgus angulation occurs at the time of fracture. Too often, roentgenograms of these fractures are taken in a cast with the knee flexed, and the valgus angulation is not apparent. Furthermore, roentgenograms of the contralateral extremity are not taken for comparison, and the amount of valgus is not appreciated. Bahnson and Lovell stressed the importance of accurate initial assessment and reduction. Pollen postulated that weight-bearing before solid union of the fracture produces the valgus angulation; this concept was supported by Salter and Best.
5. Weber and others postulated that soft tissue, such as the pes anserinus, is interposed between the fragments, preventing an adequate reduction and complete healing of the fracture, which causes an exaggerated stimulation of the physis on the medial side of the tibia, resulting in overgrowth and valgus deformity (Fig. 33-170). They recommended open reduction, especially when the fracture fragments are mildly to moderately separated medially, and removal of the interposed material.
6. Others concluded that a physeal injury occurs, causing

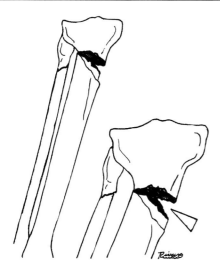

Fig. 33-170 Opening of fracture gap medially showing that periosteum or pes anserinus could be interposed. (From Weber BG, Brunner C, Freuler F, eds: *Treatment of fractures in children and adolescents*, New York, 1980, Springer-Verlag.)

premature closure of the physis laterally, leaving the physis open medially with resultant valgus angulation.

Because the incidence, etiology, and prognosis of this deformity are unknown, prevention and treatment are controversial. The fractures usually occur between the ages of 3 and 8 years, when the normal physiological valgus is at its maximum. We have treated eight children with this deformity whose ages ranged from 2 to 9 years. Like others, we are uncertain of the exact cause of the deformity or how to prevent it. However, the fracture should be treated precisely. First, the parents should be warned before treatment is begun of the possibility of valgus deformity. Second, a straight leg cast should be applied, and roentgenograms of the fractured tibia and the opposite tibia should be taken frequently and compared. If any valgus angulation does occur, the cast should be wedged into a corrected position. Robert et al. recommended reduction, with the patient under general anesthesia, of any fracture with a break in the medial cortex and even minimal valgus deformity. Third, the parents should be warned that an angular deformity can increase, even after cast treatment has been discontinued and healing is complete. Fourth, we have recently, when appropriate, tried to put the fractured tibia in slightly less valgus than the opposite tibia.

Of the eight children we treated, the deformity increased in some as late as 12 months after treatment. In some the deformity improved spontaneously for 3 years after injury (Fig. 33-171). This improvement may have been caused by the normal correction of physiological valgus seen in children between the ages of 2 and 9 years. Bracing was of some benefit in two patients. Proximal tibial osteotomy for significant deformity should be delayed because the deformity may correct spontaneously. Osteotomy will correct the deformity, but it also can stimulate the medial side of the tibia and cause the deformity to recur later, as noted in some of our children and by Pappas and others.

Some spontaneous correction occurred in most children. Skak reported that bracing was of some benefit in several children. Bracing may augment the natural correction of physiological genu valgum. Osteotomy of the proximal tibia should be performed only for significant deformity and should be correlated with the age of the child, the normal physiological valgus, the amount of deformity, cosmesis, and the parents' perception of the problem. Less than 12 degrees of increased valgus angulation (femoral-tibial angle) on a standing roentgenogram compared with the opposite leg should be treated conservatively. If more than 15 degrees of increased angulation is present, an osteotomy should be considered but with the warning that after the osteotomy the valgus deformity may recur (Fig. 33-172).

◆ Open Reduction and Removal of Interposed Tissue

According to Weber et al., if interposition of soft tissue is strongly suspected or is confirmed by appropriate valgus stress roentgenograms with gapping of the fracture, and if the fracture is not a stress fracture, then operative removal of the tissues, including the periosteum and pes anserinus, from the fracture may be necessary. Although we are not convinced that this is the cause of the valgus deformity in all patients, we do agree with Skak et al. that operative treatment is indicated when a wide medial gap persists after closed reduction.

TECHNIQUE 33-43 *(Weber et al.)*

Place the patient supine on the operating table and prepare and drape in the usual fashion. Approach the fracture site medially through a 6-cm vertical incision. Carry the soft tissue dissection down to the medial surface of the tibia and identify the fracture. Notice if the periosteum is stripped away from the medial surface of the tibia and, together with the pes anserinus, is trapped in the transverse fracture gap (Fig. 33-173, *A* and *B*). Clean all debris away from the fracture, including the hematoma. Slide a periosteal elevator under the interposed tissues and extract it from the fracture. Hold the periosteum back with forceps (Fig. 33-173, *C* and *D*) and irrigate the fracture. Suture the periosteum and the pes anserinus in their original positions if at all possible. Observe the fracture before closing to make sure that the gap is closed and that no further interposition of periosteum has occurred. Close the wound in layers and apply a long straight leg cast.

AFTERTREATMENT. Roentgenograms of both lower extremities in full extension should be taken to make sure no increased valgus is present in the injured tibia compared with the opposite tibia.

MIDDLE AND DISTAL TIBIAL SHAFT FRACTURES

Fractures of the shaft of the tibia, with or without associated fibular fractures, usually can be treated by closed reduction and

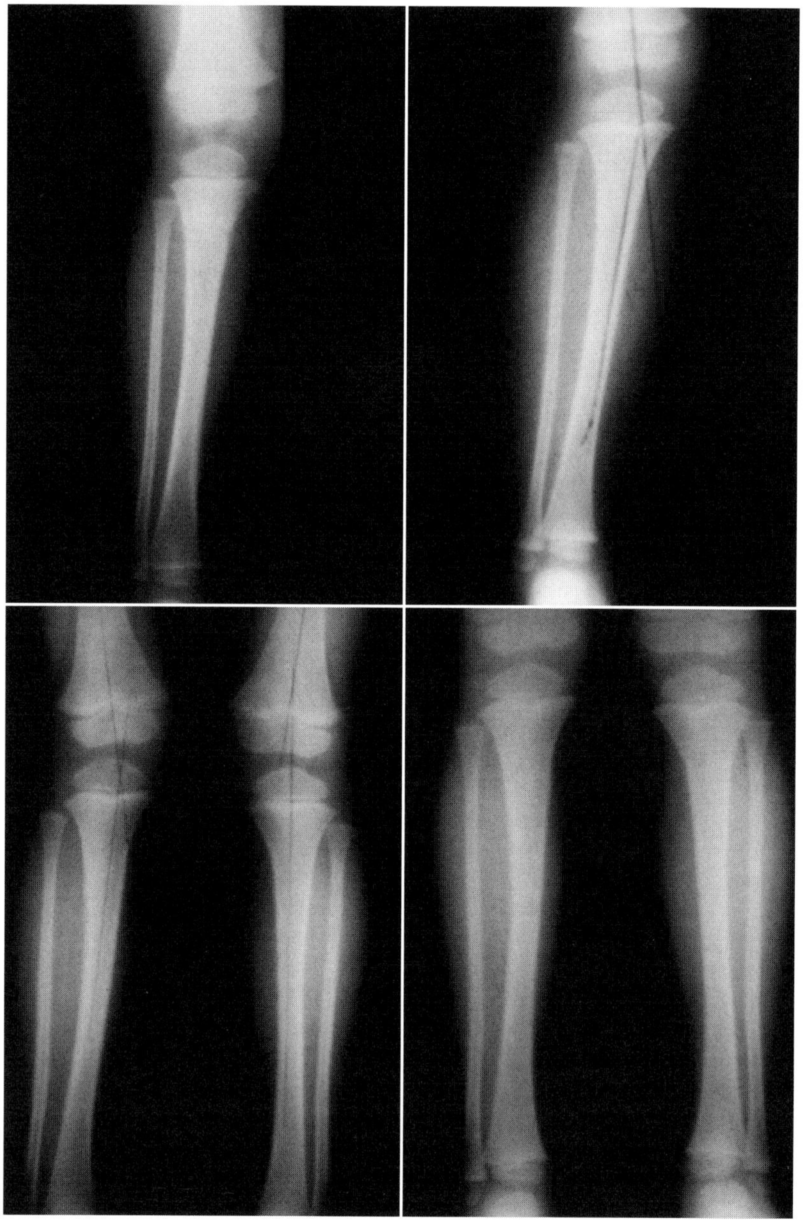

Fig. 33-171 Spontaneous correction of valgus deformity. **A,** Proximal metaphyseal fracture at time of injury with no valgus angulation while standing. **B,** At 8 months valgus angulation of 15 degrees is present. **C,** At 16 months some spontaneous correction of angulation has occurred. **D,** At 2 years' follow-up valgus angulation has almost disappeared.

casting. This also applies to distal tibial metaphyseal fractures. Shannak, in a study of 117 tibial shaft fractures treated with above-knee casts, found that (1) initial shortening of up to 10 mm was compensated wholly or partially by growth acceleration, (2) mild varus deformities corrected spontaneously, (3) valgus deformity and posterior angulation persisted to some degree, and (4) rotational deformities persisted, especially internal rotation.

Briggs et al. reported 65 tibial fractures in children, 25 of which were isolated fractures. In their patients, transverse isolated fractures did not displace either early or late while in the plaster cast, but spiral and oblique fractures were prone to displacement into varus for as long as 2 weeks after injury and required careful follow-up. Fractures manipulated at 2 weeks were still mildly malleable, but those left for 3 weeks were not.

Yang and Letts noted the same and suggested that an intact fibula acts like a splint, thus producing a bending moment that results in varus angulation.

Spontaneous correction of angular deformity after tibial fractures has been reported to occur in boys up to the age of 10 years and in girls up to the age of 8 years; however, other reports indicate that little spontaneous correction occurs regardless of the age of the child. Briggs et al., contrary to the study by Shannak, suggested that varus angulation of more than 5 degrees is unacceptable, especially in older children. They recommended careful follow-up with weekly roentgenograms and manipulation if varus displacement is more than 5 degrees during the first 2 weeks after injury.

Because of the possibility of compartment syndromes, a both-bone fracture of the lower extremity should not be treated

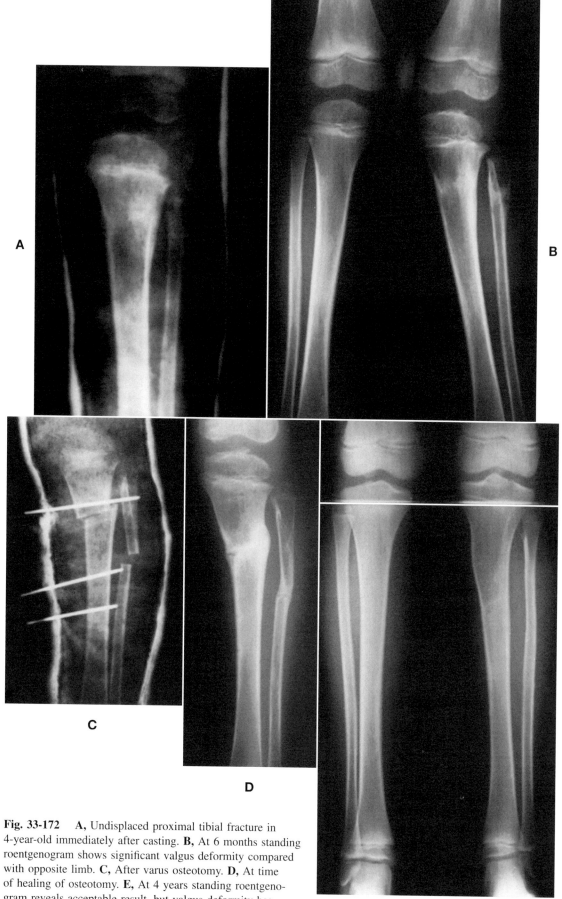

Fig. 33-172 **A,** Undisplaced proximal tibial fracture in 4-year-old immediately after casting. **B,** At 6 months standing roentgenogram shows significant valgus deformity compared with opposite limb. **C,** After varus osteotomy. **D,** At time of healing of osteotomy. **E,** At 4 years standing roentgenogram reveals acceptable result, but valgus deformity has recurred mildly.

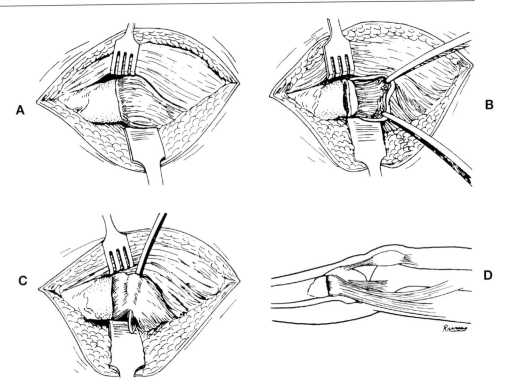

Fig. 33-173   Weber technique for removing soft tissue from proximal metaphyseal fracture. **A,** Exposure of fracture. **B** to **D,** Removal of pes anserinus and periosteum from fracture with periosteal elevator and forceps. (From Weber BG: Fractures of the proximal tibial metaphysis. In Weber BG, Brunner C, Freuler F, eds: *Treatment of fractures in children and adolescents,* New York, 1980, Springer-Verlag.)

casually. If vascular injury is suspected, an anterior compartment syndrome may be developing; then a soft tissue dressing should be applied instead of a circular cast, and the extremity should be monitored with a wick catheter or some other suitable compartment-pressure measuring device. If swelling is extreme and compartment syndrome is anticipated, an external fixator can be used to stabilize the fracture. The treatment of impending and established compartment syndromes is described elsewhere (Chapter 46).

The only indications for operative treatment of tibial and fibular fractures in a child are the following:

1. Fractures that cannot be managed by closed methods, such as those in a child with a head injury, although surgery for tibial and fibular fractures seems to be needed less frequently than for fractures of the femur.

2. Open tibial fractures, which should be treated as emergencies with irrigation and debridement. If soft tissue damage is extensive, an external fixator is used as in adults. Care should be taken not to cross the physis with pins when applying the fixator.

3. Nonunions of tibial fractures, which are rare in children and are probably more serious and more difficult to manage than in adults. We have treated several children with obvious nonunions of the tibia with no other pathological or congenital anomaly in whom internal fixation and bone grafting were required to achieve union (Fig. 33-174).

Cramer et al., in a report of 40 open diaphyseal fractures of the femur and tibia in children, refuted the general assumption that even grades II and III open diaphyseal fractures in children heal readily. Twenty-two fractures (55%) healed primarily, 12

(30%) had delayed union, and 3 (7.5%) were classified as nonunions. Three patients with Gustilo grade IIIC fractures had early amputation. Fifteen of their 40 patients (37.5%) had delayed unions or nonunions. Cramer et al. postulated that the same factors that predispose to these complications in adults (degree of displacement, comminution, soft tissue damage, and periosteal stripping) also contribute to delayed union and nonunion in children. In a study of 42 open tibial metaphyseal or diaphyseal fractures in children, Buckley et al. reported incidences of compartment syndrome, vascular injury, infection, and delayed union that were similar to those in adults. Two complications that occurred made this injury different in children: 4 developed angular deformities of more than 10 degrees, 3 of which corrected spontaneously, and 4 patients with severe fractures treated with external fixation had more than 1 cm of tibial overgrowth.

Hope and Cole reported 92 open tibial fractures in children and correlated their results with the Gustilo classification system. Extensive wounds (type III) were treated with external fixation and delayed wound closure, and less severe wounds (types I and II) were treated with primary wound closure and casting. Early complications included compartment syndrome, superficial and deep infection, delayed union, nonunion, and malunion. The incidences of these complications were similar to those reported by Cramer et al. At long-term follow-up continued pain at the fracture, restriction of sports activities, joint stiffness, cosmetic defects, and minor leg length discrepancies were common. Levy et al. noted in their series of 40 open tibial fractures that children surveyed missed an average of 4.1 months of school, and 33% had to repeat a year.

Hope and Cole concluded that open tibial fractures in

A   B   C   D   E

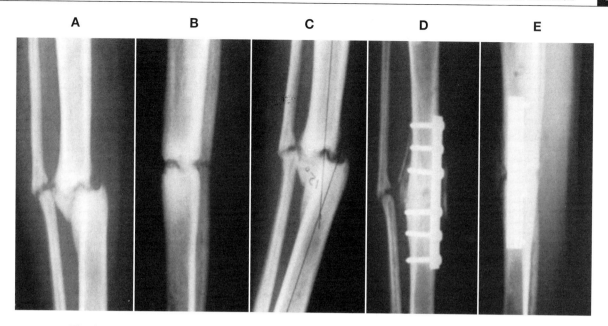

Fig. 33-174   Nonunion of tibia and fibula in child. **A** and **B,** Nonunion before treatment. **C,** Stress roentgenogram showing motion at fracture. **D** and **E,** Early union after bone grafting and compression plate fixation.

children are associated with high incidences of early and late complications, especially in those with Gustilo type III injuries, and that the Gustilo classification is useful for predicting outcome and planning treatment. Song et al. noted that children older than 11 years with open tibial fractures have nonunion and infection rates that parallel those of adult patients, but that younger children (younger than 6 years) have a more benign course. Studies by Buckley et al., Grimard et al., Blasier and Barnes, and Cullen et al. concur with these findings.

Rarely, intramedullary nailing may be indicated because of an inability to obtain or maintain reduction in an older child or for multiple pathological fractures in a younger child, such as occur in osteogenesis imperfecta or congenital pseudarthrosis of the tibia. The proximal and distal physes, if open, must be avoided. Intramedullary nailing has been reported to be successful in stabilizing severely comminuted tibial fractures so that union is obtained without angular deformity. If possible, closed techniques of nail insertion should be used, with a small incision over the fracture if necessary for adequate reduction of the fracture. Bailey-Dubow rods or larger intramedullary nails may be used, but the medullary canal of the tibia must be carefully measured, since the smallest commercially available intramedullary nail at present is 8 mm in diameter (Russell-Taylor Delta tibial nail).

DISTAL TIBIAL AND FIBULAR EPIPHYSEAL FRACTURES

Carothers and Crenshaw described the mechanism of injury of distal tibial physeal fractures using a classification of abduction, external rotation, and plantar flexion; adduction; and axial compression. Abduction, external rotation, and plantar

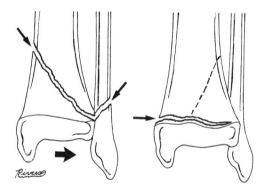

Fig. 33-175   Salter-Harris type II physeal fractures are produced by external rotation, abduction, and plantar flexion forces. (Redrawn from Ogden JA: *Skeletal injury in the child,* Philadelphia, 1982, Lea & Febiger.)

flexion frequently produce Salter-Harris type I or II physeal fractures (Fig. 33-175); adduction produces type III or IV fractures (Fig. 33-176); and axial compression produces type V fractures. Since this original study, we have reviewed 100 ankle fractures in children. The most common were Salter-Harris type II fractures (26). Type III fractures were more common than anticipated (19), and type I fractures (9) and type IV fractures (6) were relatively rare. Also studied were 6 triplane and 6 Tillaux fractures. The remaining were distal fibular fractures, and all were Salter-Harris type I or II except for one Salter-Harris type IV fracture. Most fractures of the fibular physis occur in conjunction with distal tibial fractures; Salter-Harris type III fractures usually are isolated injuries.

Fibular physeal fractures are treated for 3 to 6 weeks in a short leg cast. Salter-Harris types I and II fractures of the distal tibial physis usually are treated by closed reduction and the application of a bent-knee, long leg cast. In young children, moderate displacement after closed reduction, especially in the anteroposterior plane, can be accepted. However, varus or valgus angulation in older children with type I or II fractures will not correct spontaneously, and excessive angulation should not be accepted (Fig. 33-177). Because the foot tolerates these positions poorly, the result will be unacceptable. Two of our

patients had open reduction because such a deformity could not be reduced closed (Fig. 33-178).

Most Salter-Harris types III and IV fractures, as well as triplane and Tillaux fractures, require open reduction and internal fixation. The amount of displacement acceptable for closed treatment has not been defined. If after a closed reduction the surgeon believes that the amount of displacement can be reduced operatively, open reduction and internal fixation are justified (Fig. 33-179). Surgery has been recommended for 2 to 3 mm or more of displacement. However, as mentioned in the discussion of proximal tibial physeal and distal femoral physeal injuries, tomograms and CT scans are now being used, and standards for acceptable displacement using these techniques have not been refined or defined.

Salter-Harris types III and IV fractures are almost always medial and occur at the plafond, with the exception of Tillaux and triplane fractures. Quite often, a tiny triangular piece of bone is present on the metaphyseal side in the type IV fracture (Fig. 33-180). At the time of open reduction we, as do others, remove this piece of bone in an effort to see the physis better and to try to prevent the formation of a peripheral bony bridge in this area. As noted by Stanitski and Micheli, symptomatic ossification centers in the medial malleolus should not be mistaken for Salter-Harris type III fractures.

Kling et al. reported that in some types III and IV fractures fixed with pins—even smooth pins—that crossed the physis,

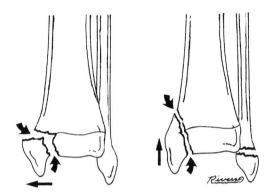

Fig. 33-176 Salter-Harris types III and IV fractures are produced by adduction forces (supination inversion). (Redrawn from Ogden JA: *Skeletal injury in the child*, Philadelphia, 1982, Lea & Febiger.)

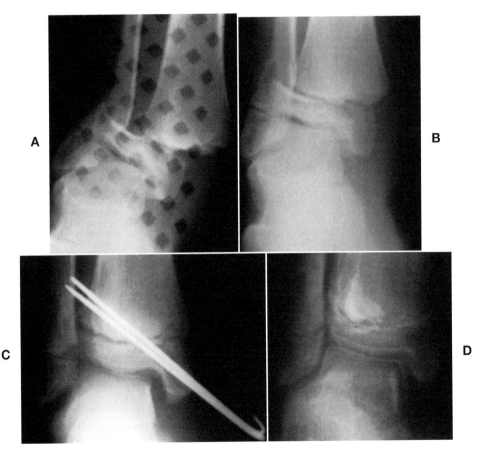

Fig. 33-177 Open reduction of Salter-Harris type I fracture. **A,** Before treatment. **B,** After closed reduction, residual angulation is 17 degrees in this older child. **C,** After open reduction and internal fixation with smooth pins, flap of periosteum was found caught in fracture. **D,** At early follow-up, no evidence of bony bridge is seen.

the physis closed prematurely by forming a bony bridge in the area where the pins crossed the plate. Thus it is best not to cross the physis with any kind of pin unless absolutely necessary for fixation.

The perichondral ring, according to Rang and to Weber and Sussenbach, can be avulsed in this area, just as from the distal femoral physis, from a minor fracture or ligamentous or other injury, and may cause peripheral growth arrest with resultant angular deformity.

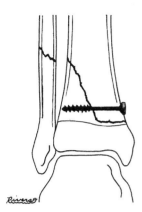

Fig. 33-178 Cancellous screw fixing large metaphyseal spike of Salter-Harris type II fracture. (Redrawn from Weber BG, Sussenbach F: Malleolar fractures. In Weber BG, Brunner C, Freuler F, eds: *Treatment of fractures in children and adolescents,* New York, 1980, Springer-Verlag.)

Of our 100 ankle fractures, the result was poor in 4 type III tibial injuries and 1 type IV tibial injury because of varus or valgus deformity secondary to growth arrest and in 1 type II tibial injury because of refracture. Supramalleolar osteotomy was necessary in 2.

Hynes and O'Brien, in a study of 26 Salter-Harris types II and III distal tibial physeal fractures, noted the development of a sclerotic line of growth disturbance that appeared 6 to 12 weeks after fracture, and they suggested that the likelihood of growth arrest can be determined from the presence and displacement of the line. In their series, if the line extended across the whole width of the metaphysis in both planes, and if the line continued to grow away from the physis remaining parallel to it, growth disturbance did not occur. Patients without this formation and displacement of the line had abnormal growth resulting in varus or valgus angulation. They pointed out that previous reports indicated that growth arrest cannot be determined before 18 months after injury, and they suggested that their method can predict function of the physis as early as 3 months after injury.

High-velocity motor vehicle accidents or lawn mower injuries often produce severe open ankle fractures. These injuries may involve the distal tibial physis, and a shearing fracture of the body of the talus also can be present. The result is physeal arrest and joint roughening. After an open fracture, infection can develop. External fixators can be used in the initial management until the wound is clean. Bony bridge resection may be necessary later, as well as osteotomy for angular deformity. If infection develops or joint involvement is

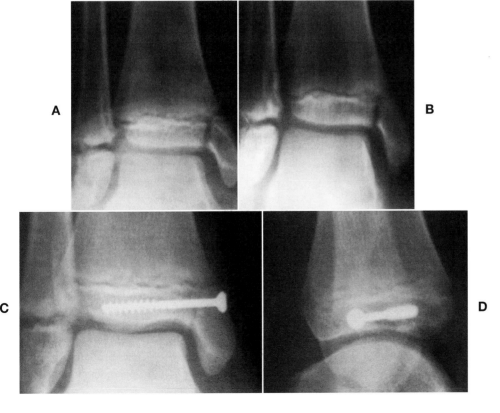

Fig. 33-179 **A** and **B,** Anteroposterior roentgenogram and tomogram of displaced Salter-Harris type III fracture of medial malleolus and Salter-Harris type I fracture of lateral malleolus. **C** and **D,** After open reduction and internal fixation of medial malleolar fracture with threaded screw through epiphysis.

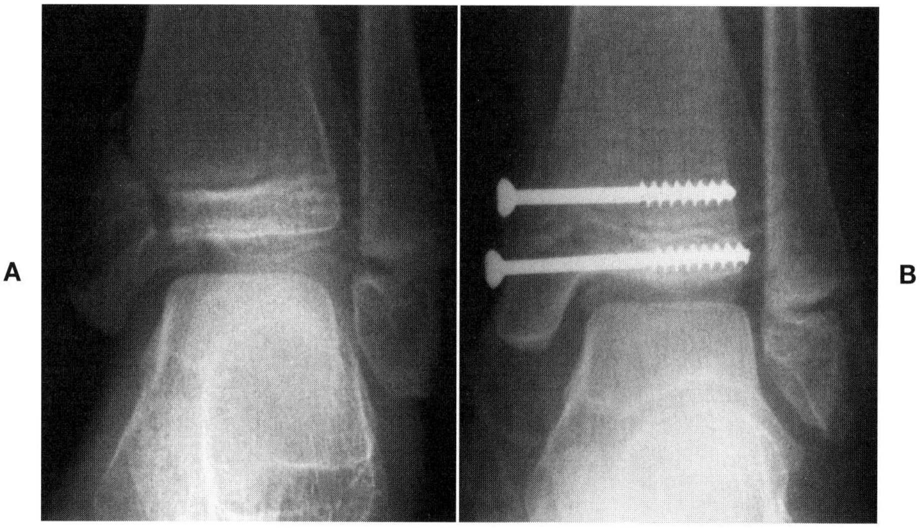

Fig. 33-180 **A,** Salter-Harris type IV fracture of medial malleolus. **B,** After open reduction and internal fixation with threaded cancellous screws in metaphysis and physis, avoiding physis.

severe, ankle fusion may be necessary (Fig. 33-181). At the time of fusion, the physis should be preserved and compression clamps should be used to hasten fusion. An interposed iliac bone graft, as described by Chuinard and Peterson for ankle fusion, can be used (Chapter 3).

◆ **Open Reduction and Internal Fixation**

TECHNIQUE 33-44

Place the patient supine on the operating table; prepare and drape in the usual fashion and use a tourniquet. Make a straight longitudinal incision over the medial malleolus, anteriorly and slightly laterally, for approximately 4 cm. Carry the soft tissue dissection down to the fracture. Clear all soft tissue from the area, but preserve the periosteum if possible. Gently expose the fracture. Remove any interposed soft tissue from within the fracture, especially periosteum and small bony fragments. Expose the ankle joint anteriorly, and with the aid of a bone holder, reduce the fracture anatomically. If the fracture is a Salter-Harris type IV with a small metaphyseal spike, remove the spike to better see the reduction and prevent a later bony bridge at the periphery. Insert small, parallel, smooth Steinmann pins horizontally across the fracture. Do not cross the physis unless necessary. Use a cannulated or cancellous screw if desired, making sure, however, that the threads do not damage the physis and the screw is horizontal across the fracture (Fig. 33-182). Check the reduction and pin or screw placement with roentgenograms. Reduce manually any fibular fracture, close the wound, and apply a long leg, bent-knee cast with the ankle in neutral position.

AFTERTREATMENT. Weight-bearing is not permitted for 4 to 6 weeks, depending on the age of the patient. Then a short leg, weight-bearing cast is worn for 3 weeks. The pins or screw can be removed at 6 to 8 weeks.

TRIPLANE FRACTURES

Triplane fractures are caused by an external rotational force and are considered a combination of Salter Harris types II and III fractures. Marmor first coined the term "triplane fracture of the distal part of the tibia" in 1970 in his description of lesions consisting of three fragments: (1) the anterolateral portion of the distal tibial epiphysis, (2) the remainder of the epiphysis (anteromedial and posterior portions) with an attached postero-lateral spike of the distal tibial metaphysis, and (3) the remainder of the distal tibial metaphysis and tibial shaft.

The triplane fracture has been reported by Dias and Giegerich to be a two-part rather than a three-part fracture. This fracture is caused by an external rotational force and, if a three-part fracture, is considered a combination of Salter-Harris types II and III fractures. If a two-part fracture, it is then a Salter-Harris type IV fracture (Figs. 33-183 and 33-184). Cooperman, Spiegel, and Laros and others have described the mechanism of injury and have suggested the use of tomograms to determine the amount of displacement. Rapariz et al. recommended CT scans because plain roentgenograms alone did not demonstrate the configuration of the fracture accurately. Usually closed reduction can be achieved by internal rotation of the foot and immobilization in a long leg cast. If a closed reduction cannot be achieved, open reduction and internal fixation are indicated. Rapariz et al. noted in 35 patients that when adequate reduction (less than 2 mm displacement) was not achieved, degenerative changes were seen at long-term follow-up. Because of the complex fracture pattern

A

B

C

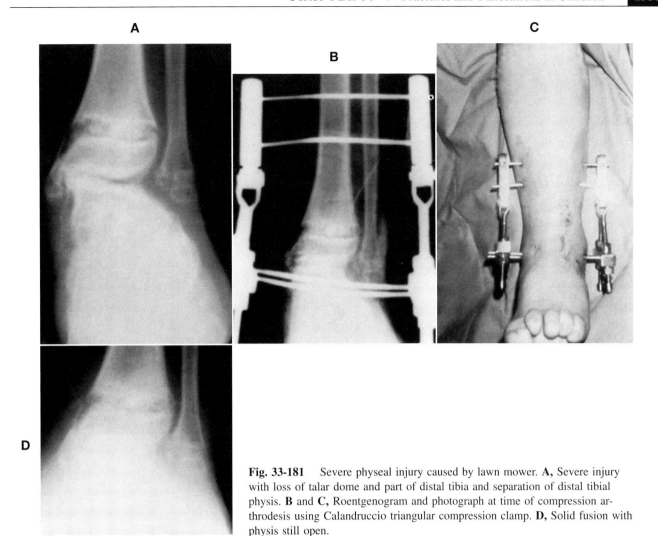

D

Fig. 33-181 Severe physeal injury caused by lawn mower. **A,** Severe injury with loss of talar dome and part of distal tibia and separation of distal tibial physis. **B** and **C,** Roentgenogram and photograph at time of compression arthrodesis using Calandruccio triangular compression clamp. **D,** Solid fusion with physis still open.

and large fragments, this fracture is not easy to reduce, and extensive dissection is quite often necessary to achieve reduction. If it is a three-part fracture, then open reduction of both the Salter-Harris type II and type III components may be necessary and adequate exposure is required.

Triplane fractures frequently occur in older children, and although physeal arrest and angular deformity can occur, they are rare.

The surgical technique for triplane fractures, according to Dias and Giegerich, depends on whether it is a two-part or a three-part fracture. Most two-fragment triplane fractures, according to them, can be treated by closed reduction. The closed reduction should be satisfactory because this is a Salter-Harris type IV fracture with possible joint incongruity and physeal arrest. When an open reduction of this intraarticular fracture is necessary, it usually is a three-part fracture. Unlike Dias and Giegerich, we approach the Salter-Harris type III component laterally first. If adequate open reduction can be achieved, the Salter-Harris type II component (medially) can be treated closed; if not, both components require open reduction.

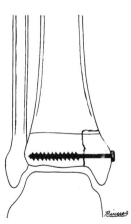

Fig. 33-182 Salter-Harris type III or IV fracture should be fixed by horizontal pins or cancellous bone screws not involving physis. (Redrawn from Weber BG, Sussenbach F: Malleolar fractures. In Weber BG, Brunner C, Freuler F, eds: *Treatment of fractures in children and adolescents*, New York, 1980, Springer-Verlag.)

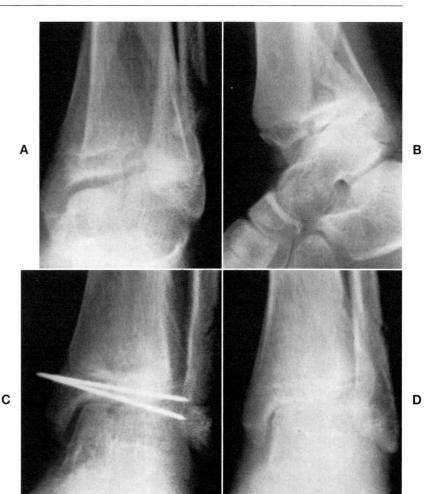

Fig. 33-183   Distal tibial triplane fracture. **A,** Anteroposterior view showing triplane fracture. **B,** Lateral view of fracture, Salter-Harris type IV (two parts of three-part fracture, type II plus type III). **C,** After open reduction and internal fixation. **D,** Satisfactory result at 2 years.

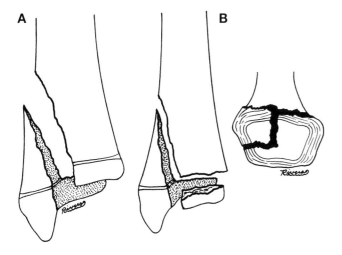

Fig. 33-184   A, Example of two-fragment triplane fracture, which is Salter-Harris type IV fracture. **B,** Example of three-fragment triplane fracture, consisting of Salter-Harris types II and III fractures. (Redrawn from Rockwood CA Jr, Wilkins KE, King RE, eds: *Fractures in children*, Philadelphia, 1984, JB Lippincott.)

◆ Open Reduction and Internal Fixation

TECHNIQUE 33-45 *(Dias and Giegerich)*

Make a medial longitudinal incision over the distal metaphyseal area of the tibia down to the ankle joint. Expose the fracture fragments but do not resect any periosteum. Examine the fracture gap and make sure that no periosteum is inverted into it. Reduce the metaphyseal fragment. If the reduction is not anatomical, do not use internal fixation at this time but proceed to the lateral fragment. However, if the reduction is satisfactory, insert two cancellous screws parallel and transverse across the metaphyseal fragment. The triplane fracture has now been converted to a Tillaux fracture, or a Salter-Harris type III fracture laterally. Make an anterolateral longitudinal incision, expose the lateral fragment, and reduce it anatomically, making sure no periosteum is caught within the fracture. Insert smooth pins transversely across the fracture, or use a cancellous bone screw making sure the threads do not

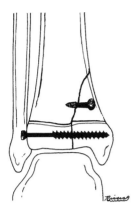

Fig. 33-185 Example of triplane fracture with medial metaphyseal spike and lateral Tillaux fracture both fixed with transverse screws.

damage the physis (Fig. 33-185). Confirm the reduction by inspecting the joint. Also confirm the reduction and the placement of the pins by roentgenograms. Close the wounds and apply a long leg cast.

AFTERTREATMENT. Weight-bearing is not permitted for 8 weeks. At 6 weeks the long leg cast is removed, and a short leg, non-weight-bearing cast is applied. The pins are removed at 8 weeks if necessary.

TILLAUX FRACTURE

A special fracture occurring in older adolescents was originally described by Tillaux. The mechanism of injury is an external rotational force with stress placed on the anterior tibiofibular ligament, causing avulsion of the distal tibial physis anterolaterally (Fig. 33-186). This occurs after the medial part of the physis has closed (Fig. 33-187) but before the lateral part closes. The resultant fracture through the physis runs across the epiphysis and distally into the joint, creating a Salter-Harris type III or IV fracture. Open reduction and internal fixation are indicated if the fracture is displaced (Fig. 33-188). We have treated six of these fractures: two were basically undisplaced and healed uneventfully, two had prompt open reduction and internal fixation, and two displaced fractures had open reduction and internal fixation because of delayed union.

The fracture fragment, because it is pulled off by the anterior tibiofibular ligament, is almost always anterior and the fibula need not be osteotomized or "taken down" to expose the fracture fragment. In one child, using the Gatellier approach (Chapter 1), we osteotomized the fibula and, while pulling it distally, created a Salter-Harris type I fracture at the distal fibular physis. This approach should be avoided in children, and it is unnecessary here because the fracture can be seen

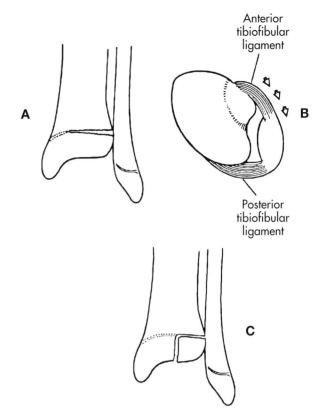

Fig. 33-186 Mechanism of injury in Tillaux fracture. **A,** Physis in older child closing medially but still open laterally. **B,** External rotational force causes anterior tibiofibular ligament to avulse physis anterolaterally. **C,** Avulsion produces Salter-Harris type III fracture because medial part of physis is closed. (From Rang M: *Children's fractures*, ed 2, Philadelphia, 1983, JB Lippincott.)

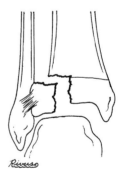

Fig. 33-187 Tillaux fracture. See Fig. 33-186 for mechanism of injury. (Redrawn from Weber BG, Sussenbach F: Malleolar fractures. In Weber BG, Brunner C, Freuler F, eds: *Treatment of fractures in children and adolescents*, New York, 1980, Springer-Verlag.)

adequately anteriorly. Lintecum and Blasier described approaching the ankle through an anterior arthrotomy to accurately manipulate and reduce a fracture. They then placed rigid fixation percutaneously from medial or lateral under fluoroscopic control.

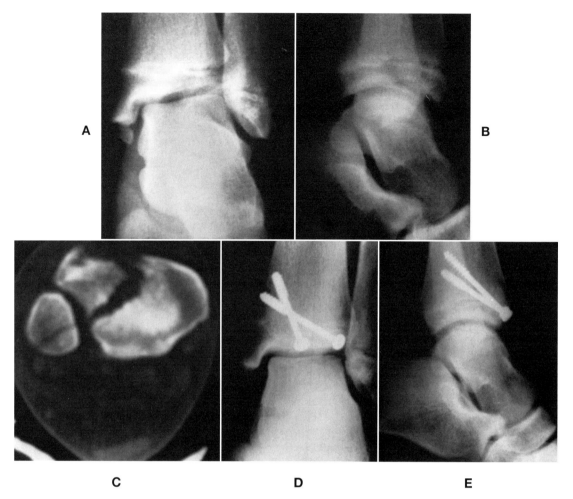

Fig. 33-188   Tillaux fracture. **A** and **B,** Seemingly undisplaced Tillaux type of Salter-Harris type III fracture. **C,** CT scan revealing significant displacement. **D** and **E,** After satisfactory open reduction and internal fixation.

◆ Open Reduction and Internal Fixation

TECHNIQUE 33-46

Expose the type III or IV fracture anterolaterally through a 6-cm anterolateral incision. Gently clean and observe the fracture fragments. Take care not to disrupt the periosteum but remove it from within the fracture. Then use a bone holder to gently reduce the fracture. Check the reduction by examining the fragment in the ankle joint. Insert two smooth pins parallel or a small cancellous screw transversely across the fracture but not penetrating the physis. Check the reduction with roentgenograms, close the wound, and apply a long leg cast with the knee bent.

AFTERTREATMENT. Weight-bearing is prohibited for 6 to 10 weeks, and any subcutaneous smooth pins should be removed at 4 to 6 weeks, depending on the age of the child.

◆ Percutaneous Reduction and Internal Fixation

Schlesinger and Wedge described a technique for percutaneous reduction and fixation of Tillaux fractures that appears to be satisfactory when closed treatment fails to restore the articular surface. We prefer a cannulated screw rather than a Kirschner wire when using this technique.

TECHNIQUE 33-47 *(Schlesinger and Wedge)*

With the patient under general anesthesia, perform a closed reduction of the fracture with the aid of image intensification. Apply (but do not inflate) a tourniquet to the lower extremity to be used if the closed reduction fails and open reduction is necessary. Prepare and drape the foot and ankle in the usual manner. Mark the skin midway between the anterior border of the lateral malleolus and peroneus tertius overlying the anteroinferior talofibular ligament (Fig. 33-189, *A*). With the aid of image intensification, insert

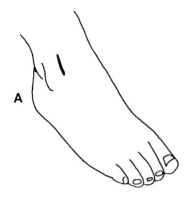
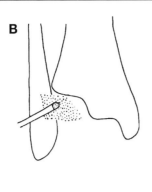
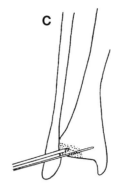

Fig. 33-189 Percutaneous reduction and fixation of displaced Tillaux fracture. **A,** Skin incision. **B,** Steinmann pin used to reduce fracture. **C,** While fracture is held reduced with pin, Kirschner wire is inserted in fragment and across fracture. (Redrawn from Schlesinger I, Wedge JH: *J Pediatr Orthop* 13:389, 1993.)

a 2-mm Steinmann pin into the fracture fragment and use it to manipulate the fragment into place (Fig. 33-189, *B*). Confirm reduction with image intensification. If reduction is satisfactory, insert a 1.6-mm Kirschner wire centrally in the fragment across the fracture (Fig. 33-189, *C*). Again, check the reduction with image intensification. If satisfactory, remove the Steinmann pin, leave the Kirschner wire protruding through the skin or bury it just beneath the skin, close the wounds, and apply a short leg weight-bearing cast.

AFTERTREATMENT. The cast is worn for 6 to 8 weeks. The pin is removed at the time of cast removal.

PERITALAR DISLOCATIONS

Dimentberg and Rosman reported peritalar dislocations in five adolescents, four of whom had acceptable functional results. They noted that this rare injury usually occurs in adolescents near skeletal maturity and that its natural history is similar to that of peritalar dislocations in adults. They recommended closed reduction initially, with open reduction indicated if the closed reduction is unsuccessful or if diagnosis has been delayed.

Foot Fractures

TALAR FRACTURES

Talar Neck Fractures

Fractures of the talus comprise three basic types: (1) fractures of the neck, (2) fractures of the body and dome, and (3) transchondral (osteochondral) fractures. We (Canale and Kelley) reviewed 71 fractures of the neck of the talus, 12 of which were in children. Most of the 12 were in older children.

It is important to be aware of the retrograde blood supply, which is present in a sling fashion around the talar head and neck. This blood supply enters the bone in three main ways: (1) through the neck, (2) through the foramina in the sinus tarsi

and tarsal canal, and (3) deep into the foramina in the medial surface of the body. We use the fracture classification proposed by Hawkins, which is based on the amount of disruption of the blood supply to the talus. A type I lesion is a fracture through the neck of the talus with minimal displacement and minimal damage to the blood supply of the talus, theoretically damaging only one vessel, the one entering through the neck. In type II lesions the subtalar joint is subluxated or dislocated and at least two of the three sources of blood supply are lost, that through the neck and that entering the tarsal canal and sinus tarsi. King described a talar neck fracture in which avascular necrosis of only the lateral portion of the neck and dome of the talus occurred, with no evidence of avascular necrosis on the medial side. This probably occurred because the blood supply through the foramina into the medial surface of the body was spared. In type III lesions the body of the talus is dislocated from the tibia and from the calcaneus, and all three of the sources of blood supply are disrupted. The incidence of avascular necrosis is high in type III fractures.

We have described a type IV fracture that is not related to the blood supply, in which the body of the talus is dislocated or subluxated at the subtalar joint, the body of the talus is dislocated at the ankle joint, the talar neck is fractured, and the head of the talus is dislocated at the talonavicular joint. Most of the fractures in our series were type I, II, or III.

We use the treatment recommended by Boyd and Knight. Closed reduction followed by non-weight-bearing is the preferred treatment for type I mildly or moderately displaced fractures. If an adequate reduction cannot be obtained or maintained, open reduction and internal fixation are recommended. A reduction of less than 5 mm of displacement and less than 5 degrees of malalignment is considered adequate. Most of the closed reductions are carried out on type I fractures. In types II, III, and IV fractures, open reduction with or without internal fixation is used frequently because of the difficulty of maintaining an adequate reduction by closed methods in significantly displaced fractures. Open fractures are treated by irrigation and debridement, and internal fixation is carried out only if required for stability of reduction. The wounds are left open. The 12 children in our series were treated in this manner.

Varus malalignment is a frequent problem. A special

roentgenographic technique is used to determine the amount of varus angulation in the anteroposterior plane. A cassette is placed directly under the foot, and the ankle is placed in maximal equinus position, the usual position after reduction of the fracture of the talar neck. This position can be maintained more easily by maximal flexion of the hip and knee. The foot is then pronated 15 degrees and the roentgen tube is directed cephalad at a 75-degree angle from the horizontal tabletop. This technique has enabled us to detect any offset or varus deformity of the head and neck of the talus.

For open reduction an anteromedial approach is used, retracting the neurovascular bundle laterally. Fixation is usually with a cancellous screw from a medial to a lateral direction. As an alternative, a cancellous lag screw can be inserted percutaneously from posterior to anterior.

Complications include avascular necrosis of the talar body, malunion, traumatic arthritis of the ankle and subtalar joint, and infection.

A subchondral lucency present 12 weeks after injury (Hawkins line) is an indication that avascular necrosis will not occur, but this is not an absolute prognosticator. Conversely, lack of a subchondral lucency at 3 months is indicative that avascular necrosis has occurred (Fig. 33-190), and bone scanning may show decreased uptake, also indicative of avascular necrosis (Fig. 33-191).

We evaluated all patients, children and adults, for a Hawkins line to determine early if avascular necrosis was present. Avascular necrosis did not occur in any patient in whom a Hawkins line was present. A large percentage of patients in whom a Hawkins line was absent at 12 weeks developed avascular necrosis. However, a few patients who were only immobilized for a short time did not have a Hawkins line and did not develop avascular necrosis. Not all the patients who developed avascular necrosis required operative treatment. Some did quite satisfactorily with patellar tendon-bearing braces. Of the 12 children, avascular necrosis developed in five, and all five healed uneventfully. The avascular process in these children was different from that in adults. They developed a sclerotic lesion in the dome and body of the talus that became a cystic lesion on roentgenograms; over a 2- to 3-year period the area resolved, and all but one at long-term follow-up were asymptomatic (Fig. 33-192). Obviously most children with avascular necrosis will not require surgery, and consequently a prolonged period of either non-weight-bearing or the use of a patellar tendon–bearing, weight-relieving brace should be tried before surgery is considered.

Malunions of talar fractures were frequent in adults; however, only 2 of the 12 children had malunion. Malunion usually occurs with the distal fragment dorsiflexed or in a varus position and with the fibula rotated more anteriorly than normal. Most of our adult patients bore an excessive amount of weight on the lateral side of the foot, and many developed traumatic arthritis in the ankle and subtalar joint. As yet, no children have had this problem.

One child had an open talar neck fracture and developed significant drainage and infection. Persistent drainage from an

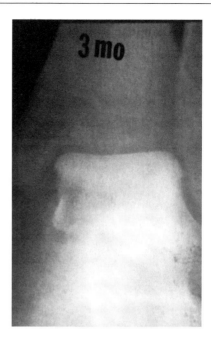

Fig. 33-190   Hawkins line is not visible in sclerotic (latent avascular necrosis) talar dome 3 months after injury.

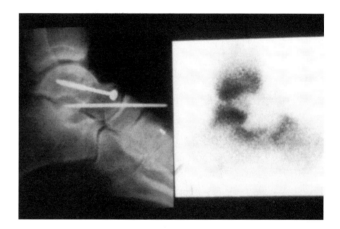

Fig. 33-191   Bone scan 8 days after open reduction of type IV talar neck fracture with talonavicular dislocation shows decreased uptake indicating area of avascular necrosis.

infection here can be a problem. Because the talus is composed almost entirely of cancellous bone, and because fracture through the neck may seriously disrupt the blood supply, an established osteomyelitis of the talus may be resistant to treatment. Repeated sequestrectomy or attempted excision and drainage of the sinus tract are not indicated in established osteomyelitis of the talus. The results of talectomy without fusion have been poor. The preferred treatment for fractures of the talus complicated by infection is excision of the affected bone followed by arthrodesis, even in children. Operations, when necessary for avascular necrosis, malunion, or infection, include triple arthrodesis (Chapter 31), ankle fusion (Chapter 3), Blair fusion (Chapter 55), and talocalcaneal fusion

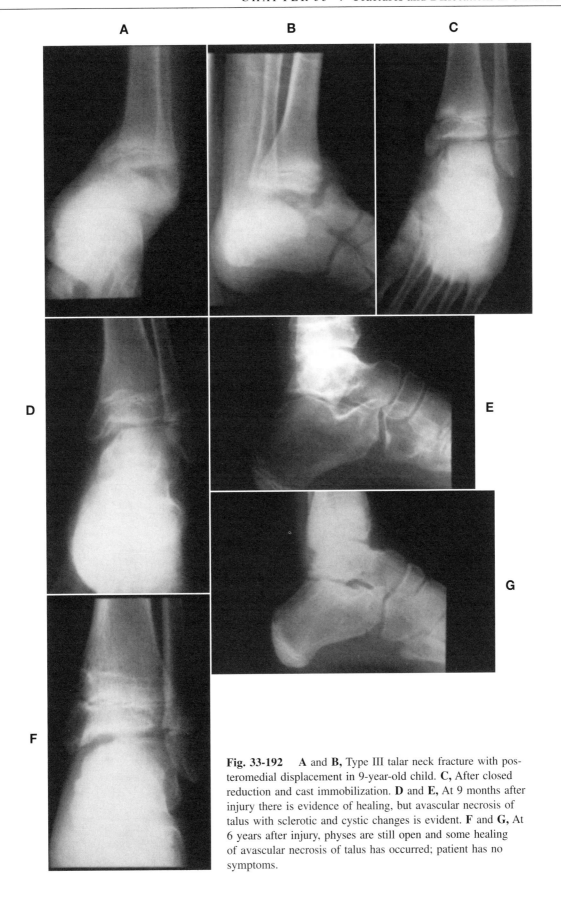

Fig. 33-192 **A** and **B,** Type III talar neck fracture with posteromedial displacement in 9-year-old child. **C,** After closed reduction and cast immobilization. **D** and **E,** At 9 months after injury there is evidence of healing, but avascular necrosis of talus with sclerotic and cystic changes is evident. **F** and **G,** At 6 years after injury, physes are still open and some healing of avascular necrosis of talus has occurred; patient has no symptoms.

(Chapter 3), all of which produce better results than talectomy alone.

Fractures of Dome and Body of Talus

Fractures of the dome and body of the talus are rare in children but do occur in shearing injuries, especially lawn mower, bicycle spoke, and "degloving" injuries. Often severe, open shearing injuries from lawn mowers and other power equipment require excision of a portion of the talus. The wound should be irrigated, debrided, and left open; delayed closure and skin grafting, if necessary, are performed later. The primary goal of treatment is to salvage as much length and function of the foot and ankle as possible. A large, nondisplaced, closed talar dome or body fracture can be treated satisfactorily by closed methods, especially in a child, and good results can be expected. If the fracture is significantly displaced, is intraarticular, and has cancellous bone attached to the fragment, open reduction and internal fixation through an anteromedial approach (Chapter 1) usually are necessary. Only rarely is osteotomy of the medial malleolus necessary for exposure.

Care should be taken to avoid the physis in this area. Oblique or transverse cancellous screws inserted across the body of the talus, usually without medial malleolar osteotomy, are all that is necessary. Smaller displaced fragments often can be removed and handled in much the same manner as osteochondral fragments.

Osteochondral Fractures of Talus

We (Canale and Belding) reviewed 31 osteochondral lesions of the talus in 29 patients treated at this clinic. Because symptoms began in the second decade of life in 21 patients, we believe this to be a lesion of adolescence progressing into early adulthood. We used the classification of Berndt and Harty: stage I, a small area of subchondral compression; stage II, a partially detached fragment; stage III, a completely detached fragment remaining in the crater; and stage IV, a fragment that is detached and also loose in the joint (Fig. 33-193).

Of the lesions 14 were medial, 15 were lateral, and 2 were central. Most patients, especially the adolescents, were treated initially by immobilization in a cast (approximately 12 weeks);

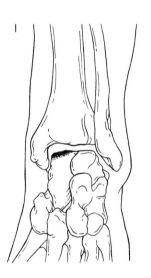
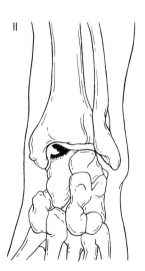
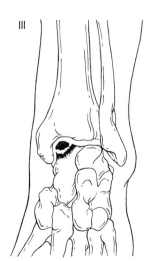
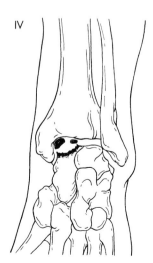

Fig. 33-193   Four types or stages of osteochondral fractures (osteochondritis dissecans of talus). Stage I, "blister"; stage II, elevated fragment but attached; stage III, fragment detached but still in crater; stage IV, displaced fragment.

double, upright, patellar tendon–bearing braces; arch supports; or leather, lace-up ankle corsets. The patients' symptoms were then reevaluated.

Almost all the lateral lesions were caused by trauma. Morphologically the lateral lesions were thin and wafer shaped and resembled osteochondral fractures. Conversely, although most patients with medial lesions had been injured, in some no history of trauma could be elicited; two older women had bilateral medial lesions unrelated to trauma. Most of the medial lesions were deep and morphologically cup shaped, not resembling a traumatic fracture (Fig. 33-194).

In our patients any operation was performed because of persistent symptoms or a loose body in the ankle joint. Fifteen of the lesions ultimately required surgery, most of them lateral stage III or IV lesions. Stage I and II lesions were treated successfully without operation. The results of nonoperative treatment of stage III medial lesions compared favorably with the results of surgical treatment; most were asymptomatic after conservative treatment. Conversely, lateral stage III lesions had better results after surgical excision than after conservative treatment. Several stage III lateral lesions did not heal, and traumatic arthritis developed after nonoperative treatment. Stage IV lesions, with the fragment loose in the joint, did well after surgery. Thus we recommend operative treatment of stage III lateral lesions and all stage IV lesions; all stages I and II lesions and stage III medial lesions can be observed for healing, especially in young children and adolescents.

Histological findings were analyzed; although morphologically the lesions were wafer shaped on the lateral side and cup shaped on the medial side, histologically they were the same. We could not definitely say that the lateral lesions were osteochondral fractures and the medial lesions were true osteochondritis dissecans. The lateral lesions had more persistent symptoms and degenerative changes than the medial lesions and required surgery more often.

Three technical operative points should be made:

1. If the osteochondral fragment appears on roentgenograms to be floating in its crater and riding high, with a flake of bone proximally that appears to be in the joint, then the fragment probably is inverted in the crater. This means that the subchondral bone is proximal in the ankle joint, and the cartilaginous portion is in the crater (Fig. 33-195). In this position the cartilaginous fragment will not heal to the bone in the crater, and excision is indicated. This elevated, apparently "floating" fragment is pathognomonic of an inverted fragment within the craters.

2. It is difficult on lateral roentgenograms to locate either a medial or lateral lesion and to determine whether it is anterior, in the middle, or posterior. We have solved this problem by the use of a CT scan in the coronal (axial) plane. Coronal sections through the dome and body of the talus reveal the exact location of the lesion and help in planning the surgical approach (Fig. 33-196).

3. Because the fibula is more posterior than the medial malleolus, osteotomy rarely is needed to reach the lateral lesions. However, if a CT scan shows the medial lesion to be in the middle or posterior part of the talus, a medial malleolar osteotomy often is necessary in skeletally mature patients. We osteotomize the medial malleolus at the plafond horizontally or obliquely. The malleolus should be predrilled to accept a cancellous screw. The malleolar fragment can be displaced with a towel clip, and the lesion is seen quite readily.

We have replaced several large fragments and held them with subchondral pins (Fig. 33-197), similar to the technique described for osteochondritis dissecans of the knee (Chapter 43). The short-term results have been variable.

The lesions in types I, II, and III are often difficult to see at surgery and can only be palpated or "ballotted" to determine its

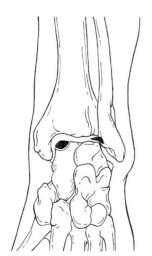

Fig. 33-194   Morphology of medial and lateral lesions (see text).

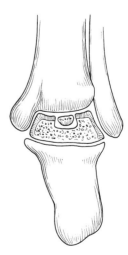

Fig. 33-195   "Floating" fragment in reality is loose fragment turned upside-down in crater.

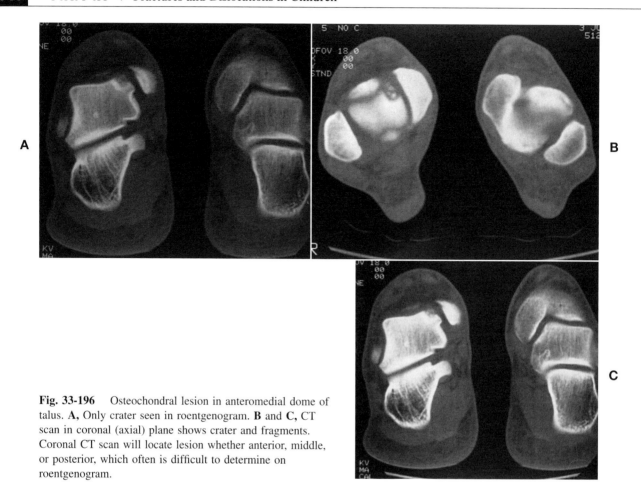

Fig. 33-196 Osteochondral lesion in anteromedial dome of talus. **A,** Only crater seen in roentgenogram. **B** and **C,** CT scan in coronal (axial) plane shows crater and fragments. Coronal CT scan will locate lesion whether anterior, middle, or posterior, which often is difficult to determine on roentgenogram.

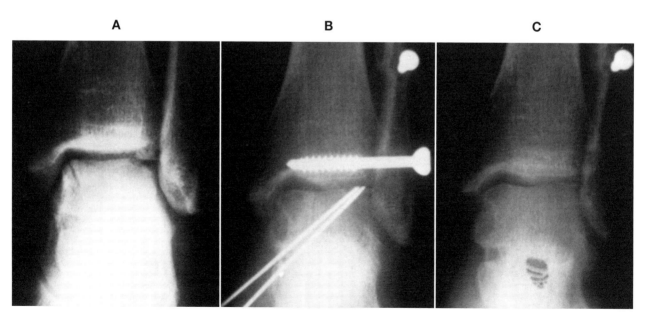

Fig. 33-197 **A,** Large osteochondral fragment in lateral talus. **B,** After retrograde pinning of fragment; osteotomy of malleolus was performed for better exposure. **C,** Healed lesion after removal of syndesmosis screw.

location. Using a Keith needle or a hemostat to "ballotte" helps outline the extent of the lesion. Arthroscopy has been used, but it is difficult to find and define the margins of occult lesions (see discussion of arthroscopy of the ankle joint in Chapter 48). Ferkel et al. and others have described the technique of arthroscopic excision of osteochondral lesions of the talus, and Parisien reported 88% good or excellent results in 18 patients.

◆ **Excision of Osteochondral Fragment of Talus**

TECHNIQUE 33-48

If osteotomy of the medial malleolus is necessary, surgery on the medial side should be delayed until after closure of the physis. Place the patient supine. Make a longitudinal incision 7 cm long over the anteromedial aspect of the ankle. Be sure to place the incision far enough medially to allow an osteotomy of the medial malleolus to be made if necessary and to allow inspection of the medial aspect of the joint. Carry the soft tissue dissection down to the ankle joint; retract the neurovascular bundle, the tibialis anterior tendon, and the common extensor tendons. Incise the capsule and expose the ankle joint. Plantar flex the foot as much as possible to try to see the lesion. If the lesion is posterior, an osteotomy usually is necessary. Predrill for a cancellous screw from distal to proximal through the medial malleolus into the distal tibia and remove the screw. Then make an osteotomy obliquely across the medial malleolus at the ankle joint level perpendicular to the predrilled hole for the cancellous screw. With a towel clip, turn the medial malleolus distally. Evert the ankle until the medial and posterior aspects of the talar dome can be seen. Ballotte for any occult lesion with a Keith needle; with a small curet remove the central necrotic area and determine the margins of the lesion. The fragment often is loose and the subchondral bone is yellowish and hard. Remove the crater and the fragment and copiously irrigate the joint; then with a small drill make four or five holes in the subchondral crater for vascular ingrowth. Realign the medial malleolar osteotomy and insert a cancellous bone screw in the predrilled hole. Take roentgenograms to check for anatomical alignment of the screw and the osteotomy, close the wound in layers, and apply a short leg cast.

AFTERTREATMENT. The patient should wear a cast or patellar tendon–bearing brace for 10 to 12 weeks, preferably non-weight-bearing, while fibrocartilaginous tissue in the crater fills in the defect.

CALCANEAL FRACTURES

Calcaneal fractures are rare in children. They differ from calcaneal fractures in adults because (1) they occur much less frequently; (2) they do not exhibit the same fracture patterns, having less intraarticular involvement; (3) they are less serious

because of the elasticity of structures in children; and (4) they will remodel (Fig. 33-198). Schmidt and Weiner reported 62 calcaneal fractures in children, which they classified using a system similar to that of Essex-Lopresti (Chapter 86). They included physeal fractures at the tuberosity and a fracture almost unique to children that involves the posterior aspect of the calcaneus with significant loss of bone that occurs in lawn mower injuries. Of the fractures 63% were extraarticular, and only 37% were intraarticular, which is the reverse of the adult fracture pattern. Displacement of the intraarticular fractures was minimal compared with adult fractures, and only two required open reduction and internal fixation. However, in several older children, the subtalar joint was obviously involved and incongruous, similar to the Essex-Lopresti type II fracture, with a decreased "crucial" angle and the presence of a joint compression fracture. Open fractures of the calcaneus occur more often in children than in adults, probably because of the increased incidence of lawn mower injuries.

Schmidt and Weiner reported that because displacement is uncommon in both extraarticular and intraarticular fractures, most calcaneal fractures in children can be expected to heal without any functional loss. According to them the prognosis in calcaneal fractures in children is good, unless a lawn mower injury results in loss of bone and soft tissue from the heel.

Harris views (ski-jump views) of the heel should be obtained, and a CT scan can be helpful, since the diagnosis can be obscure because of minimal disturbance in the bony architecture and the high percentage of cartilage in the calcaneus of children compared with adults. Operative treatment of calcaneal fractures in children is not indicated unless subtalar joint disruption is significant. A CT scan is mandatory in preoperative surgical planning. Stress fractures of the calcaneus have been reported in children, and a bone scan may be helpful in making the diagnosis. Trott noted that cysts in the triangular space of the calcaneus can become large enough for ordinary activities to produce stress or pathological fractures.

TARSAL FRACTURES

Fractures of the tarsal bones are uncommon in children because of the flexibility of the foot. Fractures especially of the navicular, cuboid, or cuneiform bones usually are part of a severe injury to the foot, such as a wringer, severe compression, or lawn mower injury. Wiley described 19 tarsometatarsal joint injuries in adults and children. He pointed out that the second metatarsal is the cornerstone of the foot and that strong ligamentous attachments are present between the metatarsals themselves and between the cuneiforms. The most relevant anatomical features are the fixed mortise position of the base of the second metatarsal and the ligamentous attachments at this base. If there is a fracture of the base of the second metatarsal, with or without a "buckle" fracture of the cuboid, significant tarsometatarsal joint injury, although occult, has occurred. Treatment recommendations included closed reduction for gross displacement or instability, with open reduction only rarely required. However, because of inherent instability

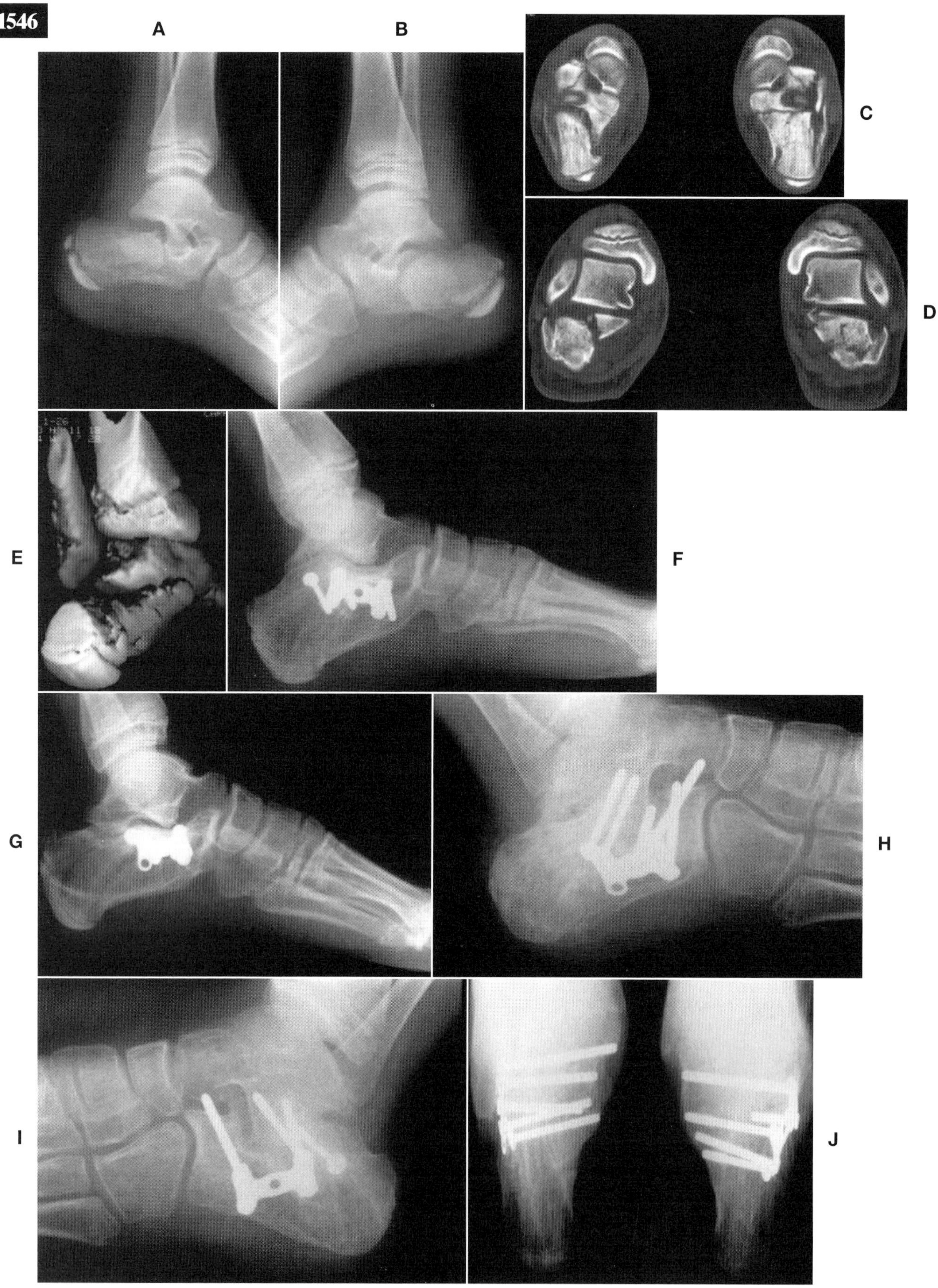

A

B

C

D

E

F

G

H

I

J

Fig. 33-198   A and B, Lateral roentgenograms of bilateral severe calcaneal fractures with depression of crucial angle in child who also had T12 compression fracture from a fall. C and D, CT scan at two different levels, revealing severe comminution and displacement. E, Three-dimensional reconstruction of lateral calcaneal fractures, bilaterally. F and G, Lateral roentgenograms after open reduction and internal fixation with contour plates and screws. H to J, Bilateral oblique and anteroposterior roentgenograms at follow-up.

percutaneous Kirschner wire fixation was used to maintain the reduction and the alignment after open or closed reduction. The wires were removed after approximately 4 weeks. In all of his patients, the reduction was maintained in the presence of known intraarticular fractures of the tarsometatarsal joints, and some inherent joint incongruity was accepted. At review, 4 of the 19 patients had persistent discomfort at fractures or fracture-dislocations of the tarsometatarsal joint; in most of these the discomfort was minor and present only during strenuous activity. Two patients with poor results had persistent angular deformity because of an incomplete reduction. From Wiley's results, it appears that some of these fractures with intraarticular components will heal if the incongruity is not severe; however, a subluxation or dislocation will not remodel. In our experience a persistent dorsal dislocation, even in the child, will produce a painful hypertrophic osseous area on the dorsum of the foot. Also, varus angulation often is present. Therefore, with the patient under general anesthesia, any dislocated tarsometatarsal joints should be reduced. If this cannot be accomplished closed, then open reduction and internal fixation of the dislocation are indicated (Fig. 33-199). Care should be taken not to violate the proximal physis of the first metatarsal.

Johnson described a pediatric Lisfranc fracture, calling it a "bunk bed" fracture. This fracture of the first tarsometatarsal area produces a subtle deformity that can be overlooked. Often, a fracture-dislocation or a fracture-subluxation of the first tarsometatarsal joint occurs, or the first and second metatarsals may be involved (Fig. 33-200). According to him the injury occurs from a twisting force when the foot is extended, such as on a bunk bed, and the soft tissue injury is more severe than is indicated by the bony injury seen on the roentgenograms.

METATARSAL AND PHALANGEAL FRACTURES

Trott and Gross both reported that metatarsal and phalangeal fractures in the child are fairly common. However, little has been written about these fractures. Perhaps this is because they usually heal uneventfully and rarely need operative treatment. Because of their strong interosseous ligaments, fractures of the proximal metatarsals usually do not become displaced significantly. Displaced fractures usually are produced by severe trauma. In addition to the fractures, the soft tissues usually are damaged considerably and swelling may be excessive. These severe injuries should be treated by elevation and observation and not by a circumferential cast. Once the swelling has resolved, a displaced fracture can be reduced closed, if necessary, by longitudinal traction. For severe trauma producing multiple fractures with significant displacement, once the swelling has subsided, open reduction and smooth pin fixation are performed if necessary. This is occasionally needed in the first metatarsal of older children, where little remodeling can be expected (Fig. 33-201). Most displaced fractures of the metatarsal neck heal and usually remodel nicely in young children; however, if displacement and deformity are significant, especially in the anteroposterior plane, and multiple neck fractures are present, then occasionally open reduction and internal fixation with longitudinal wires are necessary, especially in older children.

Stress fractures of the metatarsal shaft or neck occur in children. Bone scan may be helpful in diagnosis, and these fractures should be treated expectantly. We have seen a child as young as 10 years of age with a metatarsal stress fracture, and although they occur less frequently in children than in adults, they can be produced by chronic repetitive, stressful activity.

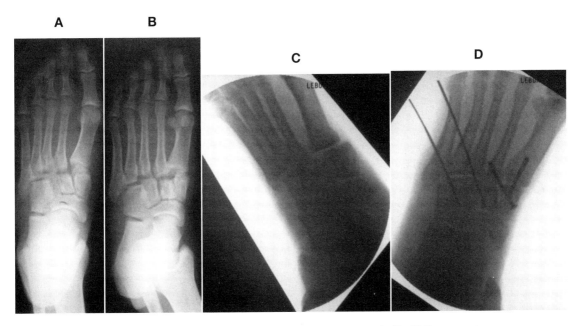

A   B   C   D

Fig. 33-199   **A,** Anteroposterior roentgenogram appears normal. **B,** Oblique roentgenogram reveals subtle subluxation of the metatarsocuneiform joint. **C,** At surgery image intensification reveals extent of involvement. **D,** Open and percutaneous reduction and fixation of Lisfranc dislocation. Physis of first metatarsal is closed.

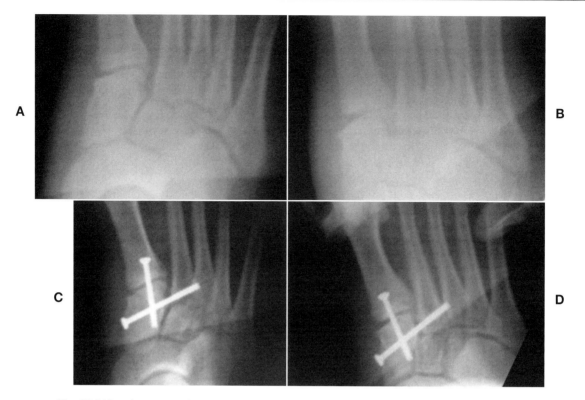

Fig. 33-200   Anteroposterior and stress roentgenograms of foot with subtle Lisfranc dislocation. **A,** Roentgenogram appears normal. **B,** With stress into everted position, metatarsals sublux laterally. **C,** Postreduction roentgenogram reveals satisfactory reduction and internal fixation. **D,** Reduction maintained on eversion stress roentgenogram.

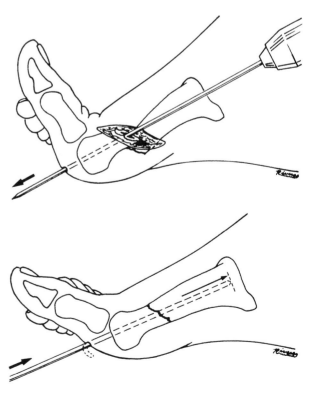

Fig. 33-201   Method of open pinning of metatarsal shaft or neck fractures in retrograde fashion through first metatarsal head. (Redrawn from Cehner J: Fractures of the tarsal bones, metatarsals, and toes. In Weber BG, Brunner C, Freuler F, eds: *Treatment of fractures in children and adolescents*, New York, 1980, Springer-Verlag.)

Fractures of the base of the fifth metatarsal have traditionally, in both children and adults, been called the Jones fracture. Kavanaugh et al. reviewed 22 Jones fractures, 16 of which were in older adolescents. They also reviewed Robert Jones' original description from 1896 and concluded that what he described was a diaphyseal fracture rather than an avulsion fracture of the base of the fifth metatarsal caused by overpull of the peroneus brevis muscle. Most of their fractures were stress fractures and were not caused by inversion and overpull of the peroneus brevis. They noted the uncertainty of healing of this diaphyseal fracture and suggested that in high-performance athletes, recreational athletes, and even nonathletes with delayed union, open reduction and internal fixation with a medullary screw be carried out. Avulsions of the most proximal base of the fifth metatarsal also occur in children and heal uneventfully, except for some bony hypertrophy at the fracture site.

Fractures of the phalanges are caused primarily by hitting a hard object or compressing the toe with a heavy weight. Dislocations usually are dorsal and can be reduced quite easily. Certain developmental disorders of the phalanges should not be confused with fractures. Lyritis pointed out that fragmentation of the proximal epiphysis of the hallux occurs quite frequently (Fig. 33-202). The epiphysis may be fissured, compressed, or fragmented. Usually the physis is not fractured.

Both fractures and dislocations of the phalanges should be reduced by longitudinal traction, and held by "buddy" taping to the next toe. Open reduction and internal fixation are only rarely indicated. If fracture of a phalanx is caused by a penetrating wound, as in stepping on a nail, *Pseudomonas* infection should be suspected. If the wound becomes infected, it should be irrigated and debrided, and intravenous antibiotic therapy should be administered. As Trott noted, for infected phalangeal fractures, debridement, wet dressing, intravenous administration of antibiotics, and delayed closure will save some toes, especially the great toe, when impending infection or gangrene has suggested amputation. Severe open fractures occur in the forefoot and the phalanges primarily in bicycle spoke or rotary lawn mower injuries. The treatment consists of adequate debridement of the wounds, leaving the wounds open, and delayed closure. The operative treatment of these injuries is similar to that for the digits of adults (Chapter 64).

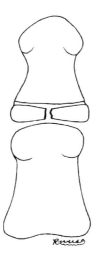

Fig. 33-202   Fissuring of physis of proximal phalanx of great toe; this is not a fracture. (Redrawn from Lyritis G: *Skeletal Radiol* 10:250, 1983.)

References

PHYSEAL INJURIES
Aitken AT: Fractures of the epiphysis, *Clin Orthop* 41:19, 1965.
Birch JG, Herring JA, Wenger DR: Surgical anatomy of selected physes, *J Pediatr Orthop* 4:224, 1984.
Blount WP: *Fractures in children*, Baltimore, 1955, Williams & Wilkins.
Böstman O, Mäkelä EA, Södergård J, et al: Absorbable polyglycolide pins in internal fixation of fractures in children, *J Pediatr Orthop* 13:242, 1993.
Boyd HB, Altenberg AR: Fractures about the elbow in children, *Arch Surg* 49:213, 1944.
Bright RW: Operative correction of partial epiphyseal plate closure by osseous ridge resection and silicone rubber implant, *J Bone Joint Surg* 56A:655, 1974.
Bright RW: Partial growth arrest: identification, classification, and results of treatment, *Orthop Trans* 6:65, 1982 (abstract).
Canale ST, Russell RA, Holcomb RL: Percutaneous epiphysiodesis: experimental study and preliminary clinical results, *J Pediatr Orthop* 6:150, 1986.
Carlson WO, Wenger DR: A mapping method to prepare for surgical excision of a partial physeal arrest, *J Pediatr Orthop* 4:232, 1984.
Chadwick CJ, Bentley G: The classification and prognosis of epiphyseal injuries, *Injury* 18:157, 1987.
Currey JD, Butler G: Mechanical properties of bone tissues in children, *J Bone Joint Surg* 57A:810, 1975.
Golz RJ, Grogan DP, Greene TL, et al: Distal ulnar physeal injury, *J Pediatr Orthop* 11:318, 1991.
Green WT, Anderson M: Skeletal age in the control of limb growth, *Instr Course Lect* 17:199, 1960.
Gustilo RB, Simpson L, Nixon R, et al: An analysis of 511 open fractures at Hennepin County General Hospital, *J Bone Joint Surg* 52A:830, 1968.
Holland CT: A radiologic note on injuries to the distal epiphyses of the radius and ulna, *Proc R Soc Med* 22:695, 1929.
Karaharju EO, Ryöppy SA, Makiner RJ: Remodeling by asymmetrical epiphyseal growth, *J Bone Joint Surg* 58B:122, 1976.
Kling TF Jr, Bright RW, Hensinger RN: Distal tibial physeal fractures in children that may require open reduction, *J Bone Joint Surg* 66A:647, 1984.
Langenskiöld A: Surgical treatment of partial closure of the growth plate, *J Pediatr Orthop* 1:3, 1981.
Loder RT, Bookout C: Fracture patterns in battered children, *J Orthop Trauma* 5:428, 1991.
Mann DC, Rajmaira S: Distribution of physeal and nonphyseal fractures in 2650 long-bone fractures in children aged 0-16 years, *J Pediatr Orthop* 10:713, 1990.
Martin RP, Parsons DL: Avascular necrosis of the proximal humeral epiphysis after physeal fracture, *J Bone Joint Surg* 79A:760, 1997.
Mendez AA, Bartal E, Grillot MB, Lin JJ: Compression (Salter-Harris type V) physeal fracture: an experimental model in the rate, *J Pediatr Orthop* 12:29, 1992.
Moseley CF: A straight-line graph for leg-length discrepancies, *J Bone Joint Surg* 59A:174, 1977.
Ogden JA: *Skeletal injury in the child*, Philadelphia, 1982, Lea & Febiger.
Peterson HA: Partial growth arrest and its treatment, *J Pediatr Orthop* 4:246, 1984.
Peterson HA: Physeal fractures. 2. Two previously unclassified types, *J Pediatr Orthop* 14:431, 1994.
Peterson HA: Physeal fractures. 3. Classification, *J Pediatr Orthop* 14:439, 1994.
Peterson HA, Burkhart SS: Compression injury of the epiphyseal growth plate: fact or fiction? *J Pediatr Orthop* 1:377, 1981.
Peterson HA, Madhok R, Benson JT, et al: Physeal fractures. 1. Epidemiology in Omsted County, Minnesota, 1979-1988, *J Pediatr Orthop* 14:423, 1994.

Phemister D: Operative assessment of longitudinal growth of bones in the treatment of deformities, *J Bone Joint Surg* 15:1, 1933.

Poland J: *Traumatic separation of the epiphyses*, London, 1898, Smith, Elder.

Poland J: Traumatic separation of the epiphysis in general, *Clin Orthop* 41:7, 1965.

Pritchett JW: Growth plate activity in the upper extremity, *Clin Orthop* 268:235, 1991.

Rang M: *The growth plate and its disorders*, Baltimore, 1969, Williams & Wilkins.

Ray TD, Tessler RH, Dell RC: Traumatic ulnar physeal arrest after distal forearm fractures in children, *J Pediatr Orthop* 16:195, 1996.

Salter RB, Harris WR: Injuries involving the epiphyseal plate, *J Bone Joint Surg* 45A:587, 1963.

Smith BG, Rand F, Jaramillo D, Shapiro F: Early MR imaging of lower-extremity physeal fracture-separations: a preliminary report, *J Pediatr Orthop* 14:526, 1994.

Weber BG, Brunner C, Freuler F, eds: *Treatment of fractures in children and adolescents*, New York, 1980, Springer-Verlag.

COMPOUND AND PATHOLOGICAL FRACTURES

Cheng JCY, Ng BKW, Ying SY, Lam PKW: A 10-year study of the changes in pattern and treatment of 6493 fractures, *J Pediatr Orthop* 19:344, 1999.

Fee NF, Dobranski A, Bisla RS: Gas gangrene complicating open forearm fractures: report of five cases, *J Bone Joint Surg* 59A:135, 1977.

Robertson P, Karol LA, Rab GT: Open fractures of the tibia and femur in children, *J Pediatr Orthop* 16:621, 1996.

Roy DR, Crawford AH: Operative management of fractures of the shaft of the radius and ulna, *Orthop Clin North Am* 21:245, 1990.

Skaggs DL, Kautz SM, Kay RM, Tolo VT: Effect of delay of surgical treatment on rate of infection in open fractures in children, *J Pediatr Orthop* 20:19, 2000.

Song KM, Sangeorzan B, Benirschke S, Browne R: Open fractures of the tibia in children, *J Pediatr Orthop* 16:635, 1996.

Walker RN, Green NE, Spindler KP: Stress fractures in skeletally immature patients, *J Pediatr Orthop* 16:578, 1996.

HAND AND WRIST FRACTURES, DISLOCATIONS, AND FRACTURE-DISLOCATIONS

Abram LJ, Thompson GH: Deformity after premature closure of the distal radial physis following a torus fracture with a physeal compression injury: report of a case, *J Bone Joint Surg* 69A:1450, 1987.

Barton NJ: Fractures of the phalanges of the hand in children, *Hand* 2:134, 1979.

Beatty E, Light TR, Belsole RJ, Ogden JA: Wrist and hand skeletal injuries in children, *Hand Clin* 6:723, 1990.

Blount WP: *Fractures in children*, Baltimore, 1955, Williams & Wilkins.

Brundy M: Fractures of the carpal scaphoid in children, *Br J Surg* 56:523, 1969.

Campbell RM: Operative treatment of fractures and dislocations of the hand and wrist region in children, *Orthop Clin North Am* 21:217, 1990.

Coonrad RW, Pohlman MH: Impacted fractures in the proximal portion of the proximal phalanx of the finger, *J Bone Joint Surg* 51A:1291, 1969.

Crick JC, Franco RS, Conner JJ: Fractures about the interphalangeal joints in children, *J Orthop Trauma* 1:318, 1988.

Cullen JC: Thiemann's disease: osteochondrosis juvenilis of the basal epiphyses of the phalanges of the hand—report of two cases, *J Bone Joint Surg* 52B:532, 1970.

Dameron TB: Traumatic dislocation of the distal radioulnar joint, *Clin Orthop* 83:55, 1972.

Dixon GL Jr, Moon NF: Rotational supracondylar fractures of the proximal phalanx in children, *Clin Orthop* 83:151, 1972.

Dykes RG: Kirner's deformity of the little finger, *J Bone Joint Surg* 60B:58, 1978.

Eaton RG: *Joint injuries of the hand*, Springfield, Ill, 1971, Charles C Thomas.

Farabeuf LHF (as quoted by Barnard HL): Dorsal dislocation of the first phalanx of the little finger: reduction by Farabeuf's dorsal incision, *Lancet* 1:88, 1901.

Gamble JG, Simmons SC: Bilateral scaphoid fractures in a child, *Clin Orthop* 162:125, 1982.

Gerard FM: Post-traumatic carpal instability in a young child, *J Bone Joint Surg* 62A:131, 1980.

Green DP: Hand injuries in children, *Pediatr Clin North Am* 24:903, 1977.

Green DP, Terry GC: Complex dislocation of the metacarpophalangeal joint, *J Bone Joint Surg* 55A:1480, 1973.

Greene MH, Hadied AM, LaMont RL: Scaphoid fractures in children, *J Hand Surg* 9A:536, 1984.

Greene WB, Anderson WJ: Simultaneous fracture of the scaphoid and radius in a child: case report, *J Pediatr Orthop* 2:191, 1982.

Griffiths JC: Bennett's fracture in childhood, *Br J Clin Pract* 20:582, 1966.

Kaplan EB: Dorsal dislocation of the metacarpophalangeal joint of the index finger, *J Bone Joint Surg* 39A:1081, 1957.

Lascombes P, Prevot J, Ligier JN, et al: Elastic stable intramedullary nailing in forearm shaft fractures in children: 85 cases, *J Pediatr Orthop* 10:167, 1990.

Leonard MH: Open reduction of fractures of the neck of the proximal phalanx in children, *Clin Orthop* 116:176, 1976.

Letts M, Esser D: Fractures of the triquetrum in children, *J Pediatr Orthop* 13:228, 1993.

Mann DC, Rajmaira S: Distribution of physeal and nonphyseal fractures in 2650 long-bone fractures in children aged 0-16 years, *J Pediatr Orthop* 10:713, 1990.

Matthews MG: Correspondence. The image intensifier as an operating table: a dangerous practice, *J Bone Joint Surg* 82B:774, 2000.

Maxted MJ, Owen R: Two cases of non-union of carpal scaphoid fractures in children, *Injury* 13:441, 1982.

McLaughlin HL: Complex locked dislocation of the metacarpal phalangeal joints, *J Trauma* 5:683, 1965.

Mintzer CM, Waters PM: Surgical treatment of pediatric scaphoid fracture nonunions, *J Pediatr Orthop* 19:236, 1999.

Nafie SAA: Fractures of the carpal bones in children, *Injury* 18:117, 1987.

O'Brien ET: Fractures of the hand and wrist region. In Rockwood CA Jr, Wilkins KE, King RE, eds: *Fractures in children*, Philadelphia, 1984, JB Lippincott.

Peiro A, Martos F, Mut T, Aracil J: Trans-scaphoid perilunate dislocation in a child: a case report, *Acta Orthop Scand* 52:31, 1981.

Perona PG, Light TR: Remodeling of the skeletally immature distal radius: a case report and review of the literature, *J Orthop Trauma* 4:356, 1990.

Rang M: *The growth plate and its disorders*, Baltimore, 1969, Williams & Wilkins.

Rasmussen LB: Kirner's deformity: juvenile spontaneous incurving of the terminal phalanx of the fifth finger, *Acta Orthop Scand* 52:35, 1981.

Salter RB, Harris WR: Injuries involving the epiphyseal plate, *J Bone Joint Surg* 45A:587, 1963.

Santoro V, Mara J: Compartmental syndrome complicating Salter-Harris type II distal radius fracture, *Clin Orthop* 223:226, 1988.

Segmüller G, Schöenberger F: Fractures of the hand. In Weber BG, Bruner C, Freuler F, eds: *Treatment of fractures in children and adolescents*, New York, 1980, Springer-Verlag.

Southcott R, Rosman MA: Nonunion of carpal scaphoid fractures in children, *J Bone Joint Surg* 59B:20, 1977.

Stahl S, Jupiter JB: Salter-Harris type III and IV epiphyseal fractures in the hand treated with tension-band wiring, *J Pediatr Orthop* 19:233, 1999.

Stark HH: Troublesome fractures and dislocations of the hand, *Instr Course Lect* 19:130, 1970.

Stühmer KG: Fractures of the distal forearm. In Weber BG, Bruner C, Freuler F, eds: *Treatment of fractures in children and adolescents*, New York, 1980, Springer-Verlag.

Vahvanen V, Westerlund M: Fracture of the carpal scaphoid in children: a clinical and roentgenographical study of 108 cases, *Acta Orthop Scand* 51:909, 1980.

Waseem M, Kenny NW: The image intensifier as an operating table—a dangerous practice, *J Bone Joint Surg* 82B:95, 2000.

Watson-Jones R: *Fractures and joint injuries*, ed 4, Baltimore, 1960, Williams & Wilkins.

Wood VE: Fractures of the hand in children, *Orthop Clin North Am* 7:527, 1976.

FOREARM FRACTURES

Aitken AP: The end results of the fractured distal radial epiphysis, *J Bone Joint Surg* 17:302, 1935.

Albert SM, Wohl MA, Rechtman AM: Treatment of the disrupted radio-ulnar joint, *J Bone Joint Surg* 45A:1373, 1963.

Almquist EE, Gordon LH, Blue AI: Congenital dislocation of the head of the radius, *J Bone Joint Surg* 51A:1118, 1969.

Alpar EK, Thompson K, Owen R, Taylor J: Midshaft fractures of forearm bones in children, *Injury* 13:153, 1981.

Aminian A, Schoenecker PL: Premature closure of the distal radial physis after fracture of the distal radial metaphysis, *J Pediatr Orthop* 15:395, 1995.

Bado JL: *The Monteggia lesion*, Springfield, Ill, 1962, Charles C Thomas.

Bado JL: The Monteggia lesion, *Clin Orthop* 50:71, 1967.

Barquet A, Caresani J: Fracture of the shaft of ulna and radius with associated dislocation of the radial head, *Injury* 12:471, 1980.

Bell Tawse AJ: The treatment of malunited anterior Monteggia fractures in children, *J Bone Joint Surg* 47B:718, 1965.

Blount WP: Forearm fractures in children, *Clin Orthop* 51:93, 1967.

Borden S: Roentgen recognition of acute plastic bowing of the forearm in children, *Am J Roentgenol* 125:524, 1975.

Boyd HB: Surgical exposure of the ulna and proximal third of the radius through one incision, *Surg Gynecol Obstet* 71:86, 1940.

Boyd HB, Boals JC: The Monteggia lesion: a review of 159 cases, *Clin Orthop* 66:94, 1969.

Bruce HE, Harvey JP Jr, Wilson JC Jr: Monteggia fractures, *J Bone Joint Surg* 56A:1563, 1974.

Campbell C, Waters MP, Emans JB: Excision of the radial head for congenital dislocation, *J Bone Joint Surg* 74A:726, 1992.

Cullen MC, Roy DR, Giza E, Crawford AH: Complications of intramedullary fixation of pediatric forearm fractures, *J Pediatr Orthop* 18:14, 1998.

Currey JD, Butler G: The mechanical properties of bone tissue in children, *J Bone Joint Surg* 57A:810, 1975.

Dameron TB: Traumatic dislocation of the distal radio-ulnar joint, *Clin Orthop* 83:55, 1972.

Daruwalla JS: A study of radioulnar movements following fracture of the forearm in children, *Clin Orthop* 139:114, 1979.

Fahmy NRM: Unusual Monteggia lesions in children, *Injury* 12:399, 1980.

Flynn JM, Waters PM: Single-bone fixation of both bone forearm fractures, *J Pediatr Orthop* 16:655, 1996.

Friberg KSI: Remodeling after distal forearm fractures in children. I. The effect of residual angulation on the spatial orientation of the epiphyseal plates, *Acta Orthop Scand* 50:537, 1979.

Friberg KSI: Remodeling after distal forearm fractures in children. II. The final orientation of the distal and proximal epiphyseal plates of the radius, *Acta Orthop Scand* 50:731, 1979.

Friberg KSI: Remodeling after distal forearm fractures in children. III. Correction of residual angulation in fractures of the radius, *Acta Orthop Scand* 50:741, 1979.

Fuller DJ, McCullough CJ: Malunited fractures of the forearm in children, *J Bone Joint Surg* 64B:364, 1982.

Galeazzi R: Di una particulare sindrome: traumatica delle sheletro dell avambraccio, *Attie Mem Soc Lombardi di Chir* 2:12, 1934.

Gupta RP, Danielsson LG: Dorsally angulated solitary metaphyseal greenstick fractures in the distal radius: results after immobilization in pronated, neutral, and supinated position, *J Pediatr Orthop* 10:90, 1990.

Hirayama T, Takemitsu Y, Yagihara K, Mikata A: Operation for chronic dislocation of the radial head in children: reduction by osteotomy of the ulna, *J Bone Joint Surg* 69B:639, 1987.

Holdsworth BJ, Sloan JP: Proximal forearm fractures in children: residual disability, *Injury* 14:174, 1982.

Holmes JR, Louis DS: Entrapment of pronator quadratus in pediatric distal-radius fractures: recognition and treatment, *J Pediatr Orthop* 14:498, 1994.

Hurst LC, Dubrow EN: Surgical treatment of symptomatic chronic radial head dislocation: a neglected Monteggia fracture, *J Pediatr Orthop* 3:227, 1983.

Irani RN, Ziegler RW, Petrucelli RC, O'Hara AE: Ulnar lengthening for negative ulnar variance in hereditary multiple exostoses, *Orthop Trans* 6:350, 1982.

Jessing P: Monteggia lesions and their complicating nerve damage, *Acta Orthop Scand* 46:601, 1975.

Jones K, Weiner DS: The management of forearm fractures in children: a plea for conservatism, *J Pediatr Orthop* 19:811, 1999.

King RE: Fractures of the shafts of the radius and ulna. In Rockwood CA Jr, Wilkins KE, King RE, eds: *Fractures in children*, Philadelphia, 1984, JB Lippincott.

Landfried MJ, Stenclik M, Susi JG: Variant of Galeazzi fracture-dislocation in children, *J Pediatr Orthop* 11:332, 1991.

Lascombes P, Prevot J, Ligier JN, et al: Elastic stable intramedullary nailing in forearm shaft fractures in children: 85 cases, *J Pediatr Orthop* 10:167, 1990.

Lee SB, Esterhai JL, Das M: Fracture of the distal radial epiphysis, *Clin Orthop* 185:90, 1984.

Letts M, Locht R, Weins J: Monteggia fracture-dislocations in children, *J Bone Joint Surg* 67B:724, 1985.

Lichter RL, Jacobsen T: Tardy palsy of posterior interosseous nerve with a Monteggia fracture, *J Bone Joint Surg* 57A:124, 1975.

Lloyd-Roberts GC, Bucknill TM: Anterior dislocation of the radial head in children, *J Bone Joint Surg* 59B:402, 1977.

Luhmann SJ, Gordon JE, Schoenecker PL: Intramedullary fixation of unstable both bone forearm fractures in children, *J Pediatr Orthop* 18:451, 1998.

Mabrey JD, Fitch RD: Plastic deformation in pediatric fractures: mechanism and treatment, *J Pediatr Orthop* 9:310, 1989.

McFarland B: Congenital dislocation of the head of the radius, *Br J Surg* 24:41, 1936.

Mikic ZD: Galeazzi fracture-dislocation, *J Bone Joint Surg* 57A:107, 1975.

Milch H: Roentgenographic diagnosis of torsional deformities in tubular bones, *Surgery* 15:440, 1944.

Monteggia GB: *Instit Chirurg* 5:130, 1814 (Translated by Helen Rang).

Müller J, Roth B, Willenegger H: Long-term results of epiphyseal fractures to the distal radius treated by percutaneous wire fixation. In Chapchal G, ed: *Fractures in children*, New York, 1981, Georg Thieme Verlag.

Nelson CA, Buchanan JR, Harrison CS: Distal ulnar growth arrest, *J Hand Surg* 9A:164, 1984.

Nielson AB, Simonsen O: Displaced forearm fractures in children treated with plates, *Injury* 15:393, 1984.

Nimityongskul P, Anderson LD, Sri P: Plastic deformation of the forearm: a review and case reports, *J Trauma* 31:1678, 1991.

O'Brien ET: Fractures of the hand and wrist region. In Rockwood CA Jr, Wilkins KE, King RE, eds: *Fractures in children*, Philadelphia, 1984, JB Lippincott.

Ogden JA: *Skeletal injury in the child*, Philadelphia, 1982, Lea & Febiger.

Onley BW, Menelaus MB: Monteggia and equivalent lesions in childhood, *J Pediatr Orthop* 9:219, 1989.

Ortega R, Loder RT, Louis DS: Open reduction and internal fixation of forearm fractures in children, *J Pediatr Orthop* 16:651, 1996.

Peiro A, Andres F, Fernandez-Esteve F: Acute Monteggia lesions in children, *J Bone Joint Surg* 59A:92, 1977.

Price CT, Scott DS, Kurzner ME, Flynn JC: Malunited forearm fractures in children, *J Pediatr Orthop* 10:705, 1990.

Rang MC: *Children's fractures*, ed 2, Philadelphia, 1983, JB Lippincott.

Ray TD, Tessler RH, Dell PC: Traumatic ulnar physeal arrest after distal forearm fractures in children, *J Pediatr Orthop* 16:195, 1996.

Reckling FW: Unstable fracture-dislocations of the forearm (Monteggia and Galeazzi lesions), *J Bone Joint Surg* 64A:857, 1982.

Richter D, Ostermann PA, Ekkernkamp A, et al: Elastic intramedullary nailing: a minimally invasive concept in the treatment of unstable forearm fractures in children, *J Pediatr Orthop* 18:457, 1998.

Salter RB, Harris WR: Injuries involving the epiphyseal plate, *J Bone Joint Surg* 45A:587, 1963.

Sanders WE, Heckman JD: Traumatic plastic deformation of the radius and ulna, *Clin Orthop* 188:58, 1984.

Shoemaker SK, Comstock CDP, Mubarak SJ, et al: Intramedullary Kirschner wire fixation of open or unstable forearm fractures in children, *J Pediatr Orthop* 19:329, 1999.

Speed JS, Boyd HB: Treatment of fractures of the ulna with dislocation of the head of the radius (Monteggia fracture), *JAMA* 115:1900, 1940.

Spinner M, Freundlich BD, Teicher J: Posterior interosseous nerve palsy as a complication of Monteggia fractures in children, *Clin Orthop* 58:141, 1968.

Stanitski CL, Micheli LS: Simultaneous ipsilateral fractures of the arm and forearm in children, *Clin Orthop* 153:218 1980.

Stein F, Grabias SL, Deffer PA: Nerve injuries complicating Monteggia lesions, *J Bone Joint Surg* 53A:1432, 1971.

Stühmer M: Fractures of the distal forearm. In Weber BG, Bruner C, Freuler F, eds: *Treatment of fractures in children and adolescents*, New York, 1980, Springer-Verlag.

Theodorou SD, Ierodiaconou MN, Roussis N: Fracture of the upper end of the ulna associated with dislocation of the head of the radius in children, *Clin Orthop* 228:240, 1988.

Thompson JL: Acute plastic bowing of bone, *J Bone Joint Surg* 64B:123, 1982.

Treadwell SJ, van Peteghem K, Clough MP: Pattern of forearm fractures in children, *J Pediatr Orthop* 4:604, 1984.

Vainionpää S, Böstman O, Pätiälä H, Rokkanen P: Internal fixation of forearm fractures in children, *Acta Orthop Scand* 58:121, 1987.

Van der Reis WL, Otsuka NY, Moroz P, and Mah J: Intramedullary nailing versus plate fixation for unstable forearm fractures in children, *J Pediatr Orthop* 18:9, 1998.

Verstreken L, Delronge G, Lamoureux J: Shaft forearm fractures in children: intramedullary nailing with immediate motion: a preliminary report, *J Pediatr Orthop* 8:450, 1988.

Vesely DG: Isolated traumatic dislocations of the radial head in children, *Clin Orthop* 50:31, 1967.

Vince KG, Miller JE: Cross-union complicating fracture of the forearm. II. Children, *J Bone Joint Surg* 69A:654, 1987.

Vittas D, Larsen E, Torp-Pedersen S: Angular remodeling of midshaft forearm fractures in children, *Clin Orthop* 265:261, 1991.

Voto SJ, Weiner DS, Leighley B: Redisplacement after closed reduction of forearm fractures in children, *J Pediatr Orthop* 10:79, 1990.

Voto SJ, Weiner DS, Leighley B: Use of pins and plaster in the treatment of unstable pediatric forearm fractures, *J Pediatr Orthop* 10:85, 1990.

Vrsansky P, Bourdelat D, Al Faour A: Flexible stable intramedullary pinning technique in the treatment of pediatric fractures, *J Pediatr Orthop* 20:23, 2000.

Walker JL, Rang M: Forearm fractures in children: cast treatment with the elbow extended, *J Bone Joint Surg* 73B:299, 1991.

Walsh HPJ, McLaren CAN, Owen R: Galeazzi fractures in children, *J Bone Joint Surg* 69B:730, 1987.

Weber BG, Brunner C, Frueler F, eds: *Treatment of fractures in children and adolescents*, New York, 1980, Springer-Verlag.

Wiley JJ, Galey JP: Monteggia injuries in children, *J Bone Joint Surg* 67B:728, 1985.

Wiley JJ, Pegington J, Horwich JP: Traumatic dislocation of the radius at the elbow, *J Bone Joint Surg* 56B:501, 1974.

Wyrsch B, Mencio GA, Green NE: Open reduction and internal fixation of pediatric forearm fractures. *J Pediatr Orthop* 16:644, 1996.

Young S, Letts M, Jarvis J: Avascular necrosis of the radial head in children, *J Pediatr Orthop* 20:15, 2000.

Zehntner MK, Jakob RP, McGanity PLJ: Growth disturbance of the distal radial epiphysis after trauma: operative treatment by corrective radial osteotomy, *J Pediatr Orthop* 10:411, 1990.

ELBOW JOINT FRACTURES AND DISLOCATIONS

Abe M, Ishizu T, Nagaoka T, Onomura T: Epiphyseal separation of the distal end of the humeral epiphysis: a follow-up note, *J Pediatr Orthop* 15:426, 1995.

Amillo S, Mora G: Surgical management of neural injuries associated with elbow fractures in children, *J Pediatr Orthop* 19:573, 1999.

Angelov A: A new method for treatment of the dislocated radial neck fracture in children. In Chapchal G, ed: *Fractures in children*, New York, 1981, Georg Thieme Verlag.

Beaty JH: Fractures and dislocations about the elbow in children, *Instr Course Lect* 41:373, 1992.

Bell SM, Morrey BF, Bianco AJ Jr: Chronic posterior subluxation and dislocation of the radial head, *J Bone Joint Surg* 73A:392, 1991.

Bernstein SM, McKeever P, Bernstein L: Percutaneous reduction of displaced radial neck fractures in children, *J Pediatr Orthop* 13:85, 1993.

Beverly HC, Fearn CB: Anterior interosseous nerve palsy and dislocation of the elbow, *Injury* 16:126, 1984.

Blatz DJ: Anterior dislocation of the elbow, *Orthop Rev* 10:129, 1981.

Blount WP: *Fractures in children*, Baltimore, 1955, Williams & Wilkins.

Boyd HB, Altenberg AR: Fractures about the elbow in children, *Arch Surg* 49:213, 1944.

Brodeur AE, Silberstein MJ, Graviss ER: *Radiology of the pediatric elbow*, Boston, 1981, GK Hall Medical.

Cappellino A, Wolfe SW, Marsh JS: Use of a modified Bell Tawse procedure for chronic acquired dislocation of the radial head, *J Pediatr Orthop* 18:410, 1998.

DeLee JC: Transverse divergent dislocation of the elbow in a child, *J Bone Joint Surg* 63A:322, 1981.

D'souza S, Vaishya R, Klenerman L: Management of radial neck fractures in children: a retrospective analysis of one hundred patients, *J Pediatr Orthop* 13:232, 1993.

Evans MC, Graham HK: Olecranon fractures in children. I. A clinical review, *J Pediatr Orthop* 19:559, 1999.

Evans MC, Graham HK: Olecranon fractures in children. II. A new classification and management algorithm, *J Pediatr Orthop* 19:559, 1999.

Fowles JV, Kassab MT: Observations concerning radial neck fractures in children, *J Pediatr Orthop* 6:51, 1986.

Fowles JV, Kassab MT, Moula T: Untreated posterior dislocation of the elbow in children, *J Bone Joint Surg* 66A:921, 1984.

Furry KL: Comminuted fractures of the radial head, *Clin Orthop* 353:40, 1998.

Futami T, Tsukamoto Y, Fujita T: Rotation osteotomy for dislocation of the radial head: 6 cases followed for 7 (3-10) years, *Acta Orthop Scand* 63:455, 1992.

Gaddy BC, Strecker WB, Schoenecker PL: Surgical treatment of displaced olecranon fractures in children, *J Pediatr Orthop* 17:321, 1997.

Gillingham BL, Wright JG: Convergent dislocation of the elbow, *Clin Orthop* 340:198, 1997.

Gillingham BL, Rang M: Advances in children's elbow fractures, *J Pediatr Orthop* 15:419, 1995 (editorial).

Gonzalez-Herranz P, Alvarez-Romera A, Burgos J, et al: Displaced radial neck fractures in children treated by closed intramedullary pinning (Metaizeau technique), *J Pediatr Orthop* 17:325, 1997.

Grantham SA, Kiernan HA: Displaced olecranon fractures in children, *J Trauma* 15:197, 1975.

Graves SC, Canale ST: Fractures of the olecranon in children: long-term follow-up, *J Pediatr Orthop* 13:239, 1993.

Gruber MA, Healy WA: The posterior approach to the elbow revisited, *J Pediatr Orthop* 16:215, 1996.

Hallet J: Entrapment of the median nerve after dislocation of the elbow, *J Bone Joint Surg* 63B:408, 1981.

Hansen PE, Barnes DA, Tullos HS: Arthroscopic diagnosis of an injury pattern in the distal humerus of an infant, *J Pediatr Orthop* 2:569, 1982.

Hassmann GC, Brunn F, Neer CS: Recurrent dislocation of the elbow, *J Bone Joint Surg* 57A:1080, 1975.

Herring JA, Sullivan JA: Instructional case: recurrent dislocation of the elbow, *J Pediatr Orthop* 9:483, 1989.

Hirayama T, Takemitsu Y, Yagihara K, Mikita A: Operation for chronic dislocation of the radial head in children: reduction by osteotomy of the ulna, *J Bone Joint Surg* 69B:639, 1987.

Jakob R, Fowles JV, Rang M, Kassab MT: Observations concerning fractures of the lateral humeral condyle in children, *J Bone Joint Surg* 57B:430, 1975.

Jeffery CC: Fracture of the head of the radius in children, *J Bone Joint Surg* 32B:314, 1950.

Kapel O: Operation for habitual dislocation of the elbow, *J Bone Joint Surg* 33A:707, 1951.

Kasser JR, Richards K, Millis M: The triceps-dividing approach to open reduction of complex distal humeral fractures in adolescents: a Cybex evaluation of triceps function and motion, *J Pediatr Orthop* 10:93, 1990.

King T: Recurrent dislocation of the elbow, *J Bone Joint Surg* 35B:50, 1953.

Letts M, Rumball K, Bauermeister S, et al: Fractures of the capitellum in adolescents, *J Pediatr Orthop* 17:315, 1997.

Leung AG, Peterson HA: Fractures of the proximal radial head and neck in children with emphasis on those that involve the articular cartilage, *J Pediatr Orthop* 20:7, 2000.

Lincoln TL, Mubarak SJ: "Isolated" traumatic radial head dislocation, *J Pediatr Orthop* 14:454, 1994.

Linscheid RL, Wheeler DK: Elbow dislocations, *JAMA* 194:113, 1965.

Lins RE, Simovitch RW, Waters PM: Pediatric elbow trauma, *Orthop Clin North Am*, 30:119, 1999.

Lloyd-Roberts GC, Bucknill TM: Anterior dislocation of the radial head in children, *J Bone Joint Surg* 59B:402, 1977.

Mäkelä EA, Böstman O, Kekomäki M, et al: Biodegradable fixation of distal humeral physeal fractures, *Clin Orthop* 283:237, 1992.

Manske PR: Unreduced isolated radial head dislocation in a child, *Orthopedics* 5:1327, 1982.

Matthews JG: Fractures of the olecranon in children, *Injury* 12:207, 1980.

Merchan ECR: Displaced fractures of the head and neck of the radius in children: open reduction and temporary transarticular internal fixation, *Orthopedics* 14:697, 1991.

Miura T: Congenital dislocation of the radial head, *J Hand Surg* 15B:477, 1990.

Mizuno K, Usui Y, Kohyama K, Mirohata K: Familial congenital unilateral anterior dislocation of the radial head: differentiation from traumatic dislocation by means of arthrography: a case report, *J Bone Joint Surg* 73A:1086, 1991.

Neviaser JS, Wickstrom JK: Dislocation of the elbow: a retrospective study of 115 patients, *South Med J* 70:172, 1977.

Newman JH: Displaced radial neck fractures in children, *Injury* 9:114, 1977.

O'Brien PI: Injuries involving the radial epiphysis, *Clin Orthop* 41:51, 1965.

Osborne G, Cotterill P: Recurrent dislocation of the elbow, *J Bone Joint Surg* 48B:340, 1966.

Papavasiliou VA, Beslikas TA, Nenopoulos S: Isolated fractures of the olecranon in children, *Injury* 18:100, 1987.

Patterson RF: Treatment of displaced transverse fractures of the neck of the radius in children, *J Bone Joint Surg* 16:695, 1934.

Pesudo JV, Aracil J, Barcelo M: Leverage method in displaced fractures of the radial neck, *Clin Orthop* 169:215, 1982.

Radomisli TE, Rosen AL: Controversies regarding radial neck fractures in children, *Clin Orthop* 353:30, 1998.

Regan W, Morrey BF: Classification and treatment of coronoid process fractures, *Orthopedics* 15:845, 1992.

Reichenheim PP: Transplantation of the biceps tendon as a treatment for recurrent dislocation of the elbow, *Br J Surg* 35:201, 1917.

Roberts PH: Dislocation of the elbow, *Br J Surg* 56:806, 1969.

Roy DR, Crawford AH: Operative fractures of the shaft of the radius and ulna, *Orthop Clin North Am* 21:245, 1990.

Sanders WE, Heckman JD: Traumatic plastic deformation of the radius and ulna, *Clin Orthop* 188:58, 1984.

Schwab GH, Bennett JB, Woods GW, Tullos HS: Biomechanics of elbow instability: the role of the medial collateral ligament, *Clin Orthop* 146:42, 1980.

Silberstein MJ, Brodeur AE, Graviss ER, Atchawee L: Some vagaries of the olecranon, *J Bone Joint Surg* 63A:722, 1981.

Skaggs DL, Mirzayan RL The posterior fat pad sign in associated with occult fracture of the elbow in children. *J Bone Joint Surg* 81A:1429, 1999.

Speed JS: An operation for unreduced posterior dislocation of the elbow, *South Med J* 18:193, 1925.

Speed JS, Boyd HB: Fractures about the elbow, *Am J Surg* 38:727, 1937.

Steinberg EL, Golomb D, Salama R, Weintroub S: Radial head and neck fractures in children, *J Pediatr Orthop* 8:35, 1988.

Symeonides PP, Paschaloglou C, Stavrou Z, Pangalides T: Recurrent dislocation of the elbow, *J Bone Joint Surg* 57A:1084, 1975.

Tibone JE, Stoltz M: Fracture of the radial head and neck in children, *J Bone Joint Surg* 63A:100, 1981.

Trias A, Comeau Y: Recurrent dislocation of the elbow in children, *Clin Orthop* 100:74, 1974.

Vesely DG: Isolated traumatic dislocations of the radial head in children, *Clin Orthop* 50:31, 1967.

Vostal O: Fracture of the neck of the radius in children, *Acta Chir Traumatol Czech* 37:294 1970.

Wedge JH, Robertson DE: Displaced fractures of the neck of the radius, *J Bone Joint Surg* 64B:256, 1982.

Wiley JJ, Pegington J, Horwich JP: Traumatic dislocation of the radius at the elbow, *J Bone Joint Surg* 56B:501, 1974.

Wiley JJ, Loehr J, McIntyre W: Isolated dislocation of the radial head, *Orthop Rev* 20:973, 1991.

Wilkins KE: Fractures and dislocations of the elbow region. In Rockwood CA Jr, Wilkins KE, King RE, eds: *Fractures in children*, Philadelphia, 1984, JB Lippincott.

Wirth CJ, Keyl W: Fractures of dislocations of the radial head. In Chapchal G, ed: *Fractures in children*, New York, 1981, Georg Thieme Verlag.

Wood SK: Reversal of the radial head during reduction of fractures of the neck of the radius in children, *J Bone Joint Surg* 51B:707, 1969.

Woods GM, Tullos HG: Elbow instability and medial epicondyle fracture, *Am J Sports Med* 5:23, 1977.

Yates C, Sullivan JA: Arthrography for pediatric elbow injury diagnosis, *Orthop Today* 4:9, 1984.

Yoo CI, Suh JT, Suh KT, et al: Avascular necrosis after fracture-separation of the distal end of the humerus in children, *Orthopedics* 15:959, 1992.

Zimmerman H: Fractures of the elbow. In Weber BG, Brunner C, Freuler F, eds: *Treatment of fractures in children and adolescents*, New York, 1980, Springer-Verlag.

LATERAL CONDYLAR FRACTURES

Badelon O, Bensahel H, Mazda K, Vie P: Lateral humeral condylar fractures in children: a report of 47 cases, *J Pediatr Orthop* 8:31, 1988.

Bast SC, Hoffer MM, Aval S: Nonoperative treatment for minimally and nondisplaced lateral humeral condyle fractures in children, *J Pediatr Orthop* 18:448, 1998.

Beaty JH, Wood AB: Lateral condylar fractures: long-term results. Paper presented at meeting of American Academy of Orthopaedic Surgeons, Las Vegas, Jan 18, 1985.

Blount WP: Unusual fractures in children, *Instr Course Lect* 7:57, 1954.

Blount WP, Schalz I, Cassidy RH: Fractures of the elbow in children, *JAMA* 146:699, 1951.

Boyd HB: Fractures about the elbow in children, *Surg Gynecol Obstet* 89:775, 1949.

Bright RW: Physeal fractures. In Rockwood CA, King RE, Wilkins KE, eds: *Fractures in children*, vol 3, Philadelphia, 1984, JB Lippincott.

Conner AN, Smith MG: Displaced fractures of the lateral humeral condyle in children, *J Bone Joint Surg* 52B:460, 1970.

Davids JR, Maguire MF, Mubarak SJ, Wenger DR: Lateral condylar fracture of the humerus following post-traumatic cubitus varus, *J Pediatr Orthop* 14:466, 1994.

Finnbogason T, Karlsson G, Lindberg L, Mortensson W: Nondisplaced and minimally displaced fractures of the lateral humeral condyle in children: a prospective radiographic investigation of fracture stability, *J Pediatr Orthop* 15:422, 1995.

Flynn JC: Nonunion of slightly displaced fractures of the lateral humeral condyle in children: an update, *J Pediatr Orthop* 9:691, 1989.

Flynn JC, Richards JF: Non-union of minimally displaced fractures of the lateral condyle of the humerus in children, *J Bone Joint Surg* 53A:1096, 1971.

Jeffery CC: Nonunion of the epiphysis of the lateral condyle of the humerus, *J Bone Joint Surg* 40B:396, 1958.

Kamegaya M, Shinohara Y, Kurakawa M, Ogata S: Assessment of stability in children's minimally displaced lateral humeral condyle fracture by magnetic resonance imaging, *J Pediatr Orthop* 19:570, 1999.

Marcus NW, Agins HJ: Articular cartilage sleeve fracture of the lateral humeral condyle, *J Pediatr Orthop* 4:620, 1984.

Marzo JM, d'Amato C, Strong M, Gillespie R: Usefulness and accuracy of arthrography in management of lateral humeral condyle fractures in children, *J Pediatr Orthop* 10:317, 1990.

Masada K, Kawai H, Kawabata H, et al: Osteosynthesis for old, established non-union of the lateral condyle of the humerus, *J Bone Joint Surg* 72A:32, 1990.

Milch H: Treatment of humeral cubitus valgus, *Clin Orthop* 6:120, 1955.

Milch H: Fractures and fracture-dislocations of humeral condyles, *J Trauma* 4:592, 1964.

Mintzer CM, Waters PM, Brown, DJ, Kasser JR: Percutaneous pinning in the treatment of displaced lateral condyle fractures, *J Pediatr Orthop* 14:462, 1994.

Roye DP, Bini SA, Infosino A: Late surgical treatment of lateral condylar fractures in children, *J Pediatr Orthop* 11:195, 1991.

Salter RB, Harris WR: Injuries involving the epiphyseal plate, *J Bone Joint Surg* 45A:587, 1963.

Silberstein JJ, Brodeur AE, Graviss ER: Some vagaries of the lateral epicondyle, *J Bone Joint Surg* 64A:444, 1981.

Speed JS: Surgical treatment of condylar fractures of the humerus, *Instr Course Lect* 7:187, 1950.

Speed JS, Macey HB: Fractures of the humeral condyles in children, *J Bone Joint Surg* 15:903, 1933.

Tachdjian MO: *Pediatric orthopedics*, ed 2, Philadelphia, 1990, WB Saunders.

Weber BG, Brunner C, Freuler F: *Treatment of fractures in children and adolescents*, New York, 1980, Springer-Verlag.

Wilkins KE: Fractures and dislocations of the elbow region. In Rockwood CA Jr, Wilkins KE, King RE, eds: *Fractures in children*, Philadelphia, 1984, JB Lippincott.

Zeier FG: Lateral condylar fracture and its many complications, *Orthop Rev* 10:49, 1981.

MEDIAL EPICONDYLAR AND MEDIAL HUMERAL CONDYLAR FRACTURES

Aitken AP, Childress HM: Intra-articular displacement of the internal epicondyle following dislocation, *J Bone Joint Surg* 20:161, 1938.

Beghin JL, Bucholz RW, Wenger DR: Intercondylar fractures of the humerus in young children, *J Bone Joint Surg* 64A:1083, 1982.

Burnstein SM, King JD, Sanderson RA: Fractures of the medial epicondyle of the humerus, *Contemp Orthop* 3:7, 1981.

Dangles C, Tylkowski C, Pankovich AM: Epicondylotrochlear fracture of the humerus before the appearance of the ossification center, *Clin Orthop* 171:161, 1982.

Fahey JJ, O'Brien E: Fracture-separation of the medial humeral condyle in a child confused with fracture of the medial epicondyle, *J Bone Joint Surg* 53A:1102, 1971.

Fowles JV, Kassab M: Displaced fractures of the medial humeral condyle in children, *J Bone Joint Surg* 62A:1159, 1980.

Fowles JV, Kassab MT, Moula T: Untreated intra-articular entrapment of the medial humeral epicondyle, *J Bone Joint Surg* 66B:562, 1984.

Grant IR, Miller JS: Osteochondral fracture of the trochlea associated with fracture dislocation of the elbow, *Injury* 6:257, 1975.

Hines RF, Herndon WA, Evans JP: Operative treatment of medial epicondyle fractures in children, *Clin Orthop* 223:170, 1987.

Holmberg L: Fractures in the distal end of the humerus in children, *Acta Chir Scand Suppl* 103, 1945.

Jarvis JD, D'Astous JL: Pediatric T-supracondylar fracture, *J Pediatr Orthop* 4:697, 1984.

Johansson J, Rosman M: Fracture of the capitulum humeri in children: a rare diagnosis, often misdiagnosed, *Clin Orthop* 146: 157, 1980.

Kasser JR, Richards K, Millis M: The triceps-dividing approach to open reduction of complex distal humeral fractures in adolescents: a Cybex evaluation of triceps function and motion, *J Pediatr Orthop* 10:93, 1990.

Kilfoyle FM: Fractures of the medial condyle and epicondyle of the elbow in children, *Clin Orthop* 41:43, 1965.

Ogden JA: *Skeletal injury in the child*, Philadelphia, 1982, Lea & Febiger.

Papavasiliou V, Nenopoulos S, Venturis T: Fractures of the medial condyle of the humerus in childhood, *J Pediatr Orthop* 7:421, 1987.

Patrick J: Fracture of the medial epicondyle with displacement into the elbow joint, *J Bone Joint Surg* 28:143, 1946.

Peterson HA: Triplane fracture of the distal humeral epiphysis, *J Pediatr Orthop* 3:81, 1983.

Schwab GH, Bennett JB, Woods GW, Tullos HG: Biomechanics of elbow instability: the role of the medial collateral ligament, *Clin Orthop* 146:42, 1980.

Silberstein JJ, Brodeur AE, Graviss ER: Some vagaries of the lateral epicondyle, *J Bone Joint Surg* 64A:444, 1982.

Weber BG, Brunner C, Freuler F, eds: *Treatment of fractures in children and adolescents*, New York, 1980, Springer-Verlag.

Woods GM, Tullos HG: Elbow instability and medial epicondyle fracture, *Am J Sports Med* 5:23, 1977.

Zimmerman H: Fractures of the elbow. In Weber BG, Brunner C, Freuler F, eds: *Treatment of fractures in children and adolescents*, New York, 1980, Springer-Verlag.

SUPRACONDYLAR FRACTURES

Abraham E, Powers T, Witt P, Ray RD: Experimental hyperextension supracondylar fractures in monkeys, *Clin Orthop* 171:309, 1982.

Akbarnia BA, Silverstein MJ, Graviss ER, Renday RJ: Arthrography for pediatric elbow injury diagnoses, *Orthop Today* 4:6, 1984.

Alburger PD, Weidner PL, Betz RR: Supracondylar fractures of the humerus in children, *J Pediatr Orthop* 12:16, 1992.

Amspacher JC, Messenbaugh JF Jr: Supracondylar osteotomy of the humerus for correction of rotational and angular deformities of the elbow, *South Med J* 57:846, 1964.

Arino VL, Lluch EE, Ramirez AM, et al: Percutaneous fixation of supracondylar fractures of the humerus in children, *J Bone Joint Surg* 59A:914, 1977.

Aronson DD, Prager BI: Supracondylar fractures of the humerus in children: a modified technique for closed pinning, *Clin Orthop* 219:174, 1987.

Barrett WP, Almquist EA, Staheli LT: Fracture separation of the distal humeral epiphysis in the newborn, *J Pediatr Orthop* 4:617, 1984.

Beals RK: The normal carrying angle of the elbow, *Clin Orthop* 119:194, 1976.

Bellemore MC, Barrett IR, Middleton RWD: Supracondylar osteotomy of the humerus with correction of cubitus varus, *J Bone Joint Surg* 66B:566, 1984.

Biyani A, Gupta SP, Sharma JC: Determination of medial epicondylar epiphyseal angle for supracondylar humeral fractures in children, *J Pediatr Orthop* 13:94, 1993.

Blount WP: Fractures in children, *Instr Course Lect* 7:194, 1950.

Bosanquet JS, Middleton RW: The reduction of supracondylar fractures of the humerus in children treated by traction-in extension, *Injury* 14:373, 1983.

Boyd DW, Aronson DD: Supracondylar fractures of the humerus: a prospective study of percutaneous pinning, *J Pediatr Orthop* 12:789, 1992.

Brown IC, Zinar DM: Traumatic and iatrogenic neurological complications after supracondylar humerus fractures in children, *J Pediatr Orthop* 15:440, 1995.

Carlson CS, Rosman MA: Cubitus varus: a new and simple technique for correction, *J Pediatr Orthop* 2:199, 1982.

Casiano E: Reduction and fixation by pinning "banderillero," *Mil Med* 125:262, 1961.

Celiker O, Pestilci FI, Tuzuner M: Supracondylar fractures of the humerus in children: analysis of the results in 142 patients, *J Orthop Trauma* 4:265, 1990.

Clement DA, Phil D: Assessment of a treatment plan for managing acute vascular complications associated with supracondylar fractures of the humerus in children, *J Pediatr Orthop* 10:97, 1990.

Culp RW, Osterman AL, Davidson RS, et al: Neural injuries associated with supracondylar fractures of the humerus in children, *J Bone Joint Surg* 72A:1211, 1990.

Dameron TB: Transverse fractures of the distal humerus in children, *Instr Course Lect* 30:224, 1981.

Danielsson L, Pettersson H: Open reduction and pin fixation of severely displaced supracondylar fractures of the humerus in children, *Acta Orthop Scand* 51:249, 1980.

Davids JR, Maguire MF, Mubarak SJ, Wenger DR: Lateral condylar fracture of the humerus following post-traumatic cubitus varus, *J Pediatr Orthop* 14:466, 1994.

De Boeck H, De Smet P, Peners W, DeRydt D: Supracondylar elbow fractures with impaction of the medial condyle in children, *J Pediatr Orthop* 15:444, 1995.

DeLee JC, Wilkins KE, Rogers LF, Rockwood CA: Fracture-separation of the distal humerus epiphysis, *J Bone Joint Surg* 62A:46, 1980.

DeRosa GP, Graziano GP: A new osteotomy for cubitus varus, *Clin Orthop* 236:160, 1988.

Dodge HS: Displaced supracondylar fractures of the humerus in children: treatment by Dunlop's traction, *J Bone Joint Surg* 54A:1408, 1972.

Eaton RG, Green WT: Epimysiotomy and fasciotomy in the treatment of Volkmann's ischemic contracture, *Orthop Clin North Am* 3:175, 1972.

Flynn JC, Matthews JG, Benoit RL: Blind pinning of displaced supracondylar fractures of the humerus in children, *J Bone Joint Surg* 56A:263, 1974.

Foster BK, Paterson DC: Difficult supracondylar elbow fractures in children: analysis of percutaneous pinning technique, *J Pediatr Orthop* 12:11, 1991.

Fowles JV, Kassab MT: Displaced supracondylar fractures of the elbow in children, *J Bone Joint Surg* 56B:490, 1974.

French PR: Varus deformity of elbow following supracondylar fractures of the humerus in children, *Lancet* 2:439, 1959.

Fuller DJ, McCullough CJ: Malunited fractures of the forearm in children, *J Bone Joint Surg* 64B:364, 1982.

Garbuz DS, Leitch K, Wright JG: The treatment of supracondylar fractures in children with an absent radial pulse, *J Pediatr Orthop* 16:594, 1996.

Gartland JJ: Management of supracondylar fractures of the humerus in children, *Surg Gynecol Obstet* 109:145, 1959.

Gelberman RH, Garfin SR, Hergenroeder PT, et al: Compartment syndromes of the forearm: diagnosis and treatment, *Clin Orthop* 161:252, 1981.

Graham B, Tredwell SJ, Beauchamp RD, Bell HM: Supracondylar osteotomy of the humerus for correction of cubitus varus, *J Pediatr Orthop* 10:228, 1990.

Graves SC, Beaty JH: Supracondylar fractures of the humerus in children: treatment by closed reduction and pinning, *Orthop Trans* 13:540, 1989.

Gruber MA, Hudson OC: Supracondylar fractures of the humerus in childhood, *J Bone Joint Surg* 46A:1245, 1964.

Haddad RJ, Saer JK, Riordan DC: Percutaneous pinning of displaced supracondylar fractures of the elbow in children, *Clin Orthop* 71:112, 1970.

Hadlow AT, Devane P, Nicol RO: A selective treatment approach to supracondylar fracture of the humerus in children, *J Pediatr Orthop* 16:104, 1996.

Hansen PE, Barnes DA, Tullos HS: Arthroscopic diagnosis of an injury pattern in the distal humerus of an infant, *J Pediatr Orthop* 2:569, 1982.

Herzenberg JE, Korseka J, Carroll NC, Rang M: Biomechanical testing of pin fixation techniques for pediatric supracondylar elbow fractures, *Orthop Trans* 12:678, 1988.

Holda ME, Manoli A, LaMont RL: Epiphyseal separation of the distal end of the humerus with medial displacement, *J Bone Joint Surg* 62A:52, 1980.

Ippolito E, Caterini R, Scola E: Supracondylar fractures of the humerus in children: analysis at maturity of fifty-three patients treated conservatively, *J Bone Joint Surg* 68A:333, 1986.

Kasser JR: Percutaneous pinning of supracondylar fractures of the humerus in children, *Instr Course Lect* 41:385, 1992.

Kekomäki M, Luoma RR, Rikalainen H, Vilkki P: Operative reduction and fixation of difficult supracondylar extension fracture, *J Pediatr Orthop* 4:13, 1984.

King D, Secor C: Bow elbow (cubitus varus), *J Bone Joint Surg* 33A:572, 1951.

Kiyoshige Y: Critical displacement of neural injuries in supracondylar humeral fractures in children, *J Pediatr Orthop* 19:816, 1999.

Kramhøft M, Keller IL, Solgaard S: Displaced supracondylar fractures of the humerus in children, *Clin Orthop* 221:215, 1987.

Kurer MHJ, Regan MW: Completely displaced supracondylar fracture of the humerus in children: a review of 1708 comparable cases, *Clin Orthop* 256:205, 1990.

Labelle H, Bunnell WP, Duhaime M, Poitras B: Cubitus varus deformity following supracondylar fractures of the humerus in children, *J Pediatr Orthop* 2:539, 1982.

Lyons JP, Ashley E, Hoffter MM: Ulnar nerve palsies after percutaneous cross-pinning of supracondylar fractures in children's elbows, *J Pediatr Orthop* 18:43, 1998.

Mapes RC, Hennrikus WL: The effect of elbow position on the radial pulse measured by Doppler ultrasonography after surgical treatment of supracondylar elbow fractures in children, *J Pediatr Orthop* 18:441, 1998.

Marion J, LaGrange J, Faysse R, Rigault P: Les fractures d l'extremite inferieure de l'humerus chez l'enfant, *Rev Chir Orthop* 48:337, 1962.

Mehserle WL, Meehan PL: Treatment of the displaced supracondylar fracture of the humerus (type III) with closed reduction and percutaneous cross-pin fixation, *J Pediatr Orthop* 11:705, 1991.

Merchan ECR: Supracondylar fractures of the humerus in children: treatment by overhead skeletal traction, *Orthop Rev* 21:475, 1992.

Mizuno K, Hirohata K, Kashiwagi D: Fracture-separation of the distal humeral epiphysis in young children, *J Bone Joint Surg* 61A:570, 1979.

Mohammad S, Rymaxzewski LA, Runciman J: The Baumann angle in supracondylar fractures of the distal humerus in children. *J Pediatr Orthop* 19:65, 1999.

O'Brien WR et al: The metaphyseal-diaphyseal angle as a guide to treating supracondylar fractures of the humerus in children. Paper presented at the Fifty-fourth Annual Meeting of The American Academy of Orthopaedic Surgeons, San Francisco, Jan 1987.

Oh CW, Park BC, Ihn JC, Kyung HS: Fracture separation of the distal humeral epiphysis in children younger than three years old, *J Pediatr Orthop* 20:173, 2000.

Oppenheim WL, Calder TJ, Smith C, et al: Supracondylar humeral osteotomy for traumatic childhood cubitus varus deformity, *Clin Orthop* 188:34, 1984.

Peiro A, Mut T, Aracil J, Martos F: Fracture-separation of the lower humeral epiphysis in young children, *Acta Orthop Scand* 52:295, 1981.

Pirone AM, Graham HK, Krajbich JI: Management of displaced extension-type supracondylar fractures of the humerus in children, *J Bone Joint Surg* 70A:641, 1988.

Rang M, Moseley CF, Roberts JM, et al: Symposium: management of displaced supracondylar fractures of the humerus, *Contemp Orthop* 18:497, 1989.

Rasool MN, Naidoo KS: Supracondylar fractures: posterolateral type with brachialis muscle penetration and neurovascular injury, *J Pediatr Orthop* 19:518, 1999.

Re PR, Waters PM, Hresko T: T-condylar fractures of the distal humerus in children and adolescents, *J Pediatr Orthop* 19:313, 1999.

Roach JW, Hernandez MA: Corrective osteotomy for cubitus varus deformity, *J Pediatr Orthop* 14:487, 1994.

Rorabeck CH: A practical approach to compartment syndromes. III. Management, *Instr Course Lect* 33:102, 1983.

Royce RO, Dutkowsky JP, Kasser JR, Rand FR: Neurologic complications after Kirschner wire fixation of supracondylar humerus fractures in children, *J Pediatr Orthop* 11:191, 1991.

Sabharwal S, Tredwell SJ, Beauchamp RD, et al: Management of pulseless pink hand in pediatric supracondylar fractures of the humerus, *J Pediatr Orthop* 17:303, 1997.

Shaw BA, Kasser JR, Emans JB, Rand FF: Management of vascular injuries in displaced supracondylar humerus fractures without arteriography, *J Orthop Trauma* 4:25, 1990.

Silberstein MJ, Brodeur AE, Graviss ER: Some vagaries of the capitellum, *J Bone Joint Surg* 61A:244, 1979.

Smith FM: Children's elbow injuries: fractures and dislocations, *Clin Orthop* 50:7, 1967.

Smith L: Deformity following supracondylar fractures of the humerus, *J Bone Joint Surg* 42A:235, 1960.

Spinner M, Schreiber SN: Anterior interosseous nerve paralysis as a complication of supracondylar fractures of the humerus in children, *J Bone Joint Surg* 51A:1584, 1969.

Swenson AL: The treatment of supracondylar fractures of the humerus by Kirschner wire fixation, *J Bone Joint Surg* 30A:993, 1948.

Thometz JG: Techniques for direct radiographic visualization during closed pinning of supracondylar humerus fractures in children, *J Pediatr Orthop* 10:555, 1990.

Topping RE, Blanco JS, Davis TJ: Clinical evaluation of crossed-pin versus lateral-pin fixation in displaced supracondylar humerus fractures, *J Pediatr Orthop* 15:435, 1995.

Uchida Y, Ogata K, Sugioka Y: A new three-dimensional osteotomy for cubitus varus deformity after supracondylar fracture of the humerus in children, *J Pediatr Orthop* 11:327, 1991.

Vasli LR: Diagnosis of vascular injury in children with supracondylar fractures of the humerus, *Injury* 9:11, 1988.

Voss FR, Kasser JR, Trepman E, et al: Uniplanar supracondylar humeral osteotomy with preset Kirschner wires for post-traumatic cubitus varus, *J Pediatr Orthop* 14:471, 1994.

Webb AJ, Sherman FC: Supracondylar fractures of the humerus in children, *J Pediatr Orthop* 9:315, 1989.

Weber BG, Brunner C, Freuler F, eds: *Treatment of fractures in children and adolescents*, New York, 1980, Springer-Verlag.

Wilkins KE: The operative management of supracondylar fractures, *Orthop Clin North Am* 21:269, 1990.

Williamson DM, Coates CJ, Miller RK, Cole WG: Normal characteristics of the Baumann (humerocapitellar) angle: an aid in assessment of supracondylar fractures, *J Pediatr Orthop* 12:636, 1992.

Worlock PH, Colton C: Severely displaced supracondylar fractures of the humerus in children: a simple method of treatment, *J Pediatr Orthop* 7:49, 1987.

Yates C, Sullivan JA: Arthrographic diagnosis of elbow injuries in children, *J Pediatr Orthop* 7:54, 1987.

FRACTURES OF SHAFT AND PROXIMAL END OF HUMERUS, ACROMIOCLAVICULAR DISLOCATIONS, AND FRACTURES AND DISLOCATIONS OF SHAFT AND EPIPHYSIS OF CLAVICLE

Beaty JH: Fractures of the proximal humerus and shaft in children, *Instr Course Lect* 41:369, 1992.

Beringer DC, Weiner DS, Noble JS, Bell RH: Severely displaced proximal humeral epiphyseal fractures: a follow-up study, *J Pediatr Orthop* 18:31, 1998.

Curtis RJ Jr: Operative management of children's fractures of the shoulder region, *Orthop Clin North Am* 21:315, 1990.

Dameron TB, Reibel DB: Fractures involving the proximal humeral epiphyseal plate, *J Bone Joint Surg* 51A:289, 1969.

Falstie-Jensen S, Mikkelsen P: Pseudodislocation of the acromioclavicular joint, *J Bone Joint Surg* 64B:368, 1982.

Havranek P: Injuries of the distal clavicular physis in children, *J Pediatr Orthop* 9:213, 1989.

Holstein A, Lewis GB: Fractures of the humerus with radial nerve paralysis, *J Bone Joint Surg* 45A:1382, 1963.

Katznelson A, Nerubay J, Oliver S: Dynamic fixation of the avulsed clavicle, *J Trauma* 16:841, 1976.

Kawam M, Sinclair J, Letts M: Recurrent posterior shoulder dislocation in children: the results of surgical management, *J Pediatr Orthop* 17:533, 1997.

Larsen CL, Kiær T, Lindequist S: Fractures of the proximal humerus in children: nine-year follow-up of 64 unoperated cases, *Acta Orthop Scand* 61:255, 1990.

Lloyd-Roberts GC, Apley AG, Owen R: Reflections upon the aetiology of congenital pseudarthrosis of the clavicle, *J Bone Joint Surg* 57B:24, 1975.

Neer CS II: Fractures of the distal third of the clavicle, *Clin Orthop* 58:43, 1968.

Neer CS, Horowitz BS: Fractures of the proximal humeral epiphyseal plate, *Clin Orthop* 41:24, 1965.

Rockwood CA: Dislocations of the sternoclavicular joint, *Instr Course Lect* 24:144, 1975.

Rockwood CA: Fractures of the outer clavicle in children and adults, *J Bone Joint Surg* 64B:642 1982.

Rockwood CA Jr: Fractures and dislocations of the shoulder. III. Fractures and dislocations of the ends of the clavicle, scapula, and glenohumeral joint. In Rockwood CA Jr, Wilkins KE, King RE, eds: *Fractures in children*, Philadelphia, 1984, JB Lippincott.

Rowe CR, Pierce DS, Clark JG: Voluntary dislocation of the shoulder, *J Bone Joint Surg* 55A:445, 1973.

Sherk HH, Probst C: Fractures of the proximal humeral epiphysis, *Orthop Clin North Am* 6:401, 1975.

Torode I, Donnan L: Posterior dislocation of the humeral head in association with obstetric paralysis, *J Pediatr Orthop* 18:611, 1998.

Visser JO, Rietberg M: Interposition of the tendon of the long head of biceps in fracture separation of the proximal humeral epiphysis, *Netherlands J Surg* 32:12, 1980.

Wagner KT, Lyne ED: Adolescent traumatic dislocations of the shoulder with open epiphysis, *J Pediatr Orthop* 3:61, 1983.

Wilkes JA, Hoffer MM: Clavicle fractures in head-injured children, *J Orthop Trauma* 1:55, 1987.

Williams DJ: The mechanisms producing fracture separation of the proximal humeral epiphysis, *J Bone Joint Surg* 63B:102, 1981.

Zenni EJ, Krieg JK, Rosen MJ: Open reduction and internal fixation of clavicular fractures, *J Bone Joint Surg* 63A:147, 1981.

SPINE FRACTURES AND DISLOCATIONS

Anderson LD, D'Alonzo RT: Fractures of the odontoid process of the axis, *J Bone Joint Surg* 56A:1663, 1974.

Bailey DK: The normal cervical spine in infants and children, *Radiology* 59:712, 1952.

Bohlman HH: Acute fractures and dislocations of the cervical spine, *J Bone Joint Surg* 61A:1119, 1979.

Carrion WV, Dormans JP, Drummond, DS, Christofersen MR: Circumferential growth plate fracture of the thoracolumbar spine from child abuse, *J Pediatr Orthop* 16:210, 1996.

Cattell HS, Filtzer DL: Pseudosubluxation and other normal variations in the cervical spine in children, *J Bone Joint Surg* 47A:1295, 1965.

Clark JE: Apophyseal fracture of the lumbar spine in adolescence, *Orthop Rev* 20:512, 1991.

Crawford AH: Operative treatment of spine fractures in children, *Orthop Clin North Am* 21:325, 1990.

Crockard HA, Rogers MA: Open reduction of traumatic atlanto-axial rotatory dislocation with use of the extreme lateral approach, *J Bone Joint Surg* 78A:431, 1996.

Edmonson AS: The spine. In Edmonson AS, Crenshaw AH, eds: *Campbell's operative orthopaedics*, ed 8, St Louis, 1992, Mosby.

Fielding JW: Normal and selected abnormal motion of the cervical spine from the second cervical vertebra to the seventh cervical vertebra based on cineroentgenography, *J Bone Joint Surg* 46A: 1779, 1964.

Fielding JW: Selected observations on the cervical spine in the child. In Ahstrom JP Jr, ed: *Current practice in orthopaedic surgery*, vol 5, St Louis, 1973, Mosby.

Fielding JW: Fractures of the spine. Part I. Injuries of the cervical spine. In Rockwood CA Jr, Wilkins KE, King RE: *Fractures in children*, Philadelphia, 1984, JB Lippincott.

Fielding JW, Hensinger RN, Hawkins RJ: Os odontoideum, *J Bone Joint Surg* 62A:376, 1980.

Gertzbein SD: Scoliosis Research Society: multicenter spine fracture study, *Spine* 17:528, 1992. Griffiths SC: Fracture of the odontoid process in children, *J Pediatr Surg* 7:680, 1972.

Henrys P, Lyne ED, Lifton C, Salciccioli G: Clinical review of cervical spine injuries in children, *Clin Orthop* 129:172, 1977.

Hensinger RN: Fractures of the spine. II. Fractures of the thoracic and lumbar spine. In Rockwood CA Jr, Wilkins KE, King RE: *Fractures in children*, Philadelphia, 1984, JB Lippincott.

Herzenberg JE, Hensinger RN, Dedrick DK, Phillips WA: Emergency transport and position of young children who have an injury of the cervical spine: the standard backboard may be hazardous, *J Bone Joint Surg* 71A:15, 1989.

Horal J, Nachemson A, Scheller S: Clinical and radiological long term follow-up of vertebral fractures in children, *Acta Orthop Scand* 43:491, 1972.

Jackson DW, Wiltse LL, Cirincione RJ: Spondylolysis in the female gymnast, *Clin Orthop* 117:68, 1976.

Jones ET, Hensinger RN: Spinal deformity in idiopathic juvenile osteoporosis, *Spine* 6:1, 1981.

Keller RH: Traumatic displacement of the cartilaginous vertebral rim: a sign of intervertebral disc prolapse, *Radiology* 110:21, 1974.

Kewalramani LS, Tori JA: Spinal cord trauma in children: neurologic patterns, radiologic features, and pathomechanics of injury, *Spine* 5:11, 1980.

Lancourt JE, Dickson JH, Carter RE: Paralytic spinal deformity following traumatic spinal-cord injury in children and adolescents, *J Bone Joint Surg* 63A:47, 1981.

Lowrey JJ: Dislocated lumbar vertebral epiphysis in adolescent children: report of three cases, *J Neurosurg* 38:232, 1973.

Marar BC, Balachandran N: Non-traumatic atlanto-axial dislocation in children, *Clin Orthop* 92:220, 1973.

Micheli LJ: Low back pain in the adolescent: differential diagnosis, *Am J Sports Med* 7:362, 1979.

Odent T, Langlais J, Glorion C, et al: Fractures of the odontoid process: a report of 15 cases in children younger than 6 years, *J Pediatr Orthop* 19:51, 1999.

Parke WW, Schiff DCM: The applied anatomy of the intervertebral disc, *Orthop Clin North Am* 2:309, 1971.

Reid AB, Letts RM, Black GB: Pediatric Chance fractures: association with intra-abdominal injuries and seat belt use, *J Trauma* 30:384, 1990.

Rumball K, Jarvis J: Seat-belt injuries of the spine in young children, *J Bone Joint Surg* 74B:571, 1992.

Scheuermann HW: The classic kyphosis dorsalis juvenilis, *Z Ortho Chir* 41:305, 1921.

Schiff DCM, Parke WW: The arterial blood supply of the odontoid process (dens), *Anat Rec* 172:399, 1972.

Sherk HH, Nicholson JT, Chung SMK: Fractures of the odontoid process in young children, *J Bone Joint Surg* 60A:921, 1978.

Sherk HH, Schut L, Lane J: Fractures and dislocations of the cervical spine in children, *Orthop Clin North Am* 7:593, 1976.

Wiltse LL, Newman PH, Macnab I: Classification of spondylolysis and spondylolisthesis, *Clin Orthop* 117:23, 1976.

Wiltse LL, Widell EH, Jackson DW: Fatigue fracture: the basic lesion in isthmic spondylolisthesis, *J Bone Joint Surg* 57A:17, 1975.

PELVIC AND HIP FRACTURES AND DISORDERS

Ablin DS, Greenspan A, Reinhart MA: Pelvic injuries in child abuse, *Pediatr Radiol* 22:454, 1992.

Alonzo JE, Horowitz M: Use of the AO-ASIF external fixator in children, *J Pediatr Orthop* 7:594, 1987.

Altenberg AR: Acetabular labrum tears: cause of hip pain and degenerative arthritis, *South Med J* 70:174, 1977.

Barquet A: Traumatic dislocation of the hip in childhood, *Injury* 13:435, 1982.

Behrens F: External skeletal fixation. Part A. Introduction to external skeletal fixation, *Instr Course Lect* 30:116, 1981.

Behrens F: External skeletal fixation. Part H. Complications of external skeletal fixation, *Instr Course Lect* 30:179, 1981.

Bennett FS, Zinar DM, Kilgus DJ: Ipsilateral hip and femoral shaft fractures, *Clin Orthop* 296:168, 1993.

Blair W, Hansen C: Traumatic closure of triradiate cartilage, *J Bone Joint Surg* 61A:144, 1979.

Boitzy A: Fractures of the proximal femur. In Weber BG, Brunner C, Freuler F, eds: *Treatment of fractures in children and adolescents*, New York, 1980, Springer-Verlag.

Bond SJ, Gotschall CS, Eichelberger MR: Predictors of abdominal injury in children with pelvic fracture, *J Trauma* 31:1169, 1991.

Bos CFA, Eulderink F, Bloem JL: Bilateral pelvitrochanteric heterotopic ossification in a child: a case report, *J Bone Joint Surg* 75A:1840, 1993.

Brooks E, Rosman M: Central fracture dislocation of the hip in the child, *J Trauma* 28:1590, 1988.

Bryan WJ, Tullos HS: Pediatric pelvic fractures: a review of 52 patients, *J Trauma* 19:799, 1979.

Bucholz RW, Ezaki M, Ogden JA: Injury to the acetabular triradiate epiphyseal cartilage, *J Bone Joint Surg* 64A:600, 1982.

Bunnell WP, Webster DA: Late reduction of bilateral traumatic hip dislocation in a child, *Clin Orthop* 147:160, 1980.

Calandruccio RA, Anderson WE III: Post-fracture avascular necrosis of the femoral head: correlation of experimental and clinical studies, *Clin Orthop* 152:49, 1980.

Canale ST: Fractures of the hip in children and adolescents, *Orthop Clin North Am* 21:341, 1990.

Canale ST, Bourland WL: Fracture of the neck and intertrochanteric region of the femur in children, *J Bone Joint Surg* 59A:431, 1977.

Canale ST, Manugian AH: Irreducible traumatic dislocations of the hip, *J Bone Joint Surg* 61A:7, 1979.

Chung SMK: The arterial supply of the developing proximal end of the human femur, *J Bone Joint Surg* 58A:961, 1976.

Colonna PC: Fractures of the neck of the femur in children, *Am J Surg* 6:793, 1929.

Davison BL, Weinstein SL: Hip fractures in children: a long-term follow-up study, *J Pediatr Orthop* 12:355, 1992.

Devas MD: Stress fractures of the femoral neck, *J Bone Joint Surg* 47B:728, 1965.

Epstein HC: *Traumatic dislocation of the hip*, Baltimore, 1980, Williams & Wilkins.

Fernbach SK, Wilkinson RH: Avulsion injuries to the pelvis and proximal femur, *Am J Radiol* 137:581, 1981.

Forlin E, Guille JT, Kumar SJ, Rhee KJ: Complications associated with fracture of the neck of the femur in children, *J Pediatr Orthop* 12:503, 1992.

Forlin E, Guille JT, Kumar SJ, Rhee KJ: Transepiphyseal fractures of the neck of the femur in very young children, *J Pediatr Orthop* 12:164, 1992.

Gartland JJ, Brenner JH: Traumatic dislocations in the lower extremity in children, *Orthop Clin North Am* 7:687, 1976.

Gaul RW: Recurrent traumatic dislocation of the hip in children, *Clin Orthop* 90:107, 1973.

Gepstein R, Weiss RE, Hallel T: Acetabular dysplasia and hip dislocation after selective premature fusion of the triradiate cartilage: an experimental study in rabbits, *J Bone Joint Surg* 66B:334, 1984.

Gerber C, Lehmann A, Ganz R: Femoral neck fractures in children: experience in 7 Swiss AO hospitals, *Orthop Trans* 9:474, 1985 (abstract).

Hall BB, Klassen RA, Ilstrup DM: Pelvic fractures in children: a long-term follow-up study, unpublished data.

Haller JA Jr, Garrett R: A new philosophy of pediatric splenic surgery: save our spleens, *Surg Rounds* 3:23, 1980.

Hamilton PR, Broughton NS: Traumatic hips dislocation in childhood, *J Pediatr Orthop* 18:691, 1998.

Harper MC, Canale ST: Angulation osteotomy: a trigonometric analysis, *Clin Orthop* 166:173, 1982.

Harper MC, Canale ST, Cobb RM: Proximal femoral osteotomy: a trigonometric analysis of effect on leg length, *J Pediatr Orthop* 3:341, 1983.

Heeg M, Klasen HJ, Visser JD: Acetabular fractures in children and adolescents, *J Bone Joint Surg* 71B:418, 1989.

Heeg M, Visser JD, Oostvogel HJM: Injuries of the acetabular triradiate cartilage and sacroiliac joint, *J Bone Joint Surg* 70B:34, 1988.

Heiser JM, Oppenheim WL: Fracture of the hip in children, *Clin Orthop* 149:177, 1980.

Hughes LO, Beaty JH: Fractures of the head and neck of the femur in children, *J Bone Joint Surg* 76A:283, 1994.

Ingram AJ, Bachynski B: Fractures of the hip in children: treatment and results, *J Bone Joint Surg* 35A:867, 1953.

Ingram AJ, Turner TC: Bilateral traumatic posterior dislocation of the hip complicated by bilateral fracture of the femoral shaft, *J Bone Joint Surg* 36A:1249, 1954.

Kane WJ: Fractures of the pelvis. In Rockwood CA Jr, Green DP, eds: *Fractures*, Philadelphia, 1975, JB Lippincott.

Kaweblum M, Lehman WB, Grant AD, Strongwater A: Avascular necrosis of the femoral head as sequela of fracture of the greater trochanter: a case report and review of the literature, *Clin Orthop* 294:193, 1993.

Key JA, Conwell HE: *Management of fractures, dislocations, and sprains*, St Louis, 1951, Mosby.

Lam SF: Fractures of the neck of the femur in children, *J Bone Joint Surg* 53A:1165, 1971.

Leenen LP, van der Werken C, Schoots F, Goris RJ: Internal fixation of open unstable pelvic fractures, *J Trauma* 35:220, 1993.

Libri R, Calderon JE, Capelli A, Soncini G: Traumatic dislocation of the hip in children and adolescents, *Ital J Orthop Traumatol* 12:61, 1986.

Liebergall M, Lowe J, Whitelaw GW, et al: The floating hip: ipsilateral pelvic and femoral fractures, *J Bone Joint Surg* 74B:93, 1992.

MacFarlane IJ: Survey of traumatic dislocation of the hip in children, *J Bone Joint Surg* 58B:267, 1976.

Magid D, Fishman EK, Ney DR, et al: Acetabular and pelvic fractures in the pediatric patient: value of two- and three-dimensional imaging, *J Pediatr Orthop* 12:621, 1992.

Mass DP, Spiegel PG, Laros GS: Dislocation of the hip with traumatic separation of the capital femoral epiphysis: report of case with successful outcome, *Clin Orthop* 146:184, 1980.

McDonald GA: Pelvic disruptions in children, *Clin Orthop* 151:130, 1980.

McIntyre RC, Bensard DD, Moore EE, et al: Pelvic fracture geometry predicts risk of life-threatening hemorrhage in children, *J Trauma* 35:423, 1993.

Mears DC, Fu F: External fixation in pelvic fractures, *Orthop Clin North Am* 11:465, 1980.

Milch H: Avulsion fracture of the tuberosity of the ischium, *J Bone Joint Surg* 8:832, 1926.

Milch H: Ischio-acetabular (Walther's) fracture, *Bull Hosp Jt Dis* 16:7, 1955.

Mody BS, Patil SS, Carty H, Klenerman L: Fracture through the bone of traumatic myositis ossificans: a report of three cases, *J Bone Joint Surg* 76B:607, 1994.

Morgan JD, Somerville EW: Normal and abnormal growth at the upper end of the femur, *J Bone Joint Surg* 42B:264, 1960.

Morgenstern L: Conservation of the injured spleen, *Surg Rounds* 3:13, 1980.

Morrissy R: Hip fractures in children, *Clin Orthop* 152:202, 1980.

Moseley CF: A straight-line graph for leg-length discrepancies, *J Bone Joint Surg* 59A:174, 1977.

Moseley CF: Fractures and dislocations of the hip, *Instr Course Lect* 41:397, 1992.

Newton PO, Mubarak SJ: The use of modified Neufeld's skeletal traction in children and adolescents, *J Pediatr Orthop* 15:467, 1995.

Nierenberg G, Volpin G, Bialik V, Stein H: Pelvic fractures in children. Part B. A follow-up in 20 children treated conservatively, *J Pediatr Orthop* 1:140, 1993.

Ogden JA: Changing patterns of proximal femoral vascularity, *J Bone Joint Surg* 56A:941, 1974.

Ogden JA, Lee KE, Rudicel SA, Pelker RR: Proximal femoral epiphysiolysis in the neonate, *J Pediatr Orthop* 4:285, 1984.

Ovesen O, Arreskov J, Bellstrøn T: Hip fractures in children: a long-term follow-up of 17 cases, *Orthopedics* 12:361, 1989.

Patterson FP: The cause of death in fractures of the pelvis, *J Trauma* 13:849, 1973.

Petrini A, Grassi G: Long-term results in traumatic dislocation of the hip in children, *Ital J Orthop Traumatol* 9:225, 1983.

Pförringer W, Rosemeyer B: Fractures of the hip in children and adolescents, *Acta Orthop Scand* 51:91, 1980.

Ponseti IV: Growth and development of the acetabulum in the normal child, *J Bone Joint Surg* 60A:575, 1978.

Quinby WC Jr: Fractures of the pelvis and associated injuries in children, *J Pediatr Surg* 1:353, 1966.

Quinlan WR, Brady PG, Regan BS: Fractures of the neck of the femur in childhood, *Injury* 11:242, 1980.

Rang M: *Children's fractures*, ed 2, Philadelphia, 1983, JB Lippincott.

Ratliff AHC: Complications after fractures of the femoral neck in children and their treatment, *J Bone Joint Surg* 52B:175, 1970.

Rieger H, Brug E: Fractures of the pelvis in children, *Clin Orthop* 336:226, 1997.

St Pierre P, Staheli LT, Smith JB, Green NE: Femoral neck stress fractures in children and adolescents, *J Pediatr Orthop* 15:470, 1995.

Salvino CK, Esposito, TJ, Smith D, et al: Routine pelvic x-ray studies in awake blunt trauma patients: a sensible policy? *J Trauma* 33:413, 1992.

Scuderi G, Bronson MJ: Triradiate cartilage injury: report of two cases and review of the literature, *Clin Orthop* 217:179, 1987.

Sundar M, Carty H: Avulsion fractures of the pelvis in children: a report of 32 fractures and their outcome, *Skel Radiol* 23:85, 1994.

Swiontkowski MF, Winquist RA: Displaced hip fractures in children and adolescents, *J Trauma* 26:384, 1986.

Theodorou SD, Ierodiaconou MN, Mitsou A: Obstetrical fracture separation of upper femoral epiphysis, *Acta Orthop Scand* 53:239, 1982.

Tile M: Fractures of the acetabulum, *Orthop Clin North Am* 11:418, 1980.

Tile M: Pelvic fractures, *Orthop Clin North Am* 11:423, 1980.

Torode I, Zieg D: Pelvic fractures in children, *J Pediatr Orthop* 5:76, 1985.

Trueta J: The normal vascular anatomy of the human femoral head during growth, *J Bone Joint Surg* 39B:358, 1957.

Vazquez WD, Garcia VF: Pediatric pelvic fractures combined with an additional skeletal injury as an indicator of significant injury, *Surg Gynecol Obstet* 177:468, 1993.

Watts HG: Fractures of the pelvis in children, *Orthop Clin North Am* 7:615, 1976.

Weber BG, Brunner C, Freuler F, eds: *Treatment of fractures in children and adolescents*, New York, 1980, Springer-Verlag.

Wojtowycz M, Starshak RJ, Sty JR: Neonatal proximal femoral epiphysiolysis, *Radiology* 136:647, 1980.

Wolfgang GL: Stress fracture of the femoral neck in a patient with open capital femoral epiphyses, *J Bone Joint Surg* 59A:680, 1977.

SLIPPED CAPITAL FEMORAL EPIPHYSIS

Aadalen RJ, Weiner DS, Hoyt W, Herndon CH: Acute slipped capital femoral epiphysis, *J Bone Joint Surg* 56A:1473, 1974.

Abraham E, Garst J, Barmada R: Treatment of moderate to severe slipped capital femoral epiphysis with extracapsular base-of-neck osteotomy, *J Pediatr Orthop* 13:294, 1993.

Aronson DD, Carlson WE: Slipped capital femoral epiphysis: a prospective study of fixation with a single screw, *J Bone Joint Surg* 74A:810, 1992.

Aronson DD, Loder RT: Slipped capital femoral epiphysis in black children, *J Pediatr Orthop* 12:74, 1992.

Aronson DD, Loder RT: Treatment of the unstable (acute) slipped capital femoral epiphysis, *Clin Orthop* 322:99, 1996.

Aronson J, Tursky EA: The torsional basis for slipped capital femoral epiphysis, *Clin Orthop* 322:37, 1996.

Asnis SE: *The Asnis guided screw system technique manual,* Rutherford, NJ, 1984, Howmedica.

Bassett GS: Bone endoscopy: direct visual confirmation of cannulated screw placement in slipped capital femoral epiphysis, *J Pediatr Orthop* 13:159, 1993.

Baynham GC, Lucie RS, Cummings RJ: Femoral neck fracture secondary to in situ pinning of slipped capital femoral epiphysis: a previously unreported complication, *J Pediatr Orthop* 11:187, 1991.

Bennet GC, Koreska J, Rang M: Pin placement in slipped capital femoral epiphysis, *J Pediatr Orthop* 4:574, 1984.

Betz RR, Steel HH, Emper WD, et al: Treatment of slipped capital femoral epiphysis, *J Bone Joint Surg* 72A:587, 1990.

Blanco JS, Taylor B, Johnston CE: Comparison of single pin versus multiple pin fixation in treatment of slipped capital femoral epiphysis, *J Pediatr Orthop* 12:384, 1992.

Bloom ML, Crawford AH: Slipped capital femoral epiphysis: an assessment of treatment modalities, *Orthopedics* 8:36, 1985.

Boyd HB, Ingram AJ, Bourkhard HO: The treatment of slipped femoral epiphysis, *South Med J* 42:551, 1949.

Boyer W, Mickelson MR, Ponseti IV: Slipped capital femoral epiphysis: long-term follow-up study of 121 patients, *J Bone Joint Surg* 63A:85, 1981.

Broughton NS, Todd RC, Dunn RM, Angel JC: Open reduction of the severely slipped upper femoral epiphysis, *J Bone Joint Surg* 70B:435, 1988.

Cameron HU, Wang M, Koreska J: Internal fixation of slipped capital femoral epiphyses, *Clin Orthop* 137:148, 1978.

Canale ST: Problems and complications of slipped capital femoral epiphysis, *Instr Course Lect* 38:281, 1989.

Canale ST, Azar F, Young J, et al: Subtrochanteric fracture after fixation of slipped capital femoral epiphysis: a complication of unused drill holes, *J Pediatr Orthop* 14:623, 1994.

Canale ST, Casillas M, Banta JV: Displaced femoral neck fractures at the bone-screw interface after in situ fixation of slipped capital femoral epiphysis, *J Pediatr Orthop* 17:212, 1997.

Carney BT, Weinstein SL: Natural history of untreated chronic slipped capital femoral epiphysis, *Clin Orthop* 322:43, 1996.

Carney BT, Weinstein SL, Noble J: Long-term follow-up of slipped capital femoral epiphysis, *J Bone Joint Surg* 73A:667, 1991.

Casey BH, Hamilton HW, Bobechko WP: Reduction of acutely slipped upper femoral epiphysis, *J Bone Joint Surg* 54B:607, 1972.

Clark CR, Southwick WO, Odgen JA: Anatomic aspects of slipped capital femoral epiphysis and correction by biplane osteotomy, *Instr Course Lect* 29:90, 1980.

Compere CL: Correction of deformity and prevention of aseptic necrosis in late cases of slipped femoral epiphysis, *J Bone Joint Surg* 32A:351, 1950.

Cowell HR: The significance of early diagnosis and treatment of slipping of the capital femoral epiphysis, *Clin Orthop* 48:89, 1966.

Crandall DG, Gabriel KR, Akbarnia BA: Second operation for slipped capital femoral epiphysis: pin removal, *J Pediatr Orthop* 12:434, 1992.

Crawford AH: Current concepts review: slipped capital femoral epiphysis, *J Bone Joint Surg* 70A:1422, 1988.

Crawford AH: The role of osteotomy in the treatment of slipped capital femoral epiphysis, *Instr Course Lect* 38:273, 1989.

Davidson RS, Weitzel P, Stanton R, et al: Slipped capital femoral epiphysis (SCFE): a multicenter review of the complications by treatment group in 432 hips. Paper presented at the annual meeting of the Pediatric Orthopaedic Society of North America, Miami, April 30, 1995.

DeRosa GP, Mullins RC, Kling TF: Cuneiform osteotomy of the femoral neck in severe slipped capital femoral epiphysis, *Clin Orthop* 322:48, 1996.

Duncan JW, Lovell WW: Anterior slip of the capital femoral epiphysis: report of a case and discussion, *Clin Orthop* 110:171, 1975.

Dunn DM: The treatment of adolescent slipping of the upper femoral epiphysis, *J Bone Joint Surg* 46B:621, 1964.

Dunn DM, Angel JC: Replacement of the femoral head by open operation in severe adolescent slipping of the upper femoral epiphysis, *J Bone Joint Surg* 60B:394, 1978.

Fairbank JT: Manipulative reduction in slipped capital femoral epiphysis, *J Bone Joint Surg* 51B:252, 1969.

Ferguson AB, Howorth MB: Slipping of upper femoral epiphysis: a study of seventy cases, *JAMA* 97:1867, 1931.

Fish JB: Cuneiform osteotomy of the femoral neck in the treatment of slipped capital femoral epiphysis, *J Bone Joint Surg* 66A:1153, 1984.

Fish JB: Cuneiform osteotomy of the femoral neck in the treatment of slipped capital femoral epiphysis: a follow-up note, *J Bone Joint Surg* 76A:46, 1994.

Futami T, Kasahara Y, Suzuki S, et al: Arthroscopy for slipped capital femoral epiphysis, *J Pediatr Orthop* 12:592, 1992.

Gage JR, Sundburg AB, Nolan DR, et al: Complications after cuneiform osteotomy for moderately or severely slipped capital femoral epiphysis, *J Bone Joint Surg* 60B:157, 1978.

Gamble JG, Lettice J, Smith JT, Rinsky LA: Transverse cervicopertrochanteric hip fracture: case report, *J Pediatr Orthop* 11:779, 1991.

Goodman WW, Johnson JT, Robertson WW: Single screw fixation for acute and acute-on-chronic slipped capital femoral epiphysis, *Clin Orthop* 322:86, 1996.

Greenough CG, Bromage JD, Jackson AM: Pinning of the slipped upper femoral epiphysis—a trouble free procedure? *J Pediatr Orthop* 5:657, 1985.

Griffith MJ: Slipping of the capital femoral epiphysis, *Ann R Coll Surg Engl* 58:34, 1976.

Herman MJ, Dormans JP, Davidson RS, et al: Screw fixation of grade III slipped capital femoral epiphysis, *Clin Orthop* 322:77, 1996.

Herndon CH: Treatment of severely slipped upper femoral epiphysis by means of osteoplasty and epiphysiodesis, *Instr Course Lect* 21:214, 1972.

Herndon CH, Heyman CH, Bell DM: Treatment of slipped capital femoral epiphysis by epiphysiodesis and osteoplasty of the femoral neck: a report of further experiences, *J Bone Joint Surg* 45A:999, 1963.

Heyerman W, Weiner D: Slipped epiphysis associated with hypothyroidism, *J Pediatr Orthop* 4:569, 1984.

Heyman CH: Treatment of slipping of the upper femoral epiphysis: a study of results of 42 cases, *Surg Gynecol Obstet* 89:559, 1949.

Heyman CH, Herndon CH: Epiphysiodesis for early slipping of the upper femoral epiphysis, *J Bone Joint Surg* 36A:539, 1954.

Howorth MB: The bone-pegging operation: for slipping of the capital femoral epiphysis, *Clin Orthop* 48:79, 1966.

Hurley JM, Betz RR, Loder RT, et al: Slipped capital femoral epiphysis: the prevalence of late contralateral slip, *J Bone Joint Surg* 78A:226, 1996.

Ingram AJ, Clarke MS, Clark CS Jr, Marshall WR: Chondrolysis complicating slipped capital femoral epiphysis, *Clin Orthop* 165:99, 1982.

Johnson CE II, Hernandez AA: Prophylactic pinning in upper slipped capital femoral epiphysis, *Orthopedics* 7:1502, 1984.

Jones JR, Paterson DC, Hillier TM, Foster BK: Remodeling after pinning for slipped capital femoral epiphysis, *J Bone Joint Surg* 72B:568, 1990.

Kallio PE, Foster BK, LeQuesne GW, Paterson DC: Remodeling in slipped capital femoral epiphysis: sonographic assessment after pinning, *J Pediatr Orthop* 12:438, 1992.

Kallio P, Lequesne GW, Paterson DC, Foster BK: Ultrasonography in slipped capital femoral epiphysis: diagnosis and assessment of severity, *J Bone Joint Surg* 73B:884, 1991.

Kennedy JP, Weiner DS: Results of slipped capital femoral epiphysis in the black population, *J Pediatr Orthop* 10:224, 1990.

Kibiloski LJ, Doane RM, Karol LA, et al: Biomechanical analysis of single- versus double-screw fixation in slipped capital femoral epiphysis at physiological load levels, *J Pediatr Orthop* 14:627, 1994.

King D: Slipping capital femoral epiphysis, *Clin Orthop* 48:71, 1966.

Koval KJ, Lehman WB, Rose D, et al: Treatment of slipped capital femoral epiphysis with a cannulated screw technique, *J Bone Joint Surg* 71A:1370, 1989.

Krahn TH, Canale ST, Beaty JH, et al: Long-term follow-up of patients with avascular necrosis after treatment of slipped capital femoral epiphysis, *J Pediatr Orthop* 13:154, 1993.

Kramer WG, Craig WA, Noel S: Compensating osteotomy of the base of the femoral neck for slipped capital femoral epiphysis, *J Bone Joint Surg* 58A:796, 1976.

Kumm DA, Schmidt J, Eisenburger SH, Hackenbroch J: Prophylactic dynamic screw fixation of the asymptomatic hip in slipped capital femoral epiphysis, *J Pediatr Orthop* 16:249, 1996.

Laplaza FJ, Burke SW: Epiphyseal growth after pinning of slipped capital femoral epiphysis, *J Pediatr Orthop* 15:357, 1995.

Lee TK, Haynes RJ, Longo JA, Chu JR: Pin removal in slipped capital femoral epiphysis: the unstability of titanium devices, *J Pediatr Orthop* 16:49, 1996.

Lehman WB, Menche D, Grant A, Norman A, Pugh J: The problem of evaluating in situ pinning of slipped capital femoral epiphysis: an experimental model and a review of 63 consecutive cases, *J Pediatr Orthop* 4:297, 1984.

Lehman WB, Menche D, Grant A, et al: A method of evaluating possible pin penetration in slipped capital femoral epiphysis using a cannulated internal fixation device, *Clin Orthop* 186:65, 1984.

Lindaman LM, Canale ST, Beaty JH, Warner WC: A fluoroscopic technique for determining the incision site for percutaneous fixation of slipped capital femoral epiphysis, *J Pediatr Orthop* 11:397, 1991.

Loder RT: The demographics of slipped capital femoral epiphysis, *Clin Orthop* 322:8, 1996.

Loder RT, Aronson DD, Greenfield ML: The epidemiology of bilateral slipped capital femoral epiphysis, *J Bone Joint Surg* 75A:1141, 1993.

Loder RT, Richards BS, Shapiro PS, et al: Acute slipped capital femoral epiphysis: the importance of physeal stability, *J Bone Joint Surg* 75A:1134, 1993.

Loder RT, Wittenberg B, DeSilva G: Slipped capital femoral epiphysis associated with endocrine disorders, *J Pediatr Orthop* 15:349, 1995.

Lyden JP: Personal communication, 1985.

MacEwen GD: Advantages and disadvantages of pin fixation in slipped capital femoral epiphysis, *Instr Course Lect* 29:86, 1980.

Mandell GA, Keret D, Harcke HT, Bowen JR: Chondrolysis: detection by bone scintigraphy, *J Pediatr Orthop* 12:80, 1980.

Matava MJ, Patton CM, Luhmann S, et al: Knee pain as the initial symptom of slipped capital femoral epiphysis: an analysis of initial presentation and treatment, *J Pediatr Orthop* 19:455, 1999.

Meier MC, Meyer LC, Ferguson RL: Treatment of slipped capital femoral epiphysis with a spica cast, *J Bone Joint Surg* 74A:1522, 1992.

Melby A, Hoyt W, Weiner D: Treatment of chronic slipped capital femoral epiphysis by bone graft epiphysiodesis, *J Bone Joint Surg* 62A:119, 1980.

Menche D, Lehman WB: In situ pinning of slipped capital femoral epiphysis, *Orthop Rev* 9:129, 1982.

Morrissy RT: Principles of in situ fixation in chronic slipped capital femoral epiphysis, *Instr Course Lect* 38:257, 1989.

Morrissy RT: Slipped capital femoral epiphysis: technique of percutaneous in situ fixation, *J Pediatr Orthop* 10:347, 1990.

Nishiyama K, Sakamaki T, Ishii Y: Follow-up study of the subcapital wedge osteotomy for severe chronic slipped capital femoral epiphysis, *J Pediatr Orthop* 9:412, 1989.

Nonweiler B, Hoffer M, Weinert C, Rosenfeld S: Percutaneous in situ fixation of slipped capital femoral epiphysis using two threaded Steinmann pins, *J Pediatr Orthop* 16:56, 1996.

O'Beirne J, McLoughlin R, Dowling F, et al: Slipped upper femoral epiphysis: internal fixation using single central pins, *J Pediatr Orthop* 9:304, 1989.

O'Brien ET, Fahey JJ: Remodeling of the femoral neck after in-situ pinning for a slipped capital femoral epiphysis, *J Bone Joint Surg* 59A:62, 1977.

Ordenberg G, Hansson IL, Sandstrom S: Slipped capital femoral epiphysis in southern Sweden: long-term result with closed reduction and hip plaster spica, *Clin Orthop* 220:148, 1987.

Orr TR, Bollinger BA, Strecker WB: Blind zone determination of the femoral head, *J Pediatr Orthop* 9:417, 1989.

Rab GT, Simon SR: An improved method for pinning chronic slipped capital femoral epiphysis, *J Pediatr Orthop* 5:212, 1985.

Rao JP, Francis AM, Siwek CW: The treatment of chronic slipped capital femoral epiphysis by biplane osteotomy, *J Bone Joint Surg* 66A:1169, 1984.

Rao SB, Crawford AH, Burger RR, Roy DR: Open bone peg epiphysiodesis for slipped capital femoral epiphysis, *J Pediatr Orthop* 16:37, 1996.

Rao SB, Crawford AH, Roy DR: Open bone peg epiphysiodesis for slipped capital femoral epiphysis: experience in 64 cases. Paper presented at the annual meeting of the Pediatric Orthopaedic Society of North America, Miami, April 30, 1995.

Rattey T, Piehl F, Wright JG: Acute slipped capital femoral epiphysis: review of outcomes and rates of avascular necrosis, *J Bone Joint Surg* 78:398, 1996.

Riley PM, Weiner DS, Gillespie R, Weiner SD: Hazards of internal fixation in the treatment of slipped capital femoral epiphysis, *J Bone Joint Surg* 72A:1500, 1990.

Rooks MD, Schmitt EW: The accuracy of subchondral placement of Knowles pins in slipped capital femoral epiphysis, *Orthop Trans* 8:45, 1984 (abstract).

Rooks MD, Schmitt EW, Dravaric DM: Unrecognized pin penetration in slipped capital femoral epiphysis, *Clin Orthop* 234:82, 1988.

Roy DR, Crawford AH: Idiopathic chondrolysis of the hip: management by subtotal capsulectomy and aggressive rehabilitation, *J Pediatr Orthop* 8:203, 1988.

Samuelson T, Olney B: Percutaneous pin fixation of chronic slipped capital femoral epiphysis, *Clin Orthop* 326:225, 1996.

Scher MA, Jakim I: Intertrochanteric osteotomy and autogenous bone-grafting for avascular necrosis of the femoral head, *J Bone Joint Surg* 75A:1119, 1993.

Schmidt R, Gregg JR: Subtrochanteric fractures complicating pin fixation of slipped capital femoral epiphysis, *Orthop Trans* 9:497, 1985.

Schmidt TL, Cimino WG, Seidel FG: Allograft epiphysiodesis for slipped capital femoral epiphysis, *Clin Orthop* 322:61, 1996.

Segal LS, Davidson RS, Robertson WW, Drummond DS: Growth disturbances of the proximal femur after pinning of juvenile slipped capital femoral epiphysis, *J Pediatr Orthop* 11:631, 1991.

Segal LS, Weitzel PP, Davidson RS: Valgus slipped capital femoral epiphysis, *Clin Orthop* 322:91, 1996.

Shaw JA: Preventing unrecognized penetration into the hip joint, *Orthop Rev* 13:122, 1984.

Siegel B, Kasser JR, Sponseller P, Gelberman RH: Slipped capital femoral epiphysis: a quantitative analysis of motion, gait, and femoral remodeling after in situ fixation, *J Bone Joint Surg* 73;659, 1991.

Southwick WO: Osteotomy through the lesser trochanter for slipped capital femoral epiphysis, *J Bone Joint Surg* 49A:807, 1967.

Southwick WO: Compression fixation after biplane intertrochanteric osteotomy for slipped capital femoral epiphysis: a technical improvement, *J Bone Joint Surg* 55A:1218, 1973.

Spero CR, Masciale JP, Tornetta P III, et al: Slipped capital femoral epiphysis in black children: incidence of chondrolysis, *J Pediatr Orthop* 12:444, 1992.

Stanitksi CL: Acute slipped capital femoral epiphysis: treatment alternatives, *J Am Assoc Orthop Surg* 2:96, 1994.

Steel HH: The metaphyseal blanch sign of slipped capital femoral epiphysis, *J Bone Joint Surg* 68A:920, 1986.

Steel HH: Non-operative treatment of slipped capital femoral epiphysis, *Orthop Trans* 5:7, 1981.

Sternling AL, Ehrlich MG, Armstrong AL, Zaleske DJ: Role of pin protrusion in the etiology of chondrolysis: a surgical model with radiographic, histologic, and biochemical analysis, *J Pediatr Orthop* 12:428, 1992.

Strong M, Lejman T, Michno P, Sulko J: Fixation of slipped capital femoral epiphysis with unthreaded 2-mm wires, *J Pediatr Orthop* 16:53, 1996.

Szypryt EP, Clement DA, Colton CL: Open reduction or epiphysiodesis for slipped upper femoral epiphysis: a comparison of Dunn's operation and the Heyman-Herndon procedure, *J Bone Joint Surg* 69B:737, 1987.

Valdiserri, L, Rubbini L, DiGennaro GL: Three-dimensional intertrochanteric osteotomy in slipped capital femoral epiphysis (SCFE) treatment. Paper presented at the annual meeting of the Pediatric Orthopaedic Society of North America, Miami, April 30, 1995.

Vresilovic EJ, Spindler KP, Robertson WW, et al: Failures of pin removal after in situ pinning of slipped capital femoral epiphysis: a comparison of different pin types, *J Pediatr Orthop* 10:764, 1990.

Vrettos BC, Hoffman EB: Chondrolysis in slipped upper femoral epiphysis, *J Bone Joint Surg* 75B:956, 1993

Volz RG, Martin MD: Illusory biplane radiographic images, *Radiology* 122:695, 1977.

Walters R, Simon SR: Joint destruction: a sequel of unrecognized pin penetration in patients with slipped capital femoral epiphysis of the hip. In *Proceedings of the Eighth Open Scientific Meeting of the Hip Society*, St Louis, 1980, Mosby.

Ward WT, Wood K: Open bone graft epiphysiodesis for slipped capital femoral epiphysis, *J Pediatr Orthop* 10:14, 1990.

Weiner DS, Weiner S, Melby A, Hoyt WA Jr: A 30-year experience with bone graft epiphysiodesis in the treatment of slipped capital femoral epiphysis, *J Pediatr Orthop* 4:145, 1984.

Weiner DS, Weiner SD, Melby A: Anterolateral approach to the hip for bone graft epiphysiodesis in the treatment of slipped capital femoral epiphysis, *J Pediatr Orthop* 8:349, 1988.

Weinstein SL, Morrissy RT, Crawford AH: Slipped capital femoral epiphysis, *Instr Course Lect* 33:310, 1984.

Wilson PD, Jacobs B, Schecter L: Slipped capital femoral epiphysis: an end-result study, *J Bone Joint Surg* 47A:1128, 1965.

Zahrawi FB, Stephens TL, Spencer GE Jr, Clough JM: Comparative study of pinning in situ and open epiphysiodesis in 105 patients with slipped capital femoral epiphysis, *Clin Orthop* 177:160, 1983.

Zionts LE, Simonian PT, Harvey JP: Transient penetration of the hip joint during in situ cannulated screw fixation of slipped capital femoral epiphysis, *J Bone Joint Surg* 73A:1054, 1991.

FEMORAL FRACTURES

Allen B, Kant A, Emery F: Displaced fractures of the femoral diaphysis in children, *J Trauma* 17:8, 1977.

Anderson WA: The significance of femoral fractures in children, *Ann Emerg Med* 11:174, 1982.

Aronson DD, Singer RM, Higgins RF: Skeletal traction for fractures of the femoral shaft in children: a long-term study, *J Bone Joint Surg* 69A:1435, 1987.

Aronson J, Tursky EA: External fixation of femur fractures in children. Paper presented at the Fifty-seventh Annual Meeting of the American Academy of Orthopaedic Surgeons, Las Vegas, Feb 10, 1990.

Aronson J, Tursky EA: External fixation of femur fractures in children, *J Pediatr Orthop* 12:157, 1992.

Banagale RC, Kuhns LR: Traumatic separation of the distal femoral epiphysis in a newborn, *J Pediatr Orthop* 3:3, 1983.

Bar On E, Sagiv S, Porat S: External fixation or flexible intramedullary nailing for femoral shaft fractures in children: a prospective, randomised study, *J Bone Joint Surg* 79B:975, 1997.

Beaty JH: Orthopedic aspects of child abuse, *Curr Opin Pediatr* 9:100, 1997.

Beaty JH, Austin SM, Warner WC, et al: Interlocking intramedullary nailing of femoral-shaft fractures in adolescents: preliminary results and complications, *J Pediatr Orthop* 14:178, 1994.

Blakemore LC, Loder RT, Hensinger RN: Role of intentional abuse in children 1 to 5 years old with isolated femoral shaft fractures, *J Pediatr Orthop* 16:585, 1996.

Blasier RD, Aronson J, Tursky EA: External fixation of pediatric femur fracture, *J Pediatr Orthop* 17:342, 1997.

Blount W: *Fractures in children*, Baltimore, 1955, Williams & Wilkins.

Bohn WW, Durbin RA: Ipsilateral fractures of the femur and tibia in children and adolescents, *J Bone Joint Surg* 73A:429, 1991.

Boman A, Gardell C, Janarv PM: Home traction of femoral shaft fractures in younger children, *J Pediatr Orthop* 18:478, 1998.

Bordelat D: Fracture of the femoral shaft in children: advantages of the descending medullary nailing, *J Pediatr Orthop* 5:110, 1996.

Bright RW: Operative correction of partial epiphyseal plate closure by osseous-bridge resection and silicone-rubber implant, *J Bone Joint Surg* 56A:655, 1974.

Brower KJ: Torsional deformities after fractures of the femoral shaft in childhood, *Acta Orthop Scand Suppl* 52, 1981.

Brower KJ, Molenaar JC, Van Linge B: Rotational deformities after femoral shaft fractures in childhood, *Acta Orthop Scand* 52:81, 1981.

Buckley SL, Sturm PF, Tosi LL, et al: Ligamentous instability of the knee in children sustaining fractures of the femur: a prospective study with knee examination under anesthesia, *J Pediatr Orthop* 16:206, 1996.

Buford D Jr, Christensen K, Weatherall P: Intramedullary nailing of femoral fractures in adolescents, *Clin Orthop* 350:85, 1998.

Canale ST, Puhl J, Watson FM, Gillespie R: Acute osteomyelitis following closed fractures, *J Bone Joint Surg* 57A:415, 1975.

Carey TP, Galpin RD: Flexible intramedullary nail fixation of pediatric femoral fractures, *Clin Orthop* 332:110, 1996.

Cassebaum WH, Patterson AH: Fractures of the distal femoral epiphysis, *Clin Orthop* 41:79, 1965.

Cheng JC, Cheung SSC: Modified functional bracing in the ambulatory treatment of femoral shaft fractures in children, *J Pediatr Orthop* 9:457, 1989.

Cheng JC, Tang N: Decompression and stable internal fixation of femoral neck fractures in children can affect the outcome, *J Pediatr Orthop* 19:578, 1999.

Clement DA, Colton CL: Overgrowth of the femur after femoral fractures in childhood, *J Bone Joint Surg* 68B:534, 1986.

Clinkscales CM, Peterson HA: Isolated closed diaphyseal fractures of the femur in children: comparison of effectiveness and cost of several treatment methods, *Orthopedics* 20:1131, 1997.

Coyte PC, Bronskill SE, Hirji ZZ, et al: Economic evaluation of two treatments for pediatric femoral shaft fractures, *Clin Orthop* 336:205, 1997.

Czertak DJ, Hennrikus WL: The treatment of pediatric femur fractures with early 90-90 spica casting, *J Pediatr Orthop* 19:229, 1999.

Czitrom AA, Salter RB, Willis RB: Fractures involving the distal femoral epiphyseal plate of the femur, *Int Orthop* 4:269, 1981.

Ehrlich MG, Strain RE Jr: Epiphyseal injuries about the knee, *Orthop Clin North Am* 10:91, 1979.

Evanoff M, Strong ML, MacIntosh R: External fixation maintained until fracture consolidation in the skeletally immature, *J Pediatr Orthop* 13:98, 1993.

Fein LH, Pankovich AM, Spero CM, Baruch HM: Closed flexible intramedullary nailing of adolescent femoral shaft fractures, *J Orthop Trauma* 3:133, 1989.

Fyodorov I, Sturm PF, Robertson WW Jr: Compression-plate fixation of femoral shaft fractures in children aged 8 to 12 years, *J Pediatr Orthop* 19:578, 1999.

Gregory P, Pevny T, Teague D: Early complications with external fixation of pediatric femoral shaft fractures, *J Orthop Trauma* 10:191, 1996.

Griffin PP, Anderson M, Green WT: Fractures of the shaft of the femur in children, *Orthop Clin North Am* 3:213, 1972.

Guttmann GG, Simon R: Three-point fixation walking spica cast: an alternative to early or immediate casting of femoral shaft fractures in children, *J Pediatr Orthop* 8:699, 1988.

Hansen ST: Internal fixation of children's fractures of the lower extremity, *Orthop Clin North Am* 21:353, 1990.

Hansen TB: Fractures of the femoral shaft in children treated with an AO-compression plate: report of 12 cases followed until adulthood, *Acta Orthop Scand* 63:50, 1992.

Heinrich SD, Drvaric D, Darr K, MacEwen GD: Stabilization of pediatric diaphyseal femur fractures with flexible intramedullary nails (a technique paper), *J Orthop Trauma* 6:452, 1992.

Heinrich SD, Drvaric DM, Darr K, MacEwen, GD: The operative stabilization of pediatric diaphyseal femur fractures with flexible intramedullary nails: a prospective analysis, *J Pediatr Orthop* 14:501, 1994.

Hennrikus WL, Kasser JR, Rand F, et al: **The function of the quadriceps muscle after a fracture of the femur in patients who are less than seventeen years old,** *J Bone Joint Surg* 75A:508, 1993.

Henderson OL, Morissy RT, Gerdes MH, McCarthy RE: Early casting of femoral shaft fractures in children, *J Pediatr Orthop* 4:16, 1984.

Herndon WA, Mahnken RF, Hygve DA, Sullivan JA: Management of femoral shaft fractures in the adolescent, *J Pediatr Orthop* 9:29, 1989.

Hinton RY, Lincoln A, Crockett MM, et al: Fractures of the femoral shaft in children: incidence, mechanisms, and sociodemographic risk factors, *J Bone Joint Surg* 81A:500, 1999.

Hoffer M, Garrett A, Brink J, et al: **The orthopaedic management of brain-injured children,** *J Bone Joint Surg* 53A:567, 1971.

Holmes SJ, Sedgwick DM, Scobie WG: Domiciliary gallow traction for femoral shaft fractures in young children, *J Bone Joint Surg* 65B:288, 1983.

Hougaard K: Femoral shaft fractures in children: a prospective study of the overgrowth phenomenon, *Injury* 20:170, 1989.

Hresko MT, Kasser JR: Physeal arrest about the knee associated with non-physeal fractures in the lower extremity, *J Bone Joint Surg* 71A:698, 1989.

Hughes BF, Sponseller PD, Thompson JD: Pediatric femur fractures: effects of spica cast treatment on family and community, *J Pediatr Orthop* 15:457, 1995.

Humberger F, Eyring E: Proximal tibial 90-90 traction in treatment of children with femoral shaft fractures, *J Bone Joint Surg* 51A:499, 1969.

Hutchins CM, Sponseller PD, Sturm P, Mosquero R: Open femur fractures in children: treatment, complications, and results, *J Pediatr Orthop* 20:183, 2000.

Illgen R II, Rodgers WB, Hresko MT, et al: Femur fractures in children: treatment with early sitting spica casting, *J Pediatr Orthop* 18:481, 1998.

Irani R, Nicholson J, Chung S: **Long-term results in the treatment of femoral-shaft fractures in young children by immediate spica immobilization,** *J Bone Joint Surg* 58A:945, 1976.

Jeng C, Sponseller PD, Yates A, Paletta G: Subtrochanteric femoral fractures in children: alignment after 90 degrees–90 degrees traction and cast application, *Clin Orthop* 341:170, 1997.

Kasser JR: Femur fractures in children, *Instr Course Lect* 41:403, 1992.

Kirby RM, Winquist RA, Hansen ST Jr: Femoral shaft fractures in adolescents, comparison between traction plus cast treatment and closed intramedullary nailing, *J Pediatr Orthop* 1:193, 1981.

Kissel EW, Miller ME: Closed-ended nailing of femur fractures in older children, *J Trauma* 29:1585, 1989.

Langenskiöld A: **An operation for partial closure of an epiphyseal plate in children and its experimental basis,** *J Bone Joint Surg* 57B:325, 1975.

Ligier JN, Metaizeau JP, Prevot J, Lescombes P: Elastic stable intramedullary nailing of femoral shaft fractures in children, *J Bone Joint Surg* 70B:74, 1988.

Limbird TJ, Cramer KE: Pediatric lower extremity open fractures: treatment results and complications. Paper presented at the Fifty-seventh Annual Meeting of the American Academy of Orthopaedic Surgeons, Las Vegas, Feb 10, 1990.

Litt R, Albassir A, Willems S, Debry R: Coxa vara: isolated growth of the greater trochanter: prevention and treatment, *Acta Orthop Belg* 56:310, 1990.

Lombardo SJ, Harvey JP Jr: **Fractures of the distal femoral epiphysis: factors influencing prognosis: a review of thirty-four cases,** *J Bone Joint Surg* 59A:742, 1977.

Mäkelä EA, Vainionpää S, Vihtonen K, et al: The effect of trauma to the lower femoral epiphyseal plate: an experimental study in rabbits, *J Bone Joint Surg* 70B:187, 1988.

Mann DC, Weddington J, Davenport K: Closed Enders nailing of femoral shaft fractures in adolescents, *J Pediatr Orthop* 6:651, 1986.

Martinez AG, Carroll NC, Sarwark JF, et al: Femoral shaft fractures in children treated with early spica cast, *J Pediatr Orthop* 11:712, 1991.

Meals R: Overgrowth of the femur following fractures in children: influence of handedness, *J Bone Joint Surg* 61A:381, 1979.

Momberger N, Stevens P, Smith J, et al: Intramedullary nailing of femoral fractures in adolescents, *J Pediatr Orthop* 20:482, 2000.

Moseley CF: A straight-line graph for leg-length discrepancies, *J Bone Joint Surg* 59A:174, 1977.

Neer C, Cadman E: Treatment of fractures of the femoral shaft in children, *JAMA* 163:634, 1957.

Newton PO, Mubarak SJ: **Financial aspects of femoral shaft fracture treatment in children and adolescents,** *J Pediatr Orthop* 14:508, 1994.

Nork SE, Bellig GW, Woll JP, Hoffinger SA: Overgrowth and outcome after femoral shaft fracture in children younger than 2 years, *Clin Orthop* 357:186, 1998.

Nork SE, Hoffinger SA: Skeletal traction versus external fixation for pediatric femoral shaft fractures: a comparison of hospital costs and charges, *J Orthop Trauma* 12:563, 1999.

Peterson HA, Burkhart SS: Compression injury of the epiphyseal growth plate: fact or fiction? *J Pediatr Orthop* 1:377, 1981.

Pollak AN, Cooperman DR, Thompson GH: Spica cast treatment of femoral shaft fractures in children—the prognostic value of the mechanism of injury, *J Trauma* 37:223, 1994.

Prevot J, Lascombes P, Mainard D, et al: Osteoarthritis in infants: follow-up and treatment, *Chir Pediatr* 26:143, 1985.

Probe R, Lindsey RW, Hadley NA, Barnes DA: **Refracture of adolescent femoral shaft fractures: a complication of external fixation—a report of two cases,** *J Pediatr Orthop* 13:102, 1993.

Rang M: *Children's fractures,* Philadelphia, 1974, JB Lippincott.

Reeves RB, Ballard RI, Hughes JL: **Internal fixation versus traction and casting of adolescent femoral shaft fractures,** *J Pediatr Orthop* 10:591, 1990.

Rejholec M, Stryhal F: Behavior of the proximal femur during the treatment of congenital dysplasia of the hip: a clinical long-term study, *J Pediatr Orthop* 11:506, 1991.

Riseborough EJ, Barrett IR, Shapiro F: Growth disturbances following distal femoral epiphyseal fracture-separations, *J Bone Joint Surg* 65A:885, 1983.

Roberts JM: **Fracture separation of the distal femoral epiphysis,** *J Bone Joint Surg* 55A:1324, 1973.

Robertson P, Karol LA, Rab GT: Open fractures of the tibia and femur in children, *J Pediatr Orthop* 16:621, 1996.

Rosenberg NM, Vraneisch P, Bottenfield G: Fractured femurs in pediatric patients, *Ann Emerg Med* 11:84, 1982.

Salter RB, Harris WR: Injuries involving the epiphyseal plate, *J Bone Joint Surg* 45A:587, 1963.

Saxer U: Fractures of the shaft of the femur. In Weber BG, Brunner C, Frueler F, eds: *Treatment of fractures in children and adolescents,* New York, 1980, Springer-Verlag.

Schneider M: The effect of growth on femoral torsion: an experimental study in dogs, *J Bone Joint Surg* 45A:1439, 1963.

Schwend RM, Werth C, Johnston A: Femur shaft fractures in toddlers and young children: rarely from child abuse, *J Pediatr Orthop* 20:475, 2000.

Searfin J, Szulc W: Coxa vara infantum, hip growth disturbances, etiopathogenesis, and long-term results of treatment, *Clin Orthop* 272:103, 1991.

Shapiro F: Fractures of the femoral shaft in children: the overgrowth phenomenon, *Acta Orthop Scand* 52:649, 1981.

Skaggs DL, Leet AI, Money MD, et al: Secondary fractures associated with external fixation in pediatric femur fractures, *J Pediatr Orthop* 19:582, 1999.

Sola J, Schoenecker PL, Gordon JE: External fixation of femoral shaft fractures in children: enhanced stability with the use of an auxiliary pin, *J Pediatr Orthop* 19:587, 1999.

Staheli L: Femoral and tibial growth following femoral shaft fracture in childhood, *Clin Orthop* 55:159, 1967.

Staheli L, Sheridan G: Early spica cast management of femoral shaft fractures in young children, *Clin Orthop* 126:162, 1977.

Stannard JP, Christensen KP, Wilkins KE: Femur fractures in infants: a new therapeutic approach, *J Pediatr Orthop* 15:461, 1995.

Stans AA, Morrissy RT, Renwick SE: Femoral shaft fracture treatment in patients age 6 to 16 years, *J Pediatr Orthop* 19:222, 1999.

Stephens DC, Louis DS, Louis E: Traumatic separation of the distal femoral epiphyseal cartilage plate, *J Bone Joint Surg* 56A:1383, 1974.

Strauss E, Nelson JM, Abdelwahab IF: Fracture of the lateral femoral condyle: a case report, *Bull Hosp Jt Dis* 44:87, 1984.

Strong ML, Wong-Chung J, Babikian G, Brody A: Rotational remodeling of malrotated femoral fractures: a model in the rabbit, *J Pediatr Orthop* 12:173, 1992.

Theologis TN, Cole WG: Management of subtrochanteric fractures of the femur in children, *J Pediatr Orthop* 18:22, 1998.

Thompson GH, Wilber JH, Marcus RE: Internal fixation of fractures in children and adolescents: a comparative analysis, *Clin Orthop* 188:10, 1984.

Thompson JD, Duehler KC, Sponseller PD, et al: Shortening in femoral shaft fractures in children treated with spica cast, *Clin Orthop* 338:74, 1997.

Thomson JD, Stricker SJ, Williams MM: Fractures of the distal femoral epiphyseal plate, *J Pediatr Orthop* 15:474, 1995.

Timmerman LA, Rab GT: Closed reamed intramedullary nail versus traction and casting in treatment of femoral shaft fractures in the 10- to 14-year old. Paper presented at the Fifty-seventh Annual Meeting of the American Academy of Orthopaedic Surgeons, Las Vegas, Feb 10, 1990.

Valdiserri L, Marchiodi L, Rubbini L: Küntscher nailing in the treatment of femoral fractures in children: is it completely contraindicated? *Ital J Orthop Traumatol* 9:293, 1983.

Vrsansky P, Bourdelat D, Al Faour A: Flexible stable intramedullary pinning technique in the treatment of pediatric fractures, *J Pediatr Orthop* 20:23, 2000.

Wallace ME, Hoffman EB: Remodeling of angular deformity after femoral shaft fractures in children, *J Bone Joint Surg* 74B:765, 1992.

Ward WT, Levy J, Kaye A: Compression plating for child and adolescent femur fractures, *J Pediatr Orthop* 12:626, 1992.

Weber BG, Brunner C, Freuler F, eds: *Treatment of fractures in children and adolescents*, New York, 1980, Springer-Verlag.

Weiss AC, Schenck RC, Sponseller PD, Thompson JD: Peroneal nerve palsy after early cast application for femoral fractures in children, *J Pediatr Orthop* 12:25, 1992.

Yandow SM, Archibeck MJ, Seevens SM, Schultc R: Femoral shaft fractures in children: a comparison of immediate casting and traction, *J Pediatr Orthop* 19:55, 1999.

Ziv I, Blackburn N, Rang M: Femoral intramedullary nailing in growing child, *J Trauma* 24:432, 1984.

Ziv I, Rang M: Treatment of femoral fracture in the child with head injury, *J Bone Joint Surg* 65B:184, 1983.

KNEE FRACTURES

Bassett FH III: Acute dislocation of the patella osteochondral fractures and injuries to the extensor mechanism of the knee, *Instr Course Lect* 25:40, 1976.

Baxter MP, Wiley JJ: Fractures of the tibial spine in children: an evaluation of knee stability, *J Bone Joint Surg* 70B:228, 1988.

Bergström R, Gillquist J, Lysholm J: Arthroscopy of the knee in children, *J Pediatr Orthop* 4:542, 1984.

Bernhang AM, Levine SA: Familial absence of the patella, *J Bone Joint Surg* 53A:1088, 1973.

Bohn WW, Durbin RA: Ipsilateral fractures of the femur and tibia in children and adolescents, *J Bone Joint Surg* 73A:429, 1991.

Christie MJ, Dvonch VM: Tibial tuberosity avulsion fracture in adolescents, *J Pediatr Orthop* 1:391, 1981.

Clanton TO, DeLee JC, Sanders B, Neidre A: Knee ligament injuries in children, *J Bone Joint Surg* 61A:1195, 1979.

Cofield RH, Bryan RS: Acute dislocation of the patella: results of conservative treatment, *J Trauma* 17:526, 1977.

Crothers OD, Johnson JTH: Isolated acute dislocation of the proximal tibiofibular joint, *J Bone Joint Surg* 55A:181, 1973.

Eilert R: Arthroscopy of the knee joint in children, *Orthop Rev* 5:61 1976.

Eiskjar S, Larsen ST: Arthroscopy of the knee in children, *Acta Orthop Scand* 58:273, 1987.

Falstie-Jensen S, Sondergard-Peterson PE: Incarceration of the meniscus in fracture of the intercondylar eminence of the tibia in children, *Injury* 15:236, 1984.

Fowler PJ: The classification and early diagnosis of knee joint instability, *Clin Orthop* 147:15, 1980.

Fujikawa K, Iseki F, Mikura Y: Partial resection of the discoid meniscus in the child's knee, *J Bone Joint Surg* 63B:391, 1981.

Fyfe IS, Jackson JP: Tibial intercondylar fractures in children: a review of the classification and the treatment of mal-union, *Injury* 13:165, 1981.

Green WT Jr: Painful bipartite patellae: a report of three cases, *Clin Orthop* 110:197, 1975.

Grönkvist H, Hirsch G, Johänsson L: Fracture of the anterior tibial spine in children, *J Pediatr Orthop* 4:465, 1984.

Hand WL, Hand CR, Dunn AW: Avulsion fractures of the tibial tubercle, *J Bone Joint Surg* 53A:1579, 1971.

Hayes AG, Nageswar M: The adolescent painful knee: the value of arthroscopy in diagnosis, *J Bone Joint Surg* 59B:499, 1977.

Heckman JD, Alkire CC: Distal patellar pole fractures: a proposed common mechanism of injury, *Am J Sports Med* 12:424, 1984.

Houghton GR, Ackroyd CE: Sleeve fractures of the patella in children: a report of three cases, *J Bone Joint Surg* 61B:165, 1979.

Hyndman JC, Brown DC: Major ligamentous injuries of the knee in children, *J Bone Joint Surg* 61B:245, 1979.

Juhl M, Boe S: Arthroscopy in children, with special emphasis on meniscal lesions, *Injury* 17:171, 1986.

Letts M, Vincent N, Gouw G: The "floating knee" in children, *J Bone Joint Surg* 68B:442, 1986.

McManus F, Rang M, Heslin DJ: Acute dislocation of the patella in children: the natural history, *Clin Orthop* 139:88, 1979.

Medlar RC, Lyne ED: Sinding-Larsen-Johansson disease: its etiology and natural history, *J Bone Joint Surg* 60A:1113, 1978.

Metcalf RW: An arthroscopic method for lateral release of the subluxating or dislocating patella, *Clin Orthop* 167:9, 1982.

Meyers MH, McKeever FM: Fracture of the intercondylar eminence of the tibia, *J Bone Joint Surg* 41A:209, 1959.

Meyers MH, McKeever FM: Follow-up notes: fracture of the intercondylar eminence of the tibia, *J Bone Joint Surg* 52A:167, 1970.

Morrissy RT, Eubanks RG, Park JP, Thompson SB Jr: Arthroscopy of the knee in children, *Clin Orthop* 162:103, 1982.

Nawata K, Teshima R, Morio Y, Hagino H: Anomalies of ossification in the posterolateral femoral condyle: assessment by MRI, *Pediatr Radiol* 29:781, 1999.

Nietosvaara Y, Aalto K: The cartilaginous femoral sulcus in children with patellar dislocation: an ultrasonographic study, *J Pediatr Orthop* 17:50, 1997.

Nietosvaara Y, Aalto K, Kallio PE: Acute patellar dislocation in children: incidence and associated osteochondral fractures, *J Pediatr Orthop* 14:513, 1994.

Ogden JA: Subluxation and dissociation of the proximal tibiofibular joint, *J Bone Joint Surg* 56A:145, 1974.

Ogden JA: *Skeletal injury in the child*, Philadelphia, 1982, Lea & Febiger.

Ogden JA, Tross RB, Murphy, MJ: Fractures of the tibial tuberosity in adolescents, *J Bone Joint Surg* 62A:205, 1980.

Osgood RB: Lesions of the tibial tubercle occurring during adolescence, *Boston Med Surg J* 148:114, 1903.

Roberts JM: Fractures and dislocations of the knee. In Rockwood CA Jr, Wilkins KE, King RE, eds: *Fractures in children*, Philadelphia, 1984, JB Lippincott.

Roberts JM, Lovell WW: Fractures of the intercondylar eminence of tibia, *J Bone Joint Surg* 52A:827, 1970.

Rorabeck CH, Bobechko WP: Acute dislocation of the patella with osteochondral fracture: review of eighteen cases, *J Bone Joint Surg* 58B:237, 1976.

Schlatter C: Verletzungen des Schnabelförmigen Fortsatzes der Oberen Tibiaepiphyse, *Beitr Klin Chir* 38:874, 1903.

Scott JE, Taor WS: The "small patella" syndrome, *J Bone Joint Surg* 61B:172, 1979.

Sijbrandij S: Instability of the proximal tibiofibular joint, *Acta Orthop Scand* 49:621, 1978.

Sinding-Larsen MF: A hitherto unknown affection of the patella in children, *Acta Radiol* 1:171, 1922.

Vahvanen V, Aalto K: Meniscectomy in children, *Acta Orthop Scand* 50:791, 1979.

Weber MJ, Janecki CJ, McLeod P, et al: Efficacy of various forms of fixation of transverse fractures of the patella, *J Bone Joint Surg* 62A:215, 1980.

Wiley JJ, Baxter MP: Tibial spine fractures in children, *Clin Orthop* 225:54, 1990.

Willis RB, Blokker C, Stoll TM, et al: Long-term follow-up of anterior tibial eminence fractures, *J Pediatr Orthop* 13:361, 1993.

TIBIAL AND FIBULAR EPIPHYSEAL FRACTURES

Aitken AP: Fractures of the proximal tibial epiphyseal cartilage, *Clin Orthop* 41:92 1965.

Blanks RH, Lester DK, Shaw BA: Flexion-type Salter II fracture of the proximal tibia: proposed mechanism of injury and two case studies, *Clin Orthop* 301:256, 1994.

Canale ST, Shelton WR: Fractures of the tibia through the proximal tibial epiphyseal cartilage, *J Bone Joint Surg* 61A:167, 1979.

de Sanctis N, Corte SD, and Pempinello C: Distal tibial and fibular epiphyseal fractures in children: prognostic criteria and long-term results in 158 patients. *J Pediatr Orthop* 9:40, 2000.

Gill JG, Chakrabarti HF, Becker SJ: Fracture of the proximal tibial epiphysis, *Injury* 14:324, 1983.

Harries TJ, Lichtman DM, Lonon WD: Irreducible Salter-Harris II fracture of the proximal tibia, *J Pediatr Orthop* 3:92, 1983.

Kendall NS, Hsu SYC, Chan KM: Fracture of the tibial spine in adults and children: a review of 31 cases, *J Bone Joint Surg* 74B:848, 1992.

Kreder HJ, Armstrong P: A review of open tibia fractures in children, *J Pediatr Orthop* 15:482, 1995.

Lee EH, Gao GX, Bose K: Management of partial growth arrest: physis, fat, or Silastic? *J Pediatr Orthop* 13:368, 1993.

McGuigan JA, O'Reilly MJG, Nixon JR: Popliteal artery thrombosis resulting from disruption of the upper tibial epiphysis, *Injury* 16:49, 1984.

Resnick D, Niwayama G: *Diagnosis of bone and joint disorders: with emphasis on articular abnormalities*, Philadelphia, 1981, WB Saunders.

Thompson GH, Gesler JW: Proximal tibial epiphyseal fracture in an infant, *J Pediatr Orthop* 4:185, 1984.

Weber BG, Brunner C, Freuler F, eds: *Treatment of fractures in children and adolescents*, New York, 1980, Springer-Verlag.

Wester W, Canale ST, Dutkowsky JP, et al: Prediction of angular deformity and leg-length discrepancy after anterior cruciate ligament reconstruction in skeletally immature patients, *J Pediatr Orthop* 14:516-521, 1994.

Wozasek GE, Moser KD, Haller H, Capousek M: Trauma involving the proximal tibial epiphysis, *Arch Orthop Trauma* 110:301, 1991.

PROXIMAL TIBIAL METAPHYSEAL AND TIBIAL SHAFTS FRACTURES

Bahnson DH, Lovell WW: Genu valgum following fractures of the proximal tibial metaphysis in children, *Orthop Trans* 4:306, 1980.

Balthazar DA, Pappas AM: Acquired valgus deformity of the tibia in children, *J Pediatr Orthop* 4:538, 1984.

Bartlett CS III, Weiner LS, Yang EC: Treatment of type II and type II tibia fractures in children, *J Orthop Trauma* 11:357, 1997.

Blasier RD, Barnes CL: Age as a prognostic factor in open tibial fractures in children, *Clin Orthop* 331:261, 1996.

Briggs TWR, Orr MM, Lightowler CDR: Isolated tibial fractures in children, *Injury* 23:308, 1992.

Buckley SL, Smith GR, Sponseller PD, et al: Severe (type III) open fractures of the tibia in children, *J Pediatr Orthop* 16:627, 1996.

Coates R: Knock-knee deformity following upper tibial "greenstick" fractures, *J Bone Joint Surg* 59B:516, 1977.

Cozen L: Knock knee deformity after fracture of the proximal tibia in children, *Orthopedics* 1:230, 1959.

Cramer KE, Limbird TJ, Green NE: Open fractures of the diaphysis of the lower extremity in children: treatment, results, and complications, *J Bone Joint Surg* 74A:218, 1992.

Cullen MC, Roy DR, Crawford AH, et al: Open fracture of the tibia in children, *J Bone Joint Surg* 78A:1039, 1996.

Dal Monte A, Manes E, Cammarota V: Post-traumatic genu valgum in children, *Ital J Orthop Traumatol* 9:5, 1983.

Engh CA, Robinson RA, Milgram J: Stress fractures in children, *J Trauma* 10:532, 1970.

Green NE: Tibial valga caused by asymmetrical overgrowth following a nondisplaced fracture of the proximal tibial metaphysis, *J Pediatr Orthop* 3:235, 1983.

Greiff J, Bergman F: Growth disturbance following fractures of the tibia in children, *Acta Orthop Scand* 51:315, 1980.

Grimard G, Naudie D, Laberge LC, Hamdy RC: Open fractures of the tibia in children, *Clin Orthop* 332:62, 1996.

Haas LM, Staple TW: Arterial injuries associated with fractures of the proximal tibia following blunt trauma, *South Med J* 62:1439, 1969.

Hansen BA, Greiff J, Bergmann F: Fractures of the tibia in children, *Acta Orthop Scand* 47:448, 1976.

Herring JA, Moseley C: Posttraumatic valgus deformity of the tibia, *J Pediatr Orthop* 1:435, 1981.

Houghton GR, Rooker GD: The role of the periosteum in the growth of long bones: an experimental study in the rabbit, *J Bone Joint Surg* 61B:218, 1979.

Ippolito E, Pentimalli G: Post-traumatic valgus deformity of the knee in proximal tibial metaphyseal fractures in children, *Ital J Orthop Traumatol* 10:103, 1984.

Jackson DW, Cozen L: Genu valgum as a complication of proximal tibial metaphyseal fractures in children, *J Bone Joint Surg* 53A:1571, 1971.

Jordan SE, Alonso JE, Cook FF: The etiology of valgus angulation after metaphyseal fractures of the tibia in children, *J Pediatr Orthop* 7:450, 1987.

Karlström G, Lönnerholm T, Olerud S: Cavus deformity of the foot after fracture of the tibial shaft, *J Bone Joint Surg* 57A:893, 1975.

Levy AS, Wetzler M, Lewars M, et al: The orthopedic and social outcome of open tibia fractures in children, *Orthopedics* 20:593, 1997.

Morton KS, Starr DE: Closure of the anterior portion of the upper tibial epiphysis as a complication of tibial-shaft fracture, *J Bone Joint Surg* 46A:570, 1964.

Mubarak SJ, Hargens AR, Owen CA, et al: The wick catheter technique for measurement of intramuscular pressure, *J Bone Joint Surg* 58A:1016, 1976.

Navascués JA, González-López JL, López-Valverde S, et al: Premature physeal closure after tibial diaphyseal fractures in adolescents, *J Pediatr Orthop* 20:193, 2000.

Ogden JA, Ogden DA, Pugh L, et al: Tibia valga after proximal metaphyseal fractures in childhood: a normal biologic response, *J Pediatr Orthop* 15:489, 1995.

Pappas AM, Anas P, Toczylowski HM Jr: Asymmetrical arrest of the proximal tibial physis and genu recurvatum deformity, *J Bone Joint Surg* 66A:575, 1984.

Pollen AG: *Fractures and dislocations in children*, Baltimore, 1973, Williams & Wilkins.

Rang M: *Children's fractures*, ed 2, Philadelphia, 1983, JB Lippincott.

Reynolds DA: Growth changes in fractures of the long bones, *J Bone Joint Surg* 63B:83, 1981.

Robert M, Khouri N, Carlioz H, Alain JL: Fractures of the proximal tibial metaphysis in children: review of a series of 25 cases, *J Pediatr Orthop* 7:444, 1987.

Salter RB, Best T: The pathogenesis and prevention of valgus deformity following fractures of the proximal metaphyseal region of the tibia in children, *J Bone Joint Surg* 55A:1324, 1973.

Skak SV: Valgus deformity following proximal tibial metaphyseal fracture in children, *Acta Orthop Scand* 53:141, 1982.

Skak SV, Jensen TT, Poulsen TD: Fracture of the proximal metaphysis of the tibia in children, *Injury* 18:149, 1987.

Steel HH, Sandrow RE, Sullivan PD: Complications of tibial osteotomy in children for genu varum or valgum, *J Bone Joint Surg* 53A:1629, 1971.

Taylor SL: Tibial overgrowth: a cause of genu valgum, *J Bone Joint Surg* 45A:659, 1963.

Visser JD, Veldhuizen AG: Valgus deformity after fracture of the proximal tibial metaphysis in childhood, *Acta Orthop Scand* 53: 663, 1982.

Weber BG: Fibrous interposition causing valgus deformity after fracture of the upper tibial metaphysis in children, *J Bone Joint Surg* 59B:290, 1977.

Weber BG, Brunner C, Freuler F, eds: *Treatment of fractures in children and adolescents*, New York, 1980, Springer-Verlag.

Whitesides TE Jr, Haney TC, Morimoto K, Harada H: Tissue pressure measurements as a determinant for the need of fasciotomy, *Clin Orthop* 113:43, 1975.

Yang JP, Letts RM: Isolated fractures of the tibia with intact fibula in children: a review of 95 patients, *J Pediatr Orthop* 17:347, 1997.

Zionts LE, Harcke T, Brooks KM, MacEwen GD: Posttraumatic tibia valga: a case demonstrating asymmetric activity at the proximal growth plate on technetium bone scan, *J Pediatr Orthop* 7:458, 1987.

DISTAL TIBIAL AND FIBULAR EPIPHYSEAL FRACTURES

Beaty JH, Linton RC: Medial malleolar fracture in a child: a case report, *J Bone Joint Surg* 70A:1254, 1988.

Bright RW: Operative correction of partial epiphyseal plate closure by osseous-bridge resection and silicone-rubber implant, *J Bone Joint Surg* 56A:655, 1974.

Buckley SL, Smith G, Sponseller PD, et al: Open fractures of the tibia in children, *J Bone Joint Surg* 72A:1462, 1990.

Busconi BD, Pappas AM: Chronic, painful ankle instability in skeletally immature athletes: ununited osteochondral fractures of the distal fibula, *Am J Sports Med* 24:647, 1996.

Carothers CO, Crenshaw AH: Clinical significance of a classification of epiphyseal injuries at the ankle, *Am J Surg* 89:879, 1955.

Cass JR, Peterson HA: Salter-Harris type IV injuries of the distal tibial epiphyseal growth plate, with emphasis on those involving the medial malleolus, *J Bone Joint Surg* 65A:1059, 1983.

Chadwick CJ: Spontaneous resolution of varus deformity of the ankle following adduction injury of the distal tibial epiphysis, *J Bone Joint Surg* 64A:774, 1982.

Chuinard EG, Peterson RE: Distraction-compression bone-graft arthrodesis of the ankle: a method especially applicable in children, *J Bone Joint Surg* 45A:1040, 1978.

Cooperman DR, Spiegel PG, Laros GS: Tibial fractures involving the ankle in children: the so-called triplane epiphyseal fracture, *J Bone Joint Surg* 60A:1040, 1978.

Crenshaw AH: Injuries of the distal tibial epiphysis, *Clin Orthop* 41:98, 1965.

Denton JR, Fischer SJ: The medial triplane fracture: report of an unusual injury, *J Trauma* 21:991, 1981.

Dias LS, Giegerich CR: Fractures of the distal tibial epiphysis in adolescence, *J Bone Joint Surg* 65A:438, 1983.

Dias LS, Tachdjian MO: Physeal injuries of the ankle in children, *Clin Orthop* 136:230, 1978.

Feldman DS, Otsuka NY, Hedden DM: Extra-articular triplane fracture of the distal tibial epiphysis, *J Pediatr Orthop* 15:479, 1995.

Grace DL: Irreducible fracture separations of the distal tibial epiphysis, *J Bone Joint Surg* 65B:160, 1983.

Hope PG, Cole WG: Open fractures of the tibia in children, *J Bone Joint Surg* 74B:546, 1992.

Hynes D, O'Brien T: Growth disturbance lines after injury of the distal tibial physis: their significance in prognosis, *J Bone Joint Surg* 70B:231, 1988.

Kärrholm J, Hansson LI, Laurin S: Pronation injuries of the ankle in children, *Acta Orthop Scand* 54:1, 1983.

Kärrholm J, Hansson LI, Selvik G: Roentgen stereophotogrammetric analysis of growth patterns after supination-adduction ankle injuries in children, *J Pediatr Orthop* 2:271, 1982.

Kärrholm J, Hansson LI, Selvik G: Roentgen stereophotogrammetric analysis of growth patterns after supination-eversion ankle injuries in children, *J Pediatr Orthop* 2:25, 1982.

Kling TF, Bright RW, Hensinger RM: Distal tibial physeal fractures in children that may require open reduction, *J Bone Joint Surg* 66A:647, 1984.

Langenskiöld A: An operation for partial closure of an epiphysial plate in children, and its experimental basis, *J Bone Joint Surg* 57B:325, 1975.

Letts RM: Hidden adolescent ankle fracture, *J Pediatr Orthop* 2:161, 1982.

Lintecum N, Blasier RD: Direct reduction and indirect fixation of distal tibial physeal fractures: a report of a technique, *J Pediatr Orthop* 16:107, 1996.

Marmor L: An unusual fracture of the tibial epiphysis, *Clin Orthop* 73:132, 1970.

Ogden JA, Lee J: Accessory ossification patterns and injuries of the malleoli, *J Pediatr Orthop* 10:306, 1990.

Peiro A, Aracil J, Martos F, Mut T: Triplane distal tibial epiphyseal fractures, *Clin Orthop* 160:196, 1981.

Peterson HA: Operative correction of post-fracture arrest of the epiphyseal plate: case report with a ten-year follow-up, *J Bone Joint Surg* 62A:1018, 1980.

Rapariz JM, Ocete G, Gonzalez-Herranz P, et al: Distal tibial triplane fractures: long-term follow-up, *J Pediatr Orthop* 16:113, 1996.

Roffman M, Moshel M, Mendes DG: Bicycle spoke fracture, *Clin Orthop* 144:230, 1979.

Salter RB, Harris WR: Injuries involving the epiphyseal plate, *J Bone Joint Surg* 45A:587, 1963.

Schlesinger I, Wedge JH: Percutaneous reduction and fixation of displaced juvenile Tillaux fractures: a new surgical technique, *J Pediatr Orthop* 13:389, 1993.

Shannak AO: Tibial fractures in children: follow-up study, *J Pediatr Orthop* 8:306, 1988.

Shin AY, Moran ME, Wenger DR: Intramalleolar triplane fractures of the distal tibial epiphysis, *J Pediatr Orthop* 17:352, 1997.

Spiegel PG, Cooperman DR, Laros GS: Epiphyseal fractures of the distal ends of the tibia and fibula: a retrospective study of 237 cases in children, *J Bone Joint Surg* 60A:1046, 1978.

Stanitski CL, Micheli LJ: Observations on symptomatic medial malleolar ossification centers, *J Pediatr Orthop* 13:164, 1993.

Weber BG, Sussenbach F: Malleolar fractures. In Weber BG, Brunner C, Freuler F, eds: *Treatment of fractures in children and adolescents,* New York, 1980, Springer-Verlag.

FOOT FRACTURES

Alexander AH, Lichtman DM: Surgical treatment of transchondral talar dome fractures (osteochondritis dissecans): long-term follow-up, *J Bone Joint Surg* 62A:646, 1980.

Anderson LD: Injuries of the forefoot, *Clin Orthop* 122:18, 1977.

Armstrong PF: Serious fractures and joint injuries involving the foot and ankle, *Instr Course Lect* 41:413, 1992.

Berndt AL, Harty M: Transchondral fractures (osteochondritis dissecans) of the talus, *J Bone Joint Surg* 41A:988, 1959.

Bonnin JG: Dislocations and fracture-dislocations of the talus, *Br J Surg* 28:88, 1940.

Boyd HB, Knight RA: Fractures of the astragalus, *South Med J* 35:160, 1942.

Brand RA, Black H: *Pseudomonas* osteomyelitis following puncture wounds in children, *J Bone Joint Surg* 56A:1637, 1974.

Canale ST, Beaty JH: Injuries of the talus. In Hamilton WC, ed: *Traumatic disorders of the ankle,* New York, 1983, Springer-Verlag.

Canale ST, Belding RH: Osteochondral lesions of the talus, *J Bone Joint Surg* 62A:97, 1980.

Canale ST, Kelly FB Jr: Fractures of the neck of the talus: long-term evaluation of 71 cases, *J Bone Joint Surg* 60A:143, 1978.

Cehner J: Fractures of the tarsal bones, metatarsals, and toes. In Weber BG, Brunner C, Freuler F, eds: *Treatment of fractures in children and adolescents,* New York, 1980, Springer-Verlag.

Chapman HG, Galway HR: Os calcis fractures in childhood, *J Bone Joint Surg* 59B:510, 1977.

Dimentberg R, Rosman M: Peritalar dislocations in children, *J Pediatr Orthop* 13:89, 1993.

Devas MB: Stress fractures in children, *J Bone Joint Surg* 45B:528, 1963.

Essex-Lopresti P: The mechanism, reduction technique, and results in fractures of the os calcis, *Br J Surg* 39:395, 1952.

Ferkel R, Guhl J, Beuken KV, et al: Complications in ankle arthroscopy: analysis of the first 518 cases, *Orthop Trans* 16:726, 1992.

Fitzgerald RH, Cowen JDE: Puncture wounds of the foot, *Orthop Clin North Am* 6:965, 1975.

Freiberg A: Infarction of the second metatarsal bone, *Surg Gynecol Obstet* 19:191, 1914.

Gross RH: Fractures and dislocations of the foot. In Rockwood CA Jr, Wilkins KE, King RE, eds: *Fractures in children,* Philadelphia, 1984, JB Lippincott.

Haliburton RA, Sullivan CR, Kelly PJ, Peterson LFA: The extra-osseous and intra-osseous blood supply of the talus, *J Bone Joint Surg* 40A:1115, 1958.

Harper MC, Ralston M: Isobutyl 2-cyanoacrylate as an osseous adhesive in the repair of osteochondral fractures, *J Biomed Mater Res* 17:167, 1983.

Hawkins LG: Fractures of the neck of the talus, *J Bone Joint Surg* 52A:991, 1970.

Hepple S, Winson IG, Glew D: Osteochondral lesions of the talus: a revised classification, *Foot Ankle* 20:789, 1999.

Johnson FG: Pediatric Lisfranc injury: bunk bed fracture, *Am J Roentgenol* 137:1041, 1981.

Kavanaugh JH, Brower TD, Mann RV: The Jones fracture revisited, *J Bone Joint Surg* 60A:776, 1978.

King RE: Personal communication, 1986.

Kling TF Jr: Operative treatment of ankle fractures in children, *Orthop Clin North Am* 21:381, 1990.

Lang AG, Peterson HA: Osteomyelitis following puncture wounds of the foot in children, *J Trauma* 16:993, 1976.

Letts RM, Gibeault D: Fractures of the neck of the talus in children, *Foot Ankle* 1:74, 1980.

Lyritis G: Developmental disorders of the proximal epiphysis of the hallux, *Stereoradiology* 10:250, 1983.

Manderson EL, Ollivierre CO: Closed anatomic reduction of a juvenile Tillaux fracture by dorsiflexion of the ankle: a case report, *Clin Orthop* 276:262, 1992.

Marti R: Fractures of the talus and calcaneus. In Weber BG, Brunner C, Freuler F, eds: *Treatment of fractures in children and adolescents,* New York, 1980, Springer-Verlag.

Matteri RE, Frymoyer JW: Fracture of the calcaneus in young children: report of three cases, *J Bone Joint Surg* 55A:1091, 1973.

McCullough CJ, Venugopal V: Osteochondritis dissecans of the talus: the natural history, *Clin Orthop* 144:264, 1979.

Mulfinger GL, Trueta J: The blood supply of the talus, *J Bone Joint Surg* 52B:160, 1970.

Parisien JS: Arthroscopic treatment of osteochondral lesions of the talus, *Am J Sports Med* 14:211, 1986.

Schmidt TL, Weiner DS: Calcaneal fractures in children: an evaluation of the nature of the injury in 56 children, *Clin Orthop* 171:150, 1982.

Trott A: Fractures of the foot in children, *Orthop Clin North Am* 7:677, 1976.

Vosburgh CL, Gruel CR, Herndon WA, Sullivan JA: Lawn mower injuries of the pediatric foot and ankle: observations on prevention and management, *J Pediatr Orthop* 15:504, 1995.

Wells D, Oloff-Solomon J: Radiographic evaluation of transchondral dome fractures of the talus, *J Foot Surg* 26:186, 1987.

Wiley JJ: The mechanism of tarsometatarsal joint injuries, *J Bone Joint Surg* 53B:475, 1971.

Wiley JJ: Tarsometatarsal joint injuries in children, *J Pediatr Orthop* 1:255, 1981.

PART **XII**
The Spine

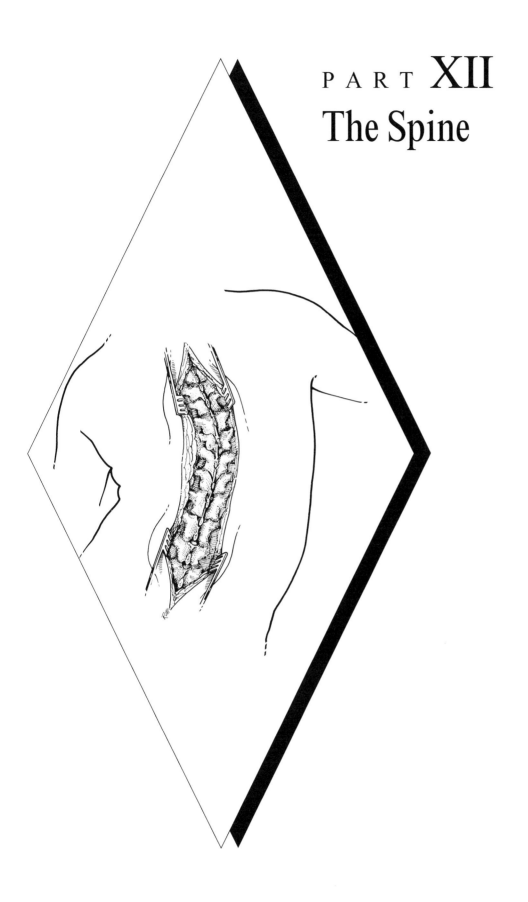

Spinal Anatomy and Surgical Approaches

Marvin R. Leventhal

Anatomy of Vertebral Column

The vertebral column is composed of alternating bony vertebrae and fibrocartilaginous discs that are connected by strong ligaments and supported by musculature that extends from the skull to the pelvis and provides axial support to the body. There are 33 vertebrae (7 cervical, 12 thoracic, 5 lumbar, 5 sacral, and 4 coccygeal) (Fig. 34-1). The sacral and coccygeal vertebrae form the sacrum and coccyx. A typical vertebra is composed of an anterior body and a posterior arch made up of two pedicles and two laminae that are united posteriorly to form the spinous process. To either side of the arch of the vertebral body is a transverse process and superior and inferior articular processes. The articular processes articulate with adjacent vertebrae to form synovial joints. The relative orientation of the articular processes accounts for the degree of flexion, extension, or rotation possible in each segment of the vertebral column. The spinous and transverse processes serve as levers for the numerous muscles attached to them. The vertebral bodies increase in size from cephalic to caudal, and this is believed to be the result of the increasing weights and stresses borne by successive segments. The intervertebral discs connecting the vertebral bodies absorb many of the stresses applied to the vertebral column. A disc consists of an outer concentric layer of fibrous tissue known as the *anulus fibrosis* and a central gelatinous portion, the *nucleus pulposus*. At birth the vertebral column is convex dorsally, which forms the predominant sagittal contour; however, when the erect position is acquired, compensatory cervical and lumbar lordotic curves develop opposite the primary thoracic and sacral kyphotic curves. The length of the vertebral column averages 72 cm in adult males and 7 to 10 cm less in adult females. The vertebral canal extends throughout the length of the column and provides protection for the spinal cord, conus medullaris, and cauda equina. Nerves and vessels pass through the intervertebral foramina formed by the superior and inferior borders of the pedicles of adjacent vertebrae.

Anatomy of Cervical, Thoracic, and Lumbar Pedicles

In recent years an increasing number of studies have documented the anatomical morphology of the cervical, thoracic, and lumbar vertebrae. Advanced internal fixation techniques, including pedicle screws, have been developed and used extensively in spine surgery, not only for traumatic injuries but also for degenerative conditions. As the role for anterior and posterior spinal instrumentation continues to evolve, understanding the morphological characteristics of the human vertebrae is critical in avoiding complications during fixation.

Placement of screws in the cervical pedicles remains controversial and carries more risk than anterior plate or lateral mass fixation. Although cervical pedicles can be suitable for

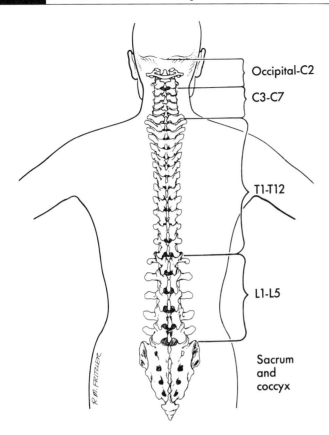

Fig. 34-1 Vertebral column: upper cervical vertebrae (occiput to C2), lower cervical vertebrae (C3-C7), thoracic vertebrae (T1-T12), lumbar vertebrae (L1-L5), sacrum, and coccyx.

screw fixation, uniformly sized cervical pedicle screws cannot be used at every level. Screw placement in the pedicles at C3, C4, and C5 require smaller screws (less than 4.5 mm) and more care in placement than those of the other cervical vertebrae. Karaikovic et al. used computed tomography (CT) measurements to study cervical pedicle morphology and found that C2 and C7 pedicles had larger mean interdiameters than all other cervical vertebrae and that C3 had the smallest mean interdiameter. The outer pedicle width to height ratio increased from C2 to C7, indicating that pedicles in the upper cervical spine (C2 through C4) are elongated, whereas pedicles in the lower cervical spine (C6 through C7) are rounded. It is also critical to know that cervical pedicles angle medially at all levels, with the most medial angulation at C5 and the least at C2 and C7. The pedicles slope upward at C2 and C3, are parallel at C4 and C5, and are angled downward at C6 and C7.

The vertebral artery from C3 to C6 is at significant risk for iatrogenic injury during pedicle screw placement. Karaikovic et al. noted that the pedicle cortex is not uniformly thick and that the thinnest portion of the cortex (the lateral cortex) protects the vertebral artery; the medial cortex toward the spinal cord is almost twice a thick as the lateral cortex. Variations in the course of the vertebral artery also place it at risk during placement of pedicle screws. At the C2 and C7 to T1 levels the vertebral artery is less at risk during pedicle screw

fixation. The vertebral artery follows a more posterior and lateral course at C2, while at C7 to T1 it is outside the transverse foramen.

Pedicle dimensions and angles change progressively from the upper thoracic spine distally. A thorough knowledge of these relationships is important when considering the use of the pedicle as a screw purchase site. Pedicle dimensions have been studied by Zindrick et al., Saillant, and others, and data obtained from these studies have added to the knowledge of pedicle morphological characteristics and provided information about the depth to which screws can be inserted safely at levels throughout the thoracolumbar spine. In 2905 pedicle measurements made from T1 to L5, pedicles were widest at L5 and narrowest at T5 in the horizontal plane (Fig. 34-2). The widest pedicles in the sagittal plane were at T11, and the narrowest were at T1. Because of the oval shape of the pedicle, the sagittal plane width was generally larger than the horizontal plane width. The largest pedicle angle in the horizontal plane was at L5. In the sagittal plane, the pedicles angle caudad at L5 and cephalad at L3 through T1. The depth to the anterior cortex was significantly longer along the pedicle axis than along a line parallel to the midline of the vertebral body at all levels, with the exception of T12 and L1.

The thoracic pedicle is a convoluted, three-dimensional structure that is filled mostly with cancellous bone (62% to 79%). Panjabi et al. showed that the cortical shell is of variable density throughout its parameter and that the lateral wall is significantly thinner than the medial wall. This appeared to be true for all levels of thoracic vertebrae. A study by Kothe et al. also demonstrated that the medial wall is thicker than the lateral wall of the thoracic pedicle, and they found that most pedicle fractures related to screw insertion occurred laterally.

The locations for screw insertion have been identified and described by Roy-Camille, Saillant, and Mazel and by Louis. The respective facet joint space and the middle of the transverse process are the most important reference points. An opening is made in the pedicle with a drill or hand-held curet, after which a self-tapping screw is passed through the pedicle into the vertebral body. The pedicles of the thoracic and lumbar vertebrae are tubelike bony structures that connect the anterior and posterior columns of the spine. Medial to the medial wall of the pedicle lies the dural sac. Inferior to the medial wall of the pedicle is the nerve root in the neural foramen. The lumbar roots usually are situated in the upper third of the foramen; therefore it is more dangerous to penetrate the pedicle medially or inferiorly as opposed to laterally or superiorly.

We use three techniques for localization of the pedicle: (1) the intersection technique, (2) the pars interarticularis technique, and (3) the mamillary process technique. It is important in preoperative planning to assess individual spinal anatomy with the use of high-quality anteroposterior and lateral roentgenograms of the lumbar and thoracic spine, as well as with axial CT scanning at the level of the pedicle. The intersection technique is perhaps the most commonly used method of localizing the pedicle. It involves dropping a line from the lateral aspect of the facet joint, which intersects a line

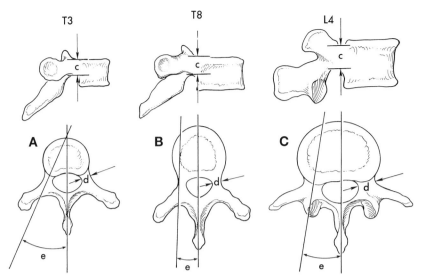

Fig. 34-2 Pedicle dimensions of T3 (**A**), T8 (**B**), and L4 (**C**) vertebrae. Vertical diameter (*c*) increases from 0.7 to 1.5 cm, horizontal diameter (*d*) increases from 0.7 to 1.6 cm with minimum of 0.5 cm in T5. Direction is almost sagittal from T4 to L4. Angle (*e*) seldom extends beyond 10 degrees. More proximally, direction is more oblique: T1 = 36 degrees, T2 = 34 degrees, T3 = 23 degrees. L5 is oblique (30 degrees) but is large and easy to drill. (Redrawn from Roy-Camille R, Saillant G, Mazel C: *Orthop Clin North Am* 17:147, 1986.)

that bisects the transverse process at a spot overlying the pedicle (Figs. 34-3 and 34-4). The pars interarticularis is that area of bone where the pedicle connects to the lamina. Because the laminae and the pars interarticularis can be easily identified at surgery, they provide landmarks by which a pedicular drill starting point can be made. The mamillary process technique is based on a small prominence of bone at the base of the transverse process. This mamillary process can be used as a starting point for transpedicular drilling. Usually the mamillary process is more lateral than the intersection technique starting point, which is also more lateral than the pars interarticularis starting point. With this in mind, a different angle must be used when drilling from these sites. With the help of preoperative CT scanning at the level of the pedicle and intraoperative roentgenograms, the angle of the pedicle to the sagittal and horizontal planes can be determined.

Circulation of Spinal Cord

The arterial supply to the spinal cord has been determined from gross anatomical dissection, latex arterial injections, and intercostal arteriography. Dommisse has contributed most significantly to our knowledge of the blood supply, stating that the principles that govern the blood supply of the cord are constant, whereas the patterns vary with the individual. He emphasizes the following factors:

1. *Dependence on three vessels.* These are the anterior median longitudinal arterial trunk and a pair of posterolateral trunks near the posterior nerve rootlets.

2. *Relative demands of gray matter and white matter.* The longitudinal arterial trunks are largest in the cervical and lumbar regions near the ganglionic enlargements and are much smaller in the thoracic region. This is because the metabolic demands of the gray matter are greater than those of the white matter, which contains fewer capillary networks.

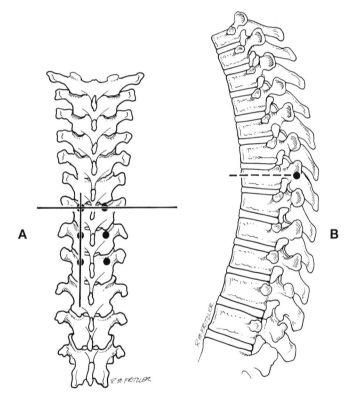

Fig. 34-3 Pedicle entrance point in thoracic spine at intersection of lines drawn through middle of inferior articular facet and middle of insertion of transverse processes (1 mm below facet joint). **A,** Anteroposterior view. **B,** Lateral view. (Redrawn from Roy-Camille R, Saillant G, Mazel C: *Orthop Clin North Am* 17:147, 1986.)

3. *Medullary feeder (radicular) arteries of the cord.* These reinforce the longitudinal arterial channels. There are from 2 to 17 anteriorly and from 6 to 25 posteriorly. The vertebral arteries supply 80 of the radicular arteries in the neck; those in the thoracic and lumbar areas arise from the aorta. The

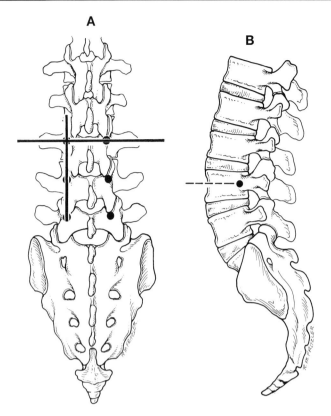

Fig. 34-4 Pedicle entrance point in lumbar spine at intersection of two lines (see Fig. 34-3). On typical bony crest it is 1 mm below articular joint. **A,** Anteroposterior view. **B,** Lateral view. (Redrawn from Roy-Camille R, Saillant G, Mazel Ch: *Orthop Clin North Am* 17:147, 1986.)

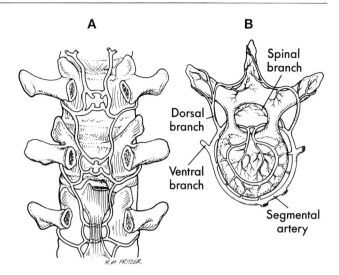

Fig. 34-5 Vertebral blood supply. **A,** Posterior view; laminae removed to show anastomosing spinal branches of segmental arteries. **B,** Cross-sectional view; anastomosing arterial supply of vertebral body, spinal canal, and posterior elements. (Redrawn from Bullough PG, Oheneba BA: *Atlas of spinal diseases,* Philadelphia, 1988, JB Lippincott.)

lateral sacral arteries, as well as the fifth lumbar, the iliolumbar, and the middle sacral arteries, are important in the sacral region.

4. *Supplementary source of blood supply to the spinal cord.* The vertebral and posteroinferior cerebellar arteries are important sources of arterial supply. Sacral medullary feeders arise from the lateral sacral arteries and accompany the distal roots of the cauda equina. The flow in these vessels seems reversible and the volume adjustable in response to the metabolic demands.

5. *Segmental arteries of the spine.* At every vertebral level a pair of segmental arteries supplies the extraspinal and intraspinal structures. The thoracic and lumbar segmental arteries arise from the aorta; the cervical segmental arteries arise from the vertebral arteries and the costocervical and thyrocervical trunks. In 60% of people an additional source arises from the ascending pharyngeal branch of the external carotid artery. The lateral sacral arteries and to a lesser extent the fifth lumbar, iliolumbar, and middle sacral arteries supply segmental vessels in the sacral region.

6. *"Distribution point" of the segmental arteries.* The segmental arteries divide into numerous branches at the intervertebral foramen, which has been termed the *distribution point* (Fig. 34-5). A second anastomotic network lies within the

spinal canal in the loose connective tissue of the extradural space. This occurs at all levels, with the greatest concentration in the cervical and lumbar regions. Undoubtedly the presence of the rich anastomotic channels offers alternative pathways for arterial flow, preserving spinal cord circulation after the ligation of segmental arteries.

7. *Artery of Adamkiewicz.* The artery of Adamkiewicz is the largest of the feeders of the lumbar cord; it is located on the left side, usually at the level of T9 to 11 (in 80% of people). It is clear that the anterior longitudinal arterial channel of the cord rather than any single medullary feeder is crucial. Equally clear is that the preservation of this large feeder does not ensure continued satisfactory circulation for the spinal cord. In principle it would seem of practical value to protect and preserve each contributing artery as far as is surgically possible.

8. *Variability of patterns of supply of the spinal cord.* The variability of blood supply is a striking feature, yet there is absolute conformity with a principle of a rich supply for the cervical and lumbar cord enlargements. The supply for the thoracic cord from approximately T4 to T9 is much poorer.

9. *Direction of flow in the blood vessels of the spinal cord.* The three longitudinal arterial channels of the spinal cord can be compared with the circle of Willis at the base of the brain, but it is more extensive and more complicated, although it functions with identical principles. These channels permit reversal of flow and alterations in the volume of blood flow in response to metabolic demands. This internal arterial circle of the cord is surrounded by at least two outer arterial circles, the first of which is situated in the extradural space and the second in the extravertebral tissue planes. It is by virtue of the latter that the spinal cord enjoys reserve sources

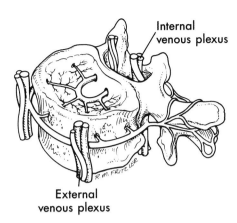

Fig. 34-6 Venous drainage of vertebral bodies and formation of internal and external vertebral venous plexuses. (Redrawn from Bullough PG, Oheneba BA: *Atlas of spinal diseases*, Philadelphia, 1988, JB Lippincott.)

of supply through a degree of anastomosis lacking in the inner circle. The "outlet points," however, are limited to the perforating sulcal arteries and the pial arteries of the cord.

In summary, the blood supply to the spinal cord is rich, but the spinal canal is narrowest and the blood supply is poorest from T4 to T9. This should be considered the critical vascular zone of the spinal cord, a zone in which interference with the circulation is most likely to result in paraplegia.

The dominance of the anterior spinal artery system has been challenged by the fact that many anterior spinal surgeries have been performed in recent years with no increase in the incidence of paralysis. This would seem to indicate that a rich anastomotic supply does exist and that it protects the spinal cord. The evidence suggests that the posterior spinal arteries may be as important as the anterior system but are as yet poorly understood. Venous drainage of the spinal cord is more difficult to clearly define than is the arterial supply (Fig. 34-6). It is well known that the venous system is highly variable. Dommisse points out that there are two sets of veins: those of the spinal cord and those that fall within the plexiform network of Batson. The veins of the spinal cord are a small component of the entire system and drain into the plexus of Batson. The Batson plexus is a large and complex venous channel extending from the base of the skull to the coccyx. It communicates directly with the superior and inferior vena cava system and the azygos system. The longitudinal venous trunks of the spinal cord are the anterior and posterior venous channels, which are the counterparts of the arterial trunks. The three components of the Batson plexus are the extradural vertebral venous plexus; the extravertebral venous plexus, which includes the segmental veins of the neck, the intercostal veins, the azygos communications in the thorax and pelvis, the lumbar veins, and the communications with the inferior vena caval system; and the veins of the bony structures of the spinal column. The venous

system plays no specific role in the metabolism of the spinal cord; it communicates directly with the venous system draining the head, chest, and abdomen. This interconnection allows metastatic spread of neoplastic or infectious disease from the pelvis to the vertebral column.

During anterior spinal surgery, we empirically follow these principles: (1) ligate segmental spinal arteries only as necessary to gain exposure; (2) ligate segmental spinal arteries near the aorta rather than near the vertebral foramina; (3) ligate segmental spinal arteries on one side only when possible, leaving the circulation intact on the opposite side; and (4) limit dissection in the vertebral foramina to a single level when possible so that collateral circulation is disturbed as little as possible.

Surgical Approaches

ANTERIOR APPROACHES

With the posterior approach for correction of spinal deformities well established, in recent years more attention has been placed on the anterior approach to the spinal column. Many pioneers in the field of anterior spinal surgery recognized that anterior spinal cord decompression was necessary in spinal tuberculosis and that laminectomy not only failed to relieve anterior pressure but also removed important posterior stability and produced worsening of kyphosis. Advances in major surgical procedures, including anesthesia and intensive care, have made it possible to perform spinal surgery with acceptable safety.

Common use of the anterior approach for spinal surgery did not evolve until the 1950s. Leaders in the anterior approach to the cervical and lumbar areas have been Cloward, Southwick and Robinson, Bailey and Badgley, Bohlman et al., and others. The transthoracic approach to the thoracic spine has developed more slowly. Nachlas and Borden, and Smith, von Lackum, and Wylie were among the first to report their experiences; however, the major proponents of this technique were Hodgson et al. of Hong Kong. Their reports of success with this method received worldwide acceptance.

In general, anterior approaches to the spine are indicated for decompression of the neural elements (spinal cord, conus medullaris, cauda equina, or nerve roots) when anterior neural compression has been documented by myelography, post-myelogram CT scanning, or magnetic resonance imaging (MRI). A number of pathological entities can cause significant compression of the neural elements, including traumatic, neoplastic, inflammatory, degenerative, and congenital lesions.

Anterior approaches to the spine generally are made by an experienced spine surgeon and, as a rule, this type of surgery is not appropriate for those who only occasionally perform spinal techniques. In many centers, a team approach is preferred to use the skill of the orthopaedic surgeon, neurosurgeon, thoracic surgeon, or head and neck surgeon. The orthopaedic surgeon still must have a working knowledge of the underlying viscera, fluid balance, physiology, and other elements of intensive care.

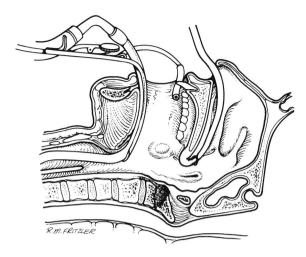

Fig. 34-7   Anterior transoral approach (see text). (Redrawn from Spetzler RF: Transoral approach to the upper cervical spine. In Evarts CM, ed: *Surgery of the musculoskeletal system*, New York, 1983, Churchill Livingstone.)

Complications of anterior spine surgery are rare; however, there is a high risk of significant morbidity, and these approaches should be used with care and only in appropriate circumstances. Potential dangers include iatrogenic injury to vascular, visceral, or neurological structures.

The exact incidence of serious complications from anterior spinal surgery is not known. A thorough understanding of anatomical tissue planes and meticulous surgical technique are necessary to prevent serious complications. The choice of approach depends on the preference and experience of the surgeon, the patient's age and medical condition, the segment of the spine involved, the underlying pathological process, and the presence or absence of signs of neural compression. Commonly accepted indications for anterior approaches are listed in Box 34-1.

Anterior Approach, Occiput to C3

The anterior approach to the upper cervical spine (occiput to C3) can be either transoral or retropharyngeal, depending on the pathological process present and the experience of the surgeon.

◆ Anterior Transoral Approach

TECHNIQUE 34-1 *(Spetzler)* (Fig. 34-7)
Position the patient supine using a Mayfield head-holding device or with skeletal traction through Gardner-Wells tongs. Monitoring of the spinal cord through somatosensory

evoked potentials is recommended. The surgeon may sit directly over the patient's head. Pass a red rubber catheter down each nostril and suture it to the uvula. Apply traction to the catheters to pull the uvula and soft palate out of the operative field, taking care not to necrose the septal cartilage by excessive pressure. Insert a McGarver retractor into the open mouth and use it to retract and hold the endotracheal tube out of the way. The operating microscope is useful to improve the limited exposure. Prepare the oropharynx with pHisoHex and Betadine. Palpate the anterior ring of C1 beneath the posterior pharynx and make an incision in the wall of the posterior pharynx from the superior aspect of C1 to the top of C3. Obtain hemostasis with bipolar electrocautery, taking care not to overcauterize, thereby producing thermal necrosis of tissue and increased risk of infection.

With a periosteal elevator subperiosteally dissect the edges of the pharyngeal incision from the anterior ring of C1 and the anterior aspect of C2. Use traction stitches to maintain the flaps out of the way. Next, under direct vision, with either the operating microscope or with magnification loupes and headlights, perform a meticulous debridement of C1 and C2 with a high-speed air drill, rongeur, or curet. When approaching the posterior longitudinal ligament, a diamond burr is safer to use in removing the last remnant of bone. Once adequate debridement of infected bone and necrotic tissue has been accomplished, decompress the upper cervical spinal cord. If the cervical spine is to be fused anteriorly, harvest a corticocancellous graft from the patient's iliac crest, fashion it to fit, and insert it. Irrigate the operative site with antibiotic solution and close the posterior pharynx in layers.

AFTERTREATMENT. An endotracheal tube is left in place overnight to maintain an adequate airway. A halo vest can then be applied or skeletal traction may be maintained before mobilization.

◆ Anterior Retropharyngeal Approach

This approach to the upper cervical spine, as described by McAfee et al., is excellent for anterior debridement of the upper cervical spine and allows placement of bone grafts for stabilization if necessary. Unlike the transoral approach, it is entirely extramucosal and is reported to have fewer complications of wound infection and neurological deficit.

TECHNIQUE 34-2 *(McAfee et al.)*

Position the patient supine, preferably on a turning frame with skeletal traction through tongs or a halo ring. Somatosensory evoked potential monitoring of cord function is suggested during the procedure. Perform fiberoptic nasotracheal intubation to prevent excessive motion of the neck and to keep the oral pharynx free of tubes that could depress the mandible and interfere with subsequent exposure.

Make a right-sided transverse skin incision in the submandibular region with a vertical extension as long as required to provide adequate exposure (Fig. 34-8, *A*). If the approach does not have to be extended below the level of the fifth cervical vertebra, there is no increased risk of damage to the recurrent laryngeal nerve.

Carry the dissection through the platysma muscle with the enveloping superficial fascia of the neck and mobilize flaps from this area. Identify the marginal mandibular branch of the seventh nerve with the help of a nerve stimulator and ligate the retromandibular veins superiorly. Keep the dissection deep to the retromandibular vein to prevent injury to the superficial branches of the facial nerve. Ligate the retromandibular vein as it joins the internal jugular vein. Next, mobilize the anterior border of the sternocleidomastoid muscle by longitudinally dividing the superficial layer of the deep cervical fascia. Feel for the pulsations of the carotid artery and take care to protect the contents of the carotid sheath. Resect the submandibular gland (Fig. 34-8, *B*) and ligate the duct to prevent formation of a salivary fistula. Identify the digastric and stylohyoid muscles and tag and divide the tendon of the former. It is important to emphasize that the facial nerve can be injured by superior retraction on the stylohyoid muscle; however, by dividing the digastric and stylohyoid muscles, the hyoid bone and hypopharynx can be mobilized medially, preventing exposure of the esophagus, hypopharynx, and nasopharynx. Next, identify the hypoglossal nerve and retract it superiorly. Continue dissection to the retropharyngeal space between the carotid sheath laterally and the larynx and pharynx medially. Increase exposure by ligating branches of the carotid artery and internal jugular vein, which prevent retraction of the carotid sheath laterally (Fig. 34-8, *C* and *D*). Identify and mobilize the superior laryngeal nerve. Following adequate retraction of the carotid sheath

laterally, divide the alar and prevertebral fascial layers longitudinally to expose the longus colli muscles. Take care to maintain the head in a neutral position and accurately identify the midline. Remove the longus colli muscles subperiosteally from the anterior aspect of the arch of C1 and the body of C2, taking care to avoid injury to the vertebral arteries. Next, meticulously debride the involved osseous structures (Fig. 34-8, *E*) and, if needed, perform bone grafting with either autogenous iliac or fibular bone.

Close the wound over suction drains and repair the digastric tendon. Close the platysma and skin flaps in layers.

AFTERTREATMENT. The patient is maintained in skeletal traction with the head of the bed elevated to reduce swelling. Intubation is continued until pharyngeal edema has resolved, usually by 48 hours. The patient can then be extubated and mobilized in a halo vest, or, if indicated, a posterior stabilization procedure can be done before mobilization.

Extended Maxillotomy and Subtotal Maxillectomy. Cocke et al. have described an extended maxillotomy and subtotal maxillectomy as an alternative to the transoral approach for exposure and removal of tumor or bone anteriorly at the base of the skull and cervical spine to C5. This approach has been used in a limited number of procedures, and the indications have not yet been firmly established. This procedure is technically demanding and requires a thorough knowledge of head and neck anatomy. It should be performed by a team of surgeons, including an otolaryngologist, a neurosurgeon, and an orthopaedist.

Before surgery the size, position, and extent of the tumor or bone to be removed should be determined, using the appropriate imaging techniques. Three to five days before the surgery, nasal, oral, and pharyngeal secretions are cultured to determine the proper antibiotics needed. Cephalosporin and aminoglycoside antibiotics are given before and after surgery if the floral cultures are normal and are adjusted if the flora is abnormal or resistant to these drugs.

◆ *Subtotal Maxillectomy*

TECHNIQUE 34-3 *(Cocke et al.)*

Position the patient on the operating table with the head elevated 25 degrees. Intubate the patient orally and move the tube to the contralateral side of the mouth. Perform a percutaneous endoscopic gastrostomy (PEG) if the wound is to be left open or if problems are anticipated. Perform a tracheostomy if the exposure may be limited or if there are severe pulmonary problems. This step usually is unnecessary.

Insert a Foley catheter and suture the eyelids closed with 6-0 nylon. Infiltrate the soft tissues of the upper lip, cheek, gingiva, palate, pterygoid fossa, nasopharynx, nasal septum,

continued

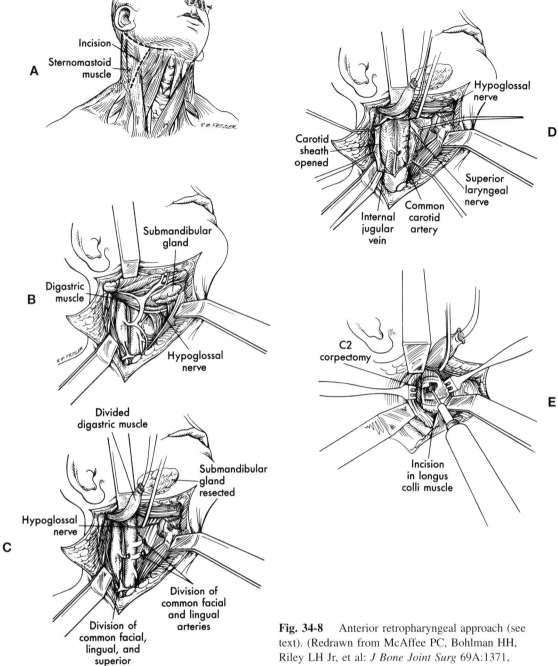

Fig. 34-8   Anterior retropharyngeal approach (see text). (Redrawn from McAffee PC, Bohlman HH, Riley LH Jr, et al: *J Bone Joint Surg* 69A:1371, 1987.)

nasal floor, and lateral nasal wall with 1% lidocaine and 1:100,000 epinephrine. Pack each nasal cavity with cottonoid strips saturated with 4% cocaine and 1% phenylephrine. Prepare the skin with Betadine, then alcohol. Drape the operative site with cloth drapes held in place with sutures or surgical clips and covered with a transparent surgical drape.

Expose the superior maxilla through a modified Weber-Ferguson skin incision (Fig. 34-9, *A*). Make a vertical incision through the upper lip in the philtrum from the nasolabial groove to the vermilion border. Extend the lower end to the midline and then vertically in the midline through the buccal mucosa to the gingivobuccal gutter. Divide the upper lip and ligate the labial arteries. Extend the external skin incision transversely from the upper end of the lip incision in the nasolabial groove to beyond the nasal ala and then superiorly along the nasofacial groove to the lower

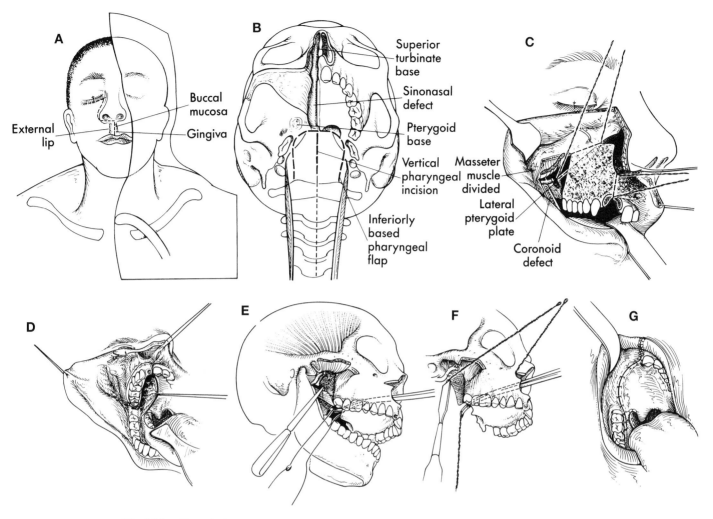

Fig. 34-9 Extended maxillotomy and subtotal maxillectomy (see text). (Redrawn from Cocke EW Jr, Robertson JH, Robertson JR, Crook JP Jr: *Arch Otolaryngol Head Neck Surg* 116:92, 1990.)

eyelid. Extract the central incisor tooth (Fig. 34-9, *B*). Make a vertical midline incision through the mucoperiosteum of the anterior maxilla from the gingivobuccal gutter to the central incisor defect and then transversely through the buccal gingiva adjacent to the teeth to the retromolar region. Elevate the skin, subcutaneous tissues, periosteum, and mucoperiosteum of the maxilla to expose the anterior and lateral walls of the maxilla, nasal bone, piriform aperture of the nose, inferior orbital nerve, malar bone, and masseter muscle. Divide the anterior margin of the masseter muscle at its malar attachment and remove a wedge of malar bone. Use this wedge to accommodate the Gigli saw as it divides the maxilla (Fig. 34-9, *C*). Make an incision in the lingual, hard palate mucoperiosteum adjacent to the teeth from the central incisor defect to join the retromolar incision. Extend the retromolar incision medial to the mandible lateral to the tonsil and to the retropharyngeal space to the level of the hyoid bone or lower pharynx, if necessary. Elevate the

mucoperiosteum of the hard palate from the central incisor defect and alveolar ridge to and beyond the midline of the hard palate. Detach the soft palate with its nasal lining from the posterior margin of the hard palate. Divide and electrocoagulate the greater palatine vessels and nerves. Pack the palatine foramen with bone wax. Retract the mucoperiosteum of the hard palate, the soft palate, anterior tonsillar pillar, tonsil, and pharynx medially from the prevertebral fascia. It is usually unnecessary to detach and retract the soft palate from the posterior or lateral pharyngeal walls. Expose the nasal cavity by detaching the nasal soft tissues from the lateral margin and base of the nasal piriform aperture (see Fig. 34-9, *B*). Remove a bony wedge of the ascending process of the maxilla to accommodate the upper Gigli saw (see Fig. 34-9, *C*). Remove the coronoid process of the mandible above the level of entrance of the inferior alveolar vessels and nerves, after dividing its temporalis muscle attachment, to expose the lateral

continued

pterygoid plate and the internal maxillary artery. Divide the pterygoid muscles with the Shaw knife or the cutting current of the Bovie cautery until the sharp, posterior bone edge of the lateral pterygoid plate is seen or palpated. Mobilize, clip, ligate, and divide the internal maxillary artery near the pterygoid plate. Position the upper Gigli saw (see Fig. 34-9, C) using a sharp-pointed, medium-size, curved, right-angle ligature carrier threaded with a no. 2 black silk suture. Direct the suture behind the lateral pterygoid plate into the nasopharynx and behind the posterior margin of the hard palate into the oropharynx. Pass a Kelly forceps through the nose to behind the hard palate to retrieve the medial end of the silk suture in the ligature carrier. Attach a Gigli saw to the lateral end of the suture. Thread the saw into position to divide the upper maxilla. Engage the medial arm of the saw into the ascending process wedge and its lateral arm into the malar wedge. Take care to position the saw as high as possible behind the pterygoid plate. Use a broad periosteal elevator beneath the saw on the pterygoid plate to maintain the elevated position (Fig. 34-9, D). Position the lower Gigli saw by passing a Kelly forceps (Fig. 34-9, E) through the nose into the nasopharynx behind the posterior nares of the hard palate. Engage the saw between the blades of the clamp and thread it through the nose into position for division of the hard palate. Divide the bony walls of the maxilla (see Fig. 34-9, E). First divide the hard palate and then the upper maxilla. Take care to avoid entangling the saws and protect the soft tissues from injury. Remove the maxilla after division of its muscle attachments. Ligate the distal end of the internal maxillary artery. Place traction sutures in the soft tissues of the lip on either side of the initial lip incision and in the mucoperiosteum of the hard and soft palates. The posterior pharynx is now fully exposed.

Infiltrate the mucous membrane covering the posterior wall of the nasopharynx, oropharynx, and the tonsillar area to the level of the hyoid bone with 1% lidocaine and epinephrine 1:100,000. Make a vertical midline incision through the soft tissues of the posterior wall of the nasopharynx extending from the sphenoid sinus to the foramen magnum. Another option is to make a transverse incision from the sphenoid to the lateral nasopharyngeal wall posterior to the eustachian tube along the lateral pharyngeal wall inferiorly posterior to the posterior tonsillar pillar behind the soft palate. Duplicate this incision on the opposite side, producing an inferiorly based pharyngeal flap (Fig. 34-9, F). Make a more extensive exposure by extending the lateral pharyngeal wall incision through the anterior tonsillar pillar to join the retromolar incision. Extend this incision into the retropharyngeal space and retract the anterior tonsillar pillar, tonsil, and soft palate toward the midline with a traction suture. It is unnecessary to completely separate the soft palate from the pharyngeal wall. Extend the pharyngeal wall incision inferiorly to the

level of the hyoid bone or beyond. Elevate, divide, and separate the superior constrictor muscle, prevertebral fascia, longus capitus muscle, and anterior longitudinal ligaments from the bony skull base and upper cervical spine ventrally. Expose the amount of bone to be operated on up to the foramen magnum to C5. Use an operating microscope or loupe magnification for improved vision. Remove the offending bone with a high-speed burr, taking care to avoid penetration of the dura.

Close the nasopharyngeal mucous membrane and the subcutaneous tissue in one layer with interrupted sutures. Use a split-thickness skin or dermal graft from the thigh to resurface the buccal mucosa and any defects in the nasal surface of the hard palate. Use a quilting stitch to hold the graft in place without packing. Replace the zygoma and stabilize it with wire if it was mobilized. Return the maxilla to its original position and hold it in place with wire or compression plates. Place a nylon sack impregnated with antibiotic into the nasal cavity. Close the oral cavity incision with vertical interrupted mattress 3-0 polyglycolic acid sutures (Fig. 34-9, G). Close the facial wound with 5-0 chromic and 6-0 nylon sutures.

◆ *Extended Maxillotomy*

TECHNIQUE 34-4

Expose the base of the skull and upper cervical spine as by the maxillectomy technique but omit the extraction of the central incisor and the gingivolingual incision. Use a degloving procedure for elevation of the facial skin over the maxilla and nose to avoid facial scars. Divide the fibromuscular attachment of the soft palate to the pterygoid plate and hard palate, exposing the nasopharynx. Place the upper Gigli saw with the aid of a ligature carrier for division of the maxilla beneath the infraorbital nerve. Elevate the mucoperiosteum of the adjacent floor of the nose from the piriform aperture to the soft palate. Extend this elevation medially to the nasal septum and laterally to the inferior turbinate. Divide the bone of the nasal floor with a Stryker saw without lacerating the underlying hard palate periosteum. Hinge the maxilla on the hard palate and nasal mucoperiosteum as well as the soft palate and rotate it medially.

AFTERTREATMENT. Continuous spinal fluid drainage is maintained and the head is elevated 45 degrees if the dura was repaired or replaced. These are omitted if there was no dural tear or defect. An ice cap is used on the cheek and temple to reduce edema. Antibiotic therapy is continued until the risk of infection is minimized. Half-strength hydrogen peroxide is used for mouth irrigations to help keep the oral cavity clean. The endotracheal tube is removed when the risk of occlusion by swelling is minimized. The nasopharyngeal cavity is cleaned with saline twice daily for 2 months after pack removal. Facial sutures are removed at 4 to 6 days and oral sutures at 2 weeks.

◆ Anterior Approach, C3 to C7

Exposure of the middle and lower cervical region of the spine is most commonly carried out through an anterior approach medial to the carotid sheath. A thorough knowledge of anatomical fascial planes, as described by Southwick and Robinson in 1957, allows a safe, direct approach to this area. The most frequent complication of the anterior approach is vocal cord paralysis caused by injury to the recurrent laryngeal nerve. Injury to the recurrent laryngeal nerve may be less common on the left side because the nerve has a more vertical course and lies in a protected position within the esophagotracheal groove. Recent work by Ebraheim, et al. determined the differences in course and location of the recurrent laryngeal nerves on both sides. On the right the nerve leaves the main trunk of the vagus nerve and passes anterior to and under the subclavian artery; whereas on the left, it passes under and posterior to the aorta at the site of origin of the ligamentum arteriosum. The nerve then runs upward, having a variable relationship with the inferior thyroid artery. These authors concluded that the recurrent laryngeal nerve on the right side is highly vulnerable to injury if the inferior thyroid vessels are not ligated as laterally as possible or if the midline structures along with the recurrent laryngeal nerve is not retracted intermittently.

Netterville et al. reported 16 patients with vocal cord paralysis after anterior cervical spine surgery; they also demonstrated that the shorter, more lateral position of the right recurrent laryngeal nerve places it at risk for injury from direct trauma or from the retraction that is necessary to expose the anterior cervical vertebrae. They suggested considering a left-sided exposure medial to the carotid artery and internal jugular vein to minimize the risk of injury. Although many spine surgeons use the right-sided approach with a low incidence of symptomatic paralysis of the recurrent laryngeal nerve, these authors suggest that the incidence of temporary, partial, or asymptomatic paralysis may go relatively unnoticed. We believe that using the left-sided approach may reduce the risk of such injuries.

TECHNIQUE 34-5 *(Southwick and Robinson)*
As with other approaches to the cervical spine, skeletal traction is suggested and spinal cord monitoring should be employed. Exposure can be carried out through either a transverse or longitudinal incision, depending on the surgeon's preference (Fig. 34-10, *A*). A left-sided skin incision is preferred because of the more constant anatomy of the recurrent laryngeal nerve and the lower risk of inadvertent injury to the nerve. In general, an incision three to four fingerbreadths above the clavicle will be needed to expose C3 to C5 and an incision two to three fingerbreadths above the clavicle will allow exposure of C5 to C7.

Center a transverse incision over the medial border of the sternocleidomastoid muscle. Infiltration of the skin and subcutaneous tissue with a 1:500,000 epinephrine solution will assist with hemostasis. Incise the platysma muscle in line with the skin incision or open it vertically for more exposure. Identify the anterior border of the sternocleidomastoid muscle and longitudinally incise the superficial layer of the deep cervical fascia and localize the carotid

continued

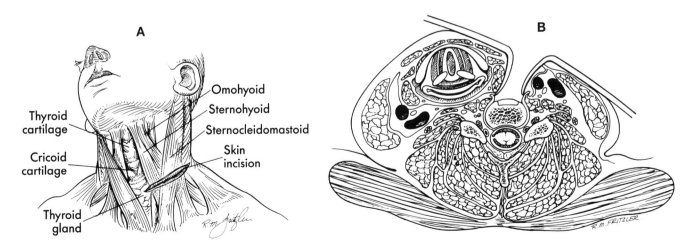

Fig. 34-10 Anterior approach to C3-C7 (see text). **A,** Incision. **B,** Thyroid gland, trachea, and esophagus have been retracted medially, and carotid sheath and its contents retracted laterally in opposite direction.

pulse by palpation. Carefully divide the middle layer of deep cervical fascia that encloses the omohyoid medial to the carotid sheath. As the sternomastoid and carotid sheath are retracted laterally, the anterior aspect of the cervical spine can be palpated. Identify the esophagus lying posterior to the trachea and retract the trachea, esophagus, and thyroid medially (Fig. 34-10, *B*). Bluntly divide the deep layers of the deep cervical fascia, consisting of the pretracheal and prevertebral fascia overlying the longus colli muscles. Subperiosteally reflect the longus colli from the anterior aspect of the spine out laterally to the level of the uncovertebral joints. The resulting exposure is sufficient for wide debridement and bone grafting.

Close the wound over a drain to prevent hematoma formation and possible airway obstruction. Approximate the platysma and skin edges in routine fashion.

Anterior Approach to Cervicothoracic Junction, C7 to T1

The cervicothoracic junction is without ready anterior access. The rapid transition from cervical lordosis to thoracic kyphosis results in an abrupt change in the depth of the wound. Also this is a confluent area of vital structures that are not readily retracted. The three approaches to this area are (1) the low anterior cervical approach, (2) the high transthoracic approach, and (3) the transsternal approach.

The low anterior cervical approach provides access to T1 at the inferior extent and the lower cervical spine at the superior extent of the dissection. Exposure is limited at the upper thoracic region but generally is adequate for placement of a strut graft if needed. Individual anatomical structure should be considered carefully in preoperative planning.

◆ Low Anterior Cervical Approach

TECHNIQUE 34-6
Enter on the left side by a transverse incision placed one fingerbreadth above the clavicle. Extend it well across the midline, taking particular care when dissecting about the carotid sheath in the area of entry of the thoracic duct. The latter approaches the jugular vein from its lateral side, but variations are not uncommon. Further steps in exposure follow those of the conventional anterior cervical approach.

◆ High Transthoracic Approach

TECHNIQUE 34-7
A kyphotic deformity of the thoracic spine tends to force the cervical spine into the chest, in which instance a high

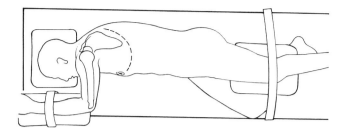

Fig. 34-11   Patient positioning and periscapular incision for high transthoracic approach.

transthoracic approach is a logical choice. Make a periscapular incision (Fig. 34-11) and remove the second or third rib; removing the latter is necessary to provide sufficient working space in a child or if a kyphotic deformity is present. This exposes the interval between C6 and T4. Excision of the first or second rib is adequate in adults or in the absence of an exaggerated kyphosis.

For equal exposure of the thoracic and cervical spine from C4 to T4, the sternal splitting approach described by Hodgson et al. and Fang, Ong, and Hodgson is recommended; it is commonly used in cardiac surgery.

◆ Transsternal Approach

TECHNIQUE 34-8
Make a Y-shaped or straight incision with the vertical segment passing along the midsternal area from the suprasternal notch to just below the xiphoid process (Fig. 34-12, *A*). Next, extend the proximal end diagonally to the right and left along the base of the neck for a short distance. To avoid entering the abdominal cavity, take care to keep the dissection beneath the periosteum while exposing the distal end of the sternum. At the proximal end of the sternal notch take care to avoid the inferior thyroid vein. By blunt dissection reflect the parietal pleura from the posterior surfaces of the sternum and costal cartilages and develop a space. Pass one finger or an instrument above and below the suprasternal space, insert a Gigli saw, and split the sternum. Now spread the split sternum and gain access to the center of the chest (Fig. 34-12, *B*). In children the upper portion of the exposure will be posterior to the thymus and bounded by the innominate and carotid arteries and their venous counter parts. Next, develop the left side of this area bluntly. In patients with kyphotic deformity the innominate vein may now be divided as it crosses the field; it may be very tense and subject to rupture. This division is recommended by Fang et al. The disadvantage of ligation is that it leaves a slight postoperative enlargement of the left upper extremity that is not apparent unless carefully assessed. This approach

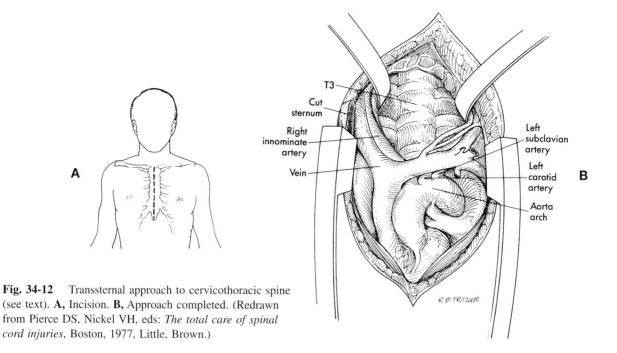

Fig. 34-12 Transsternal approach to cervicothoracic spine (see text). **A,** Incision. **B,** Approach completed. (Redrawn from Pierce DS, Nickel VH, eds: *The total care of spinal cord injuries*, Boston, 1977, Little, Brown.)

provides limited access, and its success depends on accuracy in preoperative interpretation of the deformity and a high degree of surgical precision.

◆ Modified Anterior Approach to Cervicothoracic Junction

Several authors have described an anterior approach to the cervical thoracic junction using a combined full median sternotomy and a combined cervical incision as first described by Cauchoix and Binet. Others have combined this approach with osteotomy of the clavicle or resection of the left sternoclavicular joint. Recently, Darling, McBroom, and Perrin used a modified anterior approach in four patients with metastatic disease causing cord compression at the cervical thoracic junction. Their approach provided excellent exposure from C3 to T4 without the associated morbidity related to the division of the manubrium or the innominate vein. They reported no mortality or morbidity, and all patients had posterior stabilization in 4 to 7 days. This procedure is technically simple and avoids the risk of injury to the subclavian vessels that can occur with resection of the clavicle or sternoclavicular junction.

TECHNIQUE 34-9 *(Darling et al.)*

Place the patient supine. If the neck is stable, place a sandbag transversely behind the shoulders to extend the neck and position the head in a head ring turned to the right. The left side is used to protect the left recurrent laryngeal nerve. Make an incision along the anterior border of the left sternocleidomastoid muscle to the sternal notch and continue in the midline to the level of the third costal cartilage. Divide the platysma in the line of the incision, retract the sternocleidomastoid laterally, and divide the omohyoid muscle. Retract the carotid sheath laterally, enter the prevertebral space, and develop a plane of dissection. Gently retract the esophagus, trachea, and adjacent recurrent laryngeal nerve to the right and elevate away from the vertebral column.

Incise the sternal fascia and divide the sternum in the midline from the sternal notch to the level of the second intercostal space. Retract the sternum laterally to the left through the synostosis between the manubrium and body of the sternum. Divide the strap muscles near their origin from the sternum to permit reconstruction, thus connecting the two portions of the incision. Do not divide the sternocleidomastoid muscle. Place a small chest retractor and open the partial sternotomy.

Ligate and divide the inferior thyroid artery and middle and inferior thyroid veins. Take care not to injure the recurrent laryngeal nerve or the superior laryngeal nerve through pressure or traction. Dissect the thymus and mediastinal fat away from the left innominate vein. If

continued

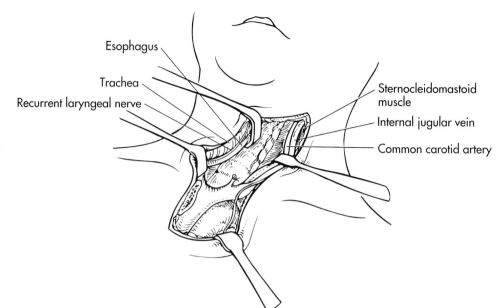

Fig. 34-13 Modified anterior approach to cervicothoracic junction. (Redrawn from Darling GE, McBroom R, Perrin R: *Spine* 20:1519, 1995.)

exposure to T3-T4 is required, divide the thymic and left innominate veins if necessary to expose the level of the aortic arch anteriorly and T4-T5 posteriorly (Fig. 34-13). In completing the dissection, take care not to injure the thoracic duct as it ascends to the left of the esophagus from the level of T4 to its junction with the left internal jugular and subclavian veins.

After the spinal decompression and stabilization are completed, close the wound by reapproximating the manubrium with two or three heavy-gauge stainless steel wires using standard techniques. Reattach the strap muscles to the sternum and close the presternal fascia. Drain the prevertebral space with a soft Silastic drain through a separate stab wound and attach to closed suction. Close the platysma and skin.

◆ Anterior Approach to Thoracic Spine

The transthoracic approach to the thoracic spine provides direct access to the vertebral bodies T2 to T12. Clearly, the midthoracic vertebral bodies are best exposed by this approach, whereas views of the upper and lower extremes of the spine are more limited. In general, a left-sided thoracotomy incision is preferred, although some surgeons favor a right-sided thoracotomy for approaching the upper thoracic spine to avoid the subclavian and carotid arteries in the left superior mediastinum. In a left-sided thoracotomy approach the heart may be retracted anteriorly, whereas in the right-sided approach the liver may present a significant obstacle to exposure. The level of the incision should be positioned to meet the level of exposure required. Ordinarily an intercostal space is selected at or just above the involved segment. If only one vertebral segment is involved, the rib at that level can be removed; however, if multiple levels are involved, the rib at the upper level of the proposed dissection should be removed. Because of the normal thoracic kyphosis, dissection is easier from proximal to distal. Exposure is improved by resection of a rib, and the rib provides a satisfactory bone graft, but resection is not necessary if a limited exposure is adequate for biopsy, decompression, or fusion. The transthoracic approach adds a significant operative risk and certainly is more hazardous than the more commonly used posterior or posterolateral approaches. The increased risk of thoracotomy must be weighed against the more limited exposure provided by alternative posterior approaches.

TECHNIQUE 34-10

Place the patient in the lateral decubitus position with the right side down; an inflatable beanbag is helpful in maintaining the patient's position, and the table may be flexed to increase exposure (Fig. 34-14, *A*). Make an incision over the rib corresponding to the involved vertebra and expose it subperiosteally. Use electrocautery to maintain hemostasis during the exposure. Disarticulate the rib from the transverse process and the hemifacets of the vertebral body. Take care to identify and preserve the intercostal nerve lying along the inferior aspect of the rib as it localizes the neural foramen leading into the spinal canal. Incise the parietal pleura and reflect it off of the spine, usually one vertebra above and one below the involved segment, to allow adequate exposure for debridement and grafting (Fig. 34-14, *B*). Identify the segmental vessels crossing the midportion of each vertebral body and ligate and divide these (Fig. 34-14, *C*). Carefully reflect the periosteum overlying the spine with elevators to expose the involved vertebrae. Use a small elevator to clearly delineate the pedicle of the vertebrae and a Kerrison rongeur to remove

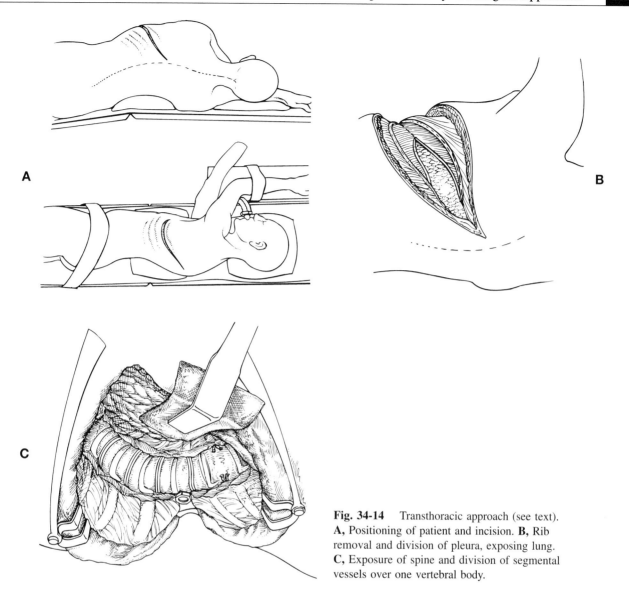

Fig. 34-14 Transthoracic approach (see text). **A,** Positioning of patient and incision. **B,** Rib removal and division of pleura, exposing lung. **C,** Exposure of spine and division of segmental vessels over one vertebral body.

the pedicle, thus exposing the dural sac. Identify the disc spaces above and below the vertebrae and incise the anulus. Remove disc material using rongeurs and curets. An entire cross section of the vertebral body is thus developed, and the anterior margin of the neural canal is identified with the posterior longitudinal ligament lying in the slight concavity on the back of the vertebral body. Expose sufficient segmental vessels and disc spaces to accomplish the intended procedure—usually corpectomy and strut grafting.

◆ Video-Assisted Thoracic Surgery

Video-assisted thoracic surgery (VATS) has been used successfully in the anterior thoracic and thoracolumbar spine and appears to have less morbidity than the standard thoracotomy, which can result in respiratory problems or pain after thoracotomy. Thoracoscopy has evolved rapidly and is capable of

providing adequate exposure to all levels of the thoracic spine from T2 to L1; however, the learning curve is significant, and the surgical team should always include a thoracic surgeon who is competent in thoracoscopy, as well as a spine surgeon who is well trained in endoscopic techniques.

Mack et al. reported 95 patients who had thoracic spine surgery using thoracoscopy. Only one patient required conversion to an open procedure because of scarring from a previous spine surgery. The mean operative time was 2 hours and 24 minutes, the average chest tube duration was 1.4 days, and the mean length of stay in the hospital was 4.82 days. Complications included intercostal neuralgia, atelectasis, excessive epidural blood loss (2500 ml), and temporary paraparesis in a scoliosis patient related to operative positioning. These authors believe that VATS offers an anterior approach to the thoracic spine that results in less morbidity.

Although the indications for the thoracoscopic approach apparently remain the same as for open thoracotomy, some procedures require extensive internal fixation and may not be suitable for this procedure. Also, patients should be informed before surgery that the thoracoscopic procedure may have to be abandoned in favor of an open procedure. Relative contraindications include preexisting pleural disease from previous surgeries.

TECHNIQUE 34-11 *(Mack et al.)*

Routine intraoperative monitoring for thoracic procedures is used, including an arterial pressure line, pulse oximeter, and end-tidal CO_2 measurement. Somatosensory evoked potentials should be monitored routinely for patients undergoing spinal deformity correction or corpectomy.

Place the initial trocar in the seventh intercostal space in the posterior axillary line. Place a 10-mm, 30-degree angled rigid telescope through the 10-mm trocar. Use a 0-degree end-viewing scope and a 30-degree scope for direct vision of the intervertebral disc space to avoid impeding surgical instrumentation or obscuring the operative field. Mack et al. recommend placing the viewing port in the posterior axillary line directly over the spine and two or three access sites for working ports in the anterior axillary line to allow better access to the spine. This "reverse L" arrangement can be moved cephalad or caudad, depending on the level of the thoracic spine to be approached. Use the portals for placement of surgical instruments (Fig. 34-15). Rotate the patient anteriorly and place him in a Trendelenburg position for the lower thoracic spine or reverse Trendelenburg for the upper thoracic spine. The lung usually will fall away from the operative field when completely collapsed, obviating the need for retraction instruments.

A departure from the standard VATS approach is the positioning of the operative team. Operative procedures routinely are performed by a spine surgeon and thoracic surgeon. In contrast to other VATS procedures in which the surgeon and assistant are positioned on opposite sides of the operating table, both surgeons are positioned on the anterior side of the patient viewing a monitor on the opposite side. In addition, the camera and therefore the viewing field is rotated 90 degrees from the standard VATS approach so that the spine is viewed horizontally.

Perform an initial exploratory thoracoscopy to determine the correct spinal level for operative intervention. Count the ribs by "palpation" with a blunt grasping instrument. Once the target level has been defined, place a 20-gauge long needle percutaneously into the disc space from the lateral aspect and confirm roentgenographically. When the correct level is ascertained, perform the specific spinal procedure.

◆ Anterior Approach to Thoracolumbar Junction

Occasionally, it may be necessary to expose simultaneously the lower thoracic and upper lumbar vertebral bodies. Technically this is a more difficult exposure because of the presence of the diaphragm and the increased risk involved in simultaneous exposure of the thoracic cavity and the retroperitoneal space. In

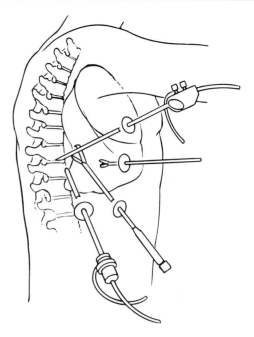

Fig. 34-15   Thoracoscopic instrument placement for thoracic spine procedures. (Redrawn from Regan JJ, McAfee PC, Mack MJ, eds: *Atlas of endoscopic spine surgery*, St Louis, 1995, Quality Medical Publishing.)

most instances thoracic lesions should be exposed through the chest, whereas lesions predominantly involving the upper lumbar spine can be exposed through an anterior retroperitoneal incision. The diaphragm is a dome-shaped organ that is muscular in the periphery and tendinous in the center. Posteriorly, it originates from the upper lumbar vertebrae through crura, the arcuate ligaments, and the twelfth ribs. Anteriorly and laterally it attaches to the cartilaginous ends of the lower six ribs and xiphoid. The diaphragm is innervated by the phrenic nerve, which descends through the thoracic cavity on the pericardium. The phrenic nerve joins the diaphragm adjacent to the fibrous pericardium, dividing into three major branches that extend peripherally in anterolateral and posterior directions. Division of these major branches may interfere with diaphragmatic function. It is best to make an incision around the periphery of the diaphragm to minimize interference with function when making a thoracoabdominal approach to the spine. We recommend a left-sided approach at the thoracolumbar junction, since the vena cava on the right is less tolerant of dissection and may result in troublesome hemorrhage and, in addition, the liver may be hard to retract.

TECHNIQUE 34-12

Place the patient in the right lateral decubitus position and place supports beneath the buttock and shoulder. Make the incision curvilinear with ability to extend either the cephalad or caudal end (Fig. 34-16, *A*). To gain the best access to the interval of T12 to L1, resect the tenth rib, which allows exposure between T10 and L2. The only

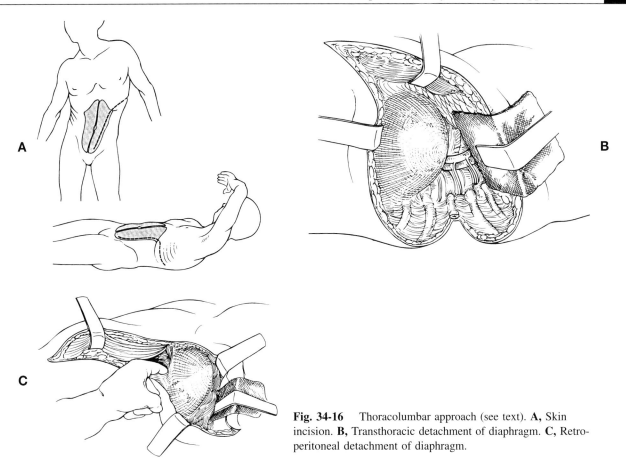

Fig. 34-16 Thoracolumbar approach (see text). **A,** Skin incision. **B,** Transthoracic detachment of diaphragm. **C,** Retroperitoneal detachment of diaphragm.

difficulty is in identifying the diaphragm as a separate structure; it tends to closely approximate the wall of the thoracic cage, allowing the edge of the lung to penetrate into the space beneath the knife as the pleura is divided (Fig. 34-16, *B*). Now take care in entering the abdominal cavity. Since the transversalis fascia and the peritoneum do not diverge, dissect with caution and identify the two cavities on either side of the diaphragm. To achieve confluence of the two cavities, reflect the diaphragm from the lower ribs and the crus from the side of the spine (Fig. 34-16, *C*). Alternatively, incise the diaphragm 2.5 cm away from its insertion and tag it with sutures for later accurate closure. Incise the prevertebral fascia. Take care to identify the segmental arteries and veins over the midportion of each vertebral body. Isolate these, ligate them in the midline, and expose the bone as previously described.

◆ **Anterior Retroperitoneal Approach, L1 to L5**

The anterior retroperitoneal approach to the lumbar vertebral bodies is a modification of the anterolateral approach commonly used by general surgeons for sympathectomy. It is an excellent approach that should be considered for extensive resection, debridement, or grafting at multiple levels in the

lumbar spine. Depending on which portion of the lumbar spine is to be approached, the incision may be varied in placement between the twelfth rib and the superior aspect of the iliac crest. The major dissection in this approach is behind the kidney in the potential space between the renal fascia and the quadratus lumborum and psoas muscles.

TECHNIQUE 34-13

Position the patient in the lateral decubitus position, generally with the right side down. The approach is made most often from the left side to avoid the liver and the inferior vena cava, which is more difficult to repair than the aorta should vascular injury occur during the approach to the spine. Flex the table to increase exposure between the twelfth rib and the iliac crest. Flex the hips slightly to release tension on the psoas muscle. Make an oblique incision over the twelfth rib from the lateral border of the quadratus lumborum to the lateral border of the rectus abdominus muscle to allow exposure of the first and second lumbar vertebrae (Fig. 34-17, *A*). Alternatively, place the incision several fingerbreadths below and parallel to the costal margin when exposure of the lower lumbar vertebrae (L3 to L5) is necessary. Use electrocautery to divide the subcutaneous tissue, fascia, and muscle of the external oblique, internal oblique, transversus abdominus, and transversalis

continued

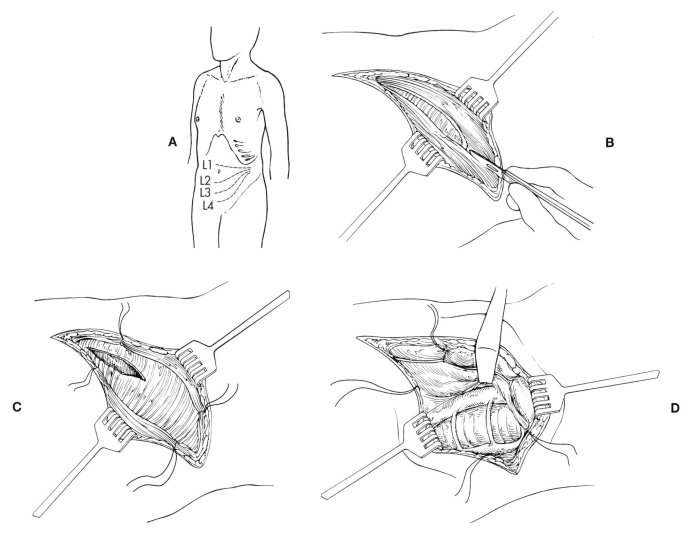

Fig. 34-17   Anterior retroperitoneal approach (see text). **A,** Skin incisions for lumbar vertebrae.
B, Incision of fibers of external oblique muscle. **C,** Incision into fibers of internal oblique muscle.
D, Exposure of spine before ligation of segmental vessels.

fascia in line with the skin incision (Fig. 34-17, *B* and *C*).
Carefully protect the peritoneum and reflect it anteriorly by
blunt dissection. If the peritoneum is entered during the
approach, it must be repaired. Identify the psoas muscle in
the retroperitoneal space and allow the ureter to fall
anteriorly with the retroperitoneal fat. The sympathetic
chain is found between the vertebral bodies and the psoas
muscle laterally, whereas the genitofemoral nerve is lying
on the anterior aspect of the psoas muscle. Place a
Finochietto rib retractor between the costal margin and the
iliac crest to aid exposure. Palpate the vertebral bodies from
T12 to L5 and identify and protect with a Deaver retractor
the great vessels lying anterior to the spine. It is important
to note that the lumbar segmental vessels are lying in the
midportion of the vertebral bodies and that the relatively
avascular discs are prominent on each adjacent side of the

vessels (Fig. 34-17, *D*). Once the appropriate involved
vertebra is identified, elevate the psoas muscle bluntly off
the lumbar vertebrae and retract it laterally to the level of the
transverse process with a Richardson retractor. Sometimes
removal of the transverse process with a rongeur is helpful
in allowing adequate retraction of the psoas muscle. Ligate
and divide the lumbar segmental vessel overlying the
involved vertebrae. Clearly delineate the pedicle of the involved vertebrae with a small elevator and locate the
neuroforamen with the exiting nerve root. Bipolar coagulation of vessels around the neuroforamen is recommended.
Then remove the pedicle with an angled Kerrison rongeur
and expose the dura.

After completion of the spinal procedure, obtain
meticulous hemostasis and close the wound in layers over a
drain in the retroperitoneal space.

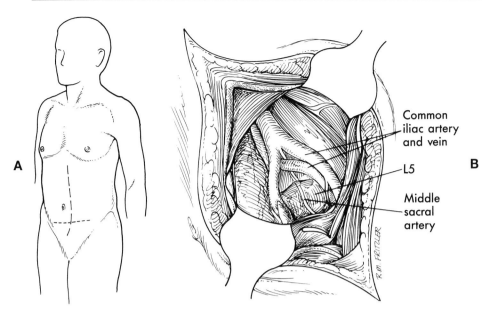

Fig. 34-18 Transperitoneal approach to lumbar and lumbosacral spine (see text). **A,** Median longitudinal or transverse Pfannenstiel incision. **B,** Dissection of middle sacral artery and vein.

Labels in figure: Common iliac artery and vein; L5; Middle sacral artery

◆ Anterior Transperitoneal Approach to Lumbosacral Junction, L5 to S1

Transperitoneal exposure of the lumbar spine is an alternative to the retroperitoneal approach. The advantage of the transperitoneal route is a somewhat more extensive exposure, especially at the L5 to S1 level. A disadvantage is that the great vessels and hypogastric nerve plexus must be mobilized before the spine is exposed. The superior hypogastric plexus contains the sympathetic function for the urogenital systems, and damage of this structure in males can cause complications such as retrograde ejaculation; however; damage to the superior hypogastric plexus should not produce impotence or failure of erection. Injury to the hypogastric plexus can be avoided by careful opening of the posterior peritoneum and blunt dissection of the prevertebral tissue from left to right and by opening the posterior peritoneum higher over the bifurcation of the aorta and then extending the opening down over the sacral promontory. In addition, electrocautery should be kept to a minimum when dissecting within the aortic bifurcation, and until the anulus of the L5 to S1 disc is clearly exposed, no transverse scalpel cuts on the front of the disc should be made.

TECHNIQUE 34-14

Position the patient supine on the operating table and make either a vertical midline or a transverse incision (Fig. 34-18, *A*). The transverse incision is cosmetically superior and gives excellent exposure; it requires transection of the rectus abduminus sheath. Identify and open the sheath and transect the rectus abduminus muscle. The posterior rectus sheath, abdominal fascia, and peritoneum are conjoined in this area. Open the posterior rectus sheath and abdominal fascia to the peritoneum. Carefully open the peritoneum to avoid damage to bowel content. Carefully pack off the abdominal contents and identify the posterior peritoneum over the sacral promontory. Palpate the aorta and the common iliac vessels through the posterior peritoneum. Make a longitudinal incision in the posterior peritoneum in the midline about the aortic bifurcation. Extend the incision distally and to the right along the right common iliac artery to its bifurcation at the external and internal iliac arteries. Identify the right ureter, crossing the right iliac artery, and curve the incision medially to avoid this structure. Avoid the use of electrocautery anterior to the L5-S1 disc space to prevent damage to the superior hypogastric plexus. The left common iliac vein often lies as a flat structure across the L5-S1 disc within the aortic bifurcation. After identification of the left common iliac artery and vein, use blunt dissection to the right of the artery and hypogastric plexus and mobilize the soft tissue from left to right. Carefully dissect the middle sacral artery and vein from left to right (Fig. 34-18, *B*). Longitudinal blunt dissection allows better mobilization of these vascular structures. If bleeding is encountered, use direct finger and sponge pressure rather than electrocautery. If electrocautery is used in this area, we recommend the bipolar rather than the unipolar machine because there is less likelihood of injuring the hypogastric plexus with a thermal burn. Following adequate exposure of the L5-S1 disc, obtain a roentgenogram after inserting a 22-gauge spinal needle into the disc space. Because the L5-S1 disc and the sacrum often are angled horizontally, the body of L5 may be mistaken for the sacrum. Further development of the exposure proceeds as in other anterior approaches to the lumbar vertebrae.

◆ Video-Assisted Lumbar Surgery

Standard anterior approaches to the lower lumbar and lumbosacral spine include the anterior transperitoneal, anterolateral extraperitoneal, and anterior retroperitoneal approaches. As with thoracoscopy, endoscopic technique is rapidly evolving in terms of its role in procedures involving the anterior aspect of the lumbar spine. Transperitoneal laparoscopic approaches, which have been used for discectomy or fusion, are true endoscopic procedures that are performed with CO_2 insufflation and may be impeded by abdominal wall adhesions. Complications include vascular and peritoneal injuries. McAffee et al. described a minimally invasive anterior retroperitoneal approach to the lumbar spine using endoscopic technique. They reported 18 patients with lumbar instability from fractures, postlaminectomy syndrome, or infection treated with minimally invasive endoscopic retroperitoneal lumbar fusions and concluded that endoscopic techniques can be used through a retroperitoneal approach with the patient in the lateral position. The morbidity was less than that reported for traditional open retroperitoneal or laparotomy techniques. No cases of injury to the great vessels causing retrograde ejaculation or implant migration were reported.

Onimus, Papin, and Gangloff described a less-invasive, standard midline, extraperitoneal approach that fully preserves the abdominal innervation and is optimized with video assistance. This procedure avoids peritoneal complications, and it is anterior and midline oriented, giving direct access to the anterior aspect of the disc. Video assistance allows for a smaller incision, improved lighting, and easier presacral dissection. In addition, good exposure of the vertebral endplates is achieved, allowing a better resection and perhaps, although not reported, an improved fusion rate. In addition, surgical assistants can observe the operation despite the small incision, and if necessary the incision can be extended cephalad or caudad if conversion to a laparotomy is necessary.

TECHNIQUE 34-15 *(Onimus et al.)*

Place the patient supine and angulate the operative table to place the lumbar spine in slight extension. Make a 4-cm vertical incision on the midline at the umbilicus for L4-L5, and halfway between the umbilicus and the pubic symphysis for the L5-S1 approach. In women, a more cosmetic horizontal suprapubic incision is available for the L5-S1 approach.

After division of the linea alba, dissect on the left side between the posterior sheath of the rectus abdominis and posterior aspect of this muscle. Then divide the posterior sheath at the lateral edge of the rectus returning to the subperitoneal fascia. The division begins at the linea arcuata. Use blunt dissection with a finger and dissecting swabs. The next landmark is the prominence of the psoas muscle and the iliac vessels. Reflect the ureter and peritoneum together. The lateral cleavage of the peritoneum can be increased by use of an inflatable balloon. Introduce a 10-mm endoscope through a lateral port between the umbilicus and anterosuperior iliac spine for exposure of L5-S1 and at the level of the umbilicus exposure of L4-L5. Introduction of the endoscope gives good exposure of the prevertebral area and allows the operation to be continued under endoscopic and direct vision. Expose the anterior aspect of the intervertebral disc by blunt dissection through the midline incision. For exposure of L5-S1, hemoclip the middle sacral vessels and divide. Retract the common iliac vessels cranially with a specially designed retractor that is introduced through the midline incision and held in position by two Steinmann pins inserted in L5 and S1. For exposure of L4-L5, retract the iliac vessels caudally. Divide the iliolumbar vein to allow caudal retraction of the left iliac vein.

More acute endoscopic exposure of the vertebral plates is possible by using a 30-degree angulated arthroscope. Intervertebral distraction allows iliac autogenous graft insertion. The procedure can be completed with disc and vertebral plate resection.

Close the wound on a retroperitoneal suction tube inserted through the endoscope's lateral port.

AFTERTREATMENT. Standing and ambulation are allowed 2 to 3 days after surgery. A body jacket orthosis is worn for 3 months.

POSTERIOR APPROACHES

The posterior approach through a midline longitudinal incision provides access to the posterior elements of the spine at all levels, including cervical, thoracic, and lumbosacral. It is the most direct access to the spinous processes, laminae, and facets and, in addition, the spinal canal can be explored and decompressed over a large area after laminectomy. Under most circumstances, the choice of approach to the spine should be dictated by the site of the primary pathological condition. Posterior approaches to the spine rarely are indicated when the anterior spinal column is the site of an infectious process or a metastatic disease. The posterior elements usually are not involved in the pathological process and provide stabilization for the uninvolved structures of the spinal column. Removal of the uninvolved posterior elements, as in laminectomy, may result in subluxation, dislocation, or severe angulation of the spine, causing increased compression of the neural elements and worsening of any neurological deficit. Posterior approaches to the spine commonly are used for degenerative or traumatic spinal disorders and allow excellent exposure to carry out a wide variety of fusion techniques, with or without internal stabilization.

◆ Posterior Approach to Cervical Spine, Occiput to C2

TECHNIQUE 34-16

Position the patient prone on a turning frame with skeletal traction through tongs, taking care to avoid excessive pressure on the eyes. Alternatively a three-point head rest can be used to provide rigid immobilization of the cervical

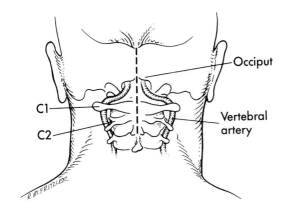

Fig. 34-19   Posterior approach to upper cervical spine (see text).

spine during surgery. After routine skin preparation, attach the drapes to the neck with stay sutures or staples. Make a midline longitudinal skin incision from the occiput to C2 (Fig. 34-19). Infiltration of the skin and subcutaneous tissue with a dilute 1:500,000 epinephrine solution is helpful to provide hemostasis. Using electrocautery and elevators, expose the posterior elements subperiosteally and insert self-retaining retractors. It is important to deepen the incision in the midline through the thin white median raphe and avoid cutting muscle tissue. The median raphe of the cervical spine is a wandering avascular ligament and does not follow a straight midline incision. In children, expose no spinal levels unnecessarily to avoid spontaneous fusion at adjacent levels, including the occiput. When exposing the upper cervical spine, take care not to carry the dissection further than 1.5 cm laterally on either side to avoid the vertebral arteries. When necessary, expose the occiput with elevators and insert the self-retaining retractors to expose the base of the skull and the dorsal spine of C2. The area in between will contain the ring of C1; this is often deep compared with the spinous process of C2. While maintaining lateral retraction of the soft tissues, identify the posterior tubercle of C1 longitudinally in the midline and begin subperiosteal dissection to the bone. Often the ring of C1 is thin, and direct pressure can fracture it or cause the instrument to slip off the ring and penetrate the atlanto-occipital membrane. The dura may be vulnerable on both the superior and inferior edges of the ring of C1. The second cervical ganglion is an important landmark on the ring of C1 laterally. It lies approximately 1.5 cm laterally on the lamina of C1 in the groove for the vertebral artery. There is little, if any, indication for dissection lateral to this groove. The vertebral artery may be damaged by penetration of the atlanto-occipital membrane off the superior border of the ring of C1 more lateral than the usually safe 1.5 cm from the midline. Below C2 the lateral margins of the facet joints are the safe lateral extent of dissection. After exposure of the posterior occiput, the ring of C1, and the posterior elements of C2, the intended surgical procedure may be

performed. After this, the wound is closed in layers over a drain.

◆ Posterior Approach to Cervical Spine, C3 to C7

TECHNIQUE 34-17
Position the patient prone on a turning frame with skeletal traction through tongs or with the head positioned in the three-point head fixation device that is attached to the table. The large spinous processes of C2 and C7 are prominent and can be identified by palpation. It is important to note on preoperative roentgenograms any posterior element deficiencies, such as an occult spina bifida, before exposure of the posterior elements. Make a midline skin incision over the appropriate vertebrae (Fig. 34-20) and inject the skin and subcutaneous tissues with a 1:500,000 epinephrine solution to aid in hemostasis. Deepen the dissection in the midline, using the electrocautery knife and staying within the thin white median raphe to avoid cutting the vascular muscle tissue (Fig. 34-21). It is helpful to maintain tension on the soft tissue by inserting self-retaining retractors. Using electrocautery and elevators, detach the ligamentous attachments to the spinous processes and expose the posterior elements subperiosteally to the lateral edge of the facet joints, which is the extent of dissection on either side of the midline. After identifying the lateral edge of the facet joint, pack each level with a taped sponge to keep blood loss to a minimum. It is helpful to expose the spinous processes distal to proximal because the muscles may then be stripped from the spinous processes in the acute angle between their insertions and the bone. If exposure in the opposite direction is attempted, the knife blade or periosteal elevator will tend to follow the direction of the fibers into the muscle and divide the vessels, thus increasing hemorrhage.

◆ Posterior Approach to Thoracic Spine, T1 to T12
The posterior approach to the thoracic spine can be made through a standard midline longitudinal exposure with reflection of the erector spinae muscle laterally to the tips of the transverse processes. Alternatively the thoracic vertebrae can be approached through a costotransversectomy when direct access to the transverse processes and pedicles of the thoracic spine and limited access to the vertebral bodies are indicated. Costotransversectomy should be considered for simple biopsy or local debridement. It should be noted, however, that this approach does not provide the working operative area or length of exposure to the thoracic vertebral bodies that is afforded by a transthoracic approach or the midlongitudinal posterior approach.

TECHNIQUE 34-18
Position the patient prone on a padded spinal operating frame. Make a long midline incision over the area to be

continued

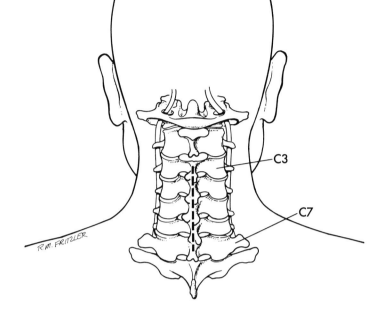

Fig. 34-20   Posterior approach to lower cervical spine (see text).

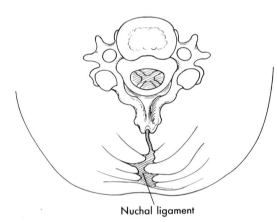

Nuchal ligament

Fig. 34-21   Posterior approach to lower cervical spine. Nuchal ligament is irregular. To maintain dry field, surgeon must stay within ligament.

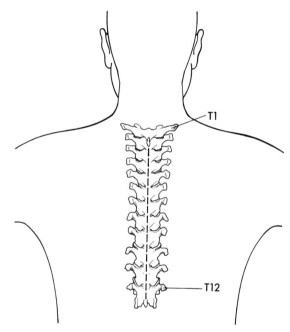

Fig. 34-22   Posterior approach to thoracic spine (see text).

exposed (Fig. 34-22). Infiltration of the skin, subcutaneous tissue, and erector spinae to the level of the laminae with a 1:500,000 epinephrine solution is helpful in providing hemostasis. Deepen the dissection in the midline using either a scalpel or the electrocautery knife through the superficial and lumbodorsal fasciae to the tips of the spinous processes. Expose subperiosteally the posterior elements by reflecting the erector spinae muscle laterally to the tips of the transverse processes distal to proximal, using periosteal elevators. Repeat the procedure until the desired number of vertebrae are exposed, and where both sides of the spine require exposure, use the same technique on each side. Pack each segment with a taped sponge immediately after exposure to lessen bleeding. After satisfactory exposure of the posterior elements, obtain a roentgenogram to confirm proper localization of the intended level. After completion of the spinal procedure, close the wound in layers over a suction drain.

◆ Costotransversectomy

TECHNIQUE 34-19
Place the patient prone on a padded spinal operating frame. Make a straight longitudinal incision about 2.5 inches (6.3 cm) lateral to the spinous processes centered over the

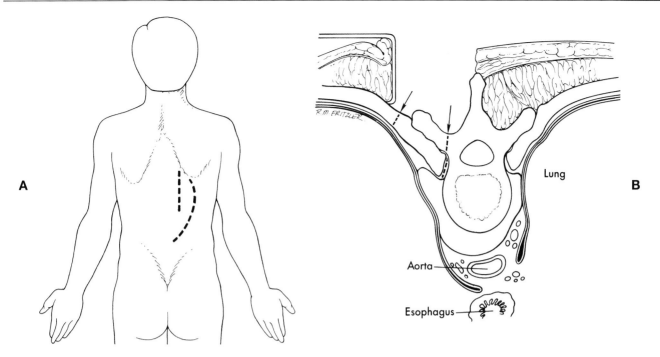

Fig. 34-23   Costotransversectomy. **A,** Straight longitudinal incision about 2.5 inches (6.3 cm) lateral to spinous processes, centered over level of vertebral dissection. **B,** Resection of costotransverse articulation.

level of the desired vertebral dissection (Fig. 34-23, *A*). (Alternatively, make a curved incision with its apex lateral to the midline.) Palpate the slight depression between the dorsal paraspinal muscle mass and the prominent posterior angle of the rib and center the incision over this groove lateral to the spinous processes. Deepen the dissection through the subcutaneous tissues and the trapezius and latissimus dorsi muscles and the lumbodorsal fasciae, which are divided longitudinally. Dissect the paraspinal muscles sharply from their insertions on the ribs and transverse processes and retract them medially. Expose the transverse process and posterior aspects of the associated rib subperiosteally and remove a section of rib 5 to 7.5 cm long at the level of involvement. The rib generally is transected with rib cutters about 3.5 inches lateral to the vertebrae at its prominent posterior angle. The costotransverse ligament and joint capsule are quite strong and increase the inherent stability of the thoracic spine. Take care to remain subperiosteal and extrapleural during this part of the exposure and to protect the intercostal neurovascular bundle. Anterior to the transverse process is the vertebral pedicle, and above and below the pedicle lie the neuroforamina. The nerve roots emerge from the superior portion of the foramina, giving off a dorsal and ventral ramus. The ventral ramus becomes the intercostal nerve and is joined by the intercostal vessels. Once the pedicles, neuroforamina, and neurovascular structures have been identified, proceed with dissection directly anteriorly on the pedicle to the vertebral body along a path that is relatively free of major

vessels or nerve (Fig. 34-23, *B*). Carefully dissect the parietal pleura with elevators anteriorly to expose the anterolateral aspect of the vertebral body, raising the sympathetic trunk and parietal pleura. Exposure may be increased by removal of the transverse process, pedicle, and facet joints as necessary. After completion of the spinal procedure, fill the wound with saline and inflate the lungs to check for air leaks. Close the wound in layers over a drain to prevent hematoma collection. Obtain a chest roentgenogram to document the absence of air in the pleural space, which may occur if the pleura is inadvertently entered during the exposure.

◆ Posterior Approach to Lumbar Spine, L1 to L5

The posterior approach to the lumbar spine provides access directly to the spinous processes, laminae, and facet joints at all levels. In addition, the transverse processes and pedicles can be reached through this approach. Recently, Wiltse and Spencer refined the paraspinal approach to the lumbar spine, which involves a longitudinal separation of the sacrospinalis muscle group to expose the posterolateral aspect of the lumbar spine. This approach is especially useful in removing far lateral disc herniation, decompressing a "far-out" syndrome, and inserting pedicle screws.

TECHNIQUE 34-20

Position the patient prone or in the kneeling position on a padded spinal frame. By allowing the abdomen to hang free,

continued

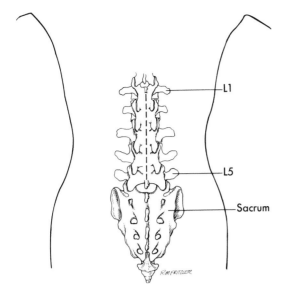

Fig. 34-24 Posterior approach to lumbar spine (see text).

intravenous pressure is decreased and blood loss is decreased as a result of collapse of the epidural venous plexus. Make a midline skin incision centered over the involved lumbar segment (Fig. 34-24). Infiltration of the skin and subcutaneous tissue with a 1:500,000 epinephrine solution aids hemostasis. Carry the dissection down in the midline through the skin, subcutaneous tissue, and lumbodorsal fascia to the tips of the spinous processes. Use self-retaining retractors to maintain tension on soft tissues during exposure. Subperiosteally expose the posterior elements from distal to proximal using electrocautery and periosteal elevators to detach the muscles from the posterior elements. Pack each segment with a taped sponge immediately after exposure to lessen bleeding. If the procedure requires exposure of both sides of the spine, use the same technique on each side. We recommend accurate localization of the involved segment with a permanent roentgenogram in the operating room. After completion of the spinal procedure, close the wound in layers over a drain.

◆ **Paraspinal Approach to Lumbar Spine**

TECHNIQUE 34-21 *(Wiltse and Spencer)*

Position the patient prone or in the kneeling position on a spinal frame. By allowing the abdomen to hang free, intravenous pressure is decreased and blood loss is decreased as a result of collapse of the epidural venous plexus. Make a midline skin incision centered over the involved lower lumbar segment (Fig. 34-25, *A*). Infiltration with 1:500,000 epinephrine solution is helpful in providing

hemostasis. Carry dissection down to the lumbodorsal fascia and retract the skin and subcutaneous tissue laterally on either side. Then make a fascial incision approximately 2 cm lateral to the midline (Fig. 34-25, *B* and *C*). Once the fascial layers have been divided, a natural cleavage plane is entered lying between the multifidus and longissimus muscles. Using blunt finger dissection between the muscle groups (Fig. 34-25, *D* and *E*), palpate the facet joints at L4-5. Place self-retaining Gelpi retractors between the two muscle groups. Using either electrocautery or an elevator, separate the transverse fibers of the multifidus from their heavy fascial attachments. Expose the lumbar transverse processes, facet joints, and lamina subperiosteally and denude them of soft tissue. Take care not to carry the dissection anterior to the transverse processes, since the exiting spinal nerves lie just in front of the transverse processes and can be injured. Use bipolar cautery to control bleeding from the lumbar arteries and veins coursing above the base of the transverse processes. Perform unilateral or bilateral decompression and fusion of the lumbosacral spine. Close the wound over a suction drain and suture the skin flaps down to the fascia to remove dead space.

◆ **Posterior Approach to Lumbosacral Spine, L1 to Sacrum**

TECHNIQUE 34-22 *(Wagoner)*

Make a longitudinal incision over the spinous processes of the appropriate vertebrae and incise the superficial fascia, the lumbodorsal fascia, and the supraspinous ligament longitudinally, precisely over the tips of the processes. With a scalpel divide longitudinally the ligament between the two spinous processes in the most distal part of the wound. Insert a small, blunt periosteal elevator through this opening so that its end rests on the junction of the spinous process with the lamina of the more proximal vertebra (Fig. 34-26, *A*). Move the handle of the elevator proximally and laterally to place under tension the muscles attached to this spinous process. Then with a scalpel moving from distal to proximal, strip the muscles subperiosteally from the lateral surface of the process. Then place the end of the elevator in the wound so that its end rests on the junction of the spinous process with the lamina of the next most proximal vertebra and repeat the procedure as described. Repeat the procedure until the desired number of vertebrae have been exposed (Fig. 34-26, *B*). For operations requiring exposure of both sides of the spine, use the same technique on each side.

This approach exposes the spinous processes and medial part of the laminae. Increase the exposure, if desired, by further subperiosteal reflection along the laminae; expose the posterior surface of the laminae and the articular facets. Pack each segment with a tape sponge immediately after exposure to lessen bleeding. Divide the supraspinous

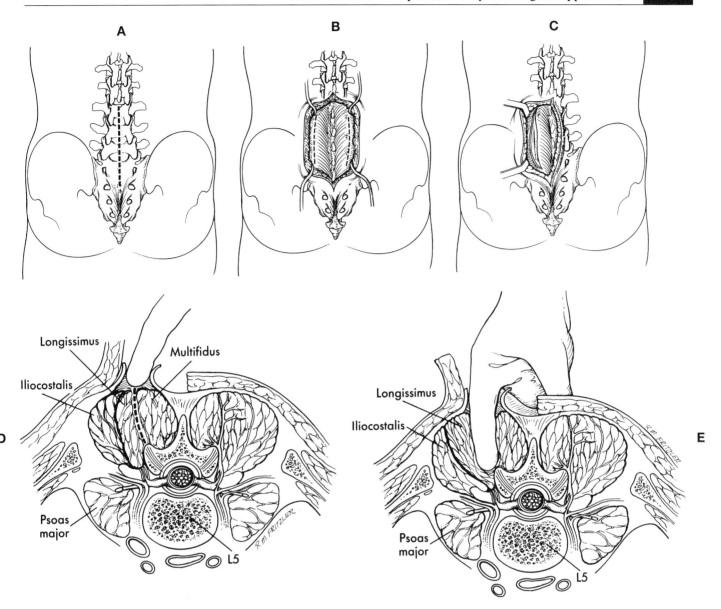

Fig. 34-25 Paraspinal approach to lumbar spine (see text). **A,** Midline skin incision. **B** and **C,** Fascial incisions. **D** and **E,** Blunt finger dissection between muscle groups to palpate facet joints. (Redrawn from Wiltse LL, Spencer CW: *Spine* 13:696, 1988.)

ligament precisely over the tip of the spinous processes and denude subperiosteally the sides of the processes because this route leads through a relatively avascular field; otherwise the arterial supply to the muscles will be encountered (see Fig. 34-26, *A*). Blood loss can be further decreased by using electrocautery and a suction apparatus. Replace blood as it is lost. Expose the spinous processes from distal to proximal as just described because the muscles can then be stripped from the spinous processes in the acute angle between their insertions and the bone. If exposure in the opposite direction is attempted, the knife blade or periosteal elevator tends to follow the direction of the fibers into the muscle and divides the vessels, thus increasing hemorrhage.

◆ Posterior Approach to Sacrum and Sacroiliac Joint

The posterior sacrum and sacroiliac joint are most commonly approached through a standard posterior exposure; however, the access to the sacroiliac joint is somewhat limited. Ebraheim et al. described a transosseous approach to the sacroiliac joint that they believe improves access for debridement and arthrodesis with only minimal soft tissue dissection and iliac bone

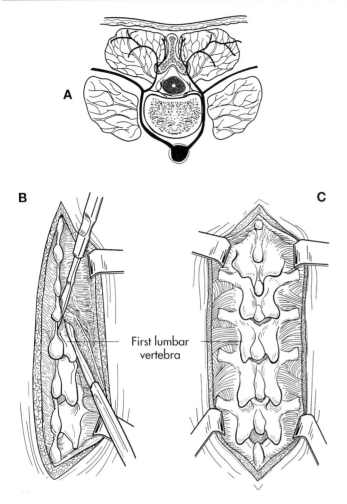

Fig. 34-26 Approach to posterior aspect of spine. **A,** Courses of arteries supplying posterior spinal muscles, showing proximity of internal muscular branches to spinous processes. **B,** Muscle insertions are freed subperiosteally from lateral side of spinous processes and interspinous ligaments; dissection proceeds proximally, with periosteal elevator being held against bases of spinous processes. **C,** Spinous processes, laminae, and articular facets exposed. (Modified from Wagoner G: *J Bone Joint Surg* 19:469, 1937.)

resection. Indications include trauma, infection, degenerative disease, and inflammatory processes. This approach allows direct exposure of the corresponding sacral articular surfaces.

TECHNIQUE 34-23 *(Ebraheim et al.)*

Place the patient prone on padded bolsters or spinal frame. Make an incision beginning at the level of the posterosuperior iliac spine and extending distal to the midpoint between the posterosuperior iliac spine and the posteroinferior iliac spine. Extend the incision laterally and distally approximately 5 cm (Fig. 34-27, *A*). Divide the superficial fascia and incise the gluteus medius muscle along the line of the skin incision. Sharply dissect the origin of the gluteus maximus from the posterior ilium. Subperiosteally elevate the gluteal musculature laterally and identify the superior border of the greater sciatic notch. Insert one or two Steinmann pins into the ilium to assist in retracting the gluteus maximus laterally and distally. It is important not to injure the superior gluteal neurovascular bundle. Expose the posterior external surface of the ilium between the posterosuperior iliac spine above and the superior border of the greater sciatic notch below. Next, elevate a right-angle, triangular-shape bone window from the posterior ilium using an osteotome or power saw and remove the articular cartilage from the sacrum and ilium (Fig. 34-27, *B*). Debride the joint with curets. After removal of the articular cartilage, place the previously elevated bone window into its original position and carefully tamp back into place.

Accurate localization of the bone window in the iliac crest is important to avoid laceration to the superior gluteal artery, which may retract into the pelvis making hemostasis difficult. Injury to the superior gluteal nerve may denervate the gluteus medius, leading to dysfunction in hip abduction. The dimensions of the right-angle triangle in the outer table of the posterior ilium are illustrated in Fig. 34-27, *B*.

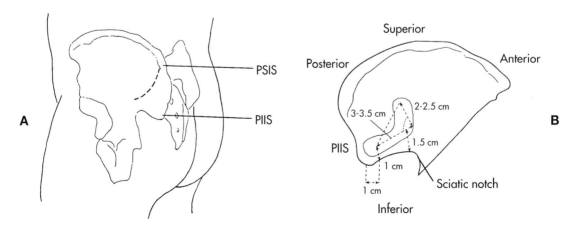

Fig. 34-27 Posterior approach to sacroiliac joint. **A,** Skin incision. **B,** Right triangle on outer table of posterior ilium. (Redrawn from Ebraheim NA, Lu J, Biyani A, Yeasting RA: *Spine* 21:2709, 1996.)

References

ANATOMY AND BIOMECHANICS

Abou-Madawi A, Solanki G, Casey AT, Crockard HA: Variation of the groove in the axis vertebra for the vertebral artery. Implications for instrumentation, *J Bone Joint Surg* 79B:820, 1997.

Amonoo-Kuofi HS: Age-related variations in the horizontal and vertical diameters of the pedicles of the lumbar spine, *J Anat* 186:321, 1995.

Aspden RM: The spine as an arch: a new mathematical model, *Spine* 14:266, 1989.

Bailey AS, Stanescu S, Yeasting RA, et al: Anatomic relationships of the cervicothoracic junction, *Spine* 20:1431, 1995.

Bullough PG, Oheneba BA: *Atlas of spinal diseases*, Philadelphia, 1988, JB Lippincott.

Carlson GD, Warden KE, Barbeau JM, et al: Viscoelastic relaxation and regional blood flow response to spinal cord compression and decompression, *Spine* 22:1285, 1987.

Dickson RA, Deacon P: Annotation: spinal growth, *J Bone Joint Surg* 69B:690, 1987.

Dommisse GF: The blood supply of the spinal cord: a critical vascular zone in spinal surgery, *J Bone Joint Surg* 56B:225, 1974.

Ebraheim NA, Jabaly G, Xu R, Yeasting RA: Anatomic relations of the thoracic pedicle to the adjacent neural structures, *Spine* 22:1553 1997.

Ebraheim NA, Lu J, Biyani A, Yeasting RA: Anatomic considerations for posterior approach to the sacroiliac joint, *Spine* 21:2709, 1996.

Ebraheim NA, Xu R, Darwich M, Yeasting RA: Anatomic relations between the lumbar pedicle and the adjacent neural structures, *Spine* 22:2338, 1997.

Ebraheim NA, Xu R, Knight T, Yeasting RA: Morphometric evaluation of lower cervical pedicle and its projection, *Spine* 22:1, 1997.

Ebraheim NA, Yeasting RA, Wong FY, Jackson WT: Morphometric evaluation of the first sacral vertebra and the projection of its pedicle on the posterior aspect of spine, *Spine* 20:936, 1995.

Esses SI, Bednar DA: The spinal pedicle screw: techniques and systems, *Orthop Rev* 18:676, 1989.

Jespersen SM, Christensen K, Svenstrup L, et al: Spinal cord and nerve root blood flow in acute double level spinal stenosis, *Spine* 22:2900, 1997.

Karaikovic EE, Daubs MD, Madsen RW, Gaines RW: Morphologic characteristics of human cervical pedicles, *Spine* 22:493, 1997.

Karlström G, Olerud S, Sjöstrom L: Transpedicular fixation of thoracolumbar fractures, *Contemp Orthop* 20:285, 1990.

Kolenda H, Steffens H, Gefeller O, et al: Critical levels of spinal cord blood flow and duration of ischemia for the acute recovery of segmental spinal cord responses in cats, *J Spinal Disord* 10:288, 1997.

Kothe R, O'Holleran JD, Liu W, Panjabi MM: Internal architecture of the thoracic pedicle: an anatomic study, *Spine* 21:264, 1996.

Louis R: Single-staged posterior lumbosacral fusion by internal fixation with screw plates. Paper presented at the annual meeting of the International Society for the Study of the Lumbar Spine, Sydney, Australia, 1985.

Lu J, Ebraheim NA, Yang H, et al: Anatomic bases for anterior spinal surgery: surgical anatomy of the cervical vertebral body and disc space, *Surg Radiol Anat* 21:235, 1999.

Mazzara JT, Fielding JW: Effect of C1-C2 rotation on canal size, *Clin Orthop* 237:115, 1988.

McCormick PC: Retropleural approach to the thoracic and thoracolumbar spine, *Neurosurgery* 37:908, 1995.

Mirkovic SR, Schwartz DG, Glazier KD: Anatomic considerations in lumbar posterolateral percutaneous procedures, *Spine* 20:1965, 1995.

Oh SH, Perin NI, Cooper PR: Quantitative three-dimensional anatomy of the subaxial cervical spine: implication for anterior spinal surgery, *Neurosurgery* 38:1139, 1996.

Panjabi MM, O'Holleran JD, Crisco JJ III, Kothe R: Complexity of the thoracic spine pedicle anatomy, *Eur Spine J* 6:19, 1997.

Prescher A: Anatomy and pathology of the aging spine, *Eur J Radiol* 27:181, 1998.

Roy-Camille R, Saillant G, Mazel CH: Plating of thoracic, thoracolumbar, and lumbar injuries with pedicle screw plates, *Orthop Clin North Am* 17:147, 1986.

Saillant G: Anatomic study of vertebral pedicles: surgical application, *Rev Chir Orthop* 62:151, 1976.

Vraney RT, Phillips FM, Wetzel FT, Brustein M: Peridiscal vascular anatomy of the lower lumbar spine: an endoscopic perspective, *Spine* 24:2183, 1999.

Xu R, Ebraheim NA, Robke J, Huntoon M, Yeasting RA: Radiologic and anatomic evaluation of the anterior sacral foramens and nerve grooves, *Spine* 21:407, 1996.

Zindrick MR, Wiltse LL, Doornik A, et al: Analysis of the morphometric characteristics of the thoracic and lumbar pedicles, *Spine* 12:160, 1987.

Zindrick MR, Wiltse LL, Widell EH, et al: A biomechanical study of intrapeduncular screw fixation in the lumbosacral spine, *Clin Orthop* 203:99, 1986.

SURGICAL APPROACHES

Bailey RW, Badgley CE: Stabilization of the cervical spine by anterior fusion, *J Bone Joint Surg* 42A:565, 1960.

Barone GW, Eidt JF, Webb JW, et al: The anterior extrapleural approach to the thoracolumbar junction revisited, *Am Surg* 64:372, 1998.

Bell GR: The anterior approach to the cervical spine, *Neuroimaging Clin N Am* 5:465, 1995.

Bohlman HH, Ducker TB, Lucas JT: Spine and spinal cord injuries. In Rothman RH, Simeone FA, eds: *The spine*, ed 2, Philadelphia, 1982, WB Saunders.

Bohlman HH, Eismont FJ: Surgical techniques of anterior decompression and fusion for spinal cord injuries, *Clin Orthop* 154:57, 1981.

Bonney G, Williams JPR: Transoral approach to the upper cervical spine: a report of 16 cases, *J Bone Joint Surg* 67B:691, 1985.

Cauchoix J, Binet JP: Anterior surgical approaches to the spine, *Ann R Coll Surg* 21:237, 1957.

Charles R, Govender S: Anterior approach to the upper thoracic vertebrae, *J Bone Joint Surg* 71B:81, 1989.

Cloward RB: The anterior approach for ruptured cervical discs, *J Neurosurg* 15:602, 1958.

Cocke EW Jr, Robertson JH, Robertson JR, Crook JP Jr: The extended maxillotomy and subtotal maxillectomy for excision of skull base tumors, *Arch Otolaryngol Head Neck Surg* 116:92, 1990.

Codivilla A: Sulla scoliosi congenita, *Arch di Ortop* 18:65, 1901.

Colletta AJ, Mayer PJ: Chylothorax: an unusual complication of anterior thoracic interbody spinal fusion, *Spine* 7:46, 1982.

Compere EL: Excision of hemivertebrae for correction of congenital scoliosis: report of two cases, *J Bone Joint Surg* 14:555, 1932.

Darling GE, McBroom R, Perrin R: Modified anterior approach to the cervicothoracic junction, *Spine* 20:1519, 1995.

Ebraheim NA, Skie M, Heck BE, Yeasting RA: Vulnerability of the recurrent laryngeal nerve in the anterior approach to the lower cervical spine, *Spine* 22:2664, 1997.

Fang HSY, Ong GB: Direct anterior approach to the upper cervical spine, *J Bone Joint Surg* 44A:1588, 1962.

Fang HSY, Ong GB, Hodgson AR: Anterior spinal fusion: the operative approaches, *Clin Orthop* 35:16, 1964.

Fraser RD: A wide muscle-splitting approach to the lumbosacral spine, *J Bone Joint Surg* 64B:44, 1982.

Freeman BL: The pediatric spine. In Canale ST, Beaty JH, eds: *Operative pediatric orthopaedics*, St Louis, 1991, Mosby.

Graham AW III, Macmillan M, Fessler RG: Lateral extracavitary approach to the thoracic and thoracolumbar spine, *Orthopedics* 20:605, 1997.

Hodgson AR, Stock FE, Fang HYS, Ong GB: Anterior spinal fusion: the operative approach and pathological findings in 412 patients with Pott's disease of the spine, *Br J Surg* 48:172, 1960.

Johnson RM, McGuire EJ: Urogenital complications of anterior approaches to the lumbar spine, *Clin Orthop* 154:114, 1981.

Johnson RM, Southwick WO: Surgical approaches to the cervical spine. In Rothman RH, Simeone FA, eds: *The spine*, ed 2, Philadelphia, 1982, WB Saunders.

Koriwchak MJ, Courey MS, Winkle M, Ossoff RH: Vocal fold paralysis following the anterior approach to the cervical spine, *Ann Otol Rhinol Laryngol* 105:85, 1996.

Lehman RM, Grunberg B, Hall T: Anterior approach to the cervicothoracic junction: an anatomic dissection, *J Spinal Disord* 10:33, 1997.

Leventhal MR: Surgical approaches in the treatment of spinal infections. In Wood GW, ed: *Spine: State of the art reviews* 3:385, 1989.

Maciejczak A, Radke A, Kowalewski J, Palewicz A: Anterior transsternal approach to the upper thoracic spine, *Acta Chir Hung* 38:83, 1999.

Mack MJ, Regan JJ, McAfee PC, et al: Video-assisted thoracic surgery for the anterior approach to the thoracic spine, *Ann Thorac Surg* 59:1100, 1995.

McAfee PC, Bohlman HH, Riley LH Jr, et al: The anterior retropharyngeal approach to the upper part of the cervical spine, *J Bone Joint Surg* 69A:1371, 1987.

McAfee PC, Regan JJ, Geis WP, Fedder IL: Minimally invasive anterior retroperitoneal approach to the lumbar spine: emphasis on the lateral BAK, *Spine* 23:1476, 1998.

McCormick PC: Retropleural approach to the thoracic and thoracolumbar spine, *Neurosurgery* 37:908, 1995.

Micheli LJ, Hood RW: Anterior exposure of the cervicothoracic spine using a combined cervical and thoracic approach, *J Bone Joint Surg* 65A:992, 1983.

Nachlas IW, Borden JN: The cure of experimental scoliosis by directed growth control, *J Bone Joint Surg* 33A:24, 1951.

Netterville JL, Koriwchak MJ, Winkle M, et al: Vocal cord paralysis following the anterior approach to the cervical spine, *Ann Otol Rhinol Laryngol* 105:85, 1996.

Onimus M, Papin P, Gangloff S: Extraperitoneal approach to the lumbar spine with video assistance, *Spine* 21:2491, 1996.

Pierce DS, Nickel WH, eds: *The total care of spinal cord injuries*, Boston, 1977, Little, Brown.

Rapport RL II, Ferguson GS: Dorsal approach to presacral biopsy: technical case report, *Neurosurgery* 40:1087, 1997.

Rothman RH, Simeone FA, eds: *The spine*, ed 2, Philadelphia, 1982, WB Saunders.

Royle ND: The operative removal of an accessory vertebra, *Med J Australia* 1:467, 1928.

Smith AD, von Lackum WH, Wylie R: An operation for stapling vertebral bodies in congenital scoliosis, *J Bone Joint Surg* 36A:342, 1954.

Southwick WO, Robinson RA: Surgical approaches to the vertebral bodies in the cervical and lumbar regions, *J Bone Joint Surg* 39A:631, 1957.

Spetzler RF: Transoral approach to the upper cervical spine. In Evarts CM, ed: *Surgery of the musculoskeletal system*, vol 4, New York, 1983, Churchill Livingstone.

Sundaresan N, Shah J, Feghali JG: A transsternal approach to the upper thoracic vertebrae, *Am J Surg* 148:473, 1984.

Turner PL, Webb JK: Surgical approach to the upper cervical spine, *J Bone Joint Surg* 69B:542, 1987.

von Lackum HL, Smith AF: Removal of vertebral bodies in the treatment of scoliosis, *Surg Gynecol Obstet* 57:250, 1933.

Wagoner G: A technique for lessening hemorrhage in operations on the spine, *J Bone Joint Surg* 19:469, 1937.

Warner WC: Cervical spine anomalies. In Canale ST, Beaty JH, eds: *Operative pediatric orthopaedics*, St Louis, 1991, Mosby.

Watkins RG: *Surgical approaches to the spine*, New York, 1983, Springer-Verlag.

Weisberg NK, Spengler DM, Netterville JL: Stretch-induced nerve injury as a cause of paralysis secondary to the anterior cervical approach, *Otolaryngol Head Neck Surg* 116:317, 1997.

Wiltse LL: The paraspinal sacrospinalis-splitting approach to the lumbar spine, *Clin Orthop* 91:48, 1973.

Wiltse LL, Spencer CW: New uses and refinements of the paraspinal approach of the lumbar spine, *Spine* 13:696, 1988.

Wood GW: Anatomic, biologic, and pathophysiologic aspects of spinal infections. In Wood GW, ed: *Spine: State of the art reviews* 3:385, 1989.

C H A P T E R

35

Fractures, Dislocations, and Fracture-Dislocations of Spine

Marvin R. Leventhal

Fractures and dislocations of the spine are serious injuries that most commonly occur in young people. Nearly 43% of patients with spinal cord injuries sustain multiple injuries. Kraus et al. estimated that each year 50 people in 1 million sustain a spinal cord injury. Of those who die within 1 year of their accidents, 90% die en route to the hospital. With the development of regional trauma centers and increased training of paramedics and emergency medical technicians, the chances of survival after serious spinal cord injury have increased. Overall, 85% of patients with a spinal cord injury who survive the first 24 hours are still alive 10 years later compared with 98% of patients of similar age and sex without spinal cord injury. The National Institute of Disability and Rehabilitation Research estimates that 14,000 Americans suffer spinal cord injury each year, that about 8000 to 10,000 are left paralyzed, and that in the United States alone there are approximately 250,000 to 400,000 individuals living with spinal cord injury or spinal dysfunction. According to the National Spinal Cord Injury Association, the most common cause of death is respiratory failure whereas in the past it was renal failure. An increasing number of people with spinal cord injury are dying of unrelated causes, such as cancer or cardiovascular disease, similar to that of the general population. Mortality rates are significantly higher during the first year after injury than during subsequent years. The monetary cost of these devastating injuries has not been calculated accurately, but estimates are as high as 4 billion dollars per year in health care costs and lost productivity.

Evaluation of Spinal Injury

HISTORY

A detailed history of the mechanism of injury is important but frequently is unobtainable at the initial examination. The most common causes of severe spinal trauma are motor vehicle accidents, falls, diving accidents, and gunshot wounds. In a review of over 300 cervical spinal injuries Bohlman found that delays in diagnosis were common and that one in three severe cervical spinal injuries was not recognized initially. The most common causes of misdiagnosis were head trauma, acute alcoholic intoxication, and multiple injuries. Patients with

1597

decreased levels of consciousness or comatose patients often do not complain of neck pain. Profuse bleeding from severe facial or scalp lacerations may divert attention from the cervical spinal injury. A Brown-Séquard type of hemiparesis may be mistaken for a stroke. Spinal injury should be suspected in any patient with a head injury or severe facial or scalp lacerations.

PHYSICAL EXAMINATION

A general physical examination is performed with the patient supine. The head should be examined for lacerations and contusions and palpated for facial fractures. The ear canals should be inspected to rule out leakage of spinal fluid or blood behind the tympanic membrane, suggestive of a skull fracture. The spinous processes should be palpated from the upper cervical to the lumbosacral region. A painful spinous process may indicate a spinal injury. Palpable defects in the interspinous ligaments may indicate disruption of the supporting ligamentous complex. Careful and gentle rotation of the head may elicit pain; however, excessive flexion and extension of the neck should be avoided. The elbows may be flexed if a spinal cord injury causes loss of function below the biceps, or they may be extended if the paralysis is higher. Penile erection and incontinence of the bowel or bladder suggest a significant spinal injury. Quadriplegia is indicated by flaccid paralysis of the extremities. Initial blood pressure may be decreased without a compensatory increase in pulse because of spinal cord shock. The chest, abdomen, and extremities should be examined for occult injuries. The spine should be protected during this initial assessment; however, once spinal cord injury has been identified and the appropriate precautions taken, the patient should be moved from the spine board as soon as possible to decrease the risk of decubitus ulcers.

NEUROLOGICAL EVALUATION

Bohlman, Stauffer et al., and Meyer all emphasize the importance of accurate and detailed neurological evaluation of patients with spinal cord injuries. The level of consciousness should be determined quickly, including pupillary size and reaction. Epidural or subdural hematoma, a depressed skull fracture, or other intracranial pathological conditions may cause progressive deterioration in neurological function. The Glasgow coma scale (Table 35-1) is useful in determining the level of consciousness. A detailed initial neurological examination, including sensory, motor, and reflex function, is important in determining prognosis and treatment (Table 35-2). The presence of an incomplete or complete spinal cord injury must be determined and documented by meticulous neurological examination. Sensory examination is performed with pinpricks, beginning at the head and neck and progressing distally, to examine specific dermatome distributions (Fig. 35-1). Important dermatome landmarks are the nipple line (T4), xiphoid process (T7), umbilicus (T10), and inguinal region (T12, L1), as well as the perineum and perianal region (S2, S3, and S4). The skin should be marked where sensation

Table 35-1   Glasgow Coma Scale

Eyes Open	
Spontaneous	4
To sound	3
To pain	2
Never	1
Best Verbal Response	
Oriented	5
Confused conversation	4
Inappropriate words	3
Incomprehensible words	2
None	1
Best Motor Response	
Obeys commands	6
Localizes pain	5
Flexion withdrawal	4
Abnormal	3
Extension	2
None	1

From Teasdale G, Jennett B: *Acta Neurochirurg* 34:45, 1976.

Table 35-2   Muscle Grading Chart

Grade	Muscle Action
0 = zero	Total paralysis
1 = trace	Visual or palpable contraction
2 = poor	Active movement, gravity eliminated
3 = fair	Active movement against gravity
4 = good	Active movement against resistance
5 = normal	Active movement against full resistance

From Connolly P, Yuan HA: Cervical spine fractures. In White AH, ed: *Spine care: diagnosis and conservative treatment*, St Louis, 1995, Mosby.

is present before proceeding to motor examination. Evidence of sacral sensory sparing can establish the diagnosis of an incomplete spinal cord injury. The only area of sensation distal to an obvious cervical lesion in a quadriplegic patient may be in the perianal region (Fig. 35-2). Motor examination should be systematic, beginning with the upper extremities. During motor examination it is important to differentiate between complete and incomplete spinal cord injuries and pure nerve root lesions. A protruded cervical disc or a unilateral dislocated facet may produce an isolated nerve root paralysis. Some lumbar spine injuries may present as isolated root injuries with weakness of the foot or leg, depending on the specific root involved. Table 35-3 shows key muscle groups and their corresponding nerve root levels that should be evaluated in a patient with spinal cord injury. After examination of the extremities and trunk, the presence or absence of sacral motor sparing should be determined by voluntary rectal sphincter or toe flexor contractions. If voluntary contraction of the sacrally innervated

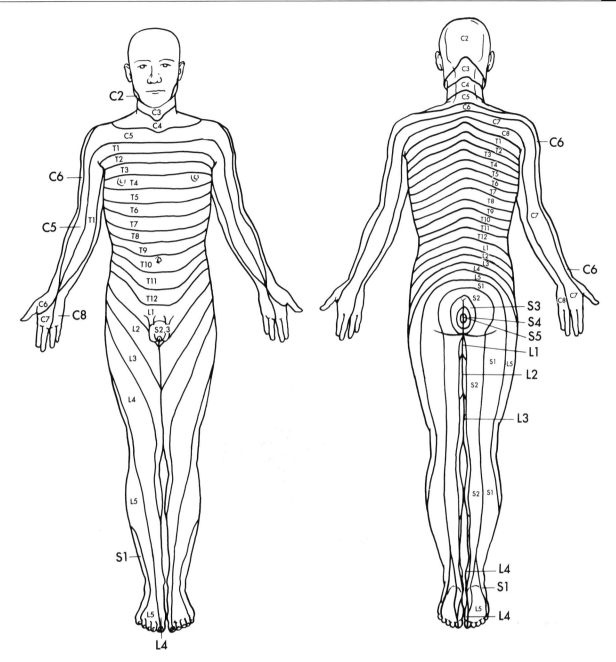

Fig. 35-1   Dermatome distributions (see text).

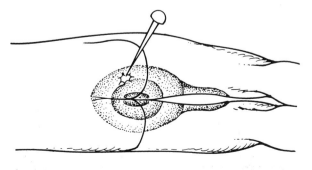

Fig. 35-2   Examination of perianal skin for sensation in cervical cord injury. Discrimination between sharpness and dullness may be only indication of incomplete injury. (Redrawn from Stauffer ES: *Clin Orthop* 112:9, 1975.)

Table 35-3 Key Muscle Groups Used in ASIA Motor Source Evaluation of Spinal Cord Injury

Level	Muscle Group
C5	Elbow flexors (biceps, brachialis)
C6	Wrist extensors (extensor carpi radialis longus and brevis)
C7	Elbow extensors (triceps)
C8	Finger flexors (flexor digitorum profundus to the middle finger)
T1	Small finger abductors (abductor digiti minimi)
L2	Hip flexors (iliopsoas)
L3	Knee extensors (quadriceps)
L4	Ankle dorsiflexors (tibialis anterior)
L5	Long toe extensors (extensor hallucis longus)
S1	Ankle plantarflexors (gastrocnemius, soleus)

From Beaty JH, ed: *Orthopaedic knowledge update home study syllabus 6,* Rosemont, Ill, 1999, American Academy of Orthopaedic Surgeons, p 654.

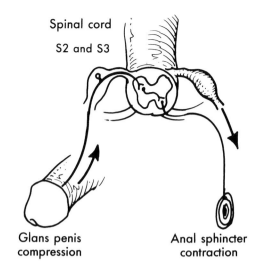

Fig. 35-3 Bulbocavernosus reflex (see text). (Redrawn from Stauffer ES: *Clin Orthop* 112:9, 1975.)

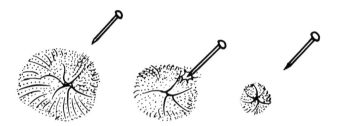

Fig. 35-4 Anal wink. Contracture of external sphincter caused by pinprick (see text). (Redrawn from Stauffer ES: *Clin Orthop* 112:9, 1975.)

muscles is present, then the prognosis for recovery of motor function is good. Finally, reflexes should be documented. Paralyzed patients usually are areflexic, and flexion withdrawal of the legs to pinprick does not indicate voluntary motion.

Although spinal shock rarely lasts longer than 24 hours, it may last for days or weeks. A positive bulbocavernosus reflex (Fig. 35-3) or return of the anal wink reflex (Fig. 35-4) indicates the end of spinal shock. If no motor or sensory function below the level of injury can be documented when spinal shock ends, a complete spinal cord injury is present and the prognosis is poor for recovery of distal motor or sensory function.

ROENTGENOGRAPHIC EXAMINATION

The initial roentgenograms should include a lateral view of the cervical spine and anteroposterior views of the chest and pelvis. The most frequently missed cervical spine fractures on roentgenograms involve the odontoid process or the cervicothoracic junction. Roentgenographic views of the injured neck should include standard anteroposterior, lateral, and right and left oblique projections with the patient immobilized and unmoved during examination. In a study of 360 normal adults Weir established the criteria for roentgenographic evaluation of the cervical spine. One of these criteria is the prevertebral soft tissue shadow, which should not exceed 5 mm in width at the level of the anteroinferior border of the third cervical vertebra. A width of more than 5 mm is strongly suggestive of injury with soft tissue swelling. Recently, the sensitivity of prevertebral soft tissue swelling measurements for the detection of cervical spine fractures and dislocations has been questioned. In a study of 212 patients Herr et al. showed that prevertebral soft tissue measurement at C3 is an insensitive marker of cervical spine fracture or dislocation and does not correlate with the location or mechanism of injury. Loss of the cervical

lordotic curve is not in itself evidence of cervical spine injury with resultant muscle spasm but may be simply a normal variant. Lateral flexion and extension views can be made to determine the stability of the cervical spine, but these are not routinely recommended in the initial examination. If flexion and extension views are made, they should be obtained under the supervision of a physician, and the patient should be carefully observed for pain response or any change in neurological status. Determining whether or not a cervical spine injury is present is extremely difficult in obtundent patients. They should be kept immobilized in a cervical brace even if roentgenograms are normal. Recently, Davis, Parks, and Detlefs have advocated the use of dynamic fluoroscopy to assess the cervical spine. They recommend early removal of the collar to decrease the incidence of decubitus ulcers, which in their study occurred in 44% of patients who had the cervical collar in place for longer than 5 days. Fluoroscopic evaluations were done in 116 patients; 110 had a negative examination. Two patients had facet fractures not diagnosed on cervical roentgenograms, but with no instability fluoroscopically. One patient had a positive examination with 2 mm of subluxation. They reported no neurological complications. If the cervico-

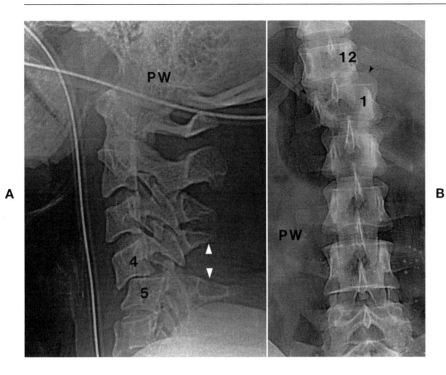

Fig. 35-5 **A,** Fracture-dislocation of cervical spine at C4-5 and complete spinal cord injury in 38-year-old woman. **B,** Anteroposterior view of thoracolumbar spine shows noncontiguous translation injury at T12-L1 level. This combination of injuries is consistent with pattern A described by Calenoff et al.

thoracic junction cannot be seen adequately on lateral views, a swimmer's view or computed tomography (CT) scans should be obtained. The cervical spine is the most easily examined because the thoracic and lumbar areas are less accessible with the patient supine. Fractures of the thoracic spine and at the cervicothoracic or thoracolumbar junction are easily overlooked, but with sophisticated imaging techniques, including tomography, water-soluble contrast myelography, postmyelogram CT with sagittal reconstructions, and magnetic resonance imaging (MRI), injuries to osseous, ligamentous, and neurological structures can be evaluated accurately. Tomography can be used to clarify questionable findings on plain roentgenograms, to reveal an otherwise occult injury, and to further evaluate a known fracture or fracture-dislocation. Excellent bony detail of the fracture pattern usually can be obtained with routine tomography. CT is helpful in evaluating the degree of compromise of the spinal canal. The addition of water-soluble contrast material to the subarachnoid space improves the contrast between bone fragments and neural elements. We prefer routine CT to standard tomography for the initial evaluation of spinal injuries. MRI has the advantages of being noninvasive, of having no risk of ionizing radiation, and of not requiring the frequent repositioning that routine myelography does. MRI allows examination of the intervertebral discs, supporting ligamentous structures, and neural elements. Its role in spinal trauma is still evolving, but it appears to provide superior images of lesions of the craniocervical and cervicothoracic regions. Several studies have suggested that MRI can help determine the prognosis for neurological recovery.

Spinal cord injuries without roentgenographic abnormalities (SCIWORA) have been reported by Dickmen et al. to occur predominantly in children. Spinal cord injuries in children frequently occur without fracture-dislocation. Because of the inherent elasticity of the juvenile spine, the spinal cord is vulnerable to injury even though the vertebral column is not disrupted. SCIWORA is most common in children younger than 8 years of age. In a review of 159 pediatric patients with cervical spine injuries, Dickman et al. reported that 16% had sustained SCIWORA. The recovery of neurological function depends on the patient's neurological status at presentation. Patients with incomplete injuries tend to recover, and those with complete injuries have a poor prognosis for recovery of neurological function.

MULTIPLE SPINAL FRACTURES

If a spinal fracture is identified at any level, the entire spine should be examined with anteroposterior and lateral views to document the presence or absence of spinal fractures at other levels. Multiple-level spinal fractures, which may be contiguous or separated, are estimated to occur in 3% to 5% of patients with spinal fractures (Fig. 35-5). Multiple noncontiguous spinal fractures rarely occur without injury to the spinal cord. Calenoff, Chessare, and Rogers reported an incidence of 4.5% in 710 patients admitted to a regional spinal cord injury unit. They described three patterns of injury (Fig. 35-6). In pattern A the primary lesion occurs between C5 and C7, with secondary injuries at T12 or the lumbar spine. In pattern B the primary injury occurs at T2 and T4, with secondary injuries in the cervical spine. In pattern C the primary injury occurs between T12 and L2, with secondary injuries from L4 to L5. They noted that patients with multiple-level, noncontiguous fractures had a disproportionate number of primary vertebral injuries in the middle and upper thoracic spine. If a fracture is identified at this level, a secondary vertebral injury should be suspected. The secondary lesions tended to cluster at L4 and L5 and at C1 and C2; approximately 43% of the secondary fractures occurred at the extremes of the spine. Recognition of these secondary

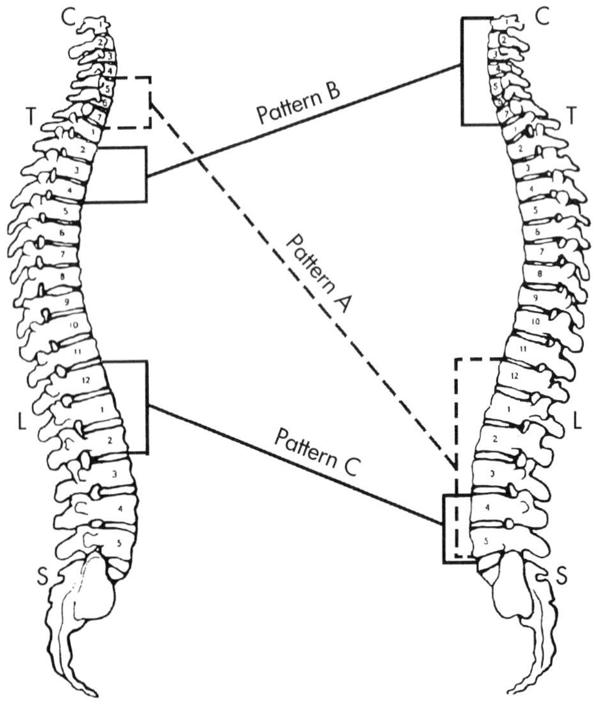

Fig. 35-6 Three patterns of multiple-level injury described by Calenoff et al. (From Calenoff L, Chessare JW, Rogers LF, et al: *Am J Roentgenol* 130:665, 1978.)

injuries is important to prevent increasing neurological deficit, chronic pain, or progressive deformity.

Spinal Cord Syndromes

Spinal cord syndromes resulting from incomplete traumatic lesions have been described by Schneider and Kahn and by Bosch, Stauffer, and Nickel. The following generalizations can be made from their investigations: (1) the greater the sparing of motor and sensory functions distal to the injury, the greater the expected recovery; (2) the more rapid the recovery, the greater the amount of recovery; and (3) when new recovery ceases and a plateau is reached, no further recovery can be expected. The importance of determining whether a patient has a complete or incomplete cord injury cannot be overemphasized in the overall prognosis (Tables 35-4 to 35-6). By definition, an incomplete spinal cord injury is one in which some motor or sensory function is spared distal to the cord injury. A complete spinal cord injury is manifested by total motor and sensory loss distal to the injury. When the bulbocavernosus reflex is positive and no sacral sensation or motor function has returned, the paralysis will be permanent and complete in most patients. An incomplete spinal cord syndrome may be a Brown-Séquard syndrome, central cord syndrome, anterior cord syndrome, posterior cord syndrome, or rarely monoparesis of the upper extremity. Ninety percent of incomplete lesions produce either a central cord syndrome, a Brown-Séquard syndrome, or an anterior cervical cord syndrome (Fig. 35-7).

Central cord syndrome is the most common. It consists of destruction of the central area of the spinal cord, including both gray and white matter (Fig. 35-7, *B*). The centrally located arm tracts in the cortical spinal area are the most severely affected,

---

Table 35-4 Function Attained after Central Cord Lesion*

	Admission (%)	Present at Discharge (%)	Follow-up (%)
Ambulation	33.3	77	59
Hand function	26	42	56
Bladder function	17	—	53
Bowel function	9.5	—	53

From Bosch A, Stauffer ES, Nickel VL: *JAMA* 216:473, 1971.
*Chronic sequelae of central cord damage: (1) increased spasticity and pyramidal tract involvement, (2) incidence of 23.8%, and (3) prognosis poor with progressive neurological loss.

Table 35-5 Function Attained after Hemisection Cord Lesion

	Admission (%)	Present at Discharge (%)	Follow-up (%)
Ambulation	60	100	80
Hand function	60	80	100
Bowel function	80	80	100
Bladder function	100	100	100

From Bosch A, Stauffer ES, Nickel VL: *JAMA* 216:473, 1971.

and the leg tracts are affected to a lesser extent. Generally patients have a quadriparesis involving the upper extremities to a greater degree than the lower. Sensory sparing is variable, but usually sacral pinprick sensation is preserved. Frequently these patients show immediate partial recovery after being placed in skeletal traction through skull tongs. Prognosis is variable, but more than 50% of patients have return of bowel and bladder control, become ambulatory, and have improved hand function. This syndrome usually results from a hyperextension injury in an older person with preexisting osteoarthritis of the spine. The spinal cord is pinched between the vertebral body anteriorly and the buckling ligamentum flavum posteriorly (Fig. 35-7, *A*). It also may occur in younger patients with flexion injuries.

Brown-Séquard syndrome is an injury to either half of the spinal cord (Fig. 35-7, *C*) and usually is the result of a unilateral laminar or pedicle fracture, penetrating injury, or a rotational injury resulting in a subluxation. It is characterized by motor weakness on the side of the lesion and the contralateral loss of pain and temperature sensation. Prognosis for recovery is good, with significant neurological improvement often occurring.

Anterior cord syndrome usually is caused by a hyperflexion injury in which bone or disc fragments compress the anterior spinal artery and cord. It is characterized by complete motor loss and loss of pain and temperature discrimination below the level of injury. The posterior columns are spared to varying degrees (Fig. 35-7, *D*), resulting in preservation of deep touch, position sense, and vibratory sensation. Prognosis for significant recovery in this injury is poor.

Posterior cord syndrome involves the dorsal columns of the spinal cord and produces loss of proprioception vibrating sense while preserving other sensory and motor functions. This syndrome is rare and usually is caused by an extension injury.

A *mixed syndrome* usually is an unclassifiable combination of several syndromes. It describes the small percentage of

Table 35-6   Function Attained after Anterior Cord Lesion

	Admission (%)	Present at Discharge (%)	Follow-up (%)
Ambulation	0	0	0
Hand function	16	16	16
Bladder function	0	0	0
Bowel function	0	0	0

From Bosch A, Stauffer ES, Nickel VL: *JAMA* 216:473, 1971.

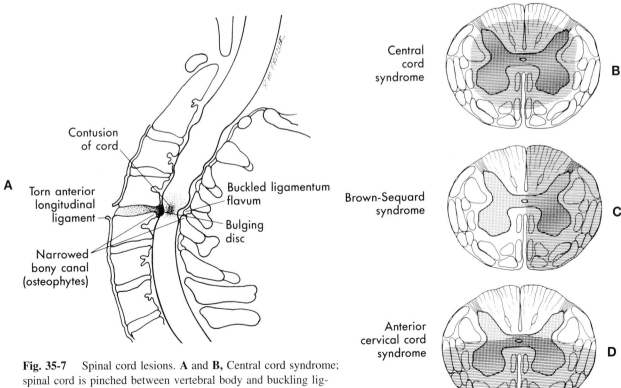

Fig. 35-7   Spinal cord lesions. **A** and **B**, Central cord syndrome; spinal cord is pinched between vertebral body and buckling ligamentum flavum. **C**, Brown-Séquard syndrome. **D**, Anterior cervical cord syndrome.

incomplete spinal cord injuries that do not fit one of the previously described syndromes.

Conus medullaris syndrome, or injury of the sacral cord (conus) and lumbar nerve roots within the spinal canal, usually results in areflexic bladder, bowel, and lower extremities. Most of these injuries occur between T11 and L2 and result in flaccid paralysis in the perineum and loss of all bladder and perianal muscle control. The irreversible nature of this injury to the sacral segments is evidenced by the absence of the bulbocavernosus reflex and the perianal wink. Motor function in the lower extremities between L1 and L4 may be present if nerve root sparing occurs.

Cauda equina syndrome, or injury between the conus and the lumbosacral nerve roots within the spinal canal, also results in areflexic bladder, bowel, and lower limbs. With a complete cauda equina injury, all peripheral nerves to the bowel, bladder, perianal area, and lower extremities are lost, and the bulbocavernosus reflex, anal wink, and all reflex activity in the lower extremities are absent, indicating absence of any function in the cauda equina. It is important to remember that the cauda equina functions as the peripheral nervous system, and there is a possibility of return of function of the nerve rootlets if they have not been completely transected or destroyed. Most often the cauda equina syndrome presents as a neurologically incomplete lesion.

Emergency Room Management

The initial examination of a trauma patient with suspected spinal injury is performed by general surgery, anesthesia, respiratory, neurosurgery, and orthopaedic specialists. Although cardiovascular, respiratory, and neurological functions generally are evaluated by the appropriate specialists, the orthopaedist should remember three changes in vital signs that suggest a cervical or upper thoracic fracture with spinal cord injury above the level of T6: hypotension, hypothermia, and bradycardia.

A National Acute Spinal Cord Injury study reported the results of a double-blind, randomized, controlled clinical trial of very high-dose methylprednisolone in the treatment of acute spinal cord injury. Compared with a control group, patients who received methylprednisolone infusion within 8 hours of injury showed significantly more improvement in motor function and pinprick and touch sensation at 6 weeks and at 6 months after injury. Interestingly, methylprednisolone infused 8 hours or more after injury appeared to be of no benefit. In fact, at 1-year follow-up the scores for sensitivity to pinprick, soft touch, and motor function were slightly lower in patients who had received methylprednisolone treatment after 8 hours of injury than in those who had received a placebo. At this time, all patients seen at our level 1 trauma center who have a confirmed acute spinal cord injury and have no contraindications for administration of a corticosteroid are treated with a protocol of methylprednisolone administration consisting of a bolus dose of 30 mg/kg of body weight administered over 15 minutes,

followed by a 45-minute pause, and then a 23-hour continuous infusion of 5.4 mg/kg/hr. Bracken et al. reported 55% overall improvement in motor function, with more significant improvement if methylprednisolone therapy was begun within 8 hours of injury. Because of the massive dose of steroid administered over a 24-hour period, there is the potential for increased incidence of wound infection and gastrointestinal hemorrhage. Currently, new pharmacological agents for resuscitating acutely traumatized spinal cords are undergoing investigation. A number of spinal cord injury centers are studying the results of using GM-1 ganglioside, naloxone (an opiate antagonist), and monosialganglioside (Sygen) to stimulate neural regeneration. These pharmacological agents are believed to be of benefit in the treatment of acute spinal cord injury; however, experimental protocols differ considerably, and transforming experimental animal results into clinical practice is difficult.

Cervical Spine Injuries

The cervical spinal column is extremely vulnerable to injury. The seven cervical vertebrae, whose specific facet joint articulations allow movement in the planes of flexion, extension, lateral bending, and rotation, have attached at the cephalic aspect the skull and its contents. Injury occurs when forces applied to the head and neck result in loads that exceed the ability of the supporting structures to dissipate energy. Many cervical spine injuries are caused by hyperextension in older patients with spondylolytic disease or in younger patients with congenitally narrowed spinal canals.

Jefferson found that injuries to the cervical spine involve two particular areas: C1 to C2 and C5 to C7. Meyer identified C2 and C5 as the two most common areas of cervical spine injury. Injuries of the cervical spine produce neurological damage in approximately 40% of patients. Approximately 10% of traumatic cord injuries have no obvious roentgenographic evidence of vertebral injury.

CLASSIFICATION

Numerous classifications of cervical spine injuries have been formulated, but the mechanistic classification proposed by Allen et al. appears to be the most complete. In a review of 165 lower cervical spine injuries, they identified the following six common patterns of injury, each of which is subdivided into stages based on the degree of injury to osseous and ligamentous structures.

Compressive Flexion (CF)—Five Stages
- CF Stage 1: blunting of the anterosuperior vertebral margin to a rounded contour, with no evidence of failure of the posterior ligamentous complex.
- CF Stage 2: obliquity of the anterior vertebral body with loss of some anterior height of the centrum, in addition to the changes seen in Stage 1. The anteroinferior vertebral body has a "beak" appearance, concavity of the inferior

end plate may be increased, and the vertebral body may have a vertical fracture.

- CF Stage 3: fracture line passing obliquely from the anterior surface of the vertebra through the centrum and extending through the inferior subchondral plate, and a fracture of the beak, in addition to the characteristics of a Stage 2 injury.
- CF Stage 4: deformation of the centrum and fracture of the beak with mild (less than 3 mm) displacement of the inferoposterior vertebral margin into the spinal canal.
- CF Stage 5: bony injuries as in Stage 3 but with more than 3 mm of displacement of the posterior portion of the vertebral body posteriorly into the spinal canal. The vertebral arch remains intact, the articular facets are separated, and the interspinous process space is increased at the level of injury, suggesting a posterior ligamentous disruption in a tension mode.

Vertical Compression (VC)—Three Stages

- VC Stage 1: fracture of the superior or inferior end plate with a "cupping" deformity. Failure of the end plate is central rather than anterior, and posterior ligamentous failure is not evident.
- VC Stage 2: fracture of both vertebral end plates with cupping deformities. Fracture lines through the centrum may be present, but displacement is minimal.
- VC Stage 3: progression of the vertebral body damage described in Stage 2. The centrum is fragmented, and the displacement is peripheral in multiple directions. Most commonly the centrum fails, with significant impaction and fragmentation. The posterior aspect of the vertebral body is fractured and may be displaced into the spinal canal. The vertebral arch may be intact with no evidence of ligamentous failure, or it may be comminuted with significant failure of the posterior ligamentous complex; the ligamentous disruption is between the fractured vertebra and the one below it.

Distractive Flexion (DF)—Four Stages

- DF Stage 1: failure of the posterior ligamentous complex, as evidenced by facet subluxation in flexion, with abnormal divergence of the spinous process.
- DF Stage 2: unilateral facet dislocation (the degree of posterior ligamentous failure ranges from partial failure sufficient only to permit the abnormal displacement to complete failure of both the anterior and posterior ligamentous complexes, which is uncommon). Subluxation of the facet on the side opposite the dislocation suggests severe ligamentous injury. In addition, a small fleck of bone may be displaced from the posterior surface of the articular process, which is displaced anteriorly. Widening of the uncovertebral joint on the side of the dislocation and displacement of the tip of the spinous process toward the side of the dislocation may be seen. Beatson serially divided the posterior interspinous ligaments, facet capsule, posterior longitudinal ligament,

annulus fibrosus, and anterior longitudinal ligament and found that unilateral facet dislocation can occur with rupture of only the posterior interspinous ligament and the facet capsule.

- DF Stage 3: bilateral facet dislocations, with approximately 50% anterior subluxation of the vertebral body. Blunting of the anterosuperior margin of the inferior vertebra to a rounded corner may or may not be present. Beatson demonstrated that rupture of the interspinous ligament, the capsules of both facet joints, the posterior longitudinal ligament, and the annulus fibrosus of the intervertebral disc was necessary to create this lesion.
- DF Stage 4: full vertebral body width displacement anteriorly or a grossly unstable motion segment, giving the appearance of a "floating" vertebra.

Compression Extension (CE)—Five Stages

- CE Stage 1: unilateral vertebral arch fracture with or without anterorotatory vertebral displacement. Posterior element failure may consist of a linear fracture through the articular process, impaction of the articular process, and ipsilateral pedicle and lamina fractures, resulting in the "transverse facet" appearance on anteroposterior roentgenograms, or a combination of ipsilateral pedicle and articular process fractures.
- CE Stage 2: bilaminar fractures without evidence of other tissue failure. Typically the laminar fractures occur at multiple contiguous levels.
- CE Stage 3: bilateral vertebral arch fractures with fracture of the articular processes, pedicles, lamina, or some bilateral combination, without vertebral body displacement.
- CE Stage 4: bilateral vertebral arch fractures with partial vertebral body width displacement anteriorly.
- CE Stage 5: bilateral vertebral arch fracture with full vertebral body width displacement anteriorly. The posterior portion of the vertebral arch of the fractured vertebra does not displace, and the anterior portion of the arch remains with the centrum. Ligament failure occurs at two levels: posteriorly between the fractured vertebra and the one above it and anteriorly between the fractured vertebra and the one below it. Characteristically, the anterosuperior portion of the vertebra below is sheared off by the anteriorly displaced centrum.

Distractive Extension (DE)—Two Stages

- DE Stage 1: either failure of the anterior ligamentous complex or a transverse fracture of the centrum. The injury usually is ligamentous, and there may be a fracture of the adjacent anterior vertebral margin. The roentgenographic clue to this injury is abnormal widening of the disc space.
- DE Stage 2: evidence of failure of the posterior ligamentous complex, with displacement of the upper vertebral body posteriorly into the spinal canal, in addition to the changes seen in Stage 1 injuries. Because

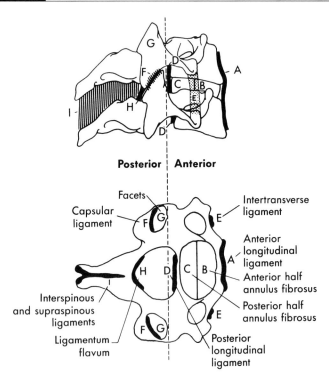

Fig. 35-8 Important anterior and posterior supporting structures of spine. (Redrawn from White AA, Southwick WO, Panjabi MM: *Spine* 1:15, 1976.)

Table 35-7 Checklist for Diagnosis of Clinical Instability in Lower Cervical Spine*

Element	Point Value
Anterior elements destroyed or unable to function	2
Posterior elements destroyed or unable to function	2
Relative sagittal plane translation >3.5 mm	2
Relative sagittal plane rotation >11 degrees	2
Positive stretch test	2
Medullary (cord) damage	2
Root damage	1
Abnormal disc narrowing	1
Dangerous loading anticipated	1

From White AA, Southwick WO, Panjabi MM: *Spine* 1:15, 1976.
*Total of 5 or more = unstable.

displacement of this type tends to reduce spontaneously when the head is placed in a neutral position, roentgenographic evidence of the displacement may be minimal, rarely greater than 3 mm on initial films with the patient supine.

Lateral Flexion (LF)—Two Stages

• LF Stage 1: asymmetrical compression fracture of the centrum and ipsilateral vertebral arch fracture, without displacement of the arch on the anteroposterior view. Compression of the articular process or comminution of the corner of the vertebral arch may be present.

• LF Stage 2: lateral asymmetrical compression of the centrum and either ipsilateral displaced vertebral arch fracture or ligamentous failure on the contralateral side with separation of the articular processes. Both ipsilateral and compressive and contralateral disruptive vertebral arch injuries may be present.

INSTABILITY

White and Panjabi defined clinical instability as the loss of the ability of the spine under physiological loads to maintain relationships between vertebrae in such a way that the spinal cord or nerve roots are not damaged or irritated and deformity or pain does not develop. Clinical instability may be caused by

trauma, neoplastic or infectious disorders, or iatrogenic causes. Instability may be acute or chronic. Acute instability is caused by bone or ligament disruption that places the neural elements in danger of injury with any subsequent loading or deformity. Chronic instability is the result of progressive deformity that may cause neurological deterioration, prevent recovery of injured neural tissue, or cause increasing pain or decreasing function.

In a series of cadaver studies White and Panjabi systematically cut the various supporting structures and noted the resulting instabilities of the spine. The supporting structures of the lower cervical spine can be divided into two groups: anterior and posterior (Fig. 35-8). A motion segment is made up of two adjacent vertebrae and the intervening soft tissues. If a motion segment has all the anterior elements and one posterior element intact, or all the posterior elements and one anterior element intact, it will remain stable under physiological loads. White and Panjabi suggest that a motion segment should be considered unstable if all the anterior or posterior elements are not functional. They developed a checklist for the diagnosis of clinical instability of the lower cervical spine (Table 35-7), in which a score of 5 or more indicates instability.

Roentgenographically, cervical spine instability is indicated by the horizontal translation of one vertebra relative to an adjacent vertebra in excess of 3.5 mm on the lateral flexion-extension view (Fig. 35-9). Instability also is indicated by more than 11 degrees of angulation of one vertebra relative to another (Fig. 35-10).

◆ Stretch Test

The stretch test (Fig. 35-11) may be useful for determining clinical instability in the lower cervical spine, but it is contraindicated in an obviously unstable injury. This test measures the displacement patterns of the spine under carefully controlled conditions and identifies anterior or posterior

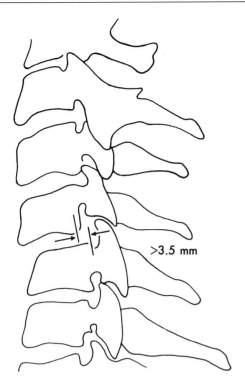

Fig. 35-9 Sagittal plane translation of more than 3.5 mm suggests clinical instability. (Redrawn from White AA, Johnson RM, Panjabi MM: *Clin Orthop* 109:85, 1975.)

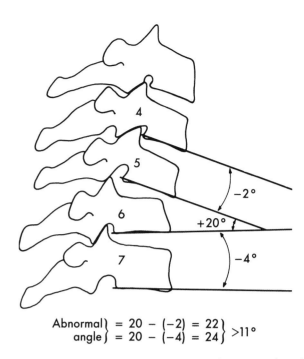

$$\text{Abnormal} \atop \text{angle} \Big\} = {20 - (-2) = 22 \atop 20 - (-4) = 24} \Big\} > 11°$$

Fig. 35-10 Significant sagittal plane rotation (more than 11 degrees) suggests instability. (Redrawn from White AA, Johnson RM, Panjabi MM: *Clin Orthop* 109:85, 1975.)

disrupted ligaments. The stretch test should always be done under supervision of the attending physician.

TECHNIQUE 35-1

Apply traction through secured skeletal traction or a head halter. If the latter is used, place a small piece of gauze sponge between the molars for patient comfort. Place a roller under the patient's head. Place the roentgenographic film as close as possible to the patient's neck, position the roentgen tube 72 inches from the film, and make a lateral exposure. Add weight up to 10 pounds and increase traction in 5-pound increments, repeating the lateral views after each addition until either one third of the body weight or 65 pounds is reached. After each addition of weight, check for any change in neurological status. The test is considered positive and should be discontinued if any neurological changes occur or if any abnormal separation of the anterior or posterior vertebral elements occurs. Allow at least 5 minutes between incremental weight applications for developing the film, evaluating neurological status, and checking for creep of the viscoelastic structures involved. White, Southwick, and Panjabi suggest that a stretch test is abnormal if differences in interspace separation are more than 1.7 mm or if the angle between the prestretched condition and that after application of maximal weight is more than 7.5 degrees.

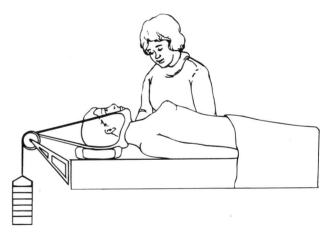

Fig. 35-11 Stretch test to determine cervical spine instability. This test must be closely monitored by the physician and is contraindicated when the spine is obviously unstable. (Redrawn from White AA III, Panjabi MM: *Clinical biomechanics of the spine,* Philadelphia, 1978, JB Lippincott.)

TREATMENT

The goals of treatment of cervical spine injuries are (1) to realign the spine, (2) to prevent loss of function of undamaged neurological tissue, (3) to improve neurological recovery, (4) to obtain and maintain spinal stability, and (5) to obtain early

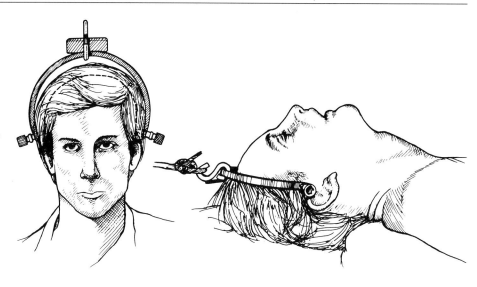

Fig. 35-12 Gardner-Wells tongs placed just above ears, below greatest diameter of skull. (From Stauffer ES: Surgical management of cervical spine injuries. In Evarts CM, ed: *Surgery of the musculoskeletal system,* New York, 1983, Churchill Livingstone.)

functional recovery. After initial medical stabilization and documentation of neurological function, spinal alignment can be obtained by skeletal traction through spring-loaded Gardner-Wells tongs or a halo ring. Continuous monitoring during reduction is essential to prevent iatrogenic injury from over-distraction of an unstable motion segment. Ten pounds of traction weight is applied, then weight is added in 5-pound increments, with lateral roentgenograms after each addition, until the spine is realigned (Fig. 35-12). Although there is no agreement on the safe upper limit of traction, most surgeons do not apply more than 40 to 50 pounds of traction. A general guideline is 10 pounds for the head and 5 pounds for each additional level of injury (Table 35-8). If spinal realignment cannot be obtained by traction, open reduction and stabilization, usually through a posterior approach, are indicated. If spinal realignment is obtained with traction and is documented roentgenographically, weight is reduced by 50% to maintain alignment and the course of treatment is determined. Usually tomograms, CT scanning, and MRI provide additional information about ligamentous, intervertebral disc, and osseous injuries. The pathological anatomy must be carefully defined before treatment is determined. Arena, Eismont, and Green reported that 8.8% of patients had extrusion of a cervical disc in addition to cervical facet subluxations or dislocations. They recommended preoperative evaluation with myelography, CT scanning, or MRI. If a disc is herniated, anterior discectomy and interbody fusion should be performed before posterior cervical wiring and fusion to avoid neurological deterioration.

Nonoperative Treatment

Many cervical spine injuries can be treated without surgery. Immobilization in a rigid cervical orthosis for 8 to 12 weeks may be sufficient. For a stable cervical spine injury with no compression of the neural elements, a rigid cervical brace or halo for 8 to 12 weeks usually produces a stable, painless spine without residual deformity. Stable compression fractures of the vertebral bodies and undisplaced fractures of the laminae,

Table 35-8	Traction Recommended for Levels of Injury	
Level	Minimum Weight in Pounds (kg)	Maximum Weight in Pounds (kg)
First cervical vertebra	5 (2.3)	10 (4.5)
Second cervical vertebra	6 (2.7)	10-12 (4.5-5.4)
Third cervical vertebra	8 (3.6)	10-15 (4.5-6.8)
Fourth cervical vertebra	10 (4.5)	15-20 (6.8-9.0)
Fifth cervical vertebra	12 (5.4)	20-25 (9.0-11.3)
Sixth cervical vertebra	15 (6.8)	20-30 (9.0-13.5)
Seventh cervical vertebra	18 (8.1)	25-35 (11.3-15.8)

lateral masses, or spinous processes also can be treated with immobilization in a cervical orthosis. Unilateral facet dislocations that are reduced in traction may be immobilized in a halo vest for 8 to 12 weeks. Patients with spinal fractures that are treated nonoperatively must be observed closely. Serial roentgenograms should be obtained weekly for the first 3 weeks, and then at 6 weeks, 3 months, 6 months, and 1 year. Herkowitz and Rothman demonstrated subacute instability of the cervical spine after initial roentgenographic evaluation that showed no bony or soft tissue abnormalities. The elastic and plastic deformation of the ligamentous structures and discs of the cervical spine is believed to be responsible for this subacute instability. Because subacute instability may occur despite adequate initial physical and roentgenographic examinations, a second complete evaluation should be performed within 3 weeks of injury.

Halo Vest Immobilization. The halo orthosis was first used by Perry and Nickels in 1959 for stabilization after cervical spine fusion in patients with poliomyelitis. Use of the halo vest

Table 35-9   Complications with Halo Immobilization

Complication	Patients (%)
Pin loosening	36
Pin infection	20
Pin site pain	18
Pressure sores under vest or cast	11
Disfiguring scars	9
Nerve injury	2
Dysphagia	2
Bleeding at pin site	1
Dural puncture	1

From Garfin SR, ed: *Complications of spine surgery,* Baltimore, 1989, Williams & Wilkins.

has expanded considerably since then, and it is used in the treatment of many cervical spine injuries.

Complications of halo immobilization have been reported to occur in as many as 30% of patients (Table 35-9). Recurrence of the spinal deformity secondary to loss of reduction also has been reported. Garfin and others suggest that many of the complications of halo use can be avoided or minimized by the following measures:

1. Before insertion of the anterolateral pins, the patient should be requested to close his eyes tightly; if not, traction on the skin and muscles of the eyelids may prevent full closure of the eyes.
2. The pins should be routinely retightened after 24 to 48 hours. A loose pin should be retightened only once. Retightening efforts should be discontinued if no resistance is met during this procedure.
3. If a pin is to be replaced, a new pin should be inserted satisfactorily before the loose pin is removed to maintain the position of the halo ring and the alignment of the spine.
4. The recommended torque for insertion of the four halo pins is 8 inch-pounds instead of 4 or 6 inch-pounds. Increasing the insertional torque to 10 pounds increases the penetration of the pin but does not significantly improve the structural properties of the pin-bone interface. Ballock, Botte, and Garfin noted marked reductions in pin loosening and pin infection rates when the pins were inserted at 8 inch-pounds compared with 6 inch-pounds.
5. The risk of dislodgment of the halo ring is minimized by proper placement of the ring above the orbit but below the greatest circumference of the calvarium.
6. Local pin care should be meticulous to prevent pin site infection. The pin site should be cleaned daily with povidone-iodine or hydrogen peroxide. If pin site infection occurs, the wound should be cultured, antibiotic sensitivities should be obtained, and appropriate antibiotic therapy should be initiated.
7. The most commonly injured nerves are the supraorbital

and supratrochlear. These injuries may be avoided by not placing pins over the medial third of the orbit.

8. Inserting the anterolateral pins behind the hairline in hopes of obtaining a more cosmetically acceptable scar should be avoided if possible. This location places the pin within the temporal fossa where the skull is the thinnest. Pins located in the temporal fossa also pierce the temporalis muscle and often lead to painful mastication.
9. Application of a well-molded plaster body jacket attached to the halo, which may be extended down over the iliac crest for additional support, may be substituted for the premolded polyethylene vest if increased stability is desired.

Kerwin et al. investigated the effects of different halos on pin forces and concluded that identical torques applied to different halos resulted in different magnitudes of pin force for halo fixation. They noted that the difference in pin forces was the result of increased friction at the pin-halo interface from different bending capabilities of the halos. Therefore it is important to consider halo size and composition when specifying appropriate levels of torque because these factors affect bending and produce disparities in pin force.

Many trauma patients with unstable cervical spinal injuries are initially managed with cervical traction through a halo ring. The potential for loss of cervical alignment when applying the halo vest is of some concern. We agree with Goldstein et al. that preapplication of the back of the halo vest is helpful in facilitating halo application in certain patients. Once alignment of the cervical spine is achieved, application of the halo vest may be completed without lifting the patient or discontinuing the cervical traction.

◆ Halo Application

TECHNIQUE 35-2

Place the patient supine with his head supported just over the end of the stretcher by an assistant or by an application device that is attached to the stretcher and that will also hold the halo ring. Prepare the skin and scalp by washing the hair with a surgical preparation such as povidone-iodine. Have an assistant hold a halo of appropriate size about the patient's head or place the halo in the application device. Hold the halo below the area of greatest diameter of the skull, about at the level of the eyebrows and approximately 1 cm above the tips of the ears (Fig. 35-13). Inject a local anesthetic into the four areas selected for pin insertion and place the two anterior pins in bare skin and not within the hairline. The bone is extremely thin just anterior to the ears, and anchorage here is not good. Also, the supraorbital nerve should be avoided. Posteriorly the central channels usually are the best sites. Introduce the pins and tighten two diagonally opposed pins simultaneously. Be certain that the patient closes his eyes during the insertion of the two

continued

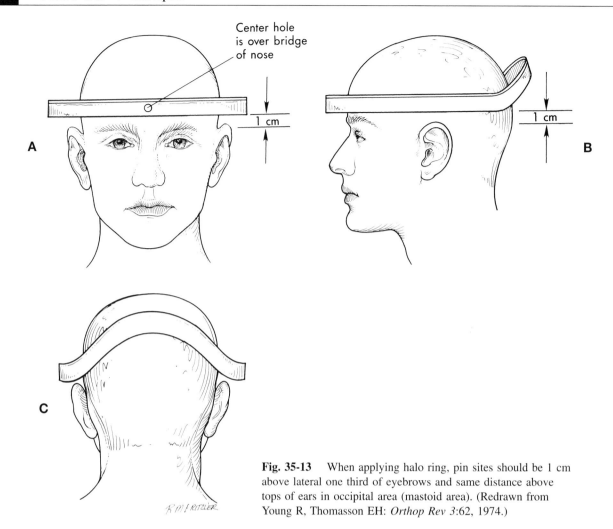

Center hole
is over bridge
of nose

1 cm

A

1 cm

B

C

Fig. 35-13   When applying halo ring, pin sites should be 1 cm above lateral one third of eyebrows and same distance above tops of ears in occipital area (mastoid area). (Redrawn from Young R, Thomasson EH: *Orthop Rev 3*:62, 1974.)

anterolateral pins. Continue to tighten the pins until all four engage the skin and bone. Continue tightening diagonal pairs of pins with a torque screwdriver. Alternate tightening of the pins to prevent migration of the halo to an asymmetrical position. Tighten all pins to 8 inch-pounds. Secure the pins to the halo with appropriate lock nuts or set screws. Attach the halo ring to the halo vest through the anterior and posterior uprights or attach the halo ring to a well-molded plaster body jacket. Anteroposterior and lateral roentgenograms should be obtained to document the alignment of the spine.

Operative Treatment

Unstable injuries of the cervical spine, with or without neurological deficit, generally require operative treatment. In most patients early open reduction and internal fixation are indicated to obtain stability and allow early functional rehabilitation. Cervical spine fractures may be stabilized through an anterior, posterior, or combined approach. This allows rapid mobilization of the patient in a cervical orthosis,

and healing usually occurs within 8 to 12 weeks. If the spinal cord or nerve roots have been compressed by retropulsed bone fragments or disc material, anterior decompression, with or without internal fixation, may be indicated to improve neurological recovery. Stauffer and Kelly, however, reported instability and recurrent deformity after anterior decompression and strut grafting in posteriorly unstable fractures. The addition of anterior internal fixation appears to prevent some of the complications of anterior strut grafting in highly unstable cervical spine injuries. In general, posterior stability should be obtained first, followed by anterior decompression and fusion if indicated. Arena et al. and other authors emphasize the importance of documenting the presence or absence of a herniated intervertebral disc in patients with subluxation or dislocation that cannot be reduced by traction and that produces minimal or no neurological symptoms. Imaging studies such as MRI, myelography, and postmyelogram CT scanning should be performed to determine if a disc is herniated. Iatrogenic neurological injuries have been documented in patients in whom reduction and posterior stabilization were carried out before anterior decompression. These authors recommended discectomy and interbody fusion with anterior internal fixation,

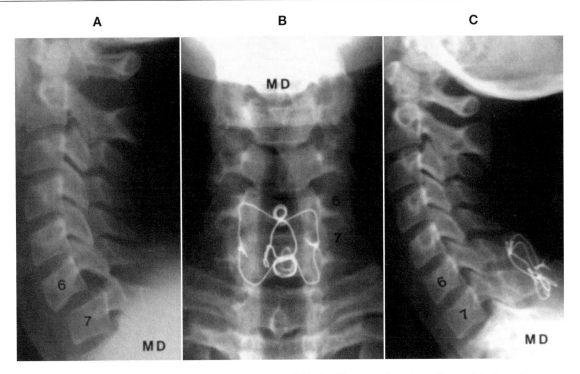

Fig. 35-14 **A,** Distraction flexion lesion at C6-7 in 18-year-old patient. Note widening of interspinous process space, moderate anterior subluxation at C6-7, and perched facets bilaterally. **B** and **C,** After posterior stabilization with triple-wire technique and autogenous iliac bone graft, spinal alignment is restored. Patient was mobilized early in rigid cervical orthosis and had full functional recovery.

followed by posterior stabilization, as optimal treatment. Bohlman, Anderson, and Freehafer reported improved neurological recovery in patients with both incomplete and complete cord injuries after anterior decompression and fusion.

When decompression or stabilization is indicated, several basic principles should be followed:

1. The injury must be clearly defined before surgery by plain roentgenograms, high-resolution CT scanning with sagittal and coronal reconstruction, or MRI.
2. Laminectomy has a limited role in the treatment of cervical fractures or dislocations and may contribute to clinical instability and neurological deficit. It occasionally may be indicated if posterior bone fragments from the neural arch are compressing the neural elements.
3. Compression of the cervical cord or roots by retropulsed bone fragments or disc material usually is anterior; therefore anterior decompression and fusion, with or without internal fixation, are indicated.
4. For posterior ligamentous or bony instability, posterior stabilization with internal fixation and bone grafting are indicated.

The choice of surgical approaches depends on the pattern of injury. Posterior stabilization procedures usually are indicated for posterior ligamentous instability (Fig. 35-14). Anterior decompression and fusion, with or without internal fixation, are most often indicated for burst fractures of the cervical spine with documented compression of the neural elements by retropulsed bone or disc fragments and an incomplete neurological deficit (Fig. 35-15). Combined anterior decompression and posterior fusion are indicated for patients who have severe instability and a significant neurocompressive pathological condition (Fig. 35-16). The advent of rigid anterior and posterior spinal internal fixation has reduced the complications related to graft extrusion and the development of deformity. The complex pathology that is present with spinal trauma necessitates exposure of both the anterior and posterior portions of the spine. As surgical techniques for the spine continue to evolve, numerous approaches have been advocated by various authors, including posterior, anterior, or combined procedures done in a staged manner or sequentially in one procedure under a single anesthetic. Staged procedures offer a period of recovery between the two surgeries, but there appears to be a statistically higher complication rate when compared with sequential procedures. Recently, authors such as Pascal-Moussellard et al. have advocated simultaneous anterior and posterior approaches to the spine. The development of special surgical tables has facilitated patient positioning and intraoperative patient adjustments to allow operative exposure for the anterior and posterior surgical teams. With this technique, which appears to be technically demanding, the proposed advantage is not having to move the patient throughout the entire procedure, thus eliminating the risk of acute instability during the two stages. In addition, it combines the advantages of solid posterior instrumentation with the benefits of an

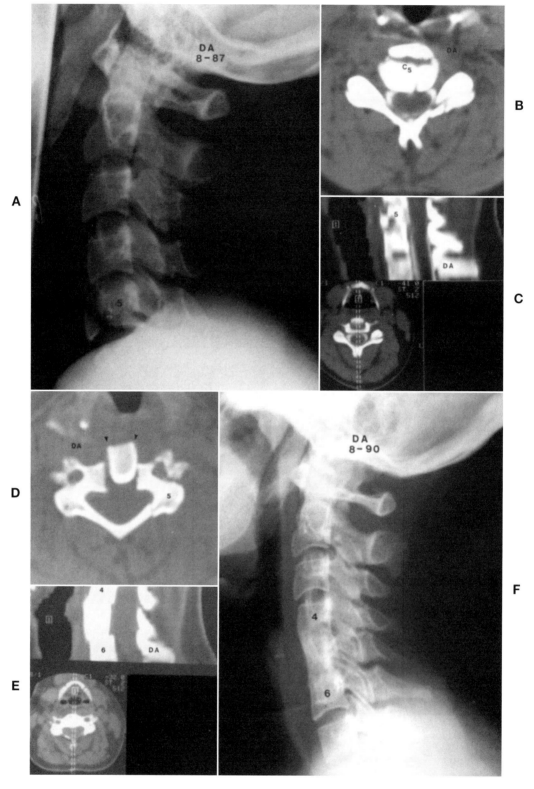

Fig. 35-15   A, Compressive flexion injury in 20-year-old woman with complete C5 quadriplegia. **B,** CT scan shows encroachment on subarachnoid space and flattening of cervical cord, with fractures of left lateral mass. **C,** CT scan with sagittal reconstruction shows fracture of C5 vertebral body with mild displacement of posterior vertebral margin into spinal canal; no widening of interspinous process space, suggestive of posterior ligamentous instability, is apparent. **D,** CT scan after anterior decompression and iliac crest strut grafting. **E,** CT scan with sagittal reconstruction shows adequate decompression of spinal cord and proper position of graft from C4 to C6. **F,** Three years after surgery, lateral roentgenogram shows incorporation of graft and solid arthrodesis from C4 to C6. Patient had single-level root recovery and is a functional C6 quadriplegic.

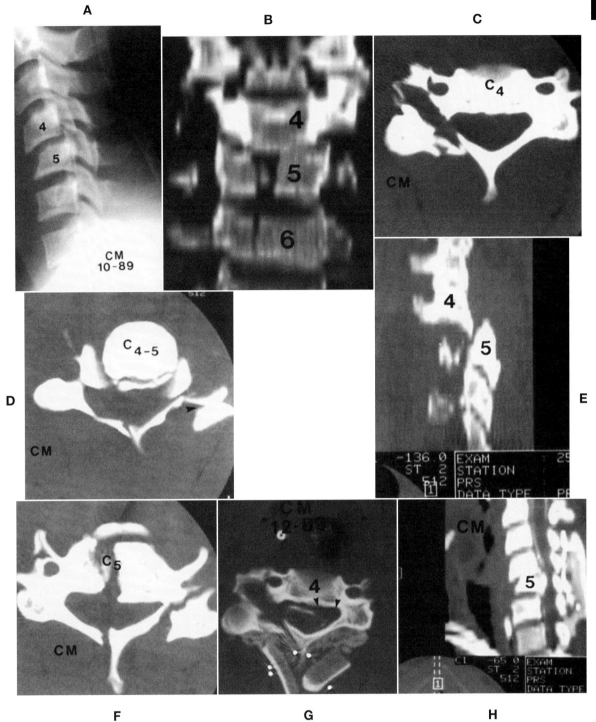

Fig. 35-16 Collegiate football defensive back sustained axial loading injury to cervical spine while making tackle; he was rendered a complete C5 quadriplegic. **A,** Lateral roentgenogram shows mild anterior subluxation of C4 and C5 caused by left unilateral facet dislocation. **B,** CT scan with coronal reconstruction shows significant fractures of bodies of C5 and C6 that were not noted on lateral roentgenogram. **C,** CT scan through C4 vertebral body shows fractures through ipsilateral right pedicle and lamina with free-floating lateral mass at this level. **D,** CT scan through C4 and C5 shows unilateral left-sided C4-5 facet dislocation *(arrow).* **E,** CT scan with sagittal reconstruction shows left-sided unilateral C4-5 facet dislocation. **F,** CT scan through C5 vertebral body shows significant fractures of anterior and posterior elements and marked narrowing of spinal canal. **G,** CT scan with sagittal reconstruction shows significant narrowing of spinal canal resulting from retropulsed bone and disc material. **H,** CT scan with contrast in subarachnoid space shows disc material retropulsed into spinal canal to left of midline behind body of C4. This was believed to impair function of left C4 nerve root and cause paralysis of left hemidiaphragm. Note also large, cortical cancellous bone graft wired into place posteriorly.

Continued

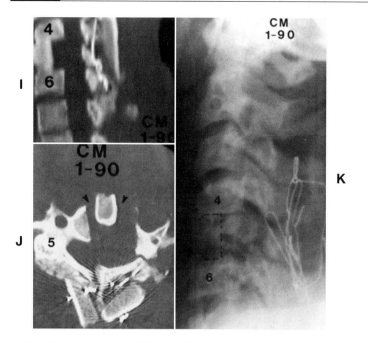

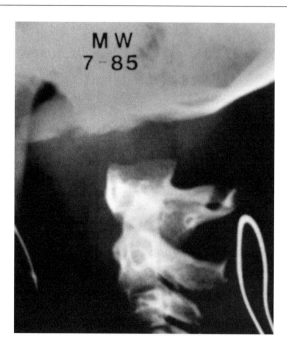

Fig. 35-16, cont'd **I,** CT scan with sagittal reconstruction shows adequate decompression at C5 and placement of iliac strut graft from C4 to C6. **J,** Axial scan confirms adequate anterior decompression and proper placement of strut grafts *(arrow).* Spinal alignment has been restored and stability achieved. **K,** Lateral roentgenogram shows final alignment of spine after combined anterior and posterior fusions; note oblique facet wire used for additional rotational stability.

Fig. 35-17 Lateral roentgenogram of pedestrian struck by car who sustained fatal atlantooccipital dislocation. Note marked widening of space between base of skull and atlas.

anterior decompression and circumferential bone grafting. Two well-trained spinal surgery teams need to be involved when considering a simultaneous anterior and posterior approach to the spine, and a special operating table should be available to allow simultaneous access to the anterior and posterior spine. Additional prospective series will have to be conducted to define the advantages of one approach over the other.

Injuries to Upper Cervical Spine (Occiput to C2)
◆ Dislocations of Atlantooccipital Joint

Dislocations of the atlantooccipital joint are uncommon (Fig. 35-17). The injury may be either anterior or posterior and usually is fatal. Davis et al., in an extensive study of fatal cranial spinal injuries, demonstrated that many spinal injuries occurred between the occiput and C3. For this injury to occur, the alar and apical ligaments, the tectorial membrane, and the posterior atlantooccipital ligaments must be disrupted. Fractures of the atlantooccipital joint may accompany the dislocation. Although many patients die immediately of complete respiratory arrest caused by brainstem compression, there are reports in the literature of patients who survived this injury. Treatment consists of reduction of the dislocation and stabilization of the atlantooccipital joint. Cervical traction is contraindicated because of severe instability. Immediate application of a halo vest is recommended to stabilize the joint. The patient's respiratory and neurological status must be carefully monitored. We recommend early surgical stabilization of the atlantooccipital joint because ligamentous healing in a halo vest is not predictable, and many of these injuries are so unstable that displacement may occur even in the halo vest. Stabilization is obtained by posterior cervical arthrodesis using large cortical cancellous bone grafts wired in place, as described by Wertheim and Bohlman (Fig. 35-18). Reports by Anderson et al. showed good results without severe complications when plates and screw fixation are used to achieve occipital cervical fusion.

TECHNIQUE 35-3 *(Wertheim and Bohlman)*

After careful fiberoptic nasal tracheal intubation and with somatosensory evoked potential monitoring equipment in place, position the patient prone on a Stryker frame with a previously applied halo vest in place. The posterior shell of the halo vest and the uprights may be removed for exposure of the neck. Prepare and drape the patient in the usual manner. Infiltrate the skin and subcutaneous tissues with a 1:500,000 epinephrine solution to aid hemostasis and make a midline skin incision from the occiput to C3. Carry dissection down in the midline from the inion distally to the level of the third cervical spinous process. Subperiosteally, expose the posterior elements from the occiput to C2 using periosteal elevators and electrocautery to reduce interfascial and periosteal bleeding. Take care not to extend the dissection farther than 1.5 cm laterally at the level of the C1 vertebra to avoid injury to the vertebral arteries. Using a high-speed burr, drill a transverse hole across the keel region of the occiput below the inion in the midline overlying the

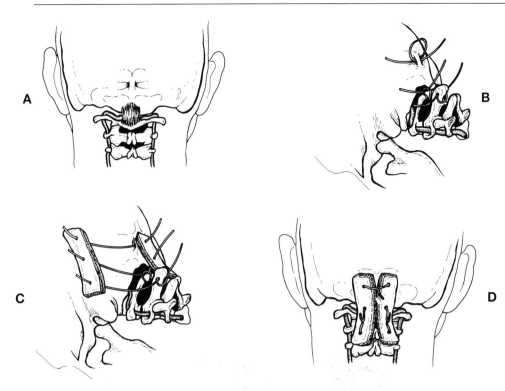

Fig. 35-18 Wertheim and Bohlman method of occipitocervical fusion. **A,** Burr is used to create ridge in external occipital protuberance, and then hole is made in ridge. **B,** Wires are passed through outer table of occiput, under arch of atlas, and through spinous process of axis. **C,** Grafts are placed on wires. **D,** Wires are tightened to secure grafts in place. (Redrawn from Wertheim SB, Bohlman HH: *J Bone Joint Surg* 69A:833, 1987.)

cerebellum (Fig. 35-18, *A*) and place a wire for fixation of the bone graft to the calvaria. If this bony prominence, the inion, does not exist, drill the hole closer to the border of the foramen magnum. Drill a second hole through the base of the spinous process of C2 and place a 20-gauge wire through the transverse hole beneath the inion and loop it on itself to fix the bone graft to the base of the skull. Place additional 20-gauge wires sublaminally beneath the ring of C1 and through the hole in the base of C2 and loop each around the inferior aspect of the spinous process (Fig. 35-18, *B*). Remove a thick, unicortical, cancellous bone graft from the posterior aspect of the ilium. The shape of the iliac wing allows the graft to curve and more nearly match the area to be spanned across the occipitocervical junction.

Lightly decorticate with a Hall high-speed burr. Drill matching holes in the graft for the insertion of the wires and tighten the graft into place with the cancellous portion of the graft adjacent to the posterior elements of the occiput and C1-2 (Fig. 35-18, *C* and *D*). Tighten the wire through the base of the occiput to its adjacent free end, the free ends of the sublaminar wire beneath the ring of C1, and the wires through the base of the spinous process of C2 to lock the bone grafts in place. Thoroughly irrigate the wound with antibiotic solution, insert a closed suction drain, and close the wound in layers.

AFTERTREATMENT. Halo traction may be used after surgery, or the posterior shell of the halo vest may be reapplied.

Consolidation of the bone grafts generally occurs by 12 to 16 weeks.

Atlas Fractures. Jefferson first described burst fractures of the atlas in 1920, attributing the fracture to axial loading to the top of the head. Levine and Edwards, in a review of 144 patients with 163 injuries of the C1-2 complex, found that 53% of patients with fractures of the atlas also had other cervical spinal fractures, most commonly type I traumatic spondylolisthesis of the axis and posteriorly displaced type II and type III dens fractures. They also emphasized the difficulty of accurate roentgenographic diagnosis of these injuries. The lateral cervical spine view usually shows fractures through the posterior arch of C1. However, when the fracture is extremely anterior to the junction of the lateral mass of C1, the fracture may not be visible on the lateral view. They found anteroposterior and lateral tomography to be accurate in detecting fractures in both the anterior and posterior portions of the ring of C1, but CT scans failed to demonstrate all fractures in 6 of 11 patients.

Three primary types of fractures of the ring of C1 have been identified: (1) posterior arch fracture, which usually occurs at the junction of the posterior arch and the lateral mass; (2) lateral mass fracture, which usually occurs on one side only with the fracture line passing either through the articular surface or just anterior and posterior to the lateral mass on one side; a fracture through the posterior arch on the opposite side sometimes occurs; and (3) burst fracture (Jefferson fracture), which is characterized by four fractures, two in the posterior arch and two in the anterior arch.

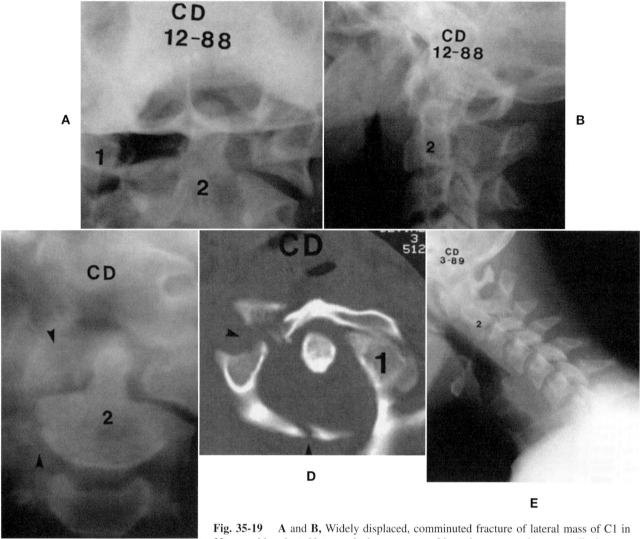

Fig. 35-19   **A** and **B,** Widely displaced, comminuted fracture of lateral mass of C1 in 22-year-old patient. Note marked asymmetry of lateral masses and extreme displacement of right lateral mass on anteroposterior open-mouth odontoid view. **C** and **D,** Anteroposterior tomogram and CT scan show associated fracture of lateral mass of C2, comminuted fracture of atlas involving right lateral mass and posterior arch. **E,** Flexion lateral view shows stability of C1-2 complex after 3 months of immobilization in halo vest.

Most fractures of the atlas can be treated with immobilization in a rigid cervical orthosis or a halo vest. Isolated posterior arch fractures are stable injuries that can be treated in a cervical collar for 8 to 12 weeks. In the 53% of patients with additional cervical spinal injuries in their series, Levine and Edwards reported loss of reduction of some C2 fractures after surgery because of a failure to recognize a fracture in the posterior arch of C1. In some patients an occiput to C2 stabilization resulted in severe restriction of cervical spine motion. We agree with Levine and Edwards that external immobilization of the cervical spine until healing of the C1 ring fracture occurs should be done before proceeding with surgical stabilization of the C2 fracture.

Nondisplaced or minimally displaced fractures of the lateral mass and Jefferson fractures can be treated by collar immobilization to prevent displacement and allow fracture healing. Fractures in which the lateral mass of the atlas is displaced laterally more than 7 mm beyond the articular surfaces of the axis should be reduced with halo traction (Fig. 35-19). Halo traction should be maintained for 3 to 6 weeks before application of a halo vest if the lateral mass is severely displaced, since displacement may recur if a halo vest is applied immediately after reduction. Spence, Decker, and Sell determined that if the lateral mass overhangs the articular surfaces of the axis more than 7 mm, a tear of the transverse ligament is likely, resulting in clinical C1-2 instability (Fig. 35-20). In axial loading of the C1-2 complex, the supporting alar ligaments, apical ligaments, and facet capsules usually remain intact and significant instability is prevented by these intact structures. Fielding et al. have shown that in severe

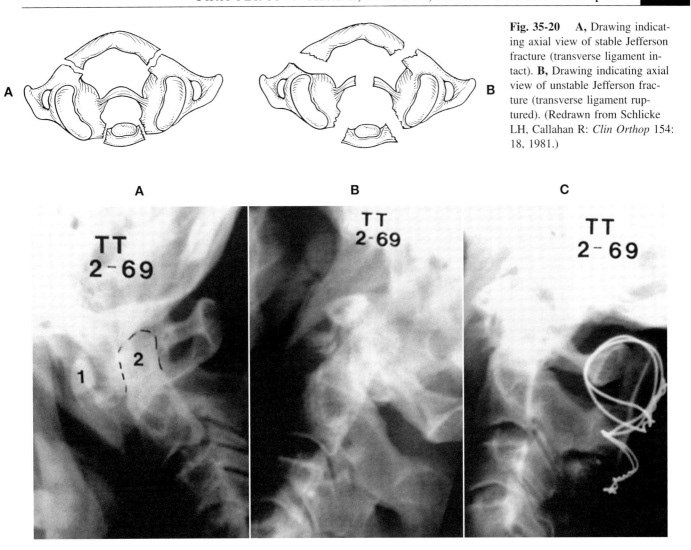

Fig. 35-20 **A,** Drawing indicating axial view of stable Jefferson fracture (transverse ligament intact). **B,** Drawing indicating axial view of unstable Jefferson fracture (transverse ligament ruptured). (Redrawn from Schlicke LH, Callahan R: *Clin Orthop* 154: 18, 1981.)

Fig. 35-21 Patient sustained severe blow to back of head, resulting in instability of C1-2 complex because of torn transverse ligament. Note widening of atlanto-dens interval in flexion **(A)** and reduction in extension **(B). C,** After Gallie type of posterior C1-2 arthrodesis, lateral roentgenogram shows anatomical reduction of atlanto-dens interval.

flexion injuries with isolated transverse ligament ruptures, the alar ligament, facet capsules, and transverse ligament are rendered incompetent, resulting in gross clinical instability. However, on flexion and extension views of all their patients with lateral mass and Jefferson fractures, Levine and Edwards found no significant C1-2 instability after fracture healing.

Rupture of Transverse Ligament. This injury is a purely ligamentous injury and is different from other injuries involving the C1-2 complex. It most commonly results from a fall with a blow to the back of the head. The transverse ligament may be avulsed with a bony fragment from the lateral mass on either side, or it may rupture in its mid substance. Dickman, Greene, and Sonntag classified injuries of the transverse atlantal ligament or its osseous insertions into two types: type I, disruptions of the substance of the ligament; and type II, fractures and avulsions involving the tubercle insertion of the transverse ligament on the lateral masses of C1. These two

types of injuries had distinctly different clinical characteristics that were useful in determining treatment. According to these authors, type I injuries are incapable of healing without internal fixation, and they should be treated with early surgery. Type II injuries, which render the transverse ligament physiologically incompetent even if the ligament substance is not torn, should be treated initially with a rigid cervical orthosis. They had a 74% success rate with nonoperative treatment of type II injuries, reserving surgery for patients who had a nonunion and persistent instability after 3 to 4 months with immobilization. Conversely, 26% of type II injuries in this study failed to heal after immobilization, suggesting that close follow-up is needed to determine which patients will require delayed surgical intervention. Usually the anterior subluxation of the ring of C1 can be detected on flexion films, and the instability can be reduced in extension (Fig. 35-21). Lateral views should be carefully checked for retropharyngeal hematoma, which

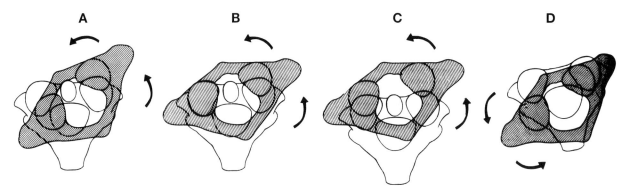

Fig. 35-22 Fielding and Hawkins classification of rotary displacement. **A,** Type I: simple rotary displacement without anterior shift; odontoid acts as pivot. **B,** Type II: rotary displacement with anterior displacement of 3 to 5 mm; lateral articular process acts as pivot. **C,** Type III: rotary displacement with anterior displacement of more than 5 mm. **D,** Type IV: rotary displacement with posterior displacement. (Redrawn from Fielding JW, Hawkins RJ: *J Bone Joint Surg* 59A:37, 1977.)

suggests an acute injury, and for small flecks of bone avulsed off the lateral masses of C1, which may indicate avulsion of the ligament. The primary indication of this injury is instability at C1-2 on flexion and extension films. Anterior widening of the atlanto-dens interval of more than 5 mm on the flexion view suggests that the transverse ligament is incompetent. Flexion and extension views should be made under the supervision of the physician, and the patient must be closely monitored for alterations in neurological or respiratory function.

Because rupture of the transverse ligament is primarily a ligamentous injury, nonoperative treatment is ineffective in obtaining stability. Surgical stabilization of the C1-2 complex is the treatment of choice. Initial treatment consists of immobilization through skull traction and then posterior stabilization of the C1-2 complex with a Gallie type of fusion. This type of fusion directs a vector force posteriorly to pull C1 into a reduced position in reference to C2. The dens prevents C1 from being pulled too far posteriorly, and therefore overreduction is impossible. If a bone block technique, such as the Brooks and Jenkins fusion, is performed, the ring of C1 may redisplace anteriorly. If the posterior arch of C1 is fractured, a halo vest should be used for 8 to 12 weeks to allow healing of the posterior arch before proceeding with a standard C1-2 posterior arthrodesis. In 12 patients with ruptures of the transverse ligament, Levine and Edwards found an average loss of correction of 4 mm after bone block techniques and 1 mm after Gallie wiring.

Rotary Subluxation of C1 on C2. This injury is uncommon in adults and is a different entity from rotary subluxation in children (Fig. 35-22). The injury in adults usually is caused by motor vehicle accidents and often is not recognized at initial evaluation because the patient presents with torticollis and restricted neck motion. An open-mouth odontoid roentgenogram may reveal the "wink sign" caused by overriding of the C1-2 joint on one side and a normal configuration on the other side. CT and routine anteroposterior tomography are helpful in clearly defining the osseous injury. Acute rotary subluxation of

C1-2 can be reduced by closed means once the direction of the dislocation has been determined (Fig. 35-23). With the patient awake and spinal cord monitoring in place, a halo ring is applied for control of the head. Using gentle traction, the halo ring is used to derotate the skull and C1 while an assistant pushes on the anteriorly displaced lateral mass through the posterior pharynx. Topical anesthesia applied to the posterior pharynx is helpful in diminishing the gag reflex. If stable reduction is obtained and satisfactory alignment is demonstrated by roentgenogram and CT scan, the patient is immobilized in a halo vest. If closed reduction is unsuccessful, or if the injury has not been detected until late, open reduction may be attempted. With the patient prone, a midline posterior incision is made to subperiosteally expose the ring of C1 and the spinous process and lamina of C2. A wire is passed beneath the posterior arch of C1 and is used to manually derotate the ring of C1. Stabilization of the C1-2 complex can then be obtained with a posterior cervical arthrodesis using autogenous iliac bone grafting. An oblique wire from the base of the anteriorly displaced lateral mass of C1 to the spinous process of C2 may be helpful in maintaining the reduction. Immobilization in a halo vest is recommended for 8 to 12 weeks to allow consolidation of the bone graft.

Occipital Condyle Fractures. Occipital condylar fractures are rare and are frequently missed on initial evaluation. Palsies of lower cranial nerves can be the only symptom of the fracture. Demisch et al. reported a case of delayed hypoglossal nerve palsy caused by fracture of the occipital condyle. These injuries usually result from axial loading and lateral bending during which force is applied to the head and neck. Anderson and Montesano described three types of occipital condylar fractures (Fig. 35-24): type I—impaction; type II—basilar skull fracture; and type III—avulsion fracture. Types I and II occipital condylar fractures are stable and can be treated in a rigid cervical orthosis or halo vest. Type III fractures are potentially unstable because of avulsion of the alar ligaments, and immobilization for 12 weeks in a halo vest is recommended. If

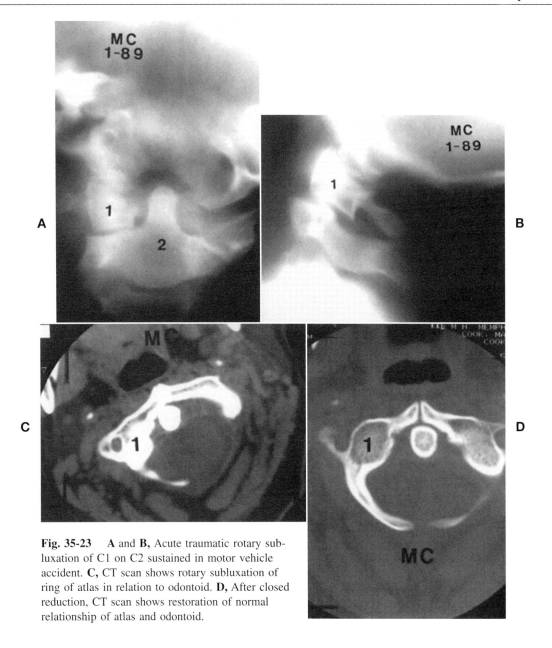

Fig. 35-23   **A** and **B,** Acute traumatic rotary sub-luxation of C1 on C2 sustained in motor vehicle accident. **C,** CT scan shows rotary subluxation of ring of atlas in relation to odontoid. **D,** After closed reduction, CT scan shows restoration of normal relationship of atlas and odontoid.

instability is indicated on flexion and extension films after an adequate period of immobilization in a halo vest, then occipital to C2 fusion may be necessary. CT and routine anteroposterior and lateral tomography of the base of the skull will most likely show this fracture.

◆ Dens Fracture

Anderson and D'Alonzo classified odontoid fractures into three types (Fig. 35-25). Type I fractures are uncommon, and even if nonunion occurs after inadequate immobilization, no instability results. Type II fractures are the most common and in the study of Anderson and D'Alonzo had a 36% nonunion rate for both displaced and nondisplaced fractures. Type III fractures have a large cancellous base and heal without surgery in 90% of patients. It also is helpful to consider the amount of displacement and angulation when determining prognosis and treatment. Clark and Whitehill, in a multicenter study of odontoid fractures, found that type II fractures united in 68% of patients treated in a halo vest and that posterior cervical fusion of the C1-2 complex was successful in 98% of patients. Treatment with orthoses was less successful. Significant displacement of more than 5 mm was evident in patients who had nonunions of type II odontoid fractures. Type III dens fractures united in 86% of patients, and the authors recommended halo vest immobilization for all displaced type III fractures because less rigid immobilization led to increased rates of nonunion and malunion. Several factors have been found to be important in union of dens fractures. The degree of initial displacement is crucial; patients with displacement of

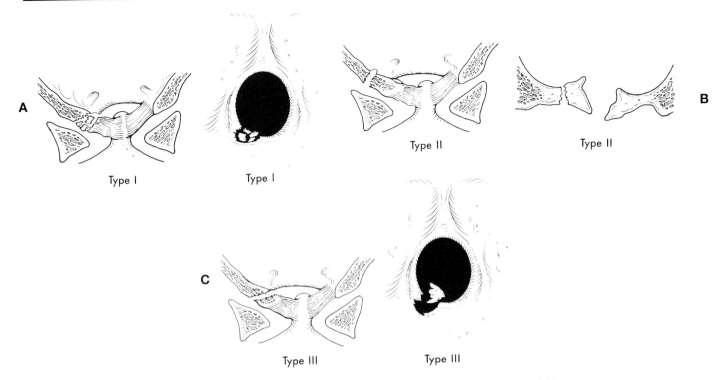

Fig. 35-24   Three types of occipital condylar fractures as described by Anderson and Montesano. **A,** Type I: impacted fracture. **B,** Type II: basilar skull fracture. **C,** Type III: avulsion fracture. (Redrawn from Anderson PA, Montesano PX: *Spine* 7:731, 1988.)

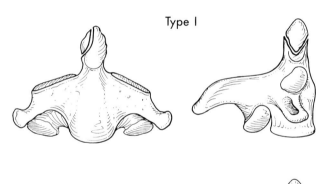

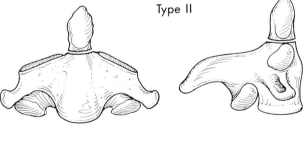

Fig. 35-25   Three types of odontoid process fractures as seen in anteroposterior and lateral planes. Type I is oblique fracture through upper part of odontoid process. Type II is fracture at junction of odontoid process and body of second cervical vertebra. Type III is fracture through upper body of vertebra. (Redrawn from Anderson LD, D'Alonzo RT: *J Bone Joint Surg* 56A:1663, 1974.)

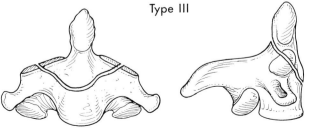

more than 5 mm appear to have more nonunions. Other factors include the regional anatomy, the adequacy of reduction, the age of the patient, and the type of immobilization.

The reported rates of fusion between the atlas and the axis vary widely in the literature. Schatzker, Rorabeck, and Waddell reported union in 13 of 15 patients treated with primary wiring and fusion, and McGraw and Rusch reported union in 14 of 15 fractures. Because most reports have similarly good results, surgical stabilization seems a more reliable means of treating displaced fractures through the base of the odontoid.

In type II fractures of the dens, it is important to determine if the displacement is anterior or posterior. Patients with posteriorly displaced dens fractures are more likely to have fractures of the ring of C1. If a fracture in the posterior arch of C1 is not recognized, reduction may be lost after surgery or the fusion may have to be extended to include the occipitocervical joint, increasing morbidity and resulting in significant restriction of cervical motion. In addition, posteriorly displaced type II dens fractures have been found to be more unstable when treated with a Gallie type of wiring as compared to a bone block technique, such as the Brooks and Jenkins procedure. In the Gallie technique a wire passed around the ring of C1 and around the spinous process of C2 results in a posteriorly directed vector force that maintains reduction by a tension band. This posteriorly directed force may result in loss of reduction of the fracture. A bone block technique decreases the posterior vector force and maintains reduction of posteriorly displaced odontoid fractures (Fig. 35-26).

Type III fractures through the body of the axis may be nondisplaced or displaced. Nondisplaced fractures are stable injuries that heal with 8 to 12 weeks of immobilization in either a halo vest or cervical collar. Levine and Edwards, in their 23 patients with displaced type III fractures through the body of the axis, found multiple combinations of angulation and translation. Although most fractures could be reduced with halo traction, continuous traction with extension was required to maintain reduction. They noted frequent loss of reduction when a halo vest was applied after only a short period of traction, but all fractures united. The goal of treatment of type III displaced dens fractures is correction of angulation in a halo vest while allowing the fracture to settle until union occurs. No late sequelae have been demonstrated from the residual translation, although significant residual anterior angulation of the dens narrows the cervical spinal canal and may compress the spinal cord.

TECHNIQUE 35-4 (Gallie)

Carefully intubate the patient in the supine position and then turn him prone on a Stryker frame with either tong or halo traction in place. In turning the patient take care to maintain the head-thoracic relationship. Then make cervical spine roentgenograms while the patient is on the operating table to be certain of the status of the fracture.

Prepare and drape the operative field in the usual fashion. Inject a 1:500,000 epinephrine solution intradermally to

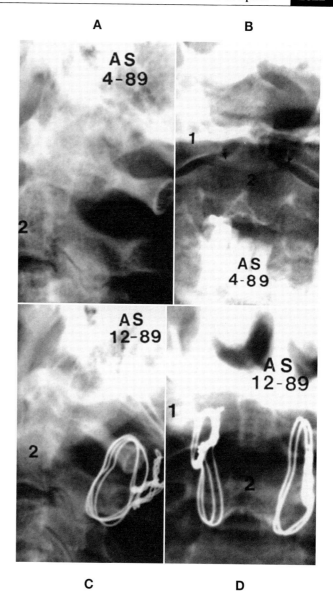

Fig. 35-26 **A** and **B,** Posteriorly displaced type II odontoid fracture in 50-year-old man. **C** and **D,** After stabilization of C1-2 complex by Brooks and Jenkins type of fusion.

help with hemostasis. Then make a midline incision from the occiput to the fourth or fifth cervical vertebra. Using electrocautery and sharp dissection subperiosteally, expose the posterior arch of the atlas and the laminae of C2 and gently remove all soft tissue from the bony surfaces. The upper surface of the arch of C1 should be exposed no farther laterally than 1.5 cm from the midline in adults and 1 cm in children to avoid the vertebral arteries. Decortication of C1 and C2 is generally not needed. Pass a 20-gauge wire loop from below upward under the arch of the atlas either directly or with the aid of a Mersilene suture; the suture can be passed using an aneurysm needle if necessary. Pass the free

continued

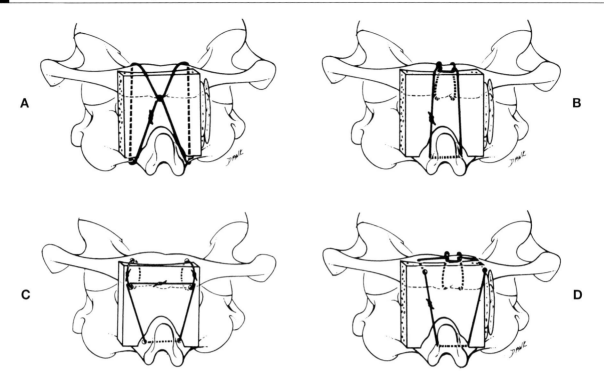

Fig. 35-27   Various methods of using wire to hold graft in place. **A,** Wire passes under lamina of atlas and axis and is tied over graft. **B,** Wire passes under lamina of atlas and through spine of axis and is tied over graft. We use this method most frequently. **C,** Wire passes through holes drilled in lamina of atlas and through spine of axis; holes are drilled through graft. **D,** Wire passes under lamina of atlas and through spine of axis; holes are drilled through graft. (From Fielding JW, Hawkins RJ, Ratzan SA: *J Bone Joint Surg* 58A:400, 1976.)

ends of the wire through the loop, thus grasping the arch of C1 in the loop (Fig. 35-27). Take a corticocancellous graft from the iliac crest and place it against the lamina of C2 and the arch of C1 beneath the wire. Then pass one end of the wire through the spinous process of C2 and twist the wire on itself to secure the graft in place. Irrigate the wound and close it in layers over suction drainage tubes.

AFTERTREATMENT. The patient is mobilized as soon as possible in either a halo vest or a rigid cervicothoracic spinal orthosis. For patients with a C1-2 arthrodesis, we prefer immobilization in a halo vest for about 12 weeks to allow consolidation of the bone grafts because biomechanical studies have shown the vest superior to cervicothoracic braces in maintaining stabilization. At 12 weeks, flexion and extension cervical roentgenograms should be made to document fusion.

TECHNIQUE 35-5 *(Brooks and Jenkins)*
Intubate and turn the patient on the operating table as in the Gallie fusion just described. Prepare and drape the patient in the same manner. Expose the C1-2 level through a midline incision, as in the Gallie fusion. Using an aneurysm needle,

pass a 2-0 Mersilene suture on each side of the midline in a cephalad-to-caudad direction, first under the arch of the atlas and then under the lamina of the axis (Fig. 35-28, *A*). These serve as guides to introduce two doubled 20-gauge stainless steel wires into place. As an alternative, braided cables may be passed in place of the wires to increase flexibility and strength significantly. Obtain two full-thickness rectangular bone grafts approximately 1.25 to 3.5 cm from the iliac crest. Bevel the grafts to fit in the interval between the arch of the atlas and each lamina of the axis (Fig. 35-28, *B*). While holding the grafts in position on each side of the midline and maintaining the width of the interlaminal space, tighten the doubled wires over them and twist and tie the wires to secure the grafts (Fig. 35-28, *C* and *D*). Irrigate and close the wound in layers over suction drains.

AFTERTREATMENT. The aftertreatment is the same as that for the Gallie fusion.

Internal Fixation of Upper Cervical Spine. Recent advances in internal fixation have allowed its use in the cervical spine. Although considerable data concerning the biomechanics

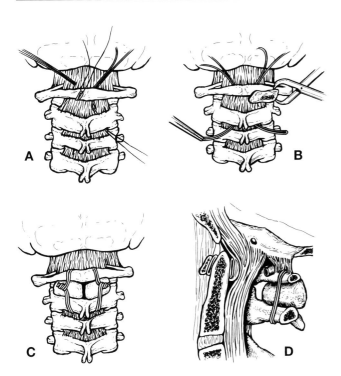

Fig. 35-28   Brooks and Jenkins technique of atlantoaxial fusion. **A,** Insertion of wires under atlas and axis. **B,** Wire in place with graft being inserted. **C** and **D,** Bone grafts secured by wires (anteroposterior and lateral views). (Redrawn from Brooks AL, Jenkins EB: *J Bone Joint Surg* 60A:279, 1978.)

of internal fixation of the spine have been accumulated, indications for rigid internal fixation of specific spinal fractures are still evolving. With the advent of more sophisticated internal fixation techniques, however, comes an increased risk of anatomical or mechanical complications. Increasing complication rates may be anticipated as use of these new techniques increases. Future outcome studies will help define the indications and contraindications for use of these procedures. For this reason, we recommend that more aggressive internal fixation techniques be used only by experienced spinal surgeons.

◆ Transarticular C1-2 Screw Fixation

Indications for this technique include C1-2 instability and odontoid fractures, which require surgical treatment. The technique requires a thorough understanding of the anatomy of the C1-2 articulation to prevent complications during screw fixation. Although the posterior arch of C1 must be intact for traditional C1-2 posterior fusion techniques, the integrity of the ring of C1 is not necessary for transarticular screws. This technique is exacting and requires image intensification intraoperatively. Stereotactic imaging intraoperatively is rapidly evolving and may in the future be extremely useful when implanting fixation devices in the complex anatomy of the upper cervical spine. The principle limitation of posterior C1-2 transarticular screw fixation appears to be the location of

the vertebral artery. Anatomical studies have been performed to better define the trajectory of the screw necessary to allow for safe placement. Recently, Dickman and Sonntag in a prospective study compared clinical outcomes of 121 patients treated with posterior C1-2 transarticular screws with wired posterior C1-2 autologous bone grafts. Long-term follow-up in 114 patients demonstrated a 98% fusion rate with transarticular screw fixation compared with an 86% union rate with C1-2 fixation using wires and autograft. They concluded that the risks of screw malpositioning, catastrophic vascular injury, or neural injury are small. These risks can be minimized by preoperative CT assessment of the transverse foramen, which contains vertebral artery, or by using high-quality intraoperative fluoroscopy or frameless stereotaxy to guide the screw insertion; 2% of the 121 screws that were inserted were malpositioned, but none were associated with clinical sequelae.

Wright and Lauryssen reported in a retrospective study that the risk of vertebral artery injury was 4.1% per patient or 2.2% per screw inserted. The risk of neurological deficit from vertebral artery injury was 0.2% per patient or 0.1% per screw; the mortality rate was 0.1%. The management of intraoperative vertebral artery injuries was either observation or immediate postoperative angiography with possible balloon occlusion.

TECHNIQUE 35-6 *(Magerl, Seemann)*

Position the patient prone. Use lateral image intensification to check the reduction of the C1-2 complex. Perform midline posterior cervical exposure in the routine fashion from C1 to C3. Identify the landmarks for the entry portal of the transarticular screw at the lower inner edge of the inferior articular process of C2 (Fig. 35-29, *A*). Using a 2-mm bit, drill through the isthmus near its posteromedial surface, exiting from the articular mass of C2 at the posterior aspect of the superior articular surface and entering the lateral mass of the atlas. The drill bit should perforate the cortex of the lateral mass of C1 (Fig. 35-29, *B*). Determine the appropriate screw length (Fig. 35-29, *C*). Use a 3.5-mm cortical tap to cut threads in the drill hole and insert the appropriate 3.5-mm cortical screw across the C1-2 joint. As an alternative, cannulated screws may be used after insertion of Kirschner wires under image intensification control. During insertion of the screws, take care to avoid injuring the vertebral arteries. After placing the C1-2 transarticular screws, perform a traditional posterior C1-2 fusion using either the Gallie or Brooks technique (Fig. 35-29, *D*). If the posterior arch of C1 is incompetent, decorticate the facet joints at C1-2 and pack cancellous bone into the joint before inserting the screws.

AFTERTREATMENT. Because this technique provides excellent rotational stability, postoperative immobilization with a halo vest usually is unnecessary, and a cervical collar may be worn for 8 to 12 weeks.

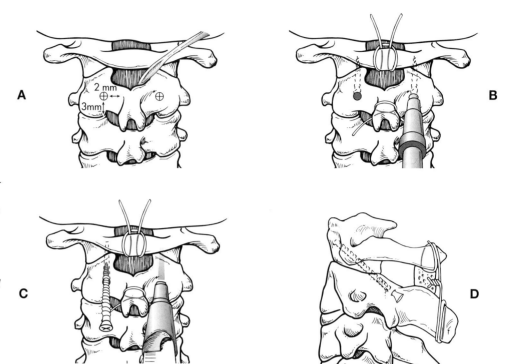

Fig. 35-29   C1-2 transarticular screw fixation (Magerl and Seemann). **A,** Landmarks for entry point of transarticular screw. **B,** Wires are brought around arch of C1 and spinous process of C2 to manipulate these two vertebrae. Screw holes are drilled through isthmus near its posterior and medial surface of C2 and enter lateral mass of atlas. **C,** Measuring screw length and tapping with 3.5-mm cortical tap. **D,** Proper screw placement for C1-2 fusion. (Redrawn from Leventhal MR: *Op Tech Sports Med* 1:199, 1993.)

◆ *Anterior Screw Fixation of Dens Fractures*

Internal fixation of dens fractures with a cannulated screw system has been described by Etter et al. This technique combines anatomical reduction of the fracture with stable internal screw fixation using the principles established by the AO/ASIF. They note that complications are common when this technique is not carried out properly or is used in contraindicated situations. In their series 23 patients were treated with direct screw fixation, with an overall union rate of 92.3%. They reported a 17% major complication rate from inappropriate use of the technique. Important contraindications to anterior screw fixation include an oblique fracture configuration (paralleling the direction of the intended screw fixation), an associated unstable fracture of the atlas, and pathological fractures and nonunions of the dens in which bone stock is inadequate for internal screw fixation.

TECHNIQUE 35-7 (Etter et al.)

After general endotracheal anesthesia has been induced and the patient has been positioned supine on the operating table, reduce displaced fractures in skeletal traction with either Gardner-Wells tongs or a halo ring (Fig. 35-30). Anatomical reduction must be obtained before internal fixation with the cannulated screw system. Insert a large nasogastric tube to allow localization of the esophagus and to prevent perforation. Use a padded occipital ring attached to the operating table to stabilize the patient's head. The head and neck must be positioned to allow maximal access to the anterior cervical spine. A large vertical mandibular-

sternal distance is required because of the size of the instrumentation and the steep inferior angle of approach necessary for screw placement. High-resolution fluoroscopic image intensification in both the anteroposterior and lateral planes is necessary for insertion of the screws. Before beginning the surgical procedure, confirm a free working path for the instrumentation by placing a long Kirschner wire along the side of the neck in the direction of the intended screw placement and viewing it with image intensification. If clearance of the sternum is not adequate, modify the patient's position. Prepare and drape the operative field in a sterile fashion, with sterile draping of the image intensifier. Make an anteromedial approach to the cervical spine through a transverse skin incision approximately 6 to 7 cm long at the level of the C5-6 disc space. Because of the steep angle of inclination required relative to the anterior plane of the neck, undermine the skin and split the platysma muscle longitudinally in line with its fibers along the anteromedial border of the sternocleidomastoid muscle. Bluntly dissect the interval between the carotid sheath laterally and the trachea and esophagus medially. Proceed anteriorly along the front of the cervical spine until the anteroinferior margin of the C2 body is reached. Place an 8-mm wide Hohmann retractor along the lateral mass of C2. Delineate the C2-3 intervertebral disc space and vertically incise the anterior longitudinal ligament at this level. Ligation of the superior thyroid artery may be necessary for exposure of the C2-3 level. Identify with image intensification the entry site at the anteroinferior head of the C2 body. Using a small drill sleeve, insert two 1.2-mm Kirschner wires with their sagittal orientations toward the posterior apex of the dens and their coronal orientation angled toward the midline (Fig. 35-30, *A*). Verify penetration of the dens cortex and appropriate wire alignment by image intensification in two planes. Measure directly the guide wire insertion depth. Insert the 3.5-mm cannulated drill bit over each guide wire and drill a screw starter hole to a depth of 5 mm (Fig. 35-30, *A*). Insert self-tapping 3.5-mm screws of appropriate length over each guide wire and advance them with the cannulated screwdriver until the opposing apical cortical bone is secured (Fig. 35-30, *B*). Observe the progression of each screw under image control to ensure that the guide wire does not bind and migrate proximally into the foramen magnum (Fig. 35-30, *C*). The screw heads tend to encroach on the anterior margin of the C2-3 intervertebral disc, frequently requiring removal of a small amount of annulus to create a recess. Always use tissue protection guards during drilling to avoid damage to neurovascular structures.

AFTERTREATMENT. The patient is observed closely for respiratory status in an intensive care unit for the 24 hours after surgery. Then a rigid cervical orthosis is applied and is worn for 6 weeks. The orthosis may be removed for bathing and resting. Clinical and roentgenographic evaluations are performed at 6, 12, and 24 weeks (Fig. 35-31).

◆ *Internal Fixation and Posterior Plating of Occiput to C2*

TECHNIQUE 35-8

Use two one-third tubular AO plates or two 3.5 AO reconstruction plates for this procedure, with one plate on each side, spanning the occiput to C2. The plates are prebent according to the posterior angle of the occipitocervical junction. Extend internal fixation beyond C2 if necessary to achieve rigid internal fixation. Insert a 1.2-mm Kirschner wire into the lateral mass of C2, using the technique described by Magerl and Seemann (p. 1623), or insert the Kirschner wire into the pedicle of C2. It is critical that the position of the Kirschner wires be checked with biplanar image intensification. Insert the prebent plate over the Kirschner wires on each side and place on the occiput, determining the points for screw insertion into the occiput (Fig. 35-32, *A*). Attach the plate to the occiput with two 3.5-mm cortical screws, usually 10 mm long on each side. Use a 2-mm tap for the outer and inner tables of the occipital bone. Use a drill guide with a stopper to perforate the dura mater at the desired depths (Fig. 35-32, *B*). Adjust the depths of the screw holes and screws gradually until the inner table

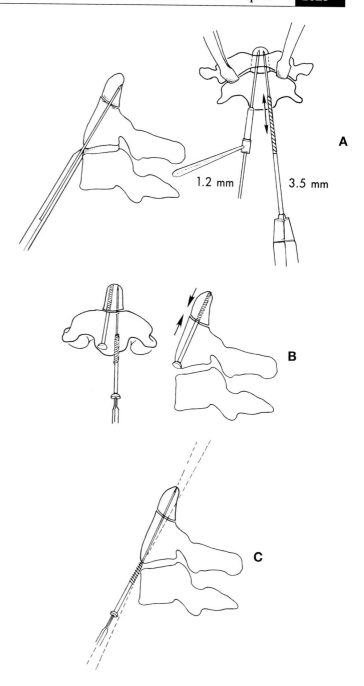

Fig. 35-30 Anterior fixation of dens fracture with cannulated screws, as described by Etter et al. **A,** Two Kirschner wires are inserted, and depth is measured; 5-mm screw starter hole is drilled. **B,** Threaded cannulated screws are inserted over wires. **C,** Screw insertion is monitored with image intensification to ensure that guide wires do not bind and migrate proximally into foramen magnum. (Redrawn from Etter C, Coscia M, Jaberg H, Aebi M: *Spine* 16:25, 1991.)

continued

A   B   C

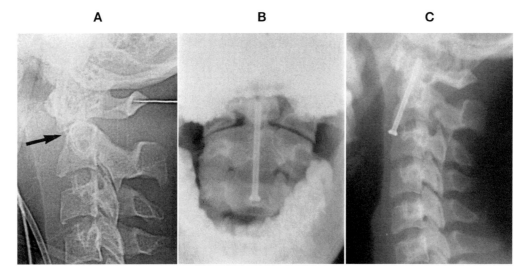

Fig. 35-31 **A,** Lateral roentgenogram showing anteriorly displaced odontoid fracture. **B** and **C,** Anteroposterior and lateral roentgenograms after internal fixation of dens fracture with single cannulated screw.

Fig. 35-32 Posterior plating of upper cervical spine, with fixation from occiput to C3. **A,** Prebent 3.5 AO reconstruction plate inserted over Kirschner wires in lateral mass of C2 and C3 to determine position of screws in occiput. **B,** Drilling of external and internal tables of occiput using drill guide with stopper at intended depths. (Redrawn from Aebi M: Surgical treatment of cervical spine fractures by AO spine techniques. In Bridwell KH, DeWald RL: *Textbook of spinal surgery*, vol 2, Philadelphia, 1991, Lippincott-Raven.)

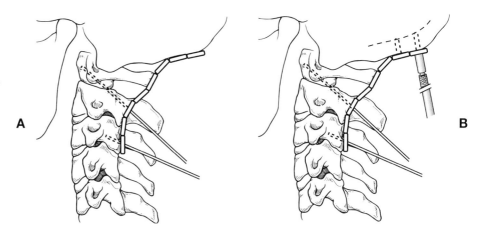

is perforated. Remove the Kirschner wires from the C2 lateral masses and place two screws holes and screws, or as an alternative use cannulated self-tapping screws over the Kirschner wires. For additional fixation to the arch of C1, use a sublaminar wire and tighten through an open screw hole of the plate. Perform a midline fusion using corticocancellous bone graft between the occiput and spinous processes of C2, as well as additional bone graft around the plates (Fig. 35-33, *A* to *C*).

AFTERTREATMENT. Immobilization in a cervical orthosis is recommended until cervical arthrodesis has occurred, which usually is at 8 to 12 weeks. In most patients halo vest immobilization is not necessary unless screw purchase is not satisfactory.

Traumatic Spondylolisthesis of the Axis (Hangman Fractures). Hangman fractures were originally those neck injuries incurred during the hanging of criminals. Their most common cause now is motor vehicle accidents with hyperextension of the head on the neck. The occiput is forced down against the posterior arch of the atlas, which in turn is forced against the pedicles of C2. Levine and Edwards reviewed 52 traumatic spondylolistheses of the axis and classified these fractures into four types (Fig. 35-34). Type I fractures are minimally displaced and are believed to be caused by hyperextension and axial loading with failure of the neural arch in tension. Because ligamentous injury is minimal, these fractures are stable and usually heal with 12 weeks of immobilization in a rigid cervical orthosis. Type II fractures have more than 3 mm of anterior translation and significant angulation. These injuries result from hyperextension and axial loading that cause the neural arch to fail with a predominantly

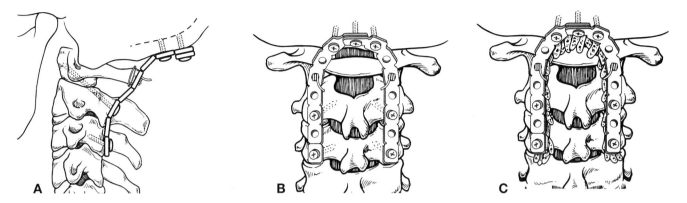

Fig. 35-33 A left- and right-sided plate, overlapping in midline of occiput, in place and fixed with screws and sublaminar wires at arch of C1. **A,** Lateral view. **B,** Posterior view. **C,** Arches and lateral mass are decorticated when corticocancellous bone graft is added from occiput to C3. (Redrawn from Aebi M: Surgical treatment of cervical spine fractures by AO spine techniques. In Bridwell KH, DeWald RL: *Textbook of spinal surgery*, vol 2, Philadelphia, 1991, Lippincott-Raven.)

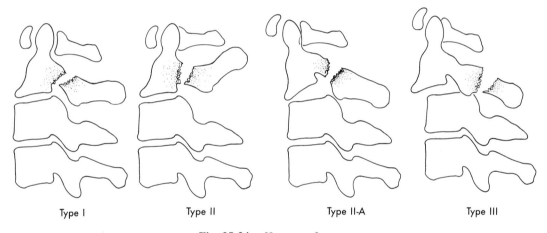

Type I   Type II   Type II-A   Type III

Fig. 35-34 Hangman fracture.

vertical fracture line, followed by significant flexion resulting in stretching of the posterior annulus of the disc and significant anterior translation and angulation. The C2-3 disc may be disrupted by the sudden flexion component involved in this injury. Treatment consists of application of skull traction through tongs or a halo ring with slight extension of the neck over a rolled-up towel. Immobilization in a halo vest does not achieve or maintain reduction, and halo traction with slight extension may be necessary for 3 to 6 weeks to maintain anatomical reduction. Then the patient can be mobilized in a halo vest for the rest of the 3-month period. These fractures usually unite with an initial gap in the neural arch and develop a spontaneous anterior fusion at C2-3. Type IIA fractures are a variant of type II fractures that demonstrate severe angulation between C2 and C3 with minimal translation. They usually

have a more horizontal than vertical fracture line through the C2 arch. The mechanism of injury is predominantly flexion and distraction. It is important to identify this particular fracture pattern because application of traction can cause marked widening of the C2-3 disc space and increased displacement. The recommended treatment is application of a halo vest with slight compression applied under image intensification to achieve and maintain anatomical reduction. Once reduction has been obtained, halo vest immobilization is continued for 12 weeks, until union occurs. Type III injuries combine a bipedicular fracture with posterior facet injuries. They usually have both severe angulation and translation of the neural arch fracture and an associated unilateral or bilateral facet dislocation at C2-3. Type III injuries are the only type of hangman's fracture that commonly require surgical stabiliza-

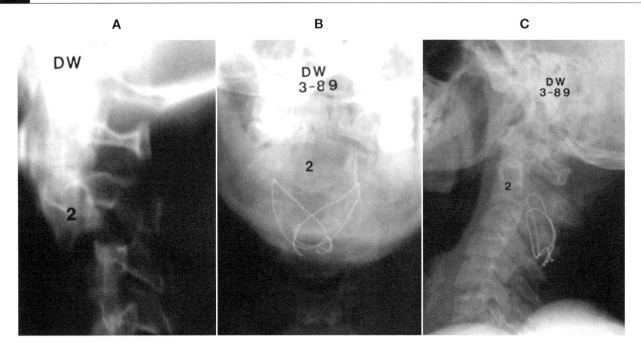

Fig. 35-35 **A,** Lateral tomogram of upper cervical spine demonstrating type III hangman fracture with dislocation of C2-3 facets. **B** and **C,** After open reduction and posterior stabilization with bilateral oblique facet wires. This 18-year-old patient was a ventilator-dependent quadriplegic after this fracture.

tion. These fractures frequently are associated with neurological deficits. Open reduction and internal fixation usually are required because of inability to obtain or maintain reduction of the C2-3 facet dislocation. Because the lamina and spinous process of C2 are a free floating fragment, bilateral oblique wiring of C2-3 is necessary for stable reduction (Fig. 35-35). After posterior cervical fusion at the C2-3 level, halo vest immobilization for 3 months is necessary for the bipedicular fracture and for consolidation of the fusion mass.

Injuries to Lower Cervical Spine (C3-7)

Injuries to the lower cervical spine are different from those involving the upper cervical region. Patients with these injuries may have isolated minor compression and avulsion fractures or severe fractures and fracture-dislocations and profound neurological deficits. The primary goals of treatment are to realign the spine, prevent loss of function of uninjured neurological tissue, improve neurological recovery, obtain and maintain spinal stability, and obtain early functional recovery.

Posterior Ligamentous Injury. Failure of the posterior ligamentous complex is caused by distraction and flexion forces and is manifested by widening of the interspinous process space during flexion (Fig. 35-36). These injuries may be difficult to diagnose. Disruption of the posterior ligamentous complex may cause unilateral or bilateral facet dislocation and can occur with or without neurological deficits. Because it is a purely ligamentous injury, healing is unlikely with external immobilization, and chronic pain, progressive deformity, or increasing neurological deficit may occur. We recommend

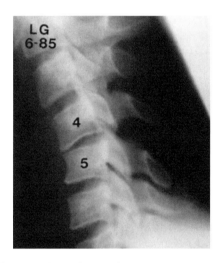

Fig. 35-36 Tearing of posterior ligamentous structures is evidenced by widening of interspinous process space, as well as widening of posterior aspect of C4-5 disc space. Patient was neurologically intact and complained only of neck pain after motor vehicle accident.

posterior cervical fusion with interspinous process wiring or oblique facet joint wiring to obtain stability, maintain alignment, prevent chronic pain or progressive deformity, and protect the neural elements.

Unilateral Facet Dislocation. Unilateral facet dislocations usually result from flexion and rotation of the cervical spine. They are considered stage 2 distractive flexion injuries (see pp. 1604 to 1606 for classification). The most common site of dislocation is at C5-6. Patients may present with an isolated nerve root injury or an incomplete neurological deficit. The injury may be purely ligamentous or may involve a facet fracture in addition to the dislocation. Unilateral facet dislocations may be difficult to reduce in skeletal traction. Closed reduction may be attempted to unlock the dislocated facet joint; however, this is successful in less than 50% of patients and we do not routinely use manipulation of the cervical spine. Rorabeck et al. reviewed 26 patients with unilateral facet dislocations and found that 12 had isolated dislocations and 14 had fractures of the facets or vertebral bodies; closed reduction was possible in only six patients. Of the other 20, 10 fractures were left unreduced and 10 had open reduction. Those patients who underwent open reduction and fusion had better results than those whose fractures were left unreduced. In our experience, open reduction and internal fixation of unilateral facet dislocations have provided consistently good results. If a unilateral facet dislocation can be reduced in skull traction, halo vest immobilization can be used for 3 months, with the possibility that stability will be obtained by spontaneous fusion. However, if skull traction does not reduce the dislocation, we prefer to proceed with open reduction and posterior cervical fusion with either triple wiring or oblique facet wiring for additional rotational control (Fig. 35-37). Postoperative treatment consists of immobilization in a rigid cervical orthosis for 6 to 8 weeks.

Often patients present with chronic pain, limitation of rotation, and radiculopathy caused by a unilateral jump facet that was either missed initially or was allowed to heal unreduced. For these patients with nerve root impingement and chronic pain, we recommend foraminotomy with decompression of the involved nerve root and posterior cervical fusion over the involved segment. Reduction with traction may be attempted, but this usually is impossible.

Bilateral facet dislocations are flexion-rotation injuries and are considered stage 3 distractive flexion lesions. These injuries produce approximately 50% anterior subluxation of one vertebral body on the vertebra below. Usually both facet capsules, the posterior longitudinal ligament, and the posterior annulus fibrosus and disc are disrupted. These injuries are more frequently associated with neurological deficits than are unilateral facet dislocations. These dislocations are more easily reduced with closed traction methods than are unilateral dislocations, but because they are so unstable, redislocation is frequent when they are treated with prolonged skeletal traction or even in a halo vest. Some bilateral facet dislocations heal with spontaneous anterior interbody fusions, but this is unpredictable and we prefer open reduction and internal fixation with an interspinous process wiring technique, such as the Bohlman triple-wire technique, or oblique wiring from the inferior facet of the upper level to the spinous process of the lower level (Fig. 35-38). Posterior cervical plating also provides stable fixation and is advantageous when laminar and spinous processes are deficient.

Studies by Arena et al. have demonstrated the association of

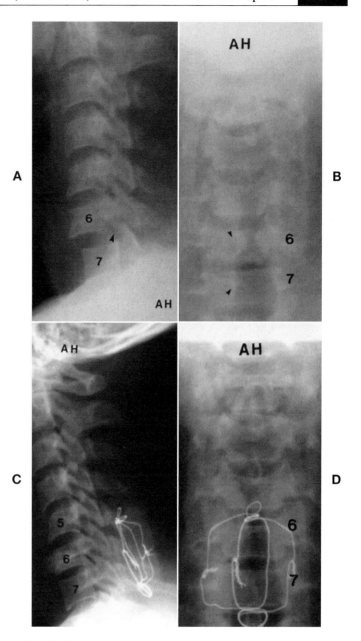

Fig. 35-37 **A** and **B,** Mild anterior subluxation of C6 on C7; spinous process fracture of C6 is visible on lateral view and malrotation of spinous process on anteroposterior view. **C** and **D,** Realignment of cervical spine after open reduction and posterior fusion from C5 to C7 with triple-wire technique.

disc herniation with unilateral and bilateral facet dislocations. Disc herniations occurred in 6 of 68 patients (8.8%) in their series, and most were identified by myelography, postmyelography CT scanning, or MRI. Vaccaro et al. reported an increased incidence of disc herniation after awake closed traction reduction for cervical spine dislocation. Two of the 11 patients had disc herniations noted on MRI before reduction; however, after reduction 5 patients were noted to have disc herniations, although none had increased neurological deficit. Although the process of closed traction reduction appears to

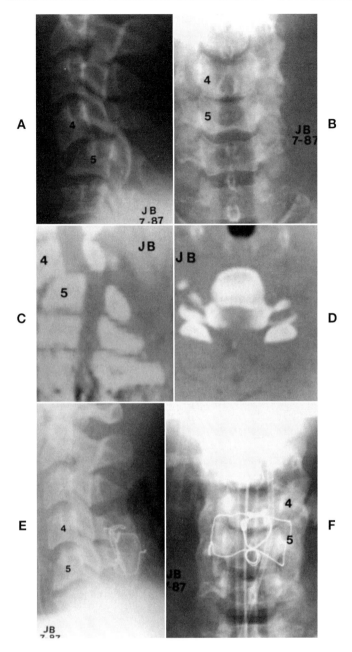

Fig. 35-38 **A** and **B,** Twenty-year-old patient with distractive flexion injury of C4-5 (bilateral facet dislocation) and complete spinal cord injury. **C** and **D,** CT scans confirm facet dislocation with marked canal stenosis. **E** and **F,** Realignment of spine after posterior cervical arthrodesis with triple-wire technique.

increase the incidence of intervertebral disc herniations, the relationship of these findings to the neurological safety of this procedure remains unclear. One roentgenographic indication of disc herniation is marked narrowing of intervertebral disc space on the plain lateral view. Failure to recognize a herniated disc associated with unilateral or bilateral facet injuries may result in increased neurological deficit when realignment of the spine with skull traction is attempted. Arena et al. recommended

anterior discectomy for removal of extruded disc material before posterior interspinous wiring and fusion.

Fractures of Vertebral Body. Vertebral body fractures may range from stable compression fractures without neurological involvement to highly unstable burst fractures with significant neurological injury. Many mechanisms of injury are possible, but most vertebral body fractures result from axial loading and flexion. Eismont et al. have shown that the sagittal dimension of the cervical spinal canal plays an important role in determining the degree of neurological deficit with these injuries. Mild compression fractures with minimal displacement and without posterior element fracture, ligament disruption, facet dislocation, or neurological injury are stable fractures that will heal with 8 to 12 weeks of external cervical orthotic immobilization. The stability of the posterior ligamentous structures should be verified by the criteria of White and Panjabi (p. 1606) or by the stretch test previously described (p. 1606). More significant body fractures, such as burst fractures with posterior element disruption and incompetent posterior ligaments, are unstable injuries and usually result in displacement of posterior fragments into the spinal canal, causing spinal cord injury. The initial treatment of these injuries is application of longitudinal skull traction to realign the spinal canal, using intact soft tissue structures to pull the retropulsed bone fragments into more acceptable alignment and decrease cord compression. Care must be taken, however, not to overdistract the cervical spine, and lateral cervical roentgenograms are mandatory after application of skeletal traction. After the patient's condition has stabilized, a decision should be made as to whether the spinal cord should be decompressed through an anterior approach and whether posterior stabilization is required. Stauffer has emphasized the problems that may be encountered in anterior vertebral body excision and strut grafting when the posterior ligaments are disrupted. If decompression is indicated and the posterior interspinous ligaments are intact, anterior vertebral body excision and grafting with an iliac bone strut can be performed and has proven useful in the management of patients with incomplete quadriplegia or those who have failure of root recovery at the level of injury (see Fig. 35-15). In patients with documented compression of the neural elements from retropulsed bone fragments and incompetent posterior elements and ligamentous structures, anterior strut grafting alone usually is inadequate. Studies from the AO/ASIF and others have indicated that anterior plate fixation is successful in the management of these injuries, but the indications for rigid internal fixation of the cervical spine are still evolving. Clearly, increased complications may occur from the use of such fixation, including iatrogenic neurological deficits and loss of reduction with loosening of the implants. More biomechanical data are necessary to define the indications for their use. For fractures that combine posterior instability with anterior compression of the cord or nerve roots, we prefer a combined procedure consisting of anterior decompression and strut grafting with posterior stabilization by interspinous wiring (see Fig. 35-16). The addition of anterior cervical plating may preclude the need for posterior stabilization in many instances; however, many highly unstable cervical spine injuries require more rigid internal fixation that is afforded by anterior plate and screw fixation. In patients in whom the spinous processes and lamina are deficient, posterior cervical plating is indicated to achieve stable fixation. These procedures may be carried out simultaneously or in stages. McAfee and Bohlman reported their experience with simultaneous anterior and posterior cervical spine procedures, and we agree that the two procedures may be successfully carried out at the same time. As others have noted, there is an extensive learning curve with these advanced surgical techniques; however, as surgeons gain experience the complication rate should decline. Postoperative immobilization generally consists of 12 weeks in a rigid cervical brace.

Other isolated fractures of the cervical spine may occur, including fractures of the lamina, lateral masses, spinous processes, and pedicles, as well as small avulsion fractures off the anterior, inferior, or superior margins of the vertebral bodies. The stability of these fractures should be determined before treatment. In general, these isolated fractures are stable injuries and require only immobilization in a rigid cervical orthosis or halo vest until union occurs.

◆ Triple-Wire Procedure for Posterior Fusion

This procedure may be done safely with the patient under general or local anesthesia. In patients with high cervical quadriplegia, local anesthesia may be preferred to avoid the respiratory complications that may be encountered with general anesthesia. Usually, the patient is intubated with an atraumatic, fiberoptic intubation technique and is then positioned prone on a Stryker turning frame. Longitudinal traction is applied to the shoulders and is maintained with tape. A permanent lateral roentgenogram is obtained in the operating room to document alignment of the cervical spine.

TECHNIQUE 35-9 *(Bohlman)*

With the patient prone on the Stryker frame, prepare and drape the posterior neck and the iliac crest. Make a midline posterior incision, usually extending one spinous process above and one below the segment to be fused. Infiltration of the skin, subcutaneous tissue, and erector spinae muscle down to the lamina with a 1:500,000 epinephrine solution is helpful in obtaining hemostasis. Carry subperiosteal exposure down to the lamina with electrocautery. Dissect laterally on either side of the lateral margin of the facet joint. With a marker on a spinous process, obtain a lateral roentgenogram to confirm accurate location.

Using either a small high-speed burr or a towel clip, drill holes in the bases of the spinous processes to be wired (Fig. 35-39, *A*). To avoid passage of the wire into the spinal canal, take care to place the holes posterior to the spinal laminar fusion line. Pass a 20-gauge wire through the hole in the superior spinous process, loop it over the top of the superior edge, pass it through and around the inferior

spinous process, and carefully twist its ends together (Fig. 35-39, *B* to *D*). Then pass 22-gauge wires through and around the holes in the spinous process of the superior and inferior vertebrae to be fused, in preparation for securing a thick unicortical cancellous bone graft. Measure the length of the area to be fused and harvest a bone graft from the posterior iliac crest of sufficient size that it can be divided into two pieces for placement on each side of the fusion. Harvest strips of cancellous bone from the pelvis and place them beneath the thick unicortical cancellous bone grafts. Make holes in the superior and inferior ends of the grafts, pass the 22-gauge wires through them, and tighten the wires to hold the grafts in place against the lamina and spinous processes. Cut off the wires and bend them to prevent protrusion into the soft tissues (Fig. 35-39, *E* and *F*). Grasp the spinous process of one vertebra and pick it up to test stability; the wired levels should move as one unit. Confirm the position of the wires and fusion of the proper segments with a lateral roentgenogram. Thoroughly irrigate the wound with an antibiotic solution and close it in layers over a suction drain.

AFTERTREATMENT. In most patients skeletal traction can be discontinued and a cervical orthosis can be applied immediately after surgery. If preferred, the patient may be kept supine with light cervical traction for 24 to 48 hours before the orthosis is allowed. Prophylactic antibiotics are recommended for 48 hours. The cervical orthosis is worn for 8 to 12 weeks, and then lateral flexion and extension roentgenograms are made. The brace is discontinued when fusion is evident and stability is documented on lateral flexion and extension views.

◆ Oblique Facet Wiring

This technique is a modification of the procedure described by Robinson and Southwick. It is indicated when the posterior elements are insufficient for spinous process wiring or additional rotational stability is needed (Fig. 35-40). The procedure may be performed when there are fractures of the lamina or spinous processes or after previous laminectomy.

TECHNIQUE 35-10

Position the patient prone on a Stryker frame with cervical alignment maintained using skeletal traction in either a halo ring or Gardner-Wells tongs. Using electrocautery, expose the posterior elements in the midline as described for the triple-wire technique. Be sure to expose the lateral margins of the facet joints to allow adequate access. After roentgenographic verification of the level to be fused, use a 7/64-inch bit to drill a hole in the lateral mass at 45 degrees off the horizontal through the inferior facet (Fig. 35-41, *A*). The facet joint can be pried open with a small Freer or a Penfield elevator. Pass a 20- or 22-gauge stainless steel wire

continued

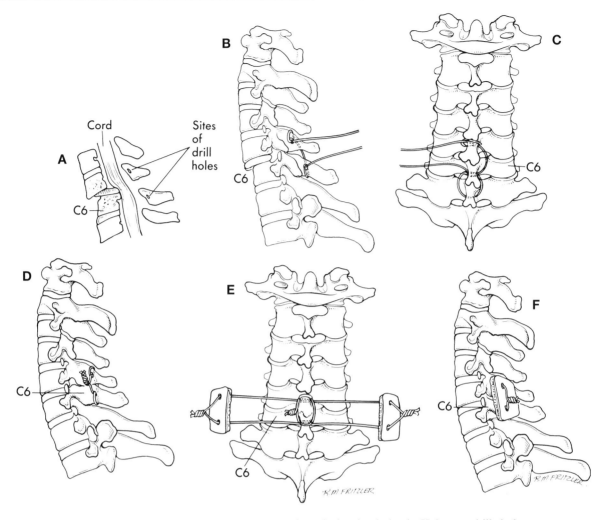

Fig. 35-39 Bohlman triple-wire technique of cervical arthrodesis. **A,** Holes are drilled above spinolaminar fusion line. **B** to **D,** Midline 20-gauge tethering wire is wrapped through and around spinous processes above and below. **E,** Two 22-gauge wires are added to secure thick unicortical cancellous bone grafts against posterior elements. **F,** Final position of graft.

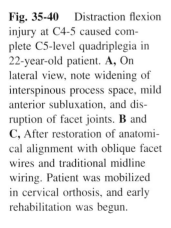

Fig. 35-40 Distraction flexion injury at C4-5 caused complete C5-level quadriplegia in 22-year-old patient. **A,** On lateral view, note widening of interspinous process space, mild anterior subluxation, and disruption of facet joints. **B** and **C,** After restoration of anatomical alignment with oblique facet wires and traditional midline wiring. Patient was mobilized in cervical orthosis, and early rehabilitation was begun.

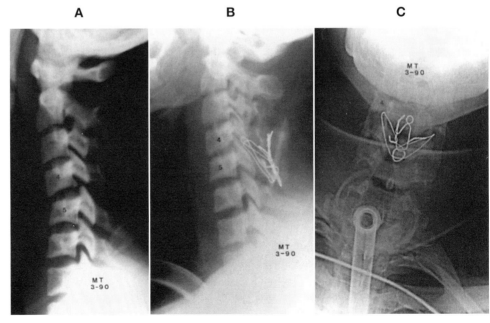

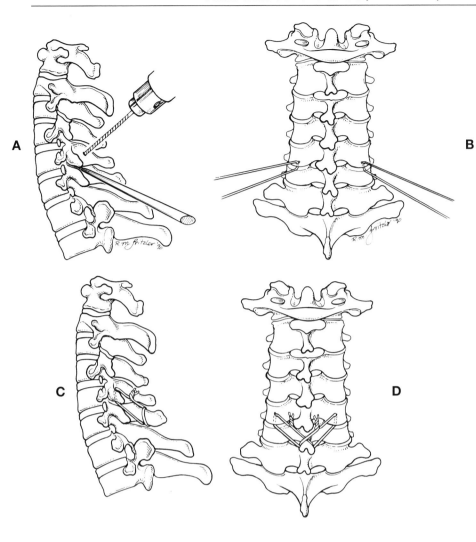

Fig. 35-41   Oblique facet wiring. **A,** Hole is drilled in lateral mass at 45-degree angle to horizontal; note placement of Penfield elevator in facet joint. **B,** Oblique facet wires are placed through holes in articular masses. **C** and **D,** Wires are tightened around intact caudal spinous process. (Modified from Robinson RA, Southwick WO: *South Med J* 53:565, 1960.)

through the hole in the facet joint and grasp it with a small hemostat. Repeat this procedure on each facet bilaterally (Fig. 35-41, *B*). Tighten the wires down and around an intact spinous process inferiorly (Fig. 35-41, *C* and *D*) or pass them through a thick, unicortical, cancellous bone graft. Close the wound in layers over a suction drain.

AFTERTREATMENT. A halo vest or rigid cervical orthosis is worn for 8 to 12 weeks or until stability is confirmed by lateral flexion and extension roentgenograms.

◆ Anterior Decompression and Fusion

The middle and lower cervical spine is most commonly exposed through an anterior approach medial to the carotid sheath. A thorough knowledge of anatomical fascial planes, as described by Robinson and Southwick, allows a safe, direct approach to this area. Reports have suggested that stability is improved with the use of anterior plates and screws, but these also increase the risk of iatrogenic neurological deficits. In our experience, anterior decompression and placement of the strut graft are safe

and effective without internal fixation. Biomechanical testing has shown that if the posterior ligaments are stable, the addition of anterior plate fixation to structural bone grafting of an injured level significantly reduces motion at that level.

TECHNIQUE 35-11

Place the patient supine with skeletal traction maintained through tongs or a halo ring. Exposure may be through either a transverse or longitudinal incision, depending on the surgeon's preference. We usually prefer a left-sided transverse incision (Fig. 35-42) because of the more constant anatomy of the recurrent laryngeal nerve and the lower risk of inadvertent injury. In general, make an incision three to five fingerbreadths above the clavicle to expose from C3-5 and two to three fingerbreadths above the clavicle to expose from C5-7. Center the transverse incision over the medial border of the sternocleidomastoid muscle. Infiltration of the skin and subcutaneous tissues with a 1:500,000 epinephrine solution aids hemostasis. Incise the platysma muscle in line with the skin incision. Identify the anterior border of the sternocleidomastoid muscle and incise longitudinally the superficial layer of the deep cervical

continued

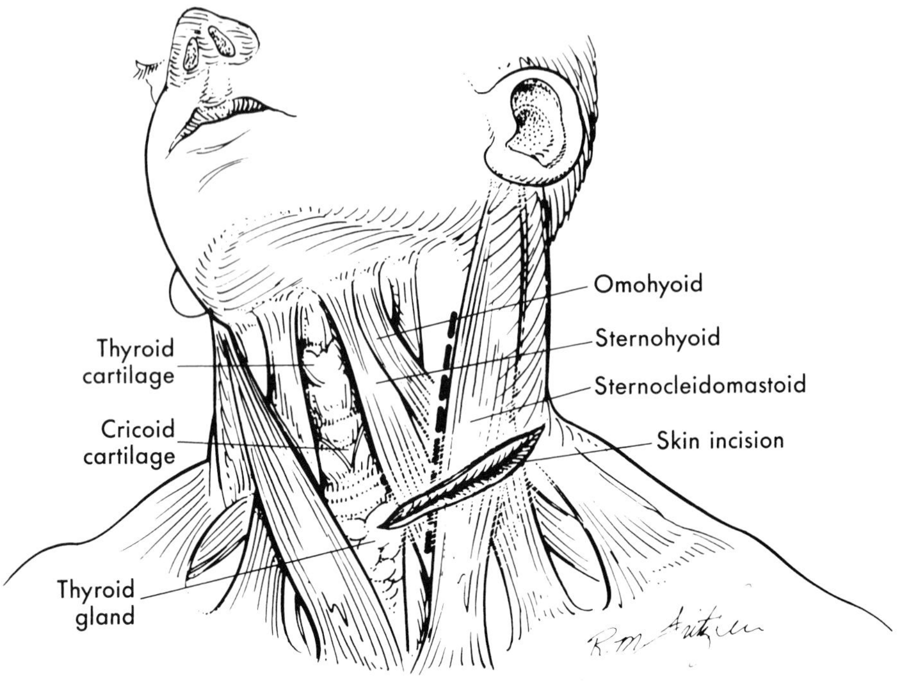

Fig. 35-42 Anterior approach to middle and lower cervical spine through left-sided transverse incision. Dissection is carried medially to carotid sheath and laterally to trachea and esophagus. (Redrawn from Southwick WO, Robinson RA: *J Bone Joint Surg* 39A:631, 1957.)

fascia while localizing the carotid pulse with finger palpation. Carefully divide the middle layer of the deep cervical fascia that encloses the omohyoid medial to the carotid sheath. Retract the sternocleidomastoid muscle and carotid sheath laterally and palpate the anterior aspect of the cervical spine. Identify the esophagus posterior to the trachea and retract medially the trachea, esophagus, and thyroid. Bluntly divide the deep layers of the deep cervical fascia, consisting of the pretracheal and prevertebral fasciae overlying the longus colli muscle. Reflect the longus colli subperiosteally from the anterior aspect of the spine laterally to the level of the uncovertebral joints (Fig. 35-43) to provide exposure for wide decompression and bone grafting. Usually the fractured vertebra can be readily identified; however, to accurately locate the area of decompression, place a needle into a disc space and obtain a lateral roentgenogram.

After identification of the level of decompression, incise the anterior longitudinal ligament and annulus overlying the adjacent disc and remove this material with curets. Using hand-held rongeurs or a high-speed drill, remove the anterior portion of the fractured vertebral body (Fig. 35-44, *A* and *B*). Remove disc material back to the posterior longitudinal ligament. Completely remove the intervertebral disc to allow identification of the posterior longitudinal ligament and to help determine the extent of the corpectomy. Next, using power burrs and hand-held curets, carefully remove the posterior aspect of the vertebral body; use pituitary forceps as the posterior cortical wall of the vertebra

is approached (Fig. 35-44, *C* and *D*). Carefully remove retropulsed bone and disc fragments from the spinal canal.

Define the lateral margin of dissection by the uncovertebral joints. Take care not to extend the dissection too far laterally because of the risk of injury to the vertebral bodies. After completion of the anterior carpectomy, expose the end plates of the superior and inferior vertebrae and make seating holes with an angled curet or small burr in preparation for placement of the tricortical iliac crest of fibular graft (Fig. 35-44, *E*). Center these seating holes in the end plate and make them large enough to allow placement of approximately half the length of the distal phalanx of the little finger. Once the holes have been made, Gelfoam can be placed over the exposed dura mater, which should expand anteriorly after complete decompression. Harvest the iliac strut graft and fashion it into a T-shape, with the cancellous portion facing anteriorly. Increase longitudinal traction and lock the graft into the seating holes. Trim the anterior aspect of the graft flush with the front of the vertebral bodies to prevent erosion into the esophagus. Obtain a lateral roentgenogram to confirm proper position of the graft. Place a drain along the anterior aspect of the spine to prevent postoperative respiratory compromise from a hematoma in the prevertebral space. Close the platysma muscle, the subcutaneous tissues, and the skin in layers.

AFTERTREATMENT. Depending on the degree of stability, a rigid cervical orthosis or halo vest is worn for 8 to 12 weeks while the bone graft incorporates.

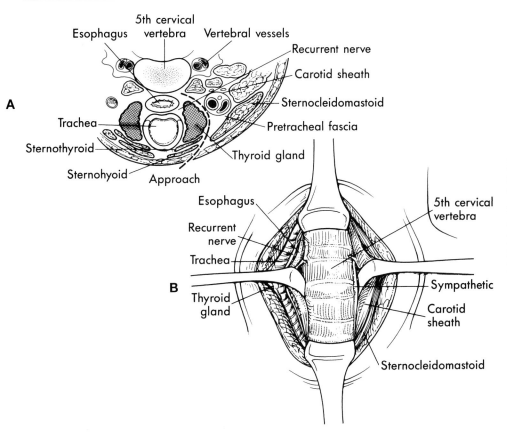

Fig. 35-43 Deep dissection to middle and lower cervical spine. Thorough knowledge of anatomical fascial planes is mandatory to gain adequate exposure of anterior aspect of cervical spine. (Redrawn from Southwick WO, Robinson RA: *J Bone Joint Surg* 39A:631, 1957.)

Posterior and Anterior Cervical Fusion with Rigid Internal Fixation. Rigid internal fixation of the cervical spine was developed because of certain inherent limitations of interspinous wiring when instability is severe or the posterior elements are deficient. Posterior stabilization of the cervical spine with rigid internal fixation devices has been described by several authors, including Roy-Camille et al.; Magerl and Seemann; Louis; Anderson, and Montesano; and Hadley et al. These implants consist of posterior plates and screws or hook plates and offer the advantage of rigid fixation of a single motion segment, thereby minimizing the extent of fusion and increasing postoperative mobility of the cervical spine. In addition, Harrington and Luque instrumentations have been modified by segmental wiring of the facet joints to obtain stability of certain fractures and dislocations.

Anterior internal fixation of the cervical spine provides stability after decompression and may make additional posterior surgery unnecessary. Anterior implants involve plating systems that depend on engaging the posterior vertebral wall (bicortical purchase) to prevent screw loosening, or unicortical screws with expansion heads locked to the plate, creating an intrinsically stable implant. Each of these techniques has advantages and disadvantages, and good results with few complications have been reported for each. Although the number of patients in whom these devices have been used is not large and the follow-up not long, these techniques offer advantages over conventional wiring techniques in certain groups of high-risk patients.

Proper patient selection and meticulous surgical technique are necessary to obtain a satisfactory result with minimal morbidity. Although internal fixation techniques have become more advanced, the expected benefits must be carefully weighed against the known risks.

◆ Posterior Cervical Plating

Lateral mass plating provides rigid internal fixation and improved fusion when spinous processes are incompetent or a laminectomy has been performed previously. Heller et al. reported on the inherent anatomical risks, variations in anatomy, morphology, and bone quality that impose limitations on this procedure.

TECHNIQUE 35-12 *(Anderson et al.)*
Place the patient prone. Expose the posterior cervical spine subperiosteally to the border of the facet joints. A thorough understanding of the anatomy of the cervical spine is required for safe insertion of lateral mass screws. Remove the facet capsules and identify the boundaries of the lateral mass, which consist of the superior articular surface, the inferior articular surface, the lateral border, and the medial sulcus (Fig. 35-45, *A*). Select an entry portal 1 mm medial

continued

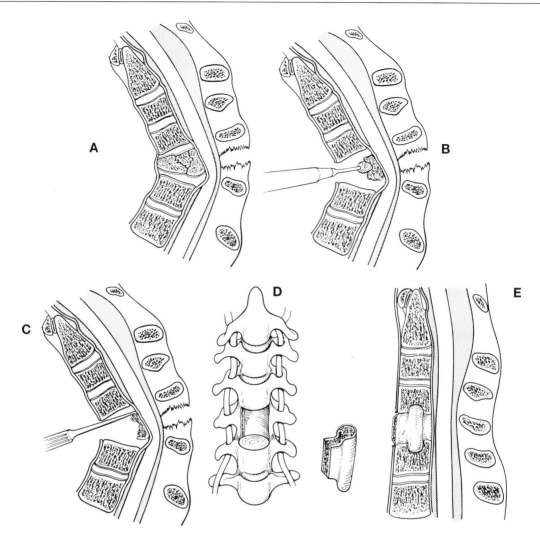

Fig. 35-44   **A,** Typical burst fracture at C5 with retropulsed bone and disc fragments in spinal canal compressing neural elements. **B,** Material above and below fractured vertebra has been removed, and high-speed power burr is used to remove bone back to level of posterior longitudinal ligament. **C,** Residual posterior vertebral margin is removed with small curet to decompress neural elements. **D,** Extent of anterior cervical corpectomy. **E,** Placement of tricortical iliac crest graft after adequate cervical decompression. (**A** redrawn from Bohlman HH: *J Bone Joint Surg* 61A:1119, 1979; **B** to **E** redrawn from Bohlman HH, Eismont FJ: *Clin Orthop* 154:57, 1981.)

to the center of the lateral mass. Drilling of the lateral mass should be 25 to 35 degrees laterally and 15 degrees cephalad (parallel to the plane of the facet joint) for C3 to C6 (Fig. 35-45, *B*). The drilling should be 10 to 25 degrees medially and 25 degrees superiorly at C2 to avoid injuring the vertebral artery (Fig. 35-45, *C*). Use a drill with a stop guide to prevent drilling of the opposite cortex. Tap the drill hole. Place and secure a contoured posterior cervical plate with cortical screws of the appropriate length. Before placing the implants, place cancellous bone grafts in the facet joints after decortication of the articular cartilage. In simple dislocations, internal fixation can be limited to one motion segment (Fig. 35-46); for more unstable fractures

and fracture-dislocations, internal fixation should be extended to two motion segments, with a screw above and below the level of injury. Potential areas of danger in posterior plate screw fixation of the cervical spine include the vertebral artery, spinal cord, and nerve roots. Obtain preoperative CT scans to scrutinize the location of the vertebral artery. The nerve exits at the anterolateral aspect of the superior articular process and may be injured inadvertently if the lateral mass screw is placed too medially or too cephalad.

AFTERTREATMENT. After posterior internal fixation, immobilization in a cervical orthosis is recommended; in most instances a halo vest is not necessary. The posterior implant

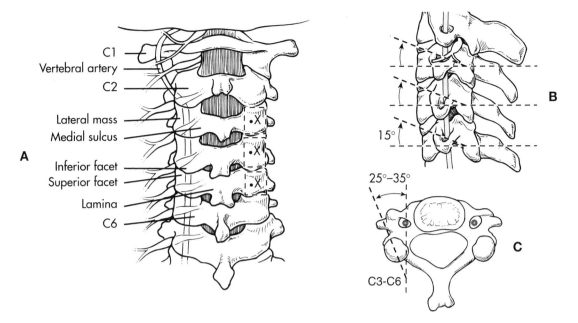

Fig. 35-45 Posterior cervical plating. **A,** Landmarks used for identifying center of lateral mass and point for drilling. **B,** Relationship of facet joints, nerve root, and drill angle. **C,** Superior view of cervical vertebra showing relationship of drill angle, foramen transversarium, and vertebral artery. (Redrawn from Leventhal MR: *Op Tech Sports Med* 1:199, 1993.)

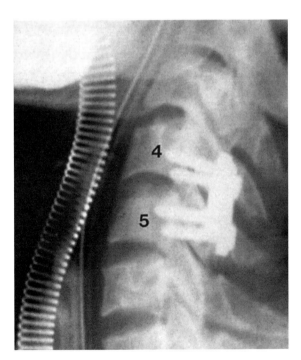

Fig. 35-46 Lateral view of cervical spine after internal fixation of C4-5 dislocation with lateral mass plates and screws. (From Leventhal MR: *Op Tech Sports Med* 1:199, 1993.)

may loosen or the screws may break if external mobilization is not used.

◆ *Anterior Cervical Plating*

The development of anterior cervical plates now allows immediate rigid internal fixation after decompression and bone grafting. The major differences in the techniques depend on the necessity of unicortical or bicortical screw purchase (Fig. 35-47).

TECHNIQUE 35-13 *(Morscher et al.)*

After positioning the patient supine, expose the anterior cervical spine medial to the carotid sheath. After anterior cervical corpectomy, restore the anterior and middle columns by placing a strut graft harvested from either the iliac crest or fibula (Fig. 35-48).

Cervical spine locking plates do not rely on screw perforation of the posterior vertebral cortex for stability. A

continued

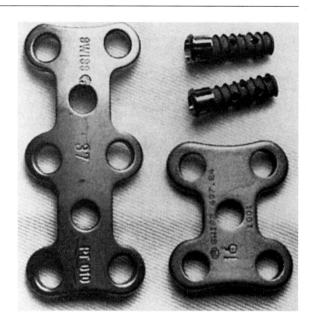

Fig. 35-47 Anterior cervical spine locking plate and screws. (From Leventhal MR: *Op Tech Sports Med* 1:199, 1993.)

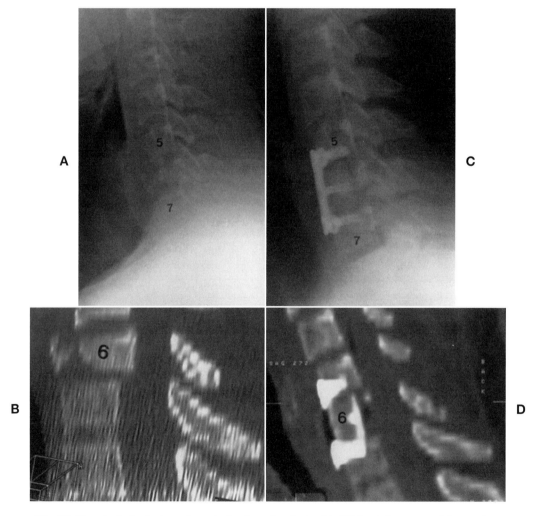

Fig. 35-48 **A,** Lateral view of cervical spine of patient with C6 burst fracture and incomplete spinal cord injury. **B,** Sagittal reconstruction of C6 burst fracture demonstrates retropulsed bone fragment into spinal canal. **C** and **D,** Postoperative lateral view and CT scan show decompression of spinal canal, strut graft, and cervical plate.

special expansion-head locking screw is used to lock the screw to the plate. The drill guide with stop ensures a safe drilling depth without roentgenographic control and reduces the risk to the spinal cord. Both smooth and plasma-sprayed screws with expansion heads are available to anchor the plate to the cervical spine. The plates are available in five- and eight-hole configurations of varying lengths.

Use the plate positioner to hold the plate against the cervical spine while drilling. Place each anchor screw before drilling any subsequent holes. Use the drill guide and a 3-mm bit. Screw penetration is 14 mm. Take care to protect soft tissue structures in the neck during drilling. Use a 4-mm tap to cut the screw thread, then place the expansion screws using a cruciform screwdriver. Insert the screw until the rim of the screw head is flush with the plate. Seat all anchor screws one at a time before placing the 1.8-mm locking screws. Insert the 1.8-mm locking screws to achieve an intrinsically stable construct between the plate and screw. Seat each locking screw into the expansion-head screw, thus compressing the sides of the screw head against the plate and locking it into the plate hole.

Anterior plate fixation with standard H-type or Caspar plates also provides satisfactory rigid internal fixation in the stabilization of fractures and dislocations of the cervical spine. These implants differ from the cervical spine locking plate in that they require bicortical screw purchase. Because the posterior vertebral body wall must be engaged, there is increased risk of injury to the neural elements. Special drill guides have been developed with stopping devices to control the depth of drilling, and careful roentgenographic control must be used when inserting these implants. Experimental studies are under way to determine if these implants are biomechanically superior or inferior to posterior fixation alone.

AFTERTREATMENT. External immobilization is recommended with a rigid cervical brace. In most instances a halo vest is not needed.

Complications. Potential complications include loosening of the screws and the plate, erosion into the esophagus, and breakage of the plate if a pseudarthrosis develops.

◆ ◆ ◆

The ORION anterior cervical plate offers certain advantages over the Morscher plating system. Screws may be placed in a convergent or divergent manner, and unicortical and bicortical screw purchase may be achieved. The amount of lordosis present in the ORION anterior cervical plate is acceptable in most instances; however, the lordosis may be altered by gentle bending if necessary. An anterior locking screw is threaded into the plate to prevent the bone screws from backing out.

TECHNIQUE 35-14 *(Lowery)*

Place the patient supine, and position the head in a stable supine position, using a headrest or traction, with slight extension of the neck. Confirm the positioning and vertebral levels with fluoroscopy. Countertraction on the arm often is helpful. For one- or two-level corpectomies, make a standard transverse incision. Dissect the fascial planes fully for longer constructs. For long reconstructions or difficult exposures, a carotid incision may be necessary. Perform corpectomy or prepare interbody fusion receptor sites. Obtain cervical lordosis or distraction, if necessary. Prepare a trapezoid strut construct or one or more trapezoidal interbody fusion wedges. Carefully position and impact the strut or interbody fusion construct. Release distraction and check the stability of the construct. Levels to be instrumented can be identified easily with fluoroscopy. Ensure that all anterior osteophytes have been removed for proper positioning of the plate.

Determine the appropriate plate length by positioning the plate screw holes close to the graft receptor site at both the cephalad and caudad ends (Fig. 35-49, *A*). This allows 15 degrees cephalad and caudad screw angulation (Fig. 35-49, *B*) and helps ensure that the plate does not extend over the adjacent disc spaces. If necessary, adjust the lordotic curvature of the plate by using the ORION plate bender to gently bend the plate over its entire length (Fig. 35-49, *C*). Avoid sharp angulations. It is important to note that plate contouring will alter the standard cephalad and caudad angulation of the end screws. Secure the plate holder to the plate by sliding the sleeve toward the handle and engaging the feet into the plate's diagonal slot. Slide the sleeve down toward the plate to lock the holder to the plate (Fig. 35-49, *D*).

Position the plate on the anterior surface of the spine. Review landmarks to ensure that the plate is centered medially and laterally on the spine (Fig. 35-49, *E*). The uncinate processes serve as excellent reference points. Seat the drill guide into the plate at the correct cranial/caudal and convergent angle (Fig. 35-49, *F*). For convergent plate constructs, the drill guide angles 6 degrees toward the midline of the plate. Once the drill guide has been correctly seated, lock it securely into the plate by applying light downward pressure on the drill guide handle. Make sure to align the handle along the longitudinal axis of the plate (Fig. 35-49, *G*). Insert the appropriate bit into the drill guide. Drill the screw holes, using either the 13-mm bit or the adjustable bit and adjustable drill stop for screws other than 13 mm long. Screw length is determined by the depth of bone purchase required. Remove the drill guide, insert the appropriate tap into the predrilled hole at the same angulation, and tap the vertebral bodies using the tap that corresponds to the length of the drill bit. A depth gauge may be used through the plate or against the bone to confirm the depth of the hole for proper screw length. Use the screw

continued

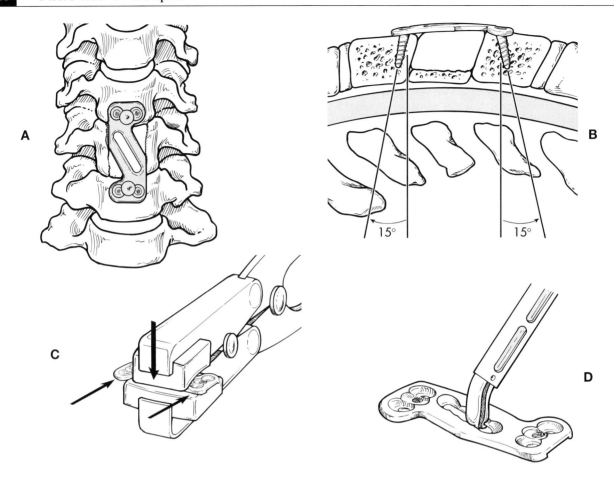

Fig. 35-49   ORION anterior cervical plate system. **A,** Bone graft and plate position. **B,** Cephalad and caudad screw angulation. **C,** Contouring of plate with plate bender. **D,** Plate holder locked into plate.   *Continued*

plate gauge to verify the appropriate screw length. Insert the screw through the plate, using a screwdriver with a tapered, self-holding tip, and tighten the screw securely but not totally (Fig. 35-49, *H*). The recommended order of screw insertion is (1) drill, tap, and place one screw securely through the plate (if necessary, obtain an anteroposterior roentgenogram before drilling the screw hole); (2) drill, tap, and place one screw securely at the opposite end of the plate, diagonally from the first screw position; and (3) drill and tap the remaining two screw implant sites, insert the screws, and secure.

The plate holder can be used throughout the entire procedure. Normally, however, the plate holder is not required after the first one or two screws have been implanted. Tighten the screws to ensure that they are seated

below the surface of the plate (Fig. 35-49, *I*). Obtain roentgenograms to ensure that screw length and screw position are appropriate. Although plate malposition can be determined from a lateral roentgenogram, an anteroposterior roentgenogram provides information for verifying the implant's position.

For multilevel interbody fusions or long strut graft reconstructions, position the drill guide in the center slot of the plate and drill the hole in a straight manner to either 11, 13, or 15 mm depths. Use the gold-colored 4.35-mm tap and adjustable tap stop to tap the hole to the appropriate depth. Use the screwdriver to insert 4.35-mm screws and firmly tighten (Fig. 35-49, *J*).

Attach the lock screw holder to the lock screw by gently squeezing the prongs, then engage the holder into the lock

continued

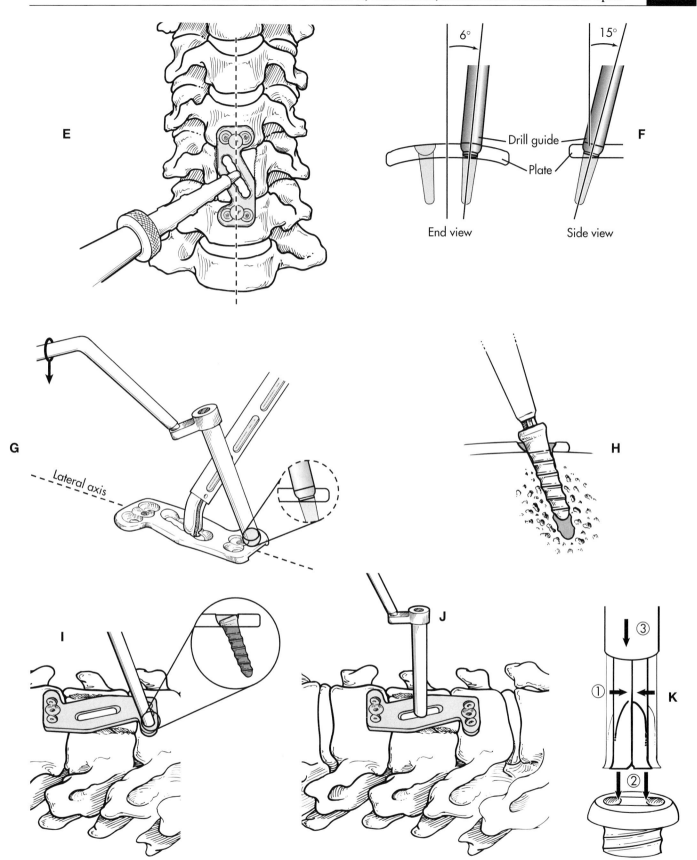

Fig. 35-49, cont'd   E, Positioning of plate medially and laterally. **F,** Angulation of drill guide in cephalad-caudad direction. **G,** Locking drill guide into plate. **H,** Screw insertion. **I,** Final tightening of bone screws. **J,** Placing screw in diagonal slot. **K,** Attaching lock screw holder to lock screw.

Continued

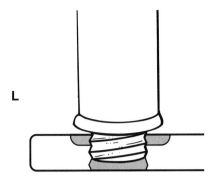

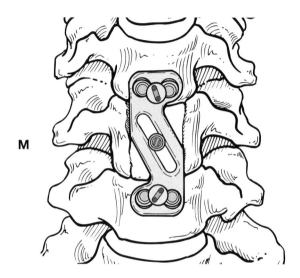

Fig. 35-49, cont'd **L,** Initial threading of lock screw into plate. **M,** Completed ORION anterior cervical plate construct. (Redrawn from Lowery GL: *ORION anterior cervical plate system, surgical technique booklet,* Memphis, 1995, Sofamor Danek.)

screw (Fig. 35-49, *K*). Slide the sleeve down toward the end of the holder. After the lock screw has been initially threaded into the plate (Fig. 35-49, *L*), detach the lock screw holder by pulling the sleeve up and tilting the holder to release it from the lock screw. Do not attempt to tighten the lock screw with the lock screw holder because this will damage the instrument. For final tightening, place the lock screwdriver firmly into the slot and turn the lock screw clockwise until the screwdriver slips out of the slot (this is a self-limiting device). The lock screw is now firmly secured (Fig. 35-49, *M*). Irrigate the wound and close it over a drain.

AFTERTREATMENT. The ORION anterior cervical plate system provides secure, selective vertebral immobilization, obviating in some the need for external brace support while allowing freedom of movement of the unaffected levels. Patients should wear some type of external support, such as a hard collar, when they are in a moving vehicle. Roentgenographic evaluation should be performed at 2, 6, and 12 weeks and then on each of the extended follow-up visits (e.g., 6 months, 12 months) (Fig. 35-50). Physical therapy usually consists of home exercises for range of motion and isometric strengthening.

Thoracic and Lumbosacral Fractures

The treatment of unstable fractures and fracture-dislocations of the thoracic and lumbar spine has long been controversial. Many authors, such as Guttmann and Bedbrook, advised nonoperative treatment, but later reports, such as those by

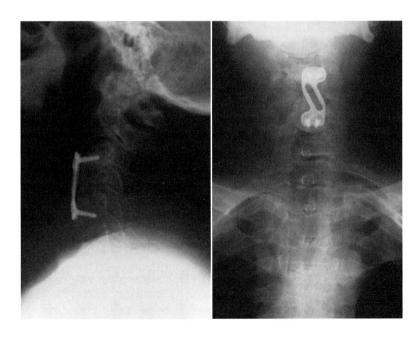

Fig. 35-50 Anteroposterior and lateral roentgenograms of C3-5 fusion with ORION anterior internal fixation device.

Levine and Edwards, Bohlman, Bradford et al., McAfee, Bohlman, and Yuan, Luque, Cassis, and Ramirez-Wiella, Eismont et al., and Cotrel, Dubousset, and Guillaumat have emphasized the advantages of open reduction and rigid internal fixation with posterior instrumentation. Paul of Aegina (625 to 690 AD) first introduced laminectomy for spinal cord injury, unaware of the controversy this would cause. The seventeenth century saw an increase in its use, which has continued to the present. Munro and Irwin, in the late 1930s, advised that laminectomy be delayed and reserved for selected patients. Guttmann condemned the routine use of early laminectomy and certain forms of internal fixation and advocated a conservative program of postural reduction by extension of the spine. Holdsworth and Hardy agreed about the dangers of a routine laminectomy and preferred early open reduction and internal fixation for certain injuries of the thoracolumbar and lumbar spine. Morgan, Wharton, and Austin pointed out that laminectomy offers little benefit in these injuries and is not without morbidity and mortality. We also believe that laminectomy alone is contraindicated in fracture-dislocations because it fails to relieve the anterior compression and increases spinal instability.

CLASSIFICATION OF THORACOLUMBAR FRACTURES

The classification of thoracolumbar fractures has evolved over the past 40 years. Nicoll described these fractures as having stable or unstable patterns. Holdsworth modified and expanded Nicoll's classification, and this modification is the basis of all subsequent classification schemes. Holdsworth classified thoracolumbar fractures into five groups according to the mechanism of injury: (1) *pure flexion,* which causes a stable wedge compression fracture; (2) *flexion and rotation,* which produce an unstable fracture-dislocation with rupture of the posterior ligament complex, separation of the spinous processes, a slice fracture near the upper border of the lower vertebra, and dislocation of the lower articular processes of the upper vertebra; (3) *extension,* which causes rupture of the intervertebral disc and the anterior longitudinal ligament and avulsion of a small bone fragment from the anterior border of the dislocated vertebra; this dislocation almost always reduces spontaneously and is stable in flexion; (4) *vertebral compression,* which causes a fracture of the end plate as the nucleus of the intervertebral disc is forced into the intervertebral body, causing it to burst, with outward displacement of fragments of the body; because the ligaments remain intact, this comminuted fracture is stable; (5) *shearing,* which results in displacement of the whole vertebra and an unstable fracture of the articular processes or pedicles. This classification system does not consider the "unstable burst fracture" described by McAfee et al.

Kelly and Whitesides described the thoracolumbar spine as consisting of two weight-bearing columns: the hollow column of the spinal canal and the solid column of the vertebral bodies. Denis developed a three-column concept of spinal injury using

a series of more than 400 CT scans of thoracolumbar injuries (Fig. 35-51). The anterior column contains the anterior longitudinal ligament, the anterior half of the vertebral body, and the anterior portion of the annulus fibrosus. The middle column consists of the posterior longitudinal ligament, the posterior half of the vertebral body, and the posterior aspect of the annulus fibrosus. The posterior column includes the neural arch, the ligamentum flavum, the facet capsules, and the interspinous ligaments. Denis noted that one or more of the three columns predictably failed in axial compression, axial distraction, or translation from combinations of forces in different planes. In a CT study of 100 consecutive patients with potentially unstable fractures and fracture-dislocations, McAfee et al. determined the mechanisms of failure of the middle osteoligamentous complex and developed a new system based on these mechanisms. We have found their simplified system useful in classifying injuries to the thoracolumbar spine.

1. *Wedge compression fractures* cause isolated failure of the anterior column and result from forward flexion. They rarely are associated with neurological deficit except when multiple adjacent vertebral levels are affected.

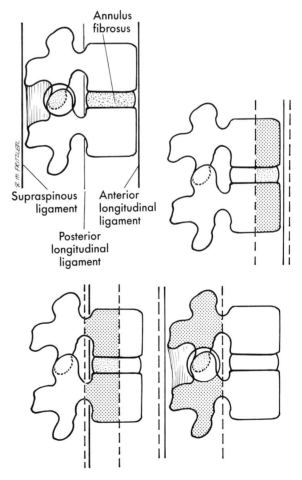

Fig. 35-51 Three-column classification of spinal instability. Illustrations of anterior, middle, and posterior columns (see text). (Redrawn from Denis F: *Spine* 8:817, 1983.)

2. In *stable burst fractures* the anterior and middle columns fail because of a compressive load, with no loss of integrity of the posterior elements.

3. In *unstable burst fractures* the anterior and middle columns fail in compression, and the posterior column is disrupted. The posterior column can fail in compression, lateral flexion, or rotation. There is a tendency for posttraumatic kyphosis and progressive neural symptoms because of instability. If the anterior and middle columns fail in compression, the posterior column cannot fail in distraction.

4. *Chance fractures* are horizontal avulsion injuries of the vertebral bodies caused by flexion about an axis anterior to the anterior longitudinal ligament. The entire vertebra is pulled apart by a strong tensile force.

5. In *flexion distraction injuries* the flexion axis is posterior to the anterior longitudinal ligament. The anterior column fails in compression while the middle and posterior columns fail in tension. This injury is unstable because the ligamentum flavum, interspinous ligaments, and supraspinous ligaments usually are disrupted.

6. *Translational injuries* are characterized by malalignment of the neural canal, which has been totally disrupted. Usually all three columns have failed in shear. At the affected level, one part of the spinal canal has been displaced in the transverse plane.

We believe the three-column classification of McAfee et al. is the best classification scheme currently available; however, not all injuries to the thoracolumbar spine can be assigned to one of the six categories. Plain roentgenograms and CT scanning provide only static images and do not demonstrate maximal displacement. Occult ligamentous injuries are not readily identified on plain films or CT scans, and flexion and extension views of the thoracolumbar spine are risky. A report by Kulkarni et al. suggested that MRI is helpful in detecting occult ligamentous injuries and hemorrhage into surrounding soft tissue structures and in determining the extent of neural damage and the degree of cord edema. They also suggested that MRI may be of value in determining the prognosis for recovery after spinal cord injuries.

Finally, many authors have noted the lack of direct correlation between the severity of neurological deficit and the degree of spinal canal compromise. Retropulsion of bone and disc fragments into the spinal canal clearly is more significant at the thoracolumbar junction than in the lumbar spine because the spinal cord and conus medullaris have a poor prognosis for recovery, whereas the cauda equina, which behaves as a peripheral nerve root lesion, carries a prognosis for neural recovery. Numerous examples of nearly complete canal compromise in patients with normal neurological function have been reported.

TIMING OF SURGERY

The timing of surgery for spinal cord injuries is controversial. Most authors agree that in the presence of a progressive neurological deficit, emergency decompression is indicated. In patients with complete spinal cord injuries or static incomplete spinal cord injuries, some authors advocate delaying surgery for several days to allow resolution of cord edema, whereas others favor early surgical stabilization. There is no conclusive evidence in the literature that early surgical decompression and stabilization improve neurological recovery or that neurological recovery is compromised by a delay of several days. Studies by Bohlman, Transfeldt et al., Bradford et al., and others have documented return of neurological function after anterior decompression done more than a year after the initial injury. For neurologically normal patients with unstable spinal injuries and those with nonprogressive neurological injuries, we believe that open reduction and internal fixation should be carried out as soon as possible. Mirza et al. in a recent study concluded that patients who sustain acute traumatic injuries to the cervical spine with associated neurologic deficit may benefit from cervical decompression and stabilization within 72 hours of injury. Surgery within 72 hours of injury is not associated with a higher complication rate. Early surgery may improve neurological recovery and decrease hospitalization time in patients with cervical spinal cord injuries.

DECOMPRESSION

The role of decompression also is controversial. Compression of the neural elements by retropulsed bone fragments can be relieved indirectly by the insertion of posterior instrumentation or directly by exploration of the spinal canal through a posterolateral or anterior approach. There is no universal agreement as to indications for each of these. The indirect approach to decompression of the spinal canal generally involves insertion of posterior instrumentation (Harrington, Edwards, Cotrell-Dubousset, or Texas Scottish Rite Hospital implants). These techniques use the distraction instrumentation and the intact posterior longitudinal ligament to reduce the retropulsed bone from the spinal canal. Excellent results with this technique have been documented by numerous authors, and it is a familiar technique to most orthopaedic surgeons. Problems with this technique occur if surgery is delayed for several weeks or more because then indirect reduction of the spinal canal cannot be achieved with posterior instrumentation alone. In addition, severely comminuted fractures with multiple pieces of bone pushed into the spinal canal may not be completely reduced by distraction instrumentation. Intraoperative myelographic documentation of reduction of the retropulsed bone fragments may be inadequate, and ultrasonography requires creation of a laminotomy defect to allow insertion of the transducer head; removal of excessive bone may increase instability.

The posterolateral technique for decompression of the spinal canal is effective at the thoracolumbar junction and in the lumbar spine. This procedure involves hemilaminectomy and removal of a pedicle with a high-speed burr to allow posterolateral decompression of the dura along its anterior aspect (Fig. 35-52). In the thoracic spine, where less room is available for the cord, this technique involves increased risk to the neural elements. The anterior approach allows direct

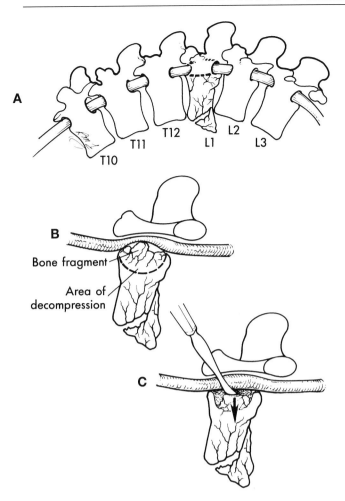

Fig. 35-52 Posterolateral decompression technique. **A,** L1 burst fracture. Pedicle, transverse process, and lateral portions of T12-L1 facet are removed after L1 root has been isolated *(dotted lines).* **B,** Area of encroachment is exposed. **C,** After fragments have been undercut, they are reduced into vertebral body. (Redrawn from McAfee PC, Yuan HA, Lasda NA: *Spine* 7:365, 1982.)

decompression of the thecal sac but is an unfamiliar approach to many surgeons. Visceral and vascular structures may be injured, and this approach carries the greatest risk of potential morbidity. In addition, anterior decompression and placement of an iliac strut graft provide no immediate stability to the fracture unless anterior internal fixation is used. The role of anterior internal fixation devices is rapidly evolving, and these devices have proved to be safe and beneficial in achieving spinal stabilization. The need for posterior stabilization procedures has been eliminated in some patients. When anterior decompression and strut grafting are performed in the face of posterior instability, posterior instrumentation and fusion can be done to improve stability. At this time, we favor early posterior instrumentation in an attempt to achieve anatomical reduction of the fracture. Decompression of the spinal canal is confirmed by intraoperative myelography or ultrasonography. If residual neural compression exists, a posterolateral decompression is carried out. Postoperatively a CT scan of the spine with sagittal reconstructions is obtained through the injured

segment to further evaluate the patency of the spinal canal. If an incomplete neurological deficit exists and significant residual neural compression is documented, we prefer to perform anterior decompression and fusion as staged procedures. In a retrospective review of 49 nonparaplegic patients who sustained an acute unstable, thoracolumbar burst fracture, Danisa et al. concluded that patients treated with posterior surgery had a statistically significant decrease in operative time and blood loss. Three treatment groups were studied. The first group of 16 patients underwent anterior decompression and fusion with instrumentation; the second group of 27 patients underwent posterior decompression and fusion; and the third group of 6 patients had combined anterior-posterior surgery. They noted no significant intergroup differences when considering postoperative kyphotic correction, neurological function, pain assessment, or the ability to return to work. Posterior surgery was found to be as effective as anterior or anteroposterior surgery when treating unstable thoracolumbar burst fractures. Of the three procedures, posterior surgery, however, takes the least time, causes the least blood loss, and is the least expensive.

DEGREE OF CANAL STENOSIS

Studies by McAfee, Denis, Trafton and Boyd, and others have demonstrated no reliable correlation between the degree of compromise of the spinal canal and the severity of the neurological deficit. Because of variations in the diameter of the spinal canal and differences in regional blood supply to the spinal cord in the thoracic and lumbar region and the cauda equina in the lumbosacral spine, the damage to the neural elements caused by fractures and fracture-dislocations is determined to some extent by the level of injury. The spinal canal in the thoracic area is small, and the blood supply is sparse; therefore significant neurological injury is common with severe fractures and dislocations in the thoracic spine. Fractures or fracture-dislocations in the lumbosacral region may result in marked displacement and still cause little or no neurological deficit. Not only is the canal large in this region, but also the spinal cord ends at approximately the first lumbar vertebra and the cauda equina is less vulnerable than the cord above. Experimental work in dogs by Delamarter et al. showed that the neurological signs and symptoms after constriction of the cauda equina occurred progressively and predictably in direct proportion to the percentage of compromise of the canal. Constriction of more than 50% of the cauda equina resulted in complete loss of cortical evoked potentials, neurological deficits, and histological abnormalities. In a recent canine study Carlson et al. found that spinal cord decompression was associated with an early recovery of regional spinal cord blood flow and somatosensory evoked potential. Although spinal cord blood flow was similar in both the compressed and decompressed groups after 3 hours of decompression, somatosensory evoked potential recovery occurred only in the decompressed group.

Denis et al. reported neurological complications in 6 (21%) of 29 patients with burst fractures treated conservatively.

Krompinger et al. reported that late CT analysis of patients with burst fractures treated conservatively showed significant resolution of bony canal compromise. The remodeling process appears to be age and time dependent and follows expected principles of bone remodeling to applied stress. Recent work reported by DeKlerk, Fontijen, and Stijnen showed that remodeling and reconstitution of the spinal canal takes place within the first 12 months after injury. They examined 42 patients who were treated conservatively for a burst fracture of the thoracic, thoracolumbar, or lumbar spine. The mean percentage of the sagittal diameter of the spinal canal was 50% of the normal diameter at the time of the fracture and 75% of the normal diameter at 1-year follow-up examination.

These authors concluded that conservative management of thoracolumbar burst fractures is followed by a marked degree of spontaneous redevelopment of the deformed spinal canal. This study supports conservative management of thoracolumbar burst fractures in selected cases. Neurological deficits have not developed in these patients. The treatment of thoracolumbar burst fractures must be individualized, and canal compromise from retropulsed bone fragments is not in itself an absolute indication for surgical decompression. Nonoperative treatment with canal compromise of up to 50% may be successful in selected patients, although some authors recommend surgical decompression of all burst fractures, regardless of neurological involvement, to prevent late neurological deterioration or progressive kyphosis. We advise patients of the risk and complications of surgery, including inadequate decompression, increased neurological deficit, failure of internal fixation, and the need for implant removal. Our indications for surgical treatment of thoracolumbar spine injuries include burst fractures with 50% or more canal compromise, 30 degrees or more of kyphosis, late neurological deficits, and clearly unstable fractures and fracture-dislocations.

The application of Harrington rods, which initially were used for scoliosis, for the treatment of thoracolumbar fractures and dislocations has resulted in disagreements concerning the number of segments to be instrumented and the length of the posterior fusion mass. Initial work by Dickson, Harrington, and Erwin; Whitesides and Shah; and Meyer suggested that two intact vertebrae above and two below the fracture should be instrumented to provide a lever arm long enough to reduce the fracture and maintain the reduction. Purcell, Markolf, and Dawson recommended hook placement in three laminae above and two below the point of instability to increase stability and reduce the tendency of the upper hook to back out because of vertebral tilting. Edwards and Levine recommended placing hooks 3 to 5 cm above and below the polyethylene rod sleeves to provide a satisfactory lever arm to obtain anatomical reduction of the fracture. Most authors agree that posterior arthrodesis should be performed in conjunction with posterior instrumentation. If the fusion is not performed, the internal fixation device will eventually fail. Kahanovitz, Bullough, and Jacobs showed that internal fixation of the spine without arthrodesis may be a predisposing factor in the development of symptomatic spinal arthritis. Internal fixation without arthrod-

esis of facet joints has been shown to result in irreversible gross and histological findings typical of osteoarthritis. The advantages of "rodding long and fusing short" are perhaps negated by the development of degenerative changes occurring at the unfused but instrumented levels. Arthritic changes have been noted in the facet joints of instrumented but unfused levels in animal models and in humans. Whether the degenerative facet joints cause significant symptoms is uncertain. However, Akbarnia et al. concluded that using long, dual-contoured Harrington distraction rods in short arthrodeses improves vertebral body height and the posttraumatic kyphosis associated with fractures of the thoracolumbar spine without endangering motion of the facets outside the level of arthrodesis. They noted that any long-term degenerative changes of the facet joint of the segments that had not been included in the arthrodesis did not seem to be clinically important. It is clear from biomechanical and clinical studies that preserving motion segments is important in the mobile lumbar spine and perhaps less important in the thoracolumbar region. Extensive research is being done and data collected to further define the appropriate levels to be instrumented, the length of fusion, and the rigidity of the implants used in the treatment of thoracolumbar fractures.

Vertebral Compression Fractures

Wedge compression fractures as defined by McAfee are the result of failure of the anterior column by forward flexion forces. They rarely are associated with neurological deficit, except when multiple adjacent vertebral levels are affected. Medical management is the mainstay of treatment for these acute, painful compression fractures and includes bed rest, analgesics, braces, and physical therapy. In general, the acute pain resolves in 4 weeks to 8 months, but a spinal deformity may be the end result. Many of these fractures are the result of osteoporosis and relatively minor trauma. It appears that many of these fractures are not painful; however, they seem to be associated in certain instances with an impaired quality of life, increased mortality, and a significant morbidity. In a recent review of the clinical consequences of vertebral compression fractures Silverman showed that with each successive fracture, pulmonary force vital capacity was reduced by an average of 9%. Lieberman in unpublished data has shown that patients with vertebral compression fractures are at a 23% increased risk of mortality compared to age-matched controls. Surgical treatment for symptomatic vertebral compression fractures has consisted in the past of reduction and internal fixation using an open anterior or posterior approach. Results have often been compromised because of osteoporosis, resulting in poor implant fixation.

As minimally invasive spinal surgery techniques have evolved, acutely painful vertebral compression fractures can be treated with a percutaneous procedure termed *vertebroplasty*. This procedure entails placing large spinal needles into the fractured vertebral body through a channel made in the pedicle and injecting bone cement into the fractured bone. Vertebroplasty requires high-pressure injection because of the structure

A   B   C

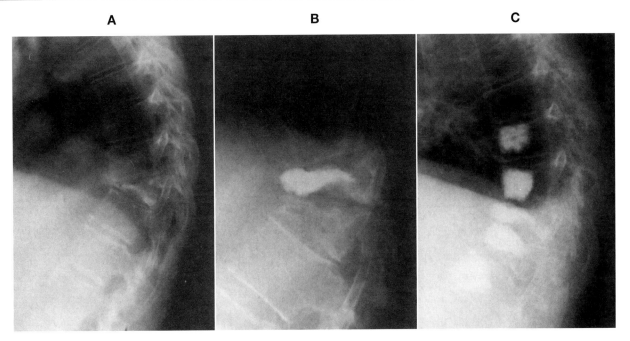

Fig. 35-53   **A,** Severely compressed T11 vertebra producing a marked kyphosis. Patient had dramatic pain reduction after percutaneous vertebroplasty of fractured vertebra. Ten days later, he had severe lower thoracic pain. **B,** Lateral roentgenogram showed new T12 fracture and worsened kyphosis. Radiopaque cement is visible within T11 vertebra. New fracture was thought to be caused by strengthening of T11 vertebra by cement and increased mechanical force exerted on osteoporotic T12 vertebra from the kyphosis. Percutaneous vertebroplasty was performed on acutely fractured T12 vertebra. Prophylactic treatment of adjacent T9, T10, L1, and L2 vertebrae also was performed. **C,** Lateral roentgenogram shows cement within the multiple vertebrae. Injection of cement into T12 was done with patient in hyperextension (although this was not routinely done in other patients). Significant height restoration and reduction in kyphosis were achieved. Patient again reported marked reduction in pain after second procedure. (From Barr JD et al: *Spine* 25:923, 2000).

of the trabeculae and the high viscosity of the bone cement as it hardens. This procedure was designed to decrease pain and strengthen the bone to prevent further collapse and not to restore vertebral body height or prevent spinal deformity. Deramond reported that vertebroplasty reduced pain in 70% to 90% of patients; Chiras reported a major complication rate of 4.5%.

◆ **Vertebroplasty** (Fig. 35-53)

TECHNIQUE 35-15 *(Barr et al.)*

Position the patient prone on a CT scanner table and use sequential images to direct an 11-gauge bone marrow biopsy needle through a posterior transpedicular approach into the vertebral body. After the tip of the needle is advanced through the pedicle, use a portable digital subtraction angiography-capable C-arm to provide lateral fluoroscopy to guide the needle into the anterior half of the vertebral body. Perform an intraosseous venogram to ensure that the needle tip does not have a direct anastomosis with the

epidural or central veins that could allow embolization of the PMMA cement.

Commercially available PMMA cement does not have adequate radiopacity to allow controlled injection with fluoroscopic monitoring. Barr et al. reported the use of 5 g of barium sulfate (E.Z.; EM, Inc., Westbury, NY) and 2 g of tungsten powder (Nycomed, Paris, France) mixed with each kit of PMMA cement (Cranioplastic; Codman and Shurtleff, Inc., Randolph, Mass.) to render the cement radiopaque. Allow the cement mixture to polymerize until it has a pastelike consistency necessary for controlled injection.

Inject the cement and continue fluoroscopic monitoring to prevent overfilling or extension into the spinal canal or neural foramen. If central venous filling is observed, stop the injection for 60 seconds and then slowly resume. Polymerization of cement within the proximal vein prevents further venous filling as the injection is resumed. If cement is observed within the posterior one third of the vertebral body or if epidural venous filling is suspected, do not continue with the injection. Use extreme caution if the posterior

continued

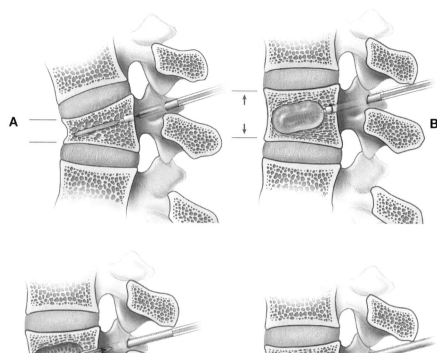

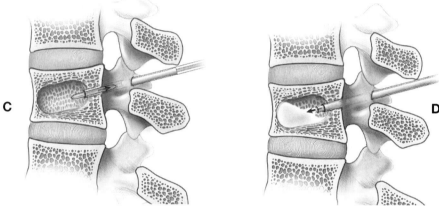

Fig. 35-54 Balloon kyphoplasty. (Redrawn from Griffin S: What the experts say: treatment options for VCF, including balloon kyphoplasty, http://kyphon.com, Kyphon, Inc, Daly City, Calif.)

vertebral cortex is not intact. Because significant cross-filling occurs in slightly more than one half of the vertebrae injected, often it is necessary to inject only one side of the vertebra.

After the procedure, most patients can be transferred to the same-day surgery unit and discharged within 24 hours.

Balloon Kyphoplasty. Balloon kyphoplasty (Fig. 35-54) has evolved as the next step in the treatment of vertebral compression fractures. This is a minimally invasive procedure that involves reduction and fixation. The procedure is performed through small instruments that are inserted into the vertebral body through the pedicle. A small balloon is inflated to restore the height of a collapsed vertebral body and create a cavity inside. The balloon is then deflated and withdrawn, and the remaining cavity is filled under low pressure with the surgeon's choice of material. Essentially, this process stabilizes the vertebrae internally and facilitates pain relief and restores function rapidly. Restoring vertebral height and spinal alignment is believed to be important in the treatment of long-term

increased morbidity and mortality that arises from vertebral compression fractures and spinal deformity. Although our experience with this technique is limited, we have used balloon kyphoplasty in the treatment of painful vertebral compression fractures that have failed medical management. Early results have been good in terms of pain relief and morbidity, but additional prospective studies are needed to refine the indications for the surgical procedure. Potential complications include extrusion of the cement into the spinal canal, resulting in neurological compromise, infection, hematoma, pulmonary embolus, failure to relieve pain, and incomplete deformity correction. A recent large series showed a significant complication rate of 0.8%. As of this writing, approximately 4000 fractures in 3000 patients have been treated by balloon kyphoplasty with good results.

SPECIFIC INSTRUMENTATION

In our experience posterior instrumentation is a safe and effective treatment for thoracolumbar instability. Numerous internal fixation devices have been developed for the treatment of thoracolumbar spinal fractures (Box 35-1). Some of these

BOX 35-1 • Internal Fixation Devices for Thoracolumbar Spinal Fractures

ANTERIOR IMPLANTS
Kaneda device
Syracuse I-plate
Z-plate
Zielke
Kostuick-Harrington
TSRH

POSTERIOR ROD IMPLANTS
Harrington
Distraction
Compression
Edwards
Jacobs locking hood rod
Luque
Harrington-Luque
Wisconsin (Drummond)

POSTERIOR PEDICLE IMPLANTS
Steffe
Luque
Roy-Camille
Wiltse
AO Fixateur Internal
TSRH
Dynalock
Cotrel-Dubousset
ISOLA
Rogozinski

implants remain investigational at this time, and their use is limited to specific spinal trauma centers. These implants have been developed because of the deficiencies of Harrington rods, such as breakage, cutting out of hooks, and loss of fixation. Biomechanical studies suggest that these newer devices offer improved fixation, but because they may be technically more difficult to insert, neurological risks are increased. Anterior instrumentation has evolved significantly, now allowing correction of a deformity, stabilization of spinal segments during decompression, and bone grafting to be performed simultaneously. These implants are useful in the treatment of thoracolumbar burst fractures. The efficacy of anterior decompression in improving the neurological status of a patient with an incomplete deficit is well documented. Anterior internal fixation devices allow treatment of mechanical instability and neurological compression in a single-stage surgical procedure. Collected data indicate that these implants generally are safe and effective compared with posterior implants. In a study of anterior spinal fixation after lumbar corpectomy in an animal model, Zdeblick noted the efficacy of anterior instrumentation. A higher percentage of fusions were obtained with anterior internal fixation compared with a strut graft alone, and biomechanically the spines that had been fixed with instrumentation were torsionally more rigid than those that had not been fixed with instrumentation. At this time most of our clinical experience has been with the Kaneda device and the Z-plate. We recognize that other anterior internal fixation devices are currently in use. The indications and contraindications for their use continue to evolve, and data on complication rates are being collected as their use becomes more widespread.

◆ Harrington Distraction Instrumentation

Harrington used his instrumentation for stabilization of thoracolumbar fractures, and numerous authors, including Flesch et al., Dickson, Harrington, and Erwin, and Bradford et al., reported satisfactory results with the use of these implants in the treatment of unstable thoracolumbar fractures. Harrington rods achieved wide acceptance but in their initial application failed to take into account the sagittal contour of the spine, especially in the lumbar spine, and they were biomechanically insufficient for unstable translational injuries. As clinical and biomechanical data were obtained, the inadequacies of conventional straight Harrington rods were documented. The most common complication was hook cut-out, which was estimated to have an incidence of 10%. McAfee et al. provided valuable data for determining the biomechanical advantages and disadvantages of various internal fixation devices. They determined that the location of ultimate failure in Harrington distraction systems was at the metal-bone interface, and they recommended segmentally wired Harrington distraction instrumentation for injuries in which resistance to axial compression was necessary and for translational injuries, including fracture-dislocations. Luque segmental spinal instrumentation more effectively stabilized the injured spinal segment against shear and torsion without risk of overdistraction. McAfee and Bohlman showed that technical problems or the improper use of Harrington instrumentation systems complicated the management of thoracolumbar fractures. They noted that serious complications can occur when decompression of the neural canal by excessive distraction force is attempted. Overdistraction, failure of fixation, and iatrogenic neurological deficits can occur if excessive posterior distraction is used in an attempt to reduce anterior fragments of bone or disc from the spinal canal. The most common complication in their series was failure of the Harrington distraction rods to decompress the spinal canal after stabilization. Ultimately the original straight Harrington rods were modified. Contouring of the rods and the use of square-ended rods and hooks allowed successful use of the implant for reduction and stabilization of thoracolumbar injuries. For successful use of the Harrington distraction system, the anterior longitudinal ligament should be intact. This system requires a three-point fixation principle for reduction of the fracture, and proper contouring of the rods, especially in the lumbar spine, is necessary to maintain the normal lumbar lordosis. We have the most experience with Harrington rods in the treatment of thoracolumbar injuries and, in general, these implants are the most familiar to spinal surgeons. We have found that early stabilization (within 48 hours) allows restoration of anatomical alignment in most patients

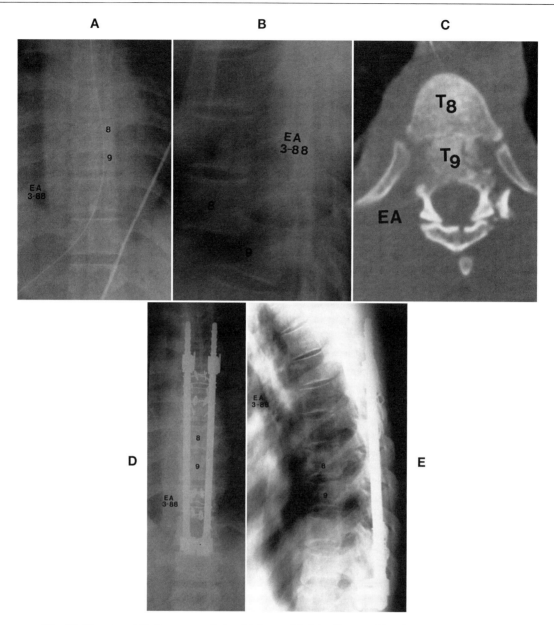

Fig. 35-55   **A** and **B,** Severe translational injury at T8-9 in 20-year-old patient involved in motor vehicle accident. Patient had complete spinal cord injury at T8 level. **C,** CT scan shows complete disruption of normal spinal alignment, with "double margin" sign at T8-9. **D** and **E,** Alignment of spine after posterior instrumentation with dual Harrington distraction rods, augmented with Wisconsin wires. Patient was mobilized in external orthosis and made rapid recovery in spinal rehabilitation program.

(Fig. 35-55). When surgery is delayed between 48 hours and 10 days, less than anatomical alignment usually is obtained, but results remain quite good. If surgery is delayed for more than 2 weeks, we have found little improvement in the canal area. In some burst fractures that have remained untreated for longer than 2 weeks, satisfactory reduction cannot be obtained by posterior Harrington distraction rods alone, and anterior decompression and strut grafting are necessary for decompression (Fig. 35-56). As a secondary procedure, Harrington instrumentation may be applied posteriorly. Alternatively,

anterior decompression, strut grafting, and anterior internal fixation may be carried out as a one-stage procedure.

TECHNIQUE 35-16
Place the patient prone on a padded spinal frame or operating table with chest rolls. Perform routine, sterile skin preparation and draping. Make a midline skin incision centered over the spinous process at the level of injury. Infiltrate the skin, subcutaneous tissues, and erector spinae

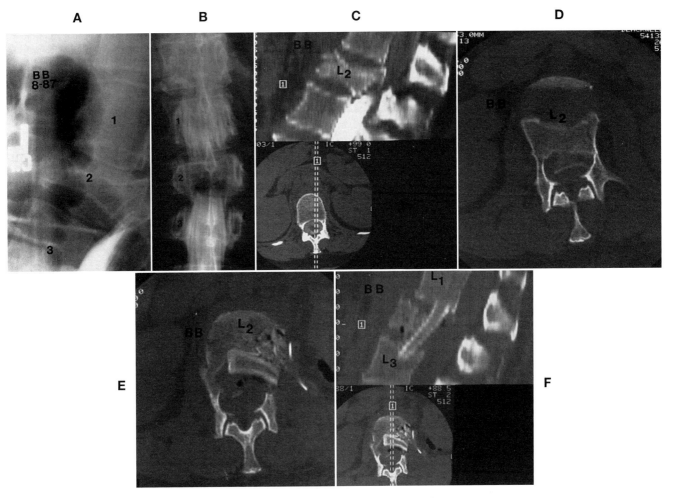

Fig. 35-56   Burst fracture of L2 in 42-year-old woman, with incomplete paraparesis, 3 weeks after injury. **A** and **B,** Myelograms show significant extradural compression at L2 level from bone retropulsed into spinal canal. **C** and **D,** CT scans show degree of canal compromise at L2 level. **E** and **F,** CT scans show adequate decompression of spinal canal and proper placement of iliac strut graft from L1 to L3. Patient made excellent neurological recovery and regained ambulatory status, with return of bowel and bladder function.

muscle down to the level of the lamina with a 1:500,000 epinephrine solution to minimize bleeding. Deepen the incision to expose posterior elements three levels above and three below the level of injury. Carry the dissection laterally to the tips of the transverse processes, maintaining meticulous hemostasis in a dry field. Confirm the level of injury with roentgenograms. Identify the facet joints of three intact lamina above the level of injury and remove the facet joint capsules. Prepare the site for insertion of the upper hooks and be certain that the inferior articular mass of the cephalic vertebra is not split with insertion of the Harrington hooks. Then insert two no. 1252 hooks in the facet joints. As an alternative, use two bifid hooks or keeled hooks to improve stability. Identify the interlaminar space of the lamina two below the level of injury and prepare the hook

sites by removing the ligamentum flavum from the superior edge of the inferior lamina and performing small laminotomies to allow seating of the inferior hooks against the lamina. Then place two no. 1254 hooks beneath the lamina. If one side of the lamina or one side of the vertebral body seems to be more involved, place the first distraction rod on the opposite side. Reduce the fracture as the Harrington rod is inserted. Insert the opposite rod, taking care not to overdistract the fracture. We recommend distracting the rods until they are snug. Somatosensory evoked potential monitoring currently is recommended during insertion of posterior instrumentation in patients who are neurologically normal or have incomplete neurological lesions. This allows physiological monitoring of the spinal cord as the fracture is reduced and distraction is applied to the spine. Obtain a

continued

cross-table lateral roentgenogram to evaluate alignment and reduction. We prefer to introduce water-soluble contrast material into the subarachnoid space and obtain a myelogram or create a small laminotomy defect, fill it with saline, and confirm decompression by ultrasonography. Complete reduction of the retropulsed bone fragments with insertion of Harrington distraction rods alone is not reliable. If the reduction is incomplete, as documented by intraoperative myelography or ultrasonography, and the lesion is neurologically incomplete, proceed with a posterolateral decompression, using a high-speed drill to remove a portion of the lamina and pedicle and reverse angled curets to remove retropulsed bone fragments from the anterior aspect of the dura (see Fig. 35-52). If, however, anatomical reduction is obtained or the residual compression is minimal and the patient is neurologically normal, proceed with posterior and posterolateral fusions spanning the entire length of the instrumentation in patients with a complete spinal cord injury or limited to one vertebra above and one vertebra below the injury in patients who are neurologically normal or have an incomplete spinal cord injury. We prefer autogenous iliac bone grafting, which may be supplemented with allografts if necessary.

Apply C-washers to the ratchet end of the rods beneath the cephalic hooks to prevent loss of reduction. Try to minimize the number of ratchets exposed below the upper hooks to decrease the chance of fracture at the junction of the rod and ratchet as a late complication. Thoroughly irrigate the wound with antibiotic solution, insert closed suction drainage, and close the wound in routine fashion.

If instrumentation is used in the lower lumbar spine, we prefer the square-ended Harrington rods, contoured into lordosis, with modified square-ended hooks. This maintains the normal lumbar lordosis and improves stability. In the thoracic region and at the thoracolumbar junction, either the traditional round-ended Harrington rods or the square-ended rods can be used.

AFTERTREATMENT. The patient is kept on bed rest initially and is fitted with a molded, bivalved thoracolumbosacral orthosis. The orthosis is worn for 12 to 16 weeks except during bed rest. Early ambulation and rehabilitation are encouraged.

Harrington Compression Instrumentation

Harrington compression instrumentation may be indicated for thoracolumbar fractures, especially when the posterior column has failed in a tension mode. Small (⅛-inch) and large (3/16-inch) threaded compression rods are available and provide rigid stabilization during fracture healing and fusion of the posterolateral arthrodesis. We have found them most useful for stabilizing flexion-distraction injuries and Chance fractures. When used in the thoracic spine, Harrington compression rods should be coupled to hooks that are placed around the base of the transverse processes. In the lumbar spine the hook should

be placed beneath the lamina to provide rigid fixation. Modifications of the Harrington compression instrumentation to include Keene hooks and bushings have made the use of this implant simpler and less time-consuming. Studies have suggested that sublaminar wiring to compression rods should not be done because the wiring may pull the sublaminar hook into the underlying neural structures, resulting in iatrogenic neurological deficits. Placing hooks in the transverse processes gives less strength than hook placement beneath the lamina; however, there is less danger of damage to the neural structures with the former technique. Biomechanical studies by Stauffer and Neil and by Pinzur et al. found compression rods to be stronger than distraction rods when subjected to a combination of flexion and rotation. Compression rods tend to fail by fracture of the transverse process during flexion and lateral bending and by hooks slipping off in extension. We have favored the Edwards reversed ratcheted compression rods over traditional Harrington compression rods; they are technically easier to insert and equally effective (Fig. 35-57).

◆ Edwards Instrumentation

Edwards and Levine developed a rod-sleeve fixation technique that appears to offer improved reduction and biomechanical fixation. The rod-sleeve reduction of spinal fractures produces indirect decompression through a relatively low-risk posterior approach (Fig. 35-58). Edwards and Levine reported 135 consecutive spinal injuries and noted that in 91% of patients treated within 3 weeks, anatomical correction was obtained in all planes; however, if surgery was delayed more than 3 weeks, anatomical alignment was obtained in only 20%. In addition, in 98% of patients with an intact anterior ligamentous complex, rod-sleeve fixation alone was sufficiently rigid to limit total motion across the instrumented segments to less than 2 mm in any plane. In patients treated within 48 hours of injury, reduction with the rod-sleeve technique restored 32% of the canal area; when surgery was delayed between 3 and 14 days, 23% of the canal area was restored; and if surgery was delayed for more than 2 weeks, there was little improvement in the canal area. In addition to increasing the canal area, the rod-sleeve technique was designed to create a relative lordosis at the level of injury and allow the cord to shift posteriorly in the canal, away from the remaining anterior fragments. They noted that relative lordosis averaged 3 degrees for patients treated with the bridging sleeve construct; 2.5 degrees for those treated with a single pair of sleeves, distraction rods, and anatomical hooks; and 0 degrees for those treated with compression rods.

The Edwards instrumentation is a modification of the Harrington instrumentation. Distraction rods, polyethylene sleeves, and the anatomical hook design provide simultaneous hyperextension and distraction forces that eliminate kyphotic deformity and restore vertebral height. The sleeves come in various sizes to accommodate the upper and lower thoracic regions, the thoracolumbar junction, and the lumbar spine. They wedge between the facets and spinous processes to

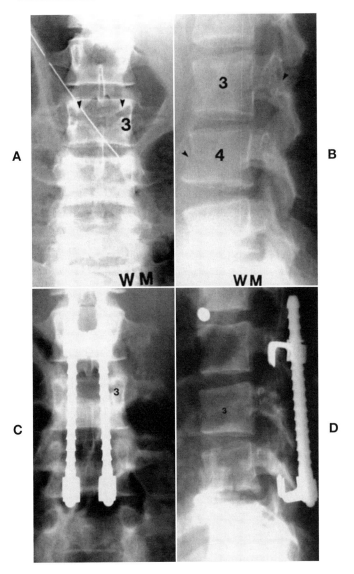

Fig. 35-57 **A** and **B,** Chance fracture of L3 and compression fracture of L4 in 20-year-old polytrauma patient without neurological deficit. **C** and **D,** After internal fixation with dual Edwards reverse ratchet compression rods and anatomical hooks. Bilateral intertransverse process fusion from L2 to L4 was performed, and patient was mobilized in external orthosis.

correct translational deformity and provide rotational stability. Edwards and Levine recommend that the polyethylene sleeve be centered over the superior facet of the most apical fractured vertebra. If an unstable lamina or a comminuted pedicle fracture is present, they recommend a bridging sleeve construct. Care should be taken not to place the polyethylene sleeve directly over an unstable lamina or pedicle to prevent injury to the neural elements. Anatomical hooks should be inserted between 3 and 5 cm on either side of the edges of the sleeves to allow sufficient corrective moments yet keep the instrumentation relatively short. Usually upper hooks are placed in the second interspace proximal to the sleeve and the first or second interspace distal to the sleeve. It is important to

select the proper-sized rod sleeve to achieve anatomical alignment. The sleeves generate corrective moments to provide simultaneous lordosis and distraction. To oppose the normal loss of rigidity caused by the gradual stretching of the anterior ligamentous structures, this method takes advantage of the normal elasticity of the stainless steel Harrington rods. A bow can be made in the rod by pressure on the sleeve between the rod and lamina. Thus, as the anterior ligamentous structures relax, the posterior rods straighten, helping to provide continuous correction (Fig. 35-59, *A*). The polyethylene sleeves and the L-shaped anatomical hooks provide increased contact surface with the lamina and minimize bone resorption, late loosening, and hook dislodgment (Fig. 35-59, *B*). With the Edwards system, the number of instrumented segments can be reduced, especially in the lumbar spine where preservation of motion segments is important. We have found this system to be effective and relatively simple to use.

TECHNIQUE 35-17

Place the patient prone on a padded spinal frame and expose the thoracolumbar spine as described for the Harrington technique (see Fig. 35-59). Confirm the level of injury with a lateral roentgenogram and remove any depressed laminar fragments. Select the correct sleeve position over the superior facets of the apical vertebra or over adjacent facets if the pedicle or lamina is comminuted. Place anatomical hooks in the interspace that lies 3 to 5 cm on either side of the intended sleeve position. Use low-profile hooks in the thoracic facets and lamina and high-profile hooks to accommodate the thicker lumbar lamina. Place a trial sleeve between the apical facet and spinous process. In general, the small (2 mm) sleeve is appropriate for the midthoracic spine, the medium (4 mm) sleeve for the distal thoracic spine, the large (6 mm) sleeve for the upper lumbar spine, and the elliptical (8 mm) sleeve for the midlumbar spine. If necessary, the polyethylene sleeves can be trimmed with a high-speed burr or scalpel to ensure a snug fit between the facet and spinous processes. Slide the sleeve over a distraction rod of sufficient length to allow at least 1 cm above the upper hook after final distraction. Pass the rod through the upper hook and then position the sleeve near the middle of the rod. Reduce the spine by pushing down on the distal end of the rod while pulling up on the lower hooks until the nipple of the rod engages the lower hook. To make reduction easier, a long rod on the opposite side can be used as a reduction lever. Place a large sleeve on the rod and position it over the apical lamina to serve as a fulcrum. Perform the reduction maneuver with a permanent rod while having an assistant push the end of the reduction lever in an anterocephalad direction. Once the rods and hooks are coupled, complete the reduction by refining the sleeve position. Use a rod clamp and Harrington spreader to push the sleeve into position over the superior facet of the fractured vertebral body, being sure it is wedged against the proximal spinous process. The correctly sized rod sleeve

continued

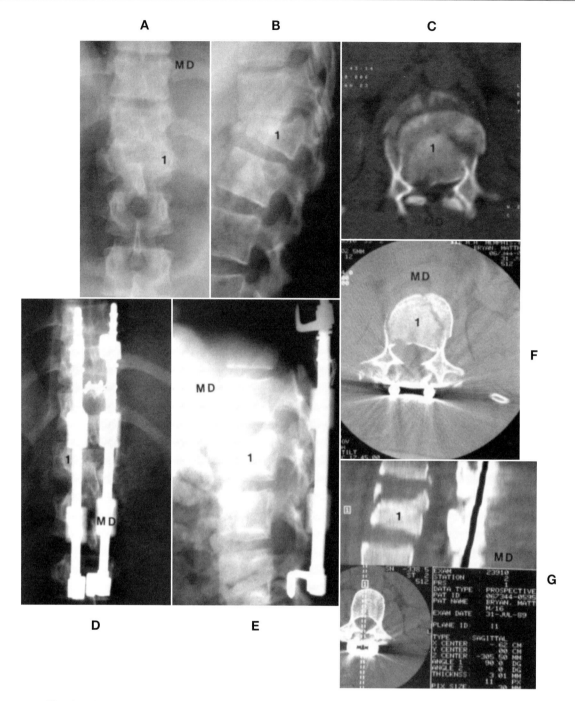

Fig. 35-58 **A** and **B,** Unstable burst fracture of L1 in 17-year-old patient, with incomplete paraparesis. **C,** CT scan shows significant canal compromise from retropulsed bone at L1 level. **D** and **E,** Realignment of spinal canal after posterior instrumentation with dual Harrington distraction rods and Edwards sleeves in bridging construct. **F** and **G,** CT scans show nearly anatomical reduction of bone fragments from spinal canal after posterior instrumentation. Patient was immobilized in thoracolumbosacral orthosis for 3 months and had complete neurological recovery.

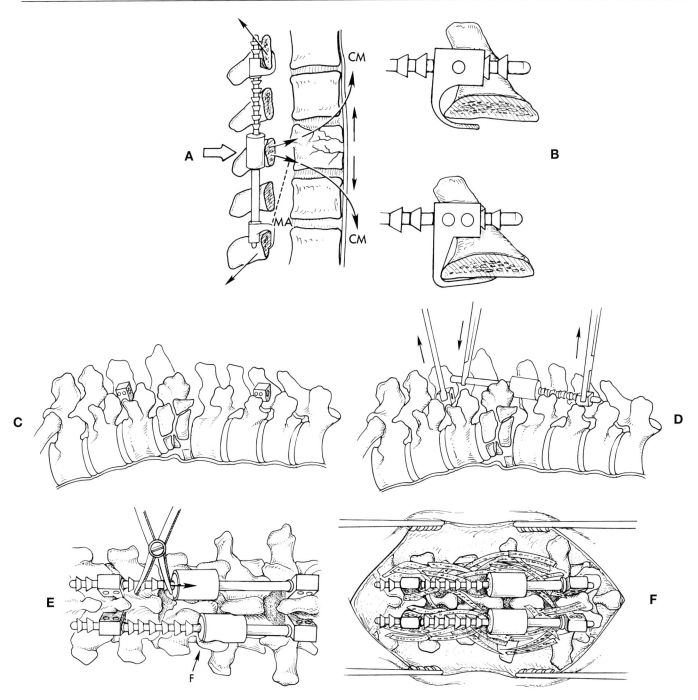

Fig. 35-59 Rod-sleeve reduction technique (see text). **A,** Sleeves generate corrective moments to provide simultaneous lordosis and distraction. **B,** C-shaped hooks provide edge contact only, anatomical hooks contact edge and undersurface. **C,** Hook placement. **D,** Reduction maneuver. **E,** Sleeve positioning. **F,** Fusion. (Redrawn from Edwards CC: *Orthopedics Today,* Dec 15, 1985, SLACK.)

should fully reduce kyphosis and leave a slight but definite bow in the rods. Apply this distraction in stages for at least 20 minutes and limit the distraction force at any one time to no more than one fingerbreadth on each side of the arm of the Harrington spreader. Obtain a lateral roentgenogram before final distraction to confirm the reduction and sleeve position.

For patients with incomplete paraplegia, we perform an intraoperative myelogram to confirm sufficient canal decompression to permit passage of dye anterior to the cord

continued

(Fig. 35-60). Inject water-soluble contrast dye distal to the injury with a spinal needle. Tilt the patient approximately 25 degrees with the head down and obtain a lateral roentgenogram. If residual compression of the thecal sac is present, perform a posterolateral decompression, as described by Erickson, Leider, and Brown and by and Garfin et al. Place two C-washers under each upper hook to prevent loss of distraction. Harvest a generous corticocancellous bone graft from the posterior ilium, lightly decorticate the posterior elements, and place posterior and posterolateral bone grafts over the instrumented segments. Thoroughly irrigate the wound with antibiotic solution, insert a closed suction drain, and close the wound in routine fashion.

AFTERTREATMENT. Patients are mobilized in a polypropylene orthosis. We recommend a postoperative CT scan to evaluate the adequacy of decompression. If decompression is, inadequate, a staged anterior decompression should be considered in selected patients to improve neurological recovery.

Jacobs Locking Hook Instrumentation

This posterior instrumentation device (Fig. 35-61) was devised by Jacobs et al. in conjunction with the AO group in an attempt to correct some of the deficiencies associated with traditional Harrington rod instrumentation. Gertzbein et al. reviewed 95 consecutive thoracolumbar injuries treated with the locking hook spinal rod and found a 38% improvement in the initial kyphotic deformity and restoration of 37% of vertebral body height. In addition, 84% of patients with incomplete neurological deficits improved by one or more grades. An instrument complication rate of 8.4% was noted. Possible disadvantages of this device are that it spans at least five motion segments, it may not provide adequate fixation for severely comminuted burst fractures because of insufficiency of the anterior and middle columns, and it is not recommended for fractures of the lower lumbar spine. This implant includes several modifications of the Harrington instrumentation. Instead of notches, both ends of the rods are threaded so that linear distraction of any distance is possible and weakening of the rod because of the narrow cross-section at the notches is avoided. The hooks are fixed with locking nuts and can be freely rotated on the rod. The rod can be contoured to the shape of the spine, even in lordosis, since rotation cannot occur. The rod maintains contact against the vertebral arch. The diameter of the rod is increased to 7 mm, and the lip of the cranial hook is tilted 15 degrees away from its axis, thus shaping the rod precisely to the anatomical shape of the anterior part of the proximal vertebral arch. In addition, the upper hook is fitted with a cover that can be pushed forward and is secured by corresponding grooves on the upper part of the hook. This allows the hook to grip firmly around the upper edge of the lamina. Jacobs et al. recommended that the implant be inserted in accordance with the three vertebrae above and three vertebrae below rule. They showed a

50% increase in the detachment force of the upper hook and a threefold increase in stiffness in flexion of the instrumented lumbar spine using this fixation. We have little experience with this implant but believe that it does offer improved stability over traditional Harrington rods.

◆ Luque Instrumentation

The Luque instrumentation system provides more rigid internal fixation and resistance to rotational forces than does traditional Harrington instrumentation. This instrumentation has been used for correction of scoliotic deformities, as well as for stabilization of thoracolumbar fractures and dislocations. McAfee has shown that the ability to resist torsion is less in the Harrington distraction rods and that the system absorbing the highest energy is the Luque segmental system. Biomechanical testing found that the Luque segmental spinal instrumentation failed by fracture-dislocation, either above or below the instrumented segment. Ferguson and Allen reported one failure at the metal-bone interface and seven losses of correction in a series of 54 fractures and dislocations treated with Luque instrumentation. Loss of translational stability or malrotation did not occur. As biomechanical testing suggests, the weak point in the Luque system is a failure to counteract axial loading; thus it does not provide rigid fixation for unstable burst fractures. This system appears to be best suited for treatment of translational injuries of the thoracic or lumbar spine with complete neurological injuries. When used in neurologically normal patients or those with incomplete neurological lesions, care must be taken in passing the sublaminar wires to avoid neurological injury. Wilber et al. reported transient sensory changes in 3 of 20 patients with Luque instrumentation and a major sensory deficit in one. They listed as factors related to increased risk for spinal cord injury the passage of sublaminar wires in the thoracic and thoracolumbar spine. We have limited experience with Luque rod instrumentation in the treatment of thoracolumbar fractures but favor either a double Luque rod or a solid Luque rectangle, segmentally wired at each level with 16-gauge wire.

TECHNIQUE 35-18

With the patient prone, expose the segment of spine to be instrumented (p. 1650). For fracture-dislocations of the thoracolumbar spine, we recommend instrumentation three levels above and three levels below, using either a solid Luque rectangle or double rods. Expose the ligamentum flavum at each level to be instrumented using a needle-nose rongeur to remove soft tissue overlying the interspace (Fig. 35-62). In the lumbar spine, because of the lordosis there is often shingling of the lamina over the interspace. Excise this bone with rongeurs. Incise the ligamentum flavum with the rongeur and excise it with a small Kerrison punch (Figs. 35-63 and 35-64). The ligamentum flavum must be excised at every interspace to be instrumented. Pass wires beneath each lamina by forming a loop of 16-gauge

continued

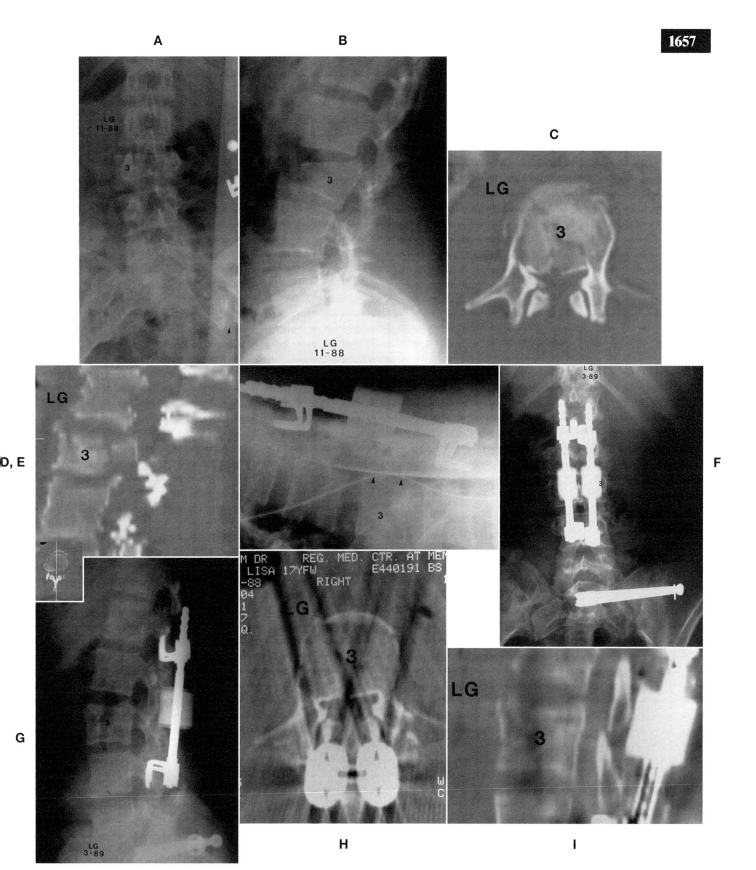

Fig. 35-60 **A** and **B,** Burst fracture of L3 in 17-year-old patient involved in motor vehicle accident. Despite significant canal compromise, patient had no neurological deficits. **C** and **D,** CT scans show canal compromise from retropulsed bone at L3 level. **E,** Intraoperative myelogram shows excellent reduction of burst fracture, with dye flowing freely past L3 level after posterior Edwards instrumentation. **F** and **G,** Restoration of spinal alignment after posterior instrumentation with elliptical sleeves to maintain lordosis. Note internal fixation of sacroiliac joint injury with multiple cannulated screws. **H** and **I,** CT scans show restoration of spinal canal.

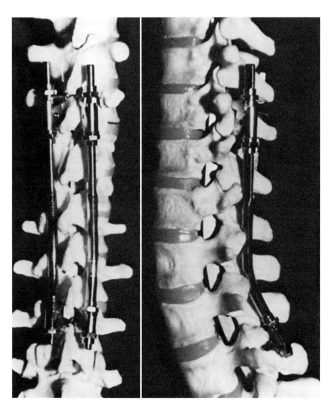

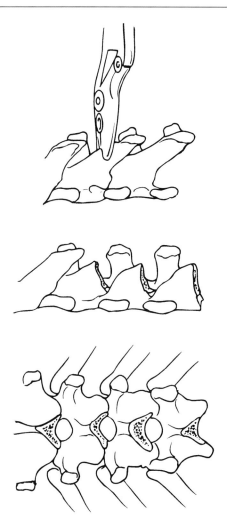

Fig. 35-61 Jacobs posterior instrumentation. Rods are thick, are threaded on upper end, and have locking device at upper end to provide rigid fixation to lamina. (From Meyer PR Jr: *Surgery of spine trauma*, New York, 1989, Churchill Livingstone.)

Fig. 35-62 Segmental spinal instrumentation (see text). Removal of caudally slanting spinous processes to expose ligamentum flavum. (Redrawn from *Segmental spinal fixation and correction using Richards L-rod instrumentation,* Memphis, Smith & Nephew.)

Fig. 35-63 Segmental spinal instrumentation (see text). Penfield No. 4 dissector is used to free deep surfaces of ligamentum flavum. (Redrawn from *Segmental spinal fixation and correction using Richards L-rod instrumentation,* Memphis, Smith & Nephew.)

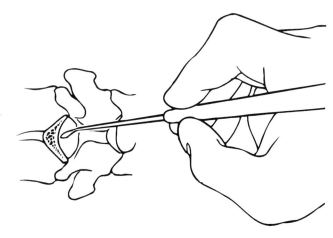

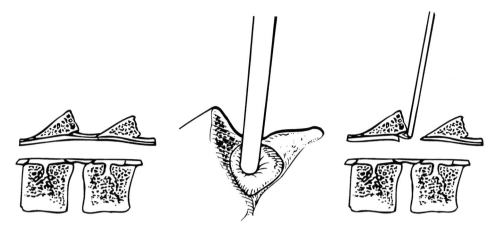

Fig. 35-64   Segmental spinal instrumentation (see text). Kerrison punch is used to remove remainder of ligamentum flavum. (Redrawn from *Segmental spinal fixation and correction using Richards L-rod instrumentation,* Memphis, Smith & Nephew.)

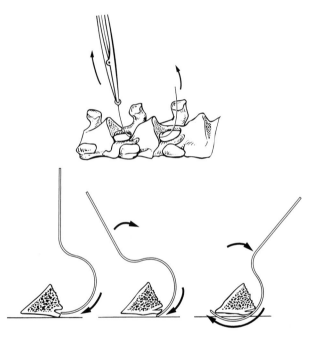

Fig. 35-65   Segmental spinal instrumentation (see text). Shape of double wire before it passes under lamina. (Redrawn from *Segmental spinal fixation and correction using Richards L-rod instrumentation,* Memphis, Smith & Nephew.)

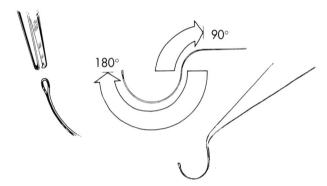

Fig. 35-66   Segmental spinal instrumentation (see text). Passage of segmental wire beneath lamina. (Redrawn from *Segmental spinal fixation and correction using Richards L-rod instrumentation,* Memphis, Smith & Nephew.)

wire and bending the loop to two right angles. The distance between the two bends should equal the width of the lamina to be instrumented. Pass the wires from a caudal to a cephalad direction (Fig. 35-65). At the upper and lower levels of instrumentation use double loops of wire (Fig. 35-66) and at the intervening levels, one loop of wire. Divide the single loop of wire in the intervening levels so that two wires lie beneath each lamina and retract these to each side of the wound. Take care not to force the wires against the thecal sac during passage. Excise the facet joints bilaterally and pack bone graft around the facet joints while the laminae are decorticated. Insert the Luque rods, taking care to place the short arm or transverse limb of each rod beneath the longitudinal or long arm to prevent rotation and subsequent migration of the implant, and carefully tighten the wires around the rod to fix the spine to the rods. We usually begin tightening in the middle of the rod and proceed toward either end. Burst fractures can be reduced by applying a Harrington outrigger and securely fixing them with a double C-rod to prevent collapse. Perform a routine posterolateral arthrodesis (Chapter 36) and close the wound in layers over a suction drain.

AFTERTREATMENT. Postoperative immobilization usually is not necessary, and rehabilitation can begin soon after surgery without the use of an external orthosis.

◆ ◆ ◆

It must be emphasized that we have little experience with this technique in neurologically normal patients or in those with incomplete neurological lesions and have limited its use to patients with neurologically complete lesions and unstable translational injuries.

Sublaminar Wiring with Harrington Distraction Instrumentation

This technique, which combines the advantages of the Harrington and Luque systems by sublaminar wiring of Harrington distraction rods, is reported to increase stability and resistance to pull-out, and it has proved effective in managing unstable thoracolumbar fractures (Fig. 35-67). Wenger et al. demonstrated that resistance to failure is greatest in intact lamina, followed in decreasing order by decorticated lamina, the transverse processes, and the spinous processes. Stability of Harrington rods therefore can be increased by sublaminar wiring at multiple sites. Sullivan noted a decreased incidence of distraction rod failure and a reduction in postoperative immobilization time. Studies suggest that sublaminar wiring to compression rods should not be done because of the risk of driving the sublaminar hook into the underlying spinal canal. We have found that sublaminar wiring increases the stability of Harrington distraction rods in those patients with neurologically complete lesions and unstable thoracolumbar spine fractures. Considerable care must be taken when passing sublaminar wires, and the risk of neurological injury must be considered when using this technique in neurologically normal patients or those with incomplete spinal cord injuries.

Wisconsin (Drummond) Interspinous Segmental Spinal Instrumentation

Drummond, Keene, and Breed developed interspinous segmental spinal instrumentation to provide the stability of Luque instrumentation without the passage of sublaminar wires. This technique has been used for the correction of scoliotic deformities and in the treatment of unstable thoracolumbar spine fractures. The base of the spinous process is readily accessible and easy to instrument and it provides a broad base of insertion for this particular implant (Fig. 35-68). The best purchase site for instrumentation with the Wisconsin system is the base of the spinous process, not the middle or tip. The anchoring hole must be created deep enough to obtain purchase in good bone stock but superficial enough to avoid penetrating the spinal canal. The button-wire implant is made of stainless steel that is 8 mm in diameter and 0.8 mm thick. The attached wire is 16- or 18-gauge stainless steel and is welded at the free end to form a smooth round bead, which eases passage of the wire through the base of the spinous process. The button has a hole in the surface large enough to allow passage of the beaded wires. Buttons are inserted on each side of the spinous processes, and a bead from each implant passes through the hole in the spinous process and then through the hole in the opposite button (Fig. 35-69). In the treatment of thoracolumbar fractures, we have used paired wires to increase

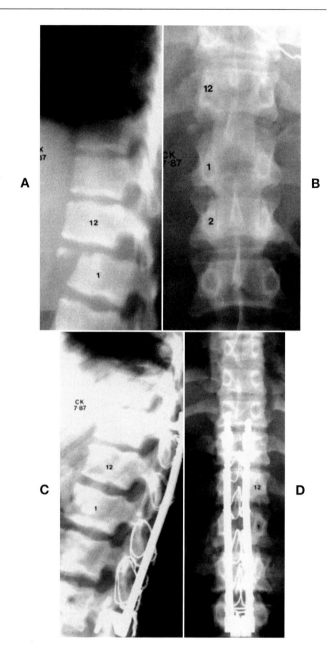

Fig. 35-67 **A** and **B,** Translational injury of T12 on L1 in 19-year-old patient with complete paraplegia. **C** and **D,** Realignment of spinal canal after internal fixation with dual Harrington distraction rods augmented with sublaminar wires. Patient was mobilized early without external orthosis.

stability when intact spinous processes are available in the intervening levels between the cephalad and caudal hooks (Fig. 35-70). This technique is safe and simple and the risk of neurological injury is low if the hole is correctly placed in the base of the spinous process.

Pedicle Screw Instrumentation

Fixation of thoracolumbar fractures with pedicle screws and plates has been performed by Roy-Camille and others as early as 1961. Pedicle screw and plate implants for spinal fractures

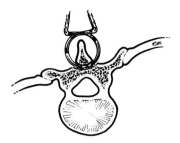

Fig. 35-68 Interspinous wiring technique (see text). Lewen clamp is used to make hole in base of spinous process for passage of wires.

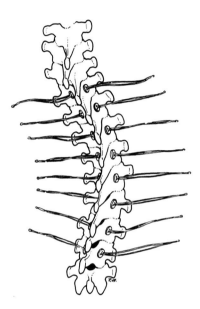

Fig. 35-69 Interspinous wiring technique (see text) with placement of buttons and wires.

were developed by Steffee and Sitkowski, Luque, Roy-Camille, and others and have been investigated in various centers. Surgeons in Europe have had widespread experience with pedicle screws, and experience with the technique is expanding rapidly in North America; however, these implants are still the subject of considerable controversy. They have not been cleared for general use by the U.S. Food and Drug Administration (FDA). Pedicle screw devices are class III implants. This category includes screws placed transfacetally within pedicles or in articular or lateral masses. The FDA has allowed class II clearance for the use of pedicle screws to supplement fusions in the treatment of grade III and grade IV spondylolistheses with the provision that the implants are to be removed after the arthrodesis has healed. Anterior vertebral body screws (cervical, thoracic, and lumbar) are class II devices and can be used as labeled in vertebral bodies. Extensive testing of posterior screw-based devices has shown them to be useful in treating fractures and other degenerative conditions of the spine. Informed consent should be obtained before implanta-

tion of these devices, and the inherent risks and benefits of the implant should be discussed in depth with the patient. In our clinical experience we have found pedicle screw instrumentation to be very effective in the treatment of fractures of the lower lumbar spine, with a high percentage of fusions and a low percentage of hardware failures. We believe these implants should be used only by experienced spinal surgeons who have a thorough knowledge of spinal anatomy so as to reduce the incidence of complications, including pedicle fracture, dural tear, nerve root injury, spinal cord injury, and vascular injuries.

◆ Luque Pedicle Screw

TECHNIQUE 35-19

We prefer to use a pedicle probe or a hand-held curet to enter the pedicle. Preoperative anteroposterior and lateral roentgenograms and CT scans through the pedicles of the vertebral body to be instrumented are studied to determine the correct angle of entry in both the coronal and sagittal planes. Insert blunt Kirschner wires into the pedicles and confirm their position with anteroposterior and lateral roentgenograms. Probe the pedicle in all four quadrants to be sure that a solid tube of bone exists and that violation into the spinal canal or inferiorly into the neuroforamen has not occurred. Once the Kirschner wires are in place, as confirmed by roentgenograms, introduce a cannulated screw tap over each wire and through the pedicle. If a wire bends or deforms in any way, replace it to prevent inadvertent advancement of the wire as the tap is passed over it. The tapping depth should be no more than the depth of the pedicle, and the tap should not enter the vertebral body so that screw purchase is maximized. In tapping the sacral pedicles, penetrate only the posterior cortex. When all wires are in proper position, select a plate of the appropriate size and contour it to maintain normal lumbar lordosis. When three or more screws are used, pass a plate ring over the plate before placing the plate over the wires. Select a cannulated screw of appropriate length so that penetration into the vertebral body is approximately 50%. Before seating the bone screws in the plate, "joy sticks" can be used to apply compression or distraction as necessary. When the screws are seated in the corresponding concavity of the plate, remove the wires at each level. Harvest a generous corticocancellous bone graft from the posterior ilium and perform a posterolateral fusion in the usual fashion. After insertion of the pedicle screws and plate, the cauda equina can be decompressed by laminectomy (Fig. 35-71). Thoroughly irrigate the wound with antibiotic solution, insert closed suction drainage, and close the wound in layers.

AFTERTREATMENT. Patients are mobilized rapidly in a lightweight lumbosacral orthosis. Routine follow-up is recommended at 3 weeks, 6 weeks, 3 months, 6 months, and 1 year.

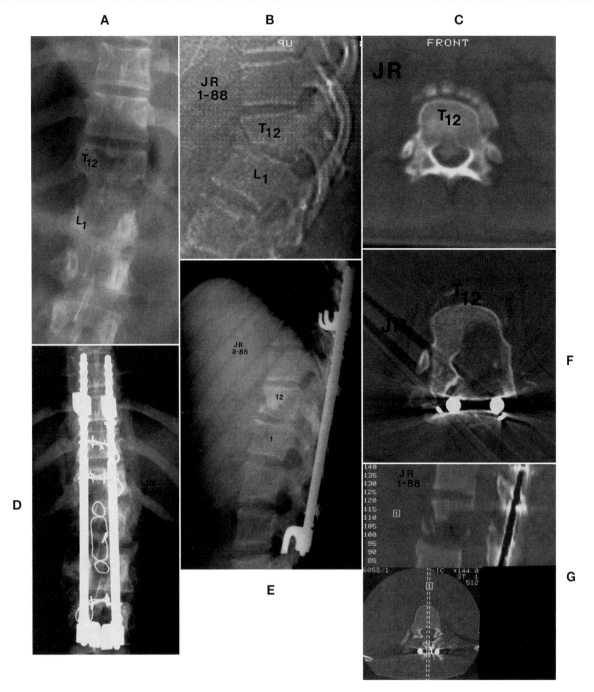

Fig. 35-70 **A** and **B,** Unstable burst fracture of T12 with complete paraplegia in 16-year-old girl. **C,** Comminution of fracture and nearly complete obliteration of spinal canal at T12 level. **D** and **E,** Realignment of spinal canal after posterior instrumentation with dual Harrington distraction rods augmented with wires. **F** and **G,** Decompression of spinal canal after removal of bone fragment through posterolateral approach.

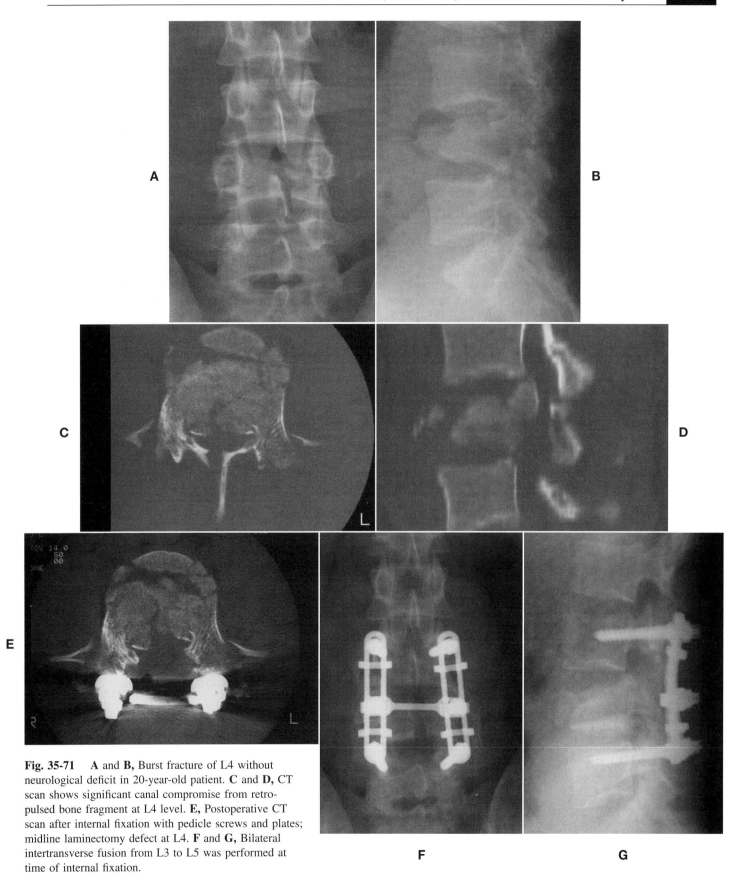

Fig. 35-71 **A** and **B,** Burst fracture of L4 without neurological deficit in 20-year-old patient. **C** and **D,** CT scan shows significant canal compromise from retropulsed bone fragment at L4 level. **E,** Postoperative CT scan after internal fixation with pedicle screws and plates; midline laminectomy defect at L4. **F** and **G,** Bilateral intertransverse fusion from L3 to L5 was performed at time of internal fixation.

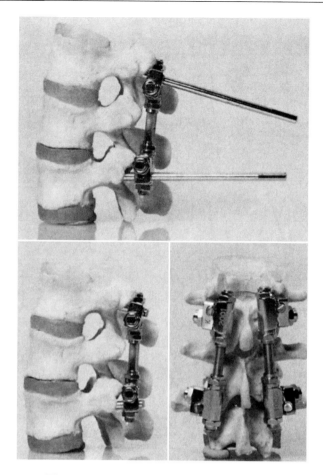

Fig. 35-72   AO spinal internal fixation system.

AO Spinal Internal Fixation System

The AO spinal internal fixation system has been used successfully in many European centers; Magerl and Dick developed and modified the instrumentation. Currently this implant system is undergoing clinical trials in the United States. The AO spinal internal fixation system uses 5-mm transpedicular Schanz screws with 7-mm fully threaded stainless steel rods (Fig. 35-72). The screws are self-tapping, and the standard size is 35 mm of threaded length. The threaded rods are flattened on two sides and come in a variety of lengths ranging from 70 to 300 mm. The coupling device is mobile in the sagittal plane and allows angulation of the Schanz screws before securing them to the rods. The nuts have a lug that can be crimped to secure them to the flattened threads. This system allows axial, angular, and rotational adjustability and permits segmental fixation of injured spinal segments. The AO internal fixator combines the advantages of the external spinal skeletal fixation device developed by Magerl and Dick with the advantage of being completely implantable. It appears to be effective in obtaining decompression of the spinal canal in burst fractures while, in most instances, limiting instrumentation to only two spinal motion segments. At this time we have no experience with this implant, but it appears to be promising for the treatment of thoracolumbar injuries.

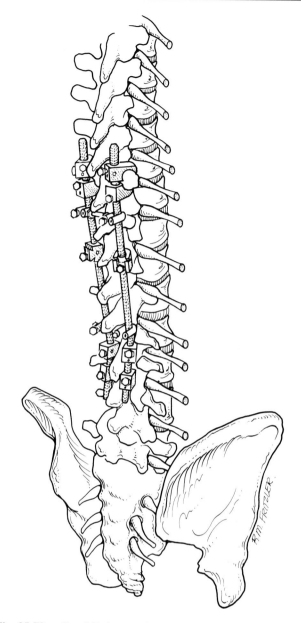

Fig. 35-73   Cotrel-Dubousset instrumentation. Type I configuration is most commonly used design and is recommended for fracture-dislocations and unstable burst fractures. (From McBride GG: *Semin Spine Surg* 2:24, 1990.)

Combined Fixation Devices

These instrumentation systems offer considerable flexibility in obtaining an extremely stable construct for thoracolumbar spine fractures. The Cotrel-Dubousset spinal instrumentation system was initially designed for scoliosis correction but has been used in the management of thoracolumbar spine injuries. The Texas Scottish Rite Hospital implant system also has been used to obtain stability and correct deformity in spinal injuries. These systems offer advantages in that multiple hooks can be inserted and segmental fixation can be obtained. In some systems, pedicle screws can be coupled to the rods for use in the lower lumbar spine and for improved sacral fixation. Spinal

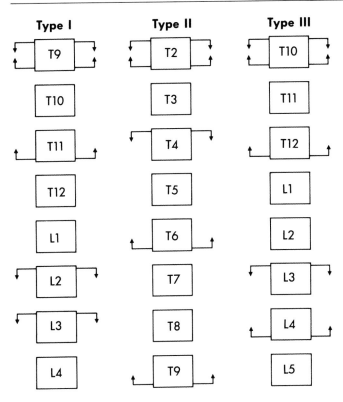

Fig. 35-74 Three configurations of Cotrel-Dubousset instrumentation for reduction and fixation of unstable spinal injuries. Type I is used for fracture-dislocations and burst fractures, type II for flexion-distraction injuries, and type III for injuries of lumbar spine, where maintenance of lordosis is important. (Redrawn from McBride GG: *Semin Spine Surg* 2:24, 1990.)

injuries can be stabilized as necessary by placement of pedicle hooks, transverse process hooks, or sublaminar hooks in either a distraction or compression mode (Fig. 35-73). Proponents of these instrumentation systems suggest that another advantage is that the stability obtained makes any form of postoperative external immobilization unnecessary, but further studies are necessary to document this. These instrumentation systems are complex and have higher incidences of neurological injury than traditional Harrington or Edwards posterior instrumentation. Insertion is technically more difficult than with traditional Harrington or Edwards instrumentation, and there appears to be a significant learning curve in their use.

Biomechanical studies suggest that cross-linking of the rods, that is, either the device for transverse traction with the Cotrel-Dubousset system or the cross-linking plates with the Texas Scottish Rite Hospital system, converts the entire construct into a stable rectangle with improved rotational stability. High fusion rates with low rates of pseudarthrosis and rod breakage have been reported in early series of scoliosis corrections. McBride reported various configurations for hook placement in the treatment of unstable spinal injuries (Fig. 35-75). The basic pattern is a claw configuration at the most cephalad vertebra with various placement of intermediate and caudal hooks either in a distraction or compression mode (Fig. 35-75). In McBride's report of 48 patients, 20 were not braced after surgery. Two patients had early lower hook loosening with loss of reduction and required revision of instrumentation. Overall there was a 4% major medical complication rate and a 6% surgical complication rate. As more

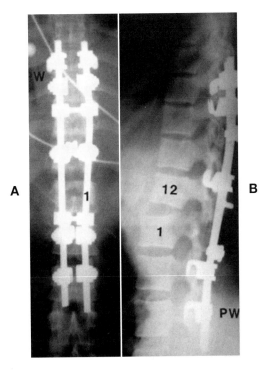

Fig. 35-75 **A** and **B**, Postoperative roentgenograms of patient shown in Fig. 35-5 with translational injury at T12-L1 level. Posterior instrumentation with Texas Scottish Rite implants with type I configuration and posterior cervical arthrodesis with triple-wire technique were performed.

experience is gained with these systems and more long-term follow-up is obtained, the indications for their use will be further defined. Recent prospective studies by Katonis et al. and Korovessis, Baikousis, and Stamatakis document the efficacy of Texas Scottish Rite Hospital instrumentation and Cotrel-Dubousset instrumentation in the treatment of thoracolumbar and lumbar injuries. With mean follow-up of 32 months, these authors concluded that Cotrel-Dubousset instrumentation and Texas Scottish Rite Hospital instrumentation provided solid internal fixation with restoration of the sagittal profile without significant loss of correction and minimal complications.

Anterior Internal Fixation Devices

As stated earlier, anterior decompression of the spinal cord or cauda equina can be safely and directly obtained through an anterior approach. Placement of an iliac strut graft provides no immediate stability if the posterior ligamentous or osseous structures are incompetent. Numerous anterior internal fixation devices have been developed, including the Z-plate, Kaneda device, Texas Scottish Rite Hospital, Zielke, modified Kostuick-Harrington instrumentation, and various plate-and-screw devices. Many studies currently are under way to evaluate the stability of anterior instrumentation without additional posterior stabilization. The disadvantages of anterior instrumentation include the increased morbidity of the surgical approach and potential vascular injuries caused by large anterior implants. If complications occur, the operation to remove implants from the anterior aspect of the spine is more difficult than for posterior implants, and adequate correction of kyphosis may be impossible with anterior instrumentation alone if the posterior supporting structures are incompetent. In addition, a large amount of bone graft material is needed to bridge the defect after an anterior decompression; therefore a large amount of iliac crest must be harvested or allograft used from the bone bank. Biomechanical studies indicate enhanced bone graft healing with the use of anterior internal fixation devices. Advantages of anterior decompression and anterior internal fixation include more adequate debridement of the spinal canal, decompression of the neural elements, avoidance of damage to the posterior muscle structures, which are important for dynamic stabilization of the spine, and avoidance of soft tissue irritation, which frequently occurs with posteriorly implanted spinal instrumentation. The chance of additional damage to the spinal cord, nerve roots, or thecal sac is avoided during an anterior approach, unlike with the posterior approach, in which iatrogenic manipulation or compression of the dural sac during a reduction maneuver may occur.

◆ Kaneda Anterior Spinal Instrumentation

The Kaneda anterior spinal instrumentation is indicated for fractures from T10 to L3 and must be used as a lateral vertebral body device only. The device is designed to span a maximum of four motion segments. In a review of 150 consecutive patients who had a single-stage anterior spinal decompression, strut grafting, and Kaneda spinal instrumentation for a burst fracture of the thoracolumbar spine and neurological deficits, Kaneda et al. reported fusion of the interspinal segment in 140 patients (93%). The percentage of canal occlusion as measured by CT improved from a preoperative mean of 47% to a postoperative mean of 2%. Despite breakage of the Kaneda device in 9 of 150 patients, removal of the implant was not necessary in any patient. None of the patients had iatrogenic neurological deficit. Kaneda et al. reported that 95% of the patients improved by at least 1 grade as measured by the Frankel scale. Seventy-two percent of the patients who had preoperative paralysis or dysfunction of the bladder recovered completely. Follow-up ranged from 5 years to 12 years and 11 months with a mean of 8 years.

TECHNIQUE 35-20 *(Kaneda and Gaines)*

Position the patient for a left retroperitoneal or combined thoracolumbar approach. Unusual anatomy or a need for extensive decompression on the right side may necessitate an approach from the right side.

Place the patient in a lateral decubitus position with the left or right side exposed. Hold the patient securely with positioners and straps. Correct any spinal deformity by careful positioning of the patient. Protect the peripheral nerves (Fig. 35-76, *A*).

Determine the surgical approach and incision by the level of the damaged segment(s). Segments above the thoracolumbar junction are reached most easily through a thoracolumbar incision over the rib, two levels above the damaged segment. Lumbar segments are more easily exposed through a retroperitoneal approach. The thoracolumbar junction can be approached through an incision over the tenth or eleventh rib.

Split the costal cartilage longitudinally and remove the corresponding rib to improve the exposure and provide autologous graft material. Separate the retroperitoneal fat and retroperitoneal structures from the iliopsoas muscle and spine by blunt dissection. Identify the great vessels by palpation. Extend the thoracic exposure by either retropleural or intrapleural dissection. Deflate the lung or bisect the diaphragm if necessary to improve exposure.

After exposing the spine one segment above and below the damaged segment(s), identify, isolate, close, and ligate the segmental vessels at all involved levels 1 cm from the aorta. Bluntly dissect the iliopsoas muscle from all involved vertebrae (Fig. 35-75, *B*). Take care to avoid damage to the genitofemoral nerve, the sympathetic nerves, the ureter, and the aorta.

Corpectomy. Remove the disc and end plate material above and below to the damaged segment(s), leaving the anterior and contralateral cortices intact if possible. Morselize bone removed from the corpectomy site(s) for use as autologous graft material. Perform any required anterior decompression (Fig. 35-76, *C*).

Placement of Spinal Plates. Tetra-spiked Kaneda SR (smooth rod) spinal plates serve as templates for placement

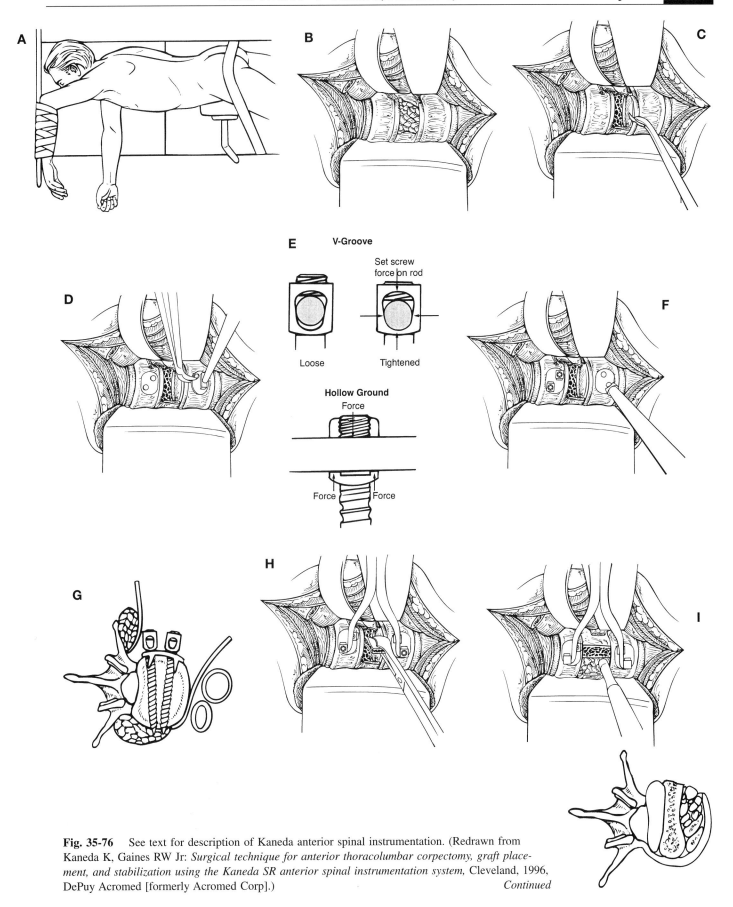

Fig. 35-76 See text for description of Kaneda anterior spinal instrumentation. (Redrawn from Kaneda K, Gaines RW Jr: *Surgical technique for anterior thoracolumbar corpectomy, graft placement, and stabilization using the Kaneda SR anterior spinal instrumentation system,* Cleveland, 1996, DePuy Acromed [formerly Acromed Corp].) *Continued*

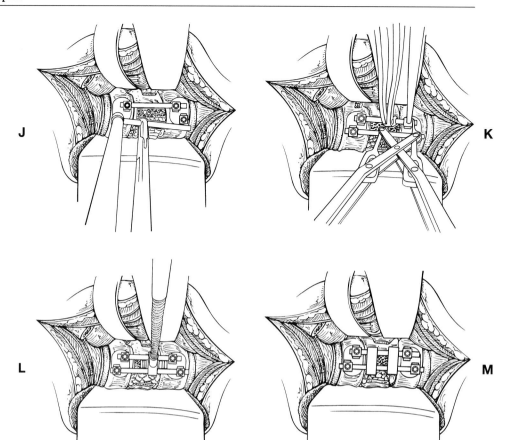

Fig. 35-76, cont'd For legend see p. 1667.

of the Kaneda SR screws and are designed to help prevent the screws from migrating through the vertebral bodies under axial load. Each plate is marked with the letters *A* (anterior), *P* (posterior), and *C/R* (caudal/rostral) to aid in correct placement. When placed correctly the plates allow the rod in the anterior location to be longer than the rod in the posterior position.

The plates are available in three sizes: small, medium, and large. Select a plate that maximizes coverage of the lateral aspect of the vertebra with all four spikes located well within the margins of the vertebral body. Do not allow the spikes to penetrate into the disc spaces above and below the body. Position and impact the plates on each vertebral body (Fig. 35-76, *D*).

Placement of Spinal Screws. The spinal screws serve as the anchors for the longitudinal rods. Each open or closed screw connects to the longitudinal rod with a VHG (V-Groove, Hollow Ground) connection and is secured with a set screw (Fig. 35-76, *E*). The screws are 6.25 mm in diameter and are available in 5-mm increments from 30 mm through 60 mm in length. Two open screws cannot be used together on the same spinal plate.

Determine screw length required by measuring preoperative images, measuring through the corpectomy site(s), or measuring across the intact body with a gauge. Position the posterior screws parallel with a vertebral end plate and angled approximately 10 degrees away from the posterior wall of the body. Place the anterior screws parallel with the same vertebral end plate and parallel with the posterior wall of the vertebral body. Use a single vertebral end plate as a reference for placement of all screws to achieve perpendicular alignment of all screws and rods.

Drive each screw until the head is recessed into the surface of the plate and the screw heads are aligned to allow rod passage (Fig. 35-76, *F*). To ensure secure bicortical purchase, allow each blunt-tipped screw to extend beyond the contralateral cortex by approximately 2 mm (Fig. 35-76, *G*). Confirm correct screw placement by direct palpation or roentgenogram.

Correction of Deformity and Grafting. Place the vertebral body spreader between the heads of the upper and lower screws. Apply distraction until the bodies have been returned to their anatomically correct location. A taut anterior or posterior longitudinal ligament indicates correct vertebral height and lordosis/kyphosis correction. The anterior longitudinal ligament can be divided if it prevents correction of a kyphotic deformity.

Measure the graft site and harvest a tricortical graft

segment of the appropriate length from the iliac crest. Correct sizing of the graft is important to ensure that the graft is placed in compression between the upper and lower vertebral bodies, the anatomical load is accepted by the graft, and the correct anatomical orientation of the vertebral bodies is maintained. Poor graft sizing can lead to hardware failure and poor clinical results.

Position the graft to place the cortical strut on the ipsilateral side and tap into place (Fig. 35-76, *H*). Protect the anterior wall of the spinal canal and place the rib struts in the anterior portion of the defect (Fig. 35-76, *I, inset*). Pack additional morselized bone into the remaining anterior defect (Fig. 35-76, *I*). Remove the distractor.

Placing the Rods. Use a gauge to measure between the upper edge of the posterior upper screw and the lower edge of the posterior lower screw. Add length to allow the rod to extend 2 mm from the edges of the screw connections. Cut a rod to the indicated length and insert it, connecting the two posterior screws.

To prevent impingement on the rods, position the set screws so that they do not protrude into the VHG connection before rod insertion. To aid in rod insertion, rotate one screw slightly away from the longitudinal axis of the construct, insert the rod, and rotate the screw back into correct orientation. Repeat the process for the anterior screw pair (Fig. 35-76, *J*).

Position all set screws to locate the rod at the opening of the VHG, but do not tighten securely. Position the posterior rod relative to either the lower or upper screw and tighten the set screw. Clamp a rod holder onto the posterior rod approximately 2 cm from the unsecured screw to serve as a compression anchor. Place a compressor across the loose screw and rod holder. Apply firm compression and tighten the set screw. Repeat the process for the anterior rod (Fig. 35-76, *K*).

Firm compression is required to ensure that the anatomical loads are passed through the graft rather than the construct. Failure to compress the graft can lead to hardware failure and poor clinical results.

Placing the Transverse Couplers. Transverse couplers stabilize the construct. Two transverse couplers are used for each construct. Load a transverse coupler of appropriate size onto a self-retaining ⅛-inch wrench and loosen the bolt. Position the upper and lower portions of the coupler so that they are perpendicular to each other and introduce the lower portion through the longitudinal rods (Fig. 35-76, *L*). Rotate the ⅛-inch wrench or Penfield to obtain final positioning of the lower portion and move the coupler to one end of the construct. Engage the lower portion onto the rod with gentle upward traction and tension the bolt loosely. Use a modular ⅛-inch wrench for final tightening. Repeat the process for the second coupler.

After the construct assembly has been completed, tension each set screw and transverse coupler bolt to a minimum of 60 inch-pounds (Fig. 35-76, *M*).

Close the wound in the routine fashion. Depending on the surgical approach used, repair of the diaphragm or placement of a chest tube may be necessary.

AFTERTREATMENT. The patient is instructed to wear a thoracolumbar spinal orthosis and to restrict activity for 4 to 6 months.

◆ **Z Plate–ATL Anterior Fixation System**

This device was developed for the management of thoracolumbar burst fractures and tumors. The plate, bolt, and screw system permits anterior loading, allows distraction for reduction and compression of the bone graft, and is relatively easy to implant. The Z plate–ATL also is compatible with MRI and CT (Fig. 35-77).

TECHNIQUE 35-21 *(Zdeblick)*

When treating thoracolumbar fractures or tumors with anterior instrumentation, position the patient so that the approach is from the left side. If indications warrant, the procedure can be done from the patient's right side.

Ensure that the patient is positioned in a true lateral position and is held secure throughout the procedure. When positioning and securing the patient, take care to prevent undue pressure points and nerve palsies. Approach the thoracolumbar junction through the bed of the tenth or eleventh rib. After exposing the spinal segments to be instrumented, excise the discs above and below the area of abnormal anatomy. Perform a corpectomy and complete canal decompression. When necessary, perform reduction at this time. Using the depth gauge, measure the coronal diameter of the vertebral body above and below the corpectomy (Fig. 35-78, *A*). This distance is used to determine the length of the bolts and screws to be used. The bolts and screws of the Z plate–ATL system are intended to engage the opposite cortex of the vertebral body.

Identify the entry points of bolts as shown in Fig. 35-78, *A*. If spinal reduction is required, use the bolt positioning guide to prepare the insertion point for the first bolt with a straight awl. The first bolt should be placed in the inferior posterior position (Fig. 35-78, *B*). Take care when determining placement of this bolt to minimize impingement of the inferior disc space. If spinal reduction is not required, use the appropriate template to determine the required plate length. Position the slots superiorly. With the template in position, use the straight awl to prepare the insertion point for the first bolt (Fig. 35-78, *C*). Place the first bolt in the inferior posterior position. Take care when determining placement of this bolt so that impingement of the inferior disc space is minimized. Once the position

continued

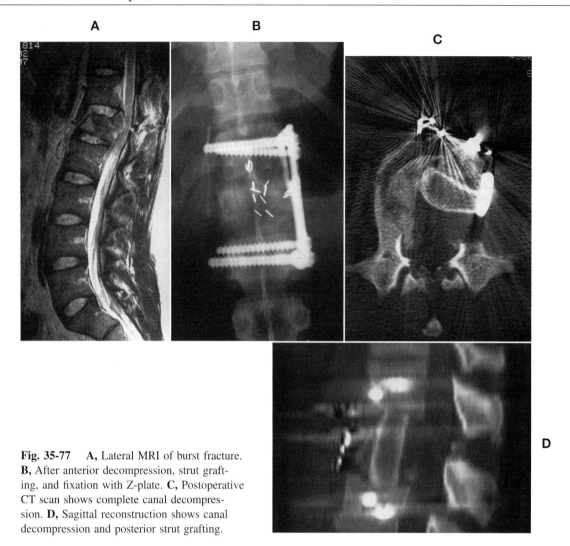

Fig. 35-77 **A,** Lateral MRI of burst fracture. **B,** After anterior decompression, strut grafting, and fixation with Z-plate. **C,** Postoperative CT scan shows complete canal decompression. **D,** Sagittal reconstruction shows canal decompression and posterior strut grafting.

for the first bolt has been marked, remove the template. Using the driver shaft and the ratcheting handle, insert the first bolt parallel to the inferior end plate and angle approximately 10 degrees anteriorly (away from the canal) (Fig. 35-78, *D*). Position the template over the bolt previously implanted with the slots positioned superiorly. Determine the superior posterior bolt location through the posterior slot. Position the bolt near the superior end plate of the vertebral body. Use a straight or curved awl to prepare the insertion point for the second bolt. Note that in patients in whom reduction is required, the template cannot be used because of abnormal anatomy. In such patients the bolt should be started using the bolt positioning guide, as described previously. With the driver shaft and the ratcheting handle, insert the second bolt parallel to the superior end plate and angle it approximately 10 degrees anteriorly (away from the canal) (Fig. 35-78, *E*). If required, perform reduction at this time.

Apply manual pressure on the posterior spine and distract against the vertebral end plates using a standard lamina spreader. Use the Z plate–ATL distractor against the two exposed bolts (Fig. 35-78, *F*). Once final distraction has been obtained, remove the lamina spreader. Measure the corpectomy with the caliper to determine the appropriate bone graft length. Prepare the vertebral body end plates for grafting and harvest the graft. Implant the bone graft into the corpectomy space while maintaining distraction against the machine thread portion of the bolts using the Z plate–ATL distractor (Fig. 35-78, *G*). (Note that the distractor is out of the corpectomy space, allowing full access to the end plates of the superior and inferior vertebral bodies.)

Using the ³⁄₁₆-inch rod/plate holder, place the appropriate-size Z plate–ATL implant over the previously implanted bolts. Place the slots superiorly (Fig. 35-78, *H*). To minimize impingement of the superior disc space and to allow maximal compression, select the shortest-length plate possible. Take special care in preparing a flat surface for the plate by removing the lateral prominence of the vertebral

continued

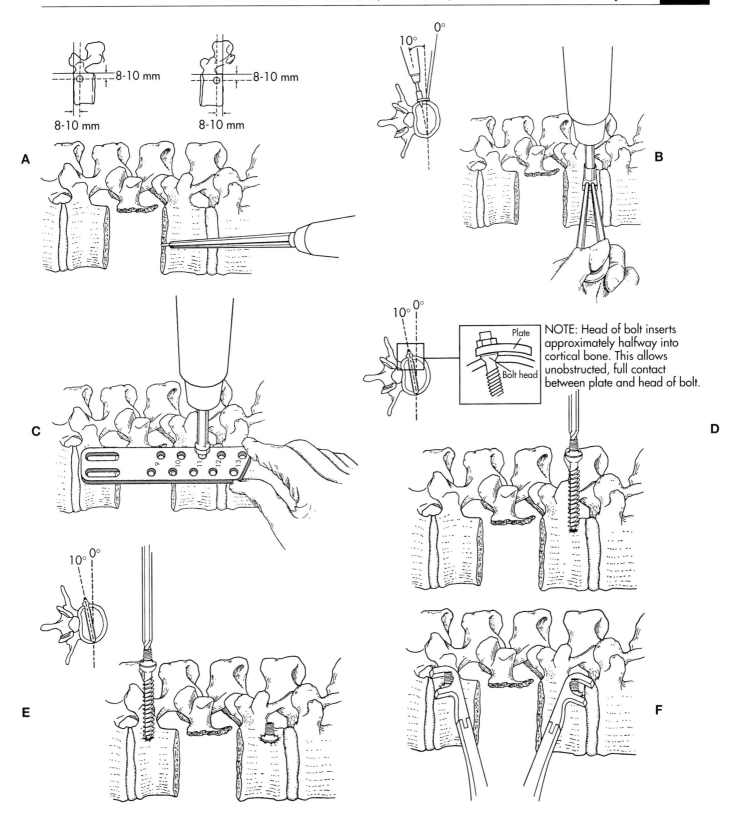

NOTE: Head of bolt inserts approximately halfway into cortical bone. This allows unobstructed, full contact between plate and head of bolt.

Fig. 35-78 Z plate–ATL anterior fixation system (see text). (From Zdeblick TA: Z plate–ATL anterior fixation system technique manual, Memphis, Danek Medical.) *Continued*

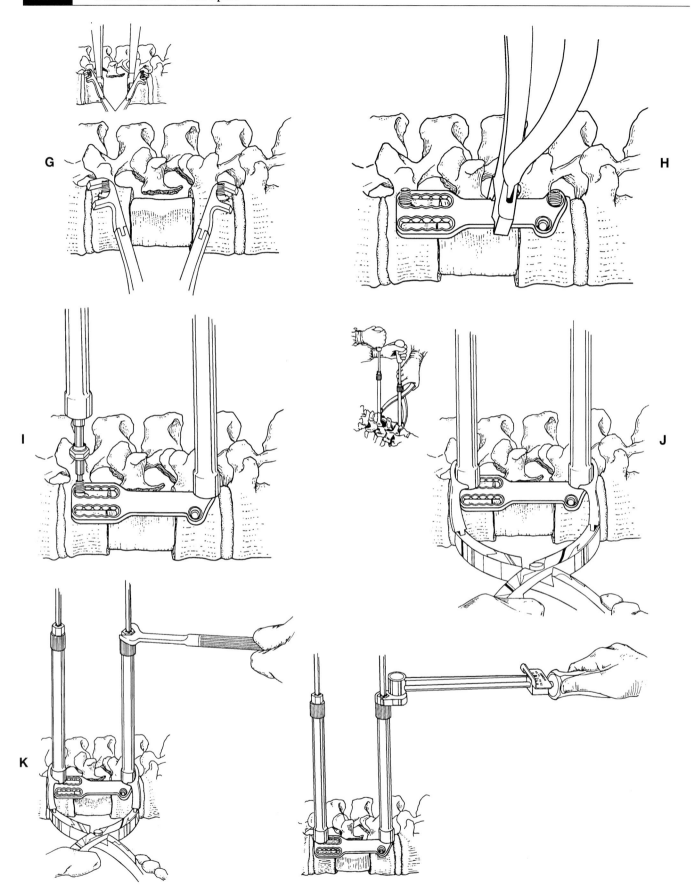

Fig. 35-78, cont'd For legend see p. 1671.

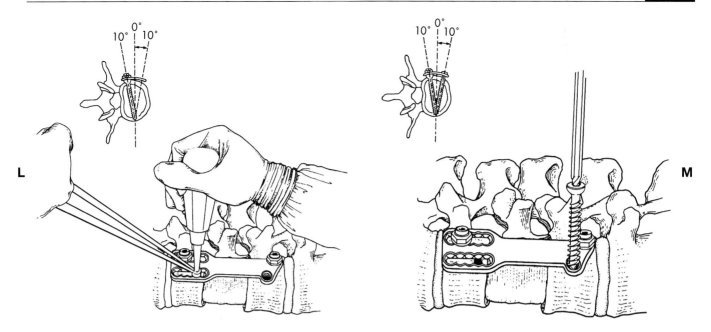

Fig. 35-78, cont'd For legend see p. 1671.

end plates; a high-speed burr or rongeur can be used. Thread the nut (removed from the previously implanted bolt) onto the nut starter shaft/socket. The collar of the nut must be directed toward the handle. Two nut starter shaft/sockets are supplied, and one nut should be threaded onto each shaft at this time. Insert the hex end of one of the nut starter shaft/sockets into the recessed hex of the inferior bolt. While holding countertorque on the handle of the shaft, turn the socket clockwise until the nut has started into the bolt. Tighten the nut using only finger pressure at this time. The nut starter shaft/socket should be held in place by the assistant, as it will be needed shortly.

Insert the hex end of the second nut starter shaft/socket into the recessed hex of the superior bolt. While holding countertorque on the handle of the shaft, turn the socket clockwise until the nut has started onto the bolt (Fig. 35-78, *I*). Do not tighten this nut. Do not remove the nut starter shaft/socket. Slip the shoes of the Z plate–ATL compressor around the base of the two nut starter shaft/sockets (Fig. 35-78, *J*). To ensure that compressive forces are distributed evenly across the disc space, an assistant must hold the handles of the shafts parallel while compression is applied and maintained. Using the nut starter wrench, tighten the superior nut while holding counter-torque on the shaft handle. Once the superior nut has been tightened, the inferior nut is tightened, using the same technique (while holding countertorque on the shaft handle) (Fig. 35-78, *K*). Note that compression must be maintained until both nuts have been tightened. Both nuts must be tightened to a minimum of 80 inch-pounds using the deflection beam torque wrench and the ⁷/16-inch open-end

crowfoot. Countertorque should be applied on the nut starter shaft/socket. Remove the compressor.

Now implant the two anterior screws. Using the awl drill guide and the straight awl, prepare the placement sites of the inferior and superior screws. These screw sites should be directed between 0 and 10 degrees posteriorly (Fig. 35-78, *L*). Using the driver shaft and the ratcheting handle, implant the screws into the previously prepared screw sites (Fig. 35-78, *M*). (To engage the opposite cortex, these screws need to be 5 mm longer than the bolt implanted.) Using the Z plate–ATL crimper, crimp the nut collars onto the flat portion of the bolts. Obtain hemostasis and close the wound in a routine manner over suction drains.

AFTERTREATMENT. Typically, a TLSO molded brace is applied on the third postoperative day. Ambulation is allowed while the patient is in the brace. Bracing is continued for 12 weeks or until solid fusion is noted on the roentgenogram.

◆ ANTERIOR VERTEBRAL BODY EXCISION FOR BURST FRACTURES

Anterior vertebral body excision and grafting, as already mentioned, may be selected primarily or may be necessary in certain burst fractures left untreated for more than 2 weeks and not believed to be candidates for posterior instrumentation and indirect decompression of the spinal canal. McAfee and Bohlman reported 70 patients with spinal cord injury secondary to thoracolumbar fractures treated by anterior decompression through a retroperitoneal approach. All had incomplete neurological deficits caused by retropulsed bone or disc

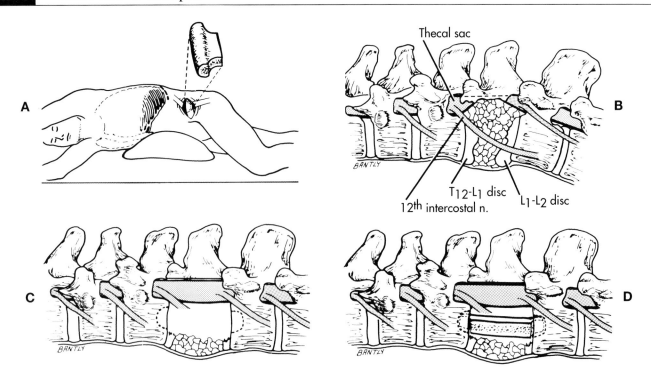

Fig. 35-79 Anterior decompression and strut graft fusion. **A,** Retroperitoneal approach. **B,** Orientation is made easier by tracing course of twelfth intercostal nerve. After removal of left pedicle and vertebra, retropulsed vertebral body fragments of burst fracture of L1 are seen compressing thecal sac. **C,** Vertebral body fragments are removed with high-speed burr until base of opposite pedicle is exposed. **D,** Iliac crest tricortical graft is locked in place using bone tamps. Each end is countersunk into vertebral body above and below. (Redrawn from McAffee PC, Bohlman HH, Yuan HA: *J Bone Joint Surg* 67A:90, 1985.)

material in the spinal canal. Motor deficits in 88% of patients improved by at least one class, and nearly 50% of patients whose quadriceps and hamstrings were impaired enough to prevent walking regained independent walking ability. Of the patients with a conus medullaris injury, 37% demonstrated recovery of neurogenic bowel and bladder function. McAfee and Bohlman concluded that the degree of neurological recovery after anterior decompression of thoracolumbar fractures was greater than after other techniques that do not decompress the spinal canal. We have done limited anterior decompression and strut-graft fusion in patients with incomplete neurological deficits and residual neural compression after posterior instrumentation and in patients whose surgery has been delayed for more than 2 weeks when indirect decompression through posterior instrumentation cannot be expected to produce satisfactory reduction of retropulsed bone and disc fragments. As a result of our increasing experience with anterior decompression and anterior internal fixation, we now perform a single-stage anterior decompression, strut grafting, and internal fixation in many patients. With the use of anterior spinal implants, staged posterior spinal instrumentation generally is not necessary. Close observation with follow-up roentgenograms is recommended. Despite the stability achieved with anterior implants, we recommend immobilization in a spinal orthosis while arthrodesis is taking place.

TECHNIQUE 35-22

Approach the spine anteriorly through a retroperitoneal or retropleural approach (Fig. 35-79, *A* and *B*). Identify the fractured vertebra and excise the intervertebral discs above and below. Next, remove the bulk of the fractured vertebral body using a rongeur and osteotome or, if necessary, a small power burr (Fig. 35-79, *C*). It is best to remove most of the vertebral body before removing the posterior cortex, which exposes the dura. If decompression of the posterior cortex is begun on the side of the body opposite the surgeon, troublesome bulging of the dura into the space created by removing the vertebral body will be minimized and the surgeon's view will be less obstructed. Control bleeding from the bone with bone wax and epidural bleeding with Gelfoam. After the decompression has been completed, cut slots into the end plates of the vertebral bodies above and below the defect; undercut the ends of the slots about 1 cm to allow the graft to be keyed in place. Place Gelfoam over the dura for protection and keep all bone grafts anterior and away from the dura itself. Obtain a tricortical iliac graft or a fibular graft. Undercut the ends of the graft and key it into place to prevent it from dislodging (Fig. 35-79, *D*). Do not place any bone deep to the graft in the area of

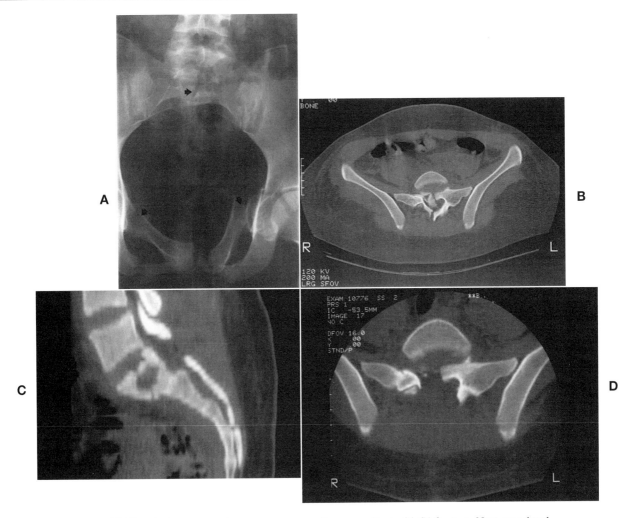

Fig. 35-80   **A,** Anteroposterior roentgenogram of trauma patient with S1 fracture. Note associated pelvic fractures. **B,** Axial CT image of bone retropulsed into sacral canal after sacral fracture (Denis type 3 fracture). **C,** Sagittal CT image after sacral laminectomy and canal clearance. **D,** Axial CT image after sacral laminectomy.

decompression. Obtain hemostasis and close the wound in a routine manner over suction drains.

AFTERTREATMENT. The patient is kept on bed rest until it is certain that wound infection or other complications are absent; then he is mobilized in a molded thoracolumbosacral orthosis. The orthosis is worn for 12 to 16 weeks. If posterior stability is questionable, posterior instrumentation or anterior internal fixation is indicated.

Sacral Fractures and Lumbosacral Dislocation

Sacral fractures and lumbosacral dislocation constitute approximately 1% of all spinal fractures. They frequently are associated with pelvic fractures and often are overlooked

(Fig. 35-80). The most common causes of these fractures are motor vehicle accidents and falls. Lafollette, Levine, and McNiesh noted that 60% of sacral fractures are missed initially. A high index of suspicion is necessary to diagnose sacral fractures in patients with multiple trauma. These patients should be carefully examined for sacral root dysfunction, suggested by decreased perianal sensation and rectal sphincter disturbance. Decreased ankle jerk reflexes and absence of a bulbocavernosus reflex also may suggest sacral root injury. Schmidek et al. classified sacral fractures into those resulting from direct trauma and those resulting from indirect trauma. Gunshots were the most common causes of direct trauma. Most of these injuries are structurally stable. Direct, severe, blunt trauma results in a comminuted sacral fracture. Sacral nerve root injuries generally accompany this injury. Low transverse fractures are caused by a direct blow to the coccyx, resulting in forward displacement of the sacrococcygeal fragment. Most fractures of the sacrum are the result of indirect injury. More than 90% are associated with pelvic fractures; 25% to 50% of these fractures have an accompanying neurological deficit

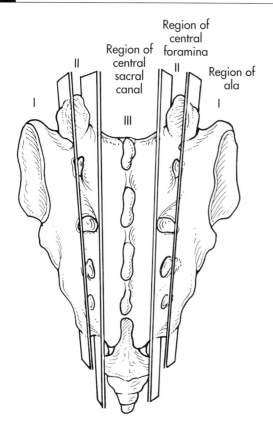

Fig. 35-81 Three zones of sacrum described by Denis: region of ala, region of sacral foramina, and region of central sacral canal. (Redrawn from Carl A: Sacral spine fractures. In Errico TJ, Bauer RD, Waugh T, eds: *Spinal trauma*, Philadelphia, 1990, JB Lippincott.)

(Box 35-2). Denis devised a classification system that divides the sacrum into three zones: (1) the region of the ala, (2) the region of the sacral foramina, and (3) the region of the central sacral canal (Fig. 35-81). In his series of 236 patients, he reported a 32% incidence of neurological deficits. Nerve root damage was present in 5.9% when fractures were in zone 1, 28% in zone 2, and 87% in zone 3. Bonnin found that the foramina is the weakest structural part of the sacrum. Aihara et al. proposed a new classification system for fracture-dislocations of the lumbosacral junction (Fig. 35-82). They

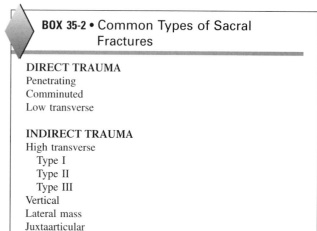

> **BOX 35-2 • Common Types of Sacral Fractures**
>
> **DIRECT TRAUMA**
> Penetrating
> Comminuted
> Low transverse
>
> **INDIRECT TRAUMA**
> High transverse
>   Type I
>   Type II
>   Type III
> Vertical
> Lateral mass
> Juxtaarticular
> Cleaving
> Avulsion

From Schmidek HH, Smith DA, Kristiansen TK: *Neurosurgery* 15:735, 1984.

Fig. 35-82 Aihara classification of fracture-dislocation of fifth lumbar vertebra (see text). (From Aihara T, Takahashi K, Yamagata M, Moriya H: *J Bone Joint Surg* 80B: 840, 1998.)

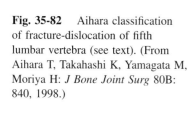

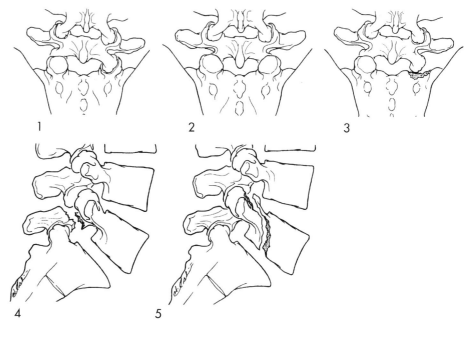

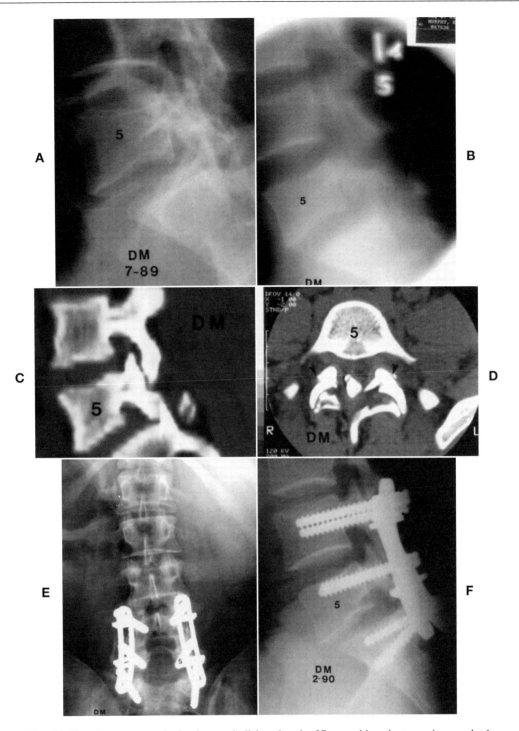

Fig. 35-83   Acute traumatic lumbosacral dislocation in 27-year-old patient causing grade 1 spondylolisthesis of L5 on sacrum. Patient had isolated left S1 nerve root injury. **A** and **B,** Lateral roentgenogram and tomogram of lumbosacral joint show spondylolisthesis and fracture of spinous process of L5. **C** and **D,** CT scans show dislocated inferior articular masses of L5 in relationship to superior articular facets of sacrum and compression of S1 nerve root by left paracentral L5-S1 disc herniation. **E** and **F,** After internal fixation with pedicle screws and plates and midline decompressive laminectomy of L5. Patient was left with only residual decreased ankle jerk reflex on left and mild back pain that did not prevent return to work.

reviewed 50 previously reported fracture-dislocations of L5 and concluded that conservative treatment generally is not effective because the injury is unstable. Their classification system includes type I, unilateral lumbosacral facet dislocation with or without facet fracture; type II, bilateral lumbosacral facet dislocation with or without facet fracture; type III, unilateral lumbosacral facet dislocation and contralateral lumbosacral facet fracture; type IV, dislocation of the body of L5 with bilateral fractures of the pars interarticularis; type V, dislocation of the body of L5 with fracture of the body or pedicle with or without injury to the lamina or facet.

Treatment of sacral fractures and lumbosacral dislocation may be difficult, and both nonoperative and operative management have been used with satisfactory results. Conservative treatment includes bed rest for 8 to 12 weeks, and the successful use of a hip spica cast has been reported. Sacral fractures with unstable pelvic injuries may be successfully treated with external or internal fixation of the pelvic fracture. Delayed neurological injury from entrapment of sacral nerve roots and fracture deformity and callus are not uncommon. Surgery is indicated for patients with neurological impairment, confirmed neural compression from fracture fragments, or sacral deformity and chronic pain. Sacral laminectomy allows exploration of the lower lumbar and upper sacral nerve roots, which innervate the distal lower extremities, and of the lower sacral nerve roots, which control the genital, bladder, anal, and rectal functions. The prognosis for return of bowel and bladder function is uncertain, and recovery depends on whether the deficits are from direct root compression, stretching, or laceration. Instrumentation and fusion with Harrington rods and pedicle screws also have been reported. We have had limited experience with open reduction and internal fixation of displaced sacral fractures; however, lumbosacral dislocation may be effectively stabilized with pedicle screws (Fig. 35-83). We have successfully treated several patients with prolonged bed rest and the use of a hip spica cast. We also have surgically treated several patients with late pain and significant neurological deficits from displaced sacral fractures. The results of sacral laminectomy, decompression, and exploration of the sacral neural elements were satisfactory, but return of bowel and bladder control was poor regardless of the type of treatment. We have found sacral laminectomy to be helpful in evacuation of hematomas, exploration of nerve roots, removal of bone fragments from the spinal canal, and improvement or correction of osseous deformity. Internal fixation of these fractures is technically demanding and depends on the quality of the bone present and the experience of the spinal surgeon. Recent reports on the operative management of displaced fractures of the sacrum by Taguchi et al., Schildhauer et al., Templeman et al., and Gorczyca et al. suggest that internal fixation with iliosacral screws, transiliac screws, or transsacral plating provides earlier mobilization and progression to full weight bearing. Long-term problems with sexual function and bowel and bladder control can be expected. We recommend that treatment be individualized for these infrequent and debilitating injuries (Fig. 35-84).

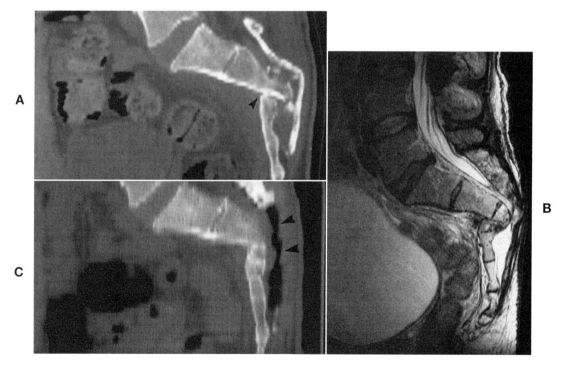

Fig. 35-84   **A,** Sagittal CT image of transverse fracture through S3 resulting in transection of sacral nerve roots. **B,** MRI of sacral fracture resulting in complete canal compromise. **C,** Postoperative CT demonstrating decompression of sacral spinal canal after laminectomy.

References

GENERAL

Amling M, Posl M, Wening VJ, et al: Structural heterogeneity within the axis—the main cause in the etiology of dens fractures: a histomorphometric analysis of 37 normal and osteoporotic autopsy cases, *J Neurosurg* 83:330, 1995.

Anderson PA: Nonsurgical treatment of patients with thoracolumbar fractures, *Instr Course Lect* 44:57, 1995.

Anderson PA, Bohlman HH: Anterior decompression and arthrodesis of the cervical spine: long-term motor improvement (two parts), *J Bone Joint Surg* 74A:671, 1992.

Apple DF, Anson C: Spinal cord injury occurring in patients with ankylosing spondylitis: a multicenter study, *Orthopedics* 18:1005, 1995.

Beard VV, Hochschuler SH: Reflex sympathetic dystrophy following spinal surgery, *Semin Spine Surg* 5:153, 1993.

Beaty JH, ed: *Orthopaedic knowledge update, home study syllabus 6,* Rosemont, Ill, 1999, American Academy of Orthopaedic Surgeons.

Bohlman HH: Pathology and current treatment concepts of acute spine injuries, *Instr Course Lect* 21:108, 1972.

Bosch A, Stauffer ES, Nickel VL: Incomplete traumatic quadriplegia: a ten-year review, *JAMA* 216:473, 1971.

Botte MJ, Byrne TP, Abrams RA, Garfin SR: Halo skeletal fixation: techniques of application and prevention of complications, *J Am Assoc Orthop Surg* 4:44, 1996.

Bracken MB, Holford TR: Effects of timing of methylprednisolone or naloxone administration on recovery of segmented and long-tract neurological function in NACSI II, *J Neurosurg* 79:500, 1993.

Bracken MB, Shepard MJ, Collins WF, et al: A randomized controlled trial of methylprednisolone or naloxone in the treatment of acute spinal cord injury: results of the second National Acute Spinal Cord Injury Study, *N Engl J Med* 322:1405, 1990.

Brightman RP, Miller CA, Rea GL, et al: Magnetic resonance imaging of trauma to the thoracic and lumbar spine: the importance of the posterior longitudinal ligament, *Spine* 17:541, 1992.

Brown MD, Eismont FJ, Quencer RM: Symposium. Intraoperative ultrasonography in spinal surgery, *Contemp Orthop* 11:47, 1985.

Chow YW, Inman C, Pollintine P, et al: Ultrasound bone densitometry and dual energy X-ray absorptiometry in patients with spinal cord injury: a cross-sectional study, *Spinal Cord* 34:736, 1996.

Clark WK: Spinal cord decompression in spinal cord injury, *Clin Orthop* 154:9, 1981.

Cody DD, Goldstein SA, Flynn MJ, Brown EB: Correlations between vertebral regional bone mineral density (rBMD) and whole bone fracture load, *Spine* 16:146, 1991.

Colterjohn NR, Bednar DA: Identifiable risk factors for secondary neurologic deterioration in the cervical spine–injured patient, *Spine* 20:2293, 1995.

Connolly P, Yuan HA: Cervical spine fractures. In White AH, ed: *Spine care: diagnosis and conservative treatment,* St Louis, 1995, Mosby.

Cooper C, Atkinson EJ, Fallon WM, Melton LJ III: Incidence of clinically diagnosed vertebral fractures: a population-based study in Rochester, Minnesota, 1985-1989, *J Bone Miner Res* 7:221, 1992.

Cotler JM, Herbison GJ, Nasti JF, et al: Closed reduction of traumatic cervical spine dislocation using traction weights up to 140 pounds, *Spine* 18:386, 1983.

Coyne TJ, Fehlings MG, Wallace MC, et al: C1-C2 posterior cervical fusion: long-term evaluation of results and efficacy, *Neurosurgery* 37:688, 1995.

Crowther ER: Missed cervical spine fractures: the importance of reviewing radiographs in chiropractic practice, *J Manipulative Physiol Ther* 18:29, 1995.

Danisa OA, Shaffrey CI, Jane JA, et al: Surgical approaches for the correction of unstable thoracolumbar burst fractures: a retrospective analysis of treatment outcomes, *J Neurosurg* 83:977, 1995.

Delamarter RB, Sherman J, Carr JB: Spinal cord injury: the pathophysiology of spinal cord damage and subsequent recovery following immediate or delayed decompression. Paper presented at Cervical Spine Research Society meeting, New York, 1993.

De La Torre JC: Spinal cord injury: review of basic and applied research, *Spine* 6:315, 1981.

Denis F: Spinal instability as defined by the three-column spine concept in acute spinal trauma, *Clin Orthop* 189:65, 1984.

Devilee R, Sanders R, deLange S: Treatment of fractures and dislocations of the thoracic and lumbar spine by fusion and Harrington instrumentation, *Arch Orthop Trauma Surg* 114:100, 1995.

Dickman CA, Zabramski JM, Hadley MN, et al: Pediatric spinal cord injury without radiographic abnormalities: report of 26 cases and review of the literature, *J Spinal Disord* 4:296, 1991.

Dorr LD, Harvey JP, Nickel VL: Clinical review of the early stability of spine injuries, *Spine* 7:545, 1982.

Ebraheim NA, Rupp RE, Savolaine ER, Brown JA: Posterior plating of the cervical spine, *J Spinal Disord* 8:111, 1995.

Eismont FJ, Arena M, Green B: Extrusion of an intervertebral disc associated with traumatic subluxation or dislocation of cervical facets, *J Bone Joint Surg* 73A:1555, 1991.

Eismont FJ, Clifford S, Goldberg M, Green B: Cervical sagittal spinal canal size in spine injury, *Spine* 9:663, 1984.

Fan RS, Schenk RS, Lee CK: Burst fracture of the fifth lumbar vertebra in combination with a pelvic ring injury, *J Orthop Trauma* 9:345, 1995.

Fontijne WPJ, DeKlerk LWL, Braakman R, et al: CT scan prediction of neurological deficit in thoracolumbar burst fractures, *J Bone Joint Surg* 74B:683, 1992.

Fowler BL, Dall BE, Rowe DE: Complications associated with harvesting autogenous iliac bone graft, *Am J Orthop* Dec 1995, p 895.

Fricker R, Gächter A: Lateral flexion/extension radiographs: still recommended following cervical spinal injury, *Arch Orthop Trauma Surg* 113:115, 1994.

Garfin SR, ed: *Complications of spine surgery,* Baltimore, 1989, Williams & Wilkins.

Geisler FH, Dorsey FC, Coleman WP: Recovery of motor function after spinal cord injury: a randomized, placebo-controlled trial with GM-1 ganglioside, *N Engl J Med* 324:1829, 1991.

Geisler FH, Dorsey FC, Coleman WP: GM-1 ganglioside in human spinal cord injury, *J Neurotrauma* 9(suppl):517, 1992.

Gertzbein SD, Court-Brown CM, Marks P et al: The neurological outcome following surgery for spinal fractures, *Spine* 13:641, 1988.

Gold DT: The clinical impact of vertebral fractures: quality of life in women with osteoporosis, *Bone* 18(suppl 3):185, 1996.

Grabb PA, Pang D: Magnetic resonance imaging in the evaluation of spinal cord injury without radiographic abnormality in children, *Neurosurgery* 35:406, 1994.

Green BA, Callahan RA, Klore KJ et al: Acute spinal cord injury: current concepts, *Clin Orthop* 154:125, 1981.

Heller JG, Silcox DH, Sutterlin CE: Complications of posterior cervical plating, *Spine* 20:2442, 1995.

Hildingsson C, Hietala SO, Toolanen G et al: Negative scintigraphy despite spinal fractures in the multiply injured, *Injury* 24:467, 1993.

Holdsworth FW: Traumatic paraplegia. In Platt H, ed: *Modern trends in orthopaedics (second series),* New York, 1956, Paul B Hoeber.

Holdsworth FW: Fractures, dislocations, and fracture-dislocations of the spine, *J Bone Joint Surg* 45B:6, 1963.

Holdsworth FW: Fractures, dislocations, and fracture-dislocations of the spine, *J Bone Joint Surg* 52A:1534, 1970.

Holdsworth SF: Review article: fractures, dislocations, and fracture-dislocations of the spine, *J Bone Joint Surg* 52B:1534, 1970.

Hopkins TJ, White AA: Rehabilitation of athletes following spine injury, *Clin Sports Med* 12:603, 1993.

Huang TJ, Hsu RWW, Fan GF, et al: Two-level burst fractures: clinical evaluation and treatment options, *J Trauma* 41:77, 1996.

Jelsma RK, Rice JF, Jelsma LF, Kirsch PT: The demonstration and significance of neural compression after spinal injury, *Surg Neurol* 18:79, 1982.

Kado DM, Browner WS, Palermo L, et al: Vertebral fractures and mortality in older women: a prospective study. Study of osteoporotic fractures research group, *Arch Intern Med* 159:1215, 1999.

Kahnovitz N, Bullough P, Jacobs RR: The effect of internal fixation without arthrodesis on human facet joint cartilage, *Clin Orthop* 189:204, 1984.

Karasick D, Huettl EA, Cotler JM: Value of polydirectional tomography in the assessment of the postoperative spine after anterior decompression and vertebral body autografting, *Skeletal Radiol* 21:359, 1992.

Kirkpatrick JS, Wilber RG, Likavec M, et al: Anterior stabilization of thoracolumbar burst fractures using the Kaneda device: a preliminary report, *Orthopedics* 18:673, 1995.

Kraus JF, Franti CE, Riggins RS, et al: Incidence of traumatic spinal cord lesions, *J Chronic Dis* 28:471, 1975.

Kreitz BG, Cote P, Cassidy JD: L5 vertebral compression fracture: a series of five cases, *J Manipulative Physiol Ther* 18:91, 1995.

Laborde JM, Bahniuk E, Bohlman HH, Samson B: Comparison of fixation of spinal fractures, *Clin Orthop* 152:303, 1980.

Leroux JL, Denat B, Thomas E, et al: Sacral insufficiency fractures presenting as acute low-back pain: biomechanical aspects, *Spine* 18:2502, 1993.

Levine AM, McAfee PC, Anderson PA: Evaluation and emergent treatment of patients with thoracolumbar trauma, *Instr Course Lect* 44:33, 1995.

Lyles KW, Gold DT, Shipp KM, et al: Association of osteoporotic vertebral compression fractures with impaired functional status, *Am J Med* 94:595, 1993.

Mann DC, Dodds JA: Spinal injuries in 57 patients 17 years or younger, *Orthopedics* 16:159, 1993.

Markel DC, Graziano G: A comparison study of treatment of thoracolumbar fractures using the ACE Posterior Segmental Fixator and Cotrel-Dubousset instrumentation, *Orthopedics* 18:679, 1995.

Markel DC, Raskas DS, Graziano GP: A case of traumatic spino-pelvic dissociation, *J Orthop Trauma* 7:562, 1993.

McAfee PC, Bohlman HH, Ducker TB, et al: One-stage anterior cervical decompression and posterior stabilization: a study of one hundred patients with a minimum of two years of follow-up, *J Bone Joint Surg* 77A:1791, 1995.

McDonnell MF, Glassman SD, Dimar JR, et al: Perioperative complications of anterior procedures on the spine, *J Bone Joint Surg* 78A:839, 1996.

McLain RF, Benson DR: Urgent surgical stabilization of spinal fractures in polytrauma patients, *Spine* 24:1646, 1999.

McPhee IB: Spinal fractures and dislocations in children and adolescents, *Spine* 6:533, 1981.

Meyer PR Jr: Emergency room assessment: management of spinal cord and associated injuries. In Meyer PR Jr, ed: *Surgery of spine trauma*, New York, 1989, Churchill Livingstone.

Modic MT, Masaryk T, Paushter D: Magnetic resonance imaging of the spine, *Radiol Clin North Am* 24:229, 1986.

Montgomery TJ, McGuire RA Jr: Traumatic neuropathic arthropathy of the spine, *Orthop Rev* 22:1153, 1993.

Nagel DA, Edwards WT, Schneider E: Biomechanics of spinal fixation and fusion, *Spine* 16(suppl):151, 1991.

Pang D, Pollack IF: Spinal cord injury without radiographic abnormality in children—the SCIWORA syndrome, *J Trauma* 29:654, 1989.

Panjabi MM, Oxland T, Takata K, et al: Articular facets of the human spine: quantitative three-dimensional anatomy, *Spine* 18:1298, 1993.

Pascal-Moussellard H, Klein JR, Schwab FJ, Farcy JP: Simultaneous anterior and posterior approaches to the spine for revision surgery: current indications and techniques, *Spinal Disord* 12:206, 1999.

Potter PJ, Hayes KC, Hsieh JT, et al: Sustained improvements in neurological function in spinal cord injured patients treated with oral 4-aminopyridine: three cases, *Spinal Cord* 36:147, 1998.

Poynton AR, O'Farrell DA, Shannon F, et al: An evaluation of the factors affecting neurological recovery following spinal cord injury, *Injury* 28:545, 1997.

Quencer RM: Intraoperative ultrasound of the spine, *Surg Rounds*, Oct 1987, p 17.

Riggs BL, Melton LJ III: The worldwide problem of osteoporosis: insights afforded by epidemiology, *Bone* 17:505S, 1995.

Rosenberg N, Lenger R, Weisz I, Stein H: Neurological deficit in a consecutive series of vertebral fracture patients with bony fragments within spinal canal, *Spinal Cord* 35:92, 1997.

Rupp RE, Ebraheim NA, Coombs RJ: Magnetic resonance imaging differentiating compression spine fractures or vertebral lesions caused by osteoporosis or tumor, *Spine* 20:2499, 1995.

Saboe LA, Reid DC, Davic LA, et al: Spine trauma and associated injuries, *J Trauma* 31:43, 1991.

Sapkas G, Korres D, Babis GC, et al: Correlation of spinal canal post-traumatic encroachment and neurological deficit in burst fractures of the lower cervical spine (C3-7), *Eur Spine J* 4:39, 1995.

Savolaine ER, Ebraheim NA, Rusin JJ, Jackson WT: Limitations of radiography and computed tomography in the diagnosis of transverse sacral fracture from a high fall, *Clin Orthop* 272:122, 1991.

Schlaich C, Minne HW, Bruckner T, et al: Reduced pulmonary function in patients with spinal osteoporotic fractures, *Osteoporos Int* 8:261, 1998.

Schlegel J, Bayley J, Yuan H, Fredrickson B: Timing of surgical decompression and fixation of acute spinal fractures, *J Orthop Trauma* 10:323, 1996.

Schneider RC, Kahn EA: Chronic neurologic sequelae of acute trauma to the spine and spinal cord. II. The syndrome of chronic anterior spinal cord injury or compression, *J Bone Joint Surg* 41A:449, 1959.

Slucky AV, Eismont FJ: Treatment of acute injury of the cervical spine, *J Bone Joint Surg* 76A:1882, 1994.

Smith MD, Johnson LJ, Perra JH, Rawlins BA: A biomechanical study of torque and accuracy of halo pin insertional devices, *J Bone Joint Surg* 78A:231, 1996.

Sobel JW, Bohlman HH, Freehafer AA: Charcot's arthropathy of the spine following spinal cord injury: a report of five cases, *J Bone Joint Surg* 67A:771, 1985.

Southwick WO: Management of fractures of the dens (odontoid process), *J Bone Joint Surg* 62A:482, 1980.

Stambough JL, Lazio BE: Unusual L5 fracture with neurologic involvement, *Orthopedics* 18:1034, 1995.

Stauffer ES, Wood RW, Kelly EG: Gunshot wounds of the spine: the effects of laminectomy, *J Bone Joint Surg* 61A:389, 1979.

Tator CH, Fehlings MG, Thorpe K, Taylor W: Current use and timing of spinal surgery for management of acute spinal cord injury in North America: results of a retrospective multi-center study, *J Neurosurg* 91:12, 1999.

Torg JS, Currier B, Douglas R, et al: Symposium: spinal cord resuscitation, *Contemp Orthop* 30:495, 1995.

Turgut M, Akpinar G, Akalan N, Ozcan OE: Spinal injuries in the pediatric age group: a review of 82 cases of spinal cord and vertebral column injuries. *Eur Spine J* 5:148:1996.

Vornanen MJ, Bostman OM, Myllynen PJ: Reduction of bone retropulsed into the spinal canal in thoracolumbar vertebral body compression burst fractures: a prospective randomized comparative study between Harrington rods and two transpedicular devices, *Spine* 20:1699, 1995.

Wilmink JT: MR imaging of the spine: trauma and degenerative disease, *Eur Radiol* 9:1259, 1999.

Xu R, Haman SP, Ebraheim NA, Yeasting RA: The anatomic relation of lateral mass screws to the spinal nerves: a comparison of the Magerl, Anderson, and An techniques, *Spine* 24:2057, 1999.

Zdeblick TA: Complications of anterior spinal instrumentation, *Sem Spin Surg* 5:101, 1993.

CERVICAL SPINE

Aebi M, Zuber K, Marchesi D: Treatment of cervical spine injuries with anterior plating: indications, techniques, and results, *Spine* 16(suppl 3):38, 1991.

Allen BL Jr, Ferguson RL, Lehmann R, O'Brian RP: Mechanistic classification of closed indirect fractures and dislocations of the lower cervical spine, *Spine* 7:1, 1982.

An HS: Internal fixation of the cervical spine: current indications and techniques, *J Am Assoc Orthop Surg* 3:194, 1995.

Anderson LD, D'Alonzo RT: Fractures of the odontoid process of the axis, *J Bone Joint Surg* 56A:1663, 1974.

Anderson PA, Bohlman HH: Anterior decompression and arthrodesis of the cervical spine: long-term motor improvement, *J Bone Joint Surg* 74A:683, 1992.

Anderson PA, Grady MS: Posterior stabilization of the lower cervical spine with lateral mass plates and screws, *Op Tech Orthop* 6:58, 1996.

Anderson PA, Henley MB, Grady MS, et al: Posterior cervical arthrodesis with AO reconstruction plates and bone grafts, *Spine* 16:572, 1991.

Anderson PA, Montesano PX: Morphology and treatment of occipital condyle fractures, *Spine* 13:731, 1988.

Aprin H, Harf R: Stabilization of atlantoaxial instability, *Orthopedics* 11:1687, 1988.

Arena MJ, Eismont FJ, Green BA: Intervertebral disc extrusion associated with cervical facet subluxation and dislocation. Paper presented at the Fifteenth Annual Meeting of the Cervical Spine Research Society, Washington, DC, Dec 2-5, 1987.

Ballock RT, Botte MJ, Garfin SR: Complications of halo immobilization. In Garfin SR, ed: *Complications of spine surgery*, Baltimore, 1989, Williams & Wilkins.

Beatson TR: Fractures and dislocations of the cervical spine, *J Bone Joint Surg* 45B:21, 1963.

Benzel EC, Hart BL, Ball PA, et al: Magnetic resonance imaging for the evaluation of patients with occult cervical spine injury, *J Neurosurg* 85:824, 1996.

Beyer CA, Cabanela ME: Unilateral facet dislocations and fracture-dislocations of the cervical spine: a review, *Orthopedics* 15:311, 1992.

Beyer CA, Cabanela ME, Berquist TH: Unilateral facet dislocations and fracture-dislocations of the cervical spine, *J Bone Joint Surg* 73B:977, 1991.

Blacksin MF, Lee HJ: Frequency and significance of fractures of the upper cervical spine detected by CT in patients with severe neck trauma, *Am J Roentgenol* 165:1201, 1995.

Bloom AI, Neeman Z, Slasky BS, et al: Fracture of the occipital condyles and associated craniocervical ligament injury: incidence, CT imaging and implications, *Clin Radiol* 52:198, 1997.

Bohlman HH: Pathology and current treatment concepts of cervical spine injuries, *Instr Course Lect* 21:108, 1972.

Bohlman HH: The pathology and current treatment concepts of cervical spine injuries: a critical review of 300 cases, *J Bone Joint Surg* 54A:1353, 1972.

Bohlman HH: Complications of treatment of fractures and dislocations of the cervical spine. In Epps CH, ed: *Complications in orthopaedic surgery*, Philadelphia, 1978, JB Lippincott.

Bohlman HH: Acute fractures and dislocations of the cervical spine, *J Bone Joint Surg* 61A:1119, 1979.

Bohlman HH: Complications and pitfalls in the treatment of acute cervical spinal cord injuries. In Tator CH, ed: *Early management of acute spinal cord injury*, New York, 1982, Raven.

Bohlman HH: Indications for late anterior decompression and fusion for cervical spinal cord injuries. In Tator CH, ed: *Early management of acute spinal cord injury*, New York, 1982, Raven.

Bohlman HH: Surgical management of cervical spine fractures and dislocations, *Instr Course Lect* 34:163, 1985.

Bohlman HH, Anderson PA: Anterior decompression and arthrodesis of the cervical spine: long-term motor improvement, *J Bone Joint Surg* 74A:671, 1992.

Bohlman HH, Anderson PA, Freehafer A: Anterior decompression and arthrodesis in patients with motor incomplete cervical spinal cord injury: long-term results of neurologic recovery in 58 patients (unpublished data).

Bohlman HH, Bahnuik E, Gield G, Raskulinecz G: Spinal cord monitoring of experimental incomplete cervical spinal cord injury, *Spine* 6:428, 1981.

Bohlman HH, Bahnuik E, Raskulinecz G, Field G: Mechanical factors affecting recovery from incomplete cervical spine injury: a preliminary report, *Johns Hopkins Med J* 145:115, 1979.

Bohlman HH, Eismont FJ: Surgical techniques of anterior decompression and fusion for spinal cord injuries, *Clin Orthop* 154:57, 1981.

Bosch A, Stauffer ES, Nickel VL: Incomplete traumatic quadriplegia: a ten-year review, *JAMA* 216:473, 1967.

Bridwell KH, DeWald RL: *Textbook of spinal surgery*, vol 2, New York, 1991, Lippincott-Raven.

Brooks AL, Jenkins EB: Atlanto-axial arthrodesis by the wedge compression method, *J Bone Joint Surg* 60A:279, 1978.

Budorick TE, Anderson PA, Rivara FP, Cohen W: Flexion-distraction fracture of the cervical spine, *J Bone Joint Surg* 73A:1097, 1991.

Campanelli M, Kattner KA, Stroink A, et al: Posterior C1-C2 transarticular screw fixation in the treatment of displaced type II odontoid fractures in the geriatric population—review of seven cases, *Surg Neurol* 51:596, 1999.

Capen D, Zigler J, Garland D: Surgical stabilization in cervical spine trauma, *Contemp Orthop* 14:25, 1987.

Capen DA, Nelson RW, Zigler JE, et al: Decompressive laminectomy in cervical spine trauma: a review of early and late complications, *Contemp Orthop* 17:21, 1988.

Carroll C, McAfee PC, Riley LH Jr: Objective findings for diagnosis of "whiplash," *J Musculoskel Med*, March 1986, p 57.

Carter DR, Frankel VH: Biomechanics of hyperextension injuries to the cervical spine in football, *Am J Sports Med* 8:302, 1982.

Caspar W: Advances in cervical spine surgery: first experiences with trapezial osteosynthetic plate and new surgical instrumentation for anterior interbody stabilization, *Orthop News* 4:1, 1982.

Castillo M, Mukherji SK: Vertical fractures of the dens, *Am J Neuroradiol* 17:1627, 1996.

Chen IH, Yang RS, Chen PQ: Plate fixation for anterior cervical interbody fusion, *J Formos Med Assoc* 90:172, 1991.

Chen JY, Chen WJ, Huang TJ, Shih CH: Spinal epidural abscess complicating cervical spine fracture with hypopharyngeal perforation, *Spine* 17:971, 1992.

Choueka J, Spivak JM, Kummer FJ, Steger T: Flexion failure of posterior cervical lateral mass screws: influence of insertion technique and position, *Spine* 21:462, 1996.

Clark CR: Dens fractures, *Semin Spine Surg* 3:39, 1991.

Ching RP, Watson NA, Carter JW, Tencer AF: The effect of post-injury spinal position on canal occlusion in a cervical spine burst fracture model, *Spine* 22:1710, 1997.

Choi WG, Vishteh AG, Baskin JJ, et al: Completely dislocated hangman's fracture with a locked C2-3 facet. Case report, *J Neurosurg* 87:757, 1997.

Clark CR, Whitehill R: Two views of the use of methylmethacrylate for stabilization of the cervical spine, *Orthopedics* 12:589, 1989.

Clausen JD, Ryken TC, Traynelis VC, et al: Biomechanical evaluation of Caspar and cervical spine locking plate systems in a cadaveric model, *J Neurosurg* 84:1039, 1996.

Cooper PR, Cohen A, Rosiello A, et al: Posterior stabilization of cervical spine fractures and subluxation using plates and screws, *Neurosurgery* 23:300, 1988.

Coric D, Branch CL Jr, Wilson JA, Robinson JC: Arteriovenous fistula as a complication of C1-2 transarticular screw fixation. Case report and review of the literature, *J Neurosurg* 85:340, 1996.

Coric D, Wilson JA, Kelly DL Jr: Treatment of traumatic spondylolisthesis of the axis with nonrigid immobilization: a review of 64 cases, *J Neurosurg* 85:550, 1996.

Coyne TJ, Fehlings MG, Wallace MC, et al: C1-C2 posterior cervical fusion: long-term evaluation of results and efficacy, *Neurosurgery* 37:688, 1995.

Crenshaw AH Jr, Wood GW, Wood MW Jr, Ray MW: Fracture and dislocation of the fourth and fifth cervical vertebral bodies with transection of the spinal cord, *Clin Orthop* 248:158, 1989.

Crisco JJ, Panjabi MM, Oda T, et al: Bone graft translation of four upper cervical spine fixation techniques in a cadaveric model, *J Orthop Res* 9:835, 1991.

Cusick JF, Yoganandan N, Pintar F, Gardon M: Cervical spine injuries from high-velocity forces: a pathoanatomic and radiologic study, *J Spinal Disord* 9:1, 1996.

Davis D, Bohlman H, Walker E, et al: The pathological findings in fatal craniospinal injuries, *J Neurol* 34:603, 1971.

Davis J: Injuries to the subaxial cervical spine: posterior approach options, *Orthopedics* 20:929, 1997.

Davis JW, Parks SN, Detlefs CL, et al: Clearing the cervical spine in obtunded patients: the use of dynamic fluoroscopy, *J Trauma* 39:435, 1995.

Deen HG, McGirr SJ: Vertebral artery injury associated with cervical spine fracture, *Spine* 17:230, 1992.

Delamarter RB: The cervical spine. III. Management of cervical spine injuries. Instructional course lecture presented at the Fifty-seventh Annual Meeting of the American Academy of Orthopaedic Surgeons, New Orleans, Feb 12, 1990.

Demisch S, Lindner A, Beck R, Zierz S: The forgotten condyle: delayed hypoglossal nerve palsy caused by fracture of the occipital condyle, *Clin Neurol Neurosurg* 100:44, 1998.

Dickman CA, Crawford NR, Paramore CG: Biomechanical characteristics of C1-2 cable fixations, *J Neurosurg* 85:316, 1996.

Dickman CA, Greene KA, Sonntag VK: Injuries involving the transverse atlantal ligament: classification and treatment guidelines based upon experience with 39 injuries, *Neurosurgery* 38:44, 1996.

Dickman CA, Sonntag VK: Posterior C1-C2 transarticular screw fixation for atlantoaxial arthrodesis, *Neurosurgery* 43:275, 1998.

Donaldson WF III, Heil BV, Donaldson VP, et al: The effect of airway maneuvers on the unstable C1-C2 segment: a cadaver study, *Spine* 22:1215, 1997.

Donaldson WF III, Lauerman WC, Heil B, et al: Helmet and shoulder pad removal from a player with suspected cervical spine injury: a cadaveric model, *Spine* 23:1729, 1998.

Ducker TB, Bellegarrigue R, Salcman M, Walleck C: Timing of operative care in cervical spinal cord injury, *Spine* 9:525, 1984.

Dull ST, Toselli RM: Preoperative oblique axial computed tomographic imaging for C1-C2 transarticular screw fixation: technical note, *Neurosurgery* 37:150, 1995.

Duncan RW, Esses SI: Dens fractures: specifications and management, *Semin Spine Surg* 8:19, 1996.

Ebraheim NA, DeTroye RJ, Rupp RE, et al: Osteosynthesis of the cervical spine with an anterior plate, *Orthopedics* 18:141, 1995.

Ebraheim NA, Hoeflinger MJ, Salpietro B, et al: Anatomic considerations in posterior plating of the cervical spine, *J Orthop Trauma* 5:196, 1991.

Ebraheim NA, Lu J, Yang H: The effect of translation of the C1-C2 on the spinal canal, *Clin Orthop* 351:222, 1998.

Ebraheim NA, Tremains MR, Xu R, et al: Lateral radiologic evaluation of lateral mass screw placement in the cervical spine, *Spine* 23:458, 1998.

Edwards CC, Matz SO, Levine AM: Oblique wiring technique for rotational injury of cervical spine, *Orthop Trans* 9:142, 1985 (abstract).

Eismont FJ, Bohlman HH: Posterior atlanto-occipital dislocation with fractures of the atlas and odontoid process, *J Bone Joint Surg* 60A:397, 1978.

Eismont FJ, Bohlman HH: Posterior methylmethacrylate fixation for cervical trauma, *Spine* 6:347, 1981.

Eismont FJ, Bora F, Bohlman HH: Complete dislocations at two adjacent levels of the cervical spine, *Spine* 9:319, 1984.

El-Khoury GY, Kathol MH: Radiographic evaluation of cervical spine trauma, *Semin Spine Surg* 3:3, 1991.

Etter C, Coscia M, Jaberg H, et al: Direct anterior fixation of dens fracture with a cannulated screw system, *Spine* 16:S25, 1991.

Fabris D, Nena U, Gentilucci G, et al: Surgical treatment of traumatic lesions of the middle and lower cervical spine with Roy-Camille plates, *Ital J Orthop Traumatol* 18:43, 1992.

Fielding JW: Selected observations on the cervical spine in the child. In Ahstrom JP Jr, ed: *Current practice in orthopaedic surgery*, vol 5, St Louis, 1973, Mosby.

Fielding JW, Cochran GVB, Lawsing JF III, et al: Tears of the transverse ligament of the atlas: a clinical and biomechanical study, *J Bone Joint Surg* 56A:1683, 1974.

Fielding JW, Francis WR, Hawkins RJ, et al: Atlantoaxial rotary deformity, *Semin Spine Surg* 3:33, 1991.

Fielding JW, Hawkins RJ: Atlanto-axial rotatory fixation: fixed rotatory subluxation of the atlanto-axial joint, *J Bone Joint Surg* 59A:37, 1977.

Fielding JW, Hawkins RJ, Ratzan SA: Spine fusion for atlanto-axial instability, *J Bone Joint Surg* 58A:400, 1976.

Fielding JW, Hensinger RN: Cervical spine surgery: past, present, and future potential, *Orthopedics* 10:1701, 1987.

Foley KT, DiAngelo DJ, Rampersaud YR, et al: The in vitro effects of instrumentation on multilevel cervical strut-graft mechanics, *Spine* 15:2366, 1999.

Fujimura Y, Nishi Y, Chiba K, et al: Prognosis of neurological deficits associated with upper cervical spine injuries, *Paraplegia* 33:195, 1995.

Gallie WE: Fractures and dislocations of the cervical spine, *Am J Surg* 46:495, 1939.

Garvey TA, Eismont FJ, Roberti LJ: Anterior decompression, structural bone grafting, and Caspar plate stabilization for unstable cervical spine fractures and/or dislocations, *Spine* 17(suppl):431, 1992.

Giacobetti FB, Vaccaro AR, Bos-Giacobetti MA, et al: Vertebral artery occlusion associated with cervical spine trauma: a prospective analysis, *Spine* 22:188, 1997.

Goldstein R, Deen HG Jr, Zimmerman RS, et al: "Preplacement" of the back of the halo vest in patients undergoing cervical traction for cervical spine injuries: a technical note, *Surg Neurol* 44:476, 1995.

Graber MA, Kathol M: Cervical spine radiographs in the trauma patient, *Am Fam Physician* 59:331, 1999.

Greene KA, Dickman CA, Marciano F, et al: Acute axis fractures: analysis of management and outcome in 340 consecutive cases, *Spine* 22:1843, 1997.

Grob D, Crisco JJ III, Panjabi MM, et al: Biomechanical evaluation of four different posterior atlantoaxial fixation techniques, *Spine* 17:480, 1992.

Gruenbert MF, Rechtine GR, Chrin AM, et al: Overdistraction of cervical spine injuries with the use of skull traction: a report of two cases, *J Trauma* 42:1152, 1997.

Guiot B, Fessler RG: Complex atlantoaxial fractures, *J Neurosurg* 91:139, 1999.

Hadley MN, Dickman CA, Browner CM, et al: Acute traumatic atlas fractures: management and long-term outcome, *Adv Orthop Surg* 12:234, 1989.

Hadley MN, Fitzpatrick BC, Volker KH, et al: Experimental and clinical studies, *Neurosurgery* 30:661, 1992.

Hamilton A, Webb JK: The role of anterior surgery for vertebral fractures with and without cord compression, *Clin Orthop* 300:79, 1994.

Hanssen AD, Cabanela ME, Cass JR: Fractures of the dens (odontoid process), *Adv Orthop Surg* 10:170, 1987.

Harris MB, Waguespack AM, Kronlage S: "Clearing" cervical spine injuries in polytrauma patients: is it really safe to remove the collar? *Orthopedics* 20:903, 1997.

Heller JG: Complications of posterior cervical plating, *Semin Spine Surg* 5:128, 1993.

Herkowitz HN, Rothman RH: Subacute instability of the cervical spine, *Spine* 9:348, 1984.

Herr CH, Ball PA, Sargent SK, et al: Sensitivity of the prevertebral soft tissue measurement of C3 for detection of cervical spine fractures and dislocations, *Am J Emerg Med* 16:346, 1998.

Holness RO, Huestis WS, Howes WJ, et al: Posterior stabilization with an interlaminar clamp in cervical injuries: technical note and review of the long-term experience with the method, *Neurosurgery* 14:318, 1984.

Huang CI, Chen IH: Atlantoaxial arthrodesis using Halifax interlaminar clamps reinforced by halo vest immobilization: a long-term follow-up experience, *Neurosurgery* 38:1153, 1996.

Illgner A, Haas N, Tscherne H: A review of the therapeutic concept and results of operative treatment in acute and chronic lesions of the cervical spine: the Hanover experience, *J Orthop Trauma* 5:100, 1991.

Jacobs B: Cervical fractures and dislocations (C3-7), *Clin Orthop* 109:18, 1975.

Jauregui N, Lincoln T, Mubarak S, et al: Surgically related upper cervical spine canal anatomy in children, *Spine* 18:1939, 1993.

Jeanneret B, Magerl F, Halter WE, et al: Posterior stabilization of the cervical spine with hook plates, *Spine* 16:556, 1991.

Jeanneret B, Magerl F, Ward JC: Overdistraction: a hazard of skull traction in the management of acute injuries of the cervical spine, *Arch Orthop Trauma Surg* 110:242, 1991.

Jefferson G: Fracture of the atlas vertebra: report of four cases and a review of those previously recorded, *Br J Surg* 7:407, 1920.

Johnson RM, Owen JR, Hart DL, et al: Cervical orthoses: a guide to their selection and use, *Clin Orthop* 154:34, 1981.

Jones ET, Haid R Jr: Injuries to the pediatric subaxial cervical spine, *Semin Spine Surg* 3:61, 1991.

Jónsson H Jr, Cesarini K, Petrén-Mallmin M, et al: Locking screw–plate fixation of cervical spine fractures with and without ancillary posterior plating, *Arch Orthop Trauma Surg* 111:1, 1991.

Jónsson H Jr, Rauschning W: Postoperative cervical spine specimens studied with the cryoplaning technique, *J Orthop Trauma* 6:1, 1992.

Jun BY: Anatomic study for ideal and safe posterior C1-C2 transarticular screw fixation, *Spine* 23:1703, 1998.

Kang JD, Figgie MP, Bohlman HH: Sagittal measurements of the cervical spine in subaxial fractures and dislocations, *J Bone Joint Surg* 76A:1617, 1994.

Kathol M, El-Khoury GY: Diagnostic imaging of cervical spine injuries, *Semin Spine Surg* 8:2, 1996.

Kaufman WA, Lunsford TR, Lunsford BR, et al: Comparison of three prefabricated cervical collars, *Orthotics Prosthetics* 39:21, 1986.

Kerwin GA, Chou KL, White DB, et al: Investigation of how different halos influence pin forces, *Spine* 19:1078, 1994.

Klein GR, Vaccaro AR, Albert TJ, et al: Efficacy of magnetic resonance imaging in the evaluation of posterior cervical spine fractures, *Spine* 24:771, 1999.

Kostuik JP: Indications of the use of halo immobilization, *Clin Orthop* 154:46, 1981.

Kraus DR, Stauffer ES: Spinal cord injury as a complication of elective anterior cervical fusion, *Clin Orthop* 112:130, 1975.

Lander P, Gardner D, Hadjipavlou A: Pseudonotch of the atlas vertebra simulating fracture with computed tomographic diagnosis, *Orthop Rev* 20:614, 1991.

Laxer EB, Aebi M: Management of subaxial cervical spine injuries with internal fixation: the anterior approach, *Semin Spine Surg* 8:27, 1996.

Lee SW, Draper ER, Hughes SP: Instantaneous center of rotation and instability of the cervical spine: a clinical study, *Spine* 22:641, 1997.

Lesoin F, Pellerin P, Villette L, et al: Anterior approach and osteosynthesis for recent fractures of the pedicles of the axis, *Adv Orthop Surg* 10:130, 1987.

Leventhal MR: Management of lower cervical spine injuries (C4-C7). In Torg JS, ed: *Athletic injuries to the head, neck, and face,* ed 2, St Louis, 1991, Mosby.

Leventhal MR: Operative management of cervical spine problems in athletes, *Op Tech Sports Med* 1:199:1993.

Levine AM, Edwards CC: Treatment of injuries in the C1-C-2 complex, *Orthop Clin North Am* 17:31, 1986.

Levine AM, Mazel C, Roy-Camille R: Management of fracture separations of the articular mass using posterior cervical plating, *Spine* 17:447, 1992.

Levine AM, Rhyne AL: Traumatic spondylolisthesis of the axis, *Semin Spine Surg* 3:47, 1991.

Louis R: *Surgery of the spine: surgical anatomy and operative approaches,* New York, 1983, Springer-Verlag.

Lowery GL: ORION anterior cervical plate system surgical technique manual, Memphis, 1995, Sofamor Danek.

Lowery GL, McDonough RF: The significance of hardware failure in anterior cervical plate fixation: patients with 2- to 7-year follow-up, *Spine* 23:181, 1998.

Lundy DW, Murray HH: Neurological deterioration after posterior wiring of the cervical spine, *J Bone Joint Surg* 79:948, 1997.

Majd ME, Vadhva M, Holt RT: Anterior cervical reconstruction using titanium cages with anterior plating, *Spine* 24:1604, 1999.

Magerl F, Grob D, Seeman P: Stable dorsal fusion of the cervical spine (C2-T1) using hook plates. In Kehr P, Weidner A, eds: *Cervical spine,* New York, 1987, Springer-Verlag.

Magerl F, Seemann PS: Stable posterior fusion of the atlas and axis by transarticular screw fixation. In Kehr P, Weidner A, eds: *Cervical spine,* New York, 1987, Springer-Verlag.

Maroon JC, Bailes JE: Athletes with cervical spine injury, *Spine* 21:2294, 1996.

Mazur JM, Stauffr ES: Unrecognized spinal instability associated with seemingly "simple" cervical compression fractures, *Spine* 8:687, 1983.

McAfee PC, Bohlman HH, Wilson WL: The triple wire fixation technique for stabilization of acute cervical fracture-dislocations: a biomechanical analysis, *Orthop Trans* 9:142, 1985 (abstract).

McClelland SH, James RL, Jarenwattananon A, et al: Traumatic spondylolisthesis of the axis in a patient presenting with torticollis, *Clin Orthop* 218:195, 1987.

McGraw RW, Rusch RM: Atlanto-axial arthrodesis, *J Bone Joint Surg* 55B:482, 1973.

McGrory BJ, Klassen RA, Chao EYS, et al: Acute fractures and dislocations of the cervical spine in children and adolescents, *J Bone Joint Surg* 75A:988, 1993.

McGuire RA Jr, Harkey HL: Modification of technique and results of atlantoaxial transfacet stabilization, *Orthopedics* 18:1029, 1995.

McLain RF, Aretakis A, Moseley TA, et al: Subaxial cervical dissociation: anatomic and biomechanical principles of stabilization, *Spine* 19:653, 1994.

Meyer PR Jr: Emergency room assessment: management of spinal cord and associated injuries. In Meyer PR Jr, ed: *Surgery of spine trauma,* New York, 1989, Churchill Livingstone.

Mirza SK, Krengel WF III, Chapman JR, et al: Early versus delayed surgery for acute cervical spinal cord injury, *Clin Orthop* 359:104, 1999.

Mitchell TC, Sadasivan KK, Ogden AL, et al: Biomechanical study of atlantoaxial arthrodesis: transarticular screw fixation versus modified Brooks posterior wiring, *J Orthop Trauma* 13:483, 1999.

Morscher E, Sutter F, Jenny H, et al: Die vordere Verplattung der Halwirbelsaule mit dem Hohlschrauben-Plattensystem aus Titanium, *Chirurg* 57:702, 1986.

Noble ER, Smoker WR: The forgotten condyle: the appearance, morphology, and classification of occipital condyle fractures, *Am J Neuroradiol* 17:507, 1996.

O'Brien PJ, Schweigel JF, Thompson WJ: Dislocation of the lower cervical spine, *J Trauma* 22:710, 1982.

Ohiorenoya D, Hilton M, Oakland CD, et al: Cervical spine imaging in trauma patients: a simple scheme of rationalising arm traction using zonal divisions of the vertebral bodies, *J Accid Emerg Med* 13:175, 1996.

Olerud C, Jónsson H Jr: Compression of the cervical spine cord after reduction of fracture dislocations, *Acta Orthop Scand* 62:599, 1991.

Osti OL, Fraser RD, Griffiths ER: Reduction and stabilization of cervical dislocations, *J Bone Joint Surg* 71B:275, 1989.

Otis JC, Burstein AH, Torg JS: Mechanisms and pathomechanics of athletic injuries to the cervical spine. In Torg JS, ed: *Athletic injuries to the head, neck, and face,* ed 2, St Louis, 1991, Mosby.

Padua L, Padua R, LoMonaco M, et al: Radiculomedullary complications of cervical spinal manipulation, *Spinal Cord* 34:488, 1996.

Pal GP, Routal RV: The role of the vertebral laminae in the stability of the cervical spine, *J Anat* 188:485, 1996.

Panjabi MM, Isomi T, Wang JL: Loosening at the screw-vertebra junction in multilevel anterior cervical plate constructs, *Spine* 15:2383, 1999.

Papadopoulos SM: C6-7 bilateral facet dislocation and herniated disc, *Spinal Frontiers,* Oct 1994, p 8.

Perry J, Nickels VL: Total cervical-spine fusion for neck paralysis, *J Bone Joint Surg* 41A:37, 1959.

Phillips WA, Hensinger RN: The management of rotatory atlanto-axial subluxation in children, *J Bone Joint Surg* 71A:664, 1989.

Pizzutillo PD: Pediatric occipitoatlantal injuries, *Semin Spine Surg* 3:24, 1991.

Reid DC, Leung P: A study of the odontoid process, *Adv Orthop Surg* 12:147, 1989.

Ricciardi JE, Whitecloud TS III: Complications of cervical spine fixation, *Semin Spine Surg* 8:57, 1996.

Richman J: Biomechanics of cervical spine fixation, *Semin Spine Surg* 8:49, 1996.

Ripa DR, Kowell MG, Meyer PR Jr, et al: Series of ninety-two traumatic cervical spine injuries stabilized with anterior ASIF plate fusion technique, *Spine* 16(suppl 3):46, 1991.

Rizzolo SJ, Vaccaro AR, Cotler JM: Cervical spine trauma, *Spine* 19:2288, 1994.

Robinson RA, Southwick WO: Indications and technics for early stabilization of the neck in some fracture dislocations of the cervical spine, *South Med J* 53:565, 1960.

Robinson RA, Southwick WO: Surgical approaches to the cervical spine, *Instr Course Lect* 17:299, 1960.

Romanelli DA, Dickman CA, Porter RW, Haynes RJ: Comparison of initial injury features in cervical spine trauma of C3-C7: predictive outcome with halo-vest management, *J Spinal Disord* 9:146, 1996.

Rorabeck CH, Rock MG, Hawkins AJ, Bourne RB: Unilateral facet dislocation of the cervical spine: an analysis of the results of treatment in 26 patients, *Spine* 12:23, 1987.

Roy-Camille R, Saillant G, Laville C, Benazet JP: Treatment of lower cervical spinal injuries C3 to C7, *Spine* 17(suppl):442, 1992.

Roy-Camille R, Saillant G, Mazel C: Internal fixation of the unstable cervical spine by a posterior-osteosynthesis with plate and screws. In Cervical Spine Research Society, eds: *The cervical spine,* ed 2, Philadelphia, 1989, JB Lippincott.

Rumana CS, Baskin DS: Brown-Sequard syndrome produced by cervical disc herniation: case report and literature review, *Surg Neurol* 45:359, 1996.

Rushton SA, Vaccaro AR, Levine MJ, et al: Bivector traction for unstable cervical spine fractures: a description of its application and preliminary results, *J Spinal Disord* 10:436, 1997.

Ryan MD, Henderson JJ: The epidemiology of fractures and fracture-dislocations of the cervical spine, *Injury* 23:38, 1992.

Sapkas G, Korres D, Babis GC, et al: Correlation of spinal canal post-traumatic encroachment and neurological deficit in burst fractures of the lower cervical spine (C3-7), *Eur Spine J* 4:39, 1995.

Schatzker J, Rorabeck CH, Waddell JP: Fractures of the dens (odontoid process): an analysis of thirty-seven cases, *J Bone Joint Surg* 53B:392, 1971.

Schlicke LH, Callahan RA: A rational approach to burst fractures of the atlas, *Clin Orthop* 154:18, 1981.

Schneider RC, Kahn EA: Chronic neurological sequelae of acute trauma to the spine and spinal cord. I. The significance of the acute-flexion or "tear-drop" fracture-dislocation of the cervical spine, *J Bone Joint Surg* 38A:985, 1956.

Schneider RC, Kahn EA: Chronic neurological sequelae of acute trauma to the spine and spinal cord. II. The syndrome of chronic anterior spinal cord injury or compression: herniated intervertebral discs, *J Bone Joint Surg* 41A:449, 1959.

Schulte K, Clark CR, Goel VK: Kinematics of the cervical spine following discectomy and stabilization, *Spine* 14:1116, 1989.

Seybold EA, Baker JA, Criscitiello AA, et al: Characteristics of unicortical and bicortical lateral mass screws in the cervical spine, *Spine* 24:2397, 1999.

Shacked I, Ram Z, Hadani M: The anterior cervical approach for traumatic injuries to the cervical spine in children, *Clin Orthop* 292:144, 1993.

Shapiro S, Snyder W, Kaufman K, Abel T: Outcome of 51 cases of unilateral locked cervical facets: interspinous braided cable for lateral mass plate fusion compared with interspinous wire and facet wiring with iliac crest, *J Neurosurg* 91:19, 1999.

Sherk HH, Schut L, Lane JM: Fractures and dislocations of the cervical spine in children, *Orthop Clin North Am* 7:593, 1976.

Slone RM, MacMillan M, Montgomery WJ: Spinal fixation. I. Principles, basic hardware, and fixation techniques for cervical spine, *Radiographics* 13:341, 1993.

Smith MD: Cervical spine surgery: fusion of the upper portion of the cervical spine, *Op Tech Orthop* 6:46, 1996.

Southwick WO, Robinson RA: Surgical approaches to the vertebral bodies in the cervical and lumbar regions, *J Bone Joint Surg* 631A:39, 1957.

Spence KF Jr, Decker S, Sell KW: Bursting atlantal fracture associated with rupture of the transverse ligament, *J Bone Joint Surg* 52A:543, 1970.

Spivak JM, Chen D, Kummer FJ: The effect of locking fixation screws on the stability of anterior cervical plating, *Spine* 24:334, 1999.

Stauffer ES: Diagnosis and prognosis of acute cervical spinal cord injury, *Clin Orthop* 112:9, 1975.

Stauffer ES: Surgical management of cervical spine injuries. In Evarts CM, ed: *Surgery of the musculoskeletal system*, New York, 1983, Churchill Livingstone.

Stauffer ES: Wiring techniques of the posterior cervical spine for the treatment of trauma, *Orthopedics* 11:1543, 1988.

Stauffer ES, Kelly EG: Fracture-dislocations of the cervical spine: instability and recurrent deformity following treatment by anterior interbody fusion, *J Bone Joint Surg* 59A:45, 1977.

Steinmann JC, Anderson PA: Subaxial cervical spine fractures with internal fixation: the posterior approach, *Semin Spine Surg* 8:35, 1996.

Suh PB, Kostuik JP, Esses SI: Anterior cervical plate fixation with the titanium hollow screw plate system, *Spine* 15:1079, 1990.

Sutterlin CE, McAfee PC, Warden KE, et al: A biomechanical evaluation of cervical spinal stabilization methods in a bovine model: static and cyclical loading, *Spine* 13:795, 1988.

Sutton DC, Vaccaro AR, Cotler JM: Halo orthosis: indications and application technique, *Op Tech Orthop* 6:2, 1996.

Swank ML, Sutterlin CE III, Bossons CR, et al: Rigid internal fixation with lateral mass plates in multilevel anterior and posterior reconstruction of the cervical spine, *Spine* 22:274, 1997.

Thalgott JS, Fritts K, Guiffre JM, et al: Anterior interbody fusion of the cervical spine with coralline hydroxyapatite, *Spine* 24:1295, 1999.

Torg JS: Cervical spinal stenosis with cord neurapraxia and transient quadriplegia, *Sports Med* 20:429, 1995.

Torg JS, Naranja RJ Jr, Pavlov H, et al: The relationship of developmental narrowing of the cervical spinal canal to reversible and irreversible injury of the cervical spinal cord in football players, *J Bone Joint Surg* 78A:1308, 1996.

Torg JS, Pavlov H, O'Neill MJ, et al: The axial load teardrop fracture: a biomechanical, clinical, and roentgenographic analysis, *Am J Sports Med* 19:355, 1991.

Torg JS, Sennett B, Pavlov H, et al: Spear tackler's spine: definition of an entity precluding participation in contact activities, *Am J Sports Med* 21:640, 1993.

Torg JS, Sennett B, Vegso JJ, et al: Axial loading injuries to the middle cervical spine segment: an analysis and classification of twenty-five cases, *Am J Sports Med* 19:6, 1991.

Torg JS, Vegso JJ, O'Neill MJ, et al: The epidemiologic, pathologic, biomechanical, and cinematographic analysis of football-induced cervical spine trauma, *Am J Sports Med* 18:50, 1990.

Torre PD, Rinonapoli E: Halo-cast treatment of fractures and dislocations of the cervical spine, *Int Orthop* 16:227, 1992.

Traynelis VC, Donaher PA, Roach RM, et al: Biomechanical comparison of anterior Caspar plate and three-level posterior fixation techniques in a human cadaveric model, *J Neurosurg* 79:96, 1993.

Tribus CFB, Corteen DP, Zdeblick TA: The efficacy of anterior cervical plating in the management of symptomatic pseudoarthrosis of the cervical spine, *Spine* 24:860, 1999.

Tuli S, Tator CH, Fehlings MG, et al: Occipital condyle fractures, *Neurosurgery* 41:368, 1997.

Vaccaro AR, Albert TJ, Cotler JM: Anterior instrumentation in the treatment of lower cervical spine injuries, *Op Tech Orthop* 6:52, 1996.

Vaccaro AR, Falatyn SP, Flanders AE, et al: Magnetic resonance evaluation of the intervertebral disc, spinal ligaments, and spinal cord before and after closed traction reduction of cervical spine dislocations, *Spine* 24:1210, 1999.

Verheggen R, Jansen J: Hangman's fracture: arguments in favor of surgical therapy for type II and III according to Edwards and Levine, *Surg Neurol* 49:253, 1998.

Walsh GS, Cusimano MD: Vertebral artery injury associated with a Jefferson fracture, *Can J Neurol Sci* 22:308, 1995.

Wang JC, McDonough PW, Endow K, et al: The effect of cervical plating on single-level anterior cervical discectomy and fusion, *J Spinal Disord* 12:467, 1999.

Waters RL, Adkins RH, Nelson R, Garland D: Cervical spinal cord trauma: evaluation and nonoperative treatment with halo-vest immobilization, *Contemp Orthop* 14:35, 1987.

Weiland DJ, McAfee PC: Enhanced immediate postoperative stability: posterior cervical fusion with triple wire strut technique. Paper presented at the Seventeenth Annual Meeting of the Cervical Spine Research Society, New Orleans, 1989.

Weir DC: Roentgenographic signs of cervical injury, *Clin Orthop* 109:9, 1975.

Weller SJ, Malek AM, Rossitch E Jr: Cervical spine fractures in the elderly, *Surg Neurol* 47:274, 1997.

Wellman BJ, Follett KA, Traynelis VC: Complications of posterior articular mass plate fixation of the subaxial cervical spine in 43 consecutive patients, *Spine* 23:193, 1998.

Wertheim SB, Bohlman HH: Occipitocervical fusion: indications, technique, and long-term results in 13 patients, *J Bone Joint Surg* 69A:833, 1987.

White AA III, Johnson RM, Panjabi MM, Southwick WO: Biomechanical analysis of clinical stability in the cervical spine, *Clin Orthop* 109:85, 1975.

White AA III, Panjabi MM: The role of stabilization in the treatment of cervical spine injuries, *Spine* 9:512, 1984.

White AA III, Panjabi MM, Posner I, et al: Spine stability: evaluation and treatment, *Instr Course Lect* 30:457, 1981.

White AA III, Southwick WO, Panjabi MM: Clinical instability in the lower cervical spine: a review of past and current concepts, *Spine* 1:15, 1976.

Whitehill R: Fractures of the lower cervical spine: subaxial fractures in the adult, *Semin Spine Surg* 3:71, 1991.

Wilson AJ, Marshall RW, Ewart M: Transoral fusion with internal fixation in a displaced hangman's fracture, *Spine* 24:295, 1999.

Wright NM, Lauryssen C: Vertebral artery injury in C1-2 transarticular screw fixation: results of a survey of the AANS/CNS section on disorders of the spine and peripheral nerves. American Association of Neurological Surgeons/Congress of Neurological Surgeons, *J Neurosurg* 88:634, 1998.

Young R, Thomasson EH: Step-by-step procedure for applying halo ring, *Orthop Rev* 3: 62, 1974.

THORACIC AND LUMBAR SPINE AND SACRUM

Abe E, Sato K, Shimada Y, et al: Thoracolumbar burst fracture with horizontal fracture of the posterior column, *Spine* 22:83, 1997.

Aebi M, Etter C, Kehl T, Thalgott J: Stabilization of the lower thoracic and lumbar spine with internal spinal skeletal fixation system: indications, techniques, and the first results of treatment, *Spine* 12:544, 1987.

Ahlgren BD, Herkowitz HN: A modified posterolateral approach to the thoracic spine, *J Spinal Disord* 8:69, 1995.

Aihara T, Takahashi K, Yamagata M, Moriya H: Fracture-dislocation of the fifth lumbar vertebra: a new classification, *J Bone Joint Surg* 80:840, 1998.

Akbarnia BA, Crandall DG, Burkus K, et al: Use of long rods and a short arthrodesis for burst fractures of the thoracolumbar spine, *J Bone Joint Surg* 76A:1629, 1994.

Akbarnia BA, Fogarth JP, Tayob AA: Contoured Harrington instrumentation in the treatment of unstable spinal fractures (the effect of supplementary sublaminar wires), *Clin Orthop* 189:186, 1984.

Akbarnia BA, Gaines R Jr, Keppler L, et al: Surgical treatment of fractures and fracture-dislocations of thoracolumbar and lumbar spine using pedicular screw and plate fixation. Paper presented at the Twenty-third Annual Meeting of the Scoliosis Research Society, Baltimore, 1988.

Allen BL, Ferguson RL: A pictorial guide to the Galveston LRI pelvic fixation technique, *Contemp Orthop* 7:51, 1983.

Allen BL Jr, Ferguson RL: The Galveston technique of pelvic fixation with L-rod instrumentation of the spine, *Spine* 9:388, 1984.

An HS, Simpson JM, Ebraheim NA: Low lumbar burst fractures: comparison between conservative and surgical treatments, *Orthopedics* 15367, 1992.

Anden U, Lake A, Norwall A: The role of the anterior longitudinal ligament and Harrington rod fixation of unstable thoracolumbar spinal fractures, *Spine* 5:23, 1980.

Anderson PA: Nonsurgical treatment of patients with thoracolumbar fractures, *Instr Course Lect* 44:57, 1995.

Anderson PA, Henley MB, Rivara FP, et al: Flexion distraction and chance injuries to the thoracolumbar spine, *J Orthop Trauma* 5:153, 1991.

Andreychik DA, Alander DH, Senica KM, et al: Burst fractures of the second through fifth lumbar vertebrae: clinical and radiographic results, *J Bone Joint Surg* 78A:1156, 1996.

Angtuaco EJC, Binet EF: Radiology of thoracic and lumbar fractures, *Clin Orthop* 189:43, 1984.

Aydin E, Solak AS, Tuzuner MM, et al: Z-plate instrumentation in thoracolumbar spinal fractures, *Bull Hosp Jt Dis* 58:92, 1999.

Baba H, Uchida K, Furusawa N, et al: Posterior limbus vertebral lesions causing lumbosacral radiculopathy and the cauda equina syndrome, *Spinal Cord* 34:427, 1996.

Barr JD, Barr MS, Lemley TJ, et al: Percutaneous vertebroplasty for pain relief and spinal stabilization, *Spine* 25:923, 2000.

Bedbrook GM: Treatment of thoracolumbar dislocation and fractures with paraplegia, *Clin Orthop* 112:27, 1975.

Been HD: Anterior decompression and stabilization of thoracolumbar burst fractures by the use of the Slot-Zielke device, *Spine* 16:70, 1991.

Benli IT, Tandogan NR, Kis M, et al: Cotrel-Dubousset instrumentation in the treatment of unstable thoracic and lumbar spine fractures, *Arch Orthop Trauma Surg* 113:86, 1994.

Benzel EC: Short-segment compression instrumentation for selected thoracic and lumbar spine fractures: the short-rod/two-claw technique, *J Neurosurg* 79:335, 1993.

Berg EE: The sternal-rib complex: a possible fourth column in thoracic spine fractures, *Spine* 18:1916, 1993.

Berlanda P, Bassi G: Surgical treatment of traumatic spinal injuries with cord damage: clinical review of 12 years of experience with the Roy-Camille technique, *Ital J Orthop Traumatol* 17:491, 1991.

Berry JL, Moran JM, Berg WS, et al: A morphometric study of human lumbar and selected thoracic vertebrae, *Spine* 12:362, 1987.

Blauth M, Tscherne H, Haas N: Therapeutic concept and results of operative treatment in acute trauma of the thoracic and lumbar spine: the Hanover experience, *J Orthop Trauma* 1:240, 1987.

Bohlman HH: Current concepts review: treatment of fractures and dislocations of the thoracic and lumbar spine, *J Bone Joint Surg* 67A:165, 1985.

Bohlman HH, Freehafer A, Dejak J: The results of acute injuries of the upper thoracic spine with paralysis, *J Bone Joint Surg* 67A:360, 1985.

Bohlman HH, Kirkpatrick JS, Delamarter RB, et al: Anterior decompression for late pain and paralysis after fractures of the thoracolumbar spine, *Clin Orthop* 300:24, 1994.

Bolesta MJ, Bohlman HH: Mediastinal widening associated with fractures of the upper thoracic spine, *J Bone Joint Surg* 73A:447, 1991.

Bonnin JG: Sacral fractures and injuries to the cauda equina, *J Bone Joint Surg* 27:113, 1945.

Bordurant FJ, Cotler HB, Kulkarni MV, et al: Acute spinal cord injury: a study using physical examination and magnetic resonance imaging, *Spine* 15:161, 1990.

Borrelli J, Koval KJ, Helfet DL: The crescent fracture: a posterior fracture dislocation of the sacroiliac joint, *J Orthop Trauma* 10:165, 1996.

Bostman OM, Myllynen PJ, Riska EB: Unstable fracture of the thoracic and lumbar spine: the audit of an 8-year series with early reduction using Harrington instrumentation, *Injury* 18:190, 1987.

Bracken MB, Shepard MJ, Collins WF, et al: A randomized, controlled trial of methylprednisolone or naloxone in the treatment of acute spinal cord injury, *N Engl J Med* 322:1405, 1990.

Bradford DS, Akbarnia BA, Winter RD, et al: Surgical stabilization of fractures and fracture-dislocations of the thoracic spine, *Spine* 2:185, 1977.

Bradford DS, McBride GG: Surgical management of thoracolumbar spine fractures with incomplete neurologic deficits, *Clin Orthop* 218:201, 1987.

Broom MJ, Jacobs RR: Update 1988: current status of internal fixation of thoracolumbar fractures, *J Orthop Trauma* 3:148, 1989.

Bryant CE, Sullivan JA: Management of thoracic and lumbar spine fractures with Harrington distraction rods supplemented with segmental wiring, *Spine* 8:532, 1983.

Calenoff L, Chessare JW, Rogers LF, et al: Multiple level spinal injuries: importance of early recognition, *Am J Roentgenol* 130:665, 1978.

Campbell SE, Phillips CD, Dubovsky E, et al: The value of CT in determining potential instability of simple wedge-compression fractures of the lumbar spine, *Am J Neuroradiol* 16:1385, 1995.

Capen DA: Classification of thoracolumbar fractures and posterior instrumentation for treatment of thoracolumbar fractures, *Instr Course Lect* 48:437, 1999.

Carl A: Sacral spine fractures. In Errico TJ, Bauer RD, Waugh T, eds: *Spinal trauma*, Philadelphia, 1990, JB Lippincott.

Carl AL, Tranmer BI, Sachs BL: Anterolateral dynamized instrumentation and fusion for unstable thoracolumbar and lumbar burst fractures, *Spine* 22:686, 1997.

Carl AL, Tromanhauser SG, Roger DJ: Pedicle screw instrumentation for thoracolumbar burst fractures and fracture-dislocations, *Spine* 17:S317, 1992.

Carlson GD, Warden KE, Barbeau JM, et al: Viscoelastic relaxation and regional blood flow response to spinal cord compression and decompression, *Spine* 22:1285, 1997.

Chan DPK, Seng NK, Kaan KT: Nonoperative treatment in burst fractures of the lumbar spine (L2-L5) without neurologic deficits, *Spine* 18:320, 1993.

Chang KW: A reduction-fixation system for unstable thoracolumbar burst fractures, *Spine* 17:879, 1992.

Chen WJ, Niu CC, Chen LH, et al: Back pain after thoracolumbar fracture treated with long instrumentation and short fusion, *J Spinal Disord* 8:474, 1995.

Chiras J, Depriester C, Weill A, et al: Percutaneous vertebral surgery. Technics and indications, *J Neuroradiol* 24:45, 1997.

Chow GH, Nelson BJ, Gebhard JS, et al: Functional outcome of thoracolumbar burst fractures managed with hyperextension casting or bracing and early mobilization, *Spine,* 21:2170, 1996.

Clark JE: Apophyseal fracture of the lumbar spine in adolescence, *Orthop Rev* 20:512, 1991.

Clohisy JC, Akbarnia BA, Bucholz RD, et al: Neurologic recovery associated with anterior decompression of spine fractures at the thoracolumbar junction (T12-L1), *Spine* 17(suppl):325, 1992.

Cotrel Y, Dubousset J: *Universal instrumentation (CD) for spinal surgery,* (technique manual), Greensburg, Penn, 1985, Stuart.

Cotrel Y, Dubousset J, Guillaumat M: New universal instrumentation for spinal surgery, *Clin Orthop* 227:10, 1988.

Court-Brown CM, Gertzbein SD: The management of burst fractures of the fifth lumbar vertebra, *Spine* 12:308, 1987.

Cresswell TR, Marshall PD, Smith RB: Mechanical stability of the AO internal spinal fixation system compared with that of the Hartshill rectangle and sublaminar wiring in the management of unstable burst fractures of the thoracic and lumbar spine, *Spine* 23:111, 1998.

Daniaux H, Seykora P, Genelin A, et al: Application of posterior plating and modifications in thoracolumbar spine injuries, *Spine* 16(suppl):126, 1991.

Danisa OA, Shaffrey CI, Jane JA, et al: Surgical approaches for the correction of unstable thoracolumbar burst fractures: a retrospective analysis of treatment outcomes, *J Neurosurg* 83:977, 1995.

Davies WE, Morris JH, Hill V: An analysis of conservative (nonsurgical) management of thoracolumbar fractures and fracture dislocations with neural damage, *J Bone Joint Surg* 62A:1324, 1980.

Davis LA, Warren SA, Reid DC, et al: Incomplete neural deficits in thoracolumbar and lumbar spine fractures: reliability of Frankel and Sunnybrook scales, *Spine* 18:257, 1993.

De Klerk LW, Fontijne WP, Stijnen T, et al: Spontaneous remodeling of the spinal canal after conservative management of the thoracolumbar burst fractures, *Spine* 23:1057, 1998.

Delamarter RB, Bohlman HH, Dodge LD, Biro C: Experimental lumbar spinal stenosis: analysis of the cortical evoked potentials, microvasculature, and histopathology, *J Bone Joint Surg* 72A:110, 1990.

Del Bigio MR, Johnson GE: Clinical presentation of spinal cord concussion, *Spine* 14:37, 1989.

Denis F: The three-column spine and its significance in the classification of acute thoracolumbar spinal injuries, *Spine* 8:817, 1983.

Denis F, Armstrong GWD, Searls K, et al: Acute thoracolumbar burst fractures in the absence of neurologic deficit (a comparison between operative and nonoperative treatment), *Clin Orthop* 189:142, 1984.

Denis F, Burkus JK: Diagnosis and treatment of cauda equina entrapment in the vertical lamina fracture of lumbar burst fractures, *Spine* 16:S433, 1991.

Denis F, Burkus JK: Shear fracture-dislocations of the thoracic and lumbar spine associated with forceful hyperextension (lumberjack paraplegia), *Spine* 17:156, 1992.

Denis F, Davis S, Comfort T: Sacral fractures: an important problem, though frequently undiagnosed and untreated: retrospective analysis of two hundred and three consecutive cases, *Orthop Trans* 11:118, 1987.

Denis F, Fuiz H, Searls K: Comparison between square-ended distraction rods and standard round-ended distraction rods in the treatment of thoracolumbar spinal injuries: a statistical analysis, *Clin Orthop* 189:162, 1984.

Devilee R, Sanders R, de Lange S: Treatment of fractures and dislocations of the thoracic and lumbar spine by fusion and Harrington instrumentation, *Arch Orthop Trauma Surg* 114:100, 1995.

DeWald RL: Burst fractures of the thoracic and lumbar spine, *Clin Orthop* 189:150, 1984.

Deyo RA, Cherkin DC, Loeser JD, et al: Morbidity and mortality in association with operations on the lumbar spine, *J Bone Joint Surg* 74A:536, 1992.

Dick W: The "fixateur interne" as a versatile implant for spine surgery, *Spine* 12:882, 1987.

Dickman CA, Yahiro MA, Lu HTC, et al: Surgical treatment alternatives for fixation of unstable fractures of the thoracic and lumbar spine: a meta-analysis, *Spine* 19(suppl):2266, 1994.

Dickson JH, Harrington PR, Erwin WD: Harrington instrumentation in the fractured, unstable thoracic and lumbar spine, *Texas Med* 69:91, 1973.

Dickson JH, Harrington PR, Erwin WD: Results of reduction and stabilization of the severely fractured thoracic and lumbar spine, *J Bone Joint Surg* 60A:799, 1978.

Dietemann JL, Runge M, Dosh JC, et al: Radiology of posterior lumbar apophyseal ring fractures: report of 13 cases, *Neuroradiology* 30:337, 1988.

Dimar JR II, Wilde PH, Glassman SD, et al: Thoracolumbar burst fractures treated with combined anterior and posterior surgery, *Am J Orthop* 25:159, 1996.

Doerr TE, Montesano PX, Burkus JK, et al: Spinal canal decompression in traumatic thoracolumbar burst fractures: posterior distraction rods versus transpedicular screw fixation, *J Orthop Trauma* 5:403, 1991.

Donovan DJ, Polly DW Jr, Ondra SL: The removal of a transdural pedicle screw placed for thoracolumbar spine fracture, *Spine* 21:2495, 1996.

Drummond D, Gaudagni J, Keene JS, et al: Interspinous process segmental spinal instrumentation, *J Pediatr Orthop* 4:397, 1984.

Drummond D, Keene J: A technique of segmental spinal instrumentation without the passing of sublaminar wires, *Mediguide Orthop* 6:1, 1985.

Drummond D, Keene JS, Breed A: The Wisconsin system: a technique of interspinous segmental spinal instrumentation, *Contemp Orthop* 8:29, 1984.

Ebelke DK, Asher MA, Neff JR, et al: Survivorship analysis of VSP spine instrumentation in the treatment of thoracolumbar and lumbar burst fractures, *Spine* 16:S432, 1991.

Ebraheim NA, Biyani A, Salpietro B: Zone III fractures of the sacrum: a case report, *Spine* 21:2390, 1996.

Edwards CC, Levine AM: Early rod-sleeve stabilization of the injured thoracic and lumbar spine, *Orthop Clin North Am* 17:327, 1986.

Edwards CC, Levine AM: Complications associated with posterior instrumentation for thoracolumbar injuries and their prevention, *Semin Spine Surg* 5:108, 1993.

Eismont FJ, Green BA, Berkowitz BM, et al: The role of intraoperative ultrasonography in the treatment of thoracic and lumbar spine fractures, *Spine* 9:782, 1984.

Elattrache N, Fadale PD, Fu F: Thoracic spine fracture in a football player, *Am J Sports Med* 21:157, 1993.

Erickson DL, Leider LC Jr, Brown WE: One-stage decompression-stabilization for thoraco-lumbar fractures, *Spine* 2:53, 1977.

Esses SI: The placement and treatment of thoracolumbar spine fractures: an algorithmic approach, *Orthop Rev* 17:571, 1988.

Esses SI: The AO spinal internal fixator, *Spine* 14:373, 1989.

Esses SI, Botsford DJ, Kostuik JP: Evaluation of surgical treatment for burst fractures, *Spine* 15:667, 1990.

Faden AI, Jacobs TP, Patrick DH, et al: Megadose corticosteroid therapy following experimental traumatic spinal injury, *J Neurosurg* 60:712, 1984.

Ferguson RL, Allen BL Jr: A mechanistic classification of thoracolumbar spine fractures, *Clin Orthop* 189:77, 1984.

Finkelstein JA, Chapman JR, Mirza S: Anterior cortical allograft in thoracolumbar fractures, *J Spinal Disord* 12:424, 1999.

Flesch JR, Leider LL, Erickson D, et al: Harrington instrumentation and spine fusion for unstable fractures and fracture dislocations of the thoracic and lumbar spine, *J Bone Joint Surg* 59A:143, 1977.

Fountain SS, Hamilton RD, Jameson RM: Transverse fractures of the sacrum: a report of six cases, *J Bone Joint Surg* 59A:486, 1977.

Francaviglia N, Bragazzi R, Maiello M, et al: Surgical treatment of fractures of the thoracic and lumbar spine via the transpedicular route, *Br J Neurosurg* 9:511, 1995.

Fredrickson BE, Yuan HA, Miller H: Burst fractures of the fifth lumbar vertebra, *J Bone Joint Surg* 64A:1088, 1982.

Gaebler C, Maier R, Kukla C, et al: Long-term results of pedicle-stabilized thoracolumbar fractures in relation to the neurological deficit, *Injury* 28:661, 1997.

Gaines RW, Breedlove RF, Munson G: Stabilization of thoracic and thoracolumbar fracture-dislocations with Harrington rods and sublaminar wires, *Clin Orthop* 189:195, 1984.

Gaines RW, Humphreys WG: A plea for judgment in management of thoracolumbar fractures and fracture-dislocations: a reassessment of surgical indications, *Clin Orthop* 189:36, 1984.

Garcia F, Florez MT, Conejero JA: A butterfly vertebra or a wedge fracture? *Int Orthop* 17:7, 1993.

Garfin S: What the experts say: treatment options for VCF, including balloon kyphoplasty, http://kyphon.com. Accessed Feb 2002.

Garfin SD, Jacobs RR, Stoll J, et al: Results of a locking-hook spinal rod for fractures of the thoracic and lumbar spine, *Spine* 15:275, 1990.

Garfin SR, Mowery CA, Guerra J Jr, et al: Confirmation of the posterolateral technique to decompress and fuse thoracolumbar spine burst fractures, *Spine* 10:218, 1985.

Gertzbein SD: Neurologic deterioration in patients with thoracic and lumbar fractures after admission to the hospital, *Spine* 19:1723, 1994.

Gertzbein SD: Spine update: classification of thoracic and lumbar fractures, *Spine* 19:626, 1994.

Gertzbein SD, Jacobs RR, Stoll J, et al: Results of a locking-hook spinal rod for fractures of the thoracic and lumbar spine, *Spine* 15:275, 1990.

Ghanayem AJ, Zdeblick TA: Anterior instrumentation in the management of thoracolumbar burst fractures, *Clin Orthop* 335:89, 1997.

Gorczyca JT, Varga E, Woodside T, et al: The strength of iliosacral lag screws and transiliac bars in the fixation of vertically unstable pelvic injuries with sacral fractures, *Injury* 27:561, 1996.

Grasland A, Pouchot J, Mathieu A, et al: Sacral insufficiency fractures: an easily overlooked cause of back pain in elderly women, *Arch Intern Med* 56:668, 1996.

Greenfield RT, Grant RE, Bryant D: Pedicle screw fixation in the management of unstable thoracolumbar spine injuries, *Orthop Rev* 21:701, 1992.

Grob D, Scheier HJG, Dvorak J, et al: Circumferential fusion of the lumbar and lumbosacral spine, *Arch Orthop Trauma Surg* 111:20, 1991.

Grootboom MJ, Govender S: Acute injuries of the upper dorsal spine, *Injury* 24:389, 1993.

Gurr KR, McAfee PC, Shih C: Biomechanical analysis of posterior instrumentation systems following decompressive laminectomy (an unstable calf spine model), NIH grant, Johns Hopkins University School of Medicine, May 8, 1987.

Gurwitz GS, Dawson JM, McNamara MJ, et al: Biomechanical analysis of three surgical approaches for lumbar burst fractures using short-segment instrumentation, *Spine* 18:977, 1993.

Guttmann L: The treatment and rehabilitation of patients with injuries of the spinal cord. In Cope Z, ed: *Medical history of the Second World War: surgery,* London, 1953, His Majesty's Stationery Office.

Guttmann L: A new turning-tilting bed, *Paraplegia* 3:193, 1965.

Guttmann L: Spinal deformities in traumatic paraplegics and tetraplegics following surgical procedures, *Paraplegia* 7:38, 1969.

Ha KI, Han SH, Chung M, et al: A clinical study of the natural remodeling of burst fractures of the lumbar spine, *Clin Orthop* 323:210, 1996.

Hack HP, Zielke K, Harms J: *Spinal instrumentation and monitoring,* (technique manual), Greensburg, Penn, 1985, Stuart.

Hanley EN Jr, Eskay ML: Thoracic spine fractures, *Orthopedics* 12:689, 1989.

Hardaker WT, Cook WA, Friedman AH, et al: Bilateral transpedicular decompression and Harrington rod stabilization in the management of severe thoracolumbar burst fractures, *Spine* 17:162, 1992.

Harkonen M, Kataja M, Keski-Nisula L, et al: Fractures of the lumbar spine: clinical and radiological results in 94 patients, *Orthop Trauma Surg* 94:43, 1979.

Harrington PR: The history and development of Harrington instrumentation (1973 Nicholas Andry Award Contribution), *Clin Orthop* 93:110, 1973.

Harris MB: The role of anterior stabilization with instrumentation in the treatment of thoracolumbar burst fractures, *Orthopedics* 15:347, 1992.

Hartman MB, Chrin AM, Rechtine GR: Nonoperative treatment of thoracolumbar fractures, *Paraplegia* 33:73, 1995.

Harvey J, Tanner S: Low back pain in young athletes: a practical approach, *Sports Med* 12:394, 1991.

Hatem SF, West OC: Vertical fracture of the central sacral canal: plane and simple, *J Trauma* 40:138, 1996.

Heggeness MH, Doherty BJ: The trabecular anatomy of thoracolumbar vertebrae: implications for burst fractures, *J Anat* 191:309, 1997.

Heinig CF, Chapman TM, Chewning SJ Jr, et al: Preliminary report on VSP spine fixation system, unpublished data, 1988.

Herring JA, Wenger DR: Segmental spine instrumentation, *Spine* 7:285, 1982.

Hitchon PW, Torner JC: Recumbency in thoracolumbar fractures, *Neurosurg Clin North Am* 8:509, 1997.

Holdsworth FW, Hardy A: Early treatment of paraplegia from fractures of the thoraco-lumbar spine, *J Bone Joint Surg* 35B:540, 1953.

Hu SS, Capen DA, Rimoldi RL, et al: The effect of surgical decompression on neurologic outcome after lumbar fractures, *Clin Orthop* 288:166, 1993.

Huang TJ, Chen JY, Shih HN, et al: Surgical indications in low lumbar burst fractures: experiences with anterior locking plate system and reduction fixation system, *J Trauma* 39:910, 1995.

Jacobs RR, Asher MA, Snider RK: Thoracolumbar spinal injuries: a comparative study of recumbent and operative treatment in 100 patients, *Spine* 5:463, 1980.

Jacobs RR, Casey MP: Surgical management of thoracolumbar spinal injuries (general principles and controversial considerations), *Clin Orthop* 189:22, 1984.

Jacobs RR, Nordwall A, Nachemson A: Reduction, stability and strength provided by internal fixation systems for thoracolumbar spinal injuries, *Clin Orthop* 171:300, 1982.

Jacobs RR, Schlaepfer F, Mathys R Jr, et al: A locking-hook spinal rod system for stabilization of fracture-dislocations and correction of deformities of the dorsolumbar spine: a biomechanical evaluation, *Clin Orthop* 189:168, 1984.

James KS, Wenger KH, Schlegel JD, et al: Biomechanical evaluation of the stability of thoracolumbar burst fractures, *Spine* 19:1731, 1994.

Jane MJ, Freehafer AA, Hazel C, et al: Autonomic dysreflexia: a cause of morbidity and mortality in orthopedic patients with spinal cord injury, *Clin Orthop* 169:151, 1982.

Jelsma RK, Kirsch PT, Jelsma LF, et al: Surgical treatment of thoracolumbar fractures, *Surg Neurol* 3:156, 1982.

Johnson JR, Leatherman KD, Holt RT: Anterior decompression of the spinal cord for neurologic deficit, *Spine* 8:396, 1983.

Johnson KD, Dadambis A, Seibert GB: Incidence of adult respiratory distress syndrome in patients with multiple musculoskeletal injuries: effect of early operative stabilization of fractures, *J Trauma* 25:375, 1985.

Johnson LP, Nasca RJ, Bonnin JM: Pathoanatomy of a burst fracture, *Surg Rounds Orthop,* Jan 1988, p 43.

Johnston CE II, Ashman RB, Sherman MC, et al: Mechanical consequences of rod contouring and residual scoliosis in sublaminar segmental instrumentation, *J Orthop Res* 5:206, 1987.

Kahanovitz N, Bullough P, Jacobs RR: The effect of internal fixation without arthrodesis on human facet joint cartilage, *Clin Orthop* 189:204, 1984.

Kaneda K, Abumi K, Fujiya M: Burst fractures with neurologic deficits of the thoracolumbar-lumbar spine: results of anterior decompression and stabilization with anterior instrumentation, *Spine* 9:788, 1984.

Kaneda K, Gaines RW: *Kaneda anterior spinal instrumentation for the thoracolumbar spine,* ed 2, Cleveland, 1990, Acromed.

Kaneda K, Taneichi H, Abumi K, et al: Anterior decompression and stabilization with the Kaneda device for thoracolumbar burst fractures associated with neurological deficits, *J Bone Joint Surg* 79A:69, 1997.

Kaplan SS, Wright NM, Yundt KD, et al: Adjacent fracture-dislocations of the lumbosacral spine: case report, *Neurosurg* 44:1134, 1999.

Karjalainen M, Aho AJ, Katevuo K: Operative treatment of unstable thoracolumbar fractures by the posterior approach with the use of Williams plates or Harrington rods, *Int Orthop* 16:219, 1992.

Katonis PG, Kontakis GM, Loupasis GA, et al: Treatment of unstable thoracolumbar and lumbar spine injuries using Cotrel-Dubousset instrumentation, *Spine* 24:2352, 1999.

Kelly RP, Whitesides TE Jr: Treatment of lumbodorsal fracture-dislocations, *Ann Surg* 167:705, 1968.

Kennedy JG, Soffe KE, McGrath A, et al: Predictors of outcome in cauda equina syndrome, *Eur Spine J* 8:317, 1999.

Kim NH, Lee HM, Chun IM: Neurologic injury and recovery in patients with burst fracture of the thoracolumbar spine, *Spine* 24:290, 1999.

King AG: Burst compression fractures of the thoracolumbar spine: pathologic anatomy and surgical management, *Orthopedics* 10: 1711, 1987.

Kirkpatrick JS, Wilber RG, Likavec M, et al: Anterior stabilization of thoracolumbar burst fractures using the Kaneda device: a preliminary report, *Orthopedics* 18:673, 1995.

Korovessis PG, Baikousis A, Stamatakis M: Use of the Texas Scottish Rite Hospital instrumentation in the treatment of thoracolumbar injuries, *Spine* 22:882, 1997.

Korovessis P, Sidiropoulos P, Dimas A: Complete fracture-dislocation of the thoracic spine without neurologic deficit: case report, *J Trauma* 36:122, 1994.

Kostuik JP: Anterior spinal cord decompression for lesions of the thoracic and lumbar spine: techniques: new methods of internal fixation, results, *Spine* 8:512, 1983.

Kraemer WJ, Schemitsch EH, Lever J, et al: Functional outcome of thoracolumbar burst fractures without neurological deficit, *J Orthop Trauma* 10:541, 1996.

Krag MH, Weaver DL, Beynnon BD, et al: Morphometry of the thoracic and lumbar spine related to transpedicular screw placement for surgical spinal fixation, *Spine* 13:27, 1988.

Kramer DL, Rodgers WB, Mansfield FL: Transpedicular instrumentation and short-segment fusion of thoracolumbar fractures: a prospective study using a single instrumentation system, *J Orthop Trauma* 9:499, 1995.

Krompinger WJ, Frederickson BE, Mino DE, et al: Conservative treatment of fractures of the thoracic and lumbar spine, *Orthop Clin North Am* 17:161, 1986.

Krueger MA, Green DA, Hoyt D, et al: Overlooked spine injuries associated with lumbar transverse process fractures, *Clin Orthop* 327:191, 1996.

Kulkarni MB, McArdle CB, Kopaniky D, et al: Acute spinal cord injury: MR imaging at 115 T1, *Neuroradiology* 164:837, 1987.

Kupferschmid JP, Weaver ML, Raves JJ, et al: Thoracic spine injuries in victims of motorcycle accidents, *J Trauma* 29:593, 1989.

Laborde JM, Bahniuk E, Bohlman HH, et al: Comparison of fixation of spinal fractures, *Clin Orthop* 152:305, 1980.

Lafollete BF, Levine MI, McNiesh LM: Bilateral fracture-dislocation of the sacrum, *J Bone Joint Surg* 68A:1099, 1986.

Levine AM, Bosse M, Edwards CC: Bilateral facet dislocations in the thoracolumbar spine, *Spine* 13:630, 1988.

Levine AM, Edwards CC: Low lumbar burst fractures: reduction and stabilization using the modular spine fixation system, *Orthopedics* 1:9, 1988.

Limb D, Shaw DL, Dickson RA: Neurological injury in thoracolumbar burst fractures, *J Bone Joint Surg* 77B:774, 1995.

Lindahl S, Willen J, Nordwall A, et al: The crush-cleavage fracture: a "new" thoracolumbar unstable fracture, *Spine* 8:559, 1983.

Lindsey RW, Dick W: The fixateur interne in the reduction and stabilization of thoracolumbar spine fractures in patients with neurologic deficit, *Spine* 16(suppl):140, 1991.

Lindsey RW, Dick W, Nunchuck S, et al: Residual intersegmental spinal mobility following limited pedicle fixation of thoracolumbar spine fractures with the fixateur interne, *Spine* 18:474, 1993.

Louis R: Fusion of the lumbar and sacral spine by internal fixation with screw plates, *Clin Orthop* 203:18, 1986.

Luque ER, Cassis N, Ramirez-Weilla G: Segmental spinal instrumentation in the treatment of fractures of the thoracolumbar spine, *Spine* 7:312, 1982.

Macmillan M, Stauffer ES: Transient neurologic deficits associated with thoracic and lumbar spine trauma without fracture or dislocation, *Spine* 15:466, 1990.

Magerl FP: Stabilization of the lower thoracic and lumbar spine with external skeletal fixation, *Clin Orthop* 189:125, 1984.

Maiman DJ, Pintar F, Yoganandan N, et al: Effects of anterior vertebral grafting on the traumatized lumbar spine after pedicle screw-plate fixation, *Spine* 18:2423, 1993.

Mann KA, McGowan DP, Fredrickson BE, et al: A biomechanical investigation of short segment spinal fixation for burst fractures with varying degrees of posterior disruption, *Spine* 15:407, 1990.

Markel DC, Graziano GP: A comparison study of treatment of thoracolumbar fractures using the ACE Posterior Segmental Fixator and Cotrel-Dubousset instrumentation, *Orthopedics* 18:679, 1995.

McAfee PC: Biomechanical approach to instrumentation of the thoracolumbar spine: a review article, *Adv Orthop Surg* 8:313, 1985.

McAfee PC, Bohlman HH: Anterior decompression of traumatic thoracolumbar fractures with incomplete paralysis through the retroperitoneal approach, *Orthop Trans* 8:392, 1984.

McAfee PC, Bohlman HH: Complications following Harrington instrumentation for fractures of the thoracolumbar spine, *J Bone Joint Surg* 67A:672, 1985.

McAfee PC, Bohlman HH, Yuan HA: Anterior decompression of traumatic thoracolumbar fractures with incomplete neurological deficit using a retroperitoneal approach, *J Bone Joint Surg* 67A:89, 1985.

McAfee PC, Levine AM, Anderson PA: Surgical management of thoracolumbar fractures, *Instr Course Lect* 44:47, 1995.

McAfee PC, Werner FW, Glisson RR: A biomechanical analysis of spinal instrumentation systems in thoracolumbar fractures: comparison of traditional Harrington side traction instrumentation with segmental spinal instrumentation, *Spine* 10:204, 1985.

McAfee PC, Yuan HA, Frederickson BE, et al: The value of computed tomography in thoracolumbar fractures, *J Bone Joint Surg* 64A:461, 1983.

McAfee PC, Yuan HA, Lasada NA: The unstable burst fracture, *Spine* 7:365, 1982.

McBride GG: Surgical stabilization of thoracolumbar fractures using Cotrel-Dubousset rods, *Semin Spine Surg* 2:24, 1990.

McCrory BJ, VanderWilde RS, Currier BL: Diagnosis of subtle thoracolumbar burst fractures: a new radiographic sign, *Spine* 18:2282, 1993.

McFarland EG, Giangarra C: Sacral stress fractures in athletes, *Clin Orthop* 329:240, 1996.

McGuire RA Jr: The role of anterior surgery in the treatment of thoracolumbar fractures, *Orthopedics* 20:959, 1997.

McGuire RA, Freeland AE: Flexion-distraction injury of the thoracolumbar spine, *Orthopedics* 15:379, 1992.

Meldon SW, Moettus LN: Thoracolumbar spine fractures: clinical presentation and the effect of altered sensorium and major injury, *J Trauma* 39:1110, 1995.

Mermelstein LE, McLain RF, Yerby SA: Reinforcement of the thoracolumbar burst fractures with calcium phosphate cement: a biomechanical study, *Spine* 23:664, 1998.

Meyer PR: Complications of treatment of fractures and dislocations of the dorsolumbar spine. In Epps CH, ed: *Complications in orthopaedic surgery*, Philadelphia, 1978, JB Lippincott.

Miyakoshi N, Abe E, Shimada Y, et al: Anterior decompression with single segmental spinal interbody fusion for lumbar burst fracture, *Spine* 24:67, 1999.

Moorman CT, Richardson WJ, Fitch RD, Hardaker WT: Flexion-distraction injuries to the lumbar spine in children, *J South Orthop Assoc*, Nov/Dec 1992, p 296.

Morgan FH, Wharton W, Austin GN: The results of laminectomy in patients with incomplete spinal cord injuries, *Paraplegia* 9:14, 1971.

Mozes GC, Kollender Y, Sasson AA: Transpedicular screw-rod fixation in the treatment of unstable lower thoracic and lumbar fractures, *Bull Hosp Jt Dis* 53:37, 1993.

Mumford J, Weinstein JN, Spratt KF, Goel VK: Thoracolumbar burst fractures: the clinical efficacy and outcome of nonoperative management, *Spine* 18:955, 1993.

Munro AHG, Irwin CG: Interlocked articular processes complicating fracture-dislocation of the spine, *Br J Surg* 25:621, 1938.

Myllynen P, Bostman O, Riska E: Recurrence of deformity after removal of Harrington's fixation of spine fractures (seventy-six cases followed for 2 years), *Acta Orthop Scand* 59:497, 1988.

Nagai H, Shimizu K, Shikata J: Chylous leakage after circumferential thoracolumbar fusion for correction of kyphosis resulting from fracture: report of three cases, *Spine* 22:2766, 1997.

Nagel DA, Koogle TA, Piziali RL, Perkash I: Stability of the upper lumbar spine following progressive disruptions in the application of individual internal and external fixation devices, *J Bone Joint Surg* 63A:62, 1981.

Nicoll EA: Fractures of the dorso-lumbar spine, *J Bone Joint Surg* 31B:376, 1949.

Okuyama K, Abe E, Chiba M, et al: Outcome of anterior decompression and stabilization for thoracolumbar unstable burst fractures in the absence of neurologic deficits, *Spine* 21:620, 1996.

Olerud C, Sjöström L, Jónsson H, Karlström G: Posterior reduction of a pathologic spinal fracture: a case of indirect anterior dual decompression, *Acta Orthop Scand* 63:345, 1992.

Oner FC, van-Gils AP, Dhert WJ, Verbout AJ: MRI findings of thoracolumbar spine fractures: a categorisation based on MRI examinations of 100 fractures, *Skeletal Radiol* 28:433, 1999.

Oner FC, van-der-Rijt RR, Ramos LM, et al: Changes in the disc space after fractures of the thoracolumbar spine, *J Bone Joint Surg* 80B:833, 1998.

Osebold WR, Weinstein SL, Sprague BL: Thoracolumbar spine fractures: results of treatment, *Spine* 6:13, 1981.

Osti OL, Fraser RD, Cornish BL: Fractures and fractures-dislocations of the lumbar spine: a retrospective study of 70 patients, *Int Orthop* 11:323, 1987.

Panjabi MM, Oxland TR, Kifune M, et al: Validity of the three-column theory of thoracolumbar fractures: a biomechanic investigation, *Spine* 20:1122, 1995.

Panjabi MM, Oxland TR, Lin RM, McGowen TW: Thoracolumbar burst fracture: a biomechanical investigation of its multidirectional flexibility, *Spine* 19:578, 1994.

Panjabi MM, Kifune M, Wen L, et al: Dynamic canal encroachment during thoracolumbar burst fractures, *J Spinal Disord* 8:39, 1995.

Parfenchuck TA, Chambers J, Goodrich JA, Levine MI: Lumbar spine arthrodesis: a comparison of hospital costs between 1986 and 1993, *Am J Orthop* 24:854, 1995.

Pattee GA, Bohlman HH, McAfee PC: Compression of a sacral nerve as a complication of screw fixation of the sacro-iliac joint, *J Bone Joint Surg* 68A:769, 1986.

Pearch M, Protek I, Shepherd J: Three-dimensional x-ray analysis of normal movement in the lumbar spine, *Spine* 9:294, 1984.

Peh WC, Ooi GC: Vacuum phenomena in the sacroiliac joints and in association with sacral insufficiency fractures: incidence and significance, *Spine* 22:2005, 1997.

Pinzur MS, Meyer PR Jr, Lautenschlager EP, et al: Measurement of internal fixation device: a report in experimentally produced fractures of the dorsolumbar spine, *Orthopedics* 2:28, 1979.

Post MJD, Green BA, Stokes NA, et al: Value of computed tomography in spinal trauma, *Spine* 7:417, 1982.

Pringle RG: The conservative management of the spinal injured patients, *Semin Orthop* 4:34, 1989.

Purcell GA, Markolf KL, Dawson EG: Twelfth thoracic–first lumbar vertebral mechanical stability of fractures after Harrington rod instrumentation, *J Bone Joint Surg* 63A:71, 1981.

Rao S, Patel A, Schildhauer T: Osteogenesis imperfecta as a differential diagnosis of pathologic burst fractures of the spine, *Clin Orthop* 289:113, 1993.

Rea GL, Zerick WR: The treatment of thoracolumbar fractures: one point of view, *J Spinal Disord* 8:368, 1995.

Rechtine GR: Nonsurgical treatment of thoracic and lumbar fractures, *Instr Course Lect* 48:413, 1999.

36 ◆ Arthrodesis of Spine

Keith D. Williams

Since the descriptions of spinal fusion by Hibbs and by Albee, arthrodesis of the spine has been performed for many spinal conditions, including tuberculosis and other infections, fractures, congenital and developmental deformities, arthritic and other degenerative diseases, and disc lesions. Although it is difficult to separate discussions of arthrodesis and the conditions for which it is performed, this section discusses various techniques of arthrodesis useful in both traumatic and nontraumatic disorders of the entire spine. Techniques of spinal arthrodesis using instrumentation, such as rods, plates and screws, and wires, are described in Chapters 35, 38, and 39.

Bone Grafts and Arthrodesis Healing

Despite significant advances in techniques and in our understanding of the physiology of the incorporation process for bone grafts, pseudarthrosis remains a significant problem. Knowledge of the required histological events and sequences brings an appreciation of successful fusion. Graft incorporation really is a partnership between the graft (autograft, allograft, or synthetic substitute) and the recipient site, and each must provide specific contributions. Age, nutritional status, and metabolic disorders in patients, as well as the mechanical environment, all have been shown to affect bone formation.

In recent years many authors have attempted to define this complex cascade of events. Boden et al. used an animal model to investigate the coupling of the membranous and enchondral mechanisms of bone formation in intertransverse process spinal fusions, which in humans remains the most common type of arthrodesis. The pioneering work by Urist and others has led to the availability of various growth factors, including platelet-derived growth factor, members of the transforming growth factor (TGF)-ß superfamily, including bone morphogenic protein (BMP) 2-7 superfamily, and growth and differentiation factor (GDF)-5, which has been of enormous benefit.

Although many questions remain, it has been shown in rabbit models that three primary phases occur with bone grafting that are different qualitatively from the healing steps that occur with fractures. In addition, different areas of fusion mass heal at different rates, depending on the distance from decortication and vascular ingrowth.

During the initial or inflammatory stage, the hematoma formed from decortication is invaded by inflammatory cells, and a fibrovascular stroma is formed. Membranous bone is formed at the decorticated surfaces, and BMP-6, BMP-4, alkaline phosphatase, and osteonectin are all increased. The middle or reparative phase consists of increased revascularization, resorption of necrotic bone, and differentiation of osteoblastic and chondroblastic cells. Enchondral ossification occurs centrally to unite the two areas forming from the adjacent transverse processes. During this phase, levels of osteocalcin and osteopontin peak, and there is a second peak in BMP-6. The late or remodeling phase begins during week 6. Minimal cartilage is noted and there is marked remodeling and formation of a peripheral cortical rim from which trabecular bone extends. Generally, except for BMP-6, there is a return to baseline for the expression of genes. At a cellular level osteoprogenitor cells are recruited from the decorticated surfaces as well as from the graft (when autograft is used). This is followed by coupled bone resorption by osteoclasts, then osteoinduction in which osteoprogenitor cells give rise to osteoblasts. New bone matrix is formed on the trabecular scaffolding of the substrate. This process begins where vascular ingrowth occurs first (i.e., areas of decortication) and proceeds outwardly from there. The new bone so formed then is remodeled in accordance with Wolff's law.

Understanding this information makes evident the importance of surgical technique as it relates to recipient site preparation, autologous graft harvest and preparation, and the appropriate use of allograft or bone extenders.

ALLOGRAFTS AND AUTOGRAFTS

In addition to autologous bone grafts harvested most commonly from the ilium but also from the fibula, tibia, or locally, a variety of allograft types are available. These allografts have differing osteoinductive and osteoconductive properties, depending on how they are processed, and also differing biomechanical properties. Structural allografts usually are placed anteriorly as strut grafts, spanning multiple segments, or as interbody grafts. Usually, posteriorly placed grafts are morselized and are not load-bearing structures, although there are exceptions to both. Historically, autologous graft has proved to be superior with respect to fusion mass formation in essentially all grafting situations; however, the associated morbidity of graft harvesting and limited bone availability have led to development of a variety of allografts, bone graft extenders, and most recently recombinant human bone morphogenetic proteins, which ultimately may be substitutes for autograft.

Allograft bone should be considered only weakly osteoinductive but highly osteoconductive. Achieving a successful fusion using allograft bone in the spine depends on the type of allograft, the location of the fusion, and the patient's age. Butterman, Glazer, and Bradford reviewed their experience and the literature regarding the use of allografts with the following findings. In the cervical spine, freeze-dried allograft bone should not be used posteriorly. For single-level anterior cervical discectomy and fusion, both fresh frozen and freeze-dried allografts give acceptable results. However, the risk of disease transmission, although extremely small, is greater with the fresh frozen grafts. Allograft struts used in the cervical spine give satisfactory fusion rates, although healing is slower than with autograft, necessitating longer periods of immobilization or additional stabilizing procedures. Allografts should not be used for multilevel interbody fusions because the nonunion rates and subsidence rates are unacceptably high unless internal stabilization also is used. Butterman et al. found that in adults allograft bone should not be used for posterior grafts in the thoracolumbar spine; several other prospective studies have had similar findings.

Ethylene oxide–sterilized allograft should not be used. Fresh-frozen cancellous allograft gives variable results, and its use should be limited to patients with insufficient bone stock for autologous graft. Bridwell et al. found allograft suitable in paralytic patients when harvesting of autogenous graft was not feasible. There have been several reports of successful posterior fusion in children using allograft. Anteriorly, structural allografts supplemented with autologous bone provide acceptable fusion rates, although subsidence has been noted to occur in the lumbar spine in a high percentage of patients, but not in the thoracolumbar region. In patients requiring anterior strut type allografts, supplemental segmental instrumentation allows better maintenance of deformity correction and higher fusion rates.

BONE GRAFT EXTENDERS

In addition to allograft, there are a variety of commercially available products containing demineralized bone matrix (DBM). These products have been shown in animal models to enhance fusion when added to a variety of osteoconductive materials; however, Cook et al. were unable to show adequate fusion using DBM with allograft in a dog model. Well-controlled human studies remain lacking. Demineralized bone matrix is obtained by the acid abstraction of bone. The components that remain behind include bone osteoinductive growth factors (most importantly BMPs), type I collagen, and noncollagenous proteins. Demineralized bone matrix does not provide any mechanical support and is thus limited somewhat in use. In addition to DBM, various forms of ceramics are currently available. These ceramics are in the form of hydroxyapatite and tricalcium phosphate primarily and are available in block form as well as a granular form. They appear to have only osteoconductive properties. There are some reports of satisfactory use in adolescent scoliosis patients; however, this cannot be extrapolated to general use in adults, and their role in spinal fusion remains to be better defined.

Certainly the most promising bone graft extender at the present time is bone morphogenic protein (BMP), a group of low-molecular weight noncollagenous glycoproteins with the ability to induce ectopic bone formation in standard in vivo rodent assay systems. Wozney et al. first identified the specific molecules, making recombinant production possible. Several recombinant human BMPs are available, but rhBMP-2 and rhBMP-7 (also designated OP-1) have been studied most thoroughly. Data obtained from long bone studies in humans and arthrodesis models in primates appear promising. However, the determination of the specific roles of the various BMPs, as well as optimal carriers and dosages, has not been completed. Boden et al. reported the first human pilot study of rhBMP-2 for spinal fusion. This multicenter study of 14 patients using anterior threaded interbody cages compared autograft with rhBMP-soaked collagen sponge ($n = 11$). All patients receiving rhBMP-2 had fusion by 6 months, and one patient who had an autograft had a nonunion at 1 year. Studies involving local gene therapy and use of spinal fixation with bioactive substances warrant further investigation, as does the biology of healing for spinal arthrodesis.

Cervical Spine

ANTERIOR ARTHRODESIS

Anterior cervical discectomy with interbody fusion has gained wide acceptance by both orthopaedic surgeons and neurosurgeons in the management of refractory symptoms of cervical disc disease. The literature attests to a low incidence of major complications and postoperative morbidity and a high degree of success in relieving these symptoms. The fundamental difference in the many techniques is whether surgery is limited to simple discectomy and interbody fusion or whether an attempt is made to enter the spinal canal to remove osteophytes or otherwise decompress the spinal cord and nerve roots.

Extreme care must be exercised in anterior fusion of the cervical spine because of significant potential complications including injury to the cervical viscera and neurological and vascular injury. Kraus and Stauffer reported 10 patients with spinal cord injury resulting from surgery. An incomplete spinal cord injury was present in three patients, including two incomplete quadriplegias of the anterior cervical cord type and one incomplete quadriplegia of the Brown-Séquard type. Seven additional patients were reviewed from the literature and personal communications. The causes were identified in four of the last six patients as (1) operation of a drill without the protection of the drill guard, which allowed the drill to enter the spinal canal, and (2) displacement of a dowel bone graft into the spinal canal, either during surgery or postoperatively, which damaged the cervical cord. One of the other two patients sustained a transient postoperative transverse myelitis attributed to the use of electrocoagulation on the posterior longitudinal ligament. All these fusions had been performed by the drill and dowel method. The use of a tricortical iliac graft is recommended for interbody fusions.

Aronson, Bagan, and Feltzer have shown that anterior discectomy and interbody fusion have a much wider application, producing excellent results in virtually all forms of cervical disc disease and spondylosis, regardless of the objective neurological signs. Despite subtle differences in surgical technique, the intent of their procedure is still discectomy and interbody fusion with no attempt to remove osteophytes. The extent to which the posterior and posterolateral osteophytes with spondylosis contribute to the symptoms of cervical disc disease and the indications for removing them have not been completely defined. Often the discrepancy between the degree of bony spurring or other roentgenographic changes and the symptoms present is striking. Also, the level of neurological involvement does not always coincide with the site of the greatest roentgenographic findings. Because plain roentgenograms cannot provide the necessary information for

identifying the level or levels of neural compression, either CT myelography or MRI is strongly recommended in operative planning; both provide the detailed diagnostic information necessary. In descending order of frequency, the disc levels involved with degenerative changes are C5, C6, and C4. Correlation of the patient's symptoms with diagnostic studies is crucial because 14% of asymptomatic patients younger than 40 years of age and 28% of those older than 40 years have significant abnormalities as shown on MRI studies. The symptoms of the degenerative processes are related to the interplay of multiple aspects of the disease process and not solely to the amount of bony spurs present. Observation of patients who have had fusions shows that a significant percentage of osteophytes but not all will be spontaneously resorbed postoperatively in the presence of a stable interbody fusion. DePalma and Rothman concurred with this observation and noted that in the presence of a stable fusion the results were not influenced by the subsequent fate of these osteophytes.

In our experience simple discectomy and interbody fusion without removal of the posterior longitudinal ligament or osteophytes has been adequate in the treatment of neural compression caused by soft disc material. If the compression of neural tissue, especially the spinal cord, is caused by large osteophytes or an ossified posterior longitudinal ligament, direct decompression by removal of the compressing structures has given superior results and is recommended. This is especially true if the T2 sequences on MRI demonstrate cord signal abnormality. In the hands of skilled surgeons, with the use of an operating microscope, a high-speed burr, small angled curets, and small Kerrison rongeurs (Fig. 36-1), safe anterior excision of osteophytes and other offending structures from the spinal canal can be completed before grafting and stabilization. In selected instances, monitoring of somatosensory and motor evoked potentials is useful, primarily in patients with my-

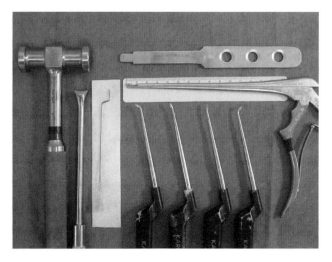

Fig. 36-1 Instruments for cervical spine surgery include cervical spanners, angled curets, cervical Kerrison ronguer, prebent spinal needle, graft impactor, and mallet.

elopathy or spinal cord signal abnormality, to minimize the risk of spinal cord injury from positioning or hypotension while the exposure and initial phase of decompression is being completed.

General Complications

Macnab summarized the complications of anterior cervical fusion extremely well. For every anatomical structure present in the neck, there is a possibility of a surgical error; however, he pointed out that poor results also occur because of poor indications and surgical technique. The following points are Macnab's, with occasional observations from our experience.

The *wrong patient* may be operated on, since the neck is a common target for psychogenic pain. Careful preoperative evaluation is essential to rule out a hysterical personality or a chronic anxiety state. In the absence of significant neurological findings to localize the level of pathological condition, great care in evaluating the patient's pain is essential. The relatively high incidence of imaging abnormalities in asymptomatic volunteers should be kept in mind. Adjunctive studies, including discography, may be of benefit. Disc degeneration may be a multifocal disease in the cervical and lumbar spine; therefore even if an examination seems to point to a single level, it is possible that within a short time other segments will become symptomatic and surgery will be of no long-term benefit. With multilevel disc degeneration, results have not been gratifying. The best results are obtained with a single segment discectomy and fusion for definite nerve root impairment, spinal cord compression, or less commonly for localized disc disease without root compression. Fusions of more than two segments performed for pain relief alone produce fair or poor results; improvement, not cure, is the best possible result.

The operation can be done at the *wrong level* if an incorrect vertebral count is made at surgery. Use of a localization film with a metal marker is mandatory, and the first or second cervical vertebra should always be shown on this check film. The marker needle should be directed cranially so that the tip butts the vertebra above and avoids the theca. Additionally, by placing two right-angle bends, beginning 1 cm proximal to the tip of the spinal needle, penetration of the needle beyond a depth of 1 cm is prevented.

The operation may be performed in the *wrong way*; for example, the recurrent laryngeal nerve, esophagus, or pharynx can be injured by retractors. Sympathetic nervous system injuries are avoided by dissecting in the correct planes. Keeping the dissection medial to the carotid avoids the sympathetic nervous system. An approach from the left is less likely to damage the recurrent laryngeal nerve. In an approach from the right, the recurrent laryngeal nerve is in jeopardy from C6 caudally, and it should be specifically identified and protected. This nerve enters the groove between the trachea and the esophagus at the point where the inferior thyroid artery enters the lower pole of the thyroid gland. Apfelbaum, Kriskovich, and Haller presented a large series that suggested that

compression of the recurrent laryngeal nerve may well be caused by endotracheal tube position combined with tracheal retraction. Their series included 900 patients, and the incidence of recurrent laryngeal nerve palsy was decreased by deflating and reinflating the endotracheal tube cuff after retractor placement to allow the tube to reposition itself within the trachea. Instruments can tear the dura or compress neural tissue and must be used with extreme caution in removing the posterior disc fragments and osteophytes. Small, angled curets and Kerrison rongeurs should be sharp to prevent the need for excessive force and loss of control of the instruments. Grafts must be accurately measured and tightly fitted under compression.

The operation may be done at the *wrong time*. Timing of an operation is important; surgery should not be delayed if root conduction is significantly impaired. In patients in whom the clinical findings are purely subjective, consideration usually is given to delaying surgery until any possible litigation is settled. However, this can lead to chronic pain patterns that are difficult to eradicate. If such a patient has been significantly disabled for more than a year and has shown no improvement over the past 6 months, Macnab advised a thiopental pain study and discography. If a significant physiogenic basis for the pain is demonstrated, prompt anterior cervical discectomy and fusion should be carried out without awaiting the results of litigation. We rarely treat surgically patients who do not have objectively demonstrated neural compression or neurological deficits. Otherwise results seem, at best, unpredictable.

Postoperative Complications

All anterior surgical wounds are best drained to decrease the risks of a retropharyngeal hematoma, which can produce obstruction of the airway with its subsequent complications. A soft, closed suction drainage system usually is inserted deep into the wound. Airway obstruction, although rare, typically occurs 12 to 36 hours postoperatively.

Extrusion of a graft is most commonly seen in the treatment of fracture-dislocations of the neck with posterior instability. This is not commonly seen in fusions for disc degeneration when posterior stability of the ligamentous structures is not impaired. At this clinic anterior plate stabilization or posterior internal fixation is a routine adjunct when posterior ligamentous stability is lost for any reason and the anterior approach for arthrodesis is necessary. Generally, with anterior instrumentation, immobilization with a cervical orthosis is all that is necessary, although halo-vest external fixation sometimes is used. Use of the halo-vest may preclude the need for posterior internal fixation, which is reserved for patients in whom use of the halo-vest is complicated by other injuries, the patient's general debility, or the patient's body habitus. We have found the combination of stable anterior graft reconstruction and anterior instrumentation to be effective in most patients, and the use of additional posterior instrumentation or halo-vest immobilization in this situation is infrequent. A rectangular graft provides better stability than a circular Cloward graft.

Unless the graft extrudes more than 50% of its depth or unless it causes dysphagia, revision surgery usually is not indicated. The extruded portion will be resorbed and the graft will ossify as the arthrodesis heals. If healing time is protracted, external immobilization time should be adjusted accordingly. Whitehill et al. reported a late esophageal perforation from a corticocancellous strut graft from the iliac crest. The first symptoms of dysphagia occurred 2½ months after the surgery, and an "inferior osseous spike" on the graft apparently eroded into the esophagus.

Complications related to anterior instrumentation have been reported. Locking-type plate devices minimize the risk of screws backing out and esophageal or tracheal perforation. This type of device also precludes the need for bicortical drilling and thereby decreases the risk for spinal cord injury during drilling or screw placement.

Postoperative collapse of a vertebral body is seen on occasion with a multilevel dowel technique, which jeopardizes the vertebral blood supply. This is caused by excessive thinning of the vertebral body at its midpoint, where adjacent dowel holes are closest. This technique has not been used in many years.

Nonunion of an anterior cervical fusion is unusual. With multilevel interbody fusions, however, the pseudarthrosis rate increases in a nonlinear fashion. For single-level fusions the literature reports a 3% to 7% nonunion rate even with autograft bone. Similar pseudarthrosis rates are noted with single-level fusions using allograft. With autogenous iliac tricortical grafts, the nonunion rate in two-level interbody fusions without anterior instrumentation ranges from 12% to 18%. However, the addition of stable internal fixation reduces this significantly. This also is true for three or more level fusions. Allograft bone should not be used for multilevel interbody fusions without anterior plating because of a high nonunion rate. Multilevel anterior fusions using adjunctive anterior plate fixation with allograft bone can provide satisfactory fusion rates, although the results are not as good as with autograft. This situation may be reversed when bone graft extenders such as BMP-2 or BMP-7 are used with the allograft. When nonunions occur, typically they occur at the caudalmost segment.

If a cervical pseudarthrosis is determined to be symptomatic, usually it is best managed by posterior cervical fusion. If a significant anterior pathological condition persists, satisfactory revision anterior surgery can be performed. Zdeblick et al. performed repeat anterior decompression and autogenous bone grafting in 35 patients who had nonunion after failure of anterior cervical discectomy and arthrodesis. They concluded that an excellent result can be achieved with reoperation in patients who have persistent symptoms after anterior cervical arthrodesis (Fig. 36-2).

When anterior cervical arthrodesis is being performed for traumatic disorders with resultant instability from ligamentous tears or posterior element fractures, postoperative treatment must be planned to accommodate this added factor. The aftertreatment described here usually applies to arthrodesis for "stable" degenerative or other nontraumatic conditions. If cervical instability is present, or if two or more disc levels are fused, such as with corpectomy, anterior internal fixation and immobilization for up to 3 months is routinely used.

◆ Types of Anterior Arthrodesis of Cervical Spine

Of the three commonly used techniques for anterior cervical spine fusion—those of Robinson and Smith, Bailey and Badgley, and Cloward—White et al. found the Robinson and Smith configuration to be the strongest in compressive loading. These grafts could all bear loads of 2½ to 5 times the body weight, much more than the loads the cervical spine is normally expected to bear. Thus the limiting factor was not the graft itself but the graft vertebral construct (Fig. 36-3). The major load on the vertebrae in vivo is that of axial compression, but Simmons, Bhalla, and Butt directed attention to the rotary displacement taking place in the spine and its relationship to the various constructs of the bone grafts. The strong configuration of the Robinson and Smith arthrodesis is the result of leaving intact the cortical shell of the vertebral body. Since it has been shown that 40% to 75% of the strength of the vertebra comes from the cortical bone, preserving the endplate is very important because it prevents collapse into the cancellous portion of the body with subsequent displacement.

In our experience removal of the posteriormost portion of the vertebral endplates to accomplish more complete anterior decompression when the offending osteophyte is large has not created a serious problem unless the bone was very osteoporotic. Even then, only a partial collapse of the interspace has occurred during healing. We believe that thorough decompression is more important for relief of neural symptoms than strict preservation of the endplates, especially posteriorly. Removal of the most anterior portion of the inferior endplate of the cephalad vertebra is routinely carried out to improve exposure of the disc space and ensure adequate removal of the cartilaginous endplate that would impede fusion. This also allows the endplates to be parallel. If wider than usual resection is necessary, our technique becomes more like the Simmons "keystone" graft and less like the Smith-Robinson technique. Bailey and Badgley, Robinson et al., Simmons et al., Macnab, and others have fused the cervical spine anteriorly for instability after extensive laminectomy, fractured posterior arch elements, certain fracture-dislocations, and destructive lesions. Robinson et al., Williams, Allen, and Harkess, and many others have combined excision of cervical intervertebral discs with anterior fusion. The various approaches to the anterior aspect of the cervical spine are described in Chapter 34.

Robinson et al. have arthrodesed the cervical spine anteriorly for intervertebral disc degeneration by excising the disc and the cartilaginous plates from the selected disc space or spaces and inserting tricortical blocks of iliac bone.

Smith-Robinson fusions are made easier by using a system of retractors and instrumentation designed specifically for this purpose. However, we believe that the distraction pins should

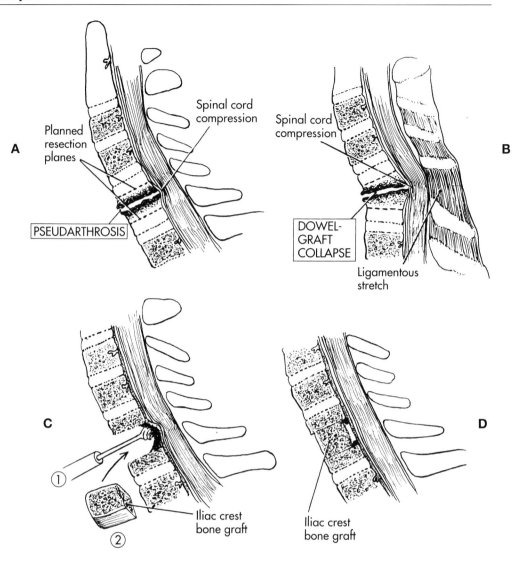

Fig. 36-2 **A,** Typical nonunion with fibrocartilage compromising canal. **B,** Collapse of graft leads to sharp angular kyphosis, which, combined with nonunion, causes compression of cord. **C,** Decompression through anterior approach. Hemicorporectomy performed cephalad and caudad to disc space with high-speed burr to create parallel surfaces of cancellous bone. Decompression completed with angled curets. **D,** Anterior bone grafting performed with tricortical Smith-Robinson bone graft countersunk into position. (From Zdeblick TA, Hughes SS, Riew D, et al: *J Bone Joint Surg* 79A:523, 1997.)

not be used in patients in whom anterior plate fixation is planned because these pins can cause microfractures that compromise screw purchase; in this situation we prefer to use halter traction.

TECHNIQUE 36-1 *(Robinson et al.)*

Place the patient supine on the operating table with a small roll in the interscapular area. Apply a head halter if anterior plate fixation is to be used. Apply 5 to 10 pounds of traction to the head halter if so desired. Otherwise, the halter is not necessary because the distraction pins and the retraction set can be used to open the disc space and allow exposure.

Rotate the patient's head slightly to the side opposite the planned approach. Mark the anterior cervical skin, preferably using an existing curved skin crease, before placing the adhesive surgical field drape. The hyoid (C3), thyroid cartilage (C4-5), and cricoid cartilage (C6) are useful landmarks. The transverse-type skin incision can be used, even for three-level corpectomies if it is well placed;

otherwise, an incision along the sternocleidomastoid border is useful. Throughout the exposure meticulous hemostasis should be maintained to allow better identification of dissection planes and important anatomic structures. After sharply dividing the skin, sharply dissect the subcutaneous layer off the anterior fascia of the platysma to allow mobility of the wound to the desired level. Divide the platysma vertically near the midline by lifting it between two pairs of forceps and dividing it sharply in the cephalad and caudad directions. This allows exposure of the sternocleidomastoid border. Develop the interval just medial to the sternocleidomastoid to allow palpation and exposure of the carotid sheath and the overlying omohyoid muscle. Mobilize the omohyoid and retract caudally for access cephalad to C5 or mobilize cranially for access to C5 or caudal levels. Sharply divide the pretracheal fascia medial to the carotid sheath. Take care to avoid any dissection lateral to the carotid sheath that would place the sympathetic chain at risk. Once the

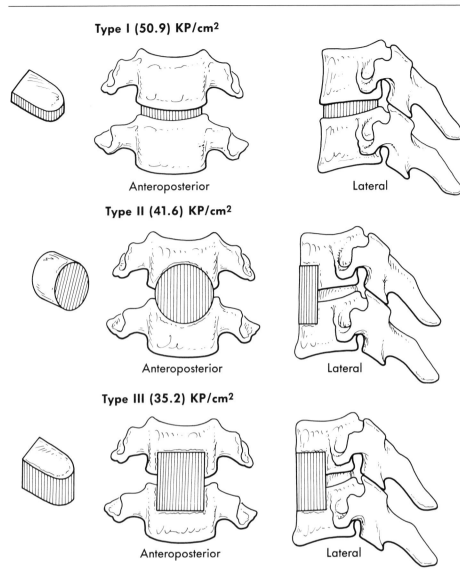

Type I (50.9) KP/cm²

Anteroposterior   Lateral

Type II (41.6) KP/cm²

Anteroposterior   Lateral

Type III (35.2) KP/cm²

Anteroposterior   Lateral

Fig. 36-3 Types (configurations) of grafts used in anterior arthrodesis of cervical spine. *Type I,* Robinson and Smith; *Type II,* Cloward; *Type III,* Bailey and Badgley. Numbers are means for load-bearing capacity for each. (Redrawn from White AA III, Jupiter J, Southwick WO, et al: *Clin Orthop* 91:21, 1973.)

pretracheal fascia has been incised, adequately develop the prevertebral space using blunt finger dissection directed medially and posteriorly. Place blunt hand-held retractors medially to view the paired longus colli muscles. To avoid injury to the midline structures, use bipolar cautery and small key-type elevators to subperiosteally elevate the longus colli so that self-retaining retractors can be placed deep to the medial borders of these muscles. Obtain a localization roentgenogram using a prebent spinal needle to mark the disc space before proceeding with disc excision or corpectomy. If the superior or inferior thyroid vessels limit exposure, ligate and divide the vessels. When elevating the longus colli muscles do not extend laterally to the transverse processes to avoid the sympathetic chain and the vertebral artery. This dissection, however, must extend laterally enough to expose the anterior aspect of the uncovertebral joints bilaterally. Place self-retaining retractor blades deep to the longus colli bilaterally and attach to the self-retaining

retractor. For single-level discectomy, distraction pins can be inserted. For multiple-level procedures or if screw fixation is planned, the distraction pins are best avoided because of potential microfracture at the pin sites that will compromise screw purchase. Once all levels are adequately exposed, use a no. 11 blade scalpel to remove the anterior annulus at each level, cutting toward the midline from each uncovertebral joint. Remove the annulus with pituitary rongeurs and curets to allow exposure of each uncinate process, which appears as a slight upward curve of the endplate of the caudal segment. This marks the safe extent of lateral dissection to avoid the vertebral artery. Remove the anterior one half to two thirds of the disc at each level in this way. Use an operating microscope for safe removal of the posterior disc, osteophytes, or posterior longitudinal ligament as needed. With a high-speed burr, remove the anterior lip of the cephalad vertebra to a level matching the subchondral bone at midbody level (Fig. 36-4). This forms

continued

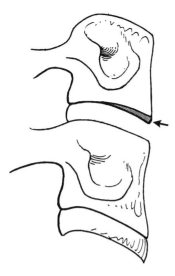

Fig. 36-4   Diagram of bone removal with high-speed burr of anterior lip of cephalad vertebra to level matching subchondral bone at midbody level.

a completely flat surface and enhances visibility for removing the remaining disc material and the cartilaginous endplates to the level of the posterior longitudinal ligament. If preoperative imaging demonstrates a soft disc fragment and this is found without violation of the posterior longitudinal ligament, further exploration of the canal is not warranted. If necessary, perform foraminotomy to remove uncovertebral tissue with small Kerrison rongeurs. If a defect through the posterior longitudinal ligament is found, enlarge it and explore the canal for additional fragments. If the surgical plan calls for complete removal of the posterior longitudinal ligament, complete all corpectomies first. To perform the corpectomies use a high-speed burr to create a lateral gutter at the level of the uncinate process bilaterally that extends from one disc space to the next. Remove the midline bone to the same depth as the gutters and continue posteriorly until the brisk bleeding of cancellous bone gives way to cortical bone. Usually there will be significant bleeding from the posterior midpoint of the body that can be easily controlled with bipolar cautery once the cortical bone has been drilled away. Do not use unipolar cautery in close proximity to neural tissue. Thin the cortical bone with the high-speed burr and remove with angled curets, or remove carefully with the burr. If necessary, remove the posterior longitudinal ligament by lifting it anteriorly with a small blunt hook and opening the epidural space with a 1-mm Kerrison rongeur. This must be done with excellent visualization and care to avoid dural injury. Once the epidural space is entered, remove the posterior longitudinal ligament entirely if needed. If the canal is significantly compromised, carefully free it from the underlying dura with blunt dissection. Perform foraminotomies at this time

and remove osteophytes if necessary. A small blunt probe should pass easily anterolaterally after foraminotomy. When possible, preserve the posterior longitudinal ligament to enhance construct stability. Carefully prepare the adjacent endplates so that all cartilage is removed, subchondral bone is preserved, the entire decompression is the width of the endplate between the uncinate processes, and the endplates are parallel to one another. Carefully measure the anterior to posterior dimension at each endplate. The graft depth should be 3 to 4 mm less than the shorter of the two to allow the graft to be recessed 2 mm anteriorly and not compromise the spinal canal posteriorly. Also, carefully measure the length of graft needed in the cephalad to caudad dimension. Remember to measure with and without traction being applied through the head halter so that the graft will be under proper compression. Also, make sure at this point that endplates are parallel to one another.

Remove the disc laterally to allow visualization of the uncinate process bilaterally, which will appear as a slight upturning of the endplate and marks the safe extent of lateral decompression.

Obtain a tricortical iliac graft using a small oscillating saw (Fig. 36-5), as described in Technique 1-3. During preparation of the endplate, take care to preserve the anterior cortex of the cephalad and caudad vertebrae. Fashion the bone graft to the appropriate depth. Position the graft with the cancellous surface directed posteriorly and bevel the cephalad and caudad posterior margins slightly to facilitate impaction. With traction applied, impact the graft into place so that the cortical portion is recessed 1 to 2 mm posterior to the anterior cortex of the vertebral bodies. There should be 2 mm of free space between the posterior margin of the graft and the spinal canal. The graft should fit snugly even when traction is being applied. Release traction and check the fit of the graft using a Kocher clamp to grasp it. Repeat this procedure for each additional disc space. Now apply anterior cervical plate instrumentation if necessary with all traction released. Various systems are available and should be placed according to the manufacturer's recommendations. Obtain intraoperative roentgenograms to verify graft and hardware position. Close the platysmal layer over a soft, closed-suction drain and close the skin and subcutaneous layers. Apply a thin dressing. Place the patient in a cervical orthosis before extubation.

AFTERTREATMENT. The patient is allowed to be up out of bed later on the day of surgery or the next morning. The drain is removed on the first postoperative day. The cervical orthosis is continued 4 to 6 weeks for discectomy patients and 8 to 12 weeks for patients undergoing corpectomies, depending on patient compliance and roentgenographic appearance of the graft. Occasionally a soft collar is helpful for an additional week or two. Flexion and extension lateral cervical spine roentgenograms should reveal no evidence of motion at the

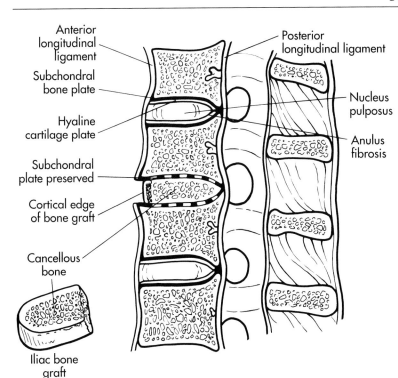

Anterior longitudinal ligament

Subchondral bone plate

Hyaline cartilage plate

Subchondral plate preserved

Cortical edge of bone graft

Cancellous bone

Iliac bone graft

Posterior longitudinal ligament

Nucleus pulposus

Anulus fibrosis

Fig. 36-5 Technique of Robinson et al. for anterior fusion of cervical spine (see text). (Modified from Robinson RA, Walker EA, Ferlic DC, et al: *J Bone Joint Surg* 44A:1569, 1962.)

fusion site, and trabeculation should be present before discontinuation of the rigid cervical orthosis.

◆ ◆ ◆

Bloom and Raney recommended reversing the orientation of the iliac graft as it is inserted so that the rounded cortical edge of the iliac cortex is placed posteriorly and the cancellous edge is anterior. They claimed that protruding portions of the graft can be trimmed off easily with a rongeur without sacrificing the cortical portion and decreasing the strength of the graft. We have experienced collapse of the anterior noncortical edge of the graft and a resulting slight kyphotic deformity at the fused level when the graft is "reversed." This has been noted especially in older women whose pelvic bone cortices were thinned from osteoporosis.

TECHNIQUE 36-2 *(Bailey and Badgley)*

This technique is altered as the specific pathological problem demands. The operation is done with the patient on a Stryker frame or operating table with skull-tong traction in place. Endotracheal anesthesia is used. Fielding, Lusskin, and Batista found the method of Bailey and Badgley satisfactory in fusing several segments for instability after multiple laminectomies; in this situation in children, Cattell and Clark used a strut graft of tibial bone as described by Robinson.

Place a folded towel beneath the interscapular region to hold the neck in moderate extension. Rotate the patient's head about 15 degrees to the right and approach the cervical spine anteriorly from the left as described above. When the

prevertebral fascia is reached but before it is incised, insert a drill as a marker in one of the vertebral bodies and identify it with a lateral roentgenogram. After this orientation, incise the prevertebral fascia longitudinally in the exact midline. Place heavy silk sutures in the fascia to facilitate retraction and later to use in closure. Mobilize the fascia from the anterior surfaces of the vertebral bodies and control bleeding from the bone with electrocautery or bone wax. Identify the vertebrae to be fused and cut a trough in the anterior aspect of the vertebral bodies about 1.2 cm wide and 4.7 mm deep from near the top of the upper vertebra to near the bottom of the lower one. Use of a small power saw or drill is less traumatic than use of an osteotome and a mallet. Clean out the intervertebral disc spaces with a rongeur and remove the cartilaginous endplates on the inferior and superior aspects of the bodies to be fused. Disc removal should be carried out to the uncinate process bilaterally. Once the cartilaginous endplates have been removed, obtain and gently pack chips of cancellous iliac bone into the cleaned intervertebral disc spaces, trim an iliac graft to fit, and mortise it into the trough in the vertebrae (Fig. 36-6). Now decrease the extension of the cervical spine by raising the line of pull of the traction, thus wedging the graft more securely in the trough. The graft must not project farther anteriorly than the anterior surface of the vertebral bodies.

Once the graft is properly seated, tie the sutures previously placed in the prevertebral fascia; the fascia maintains the graft in its bed. Place a large Penrose drain or

continued

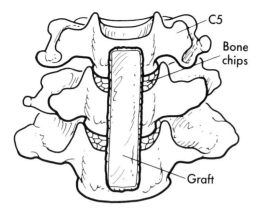

Fig. 36-6   Anterior fusion of cervical spine. Trough has been cut in anterior aspect of vertebral bodies, intervertebral disc spaces have been cleared and filled with iliac bone chips, and iliac graft has been mortised into trough. (Redrawn from Bailey RW, Badgley CE: *J Bone Joint Surg* 42A:565, 1960.)

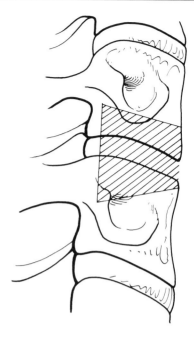

Fig. 36-7   Placement of keystone graft shown in lined area. (Redrawn from Simmons EH, Bhalla SK, Butt WP: *J Bone Joint Surg* 51B:225, 1969.)

suction drainage tube in the retropharyngeal space and bring it out through the lower portion of the incision. Close the wound in layers with interrupted sutures.

AFTERTREATMENT. Traction is maintained on a Stryker frame or Foster bed. The drain is removed in 24 hours. After 6 weeks in traction, the patient is allowed to get up with the neck immobilized in a Taylor back brace with an attached Forrester collar. The brace is worn until fusion is complete, usually for 4 to 6 months.

A halo-vest is almost always used rather than 6 weeks of traction. This allows much earlier ambulation and consequently much earlier hospital discharge. With proper supervision and maintenance of the halo-vest, the results should be equally satisfactory. When this technique has been used a halo-vest is kept in place for about 3 months. A cervical collar is used during the next 4 to 6 weeks as immobilization is gradually decreased and as rehabilitation progresses. Serial roentgenographic evaluations and support are continued until healing is complete. Our experience with this technique is very limited.

◆ ◆ ◆

The cervical arthrodesis with discectomy described by Simmons, Bhalla, and Butt produced excellent results in 80.8% of their patients. Our experience with this technique has been with trauma and has been minimal, but it does provide a stable configuration.

TECHNIQUE 36-3 *(Simmons et al.)*
Use endotracheal anesthesia. Place the patient on the operating table and strap the ankles to the table. Apply a head halter and drape the patient. Using a left-sided approach, make a transverse skin incision along the line of the skin creases as previously described to expose the spine. Remove a keystone square or rectangle of tissue, beveling it upward into the vertebra above and downward into the vertebra below using special osteotomes and chisels of Simmons' design, with a depth of 1.2 cm each and with widths of 1.27, 1.1, and 0.95 cm. Exercise care to avoid outward progression of the chisel while keeping the cut in the true anteroposterior plane. Remove a 1.27-cm square of tissue for the one-level fusion in most patients. When this material is completely removed with rongeurs and by curettage, remove the disc from posteriorly to anteriorly. At the final stage of cleansing of this space, ask the anesthetist to apply strong head halter traction, which opens the disc space and allows discectomy to be carried out well to the neurocentral joints. Deepen the trough to the posterior cortex of the vertebrae. Next carefully cut the corners squarely. Measure the length of the rectangle while forceful traction is placed on the head halter to allow opening of the space at least 3 mm. Obtain a rectangular graft from the iliac crest and shape it to fit the trough. Bevel the ends upward and downward to approximately 14 to 18 degrees. Now distract the neck fully by forceful traction and place the graft into the defect. Release the traction; the graft is thus locked firmly into position, maintaining fixed distraction and immobilization (Fig. 36-7). In a two-level fusion extend the trough and graft through the intervening vertebra into the one above and below.

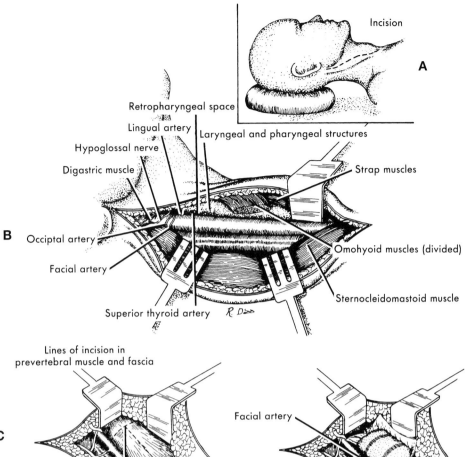

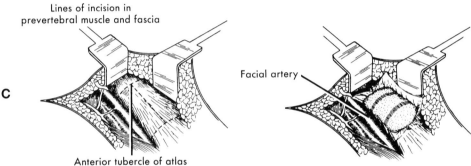

Fig. 36-8 Technique of de Andrade and Macnab for anterior occipito-cervical arthrodesis (see text). (Redrawn from de Andrade JR, Macnab I: *J Bone Joint Surg* 51A:1621, 1969.)

AFTERTREATMENT. Early mobilization is allowed in a brace until union is achieved. Because grafting under distraction is quite stable, postoperative pain is relatively mild.

◆ ANTERIOR OCCIPITOCERVICAL ARTHRODESIS BY EXTRAPHARYNGEAL EXPOSURE

Rarely an anterior occipitocervical fusion is required for a grossly unstable cervical spine when posterior fusion is not feasible. It was used by de Andrade and Macnab in patients who had extensive laminectomies and for rheumatoid arthritis, traumatic quadriparesis, neoplastic metastasis to the spine, and congenital abnormalities. This operation is a cranial extension of the approach described by Robinson and Smith and by Bailey and Badgley; it permits access to the base of the occiput and the anterior aspect of all the cervical vertebrae.

TECHNIQUE 36-4 *(de Andrade and Macnab)*
Maintain initial spinal stability by applying a cranial halo with the patient on a turning frame. Keep the patient on the

frame and maintain the traction throughout the operation. Make the exposure from the right side with an incision coursing along the anterior border of the sternocleidomastoid muscle from above the angle of the mandible to below the cricoid cartilage (Fig. 36-8). Divide the platysma and deep cervical fascia in line with the incision and expose the anterior border of the sternocleidomastoid. Take care not to injure the spinal accessory nerve as it enters the anterior aspect of the sternocleidomastoid at the level of the transverse process of the atlas. Retract the sternocleidomastoid laterally and the pretracheal strap muscles anteriorly and palpate the carotid artery in its sheath. Expose the latter. Divide the omohyoid muscle as it crosses at the level of the cricoid cartilage. Identify the digastric muscle and hypoglossal nerve at the cranial end of the wound. Bluntly dissect the retropharyngeal space and enter it at the level of the thyroid cartilage. Now divide the superior thyroid, lingual, and facial arteries and veins to gain access to the retropharyngeal space in the upper part of the wound. Continue

continued

blunt dissection in the retropharyngeal space and palpate the anterior arch of the atlas and the anterior tubercle in the midline. Continue above this area with the exploring finger and enter the hollow at the base of the occiput. Dissection cannot be carried farther cephalad because of the pharyngeal tubercle, to which the pharynx is attached. Insert a broad right-angled retractor under the pharynx and displace it anterosuperiorly. Use intermittent traction on the pharyngeal and laryngeal branches of the vagus nerve during this maneuver to minimize the risk of hoarseness. The anterior aspect of the upper cervical spine and the base of the occiput are now exposed. Coagulate the profuse plexus of veins under the anterior border of the longus colli. Separate the muscles from the anterior aspect of the spine by incising the anterior longitudinal ligament vertically and transversely and expose the anterior arch of C1 and the bodies of C2 and C3. The working space is approximately 4 cm because the hypoglossal nerve exits from the skull through the anterior condyloid foramen about 2 cm lateral to the midline. Roughen the anterior surface of the base of the occiput and upper cervical vertebrae with a curet. Obtain from the iliac crest slivers of fresh autogenous cancellous bone and place them on the anterior surface of the vertebrae to be fused. Make the slivers no thicker than 4.2 mm to prevent excessive bulging into the pharynx. Close the wound by suturing the platysma and skin only with a suction drain left in the retropharyngeal space for 48 hours.

AFTERTREATMENT. The patient is kept on a turning frame, and traction is maintained for 6 weeks. A tracheostomy set must be kept by the bedside in case upper airway obstruction occurs. For earlier ambulation a halo-vest can be applied; the halo is removed 16 weeks after the operation. Consolidation of the graft should occur by this time.

◆ ANTERIOR UPPER CERVICAL ARTHRODESIS

TECHNIQUE 36-5 *(Robinson and Riley)*

Perform a tracheostomy and maintain anesthesia via this route. Begin the incision just to the left of the midline in the submandibular region and carry it posteriorly to the angle of the mandible. Then gently curve it lateral to the posterior border of the sternocleidomastoid muscle to the base of the neck; finally curve it anteriorly and inferiorly across the clavicle and end it in the suprasternal space (Fig. 36-9). Develop the incision through the platysma muscle and retract the myocutaneous flap so outlined medially to expose the sternocleidomastoid and strap muscles, the pharynx, the

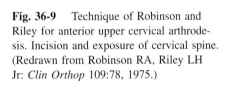

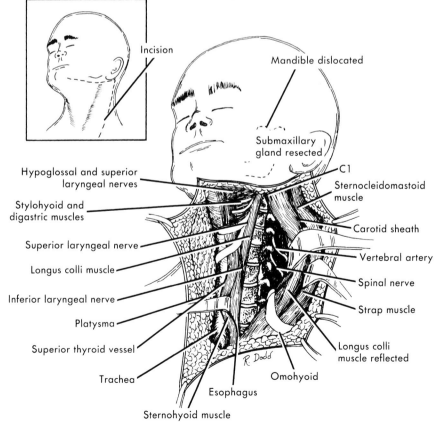

Fig. 36-9   Technique of Robinson and Riley for anterior upper cervical arthrodesis. Incision and exposure of cervical spine. (Redrawn from Robinson RA, Riley LH Jr: *Clin Orthop* 109:78, 1975.)

Incision

Mandible dislocated

Submaxillary gland resected

C1

Sternocleidomastoid muscle

Carotid sheath

Vertebral artery

Spinal nerve

Strap muscle

Longus colli muscle reflected

Hypoglossal and superior laryngeal nerves

Stylohyoid and digastric muscles

Superior laryngeal nerve

Longus colli muscle

Inferior laryngeal nerve

Platysma

Superior thyroid vessel

Trachea

Sternohyoid muscle

Esophagus

Omohyoid

R. Dodd

thyroid gland, the edge of the mandible, and the submaxillary triangle. Identify the anterior surface of the lower cervical spine by retracting the sternocleidomastoid muscle and carotid sheath laterally and transecting the tendinous portion of the omohyoid muscle. Incise the prevertebral fascia in the midline and retract the thyroid gland, esophagus, and trachea medially. Now note that the continuation of this plane superiorly is impeded by the superior thyroid artery, the superior laryngeal neurovascular bundle, the hypoglossal nerve, the stylohyoid muscle, and the digastric muscle. Ligate and divide the superior thyroid artery. Divide and reflect the stylohyoid muscle and digastric muscle; identify and protect the superior laryngeal and hypoglossal nerves. Retract the larynx and the pharynx medially and the external carotid artery laterally and identify the floor of the submaxillary triangle. Maintain superior retraction so that the base of the skull and the anterior arch of the first cervical vertebra are visible. To gain additional exposure, excise the submaxillary gland and dislocate the temporomandibular joint anteriorly by rotating the mandible superiorly and toward the right. The anterior arch of the first cervical vertebra, the odontoid process, and both vertebral arteries are now visible. Cut a trough in the anterior aspect of the second and third vertebral bodies to the level of the posterior cortex of the odontoid process. Remove cancellous bone from the odontoid process with a small curet and convert it to a hollow shell. Shape a bone graft removed from the anterior iliac crest to the dimensions of the previously constructed trough. Shape the superior end of the graft to resemble a saddle and fit one protrusion into the odontoid process and leave the other protrusion abutting the anterior arch of the first cervical vertebra. With the saddle supporting the anterior cortex of the odontoid and the inferior portion of the anterior arch of the first cervical vertebra, secure the inferior end of the graft with a loop of wire or heavy suture material through the cortex of the inferior vertebral body. If a twisted wire loop has been placed, use a small amount of methylmethacrylate bone cement to cover its sharp edges and avoid wire protrusion into the posterior pharynx.

AFTERTREATMENT. The aftertreatment is the same as for the Bailey and Badgley technique (Technique 36-2).

◆ FIBULAR STRUT GRAFT IN CERVICAL SPINE ARTHRODESIS WITH CORPECTOMY

TECHNIQUE 36-6 (Whitecloud and LaRocca)

Use the surgical approach of Robinson et al. (Technique 36-1). As described in that technique, self-retaining retractors are helpful. These can be placed for cephalad and caudad retraction, as well as midline retraction achieved by placing the blades deep to the longus colli muscles that have been elevated.

Remove a rectangular segment of the anterior longitudinal ligament and remove the anterior annulus at each disc level that is to be excised. Remove the anterior half to two thirds of the disc with a curet and pituitary rongeurs and identify the uncovertebral joints at each level laterally. With the uncovertebral joints clearly identified with the operating microscope, use a high-speed burr, small curets, and small Kerrison rongeurs to remove the remaining disc material back to the posterior longitudinal ligament at each disc level and remove the intervening vertebral bodies as described in the technique of Robinson. The width of the trough should be maintained at the width between the uncinate processes. The medial portion of the uncinate process can be removed, but removal should not be carried lateral to the uncinate process because this endangers the vertebral artery. Carry the dissection through the vertebral body until the posterior cortex is encountered. The bleeding pattern of the bone will change from a cancellous pattern to a cortical pattern at this point. Perform the vertebrectomy and the posterior discectomy at each level with the aid of the operating microscope or loupe magnification with the use of a headlight. Maintain meticulous hemostasis and use bipolar cautery on the posterior soft tissue structures, such as the posterior longitudinal ligament. Apply bone wax to the cancellous surfaces laterally on the edges of the trough. Maintain the sides of the trough in a parasagittal plane. Once the posterior cortex has been reached and thinned to paper thickness, use a small curet to pull the bone anteriorly, detaching it from the posterior longitudinal ligament. In this fashion the posterior longitudinal ligament can be thinned, and pathological processes, such as ossification of the posterior longitudinal ligament where spinal cord compression occurs, can be treated. Remove the posterior longitudinal ligament by thinning the posterior longitudinal ligament and developing a plane just ventral to the dura. The dura can be quite attenuated in some circumstances and is easily torn. Exercise great caution during this portion of the procedure. Small curets, small Kerrison rongeurs, and micro blunt hook and micro blunt dissector are quite useful in removing the posterior longitudinal ligament and osteophytes at the posterior aspect of the uncovertebral joints.

On completion of the decompression use a full segment of fibula for strut graft placement. Place the fibular graft into prepared notches in the vertebra at both ends of the segment to be spanned. Notch the fibular graft at each end so that it will key into the prepared notch in each endplate. Place the endplate recess at the cephalad endplate slightly more posterior than the recess through the endplate at the caudal end to make graft insertion easier. Prepare the superior and inferior endplates to accept the graft by removing the cartilaginous endplate and preparing the notches. Preserve the anterior portion of the vertebral cortex to prevent graft dislodgment anteriorly. Once the fibular graft has been cut

continued

and shaped to appropriate dimensions, increase the traction on the head and insert the graft into the superior vertebra, using an impactor to sink the inferior portion of the graft into the endplate recess, and pull distally, locking it into place. Two thirds of the graft then comes to lie posterior to the anterior aspect of the vertebral column. Anterior cervical plate fixation can be added if desired. Take care in selecting proper plate length so that the screws will not be too close to the graft-recipient site interface. Check the graft position by roentgenogram and close the wound over soft, closed suction drains in layers.

An alternative technique was described previously in the Robinson technique, consisting of an autologous iliac graft and anterior cervical plating. This provides adequate stability so that only a cervical orthosis is needed after surgery. However, if screw purchase is not acceptable, halo-vest immobilization should be used with the uninstrumented fibular technique. Without instrumentation halo-vest immobilization should be used for 3 months. Postoperative immobilization may be necessary for longer than 3 months, especially with fibular allografts, because incorporation of the cortical bone will be somewhat slower than with iliac bone. However, Hughes et al. reported excellent results with the use of fibular grafts in the treatment of cervical spondylolytic myelopathy.

AFTERTREATMENT. Depending on the type of internal fixation, initial immobilization is continued by skeletal traction, a halo-vest, a plastic collar, a Philadelphia brace, or a cervicodorsal brace. The time required for fusion will understandably be longer with cortical bone than with a corticocancellous bone graft. Whitecloud and LaRocca kept their patients immobilized in a hard cervical collar, Philadelphia brace, or cervicodorsal brace for an average of 15 weeks. They concluded that this is too short a time; perhaps, like the canine fibular transplantation studied by Enneking et al., the graft may require a year for incorporation in humans. Therefore prolonged immobilization is necessary. We usually use anterior iliac crest grafts and anterior instrumentation with a cervical orthosis for postoperative immobilization for 8 to 12 weeks.

POSTERIOR ARTHRODESIS

The techniques of posterior arthrodesis of the cervical spine are discussed in the section on fractures, dislocations, and fracture-dislocations of the cervical spine (Chapter 35).

Dorsal and Lumbar Spine

The indications for arthrodesis of the lumbar spine are now considerably different from in the days of Hibbs and Albee. Fusion of the lumbosacral region for degenerative, traumatic, and congenital lesions is now more common. Indications for

and techniques of spinal fusion and care after surgery vary from one orthopaedic center to another. Many orthopaedists prefer posterior arthrodesis, usually some modification of the intertransverse process type fusion, using a large quantity of autogenous iliac bone. Internal fixation can be used with posterior arthrodesis. Before the use of instrumentation, the current status of the implant—its risks and indications and approval by the FDA—should be reviewed carefully and completely with the patient. Posterolateral or intertransverse process fusions are used most frequently, either alone or occasionally in combination with an anterior fusion and with or without posterior internal fixation. Interbody fusions from posterior, anterior, retroperitoneal, or transperitoneal approach are preferred by other orthopaedic surgeons.

For lumbar fusion, the best technique for a particular patient remains controversial. The decision should be based on the pathological entity being treated, expected applicable biomechanics and healing potential of different constructs, and the surgeon's experience. With regard to the pathological entity, consideration must be given to the spinal column and the neural elements. In this way the proper balance can be obtained between the need for possible increased instability from neural decompression and strategies to increase stability to promote fusion. After determining the optimal operative plan for a particular patient, additional controversy exists regarding the best technique to execute the plan, that is, an open technique versus a minimally invasive approach.

POSTERIOR ARTHRODESIS

Posterior arthrodeses of the spine generally are based on the principles originated by Hibbs in 1911. In the Hibbs operation fusion of the neural arches is induced by overlapping numerous small osseous flaps from contiguous laminae, spinous processes, and articular facets. In the thoracic spine the arthrodesis is generally extended laterally out to the tips of the transverse processes so that the posterior cortex and cancellous bone of these portions of the vertebrae are used to widen the fusion mass. Accurate visual identification of a specific vertebral level is always difficult except when the sacrum can be exposed and thus identified. At any other level, despite the fact that identification of a given vertebra may be possible because of the anatomical peculiarities of spinous processes, laminae, and articular facets, it is always advisable to make marker roentgenograms at surgery. Marker films occasionally are made before surgery, using a metal marker on the skin with a scratch on the skin to identify the level. We recommend a method consisting of the roentgenographic identification of a marker of adequate size clamped to a spinous process within the operative field. The closer to the base of the spinous process the marker can be inserted, the more accurate and easier the identification. Cross-table lateral roentgenograms or anteroposterior roentgenograms taken on the operating table to compare with good-quality preoperative roentgenograms usually are sufficient for accurate identification of the vertebral level, although the quality of the portable roentgenograms may at times make this difficult. Patient positioning to maintain lumbar lordosis also is important.

◆ Hibbs Fusion of Spine

With the Hibbs technique, fusion is attempted at four different points—the laminae and articular processes on each side. The procedure has been modified slightly over the years.

TECHNIQUE 36-7 *(Hibbs, As Described by Howorth)*

Incise the skin and subcutaneous tissues in the midline along the spinous processes and attach towels to the skin edges with clips or use an adhesive plastic drape. Divide the deep fascia and supraspinous ligament in line with the skin incision. With a Kirmisson or Cobb elevator remove the supraspinous ligament from the tips of the spines. Next strip the periosteum from the sides of the spines and the dorsal surface of the laminae with a curved elevator. Control bleeding with long thin sponge packs (Hibbs sponges). Incise the interspinous ligaments in the direction of their length, making a continuous longitudinal exposure. Now elevate the muscles from the ligamentum flavum and expose the fossa distal to the lateral articulation overlying the pars interarticularis and transverse process base. Excise the fat pad in the fossa with a scalpel or curet. Thoroughly denude the spinous processes of periosteum and ligament with an elevator and curet, split them longitudinally and transversely with an osteotome, and remove them with the Hibbs biting forceps. Using a thick chisel elevator, strip away the capsules of the lateral articulations. Free with a curet the posterior layer (about two thirds) of the ligamentum flavum from the margins of the distal and proximal laminae in succession and peel it off the anterior layer; leave the latter to cover the dura. Excise the articular cartilage and cortical bone from the lateral articulations with special thin osteotomes, either straight or angled at 30, 45, or 60 degrees as required. A.D. Smith emphasized that the lateral articulations of the vertebra above the area of fusion must not be disturbed, since this may cause pain later. However, it is important to include the lateral articulations within the fusion area, because if they are not obliterated, the entire fusion is jeopardized. After curetting the lateral articulations in the fusion area, he narrowed the remaining defect by making small cuts into the articular processes parallel with the joint line so that these thin slices of bone separate slightly and fill the space. This, he believed, is preferable to packing the joint spaces with cancellous bone chips.

Using a gouge, cut chips from the fossa below each lateral articulation and turn them into the gap left by the removal of the articular cartilage or insert a fragment of spinous process into the gap. Denude the fossa of cortical bone and pack it fully with chips. Also with a gouge remove chips from the laminae and place them in the interlaminar space in contact with raw bone on each side. Use fragments from the spinous processes to bridge the laminae. Also use additional bone from the ilium near the posterosuperior spine or from the spinous processes beyond the fusion area. When large or extensive grafts are taken from the posterior ilium, postoperative pain or sensitivity of the area may be marked. Care should be taken to avoid injury to the cluneal nerves with subsequent neuroma formation. Bone from the bone bank can be used, especially if the bone available locally is scant because of spina bifida. The bone grafts should not extend beyond the laminae of the end vertebrae because the projecting ends of the grafts can cause irritation and pain. If the nucleus pulposus is to be removed, the chips are cut before exposure of the nucleus and are kept until needed. The remaining layer of the ligamentum flavum is freed as a flap with its base at the midline, is retracted for exposure of the nerve root and nucleus, and after removal of the nucleus is replaced to protect the dura.

Suture the periosteum, ligaments, and muscles snugly over the chips with interrupted sutures. Then suture the subcutaneous tissue carefully to eliminate dead space and close the skin either with a subcuticular suture or nonabsorbable skin suture technique.

At this clinic we routinely use an adhesive plastic film material to isolate the skin surface from the wound rather than attaching towels to skin edges with clips because clips have an unfortunate tendency to become displaced and can get lost within the wound. We routinely use modified Cobb elevators, which when sharp are efficient in stripping away the capsules of the lateral articulations. The most important single project at the time of surgery is preparing an extensive fresh cancellous bed to receive the grafts. This means denuding the facet joints, articular processes, pars interarticularis, laminae, and spinous processes. Subcuticular wound closure routinely is used to improve patient comfort.

AFTERTREATMENT. We routinely use closed wound suction for 12 to 36 hours, with removal mandatory by 48 hours. Depending on the level of the arthrodesis, the age of the patient, and the presence or absence of internal fixation, walking is allowed in 24 to 48 hours when pain permits. For obese patients all types of external fixation or support likely will be inadequate, and limitation of activity may be the only reasonable alternative. The appropriateness of bracing remains controversial. Generally, for fusions with marked preoperative instability (e.g., burst fractures), rigid bracing is continued for 12 weeks. For fusions without marked instability (e.g., degenerative spondylolisthesis), bracing generally, if used, is less rigid and of shorter duration.

◆ Posterolateral or Intertransverse Fusions

In 1948 Cleveland, Bosworth, and Thompson described a technique for repair of pseudarthrosis after spinal fusion in which grafts are placed posteriorly on one side over the laminae, lateral margins of the articular facets, and base of the transverse processes. Watkins described what he called a posterolateral fusion of the lumbar and lumbosacral spine in which the facets, pars interarticularis, and bases of the transverse processes are fused with chip grafts and a large graft is placed posteriorly on the transverse processes. When the lumbosacral joint is included, the grafts extend to the posterior aspect of the first sacral segment.

We, like many others, use this operation and its modifications for primary lumbar and lumbosacral fusions and in patients with pseudarthrosis, laminar defects either congenital or surgical, or spondylolisthesis with chronic pain from instability. The operation may be unilateral or bilateral but usually is bilateral, covering one or more joints depending on the stability of the area to be fused. The retraction instruments designed by McElroy and others are useful. However, one should be mindful of the ischemia caused by retractors, and they should be periodically released to allow perfusion of the paraspinal musculature. When placing the retractors, minimal retractor bulk and tension should be employed. The technique described by Watkins allows exposure for a posterolateral fusion without much need for soft tissue retraction.

TECHNIQUE 36-8 *(Watkins)*

Make a longitudinal skin incision along the lateral border of the paraspinal muscles, curving it medially at the distal end across the posterior crest of the ilium (Fig. 36-10, *A*). Alternatively, a single midline skin incision can be used with bilateral fascial incisions. Divide the lumbodorsal fascia and establish the plane of cleavage between the border of the paraspinal muscles and the fascia overlying the transversus abdominis muscle. The tips of the transverse processes can now be palpated in the depths of the wound (Fig. 36-10, *B*). Release the iliac attachment of the muscles

with an osteotome, taking a thin layer of ilium. Continue the exposure of the posterior crest of the ilium by subperiosteal dissection and remove the crest almost flush with the sacroiliac joint, taking enough bone to provide one or two grafts. Removal of the iliac crest increases exposure of the spine. Retract the sacrospinalis muscle toward the midline and denude the transverse processes of the dorsal muscle and ligamentous attachments; expose the articular facets by excising the joint capsule. Remove the cartilage from the facets with an osteotome and level the area down to allow the graft to fit snugly against the facets, pars interarticularis, and base of the transverse process at each level. Comminute the facets with a small gouge or osteotome and turn bone chips up and down from the facet area, upper sacral area, and transverse processes. Now split the resected iliac crest longitudinally into two grafts. Shape one to fit into the prepared bed and impact it firmly in place with its cut surface against the spine (Fig. 36-10, *B*). Preserve the remaining graft for use on the opposite side with or without additional bone from the other iliac crest. Now pack additional ribbons and chips of cancellous bone from the ilium about the graft. Allow the paraspinal muscles to fall in position over the fusion area, and close the wound.

AFTERTREATMENT. Aftertreatment is the same as that described for posterior arthrodesis (p. 1705).

◆ ◆ ◆

Wiltse in 1961, Truchly and Thompson in 1962, Rombold in 1966, and Wiltse et al. in 1968 described modifications of the Watkins technique. Wiltse et al. split the sacrospinalis muscle longitudinally and included the laminae, as well as the articular facets and transverse processes, in the fusion (Figs. 36-11 and 36-12). Some members of our staff combine the pos-

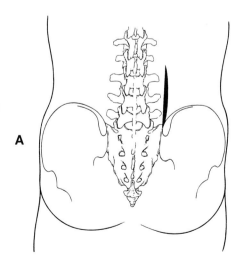
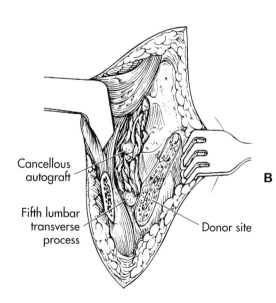

Fig. 36-10   Watkins posterolateral fusion. **A,** Incision. **B,** Lumbothoracic fascia has been incised, paraspinal muscles have been retracted medially, and tips of transverse processes are now palpable. Split iliac crest and smaller grafts have been placed against spine.

A

Cancellous autograft

Fifth lumbar transverse process

Donor site

B

terolateral fusion using a midline approach with a modified Hibbs type fusion in routine lumbar and lumbosacral fusions (Fig. 36-13); they add autologous grafts obtained from the ilium. DePalma and Prabhakar also combined posterior and posterolateral fusions.

Adkins used an intertransverse or alar transverse fusion in which tibial grafts are inserted between the transverse processes of L4 and L5 and between that of L5 and the ala of the sacrum on one or both sides.

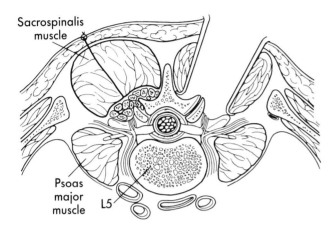

Fig. 36-11   Technique of posterolateral fusion in which sacrospinalis muscle is split longitudinally, and laminae, articular facets, and transverse processes are all included in fusion. (Modified from Wiltse LL, Bateman JG, Hutchinson RH, et al: *J Bone Joint Surg* 50A:919, 1968.)

TECHNIQUE 36-9 *(Adkins)*

Dissect the erector spinae muscles laterally from the pedicles, exposing the transverse processes and ala of the sacrum. This is easier when the facets have been removed, but if these are intact, exposure can be obtained without disturbing them. Cut a groove in the upper or lower border of each transverse process with a sharp gouge or forceps. Take care not to fracture the transverse process. In the ala of the sacrum, first make parallel cuts in its posterosuperior border with an osteotome. Then drive a gouge across the ends of these cuts, and lever the intervening bone out of the slot so made. For fusions of the fourth to the fifth lumbar vertebrae, cut a tibial graft with V-shaped ends; insert it obliquely between the transverse processes and then rotate it into position so that it causes slight distraction of the processes and becomes firmly impacted between them. For the lumbosacral joint cut the graft so that it is V-shaped at its upper end and straight but slightly oblique at its lower end. Insert one arm of the V in front of the transverse process and punch the lower end into the slot in the sacrum. If only one side is grafted, arrange the patient so that there is a slight convex curve of the spine on the operated side; thus firm impaction occurs when the spine is straightened. Bilateral grafts are preferred. The grafts should be placed as far laterally as possible to avoid the nerve roots and to gain maximal stability.

Alternatively, strips of iliac wing cortex no more than 2 to 3 mm thick are placed anterior to the transverse processes

continued

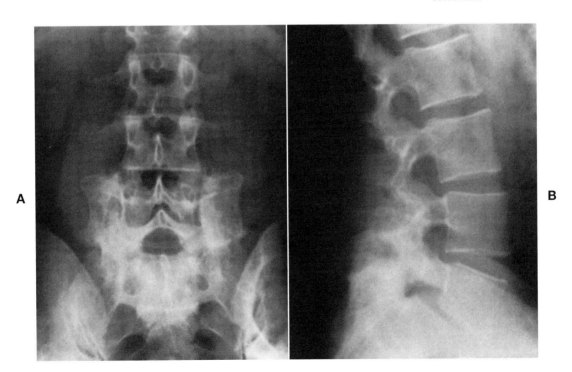

Fig. 36-12   Bilateral posterolateral fusion for spondylolisthesis in adult. Anteroposterior (**A**) and lateral (**B**) roentgenograms 6 months after surgery.

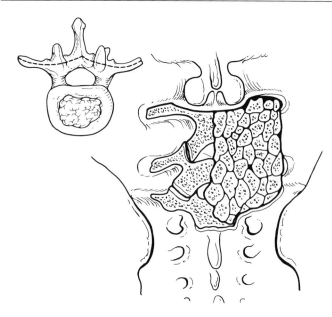

Fig. 36-13 Slocum technique combining posterior (modified Hibbs) and posterolateral fusions. Midline incision is used. *Inset,* All bone posterior to broken line is removed. (Redrawn from Wiltse LL: *Clin Orthop* 21:156, 1961.)

of L4 and L5 to bridge the gap and lie on the intertransverse fascia. Similarly, another strip is placed between the ala of the sacrum and L5 by wedging it into the space after the ala has been slotted and decorticated. Care must be taken that these grafts do not protrude too far anterior to the plane of the transverse processes. This modification does not require a tibial graft and is recommended.

AFTERTREATMENT. Aftertreatment is the same as that described for posterior arthrodesis (p. 1705).

Internal Fixation in Spinal Fusion

Various types of internal fixation have been used in spinal fusion. The object is to immobilize the joints during fusion and thus hasten consolidation and reduce pain and disability after surgery. Additionally, the instrumentation maintains correction of deformity and normal contours during the consolidation of the fusion mass. For many years surgeons fixed the spinous processes of the lumbar spine with heavy wire loops, as described by Rogers for fracture-dislocation of the cervical spine (Chapter 35).

McBride reported a method of fixing the articular facets with bone blocks. Later he used cylindrical bone grafts to transfix the facets, particularly at the lumbosacral joint. Still later he elevated subperiosteally the soft tissue attachments to the spinous processes and laminae, removed the spinous processes of L4, L5, and S1 at their bases, and with special trephine cutting tools cut mortise bone grafts from them. The laminae are then spread forcibly with laminae distractors, and,

again with the use of special trephine cutting tools, a round hole is made across each facet joint into the underlying pedicle. The bone grafts are then impacted firmly across each joint into the pedicle, and the distractors are removed.

Overton also fixed the articular facets with bone grafts, but in addition he used H grafts between the spinous processes and added bone chips about the fusion area. Of 187 patients treated by his method, 174 (or 93%) obtained solid fusion as judged by roentgenograms. This technique has not been used at this clinic.

Internal fixation (such as pedicle screws and plates) are described in Chapter 35. Again, however, before using these techniques the indications and current status of the use of these implants as approved by the FDA should be reviewed carefully with the patient. A special consent form should be signed by the patient if these devices are being used for anything other than the strictly approved indications.

Treatment After Posterior Arthrodesis

Opinions vary as to the proper treatment after spinal fusion. Usually the patient is placed on bed rest for a period of 12 to 24 hours; mobilization is then begun. No clear consensus exists on the duration of bed rest or the type of external support that should be used or even whether external support should be used. This depends on the pathological condition being treated and on the location and extent of the fusion. Surgeon preference also is important in this decision and often is based more on the patient's comfort rather than immobilization for promotion of fusion, especially if instrumentation has been used for a degenerative process rather than for treatment of traumatic instability. If the lumbosacral area is fused and postoperative immobilization is a primary goal, a well-molded body cast or plastic jacket can be applied a few days after fusion. Additionally, thigh extension can be added on one side; however, it has been shown that even with this degree of brace support the lumbosacral junction is not truly immobilized. Immobilization is continued until the patient is comfortable or until consolidation of the fusion mass occurs as seen on roentgenograms. Anteroposterior roentgenograms are made with the patient supine and in right and left bending positions, and a lateral roentgenogram is made with the patient in flexion and extension between 3 and 4 months postoperatively to confirm consolidation of the fusion mass. A longer period may be needed, especially in uninstrumented fusions. However, even with instrumentation the fusion mass may require a year or more to mature.

Pseudarthrosis After Spinal Fusion

The possibility of pseudarthrosis after spinal arthrodesis should be remembered from the time the operation is proposed until the fusion mass is solid. A frank discussion of this problem with each patient before operation is important.

In a study of lumbosacral spine fusions performed on 594 patients, Cleveland et al. found pseudarthrosis in 119, an incidence of 20%. When calculated on the basis of the number of intervertebral spaces fused, the incidence was 12.1%. There was a definite relationship between the extent of fusion and the incidence of pseudarthrosis. When the fifth lumbar vertebra was fused to the sacrum, the pseudarthrosis rate was 3.4%; when the fourth lumbar vertebra was included, the rate was 17.4%; and when the fusion extended up to the third or second lumbar vertebra, one third of the patients showed one or more pseudarthroses. Bosworth recommended that in the lumbosacral region arthrodesis should extend only from the fourth lumbar vertebra to the sacrum as a maximum at one stage, unless the situation at the time of surgery requires more extensive fusion. Other segments to be included in the final fusion area are added later. Ralston and Thompson, in a study of 1096 patients after spinal fusion, found an overall pseudarthrosis rate of 16.6%. Prothero, Parkes, and Stinchfield, in a review of 430 fusions, found a rate of 15.1%; as in the study of Cleveland et al., the rate varied with the extent of the fusion: when the fifth lumbar vertebra was fused to the sacrum, the rate was 8.3%; when the fourth lumbar vertebra was included, the rate was 15.8%; and when the fusion extended to the third lumbar vertebra, the rate was 26.6%. In contrast, DePalma and Rothman, in a review of 448 patients 5 to 17 years after spinal fusion, found an overall pseudarthrosis rate of only 8.7%.

In addition to these studies, the literature contains multiple studies with single-level pseudarthrosis rates as high as 30%. Meticulous technique in preparing the recipient site and in harvesting and preparing autologous bone is required to optimize fusion rates regardless of any other techniques that may be used.

It has been estimated that 50% of patients with pseudarthrosis have no symptoms. Bosworth, in a review of 101 patients with pseudarthrosis, found 43 who had no pain. DePalma and Rothman matched 39 patients with pseudarthrosis against 39 otherwise similar patients without pseudarthrosis. The results were a little better when the fusions were solid, but the difference was not marked. In each group some patients had pain and some did not. We have presumed that persistent pain after spinal fusion with no other identifiable cause is caused by pseudarthrosis when this condition is present. Yet, in some instances pain has continued after a successful repair. Even though pain can persist, repair of a pseudarthrosis is indicated when disabling pain persists; repair is contraindicated when pain is slight or absent.

The following findings are helpful in making a diagnosis of pseudarthrosis: (1) discretely localized pain and tenderness over the fusion area, (2) progression of the deformity or disease, (3) localized motion in the fusion mass, as found in biplane bending roentgenograms, and (4) motion in the fusion mass found on exploration. Cobb and others pointed out that exploration is the only way one can be absolutely certain that a fusion mass is completely solid. Technetium bone scanning may show increased uptake over a pseudarthrosis but is not always reliable, as pointed out by Bohnsack et al. Anteroposterior tomography has been used to evaluate bilateral lateral fusions. The addition of spinal instrumentation significantly hinders imaging of the fusion mass.

◆ Pseudarthrosis Repair

TECHNIQUE 36-10 *(Ralston and Thompson)*

Expose the entire fusion plate subperiosteally through the old incision; should the defect be wide and filled with dense fibrous tissue, subperiosteal stripping in that area can be difficult. On the other hand, a narrow defect often is difficult to locate because the surface of the plate usually is irregular, and the line of pseudarthrosis may be sinuous in both coronal and sagittal planes. In our experience, adherence of the overlying fibrous tissue has been the key factor that aids in identifying a pseudarthrosis. The characteristic smooth cortical surface and easily stripped fibrous "periosteum" of a solid, mature fusion mass are quite different from the adherent fibrous tissue overlying a pseudarthrosis. Meticulous inspection of the region of the facet joint is needed. Often a mature and solid fusion mass extends across the transverse processes, but motion is detectable at the facet joint, indicating the fusion mass did not incorporate to the fusion bed, that is, the transverse processes. Thoroughly clean the fibrous tissue from the fusion mass in the vicinity of the pseudarthrosis. The adjacent superior and inferior borders of the fusion mass on either side of the pseudarthrosis usually will be seen to move when pressure is applied with a blunt instrument, such as a curet. As the defect is followed across the fusion mass, it will be found to extend into the lateral articulations on each side. Carefully explore these articulations and excise all fibrous tissue and any remaining articular cartilage down to bleeding bone. Should the defect be wide, excise the fibrous tissue that fills it to a depth of 3 to 6 mm across the entire mass and protect the underlying spinal dura. Thoroughly freshen the exposed edges of the defect. When the defect is narrow and motion is minimal, limit the excision of the interposed soft tissue to avoid loss of fixation. Now fashion a trough 6 mm wide and 6 mm deep on each side of the midline, extending longitudinally both well above and well below the defect. "Fish scale" the entire fusion mass on both sides of the defect, the bases of the bone chips raised being away from the defect. Now obtain both strip and chip bone grafts either from the fusion mass above or below or from the ilium, preferably the latter. Pack these grafts tightly into the lateral articulations, into the pseudarthrosis defect, and into the longitudinal troughs. Then place small grafts across the pseudarthrosis line and wedge the edge of each transplant beneath the fish-scaled cortical bone chips. Use all remaining graft material to pack neatly in and about the grafts.

Internal fixation (Chapter 35) can be used to improve the rate of healing after pseudarthrosis repair but often is not necessary, and removal of loose hardware improves postoperative imaging capability.

Minimally Invasive Posterior Lumbar Fusion

Multiple investigators have developed techniques for endoscopically assisted posterior fusions. Results using bone graft extenders such as BMPs in animal models are encouraging. Other techniques may have less utility, but continued study is warranted. We have no significant experience with these various techniques, although if efficacy and safety can be demonstrated, they will offer significant advantages over current techniques.

LUMBAR INTERBODY ARTHRODESIS

Numerous indications for anterior arthrodesis of the lumbar spine are reported in the literature. At this clinic the indications include debridement of infection, tuberculosis, excision of tumors, correction of kyphosis, scoliosis, neural decompression after fracture, and to achieve stability when posterior arthrodesis is not feasible. Less frequently we have used this technique in the treatment of spondylolisthesis or internal intervertebral disc derangements. The surgical approach used in tuberculosis by Hodgson and Stock should be applicable in most instances (see Chapter 40).

◆ Anterior Disc Excision and Interbody Fusion

The rationale of management of lower back pain must be based on an accurate diagnosis. The pain syndromes in this area are many, and diagnostic pitfalls are ever present. Treatment varies according to the physical and emotional profile of the patient and the experience of the surgeon involved. Hemilaminectomy and decompression of nerve roots still constitute the most widely used surgical procedure for unremitting lower back pain. With continued instability of the anterior and posterior elements, supplemental posterior or posterolateral fusion usually proves satisfactory. Rothman found only a 5% decrease in residual back pain and sciatica when disc excision is combined with spinal fusion, but this was not statistically significant. There also was no difference in postoperative evaluation between patients with solid fusion and those with pseudarthrosis.

A group of patients remains for whom the aforementioned standard surgical procedures have been unsuccessful. Stauffer and Coventry emphasized the following causes of persistent symptoms after disc surgery:

1. Mistaken original diagnosis
2. Recurrent herniation of disc material (also incomplete removal)
3. Herniation of disc at another level
4. Bony compression of nerve root
5. Perineural adhesions
6. Instability of vertebral segments
7. Psychoneurosis

In this group improved diagnostic accuracy currently can be obtained with the use of electromyography, a psychological profile assessment, postmyelographic CT, MRI with and without gadolinium contrast, and possibly discography. Finally, differential spinal anesthesia is helpful in discriminating between the various pain types.

As a rule, failure of the usual posterior methods of fusion to relieve pain in the presence of a solid arthrodesis and in the absence of other pathology as listed above dictates *consideration* of anterior intervertebral disc excision and interbody spinal fusion. Goldner, Urbaniak, and McCollum used this criterion and found moderate or complete relief of lower back pain in 78% of patients and complete or moderate relief of lower extremity pain in 85%; no patients had pain worse than before surgery. The Mayo Clinic, on the other hand, reported an overall satisfactory result incidence of only 36%, the difference being attributed chiefly to interpretation of clinical factors and patient type; they also recommended its use primarily as a salvage procedure.

Sacks, polling 15 surgeons in nine different countries, found variations of opinion, no adequate follow-up, and therefore inconclusive long-term results. Conversely, Freebody, Bendall, and Taylor performed 466 operations, the first 243 (1956 to 1967) showing satisfactory results in 90%. Their indications include (1) instability causing backache and sciatica, (2) spondylolisthesis of all types, (3) pain following multiple posterior explorations, and (4) failed posterior fusions. They use three iliac wedge grafts for degenerative disease and a block graft for spondylolisthesis (Fig. 36-14).

Flynn and Hoque in Florida, Fujimake, Crock, and Bedbrook in Australia, and van Rens and van Horn in the Netherlands reported a total of 435 patients who had anterior interbody fusion. Flynn and Hoque and van Rens and van Horn had no male patients with retrograde ejaculation, and in both studies the authors suggested that the incidence of this complication may be exaggerated.

TECHNIQUE 36-11 *(Goldner et al.)*

Administer general anesthesia and place the patient in the Trendelenburg position. Develop the retroperitoneal approach to the vertebral bodies and identify the psoas muscle, the iliac artery and vein, and the left ureter. If more than three interspaces are to be fused, retract the ureter toward the left. Identify the sacral promontory by palpation. Inject saline solution under the prevertebral fascia over the lumbar vertebra and lift the sympathetic chain for easier dissection. Expose the lumbosacral disc space by retracting the left iliac artery and vein to the left. In exposing the fourth lumbar interspace, displace the left artery and vein and ureter to the right side. Elevate the anterior longitudinal ligament as a flap with the base toward the left. Tag the flap with sutures and retract it to give additional protection to the vessels. Separate the intervertebral disc and annulus from the cartilaginous endplates of the vertebrae with a thin osteotome and remove them with pituitary rongeurs and large curets. Clean the space thoroughly back to the posterior longitudinal ligament without removing bone, thereby keeping bleeding to a minimum until the site is ready for grafting. Finally, remove the cartilaginous endplates from the vertebral bodies with an osteotome until bleeding bone is encountered. Cut shallow notches in the opposing surfaces of the vertebrae and measure the dimensions of the notches carefully with a caliper. Cut grafts from the iliac wing, making them larger than the notches

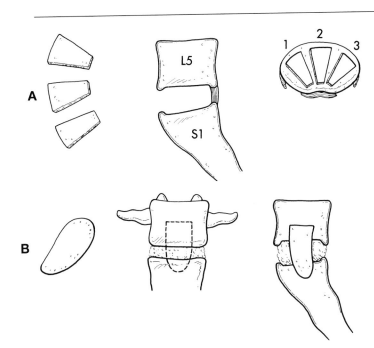

Fig. 36-14   Freebody technique for anterior interbody fusion in lower lumbar spine. **A,** Technique for degenerative disease. **B,** Technique for spondylolisthesis. (Redrawn from Sacks S: *Orthop Clin North Am* 6:272, 1975.)

for later firm impaction (Fig. 36-15). Hyperextend the spine, insert multiple grafts, and relieve the hyperextension. Bipolar electrocautery is useful in obtaining hemostasis, but take care not to coagulate the sympathetic fibers over the anterior aspect of the lumbosacral joint. Use of silver clips in this area is preferred. After completion of the fusion, close all layers with absorbable sutures. Estimate the amount of blood lost and replace it.

AFTERTREATMENT. Nasogastric suction may be necessary for gastric decompression for about 36 hours. Attention must be paid to mobilization of the lower extremities to prevent dependency and blood pooling. Thigh-length TED hose, intermittent compression boots, and low-molecular-weight heparin all are used for deep vein thrombosis prophylaxis. In-bed exercises with straight-leg raising are started on the first postoperative day and continued indefinitely. The patient is allowed to sit and walk with a low back corset used for postoperative immobilization as tolerated. Postoperative roentgenograms are made before discharge from the hospital to serve as a baseline for judging graft appearance. Three months later, side-bending and flexion and extension roentgenograms are made in the standing position to provide information about the success of arthrodesis. Roentgenograms are then repeated at 6 and 12 months after surgery, with the solid fusion not confirmed until 1 year after surgery. Tomograms may be useful in evaluating suspected pseudarthrosis.

◆ ◆ ◆

We have used a retroperitoneal approach to L2, L3, L4, and L5 discs. For the L5 or lumbosacral disc, some prefer a transperitoneal approach if good anterior access is needed. The

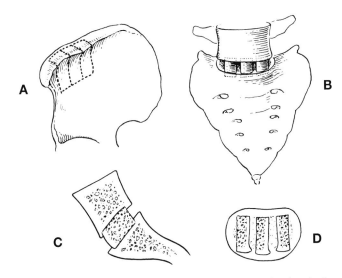

Fig. 36-15   Technique of Goldner et al. for anterior interbody fusion of lumbosacral joint. (From Goldner JL, Urbaniak JR, McCollum DE: *Orthop Clin North Am* 2:543, 1971.)

incidence of deep venous thrombosis after these approaches, especially the midline transperitoneal approach, is much higher than after ordinary spinal surgery. Suitable prophylaxis is indicated, even though it may not be successful in preventing this complication.

Minimally Invasive Anterior Fusion

In the fields of general surgery and thoracic surgery, the development of laparoscopic surgical techniques and video-assisted thoracic surgery (VATS) has allowed significant improvements to be made with respect to decreasing pain, duration of hospitalization, and recovery times for a variety

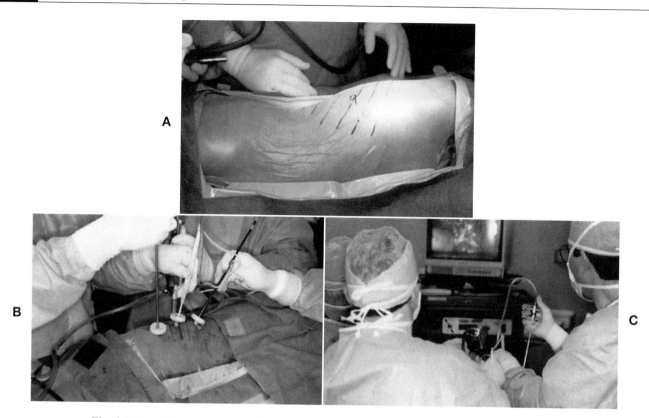

Fig. 36-16 Video-assisted thoracic surgery (VATS) is used for anterior release and interbody fusion. **A,** Patient positioned in left lateral decubitus position and portal positions marked. **B,** Three portals allow two working portals and one portal for camera placement. **C,** VATS techniques have a steep learning curve.

of procedures (Fig. 36-16). Similarly, laparoscopic and VATS techniques have been applied to anterior spine surgery with significant improvements in these same areas. Video-assisted thoracic surgery is discussed in the chapter on scoliosis. We have limited experience with this technique; however, it does appear to provide an excellent way to perform anterior release and discectomy with anterior interbody fusion.

Laparoscopic transperitoneal lumbar instrumentation and fusion also has been developed, and several systems are currently available. These systems allow disc removal and insertion of threaded cylindrical devices, as well as trapezoidal cages packed with autogenous bone into the disc spaces, typically at the L5, S1, and the L4, L5 levels. McAfee et al. and Zdeblick reported series using such systems. The report by McAfee et al. was of a multicenter trial and included 200 cases. Although other reports have been of relatively small series, these techniques do provide an effective means of achieving anterior interbody fusion with maintenance of disc space distraction. However, these techniques appear to require a significant learning curve. Both the VATS and laparoscopic techniques should be performed by surgeons experienced in these techniques to minimize potentially catastrophic complications. The ultimate success of the procedure depends on the proper diagnosis and patient selection. Each device has a technique guide specific to it, and the reader is referred there for specific device use.

References

Adkins EWO: Lumbosacral arthrodesis after laminectomy, *J Bone Joint Surg* 37B:208, 1955.

Albee FH: A report of bone transplantation and osteoplasty in the treatment of Pott's disease of spine, *NY Med J* 95:469, 1912.

Alden TD, Pittman DD, Beres EJ, et al: Percutaneous spinal fusion using bone morphogenic protein-2 gene therapy, *J Neurosurg* 90:109, 1999.

An HS, Lynch, K, Toth J: Prospective comparison of autograft vs. allograft for adult posterolateral lumbar spine fusion: differences among freeze-dried, frozen, and mixed grafts, *J Spinal Disord* 8:131, 1995.

Apfelbaum RI, Kriskovich MD, Haller JR: On the incidence, cause, and prevention of recurrent laryngeal nerve palsies during anterior cervical spine surgery, *Spine* 25:2906, 2000.

Aronson N, Bagan M, Feltzer DL: Results of using the Smith-Robinson approach for herniated and extruded cervical discs, *J Neurosurg* 32:721, 1970.

Aurori BF, Weierman RJ, Lowell HA, et al: Pseudarthrosis after spinal fusion for scoliosis, *Clin Orthop* 199;153, 1985.

Bailey RW, Badgley CE: Stabilization of the cervical spine by anterior fusion, *J Bone Joint Surg* 42A:565, 1960.

Bloom MH, Raney FL Jr: Anterior intervertebral fusion of the cervical spine: a technical note, *J Bone Joint Surg* 63A:842, 1981.

Boden SD, Moskovitz PA, Morone MA, Toribitake Y: Video-assisted lateral intertransverse process arthrodesis: validation of a new minimally invasive lumbar spinal fusion technique in the rabbit in nonhuman primate (Rhesus) models, *Spine* 21:2689, 1996.

Boden SD, Schimandle JH, Hutton WC: An experimental lumbar intertransverse process spinal fusion model: radiographic, histologic, and biomechanical healing characteristics, *Spine* 20:412, 1995.

Boden SD, Schimandle JH, Hutton WC, et al: 1995 Volvo Award in Basic Sciences. The use of an osteoinductive growth factor for lumbar spinal fusion. I. Biology of spinal fusion, *Spine* 20:2626, 1995.

Boden SD, Titus L, Hair G, et al: Lumbar spine fusion by local gene therapy with cDNA encoding a novel osteoinductive protein (LMP-1), *Spine* 23:2486, 1998.

Bohnsack M, Gossé F, Rühmann O, et al: The value of scintigraphy in the diagnosis of pseudarthrosis after spinal fusion surgery, *J Spinal Disord* 12:482, 1999.

Bosworth DM: Clothespin graft of the spine for spondylolisthesis and laminal defects, *Am J Surg* 67:61, 1945.

Bosworth DM: Surgery of the spine, *Instr Course Lect* 14:39, 1957.

Bouchard JA, Koka A, Bensusan JS, et al: Effects of irradiation on posterior spinal fusions: a rabbit model, *Spine* 19:1836, 1994.

Bridwell KH, Lenke LG, McEnery KW, et al: Anterior fresh-frozen structural allografts in the thoracic and lumbar spine: do they work if combined with posterior fusion and instrumentation in adult patients with kyphosis or anterior column defects? *Spine* 20:1410, 1995.

Bridwell KH, O'Brien MF, Lenke LG, et al: Posterior spinal fusion supplemented with only allograft bone in paralytic scoliosis: does it work? *Spine* 19:2658, 1994.

Brigham CD, Tsahakis PJ: Anterior cervical foraminotomy and fusion: surgical technique and results, *Spine* 20:766, 1995.

Brodke DS, Zdeblick TA: Modified Smith-Robinson procedure for anterior cervical discectomy and fusion, *Spine* 17:427, 1992.

Buttermann GR, Glazer PA, Bradford DS: The use of bone allografts in the spine, *Clin Orthop* 324:75, 1996.

Cattell HS, Clark GL Jr: Cervical kyphosis and instability following multiple laminectomies in children, *J Bone Joint Surg* 49A:713, 1967.

Cleveland M, Bosworth DM, Fielding JW, Smyrnis P: Fusion of the spine for tuberculosis in children: a long-range follow-up study, *J Bone Joint Surg* 40A:91, 1958.

Cleveland M, Bosworth DM, Thompson FR: Pseudarthrosis in the lumbosacral spine, *J Bone Joint Surg* 30A:302, 1948.

Cloward RB: Vertebral body fusion for ruptured cervical discs: description of instruments and operative technic, *Am J Surg* 98: 722, 1959.

Cloward RB: Lesions of the intervertebral disks and their treatment by interbody fusion methods: the painful disk, *Clin Orthop* 27:51, 1963.

Cobb JR: Technique, aftertreatment, and results of spine fusion for scoliosis, *Instr Course Lect* 9:65, 1952.

Connolly PJ, Grob D: Controversy. Bracing of patients after fusion for degenerative problems of the lumbar spine—yes or no? *Spine* 23:1426, 1998.

Connor PM, Darden BV: Cervical discography complications and clinical efficacy, *Spine* 18:2035, 1993.

Cook SD, Dalton JE, Prewett AB, et al: In vivo evaluation of demineralized bone matrix as a bone graft substitute for posterior spinal fusion, *Spine* 20:877, 1995.

Cook SD, Rueger DC: Osteogenic protein-1, *Clin Orthop* 324:29, 1996.

Cook SD, Salkeld S, Prewett AB: Simian immunodeficiency virus (human HIV-II) transmission in allograft bone procedures, *Spine* 20:1338, 1995.

Crock HV: Observations on the management of failed spinal operations, *J Bone Joint Surg* 58B:193, 1976.

David SM, Gruber HE, Meyer RA, et al: Lumbar spinal fusion using recombinant human bone morphogenetic protein in the canine: a comparison of three dosages and two carriers, *Spine* 24:1973, 1999.

de Andrade JR, Macnab I: Anterior occipito-cervical fusion using an extrapharyngeal exposure, *J Bone Joint Surg* 51A:1621, 1969.

DePalma AF Prabhakar M: Posterior-posterobilateral fusion of the lumbosacral spine, *Clin Orthop* 47:165, 1966.

DePalma AF, Rothman RH: The nature of pseudarthrosis, *Clin Orthop* 59:113, 1968.

DePalma AF, Rothman RH: *The intervertebral disc*, Philadelphia, 1970, WB Saunders.

Dickman CA, Mican CA: Multilevel anterior thoracic discectomies and anterior interbody fusion using a microsurgical thoracoscopic approach, *J Neurosurg* 84:104, 1996.

Dodd CAF, Ferguson CM, Freedman L, et al: Allograft versus autograft bone in scoliosis surgery, *J Bone Joint Surg* 70B:431, 1988.

Duncan RW, McGuire RA, Meydrech EF: Pneumatic gouge versus standard method for iliac crest harvesting, *Orthop Rev* 8:672, 1994.

Emery SE, Hughes SS, Junglas WA, et al: The fate of anterior vertebral bone grafts in patients irradiated for neoplasm, *Clin Orthop* 300:207, 1994.

Enneking WF, Burchardt H, Puhl J, et al: Physical and biological aspects of repair in dog cortical-bone transplants, *J Bone Joint Surg* 57A:237, 1975.

Esses SI, Natout N, Kip P: Posterior interbody arthrodesis with a fibular strut graft in spondylolisthesis, *J Bone Joint Surg* 77A:172, 1995.

Fabry G: Allograft versus autograft bone in idiopathic scoliosis surgery: a multivariate statistical analysis, *J Pediatr Orthop* 11:465, 1991.

Farey ID, McAfee PC, Davis RF, et al: Pseudarthrosis of the cervical spine after anterior arthrodesis: treatment by posterior nerve-root decompression, stabilization, and arthrodesis, *J Bone Joint Surg* 72A:1171, 1990.

Feiertag MA, Boden SD, Schimandle JH, et al: A rabbit model for nonunion of lumbar intertransverse process spine arthrodesis, *Spine* 21:27, 1996.

Fielding JW, Lusskin R, Batista A: Multiple segment anterior cervical spinal fusion, *Clin Orthop* 54:29, 1967.

Flynn JC, Hoque A: Anterior fusion of the lumbar spine: end-result study with long-term follow-up, *J Bone Joint Surg* 61A:1143, 1979.

Freebody D, Bendall R, Taylor RD: Anterior transperitoneal lumbar fusion, *J Bone Joint Surg* 53B:617, 1971.

Friedlaender GE: Current concepts review: bone grafts, *J Bone Joint Surg* 69A:786, 1987.

Fujimake A, Crock HV, Bedbrook GM: The results of 150 anterior lumbar interbody fusion operations performed by two surgeons in Australia, *Clin Orthop* 165:164, 1982.

Gill K, O'Brien JP: Observations of resorption of the posterior lateral bone graft in combined anterior and posterior lumbar fusion, *Spine* 18:1885, 1993.

Glassman SD, Anagnost SC, Parker A, et al: The effect of cigarette smoking and smoking cessation on spinal fusion, *Spine* 25:2608, 2000.

Goldner JL, Urbaniak JR, McCollum DE: Anterior disc excision and interbody spinal fusion for chronic low back pain, *Orthop Clin North Am* 2:543, 1971.

Grob D, Scheier HJG, Dvorak J, et al: Circumferential fusion of the lumbar and lumbosacral spine, *Arch Orthop Trauma Surg* 111:20, 1991.

Hibbs RA: An operation for progressive spinal deformities, *NY Med J* 93:1013, 1911.

Hibbs RA, Risser JC: Treatment of vertebral tuberculosis by the spine fusion operation: a report of 286 cases, *J Bone Joint Surg* 10:805, 1928.

Hodgson AR, Stock FE: Anterior spine fusion for treatment of tuberculosis of the spine: the operative findings and results of treatment of the first 100 cases, *J Bone Joint Surg* 42A:295, 1960.

Holliger EH, Trawick RH, Boden SD, et al: Morphology of the lumbar intertransverse process fusion mass in the rabbit model: a comparison between two bone graft materials—rhBMP-2 and autograft, *J Spinal Disord* 9:125, 1996.

Howorth MB: Evolution of spinal fusion, *Ann Surg* 117:278, 1943.

Hu RW, Bohlman HH: Fracture at the iliac bone graft harvest site after fusion of the spine, *Clin Orthop* 309:208, 1994.

Hughes SS, Pringle T, Phillips MM, et al: Multilevel cervical corpectomy and fibular strut grafting, *Orthop Trans* 20:432, 1996.

Ido K, Shimizu K, Nakayama Y, et al: Anterior decompression and fusion for ossification of posterior longitudinal ligament in the thoracic spine, *J Spinal Disord* 8:317, 1995.

Jenis LG, Leclair W: Late vascular complication with anterior cervical discectomy and fusion, *Spine* 19:1291, 1994.

Jones AAM, McAfee PC, Robinson RA, et al: Failed arthrodesis of the spine for severe spondylolisthesis: salvage by interbody arthrodesis, *J Bone Joint Surg* 70A:25, 1988.

Jorgenson SS, Lowe TG, France J, et al: A prospective analysis of autograft versus allograft in posterolateral lumbar fusion in the same patient: a minimum of 1-year follow-up in 144 patients, *Spine* 19:2048, 1994.

Kraus DR, Stauffer ES: Spinal cord injury as a complication of elective anterior cervical fusion, *Clin Orthop* 112:130, 1975.

Kumar A, Kozak JA, Doherty BJ, et al: Interspace distraction and graft subsidence after anterior lumbar fusion with femoral strut allograft, *Spine* 18:2393, 1993.

Kurz LG, Garfin SR, Booth RE: Harvesting autogenous iliac bone grafts, *Spine* 14:1324, 1989.

Lindholm TS, Ragni P, Lindholm TC: Response of bone marrow stroma to demineralized cortical bone matrix in experimental spinal fusion in rabbits, *Clin Orthop* 230:296, 1988.

Lovell TP, Dawson EG, Nilsson OS, et al: Augmentation of spinal fusion with bone morphogenetic protein in dogs, *Clin Orthop* 243:266, 1989.

Ludwig SC, Boden SD: Osteoinductive bone graft substitutes for spinal fusion, *Orthop Clin North Am* 30:635, 1999.

Macnab I: The blood supply of the lumbar spine and its application to the technique of intertransverse lumbar fusion, *J Bone Joint Surg* 53B:628, 1971.

Macnab I: Complications of anterior cervical fusion, *Orthop Rev* 1:29, 1972.

Mahvi DM, Zdeblick TA: A prospective study of laparoscopic spinal fusion: technique and operative complications, *Ann Surg* 224:85, 1996.

Mathews HH, Evans MT, Molligan HJ, et al: Laparoscopic discectomy with anterior lumbar interbody fusion: a preliminary review, *Spine* 20:1797, 1995.

McAfee PC, Regan JR, Zdeblick T, et al: The incidence of complications in endoscopic anterior thoracolumbar spinal reconstructive surgery: a prospective multicenter study comprising the first 100 consecutive cases, *Spine* 20:1624, 1995.

McBride ED: A mortised transfacet bone block for lumbosacral fusion, *J Bone Joint Surg* 31A:385, 1949.

Meril AJ: Direct current stimulation of allograft in anterior and posterior lumbar interbody fusions, *Spine* 19:2393, 1994.

Minamide A, Tamaki T, Kawakami M, et al: Experimental spinal fusion using sintered bovine bone coated with type I collagen and recombinant human bone morphogenetic protein-2, *Spine* 24:1863, 1999.

Mooney V, McDermott KL, Song J: Effects of smoking and maturation on long-term maintenance of lumbar spinal fusion success, *J Spinal Disord* 12:380, 1999.

Morone MA, Boden SD: Experimental posterolateral lumbar spinal fusion with demineralized bone matrix gel, *Spine* 23:159, 1998.

Morone MA, Boden SD, Hair G, et al: Gene expression during autograft lumbar spine fusion and the effect of bone morphogenetic protein-2, *Clin Orthop* 351:252, 1998.

Nymberg SM, Crawford AH: Video-assisted thoracoscopic releases of scoliotic anterior spines, *AORN J* 63:561, 1996.

Overton LM: Arthrodesis of the lumbosacral spine, *Clin Orthop* 5:97, 1955.

Overton LM: Lumbosacral arthrodesis: an evaluation of its present status, *Am Surg* 25:771, 1959.

Prothero SR, Parkes JC, Stinchfield FE: Complications after low-back fusion in 1000 patients: a comparison of two series one decade apart, *J Bone Joint Surg* 48A:57, 1966.

Ralston EL, Thompson WAL: The diagnosis and repair of pseudarthrosis of the spine, *Surg Gynecol Obstet* 89:37, 1949.

Regan JJ, Mack MJ, Picetti GD: The technical report on video-assisted thoracoscopy in thoracic spinal surgery: preliminary description, *Spine* 20:831, 1995.

Riley EH, Lane JM, Urist MR, et al: Bone morphogenetic protein-2, *Clin Orthop* 324:39, 1996.

Robinson RA: Anterior and posterior cervical spine fusions, *Clin Orthop* 35:34, 1964.

Robinson RA, Riley LH Jr: Techniques of exposure and fusion of the cervical spine, *Clip Orthop* 109:78, 1975.

Robinson RA, Smith GW: Anterolateral cervical disc removal and interbody fusion for cervical disc syndrome, *Bull Johns Hopkins Hosp* 96:223, 1955 (abstract).

Rogers WA: Fractures and dislocations of the cervical spine: an end-result study, *J Bone Joint Surg* 39A:341, 1957.

Rombold C: Treatment of spondylolisthesis by posterolateral fusion, resection of the pars interarticularis, and prompt mobilization of the patient: an end-result study of seventy-three patients, *J Bone Joint Surg* 48A:1282, 1966.

Rothman RH: New developments in lumbar disk surgery, *Orthop Rev* 4:23, 1975.

Rothman RH, Booth R: Failures of spinal fusion, *Orthop Clin North Am* 6:299, 1975.

Sacks S: Anterior interbody fusion of the lumbar spine, *J Bone Joint Surg* 47B:211, 1965.

Sacks S: Anterior interbody fusion of the lumbar spine: indications and results in 200 cases, *Clin Orthop* 44:163, 1966.

Sacks S: Present status of anterior interbody fusion in the lower lumbar spine, *Orthop Clin North Am* 6:275, 1975.

Sandhu H, Grewal HS, Parvataneni H: Bone grafting for spinal fusion, *Orthop Clin North Am* 30:685, 1999.

Sandhu HS, Kanim LE, Kabo JM, et al: Evaluation of rhBMP-2 with an OPLA carrier in a canine posterolateral transverse process spinal fusion model, *Spine* 20:2669, 1995.

Schimandle JH, Boden SD, Hutton WC: Experimental spinal fusion with recombinant human bone morphogenetic protein-2, *Spine* 20:1326, 1995.

Simmons EH, Bhalla SK, Butt WP: Anterior cervical discectomy and fusion: a clinical and biomechanical study with eight-year follow-up, *J Bone Joint Surg* 51B:225, 1969.

Smith AD: Lumbosacral fusion by the Hibbs technique, *Instr Course Lect* 9:41, 1952.

Smith AD: Tuberculosis of the spine: results in 70 cases treated at the New York Orthopaedic Hospital from 1945 to 1960, *Clin Orthop* 58:171, 1968.

Smith GW, Robinson RA: The treatment of certain cervical-spine disorders by anterior removal of the intervertebral disc and interbody fusion, *J Bone Joint Surg* 40A:607, 1958.

Stauffer RN, Coventry MB: Anterior interbody lumbar spine fusion: analysis of Mayo Clinic Series, *J Bone Joint Surg* 54A:756, 1972.

Stauffer RN, Coventry MB: Posterolateral lumbar-spine fusion: analysis of Mayo Clinic series, *J Bone Joint Surg* 54A:1195, 1972.

Stinchfield FE, Sinton WA: Criteria for spine fusion with use of "H" bone graft following disc removal: results in 100 cases, *Arch Surg* 65:542, 1952.

Thompson WAL, Ralson EL: Pseudarthrosis following spine fusion, *J Bone Joint Surg* 31A:400, 1949.

Truchly G, Thompson WAL: Posterolateral fusion of the lumbosacral spine, *J Bone Joint Surg* 44A:505, 1962.

Urist MR: Bone formation by autoinduction, *Science* 150:893, 1965.

van Rens TJG, van Horn JR: Long-term results in lumbosacral interbody fusion for spondylolisthesis, *Acta Orthop Scand* 53:383, 1982.

Vazquez-Seoane P, Yoo J, Zou D, et al: Interference screw fixation of cervical grafts: a combined in vitro biomechanical and in vivo animal study, *Spine* 18:946, 1993.

Watkins MB: Posterolateral fusion in pseudarthrosis and posterior element defects of the lumbosacral spine, *Clin Orthop* 35:80, 1964.

White AA III, Hirsch C: An experimental study of the immediate load bearing capacity of some commonly used iliac bone grafts, *Acta Orthop Scand* 42:482, 1971.

White AA III, Jupiter J, Southwick WO, et al: An experimental study of the immediate load bearing capacity of three surgical constructions for anterior spine fusions, *Clin Orthop* 91:21, 1973.

Whitecloud TS III, LaRocca H: Fibular strut graft in reconstructive surgery of the cervical spine, *Spine* 1:33, 1976.

Whitehill R, Sirna EC, Young DC, et al: Late esophageal perforation from an autogenous bone graft: report of a case, *J Bone Joint Surg* 67A:644, 1985.

Williams JL, Allen MB Jr, Harkess JW: Late results of cervical discectomy and interbody fusion: some factors influencing the results, *J Bone Joint Surg* 50A:277, 1968.

Wiltse LL: Spondylolisthesis in children, *Clin Orthop* 21:156, 1961.

Wiltse LL, Bateman JG, Hutchinson RH, et al: The paraspinal sacrospinalis-splitting approach to the lumbar spine, *J Bone Joint Surg* 50A:919, 1968.

Wing KJ, Fisher CG, O'Connell JX, et al: Stopping nicotine exposure before surgery: the effect on spinal fusion in a rabbit model, *Spine* 25:30, 2000.

Wozney JM, Rosen U, Celeste AJ, et al: Novel regulators of bone formation: molecular clones and activities, *Science* 242:1528, 1988.

Young WF, Rosenwasser RH: An early comparative analysis of the use of fibular allograft versus autologous iliac crest graft for interbody fusion after anterior cervical discectomy, *Spine* 18:1123, 1993.

Zdeblick TA: A prospective randomized study of lumbar fusion: preliminary results, *Spine* 18:983, 1993.

Zdeblick TA, Ducker TB: The use of freeze-dried allograft bone for anterior cervical fusions, *Spine* 16:726, 1991.

Zdeblick TA, Hughes SS, Riew D, et al: Failed anterior cervical discectomy and arthrodesis, *J Bone Joint Surg* 79A:523, 1997.

Zdeblick TA, Cooke ME, Wilson D, et al: Anterior cervical discectomy, fusion, and plating: a comparative animal study, *Spine* 18:1974, 1993.

Zdeblick TA, Wilson D, Cooke ME, et al: Anterior cervical discectomy and fusion: a comparison of techniques in an animal model, *Spine* 17:S418, 1992.

Zeller RD, Ghanem I, Miladi L, et al: Posterior spinal fusion in neuromuscular scoliosis using a tibial strut graft: results of a long-term follow-up, *Spine* 19:1628, 1994.

Zlotolow DA, Vaccaro AR, Salamon ML, et al: The role of human bone morphogenetic proteins in spinal fusion, *J Am Acad Orthop Surg* 8:3, 2000.

Zucherman JF, Zdeblick TA, Bailey SA, et al: Instrumented laparoscopic spinal fusion: preliminary results, *Spine* 20:2029, 1995.

CHAPTER

37 Pediatric Cervical Spine

William C. Warner, Jr.

Anomalies of Odontoid

Although congenital anomalies of the odontoid are rare, they can cause significant atlantoaxial instability. These anomalies usually are detected as incidental findings after trauma or when symptoms occur. Atlantoaxial instability can cause a compressive myelopathy, vertebral artery compression, or both.

Congenital anomalies of the odontoid can be divided into three groups: aplasia, hypoplasia, and os odontoideum. Aplasia or agenesis is complete absence of the odontoid. Hypoplasia is partial development of the odontoid, and the bone varies from a small, peglike projection to almost normal size. In os odontoideum, the odontoid is an oval or round ossicle with a smooth, sclerotic border. It is separated from the axis by a transverse gap, leaving the apical segment without support (Fig. 37-1). The ossicle is of variable size and usually is located in the position of the normal odontoid (orthotopic), although occasionally it appears near the occiput in the area of the foramen magnum (dystopic). Because this lesion is frequently asymptomatic and remains undiscovered until it is brought to the physician's attention by trauma or the onset of symptoms, the exact incidence of os odontoideum is not known but is probably more common than appreciated. Odontoid anomalies have been reported to be more common in patients with Down syndrome, Klippel-Feil syndrome, Morquio syndrome, and spondyloepiphyseal dysplasia.

Knowledge of the embryology and vasculature of the odontoid is essential to understanding the etiological theories of congenital anomalies of the odontoid. The odontoid is derived from mesenchyme of the first cervical vertebra. During development it becomes separated from the atlas and fuses with the axis. A vestigial disc space between C1 and C2 forms a synchondrosis within the body of the axis. The apex, or tip, of the odontoid is derived from the most caudal occipital sclerotome, or proatlas. This separate ossification center, called *ossiculum terminale*, appears at age 3 years and fuses by age 12 years. Anomalies of this terminal portion rarely are of clinical significance (Fig. 37-2).

The arterial blood supply to the odontoid is derived from the vertebral and carotid arteries (Fig. 37-3). The vertebral artery gives off an anterior ascending artery and a posterior ascending artery that begin at the level of C3 and ascend anterior and posterior to the odontoid, meeting superiorly to form an apical arcade. The most rostral portion of the extracranial internal carotid artery gives off "cleft perforators," which supply the superior portion of the odontoid. This peculiar arrangement of blood supply is necessary because of the embryological development and anatomical function of the odontoid. The synchondrosis prevents direct vascularization of the odontoid from C2, and vascularization from the blood supply of C1 cannot occur because of the synovial joint cavity surrounding the odontoid.

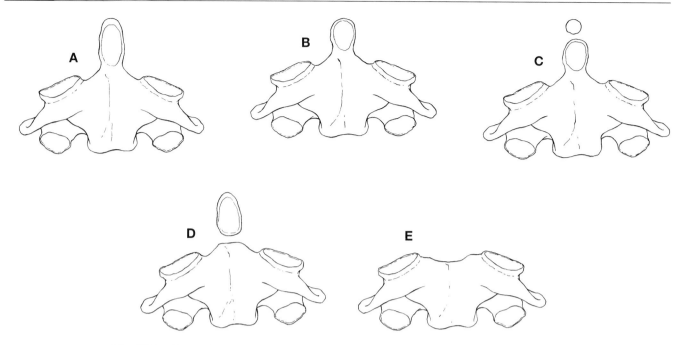

Fig. 37-1   Types of odontoid anomalies. **A,** Normal odontoid. **B,** Hypoplastic odontoid. **C,** Ossiculum terminale. **D,** Os odontoideum. **E,** Aplasia of odontoid.

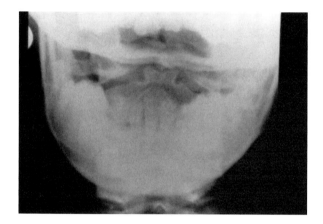

Fig. 37-2   Anteroposterior open-mouth odontoid view demonstrating V-shaped dens bicornis and ossiculum terminale.

Both congenital and acquired causes of odontoid anomalies have been suggested. The congenital causes include failure of fusion of the apex or ossiculum terminale and failure of fusion of the odontoid to the axis, neither of which explains all the findings in os odontoideum. The ossiculum terminale usually is too small to influence stability significantly, and the theory of failure of fusion of the odontoid to the axis does not explain the fact that the space between the ossicle and the axis is at the level of the articulating facets of C2 rather than below the level of the articulating facets where the synchondrosis occurs during development. Os odontoideum can be acquired after infection or trauma or can result from avascular necrosis. Several authors suggest that an unrecognized fracture at the base of the

odontoid is the most common cause. A distraction force by the alar ligament pulls the tip of the fractured odontoid away from its base to produce a nonunion. Tredwell and O'Brien documented 13 patients with acquired os odontoideum resulting from avascular necrosis after halo-pelvic traction.

DIAGNOSIS

The presentation of os odontoideum is variable. Signs and symptoms can range from minor to frank compressive myelopathy or vertebral artery compression. Presenting symptoms may include neck pain, torticollis, or headache caused by local irritation of the atlantoaxial joint. Neurological symptoms vary from transient episodes of paresis after trauma to complete myelopathy caused by cord compression. Symptoms may consist of weakness and loss of balance with upper motor neuron signs, although upper motor neuron signs may be completely absent. Proprioceptive and sphincter disturbances are common findings. Vertebral artery compression causes cervical and brainstem ischemia, resulting in seizures, syncope, vertigo, and visual disturbances. Lack of cranial nerve involvement helps differentiate os odontoideum from other occipitovertebral anomalies because the spinal cord impingement occurs below the foramen magnum.

ROENTGENOGRAPHIC FINDINGS

Odontoid anomalies can be diagnosed on routine cervical spine roentgenograms that include an open-mouth odontoid view (Fig. 37-4). Anteroposterior and lateral tomograms can be helpful in making the initial diagnosis of os odontoideum, and

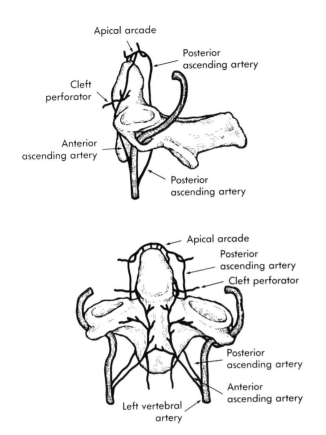

Fig. 37-3 Blood supply to odontoid: posterior and anterior ascending arteries and apical arcade. (Redrawn from Schiff DC, Parke WW: *J Bone Joint Surg* 55A:1450, 1973.)

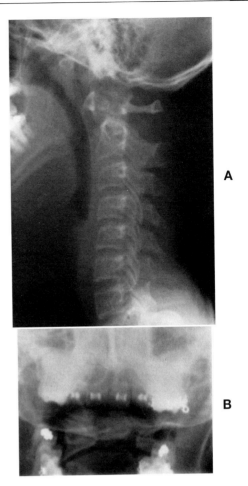

Fig. 37-4 Lateral roentgenogram (**A**) and open-mouth odontoid roentgenogram (**B**) demonstrating os odontoideum.

lateral flexion and extension roentgenograms and tomograms can detect any instability. Odontoid aplasia appears as a slight depression between the superior articulating facets on the open-mouth odontoid view. Odontoid hypoplasia is seen as a short, bony remnant. With os odontoideum a space is present between the body of the axis and a bony ossicle. The free ossicle of os odontoideum usually is half the size of a normal odontoid and is oval or round with smooth, sclerotic borders. The space differs from that of an acute fracture, in which the space is thin and irregular instead of wide and smooth. This space should not be confused with the neurocentral synchondrosis in children younger than 5 years.

The amount of instability can be documented by lateral flexion and extension plain films or tomograms that allow measurement of the amount of anterior and posterior displacement of the atlas on the axis. In children, motion between the odontoid and the body of the axis must be demonstrated before instability with os odontoideum can be diagnosed because the ossicle is fixed to the anterior arch of C1 and moves with it during flexion and extension. Measurement of the relation of

C1 to the free ossicle is of little value because this moves as one unit. A more significant measurement is made by projecting a line superiorly from the body of the axis to a line projected inferiorly from the posterior border of the anterior arch of the atlas. Measurements greater than 3 mm in adults and 4 to 5 mm in children indicate significant in stability.

The space available for the spinal cord also is a helpful measurement. This is determined by measuring the distance from the posterior aspect of the odontoid or axis to the nearest posterior structure. Fielding reported that most symptomatic patients in his study had an average of 1 cm of movement. Cineradiography also can be helpful in determining motion around the C1-C2 articulation.

Watanabe, Toyama, and Fujimura described two roentgenographic measurements that correlate with neurological signs and symptoms. They found that if there is a sagittal plane rotation angle of more than 20 degrees or an instability index of more than 40%, a patient is likely to have neurological signs and symptoms. The instability index is measured from both lateral flexion and extension roentgenograms. Minimum and

Fig. 37-5 Roentgenographic parameters. Minimal (**A**) and maximal (**B**) distance from posterior border of body of C2 to posterior atlantal arch. **C,** Change of atlantoaxial angle between flexion and extension position. *a,* Sagittal plane rotation. (Redrawn from Watanabe M, Toyama Y, Fujimura Y: *Spine* 21:1435, 1996.)

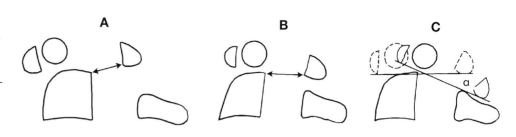

maximum distances are measured from the posterior border of the C2 body to the posterior arc of the atlas. The instability index is calculated by the following equation:

$$\text{Instability index} = \text{Maximum distance} - \text{Minimum distance} + \text{Maximum distance} \times 100(\%)$$

The sagittal plane rotation angle is measured by the change in the atlantoaxial angle between flexion and extension (Fig. 37-5). Magnetic resonance imaging can be useful in identifying reactive retrodental lesions that can occur with chronic instability. This reactive tissue will not be seen on routine roentgenograms but can be responsible for a decrease in the space available for the spinal cord and compressive myelopathy. The prognosis of os odontoideum depends on the clinical presentation. The prognosis is good if only mechanical symptoms (torticollis or neck pain) or transient neurological symptoms exist. It is poor if neurological deficits slowly progress.

TREATMENT

The primary concern in congenital anomalies of the odontoid is that an already abnormal atlantoaxial joint can subluxate or dislocate with minor trauma and cause permanent neurological damage or even death. Patients with local symptoms usually improve with conservative treatment such as cervical traction or immobilization. The indications for operative stabilization are (1) neurological involvement (even if this is transient), (2) instability of more than 5 mm anteriorly or posteriorly, (3) progressive instability, and (4) persistent neck complaints associated with atlantoaxial instability and not relieved by conservative treatment (Box 37-1).

Prophylactic operative stabilization of asymptomatic patients with instability less than 5 mm is controversial. Because it may be difficult or impossible to restrict a child's activities, the safety of stability without restriction of activity must be weighed against the possible complications of surgery. The decision concerning prophylactic fusion must be made after discussion with the patient and family concerning potential risks of both operative and nonoperative treatment.

In patients with neurological deficits, skull traction should be used before surgery to achieve reduction, allow recovery of neurological function, and decrease spinal cord irritation.

BOX 37-1 • Indications for Operative Stabilization of Os Odontoideum

Neurological involvement (even transient)
Instability of more than 5 mm posteriorly or anteriorly
Progressive instability
Persistent neck complaints

Achieving and maintaining reduction are probably the most important aspects in the treatment of this anomaly.

Before C1-C2 fusion the integrity of the posterior arch of C1 must be documented. Incomplete development of the posterior ring of C1 is uncommon (3 cases in 1000) but is reported to occur with increased frequency in patients with os odontoideum.

◆ Atlantoaxial Fusion

There are many variations of two basic techniques of atlantoaxial fusion (Box 37-2). The Gallie and the Brooks and Jenkins techniques have been the most frequently used for posterior atlantoaxial fusion. The Gallie technique has the advantage of using only one wire passed beneath the lamina of C1, but tightening the wire can cause the unstable C1 vertebra to displace posteriorly and fuse in a dislocated position (Fig. 37-6). The Brooks technique has the disadvantage of requiring sublaminar wires at C1 and C2 but gives greater resistance to rotational movement, lateral bending, and extension. The size of the wire used varies from 22 to 18 gauge, depending on the age of the patient and the size of the spinal canal. In children younger than 6 years of age, wire fixation may not be used; instead the graft is placed along the decorticated fusion site, and a halo or Minerva cast is used for postoperative immobilization.

TECHNIQUE 37-1 *(Gallie)*

Carefully intubate the patient in the supine position while the patient is on a stretcher. Place the patient on the operating table in a prone position with the head supported by traction, maintaining the head-thorax relationship at all

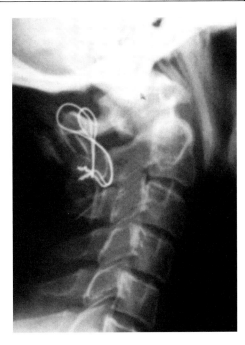

Fig. 37-6   Posterior translation of atlas after C1-C2 posterior Gallie fusion.

times during turning. Make a lateral cervical spine roentgenogram to ensure proper alignment before surgery.

Prepare and drape the skin in a sterile fashion and inject a solution of epinephrine (1:500,000) intradermally to aid hemostasis. Make a midline incision from the lower occiput to the level of the lower end of the fusion, extending it deeply within the relatively avascular midline structures, the intermuscular septum, or ligamentum nuchae. Take care not to expose any more than the area to be fused to decrease the chance of spontaneous extension of the fusion. By subperiosteal dissection, expose the posterior arch of the atlas and the lamina of C2. Remove the muscular and ligamentous attachments from C2 with a curet, taking care to dissect laterally along the atlas to prevent injury to the vertebral arteries and vertebral venous plexus that lie on the superior aspect of the ring of C1, less than 2 cm lateral to the midline. Expose the upper surface of C1 no farther laterally than 1.5 cm from the midline in adults and 1 cm in children. Decortication of C1 and C2 generally is not necessary. From below, pass a wire loop of appropriate size upward under the arch of the atlas either directly or with the aid of a Mersilene suture, which can be passed with an aneurysm needle. Pass the free ends of the wire through the loop, grasping the arch of C1 in the loop.

Take a corticocancellous graft from the iliac crest and place it against the lamina of C2 and the arch of C1 beneath the wire. Then pass one end of the wire through the spinous process of C2 and twist the wire on itself to secure the graft in place. Irrigate the wound and close it in layers with suction drainage tubes.

Fielding has described several modifications of the Gallie fusion, as shown in Fig. 37-7.

AFTERTREATMENT. The patient is immobilized in a Minerva cast, halo vest or cast, or a cervicothoracic orthosis. Immobilization usually is continued for 12 weeks.

TECHNIQUE 37-2 *(Brooks and Jenkins)*
Intubate and turn the patient onto the operating table as for the Gallie technique. Prepare and drape the operative site as described. Expose C1 and C2 through a midline incision. Using an aneurysm needle, pass a Mersilene suture from cephalad to caudad on each side of the midline under the arch of the atlas and then beneath the lamina of C2 (Fig. 37-8, *A*). These serve as guides to introduce two doubled 20-gauge wires. The size of the wire used varies depending on the size and age of the patient. Obtain two full-thickness bone grafts approximately 1.25 × 3.5 cm from the iliac crest and bevel them so that the apex of the graft fits in the interval between the arch of the atlas and the lamina of the axis (Fig. 37-8, *B*). Fashion notches in the upper and lower cortical surfaces to hold the circumferential wires and prevent them from slipping. Tighten the doubled wires over the graft and twist them on each side (Fig. 37-8, *C* and *D*). Irrigate and close the wound in layers over suction drains.

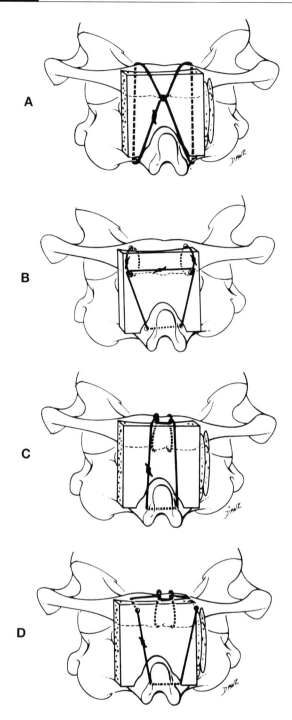

Fig. 37-7   Fielding's modifications of wire techniques for holding graft in place. **A,** Wire passes under lamina of atlas and axis and is tied over graft. **B,** Wire passes through holes drilled in lamina of atlas and through spine of axis; holes are drilled through graft. **C,** Wire passes under lamina of atlas and through spine of axis and is tied over graft. This method is most frequently used. **D,** Wire passes under lamina of atlas and through spine of axis; holes are drilled through graft. (From Fielding JW, Hawkins RJ, Ratzan SA: *J Bone Joint Surg* 37A:400, 1976.)

AFTERTREATMENT. The aftertreatment is the same as that for the Gallie technique.

C1-C2 Transarticular Screw Fixation. Wang et al. reported good results in the management of pediatric atlantoaxial instability with C1-C2 transarticular screw fixation and fusion, using a 3.5-mm screw in children as young as 4 years of age. The technique was originally described by Magrel and Seeman in 1987 for adult patients. It is technically demanding and requires fluoroscopic or stereotactic assistance for the proper placement of the transarticular screw.

◆ Occipitocervical Fusion

When other bony anomalies occur at the occipitocervical junction, such as absence of the posterior arch of C1, the fusion can extend up to the occiput. The following technique for occipitocervical fusion includes features of techniques described by Cone and Turner, Rogers, and Willard and Nicholson.

TECHNIQUE 37-3

Approach the base of the occiput and the spinous processes of the upper cervical vertebrae through a longitudinal midline incision, extending it deeply within the relatively avascular intermuscular septum. Expose the entire field subperiosteally. Dissect the posterior occiput laterally to the level of the external occipital protuberance. Make two burr holes in the posterior occiput about 7 mm from the foramen magnum and 10 mm lateral to the midline (Fig. 37-9). Separate the dura from the inner table of the skull by blunt dissection with a right-angle dissector. Pass short lengths of wire through the holes in the occiput and through the foramen magnum. Next pass wires beneath the posterior arch of C1 on either side if the arch is intact. Drill holes in the outer table of the spinous processes of C2 and C3, completing them with a towel clip or Lewin clamp, and pass short lengths of wire through the holes.

Obtain a corticocancellous graft from the iliac crest and make holes at appropriate intervals to accept the ends of the wires. Pass the wires through the holes in the graft and lay the graft against the occiput and the lamina of C2 and C3. Tighten the wires to hold the graft firmly in place (Fig. 37-9, *inset*). Lay thin strips of cancellous bone around the cortical grafts to aid in fusion. Inspect the graft and wires to ensure that they do not impinge on the dura or vertebral arteries. Irrigate and close the wound in layers over suction drains.

Robinson and Southwick pass individual wires beneath the lamina of C2 and C3 instead of through the spinous processes.

AFTERTREATMENT. Some form of external support is recommended. This may vary from a Minerva cast or halo vest

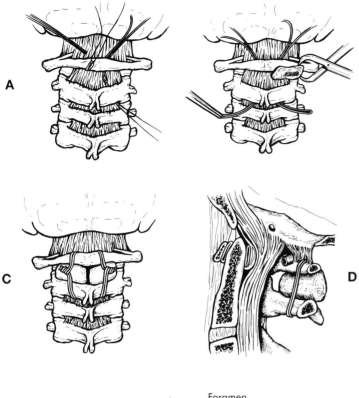

Fig. 37-8   Brooks-Jenkins technique of atlantoaxial fusion. **A,** Insertion of wires under atlas and axis. **B,** Wires in place with graft being inserted. **C** and **D,** Bone grafts secured by wires (anteroposterior and lateral views). (Redrawn from Brooks AL, Jenkins EB: *J Bone Joint Surg* 60A:279, 1978.)

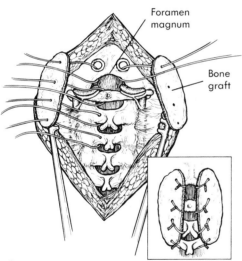

Foramen magnum

Bone graft

Fig. 37-9   Robinson and Southwick method of occipitocervical fusion. (Redrawn from Robinson RA, Southwick WO: Surgical approaches to the cervical spine. In The American Academy of Orthopaedic Surgeons: *Instructional course lectures,* vol 17, St Louis, 1960, Mosby.)

or cast to a cervicothoracic brace, depending on the degree of preoperative instability and the stability of fixation.

◆ ◆ ◆

Wertheim and Bohlman described a technique of occipitocervical fusion similar to that described by Grantham et al. in which wires are passed through the outer table of the skull at

the occipital protuberance instead of through both the inner and outer tables of the skull near the foramen magnum. Superior to the foramen magnum the occipital bone is very thin, but at the external occipital protuberance it is thick and allows passage of wires without passing through both tables. The transverse and superior sagittal sinuses are cephalad to the protuberance and thus are out of danger.

TECHNIQUE 37-4 *(Wertheim and Bohlman)*

Stabilize the spine preoperatively with cranial skeletal traction with the patient on a turning frame or cerebellar head rest. Place the patient prone and obtain a lateral roentgenogram to document proper alignment. Prepare the skin and inject the subcutaneous tissue with a solution of epinephrine (1:500,000). Make a midline incision extending from the external occipital protuberance to the spine of the third cervical vertebra. Sharply dissect the paraspinous muscles subperiosteally with a scalpel and a periosteal elevator to expose the occiput and cervical laminae, taking special care to stay in the midline to avoid the paramedian venous plexus. At a point 2 cm above the rim of the foramen magnum, use a high-speed diamond burr to create a trough on either side of the protuberance, making a ridge in the center (Fig. 37-10, *A*). With a towel clip, make a hole in this ridge through only the outer table of bone. Loop a 20-gauge wire through the hole and around the ridge and then loop another 20-gauge wire around the arch of the atlas. Pass a third wire through a drill hole in the base of the spinous process of the axis and around this structure; thus three

continued

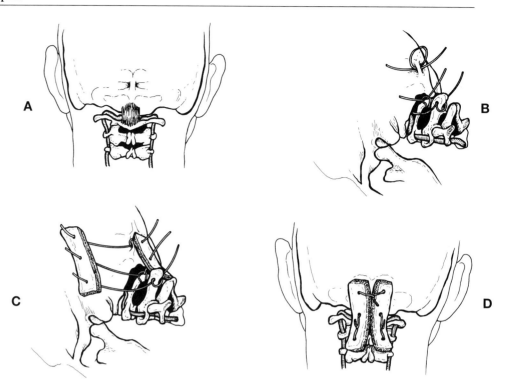

Fig. 37-10 Wertheim and Bohlman method of occipitocervical fusion. **A,** Burr is used to create ridge in external occipital protuberance; then hole is made in ridge. **B,** Wires are passed through outer table of occiput, under arch of atlas, and through spinous process of axis. **C,** Grafts are placed on wires. **D,** Wires are tightened to secure grafts in place. (Redrawn from Wertheim SB, Bohlman HH: *J Bone Joint Surg* 69A:833, 1987.)

separate wires are used to secure the bone grafts on each side of the spine (Fig. 37-10, *B*).

Expose the posterior iliac crest and obtain a thick, slightly curved graft of corticocancellous bone of premeasured length and width. Divide this horizontally into two pieces and place three drill holes in each graft (Fig. 37-10, *C*). Decorticate the occiput and anchor the grafts in place with the wires on both sides of the spine (Fig. 37-10, *D*). Pack additional cancellous bone around and between the two grafts. Close the wound in layers over suction drains.

AFTERTREATMENT. Either a rigid cervical orthosis or a halo cast is worn for 6 to 16 weeks, followed by a soft collar that is worn for an additional 6 weeks.

◆ ◆ ◆

Koop, Winter, and Lonstein described a technique of occipitocervical arthrodesis without internal fixation for use in children. The spine is decorticated and autogenous corticocancellous iliac bone is placed over the area to be fused. In children with vertebral arch defects, an occipital periosteal flap is reflected over the bone defect to provide an osteogenic tissue layer for the bone grafts. A halo cast is used for postoperative stability.

TECHNIQUE 37-5 *(Koop et al.)*
After the administration of endotracheal anesthesia, apply a halo with the child supine. Turn the child prone and secure the head with the neck in slight extension by securing the

halo to a traction frame. Make a midline incision. In patients with intact posterior elements, expose the vertebrae by sharp dissection. Decorticate the exposed vertebral elements and lay strips of autogenous cancellous iliac bone over the decorticated bone. Take care to expose just the vertebrae to be included in the fusion. In patients with defects in the posterior elements, take care not to expose the dura, if possible. At the level of the occiput, dissect the nuchal tissue from the periosteum and retract it laterally (Fig. 37-11, *A*). Then elevate the occipital periosteum in a triangular-based flap attached near the margin of the foramen magnum. Reflect this flap caudally to cover the defects in the posterior vertebral elements and suture it in place (Fig. 37-11, *B*). Decorticate the occiput and the remaining exposed vertebral elements with an air drill (Fig. 37-11, *C*). Lay strips of autogenous cancellous bone in place over the entire area (Fig. 37-11, *D*). Close the wound in layers over a suction drain. Turn the child supine and apply a halo cast.

AFTERTREATMENT. The halo cast is worn until union is roentgenographically evident, usually about 5 months. When union is documented by lateral flexion and extension roentgenograms, the halo cast is removed and a soft collar is worn for 1 month.

◆ ◆ ◆

Dormans et al. described occipitocervical fusion using a new wiring technique in 16 children with an average age of 9.6 years (2.5 years to 19.3 years). Fusion was achieved in 15 pa-

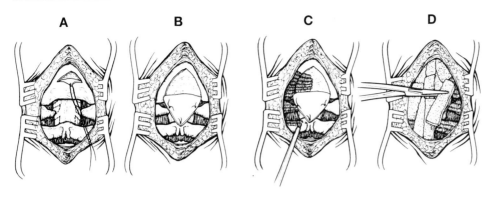

Fig. 37-11 Koop, Winter, and Lonstein method of occipitocervical fusion used when posterior arch of C1 is absent. **A,** Exposure of occiput, atlas, and axis. **B,** Reflection of periosteal flap to cover defect in atlas. **C,** Decortication of exposed vertebral elements. **D,** Placement of autogenous cancellous iliac bone grafts. (Redrawn from Koop SE, Winter RB, Lonstein JE: *J Bone Joint Surg* 66A:403, 1984.)

tients. Complications included pin track infection (4 patients), pneumonia (1 patient), additional level of fusion (1 patient), and graft fracture and nonunion (1 patient). The use of wire fixation, combined with inherent stability of the bone-graft construct, allowed for removal of the halo device relatively early (6 to 12 weeks).

TECHNIQUE 37-6 *(Dormans et al.)*

After halo ring application, place the patient prone and secure the halo to the operating table. Confirm alignment of occiput and cervical spine with lateral roentgenogram. Expose the midline from the occiput to the second or third cervical vertebrae. Take care to limit the lateral dissection to avoid damaging the vertebral arteries. In patients who require decompression because of cervical stenosis or for removal of a tumor, remove the arch of the first or second cervical vertebra, or both, with or without removal of a portion of occipital bone to enlarge the foramen magnum.

Use a high-speed drill to make four holes through both cortices of the occiput, aligning them transversely with two on each side of the midline and leaving a 1-cm osseous bridge between the 2 holes of each pair. The holes are placed caudal to the transverse sinuses (Fig. 37-12, *A*). Fashion a trough into the base of the occiput to accept the cephalad end of the bone graft. Obtain a corticocancellous graft from the iliac crest and shape it into a rectangle, with a notch created in the inferior base to fit around the spinous process of the second or third cervical vertebra (Fig. 37-12, *B*). The caudal extent of the intended arthrodesis (the second or third cervical vertebra) is determined by the presence or absence of a previous laminectomy, congenital anomalies, or the level of instability. Pass a looped 16- or 18-gauge Luque wire through the burr holes on each side and loop onto itself. Pass Wisconsin button wires (Zimmer, Warsaw, Ind.) through the base of the spinous process of either the second or third cervical vertebra (Fig. 37-12, *C*). Pass the wire that is going into the left arm of the graft through the spinous process from right to left. Place the graft into the occipital trough superiorly and about the spinous process of the vertebra that is to be at the caudal level of the arthrodesis (the second or third cervical vertebra). Contour the graft precisely so that it fits securely into the occipital trough and around the inferior spinous process before the wires are tightened. Cross the wires, twist, and cut (Fig. 37-12, *D*). Obtain a roentgenogram at this point to assess the position of the graft and wires, as well as the alignment of the occiput and cephalad cervical vertebrae. Extension of the cervical spine can be controlled by positioning of the head with the halo frame, by adjustment of the size and shape of the graft, and to a lesser extent by appropriate tightening of the wires.

For patients who have not had a decompression, pass the sublaminar wire caudal to the ring of the first cervical vertebra to secure additional fixation. In young children, however, this may be difficult or undesirable because of the small size of the ring of the first cervical vertebra or the failure of formation of the posterior arch of the first cervical vertebra.

AFTERTREATMENT. A custom halo orthosis or cast is worn until a solid fusion is obtained; thereafter a cervical collar is worn for 1 month.

◆ ◆ ◆

Occipitocervical fusion using a contoured rod and segmental wire or cable fixation, which has been described by several authors, has the advantage of achieving immediate stability of the occipitocervical junction. This allows the patient to move in a cervical collar after surgery, avoiding the need for halo immobilization. Smith et al. described occipitocervical arthrodesis using a contoured plate instead of a rod for fixation.

◆ Contoured Rod and Segmental Rod Fixation

TECHNIQUE 37-7 (Fig. 37-13)

Approach the base of the occiput and the spinous processes of the upper cervical vertebrae through a longitudinal midline incision, extending it deeply within the relatively avascular intermuscular septum. Expose the entire field subperiosteally. Carry the dissection proximally above the

continued

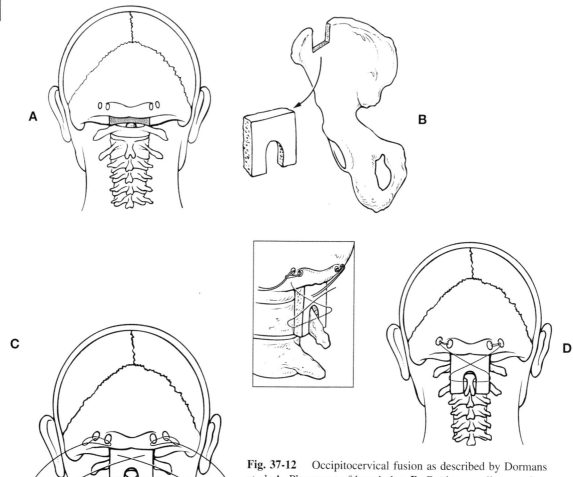

Fig. 37-12 Occipitocervical fusion as described by Dormans et al. **A,** Placement of burr holes. **B,** Corticocancellous graft obtained from iliac crest. **C,** Looped 16- or 18-gauge wires passed through burr holes and looped on itself. Graft positioned into occipital trough and around spinous process of cervical vertebrae at caudal extent of fusion and locked into place by precise contouring of bone. **D,** Wires cross, twisted, and cut. (Redrawn from Dormans et al: *J Bone Joint Surg* 77A: 1234, 1995.)

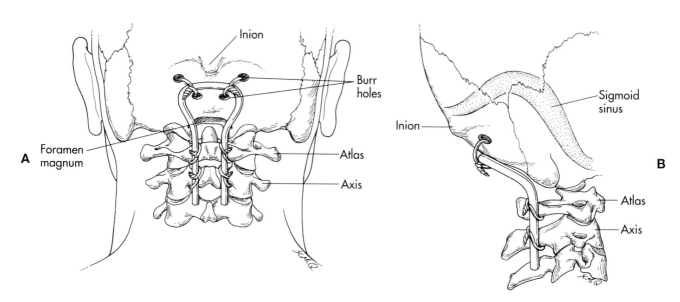

Fig. 37-13 Occipitocervical fusion using contoured rod and segmental wire or cable fixation.

BOX 37-3 • Anterior Cervical Approaches

Transoral (Fang et al.)
High incidence of wound complications and infection

Transoral Mandible- and Tongue-Splitting (Hall, Denis, and Murray)
More extensive exposure of upper cervical spine

Subtotal Maxillectomy (Cocke et al.)
Extended maxillotomy and subtotal maxillectomy are used when exposure of base of skull is necessary and cannot be obtained by other approaches

Lateral Retropharyngeal (Whitesides and Kelly)
Extension of classic Henry approach to vertebral artery
Sternocleidomastoid muscle everted and retracted posteriorly
Dissection in plane posterior to carotid sheath
Potential for postoperative edema and airway obstruction

Modifications of Robinson and Southwick Approach (deAndrade and Macnab)
Anterior to sternocleidomastoid muscle
Dissection anterior to carotid sheath
Risk of injury to superior laryngeal nerve

McAfee et al.
Exposure from atlas to body of C3
No posterior dissection of carotid sheath
No entrance into oral cavity
Adequate for insertion of iliac or fibular strut grafts

---

inion and laterally to the level of the external occipital protuberance. Make a template of the intended shape of the stainless steel rod with the appropriate length of Luque wire. Make two burr holes on each side, about 2 cm lateral to the midline and 2.5 cm above the foramen magnum. Take care to avoid the transverse and sigmoid sinus when making these burr holes. Leave at least 10 mm of intact cortical bone between the burr holes to ensure solid fixation. Pass Luque wires or Songer cables in an extradural plane through the two burr holes on each side of the midline. Pass the wires or cables sublaminar in the upper cervical spine. Bend the rod to match the template; this usually will have a head-neck angle of about 135 degrees and slight cervical lordosis. A Bend Meister (Sofamor/Danek, Memphis) may be helpful in bending the rod. Secure the wires or cables to the rod. Decorticate the spine and occiput and perform autogenous cancellous bone grafting.

AFTERTREATMENT. A Philadelphia collar or an occipitocervical orthosis is worn until the fusion is stable.

Anterior Cervical Approaches (Box 37-3)

C1-C2 subluxation or dislocation sometimes cannot be reduced with traction. If a patient has no neurological deficits, a simple in situ posterior fusion can be done with little increase

in risk. Posterior decompression by laminectomy has been associated with increased morbidity and mortality. Posterior decompression increases C1-C2 instability unless accompanied by fusion from the occiput to C2 or C3. If reduction of the C1-C2 dislocation is necessary or if posterior stabilization cannot be performed because of the clinical situation, an anterior approach should be considered. A lateral retropharyngeal or a transoral approach can be used. The retropharyngeal approach usually is preferred because of the high incidence of wound complications and infection associated with the transoral approach.

◆ Transoral Approach

TECHNIQUE 37-8 (Fang and Ong)

Parenteral prophylactic antibiotics are given based on preoperative nasopharyngeal cultures. Endotracheal intubation is achieved using a noncollapsible tube and cuff. If extensive dissection is anticipated a tracheostomy should be performed.

Place the patient in the Trendelenburg position and insert a mouth gag to provide retraction. Identify the vertebral bodies by palpation. The ring of the first vertebra has a midline anterior tubercle, and the disc between the second and third vertebrae is prominent, providing another localizing landmark. Make a longitudinal incision in the midline of the posterior pharynx (Fig. 37-14, A). The soft palate can be divided in the midline, making postretraction paresis less likely, or it can be folded back on itself. Continue the midline dissection down to bone and reflect the tissue laterally to the outer margin of the lateral masses of the axis (Fig. 37-14, B). Beyond these margins are the vertebral arteries, and care should be taken not to harm them. The soft tissue flap can be retracted using long stay sutures. After the procedure is complete, irrigate and close the wound loosely with interrupted absorbable sutures. Continue antibiotics for at least 3 days after surgery.

Fang and Ong achieved fusion by placing rectangular grafts into similarly shaped graft beds extending from the lateral mass of the atlas to the lateral mass and body of the axis. If only an anterior decompression is performed, it should be followed by a posterior fusion.

Hall, Denis, and Murray described a mandible- and tongue-splitting transoral approach to the cervical spine that gives more extensive exposure of the upper cervical spine than the approach of Fang and Ong.

◆ Transoral Mandible- and Tongue-Splitting Approach

TECHNIQUE 37-9 (Hall, Denis, and Murray)

Apply a halo cast preoperatively and perform tracheostomy through the fourth tracheal ring. Then, with the patient under

continued

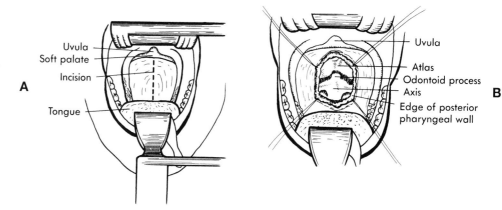

Fig. 37-14 Transoral approach to upper cervical spine for exposure of anterior aspect of atlas and axis (see text). (Redrawn from Fang HSY, Ong GB: *J Bone Joint Surg* 44A:1378, 1962.)

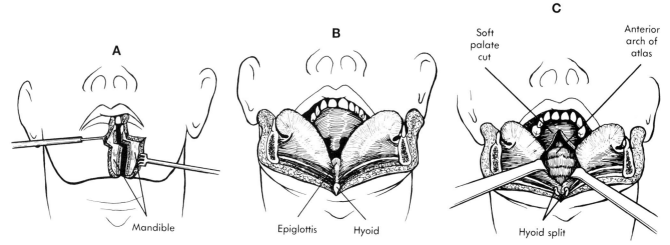

Fig. 37-15 Mandible- and tongue-splitting transoral approach (see text). (Redrawn from Sherk HH, Pratt L. In Cervical Spine Research Society: *The cervical spine,* Philadelphia, 1983, JB Lippincott; original by Bernie Kida.)

general anesthesia, prepare the operative field with povidone-iodine (Betadine) and drape it to exclude the halo cast and tracheostomy tube. Make an incision from the anterior gum margin through both surfaces of the lower lip and down over the middle of the mandible to the hyoid cartilage (Fig. 37-15, *A*). Divide the tongue in the midline with electrocautery. Place traction sutures to allow better exposure of the midline raphe. Remove the lower incisor and make a step cut with an oscillating saw in the mandible. Split the tongue longitudinally to the epiglottis through its central raphe (Fig. 37-15, *B*). Fold the uvula on itself and suture it to the roof of the soft palate; retract the mandible and tongue down on each side to improve exposure. Open the mucosa over the posterior wall of the oral pharynx to expose the anterior cervical spine from the first cervical vertebra to the upper portion of the fifth cervical vertebra (Fig. 37-15, *C*). Divide the anterior longitudinal ligament in the midline and reflect it laterally to allow enough exposure

for removal of the anterior portion of the cervical spine and placement of bone grafts for fusion. Fix the posterior pharyngeal flap with 3-0 chromic suture. Thread a suction drain through the nose and insert it deep into the pharyngeal flap. Repair the tongue with 2-0 and 3-0 chromic sutures and fix the mandible with wires inserted through drill holes on each side of the osteotomy. Close the infralingual mucosa with 3-0 chromic sutures and close the subcutaneous tissue and skin. Preoperative and postoperative antibiotics are recommended.

AFTERTREATMENT. A halo cast is worn until fusion is evident on roentgenograms. Then the halo cast is removed and a soft collar is worn for 1 month.

◆ ◆ ◆

Cocke et al. described an extended maxillotomy with subtotal maxillectomy as an alternative to the transoral approach for exposure anteriorly at the base of the skull and upper cervical spine. The indications for this approach are very limited; it can be used when exposure of the base of the skull is needed and cannot be obtained by other approaches. This approach is technically demanding and requires a thorough knowledge of head and neck anatomy. A team of surgeons, including an otolaryngologist, a neurosurgeon, and an orthopaedist, should perform this surgery.

◆ Subtotal Maxillectomy

TECHNIQUE 37-10 *(Cocke et al.)*

Position the patient on the operating table with the head elevated 25 degrees. Intubate the patient orally and move the tube to the contralateral side of the mouth. A percutaneous endoscopic gastrostomy and tracheostomy usually are unnecessary but may be required if an extensive dissection is expected.

Insert a Foley catheter and suture the eyelids closed with 6-0 nylon. Infiltrate the soft tissues of the upper lip, cheek, gingiva, palate, pterygoid fossa, nasopharynx, nasal septum, nasal floor, and lateral nasal wall with 1% lidocaine with 1:100,000 epinephrine. Pack each nasal cavity with cottonoid strips saturated with 4% cocaine and 1% phenylephrine. Prepare the skin with povidone-iodine (Betadine) and dry with alcohol. Drape the operative site with cloth drapes held in place with sutures or surgical clips and cover with a transparent surgical drape.

Expose the superior maxilla through a modified Weber-Ferguson skin incision (Fig. 37-16, *A*). Make a vertical incision through the upper lip in the philtrum from the nasolabial groove to the vermilion border. Extend the lower end to the midline and then vertically in the midline through the buccal mucosa to the gingivobuccal gutter.

Divide the upper lip and ligate the labial arteries. Extend the external skin incision transversely from the upper end of the lip incision in the nasolabial groove to beyond the nasal ala and then superiorly along the nasofacial groove to the lower eyelid. Extract the central incisor tooth (Fig. 37-16, *B*). Make a vertical midline incision through the mucoperiosteum of the anterior maxilla from the gingivobuccal gutter to the central incisor defect and then transversely through the buccal gingiva adjacent to the teeth to the retromolar region.

Elevate the skin, subcutaneous tissues, periosteum, and mucoperiosteum of the maxilla to expose the anterior and lateral walls of the maxilla, nasal bone, piriform aperture of the nose, inferior orbital nerve, malar bone, and masseter muscle. Divide the anterior margin of the masseter muscle at its malar attachment and remove a wedge of malar bone. Use this wedge to accommodate the Gigli saw as it divides the maxilla (Fig. 37-16, *C*).

Make an incision in the lingual, hard palate mucoperiosteum adjacent to the teeth from the central incisor defect to join the retromolar incision. Extend the retromolar incision medial to the mandible lateral to the tonsil and to the retropharyngeal space to the level of the hyoid bone or lower pharynx, if necessary. Elevate the mucoperiosteum of the hard palate from the central incisor defect and alveolar ridge to and beyond the midline of the hard palate. Detach the soft palate with its nasal lining from the posterior margin of the hard palate. Divide and electrocoagulate the greater palatine vessels and nerves.

Pack the palatine foramen with bone wax. Retract the mucoperiosteum of the hard palate, soft palate, anterior tonsillar pillar, tonsil, and pharynx medially from the prevertebral fascia. It is usually unnecessary to detach and retract the soft palate from the posterior or lateral pharyngeal walls. Expose the nasal cavity by detaching the nasal soft tissues from the lateral margin and base of the nasal piriform aperture (Fig. 37-16, *B*). Remove a bony wedge of the ascending process of the maxilla to accommodate the upper Gigli saw (Fig. 37-16, *C*). Remove the coronoid process of the mandible above the level of entrance of the inferior alveolar vessels and nerves, after dividing its temporalis muscle attachment, to expose the lateral pterygoid plate and the internal maxillary artery.

Divide the pterygoid muscles with a Shaw knife or the cutting current of a Bovie cautery until the sharp, posterior bone edge of the lateral pterygoid plate is seen or palpated. Mobilize, clip, ligate, and divide the internal maxillary artery near the pterygoid plate. Position the upper Gigli saw (Fig. 37-16, *C*) using a sharp-pointed, medium-sized, curved, right-angle ligature carrier threaded with a 2-0 black silk suture. Direct the suture behind the lateral pterygoid plate into the nasopharynx and behind the posterior margin of the hard palate into the oropharynx. Pass a Kelly forceps through the nose to behind the hard palate to retrieve the medial end of the silk suture in the ligature carrier. Attach a Gigli saw to the lateral end of the suture. Thread the saw into position to divide the upper maxilla. Engage the medial arm of the saw into the ascending process wedge and its lateral arm into the malar wedge. Take care to position the saw as high as possible behind the pterygoid plate. Use a broad periosteal elevator beneath the saw on the pterygoid plate to maintain the elevated position (Fig. 37-16, *D*). Position the lower Gigli saw by passing a Kelly forceps (Fig. 37-16, *E*) through the nose into the nasopharynx behind the posterior nares of the hard palate. Engage the saw between the blades of the clamp and thread it through the nose into position for division of the hard palate.

Divide the bony walls of the maxilla (Fig. 37-16, *E*). First divide the hard palate and then the upper maxilla. Take care to avoid entangling the saws and protect the soft tissues from injury. Remove the maxilla after division of its muscle attachments. Ligate the distal end of the internal maxillary artery. Place traction sutures in the soft tissues of the lip on either side of the initial lip incision and in the

continued

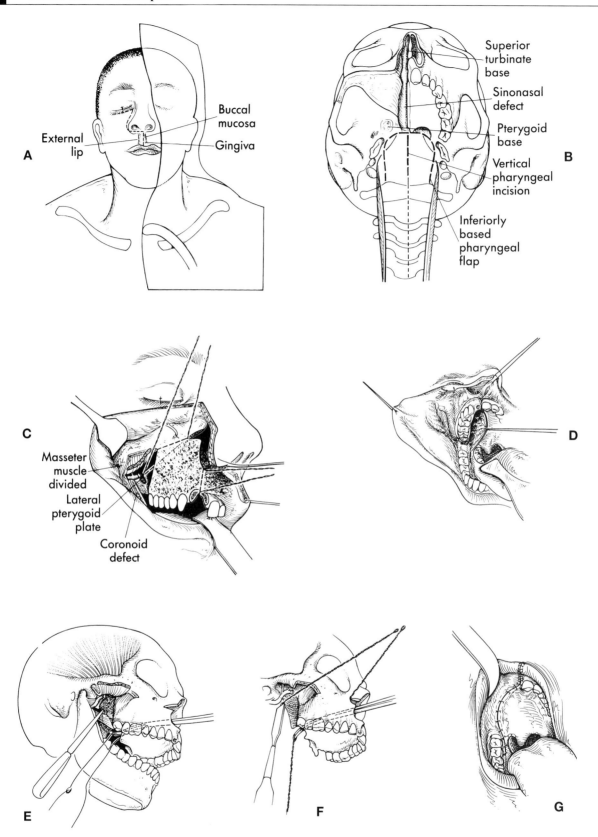

Fig. 37-16 Subtotal maxillectomy and extended maxillotomy (see text). (Redrawn from Cocke EW Jr, Roberston JH, Robertson JR, et al: *Arch Otolaryngol Head Neck Surg* 116:92, 1990.)

mucoperiosteum of the hard and soft palates. The posterior pharynx is now fully exposed.

Infiltrate the mucous membrane covering the posterior wall of the nasopharynx, oropharynx, and the tonsillar area to the level of the hyoid bone with 1% lidocaine and epinephrine 1:100,000. Make a vertical midline incision through the soft tissues of the posterior wall of the nasopharynx extending from the sphenoid sinus to the foramen magnum. Another option is to make a transverse incision from the sphenoid to the lateral nasopharyngeal wall posterior to the eustachian tube along the lateral pharyngeal wall inferiorly posterior to the posterior tonsillar pillar behind the soft palate. Duplicate this incision on the opposite side, producing an inferiorly based pharyngeal flap (Fig. 37-16, *F*). Make a more extensive exposure by extending the lateral pharyngeal wall incision through the anterior tonsillar pillar to join the retromolar incision. Extend this incision into the retropharyngeal space and retract the anterior tonsillar pillar, tonsil, and soft palate toward the midline with a traction suture. It is unnecessary to separate the soft palate completely from the pharyngeal wall. Extend the pharyngeal wall incision inferiorly to the level of the hyoid bone or beyond. Elevate, divide, and separate the superior constrictor muscle, prevertebral fascia, longus capitus muscle, and anterior longitudinal ligaments from the bony skull base and upper cervical spine ventrally. Expose the bone from the foramen magnum and distally along the upper cervical spine. Remove the offending bone with a high-speed burr, taking care to avoid penetration of the dura.

Close the nasopharyngeal mucous membrane and the subcutaneous tissue in one layer with interrupted sutures. Use a split-thickness skin or dermal graft from the thigh to resurface the buccal mucosa and any defects in the nasal surface of the hard palate. Use a quilting stitch to hold the graft in place without packing. Replace the zygoma and stabilize it with wire if it was mobilized. Return the maxilla to its original position and hold it in place with wire or compression plates. Place a nylon sack impregnated with antibiotic into the nasal cavity. Close the oral cavity incision with vertical interrupted mattress 3-0 polyglycolic acid sutures (Fig. 37-16, *G*). Close the facial wound with 5-0 chromic and 6-0 nylon sutures.

◆ Extended Maxillotomy

TECHNIQUE 37-11

Expose the base of the skull and upper cervical spine as by the maxillectomy technique but omit the extraction of the central incisor and the gingivolingual incision. Use a degloving procedure for elevation of the facial skin over the maxilla and nose to prevent facial scars. Divide the fibromuscular attachment of the soft palate to the pterygoid plate and hard palate, exposing the nasopharynx. Place the upper Gigli saw with the aid of a ligature carrier for division of the maxilla beneath the infraorbital nerve. Elevate the mucoperiosteum of the adjacent floor of the nose from the piriform aperture to the soft palate. Extend this elevation medially to the nasal septum and laterally to the inferior turbinate. Divide the bone of the nasal floor with a Stryker saw without lacerating the underlying hard palate periosteum. Hinge the maxilla on the hard palate and nasal mucoperiosteum as well as the soft palate and rotate it medially.

AFTERTREATMENT. Continuous spinal fluid drainage is maintained, and the head is elevated 45 degrees if the dura was repaired or replaced. These measures are omitted if there was no dural tear or defect. An ice cap is used on the cheek and temple to reduce edema. Antibiotic therapy is continued until the risk of infection has been minimized. Half-strength hydrogen peroxide is used for mouth irrigations to help keep the oral cavity clean. The endotracheal tube is removed when the risk of occlusion by swelling has been minimized. The nasopharyngeal cavity is cleaned with saline twice daily for 2 months after removal of the pack. Facial sutures are removed at 4 to 6 days and oral sutures at 2 weeks.

The lateral retropharyngeal approach described by Whitesides and Kelly is an extension of the classic approach of Henry to the vertebral artery. In this approach the sternocleidomastoid muscle is everted and retracted posteriorly. The remainder of the dissection follows a plane posterior to the carotid sheath.

◆ Lateral Retropharyngeal Approach

TECHNIQUE 37-12 *(Whitesides and Kelly)*

Make a longitudinal incision along the anterior margin of the sternocleidomastoid muscle. At the superior end of the muscle, carry the incision posteriorly across the base of the temporal bone. Divide the muscle at its mastoid origin. Partially divide the splenius capitis muscle at its insertion in the same area. At the superior pole of the incision is the external jugular vein, which crosses the anterior margin of the sternocleidomastoid; ligate and divide this vein. Branches of the auricular nerve also may be encountered and may require division. Evert the sternocleidomastoid muscle and identify the spinal accessory nerve as it approaches and passes into the muscle. Divide and ligate the vascular structures that accompany the nerve. Develop the approach posterior to the carotid sheath and anterior to

continued

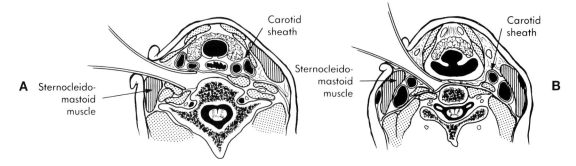

Fig. 37-17   Anterior approach to cervical spine. **A,** Whitesides and Kelly approach anterior to sternocleidomastoid muscle and posterior to carotid sheath. **B,** Approach anterior to sternocleido-mastoid muscle and anteromedial to carotid sheath. (Redrawn from Whitesides TE Jr, Kelly RP: *South Med J* 59:879, 1966.)

the sternocleidomastoid muscle (Fig. 37-17, *A*). The transverse processes of all the exposed cervical vertebrae are palpable in this interval.

Using sharp and blunt dissection, develop the plane between the alar and prevertebral fascia along the anterior aspect of the transverse processes of the vertebral bodies. The dissection plane is anterior to the longus colli and capitis muscles, as well as the overlying sympathetic trunk and superior cervical ganglion. (An alternative approach is to elevate the longus colli and capitis muscles from their bony insertion on the transverse processes and retract the muscles anteriorly, but this approach can disrupt the sympathetic rami communications and cause Horner syndrome.)

When the vertebral level is identified, make a longitudinal incision to bone through the anterior longitudinal ligament. Dissect the ligament and soft tissues subperiosteally to expose the vertebral bodies. For fusion, place corticocancellous strips in a longitudinal trough made in the vertebral bodies. Irrigate and close the wound in layers over a suction drain in the retropharyngeal space.

AFTERTREATMENT. Because of the potential for postoperative edema and airway obstruction, the patient should be monitored closely. Traction may be required for 1 to 2 days after surgery. When the traction is removed, the patient is immobilized in a cervicothoracic brace or halo vest or cast.

◆   ◆   ◆

deAndrade and Macnab described an approach to the upper cervical spine that is an extension of the approach described by Robinson and Southwick and Bailey and Badgley. This approach is anterior to the sternocleidomastoid muscle (Fig. 37-17, *B*), but the dissection is anterior to the carotid sheath rather than posterior. This approach carries an increased risk of injury to the superior laryngeal nerve.

McAfee et al. used a superior extension of the anterior approach of Robinson and Smith to the cervical spine. This approach provides exposure from the atlas to the body of the third cervical vertebra without the need for posterior dissection of the carotid sheath or entrance into the oral cavity and gives adequate exposure for insertion of iliac or fibular strut grafts.

◆ Anterior Retropharyngeal Approach

TECHNIQUE 37-13 *(McAfee et al.)*

Place the patient supine on an operative wedge turning frame and perform a neurological examination. Monitor the spinal cord during the operation using cortically recorded somatosensory evoked potentials. Apply Gardner-Wells tongs with 4.5 kg of traction, if not already in place. Carefully extend the neck with the patient awake. Mark the maximal point of safe extension and do not exceed this at any time during the operative procedure.

Perform fiberoptic nasotracheal intubation with the patient under local anesthesia. When the airway has been secured, place the patient under general anesthesia. Keep the patient's mouth free of all tubes to prevent any depression of the mandible inferiorly that may compromise the operative exposure.

Make a modified transverse submandibular incision (the incision can be made on the right or left side depending on the surgeon's preference) (Fig. 37-18, *A*). As long as the dissection does not extend caudal to the fifth cervical vertebra, this exposure is sufficiently superior to the right recurrent laryngeal nerve to prevent damage to this structure. Carry the incision through the platysma muscle and mobilize the skin and superficial fascia in the subplatysmal plane of the superficial fascia.

Locate the marginal mandibular branch of the facial nerve with the aid of a nerve stimulator and by ligating and dissecting the retromandibular veins superiorly. Branches of

continued

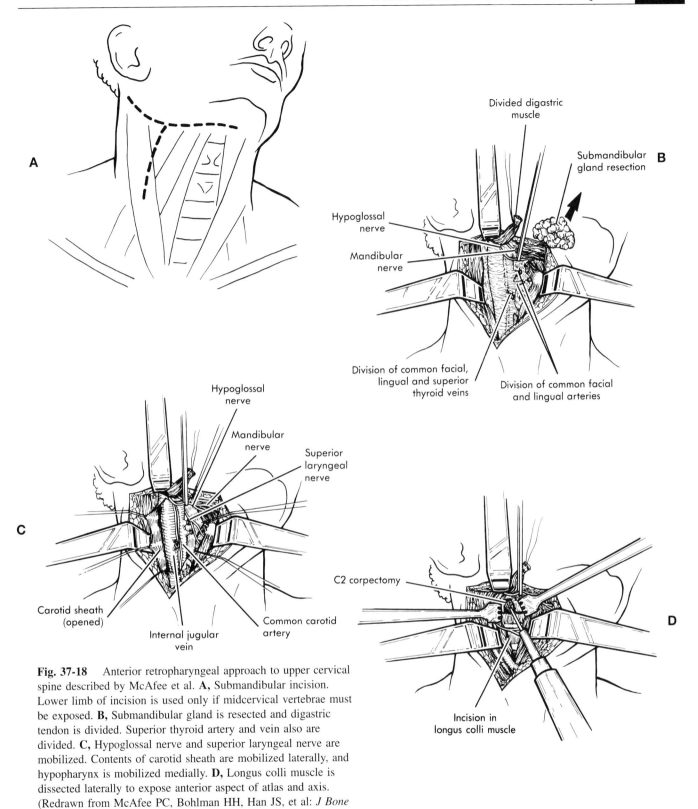

Fig. 37-18 Anterior retropharyngeal approach to upper cervical spine described by McAfee et al. **A,** Submandibular incision. Lower limb of incision is used only if midcervical vertebrae must be exposed. **B,** Submandibular gland is resected and digastric tendon is divided. Superior thyroid artery and vein also are divided. **C,** Hypoglossal nerve and superior laryngeal nerve are mobilized. Contents of carotid sheath are mobilized laterally, and hypopharynx is mobilized medially. **D,** Longus colli muscle is dissected laterally to expose anterior aspect of atlas and axis. (Redrawn from McAfee PC, Bohlman HH, Han JS, et al: *J Bone Joint Surg* 69A:1371, 1987.)

the mandibular nerves usually cross the retromandibular vein superficially and superiorly. By ligating this vein as it joins the internal jugular veins and by keeping the dissection deep and inferior to the vein as the exposure is extended superiorly, the superficial branches of the facial nerve are protected.

Free the anterior border of the sternocleidomastoid muscle by longitudinally transecting the superficial layer of deep cervical fascia. Locate the carotid sheath by palpation. Resect the submandibular salivary gland and suture its duct to prevent a salivary fistula. Identify the posterior belly of the digastric muscle and the stylohyoid muscle. Divide and tag the digastric tendon for later repair. Division of the digastric and stylohyoid muscles allows mobilization of the hyoid bone and the hypopharynx medially (Fig. 37-18, *B*). Free the hypoglossal nerve from the base of the skull to the anterior border of the hypoglossal muscle and retract it superiorly throughout the remainder of the procedure (Fig. 37-18, *C*).

Continue the dissection between the carotid sheath laterally and the larynx and pharynx anteromedially. Beginning inferiorly and progressing superiorly, the following arteries and veins may need to be ligated for exposure: the superior thyroid artery and vein, the lingual artery and vein, and the facial artery and vein. Free the superior laryngeal nerve from its origin near the nodose ganglion to its entrance into the larynx.

Transect the alar and prevertebral fascia longitudinally to expose the longus colli muscles (Fig. 37-18, *D*). Ensure orientation to the midline by noting the attachment of the right and left longus colli muscles as they converge toward the anterior tubercle of the atlas. Then detach the longus colli muscles from the anterior surface of the atlas and axis. Divide the anterior longitudinal ligament and expose the anterior surface of the atlas and axis. Take care not to carry the dissection too far laterally and damage the vertebral artery.

McAfee et al. shape a fibular or bicortical iliac strut graft into the shape of a clothespin. The anterior body of C2 and the discs of C2 and C3 can be removed. Place the two prongs of the clothespin superiorly to straddle the anterior arch of the atlas. Tamp the inferior edge of the graft into the superior aspect of the body of C3, which is undercut to receive the graft. If the anterior aspect of the atlas must be removed, the superior aspect of the graft can be secured to the clivus.

Begin closure by approximation of the digastric tendon. Place suction drains in the retropharyngeal space and the subcutaneous space. Then suture the platysma and skin in the standard fashion. If the spine has been made unstable by the anterior decompression, perform a posterior cervical or occipitocervical fusion. If the hypopharynx has been inadvertently entered, have the anesthesiologist insert a nasogastric tube intraoperatively. Close the hole in two layers with absorbable sutures.

AFTERTREATMENT. Parenteral antibiotics effective against anaerobic organisms should be added to the routine postoperative prophylactic antibiotics. The nasogastric tube is left in place for 7 to 10 days. Skull traction is maintained with the head elevated 30 degrees to reduce hypopharyngeal edema. Nasal intubation is maintained for 48 hours. If extubation is not possible in 48 to 72 hours, then a tracheostomy can be performed. Two or 4 days after surgery the Gardner-Wells tongs are removed and a halo vest is applied and is worn for about 3 months. When the halo vest is removed, a cervical collar is worn for an additional month.

Halo Vest Immobilization

The halo device, introduced by Perry and Nickel in 1959, provides immobilization for an unstable cervical spine and also can be used for preoperative traction in certain situations. Successful use of the halo has been demonstrated in infants and children with instabilities caused by injuries or by cervical malformations. Baum et al. and Dormans et al. noted that complications from the use of the halo device occur more frequently in children than in adults.

Most authors agree that the halo device provides the best immobilization of the cervical spine of all external immobilization methods, but reports have shown increased spinal motion and loss of reduction while in the halo. Lind, Sihlbom, and Nordwall reported that the halo allowed 70% of normal motion, and Koch and Nickel reported that it allowed 31%.

The halo vest has been well accepted by adult patients, and the vest usually can be easily fitted; in children, however, proper fit rarely is achieved with a prefabricated halo vest, and the use of a halo cast or custom-molded halo vest is a better choice.

Mubarak et al. recommended the following steps in the fabrication of a custom halo for a child: (1) the size and configuration of the head are obtained with the use of a flexible lead wire placed around the head; (2) the halo ring is fabricated by constructing a ring 2 cm larger in diameter than the wire model; (3) a plaster mold of the trunk is obtained for the manufacture of a custom bivalved polypropylene vest; and (4) linear measurements are made to ensure appropriate length of the superstructure. CT scanning helps determine bone structure to plan pin sites to avoid suture lines or congenital malformations.

Letts, Kaylor, and Gouw found that skull thickness in children varies greatly up to the age of 6 years; skull thickness increases between the ages of 10 and 16 years, after which the thickness is similar to that in adults. They also found that a 2-mm skull could be completely penetrated with a 160-pound load, which is below the recommended torque pressure for adult skulls.

Mubarak et al. described a technique for the application of a halo in infants younger than 2 years of age. This multiple pin technique differs from previously accepted recommendations in older children regarding pin number, pin placement, and torque. With multiple pins, significantly less torque can be used, allowing a greater range of pin placement sites in areas where the skull might otherwise be considered too thin. Skull development is important to consider in halo application in patients under 2 years of age. Cranial suture interdigitation may be incomplete, and fontanels may be open anteriorly in patients younger than 18 months of age and posteriorly in patients younger than 6 months of age. Because of this, the halo probably should not be used in children younger than 18 months.

◆ Application of Halo Device

TECHNIQUE 37-14 *(Mubarak et al.)*
Halo applications for children in this age group require a custom-made halo ring and plastic jacket. Ten to twelve standard halo skull pins can be used.

Once constructed, the halo ring is applied with the patient under general anesthesia. In older children and adolescents, local anesthesia can be used. Place the patient supine, with the head supported by an assistant or a cupped metal extension that cradles the head. If a metal extension is used, take care not to place the neck in flexion; a child's head is relatively large in proportion to the body. Shave the immediate areas of pin insertion and prepare the skin with antiseptic solution. Infiltrate the skin and the periosteum in the selected areas with local anesthetic. Support the halo around the patient's head with the application device or the help of an assistant. Hold the halo below the area of greatest diameter of the skull, just above the eyebrows, and about 1 cm above the tips of the ears. Select the pin sites carefully so that the pins enter the skull as nearly perpendicular as possible. The best position for the anterior pins is in the anterolateral aspect of the skull, above the lateral two thirds of the orbit, and below the greatest circumference of the skull; this area is a relatively safe zone. Avoid the temporalis muscle because penetration of this muscle by the halo pin can be painful and may impede mandibular motion during mastication or talking; the bone in this area also is very thin, and pin loosening is likely.

Place the posterior pins directly diagonal from the anterior pins, if possible, and inferior to the equator of the skull. Introduce the pins through the halo and tighten two diagonally opposed pins simultaneously. Make sure that the patient's eyes are closed while the pins are tightened to ensure that the forehead skin is not anchored in such a way as to prevent the eyelids from closing after application of the halo.

In an infant or young child, insert 10 pins to finger tightness or 2 inch-pounds anterolaterally and posteriorly (Fig. 37-19, *A*). If the skull thickness is of great concern, use finger tightness only to prevent penetrating the skull. In slightly older children, use 2 inch-pounds of torque. In adolescents near skeletal maturity whose skull thickness is nearly that of an adult (as determined by CT scan), torque pressure can be increased up to 6 to 8 inch-pounds. Secure

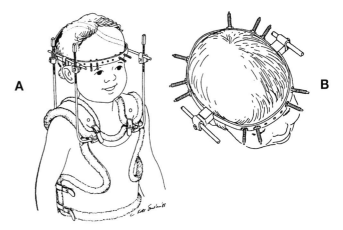

Fig. 37-19 **A,** Custom halo vest and light superstructure. **B,** Ten pin placement sites for infant halo ring attachment using multiple-pin, low-torque technique. Usually, four pins are placed anteriorly, avoiding temporal area, and remaining six pins are placed in occipital area. (From Mubarak SJ, Camp JF, Vuletich W, et al: *J Pediatr Orthop* 9:612, 1989.)

the pins to the halo with the appropriate lock nuts or set screws. Apply the polypropylene vest and superstructure after the halo ring and pins are in place (Fig. 37-19, *B*).

AFTERTREATMENT. The pins are cleansed daily at the skin interface with hydrogen peroxide or a small amount of povidone-iodine (Betadine) solution. The pins are retightened once 48 hours after application.

Complications include pin loosening, infection, pin site bleeding, and dural puncture. If a pin becomes loose, it can be retightened as long as resistance is met. If no resistance is met, the pin should be removed and another pin inserted in an alternative site. If drainage develops around a pin, oral antibiotics and local skin care is begun. If the drainage does not respond to these measures or if cellulitis or an abscess develops, the pin should be removed and another pin inserted at an alternative site. If dural puncture occurs, the pin should be removed and another pin inserted at an alternative site; the patient should receive prophylactic antibiotic therapy. The dural tear usually will heal in 4 or 5 days, at which time antibiotics can be discontinued.

Basilar Impression

Basilar impression (basilar invagination) is a rare deformity in which the tip of the odontoid is more cephalad than normal. The odontoid may protrude into the foramen magnum and encroach on the brainstem, causing neurological symptoms because of the limited space available for the brainstem and spinal cord. Neurological damage can be caused by direct pressure from the odontoid or from other constricting structures around the

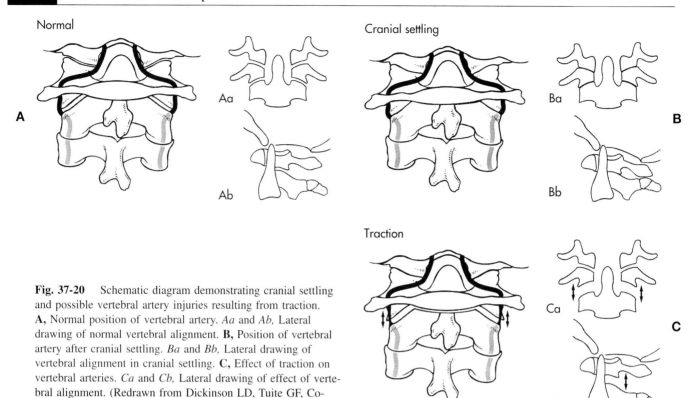

Normal

A

Aa

Ab

Cranial settling

Ba

B

Bb

Traction

Ca

C

Cb

Fig. 37-20 Schematic diagram demonstrating cranial settling and possible vertebral artery injuries resulting from traction. **A,** Normal position of vertebral artery. *Aa* and *Ab,* Lateral drawing of normal vertebral alignment. **B,** Position of vertebral artery after cranial settling. *Ba* and *Bb,* Lateral drawing of vertebral alignment in cranial settling. **C,** Effect of traction on vertebral arteries. *Ca* and *Cb,* Lateral drawing of effect of vertebral alignment. (Redrawn from Dickinson LD, Tuite GF, Colon GP, Papadoupoulos SM: *Neurosurgery* 36:835, 1995.)

foramen magnum, circulatory compromise of the vertebral arteries, or impairment of cerebrospinal fluid flow. It is important that the orthopaedist be familiar with basilar impression and its presentation because this spinal deformity often goes unrecognized or is misdiagnosed as a posterior fossa tumor, bulbar palsy of polio, syringomyelia, amyotrophic lateral sclerosis, spinal cord tumor, or multiple sclerosis.

Basilar impression can be either primary (congenital) or secondary (acquired). Primary basilar impression is a congenital structural abnormality of the craniocervical junction that often is associated with other vertebral defects (atlantooccipital fusion, Klippel-Feil syndrome, Arnold-Chiari malformation, syringomyelia, odontoid anomalies, hypoplasia of the atlas, and bifid posterior arch of the atlas); these associated conditions can cause the predominant symptoms. Secondary basilar impression is an acquired deformity of the skull resulting from systemic disease that causes softening of the osseous structures at the base of the skull, such as Paget disease, osteomalacia, rickets, osteogenesis imperfecta, rheumatoid arthritis, neurofibromatosis, and ankylosing spondylitis. Secondary basilar impression occurs more commonly in types III and IV than in type I osteogenesis imperfecta.

Basilar impression causes neurological symptoms because of crowding of the neural structures as they pass through the foramen magnum. Clinical presentation is varied, and patients with severe basilar impression may be totally asymptomatic. Symptoms usually appear during the second and third decades of life, probably because of increased ligamentous laxity and

instability with age and decreased tolerance to compression of the spinal cord and vertebral arteries.

Most patients with basilar impression have short necks, asymmetry of the face or skull, and torticollis, but these findings are not specific for basilar impression and can be seen in patients with other congenital vertebral anomalies. Headache in the distribution of the greater occipital nerve is a frequent complaint. DeBarros et al. (1968) divided the signs and symptoms into two categories: those caused by pure basilar impression and those caused by the Arnold-Chiari malformation. They found that symptoms caused by pure basilar impression were primarily motor and sensory disturbances, such as weakness and paresthesia in the limbs, whereas patients with Arnold-Chiari malformation had symptoms of cerebellar and vestibular disturbances, such as ataxia, dizziness, and nystagmus. Involvement of the lower cranial nerves also occurs in basilar impression. The trigeminal, vagus, glossopharyngeal, and hypoglossal nerves may be compressed as they emerge from the medulla oblongata. DeBarros et al. (1975) also noted sexual disturbances, such as impotence and reduction in libido, in 27% of their patients.

Compression of the vertebral arteries as they pass through the foramen magnum is another source of symptoms. Bernini et al. found a significantly higher incidence of vertebral artery anomalies in patients with basilar impression and atlantooccipital fusion. Symptoms caused by vertebral artery insufficiency, such as dizziness, seizures, mental deterioration, and syncope, can occur singly or in combination with other symptoms of

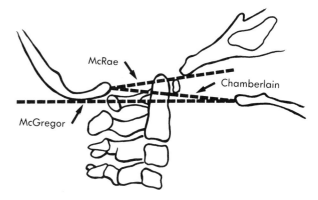

Fig. 37-21 Base of skull and upper cervical spine showing location of McRae, McGregor, and Chamberlain lines. (Redrawn from Hensinger RN: Cervical spine: pediatric. In American Academy of Orthopaedic Surgeons: *Orthopaedic knowledge update I. Home study syllabus,* Chicago, 1984, The Academy.)

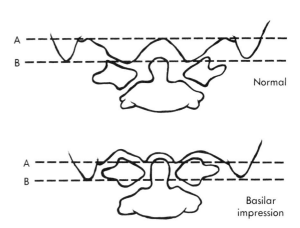

Fig. 37-22 Fischgold and Metzger lines. Line was originally drawn from lower pole of mastoid process *(B),* but because of variability in size of mastoid processes, these researchers recommend drawing line between digastric grooves *(A).* (Redrawn from Fielding JW, Hensinger R, Hawkins RJ: The cervical spine. In Lovell WW, Winter RB, eds: *Pediatric orthopaedics,* Philadelphia, 1978, JB Lippincott.)

basilar impression. Children with occipitocervical anomalies may be more susceptible to vertebral artery injury and brainstem ischemia if skull traction is applied (Fig. 37-20).

ROENTGENOGRAPHIC FINDINGS

Numerous measurements have been suggested for diagnosing basilar impression (Box 37-4), reflecting the difficulty of evaluating this area of the spine roentgenographically, and several methods of evaluation (plain roentgenography, tomography, CT scan, and MRI) may be needed to confirm the diagnosis. The most commonly used measurements are the lines of Chamberlain; McGregor; McRae; and Fischgold and Metzger. The Chamberlain, McGregor, and McRae lines are made on lateral roentgenograms of the skull (Fig. 37-21); the Fischgold and Metzger lines are made on an anteroposterior view (Fig. 37-22).

The Chamberlain line is drawn from the posterior edge of the hard palate to the posterior border of the foramen magnum. Symptomatic basilar impression can occur when the odontoid tip extends above this line. There are two disadvantages to the Chamberlain line: the posterior tip of the foramen magnum is difficult to define on the standard lateral view, and the posterior tip of the foramen magnum is often invaginated. McGregor modified the Chamberlain line by drawing a line from the upper

surface of the posterior edge of the hard palate to the most caudal point of the occipital curve, which is much easier to identify on a standard lateral roentgenogram. The position of the tip of the odontoid is measured in relation to the McGregor line, and a distance of 4.5 mm above this line is considered the upper limit of normal. The McRae line determines the anteroposterior dimension of the foramen magnum and is formed by drawing a line from the anterior tip of the foramen magnum to the posterior tip. McRae observed that if the tip of the odontoid is below this line, the patient usually is asymptomatic.

The lateral lines of McGregor and Chamberlain have been criticized because the anterior reference point (the hard palate) is not part of the skull, and measurements can be distorted by an abnormal facial configuration or a high-arched palate. To resolve these problems, Fischgold and Metzger describe a method of assessing basilar impression that uses an anteroposterior tomogram (see Fig. 37-22). This assessment is based on a line drawn between the two digastric grooves (the junction of the medial aspect of the mastoid process at the base of the skull). Normally the digastric line passes above the odontoid tip (10.7 mm) and the atlantooccipital joint (11.6 mm).

The McGregor line is used as a routine screening test because the landmarks for this line can be defined easily on a standard lateral roentgenogram. If more information is needed, an MRI of the craniovertebral junction is used to confirm the diagnosis of basilar impression. McAfee et al. recommend CT scanning and MRI for evaluation of spinal cord compression of the upper cervical spine. They state that these are complementary studies, the CT scan providing better osseous detail and the MRI providing superior soft tissue resolution. A "functional" MRI obtained with the cervical spine in flexion and then extension shows the dynamics of spinal cord compression caused by vertebral instability or anomaly.

TREATMENT

Conservative treatment of symptomatic patients with a collar or cervical orthosis has not been successful. Many patients with basilar impression have no neurological symptoms, and some have minimal symptoms with no sign of progressive neurological damage. These patients should be observed and examined periodically; surgery is indicated only if the clinical picture becomes worse. The indications for surgery are based on the clinical symptomatology and not on the degree of basilar impression. Once a patient becomes symptomatic, progression of the disease and symptoms are likely.

If symptoms are caused by anterior impingement from the odontoid, stabilization in extension by an occipital C1-C2 fusion is indicated. If symptoms and impingement persist, anterior excision of the odontoid can be done after posterior stabilization. Posterior impingement requires suboccipital craniectomy and laminectomy of C1 and possibly C2 to decompress the brainstem and spinal cord. The dura should be opened during this procedure to check for a tight posterior dural band that may be causing the symptoms instead of the bony abnormalities. Posterior fusion is recommended in addition to decompression if stability is in question.

Atlantooccipital Fusion

Atlantooccipital fusion (occipitalization) is a partial or complete congenital fusion between the atlas and the base of the occiput ranging from a complete bony fusion to a bony bridge or even a fibrous band uniting one small area of the atlas and occiput. Occipitalization is a failure of segmentation between the fourth occipital sclerotome and the first spinal sclerotome. This condition can lead to chronic atlantoaxial instability or basilar invagination and can produce a wide range of symptoms because of spinal cord impingement and vascular

compromise of the vertebral arteries. The incidence of atlantooccipital fusion has been reported to be 1.4 to 2.5 per 1000 children, affecting males and females equally. Symptoms usually appear in the third and fourth decades of life. Atlantooccipital fusion frequently is associated with congenital fusion between C2 and C3 (reportedly in as many as 70% of patients). Approximately half of patients with atlantooccipital fusion develop atlantoaxial instability. Kyphosis and scoliosis also are frequently associated with this deformity. Other associated congenital anomalies, such as anomalies of the jaw, incomplete cleft of the nasal cartilage, cleft palate, external ear deformities, cervical ribs, and urinary tract anomalies, occur in 20% of patients with atlantooccipital fusion.

Patients with atlantooccipital fusion commonly have low hairlines, torticollis, short necks, and restricted neck movement. Spillane et al. found that none of their patients with atlantooccipital fusion had a normal-appearing neck. Many patients complain of a dull, aching pain in the posterior occiput and the neck, with episodic neck stiffness, but symptoms vary depending on the area of spinal cord impingement. If the impingement is anterior, pyramidal tract signs and symptoms predominate; if the impingement is posterior, posterior column signs and symptoms predominate.

McRae and Barnum believe that the shape and position of the odontoid are the keys to neurological symptoms. When the odontoid lies above the foramen magnum, a relative or actual basilar impression is present. If the odontoid lies below the foramen magnum, the patient usually is asymptomatic. McRae found that in this condition, the odontoid was excessively long and angulated posteriorly, thus decreasing the anteroposterior diameter of the spinal canal. Autopsy findings showed that the brainstem was indented by the abnormal odontoid. Anterior spinal cord compression with pyramidal tract irritation causes muscle weakness and wasting, ataxia, spasticity, pathological reflexes (Babinski and Hoffman), and hyperreflexia. Posterior compression causes loss of deep pain, light touch, proprioception, and vibratory sensation. Nystagmus is a common finding. Cranial nerve involvement can cause diplopia, dysphagia, and auditory disturbances. Disturbances of the vertebral artery result in syncope, seizures, vertigo, and an unsteady gait.

Neurological symptoms generally begin in the third and fourth decades of life, possibly because the older patient's spinal cord and vertebral arteries become less resistant to compression. Symptoms may be initiated by trauma or infection in the pharynx or nasopharynx.

ROENTGENOGRAPHIC FINDINGS

Because this anomaly ranges from complete incorporation of the atlas into the occiput to a small fibrous band connecting part of the atlas to the occiput, routine roentgenograms usually are difficult to interpret, and tomograms may be needed to demonstrate the occipitocervical fusion (Fig. 37-23). Most commonly the anterior arch of the atlas is assimilated into the occiput and displaced posteriorly relative to the occiput. About half of the patients have a relative basilar impression caused by

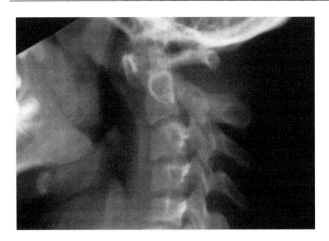

Fig. 37-23   Lateral roentgenogram of patient with occipital cervical synostosis.

loss of height of the atlas. Posterior fusion usually is a small bony fringe or a fibrous band that frequently is not evident on a roentgenogram. This fringe is directed downward and into the spinal canal and can cause neurological symptoms. Flexion and extension lateral cervical spine views should be part of the initial evaluation because of the frequency of atlantoaxial instability. McRae and Barnum measured the distance from the posterior aspect of the odontoid to the posterior arch of the atlas or the posterior lip of the foramen magnum, whichever was closer. When the distance was 19 mm or less, a neurological deficit usually was present. This measurement should be made on a flexion view because maximal narrowing of the canal usually occurs in flexion. Myelography or MRI can detect areas of encroachment on the spinal cord or medulla and is especially useful when a constricting fibrous band occurs posteriorly.

TREATMENT

Patients who have minor symptoms or become symptomatic after minor trauma or infection can be treated nonoperatively with immobilization in plaster, traction, or a cervical orthosis. When neurological symptoms occur, cervical spine fusion or decompression is indicated. Anterior symptoms usually are caused by a hypermobile odontoid; preliminary reduction of the odontoid with traction, followed by fusion from the occiput to C2, relieves the symptoms. If the odontoid is irreducible, then the appropriateness of either in situ fusion without reduction or fusion with excision of the odontoid, with its associated risks and complications, must be determined. Posterior signs and symptoms usually are caused by bony compression or compression from a dural band. When this is documented by MRI or myelography, suboccipital craniectomy, excision of the posterior arch of the atlas, and removal of the dural band are indicated. This may need to be combined with a posterior fusion to prevent instability. Surgical results have been variable.

Klippel-Feil Syndrome

Klippel-Feil syndrome is a congenital fusion of the cervical vertebrae that may involve two segments, a congenital block vertebra, or the entire cervical spine. Congenital cervical fusion is a result of failure of normal segmentation of the cervical somites during the third to eighth week of life. The skeletal system may not be the only system affected during this time, and cardiorespiratory, genitourinary, and auditory systems frequently are involved. In most patients the exact cause is not known. One proposed cause is a primary vascular disruption during embryonic development that results in fusion of the cervical vertebrae and other associated anomalies. Beals and Rolfe suggested that a global insult with variable effects on different tissues or multiple separate insults could explain the fusions of the cervical vertebrae and other associated anomalies. Gunderson et al. showed that in a few patients this is an inherited condition. His study suggests that fusion of C2-C3 may be an autosomal dominant inheritance, but the inheritance pattern of other cervical vertebral fusion patterns could not be determined. Maternal alcoholism also has been suggested as a causative factor. Tredwell et al. found a 50% incidence of cervical vertebral fusions in roentgenograms of patients with fetal alcohol syndrome.

Occipitalization of the atlas, hemivertebrae, and basilar impression occur frequently in patients with Klippel-Feil syndrome, but their isolated occurrence is not considered part of this syndrome. The classic features of Klippel-Feil syndrome are a short neck, low posterior hairline, and limited range of neck motion. Patients may consult an orthopaedist because of neurological problems, signs of instability of the cervical spine, or for cosmetic reasons. Because many patients are asymptomatic, the actual incidence of this condition is not known, but estimates in the literature range from 1 in 42,400 births to 3 in 700. There is a slight male predominance (1.5:1). Feil classified the syndrome into three types: type I, block fusion of all cervical and upper thoracic vertebrae; type II, fusion of one or two pairs of cervical vertebrae; and type III, cervical fusion in combination with lower thoracic or lumbar fusion. Minimally involved patients with Klippel-Feil syndrome lead normal, active lives with no significant restrictions or symptoms. More severely involved patients have a good prognosis if genitourinary, cardiopulmonary, and auditory problems are treated early.

In patients with Klippel-Feil syndrome, neurological compromise, ranging from radiculopathy to quadriplegia to death, can occur. The neurological symptoms are caused by occipitocervical anomalies, instability, or degenerative joint and disc disease. Instability and degenerative joint disease are common when two fused areas are separated by a single open interspace. Patients with multiple short areas of fusion (three or more vertebrae) separated by more than one open interspace do not develop instability or degenerative joint disease as frequently, possibly because of a more equal distribution of stress in the cervical spine. Fielding et al. and Hensinger et al. identified three patterns of cervical spine fusion with a potentially poor prognosis because of late instability or degenerative joint disease. Pattern 1 is fusion of C1 and C2 with occipitalization of the atlas. This pattern concentrates the motion of flexion and extension at the atlantoaxial joint; the odontoid becomes hypermobile and may dislocate posteriorly, narrowing the spinal canal and causing neurological compromise. Pattern 2 is a long fusion with an abnormal occipitocervical junction, concentrating the forces of flexion, extension, and rotation through an abnormal odontoid or poorly developed C1 ring; with time, this abnormal articulation becomes unstable. This pattern should be differentiated from a long fusion with a normal C1-C2 articulation and occipitocervical junction. Patients with pattern 2 fusions are not at high risk for instability and neurological problems and have a normal life expectancy. Pattern 3 is a single open interspace between two fused segments with cervical spine motion concentrated at the single open interspace, which becomes hypermobile and causes instability and degenerative joint disease. On lateral roentgenogram the cervical spine with this pattern appears to hinge at an open segment.

ASSOCIATED CONDITIONS

Several congenital problems have been associated with congenital fusion of the cervical vertebrae, most commonly scoliosis, renal abnormalities, Sprengel deformity, deafness, synkinesis, and congenital heart defects (Box 37-5).

Scoliosis

The most common orthopaedic anomaly is scoliosis. Studies have shown that 60% to 70% of patients with Klippel-Feil syndrome have scoliosis (curves greater than 15 degrees), kyphosis, or both. Most of these patients require treatment and should be followed closely until growth is complete. Two types of scoliosis have been identified. The first is congenital scoliosis caused by vertebral anomalies. The second occurs in a normal-appearing spine below an area of congenital scoliosis or cervical fusion; this type of curve tends to be progressive. Progression may be controlled with a brace. Surgery may be required to prevent progression in both types of scoliosis associated with Klippel-Feil syndrome. Roentgenograms of the entire spine should be obtained because a progressive curve may not be appreciated until significant deformity has occurred if attention is focused just on the congenital scoliosis or cervical fusion.

Renal Anomalies

About one third of patients with Klippel-Feil syndrome have urogenital anomalies. Because the cervical vertebrae and genitourinary tract differentiate at the same time and location in the embryo, fetal maldevelopment between the fourth and eighth weeks of development may produce both genitourinary anomalies and Klippel-Feil syndrome. These renal anomalies usually are asymptomatic, and children with Klippel-Feil syndrome should be evaluated with an ultrasound or intravenous pyelogram because the renal problems can be life threatening. The most common renal anomaly is unilateral

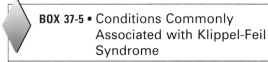

BOX 37-5 • Conditions Commonly Associated with Klippel-Feil Syndrome

Scoliosis
Most frequent orthopaedic complication (60% of cases)
Obtain roentgenograms of entire spine

Renal Abnormalities
Approximately 30% of cases
Usually asymptomatic
Obtain ultrasound or intravenous pyelogram

Cardiovascular Anomalies
Approximately 4% to 14% of cases
Ventricular septal defects most common

Deafness
Approximately 30% of cases
Obtain audiometric testing

Synkinesis (Mirror Movements)
Approximately 20% of cases
May restrict bimanual activities
Usually decreases with age

Respiratory Anomalies
Failure of lobe formation
Ectopic lungs
Restriction of lung function by shortened trunk, scoliosis, rib fusion, or deformed costovertebral joints

Sprengel Deformity
Approximately 20% of cases
Unilateral or bilateral
Increases unsightly appearance
May affect shoulder motion

absence of the kidney. Other anomalies include malrotation of kidneys, ectopic kidney, horseshoe kidney, and hydronephrosis from ureteral pelvic obstruction.

Cardiovascular Anomalies

The reported incidence of cardiovascular anomalies in children with Klippel-Feil syndrome ranges from 4.2% to 29%. Ventricular septal defects, either alone or in combination, are the most common anomaly. Patients may have significant dyspnea and cyanosis. Other reported cardiovascular anomalies include mitral valve insufficiency, coarctation of the aorta, right-sided aorta, patent ductus arteriosus, pulmonic stenosis, dextrocardia, atrial septal defect, aplasia of the pericardium, patent foramen ovale, single atrium, single ventricle, and bicuspid pulmonic valve.

Deafness

Approximately 30% of children with Klippel-Feil syndrome have some degree of hearing loss. McGaughran, Kuna, and Das reported that 80% of the 44 patients he studied had some type

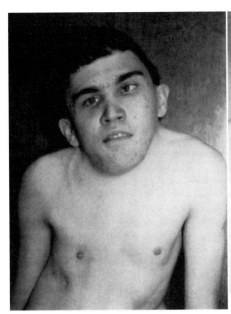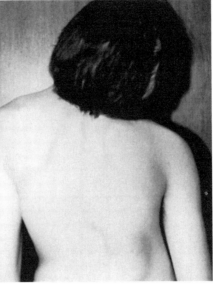

Fig. 37-24 Clinical features of Klippel-Feil syndrome in adolescent male.

of audiologic abnormalities. Several reports document conduction defects with ankylosis of the ossicles, foot plate fixation, or absence of the external auditory canal. Other reports suggest a sensorineural defect. There is no common anatomical lesion, and the hearing loss may be conductive, sensorineural, or mixed. All patients with Klippel-Feil syndrome should have audiometric testing. Early detection of hearing defects in a young child may improve speech and language development by permitting early initiation of speech and language training.

Synkinesis

Synkinesis (mirror movements) is involuntary paired movements of the hands and occasionally of the arms. One hand is unable to move without a similar reciprocal motion of the opposite hand. Synkinesis can be observed in normal children younger than 5 years and is present in 20% of patients with Klippel-Feil syndrome. Synkinesis may be so severe as to restrict bimanual activities. The mirror movements become less obvious with increasing age and usually are not clinically obvious after the second decade of life.

In autopsy studies Gunderson et al. observed incomplete decussation of the pyramidal tract in the upper cervical spinal cord, suggesting that an alternate extrapyramidal path is required to control motion in the upper extremity. Using electromyography, Baird et al. showed that clinically normal patients with Klippel-Feil syndrome had electrically detectable paired motion in the opposite extremity. These patients may be clumsier in two-handed activities. Occupational therapy can help the child disassociate the mirror movements and improve bimanual dexterity.

Respiratory Anomalies

Pulmonary complications involving failure of lobe formation, ectopic lungs, or restrictive lung disease resulting from a shortened trunk, scoliosis, rib fusion, and deformed costovertebral joints have been reported.

Sprengel Deformity

Sprengel deformity occurs in about 20% of patients with Klippel-Feil syndrome and can be unilateral or bilateral. Descent of the scapula coincides with the period of development of Klippel-Feil anomalies, and maldevelopment during this time (third to eighth week of gestation) can cause both anomalies. Sprengel deformity increases the unsightly appearance of an already short neck and can affect the range of shoulder motion.

Cervical Ribs

Cervical ribs occur in 12% to 15% of patients with Klippel-Feil syndrome. When evaluating a patient with neurological symptoms, the presence of a cervical rib and associated thoracic outlet syndrome should be investigated.

CLINICAL FINDINGS

The classic clinical presentation of Klippel-Feil syndrome is the triad of a low posterior hairline, a short neck, and limited neck motion (Fig. 37-24). This triad indicates almost complete cervical involvement and may be clinically evident at birth; however, fewer than half of patients with Klippel-Feil syndrome have all parts of the triad. Many patients with Klippel-Feil syndrome have a normal appearance, and the syndrome is diagnosed through incidental roentgenograms. Shortening of the neck and a low posterior hairline are not constant findings and may be overlooked; webbing of the neck (pterygium colli) is seen in severe involvement. The most constant clinical finding is limitation of neck motion. Rotation and lateral bending are affected more than flexion and

A   **C**   **D**

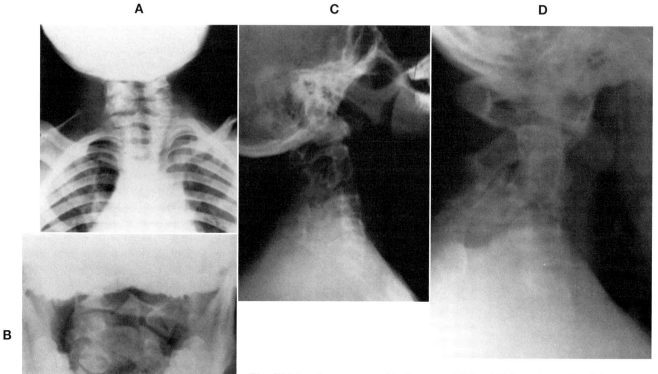

B

Fig. 37-25   Roentgenographic features of Klippel-Feil syndrome in adolescent. **A,** Posteroanterior view shows congenital anomalies of cervical spine and left Sprengel deformity. **B,** Open-mouth odontoid view shows bony anomalies of cervical spine. **C,** Extension view shows odontoid in normal position. **D,** Flexion view shows increased atlantodens interval.

extension. If fewer than three vertebrae are fused or if the lower cervical vertebrae are fused, motion is only slightly limited. Hensinger reported that some of his patients had almost full flexion and extension through only one open interspace.

Symptoms usually are not caused by the fused cervical vertebrae but by open segments adjacent to areas of synostosis that become hypermobile in response to increased stress placed on the area. Symptoms can be caused by mechanical or neurological problems. Mechanical problems are caused by stretching of the capsular and ligamentous structures near the hypermobile segment, resulting in early degenerative arthritis with pain localized to the neck. Neurological problems result from direct irritation of or impingement on a nerve root or from compression of the spinal cord. Involvement of the nerve root alone causes radicular symptoms; spinal cord compression can cause spasticity, hyperreflexia, muscle weakness, and even complete paralysis.

ROENTGENOGRAPHIC FINDINGS

Routine roentgenograms, tomograms, cineradiograms, CT scans, and MRI may be useful in evaluation of Klippel-Feil syndrome. Adequate roentgenograms can be difficult to obtain in severely involved children, but initial examination should include anteroposterior, odontoid, and lateral flexion and extension views of the cervical spine. Lateral flexion-extension views are the most important to identify atlantoaxial instability or instability near an open segment between two congenitally fused areas (Fig. 37-25). If routine lateral roentgenograms are difficult to interpret, lateral flexion-extension tomograms can be obtained. Spinal canal narrowing can occur from degenerative osteophytes or from congenital spinal stenosis. If enlargement of the spinal canal is evident on roentgenograms, syringomyelia, hydromyelia, or Arnold-Chiari malformation should be suspected. In young patients with Klippel-Feil syndrome, serial lateral flexion-extension views should be obtained to evaluate instability at the atlantoaxial joint or at an open interspace between fused areas. Development of congenital or idiopathic scoliosis should be documented by roentgenographic examination of the entire spine. Cineradiography also is helpful in determining the amount of vertebral instability. Besides vertebral fusion, flattening and widening of involved vertebral bodies and absent disc spaces are common findings. In young children the spine may appear normal because of the lack of ossification. The posterior elements usually are the first to ossify and fuse, which aids in early diagnosis of Klippel-Feil syndrome. CT is helpful in diagnosing nerve root and spinal cord impingement by osteophyte formation. To evaluate instability and the risk of neurological compromise, a flexion and extension MRI may be needed to give the soft tissue definition necessary to demonstrate instability or spinal cord compromise.

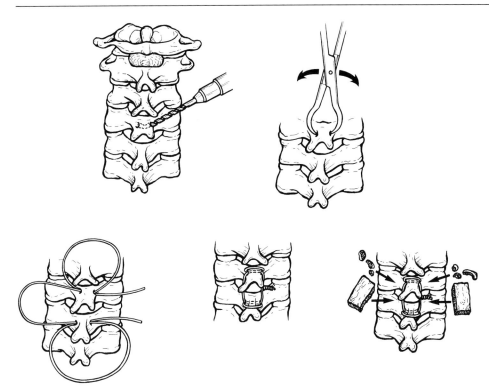

Fig. 37-26 Modified Rogers wiring of cervical spine (see text). (Redrawn from Murphy MJ, Southwick WO: Posterior approaches and fusions. In Cervical Spine Research Society: *The cervical spine,* Philadelphia, 1983, JB Lippincott.)

TREATMENT

Mechanical symptoms caused by degenerative joint disease usually respond to traction, a cervical collar, and analgesics. Neurological symptoms should be carefully evaluated to locate the exact pathological condition; surgical stabilization with or without decompression may be required. Prophylactic fusion of a hypermobile segment is controversial. The risk of neurological compromise must be weighed against the further reduction in neck motion, and this decision must be made for each patient individually. Cosmetic improvement after surgery has been limited, but surgical correction of Sprengel deformity can significantly improve appearance, and occasionally soft tissue procedures such as Z-plasty and muscle resection improve cosmesis. Bonola described a method of rib resection to obtain an apparent increase in neck length and motion, but this is an extensive procedure with significant risk. Partial thoracoplasty is performed as a two-stage procedure: removal of the upper four ribs on one side and, after the patient has recovered from the first surgery, removal of the upper four ribs on the other side.

◆ Posterior Fusion of C3 to C7

TECHNIQUE 37-15 (Fig. 37-26)

Administer general anesthesia with the patient in a supine position. Turn the patient prone on the operating table, taking care to maintain traction and proper alignment of the head and neck. The head may be positioned in a head rest or

maintained in skeletal traction. Obtain roentgenograms to confirm adequate alignment of the vertebrae and to localize the vertebrae to be exposed. There is a high incidence of extension of the fusion mass when extra vertebrae or spinous processes are exposed in the cervical spine. Make a midline incision over the chosen spinous processes and expose the spinous process and lamina subperiosteally to the facet joints. If the spinous process is large enough, make a hole in the base of the spinous process with a towel clip or Lewin clamp. Pass an 18-gauge wire through this hole, loop it over the spinous process, and pass it through the hole again. Make a similar hole in the base of the spinous process of the inferior vertebra to be fused. Pass the wire through this hole, loop it under the inferior aspect of the spinous process, and then pass it back through the same hole. Tighten the wire and place corticocancellous bone grafts along the exposed lamina and spinous processes. Close the wound in layers. If the spinous process is too small to pass wires, then an in situ fusion can be performed and external immobilization used.

AFTERTREATMENT. The patient should wear a rigid cervical orthosis until a solid fusion is documented roentgenographically.

TECHNIQUE 37-16 *(Hall)*

Hall et al. described a technique using a 16-gauge wire and threaded Kirschner wires. Pass the threaded Kirschner wires

continued

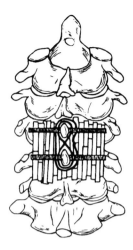

Fig. 37-27 Hall technique of fixation for posterior arthrodesis of cervical spine. (From Hall JE, Simmons ED, Danylchuk K, et al: *J Bone Joint Surg* 72A:460, 1990.)

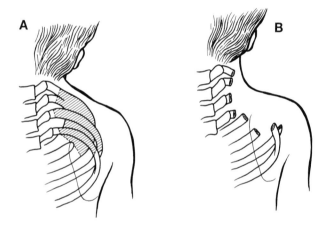

Fig. 37-28 Bonola partial thoracoplasty for treatment of short neck in Klippel-Feil syndrome (see text). (Redrawn from Bonola A: *J Bone Joint Surg* 38B:440, 1956.)

through the bases of the spinous processes of the vertebrae to be fused. This is followed by a figure-eight wiring with a 16-gauge wire. After the 16-gauge wire has been tightened about the threaded Kirschner wires, pack strips of corticocancellous and cancellous bone over the posterior arches of the vertebrae to be fused. Exposure and postoperative care are similar to those described for a Rogers posterior fusion and wiring (Fig. 37-27).

◆ Rib Resection

TECHNIQUE 37-17 *(Bonola)*
Bonola performed a partial thoracoplasty with the use of local anesthesia, but general anesthesia can be used. Through a right paravertebral incision midway between the

spinous processes and the medial margin of the scapula, divide the trapezius and rhomboid muscles to expose the posterior aspect of the first four ribs (Fig. 37-28, *A*). Cut these ribs with a rib cutter a few centimeters from the costovertebral joint. Continue dissection anteriorly along the ribs, dividing and removing the ribs as far anteriorly as dissection allows (Fig. 37-28, *B*). Close the wound in layers.

AFTERTREATMENT. A cervical collar is fitted to help mold the resected area. The second stage of the procedure is performed on the opposite side after the patient has recovered from the initial surgery.

Atlantoaxial Rotatory Subluxation

Atlantoaxial rotatory subluxation is a common cause of childhood torticollis, but the subluxation and torticollis usually are temporary. Rarely do they persist and become what is best described as atlantoaxial rotatory "fixation." Atlantoaxial rotatory subluxation occurs when normal motion between the atlas and axis becomes limited or fixed, and it can occur spontaneously, can be associated with minor trauma, or can follow an upper respiratory tract infection. The cause of this subluxation is not completely understood. Watson-Jones suggested that hyperemic decalcification of the arch of the atlas causes attachments of the transverse ligaments to be inadequate, thus allowing rotatory subluxation. Coutts believes that synovial fringes become inflamed and act as an obstruction to reduction of subluxation. Firrani-Gallotta and Luzzatti believe that subluxation is caused by disruption of one or both of the alar ligaments with an intact transverse ligament. Kawabe, Hirotani, and Tanaka reported a meniscus-like synovial fold in the C1-C2 facet joints that caused subluxation. They believe anatomical differences in the dens facet angle in children and adults account for this condition's appearance primarily in children. Most authors now agree that the subluxation is related to increased laxity of ligaments and capsular structures caused by inflammation or trauma.

Fielding and Hawkins classified atlantoaxial rotatory subluxation into four types (Fig. 37-29): type I, simple rotatory displacement without anterior shift of C1; type II, rotatory displacement with an anterior shift of C1 on C2 of 5 mm or less; type III, rotatory displacement with an anterior shift of C1 on C2 greater than 5 mm; and type IV, rotatory displacement with a posterior shift. Type I displacement is the most common and occurs primarily in children. Type II is less common but has greater potential for neurological damage. Types III and IV are rare but have high potential for neurological damage.

Atlantoaxial rotatory subluxation usually occurs in children after an upper respiratory tract infection or minor or major trauma. The head is tilted to one side and rotated to the opposite side with the neck slightly flexed (the "cock robin" position). The sternocleidomastoid muscle on the long side is often in spasm in an attempt to correct this deformity. When the

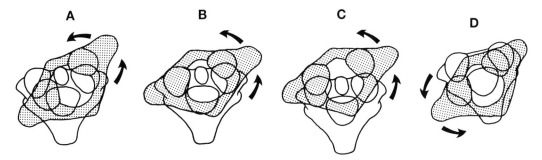

Fig. 37-29   Fielding and Hawkins classification of rotatory displacement. **A,** Type I, simple rotatory displacement without anterior shift; odontoid acts as pivot. **B,** Type II, rotatory displacement with anterior displacement of 3 to 5 mm; lateral articular process acts as pivot. **C,** Type III, rotatory displacement with anterior displacement of more than 5 mm. **D,** Type IV, rotatory displacement with posterior displacement. (Redrawn from Fielding JW, Hawkins RJ, Jr: *J Bone Joint Surg* 59A:37, 1977.)

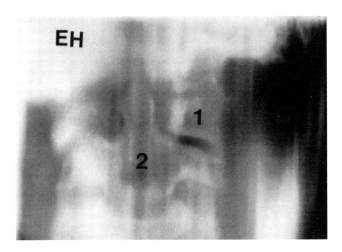

Fig. 37-30   Atlantoaxial rotatory subluxation. Note lateral masses.

> **BOX 37-6 • Treatment Plan for Rotatory Subluxation (Phillips and Hensinger)**
>
> Present <1 week: immobilization in soft collar, analgesics, bed rest for 1 week; no spontaneous reduction: hospitalization, traction
> Present >1 week but <1 month: hospitalization, cervical traction (head halter), cervical collar 4 to 6 weeks
> Present >1 month: hospitalization, cervical traction (skeletal), cervical collar 4 to 6 weeks
> Nonoperative treatment is used only if roentgenogram shows no significant anterior displacement or instability

subluxation is acute, attempts to move the head cause pain. Patients are able to increase the deformity but cannot correct the deformity past the midline. With time, muscle spasms subside and the torticollis becomes less painful, but the deformity persists. A careful neurological examination should determine any neurological compression or vertebral artery compromise.

ROENTGENOGRAPHIC FINDINGS

Adequate roentgenograms of the cervical spine can be difficult to obtain in children with torticollis. Initial examination should include anteroposterior and odontoid views of the cervical spine. On the open-mouth odontoid view the lateral mass that is rotated forward appears wider and closer to the midline, and the opposite lateral mass appears narrower and farther away from the midline (Fig. 37-30). One of the facet joints of the atlas and axis may be obscured by apparent overlapping. On the lateral view the anteriorly rotated lateral mass appears wedge shaped in front of the odontoid. The posterior arch of the atlas

may appear to be assimilated into the occiput because of the head tilt. A lateral roentgenogram of the skull may show the relative position of C1 and C2 more clearly than a lateral roentgenogram of the cervical spine. Lateral flexion and extension views should be obtained to document any atlantoaxial instability. If the atlantoaxial articulation cannot be seen on routine roentgenograms, tomograms can be obtained. Cineradiography confirms the diagnosis by demonstrating the movement of atlas and axis as a single unit but is difficult to perform during the acute stage because movement of the neck is painful. Cineradiography is not routinely used because of the increased radiation exposure. CT with the head rotated as far to the left and right as possible during scanning to confirm the loss of normal rotation at the atlantoaxial joint confirms the diagnosis of rotatory subluxation.

TREATMENT

Phillips and Hensinger base their treatment plan on the duration of the subluxation (Box 37-6). If rotatory subluxation has existed less than 1 week, immobilization in a soft collar, analgesics, and bed rest for 1 week are recommended. If reduction does not occur spontaneously, hospitalization and

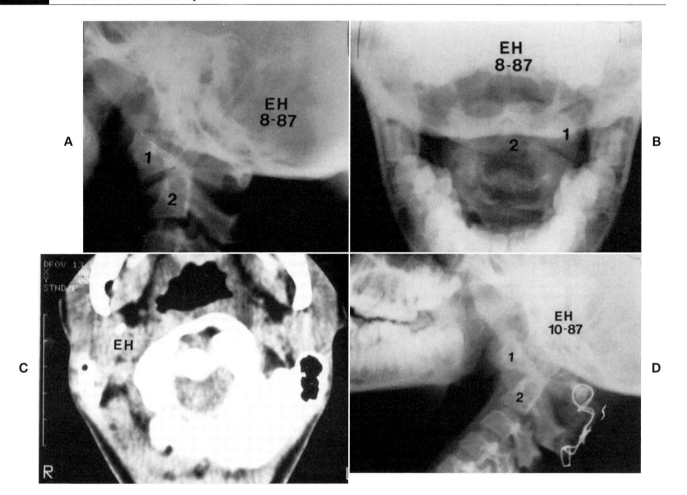

Fig. 37-31   Atlantoaxial rotatory fixation. **A,** Lateral roentgenogram shows wedge-shaped mass anterior to odontoid. **B,** Open-mouth odontoid view. **C,** CT scan. **D,** After C1-C2 in situ fusion.

traction are indicated. If rotatory subluxation is present for longer than 1 week but less than 1 month, hospitalization and cervical traction are indicated. Head halter traction generally is used, but when torticollis persists longer than 1 month, skeletal traction may be required. Traction is maintained until the deformity corrects, and then a cervical collar is worn for 4 to 6 weeks. Nonoperative treatment should be used only if no significant anterior displacement or instability is seen on roentgenographic evaluation.

Fielding listed the following as indications for operative treatment: (1) neurological involvement, (2) anterior displacement, (3) failure to achieve and maintain correction if the deformity exists for longer than 3 months, and (4) recurrence of the deformity after an adequate trial of conservative management consisting of at least 6 weeks of immobilization. If operative treatment is indicated, a C1-C2 posterior fusion is performed (Fig. 37-31). Fielding and Hawkins recommended preoperative traction for 2 to 3 weeks to correct the deformity as much as possible. Fusion is performed with the head in a neutral position. Fielding and Hawkins recommended 6 weeks of traction after surgery to maintain correction while the fusion becomes solid. This also can be accomplished with a halo cast

or vest. Immobilization is continued until there is roentgenographic evidence of fusion.

Cervical Instability in Down Syndrome

In children with Down syndrome, generalized ligamentous laxity caused by the underlying collagen defect can result in atlantoaxial and atlantooccipital instability. Atlantoaxial instability, first described by Spitzer, Rabinowitch, and Wybar in 1961, occurs in approximately 10% to 20% of children with Down syndrome. Instability can occur at more than one level and in more than one plane. Atlantooccipital instability also can occur in patients with Down syndrome; the incidence has been reported to be as high as 60%. Despite these reports of atlantoaxial and atlantooccipital instability in patients with Down syndrome, the exact natural history related to this instability is unknown.

The cervical spine instability in children with Down syndrome may be associated with congenital anomalies of the

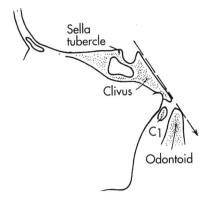

Fig. 37-32 Drawing of Wackenheim clivus-canal line. This line is drawn along the clivus into the cervical spinal canal and should pass just posterior to the tip of the odontoid. (From Menezes AH, Ryken TC: Craniovertebral junction abnormalities. In Weinstein SL, ed: *The pediatric spine: principles and practice,* New York, 1994, Raven.)

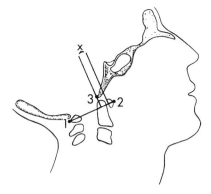

Fig. 37-33 Method of measuring atlantooccipital instability according to Wiesel and Rothman. These lines are drawn on flexion and extension lateral roentgenograms, and the translation should be no more than 1 mm. (From Gabriel KR, Mason DE, Carango P: *Spine* 15:997, 1990.)

upper cervical spine. Pueschel et al. (1990) reported that 45 of their 78 patients with Down syndrome had cervical spine anomalies and that the defects were more common in patients with atlantoaxial instability. However, whether the cervical anomalies are the cause or the result of ligamentous laxity is still controversial.

NEUROLOGICAL FINDINGS

Neurological symptoms are present in only 1% to 2.6% of patients with cervical instability, and the instability usually is discovered on routine screening examinations or on cervical roentgenograms obtained for other reasons. Burke et al. noted that progressive instability leading to neurological symptoms is most common in boys older than 10.5 years of age. Involvement of the pyramidal tract usually results in gait abnormalities, hyperreflexia, and motor weakness. Other neurological symptoms include neck pain, occipital headaches, and torticollis. Detailed neurological examination often is difficult in patients with Down syndrome, and Pueschel et al. recommended the use of somatosensory evoked potentials (SSEP) to document neurological involvement.

ROENTGENOGRAPHIC FINDINGS

Roentgenographic examination should include anteroposterior, flexion and extension lateral, and odontoid views. An atlantodens interval (ADI) of more than 4 to 5 mm is indicative of instability. If the ADI is more than 6 to 7 mm, MRI or CT scanning in flexion and extension is necessary to evaluate the space available for the spinal cord. Roentgenographic evidence of atlantooccipital instability is not as well defined as that for atlantoaxial instability, but the measurements described by Wackenheim (Fig. 37-32), Wiesel and Rothman (Fig. 37-33), Powers (Fig. 37-34), and Tredwell et al. are helpful. A Powers ratio of more than 1:0 is indicative of abnormal anterior

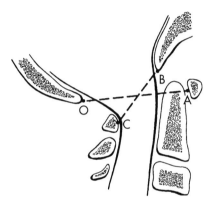

Fig. 37-34 Powers ratio is determined by drawing a line from the basion *(B)* to the posterior arch of the atlas *(C)* and a second line from the opisthion *(O)* to the anterior arch of the atlas *(A)*. The length of line *BC* is divided by the length of line *OA*. A ratio greater than 1 is diagnostic of anterior atlantooccipital translation, and a ratio less than 0.55 is diagnostic of posterior translation. (From Parfenchuck TA, Bertrand SL, Powers MJ, et al: *J Pediatr Orthop* 14:305, 1994.)

translation of the occiput, and, according to Parfenchuck et al., a ratio of less than 0:55 indicates posterior translation.

TREATMENT

Restriction of high-risk activities usually is sufficient in children with Down syndrome and ADIs of 4 to 5 mm. However, if the ADI is 6 to 7 mm, MRI or CT should be used to evaluate the risk of neurological compromise. If the ADI is 10 mm or more, posterior fusion and wiring are recommended. Before fusion and passage of the wire, the unstable C1-C2 joint should be reduced by traction. If reduction cannot be obtained, an in situ fusion reduces the risk of neurological compromise that may occur if intraoperative reduction is performed and the wires are passed through a narrowed space available for the spinal cord.

Complications are relatively common after cervical fusions in children with Down syndrome. Segal et al. reported frequent graft resorption after 10 posterior fusions and suggested as causes inadequate inflammatory response and collagen defects. Msall et al. reported the frequent development of instability above and below C1-C2 fusion in patients with Down syndrome. Postoperative immobilization in a halo cast or vest should be continued for up to 6 months because graft resorption as late as 6 months after fusion has been reported.

Familial Cervical Dysplasia

Saltzman et al. described a familial cervical dysplasia that affects the first cervical vertebra. Nine of twelve family members from three generations were affected by this inherited form of cervical vertebral dysplasia. The mode of transmission of this disorder is autosomal dominant, with apparently complete penetrance and variable expressivity. Most patients are asymptomatic, and clinical presentation varies from an incidental finding on roentgenographic examination to a passively correctable head tilt. Symptoms such as suboccipital headaches or decreased cervical motion may be present. CT scan and 3-D reconstructions best delineate the anatomical pathology. MRI is useful in identifying the potential for neurological compromise and the need for surgical stabilization. If surgery is required for stabilization, an occiput to C2 fusion usually is needed.

Congenital Anomalies of Atlas

Both Dubousset and Winter et al. described congenital hemiatlas or hypoplasia of the atlas that can cause marked torticollis if left untreated. Dubousset reported 17 patients with absence of the facet of C1 that led to severe, progressive, fixed torticollis. Initially the deformity or torticollis was flexible, but with time it became fixed.

In most patients the deformity is noted at birth as a lateral translation of the head on the trunk, with some degree of lateral tilt and rotation. The diagnosis is made by tomography or CT scans. Other spinal cord anomalies may be detected by MRI evaluation such as Arnold-Chiari malformations and stenosis of the foramen magnum. Angiography should be obtained preoperatively because vertebral arterial anomalies may occur on the aplastic side. This disorder has been classified into three types: type I is an isolated hemiatlas; type II is a partial or complete aplasia of one hemiatlas with other associated anomalies of the cervical spine; and type III is a partial or complete atlantooccipital fusion and symmetrical or asymmetrical hemiatlas aplasia, with or without anomalies of the odontoid and lower cervical spine. Dubousset recommended using a halo cast to correct the torticollis and obtain an acceptable position of the head and neck, followed by posterior

fusion from occiput to C2. Seven of his 17 patients required surgical correction. Although the age at which the torticollis could be corrected was not specified, Dubousset obtained good results in patients aged 13 and 15 years.

Intervertebral Disc Calcification

Intervertebral disc calcification is uncommon in children but does occur. This syndrome is characterized by an acute onset of cervical pain associated with torticollis and limited motion of the cervical spine. Although no definite cause has been identified, suggested causes include metabolic disease, local infection, and trauma. Most children with vertebral disc calcification are between the ages of 5 months and 11 years, and males are more frequently affected. Symptomatic disc calcification occurs most commonly in the lower cervical spine, usually at the C6-C7 level, and approximately one third of patients have multiple levels involved. In children, calcification involves the nucleus pulposus, in contrast to the process in adults, which involves the annulus fibrosus.

The most common symptoms of intervertebral disc calcification are neck pain, limitation of motion, and torticollis. Radicular pain or signs of nerve root compression are rare. Approximately 25% of patients have fever; 30% of patients have histories of trauma, and 15% have histories of upper respiratory tract infections. Pain usually begins suddenly and persists for 2 to 3 weeks; 75% of children are asymptomatic by 3 weeks, and 95% are asymptomatic within 6 months. Neurological deficits, if present, improve in 90% of patients. Disc herniation is rare, but posterior herniations can cause spinal cord compression, and anterior herniations may result in dysphagia.

Appropriate treatment consists of rest, cervical immobilization, and analgesics. Rarely, symptomatic nerve root or spinal cord impingement requires anterior discectomy and fusion. The long-term effects of intervertebral disc calcification are unknown, but Wong, Pereira, and Pho reported permanent changes about the adjacent vertebral bodies that may be associated with early degenerative changes in young adults.

References

SURGICAL APPROACHES
Bailey RW, Badgley CE: Stabilization of the cervical spine by anterior fusion, *J Bone Joint Surg* 42A:565, 1960.
Bonney G, Williams JPR: Transoral approach to the upper cervical spine: a report of 16 cases, *J Bone Joint Surg* 67B:691, 1985.
Brockmeyer DL, York JE, Apfelbaum RI: Anatomical suitability of C1-2 transarticular screw placement in pediatric patients, *J Neurosurg* 92:7, 2000.
Brooks AL, Jenkins EB: Atlantoaxial arthrodesis by the wedge compression method, *J Bone Joint Surg* 60A:279, 1978.
Cocke EW Jr, Robertson JH, Robertson JR, et al: The extended maxillotomy and subtotal maxillectomy for excision of skull base tumors, *Arch Otolaryngol Head Neck Surg* 116:92, 1990.
Cone W, Turner WG: The treatment of fracture-dislocation of the cervical vertebrae by skeletal traction and fusion, *J Bone Joint Surg* 19:584, 1937.

Coyne TJ, Fehlings MG, Wallace MC, et al: C1-C2 posterior cervical fusion: long-term evaluation of results and efficacy, *Neurosurgery* 37:688, 1995.

deAndrade JR, Macnab I: Anterior occipitocervical fusion using an extrapharyngeal exposure, *J Bone Joint Surg* 51A:1621, 1969.

Dickman CA, Sonntag VKH: Posterior C1-C2 transarticular screw fixation for atlantoaxial arthrodesis, *Neurosurgery* 43:275, 1998.

Fehlings MG, Errico T, Cooper P, et al: Occipitocervical fusion with a five-millimeter malleable rod and segmental fixation, *Neurosurgery* 32:198, 1993.

Gallie WE: Fractures and dislocations of the cervical spine, *Am J Surg* 46:495, 1939.

Hall JE, Denis F, Murray J: Exposure of the upper cervical spine for spinal decompression by a mandible and tongue-splitting approach: case report, *J Bone Joint Surg* 59A:121, 1977.

Hall JE, Simmons ED, Danylchuk K, et al: Instability of the cervical spine and neurological involvement in Klippel-Feil syndrome, *J Bone Joint Surg* 72A:460, 1990.

Henry AK: *Extensile exposure,* ed 2, Baltimore, 1957, Williams & Wilkins.

Itoh T, Tsuji H, Katoh Y, et al: Occipito-cervical fusion reinforced by Luque's segmental spinal instrumentation for rheumatoid disease, *Spine* 13:1234, 1988.

Letts M, Kaylor D, Gouw G: A biomechanical analysis of halo fixation in children, *J Bone Joint Surg* 70B:277, 1988.

Marks DS, Roberts P, Wilton PJ, et al: A halo jacket for stabilisation of the paediatric cervical spine, *Arch Orthop Trauma Surg* 112:134, 1993.

McAfee PC, Bohlman HH, Riley LH, et al: The anterior retropharyngeal approach to the upper part of the cervical spine, *J Bone Joint Surg* 69A:1371, 1987.

Menezes AH, Van Gilder JC: Transoral-transpharyngeal approach to the anterior craniocervical junction, *J Neurosurg* 69:895, 1988.

Merwin GE, Post JC, Sypert GW: Transoral approach to the upper cervical spine, *Laryngoscope* 101:780, 1991.

Ransford AO, Crockard HA, Pozo JL, et al: Craniocervical instability treated by contoured loop fixation, *J Bone Joint Surg* 68B:173, 1986.

Robinson RA, Smith GW: Anterolateral cervical disc removal and interbody fusion for cervical disc syndrome, *Bull Johns Hopkins Hosp* 96:223, 1955 (abstract).

Robinson RA, Southwick WO: Indications and technics for early stabilization of the neck in some fracture dislocations of the cervical spine, *South Med J* 53:565, 1960.

Rogers WA: Treatment of fracture-dislocation of the cervical spine, *J Bone Joint Surg* 24:245, 1942.

Rogers WA: Fractures and dislocations of the cervical spine: an end result study, *J Bone Joint Surg* 39A:341, 1957.

Smith MD, Anderson P, Grady MS: Occipitocervical arthrodesis using contoured plate fixation: an early report on a versatile fixation technique, *Spine* 18:1984, 1993.

Smith MD, Phillips WA, Hensinger RN: Fusion of the upper cervical spine in children and adolescents, *Spine* 16:695, 1990.

Sonntag KH, Kalfas I: Innovative cervical fusion and instrumentation techniques, *Clin Neurosurg* 37:636, 1989.

Tuite GF, Veres R, Crockard A, Sell D: Pediatric transoral surgery: indications, complications, and long-term outcome, *J Neurosurg* 84:573, 1996.

Whitesides TE Jr, Kelly RP: Lateral approach to the upper cervical spine for anterior fusion, *South Med J* 59:879, 1966.

Willard D, Nicholson JT: Dislocation of the first cervical vertebra, *Ann Surg* 113:464, 1941.

ANOMALIES OF ODONTOID

Baum JA, Hanley EN Jr, Pullekines J: Comparison of halo complications in adults and children, *Spine* 14:251, 1989.

Bhatnagar M, Sponseller PD, Carroll C, Tolo VT: Pediatric atlantoaxial instability presenting as cerebral and cerebellar infarcts, *J Pediatr Orthop* 11:103, 1991.

Brooks AL, Jenkins EB: Atlantoaxial arthrodesis by the wedge compression method, *J Bone Joint Surg* 60A:279, 1978.

Burke SW, French HG, Roberts JM, et al: Chronic atlantoaxial instability in Down syndrome, *J Bone Joint Surg* 67A:1356, 1985.

Callahan RA, Lockwood R, Green B: Modified Brooks fusion for an os odontoideum associated with an incomplete posterior arch of the atlas: case report, *Spine* 8:107, 1983.

Chang H, Park JB, Kim KW, Choi WS: Retro-dental reactive lesions related to development of myelopathy in patients with atlantoaxial instability secondary to os odontoideum, *Spine* 25:2777, 2000.

Davidson RG: Atlantoaxial instability in individuals with Down's syndrome: a fresh look at the evidence, *Pediatrics* 81:857, 1988.

Dormans JP, Criscitiello AA, Drummond DS, Davidson RS: Complications in children managed with immobilization in a halo vest, *J Bone Joint Surg* 77A:1370, 1995.

Fang HSY, Ong GB: Direct anterior approach to the upper cervical spine, *J Bone Joint Surg* 44A:1588, 1962.

Fielding JW: Disappearance of the central portion of the odontoid process, *J Bone Joint Surg* 47A:1228, 1965.

Fielding JW: The cervical spine in the child, *Curr Pract Orthop Surg* 5:31, 1973.

Fielding JW, Hawkins RJ, Ratzan S: Fusion for atlantoaxial instability, *J Bone Joint Surg* 58A:400, 1976.

Fielding JW, Hensinger RN, Hawkins RJ: Os odontoideum, *J Bone Joint Surg* 62A:376, 1980.

Forlin E, Herscovici D, Bowen JR: Understanding the os odontoideum, *Orthop Rev* 21:1441, 1992.

French HG, Burke SW, Roberts JM, et al: Upper cervical ossicles in Down syndrome, *J Pediatr Orthop* 7:69, 1987.

Gamble JG, Rinsky LA: Combined occipitoatlantoaxial hypermobility with anterior and posterior arch defects of the atlas in Pierre-Robin syndrome, *J Pediatr Orthop* 5:475, 1985.

Granger DK, Rechtine GR: Os odontoideum: a review, *Orthop Rev* 16:909, 1987.

Grantham SA, Dick HM, Thompson RC, et al: Occipitocervical arthrodesis: indications, technic, and results, *Clin Orthop* 65:118, 1969.

Hensinger RN: Osseous anomalies of the craniovertebral junction, *Spine* 11:323, 1986.

Hosono N, Honenobu K, Ebara S, et al: Cineradiographic motion analysis of atlantoaxial instability in os odontoideum, *Spine* 16:480, 1991.

Jun BY: Complete reduction of retro-odontoid soft tissue mass in os odontoideum following the posterior C1-C2 transarticular screw fixation, *Spine* 24:1961, 2000.

Koch RA, Nickel VL: The halo vest: an evaluation of motion and forces across the neck, *Spine* 3:103, 1978.

Koop SE, Winter RB, Lonstein JE: The surgical treatment of instability of the upper part of the cervical spine in children and adolescents, *J Bone Joint Surg* 66A:403, 1984.

Kuhns LR, Loder RT, Farley FA, Hensinger RN: Nuchal cord changes in children with os odontoideum: evidence for associated trauma, *J Pediatr Orthop* 18:815, 1998.

Lind B, Sihlbom H, Nordwall A: Forces and motion across the neck in patients treated with a halo vest, *Spine* 13:162, 1988.

Magerl F, Seeman PS: Stable posterior fusion of the atlas and axis by transarticular screw fixation. In Kehr P, Weidner A, eds: *Cervical spine,* Berlin, 1986, Springer-Verlag.

Mubarak SJ, Camp JF, Vuletich W, et al: Halo application in the infant, *J Pediatr Orthop* 9:612, 1989.

Perry J, Nickel VL: Total cervical-spine fusion for neck paralysis, *J Bone Joint Surg* 41A:37, 1959.

Pueschel SM, Scola FH: Atlantoaxial instability in individuals with Down's syndrome: epidemiologic, radiographic, and clinical studies, *Pediatrics* 80:555, 1987.

Robinson RA, Southwick WO: Surgical approaches to the cervical spine. In The American Academy of Orthopaedic Surgeons: *Instructional course lectures,* vol 17, St Louis, 1960, Mosby.

Sasaki H, Itoh T, Takei H, Hayashi M: Os odontoideum with cerebellar infarction: a case report, *Spine* 9:1178, 2000.

Schuler TC, Kurz L, Thompson DE, et al: Natural history of os odontoideum, *J Pediatr Orthop* 11:222, 1991.

Sherk HH, Pratt L: Transoral approaches. In Cervical Spine Research Society: *The cervical spine,* Philadelphia, 1983, JB Lippincott.

Spierings ELH, Braakman R: The management of os odontoideum: analysis of thirty-seven cases, *J Bone Joint Surg* 64B:442, 1982.

Tredwell SJ, O'Brien JP: Avascular necrosis of the proximal end of the dens: a complication of halo-pelvic distraction, *J Bone Joint Surg* 57A:332, 1975.

VanGilder JC, Menezes AH: Craniovertebral abnormalities and their treatment. In Schmidek HH, Sweet WH, eds: *Operative neurosurgical techniques,* ed 2, New York, 1988, Grune & Stratton.

Verska JM, Anderson PA: Os odontoideum: a case report of one identical twin, *Spine* 22:706, 1997.

Watanabe M, Toyama Y, Fujimura Y: Atlantoaxial instability in os odontoideum with myelopathy, *Spine* 21:1435, 1996.

Wertheim SB, Bohlman HH: Occipitocervical fusion: indications, technique, and long-term results in thirteen patients, *J Bone Joint Surg* 69A:833, 1987.

Whitesides TE Jr, Kelly RP: Lateral approach to the upper cervical spine for anterior fusion, *South Med J* 59:879, 1966.

BASILAR IMPRESSION

Adam AM: Skull radiograph measurements of normals and patients with basilar impression: use of Landzert's angle, *Surg Radiol Anat* 9:225, 1987.

Bernini F, Elefante R, Smaltino F, et al: Angiographic study on the vertebral artery in cases of deformities of the occipitocervical joint, *Am J Roentgenol* 107:526, 1969.

Chamberlain WE: Basilar impression (platybasia): a bizarre developmental anomaly of the occipital bone and upper cervical spine with striking and misleading neurologic manifestations, *Yale J Biol Med* 11:487, 1939.

DeBarros MC, daSilva WF, Filho HD, et al: Disturbances of sexual potency in patients with basilar impression and Arnold-Chiari malformation, *J Neurol Neurosurg Psychiatry* 38:598, 1975.

DeBarros MC, Farias W, Ataide L, et al: Basilar impression and Arnold-Chiari malformation: a study of 66 cases, *J Neurol Neurosurg Psychiatry* 31:596, 1968.

Dickinson LD, Tuite GF, Colon GP, Papadoupoulos SM: Vertebral artery dissection related to basilar impression: case report, *Neurosurgery* 36:835, 1995.

Engelbert RHH, Gerver WJM, Breslau-Siderius LJ: Spinal complications in osteogenesis imperfecta, *Acta Orthop Scand* 69:283, 1998.

Fielding JW, Hensinger R, Hawkins RJ: The cervical spine. In Lovell WW, Winter RB, eds: *Pediatric orthopaedics,* ed 2, Philadelphia, 1986, JB Lippincott.

Fischgold H, Metzger J: Etude radiotomographique de l'impression basilaire, *Rev Rheum Mal Osteoartic* 19:261, 1952.

Harkey HL, Crockard HA, Stevens JM, et al: The operative management of basilar impression in osteogenesis imperfecta, *Neurosurgery* 27:782, 1990.

Hayes M, Parker G, Ell J, Sillence D: Basilar impression complicating osteogenesis imperfecta type IV: the clinical and neuroradiological findings in four cases, *J Neurol Neurosurg Psychiatry* 66:357, 1999.

Hensinger RN: Osseous anomalies of the craniovertebral junction, *Spine* 11:323, 1986.

Hensinger RN, MacEwen GD: Congenital anomalies of the spine. In Rothman RH, Simeone FA, eds: *The spine,* ed 2, Philadelphia, 1982, WB Saunders.

Kohno K, Sakaki S, Nakamur H, et al: Foramen magnum decompression for syringomyelia associated with basilar impression and Chiari I malformation, *Neurol Med Chir* 31:715, 1991.

Kulkarni MV, Williams JC, Yeakley JW, et al: Magnetic resonance imaging in the diagnosis of the craniocervical manifestations of the mucopolysaccharidoses, *Magn Reson Imaging* 5:317, 1987.

Lee CK, Weiss AB: Isolated congenital cervical block vertebrae below the axis with neurological symptoms, *Spine* 6:118, 1981.

McAfee PC, Bohlman HH, Han JS, et al: Comparison of nuclear magnetic resonance imaging and computed tomography in the diagnosis of upper cervical spinal cord compression, *Spine* 11:295, 1986.

McGregor M: The significance of certain measurements of the skull in the diagnosis of basilar impression, *Br J Radiol* 21:171, 1948.

McRae DL: The significance of abnormalities of the cervical spine, *Am J Roentgenol* 84:3, 1960.

Raynor RB: Congenital malformations of the base of the skull. In Cervical Spine Research Society: *The cervical spine,* Philadelphia, 1983, JB Lippincott.

Rush PJ, Berbrayer D, Reilly BJ: Basilar impression and osteogenesis imperfecta in a three-year-old girl: CT and MRI, *Pediatr Radiol* 19:142, 1989.

Teodori JB, Painter MJ: Basilar impression in children, *Pediatrics* 74:1097, 1984.

Wong V, Fung CF: Basilar impression in a child with hypochondroplasia, *Pediatr Neurol* 7:62, 1990.

ATLANTOOCCIPITAL FUSION

Hensinger RN: Atlantooccipital fusion. In Cervical Spine Research Society: *The cervical spine,* Philadelphia, 1983, JB Lippincott.

Kalla AK, Khanna S, Singh IP, et al: A genetic and anthropological study of atlanto-occipital fusion, *Hum Genet* 81:105, 1989.

McRae DL: Bony abnormalities in the region of the foramen magnum: correlation of the anatomic and neurologic findings, *Acta Radiol* 40:335, 1953.

McRae DL: The significance of abnormalities of the cervical spine, *Am J Roentgenol* 84:3, 1960.

McRae DL, Barnum AS: Occipitalization of the atlas, *Am J Roentgenol* 70:23, 1953.

Sakou T, Kawaida H, Morizono Y, et al: Occipitoatlantoaxial fusion utilizing a rectangular rod, *Clin Orthop* 239:137, 1989.

Spillane JD, Pallis C, Jones AM: Developmental abnormalities in the region of the foramen magnum, *Brain* 80:11, 1957.

Watson AG, Mayhew IG: Familial congenital occipitoatlantoaxial malformation (OAAM) in the Arabian horse, *Spine* 11:334, 1986.

KLIPPEL-FEIL SYNDROME

Al-Rajeh S, Chowdhary UM, Al-Freihi H, et al: Thoracic disc protrusion and situs inversus in Klippel-Feil syndrome, *Spine* 15:1379, 1987.

Baird PA, Robinson CG, Buckler WSJ: Klippel-Feil syndrome, *Am J Dis Child* 113:546, 1967.

Beals RK, Rolfe B: VATER association: a unifying concept of multiple anomalies, *J Bone Joint Surg* 71A:948, 1989.

Bhagat R, Pant K, Singh VK, et al: Pulmonary developmental anomaly associated with Klippel-Feil syndrome and anomalous atrioventricular conduction, *Chest* 101:1157, 1992.

Bonola A: Surgical treatment of the Klippel-Feil syndrome, *J Bone Joint Surg* 38B:440, 1956.

Born CT, Petrik M, Freed M, et al: Cerebrovascular accident complicating Klippel-Feil syndrome: a case report, *J Bone Joint Surg* 70A:1412, 1988.

Drvaric DM, Ruderman RJ, Conrad RW, et al: Congenital scoliosis and urinary tract abnormalities: are intravenous pyelograms necessary? *J Pediatr Orthop* 7:441, 1987.

Dubey SP, Ghosh LM: Klippel-Feil syndrome with congenital conductive deafness: report of a case and review of the literature, *Int J Pediatr Otorhinolaryngol* 25:201, 1993.

Dubousset J: Torticollis in children caused by congenital anomalies of the atlas, *J Bone Joint Surg* 68A:178, 1986.

Farmer SF, Ingram DA, Stephens JA: Mirror movements studied in a patient with Klippel-Feil syndrome, *J Physiol* 428:467, 1990.

Feil A: L'absence et la dimunution des vertebres cervicales (etude clinique et pathogenique): le syndrome de reduction numerique cervicale, *Theses de Paris,* 1919.

Fielding JW, Hensinger RN, Hawkins RJ: The cervical spine. In Lovell WW, Winter RB, eds: *Pediatric orthopaedics,* ed 2, Philadelphia, 1986, JB Lippincott.

Guille JT, Miller A, Bowen JR, et al: The natural history of Klippel-Feil syndrome: clinical, roentgenographic, and magnetic resonance imaging findings at adulthood, *J Pediatr Orthop* 15:617, 1995.

Gunderson CH, Greenspan RH, Glaser GH, et al: Klippel-Feil syndrome: genetic and clinical reevaluation of cervical fusion, *Medicine* 46:491, 1967.

Gunderson CH, Soltaire GB: Mirror movements in patients with the Klippel-Feil syndrome: neuropathic observations, *Arch Neurol* 18:675, 1968.

Hall JE, Simmons ED, Danylchuk K, et al: Instability of the cervical spine and neurological involvement in Klippel-Feil syndrome: a case report, *J Bone Joint Surg* 72A:460, 1990.

Hensinger RN: Congenital anomalies of the atlantoaxial joint. In Cervical Spine Research Society: *The cervical spine,* Philadelphia, 1983, JB Lippincott.

Hensinger RN: Congenital anomalies of the odontoid. In Cervical Spine Research Society: *The cervical spine,* Philadelphia, 1983, JB Lippincott.

Hensinger RN, Fielding JW, Hawkins RJ: Congenital anomalies of the odontoid process, *Orthop Clin North Am* 9:901, 1978.

Hensinger RN, Lang JR, MacEwen EG: Klippel-Feil syndrome: a constellation of associated anomalies, *J Bone Joint Surg* 56A:1246, 1974.

Herring JA, Bunnell WP: Klippel-Feil syndrome with neck pain, *J Pediatr Orthop* 9:343, 1989.

Johnson MC: Klippel-Feil syndrome revisited: diagnostic pitfalls impacting neurosurgical management, *Childs Nerv Syst* 8:322, 1991.

Klippel M, Feil A: Un cas d'absence des vertebres cervicales avec cage thoracique remontant jusqu'a la base du crane, *Nouv Icon Salpetriere* 25:223, 1912.

Kulkarni MV, Williams JC, Yeakley JW, et al: Magnetic resonance imaging in the diagnosis of the craniocervical manifestations of the mucopolysaccharidoses, *Magn Reson Imaging* 5:317, 1987.

Lee CK, Weiss AB: Isolated congenital cervical block vertebrae below the axis with neurological symptoms, *Spine* 6:118, 1981.

McBride WZ: Klippel-Feil syndrome, *Am Fam Physician* 45:633, 1992.

McGaughran JM, Kuna P, Das V: Audiological abnormalities in the Klippel-Feil syndrome, *Arch Dis Child* 79:352, 1998.

Patel PR, Lauerman WC: Historical perspective of Maurice Klippel, *Spine* 20:2157, 1995.

Pizzutillo PD: Klippel-Feil syndrome. In Cervical Spine Research Society: *The cervical spine,* Philadelphia, 1983, JB Lippincott.

Pizzutillo PD, Woods M, Nicholson L, MacEwen GD: Risk factors in Klippel-Feil syndrome, *Spine* 19:2110, 1994.

Prusick VR, Samberg LC, Wesolowski DP: Klippel-Feil syndrome associated with spinal stenosis, *J Bone Joint Surg* 67A:161, 1985.

Raynor RB: Congenital malformations of the base of the skull. In Cervical Spine Research Society: *The cervical spine,* Philadelphia, 1983, JB Lippincott.

Ritterbusch JF, McGinty LD, Spar J, et al: Magnetic resonance imaging for stenosis and subluxation in Klippel-Feil syndrome, *Spine* 16:539, 1991.

Roach JW, Duncan D, Wenger D, et al: Atlantoaxial instability and spinal cord compression in children: diagnosis by computerized tomography, *J Bone Joint Surg* 66A:708, 1984.

Rock JP, Spickler EM: Anomalous rib presenting as cervical myelopathy: a previously unreported variant of Klippel-Feil syndrome, *J Neurosurg* 75:465, 1991.

Ross CA, Curnes JT, Greenwood RS: Recurrent vertebrobasilar embolism in an infant with Klippel-Feil anomaly, *Pediatr Neurol* 3:181, 1987.

Sherk HH, Dawoud S: Congenital os odontoideum with Klippel-Feil syndrome and fatal atlantoaxial instability: report of a case, *Spine* 6:42, 1981.

Sherk HH, Shut L, Chung S: Iniencephalic deformity of the cervical spine with Klippel-Feil anomalies and congenital elevation of the scapula: report of three cases, *J Bone Joint Surg* 56A:1254, 1974.

Smith BA, Griffen C: Klippel-Feil syndrome, *Ann Emerg Med* 21:876, 1992.

Southwell RB, Reynolds AF, Badger VM, et al: Klippel-Feil syndrome with cervical cord compression resulting from cervical subluxation in association with an omovertebral bone, *Spine* 5:480, 1980.

Spierings ELH, Braakman R: The management of os odontoideum: analysis of 37 cases, *J Bone Joint Surg* 64B:422, 1982.

Theiss SM, Smith MD, Winter RB: The long-term follow-up of patients with Klippel-Feil syndrome and congenital scoliosis, *Spine* 22:1219, 1997.

Thomsen MN, Schneider U, Weber M, Johannisson R: Scoliosis and congenital anomalies associated with Klippel-Feil syndrome types I and II, *Spine* 22:396, 1997.

Tori JA, Dickson JH: Association of congenital anomalies of the spine and kidneys, *Clin Orthop* 148:259, 1980.

Tredwell SJ, Smith DF, MacLeod PJ, et al: Cervical spine anomalies in fetal alcohol syndrome, *Spine* 7:331, 1982.

Ulmer JL, Elster AD, Ginsberg LE, et al: Klippel-Feil syndrome: CT and MR of acquired and congenital abnormalities of cervical spine and cord, *J Comput Assist Tomogr* 17:215, 1993.

VanRijn PM, Cremers CW: Surgery for congenital conductive deafness in Klippel-Feil syndrome, *Ann Otol Rhinol Laryngol* 97:347, 1988.

Whittle IR, Besser M: Congenital neural abnormalities presenting with mirror movements in a patient with Klippel-Feil syndrome: case report, *J Neurosurg* 59:891, 1983.

Winter RB, Lonstein JE, Leonard AS: *Congenital deformities of the spine,* New York, 1983, Thieme-Stratton.

Yousefzadeh DK, El-Khoury GY, Smith WL: Normal sagittal diameter and variation in the pediatric cervical spine, *Pediatr Radiol* 144:319, 1982.

ATLANTOAXIAL ROTATORY SUBLUXATION

Burkus JK, Deponte RJ: Chronic atlantoaxial rotatory fixation correction by cervical traction, manipulation, and bracing: case report, *J Pediatr Orthop* 6:631, 1986.

Coutts MB: Atlantooccipital subluxations, *Arch Surg* 29:297, 1934.

Fielding JW: The cervical spine in the child, *Curr Pract Orthop Surg* 5:31, 1973.

Fielding JW, Francis WR, Hawkins RJ, et al: Atlantoaxial rotary deformity, *Semin Spine Surg* 3:33, 1991.

Fielding JW, Hawkins RJ: Atlantoaxial rotatory fixation (fixed rotatory subluxation of the atlantoaxial joint), *J Bone Joint Surg* 59A:37, 1977.

Fielding JW, Hawkins RJ, Ratzan S: Fusion for atlantoaxial instability, *J Bone Joint Surg* 58A:400, 1976.

Firrani-Gallotta G, Luzzatti G: Sublussazione laterale e sublussazione rotatorie dell'atlante, *Arch Orthop Trauma Surg* 70:467, 1957.

Georgopoulos G, Pizzutillo PD, Lee MS: Occipitoatlantal instability in children: a report of five cases and review of the literature, *J Bone Joint Surg* 69A:429, 1987.

Hensinger RN, DeVito PD, Ragsdale CG: Changes in the cervical spine in juvenile rheumatoid arthritis, *J Bone Joint Surg* 68A:189, 1986.

Kawabe N, Hirotani H, Tanaka O: Pathomechanism of atlantoaxial rotatory fixation in children, *J Pediatr Orthop* 9:569, 1989.

Phillips WA, Hensinger RN: The management of rotatory atlantoaxial subluxation in children, *J Bone Joint Surg* 71A:664, 1989.

Subach BR, McLaughlin MR, Albright AL, Pollack IF: Current management of pediatric atlantoaxial rotatory subluxation, *Spine* 23:2174, 1998.

Wackenheim A: *Roentgen diagnosis of the craniovertebral region,* New York, 1974, Springer-Verlag.

Wang J, Vokshoor A, Kim S, et al: Pediatric atlantoaxial instability: management with screw fixation, *Pediatr Neurosurg* 30:70, 1999.

Watson-Jones R: Spontaneous hyperaemic dislocation of the atlas, *Proc R Soc Med* 25:586, 1931.

CERVICAL INSTABILITY IN DOWN SYNDROME

Burke SW, French CHG, Roberts JM, et al: Chronic atlantoaxial instability in Down syndrome, *J Bone Joint Surg* 67A:1356, 1985.

Committee on Sports Medicine: Atlantoaxial instability in Down syndrome, *Pediatrics* 74:152, 1984.

Dormans JP, Drummond DS, Sutton LN, et al: Occipitocervical arthrodesis in children, *J Bone Joint Surg* 77A:1234, 1995.

Dubousset J: Torticollis in children caused by congenital anomalies of the atlas, *J Bone Joint Surg* 68A:178, 1986.

Gabriel KR, Mason DE, Carango P: Occipitoatlantal translation in Down's syndrome, *Spine* 15:997, 1990.

Loder RT, Hensinger RN: Developmental abnormalities of the cervical spine. In Weinstein SL, ed: *The pediatric spine,* vol 1, New York, 1994, Raven.

Menezes AH, Ryken TC: Craniovertebral abnormalities in Down's syndrome, *Pediatr Neurosurg* 18:24, 1992.

Menezes AH, Ryken TC: Craniovertebral junction abnormalities. In Weinstein SL, ed: *The pediatric spine,* vol 1, New York, 1994, Raven.

Msall M, Rogers B, DiGaudio K, et al: Long-term complications of segmental cervical fusion in Down syndrome, *Dev Med Child Neurol* 33:5, 1991.

Nordt JC, Stauffer ES: Sequelae of atlantoaxial stabilization of two patients with Down's syndrome, *Spine* 6:437, 1981.

Parfenchuck TA, Bertrand SL, Powers MJ, et al: Posterior occipitoatlantal hypermobility in Down syndrome: an analysis of 199 patients, *J Pediatr Orthop* 14:304, 1994.

Pueschel SM: Should children with Down syndrome be screened for atlantoaxial instability? *Arch Pediatr Adolesc Med* 152:123, 1998.

Pueschel SM, Findley TW, Furia J, et al: Atlantoaxial instability in Down syndrome: roentgenographic, neurologic, and somatosensory-evoked potential studies, *J Pediatr* 110:515, 1987.

Pueschel SM, Herndon JH, Gelch MM, et al: Symptomatic atlantoaxial subluxation in persons with Down syndrome, *J Pediatr Orthop* 4:682, 1984.

Pueschel SM, Scola FH, Perry CD, et al: Atlantoaxial instability in children with Down syndrome, *Pediatr Radiol* 10:129, 1981.

Pueschel SM, Scola FH, Pezzullo JC: A longitudinal study of atlantodens relationships in asymptomatic individuals with Down syndrome, *Pediatrics* 89:1194, 1992.

Pueschel SM, Scola FH, Tupper TB, et al: Skeletal anomalies of the upper cervical spine in children with Down syndrome, *J Pediatr Orthop* 10:607, 1990.

Segal LS, Drummond DS, Zanotti RM, et al: Complications of posterior arthrodesis of the cervical spine in patients who have Down syndrome, *J Bone Joint Surg* 73A:1547, 1991.

Smith MD, Phillips WA, Hensinger RN: Complications of fusion to the upper cervical spine, *Spine* 16:702, 1991.

Smith MD, Phillips WA, Hensinger RN: Fusion of the upper cervical spine in children and adolescents: an analysis of 17 patients, *Spine* 16:695, 1991.

Spitzer R, Rabinowitch JY, Wybar KC: A study of the abnormalities of the skull, teeth, and lenses in mongolism, *Can Med Assoc J* 84:567, 1961.

Tredwell SJ, Newman DE, Lockitch G: Instability of the upper cervical spine in Down syndrome, *J Pediatr Orthop* 10:602, 1990.

Van Dyke DC, Gahagan CA: Down syndrome, cervical spine abnormalities, and problems, *Clin Pediatr* 27:415, 1988.

Wiesel SW, Rothman RH: Occipitoatlantal hypermobility, *Spine* 4:187, 1979.

Winter RB, Lonstein JE, Leonard AS: *Congenital deformities of the spine*, New York, 1983, Thieme-Stratton.

FAMILIAL CERVICAL DYSPLASIA

Saltzman CL, Hensinger RN, Blane CE, Phillips WA: Familial cervical dysplasia, *J Bone Joint Surg* 73A:163, 1991.

INTERVERTEBRAL DISC CALCIFICATION

Ginalski JM, Landry M, Gudinchet F, Schnyder P: Is tomography of intervertebral disc calcification useful in children? *Pediatr Radiol* 22:59, 1992.

Hahn YS, McLone DG, Uden D: Cervical intervertebral disc calcification in children, *Childs Nerv Syst* 3:274, 1987.

Herring JA, Hensinger RN: Cervical disc calcification, *J Pediatr Orthop* 8:613, 1988.

Oda J, Tanaka H, Tsuzuki N: Intervertebral disc changes with aging of human cervical vertebra from the neonate to the eighties, *Spine* 13:1205, 1988.

Pattisapu JV, Evans OB, Blumenthal BI: Intervertebral disc calcification in children, *Pediatr Neurol* 3:108, 1987.

Sonnabend DH, Taylor TKF, Chapman GK: Intervertebral disc calcification syndromes in children, *J Bone Joint Surg* 64B:25, 1982.

Wong CC, Pereira B, Pho RW: Cervical disc calcification in children: a long-term review, *Spine* 17:139, 1992.

C H A P T E R

38 Scoliosis and Kyphosis

Barney L. Freeman III

SCOLIOSIS

The Scoliosis Research Society (SRS) recommends that idiopathic scoliosis be classified according to the age of the patient when the diagnosis is made. Infantile scoliosis occurs from birth to 3 years of age, juvenile idiopathic scoliosis between the ages of 4 and 10 years, and adolescent idiopathic scoliosis between 10 years of age and skeletal maturity. This traditional chronological definition of scoliosis is important because major differences exist between the subtypes (Table 38-1).

Conner, Dickson et al., and Davies and Reid advocated a distinction between early-onset and late-onset scoliosis because of the effects of the deformity on cardiopulmonary development. During childhood, not only do the lungs grow in size, but also the alveoli and arteries multiply and the pattern of vascularity changes. The alveoli in the pulmonary tree increase by about tenfold between infancy and 4 years of age and are not completely developed until 8 years of age. Scoliotic deformity limits the space available for lung growth, and children who develop significant scoliosis before the age of 5 years generally have disabling dyspnea or cardiorespiratory failure.

Infantile Idiopathic Scoliosis

Infantile idiopathic scoliosis is a structural, lateral curvature of the spine occurring in patients younger than 3 years of age. James, who first used the term *infantile idiopathic scoliosis*, noted that these curves occurred before 3 years of age, were more frequent in boys than in girls, and were primarily thoracic and convex to the left.

Wynne-Davies noted plagiocephaly in 97 children in whom curves developed in the first 6 months of life; the flat side of the head was on the convex side of the curve. She also found mental retardation in 13%, inguinal hernias in 7.4% of boys with progressive scoliosis, congenital dislocation of the hip in 3.5%, and congenital heart disease in 2.5% of all patients. This led her to believe that the etiological factors of infantile idiopathic scoliosis are multiple, with a genetic tendency that is either "triggered" or prevented by external factors.

McMaster and Macnicol suggested that infantile idiopathic scoliosis is preventable and that the position in which an infant is laid may be the causative factor. Brown et al. and Mau observed that during the first few months of life all infants have a natural tendency to turn toward their right side when laid supine. McMaster et al. postulated that when an infant is laid supine and partially turned toward the right side, gravity causes plastic deformation of the immature thorax. The uppermost hemithorax tends to fall backward, causing the thoracic vertebrae to rotate backward on their long axes (Fig. 38-1). Biomechanical coupling of axial rotation and lateral bending then produces a lateral curvature of the spine with a left-sided thoracic scoliosis in infants lying on their right sides. If laid in the prone position, a child cannot roll onto its side, and this prevents asymmetrical molding of the thorax and promotes early maturation of the spinal extensor muscles. McMaster et al. found that no infants in Edinburgh who were laid prone subsequently developed infantile idiopathic scoliosis and suggested that the ideal treatment for this condition is prevention by laying infants prone.

Infantile scoliosis may be progressive, usually increasing rapidly, or resolving (structural resolving) spontaneously within a few years with or without treatment. The resolving type occurs in 70% to 90% of patients with infantile idiopathic scoliosis. Unfortunately, when a curve is mild, no absolute

Table 38-1 Classification of Idiopathic Scoliosis by Age

	Infantile	Juvenile	Adolescent
Age at presentation	Birth to 3 yr	4 to 9 yr	10 to 20 yr
Male:female	1:1 to 2:1	<6 yr: 1:3 >6 yr: 1:6	1:6
Incidence	United States: 2% to 3% Great Britain: 30%	United States: 12% to 15% Great Britain: 12% to 15%	United States: 85% Great Britain: 55%
Curve types	Left thoracic L:R (2:1) Left thoracic/right lumbar	Right thoracic R:L (6:1)	Right thoracic R:L (8:1)
Associated findings	Mental deficiency, CDH, plagiocephaly, congenital heart defects	None	None
Risk of cardiopulmonary compromise	High	Intermediate	Low
Risk of curve progression	<6 mo: low >1 yr: high	67%	23%

Risk of curve progression	Gradual progression:
	  2 to 3 degrees/yr
	Malignant progression:
	  10 degrees/yr
		Progression at puberty:
		  6 degrees/yr
		Malignant progression:
		  10 degrees/yr
			Rate of progression 1 to 2 degrees/mo during puberty

Curve resolution	<1 yr: 90% >1 yr: 20%	20%	Rare
Curve magnitude and maturity	Gradual progression: 70 to 90 degrees Malignant progression: >90 degrees	Progression at puberty: 50 to 90 degrees Malignant progression: >90 degrees	Curves over 90 degrees rare
Orthotic management	Effective at delaying and slowing rate of progression Ultimate progression 100%	Decreases rate of progression until puberty (failure rate 30% to 80%)	Effectively controls curves <40 degrees (success rate 75% to 80%)
Surgical treatment	Instrumentation without fusion <8 yr After 8 yr: ASF/PSF After 11 yr: PSF	Instrumentation without fusion <8 yr After 8 yr: ASF/PSF After 11 yr: PSF	PSF with instrumentation ASF if under 11 yr with open triradiate cartilage
Risk of crankshaft	High	High	Low

From Mardjetko SM: Infantile and juvenile scoliosis. In Bridwell KH, DeWald RL, eds: *The textbook of spinal surgery,* ed 2, Philadelphia, 1997, Lippincott-Raven.
ASF, Anterior spinal fusion; *PSF,* posterior spinal fusion; *CDH,* congenital hip dysplasia.

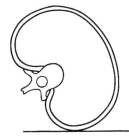 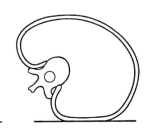

Fig. 38-1 Diagram illustrates postural moulding of thorax when baby is laid supine and partly turned toward its side. (From McMaster MJ: *J Bone Joint Surg* 65B:612, 1983.)

criteria are available for differentiating the two types. James et al. analyzed 212 children with juvenile idiopathic scoliosis and found that those with resolving scoliosis generally had a deformity that was noted before 1 year of age; most had smaller curves at presentation, and none had compensatory curves. Lloyd-Roberts and Pilcher found that curves associated with plagiocephaly or other molding abnormalities were more likely to be resolving, indicating an intrauterine positioning cause for this scoliosis. According to James, when compensatory or secondary curves develop or when the curve measures more than 37 degrees by the Cobb method when first seen, the scoliosis probably is progressive.

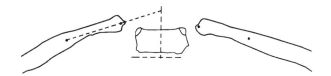

Fig. 38-2 Construction of rib-vertebral angle (RVA). (From Mehta MH: *J Bone Joint Surg* 54B:232, 1972.)

Mehta developed a method for differentiating resolving from progressive curves in infantile idiopathic scoliosis based on measurement of the rib-vertebral angle (RVA). She evaluated the relationship of the convex rib head and vertebral body of the apical vertebra by drawing one line perpendicular to the apical vertebral endplate and another from the midneck to the midhead of the corresponding rib; the angle formed by the intersection of these lines is the RVA (Fig. 38-2). The RVA difference (RVAD) is the difference between the values of the RVAs on the concave and convex sides of the curve. If the convex apical rib head does not overlap the apical vertebral body, a curve with an initial RVAD of 20 degrees or more is considered progressive. If the convex apical rib head overlaps the apical vertebral body on the anteroposterior roentgenogram, progression is highly likely. This measurement is helpful in predicting curve progression, but the curves must be monitored closely to prevent severe progression with the resultant risk of restricted pulmonary disease.

TREATMENT

Treatment options for children with infantile idiopathic scoliosis include (1) serial casting, progressing to bracing and later fusion, (2) preoperative traction to correct the curve followed by fusion, and (3) subcutaneous instrumentation without fusion. If the RVAD is more than 20 degrees and the curve is not flexible on clinical examination, it is considered progressive until proved otherwise. A competent orthotist can make a satisfactory thoracic-lumbar-sacral-orthosis (TLSO) or cervical-thoracic-lumbar-sacral orthosis (CTLSO) for curves that are not too large. Progression of many infantile curves can be prevented and significant improvement can be obtained with the use of a well-fitting orthosis during the early period of skeletal growth. In a very young child, serial casting with general anesthesia may be required until the child is large enough for a satisfactory orthosis. The interval between cast changes is determined by the rate of the child's growth, but usually a cast change is required every 2 to 3 months. Brace wear is continued full time until the curve stability has been maintained for at least 2 years. At that point brace wear can be gradually reduced. McMaster reported control of the curves of 22 children with infantile scoliosis with an average brace time of more than 6 years.

If a curve is severe or increases despite the use of an orthosis, surgical stabilization is needed. Ideally, surgery should not only stop progression of the curve but also allow continued growth of the thorax and development of the pulmonary tree. When surgical fusion is necessary, a relatively short anterior and posterior arthrodesis should be considered, including only the structural or primary curve. Combined anterior and posterior arthrodesis is necessary to prevent the "crankshaft" phenomenon (p. 1755). If technically possible, subcutaneous growth rods should be considered (Technique 38-1).

Juvenile Idiopathic Scoliosis

Juvenile idiopathic scoliosis appears between the ages of 4 and 10 years. Multiple patterns can occur, but the convexity of the thoracic curve usually is to the right. The natural history of juvenile idiopathic scoliosis is considered to be more progressive than that of adolescent idiopathic scoliosis. Lonstein found that 67% of patients younger than 10 years of age demonstrated curve progression and that the risk of progression was 100% in patients younger than 10 years of age who had curves of more than 20 degrees.

Lewonowski et al. recommended routine magnetic resonance imaging (MRI) for patients under the age of 11 years with idiopathic scoliosis. The necessity of MRI in every child with scoliosis who is younger than 11 years of age has not yet been substantiated, but specific factors that indicate a need for further evaluation include (1) pain, (2) rapid progression, (3) left thoracic deformity, (4) neurological abnormalities (alteration in the superficial abdominal reflex), and (5) other neurological findings, such as loss of bowel or bladder control.

TREATMENT

Although likely to progress and require surgery, juvenile idiopathic scoliosis is treated according to guidelines similar to those for adolescent idiopathic scoliosis. For curves of less than 20 degrees, observation is indicated, with examination and standing posteroanterior roentgenograms every 4 to 6 months. Evidence of progression on the roentgenograms as indicated by a change of at least 5 to 7 degrees warrants brace treatment. If the curve is not progressing, observation is continued until skeletal maturity.

Although much of the literature concerning orthotic treatment of juvenile idiopathic scoliosis has emphasized the Milwaukee brace, a TLSO often is used for thoracic curves with the apex at T8 or below. Initially, the brace is worn full time (22 out of 24 hours). If the curve improves after at least 1 year of full-time brace bracing, the hours per day of brace wear can be decreased gradually to a nighttime-only bracing program, which is much more tolerable, especially when the child reaches puberty. However, the patient is carefully followed for any sign of curve progression during this weaning process. If curve progression is noted, a full-time brace program is resumed.

The success of nonoperative treatment is variable. In the series of Figueiredo and James, 44% of patients were successfully managed conservatively; 56% required spinal

BOX 38-1 • Evaluation of Brace Treatment
of Juvenile Idiopathic Scoliosis
Using the RVAD

If the RVAD progresses above 10 degrees during brace wear, progression can be expected.

If the RVAD values decline as treatment continues, part-time Milwaukee brace wear should be adequate.

Those curves with RVAD values near or below 0 degrees at the time of diagnosis generally will require only a short period of full-time brace wear before part-time brace wear is begun.

fusion. In Tolo and Gillespie's series, 27% of patients required surgical fusion for progressive curves. Tolo and Gillespie found that it was not possible to predict which curves would increase from the curve pattern, the degree of curvature, or the patient's age at the time of diagnosis. Although they found the initial RVAD measurement of only limited value, serial measurements were useful to evaluate brace treatment. Several guidelines can be formulated for evaluating brace treatment (Box 38-1).

Tolo and Gillespie recommended that, unless the curve is greater than 30 degrees when the juvenile patient is first seen, evidence of progression be obtained before a Milwaukee brace is applied because some curves, even in the range of 20 to 30 degrees, did not progress over a period of several months. Mannherz et al. confirmed that the RVAD was helpful in predicting progression in most juvenile idiopathic scoliosis curves. The initial RVAD was not helpful, but progressive RVAD to greater than 10 degrees over time was associated with curve progression. A higher incidence of curve progression also was noted in patients with less than 20 degrees of thoracic kyphosis. Double major curves tended to progress most often.

Kahanovitz, Levine, and Lardone found that patients with curves of less than 35 degrees and RVADs of less than 20 degrees had excellent prognoses when treated in a part-time Milwaukee brace program. Patients with curvatures of greater than 45 degrees at the onset of bracing and whose RVADs exceeded 20 degrees all eventually underwent spinal fusion. Patients with curvatures from 35 to 45 degrees at the onset of bracing had much less predictable prognoses. The part-time brace program consisted of wearing the brace after school and all night for approximately a year. The patients were then kept in the brace at night only for another 2.5 years. The brace was at that point worn every other night for an average of 1.2 years. Bracing generally was discontinued completely at an average of about 14 years of age. Individually, however, the numbers of hours spent wearing the brace depended on the amount of improvement and stability of the curvature. Part-time brace treatment may afford these children the social and psychological benefits not provided by a full-time Milwaukee brace program. The Milwaukee brace may be preferred because it does not cause chest wall compression in these young patients. A total contact TLSO often is prescribed, but rib cage distortion is possible because of the lengthy time the child must wear the brace. Early reports of the part-time Charleston bending brace were encouraging, but its usefulness has not been established (see p. 1771).

(see p. 1771).

Even if the curve progresses, bracing may slow progression and delay surgery until the child is older, which may avoid a short trunk and lessen the possibility of a crankshaft phenomenon. If orthotic treatment fails, either a subcutaneous rod or multihook segmental system or spinal fusion should be considered. If the child is younger than 8 years of age and small, the ideal treatment is subcutaneous rod insertion, with or without an anterior apical growth arrest procedure. If the child is larger and 9 or 10 years of age, fusion may be appropriate, but combined anterior and posterior spinal fusions should be considered to avoid a crankshaft phenomenon.

Dimeglio found that during the first 5 years of life the spine from T1 to S1 grows more than 2 cm a year. Between the ages of 5 and 10 years, it grows 0.9 cm a year, and then 1.8 cm a year during puberty (Fig. 38-3). In 24 children with infantile or juvenile idiopathic scoliosis, Hefti and McMaster found that a solid spinal fusion stopped the longitudinal growth in the posterior elements, but the vertebral bodies continued to grow anteriorly. The anterior growth causes the vertebral bodies and discs to bulge laterally toward the convexity and to pivot on the posterior fusion, causing loss of correction, increasing vertebral rotation, and recurrence of the rib hump. Dubousset, Herring, and Shufflebarger have confirmed this crankshaft phenomenon (Fig. 38-4). If the child is 9 or 10 years old when fusion is considered, if the iliac crest apophysis has not yet appeared, and if the child is premenarchal with a great deal of growth potential left, consideration should be given to combined anterior and posterior fusions to prevent this crankshaft deformity (Fig. 38-5). The exact parameters to determine which children require anterior and posterior fusions have not yet been established, but this crankshaft phenomenon should always be considered in preoperative planning for patients with infantile and juvenile idiopathic scoliosis. Shufflebarger and Clark recommended that patients in the "at-risk" group (those with a Risser sign of 0 to 1, Tanner grade less than 2, and a significant three-dimensional deformity) have preliminary anterior periapical growth arrest and fusion before posterior instrumentation and fusion to prevent the crankshaft phenomenon. Sanders, Herring, and Browne believe that an open triradiate physis in the pelvis also is an important risk factor.

Subcutaneous Harrington Instrumentation
Moe et al. described the use of a subcutaneous Harrington rod without fusion, followed by a full-time external orthosis, in certain flexible curves in growing children. With the use of the "shortening formula" (0.07 cm multiplied by the number of segments fused multiplied by the number of years' growth), the average shortening in their patients would have been 4.5 cm had fusion been done. The authors noted an average length gain in the instrumented area of 3.8 cm for nine patients who ultimately underwent fusion. Complications, most frequently hook dislocation and rod breakage, occurred in 50% of patients. Careful attention to details, especially fusion around the hooks

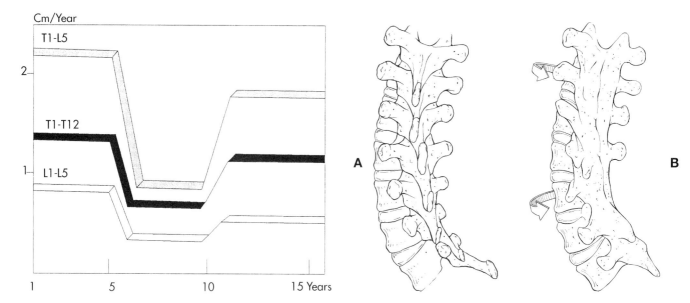

Fig. 38-3   Growth velocity of T1-L5 segment, thoracic segment T1-T12, and lumbar segment L1-L5. (From Dimeglio A: *J Pediatr Orthop* 1:102, 1993.)

Fig. 38-4   Crankshaft phenomenon. **A,** Spine with scoliosis. **B,** Despite solid posterior fusion, continued anterior growth causes increase in deformity. (From Warner WC: Juvenile idiopathic scoliosis. In Weinstein SL: *Pediatric spine*, Philadelphia, 1994, Raven.)

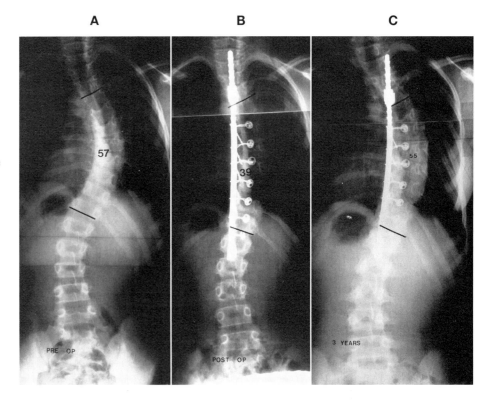

Fig. 38-5   Fifty-seven-degree curve **(A)** was corrected to 39 degrees with posterior fusion and instrumentation **(B). C,** Three years after surgery deformity has recurred because of crankshaft phenomenon.

and routine rod lengthening every 6 months, can help lessen these complications.

The subcutaneous rodding technique should be considered only for a cooperative patient who has a stable family unit. Surgery is required every 6 months to lengthen the construct, and a TLSO is necessary for at least the first 6 months to protect the instrumentation. Ultimately, a definitive spinal fusion is required.

Several different techniques of subcutaneous instrumentation have been described, including Moe's technique with a subcutaneous Harrington rod, sublaminar wires with smooth rods, and the McCarthy technique of dual rods with proximal and distal hook claws. Our preferred technique at this time is the McCarthy technique.

The McCarthy technique combines Moe's original concept of intermittent distraction lengthening with a dual rod segmental hook-rod construct. Subsequent lengthenings are done at 6- to 9-month intervals. To improve correction McCarthy adds an anterior release and annulotomy across three to five apical segments. Patterson et al. prefer apical growth arrest to deal with the apical lordosis often considered the essential lesion in this condition. The upper and lower claws are augmented with intervertebral fusion to improve hook stability. The fusion is protected with an orthosis until solid.

◆ Subcutaneous Dual Rod Instrumentation Without Fusion

A multihook segmental instrumentation system such as the CD Horizon system is used. An infant spinal set may be necessary in children under 30 pounds. This set uses a ⅛-inch smooth rod, which is quite flexible. Therefore protection by some form of external immobilization is necessary until the system can be converted to a pediatric rod system of a larger diameter.

TECHNIQUE 38-1 *(McCarthy)*

Place the patient prone on the operating table or frame; prepare and drape the back in the routine sterile fashion. Take care to select the neutral vertebrae at both ends of the curve and make a single, long, straight incision into the subcutaneous tissue from the upper to the lower neutral vertebrae. Confirm appropriate levels with a roentgenogram. Carry the dissection down to the lamina and spinous process of the end vertebrae. Strip the periosteum from the concave and convex lamina out to the facet joint of the two vertebrae selected for hooks at each end of the curve.

To form the upper "claw," insert a pedicle hook onto the lower of the two vertebrae and a superior transverse process hook on the upper of the two vertebrae on both the concave and convex sides. Form the lower "claw" by placing a supralaminar hook on the upper vertebra and an infralaminar hook on the lower vertebra. Use two rods on the concave side and two rods on the convex side. Contour the rods to the natural contours of thoracic kyphosis and lumbar lordosis.

Insert the rods under direct vision and use appropriate set screws to hold the rods in the hooks. Join the rods in the middle in an overlapping configuration with a low profile growth rod connector (Fig. 38-6). Use bone chips to pack around the upper and lower hook sites. Do not attempt subperiosteal dissection between the hook sites.

AFTERTREATMENT. The child is placed in an orthosis for the first 6 months, at which time it can be discontinued if the hook sites are solidly fused. The rod is then routinely lengthened at 6 months. If necessary, the entire rods can be exposed and longer rods can be inserted and then joined again with the growth connector.

Instrumentation with Fusion

If a child is older than 9 or 10 years of age or is unable to cooperate with the demands of subcutaneous rod insertion, combined anterior and posterior spinal fusion should be considered. The combined procedure is necessary to avoid the crankshaft phenomenon (see Figs. 38-4 and 38-5).

Preferably anterior release and fusion are done without sacrificing the segmental vessels. Anterior instrumentation is not used if posterior instrumentation is scheduled as a second procedure. Posteriorly, a multihook segmental system is used. Many of these systems, such as the Cotrel-Dubousset system, have a variety of different size hooks and rods, depending on the size of the child. Although autologous bone from the posterior iliac crest is recommended, it may have to be augmented with allograft bone in a smaller child. The technique of insertion of posterior multihook segmental instrumentation is described on p. 1882.

Adolescent Idiopathic Scoliosis

ETIOLOGY

The characteristics of adolescent idiopathic scoliosis include a three-dimensional deformity of the spine with lateral curvature plus rotation of the vertebral bodies. Most idiopathic curves are lordotic or hypokyphotic in the thoracic region, and this may represent an important factor in the etiology. The etiology also may be different for different types of curves. Lowe and Peters noted that current research into the etiology of idiopathic scoliosis has identified a number of possible causative factors (Fig. 38-7). Many observers, including Beals, Cowell et al, Dickson, and Harrington noted the role of genetics in the development of idiopathic scoliosis. Lowe et al. concluded that current population studies characterize idiopathic scoliosis as a single gene disorder that follows the pattern of Mendelian genetics, including variable penetrance and heterogeneity. Dubousset and Machida studied the association of low melatonin levels with progressive scoliosis and concluded that

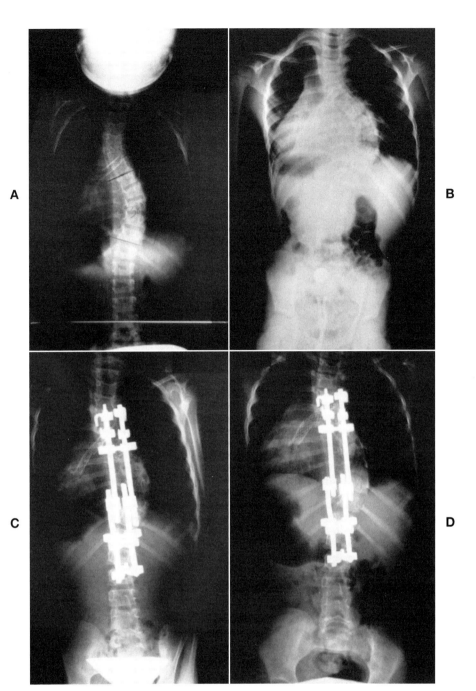

Fig. 38-6 **A** and **B,** Standing posteroanterior roentgenogram of spine in 6-year-old with neurofibromatosis. Despite bracing, her curve increased from 38 degrees (**A**) to 67 degrees (**B**). **C,** Patient has unresectable neurofibroma virtually occluding one lung. It was thought that every effort should be made to allow for continued chest cavity growth and lung expansion. Dual growth rods were inserted per technique of McCarthy. **D,** Standing posteroanterior roentgenogram after routine rod lengthening 6 months later. Curve measurement is now 45 degrees.

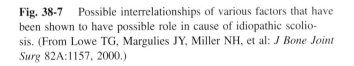
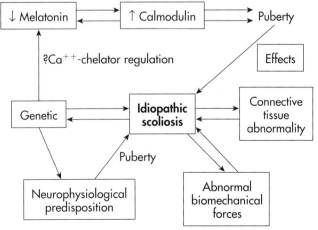

Fig. 38-7 Possible interrelationships of various factors that have been shown to have possible role in cause of idiopathic scoliosis. (From Lowe TG, Margulies JY, Miller NH, et al: *J Bone Joint Surg* 82A:1157, 2000.)

a simple lack of melatonin is not the cause, but rather that melatonin may act as a preventive measure against progression of the curve.

Because scoliosis is common in patients with connective tissue diseases, such as Marfan syndrome, many authors, including Pedrini et al., Taylor et al., Oegema et al., and Roberts et al., have studied the composition of collagen in the intervertebral disc. Echenne et al. and Hadley-Miller et al. also have studied the elastic fiber system. Most authors now believe that any changes in the connective tissue are the result of the deformity rather than the cause. Likewise, studies of skeletal muscle abnormalities seem to indicate that the changes are secondary to the idiopathic scoliosis.

Yarom and Robin demonstrated increased calcium content in the paraspinous muscles of patients with idiopathic scoliosis. This may represent a generalized membrane defect of the calcium pump mechanism. Kindsfater et al. noted markedly increased levels of calmodulin (calcium-binding receptor protein) in patients with progressive idiopathic scoliosis, which also may indicate the possibility of a cell membrane defect.

Although scoliosis often occurs in patients with various neurological disorders, multiple investigations into possible neurological etiologies have not identified any definitive neurological test for the diagnosis or prediction of progression of idiopathic scoliosis. Nevertheless, some form of central nervous system defect may play a role in the development or progression of idiopathic scoliosis.

Various mechanical etiologies also have been proposed. Because idiopathic scoliosis usually is associated with hypokyphosis, the relative imbalance of anterior and posterior growth has been suggested as a cause. The control mechanisms for growth in general still are not totally understood, and the effects on the development of idiopathic scoliosis are still being investigated.

The exact etiology of idiopathic scoliosis, however, remains unknown at this time. The general consensus is that there is a hereditary predisposition and its actual cause is multifactorial.

NATURAL HISTORY

A knowledge of the natural history and prevalence of idiopathic scoliosis is essential to determine if and when treatment is necessary. Three important questions need to be answered:

1. What is the prevalence of idiopathic scoliosis in the general population?
2. What is the likelihood of curve progression necessitating treatment in a child with scoliosis?
3. What problems may occur in adult life if scoliosis is left untreated and the curve progresses?

Idiopathic scoliotic curves of more than 10 degrees are estimated to occur in 2% to 3% of children younger than 16 years of age. Weinstein created a table of calculations that show the decreasing prevalence with increasing curve magnitude (Table 38-2). The importance of these prevalence studies is that small degrees of scoliosis are very common but larger curves

Table 38-2   Adolescent Idiopathic Scoliosis Prevalence

Cobb Angle (Degrees)	Female : Male	Prevalence (%)
>10	1.4-2 : 1	2-3
>20	5.4 : 1	0.3-0.5
>30	10 : 1	0.1-0.3
>40		<0.1

From Weinstein SL: Adolescent idiopathic scoliosis: prevalence and natural history. In Weinstein SL, ed: *The pediatric spine: principles and practice,* New York, 1994, Raven.

BOX 38-2 • Factors Related to Progression of Adolescent Idiopathic Scoliosis

Girls > boys
Premenarchal
Risser sign of 0
Double curves > single curves
Thoracic curves > lumbar curves
More severe curves

---

occur much less frequently. Fewer than 10% of children with curves of 10 degrees or more require treatment.

Once scoliosis has been discovered in a child, the curve must be evaluated for the probability of progression. Most authors define progression as an increase of 5 degrees or more measured by the Cobb measurement over two or more visits. What is unknown is whether this progression will continue and what the final curve will be. Spontaneous improvement can occur in 3% of adolescents with idiopathic scoliosis, most of whom have curves of less than 11 degrees. Certain factors have been found to be related to curve progression (Box 38-2). Progression is more likely in girls than in boys. The time of curve progression in adolescent idiopathic scoliosis generally is during the rapid adolescent growth spurt before the onset of menses. The incidence of progression decreases as the child gets older. Lonstein and Carlson showed that 36% of patients with Risser signs of 0 (no iliac apophyses ossified) showed progression, the incidence of progression falling to 11% for those with Risser signs of 4. Bunnell found that 68% of children in his series with Risser signs of 0 had curves that progressed 10 degrees or more, with the incidence falling to 18% in those with Risser signs of 3 or 4. The incidence of progression also has been found to be related to curve patterns. In general, double curves are more likely to progress than single curves, and single thoracic curves tend to be more progressive than single lumbar curves. The incidence of progression also increases with the curve magnitude. Bunnell estimated that the risk of progression for a 20-degree curve is approximately 20% and the risk for a 50-degree curve is 90%.

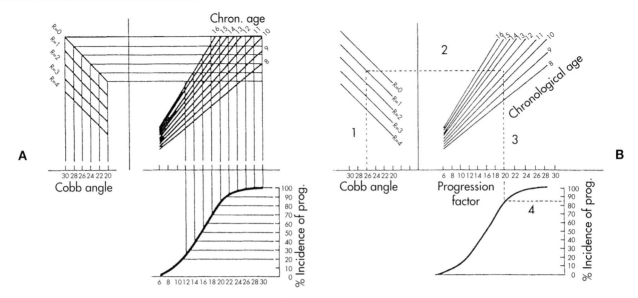

Fig. 38-8   A, Nomogram for prediction of progression of scoliotic curve. **B,** Nomogram constructed for 11.5-year-old child with 26-degree curve and Risser sign of 1. Vertical line *(1)* is drawn from Cobb angle to intercept Risser sign lines, and horizontal line *(2)* is drawn from intersection of this vertical line and Risser sign 1 *(R=1)*. Another vertical line *(3)* is drawn from intersection of line *2* and chronological age of 11.5 years and is extended to intersect progression-factor graph. At intersection of line *3* and graph curve, horizontal line *(4)* is drawn to incidence-of-progression axis and value *(85)* is read. This indicates 85% chance that curve will progress. (From Lonstein JE, Carlson JM: *J Bone Joint Surg* 66A:1038, 1984.)

Lonstein and Carlson developed a nomogram to predict progression of a curve when a patient is first seen (Fig. 38-8).

Suh and MacEwen studied the natural history of idiopathic scoliosis in males only, since they have a much higher prevalence of thoracic curves than do females. The Risser sign was an important indicator of skeletal maturity. The mean rate of curve progression from presentation to Risser 4 maturation was 3 degrees a year. Curves continued to progress until a Risser 5 (complete closure of the iliac crest apophysis) was reached, which may not occur until age 18 or 19 years in some patients. In females, idiopathic scoliosis beyond Risser 4 is considered to be an adult curve. Males with 40-degree to 50-degree curves showed no evidence of continued curve progression beyond Risser 5, contrary to other studies showing that these curves tend to progress 1 degree a year throughout life.

The effect of progressive curves on adults with untreated scoliosis has been studied by several investigators, including Ponseti and Friedman, Nilsonne and Lundgren, Nachemson, Ascani et al., and Weinstein and Ponseti. Five major considerations in the natural history of untreated adolescent idiopathic scoliosis in adults are (1) back pain, (2) pulmonary function, (3) psychosocial effects, (4) mortality, and (5) curve progression.

The incidence of back pain in the general population is between 60% and 80%, and the incidence in patients with idiopathic scoliosis is comparable. Weinstein et al., in a long-term follow-up study of over 40 years, found that 80% of scoliotic patients complained of some backache. In a control group of 100 patients who were age and sex matched and did not have scoliosis, 86% reported backache. The incidence of frequent daily backache was slightly higher in the scoliosis group than in the control group. Patients with lumbar or thoracolumbar curves, especially those with translatory shifts at the lower end of the curves, had a slightly greater incidence of backache than did patients with other curve patterns; the backache in this population was never disabling and was unrelated to the presence of osteoarthritic changes on roentgenogram. Back pain rarely was disabling in any patient with scoliosis, although it was more severe than in adults without scoliosis.

In a recent 50-year follow-up of these same patients, Weinstein et al. used a more detailed and validated questionnaire and found the incidence of back pain in the scoliosis patients was 77% compared with 37% in control subjects. Chronic back pain was reported by 61% of the scoliosis group and 35% of the control subjects. However, the ability of scoliosis patients to perform activities of daily living and work was similar to that of the control subjects. Long-term follow-up studies of Swedish patients, with more than 90% of the patients traced by Kolind-Sörensen, Machemson, and Nilsonne and Lundgren, showed that the most common symptom of patients with scoliosis was backache at the end of a strenuous day or after unusual activities. Pain generally was relieved by rest. The location of pain was variable and generally unrelated to the location or magnitude of the curve.

Table 38-3   Progression Factors in Curves More Than 30 Degrees at Skeletal Maturity

Thoracic	Lumbar	Thoracolumbar
Cobb > 50 degrees	Cobb > 30 degrees	Cobb > 30 degrees
Apical vertical rotation > 30 degrees	Apical vertical rotation > 30 degrees	Apical vertical rotation > 30%
Mehta angle > 30 degrees	Curve direction	Translatory shifts
	Relation L5 to intercrest line	
	Translatory shifts	

From Weinsten SL: *Spine* 24:2592, 1999.

As demonstrated by Kostuik and Bentivoglio and Robin et al., lumbar and thoracolumbar curves may arise in adult life and cause severe pain and discomfort. This degenerative type of scoliosis should not be confused with the natural history of untreated adolescent idiopathic scoliosis. Ultimately, it is important to determine whether the pain is related to scoliosis before treatment determinations are made.

Weinstein et al. found that pulmonary function was affected only in patents with thoracic curves; a direct correlation was found between decreasing vital capacity and increasing curve severity. The pulmonary problem was uniformly restrictive lung disease. Smokers were affected much more severely than nonsmokers. Significant limitations of forced vital capacity in nonsmokers did not occur until the curve approached 100 to 120 degrees.

Weinstein et al. also found that mortality in patients with adult idiopathic scoliosis seemed to be related to thoracic curves greater than 100 degrees, with resultant cor pulmonale. In their 40-year, long-term study, the mortality rate was 15%, but only in 1 patient was cor pulmonale secondary to scoliosis the cause of death. In their subsequent 50-year follow-up, the number of deaths increased as expected but was no different from actuarially predicted rates for patients born in the same year. In the study by Pehrsson et al, no patient with adolescent-onset idiopathic scoliosis died of respiratory failure. Most severe pulmonary effects of idiopathic scoliosis occur in curves that develop before the age of 5 years (p. 1752).

The psychological impact of scoliosis has been studied by numerous authors, including Apter et al., Clayson et al., Eliason and Richman, Fallstrom et al., and Nathan. The unhappiness with the appearance often is correlated with the size of the rib prominence. Weinstein et al. found that middle-aged patients tolerate the psychological effects of scoliosis better than teenagers; however, many adult patients seeking treatment for untreated adolescent idiopathic scoliosis are most concerned with the cosmetic aspects of the disorder.

Studies by Ascani et al., Edgar and Mehta, and Weinstein et al. have demonstrated that curves may continue to progress throughout adult life. Based on the results of their 50-year longitudinal study, Weinstein et al. identified multiple factors that predict the likelihood of curve progression after maturity (Table 38-3). In general, curves in any area of less than 30 degrees at skeletal maturity did not tend to progress in adult life. Larger curves were more likely to progress throughout

adult life, especially thoracic curves between 50 and 75 degrees.

PATIENT EVALUATION

The initial evaluation of the patient should include a thorough history, complete physical and neurological examinations, and roentgenograms of the spine. After the general physical examination, the spine should be examined carefully, and the characteristics of the deformity should be recorded. The height of the patient while standing and while sitting should be measured and recorded; these measurements are compared with later ones to determine changes in the patient's total height and whether any change is caused by growth of the lower extremities or by an increase or a decrease in the height of the trunk. A thorough neurological examination should be done to determine if an intraspinal neoplasm or a neurological disorder is the cause of scoliosis. Particular attention should be given to the abdominal reflexes, as often they are the only neurological abnormality found with some intraspinal disorders.

ROENTGENOGRAPHIC EVALUATION

Posteroanterior and lateral roentgenograms of the spine, including the iliac crest distally and most of the cervical spine proximally, should be made with the patient standing. Inclusion of the iliac crest and the cervical spine generally requires 14 × 36 inch cassettes. The organs most at risk from radiation are the maturing breasts, and radiation is decreased by a factor of 5 to 11 by using the posteroanterior view. Faster roentgenographic film and rare earth screens also reduce the patient's exposure to radiation. Right and left bending films usually are obtained only when the patient is being evaluated for surgery or bracing. If the lumbosacral junction is not well seen on the standing lateral roentgenogram, a spot lateral roentgenogram of the lumbosacral joint should be made to screen for spondylolisthesis.

Deacon et al. demonstrated that standard anteroposterior views of scoliosis curves significantly underestimate the magnitude of the curve. Also, true lateral views demonstrate a lordosis when the more standard lateral views give the erroneous impression of kyphosis (Fig. 38-9). Stagnara described a roentgenographic technique to eliminate this rotational component of the curve. In this technique an oblique roentgenogram is made with the cassette parallel to the medial

A   B   C   D

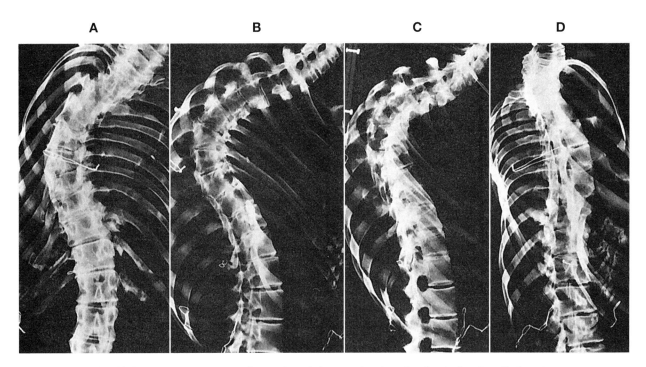

Fig. 38-9 Roentgenograms at four points during rotational cycle of articulated scoliotic spine show changes in Cobb angle with rotation. On anteroposterior view, apparent Cobb angle of 87 degrees **(A)** and true Cobb angle of 128 degrees **(B)**. On lateral view, apparent kyphosis of 61 degrees **(C)** and true apical lordosis of 14 degrees **(D)**. (From Deacon P, Flood BM, Dickson RA: *J Bone Joint Surg* 66B:509, 1984.)

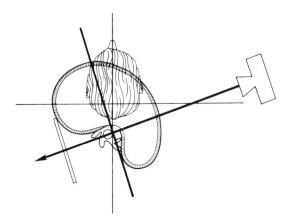

Fig. 38-10 Diagram of Stagnara derotation view. (From Bradford DS et al: *Moe's textbook of scoliosis and other spinal deformities*, ed 2, Philadelphia, 1987, WB Saunders.)

aspect of the rotational rib prominence and the roentgen beam positioned at right angles to the cassette (Fig. 38-10). A film made at 90 degrees to this provides the true lateral view, allowing a much more accurate measurement of the curve size and better evaluation of vertebral anatomy (Fig. 38-11).

Although no absolutely accurate method is available for determining skeletal maturity as an adolescent progresses

through puberty, various roentgenographic parameters can be used to assess maturity, the most common being assessment of bone age at the hand and wrist or the development of the iliac apophysis (Risser sign). Another method is maturation of the vertebral ring apophysis, but this is difficult to see and quantify on routine standing roentgenograms. Little and Sussman found that the Risser sign was less accurate than chronological age as a predictor of skeletal age and recommended that it not be used as a substitute for a hand and wrist roentgenogram in most patients. Biondi et al. and Scoles et al. concluded that by using the Risser sign combined with clinical observations of secondary sexual characteristics, an accurate measure of skeletal maturity can be made without the hand films. Because the normal standing posteroanterior roentgenogram for scoliosis often does not show the full excursion of the iliac apophysis, we combine the hand and wrist films for bone age with the Risser sign and physical signs of maturity, such as breast development and pubic hair. In a younger child, the triradiate apophysis also is a useful sign for indicating skeletal immaturity.

The peak height velocity (PHV) has been reported by several authors to be a better maturity indicator than the Risser sign, chronological age, or menarchal age. PHV is calculated from serial height measurements and is expressed as centimeters of growth per year. Average values of PHVs are 8 cm per year in girls and 9.5 cm per year in boys. Little et al. in a study

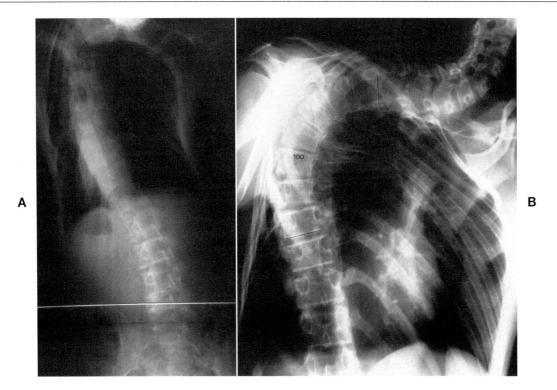

Fig. 38-11 **A,** Standard posteroanterior roentgenogram of large scoliosis. **B,** Stagnara view showing better detail of curve, size, and vertebral anatomy.

of 120 girls with scoliosis found that PHV reliably predicted cessation of growth (3.6 years after PHV in 90%) and likelihood of curve progression. Of 60 patients with curves of more than 30 degrees at PHV, 50 (83%) had curve progression to 45 degrees or more; of 28 with curves of 30 degrees or less at PHV, only 1 (4%) progressed to 45 degrees or more. Little et al. found similar results in boys with scoliosis and reported at 91% accuracy for predicting progression to 45 degrees or more. On both girls and boys, they found the PHV to be superior to the Risser sign, chronological age, and menarchal age as maturity indicator. Sanders et al. evaluated the relationship of the PHV with the occurrence of the crankshaft phenomenon after posterior arthrodesis and instrumentation. They found that in patients with open triradiate cartilages surgery done before or during the time of PHV was a strong predictor of the crankshaft phenomenon.

Measurement of Curves

The Cobb method of measurement recommended by the Terminology Committee of the Scoliosis Research Society (Fig. 38-12) consists of three steps: (1) locating the superior end vertebra, (2) locating the inferior end vertebra, and (3) drawing intersecting perpendicular lines from the superior surface of the superior end vertebra and from the inferior surface of the inferior end vertebra. The angle of deviation of these perpendicular lines from a straight line is the angle of the curve. If the endplates are obscured, the pedicles can be used instead. The end vertebra of the curve is the one that tilts the

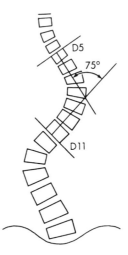

Fig. 38-12 Diagram of Cobb method. (Redrawn from Cobb JR. In The American Academy of Orthopaedic Surgeons: *Instructional course lectures,* vol 5, Ann Arbor, Mich, 1948, JW Edwards.)

most into the concavity of the curve being measured. Generally, when moving away from the apex of the curve, the next intervertebral space below the inferior end vertebra or above the superior end vertebra is wider on the concave side of the curve. Within the curve the intervertebral spaces usually are wider on the convex side and narrower on the concave side. When significantly wedged, the vertebrae themselves, rather than the intervertebral disc spaces, may be wider on the convex

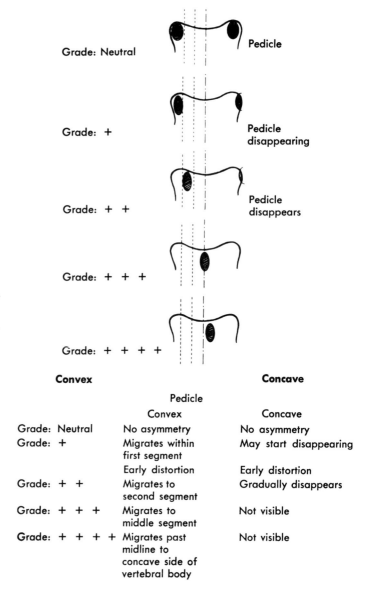

Fig. 38-13 Pedicle method of determining vertebral rotation. Vertebral body is divided into six segments and grades from 0 to 4+ are assigned, depending on location of pedicle within segments. Because pedicle on concave side disappears early in rotation, pedicle on convex side, easily visible through wide range of rotation, is used as standard. (From Nash CL Jr, Moe JH: *J Bone Joint Surg* 51A:223, 1969.)

side of the curve and narrower on the concave side. Carman et al. and Morrissy et al. found that interobserver and intraobserver variations in Cobb measurements average 5 to 7 degrees. These figures should be taken into account when determining whether a curve is truly progressing.

Vertebral Rotation

The two most commonly used methods of determining vertebral rotation are those of Nash and Moe and of Perdriolle and Vidal. In the method of Nash and Moe, if the pedicles are equidistant from the sides of the vertebral bodies, no vertebral rotation is present (0 rotation). The grades progress up to grade IV rotation, in which the pedicle is past the center of the vertebral body (Fig. 38-13). The Perdriolle torsion meter is a template that measures the amount of vertebral rotation on a spinal roentgenogram. The vertebra's pedicle shadow-offset and the edges of the vertebral body are marked and then measured with the torsion meter (Fig. 38-14). The advent of multihook segmental instrumentation systems and awareness of the rotational component of scoliosis increased interest in postoperative measurement of rotation. Because both methods are subject to measurement errors, care must be taken in evaluating postoperative rotation information based on either the Nash and Moe or Perdriolle technique. Theoretically a CT scan is much more accurate in evaluation of vertebral rotation, but CT scanning is inappropriate in routine scoliosis evaluation. Sanders et al. found that changes in the convex rib-vertebral angle were the most consistent findings when monitoring patients postoperatively for increasing rotational deformity caused by the crankshaft phenomenon.

Sagittal Balance

In the past 20 years, the importance of normal sagittal alignment has become recognized in the management of

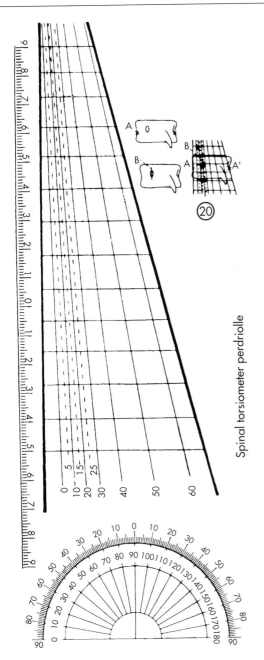

Fig. 38-14 Perdriolle torsion meter for measuring vertebral rotation.

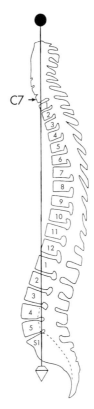

Fig. 38-15 C7 sagittal plumb line is useful measurement of sagittal balance. Plumb line dropped from middle of C7 vertebral body falls close to posterosuperior corner of S1 vertebral body. (From Bernhardt M: Normal spinal anatomy: normal sagittal plane alignment. In Bridwell KH, DeWald RL, eds: *The textbook of spinal surgery,* ed 2, Philadelphia, 1997, Lippincott-Raven.)

patients with spinal deformity. Sagittal alignment can be considered on a segmental, regional, or global basis. Segmental analysis refers to the relationships between two vertebral bodies and the intervening disc. Regional sagittal balance includes that of the cervical, thoracic, or lumbar spines; the thoracolumbar junction often is considered separately. Global spinal alignment generally is considered to be an indication of overall sagittal balance.

Overall spinal sagittal balance is determined by a plumb line dropped from the dens. This plumb line usually falls anterior to the thoracic spine, posterior to the lumbar spine, and through the posterior corner of S1 (Fig. 38-15). On the standing long lateral films generally used in spinal deformity evaluation, the dens is not easily seen. The plumb line, therefore, usually is dropped from the middle of the C7 vertebral body. This plumb line is called the *sagittal vertebral axis* (SVA). A positive SVA is considered present when the plumb line is anterior to the anterior aspect of S1. A negative SVA occurs when this plumb line passes posterior to the anterior body of S1 (Fig. 38-16). In a study of 88 adolescents, Vedantam et al. found that the average SVA was -5.7 ± 3.5 cm. The overall sagittal balance is probably a more important measurement than regional and segmental measurements. Generally to maintain sagittal balance, lumbar lordosis should measure 20 to 30 degrees more than the kyphosis. If overall sagittal balance is not considered, correction to the normal range of lordosis without similar correction of the kyphotic thoracic spine can lead to significant sagittal imbalance (Fig. 38-17).

In the thoracic spine the normal sagittal curvature is kyphotic. The kyphosis begins at the first thoracic vertebra and reaches its maximal segmental kyphosis at T6 or T7. Ranges of thoracic kyphosis in normal patients, both adults and children, have been reported (Table 38-4). Although the kyphosis begins at T1, this vertebra usually cannot be seen on standing long-cassette lateral films. The T4 or T5 vertebra is more easily

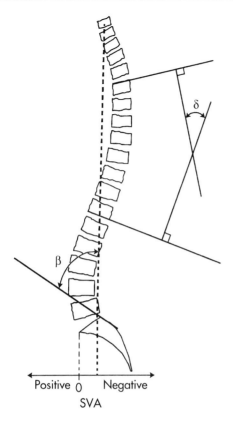

Fig. 38-16 Method of measurement of various parameters of sagittal spinal alignment. Sagittal vertical axis is horizontal distance from C7 plumb line to front corner of sacrum. Positive values indicate position anterior to sacrum; negative values are through or behind sacrum. β, Angle of sacral inclination, is angle subtended by tangent to posterior border of S1 and vertical axis. δ, Cobb angle between two vertebrae. (From Gelb DE, Lenke LG, Bridwell KH, et al: *Spine* 20:1351, 1995.)

seen and measured. Gelb et al. found that the upper thoracic kyphosis T1 to T5 in 100 adults averaged 14 ± 8 degrees. Adding this number to the kyphosis measured from T5 to T12 provides a reasonable estimate of overall regional kyphosis.

The normal regional lumbar sagittal alignment is lordotic. The normal apex of this lordosis is at the vertebral body of L3 or L4 or the disc space itself. The segments at L4-L5 and L5-S1 account for 60% of the overall lumbar lordosis. Wamboldt and Spencer reported that the lumbar discs account for −47 degrees of the lordosis, while the vertebral bodies themselves account for only −12 degrees. This emphasizes the importance of preserving disc height during anterior procedures for the treatment of spinal deformities. Since 40% of the total lumbar lordosis is in the L5-S1 segment, it is important to measure to the top of the sacrum, although this can be difficult on standing lateral images. The lumbar lordosis is a dependent variable based on the amount of kyphosis. To maintain sagittal balance, lordosis generally is 20 to 30 degrees larger than thoracic kyphosis.

The thoracolumbar junction is the transition area from a relatively rigid kyphotic thoracic spine to a relatively mobile lordotic lumbar spine. Bernhardt and Bridwell showed that the thoracolumbar junction is nearly straight. This relationship must be maintained during reconstructive procedures to prevent a junctional kyphosis.

Curve Patterns
Ponseti and Friedman Classification. Idiopathic scoliosis curves were first classified by Ponseti and Friedman into five main patterns (Fig. 38-18). A sixth curve pattern was described by Moe.

1. *Single major lumbar curve.* The lumbar curve has its apex between the L1-L2 disc and L4. These curves

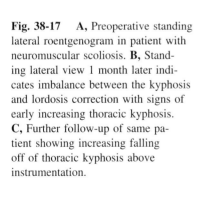

Fig. 38-17 **A,** Preoperative standing lateral roentgenogram in patient with neuromuscular scoliosis. **B,** Standing lateral view 1 month later indicates imbalance between the kyphosis and lordosis correction with signs of early increasing thoracic kyphosis. **C,** Further follow-up of same patient showing increasing falling off of thoracic kyphosis above instrumentation.

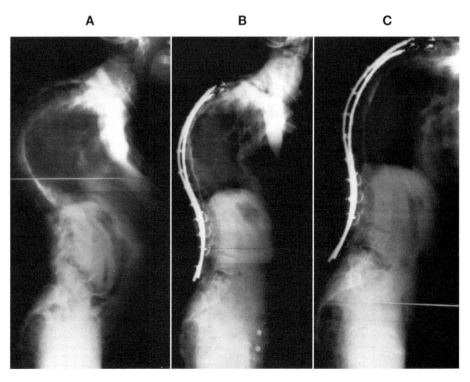

A B C

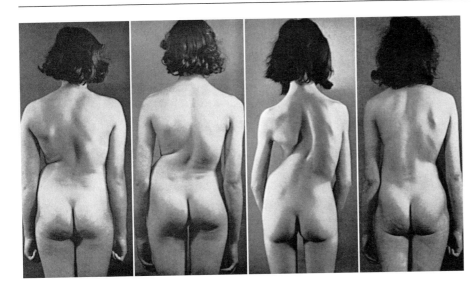

Fig. 38-18 Scoliosis deformity varies with pattern of curve. In each patient shown, angle of primary curve(s) is 70 degrees, but pattern of curve is different. *Left to right*, Lumbar, thoracolumbar, thoracic, and combined thoracic and lumbar curves. (From James JIP: *J Bone Joint Surg* 36B:36, 1954.)

Table 38-4 Mean Global Measures for Thoracic Kyphosis and Lumbar Lordosis in Normal Patients

Study	Patient Age (Yr)	Thoracic End Vertebrae	Mean Thoracic Kyphosis	Lumbar End Vertebrae	Mean Lumbar Lordosis	SVA
Bernhardt and Bridwell	12.8 (5-30)	T3-T12 apex T6-T7 disk	36 ± 10° (9-53°)	T12-L5 apex L3-L4 disk	−44 ± 12° (−14-69°)	
Fon et al	(2-77)	T2-T12	21-45° (5-66°)*			
Gelf et al	57 ± 11 (40-82)	T5-12 apex T7	34 ± 11° (9-66°)	T12-S1 apex L4	−64 ± 10° (−38-84°)	−3.2 ± 3.2 cm
Jackson and McManus	38.9 ± 9.4 (20-63)	T1-T12 apex T7-T8	42.1 ± 8.9° (22-68°)	L1-S1	−60.9 ± 12° (−31-88°)	−0.05 ± 2.5 cm (−6-6.5 cm)
Propst-Proctor and Bleck	Children 2->19	T5-T12	27° (21-33°)	L1-L5	−40° (−31-49.5°)	
Stagnara et al	20-29	T4-IVB†	37° (7-63°)	IVB-S1†	−50° (−32-84°)	
Voutsinas and MacEwen‡	5-20	T2-T12	36.7-38.5°	L1-S1	52.2-56.6°	
Wambolt and Spencer	18			T12-S1	−59° (−31-79°)	
Vedantam et al‡	14.3 (10-18)	T3-T12 apex T6	38 ± 9.8°	T12-S1 apex L4	−64° ± 12°	−5.7 ± 3.5 cm

From Lenke LG, Linville DA, Bridwell KH. In Margulies J, Aebi M, Farcy PC, eds: *Revision spine surgery*, St Louis, 1999, Mosby.
*Range is that of means for all ages male and female; range in parentheses is that of minimum and maximum values for all ages, male and female.
†*IVB*, Intermediate vertebral body, that is, transitional vertebra at thoracolumbar junction (L1, one third; T12, one fifth; L2, one fifth).
‡Values reported were means for three groups of patients grouped by age; ranges reported are upper and lower means for these groups.

produce an asymmetry of the waistline with prominence of the contralateral hip that parents often assume is caused by a short leg on the side of the curve (Fig. 38-19).

2. *Single major thoracolumbar curve.* The thoracolumbar curve apex is at T12 or L1. This curve tends to produce more trunk imbalance than other curves. This decompensation from the midline often produces a severe cosmetic deformity (Fig. 38-20).

3. *Combined thoracic and lumbar curves (double major curves).* Symmetrical double major curves generally cause less visible deformities because the curves are nearly the same degree in size and the trunk usually is well balanced (Fig. 38-21).

4. *Single major thoracic curve.* This curve pattern generally is a convex right pattern (Fig. 38-22). Because of the thoracic location of the curve, rotation of the involved vertebrae may be obvious. The curve produces

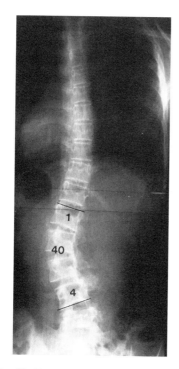

Fig. 38-19   Single major lumbar curve.

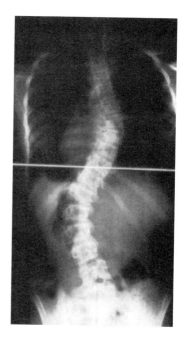

Fig. 38-21   Combined thoracic and lumbar curves with thoracic curve convex to right and lumbar curve convex to left.

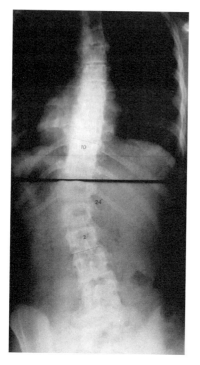

Fig. 38-20   Single major thoracolumbar curve.

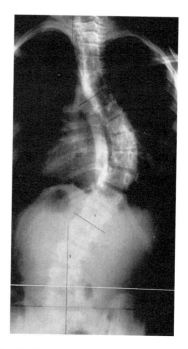

Fig. 38-22   Single major thoracic curve.

prominence of the ribs on the convex side, depression of the ribs on the concave side, and elevation of one shoulder, resulting in an unsightly deformity.

5. *Single major high thoracic curve.* There were only five patients with this curve pattern in the series of Ponseti

and Friedman; although none of these curves became large, the deformity was unsightly because of the elevated shoulder and the deformed thorax. The apex of the curve usually was at T3 with the curve extending from C7 or T1 to T4 or T5.

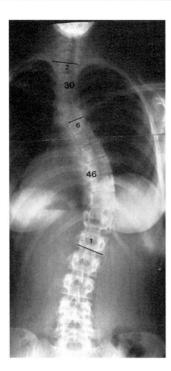

Fig. 38-23 Double major thoracic curve.

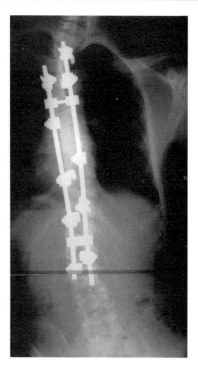

Fig. 38-24 Double major thoracic curve. Lower curve was corrected by fusion and TSRH instrumentation, but rigidity of upper curve caused unsightly shoulder elevation.

6. *Double major thoracic curve.* This pattern was described by Moe and consists of a short upper thoracic curve, often extending from T1 to T5 or T6, with considerable rotation of the vertebrae and other structural changes in combination with the lower thoracic curve extending from T6 to T12 or L1. The upper curve usually is convex to the left, and the lower usually is convex to the right (Fig. 38-23). Deformities in patients with this curve pattern usually are not as severe as in those with a single thoracic curve, but because of asymmetry of the neckline produced by the upper curve, this pattern is more deforming than combined thoracic and lumbar curves. In this curve pattern the highly structural upper curve may be overlooked if the roentgenograms are not made on 14 × 36 inch cassettes and do not include the lower part of the cervical spine. If only the lower thoracic curve is corrected by fusion and instrumentation, the upper curve may not be flexible enough to allow for correct posture and may lead to a cosmetically unacceptable result (Fig. 38-24).

King Classification. The classification system of King et al. is used to describe thoracic curves. Cummings et al. and Lenke et al. found significant interobserver and intraobserver variability in the use of this classification. Identification of curve types using the King classification begins with a careful physical examination. The location and magnitude of the thoracic rib hump and lumbar rotational prominence should be noted, as well as any elevation of the shoulder. Roentgenographic evaluation should include standing posteroanterior, lateral, and

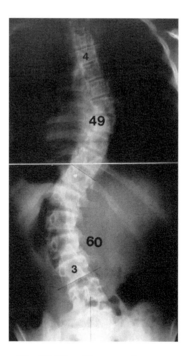

Fig. 38-25 King type I curve.

side-bending roentgenograms. The side-bending films are used to determine flexibility of the individual curves.

1. A King type I curve is recognized easily because the lumbar curve is larger than the thoracic curve (Fig. 38-25). Occasionally, the thoracic and lumbar curves are nearly

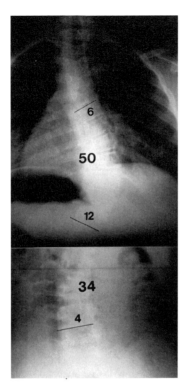

Fig. 38-26   King type II curve.

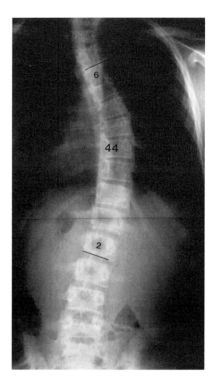

Fig. 38-27   King type III curve.

equal, but the lumbar curve is less flexible on side bending. Clinically, the lumbar rotational prominence is larger than the rib hump.

2. Type II curves have created more confusion than any other curve pattern. As defined by King, type II thoracic scoliosis is a combined thoracic and lumbar curve pattern. On roentgenograms the thoracic curve is larger than or equal to the lumbar curve (Fig. 38-26). The lumbar curve must cross the center sacral line. On supine side-bending roentgenograms the lumbar curve is more flexible than the thoracic curve. On clinical examination the thoracic rib hump is larger than the lumbar rotational prominence.

3. A type III curve is a thoracic scoliosis with the lumbar curve not crossing the midline. The lumbar curve is very flexible on side-bending roentgenograms (Fig. 38-27). On clinical examination the thoracic rib hump is quite apparent, and the lumbar prominence may be quite small or nonexistent.

4. A type IV curve is a single long thoracic curve, with L4 tilted into the curve and L5 balanced over the pelvis (Fig. 38-28).

5. A type V curve is a double structural thoracic curve (Fig. 38-29). On roentgenograms the first thoracic vertebra is tilted into the concavity of the upper curve, which is structural on side-bending films. Clinical examination frequently demonstrates an elevation of the left shoulder. On forward bending there is an upper left thoracic rib hump and a lower right thoracic rib prominence.

Lenke Classification. Lenke et al. proposed a classification based on coronal, sagittal, and axial considerations. The curves are classified according to the region of the structural curve in the coronal plane. A lumbar curve modifier is added based on the relationship of the center sacral line to the apex of the lumbar curve. Finally, a sagittal thoracic modifier is added, and the combination of the curve type, lumbar curve modifier, and sagittal thoracic modifier is the classification of a specific curve to indicate the thoracic sagittal profile (Fig. 38-30).

NONOPERATIVE TREATMENT

Various methods have been used to treat adolescent idiopathic scoliosis over the years, including physical therapy, manipulation, and electrical stimulation, but there is no scientific evidence supporting their effectiveness. Although some doubt the effectiveness of brace treatment, the two most widely accepted nonoperative techniques for idiopathic scoliosis are observation and bracing.

Observation

Although some degree of scoliosis is frequent in the general population, few individuals have curves that require treatment. Unfortunately, no method is reliable for accurately predicting at the initial evaluation which curves will progress; thus observation is the primary treatment of all curves. Currently a roentgenogram of the spine is the only definitive documentation of curve size and curve progression. Attempts have been made to monitor external contours with measurement of the rib hump, measurement of the trunk rotation angle with a

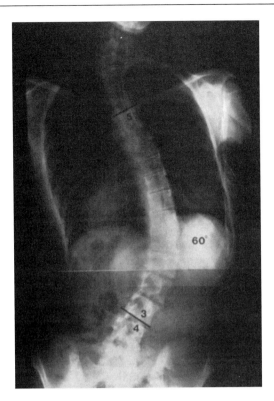

Fig. 38-28   King type IV curve.

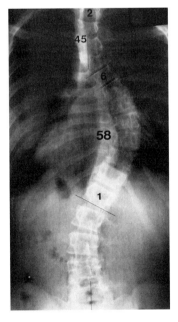

Fig. 38-29   King type V curve.

"scoliometer," and use of contour devices such as moiré topography and ISIS scanning. These methods may be useful in certain small curves and for low-risk patients, but periodic evaluation of the spine with roentgenograms still is necessary.

In general, young patients with mild curves of less than 20 degrees can be examined every 6 to 12 months. Adolescents with larger degrees of curvature should be examined every 3 to

4 months. Skeletally mature patients with curves of less than 20 degrees generally do not require further evaluation. A curve of more than 20 degrees in a patient who has not reached skeletal maturity demands more frequent examination, usually every 3 to 4 months, with standing posteroanterior roentgenograms. If progression of the curve (an increase of 5 degrees over 6 months) beyond 25 degrees is noted, orthotic treatment is considered. For curves of 30 to 40 degrees in a skeletally immature patient, orthotic treatment is recommended at the initial evaluation. Curves of 30 to 40 degrees in skeletally mature patients generally do not require treatment, but because studies indicate a potential for progression in adult life, these patients should be followed with yearly standing posteroanterior roentgenograms for 2 to 3 years after skeletal maturity, then every 5 years throughout life.

Orthotic Treatment

For many years, the accepted orthotics treatment for adolescent idiopathic scoliosis was the Milwaukee brace worn full-time (23 hours a day), but with the success of newer underarm orthotics, it now rarely is used. Numerous types of underarm orthosis (TLSOs) are available, including the Boston brace and the Wilmington plastic jacket. A basic principle of bracing for scoliosis is to control lumbar lordosis by producing a forward pelvic tilt. Loads can be applied to the spine with this flattening of the lumbar lordosis, together with pad pressure either on the paravertebral muscles or the ribs articulating with the vertebral bodies. The actual biological effects of these loads and how they alter the natural history of the curves has not yet been determined.

Studies of Milwaukee brace treatment found that approximately 50% improvement in the curve was obtained after about 6 months in the brace, after which improvement gradually lessened. When the brace was discontinued, the average curve was slightly better than before bracing, but at 5-year follow-up, the average curve is about the same as at the start of the treatment.

Results of TLSO treatment have been similar. Emans et al. found that the Boston brace controlled idiopathic scoliosis in 80% of patients in whom the apex of the curve was at T7 or below. Wiley et al. reported 50 patients with adolescent idiopathic curves measuring 35 to 45 degrees who were treated with a Boston brace. At a mean follow-up of 9.8 years, results indicated that the Boston brace, when used 18 or more hours a day, was effective in preventing progression of these larger curves. Bunnell, Bassett and Bunnell, and Hanks et al. found similar success rates with the Wilmington TLSO. Piazza and Bassett, in a follow-up study, found that 21% of their patients progressed 5 degrees after the brace was discontinued. Double structural curves that progressed during brace treatment were most likely to progress after bracing was discontinued.

The Charleston bending brace is a low-profile, anterior-opening, lightweight, thermoplastic orthosis that is worn only during nighttime sleeping hours and is used mostly for single curves. The orthosis bends the spine toward the convexity of the curve to "overcorrect" the scoliotic curve. Katz et al. in a study of 319 patients treated with either a Boston brace or a

Curve type

Type	Proximal thoracic	Main thoracic	Thoracolumbar/lumbar	Curve type
1	Nonstructural	Structural (major)	Nonstructural	Main thoracic (MT)
2	Structural	Structural (major)	Nonstructural	Double thoracic (DT)
3	Nonstructural	Structural (major)	Structural	Double major (DM)
4	Structural	Structural (major)	Structural	Triple major (TM)
5	Nonstructural	Nonstructural	Structural (major)	Thoracolumbar/lumbar (TL/L)
6	Nonstructural	Structural	Structural (major)	Thoracolumbar/lumbar—structural MT (Lumbar curve > thoracic by ≥ 10°)

Structural Criteria

Proximal thoracic: Side-bending Cobb ≥ 25°
T2-T5 kyphosis ≥ +20°

Main thoracic: Side-bending Cobb ≥ 25°

Thoracolumbar/lumbar: Side-bending Cobb ≥ 25°
T10-L2 kyphosis ≥ +20°

Location of Apex
(SRS definition)

Curve	Apex
Thoracic	T2-T11-12 Disc
Thoracolumbar	T12-L1
Lumbar	L1-2 Disc-L4

Modifiers

Lumbar Spine Modifier	CSVL to Lumbar Apex
A	CSVL between pedicles
B	CSVL touches apical body(ies)
C	CSVL completely medial

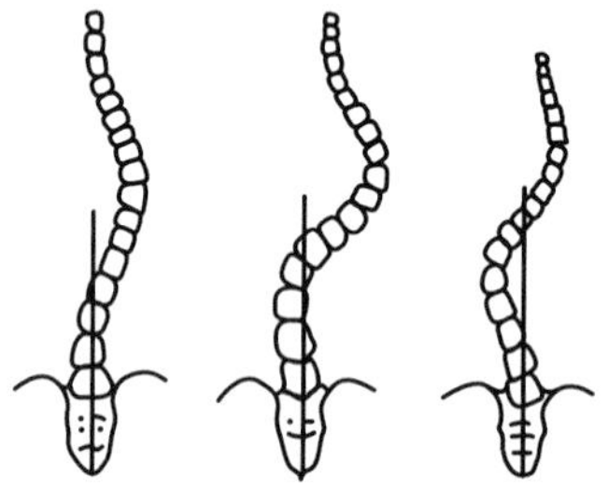

A   B   C

Thoracic Sagittal Profile T5-T12		
−	(Hypo)	< 10°
N	(Normal)	10°-40°
+	(Hyper)	> 40°

Curve type (1-6) + Lumbar spine modifier (A, B, or C) + Thoracic sagittal modifier (−, N, or +)
Classification (e.g., 1 B +): _____

Fig. 38-30 Curve types and the criteria for structural curves and location of apex. (From Lenke LG, Betz RR, Harris J, et al: *J Bone Joint Surg* 83A:1169, 2001.)

Charleston bending brace found the Boston brace to be more effective than the Charleston brace in both preventing curve progression and avoiding the need for surgery. The difference was most notable in patients with curves of 36 to 45 degrees: 83% of patients with curves of 36 to 45 degrees treated with a Charleston brace had curve progression of more than 5 degrees, compared with 43% of those treated with a Boston brace. The authors concluded that the Charleston brace should be used only in the treatment of small, single thoracolumbar or single lumbar curves.

Some authors have questioned whether bracing is effective at all in the treatment of progressive idiopathic scoliosis. Leatherman and Dickson suggested that the forces operating in idiopathic scoliosis produce primary lordosis and a resultant lateral curve. An orthosis that does not act in the appropriate plane cannot reverse the process. Goldberg et al. compared the results of brace treatment in 32 females with a similar group of 32 females treated without bracing in Dublin, Ireland. All patients were Risser 0 at diagnosis. No statistically significant difference was found between the groups on any parameter of curve progression. Other authors, however, are convinced of the effectiveness of bracing. Lonstein and Winter compared the results of 1020 patients treated with a Milwaukee brace with those of 729 patients without brace treatment. They found with statistical certainty that bracing had a positive effect on the natural history of adolescent idiopathic scoliosis. In the critical high-risk group of Risser 0-I females with thoracic curves of 20 to 40 degrees, there was a failure rate of 43% with bracing compared with a 68% expected failure rate based on the natural history. Rowe et al. in a meta-analysis of the literature also found bracing to be effective.

Patient and family compliance with brace treatment is important in evaluating the success of a device; compliance with orthotic wear has been reported to be as low as 20% (DiRaimondo and Green). Compliance generally is better with TLSOs than with the more cumbersome CTLSOs. Many other factors, however, enter into the compliance problem, such as the family situation, ineffectual parents, a family history of psychiatric problems, and alcohol and drug use.

Originally the orthoses were intended to be worn 23 hours a day, but concern about compliance has led to part-time bracing regimens. Most part-time bracing protocols call for approximately 16 hours or less of brace wear each day. Kahanovitz et al., Price et al., and Green reported that part-time brace wear controlled curve progression as well as full-time brace programs, although no long-term results were available. Rowe et al., in a more recent study, found that 23-hour brace treatment was significantly more successful than other brace regimens. However, a part-time brace program does not require an adolescent to wear the brace to school, and therefore the patient may be more likely to comply with the recommendations for brace wear. If the curve is less than 35 degrees and does not demonstrate significant vertebral wedging, part-time brace wear is certainly reasonable to attempt first. If significant progression of the curvature is noted during use of the part-time protocol, full-time bracing can then be instituted.

Orthotic treatment of adolescent idiopathic scoliosis is indicated for a flexible curve of 20 to 30 degrees in a growing child with documented progression of 5 degrees or more. Curves in the 30- to 40-degree range in growing children are treated at initial evaluation. Although surgery usually is indicated for curves in the 40- to 50-degree range in growing children, orthotic treatment may be considered for some curves, such as a cosmetically acceptable double major curve of 40 to 45 degrees. Orthotic treatment is not used in patients with curves of more than 50 degrees.

Traction

With improved spinal instrumentation and spinal cord monitoring, the need for supplemental traction correction of severe stiff curves and for monitoring spinal and pulmonary function of an unanesthetized patient has been greatly diminished. In 1959 Perry and Nickel introduced the halo, a device that provides stable fixation and comfort for the patient. The halo device may still be useful in a few selected patients: (1) for added external immobilization in patients with cervical

and upper thoracic deformities for which surgery does not offer sufficient stability to maintain correction until fusion occurs and (2) in patients with cervical spine fractures.

Mubarak et al. described a technique for the application of a halo in infants. This multiple pin technique differs significantly from recommendations for older children regarding pin number, pin placement, and torque. With multiple pins, significantly less torque can be used, allowing a greater range of pin placement sites in areas where the skull might otherwise be considered too thin. Skull development is important to consider in halo application in patients younger than 2 years of age. Cranial suture interdigitation may be incomplete, and fontanels may be open anteriorly in patients younger than 18 months of age and posteriorly in patients younger than 6 months of age. Techniques for application of halo traction are described in Chapter 37.

Halo Gravity Traction. Halo traction has been provided in the past by means of halo-femoral traction or halo-pelvic traction, but these are no longer in widespread use. Halo gravity traction currently is the primary method of applying halo traction. A possible indication for this type of traction is severe spinal deformity with secondary cor pulmonale. If correction of the curvature reverses the pulmonary failure, spinal stabilization is indicated.

Casting

Underarm Casts. With newer instrumentation systems, postoperative casting seldom is used. If postoperative immobilization is needed, an orthotist often can make a TLSO that is comparable to a postoperative cast. Unlike a cast, a TLSO allows tightening or loosening as necessary and also trimming to relieve pressure areas. If an orthotist is not available, however, a postoperative underarm cast can be used if postoperative immobilization is necessary.

◆ *Application of Underarm Cast*

TECHNIQUE 38-2

Place the patient on a Risser table and apply a stockinette to extend from over the head to the knees. Position the removable cross-bar at the level of the upper portion of the shoulders. Use felt to pad the canvas strap on which the patient is resting. Pass muslin straps around the waist over the stockinette and tie them at the level of the greater trochanter on the opposite side. Then pass the straps through the windlass at the end of the table and apply a slight amount of traction. Pad the iliac crest with felt. Use extra-strong, resin-reinforced plaster and extend the cast to the sternum anteriorly and the upper portion of the back posteriorly. Mold the cast well around the pelvis and iliac crest. As the cast dries, trim it at the level of the pubic symphysis anteriorly, extending proximally to about the level of the anterior superior iliac spine to allow 100 degrees of hip

continued

flexion. Posteriorly, trim low over the buttocks at the level of the greater trochanters. Then trim proximally to relieve pressure over the sacral prominence. Remove an abdominal window to free the upper portion of the abdomen, the lower costal margin, and the xiphoid process.

OPERATIVE TREATMENT

The surgical treatment of adolescent idiopathic scoliosis has changed dramatically over the past 10 years. Our understanding of the natural history of the condition, problems associated with the deformity, and the three-dimensional aspects of the deformity, as well as the development of newer instrumentation has contributed to this change. The accepted indications for surgical correction of spinal deformity are based on the natural history of the deformity and the potential consequences of the deformity for the patient in adult life. Natural history studies, such as those by Edgar and Mehta and Weinstein, have been used to demonstrate the potential consequences of significant deformity and pain. It is now believed that pulmonary complications result mainly from unusual deformities and early onset of the disease. In children and adolescents, surgery is considered if the curve is likely to reach a magnitude that can be expected to become troublesome in adulthood. Although most authors recommend surgery when the curve reaches 50 degrees, other factors need to be considered. Smaller lumbar and thoracolumbar curves may cause significant trunk shift, coronal decompensation, and cosmetic deformity. Double 50-degree curves are not as cosmetically unacceptable as single curves, and if progression occurs in skeletally mature patients, it is likely to be gradual. In an immature patient, on the other hand, surgery may be considered for curves between 40 and 50 degrees depending on the clinical appearance. Surgery is more likely required in a patient with a curve that progresses despite brace treatment than in a patient who has had no brace treatment. Back pain in young children and adolescents with scoliosis is an indication for an extensive evaluation; if no other cause is found, spinal fusion may be indicated. Dickson et al. emphasized the importance of lordosis in treatment decision making. Thoracic lordosis has a detrimental effect on pulmonary function, and bracing worsens thoracic lordosis. Therefore surgery is more likely to be indicated for an adolescent with a progressive curve associated with significant thoracic lordosis. The general indications for operative treatment are summarized Box 38-3.

Preoperative Preparation

Once the decision to perform spinal fusion has been made, certain preliminary precautions should be taken and tests done to ensure that the patient is properly prepared for the operative procedure. Aspirin-containing products or nonsteroidal antiinflammatory agents should be discontinued before surgery because these medications may increase blood loss during surgery. Birth control pills should be discontinued 1 month

---

> **BOX 38-3 •** Indications for Operative Treatment of Idiopathic Scoliosis
>
> Increasing curve in growing child
> Severe deformity (>50 degrees) with asymmetry of trunk in adolescent
> Pain uncontrolled by nonoperative treatment
> Thoracic lordosis
> Significant cosmetic deformity

before surgery because they have been shown to increase the possibility of thrombophlebitis in the postoperative period. Preoperative roentgenographic evaluation of the spinal levels to be fused is essential. Special imaging techniques, such as computed tomography (CT), magnetic resonance imaging (MRI), and myelography, occasionally are needed to rule out conditions such as syringomyelia, diastematomyelia, and tethered cord.

Pulmonary function studies usually are indicated in patients with paralytic scoliosis or those with idiopathic or congenital scoliosis who have severe curves or significant kyphosis or lordosis. We do not routinely obtain special pulmonary function studies in patients with idiopathic curves of less than 50 to 60 degrees as measured by the Cobb method unless they are warranted by special circumstances. Nickel et al. advocated tracheostomy before surgery in any patient with paralytic scoliosis and a vital capacity of less than 30% of predicted normal. We have found that the indications for tracheostomy can be safely narrowed if the patient spends several days after surgery in an adequately staffed intensive care unit in which the patient can remain intubated, respiratory functions can be constantly supervised, and mechanical aids for respiration are readily available. If, however, any doubt remains as to the patient's pulmonary status with these measures, a tracheostomy is better done at the time of surgery.

Preoperative autologous blood donations are recommended for all patients who qualify. The risks of homologous blood transfusion include transmitted diseases, such as hepatitis (particularly non-A, non-B), malaria, cytomegalovirus infection, and HIV infection, as well as alloimmunization and graft-versus-host reactions. Bailey and Mahoney demonstrated that 85% of patients undergoing elective scoliosis surgery can avoid receiving homologous blood by using autologous blood transfusion. MacEwen et al. showed that autologous blood transfusions in children weighing less than 45.5 kg (100 pounds) was a safe method of blood replacement; 63% of children did not require any homologous blood. Patients are given oral iron supplements three times a day. Larger children are allowed to donate one unit of blood a week. The patient's hematocrit level is checked before each donation and must be at least 34%. If the level is low, the patient is asked to return the following week. MacEwen et al. recommended obtaining a lesser volume of blood at each visit for smaller patients (Table 38-5). With improved collection and storage techniques,

Table 38-5   Quantity of Blood Taken at First Phlebotomy Based on Patient Body Weight

Patient Weight (kg)	Volume of Blood (ml)*
23.0-29.5	125-175
30.0-42.5	175-275
43.0-50.0	400-450
≥50.0	450-500

From MacEwen GD, Bennett E, Guille JT: *J Pediatr Orthop* 10:751, 1990.
*If hematocrit level remained satisfactory, the quantity of blood to be withdrawn was increased within the range at subsequent phlebotomy.

the blood can be stored in a liquid state for up to 45 days. Oga et al. showed that cryopreserved autologous blood also is an effective method for storing a sufficient volume of blood for scoliosis surgery. Cryopreserving of blood requires it to be stored at −85° C with glycerol as a cryoprotective agent and requires expensive equipment that may not be universally available. Also, after the blood is thawed, the glycerol must be removed. Once the blood is thawed and washed, it must be used within 24 hours. Cryopreserved blood donation offers much more leeway in obtaining the amount of blood necessary for surgery. Roye et al. showed that erythropoietin is an effective means of increasing red cell mass and decreasing the need for homologous blood products. The difficulty with erythropoietin use in our hospital is the cost, and we do not use it routinely.

Intraoperative Considerations

Whether the surgery is done anteriorly, posteriorly, or both, certain intraoperative considerations are important. Because spinal surgery requires extensive dissection that may result in severe blood loss, a large-bore intravenous line is necessary. An arterial line is helpful for continuous monitoring of blood pressure. An indwelling urinary catheter is used to monitor urinary output. Electrocardiogram leads, blood pressure cuff, and esophageal stethoscope also are routine monitors. A pulse oximeter is a useful adjunct to the arterial line.

Nash et al. reported the use of somatosensory evoked potentials (SSEP) in 1977, and the interest in and use of electrical spinal cord monitoring have been increasing since. Stimulation of distal sensory nerves while recording proximal to the surgical area with either high cervical or cortical leads can alert the surgeon to possible alteration of spinal cord transmission. Preoperative monitoring for a "baseline" is helpful for comparison during the operative procedure. When using these SSEPs, certain inhalation agents, such as halothane or isoflurane, should be avoided, as should diazepam and droperidol. SSEP is a useful adjunct for monitoring spinal cord function, but it is not infallible, and false-positive and false-negative results have been reported. An important limitation of SSEP is that it measures only the integrity of the sensory system.

Generally if SSEPs are used, multiple recording sites must be used, including cortical, subcortical, and peripheral sites. In

recent years the use of motor evoked potentials (MEP) has increased. The combination of MEPs and SSEPs can provide important information regarding the primary motor and sensory tracts within the spinal cord. If information is desired about individual nerve root functions, alternative neurophysiological methods are necessary. We routinely monitor SSEPs as well as MEPs in our surgeries for both adolescent idiopathic spinal deformities and neuromuscular spinal deformities.

The first available spinal cord monitoring technique was the Stagnara wake-up test, described by Vauzell, Stagnara, and Jouvinroux in 1973. In this test, the anesthesia is decreased or reversed after correction of the spinal deformity. The patient is brought to a conscious level and asked to move both lower extremities. Once voluntary movement is noted, anesthesia is returned to the appropriate level, and the surgical procedure is completed. Engler et al. pointed out possible hazards in arousing a prone, intubated patient from anesthesia, and Brown and Nash stressed that this test only documents that spinal cord function has not suffered a major compromise at the time the test is done. It also does not allow continuous spinal cord monitoring. We routinely do the wake-up test at the completion of the procedure in all patients or if readings change or diminish during surgery. In patients who are considered extremely high risks for neurological injuries, the wake up test is considered even if the signals do not change. The combination of the SSEPs and MEPs have made use of the wake-up test much less frequent.

Hypotensive anesthesia, in which arterial blood pressure is kept at 65 mm Hg, has been advocated as an effective way to decrease intraoperative blood loss. An arterial line is essential during this type of anesthesia. Care also must be taken when reducing blood pressure so that it does not lead to ischemia of the spinal cord. Hypotensive anesthesia should not be considered in patients with a heart condition or in patients with spinal cord compression in whom a decrease in arterial blood supply might restrict already compromised spinal cord blood flow.

The cell saver has been shown to save approximately 50% of the red cell mass, thereby reducing the need for intraoperative blood transfusions. The cell saver saves only healthy blood, filtering out old and fragile cells. The cell saver does add to the expense of the procedure, but if enough blood loss is anticipated, it is a reasonable option. Mann et al. reported a 40% red cell mass salvage in spinal surgery. The salvage rate was lower than in other procedures because spinal surgery does not allow pooling of lost blood. The surgical technique involves liberal use of sponges to tamponade vessels. The need for a narrow-diameter tip suction results in greater cell damage and thus a lower salvage. The cell saver is contraindicated in patients with malignancy or infection. The surgeon should try to estimate preoperatively if enough blood will be salvaged to make the cell saver cost effective. At our institution the cost of using the cell saver is equal to the cost of two units of autologous blood.

Acute normovolemic hemodilution also has been used to decrease the loss of red cell mass. The patient is phlebotomized

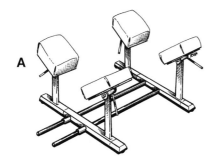

A

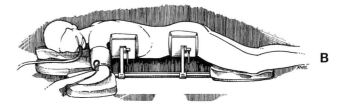

B

Fig. 38-31 **A,** Relton-Hall frame for reduction of intra-abdominal pressure. **B,** Positioning of patient on Relton-Hall frame with hips in extension to maintain lumbar lordosis.

in the operating room, and the maximal quantity of blood is withdrawn that will produce a reduction in hemoglobin to a level of 9 g/dl or higher after hemodilution. Circulating volume is maintained by crystalloid replacement. The operation is done at normal blood pressure. At the end of the procedure the patient is diuresed of excess fluid, and his own blood is retransfused. Despite the lower oxygen-carrying capability of the diluted blood, its decreased viscosity allows better tissue perfusion and tissue oxygenation is maintained. This hemodilution technique requires an anesthesiologist interested and skilled in its use.

At our institution the most commonly used methods for reducing the need for hemologous blood transfusion include meticulous surgical technique, intraoperative blood collection, and the use of predeposited autologous blood. Other techniques are used as needed.

Surgical Goals

The goals of surgery for spinal deformity are to correct or improve the deformity while maintaining sagittal balance, preserving or improving pulmonary function, minimizing morbidity or pain, maximizing postoperative function, and improving or at least not harming the function of the lumbar spine. To accomplish these goals in patients with idiopathic scoliosis, surgical techniques may include anterior, posterior, or combined anterior and posterior procedures. The surgical indications, techniques, and procedures are divided into anterior and posterior sections.

◆ Posterior Approach

The posterior approach to the spinal column is the most commonly used. It is familiar to all orthopaedic surgeons and offers a safe and extensile approach that exposes the entire vertebral column.

TECHNIQUE 38-3

Position the patient prone on a Relton-Hall frame with the arms carefully supported and the elbows padded. Proper positioning of the patient on the operating table is extremely important. Relton and Hall were first to emphasize the role of intraabdominal pressure in blood loss, and they designed a frame to eliminate some of this pressure and reduce blood

loss (Fig. 38-31, *A*). Do not abduct the shoulders more than 90 degrees to prevent pressure or stretch on the brachial plexus. Carefully pad the pressure points. The upper pads of the frame should rest on the chest and not in the axilla to avoid pressure on any nerves from the brachial plexus (Fig. 38-31, *B*). When the patient is positioned on the frame with the hips flexed, lumbar lordosis is partially eliminated. If the fusion is to be extended into the lower lumbar spine, elevate the knees and thighs so that the patient lies with the hip joints extended to maintain normal lumbar lordosis.

Scrub the patient's back with a surgical soap solution for 5 to 10 minutes and prepare the skin with an antiseptic solution. Drape the area of the operative site and use a plastic Steri-drape to seal off the skin. Make the skin incision in a straight line from one to two vertebrae superior to the proposed fusion area to one vertebra inferior to it. A straight scar improves the postoperative appearance of the back (Fig. 38-32, *A*). Make the initial incision through the dermal layer only. Infiltrate the intradermal and subcutaneous areas with an epinephrine solution (1:500,000). Deepen the incision to the level of the spinous processes and use self-retaining Weitlaner retractors to retract the skin margins. Control bleeding with an electrocautery. Identify the interspinous ligament between the spinous processes; this often appears as a white line. As the incision is deepened, keep the Weitlaner retractors tight to help with exposure and minimize bleeding. Now incise the cartilaginous cap overlying the spinous processes as close to the midline as possible (Fig. 38-32, *B*). This midline may vary because of rotation of the spinous processes. Using a Cobb elevator, expose the spinous processes subperiosteally after the cartilaginous caps have been moved to either side. After several of the spinous processes have been exposed, move the Weitlaner retractors to a deeper level and maintain tension for retraction and hemostasis. After exposure of all spinous processes, a localizing roentgenogram can be obtained. Alternatively, the T12 rib and the L1 transverse process can be used to localize the levels. While the roentgenogram is being developed, reopen the wound and continue subperiosteal exposure of the entire area to be fused, keeping the retractors tight at all times (Fig. 38-32, *C*). It is easier to dissect from caudad to

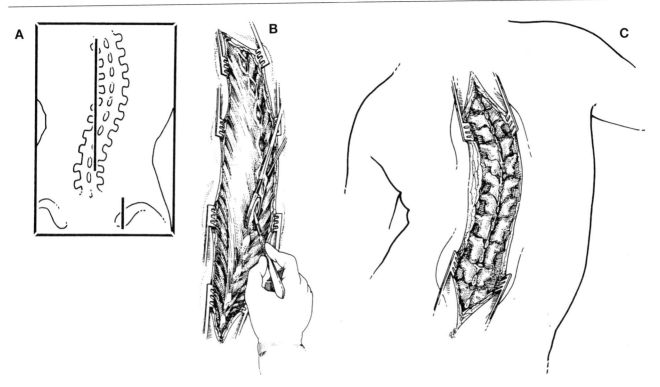

Fig. 38-32   **A,** Skin incisions for posterior fusion and autogenous bone graft. **B,** Incisions over spinous processes and interspinous ligaments. **C,** Weitlaner retractors used to maintain tension and exposure of spine during dissection.

cephalad because of the oblique attachments of the short rotator muscles and ligaments of the spine. Extend the subperiosteal dissection first to the facet joints on one side and then the other side, deepening the retractors as necessary. Continue the dissection laterally to the ends of the transverse processes on both sides. Coagulate the branch of the segmental vessel just lateral to each facet (Fig. 38-33). Place the self-retaining retractors deeper to hold the entire incision open and exposed. Sponges soaked in the 1:500,000 epinephrine solution can be used to maintain hemostasis. Use a curet and pituitary rongeur to completely clean the interspinous ligaments and the facets of all ligamentous attachments and capsule, proceeding from the midline laterally (Fig. 38-34) to decrease the possibility of the curet slipping and penetrating the spinal canal. The entire spine is now exposed from one transverse process to another, all soft tissue has been removed, and the spine is ready for instrumentation and arthrodesis as indicated by the procedure chosen.

Posterior Fusion

The long-term success of any operative procedure for scoliosis depends on a solid arthrodesis. The classic extraarticular Hibbs technique has been replaced by intraarticular fusion techniques that include the facet joints. The success of spinal arthrodesis depends on (1) the surgical preparation of the

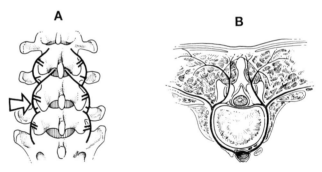

Fig. 38-33   **A,** Posterior view of segmental vessels just lateral to each facet joint. **B,** Axial view of arteries supplying posterior spinal muscles. (**A** redrawn from MacNab I, Dall D: *J Bone Joint Surg* 53B:628, 1971; **B** redrawn from Wagoner G: *J Bone Joint Surg* 19B:469, 1937.)

fusion site, (2) systemic and local factors, (3) the ability of the graft material to stimulate a healing process, and (4) the biomechanical features of the graft positioning. To obtain the best field for the fusion, soft tissue trauma should be minimal. Avascular tissue should be removed from the graft bed. The surface of the bone and the facets should be decorticated to provide a large maximally exposed surface area for vascular ingrowth and allow delivery of more osteoprogenitor cells. The patient's condition should be improved as much as possible by nutrition and control of any medical problems. Smoking has been found to inhibit fusion significantly and should be discontinued before surgery. We believe autogenous bone graft from the iliac crest remains the single best source of graft material, combining osteogenic, osteoconductive, and osteoinductive properties. Another excellent source of autogenous bone is rib obtained from a thoracoplasty. Allografts provide osteoconductive and osteoinductive properties and have been shown to produce results nearly as good as those of autogenous iliac crest graft in young patients. In certain conditions, such as paralytic scoliosis, in which large amounts of bone graft are needed and the iliac crests often are small or are used for instrumentation, allografts are used routinely. Several alternative graft materials, including tricalcium phosphate, hydroxyapatite, and demineralized bone matrix, have osteoconductive properties and are under investigation. Bone morphogenic protein can supply osteoinductive properties and also is under investigation. The future of these substances probably will be in combined osteoconductive and osteoinductive agents. In positioning the bone graft material, it should be remembered that bone graft generally does better under compression and is less effective with distraction. The farther fusion is from the instantaneous axis of rotation, the better the fusion will prevent or minimize movement of that axis of rotation.

With improvements in surgical techniques and the inclusion of intraarticular fusion, together with meticulous dissection around the transverse processes, the pseudarthrosis rate has been decreased to 2% or less in adolescents with idiopathic scoliosis.

◆ **Facet Fusion**

TECHNIQUE 38-4 *(Moe)*

Expose the spine to the tips of the transverse processes as previously described (Technique 38-3). Begin a cut over the cephalad articular processes at the base of the lamina and

carry it along the transverse process almost to its tip. Bend this fragment laterally to lie between the transverse processes, leaving it hinged if possible. Thoroughly remove the cartilage from the superior articular process. Make another cut in the area of the superior articular facet with the Cobb gouge, beginning medially and working laterally to produce another hinged fragment. Place cancellous bone graft in the defect created (Fig. 38-35). In the lumbar spine the facet joints are oriented in a more sagittal direction, and a facet fusion is best accomplished by removing the adjoining joint surface with a small osteotome or a needle-nose rongeur. This creates a defect that is packed with cancellous bone (Fig. 38-36).

Decorticate the entire exposed spine with Cobb gouges from the midline, progressing laterally so that if the gouge were to slip, it would be moving away from the spinal canal. Then add cancellous bone graft. If the fusion is done for

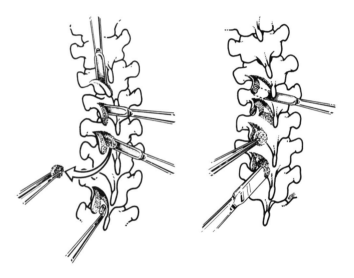

Fig. 38-35   Moe technique of thoracic facet fusion. (From Bradford DS et al: *Moe's textbook of scoliosis and other spinal deformities*, ed 2, Philadelphia, 1987, WB Saunders.)

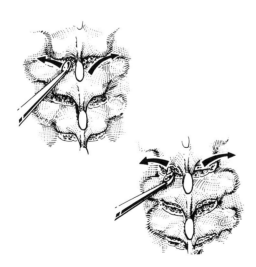

Fig. 38-34   Cobb curets used to clean facets of ligament attachments.

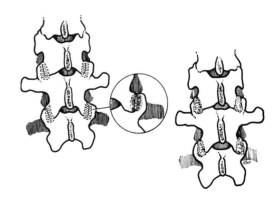

Fig. 38-36   Moe technique for lumbar facet fusion.

scoliosis and the amount of bone available is limited, concentrate the bone graft on the concave side of the curve because this bone will be subjected to compressive forces as opposed to tension forces on the convex side. The thoracolumbar and lumbar areas are the areas associated with the highest incidence of pseudarthrosis.

TECHNIQUE 38-5 *(Hall)*

First, sharply cut the inferior facet with a gouge and remove this bone fragment to expose the superior facet cartilage. Remove this cartilage with a sharp curet. Create a trough by removing the outer cortex of the superior facet and add cancellous bone grafts (Fig. 38-37). Proceed with decortication as described in the Moe technique.

At the completion of fusion, close the deep tissues with absorbable suture. Place a drain in the subcutaneous tissue or the deep layer, keeping the reservoir for this drain separate from the reservoir for the bone graft to allow monitoring of bleeding from the incision sites. Approximate the subcutaneous tissues with 2-0 absorbable sutures and the skin edges with skin staples or a running subcuticular absorbable stitch. Apply a bulky sterile dressing.

AFTERTREATMENT. The patient is transferred to the bed from the operating table. Intravenous fluids are continued until the patient is able to tolerate oral intake and no longer requires any intravenous medication. Prophylactic pre-operative, intraoperative, and postoperative intravenous antibiotics are given. Most patients have a Foley catheter inserted at the time of surgery; this is removed about 48 to 72 hours after surgery. Other postoperative treatment, such as casting, bracing, or ambulation, depends on the type of internal fixation, if any, used with the individual procedure.

◆ Bone Grafting

TECHNIQUE 38-6

Make an incision over the iliac crest to be used (Fig. 38-38, *A*). If the original incision extends far enough distally into the lumbar spine, the iliac crest can be exposed through the same incision by subcutaneous dissection. Infiltrate the intradermal and subcutaneous areas with 1:500,000 epinephrine solution. Expose the cartilaginous apophysis overlying the posterior iliac crest and split it in

continued

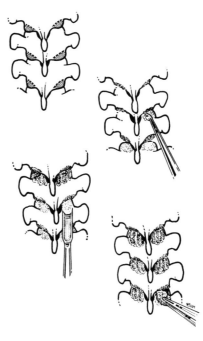

Fig. 38-37   Hall technique of facet fusion. (Redrawn in part from Bradford DS et al: *Moe's textbook of scoliosis and other spinal deformities*, ed 2, Philadelphia, 1987, WB Saunders.)

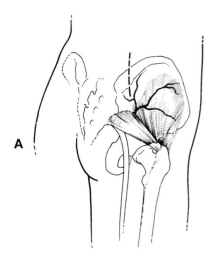
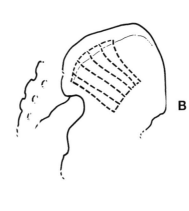

Fig. 38-38   **A,** Superior gluteal artery as it emerges from area of sciatic notch. **B,** Cortical and cancellous strips removed from outer table of ilium for autogenous bone graft.

the middle. Using a Cobb elevator, expose the ilium subperiosteally. The superior gluteal artery emerges from the area of the sciatic notch (Fig. 38-38, *A*) and should be carefully avoided during the bone grafting procedure. If bicortical grafts are desired, expose the posterior crest of the ilium on the inner side and obtain two or three strips of bicortical graft with a large gouge. Otherwise, take cortical and cancellous strips from the outer table of the ilium (Fig. 38-38, *B*). Place these bone grafts in a kidney basin and cover them with a sponge soaked in saline or blood. Control bleeding from the iliac crest with bone wax or Gelfoam. Approximate the cartilaginous cap of the posterior iliac crest with an absorbable stitch. Place a suction drain at the donor site and connect it to a separate reservoir to monitor postoperative bleeding here separately from the spinal fusion site.

Complications of Bone Grafting. The most common complication associated with bone graft harvesting from the posterior iliac crest is transient or permanent numbness over the skin of the buttock caused by injury of the superior cluneal nerves (Fig. 38-39, *A*). The superior cluneal nerves supply sensation to a large area of the buttocks. They pierce the lumbodorsal fascia and cross the posterior iliac crest beginning 8 cm lateral to the posterior superior iliac spine. Kurz et al. recommended a limited incision, staying within 8 cm of the posterior superior iliac spine, which will avoid the superior cluneal nerves.

The superior gluteal artery exits the pelvis, enters the gluteal region through the superiormost portion of the sciatic notch, and sends extensive branches to the gluteal muscles. Care should be taken when inserting a retractor into the sciatic notch. Injury to the superior gluteal artery will cause massive hemorrhage, and the artery generally retracts proximally into the pelvis. Control of the bleeding frequently requires bone removal from the sciatic notch to obtain sufficient exposure. It may be necessary to pack the wound, turn the patient, and have a general surgeon locate and ligate the hypogastric artery. Ureteral injury also can occur in the sciatic notch from the sharp tip of a retractor.

Most of the stability of the sacroiliac joint is provided by the posterior ligamentous complex (Fig. 38-39, *B*). Injury to the sacroiliac joint from removal of these ligaments can range from clinical symptoms of instability to dislocation. Coventry and Topper, as well as Lichtblau, described dislocation of the sacroiliac joint as a complication of full-thickness graft removal from the posterior ilium. If a full-thickness graft is obtained, it should not be obtained too close to the sacroiliac joint (Fig. 38-40).

POSTERIOR SPINAL INSTRUMENTATION

The goals of instrumentation in scoliosis surgery are to correct the deformity as much as possible and to stabilize the spine in the corrected position while the fusion mass becomes solid. The fusion mass in a well-corrected spine is subjected to much lower bending moments and tensile forces than the fusion mass in an uncorrected spine (Fig. 38-41).

The ideal spinal instrumentation system is safe and reliable, with infrequent instrument failure and breakage. It should be

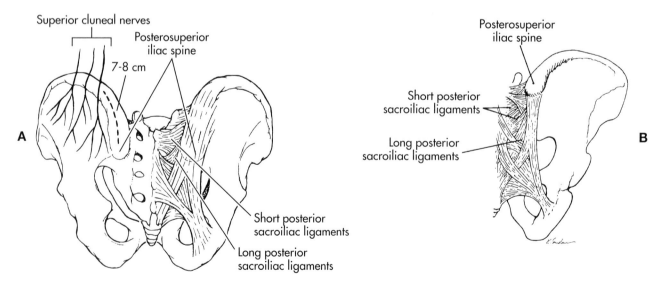

Fig. 38-39 **A,** Superior cluneal nerve may be injured during harvest of bone graft from iliac crest. Limited incision *(dotted line),* staying within 8 cm of posterior superior iliac spine, avoids nerve. **B,** Posterior ligament complex provides most of stability of sacroiliac joint. (**A** redrawn from Fernyhough JC, Schimandle JJ, Weigel MC, et al: *Spine* 17:1474, 1992; **B** redrawn from Kurz LT, Garfin SR, Booth RE Jr: Iliac bone grafting: techniques and complications of harvesting. In Garfin SR: *Complications of spine surgery,* Baltimore, 1989, Williams & Wilkins.)

strong enough to resist load from all directions without external support, be easy to use with little increase in operative time, and restore normal spinal contours in the coronal, sagittal, and transverse planes; it should not create new deformities as the instrumentation is applied. It also should be a cost-effective

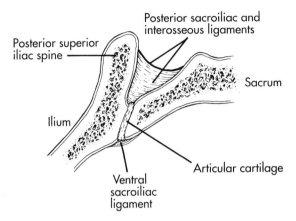

Fig. 38-40 Full-thickness graft should not be obtained too close to sacroiliac joint to avoid damage to posterior ligamentous complex. (Redrawn from Kurz LT, Garfin SR, Booth RE Jr: Iliac bone grafting: techniques and complications of harvesting. In Garfin SR: *Complications of spine surgery,* Baltimore, 1989, Williams & Wilkins.)

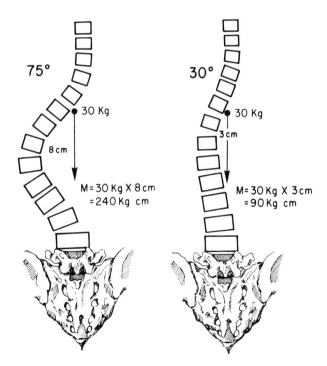

Fig. 38-41 Comparative bending forces exerted at apexes of 75-degree curve and 30-degree curve. (From Dunn HK. In The American Academy of Orthopaedic Surgeons: *Instructional course lectures,* vol 32, St Louis, 1983, Mosby.)

system. Numerous implants are available, although none meets all of the criteria for an ideal system. No one device is the best choice for every surgeon or every patient.

In 1962 Harrington introduced the first effective instrumentation system for scoliosis. For more than 30 years, use of the Harrington distraction rod, combined with a thorough posterior arthrodesis and immobilization in a cast or brace for 6 to 9 months, has been the standard surgical treatment for adolescent idiopathic scoliosis. The incidence of neurological injury with this technique is less than 1%, and the pseudarthrosis rate is less than 10%. The major correcting force with the Harrington instrumentation is distraction.

Despite its success, the Harrington instrumentation system has several disadvantages. The average curve correction in adolescent idiopathic scoliosis is approximately 50%. As the curve is corrected with distraction, the efficiency of correction is decreased. Dunn showed that in a 90-degree scoliotic deformity, about 70% of the distraction forces act to correct the curve; in a 45-degree curve, only 35% of the force is corrective. With the Harrington distraction rods the distraction force is applied only at the two laminae where the hooks are seated. If a load exceeds the strength of the lamina, fracture and loss of correction can result.

As distraction is applied, elongation of the spine results in reduction of spinal curves in both the coronal and sagittal planes. The coronal plane curve (scoliosis) is pathological, whereas the sagittal plane curve is physiological. If the spine is instrumented to the lower lumbar region with a straight distraction rod, normal lumbar lordosis is reduced (Fig. 38-42). To overcome this problem of flattening of the lumbar lordosis, Moe modified the Harrington rod by making the inferior end of the rod and the corresponding hole in the lower hook square. This allows the rod to be contoured to help preserve lumbar lordosis while preventing unwanted rotation of the rods. In addition, the spinous processes of the two lower vertebrae can be wired together (as described by Lagrone) to help maintain lordosis as distraction is applied (Fig. 38-43). In spite of these techniques, distraction across the lumbar spine inevitably leads to the loss of some degree of lumbar lordosis. The Harrington distraction rod did not deal with the problem of thoracic hypokyphosis or the rotational deformity associated with adolescent idiopathic scoliosis.

Posterior segmental spinal instrumentation systems provide multiple points of fixation to the spine and apply compression, distraction, and rotation forces through the same rod. These systems generally do not require any postoperative immobilization. They provide somewhat better coronal plane correction and better control in the sagittal plane. Hypokyphosis in the thoracic spine can be reduced and lumbar lordosis preserved when the instrumentation extends to the lower lumbar spine. The effects of segmental systems on the transverse plane axis (vertebral rotation) are more controversial. Gray et al. found insignificant changes in vertebral rotation after instrumentation with Cotrel-Dubousset (CD) rods and hooks. Lenke et al. postulated that at the apex of the curve, the derotation maneuver may be more of a translation maneuver. These

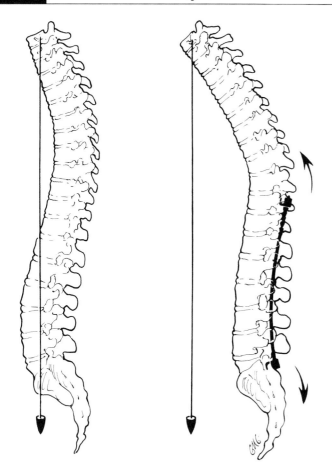

Fig. 38-42 Effects of distraction rod in lumbar spine. If contouring for lordosis is inadequate, lumbar spine can be flattened by distracting force. Also note kyphotic deformity just superior to distraction rod. (From LaGrone MO: *Orthop Clin North Am* 19:383, 1988.)

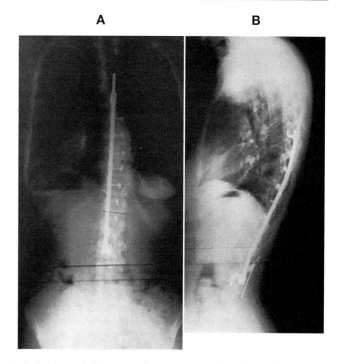

Fig. 38-43 **A,** Postoperative posteroanterior view of instrumentation and fusion into lumbar spine for idiopathic scoliosis. **B,** Lateral view of contoured Moe rod with wiring of spinous processes of lower two vertebrae to maintain lumbar lordosis.

systems generally have a lower implant failure and pseudarthrosis rates than Harrington instrumentation. The potential disadvantages of segmental systems compared with Harrington rods include the bulk of the implants, the complexity of the systems, and the surgical learning curve required. They also are more expensive than the traditional Harrington rod distraction system. In addition, it is debatable whether correction in the transverse plane axis is significantly improved compared with that obtained with Harrington rods. The advantages of these new systems, however, appear to outweigh the disadvantages, and we routinely use them instead of the Harrington rod distraction system for surgical treatment of adolescent idiopathic scoliosis.

Three kinds of devices are available for fixation of posterior segmental instrumentation: wires or cables, hooks, and screws. In the past, most systems have used wires and cables or hooks. More recently, the advantages of secure fixation to the spine with screws through the pedicles have led to an increased use of pedicle screws.

MULTIHOOK SEGMENTAL INSTRUMENTATION

General Principles of Surgical Technique

The general sequence of operative correction of idiopathic scoliosis using a multihook segmental instrumentation is as follows:

1. Exposure
2. Level identification
3. Hook site preparation
4. Facetectomy on the side of rod insertion
5. Rod contouring
6. Hook insertion and placement of the first rod
7. Seating of the hooks without attempting to correct the curve
8. Rotation of the rod to correct the curve
9. Distraction or compression of the hooks on the first rod
10. Contouring of the second rod
11. Facetectomy on the second side
12. Insertion of the second rod
13. Distraction or compression of the hooks on the second rod
14. Cross linking of the rods
15. Decortication
16. Placement of autogenous iliac bone graft
17. Closure

Alternatively, complete decortication can be done before insertion of the rods, but we have found that blood loss can be a problem while these rods are being inserted and derotated, and we prefer to decorticate after rod insertion. If the facet joints have been destroyed before rod insertion, the lamina usually can be decorticated by working around the rods.

There are basically two types of hooks: pedicle and laminar. The pedicle hooks are designed for secure fixation in the thoracic spine by insertion into the facet and impingement on the thoracic pedicle. Pedicle hooks are used in an upgoing direction at T10 or higher. The laminar hooks are for most other areas of the spine. These can be placed around either the superior or inferior edge of the lamina or transverse process according to the desired direction and point of application of forces.

◆ **Pedicle Hook Implantation**

TECHNIQUE 38-7

The pedicle hook generally is implanted in an upgoing direction from T1 to T10. Proper seating of the pedicle hook is crucial if it is to move the vertebra in three dimensions. Remove a portion of the inferior articular facet to introduce the bifid hook of the pedicle hook (Fig. 38-44, *A*), leaving 7 mm between the longitudinal osteotomy and the axis of the spinous process. Make the transverse osteotomy 4 mm caudad to the line, joining the inferior aspects of the two transverse processes. After removal of the fragment of facet, use a curet to remove the hyaline cartilage from the facet joint. Then introduce a pedicle finder into the space and push it gently against the pedicle (see Fig. 38-44, *A*). Take care in using this instrument to be sure it is introduced into the interarticular space and not into the bone of the inferior articular facet. It must find its way, sliding along the superior articular facet. Once the pedicle finder is in place, check the position by a lateral translation of the tip of the pedicle elevator. If the vertebra moves laterally when the elevator is translated, the pedicle finder is in the correct place. Insert the pedicle hook with a hook inserter and holder if needed (Fig. 38-44, *B*). In this maneuver, be certain that the horns of the bifid hook remain in the facet joint and do not hook into the remaining bone of the inferior facet. After the pedicle hook has been inserted into place, tap it further against the pedicle with a mallet.

◆ **Transverse Process Hook Implantation**

TECHNIQUE 38-8

The transverse process hook is part of a pediculotransverse claw system. In most scoliosis procedures, use this claw at the upper end of the convex side. In rigid scoliosis, if two rods on the concave side are used, use pediculotransverse claws at the upper end on both the convex and concave sides.

Place the transverse process hook over the cephalad edge of the transverse process. Prepare the area with a transverse process elevator, using the sharp edges of the elevator to divide the costotransverse ligament. Apply the transverse process hook and inspect its alignment with the pedicle hook.

◆ **Laminar Hook Implantation**

TECHNIQUE 38-9

Place laminar hooks around either the superior or inferior edge of the lamina, according to the desired direction of forces. Carefully match the type of laminar hook to the shape of the lamina and obtain the closest possible fit to avoid the possibility of hook impingement on the spinal canal (Fig. 38-45). To insert the supralaminar hook, remove the ligamentum flavum with Kerrison rongeurs and curets (Fig. 38-44, *C*). In the lumbar area, generally enough room exists between vertebrae to allow implantation of the hook without removing bone. In the thoracic area, however, the spinous process of the superior vertebra must be removed first. After the canal is open, obtain lateral extension of the area by excising the medial portion of the inferior articular facet of the superior vertebra. This will allow sufficient room for insertion of the thoracic laminar hook. At the thoracolumbar junction, the hooks usually are applied in compression. Use the smallest hook that can be fit around the lamina to prevent the blade from pushing too deeply into the spinal canal (see Fig. 38-45).

Be very careful when inserting the laminar hook in the infralaminar position. If necessary, remove a piece of the inferior border of the lamina to allow proper seating of the hook on the lamina (Fig. 38-44, *D*). Take care to preserve the lateral wall of the inferior facet to avoid lateral dislodgement of the hook. When inserting the inferiormost laminar hook, preserve the interspinous ligament and facet capsule to prevent kyphosis distal to the rods. Do not include the facet joint at this level in the fusion.

Multihook Segmental Instrumentation Systems

Several types of multihook segmental instrumentation systems are available, including Cotrel-Dubousset, Texas Scottish Rite Hospital, Cotrel-Dubousset Horizon, ISOLA, Moss-Miami, and others. These systems are constantly evolving. Although the surgical technique of using the various instrumentation systems vary, depending on the implants and instrumentation available, the basic principles of these systems are similar and are illustrated in the technique for use of the CD Horizon M-8 system, which we are currently using. The surgeon is referred to the technique manuals of the individual systems for up-to-date information about hook types and instrumentation available with each system.

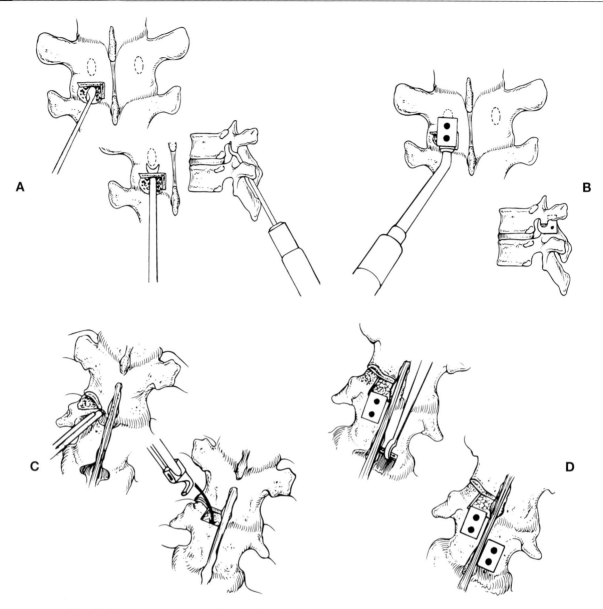

Fig. 38-44 **A,** Insertion of pedicle hook. Inferior facet is excised. Curet is used to clean cartilage. Pedicle finder rides over pedicle and indicates whether more bone should be taken off. It is moved sideways to determine stability of pedicle purchase. Beware in this sideways movement of "plunging" into the spinal canal. **B,** Pedicle hook is pushed into place by hook inserter. If necessary, plug can be introduced into hook to maintain control of hook inserter over hook as hook is inserted; plug is then removed. **C,** Supralaminar hook insertion. This insertion applies to lower two concave hooks in single thoracic curve instrumentation. Laminotomy is kept as small as possible to minimize risk of deep penetration into spinal canal during rod insertion. Tight fit is necessary, and thoracic laminar hook is used if laminar thickness is too small to allow lumbar laminar hook to be stable in anteroposterior plane. **D,** Infralaminar hook insertion. Lower convex hook in right thoracic curve is inserted in this manner. Ligamentum flavum is dissected off underside of lamina. Small inferior laminotomy provides horizontal purchase site for hook. Adjacent facet capsule should be spared because it is not included in fusion. (Redrawn from Dennis F: *Orthop Clin North Am* 19:294, 1988.)

◆ CD Horizon Instrumentation

TECHNIQUE 38-10

Patient positioning, surgical exposure, and hook site selection are as described on p. 1776. The appropriate top-loading CD Horizon hooks are inserted at the hook sites selected in the preoperative plan.

Measure the appropriately-sized rod and cut it to length outside the operative field. To achieve correct rod contour, bend the rod in small incremental steps using a French bender. Place the rod into the top-loading hooks from either

a cephalad or caudad direction. Insert the break-off set screw or plug into the hook, either by free hand or using the plug starter or plug introducer. Several methods can be used to insert the plug into the hook.

Method 1. If the rod is lying in the bottom of the hook groove, place the plug on the plug starter and turn the plug starter counterclockwise until an audible "click" occurs. Tighten the plug clockwise. Even with the audible "click," take care that the plug is not cross-threaded (Fig. 38-46, *A*). If the hook needs to be controlled during the rod insertion process, use the lateral hook holder and the plug starter to place the plug into the hook (Fig. 38-46, *B*).

Method 2. If a slight height difference exists between the rod and the hook, use the rocker instrument. Grasp the hook from the sides with the rocker cam above the rod (Fig. 38-47, *A*). Rotate the rocker backward, levering the rod into the hook groove (Fig. 38-47, *B*). Use the plug starter to insert the plug.

Method 3. If the height difference between the hook and the rod is such that the rocker cannot be used, use the plug introducer instrument. Place the instrument over the rod with its phalanges parallel to the rod. Position the tines of the plug introducer over the rod and the hook. Turn the sleeve of the plug introducer clockwise to secure the hook to the instrument (Fig. 38-48, *A*). Attach either one or two corkscrew devices to the phalanges of the plug introducer and drive the rod into the top-loading hook (Fig. 38-48, *B*). At this point it is difficult to determine when the rod is fully seated. If it cannot be determined

continued

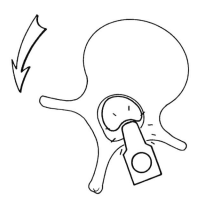

Fig. 38-45 Laminar hook should be chosen carefully to match shape of lamina and obtain closest possible fit to prevent hook impingement on spinal canal. (Redrawn from Chopin D: Cotrel-Dubousset instrumentation for adolescent idiopathic scoliosis. In Bridwell KH, DeWald RL, eds: *The textbook of spinal surgery*, Philadelphia, 1991, JB Lippincott.)

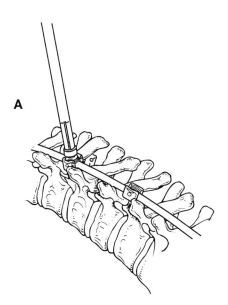
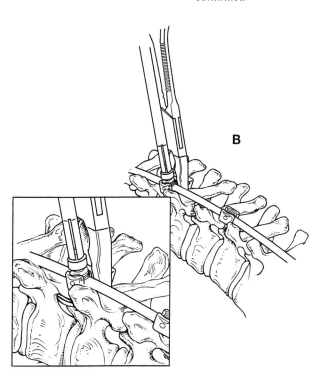

Fig. 38-46 Method 1, rod insertion. See text for description. (Redrawn from Laufer SJ, Bowe JA: Horizon spinal system surgical technique manual, Memphis, 1999, Sofamor Danek.)

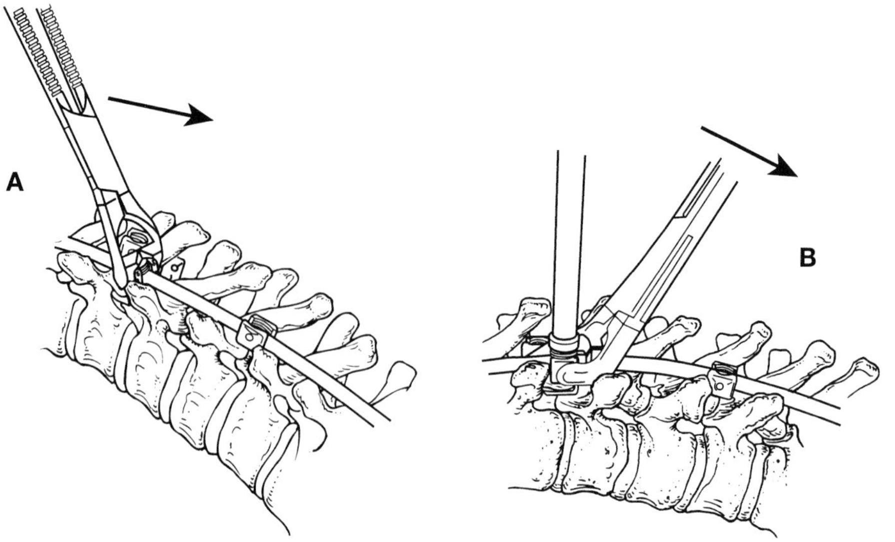

Fig. 38-47   Method 2, rod insertion. See text for description. (Redrawn from Laufer SJ, Bowe JA: Horizon spinal system surgical technique manual, Memphis, 1999, Sofamor Danek.)

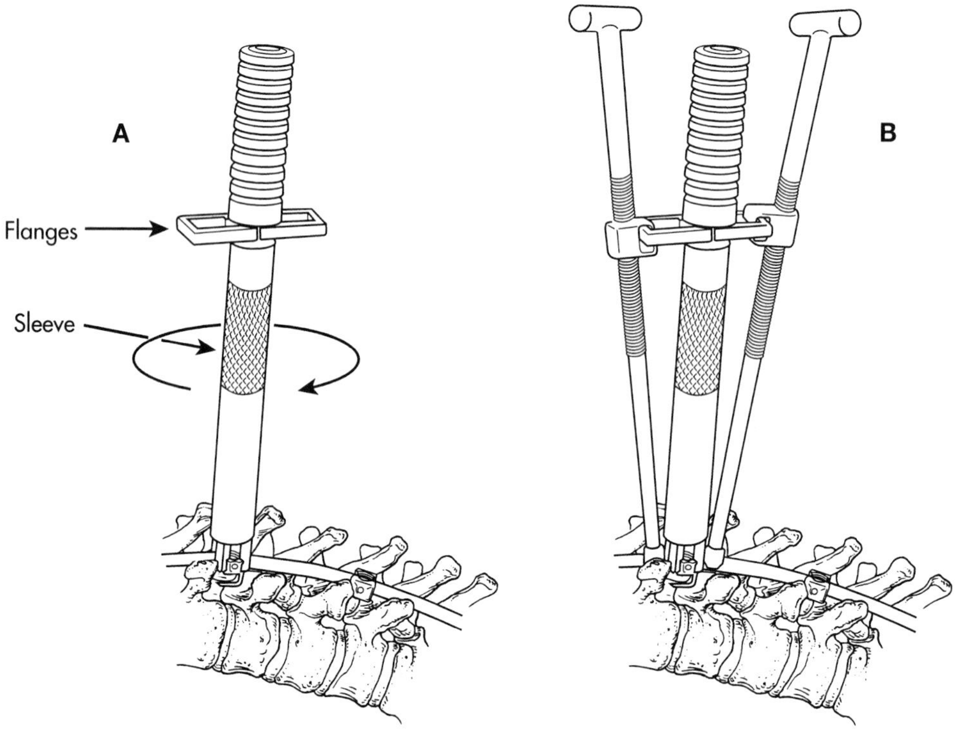

Fig. 38-48   Method 3, rod insertion. See text for description. (Redrawn from Laufer SJ, Bowe JA: Horizon spinal system surgical technique manual, Memphis, 1999, Sofamor Danek.)   *Continued*

Flanges

Sleeve

visually, place the provisional plug driver into the cannulation of the plug introducer. Check to see if the uppermost etching mark on the shaft of the plug driver is completely inside the cannulation of the plug introducer. If the etching mark is not completely inside the introducer, then the corkscrews must be turned further to fully seat the rod (Fig. 38-48, *C*). Once the etching mark is confirmed to be entirely inside the introducer, remove the driver from the cannulation, and place the plug into the cannulation and secure it with the provisional plug driver (Fig. 38-48, *D*). Match the plug driver instrument to the hex head of the plug. Turn the provisional plug driver counter clockwise until an audible "click" is heard and a palpable slight dropping of the instrument is noted. This indicates that the thread of the plug is lined up with the thread of the hook and limits the possibility of cross threading. Alternatively, the plug can be placed on the plug starter instrument, and then the instrument with the plug is placed into the cannulation of the plug introducer.

Method 4. Occasionally the rod lies medial or lateral to the hook channel and controlled translation is necessary. Use the rod reducer instrument and the accompanying lever

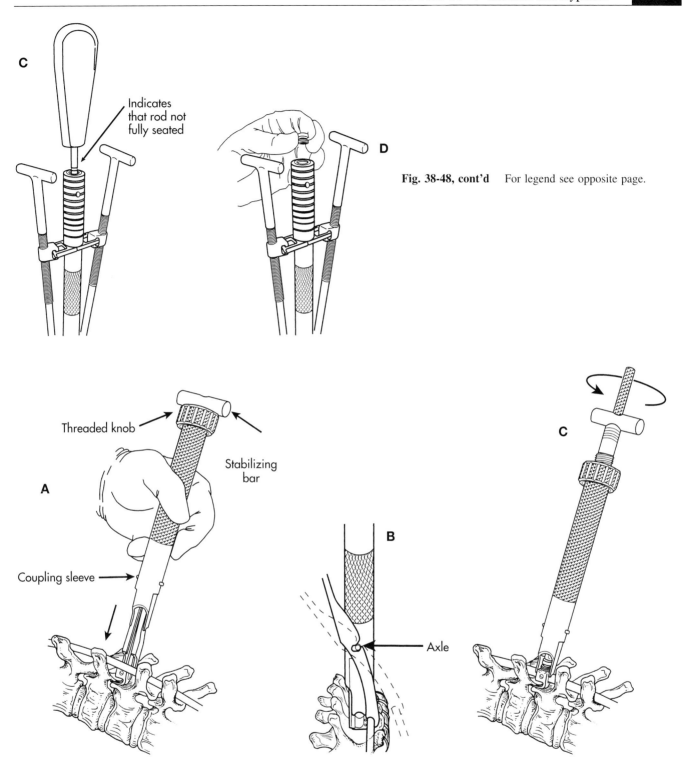

C

Indicates that rod not fully seated

D

Fig. 38-48, cont'd For legend see opposite page.

Threaded knob

Stabilizing bar

A

Coupling sleeve

B

Axle

C

Fig. 38-49 Method 4, rod insertion. See text for description. (Redrawn from Laufer SJ, Bowe JA: Horizon spinal system surgical technique manual, Memphis, 1999, Sofamor Danek.)

arm in these situations. Attach the tines of the rod reducer to a side of the hook in a manner similar to that of the lateral implant holder. By holding the coupling sleeve and stabilizing bar, position the tines of the instrument over the side of the hook body with the open side facing the rod. Once the tines are in position, hold the rod reducer steady with the stabilizing bar and slide the coupling sleeve downward until the hook is properly engaged (Fig. 38-49, *A*). With the hook contained, turn the threaded knob at least one full clockwise revolution. The

continued

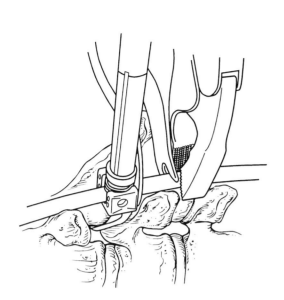

Fig. 38-50 Force application and rod rotation. See text for description. (Redrawn from Laufer SJ, Bowe JA: Horizon spinal system surgical technique manual, Memphis, 1999, Sofamor Danek.)

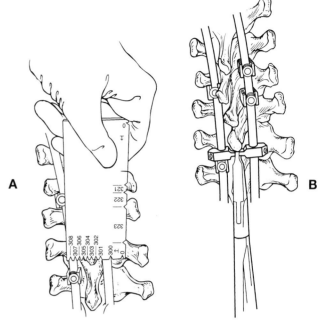

Fig. 38-51 Bone grafting and cross-link plating. See text for description. (Redrawn from Laufer SJ, Bowe JA: Horizon spinal system surgical technique manual, Memphis, 1999, Sofamor Danek.)

hook can now be manipulated by the rod reducer. For translation of a laterally positioned rod, attach the lever arm to the coupling sleeve axles. Turn the threaded knob while manipulating the lever arm with a sweeping motion to capture the rod (Fig. 38-49, *B*). Translate the rod with this lever arm until it is above the channel of the hook. Turn the threaded knob in a clockwise manner until the rod is captured in the hook channel. The lever arm can now be removed. Continue tightening the threaded knob until complete rod reduction is achieved. Use the provisional plug driver to confirm the rod position in the hook channel. Use the plug starter to introduce the plug into the implant channel (Fig. 38-49, *C*). Turn the plug starter counter clockwise until an audible "click" is noted and then turn it clockwise to insert the plug and temporarily lock the rod within the hook.

If desired at this point, compression or distraction forces can be applied to the hooks. These forces are achieved by use of the curved compressor or curve spreader instruments. Take care to ensure that the feet of either instrument are placed against the hook body and not against the plug (Fig. 38-50). Loosen the plug during application of this force and then tighten slightly to maintain temporary locking of the rod and hook construct. If the plug has been tightened in the cross-threaded position, remove and replace it. If desired, the rod can now

be rotated with the power grip or hex rotation instruments. Check the hook position carefully during these rotation maneuvers and apply necessary compression or distraction to resecure the hooks if needed. Tighten the plugs securely at this time.

Determine the appropriate sized cross-link plate with the measuring template (Fig. 38-51, *A*). Spread or compress the rods for appropriate fit. Press the cross-link plate down onto the rods (Fig. 38-51, *B*). Use plate benders to contour the cross-link plates if the rods are not exactly parallel; however, do not exceed a 20-degree bend in any single plane. Advance the set screws and the cross link, using the hex-head screwdriver. Use two screwdrivers simultaneously to advance the set screws for uniform closure. When all the hooks are securely seated, perform final tightening and break off the head of the plug. Place the counter torque device over the implant and rod (Fig. 38-52, *A*). Insert the final plug driver through the cannulation of the counter torque into the hex head of the plug. Hold the handle of the counter torque device to prevent torquing of the construct while the plug is broken (Fig. 38-52, *B*). Once the hex head has been removed, if any changes are needed, the internal plug can be removed using a modular device (Fig. 38-52, *C*).

Decortication and bone grafting can now be done as needed. Close the wound in the usual manner.

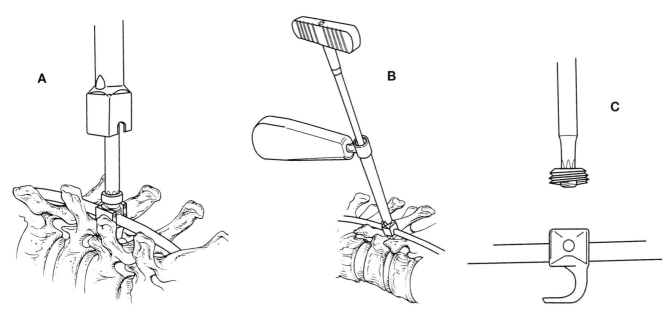

Fig. 38-52 Final tightening and closure. See text for description. (Redrawn from Laufer SJ, Bowe JA: Horizon spinal system surgical technique manual, Memphis, 1999, Sofamor Danek.)

◆ Sublaminar Wires

Sublaminar wires generally are not used alone as anchors at the upper or lower instrumented vertebrae because they provide no axial stability. We have found sublaminar wires and cables useful in and around the apex of curves to aid in translation maneuver in which the spine can be pulled to a precontoured rod, thus minimizing the need for derotational maneuvers. The more rigid the curve is, the more helpful these sublaminar wires or cables are (Fig. 38-53).

TECHNIQUE 38-11

Expose the spine as described on p. 1776. Using a needle-nose rongeur, gradually thin the ligamentum flavum until the midline cleavage plane is visible. In the thoracic spine the spinous processes slant distally and must be removed before the ligamentum flavum can be adequately seen (Fig. 38-54). Once the midline cleavage is visible, carefully sweep a Penfield no. 4 dissector across the deep surface of the ligamentum flavum on the right and left sides (Fig. 38-55). Use a Kerrison punch to remove the remainder of the ligamentum flavum (Fig. 38-56). Take care during this step to avoid damaging the dura or epidural vessels.

Johnston et al. showed that wire penetration into the neural canal during wire passage is substantial (up to 1 cm). This depth of penetration varies by level, decreasing as the wires are passed more caudally. Because the depth of penetration is less when a semicircular-shaped wire is used, shape the wire as shown in Fig. 38-57. The largest diameter of the bend should be slightly larger than the lamina. Always pass the wire in the midline and not laterally, and remove the spinous processes before wire passage. It is important that both the surgeon and the assistant be completely prepared for each step before passage of the wire and that they are careful about sudden movements and inadvertent touching or hitting of the wires that have already been passed.

Passing of the wire is divided into four steps: (1) introduction, (2) advancement, (3) roll-through, and (4) pull-through. Pass the more cephalad wires first and progress caudally. Gently place the tip of the wire into the neural canal at the inferior edge of the lamina in the midline. Hold the long end of the doubled wire in one hand and advance the tip with the other. Rest the hand that is advancing the tip firmly on the patient's back. Lift the tails of the wire slightly, pulling them to keep the wire snugly against the undersurface of the lamina. Once the wire has been introduced, advance it 5 to 6 mm. Beginning roll-through too soon will cause the tip of the wire to strike the inferior portion of the vertebral arch, and the wire can be pushed more deeply into the neural canal (Fig. 38-58, *B*). After advancement, roll the tip of the wire so that it emerges on the upper end of the lamina (Fig. 38-58, *C*). As the tip of the wire emerges, use a nerve hook to pull the end farther up from the lamina to allow enough room for a needle holder, wire holder, or Kocher clamp to be placed into the loop of the wire by the assistant. Take the clamp from the assistant and pull the wire with the clamp until it is positioned beneath the lamina, with half its length protruding above and half below the lamina.

continued

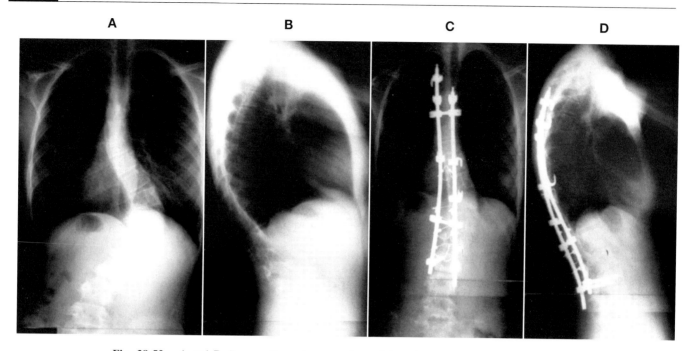

Fig. 38-53   **A** and **B,** Preoperative anteroposterior and lateral standing scoliosis films. Thoracolumbar curve measures 77 degrees. **C** and **D,** Postoperative correction using hooks with sublaminar cables, correcting thoracolumbar curve to 22 degrees.

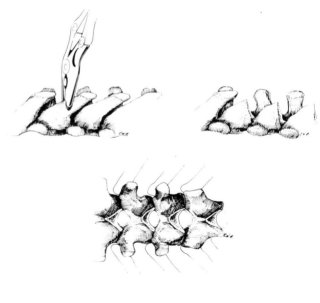

Fig. 38-54   Removal of caudally slanting spinous processes to expose ligamentum flavum. (From Segmental spinal fixation and correction using Richards' L-rod instrumentation, Memphis, Smith & Nephew Richards.)

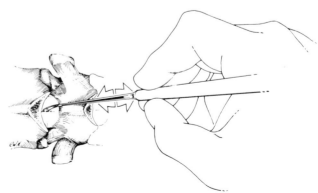

Fig. 38-55   Penfield no. 4 dissector for freeing deep surfaces of ligamentum flavum. (From Segmental spinal fixation and correction using Richards' L-rod instrumentation, Memphis, Smith & Nephew Richards.)

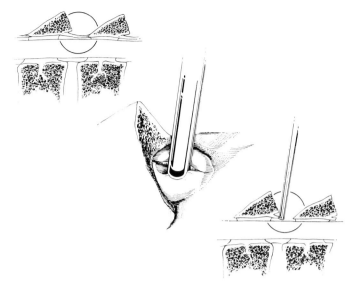

Fig. 38-56   Kerrison punch for removing remainder of ligamentum flavum. (From Segmental spinal fixation and correction using Richards' L-rod instrumentation, Memphis, Smith & Nephew Richards.)

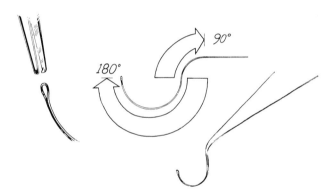

Fig. 38-57   Shape of double wire before it passes under lamina (see text). (From Segmental spinal fixation and correction using Richards' L-rod instrumentation, Memphis, Smith & Nephew Richards.)

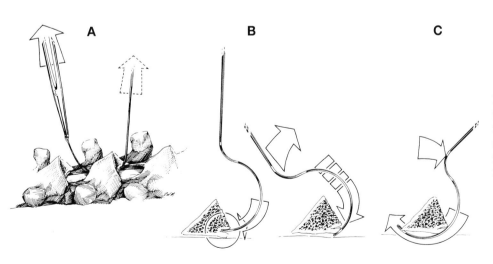

Fig. 38-58   Passage of segmental wire beneath lamina. (From Segmental spinal fixation and correction using Richards' L-rod instrumentation, Memphis, Smith & Nephew Richards.)

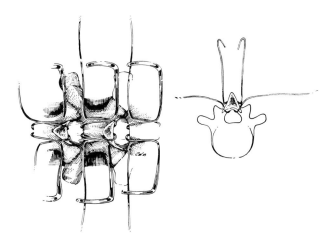

Fig. 38-59 Following division of wire, wire is crimped on laminar surface of each side of spinous process. (From Segmental spinal fixation and correction using Richards' L-rod instrumentation, Memphis, Smith & Nephew Richards.)

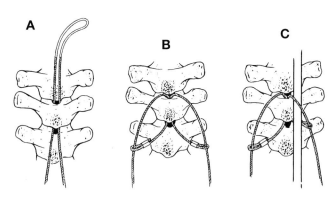

Fig. 38-60 Sublaminar cable technique. **A,** C-shaped cable leader is passed through lamina. **B,** Cable ends are passed through inferior loops to lasso lamina. **C,** Rod in place beneath cable.

As the clamp is pulled, gently feed the wire superiorly from the long end. This must be a coordinated maneuver and must be done by the surgeon. Once the wire has been pulled through, cut off the tip of the wire and place one length of the wire on the right side and the other length on the left side of the lamina. As an alternative, leave double wires on one side and pass another wire so that double wires are present on both sides. Crimp each wire into the surface to the lamina to prevent any wire from being pushed accidentally into the neural canal (Fig. 38-59). As more wires are passed, accidentally hitting the other wires becomes more likely. Even though the wires are crimped over the lamina, hitting them can be dangerous, and care must be taken to avoid these previously placed wires. Crimp the superior wire toward the midline and crimp the inferior wire laterally.

◆ Sublaminar Cables

Songer et al. recommended the use of sublaminar cables instead of monofilament stainless steel wire because wire breakage and migration have been serious complications of sublaminar wiring. They also believe that cable flexibility prevents repeated contusions to the spinal cord that can occur during insertion of the rod and tightening of the wire. We now routinely use these cables rather than monofilament sublaminar wire.

TECHNIQUE 38-12
Remove the spinous processes and ligamentum flavum (see Figs. 38-54 to 38-58). Contour the monofilament cable leader into a C shape and pass it beneath the lamina. Grasp the leader and pull it through, leaving equal amounts of wire above and below the lamina (Fig. 38-60, *A*). Cut the tip of

the leader and separate the two cables. Pass one arm of the cable through the inferior loop to "lasso" the lamina (Fig. 38-60, *B*). After the cables have been passed, contour the rods as indicated. Place the rods through the noose of the cable and use the cable to "lasso" the rod into position (Fig. 38-60, *C*). The cables currently have an integral crimp. Pass a provisional crimp (Fig. 38-61, *A*) over the cable. Prepare the cable tensioner by depressing the release lever and sliding the release button, which allows the tension to fully retract (Fig. 38-61, *B*). Insert the cable through the tensioner. The cable leader must be straight and short (Fig. 38-62, *A*). Once the cable has been threaded through the tensioner, lift the cam lever to lock the cable (Fig 38-62, *B*). Depress the tension arm repeatedly until the desired tension is obtained. After appropriate tension is obtained, lock the provisional crimp into place (Fig. 38-62, *C*). The tension on any other cables can be adjusted and retightened using the provisional crimp and tensioner. After all cables have been tightened, the integral crimp is compressed (Fig. 38-61, *D*).

Complications and Pitfalls in Multihook Segmental Instrumentation Systems

In addition to the complications inherent in any spinal arthrodesis, multihook segmental instrumentation systems have several potential pitfalls. These generally can be divided into strategic mistakes and technical mistakes.

One of the more common strategic mistakes is stopping the instrumentation at the middle of a sagittal or frontal pathological curve. If the instrumentation is stopped at the level of a thoracolumbar kyphosis, as may occur in a King type II thoracic curve, a postoperative junctional kyphosis often occurs (Fig. 38-63). This mistake is prevented by closely following the principles of hook site selection (p. 1795). Another common strategic mistake is failure to recognize the significance of the

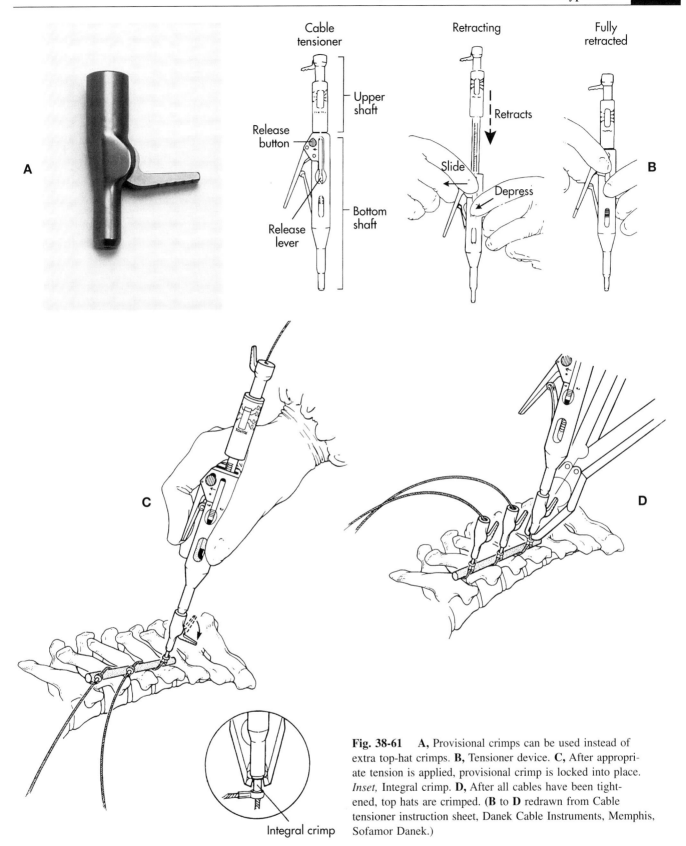

Fig. 38-61 A, Provisional crimps can be used instead of extra top-hat crimps. **B,** Tensioner device. **C,** After appropriate tension is applied, provisional crimp is locked into place. *Inset,* Integral crimp. **D,** After all cables have been tightened, top hats are crimped. (**B** to **D** redrawn from Cable tensioner instruction sheet, Danek Cable Instruments, Memphis, Sofamor Danek.)

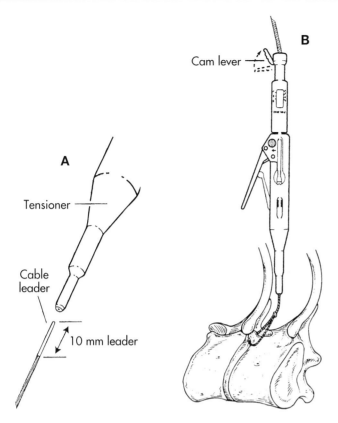

Cam lever

B

A

Tensioner

Cable
leader

10 mm leader

Fig. 38-62   **A** and **B,** Insertion and locking of cable. (Redrawn from Cable tensioner instruction sheet, Danek Cable Instruments, Memphis, Sofamor Danek.)

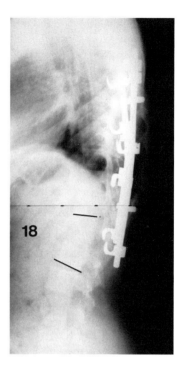

18

Fig. 38-63   Postoperative junctional kyphosis in King type II thoracic curve; instrumentation stopped at level of thoracolumbar kyphosis.

upper thoracic curve preoperatively. If the upper thoracic curve does not correct on supine bending films to the predicted correction of the lower thoracic curve, elevation of the left shoulder and an unsightly deformity will occur (p. 1801). This mistake is prevented by carefully evaluating the clinical appearance of the shoulders and the bending films, as well as the standing roentgenograms, with special attention to this upper curve. The other problem frequently described in the coronal plane is decompensation with selective fusion of the thoracic curve (Fig. 38-64). Techniques to prevent this complication are discussed on p. 1800.

Several potential technical problems should be avoided during the surgical procedure. During insertion of the pedicle hooks, the hooks should not be inserted too horizontally or else the inferior facet of the superior vertebra may be fractured; if the hooks are inserted too vertically, the superior facet of the inferior vertebra may be fractured. The pedicle hook should be carefully inserted into the intraarticular space, and care should be taken to be certain that the pedicle is incorporated into the bifid area of the hook. During insertion of the laminar hooks the most frequent problem is insufficient insertion of the hook under the lamina. If this hook is not well seated, when the rod is applied and rotated and a posterior-directed force is applied, the hook often pulls out and the lamina breaks. When inserting infralaminar hooks in the lumbar spine, it must be remembered that the lower laminar edge runs in a backward and downward

direction; therefore the hooks must be inserted in the same direction. Often, shaving down of the lamina is required to allow the hook to be well seated.

In contouring the rod, it should be remembered that the goal of the surgery is to restore normal sagittal contours. Excessive bending of the rod should be avoided if possible. If a large lumbar curve is present and the rod is contoured in the coronal plane to correspond exactly to the lumbar curve, as the rod is rotated, an excessive posterior force is applied to the lower hooks and these hooks can then cut out posteriorly (Fig. 38-65). If, however, the distance between the rod and hook is too large, the lamina can break as the rod is being inserted into the hook. In this case it may be necessary to contour the rod further.

As the rod rotation maneuver is done, the intermediate hooks of the thoracic spine tend to unload and can pull out with rotation. These hooks generally have to be reseated at least once during the rod rotation maneuver. Also, when a lordotic rod bend with a reverse hook pattern is applied at the thoracolumbar junction, the infralaminar hook at the distal end often needs to be reset with rod rotation. As the rod is rotated, the upper end vertebra hook tends to medially rotate into the canal and may cause neurological injury, such as a Brown-Séquard syndrome. This hook should be watched carefully during the rotation maneuver.

The lower intermediate hook on the concave side can be forced accidentally into the spinal canal during rod insertion.

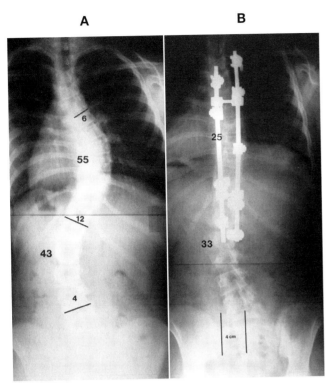

Fig. 38-64 **A,** King type II curve. **B,** Decompensated lumbar curve after fusion of thoracic curve only.

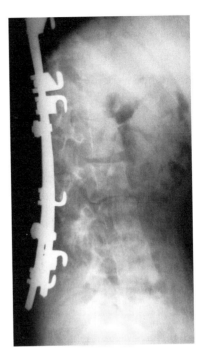

Fig. 38-65 Cut-out of lower hooks caused by improper contouring of rods.

The spinal cord generally is shifted toward the concave side of the scoliosis curve, and therefore extreme caution should be exercised when the rod is inserted. When the rod is rotated, however, the lower intermediate hook is pulled backward and away from the spinal cord. Therefore the lower intermediate hook is of more concern during rod insertion, whereas the upper end vertebra hook is of more concern during rod rotation.

When the convex rod is applied, a downward force is applied to the apical vertebra. Therefore this hook should be a pedicle hook and not a laminar hook. Generally the upper end vertebra in scoliosis should be instrumented on both sides with at least one pedicle transverse process claw. Because compression is applied to the convex rod, the pedicle transverse process claw generally is used on the convex side. The hook that most frequently dislodges is the inferior, convex, cranially directed hook. An additional caudally directed hook at the level above can give a two-level claw configuration to this hook and decrease the possibility of hook cut out.

Fusion Levels and Hook Site Placement

In determining fusion levels for multihook segmental hook instrumentation, several basic principles must be considered.

1. Anteroposterior, lateral, and bending films are essential. Because standing bending films are not nearly as revealing, supine bending films are always recommended.
2. In the sagittal plane all pathological curves must be included. The goal of multihook systems is to produce normal sagittal contours of the spine, if possible. The instrumentation should not be stopped in the middle of a pathological sagittal curve, such as a thoracolumbar junctional kyphosis. The upper hook should not stop at the apex of the kyphosis proximally. These levels are determined on standing lateral films.
3. In the transverse plane, the instrumentation should extend to a rotational neutral vertebra if possible. This is determined on standing posteroanterior or bending films.
4. The instrumentation should be stopped at the level above disc space neutralization, as determined on bending films, as long as this level does not conflict with the sagittal and transverse plane requirements. In other words the disc height should be equal on the right and left sides and should open on both the right and left sides with supine bending films. The rigid segment of the thoracic curve also is determined on coronal bending films and dictates the placement of intermediate hooks.
5. The distal level should fall within the stable zone of Harrington (Fig. 38-66). The inferior vertebra ideally is bisected by the center sacral line, but this is necessary on bending films, not on the upright standing posteroanterior film.

Once the proximal and distal levels of the fusion have been determined, hook placement patterns must be determined. To

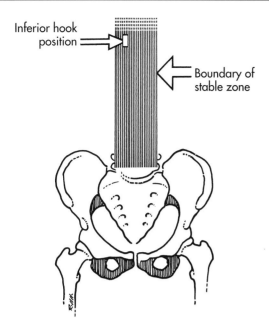

Inferior hook position

Boundary of stable zone

Fig. 38-66   Stable zone for inferior vertebra as described by Harrington.

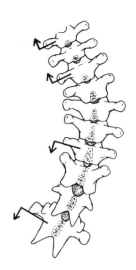

Fig. 38-67   Four-hook construct for insertion of concave rod for correction of King type III curve without junctional kyphosis.

determine the appropriate hook patterns, the type of force that must be generated on the spine and what that force will do to the sagittal plane must be determined. The basic principles are (1) distraction forces (forces directed away from the apex of the curve) decrease lordosis or contribute to kyphosis; (2) compression forces (towards the apex of the curve) decrease kyphosis or create lordosis; (3) to create kyphosis, the concave side must be approached first; (4) to create lordosis the convex side must be approached first, and the forces must be directed toward the apex of the curve; and (5) at the thoracolumbar junction, distractive forces should not be applied, and in rod bending, the lordotic bend of the rod should be initiated at the T12-L1 interspace.

Hook Site Selection in Thoracic Curves

Proper selection of fusion levels in thoracic idiopathic scoliosis is controversial. The basic hook site selection for multihook segmental instrumentation systems is described for the various types of curves based on the King classification.

Type III Thoracic Curves. The hook pattern for type III curves is the basic instrumentation; other hook patterns for types I, II, IV, and V are built on this pattern.

Type III thoracic curves are not associated with significant rotation of the distal lumbar segments. The stable vertebra usually is L1 or L2. Type III is basically a single thoracic hypokyphotic scoliosis, but the thoracolumbar junction should be evaluated carefully to be certain there is no kyphotic segment. High left thoracic curves should be carefully evaluated if present.

Type III curves without junctional kyphosis generally are corrected by rotation of a concave rod with a four-hook construct (Fig. 38-67). The upper neutral vertebra with a disc

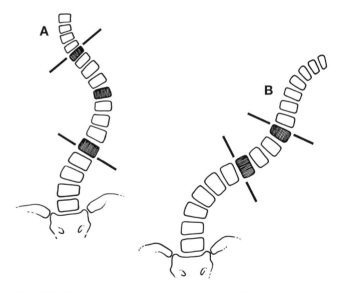

Fig. 38-68   **A,** Anteroposterior diagrams of uppermost and lowermost instrumented vertebrae. **B,** Upper and lower rigid vertebral bodies are shown on bending films.

space that is not wedged generally is chosen for the most proximal hook. The lower end vertebra should be in the stable zone of Harrington on bending films. The end vertebra should be neutral on bending films, and the disc below the end vertebra should open on both sides on bending films. Again, the lateral roentgenogram must be evaluated carefully to be certain the lower vertebra is not at the apex of a junctional kyphosis.

The apical vertebra of the deformity is identified. The rigid segment of the curve is identified on bending films (Fig. 38-68).

The intermediate curve is the stiffest zone of the deformity. On the convex bending film the discs are still closed on the concave side. The limits of this area are the upper and lower intermediate vertebrae. The apical vertebra is the most rotated and most horizontal vertebra.

◆ Hook and Rod Insertion for Type III Thoracic Curve

TECHNIQUE 38-13

On the concave side place a pedicle hook in an upgoing direction on the upper vertebra and place a laminar hook in a downgoing direction on the lower end vertebra. Place a pedicle hook in an upgoing manner on the upper intermediate vertebra and a laminar hook in a downgoing direction on the lower intermediate vertebra.

The hook sites on the convex side are illustrated in Fig. 38-69. The upper end vertebra should be instrumented by a "claw" configuration. Place a transverse process hook facing caudally and create a claw by placing a pedicle hook cranially either at that level or the next distal level. Splitting the claw over two levels increases the strength of fixation. At the apical vertebra, insert an upgoing pedicle hook for compression. Place a final upgoing laminar hook at the lower end vertebra to apply compression also.

If a junctional kyphosis is present, apply a lordotic bend to the concave rod to allow more normal transition from thoracic kyphosis to lumbar lordosis. Apply compression across the thoracolumbar junction to achieve this lordosis by adding an additional upgoing hook at the lower level of the concave rod. Also apply an additional downgoing hook to the convex rod (Fig. 38-70). Prepare hook sites and insert the hooks. Insert the concave rod first, seat the hooks, and rotate the rod to 90 degrees to convert the thoracic hypokyphosis to kyphosis. An additional lordotic bend, if necessary, will apply an opposite rotational effect at the thoracolumbar junction to cause a lordosing effect. Insert the hooks for the convex rod. Decorticate the facets and apply the convex rod. Apply compression across the convexity of the thoracic curve. If an additional lordotic bend was used, apply distraction to the fractional curve beginning at the thoracolumbar junction.

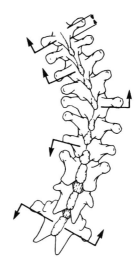

Fig. 38-69   Hook placement sites for instrumentation of King type III thoracic curve.

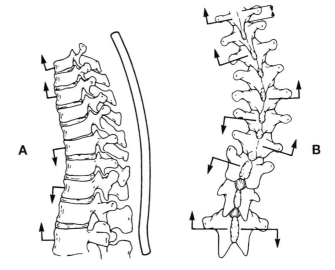

Fig. 38-70   If junctional kyphosis is present, lordotic bend is applied to concave rod (**A**), and additional downgoing hook is used on convex rod (**B**).

Double Major Curves. In double major curve patterns, both the lumbar and thoracic curves are roughly equal, and both are significantly structural. Even if the lumbar curve is slightly bigger, it often is more flexible on the side-bending films. This should not be confused with a King type II curve pattern. In treating double major curves, preservation of lumbar segments and maintenance of lumbar lordosis are important because of their possible role in back pain after fusion. As many lumbar motion segments as possible should be preserved. In double major curves, if L3 is neutral in the transverse plane (rotation) and is intersected by the center sacral line on standing roentgenograms and the curve from L3 to the sacrum bends out

completely on side-bending films, fusion may extend only to L3 instead of to L4. In our experience, however, most double major curves require fusion to L4.

King type I curves have lumbar curves greater than the thoracic curves. When the thoracic curve is small, the curve can be treated as a single lumbar curve (p. 1805). Usually the thoracic curve is large and has become significantly structural by the time surgery is considered, and the hook pattern and technique are the same as for double major curves.

The hook sites for the thoracic portion of the curve are the same as for the right thoracic lordoscoliosis without a thoracolumbar junctional kyphosis (p. 1796). In the lumbar spine the convex side hooks should be applied to provide compres-

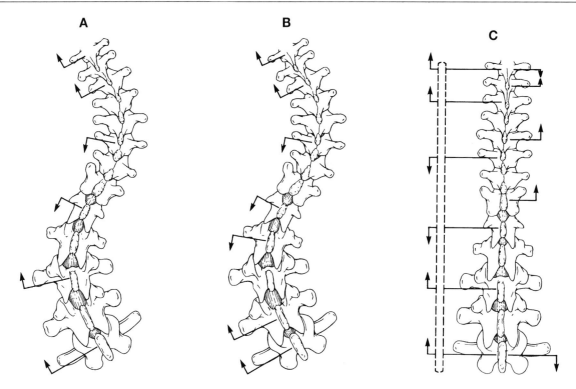

Fig. 38-71   Instrumentation of double major curve (see text). **A,** Hook placement for left rod. **B,** Two apical lumbar hooks can be used to apply compression at apex of lumbar curve. **C,** Hook placement for right rod after left rod rotation.

sion, which will restore the lumbar lordosis. We prefer to place a cranially directed infralaminar hook on the convex side of the lumbar curve at the apical vertebra (Fig. 38-71, *A*). A cranially directed inferior hook is then placed at the lowermost end of the vertebra. Alternatively, two apical lumbar hooks can be placed facing each other one segment apart to apply compression at the apex of the lumbar curve (Fig. 38-71, *B*). On the concave portion of the lumbar curve, a caudal-directed hook is applied to the end vertebra (Fig. 38-71, *C*). We prefer three cross links in these double major curves.

◆ *Hook and Rod Insertion for Double Major Curves*

TECHNIQUE 38-14

Decorticate the facets on the left side and then insert the left rod first after contouring it into an S shape to match the normal sagittal contours. Insert the rod into the hooks and seat the hooks. Rotate the rod 90 degrees in a counterclockwise direction to provide kyphosis in the thoracic spine and lordosis in the lumbar spine. Once the rod has been rotated, seat the hooks again. Contour the right rod and decorticate the facet joints. Insert the right rod and tighten the upper claw configuration first. Compress the apical thoracic hook toward the upper claw and tighten it. Then compress the lower convex thoracic hook toward the upper claw and

tighten it. Distract the lower lumbar hook away from the upper claw and tighten it (Fig. 38-71, *C*). Apply the appropriate cross links, placing two links as close as possible to the end vertebra proximally and distally and one in the middle (Fig. 38-72). Decorticate and add bone graft to complete the procedure.

Type IV Thoracic Curves. Type IV curves extend down to L4, which is the stable vertebra. Lateral roentgenograms should be carefully evaluated because some type IV curves have a sagittal malalignment consisting of a thoracic lordosis and a thoracolumbar kyphosis, whereas others have a more normal sagittal contour from top to bottom. In patients without thoracolumbar kyphosis, Bridwell et al. reported saving one or two levels if (1) L2 falls within the center sacral line, (2) all segments from L2 to the sacrum derotate and level off on bending films, (3) the thoracic curve is flexible enough for the derotation maneuver, and (4) the most caudal segment instrumented is neutral in rotation. Physical and roentgenographic examinations also must evaluate for a high thoracic curve, which could be worsened if not detected preoperatively. If, however, significant thoracolumbar kyphosis and thoracic lordosis are present, the two sagittal curves must be treated separately. Representative hook sites are shown in Fig. 38-73, *C*.

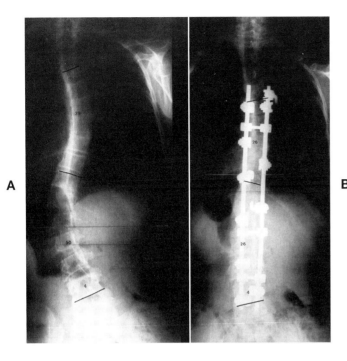

Fig. 38-72   **A,** King type I double major curve. **B,** After fusion and instrumentation with TSRH rods and cross links.

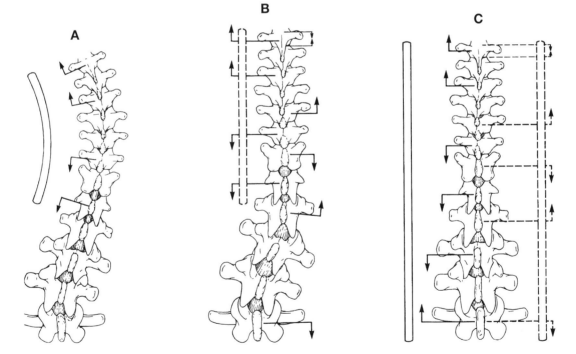

Fig. 38-73   Instrumentation of King type IV thoracic curve (see text). **A,** Thoracic curve is distracted with short rod, and rod is rotated to correct thoracic lordosis. **B,** Long right thoracic rod is inserted, and thoracic curve and thoracolumbar junction are compressed; hook on L4 is left loose. **C,** Short left rod is replaced with longer rod, and appropriate compression and distraction are applied.

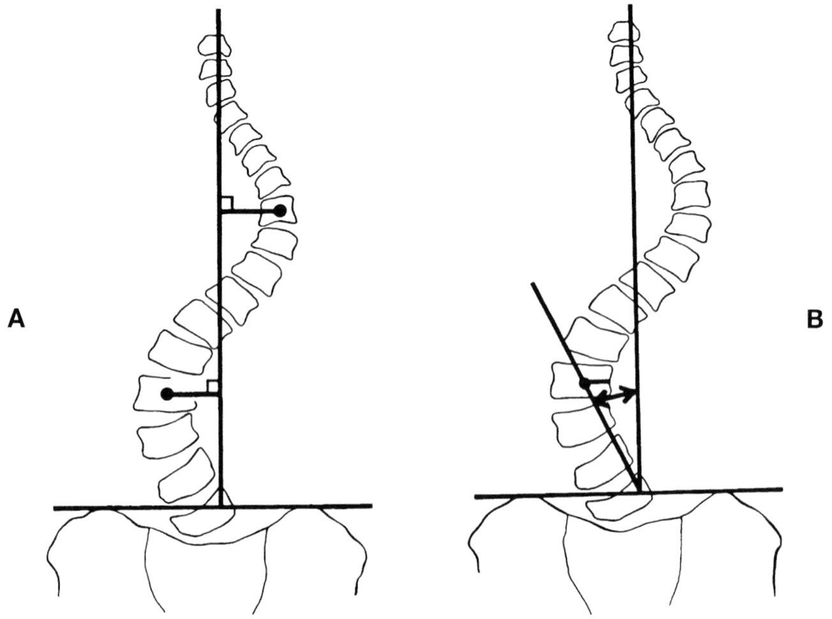

Fig. 38-74 King type II (false double major) curve. **A,** Distance of apical vertebra from plumb line is helpful in distinguishing King II curve from double major curve. **B,** Lumbosacral angle of apical vertebra is demonstrated here.

◆ *Hook and Rod Insertion for Type IV Thoracic Curve*

TECHNIQUE 38-15

To correct the thoracic hypokyphosis, approach the segment from T4 to T12 from the left side first. To correct the short segment kyphosis from T11 to L1, the right side must be approached first. To accomplish this, apply a left-sided distraction rod from T4 to T12 with hooks in the distraction mode (Fig. 38-73, *A*). Perform the derotation maneuver to correct the thoracic lordosis. Next, place a longer right-sided rod from T5 to L4 (Fig. 38-73, *B*). Contour normal thoracic kyphosis and lordosis into the rod. The hooks apply compression forces between T11 and L1 to achieve upper lumbar lordosis. Next, remove the left-sided rod and replace it with a longer rod from T4 to L4 (Fig. 38-73, *C*). Place the hooks in a distraction mode from T4 to T12 and in a compression mode from L2 to L4. Apply the compression forces between L2 and L4 on the left before applying any distraction force on the right.

Type II Thoracic Curves. Type II curves also are called false double major curves. The lumbar curve below deviates from the plumb line somewhat and is rotated. King used the flexibility index to distinguish type II curves from double major curves. Lumbar curves, however, usually are more flexible than thoracic curves even in true double major patterns, and type II curves must be carefully distinguished from double major curves. If the thoracic curve is bigger and more structural than the lumbar curve, it can be selectively instrumented. When using multihook segmental instrumentation, other factors must be considered in distinguishing a type II from a double major curve. The relationship between the rotation of the thoracic and the lumbar curves and the relative deviation of the apices of

these curves from the plumb line and the center sacral line must be considered (Fig. 38-74, *A*). In a type II curve the thoracic curve is larger, more rotated, and deviates farther from the plumb line than the lumbar curve. On clinical examination the thoracic curve is the curve producing most of the deformity, the waistline is symmetrical, and the lumbar muscle hump is minimal on forward bending.

Benson et al. divided type II curves into two subgroups. Type A includes lumbar curves that (1) are less structural, (2) are less than 35 degrees, (3) correct 70% on side bending, (4) have a lumbar apical vertebra that is crossed by the midsacral line, and (5) have a lumbosacral angle of 12 degrees or less (Fig. 38-74, *B*). Type B curves have no more than two of these characteristics. In their study, type A curves generally had excellent results after limited thoracic fusion, but two of four type B curves with limited thoracic fusion developed decompensation.

According to Bridwell et al. the criteria for type II curves are: (1) a thoracic curve 1.2 times larger than the lumbar curve (T curve degrees/L curve degrees = 1.2); (2) thoracic curve apical rotation, as measured by the Nash and Moe method, greater than the lumbar (thoracic rotation/lumbar rotation >1); and (3) thoracic curve apical vertebral body translation (AVT) from the plumbline of the body 1.2 times the lumbar AVT (thoracic AVT/lumbar AVT >1.2). Important exceptions include lumbar curves over 60 degrees, lumbar rotation over grade 2.5, and lumbar apical vertebral translation over 4 cm. In these situations, even if the other criteria are met, the curve pattern is treated as a double major.

Decompensation of the spine caused by the lumbar curve after selected thoracic fusion has been reported in as many as 22% of patients, and several methods have been proposed to prevent this decompensation. Bridwell and J.P. Thompson et al. recommended a shorter thoracic fusion to exclude the mobile

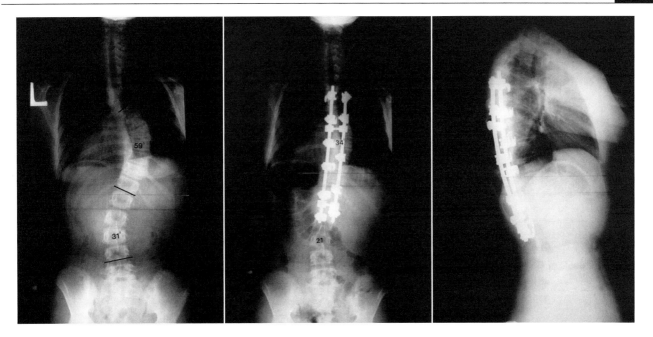

Fig. 38-75   Reverse bend and reverse hook orientation recommended by Shufflebarger et al. to prevent junctional kyphosis.

transition segment between the thoracic and lumbar curves. If the short thoracic fusion is done, however, a junctional kyphosis may be created. Lonstein et al. emphasized that the thoracic curve should not be corrected more than the flexibility of the lumbar curve or else decompensation to the left will occur. They recommended minimizing concave rod rotation and obtaining an intraoperative roentgenogram on a long 14 × 36 inch cassette. Shufflebarger and Clark described a reversal of the distal hook pattern at the thoracolumbar junction (Fig. 38-75).

In summary, the best treatment for trunk decompensation in type II curves is prevention. Careful analysis before surgery suggests that decompensation is a possibility; it is important to avoid overcorrection of the thoracic curve. An intraoperative roentgenogram that includes the thoracic and lumbar curves should be obtained. A reverse rod bend and reverse hook technique can be considered if it does not require extension of the instrumentation to several levels into the lumbar spine. The thoracic curve can be corrected with a translation maneuver rather than a derotation maneuver (Technique 38-13).

Type V Thoracic Curves. King type V curves are double thoracic curves that can cause considerable problems if only the lower curve is corrected and fused and the upper curve is ignored or overlooked. If a lower thoracic curve is corrected and a large upper left thoracic curve is left unchanged, the clinical result is an asymmetrical lower neckline, prominence of the left trapezius region, and elevation of the left shoulder. Most patients believe they look worse than before surgery. Normally the upper curve end vertebra is either T1 or T2 and

the lower end vertebra is T5 or T6. The upper curves usually are convex to the left.

Often clinical examination is more helpful than roentgenographic evaluation in recognizing this double thoracic curve pattern. The patient's hair should be moved aside to expose the shoulder and trapezius region for careful evaluation of shoulder levels. On forward bending, upper thoracic rib prominence may be present on the left.

If careful clinical examination is combined with correct roentgenographic evaluation, the upper thoracic curve should not be overlooked. Full length, 36-inch spine films are mandatory. All curves should be measured, not just the more obvious right thoracic curve. As noted by Winter, the upper end vertebra of the upper thoracic curve must be evaluated to determine if it is horizontal or is tilted, with the left upper corner of the vertebra higher than the right upper corner. When this tilt is present, the upper left ribs are higher than the upper right ribs. The apex of the curve also should be evaluated; if it is to the left of the midline, the curve probably is structural. The vertebral bodies should be evaluated for rotation and wedging, which also are signs of a structural curve. Specific left thoracic bending films of the upper curve should be obtained. In our experience, even if the roentgenographic evaluation is questionable, obvious clinical deformity with elevation of the left shoulder is an indication that both curves should be instrumented and fused.

O'Brien et al. reported that multihook segmental instrumentation with a 90-degree rod rotation maneuver may lead to shoulder imbalance when the shoulders are level or even when the right shoulder is elevated. They emphasize the importance

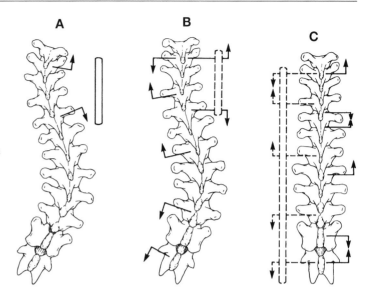

Fig. 38-76   Instrumentation of King type V double thoracic curves with temporary upper rod (see text). **A,** Hook placement for insertion of short segment rod in concavity of high thoracic curve. **B,** Gentle distraction is applied and rod is locked in place. **C,** Left rod is inserted to include both curves; compression is applied to convexity of upper curve, and distraction is applied to concavity of lower curve. Short rod is removed, and long rod is contoured with in situ benders.

of recognizing a structural upper thoracic curve when the pattern is not typical of type V. They established the following criteria for a structural upper thoracic curve: (1) a proximal thoracic curve greater than 35 degrees that corrects to no less than 20 degrees on side bending, (2) greater than grade I (Nash and Moe) rotation at the apex with more than 5 mm of apical deviation from the midline, (3) any elevation of the left first rib or any tilt of T1 into the concavity of the upper thoracic curve, and (4) transitional vertebra located between the two curves at T6 or below.

◆ *Multihook Instrumentation of Type V Thoracic Curve with Short Distraction Rod*

TECHNIQUE 38-16

Hook placement sites are as shown in Fig. 38-76. Place a short segment rod in the concavity of the high thoracic curve and gently apply distraction (Fig. 38-76, *A* and *B*). Do not attempt derotation. Lock the rod in place (Fig. 38-76, *B*). Now insert the left rod to include both curves. Because the upper hook is on the convex side of the left high thoracic curve, establish a claw on the upper vertebra, usually T2. Contour the appropriate length rod and insert it into the hooks. Adjust the rod so that as little of the rod as possible protrudes beyond the uppermost left hook. Apply compression to the convexity of the upper curve and distraction to the concavity of the lower curve. Remove the short upper right rod and contour the left rod into normal thoracic kyphosis using in situ rod benders (Fig. 38-76, *C*).

When this technique is used, no rotational maneuver is applied. Conversely, if the short distraction rod significantly improves the upper thoracic curve, the rod can be contoured into a normal thoracic kyphosis and inserted, and a derotational maneuver can be applied rather than using the in situ benders. The rod is then locked in place.

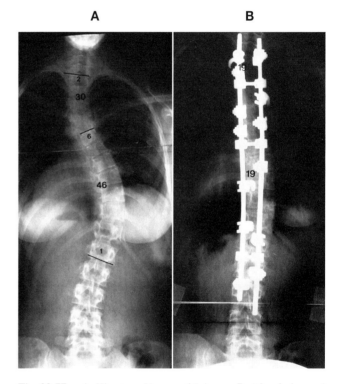

Fig. 38-77   **A,** King type V curve, 85 degree. **B,** After fusion and instrumentation with Texas Scottish Rite Hospital (TSRH) rods and cross links.

After locking in the left rod and removing the upper rod, insert the right rod in the hook pattern shown in Fig. 38-76, *C.* This rod is used more for additional support than for additional correction. Apply appropriate cross links (Fig. 38-77).

If a significant curvature of the upper thoracic spine is present before rotation, 90 degrees of rotation of the left rod

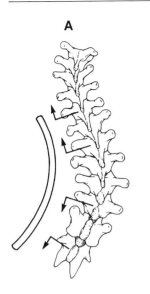

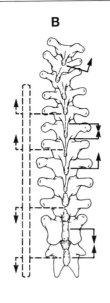

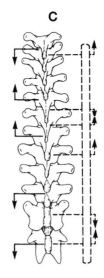

Fig. 38-78 **A,** Concave left rod is inserted for instrumentation of thoracic curve; rod is rotated to correct coronal curve and produce kyphosis in sagittal plane. **B,** Longer right rod is inserted in hook pattern shown for instrumentation of both thoracic curves; concavity of upper curve is distracted, and convexity of lower curve is compressed. **C,** Left rod is replaced with longer rod with hook pattern shown for instrumentation of both curves.

will dramatically increase the lordosis of the upper thoracic curve. The rotational maneuver of the left upper rod therefore can be done only if enough correction of the upper thoracic curve is obtained with the short distraction rod to allow the upper end of the rod to be straight while it is inserted into the hooks. If this cannot be done, the rod should be inserted and bent in situ or the following technique should be used.

◆ *Multihook Instrumentation of Type V Thoracic Curve with Temporary Lower Rod*

TECHNIQUE 38-17

Use the usual thoracic hook pattern in the lower thoracic curve (Fig. 38-78, *A*) and apply a derotational maneuver as for a King type III curve. Insert a long right rod (Fig. 38-78, *B*), applying distraction to the concavity of the high left thoracic curve and compression to the convexity of the lower curve. Lock this rod in place, remove the lower temporary rod, and replace it with a longer left rod that includes both curves (Fig. 38-78, *C*).

◆ *Multihook Instrumentation of Type V Thoracic Curve with Two Left Rods*

TECHNIQUE 38-18

Correct the left lower thoracic curve in the routine manner for a single King type III thoracic curve (p. 1797). Derotate this rod and lock it in place (Fig. 38-79, *A*). On the left side, use a short rod, usually from T2 to T5, and apply compression. Do not use a rotational maneuver on this rod. Use claw fixation on the upper vertebra. Connect the upper

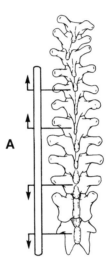

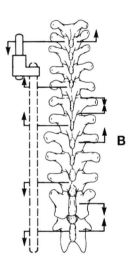

Fig. 38-79 Instrumentation of King type V curve with two rods on left side (see text). **A,** Lower rod is inserted, derotated, and locked in place. **B,** Upper rod is connected with domino or axial cross link before right rod is inserted.

rod to the lower rod with a domino or an axial cross link (Fig. 38-79, *B*). Insert the right rod and apply the cross links.

Thoracolumbar Curves. Posterior instrumentation of thoracolumbar curves produces the problem of trying to achieve normal sagittal alignment—thoracic kyphosis and lumbar lordosis—while having only one curve in the frontal plane. It is impossible to produce a normal sagittal contour across the thoracolumbar junction and correct a single frontal plane curve by rotation of the rod from the concavity. The hook sites for a normal left thoracolumbar scoliosis are shown in Fig. 38-80, *B*.

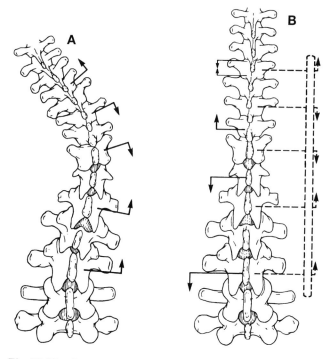

Fig. 38-80 Instrumentation of thoracolumbar curve: convex rod technique (see text). **A,** Hook pattern for insertion of convex rod; hooks are compressed, and rod is rotated to obtain normal sagittal contour. **B,** Concave rod is inserted and seated with distraction, and cross links are applied.

◆ *Multihook Segmental Instrumentation of Thoracolumbar Curve with Convex Rod*

TECHNIQUE 38-19

Insert the convex rod first to allow compression forces to be applied across the thoracolumbar junction before any distraction forces are applied. Place the apical hooks about two segments apart. Contour the convex rod for normal physiological thoracic kyphosis and lumbar lordosis and insert it. Compress the hooks and rotate the rod to achieve normal sagittal contour (Fig. 38-80, *A*). Insert the concave side rod, use distraction to seat the hooks (Fig. 38-80, *B*), and cross link the rods. Make sure the hook sites extend proximal enough into the thoracic spine to ensure adequate thoracic kyphosis.

◆ ◆ ◆

Johnston et al. described a technique in which the concave rod is inserted first. This technique is possible with the Texas Scottish Rite Hospital (TSRH) instrumentation because all hooks in this system are open hooks. The correction is produced by a cantilever mechanism (Fig. 38-81).

◆ *Multihook Segmental Instrumentation of Thoracolumbar Curve with Concave Rod*

TECHNIQUE 38-20 *(Johnston et al.)*

Contour the concave rod for the sagittal contours desired. Insert the rod into the caudal two or three hooks and distract the hooks to seat them. Rotate the rod so that the sagittal

Fig. 38-81 Instrumentation of thoracolumbar curve with concave rod technique in which correction is produced by cantilever mechanism (see text). **A,** Concave rod is inserted and rotated to convert lumbar scoliosis into lordosis as it is sequentially seated in each more-cephalad hook. **B,** Convex rod is inserted in hook pattern shown.

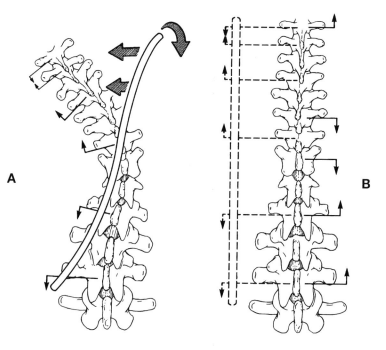

lordosis fits the lumbar scoliosis deformity in the coronal plane. This requires displacement of the cephalad portion of the rod well to the right of the upper spine. Rotate the rod to convert lumbar scoliosis into lordosis. As this is done, progressively translate the rod to the next most-cephalad hooks (Fig. 38-81, *A*). Since all the hooks are open, the rod can be sequentially seated in each more cephalad hook. Gradually correct the spine by this cantilever maneuver using rod pushers and corkscrews to translate the rod into the hooks. The rod is fully rotated into the sagittal plane contours by the time the most cephalad hook is seated.

Contour the convex rod into appropriate sagittal curves and insert it (Fig. 38-81, *B*). The lumbar hooks on the concave side have been distracted for seating of the hooks, and this distraction leads to kyphosis across the thoracolumbar junction. Release these concave hooks once the convex rod is seated. Then compress the convex hooks across the thoracolumbar junction. Gently redistract the concave hooks to seat them properly, but avoid distraction beyond this point. Add the cross links as the last step before decortication and bone grafting.

◆ ◆ ◆

Wood et al. and Sorenson and Asher described the use of pedicle screws and sublaminar wires to better derotate the vertebrae of the lumbar spine. They reported improved correction of the lateral-to-medial translation of the apical vertebra, as well as better correction and maintenance of correction of the rotational component of the deformity when compared with the use of hooks alone. Richards et al. reported less correction of lumbar curves in double major curves and an 18% loss of correction with the use of hooks alone (see p. 1797).

Primary Lumbar Curves. The most important principles in the treatment of primary lumbar curves are maintenance of lumbar lordosis and fusion of as few motion segments as possible. Lumbar curves can be instrumented both anteriorly and posteriorly. In carefully selected patients, anterior instrumentation can save lumbar motion segments and provide better curve correction and derotation. In our experience the derotational effects of posterior multihook segmental instrumentation on the lumbar spine are not as dramatic as on the thoracic spine because the apical lumbar vertebra does not seem to translate toward the midline of the body as well as the apical thoracic vertebra, or as well as the apical lumbar vertebra does with anterior instrumentation. Anterior instrumentation does, however, tend to reduce lumbar lordosis, even when the techniques described on pp. 1818 to 1825 are used. Posterior multihook segmental systems can be used for preserving and even improving lumbar lordosis, and they provide a much more rigid instrumentation system that does not require postoperative immobilization. When posterior instrumentation systems are used the sagittal plane must be carefully evaluated. Occasion-

ally, an increased kyphosis is present above the top of the instrumentation of lumbar curves. If this is a concern, fusion may extend farther into the thoracic spine.

◆ *Multihook Segmental Instrumentation of Lumbar Curves*

TECHNIQUE 38-21

The principles of hook site selection for thoracolumbar curves are applicable for lumbar curves. The basic principle is compression on the convex side of the apical vertebra. For upper hook placement, the sagittal contours must be considered. Place the top of the instrumentation well within or above any area of kyphosis seen on the lateral roentgenogram. Contour the convex rod into the desired sagittal plane alignment and place it into the hooks. Then perform rotation. Tighten the hooks sequentially about the apex to achieve apical compression, first from those hooks nearest the apex and finally to those hooks farthest from the apex. Seat the upper hook in distraction. Insert the second stabilizing rod on the concave side and seat the hooks. Apply the cross links.

◆ ◆ ◆

Pedicle screw fixation and sublaminar wires may improve correction and maintain correction.

Rigid Thoracic Curves. A severe and rigid curve cannot be corrected by rotation of a contoured rod; trying to rotate the rod actually will increase the thoracic rib hump. These curves are best corrected by a two concave rod technique. A short apical rod is used in the concavity of the most structural portion of the curve, and then a long rod is used to bridge from the upper end vertebra to the lower end vertebra. The typical hook placement for these curves is shown in Fig. 38-82.

◆ *Multihook Segmental Instrumentation of Rigid Thoracic Curves*

TECHNIQUE 38-22

Identify the apex of the curve and the rigid portion of the curve. The short apical rod generally spans three or four vertebrae. Insert the short rod and apply a distraction force to the hooks (Fig. 38-82, *A*). Do not try to rotate the short rod. Contour the long concave rod according to the desired sagittal plane and place it straight in the frontal plane (Fig. 38-82, *B*). To prevent translation, secure the rod at the upper vertebra with a claw. Approximate the short rod to the long rod and connect the rods with cross links or devices for transverse traction (DTTs) (Fig. 38-82, *C*). This maneuver translates the short rod posteriorly and medially. Apply the

continued

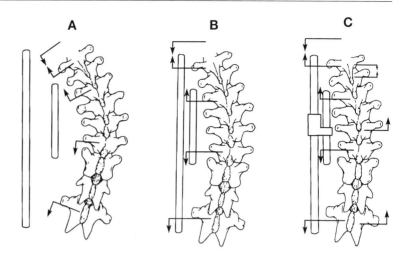

Fig. 38-82   Instrumentation of rigid thoracic curve with two concave rod technique (see text). **A,** Short apical rod spanning three or four vertebrae is inserted and distraction is applied. **B,** Long concave rod is inserted. **C,** Rods are connected with cross link or DDT.

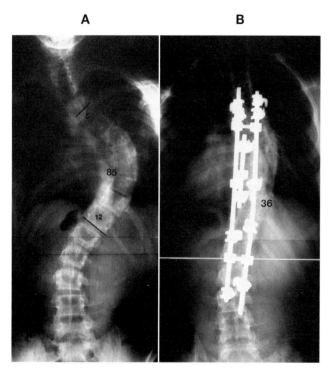

Fig. 38-83   **A,** Rigid 85-degree thoracic curve. **B,** After anterior release and posterior fusion with short-segment rod.

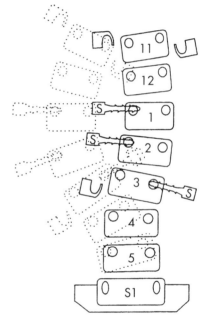

Fig. 38-84   Diagram demonstrating overcorrection of lumbar curve. When appropriate, overcorrection of instrumented lumbar curve is sought to effect correction and reduction of lateral tilt of uninstrumented, unfused spine. (From Barr SJ, Schuette AM, Emans JB: *Spine* 22:1369, 1997.)

convex rod, carefully observing the apical hook to be sure it is not pushed into the canal. If necessary, it can be eliminated. Apply two more cross links between the two long rods for additional support (Fig. 38-83).

PEDICLE FIXATION

Instrumentation that uses the pedicle as a source of purchase for bone screws from the posterior approach into the vertebral

body has become an increasingly popular form of spinal fixation. Hamill et al. compared correction of double major curves in 22 patients treated with hook configurations to 22 patients treated with pedicle fixation on the convex side of the lumbar spine. They found that pedicle screws on the convex side of the lumbar spine improved coronal and sagittal correction, allowed the lower instrumented vertebra to be translated to the midline and brought to a horizontal position, and allowed improved restoration of segmental lordosis. In a similar study, Barr et al. found that the pedicle screws provided greater lumbar curve correction, better maintenance of cor-

A   B   C   D

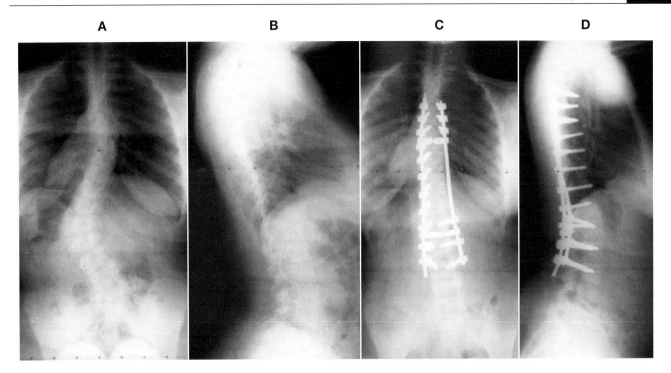

Fig. 38-85 **A** and **B,** Preoperative posteroanterior and lateral roentgenograms of patient with idiopathic scoliosis treated with lumbar and thoracic pedicle screws. **C** and **D,** Postoperative posteroanterior and lateral roentgenograms of amount of correction and restoration of sagittal balance possible with this type of instrumentation.

rection, and greater correction of the uninstrumented spine below double major curves. Neither study reported any complications associated with the placement of pedicle screws.

An important concept in the use of pedicle screws is overcorrection of the lumbar curve if possible (Fig. 38-84). Barr et al. found that because of the lateral placement of the pedicle screw, distraction on the concave side of the lumbar curve provided substantial correction of the tilt of the end vertebra in the coronal plane and helped produce a net overcorrection of the lumbar curve. In theory, overcorrection of the lower instrumented vertebra may reduce the number of levels in the fusion. However, Barr et al. noted no significant differences in the lowest vertebra fused in the hook and screw groups. They did suggest that the levels below the instrumentation were more normally oriented with screw instrumentation than hook instrumentation. Whether this improved correction and orientation of the lower levels below the fusion will decrease the incidence of low back symptoms or degenerative disc disease remains to be proved in long-term studies.

More controversial is the use of thoracic pedicle screws in the treatment of adolescent idiopathic scoliosis (Fig. 38-85). Suk et al. compared correction with hook fixation to that with thoracic pedicle screw fixation. Correction was 55% with hooks and 72% with segmental thoracic pedicle screws. They reported a 3% malposition rate for the thoracic pedicle screws based on plain roentgenograms. There were no medial intracanal malpositions, nor were there any neurological complications.

Liljenqvist et al. used CT to evaluate 120 thoracic pedicle screws. Twenty-five percent of the screws penetrated the

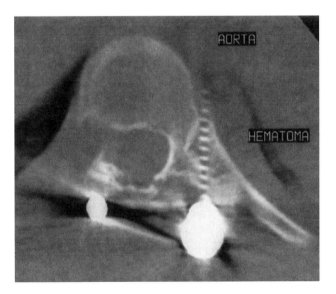

Fig. 38-86 Complete lateral pedicle screw penetration at T10 on the concave side of King-II scoliosis. Small hematoma probably was result of injury of segmental vessels. (From Liljenqvist UR, Halm HFH, Link TM: *Spine* 22:2239, 1997.)

pedicle cortex or the anterior cortex of the vertebral body. There were no neurological complications. Curve correction was only slightly better with screws than with hooks. They noted that anterior penetration of the vertebral body cortex by a pedicle screw in the thoracic spine had the most clinical relevance because of the proximity of the thoracic aorta (Fig. 38-86).

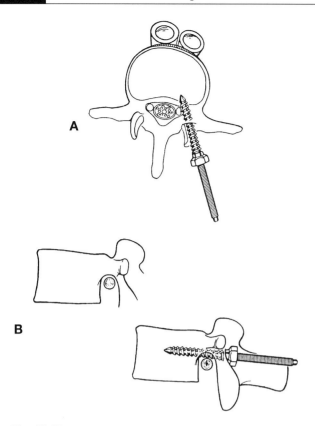

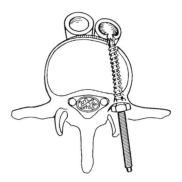

Fig. 38-88   Vascular damage by insertion of screw beyond anterior cortex. (From Pinto MR: *Spine: State of the Art Reviews* 6:45, 1992.)

Fig. 38-87   Errors in pedicle screw placement. **A,** Nerve root impingement by screw violating medial pedicle wall. **B,** Pedicle screw out inferiorly. (From Pinto MR: *Spine: State of the Art Reviews* 6:45, 1992.)

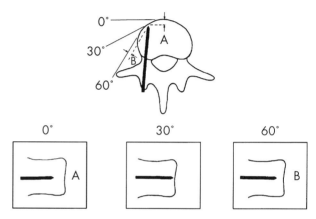

Fig. 38-89   "Near approach" roentgenographic view to decrease likelihood of anterior screw penetration. When drill (or screw or probe) tip is actually at anterior cortex, lateral view (0 degrees) misleadingly shows tip still to be some distance *(A)* away from cortex. At too oblique an angle of view (60 degrees), tip appears to be some distance *(B)* from cortex. Only when view is tangent to point of penetration (30 degrees in this illustration) does tip appear most nearly to approach actual breakthrough. (From Krag MH: *Spine* 16:84, 1991.)

A thorough knowledge of the anatomy of the pedicles is necessary for the use of pedicle fixation. The pedicle connects the posterior elements to the vertebral body. Medial to the pedicle are the epidural space, nerve root, and dural sac. The exiting nerve root at the level of the pedicle is close to the medial and caudal cortex of the pedicle (Fig. 38-87). Close to the lateral and superior aspects of the pedicle cortex is the nerve root from the level above. At the L3 and L4 vertebral bodies the common iliac artery and veins lie directly anterior to the pedicles (Fig. 38-88). In the sacral region the great vessels and their branches lie laterally along the sacral ala. In the midline of the sacrum a variable middle sacral artery can lie directly anterior to the S1 vertebral body. Anterior penetration of a vertebral body can occur without being apparent on roentgenogram unless a "near approach" view is obtained (Fig. 38-89).

Zindrick et al. studied the size of pedicles in mature and immature spines. They found that the transverse pedicle width at the L5 and L4 levels reached 8 mm or more in children 6 to 8 years of age, but transverse width at L3 approaching 8 mm was not seen until 9 to 11 years of age (Fig. 38-90). The distance to the anterior cortex increased dramatically from the youngest age group until adulthood at all levels (Fig. 38-91). They concluded that these data confirmed previous studies that

pedicle fixation can be used in adolescents in the lumbar spine before other areas of the spine. In older adolescents the thoracolumbar spine may be large enough for pedicle fixation. In patients with spinal deformities the pedicles, especially the concave pedicles, often are deformed, and great care must be taken in insertion of any pedicle fixation.

Various methods have been described for identifying the pedicle and placing the pedicle screw, but basic steps include (1) clearing the soft tissue, (2) exposing the cancellous bone of the pedicle canal by decortication at the intersection of the base of the facet and the middle of the transverse process, (3) probing the pedicle, (4) verifying the four walls of the pedicle canal by probing or obtaining roentgenographic confirmation, (5) tapping the pedicle, and (6) placing the screw.

In the lumbar spine, pedicle screws are commonly inserted using anatomical landmarks, and confirmatory roentgenograms

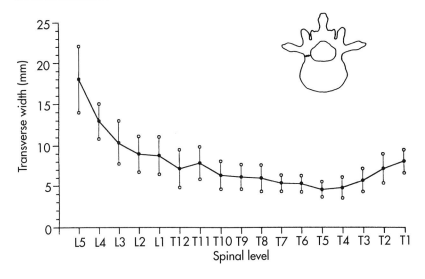

Fig. 38-90   Transverse pedicle isthmus widths. (From Zindrick MR, Wiltse LL, Doornik A, et al: *Spine* 12:160, 1987.)

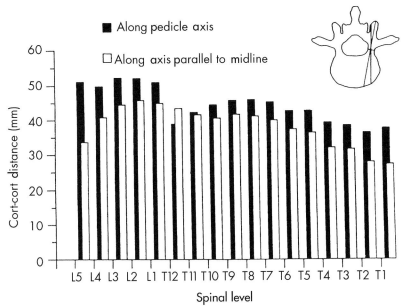

Fig. 38-91   Distance to anterior cortex through pedicle angle axis versus through line parallel to midline axis of vertebra. (From Zindrick MR, Wiltse LL, Doornik A, et al: *Spine* 12:160, 1987.)

are obtained. Because of the deformed pedicles associated with scoliosis, many surgeons use fluoroscopic guidance. Although Suk et al. used anatomical landmarks and confirmed the position of guide pins with plain roentgenograms, most surgeons believe that because of the tight confines of the pedicle in the thoracic spine, intraoperative fluoroscopy is indicated. When multiple thoracic pedicle screws are used, fluoroscopy time can be quite significant. Polly found that the average fluoroscopy time per thoracic screw was about 10 seconds. Frameless stereotactic technology is available that allows three-dimensional navigation but requires time-consuming segmental registration and preoperative CT data. Investigations are currently under way using stereotactic technology combined with fluoroscopy (fluoroNav, Medtronic Sofamor Danek, Inc., Memphis). This technology has the potential to greatly diminish radiation exposure to both the

surgeon and the patient and to allow spontaneous viewing of instrument positions in as many projections as desired.

Lumbar Pedicle Screws

Zindrick described a "pedicle approach zone" (Fig. 38-92) that is decorticated before the pedicle is cannulated with either a drill or a probe. Most surgeons prefer to use a probe rather than any type of power instrumentation. Great care is taken to advance the instrument slowly and carefully. If resistance is encountered, the probe is repositioned. An intraoperative roentgenogram or C-arm image can be used to verify correct position. Instruments should pass relatively easily and should not be forced into the pedicle. In addition to roentgenograms or image intensification, laminotomy and medial pedicle wall exposure help confirm the intrapedicular passage of the instrument. Once satisfactory entry into the pedicle has been achieved and palpation from within the pedicle demonstrates solid bone margins along the pedicle wall throughout 360 degrees, the screw can be inserted. If the screws are self-tapping, the screw itself is inserted. If the screws require tapping, the tap is inserted first and then the screw. The common entry points in the lumbar spine are shown in Fig. 38-93. The position of the pedicle in the sacrum is shown in Fig. 38-94. In the lumbar spine a medially directed screw allows the use of a longer screw and spares the facet joint, with less chance of injury to the common iliac vessels. Similarly a medially directed sacral screw reduces the possibility of injury to anterior structures if the screw penetrates the anterior cortex.

There is no uniformly accepted screw pattern for use in the lumbar spine in a double major curve. Chopin and Morin proposed that better three-dimensional correction can be achieved by using bilateral vertebral screws at the lumbar levels. Barr et al. recommended the use of one or two convex apical screws with a concave pedicle screw on the inferior lumbar vertebra (Fig. 38-95). Hamill et al., on the other hand, found that pedicle screws on the convex side combined with one laminar hook on the distal instrumented vertebra on the concave side provided sufficient correction and allowed increased surface area for bone grafting on the concave side. Barr et al. recommended choosing the lowest instrumented lumbar vertebra on bending films. Instrumentation is stopped at the vertebra just above the first disc space that opens in the concavity of the lumbar curve on the bending film away from the concavity.

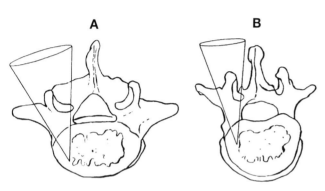

Fig. 38-92 **A,** Funnel-shaped pedicle approach zone in upper lumbar region (L1). **B,** Funnel-shaped pedicle approach zone in lower lumbar region (L5). With increased pedicle size, pedicle approach zone funnel increases, especially in lower lumbar spine, allowing more latitude in pedicle screw insertion than in smaller upper lumbar and thoracic pedicles. (From Zindrick MR: *Spine: State of the Art Reviews* 6:27, 1992.)

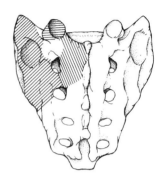

Fig. 38-94 Coronal posterior view of contribution of sacrum and posterior element to pedicle approach zone. (Redrawn from Zindrick MR: *Spine: State of the Art Reviews* 6:27, 1992.)

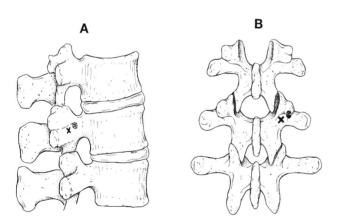

Fig. 38-93 Entrance points for pedicle screw placement in lumbar spine as described by Roy-Camille *(X)* and Weinstein (•). **A,** Lateral view. **B,** Posterior view. Weinstein approach reduces interference with upper uninvolved lumbar motion segment. (Redrawn from Weinstein JN, Spratt KF, Spengler D, et al: *Spine* 13:1012, 1988.)

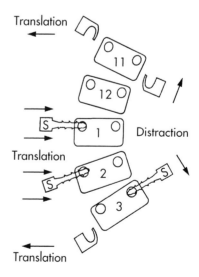

Fig. 38-95 Common pedicle screw and hook construct used in Barr's series. (From Barr SJ, Schuette AM, Emans JB: *Spine* 22:1369, 1997.)

Derotation of the spine is better with screw fixation than with hook fixation because the vertebral screws grasp the vertebral body and are more laterally situated. Hooks do not achieve as much rotation because they are too close to the spinous process and the spine does not follow the movement of the hooks (Fig. 38-96). Hooks also may rotate on the lamina and lose some of the rotation correction. With screw fixation the first stage is still done on the convex side in the lumbar spine, with the same rotation of the contoured rod. No compression or distraction is applied at the first stage. The concave rod is then inserted and introduced into the intermediate screws. As the intermediate screws are approximated to the rod, more correction of rotation can be obtained with the rod introducer. Frontal alignment is then achieved with adequate compression on the convex side and distraction on the concave side at each level.

Thoracic Pedicle Screws

The diameter of the thoracic pedicles increases from cephalad to caudad (see Fig. 38-90). Suk et al. described placing pedicle screws at all levels in the thoracic spine. Even surgeons with a great deal of experience in the placement of thoracic screws have found a significant percentage to be malpositioned and therefore use fluoroscopy, which increases radiation exposure for both the patient and the surgeon. In

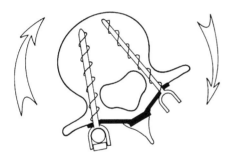

Fig. 38-96 Use of bilateral vertebral screws at lumbar level, as recommended by Chopin for better derotation of spine. (From Chopin D. In Bridwell KH, DeWald RL, eds: *The textbook of spinal surgery*, Philadelphia, 1991, JB Lippincott.)

addition, thoracic pedicle screws at every level add greatly to the expense of the instrumentation system. Whether the benefits of thoracic pedicle fixation in adolescent idiopathic scoliosis outweigh the potential risks and costs has not been proved at this time.

The thoracic pedicle is located at the base of the transverse process just medial to the lateral aspect of the pars intraarticularis (Fig. 38-97). A high-speed burr is used to remove the outer cortical bone in this area, and fluoroscopy is used to confirm placement of a guide wire before final screw placement. Because of the smaller size of the thoracic pedicles, smaller diameter pedicle screws may be necessary.

COMPLICATIONS OF POSTERIOR SCOLIOSIS SURGERY

Early Complications

Neurological Injury. The most feared and unpredictable complication in scoliosis surgery remains neurological injury. It may be caused by inadvertent entry of the instrumentation into the spinal canal. Newer and more complex instrumentation systems require the surgeon to be very aware of potential problems with instrumentation (p. 1792). Other possible causes of neurological injury during surgery are unrecognized spinal cord tethers or other spinal anomalies and vascular damage as the spine is lengthened during the correction procedure. (Spinal cord monitoring and the wake-up test are discussed on p. 1775.)

Infection. Moe et al. reported two types of wound infections after scoliosis surgery. The first is obvious because a high fever develops, usually within 2 to 5 days after surgery, and the wound almost always appears infected. In the second type the temperature is elevated only slightly or moderately, and the wound appears relatively normal. Diagnosis of this latter type of wound sepsis may be difficult. Patients often have postoperative temperature elevation of up to 102° F, which should decline gradually during the first 4 postoperative days. Any spike of temperature above 102° F should raise strong suspicion of a deep wound infection, especially if the patient's general condition does not steadily improve. The appearance of the wound can be deceiving, with no significant erythema or tenderness. Moe et al. recommended prompt aspiration of the

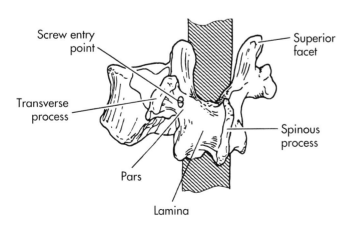

Screw entry point

Transverse process

Pars

Lamina

Superior facet

Spinous process

Fig. 38-97 Slight oblique drawing of typical lower thoracic vertebral segment showing entry point for thoracic pedicle screw. (From Lenke LG: Basic techniques of posterior segmental spine internal fixation. In Bridwell KH, DeWald RL, eds: *The textbook of spinal surgery*, ed 2, Philadelphia, 1997, Lippincott-Raven.)

wound in several sites. Cultures should be submitted, but results should not be awaited, and reoperation should be planned immediately.

The most common organism associated with postoperative infection is *Staphylococcus aureus*. When the wound infection is diagnosed, the wound is opened widely and thorough irrigation and debridement are done. The implants and most of the bone graft are left in, and the wound is closed over drains. Appropriate antibiotics are used for 3 to 6 weeks, depending on the severity of the infection. If the wound infection is discovered late, it may be necessary to debride the wound, irrigate copiously, and pack the wound open. The patient is brought back to the operating room in 3 to 5 days, and the wound is closed over suction tubes. In severe infections or gram-negative infections, such as those caused by *Pseudomonas* or *Escherichia coli*, it may be necessary to leave the wound packed open for prolonged periods and allow it to granulate in from the bottom. This also is occasionally necessary if the infection recurs a few days after the wound is closed over suction drains.

With the use of prophylactic preoperative, intraoperative, and postoperative antibiotics, the incidence of postoperative wound infections in surgery for idiopathic scoliosis is less than 1%.

Ileus. Ileus is a common complication after both anterior and posterior spinal fusion. Oral feedings are withheld until bowel sounds return, usually in 36 to 72 hours after surgery. Until that time, intravenous fluids must be administered. Malnutrition is uncommon in teenagers with idiopathic scoliosis, but patients requiring a two-stage corrective procedure may become malnourished as a result of the limited oral caloric intake associated with closely spaced surgical procedures. Combined anterior and posterior procedures also are more likely to be done in patients with neuromuscular disorders, and parenteral hyperalimentation should be considered for these patients.

Atelectasis. Atelectasis is a common cause of fever after scoliosis surgery. Frequent turning of the patient and deep breathing and coughing usually control or prevent serious atelectasis. Inhalation therapy with intermittent positive pressure breathing may be beneficial in cooperative patients, but inflation of the stomach during this type of treatment must be avoided. Incentive spirometry now is commonly used instead. The atelectasis and the temperature secondary to the atelectasis generally resolve rapidly once the patient is mobilized.

Pneumothorax. At the time of subperiosteal posterior spine exposure, the pleura may be entered inadvertently between the transverse processes on the concave side of the scoliosis. If a thoracoplasty is done at the same time, a pneumothorax is more likely to occur. Observation of the pneumothorax is probably appropriate if it is less than 20%, but chest tube insertion is needed for larger pneumothoraces.

Dural Tear. If a dural tear occurs during removal of the ligamentum flavum or insertion of a hook or wire, repair should be attempted. Often the laminotomy must be enlarged to allow access to the ends of the dural tear. If repair is not done,

drainage of the cerebrospinal fluid through the wound can cause problems postoperatively.

Wrong Levels. Care should be taken in the operating room to correctly identify the vertebral levels. If the fusion extends to the sacrum, it can be used as a landmark and the vertebrae accurately counted. For other curves, we routinely obtain an intraoperative roentgenogram using a marker on the vertebra to be identified. Alternatively, the level can be confirmed by palpation of the T12 rib and the L1 transverse process.

Urinary Complications. A high percentage of patients undergoing spinal fusion develop the syndrome of inappropriate antidiuretic hormone in the immediate postoperative period. This causes a decline in urinary output and is maximal on the evening after surgery. If the serum osmolality is diminished and the urine osmolality is elevated, this syndrome should be considered and fluid overload should be avoided. The urinary output gradually increases in the next 2 to 3 days after surgery.

Late Complications

Pseudarthrosis. A pseudarthrosis represents a failure of the operation to accomplish its purpose. In adolescents with idiopathic scoliosis, the pseudarthrosis rate is approximately 1%; the rate is higher in patients with neuromuscular scoliosis. The most common areas of pseudarthrosis are at the thoracolumbar junction or at the distally fused segment. With more rigid and stronger implants, the pseudarthrosis may not be apparent for years. The diagnosis of pseudarthrosis usually is made by oblique roentgenograms, a broken implant, tomograms, or bone scan. After successful posterior fusion, the disc height anteriorly should diminish as the vertebral body continues to grow at the expense of the disc space. A large disc space anteriorly may indicate a posterior pseudarthrosis. Often, however, the pseudarthrosis cannot be confirmed even with the most sophisticated roentgenographic evaluation and can be detected only by surgical exploration.

If a pseudarthrosis does not cause pain or loss of correction, surgery may not be necessary. Asymptomatic pseudarthrosis is more common in the distally fused segments. A pseudarthrosis at the thoracolumbar junction is more likely to cause loss of correction and pain.

At surgical exploration the cortex is smooth and firm over the mature and intact areas of the fusion mass and the soft tissues strip away easily. Conversely, at a pseudarthrosis the soft tissues usually are adherent and continuous into the defect; however, a narrow pseudarthrosis may be difficult to locate, especially if motion is slight. In this instance, decortication of the fusion mass in suspicious areas is indicated, and a search always should be made for several pseudarthroses. An extremely difficult type of pseudarthrosis to determine is a solid fusion mass posteriorly that is not well adherent to the underlying spine and lamina. Once the pseudarthrosis has been identified, it is cleared of fibrous tissue and the curve is reinstrumented by applying compression over the pseudarthrosis. If this is not done, kyphotic deformity may worsen because of incompetent spinal extensor muscles from the previous surgical exposure. The pseudarthroses are treated as ordinary

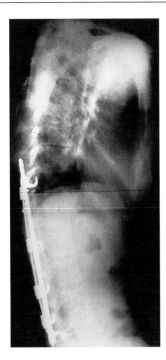

Fig. 38-98   Loss of lumbar lordosis (lumbar "flat-back").

joints to be fused: their edges are freshened and decorticated, and autogenous bone graft is applied in addition to the instrumentation.

Loss of Lumbar Lordosis. If distraction is applied across the lumbar spine, normal physiological lumbar lordosis may be diminished or eliminated, causing the patient to stand with a forward tilt that results in upper back pain, lower back pain, and even pain in the hips (Fig. 38-98). Care also must be taken in positioning the patient on the spinal frame and ensuring that the hips are not flexed (see p. 1776). Marsicano et al. demonstrated that positioning patients on a Jackson frame equipped with two chest pads, two anterior pelvic pads, and two proximal thigh pads maintained the preoperative lumbar lordosis when measured from T12 to S1 and from L1 to L5. They also confirmed the work of Hamill et al., showing that patients with pedicle screw placement to L3 or L4 had a statistically greater increase in instrumented lumbar lordosis after the completion of the instrumentation process than did patients with only hook placement from T12 to L2. The best treatment for the loss of lumbar lordosis is prevention, which includes careful patient positioning, avoidance of distraction in the lumbar spine, and the use of newer segmental instrumentation systems.

Crankshaft Phenomenon. If posterior fusion alone is done in patients with a great deal of anterior growth remaining, a crankshaft phenomenon usually occurs (p. 1755). This is prevented by combining anterior and posterior fusions in younger children.

Superior Mesenteric Artery Syndrome. Rarely, superior mesenteric artery syndrome may cause small bowel obstruction after spinal fusion. The transverse portion of the duodenum crosses the midline anterior to the spine and the aorta and posterior to the superior mesenteric artery. As the space between these structures decreases, obstruction of the duodenum can occur. The patient develops nausea and bilious vomiting. An upper gastrointestinal series is required to make the diagnosis. Initial treatment should consist of nasogastric drainage and intravenous fluid replacement, which often allows swelling in the duodenum to subside. If nonoperative treatment fails, general surgical procedures, such as release of the ligament of Trietz or duodenojejunostomy, may be necessary.

Trunk Decompensation. Problems with trunk decompensation have been noted with the newer segmental instrumentation systems in the treatment of King type II curves. If decompensation occurs (p. 1801) and is mild with minimal trunk imbalance, treatment may not be needed. The patient can be followed periodically for lumbar curve progression. For more severe decompensation cases, an orthosis can be used for treatment of the lumbar curve. If bracing is unsuccessful, it may be necessary to extend the fusion to the distal stable vertebra of the lumbar curve.

Late Infection. Dubousset et al. reported 18 patients who required late removal of their instrumentation because of pain, swelling, and spontaneous drainage. No organisms were cultured, and they concluded that this was an inflammatory response to micromotion of the components and corrosion. Clark and Shufflebarger reported 22 patients (1.7% of their series) who had a similar clinical presentation. When the wounds were cultured for 7 to 10 days, 11 were positive for low virulence skin organisms. These patients were treated with rod removal and primary wound closure, parenteral antibiotics for 48 hours, and oral antibiotics for 7 days. The infections appeared to affect soft tissue and not the bone. Richards found similar delayed deep wound infections in 10 patients who were treated with TSRH instrumentation. He suspected that several of the delayed infections resulted from intraoperative seeding and remained subclinical for an extended period.

◆ POSTERIOR THORACOPLASTY

Of all the deformities caused by idiopathic scoliosis, the posterior rib prominence is generally the patient's main concern (Fig. 38-99). With rigid curves, the trunk does not always derotate despite current advanced multihook segmental spinal instrumentation systems. If necessary for cosmetic or psychological reasons, resection of the convex ribs can improve the postoperative cosmetic result of the surgery.

The indications for a convex rib resection are not exact but are based on preoperative discussions with the patient about the magnitude of the rib deformity and the expected improvement of the deformity based on the size, the amount of rotation, and the rigidity of the curve. A preoperative rib angle on roentgenographic or clinical examination of more than 15 degrees, a thoracic curve of 60 degrees or more, curve flexibility of less than 20% on bending films, and postoperative correction of the Cobb angle of less than 50% based on intraoperative roentgenograms are all criteria that can be used to determine if rib resection is indicated. Routine scoliosis films

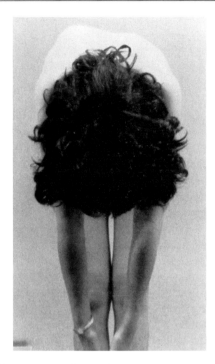

Fig. 38-99   Posterior rib prominence in adolescent patient with idiopathic scoliosis.

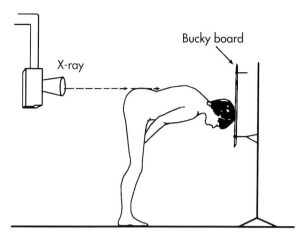

Fig. 38-100   Patient positioning for tangential roentgenographic rib view. (Redrawn from Harvey CJ, Betz, RR, Clements DH, et al: *Spine* 18:1593, 1993.)

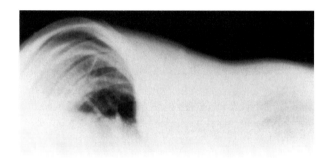

Fig. 38-101   Rib prominence on roentgenogram.

(p. 1761) and a rib prominence view (Figs. 38-100 and 38-101) can be used to assess curve flexibility and the preoperative rib angle. Of 98 patients with adolescent idiopathic scoliosis treated with Cotrel-Dubousset instrumentation, Harvey et al. found that convex rib resection was indicated in 25%.

Thoracoplasty is not appropriate for patients in whom the ribs do not protrude beyond the posterior margin of the spine, regardless of the severity of the curve. Care must be taken to verify that the patient's cosmetic complaints are caused by the rib prominence and not by trunk asymmetry, which will not be corrected by thoracoplasty. Thoracoplasty usually decreases pulmonary function in the early postoperative period. Although pulmonary function returns to normal within 2 years, thoracoplasty should not be considered in patients who have unsatisfactory preoperative pulmonary function studies.

The final decision regarding rib resection is made at the time of surgery, based on the flexibility of the curve and the rib prominence after the patient is prone under anesthesia.

TECHNIQUE 38-23 *(Betz)*
Position the patient as for a standard posterior spinal fusion for idiopathic scoliosis (Technique 38-3). Prepare and drape the patient in a standard fashion. For adequate exposure of the rib prominence, place the lateral drapes at the posterolateral axillary line or wider. Make a routine midline incision (Technique 38-3). Perform the thoracoplasty through this midline posterior incision by retracting the fascia and working under it and the latissimus dorsi or, alternatively, make a separate parallel vertical incision centered over the rib hump as described by Steel. If the single, midline posterior incision is used, extend the skin incision distally to approximately L2 or L3 for a right thoracic curve to adequately retract the thoracolumbar fascia from the midline. Stopping the skin incision at T12 does not provide adequate lateral exposure. Likewise, proximally, carry the skin incision approximately ½ to 1 inch farther. Despite the slight increase in length, this incision is much more cosmetically appealing than the two-incision technique. The advantage of the two-incision technique is easier access to the lateral rib. With newer instrumentation techniques, better translation of the apex of the curve to the midline is possible and less of the rib needs to be resected laterally than is necessary with Harrington rod techniques.

After the skin incision is made, outline the spinous processes and incise the thoracolumbar fascia off the spinous process (Fig. 38-102, *A*). In the L2-3 region, be careful to identify the very thin layer of thoracolumbar fascia. Using sharp and blunt dissection, elevate this fascia off the paravertebral muscle fascia, working laterally and proximally at the same time, to develop a plane. Sequen-

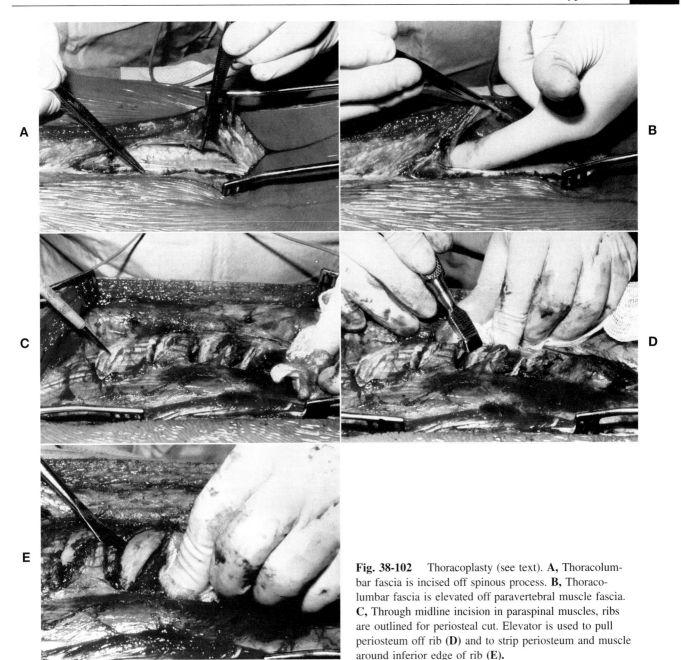

Fig. 38-102 Thoracoplasty (see text). **A,** Thoracolumbar fascia is incised off spinous process. **B,** Thoracolumbar fascia is elevated off paravertebral muscle fascia. **C,** Through midline incision in paraspinal muscles, ribs are outlined for periosteal cut. Elevator is used to pull periosteum off rib (**D**) and to strip periosteum and muscle around inferior edge of rib (**E**).

tially incise the thoracolumbar fascia off the spinous processes, proceeding proximally (Fig. 38-102, *B*). Once the fascia has been retracted laterally, palpate the ribs starting at the apex of the deformity. Starting at the apex and working distally and proximally one rib at a time, do a symmetrical resection. Mark the apical rib with an electrocautery. Make a midline incision into the paraspinal muscles medially and outline the ribs for the periosteal cut. Use an elevator to pull the periosteum off the surface of the rib to the lateral edge (Fig. 38-102, *C*). The elevator should be pulled and not pushed to prevent penetration of the pleura. Usually

between four and six ribs are outlined. Once the periosteum has been stripped to the side of the rib, use the elevator to strip the periosteum and muscle around the inferior edge of the rib (Fig. 38-102, *D*). Using a Cobb elevator, strip the periosteum from the anterior aspect of the rib in a medial to lateral direction (Fig. 38-102, *E*). This is the time the pleura is most likely to be entered.

Once the anterior aspect of the rib has been stripped with a Cobb elevator, pass a Doyen retractor circumferentially and medial to lateral on the exposed rib (Fig. 38-103). Identify the most medial attachment of the rib to the

continued

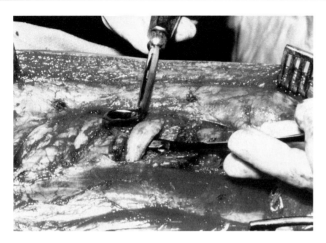

Fig. 38-103 Doyen retractor is passed circumferentially on exposed rib.

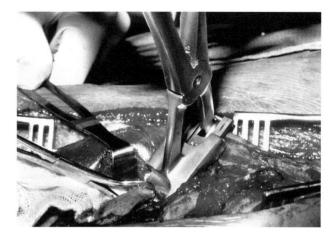

Fig. 38-104 Rib is held with Kocher clamp and is cut medially.

transverse process. Pass a rib cutter around the rib and push it as far medially as possible. Hold the rib with a towel clip or Kocher clamp to prevent it from plunging through the pleura when cut. Cut the rib medially (Fig. 38-104), keeping the cut as parallel to the floor as possible, then make the lateral cut. For a standard rib resection in a patient with a 55-degree right thoracic curve, 2 cm of rib should be cut initially (Fig. 38-105, A and B). Take care not to resect too much rib because more rib can be removed if necessary. If the thoracoplasty is done before instrumentation of the spine, the apex of the curve will translate to the midline when the curve is corrected, leaving a much larger gap than is apparent at the time of the original rib resection. Apply bone wax to the ends of the rib and pack Gelfoam into the periosteal bed (Fig. 38-105, C). Cut additional ribs in an identical fashion, but going proximally and distally from the apex, progressively removing less rib.

Once the resection has been completed, lift the edges of the wound; using a pitcher and not pressure irrigation, pour saline into the wound. Have the anesthesiologist do a Valsalva maneuver to look for a leak in the pleura. Place a suction drain over the resected rib bed. Close the thoracolumbar fascia with a running absorbable suture, starting at the distal aspect of the wound. Cut the removed segments of rib into small pieces for use as autogenous bone graft in the spinal arthrodesis.

Alternatively, the thoracoplasty procedure can be done after spinal instrumentation. This allows better evaluation of the rib hump after the instrumentation but also can lead to increased blood loss if this procedure is done after the major dissection of the spine in the midline.

AFTERTREATMENT. After skin closure and dressing application, a protective plaster shell is applied over the rib resection area. This shell is essential to help prevent a postoperative flail chest and to minimize motion of the cut ribs on top of the pleura

and the possibility of pleural effusion. The shell is made of plaster with foam underneath to protect the skin. The mold is made while the patient is prone on the operating table to prevent a plaster burn, but the shell is not applied until the patient is in the recovery room. A chest roentgenogram is obtained in the recovery room to rule out a pneumothorax, and then the shell is applied and wrapped with 6-inch elastic wraps. Alternatively, the posterior shell of a TLSO that was made preoperatively can be used. The patient's back is examined 2 days after surgery. If there is no evidence of a flail chest and the rib resection gap measures less than the width of the palm of the hand, no prolonged postoperative immobilization is needed. If there is a larger gap or a flail chest, a postoperative rib protector, such as the posterolateral half of a TLSO, is fitted. This rib protector is worn for 3 months. Alternatively, a full TLSO brace can be used for the first 3 months after surgery to protect the chest cage while the ribs regenerate.

Complications and Pitfalls

During rib resection, a hole may be made in the parietal pleura. No attempt should be made to repair the pleura. The hole in the rib bed should be gently packed with Gelfoam, and the intercostal muscles should be closed with a running suture from the most medial to the lateral aspect. As the last sutures are tightened, the anesthesiologist expands the patient's lung, expressing as much air from the pleural cavity as possible before the final sutures are tied. The purpose of closing the hole is to prevent blood from seeping into the pleural cavity. An expanding pneumothorax should not occur because only the parietal pleura is violated and not the visceral pleura. Suction drains are used routinely. Fewer than 50% of patients with pleural holes require chest tubes. Daily semierect and lateral decubitus roentgenograms are made for 3 days. A thoracentesis is done if fluid accumulation persists and the patient is symptomatic. If a second thoracentesis becomes necessary, a chest tube is considered.

Occasionally, even without a pleural hole, a pleural effusion may develop. The use of a protective shell postoperatively

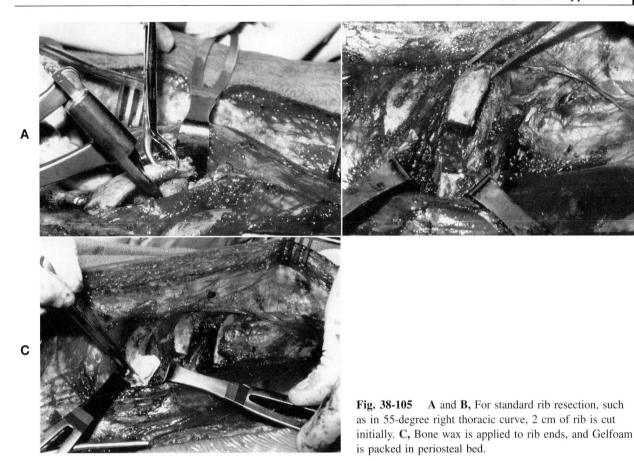

Fig. 38-105 **A** and **B,** For standard rib resection, such as in 55-degree right thoracic curve, 2 cm of rib is cut initially. **C,** Bone wax is applied to rib ends, and Gelfoam is packed in periosteal bed.

minimizes this complication. For expanding, symptomatic effusions, a thoracentesis is done; a chest tube is inserted if it occurs a second time.

Resection of too much rib will cause rib concavity. This complication is preventable, and it is better to resect too little rib than too much. Six ribs should be the maximum taken, and never more than 8 cm in length.

The most common error leading to residual rib prominence is not resecting enough ribs and not resecting the ribs medially enough. This risk must be weighed against the risk of causing a rib concavity. If a long rib deformity requires resection of more than six ribs, the risk of causing a rib concavity is high. In this situation it is better to do a second procedure later than risk a rib concavity.

◆ CONCAVE RIB OSTEOTOMIES

The concept of concave rib osteotomies was introduced by Flinchum in 1963. Kostuik, Tolo, Goldstein, and Mann et al. reported the use of concave osteotomies and their possible value as a release procedure. Halsall et al. in cadaver studies tested flexibility before and after sectioning the ribs on the tension side. They found an average increase in deflection of 53%. Flexibility increased most when five or six ribs were resected. The addition of concave rib osteotomies to instrumentation and fusion procedures increases the risk of

pulmonary morbidity. Goldstein reported 5 pleural effusions and 3 pneumothoraces in 17 patients who had resection of 5 to 6 cm of concave ribs. Mann et al. decreased the incidence of complications by performing rib osteotomies rather than rib resections. They reported 2 pleural effusions and 1 pneumothorax in 10 patients. Although concave osteotomies can increase the flexibility of rigid curves, especially those of more than 80 degrees, the exact indications for this procedure have not been defined. If concave rib osteotomies are done, a prophylactic chest tube should be inserted.

TECHNIQUE 38-24 *(Mann et al.)*

Approach the concave ribs through the midline incision used for the instrumentation and spinal fusion. Retract the paraspinous muscles lateral to the tips of the concave transverse processes. When needed, use electrocautery to incise overlying tissue along the rib axis. Incise the periosteum along the rib axis for 1.5 cm lateral to the transverse process and use small elevators to expose the rib periosteally. Protect the pleura with the elevators and use a rib cutter to section the rib approximately 1 cm lateral to the transverse process (Fig. 38-106, *A*). Lift the lateral rib segment with a Kocher clamp and allow it to posteriorly overlap the medial segment (Fig. 38-106, *B*). Rongeur any jagged ends and place a small piece of thrombin-soaked

continued

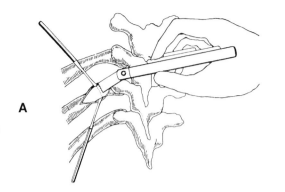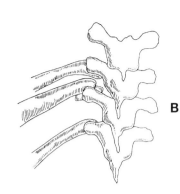

Fig. 38-106 Rib osteotomy. **A,** Rib is exposed subperiosteally 1 cm lateral to transverse process. Osteotomy is completed with microsagittal saw. **B,** Overlap of lateral rib segment. (Redrawn from Mann DC, Nash CL Jr, Wilham MR, et al: *Spine* 14:491, 1989.)

Gelfoam between the rib and pleura for protection and hemostasis. Make four to six osteotomies over the apical concave vertebrae. Approximate the paraspinous muscles with an absorbable suture. Complete the instrumentation and fusion and insert a chest tube.

ANTERIOR INSTRUMENTATION FOR IDIOPATHIC SCOLIOSIS

In 1969 Dwyer, in cooperation with Newton and Sherwood, developed instrumentation for spinal correction and fixation through an anterior approach. The Dwyer device is a cable attached to the vertebral bodies with large screws. The discs are removed and compression is applied to the convex side of the curve. This is a powerful correction device but has several disadvantages: because it is not rigid internal fixation and postoperative bracing are needed; kyphosis is caused by compression without derotation on the convex side; and pseudarthrosis and cable fractures are frequent complications.

In 1976 Zielke introduced a modification of the Dwyer device in which the vertebral body screws are connected by a 3.2-mm-diameter solid threaded rod to provide infinite adjustment in the correction force. The application of the Zielke derotation technique with the use of the solid flexible rod theoretically allows more controllable production of lordosis and lessens the tendency for kyphosis. The procedure continues to be modified in both instrumentation and technique.

Anterior instrumentation and fusion for idiopathic scoliosis is now a well-accepted procedure for certain thoracolumbar and lumbar curves. Anterior instrumentation provides better derotation and better correction of the curve in the coronal plane. Often the deformity can be corrected by fusing fewer motion segments than if the same curve were approached posteriorly. In lumbar curves, better translational correction of the apical vertebra can be obtained than with posterior multihook segmental instrumentation systems.

The ideal candidate for anterior instrumentation of thoracolumbar or lumbar curves in an adolescent or young adult with a flexible curve that corrects more than 50% on bending films (Fig. 38-107, *B*). The compensatory thoracic curve, if present, should be flexible and reducible to 20 degrees or less on the bending films. The fractional curve below the thoracolumbar or lumbar curve must be carefully evaluated because it also must be flexible enough to correct on bending films (Fig. 38-107, *C*). Even with the newer, solid rod systems, lordosis is difficult to achieve, and therefore no more than physiological thoracic kyphosis should be present above the curve. The child must be old enough for the vertebrae to be large enough to hold the screws. Caution is advised in using these systems in children younger than nine years of age.

Hall indicated that the primary method for selecting levels of anterior instrumentation and fusion involves study of the standing posteroanterior roentgenogram (Fig. 59-107, *A*). If the most horizontal element at the apex is a disc, it is necessary to instrument two vertebral bodies above and below this apical disc. If the most horizontal element is a vertebral body, one vertebral body above and below this body can be instrumented if the apical curve can be overcorrected by approximately 10 degrees. Bending films (see Figs. 38-107, *B* and *C*) also are helpful in selecting appropriate anterior fusion levels. On the convex bending film, the lower fusion level is determined by the first disc space that opens up on both sides (see Fig. 38-107, *C*). This indicates that the lower vertebra selected can be made horizontal with an anterior approach. The proximal fusion level should extend only to the neutral vertebra not into the compensatory thoracic curve above. If there is discrepancy in the levels indicated on the bending films and on the standing posteroanterior film, the method that indicates the longest segment of instrumentation and fusion should be selected.

The anterior approach for thoracolumbar and lumbar curves has several potential disadvantages: chylothorax, injury to the ureter, spleen, or great vessels, retroperitoneal fibrosis, and prominent instrumentation that must be carefully isolated from the great vessels. Without careful attention to detail, a kyphosing effect can occur even with the newer solid rod anterior instrumentation systems. The attachment to the spine is through relatively cancellous vertebral bodies, and proximal screw dislodgment also is a risk. Many orthopaedic surgeons require the assistance of a thoracic surgeon with anterior approaches.

Betz et al. formed a study group to prospectively evaluate anterior spinal instrumentation and fusion with a threaded rod

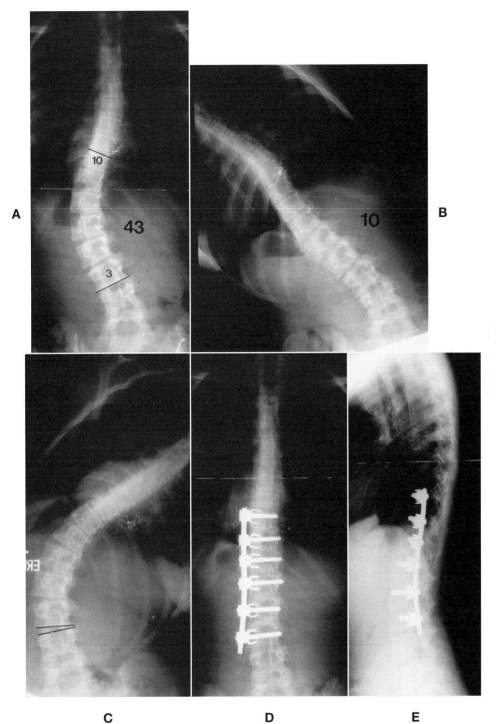

Fig. 38-107   **A,** Flexible 43-degree thoracic curve. **B,** Correction on bending film. **C,** Correction of fractional curve on bending film. **D** and **E,** After anterior fusion with TSRH instrumentation.

anterior system and compare it with posterior spinal fusion with various multisegmented hook rod systems in patients with adolescent idiopathic thoracic scoliosis. Initially, there was an unacceptably high rod breakage rate, but this was reduced by a stronger, solid rod system. Advantages of the anterior thoracic approach include (1) a more complete three-dimensional correction of the deformity because of thorough disc and annular excision, (2) curve correction by convex compression

that shortens the spinal column and avoids distraction of neural elements, (3) fusion of end vertebra to end vertebra, resulting in a shorter fusion construct than would be required posteriorly (Fig. 38-108), (4) possible reduction of the number of upper and midlumbar fusion levels, (5) avoidance of a crankshaft phenomenon in skeletally immature patients, (6) decreased frequency of decompensation in primary thoracic scoliosis with compensatory lumbar curves (King type II), (7) choice of

A   **B**   **C**

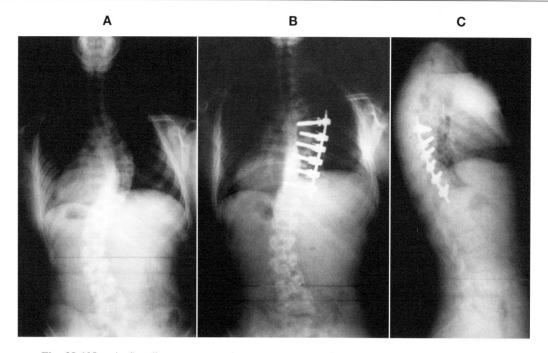

Fig. 38-108 **A,** Standing posteroanterior roentgenogram of patient with idiopathic scoliosis. If approached posteriorly, this patient would require fusion well down into the lumbar spine. **B** and **C,** Postoperative posteroanterior and lateral roentgenograms of this patient approached anteriorly. Although some loss of fixation of proximal screw is noted, patient achieved satisfactory correction and well-balanced spine in both coronal and sagittal planes by instrumenting only thoracic spine deformity.

kyphosis or lordosis of the vertebral segment to improve the sagittal profile after disc excision, and (8) avoidance of problems with prominent posterior instrumentation that occurs in thin patients even with the newer, low-profile instruments. Potential disadvantages include possible chest cage disruption, which can affect pulmonary function, the need for thoracic surgery assistance, and an increased risk of progressive kyphosis because of posterior spinal growth in skeletally immature patients (Risser 0). Currently, no long-term follow-up studies of large numbers of patients are available to confirm the effectiveness of this approach.

Surgical Approach

If the curve to be instrumented is a thoracolumbar curve, a thoracoabdominal approach is required. If the curve is purely lumbar, a lumbar extraperitoneal approach can be used.

◆ Thoracoabdominal Approach

TECHNIQUE 38-25 (see Fig. 34-14)
Place the patient in the lateral decubitus position with the convex side of the curve elevated. Make a curvilinear incision along the rib that is one level higher than the most proximal level to be instrumented. This generally is the

ninth rib in most thoracolumbar curves. Make the incision along the rib and extend it distally along the anterolateral abdominal wall just lateral to the rectus abdominus muscle. Expose and excise the rib. Enter the chest and retract the lung. Identify the diaphragm as a separate structure; it tends to closely approximate the wall of the thoracic cage. The diaphragm can be removed in two ways. We prefer to remove it from the chest cavity and then continue with retroperitoneal dissection distally. Alternatively, the retroperitoneum can be entered below the diaphragm, and then the diaphragm can be divided. To remove the diaphragm from the chest cavity, enter the chest cavity transpleurally through the bed of the rib. Then use electrocautery to divide the diaphragm close to the chest wall. Leave a small tag of diaphragm for reattachment. Once the diaphragm has been reflected, expose the retroperitoneal space. Dissect the peritoneal cavity from underneath the internal oblique muscle and the abdominal musculature. Split the internal oblique and the transverse abdominal muscles in line with the skin incisions and extend the exposure distally as far as necessary. Identify the vertebral bodies and carefully dissect the psoas muscle laterally off the vertebral disc spaces. The psoas origin usually is at about L1. Divide the prevertebral fascia in the direction of the spine. Identify the segmental arteries over the waist of each vertebral body and isolate and ligate them in the midline. Expose the bone extraperiosteally.

◆ ◆ ◆

The exposure from T10 to L2 or L3 with this approach is simple, but more distally the iliac vessels overlie the L4 and L5 vertebrae, and exposure in this area requires more meticulous dissection and displacement of these vessels.

◆ **Lumbar Extraperitoneal Approach**

TECHNIQUE 38-26

Place the patient in the lateral decubitus position with the convex side up. Make a midflank incision from the midline anteriorly to the midline posteriorly (Fig. 38-109, *A*). Divide the abdominal oblique muscles in line with the incision (Fig. 38-109, *B* and *C*). As the dissection leads laterally, identify the latissimus dorsi muscle as it adds another layer: the transversalis fascia and the peritoneum. The transversalis fascia and the peritoneum diverge posteriorly as the transversalis fascia lines the trunk wall, and the peritoneum turns anteriorly to encase the viscera. Posterior dissection in this plane allows access to the spine without entering the abdominal cavity. Repair any inadvertent entry into the peritoneum immediately because it may not be identifiable later.

Reflect all the fat-containing areolar tissue back to the transverse fascia and the lumbar fascia, reflecting the ureter along with the peritoneum (Fig. 38-109, *D*). Locate the major vessels in the midline, divide the lumbar fascia, and carefully retract the great vessels. Divide the segmental arteries and veins as they cross the waist of the vertebra in the midline and ligate them to control hemorrhage. The skin incision must be placed carefully to ensure that the most cephalad vertebra to be instrumented can be easily seen.

◆ **Disc Excision**

TECHNIQUE 38-27

Once the anterior portion of the spine has been exposed, the discs can be felt as soft, rounded, protuberant areas of the spine compared with the concave surface of the vertebral body. Divide the annulus sharply with a long-handled scalpel (Fig. 38-110) and remove it. Remove the nucleus pulposus with rongeurs and curets. It is not necessary to remove the anterior or posterior longitudinal ligaments. Once the disc excision has been completed, remove the cartilaginous endplates using either ring curets or an osteotome. The posterior aspects of the cartilaginous

endplates often are more easily removed with angled curets. Obtain hemostasis with Gelfoam soaked in thrombin unless a cell saver is in use. Usually, significant correction of the curve occurs during the discectomies, and it becomes more flexible and more easily correctable.

◆ **Anterior Instrumentation with Texas Scottish Rite Hospital System (TSRH)**

TECHNIQUE 38-28

After exposure of the spine and removal of the discs, insert TSRH bone screws into each vertebral body at the midportion. The TSRH screws come in 5.5-mm and 6.5-mm diameters. If possible, a 6.5-mm screw should be used because of the larger-diameter shank and the deeper threads, which give better pull-out strength. Alternatively, variable-angle bone screws (5.5 mm or 6.5 mm) can be used, which simplifies placement of the rod anteriorly. A 6.4-mm "flexible" rod generally is used. The diameter of the rod does not make the instrumentation any more or less prominent. Instrument the apical (most rotated) vertebra first. Place all screws in the posterior third of the vertebral body. Use the appropriate-sized staple as a template to start the hole for the vertebral body screw. Insert a staple and use an awl to make a hole in the side of the vertebral body through the hole in the staple. The legs of the staple should be placed in the vertebral endplates. If they are inserted into the disc space, they may prohibit adequate compression of that disc space. Direct the hole parallel to the endplates and slightly in a posterior to anterior direction (Fig. 38-111). Occasionally the vertebral body is too small to allow the use of a staple or circular collar, but staple fixation is recommended whenever possible to improve screw resistance to cantilever pull-out (Fig. 38-112). Impact the staple into place using the awl. Remove the awl. This is the starting hole for the vertebral body screw. It is not necessary to drill or tap a vertebral body because the screws are self-tapping. With the slotted screwdriver insert a bone screw of appropriate length through the staple. Direct the screw parallel to the endplate and to a point on the vertebral body on the other side palpable by the fingertip. Use a fingertip to guide the screw through the vertebral body (Fig. 38-113). The screw should pass completely through the opposite cortex, and the finger should be able to feel one or two threads on the opposite cortex. This screw length is critical and requires an accurate measurement of the width of the vertebral body with a caliper device or a depth gauge. The slotted or serrated side of the screws should be posterior so that the eyebolt nuts are anterior, which allows easier access for tightening the nuts. If necessary, however, the rod can be placed anterior to the screws to translate a vertebral body more anteriorly during sequential seating. The screws

continued

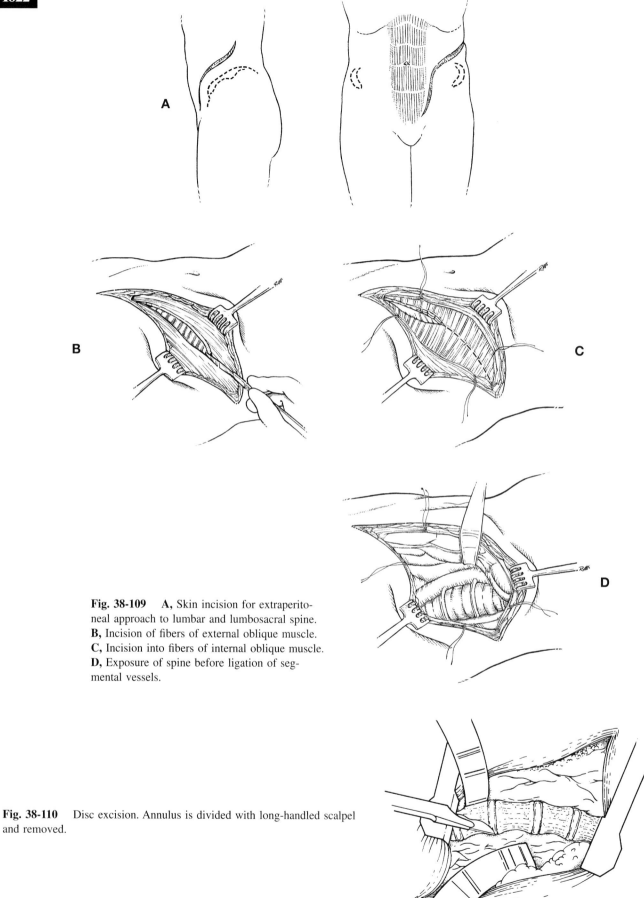

Fig. 38-109   **A,** Skin incision for extraperitoneal approach to lumbar and lumbosacral spine. **B,** Incision of fibers of external oblique muscle. **C,** Incision into fibers of internal oblique muscle. **D,** Exposure of spine before ligation of segmental vessels.

Fig. 38-110   Disc excision. Annulus is divided with long-handled scalpel and removed.

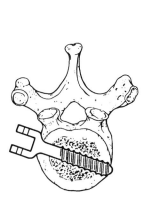

Fig. 38-111 Insertion of screw parallel to endplates and in slightly posterior to anterior direction.

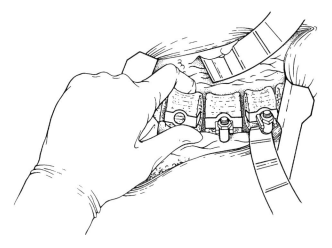

Fig. 38-113 Screw is guided through the vertebral body with a fingertip.

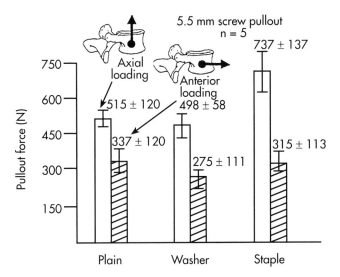

Fig. 38-112 Increased resistance to cantilever (axial) screw pullout provided by staple fixation as compared with washer fixation or no additional screw stabilizer. (From Johnston CE II, Herring JA, Ashman RB: Texas Scottish Rite Hospital (TSRH) universal spinal instrumentation system. In An HS, Cotler JM, eds: *Spinal instrumentation*, Philadelphia, 1992, Williams & Wilkins.)

should be placed in a relatively straight line, cephalad to caudal. Offsetting the screws does not produce better correction because the corrective forces imparted to the spine come from contouring of the solid rod. Cut a 6.4-mm "flexible" rod to length and contour it to maintain normal lumbar lordosis. Place eyebolts of appropriate size on the rod and use them to connect the rod to the screws. Place the rod so that the cut end is distal to avoid sharp edges against the lung. Seat the rod into the screws using the gooseneck spreader, the mini-corkscrew, or the corkscrew. Generally, because of limited exposure at the caudal level, the rod

usually is seated at the most caudal screw first and then seated successively in each more proximal screw. Tighten the eyebolts enough to hold the rod in place but still allow rotation of the rod. Rotate the rod 90 degrees (Fig. 38-114, *A* and *B*). An appropriate-size box-end wrench can be used on the hexagonal end of the rod to assist in this rotation maneuver. If the stability of these screws in the vertebral body is a concern, a smaller, 4.8-mm rod can be used with the appropriate-diameter eyebolts, which would be more flexible and exert less pull-out force on the screws. After rotation, the disc space opens up as the lordosis is increased. Place 1-cm squares of bone graft in the anterior aspect of the disc space (Fig. 38-114, *C*) to help prevent any kyphosing effect of the instrumentation. Pack the remainder of the disc space with smaller pieces of bone graft. Obtain further correction of the curve by compression toward the apical screw. This also helps to lock the bone graft into place. First tighten the apical screw and then use a compressing device to compress the screws toward the apex both proximally and distally (Fig. 38-114, *D*). Careful attention to the fit of the rod to the grooves or serrations in the screw heads is essential to secure fixation at each level (Fig. 38-115). Tighten the nuts completely to prevent any further rotation of the rod. If needed, strip the periosteum from the vertebral bodies to provide more bone area for fusion. Place remaining bone graft strips into the disc interspaces and along the area of the periosteal stripping. Suture the pleura over the upper end of the rod, repair the diaphragm, and suture the psoas origin over the lower end. Insert a chest tube if the thoracic cavity has been entered. Approximate the external oblique and latissimus dorsi muscles and close the skin incision in a routine manner.

AFTERTREATMENT. The chest tube usually is left in place for 48 to 72 hours. It is removed when the drainage decreases to less than 50 ml for two consecutive 8-hour periods. The

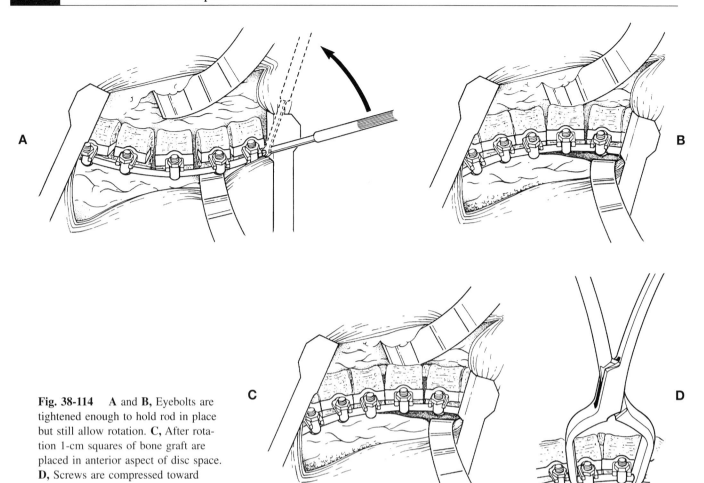

Fig. 38-114 **A** and **B,** Eyebolts are tightened enough to hold rod in place but still allow rotation. **C,** After rotation 1-cm squares of bone graft are placed in anterior aspect of disc space. **D,** Screws are compressed toward apex both proximally and distally.

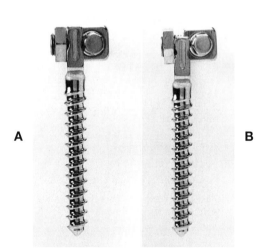

Fig. 38-115 Rod must be carefully fitted to grooves or serrations in screw head for secure fixation. **A,** Correct fit. **B,** Incorrect fit.

patient is kept on bed rest until the chest tubes are removed and then is allowed up in a TLSO. If the bone screws have good purchase and a 6.4-mm rod is used, no postoperative immobilization is needed. If there is any doubt about the stability of the fixation or cooperation of the patient, a TLSO is

used. For the first 3 to 4 days after surgery, pain relief is best managed by a patient-controlled analgesia system with an intravenous narcotic. A Foley catheter is necessary to monitor urine output because urinary retention is common. An ileus is to be expected after anterior surgery and usually lasts 2 or 3 days. Usually the patient is independent and ambulatory with or without a TLSO within 7 days of surgery. An elevated temperature consistent with atelectasis is common and usually responds to pulmonary therapy and to ambulation as soon as the patient is capable. The brace is worn for 4 to 6 months if needed.

◆ Anterior Thoracic Instrumentation

Betz et al. suggested that clinically significant hypokyphosis is an indication for anterior instrumentation in patients with thoracic idiopathic scoliosis. Another indication is the ability to save more than two distal fusion levels. The possible advantages and disadvantages of anterior thoracic instrumentation are discussed on p. 1819. In the patients reported by Betz et al., the fusion levels included all vertebrae in the Cobb angle measurement. Any vertebra that started to tilt away from the maximal angulation on the Cobb measurement was not included in the fusion. If two end vertebrae were parallel, the vertebra giving a longer fusion was selected as the end-instrumented vertebra. For King V curves, the upper thoracic curve had to bend ≤20 degrees on the left bending film; otherwise, this was considered a contraindication to anterior instrumentation. Medically significant pulmonary disease that would contraindicate a thoracotomy also was a contraindication to an anterior approach.

Numerous systems are capable of instrumenting a thoracic curve anteriorly. Threaded or solid rods can be used. We generally use solid rods.

TECHNIQUE 38-29

Approach the spine through a transthoracic incision (Technique 34-10). If instrumentation of only five to six levels is planned, do a single thoracotomy at the interspace proximal to the upper level of instrumentation (T4-T5 interspace for instrumentation up to T5). If six or more vertebrae are to be instrumented, a double thoracotomy may be required. In our experience, the second thoracotomy generally is best made at T11 to allow appropriate orientation for the instruments parallel to the disc spaces. This double entrance into the thoracic cavity is made through a single skin incision. Use a rib spreader to expose the chest cavity. Pack off the lung, and every 20 to 30 minutes irrigate the lung to remove all cyanotic spots. At this point, perform a thoracoplasty (see below) to increase mobilization and also provide bone graft material. Using blunt and sharp dissection, mobilize the soft tissue between the great vessels and the vertebral bodies. This serves as a protective layer in which to place retractors. Identify the segmental vessels as they adhere to the waist of each vertebra. Clamp and ligate each of these vessels and section them near the midline. If they are ligated too far laterally, the collateral vessels from the foramen may be disrupted and the segmental feeder vessels to the spinal cord may be damaged. Expose the spine subperiosteally and remove the annulus and discs back to the posterior longitudinal ligament.

Place bicortical screws through staples just anterior to the rib heads. Place autogenous rib graft loosely into the disc spaces that are going to be compressed to create kyphosis. Place structural grafts or cages in the discs that need to be lordosed. Cut the rod to length and contour it into the final coronal and sagittal plane alignment. Place the rod into the screws in a cantilever fashion from distal to proximal and rotate it 90 degrees counter-clockwise as necessary to recreate thoracic kyphosis. Remember to straighten out the operating table before rotating the rod if the table has been bent during thoracotomy and disc exposure.

Apply segmental compression forces from the apex to the ends of the rod. Tighten the nuts or screws to lock the rod into place. If possible, close the pleura over the implants and close the chest wall muscle layers and skin.

AFTERTREATMENT. Incentive spirometry and other respirator aids are used postoperatively. The patient is allowed up on the postoperative day. The chest tube is discontinued when chest drainage is less than 50 ml per an 8-hour shift for two consecutive shifts. If a thoracoplasty is done, we often use a lightweight, molded, elastic corset for support of the thoracoplasty for 12 weeks. No brace is required for most anterior instrumentations. Fusion usually is evident about 6 months postoperatively.

Complications and Pitfalls of Anterior Instrumentation

Pitfalls and complications may be related to poor patient selection, poor level selection, or instrument technical difficulties. A common technical problem is failure of the most proximal screw (see Fig. 38-108), which can be prevented by watching this screw carefully during the derotation maneuver. At any sign of screw loosening, the correction maneuver should be stopped. Another technical problem is encountered if the screw heads are not aligned properly and one screw head is offset from the others. If one screw is off just slightly, rod placement can be difficult. Variable-angle screws or polyaxial screws allow some adjustment to account for this offset.

A number of studies have emphasized the potential complications associated with an anterior approach to the spine, including respiratory insufficiency requiring ventilatory support, pneumonia, atelectasis, pneumothorax, pleural effusion, urinary tract infection, prolonged ileus, hemothorax, splenic injury, retroperitoneal fibrosis, and partial sympathectomy.

Neurological injury can occur during discectomy or screw insertion. The screws should be placed parallel to the vertebral endplates. When ligating the segmental vessels, the anastomosis at the intervertebral foramina should be avoided to minimize the chance of injury to the vascular supply of the spinal cord. A scoliotic deformity is approached from the convex side of the curve, and because the great vessels are inevitably on the concave side of the curve, the risk of injury to them is low. To increase purchase of the screws, however, the opposite cortex of the vertebra should be engaged by the screw, and care must be taken to be certain that the screw is not too prominent on the concave side.

◆ ANTERIOR THORACOPLASTY

The advantages of anterior thoracoplasty are the same as for posterior thoracoplasty. For the patient, reduction of the rib deformity is among the most important aspects of surgical correction and fusion. The bone graft obtained from a thoracoplasty, especially anteriorly, obviates the need for an iliac bone graft that contributes to the postoperative morbidity.

TECHNIQUE 38-30 *(Shufflebarger)*

After thoracotomy, reflect the parietal pleura over the chest wall, exposing the ribs. From within the thoracotomy, divide the periosteum in line with the rib. Use an elevator to complete circumferential subperiosteal dissection of the rib in the posterior axillary line. Divide the rib with an

continued

end-cutting instrument. Then grasp the rib and bring it into the chest. Perform circumferential dissection of the periosteum and intercostal muscles to the costotransverse articulation. Disarticulate the rib head from the costotransverse and costocorporal articulation. Remove the posterior portion of the remaining ribs in a similar manner to complete the thoracoplasty. This thoracoplasty not only improves appearance and provides bone graft but also significantly softens the chest wall to facilitate exposure in patients with rigid deformities.

VIDEO-ASSISTED THORACOSCOPY

Video-assisted thoracoscopic surgery in the treatment of pediatric spinal deformity is a relatively new and developing technique. Advantages of thoracoscopic surgery over open thoracotomy, in addition to better illumination and magnification at the site of surgery, include less injury to the latissimus muscle and chest wall with less long-term pain, decreased blood loss, better cosmesis, shorter recovery time, improved postoperative pulmonary function, and potentially shorter hospital stays. The primary disadvantages of thoracoscopy are related to a steep learning curve and the technical demands of the procedure. Newton et al. noted an average operative time for thoracoscopic procedures of 161 minutes, but this decreased as the series progressed. They found the learning curve for thoracoscopy to be substantial but not prohibitive.

Specialized equipment is required for these procedures. A general, pediatric, or thoracic surgeon familiar with thoracoscopy and open thoracotomies should be available to assist in the initial stages of the procedure and should remain scrubbed for the entire case. The anesthesiologist should be skilled in the use of double-lumen tubes with one lung ventilation.

Indications for video-assisted thoracoscopic surgery include rigid thoracic idiopathic curves that do not correct on bending, kyphotic deformities of more than 70 degrees, neuromuscular scoliosis in patients with compromised pulmonary function requiring anterior release, neurofibromatosis, and curves requiring anterior and posterior fusion. This procedure also is indicated for skeletally immature patients in whom anterior surgery is needed to prevent "crankshaft." Crawford extended his indications to include all procedures to the thoracic spine previously approached by thoracotomy.

Contraindications to the procedure include the inability to tolerate single-lung ventilation, severe or acute respiratory insufficiency, high airway pressures with positive pressure ventilation, emphysema, and previous thoracotomy.

Video-assisted thoracoscopic surgery is a technically demanding procedure. Experience should be obtained by practicing on animal or cadaver models, as well as by observing other surgeons adept in performing this procedure.

The equipment required for spinal thoracoscopic surgery is similar to that for general thoracoscopy. The basic equipment includes telescopes, light sources, cameras, monitors, and appropriate instrumentation. The most commonly used telescope is a 30-degree angled 10-mm scope. In some pediatric cases, a smaller telescope may be needed, but it does not provide the same magnitude of illumination and resolution as the 10-mm scope. Telescopes with a lens-washing and site irrigation system are useful in defogging and cleansing the end of the scope. Other equipment includes flexible portals and long-handled manual instruments, such as curets, pituitary rongeurs, fan retractors, suction irrigation systems, endoscopic clip appliers, and periosteal elevators.

Video-assisted thoracoscopic surgery is frequently used for anterior release in pediatric deformities. Mack et al., Blackman, and Picetti have all described the use of this technology in anterior instrumentation of thoracic scoliosis deformities.

◆ Video-Assisted Thoracoscopic Discectomy

Some surgeons prefer to work facing the patient with the patient in a lateral decubitus position (Fig. 38-116, *A*), whereas others prefer to work from behind the patient, therefore working away from the spinal cord (Fig. 38-116, *B*). Two monitors are positioned so that they can be seen from each side of the table. Because the traditional setup for most endoscopic procedures requires members of the surgical team to be on opposite sides of the patient and because working opposite the camera image can lead to disorientation, Horton described turning the assistant's monitor upside down. The monitor on the posterior aspect of the patient is inverted, and once the visualization port for the camera is established, the scope is inserted into the camera and rotated 180 degrees on the scope mount so that the camera is upside down. The assistant holding the inverted camera views the inverted monitor, which projects a normal monitor image as would be seen in an open thoracotomy (Fig. 38-117, *A* and *B*).

TECHNIQUE 38-31 *(Crawford)*

After general anesthesia is obtained using either a double-lumen endotracheal tube or a bronchial blocker for single lung ventilation, turn the patient into the lateral decubitus position. Prepare and drape the operative field as the anesthesiologist deflates the lung. About 20 minutes is required to obtain complete resorption atelectasis. Place the upper arm on a stand with the shoulder slightly abducted and flexed over 90 degrees to allow placement of portals higher into the axilla. Use an axillary roll to take pressure off the axillary structures. Identify the scapular borders, twelfth rib, and iliac crest and outline them with a marker. Place the first portal at or about the T6 or T7 interspace in the posterior axillary line (Fig. 38-118, *A*). Make a skin incision with a scalpel, then continue with electrocautery through the intercostal muscle to enter the chest cavity. To avoid damage to the intercostal vessels and nerves, make the incision over the top of the rib. Insert a finger to be sure the lung is deflated and that it is away from the chest wall so it will not to be injured when the trocar is inserted. Insert

continued

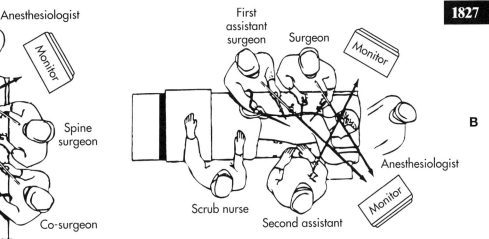

Fig. 38-116 **A,** Conventional set-up for video-assisted thoracoscopic spinal surgery. **B,** Set-up with surgeon working away from spine. (**A** redrawn from Krasna MJ, Mack MJ, eds: *Atlas of thoracoscopic surgery,* 1994, St Louis, Quality Medical Publishing; **B** redrawn from Picetti G: Endoscopic fusion technique: clinical results. Material presented at Endoscopic Approaches to the Spine, Memphis, Feb 5, 2000.)

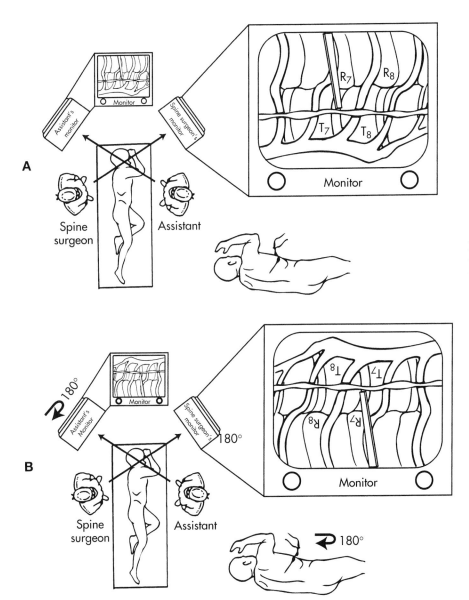

Fig. 38-117 **A,** Thoracoscopic traditional technique. **B,** Thoracoscopic inversion technique. (Redrawn from Horton, William C: Spine surgery: the technique of camera monitor inversion. Material presented at Endoscopic Approaches to the Spine. Fifth International Meeting of Advanced Spinal Techniques, Naples, Italy, May 1998; annual meeting of the Scoliosis Research Society, New York, Sept 1998.)

Fig. 38-118 **A,** First portal for anterior thoracoscopic release of spine created along posterior axillary line between T6 and T8 intercostal spaces. Subsequent portals are created along anterior axillary line. **B,** Technique of portal insertion. A 15- to 20-mm incision is made parallel to superior surface of rib. Flexible portal is inserted with trocar. **C,** Trocar is removed leaving flexible portal in place. (**A** redrawn from Krasna MJ, Mack MJ: *Atlas of thoracoscopic surgery,* St Louis, 1994, Quality Medical Publishing; **B** and **C** redrawn from Dickman CA, Mican C: *BNI Quarterly* 12:6, 1996.)

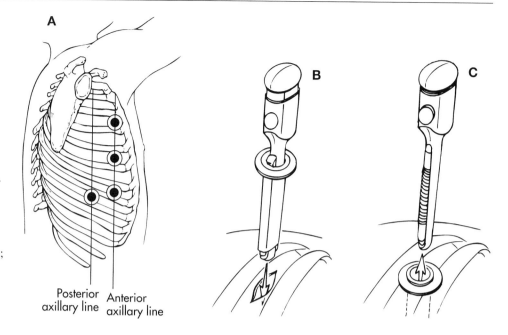

flexible portals through the intercostal spaces with a trocar (Fig. 38-118, *B* and *C*). Insert a 10-mm, 30-degree angled, rigid thoracoscope. Prevent fogging of the endoscope by prewarming it with warm irrigation solution and wiping the lens with a sterile fog reduction solution (FRED). Wipe the endoscope lens intermittently with this solution to optimize visibility. Some endoscopes have incorporated irrigating and windshield-like cleaning mechanisms to further simplify the procedure.

Evaluate the intrathoracic space to determine anatomy as well as possible sites for other portals. The superior thoracic spine usually can be seen without retraction of the lung once the lung is completely deflated; however, some retraction usually is necessary below T9-T10 because the diaphragm blocks the view. Once the spinal anatomy has been identified, continue to identify levels. The first rib usually cannot be seen, and the first visually identifiable rib is the second rib. Count the ribs sequentially to identify the levels to be released. Insert a long, blunt-tipped needle into the disc space and obtain a roentgenogram to confirm the levels intraoperatively. Select other portal sites after viewing from within. View the trocars with the endoscope as they are inserted. Take care when inserting the inferior portal to avoid perforation of the diaphragm. Use a fan retractor to retract the diaphragm but take care not to lacerate the lung.

Divide the parietal pleura with an endoscopic cautery hook. Place the hook in the parietal pleura in the region of the disc, midway between the head of the rib and the anterior spine. Pull the pleura up and cauterize in successive movements proximally and distally, avoiding the segmental vessels.

Identify the intervertebral discs as elevations on the spinal column and the vertebral bodies as depressions. For a simple anterior release, do not ligate the segmental vessels because of the risk of tearing. Bleeding can be difficult to control endoscopically. Crawford recommended coagulating any vessels that appear to be at risk for bleeding.

Once the pleura has been completely resected, proceed directly to excising the annulus at the level of the intervertebral discs to be removed. The rib heads provide excellent landmarks for localization. The rib head articulates with the base of the pedicle and the vertebral body just caudad to or at the level of the disc space; for example, the T9 rib head leads to the T8-T9 disc space (Fig. 38-119). Make a transverse cut with cautery across the vertebral body, parallel to the disc, cephalad and caudad to it. Elevate the periosteum toward the vertebral endplate to isolate the disc. Make a transverse cut across the annulus fibrosus, continuing down to the level of the nucleus pulposus. Use rongeurs, curets, and periosteal elevators as necessary to ensure complete removal of the disc materials and endplates. Control bleeding of the subchondral bone by packing the disc space with Surgicel. Stress the spinal column segment with moderate force after each release to see if mobility has been accomplished.

After the discectomies have been done, harvest rib graft through the portal sites (Fig. 38-120). The pleura can be closed or left open. Place a chest tube through the most posterior inferior portal. Use the endoscope to observe the chest tube as it is placed along the vertebral column. Connect the chest tube to a water seal. Once the anesthesiologist has inflated the lung to determine whether an air leak exists, close the portals in routine fashion.

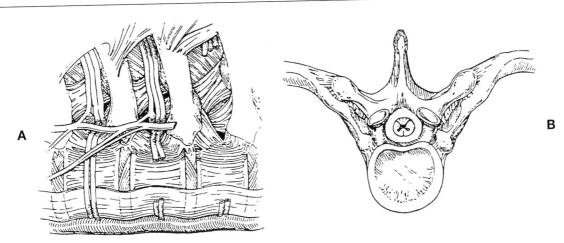

Fig. 38-119 **A,** Thoracic vertebral anatomy. Ribs attach to vertebrae via costotransverse and costovertebral ligaments. Head of ribs articulates with base of pedicle and vertebral body just below disk or at disk space. Segmental vessels cross over middle of concave surface of vertebral bodies. **B,** Cross-section of thoracic vertebrae demonstrating relationship of rib and pedicle to spinal cord. (Redrawn from Dickman CA, Mican C: *BNI Quarterly* 12:6, 1996.)

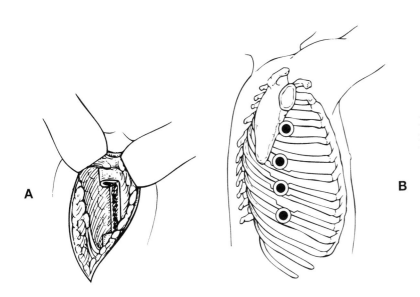

Fig. 38-120 **A** and **B,** Three to four rib sections removed and morselized until enough bone graft has been obtained. (Redrawn from Picetti GD III: CD Horizon Eclipse Spinal System surgical technique manual, Memphis, 1999, Sofamor Danek.)

Pitfalls and Complications. Bleeding can be difficult to control with endoscopic surgery. A radiopaque sponge with a heavy suture attached and loaded on a sponge stick should be available at all times to apply pressure. The suture allows later retrieval of the sponge. After application of direct pressure, electrocautery should be used for hemostasis. If necessary, endoscopic clip appliers or another hemostatic agent should be used. Instrumentation for open thoracotomy should be set up on a sterile back table to avoid delays or confusion if an immediate thoracotomy is needed to control bleeding.

Lung tissue can be damaged during the procedure. If an air leak occurs, it can be repaired with an endoscopic stapler. A dural tear can be recognized by leakage of clear cerebrospinal fluid (CSF) from the disc space. Hemostatic agents can sometimes seal small CSF leaks. If a dural tear continues to leak CSF, a thoracotomy and vertebrectomy with dural repair may be required.

Cloudy fluid in the intervertebral disc space after irrigation and suctioning may indicate a lymphatic injury, which can be closed with an endoscopic clip applier. The thoracic duct is especially vulnerable to injury at the level of the diaphragm. If a chylothorax is discovered after closure, it is treated with a low-fat diet.

The sympathetic nerve chain on the operative side often is transected. This causes little or no morbidity; however, the surgeon needs to inform the patient and family members of the possibility of temperature and skin color changes below the level of the surgery.

Postoperative pulmonary problems often involve the downside lung, in which mucous plugs can form. The anesthesiologist should suction both lungs before extubation.

Endoscopic Anterior Instrumentation of Idiopathic Scoliosis

As experience with video-assisted thoracoscopic has increased, techniques have been developed for anterior instrumentation of the thoracic spine through a thoracoscopic approach. These techniques are still developing, but their goal is to allow thoracoscopic anterior discectomy, fusion, and instrumentation that is comparable to that for open thoracotomy.

◆ CD Horizon Eclipse Spinal Instrumentation

TECHNIQUE 38-32 *(Picetti)*

Obtain appropriate preoperative roentgenograms and determine the fusion levels by Cobb angles. After general anesthesia is obtained using a double-lumen intubation technique (children weighing less than 45 kg may require selective intubation of the ventilated lung) and one lung ventilation has been achieved, place the patient into the direct lateral decubitus position, with the arms at 90/90 and the concave side of the curve down. It is imperative to have the lung completely collapsed in this procedure. If the patient's O₂ saturation drops when placed into the lateral decubitus position, have the anesthesiologist readjust the tube. Tape the hips and the shoulders to the operating table (Fig. 38-121, *A*). Have a general or thoracic surgeon assist in the first part of the procedure if necessary.

With the use of C-arm intensification, identify the vertebral levels and portal sites. A straight metallic object is used as a marker to identify the vertebral levels and portal sites. The superior and inferior access incisions are the most critical because the vertebrae at these levels are at the greatest angle in relation to the apex of the curve. View the planes with a C-arm in the posteroanterior plane and make sure the endplates are parallel and well defined. Rotate the C-arm until it is parallel to the vertebral body endplates, not perpendicular to the table (Fig. 38-121, *B*).

Position the marker posterior to the patient and align with every other vertebral body (Fig. 38-121, *C*). Obtain a C-arm image at each level. Once the marker is centered and parallel to the endplates, make a line on the patient at each portal site in line with the marker. Place incision marks two interspaces apart to allow placement of portals above and below the rib at each level and provide access to two levels through a single skin incision. Use three to five incisions, depending on the number of levels to be instrumented (Fig. 38-121, *D*). Once marks are made at all portal sites, rotate the C-arm to the lateral position. Place the marker end on each line, and adjust the marker position until the C-arm image shows the end of the marker at the level of the rib head on the vertebrae. Place a cross mark on the previous line (Fig. 38-121, *E*). This is the location of the center of the portals and will show the degree of rotation of the spine.

The spine surgeon's position at the patient's back allows all of instruments to be directed away from the spinal cord.

Exposure and Discectomy. Make a modified thoracotomy incision at the central mark. The incision can be smaller because it is used only for the central discectomies, screw placement, and viewing. The other discectomies and screw placements are done through the access portals because they provide better alignment to the end disc spaces and vertebral bodies.

Check patient positioning to confirm that he has remained in the direct lateral decubitus position, because this orientation provides a reference to gauge the anteroposterior and lateral direction of the guide wires and the screws. Prepare and drape the patient, including the axilla and scapula.

After the lung has been deflated completely, make the initial portal in the sixth or seventh interspace using the alignment marks made previously. Make sure that the portal is in line with the spine and positioned according to the amount of spinal rotation. Inserting the first portal at this level will avoid injury to the diaphragm, which normally is more caudal. Once the portal is made, use a finger to confirm that the lung is deflated and make sure there are no adhesions. Place 10.5-mm to 12.0-mm access portals under direct observation at the predetermined positions. Count the ribs to ensure the correct levels are identified based on preoperative plans.

Incise the pleura longitudinally along the entire length of the spine to be instrumented. Place a Bovie hook on the pleura over a disc and make an opening. Insert the hook under the pleura and elevate it and incise along the entire length (Fig. 38-122, *A*). Use suction to evacuate the smoke from the chest cavity. Dissect the pleura off the vertebral bodies and discs. Continue pleural dissection anteriorly off the anterior longitudinal ligament and posteriorly off the rib heads using a peanut or endoscopic grasper (Fig. 38-122, *B*).

Place a Kirschner wire into the disc space and confirm the level using C-arm intensification. With electrocautery incise the disc annulus (Fig. 38-122, *C*).

Remove the disc in standard fashion, using various endoscopic curets and pituitary, Cobb, and Kerrison rongeurs. If necessary use endoscopic shavers and rasps to assist in discectomy. Once the disc is completely removed, thin the anterior longitudinal ligament from within the disc space with a pituitary rongeur. Thin the ligament to a flexible remnant that is no longer structural but will contain the bone graft. Remove the disc and annulus posteriorly back to at least the rib head. Use a Kerrison rongeur to remove the annulus posterior to the rib heads. Leave the rib head intact at this point because it will be used to guide screw placement.

Once the disc has been evacuated, remove the endplate completely and inspect the disc space directly with the scope. Pack the disc space with Surgicel to control endplate bleeding.

Fig. 38-121 **A,** Patient positioning. **B,** Proper incision placement. Use C-arm in posteroanterior plane. **C,** Marker positioned posterior to patient and aligned with every other vertebral body. **D,** Three to five incisions are made, depending on number of levels to be instrumented. **E,** Cross mark then placed on previous line. This is location of center of portals. (Redrawn from Picetti GD III: CD Horizon Eclipse Spinal System surgical technique manual, Memphis, 1999, Sofamor Danek.)

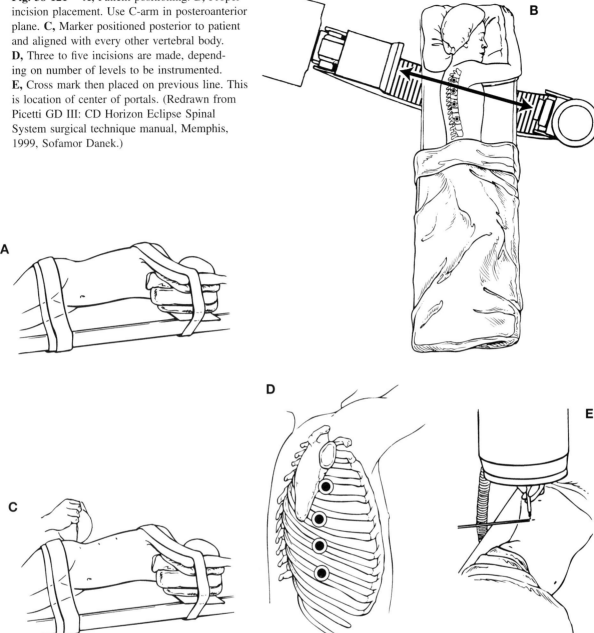

Graft Harvest. Use an Army-Navy retractor to stabilize the rib. Using a rib cutter, make two vertical cuts through the superior aspect of the rib and perpendicular to the rib extending halfway across it. Use an osteotome to connect the two cuts while using the retractor to support the rib. Remove and morselize the rib section. Remove three or four other rib sections in a similar fashion until enough bone graft has been obtained (see Fig. 38-120). If a rib is removed through an access incision, retract the portal anteriorly as far as possible. Dissect the rib subperiosteally and carry posterior dissection as far as the portal can be retracted. This technique yields an adequate amount of graft and preserves the integrity of the rib, thus protecting the intercostal nerve and decreasing postoperative pain. If the patient has a large chest wall deformity, perform thoracoplasties and use rib sections for grafting. Do not remove the rib heads at this time because they function as landmarks for screw placement.

Screw Placement. Position the C-arm at the most superior vertebral body to be instrumented. It is imperative to have the C-arm parallel to the spine to give an accurate image.

continued

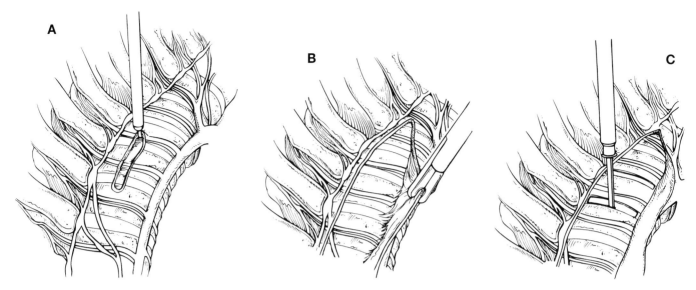

Fig. 38-122 **A,** Incision of pleura along entire length without injury to segmental vessels. **B,** Pleura is dissected off vertebral bodies and discs, anteriorly off anterior longitudinal ligament and posteriorly off rib heads using peanut or endoscopic grasper. **C,** Kirschner wire is placed into disc space, and C-arm images used to confirm level. Electrocautery is used to incise disc annulus. (Redrawn from Picetti GD III: CD Horizon Eclipse Spinal System surgical technique manual, Memphis, 1999, Sofamor Danek.)

The vessels are located in the depression or middle of the vertebral body and serve as an anatomical guide for screw placement. Grasp the segmental vessels and coagulate at the mid-vertebral body level with the electrocautery (Fig. 38-123, *A*). Hemoclip and cut larger segmental vessels if necessary. Check patient positioning again to ensure he is still in the direct lateral decubitus position.

Place the Kirschner guide wire onto the vertebral body just anterior to the rib head (Fig. 38-123, *B*). Check this position with the C-arm to verify that the wire will be parallel to the endplates and in the center of the body (Fig. 38-123, *C* and *D*). Check the inclination of the guide in the lateral plane by examining the chest wall and the rotation. The guide should be in a slight posterior to anterior inclination, directing the wire away from the canal. If there is any doubt or concern about the anterior inclination, obtain a lateral C-arm image to verify position. Once the correct alignment of the guide has been attained, insert the Kirschner wire into the cannula of the Kirschner guide that is positioned centrally on the vertebral body. Drill the guide wire to the opposite cortex, ensuring that it is parallel to the vertebral body. Confirm the position with C-arm as the wire is inserted. Take care not to drill the wire through the opposite cortex because this can injure the segmental vessels and the lung on the opposite side.

The most superior mark on the guide wire represents a length of 50 mm, and the etched lines are at 5-mm increments. The length of the Kirschner wire in the vertebral body can be determined by these marks. Start at the 50-mm

mark and subtract 5 mm for each additional mark that is showing (Fig. 38-123, *E*). For example, if there are four marks, in addition to the 50-mm mark, the length of the Kirschner wire would be 30 mm.

Remove the guide and place the tap over the Kirschner wire onto the vertebral body. To maximize fixation strength, use the largest diameter tap that will fit in the vertebral bodies, based on the preoperative roentgenograms, to maximize fixation strength. Grasp the distal end of the wire with a clamp (Fig. 38-123, *F*) and hold it as the tap is inserted so that the wire will not advance. This is important to avoid a pneumothorax in the opposite chest cavity. Tap only the near cortex (Fig. 38-123, *G*). Use the C-arm to monitor tap depth and Kirschner wire position.

Place the appropriate-sized screw, based on the Kirschner wire measurement and tap diameter, over the wire with the Eclipse screwdriver and advance it (Fig. 38-123, *H*). To ensure bicortical fixation, select a screw that is 5 mm longer than the width of the vertebral body as measured with the Kirschner wire. Grasp the wire again to avoid advancement while the screw is inserted. Remove the wire when the screw is approximately halfway across the vertebral body. Check the screw direction with the C-arm as it is advanced and seated against the vertebral body. The screw should penetrate the opposite cortex for bicortical fixation.

Instrument all Cobb levels. Use each rib head as a reference for subsequent screw placement to help ensure the screws are in line and will produce proper spinal rotation when the rod is inserted. With the screws properly aligned,

continued

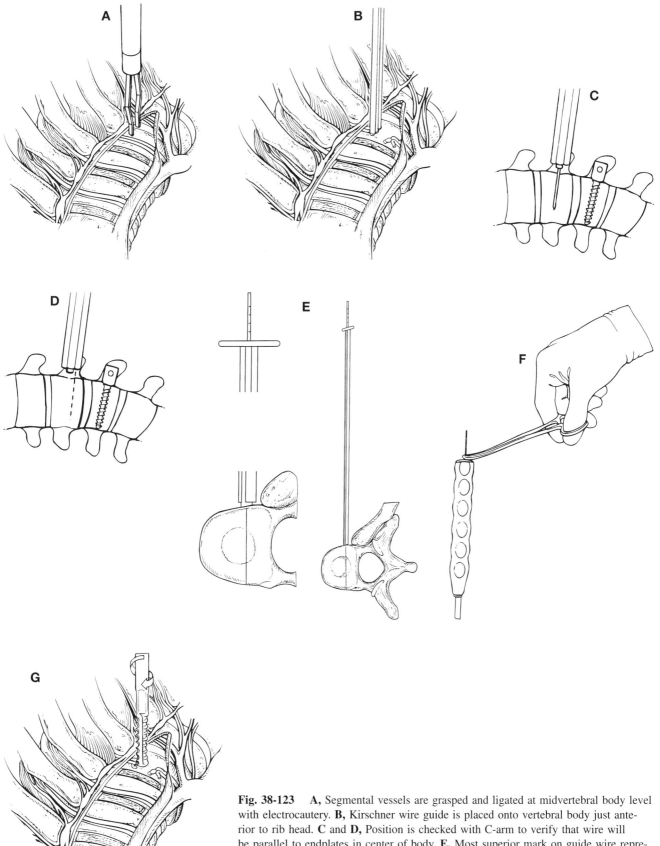

Fig. 38-123 **A,** Segmental vessels are grasped and ligated at midvertebral body level with electrocautery. **B,** Kirschner wire guide is placed onto vertebral body just anterior to rib head. **C** and **D,** Position is checked with C-arm to verify that wire will be parallel to endplates in center of body. **E,** Most superior mark on guide wire represents length of 50 mm, and etched lines are at 5-mm increments. Length of Kirschner wire is determined by these marks. **F,** Distal end of Kirschner wire grasped with clamp and held as tap is inserted. **G,** Only near cortex is tapped. *Continued*

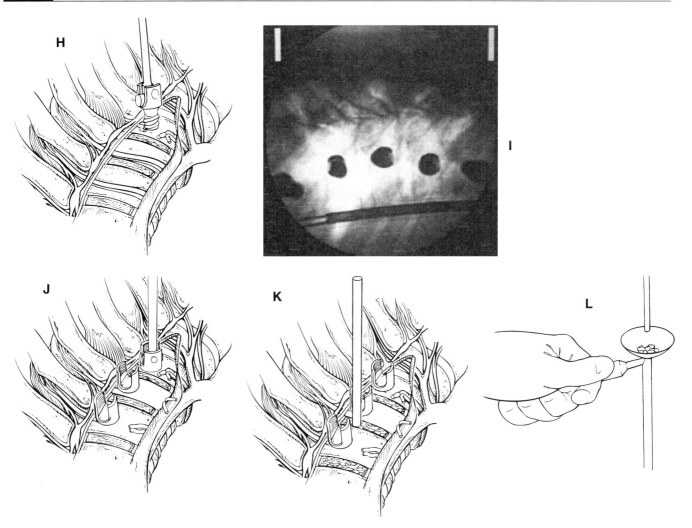

Fig. 38-123, cont'd **H,** Appropriate-sized screw is placed over Kirschner wire with Eclipse screwdriver and advanced. **I,** Alignment of screw heads verified by lateral image. **J,** Side walls of screws adjusted to be in line for receipt of rod. **K** and **L,** Graft delivered to disc space using graft funnel and plunger. Disc space should be filled all the way across to opposite side. (Redrawn from Picetti GD III: CD Horizon Eclipse Spinal System surgical technique manual, Memphis, 1999, Sofamor Danek.)

the screw heads form an arc that can be verified with a lateral image (Fig. 38-123, *I*).

Adjust the side walls of the screws (saddles) to be in line for insertion of the rod (Fig. 38-123, *J*). If a screw is sunk more than a few millimeters deeper than the rest of the screws, reduction of the rod into the screw head may be difficult. The C-arm image can confirm depth of screw placement as the screws are inserted.

Once all the screws have been placed, remove the Surgicel and use the graft funnel and plunger to deliver the graft into the disc spaces (Figs. 38-123, *K* and *L*). Fill each disc space all the way across to the opposite side.

Rod Measurement and Placement. Determine the rod length with the rod length gauge. Place the fixed ball at the end of the measuring device into the saddle of the inferior screw. Then guide the ball at the end of the cable through all of the screws with a pituitary rongeur to the most superior screw and insert it into the saddle (Fig. 38-124, *A*). Pull the wire tight and take a reading from the scale. The scale is in centimeters.

Cut the 4.5-mm diameter rod to length and insert it into the chest cavity through the thoracotomy. The rod has slight flexibility, so do not bend it before insertion. Apply anterior compression to obtain kyphosis in the thoracic spine. Do not cut the rod longer than measured because the total distance between the screws will be reduced with compression. Manipulate the rod into the inferior screw with the rod holder (Fig. 38-124, *B*). The end of the rod should be flush with the saddle of the screw to prevent the rod from protruding and irritating or puncturing the diaphragm. Once

continued

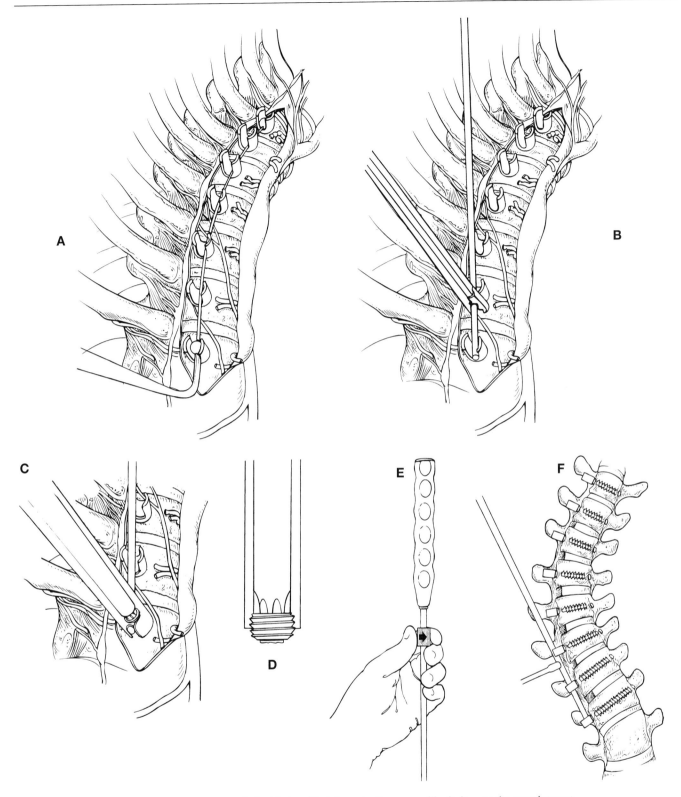

Fig. 38-124   A, Ball at end of cable is guided through all screws with pituitary to the superiormost screw and inserted into saddle. **B,** Rod manipulated into inferior screw with rod holder. **C,** Plug introduction guide placed over screw to guide plug and hold rod into position. **D,** Plug loaded onto plug-capturing T25 driver. **E,** Holding locking sleeve to prevent further rotation disengages plug from inserter as plug is inserted into screw. **F,** Rod reduced into remaining screws using rod pushers. (Redrawn from Picetti GD III: CD Horizon Eclipse Spinal System surgical technique manual, Memphis, 1999, Sofamor Danek.)

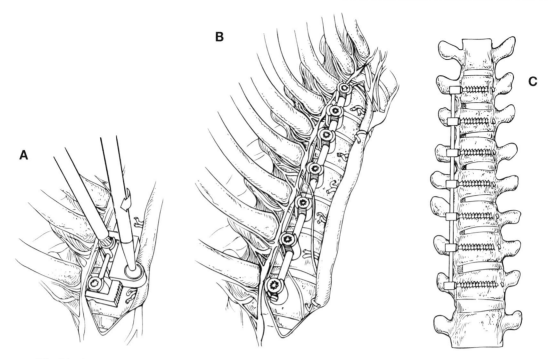

Fig. 38-125 **A,** Rack and pinion compressor fits over two screw heads on rod. **B** and **C,** Completed construct. (Redrawn from Picetti GD III: CD Horizon Eclipse Spinal System surgical technique manual, Memphis, 1999, Sofamor Danek.)

the rod is in place, remove the portal and place the plug introduction guide over the screw to guide the plug and hold the rod into position (Fig. 38-124, *C*). Place the obturator in the tube to assist in the insertion through the incision if necessary.

Load a plug onto the plug-capturing T25 driver (Fig. 38-124, *D*). Insert the plug with the flat side and the laser etching up. Once the plug is placed on the driver, turn the sleeve clockwise to engage the plug with the sleeve. Place the plug through the plug introduction guide and insert it into the screw. Do not place the plug without using the introduction guide and the plug inserter. To ensure proper threading, turn the sleeve once counter-clockwise before advancing the plug. Once the plug has been correctly started, hold the locking sleeve to prevent any further rotation. This will disengage the plug from the inserter as the plug is placed into the screw (Fig. 38-124, *E*). Remove the driver and introduction guide and torque the screw with the torque-limiting wrench. This is the only plug that is tightened completely at this time.

Sequentially insert the rod into the remaining screws using the rod pusher (Fig. 38-124, *F*). Place the rod pusher on the rod several screws above the screw that the rod is being placed into. Apply the plugs through the plug introduction guide as described. To allow compression do not fully tighten the plugs at this time.

Once the rod has been seated and all the plugs are

inserted into the screws, apply compression between the screws.

Compression—Rack and Pinion. Insert the compressor through the thoracotomy incision. Once in the thoracic cavity, manipulate it by holding the ball-shaped attachment with the compressor holder. The rack and pinion compressor fits over two screw heads on the rod; turning the compressor driver clockwise compresses the two screws (Fig. 38-125, *A*). Start compression at the inferior end of the construct with the most inferior screw's plug fully tightened. Once satisfactory compression has been obtained on a level, tighten the superior plug using the plug driver through the plug introduction guide. Apply compression sequentially superiorly until all levels have been compressed, then torque each plug to 75 in-lbs with the torque-limiting wrench. The construct is complete at this point (Figs. 38-125, *B* and *C*).

Compression—Cable Compressor. Insert each end of the cable through one of the distal holes on the side of the guide (not the larger central hole). The actuator should be in the position closest to the compressor body. Form a 3-inch loop at the end of the guide (Fig. 38-126, *A*), with the two cable ends passing through the actuator body. Engage the lever arm using one of the plug drivers through the cam mechanism (Fig. 38-126, *B*).

Place the end of the compressor through the distal portal. With the portal removed, place a plug introduction guide through the adjacent incision, through the loop and over the

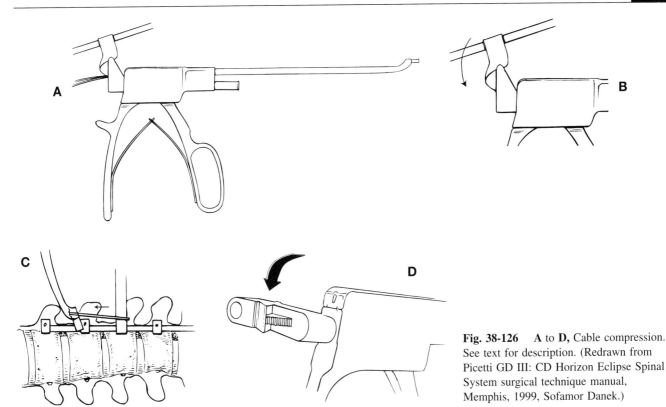

Fig. 38-126 **A** to **D,** Cable compression. See text for description. (Redrawn from Picetti GD III: CD Horizon Eclipse Spinal System surgical technique manual, Memphis, 1999, Sofamor Danek.)

next screw to be compressed. Place the foot of the compressor over the rod and against the inferior side of the end screw (Fig. 38-126, *C*). Fully tighten the plug in the end screw. Squeeze the handle of the compressor several times to compress. Once satisfactory compression has been obtained at a level, tighten the superior plug using the plug driver through the plug introduction guide.

To disengage the compressor, tilt it toward the superior screw until the foot disengages from the inferior screw. Turn the actuator mechanism 90 degrees to disengage the ratchet (Fig. 38-126, *D*). With the cable loop still around the plug introduction guide that is on the superior screw, pull the compressor until the actuator is next to the compressor body. Repeat the steps described on subsequent screws. Apply compression sequentially until all levels have been compressed and then torque each plug to 75 in-lbs with the torque-limiting wrench. The construct is complete at this point.

Place a no. 20 French chest tube through the inferior portal and close the incisions. Obtain anteroposterior and lateral roentgenograms before the patient is transferred to the recovery room.

AFTERTREATMENT. The chest tube is left in until drainage is less than 100 ml every 8 hours. Patients can be ambulatory after the first postoperative day, and they can be discharged from the hospital the day after the chest tube is removed. A brace should be worn for 3 months.

Neuromuscular Scoliosis

The specific causes of neuromuscular scoliosis are unknown, but several contributing factors are well known. Loss of muscle strength or voluntary muscle control or loss of sensory abilities, such as proprioception, in the flexible and rapidly growing spinal column of a juvenile patient are believed to be factors in development of these curves. As the spine collapses, increased pressure on the concave side of the curve results in decreased growth of that side of the vertebral body and wedging of the vertebral body itself. The vertebrae also can be structurally compromised by malnutrition or disuse osteopenia.

The Scoliosis Research Society has established a classification for neuromuscular scoliosis (Box 38-4).

Neuromuscular curves develop at a younger age than do idiopathic curves, and a larger percentage of neuromuscular curves are progressive. Unlike idiopathic curves, even small neuromuscular curves may continue to progress beyond skeletal maturity. Many neuromuscular curves are long, C-shaped curves that include the sacrum, and pelvic obliquity is common. Patients with neuromuscular scoliosis also may have pelvic obliquity from other sources, such as hip joint and other lower extremity contractures, all of which can affect the lumbar spine. The progressing neurological or muscular disease

BOX 38-4 • Classification of Neuromuscular Spinal Deformity

NEUROPATHIC
Upper Motor Neuron
Cerebral palsy
Spinocerebellar degeneration
  Friedreich ataxia
  Charcot-Marie-Tooth
  Roussy-Levy
Syringomyelia
Spinal cord tumor
Spinal cord trauma

Lower Motor Neuron
Poliomyelitis
Other viral myelitides
Traumatic
  Spinal muscle atrophy
  Werdnig-Hoffmann
  Kugelberg-Welander
Dysautonomia (Riley-Day syndrome)

MYOPATHIC
Arthrogryposis
Muscular dystrophy
  Duchenne
  Limb-girdle
  Facioscapulohumeral
Fiber-type disproportion
Congenital hypotonia
Myotonia dystrophica

also can interfere with trunk stability. These patients generally are less tolerant of orthotic management than patients with idiopathic scoliosis. Spinal surgery in this group is associated with increased bleeding, less satisfactory bone stock, longer fusions, and the necessity for fusion to the pelvis.

Many neuromuscular spinal deformities require operative intervention. The goal of treatment is to maintain a spine balanced in the coronal and sagittal planes over a level pelvis. The basic treatment methods are similar to those for idiopathic scoliosis: observation, orthotic treatment, and surgery.

NONOPERATIVE TREATMENT

Observation

Not all neuromuscular spinal deformities require immediate bracing or surgery. Small curves of less than 20 to 25 degrees can be observed carefully for progression before treatment is begun. Similarly, large curves in severely mentally retarded patients in whom the curve is not causing any functional disability or hindering nursing care can be observed. If progression of a small curve is noted, orthotic management should be considered. If the functional ability of severely mentally retarded patients is compromised by increasing curvature, treatment should be instituted.

Orthotic Treatment

Progressive neuromuscular scoliosis in very young patients is treated with an orthosis. The scoliosis may continue to progress despite orthotic treatment, but the rate of progression can be slowed and further spinal growth can occur before the definitive spinal fusion is completed. The brace also provides flaccid patients with trunk support, allowing the use of the upper extremities.

For patients who have trunk control or are ambulatory, a dynamic form of TLSO, such as a Milwaukee orthosis, can be considered. However, a custom-molded, total-contact TLSO usually is required for these children because their trunk contours do not accommodate standard braces. Most patients with neuromuscular scoliosis lack voluntary muscle control, normal righting reflexes, and the ability to cooperate with an active brace program, and therefore passive-type orthotics have been more successful in our experience in managing these neuromuscular curves. Patients with severe involvement and no head control frequently require custom-fabricated seating devices combined with orthoses or head-control devices.

A more malleable type of spinal brace, the soft Boston orthosis, is fabricated from a soft material that is well tolerated by patients, yet is strong enough to provide good trunk support. The major complaint with the use of this brace has been heat retention.

OPERATIVE TREATMENT

The goal of fusion in patients with neuromuscular scoliosis is to produce solid arthrodesis of the spine, balanced in both the coronal and sagittal planes and over a level pelvis. In doing so, the surgery should maximize function and improve the quality of life. To achieve this goal, a much longer fusion is necessary than usually is indicated for idiopathic scoliosis. Because of a tendency for cephalad progression of the deformity when fusion ends at or below the fourth thoracic vertebra, fusion should extend to T4 or above. The decision on the distal extent of the fusion generally is whether to fuse to the sacrum or to attempt to stop short of it. Occasionally the fusion can exclude the sacrum if the patient is an ambulator who requires lumbosacral motion, has no significant pelvic obliquity, and has a horizontal L5 vertebral body. Many of these patients, unfortunately, are nonambulators with a fixed spinopelvic obliquity. If the spinopelvic obliquity is fixed on bending or traction films (more than 10 to 15 degrees of L4 or L5 tilt relative to the interiliac crest line), the caudal extent of the fusion usually is the sacrum or the pelvis. Maintaining physiological lordosis in the lumbar spine is important in insensate patients who require fusion to the pelvis. This permits body weight to be distributed more equally beneath the ischial tuberosities and the posterior region of the thigh, reducing the risk of pressure sores over the coccyx. Autogenous bone almost always requires augmentation by bone-bank allograft.

Preoperative Considerations

Patients with neuromuscular scoliosis must have complete medical evaluations, including cardiac, pulmonary, and nutri-

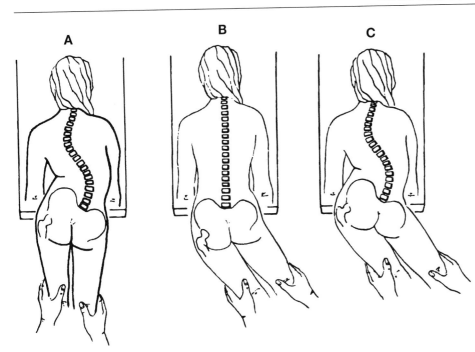

Fig. 38-127 **A,** Pelvic obliquity. **B,** If pelvic obliquity is eliminated by abduction or adduction of hips, pelvic-femoral muscle contracture is cause. **C,** If obliquity persists despite abduction or adduction of hips, fixed spinal-pelvic deformity exists. (From Shook JE, Lubicky JP: Paralytic scoliosis. In Bridwell KH, DeWald RL, eds: *The textbook of spinal surgery*, Philadelphia, ed 2, 1997, Lippincott-Raven.)

tional status. Many conditions, such as Duchenne muscular dystrophy and Friedreich ataxia, are associated with cardiac involvement. Most patients with neuromuscular scoliosis have diminished pulmonary function, and careful preoperative evaluation is essential. Nickel et al. found that their patients with vital capacities of less than 30% of predicted normal required respiratory support postoperatively, and those with a similar decrease of vital capacity and without a voluntary cough reflex required tracheostomy. Some surgeons prefer to use a nasotracheal tube for postoperative respiratory assistance as long as necessary. Preoperatively the patient should have pulmonary function studies if the patient is able to cooperate, and the vital capacity and forced expiratory volume in the first second are evaluated. This information is considered along with the patient's ability to cough and with measurements of arterial blood gas levels. Postoperative pulmonary management is then formulated in close consultation with a pulmonary specialist before surgery.

Patients with neuromuscular scoliosis often have suboptimal nutrition because of gastrointestinal problems, such as a hiatal hernia or gastroesophageal reflux. Surgery intensifies the preexisting state by raising the patient's metabolic requirements. The lack of coordination of the muscles about the mouth and pharynx often causes difficulties in swallowing. Appropriate nutritional therapy, including preoperative hyperalimentation, may help improve wound healing and decrease the possibility of postoperative infection. We have found that in many of these patients, surgical procedures, such as a gastrostomy, can be helpful in improving preoperative nutrition and decreasing the possibility of problems with gastroesophageal reflux. Procedures to control oral secretions also can be beneficial, especially in patients with cerebral palsy.

Seizure disorders are common in patients with neuromuscular scoliosis, and preoperative anticonvulsant levels should

be optimized within a therapeutic range. Osteopenia may be present because of the anticonvulsant medications.

Ambulatory status should be evaluated carefully before surgery. Often a patient with marginal ambulation capabilities and progressive scoliosis may not walk again after spinal surgery. The patient and the parents must understand this before surgery.

Techniques to minimize blood loss intraoperatively should be available, including electrocautery, hypotensive anesthesia, hemodilution techniques, and a cell saver. Because of chronic anemia and poor nutrition, most neuromuscular patients are not suitable candidates for preoperative autodonation of blood.

Most patients with neuromuscular disease have insufficient autogenous bone; therefore allograft bone must be available, which also requires preoperative planning and scheduling.

As in other scoliosis surgery, the fusion levels and instrumentation must be determined preoperatively. The source of pelvic obliquity must be determined (Fig. 38-127). Combined anterior and posterior arthrodeses may be required for severe pelvic obliquity. Other indications for a combined anterior and posterior approach include (1) necessity for an anterior release for further correction of severe kyphosis, (2) severe and rigid scoliosis that cannot be corrected by bending or traction to less than 60 degrees, and (3) deficient posterior elements, such as those in patients with myelomeningocele.

Segmental instrumentation is preferred for neuromuscular scoliosis. Broom et al. and Boachie-Adjei et al. reported acceptable results with the use of Luque segmental instrumentation in patients with neuromuscular scoliosis, and Neustadt, Shufflebarger, and Cammisa reported similar results for spinal fusions to the pelvis with Cotrel-Dubousset instrumentation. McCarthy et al. found that allograft is an acceptable alternative to autograft in spinal fusions for paralytic scoliosis.

In the past, halo-pelvic, halo-femoral, or halo-gravity traction has been used extensively in patients with neuromuscular scoliosis. Complications of traction are frequent, including pain and weakness of the neck muscles, avascular necrosis of the odontoid, cranial nerve damage, paraplegia, and pin track infections. Lonstein and Renshaw found that traction was not useful for curve correction but occasionally was useful for controlling uncooperative patients between surgical procedures and to make nursing care easier. We rarely use traction in these patients.

Finally, the patient's family should be clearly informed of the potential benefits and risks of any surgical procedure. The surgery is directed toward functional goals, such as sitting balance, pain relief, and improvement in fatigability rather than toward any cosmetic improvement. These functional goals must be weighed against the potential risks of the procedure and must be documented in the patient's medical record.

Operative Considerations

The potential for intraoperative complications in patients with neuromuscular scoliosis is great. Death can result from anesthesia problems, although more frequently it occurs from postoperative pulmonary deterioration. Relative hypothermia can easily occur in a lengthy spinal operation in which a large area of tissue is exposed and can cause myocardial depression and arrhythmias. Spinal surgery in patients with neuromuscular disease is associated with greater blood loss than in patients with idiopathic scoliosis. The anesthesiologist should be aware of both of these potential problems and should be prepared for them with an arterial blood gas line, a central venous pressure line, temperature probes, and careful management of urine output. Because the curves generally are larger, more rigid, and more difficult to instrument, neurological complications can occur during surgery. Many patients with neuromuscular scoliosis are unable or unwilling to cooperate with an intraoperative wake-up test. Spinal cord monitoring can be a valuable technique in these patients.

Surgical technique must include meticulous debridement of the soft tissue off the posterior elements of the spine. Ablation of the facet joints and a massive amount of bone graft are preferred. The bone frequently is osteopenic, and appropriate stable segmental instrumentation should be used. The Luque segmental instrumentation system is the most widely used system for neuromuscular curves at this time, although early results of spinal fusions to the pelvis with multihook segmental instrumentation systems indicate that these systems also have a role. With the newer segmental posterior instrumentation systems, anterior instrumentation frequently is unnecessary. Anterior release and fusion are useful in patients with large, fixed spinal pelvic obliquity or posterior element deficiencies or with severe and rigid curves that cannot be corrected beyond 60 degrees with bending. The role of anterior instrumentation in these curves is still being debated.

Postoperative Considerations

Pulmonary problems are the most likely complications in the immediate postoperative period, and the assistance of a pulmonary specialist is invaluable. Ventilatory support may be necessary, and such techniques as suctioning, spirometers, and intermittent positive pressure breathing may be appropriate. Possibly the best measure to prevent postoperative pulmonary problems is a spinal construct strong enough to allow early mobilization.

Fluid balance must be monitored carefully. After spinal surgery, especially in patients with neuromuscular scoliosis, antidiuretic hormone levels may be increased, leading to oliguria. If fluids are increased to overcome the oliguria, fluid overload may occur. This is especially disastrous in patients with impaired renal function, pulmonary compromise, and cardiac difficulties.

The necessity for postoperative orthotic support must be determined for each patient. If a complication, such as extremely osteopenic bone, compromises spinal fixation, or if less than ideal instrumentation is used, the use of postoperative external support may be wise. If the patient is so large, spastic, or dyskinetic that the spinal instrumentation may be excessively stressed, a postoperative orthosis should be considered.

Infection is a frequent problem in patients with neuromuscular scoliosis, probably because of the metabolically compromised host and the lengthy spinal fusions necessary. Patients with myelomeningocele and cerebral palsy have the highest infection rates. A major source of postoperative infection is the urinary tract. Any organisms found in the urine should be aggressively treated for 48 hours before surgery and for 3 months after surgery. Spinal infection is treated in the same manner as in patients with idiopathic scoliosis (see p. 1811).

Pseudarthrosis with subsequent instrumentation failure is a potential late problem. If the pseudarthrosis causes pain or loss of correction, repair probably will be necessary, but asymptomatic pseudarthrosis without curve progression or pain can be observed.

Luque Rod Instrumentation with Sublaminar Wiring

Eduardo Luque is credited with popularizing the use of long L-shaped rods and sublaminar wires in the surgical treatment of spinal deformity. The rods can be contoured, and the spine is corrected as the wires are tightened. Wenger et al. demonstrated a clear mechanical advantage of this instrumentation over traditional Harrington instrumentation because the sublaminar wires provide stability in the frontal, sagittal, and transverse planes. The technique has been developed and standardized in the United States by Allen and Ferguson.

Wilber et al. noted neurological changes in 17% of their patients with idiopathic scoliosis, but more recent studies have indicated that since surgeons have become more proficient with the technique, the incidence of neurological injury has been much lower. The neurological complications from sublaminar wires are of three types: cord injury, root injury, and dural tears. Root injuries are by far the most common and lead to hyperesthesia, but these generally resolve within 2 weeks. Johnston et al. reported delayed paraplegia in two patients who had anterior release followed by second-stage posterior fusion with sublaminar wiring. Bernard and Johnson reported a

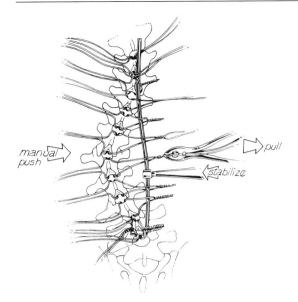

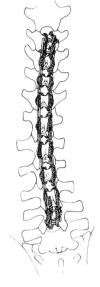

Fig. 38-128 Concave rod technique for correction of lumbar scoliosis. (From Segmental spinal fixation and correction using Richards' L-rod instrumentation, Memphis, Smith & Nephew Richards.)

neurological deficit that occurred months after surgery as a result of wire breakage. Schrader, Bethem, and Scerbin noted epidural and intramedullary hemorrhage, reactive epidural fibrosis, dural thinning and perforation, indentation of the dorsal surface of the spinal cord, and cellular destruction within the spinal cord in dogs that were subjected to sublaminar wires. They also noted a marked and uncontrolled displacement of the sharp ends of wires into the dural sac during extraction of the wires. Although sublaminar wires or cables have potential risks, we have found that for neuromuscular curves the advantages of this type of segmental instrumentation far outweigh the potential risks.

The basic instrumentation for the system consists of ³⁄₁₆-inch (4.8 mm) and ¼-inch (6.3 mm) diameter stainless steel rods. Stainless steel wires are available in diameters of 16 and 18 gauge. If desired, cables can be used instead of wires. Wenger et al. found that the ³⁄₁₆-inch diameter L-rods bend at 595 newtons of compressive loading. Because these rods are most often used in neuromuscular curves, often with instrumentation of the pelvis, the stronger ¼-inch rods should be used if possible.

◆ Luque Rod Instrumentation and Sublaminar Wires Without Pelvic Fixation

TECHNIQUE 38-33

The spine is exposed posteriorly as described in Technique 38-3. Wires or cables are passed as described in Technique 38-11. Two rods are used for most scoliosis corrections, with the first rod applied either to the convex or concave side of the curve. Lumbar scoliosis generally is more easily corrected by the concave rod technique, and because most neuromuscular curves include the lumbar spine and pelvis, the concave rod technique is most frequently used.

Bend the appropriate amount of lordosis and kyphosis

into the rods with the rod benders. Place the initial rod with its short limb passing transversely across the lamina of the lowermost vertebra to undergo instrumentation on the concave side. Pass it through the hole at the base of the spinous process if possible. Tighten the inferior double wire or cable on the concave side to supply firm fixation at the distal level. Now tighten the wires or cables to the lamina of the vertebra above the curve. Loosely attach the convex rod proximally after the short end has been placed loosely under the long limb of the concave rod. Once the concave rod has been completely tightened, it often is difficult to pass this short limb under the long limb of the concave rod. Reduce the spine to the rod, using manual correction and a wire or cable tightener. An assistant can apply appropriate manual correction by pressure on the trunk as the wires or cables are tightened beneath the apex of the curvature (Fig. 38-128). As each wire or cable is tightened, more correction is obtained, and the twisting maneuver must be repeated two or three times on each wire to ensure a tight fit. Securely fasten the convex rod, tightening wires or cables from cephalad to caudad. Once in position, both rods usually can be brought into firm contact with the lamina by squeezing them together with the rod approximator. As this is done, the concave wires or cables will again loosen and must be tightened. Trim the wires to about ½ inch in length and bend them toward the midline.

With the internal fixation device in place, very little bone is exposed for decortication and facet excision. We prefer to excise the facets if at all possible. A large volume of bone graft is necessary, and cancellous bone is harvested from the posterior iliac crest. Because the instrumentation often includes the iliac crest (p. 1847), bone-bank bone usually is necessary. Place the graft lateral to the rods on both sides of the spine and out to the tips of the transverse processes. If possible, place bone graft between the wires along the lamina.

◆ Sacropelvic Fixation

Many patients with neuromuscular problems require instrumentation and fusion to the sacrum. O'Brien described three fixation zones for sacropelvic fixation (Fig. 38-129). Examples of zone I fixation include S1 sacral screws and a McCarthy S-rod. Zone II fixation includes S2 screws and the Jackson intrasacral rod technique (see p. 1909.) Zone III fixation includes the Galveston L-rod technique and sacroiliac screws.

If fixation of the pelvis is necessary, McCarthy recommended the use of spinal fixation with an S-rod (Fig. 38-130). These two rods are cross linked at the lumbosacral junction (Fig. 38-131) and then fixed with a combination of hooks in the upper thoracic spine and multiple sublaminar wires or cables bilaterally throughout the lumbar and lower thoracic spine. The rods generally are cross linked below the fixation of the upper hooks to provide further stability against migration or rotation of the rods. We have found that if hooks are not used at the upper end, wires alone provide no support against axial loading.

The advantages of the S-rod are that firm fixation is provided around the sacral ala without crossing the sacroiliac joint and that harvesting of bone graft from the ilium is not a problem because the ilium is not violated as it is when the Galveston technique is used. Prebent S-rods are available; complex bends cannot be done effectively at the time of surgery. The rods can be further contoured with a rod bender at the time of surgery to accommodate the size of the sacrum and to provide the appropriate sagittal plane correction.

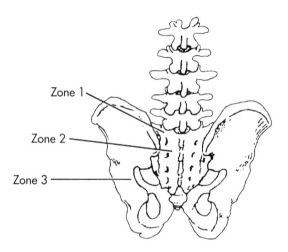

Fig. 38-129   Sacropelvic fixation zones. (Redrawn from O'Brien MF: Sacropelvic fixation in spinal deformity. Material presented at Spinal Deformity: Challenges and Solutions of Surgical Treatment, Puerto Rico, May 12-13, 2000.)

TECHNIQUE 38-34 *(McCarthy)*

Expose the spine posteriorly as described in Technique 38-3. Perform careful dissection of the sacral ala, using a curet to clean the superior edge. Use finger dissection ventrally. The rods come in different sizes and contours. In most instances, a 5-mm rod provides satisfactory fit to the sacral ala. Contour the rod to appropriate sagittal contours. If needed, place appropriate eyebolts over the rod to accommodate the area in which hooks are to be used. Place the S-rod over the sacral ala from posterior to anterior in a position adjacent to the anterior border of the sacroiliac joint. It lies posterior to the L5 nerve root and roughly parallel to it. Seat the S-portion of the rod firmly against the sacral ala by distraction between an L-4 level hook or pedicle screw. The rods then can be used as a firm fixation point for translation or correction of scoliotic deformities or by placing the right and left rods simultaneously and cross linking them, applying a strong cantilever corrective force for correction of pelvic obliquity. Cross linking the two S-rods provides stability and eliminates the increased time and difficulty of insertion of rods into the ilium. Elevate the medial aspect of the iliac apophysis and rotate it over the top of the S-rod on the sacral ala. Provide bone graft to encase the S-rod into the sacrum.

Fig. 38-130   **A** to **C,** S-rods are manufactured as a pair to fit over right and left sacral alae for fixation to sacrum without crossing sacroiliac joint. They are available in ³/₁₆-inch and ¼-inch rods. (Redrawn from McCarthy RE, Saer EH: The treatment of flaccid neuromuscular scoliosis. In Bridwell KH, DeWald RL, eds: *The textbook of spinal surgery,* ed 2, Philadelphia, 1997, Lippincott-Raven.)

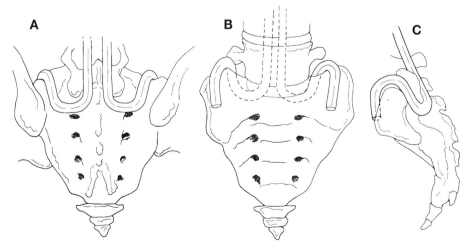

◆ ◆ ◆

Another popular method for achieving sacropelvic fixation is the Galveston technique described by Allen and Ferguson in which the pelvis is stabilized by driving a segment of the L-rod into each ilium (Fig. 38-132). The rod is inserted into the posterior iliac crest and rests between the cortices above the sciatic notch. This fixation allows immediate firm stability and is biomechanically a very stable construct. There are potential disadvantages, however, because the rod crosses the sacroiliac joint. It is postulated that motion in the sacroiliac joint is sponsible for a "halo" that is often seen around the end of the Galveston rod in the iliac wing. Whether this roentgenographic phenomenon actually results in clinical problems or not is unknown. In a biomechanical comparison of 10 lumbosacral fixation techniques, McCord et al. found that the most secure fixation of the lumbosacral joint was obtained by extending the fixation anterior to the projected lateral image of the middle column as in the Galveston technique.

TECHNIQUE 38-35 *(Allen and Ferguson)*

Expose both iliac crests from the midline incision at the level of the posterosuperior iliac spine. Expose the iliac crest to the sciatic notch. The area just proximal to the sciatic notch provides the most satisfactory fixation. Use a large,

smooth Steinmann pin corresponding to the size of the rod diameter to create a tunnel for the rod. The insertion site is just posterior to the sacroiliac joint at the level of the posteroinferior iliac spine, distal to the posterosuperior iliac spine, along the transverse bar of the ilium. The area for insertion often is difficult to identify, and the rod may be inserted too superiorly. Carefully identify the area for insertion and use a rongeur to carefully remove soft tissue and bone to expose the inner and outer tables of the ilium. Drill the Steinmann pin to a depth of approximately 6 to 9 cm.

Instead of drilling a Steinmann pin, Asher et al. described using a pedicle probe for pin insertion (Fig. 38-133, *A*). This allows for tactile perception to determine whether the probe is perforating the cortex of the ilium. Use a rongeur to remove enough cartilage and cortical bone to create a 1 × 1 cm entry site into the inferior portion of the posterosuperior iliac spine. This exposes the intramedullary space. Introduce a blunt-tipped pedicle probe into the intracortical space and advance it by gentle oscillating pressure on the handle of the probe (Fig. 38-133, *B*). Direct the probe 1 to 2 cm above the sciatic notch and advance it to the appropriate depth of the rod in the ilium (Fig. 38-133, *C*).

continued

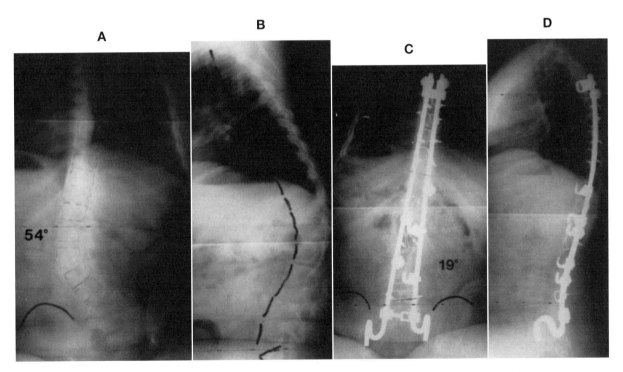

A   **B**   **C**   **D**

Fig. 38-131   Nine-year-old girl with spinal muscular atrophy and curve of 54 degrees and pelvic obliquity measuring 15 degrees. She was treated with combination of S-rods, TSRH hooks, and Songer cables. Her postoperative curve measured 19 degrees with pelvic obliquity of 0 degrees. **A** and **B,** Preoperative anteroposterior and lateral views. **C** and **D,** Postoperative anteroposterior and lateral views. (From McCarthy RE, Saer EH: The treatment of flaccid neuromuscular scoliosis. In Bridwell KH, DeWald RL, eds: *The textbook of spinal surgery,* ed 2, Philadelphia, 1997, Lippincott-Raven.)

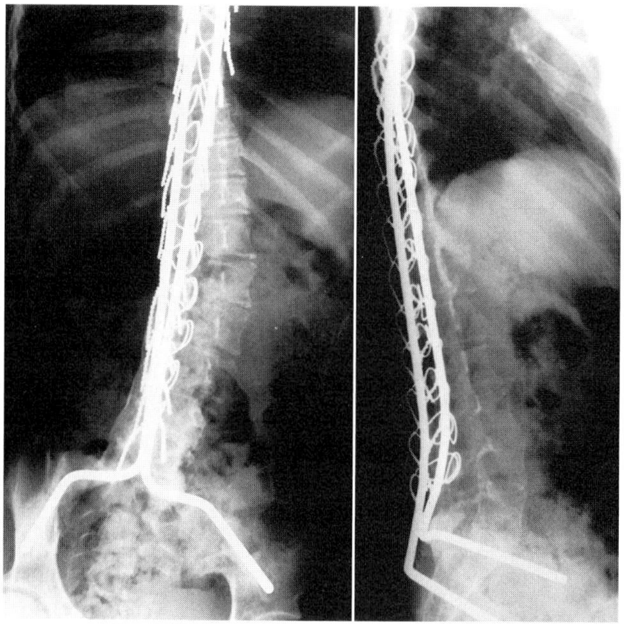

Fig. 38-132   **A** and **B,** Stabilization of pelvis with Galveston technique. Segment of rod is driven into each ilium.

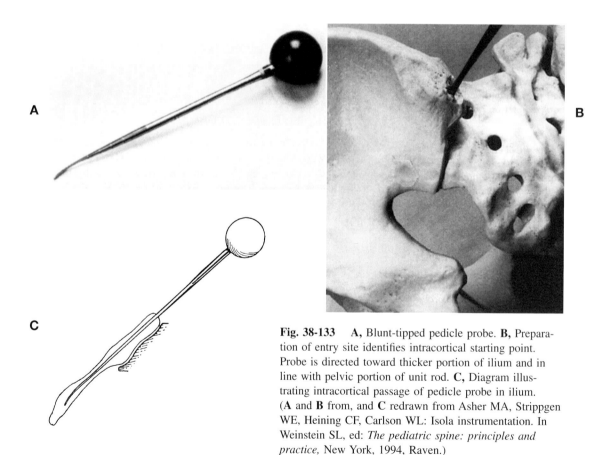

Fig. 38-133   **A,** Blunt-tipped pedicle probe. **B,** Preparation of entry site identifies intracortical starting point. Probe is directed toward thicker portion of ilium and in line with pelvic portion of unit rod. **C,** Diagram illustrating intracortical passage of pedicle probe in ilium. (**A** and **B** from, and **C** redrawn from Asher MA, Strippgen WE, Heining CF, Carlson WL: Isola instrumentation. In Weinstein SL, ed: *The pediatric spine: principles and practice,* New York, 1994, Raven.)

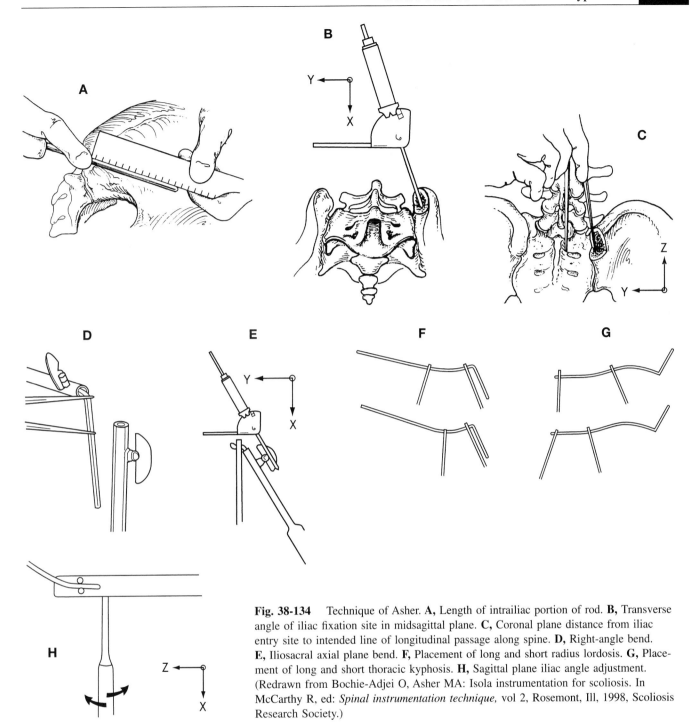

Fig. 38-134 Technique of Asher. **A,** Length of intrailiac portion of rod. **B,** Transverse angle of iliac fixation site in midsagittal plane. **C,** Coronal plane distance from iliac entry site to intended line of longitudinal passage along spine. **D,** Right-angle bend. **E,** Iliosacral axial plane bend. **F,** Placement of long and short radius lordosis. **G,** Placement of long and short thoracic kyphosis. **H,** Sagittal plane iliac angle adjustment. (Redrawn from Bochie-Adjei O, Asher MA: Isola instrumentation for scoliosis. In McCarthy R, ed: *Spinal instrumentation technique,* vol 2, Rosemont, Ill, 1998, Scoliosis Research Society.)

Now use a flexible ball-tipped pedicle probe to ensure that the hole made by the blunt-tipped probe is completely intracortical. Place the smooth Steinmann pin into the iliac hole.

Rod Contouring (Asher). Preparation of the rod is made easier by the use of a variable-radius bender set. To prepare the rod for iliac (Galveston) placement, four measurements are needed: (1) the length of the intrailiac portion of the rod (Fig. 38-134, *A*), (2) the transverse plane angle of the iliac fixation site to the midsagittal plane (Fig. 38-134, *B*), (3) the medial-lateral distance from the iliac entry site to the intended line of longitudinal passage of the rod along the spine (Fig. 38-134, *C*), and (4) the length of the rod needed from the sacrum to the most cephalad instrumentation site. A suture is laid along the spine line from the sacrum to the facet above the last instrumented vertebra, and its length plus 1 cm is the usual length for this portion of the rod. The first and third

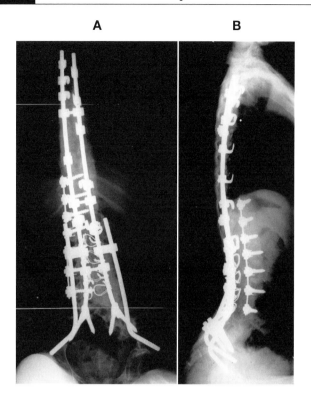

Fig. 38-135   **A** and **B,** Instrumentation with multihook segmental fixation and domino-type cross links.

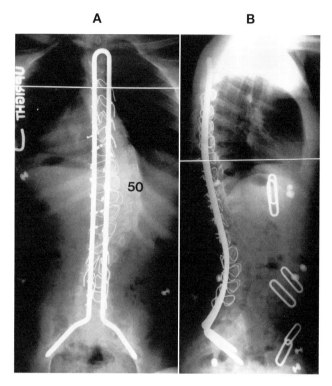

Fig. 38-136   **A** and **B,** Unit rod for neuromuscular scoliosis developed by Moseley and Koreska. Single, continuous ¼-inch stainless steel rod has U-bend at top and bullet-shaped ends for insertion into pelvis.

measurements are added, and a right-angle bend is placed at this distance from one end (Fig. 38-134, *D*); this is the iliosacral portion of the rod. The medial-lateral distance (measurement three) minus approximately 3.0 mm to allow for the bend is from the middle of the right angle bend and marked at the iliosacral portion of the rod. After verifying the right-left orientation, an angle identical to that of the iliac fixation site to the midsagittal plane is placed at this second mark (Fig. 38-134, *E*). This separates the iliosacral portion of the rod into the iliac and sacral portions.

Sagittal plane bends are added, beginning at L5-S1, thus leaving a straight portion over the sacrum. Because lordosis is not uniform but is greater in the lower lumbar spine, two contours are necessary. The contour for the entire lumbar spine is a long radius, whereas that for the lower lumbar spine is shorter (Fig. 38-134, *F*). Thoracic kyphosis is then added, again using the flat benders (Fig. 38-134, *G*). Trial placement is attempted to check whether the sagittal plane bend of the sacroiliac bend is correct. This can be determined by measuring the distance from the rod to the spine at the cephalad and caudad levels of the rod. Final sagittal plane iliac angle adjustments are made using flat bender posts and a tube bender. (Fig. 38-134, *H*).

The Galveston technique can be combined with a multihook segmental system with domino-type cross links if desired (Fig. 38-135, *A* and *B*).

Unit Rod Segmental Spinal Instrumentation

When using two unlinked L-rods, the rods may translate with respect to one another and compromise control of pelvic obliquity. Additionally, twisting within the laminar wires can result in rotation of one rod relative to another. The ¼-inch rods generally used in neuromuscular patients are difficult to bend so that they conform to the complex three-dimensional curves of the spine. In response to these problems, Bell et al. developed the unit rod. The unit rod is a single continuous ¼-inch stainless steel rod with a U bend at the top and "bullet-ended" pelvic legs for implantation into the pelvis (Fig. 38-136). The three-dimensional preshaped kyphosis, lordosis, and pelvic legs were devised from a data base of patients without spinal deformity. Eight lengths of rod are available, increasing in 20-cm increments from 310 to 450 cm. Right and left iliac guides facilitate drilling into the posterior ilia and subsequent introduction of the pelvic legs. The length of the iliac legs decreases proportionally as the rod shortens. The unit rod attempts to normalize body alignment in both the sagittal and coronal planes by establishing normal lordosis and kyphosis and correcting pelvic obliquity. We have not found the unit rod satisfactory for extremely rigid curves unless an anterior release or wedge osteotomies are done to reduce the spinal stiffness. If, however, the curves seem relatively flexible on bending films or physical examination, correcting to less

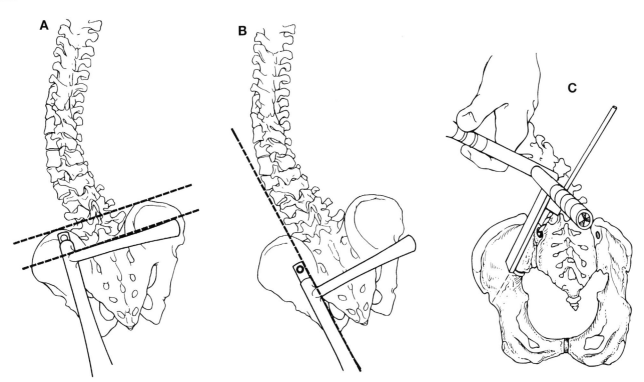

Fig. 38-137 Unit-rod instrumentation. **A,** Lateral handle of drill guide is kept parallel to pelvis. **B,** Axial handle is kept parallel to body axis. **C,** Drill hole started inferiorly on posterosuperior iliac crest. (**C** redrawn from Miller F, Dabney KW: Unit rod procedure for neuromuscular scoliosis. In McCarthy R, ed: *Spinal instrumentation technique,* vol 2, Rosemont, Ill, 1998, Scoliosis Research Society.)

than 40 degrees, we have had excellent results with the use of the unit rod.

◆ Unit Rod Instrumentation with Pelvic Fixation

TECHNIQUE 38-36

Expose the spine as described in Technique 38-3. Expose both iliac crests to the posterosuperior iliac spine and down to the sciatic notch. Mark a ¼-inch drill with a marking pen at 15 mm longer than the sciatic notch if the child's weight is over 45 kg and at 10 mm if the child weighs less than 45 kg. Place the appropriate right or left drill guide into the sciatic notch. Keep the lateral handle of the drill guide parallel to the pelvis (Fig. 38-137, *A*) and the axial handle of the drill guide parallel to the body axis (Fig. 38-137, *B*). Start the drill hole as far inferiorly on the posterosuperior iliac crest as possible (Fig. 38-137, *C*). Drill a hole in the ilium to the marked depth and check the hole with a wire to make certain the cortex has not been penetrated. Use a similar technique on the opposite iliac crest. Pass the sublaminar wires. Measure the length of the rod by placing the rod upside down, with the corner of the rod at the drilled hole on the elevated side of the pelvis. If kyphosis is severe,

choose one length shorter because the kyphotic spine shortens as it corrects. If pelvic obliquity is severe, test the length from both the high and low sides and choose an intermediate length. If the rod is placed and turns out to be too long, it may be necessary to cut off the superior end; the upper end then can be connected with a cross link. Cross the legs of the appropriate length rod and insert them first into the hole on the low side of the pelvic obliquity (Fig. 38-138, *A*). Cross the rod so that the leg going into the low side is underneath the other leg. Insert approximately one half to three fourths of the leg length into the hole. Then insert the next leg by holding it with a Harrington rod holder and guiding it into the correct direction of the hole. Use the impactor and drive the rod leg in by alternately impacting each leg (Fig. 38-138, *B*). Be certain that each rod leg is impacted in the exact direction of the hole or the cortex may be penetrated. Once the rod is firmly seated, use the proximal end of the rod as a "rudder" to bring the distal end of the rod to the spine (Fig. 38-138, *C*). Do not push the rod down completely into the wound in one move because this may pull the legs out of the pelvis or fracture the ilium. Instead, push the rod to line it up with the L5 lamina only and tie these wires down with a jet wire twister. Now push

continued

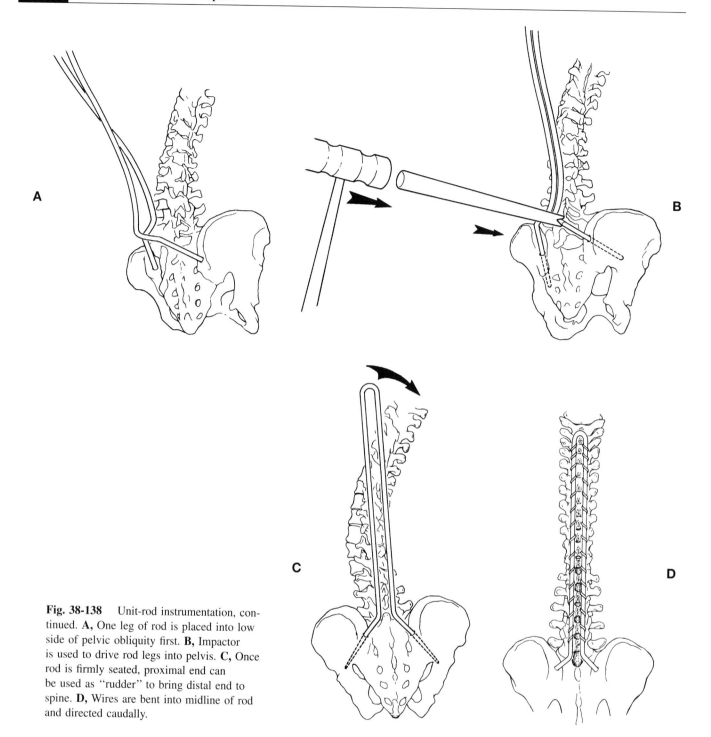

Fig. 38-138   Unit-rod instrumentation, continued. **A,** One leg of rod is placed into low side of pelvic obliquity first. **B,** Impactor is used to drive rod legs into pelvis. **C,** Once rod is firmly seated, proximal end can be used as "rudder" to bring distal end to spine. **D,** Wires are bent into midline of rod and directed caudally.

the rod to the L4 vertebra, twist the wires, and cut them off. Tighten the wires from caudad to cephalad one level at a time. Do not relax the push on the rod between the levels of the major curve or too much load may be applied to the end vertebra. Do not use the wires themselves to pull the rod down to the lamina or the wires will cut through the lamina.

After all the wires have been tightened, go back and verify that all previously tightened wires are well seated. Cut the wires at 10 to 15 mm lengths. Bend all wires into the midline of the rod and direct them caudally (Fig. 38-138, *D*). Apply bone graft. Bank bone usually is needed because the iliac crest is used for pelvic fixation.

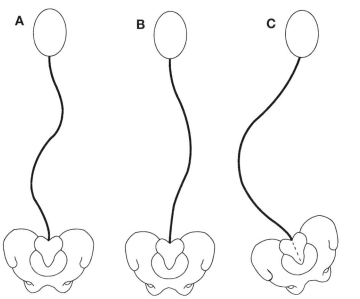
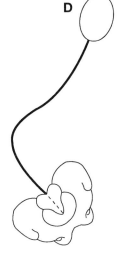

Fig. 38-139 **A** and **B**, Group I double curves with thoracic and lumbar component and little pelvic obliquity. **C** and **D**, Group II large lumbar or thoracolumbar curves with marked pelvic obliquity. (Redrawn from Lonstein JE, Akbarnia BA: *J Bone Joint Surg* 65A:43, 1983.)

AFTERTREATMENT. Initially, postoperative immobilization was not recommended after L-rod instrumentation. However, because neuromuscular curves frequently are associated with osteoporosis, spasticity, inability of the patient to cooperate, and severe curves, we advise postoperative immobilization for 4 to 6 months. This decreases the incidence of broken rods, pseudarthrosis, and loss of correction. We prefer a custom-made bivalved TLSO.

CEREBRAL PALSY

The prevalence of spinal deformities in patients with cerebral palsy varies, depending on the degree of neuromuscular involvement. Bleck found that fewer than 10% of ambulatory patients with spastic hemiplegia had scoliosis. Balmer and MacEwen found that 21% of 100 patients with cerebral palsy had scoliosis greater than 10 degrees, and 6% had scoliosis greater than 30 degrees. Madigan and Wallace found scoliosis in 65% of patients with spastic quadriplegia who required total care. Most authors agree that the severity of the curve is directly proportional to the degree of neurological impairment. Thometz and Simon demonstrated that scoliosis in patients with cerebral palsy can continue to progress into the third decade. The greatest progression was noted in patients who were unable to walk and had thoracolumbar or lumbar curves. The average progression was 0.8 degree a year in curves of less than 50 degrees and 1.4 degrees a year in curves of more than 50 degrees.

Scoliosis in patients with cerebral palsy is best managed by early recognition and control of the curve before the deformity becomes severe. Unlike idiopathic scoliosis, scoliosis caused by cerebral palsy can be painful. Bonnett et al. found that most of their patients with cerebral palsy and scoliosis complained of back pain. If the scoliosis is left untreated, function may be lost. If the patient is ambulatory, the trunk may become so distorted that standing erect becomes impossible. Sitting may become more difficult with increasing pelvic obliquity. If supplemental support by the hands is needed to sit, the patient will lose the ability to perform activities that require use of the upper extremity.

Bonnett et al. listed the following seven goals of scoliosis treatment in patients with cerebral palsy:

1. Improvement in assisted sitting to make positioning and transfer easier for nursing attendants and family
2. Relief of pain in the hips and back
3. Increased independence because of decreased need for assistance, both for the positioning required to relieve pain and to prevent pressure areas and for feeding
4. Improvement in upper extremity function and table-top activities by eliminating the need to use the upper extremities for trunk support
5. Reduction of the equipment needed, making possible the use of other equipment
6. Placement of the patient in a different facility, one in which less care is provided
7. Improved eating ability made possible by a change in position

Each patient must be evaluated individually to determine the potential for achieving these rehabilitation goals.

Classification

Lonstein and Akbarnia classified cerebral palsy curves into two groups (Fig. 38-139). Group I curves—double curves with both thoracic and lumbar components—occurred in 40% of their patients. These curves, which are similar to curves of idiopathic scoliosis, occurred more commonly in patients with only mental retardation who were ambulatory and lived at home. Group II curves were present in 58% of patients. These curves were more severe lumbar or thoracolumbar curves that extended into the sacrum, with marked pelvic obliquity.

Patients with these curves usually were nonambulatory with spastic quadriplegia, generally were not cared for at home, and were more likely to have the classic cerebral palsy rather than mental retardation alone.

Nonoperative Treatment

If the curve is small, careful observation is indicated. If the curve progresses or is more than 30 degrees in a growing child who is an independent ambulator or sitter, treatment should be instituted. If a child is skeletally mature, bracing is not likely to be effective, and surgery is indicted if the curve is 50 degrees or more. If neurological involvement is extreme in a patient who is severely mentally retarded and the curve is not causing any significant functional problems or pain, observation is appropriate.

Seating is the most common form of nonoperative treatment used for patients with cerebral palsy. Most nonambulatory patients with cerebral palsy do not have head or neck control during the first years of life. Custom seating may be quite effective in providing these patients with a straight spine and a level pelvis. Custom seating also can effectively accommodate severe spinal deformities and allow an upright posture in severely involved individuals.

Most authors believe that if the curve is progressive, an orthotic device may be helpful as a temporizing device but will not provide permanent control of the curve. Orthoses generally are used for curve control during growth in a child who is ambulatory or who has independent sitting ability. Often the orthosis provides enough trunk support to free the upper extremities for functional use. The orthosis of choice is a passive, total contact TLSO with either a one-piece, front-opening or a two-piece, bivalved design, or the soft Boston orthosis.

Operative Treatment

The operative treatment of scoliosis in cerebral palsy is complex. Determining which type of surgery is needed, and even whether any surgical procedure is warranted, is difficult. Before the introduction of newer techniques and instrumentation, the operative treatment of these patients was prone to failure, but the ability to treat these individuals has improved greatly.

The indications for surgical stabilization depend on the degree of mental involvement and the functional state of the individual with cerebral palsy. Allen and Ferguson stated that all patients who have functional abilities that would likely be lost if the scoliosis were left untreated are surgical candidates. Determining which functional abilities would be helped by surgery is not always easy. Certainly, in ambulatory children and in those of near-normal intelligence, surgical indications are similar to those for idiopathic scoliosis (curves of 40 to 45 degrees or more during adolescence, curves of over 50 to 60 degrees in young skeletally mature adults, and progressive curves that do not respond to nonoperative treatment). The decision concerning treatment of a child with total body involvement, seizure disorder, no head or trunk control, and

major nutritional problems is difficult. If a practical, functional gain is not likely, the risks of surgery probably are not acceptable.

The surgical techniques available for scoliosis in patients with cerebral palsy have improved significantly. MacEwen found a pseudarthrosis rate of 20% in patients with posterior spinal fusion and Harrington instrumentation. Bonnett et al. concluded that only combined anterior and posterior procedures with anterior and posterior instrumentation resulted in adequate correction with a low incidence of pseudarthrosis. The introduction of Luque rods and segmental instrumentation has greatly improved the results of surgery for scoliosis in cerebral palsy patients. Gersoff and Renshaw and Allen and Ferguson reported superior results with Luque rod segmental instrumentation. Swank et al. compared 10 patients treated with single-stage posterior techniques using 3/16-inch Luque rods with 21 patients treated with first-stage anterior spinal instrumentation and fusions using a Zielke apparatus followed by posterior Luque procedures to the pelvis. The pseudarthrosis rate in patients with single-stage procedures was 40%, whereas only 9.5% of those with combined procedures had pseudarthroses. Allen et al., however, questioned the need for anterior instrumentation. They suggested that anterior instrumentation actually decreases the overall correction, and they recommended an anterior release and fusion followed by a second-stage Luque procedure to the pelvis. In curves over 80 degrees, flexible anterior instrumentation systems probably do not inhibit posterior correction and increase the stability of fixation. With newer posterior instrumentation systems, anterior release and fusion without instrumentation followed by posterior instrumentation also has produced satisfactory results. Neustadt et al. reported the use of Cotrel-Dubousset instrumentation in patients with cerebral palsy and scoliosis. This instrumentation has the advantage of allowing distraction and compression along the rods in addition to bending and rotation forces. The principles, however, remain the same in that a large, stiff curve before surgery requires an anterior release, discectomy, and anterior bone grafting. Posterior instrumentation to the pelvis is done at a second stage. Neustadt et al. recommended the use of double sacral screws or iliosacral screws for fixation to the pelvis. Alternatively, a small rod can be configured as in the Galveston technique (Technique 38-35) and then dominoed to the longer rod. We have found that there is no one ideal technique for managing these complex curves. Generally speaking, we use a combination of hooks and multiple sublaminar wires. The rods are always cross linked. Our preference for pelvic fixation is the Galveston technique (Technique 38-35). If the pelvis is too small to accept Galveston fixation, we use the McCarthy S-rods (Technique 38-34) with cross linking for pelvic fixation.

The type of surgery also depends on the type of scoliosis. According to Lonstein and Akbarnia, patients with group I curves usually require only a posterior fusion, with fusion to the sacrum rarely needed (Fig. 38-140). They suggested that a combined anterior and posterior approach to group I curves is needed only when there is a significant lumbar component, in

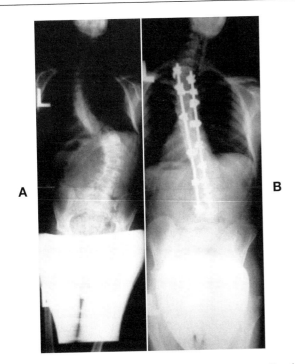

Fig. 38-140   **A,** Preoperative standing roentgenogram of patient with cerebral palsy and significant group I scoliosis. **B,** Postoperative appearance 4 years after posterior instrumentation not including the sacrum.

which case an anterior release and fusion and posterior instrumentation add correction and reduce the rate of pseudarthrosis. Group II curves usually require a long fusion to the sacrum because the sacrum is part of the curve and pelvic obliquity is present. Traction roentgenograms are made with the patient on a Risser-Cotrel frame and traction applied through a head halter, pelvic straps, and a lateral convex Cotrel strap. If a level pelvis and balanced spine can be obtained, a one-stage posterior approach is indicated. However, if the traction roentgenogram shows residual pelvic obliquity or if the torso is not balanced over the pelvis, a two-stage approach is indicated. In general, the larger the lumbar curve, the more severe the pelvic obliquity, and the more rigid the curve, the more likely a two-stage procedure will be needed.

Winter and Pinto emphasized that roentgenographic evaluation of patients with contractures about the hips can lead to erroneous conclusions. The roentgenogram often is made with the patient supine and the hips extended. If one hip has an adduction contracture and the opposite hip has an abduction contracture, then it may appear that pelvic obliquity is present. An appropriate roentgenographic evaluation should include a supine view obtained with the hips in a relaxed position, whatever the contractures dictate. This allows the spine and pelvis to assume a neutral alignment without the influence of hip contractures. Kyphosis can be caused by tight hamstrings and should be evaluated carefully because if the hamstrings are not released, the instrumentation will be severely stressed.

Several technical points should be considered when using

L-rods with segmental instrumentation in patients with cerebral palsy. The most proximal level of the fusion should be above T4 to prevent "falling off" of the kyphosis above the instrumentation. Only small portions of the ligamentum flavum on either side of the superior interspinous space to be instrumented should be removed. If possible, the supraspinous and interspinous ligaments at the superior level should be preserved to prevent an increase in kyphosis above instrumentation. We use pedicle hooks for fixation at the most proximal level to add axial load support to the system. The L-rods should be joined to prevent shifting of the rods relative to each other, especially in patients with significant preoperative pelvic obliquity. This can be accomplished with cross links or a unit rod (Technique 38-36). Although Allen and Ferguson believe a 3/16-inch rod made of MP-35-N alloy is strong enough in most patients except those with athetosis and large body mass or seizure disorders, many others prefer 1/4-inch L-rods.

Traction has not been found to improve correction of these curves either preoperatively or between anterior and posterior procedures. Lonstein and Akbarnia recommended use of halo gravity traction for selected, uncooperative patients to help control the patient or to facilitate nursing care, but not for curve correction.

Immobilization after the spinal fusion depends on the activity level of the child and the security of the internal fixation. If a child can tolerate external support without any detrimental effect on function, it can be used no matter how secure the internal fixation. Immobilization is continued until the fusion is solid, usually 9 to 12 months. If, however, external support would significantly hinder the patient's functional ability and the internal fixation is secure, it should not be used. If the bone is obviously osteopenic or instrumentation is less than ideal, postoperative external support probably should be used.

Complications

Improved techniques of instrumentation and preoperative and postoperative management have decreased complications, but a much higher complication rate should be expected after surgery for this type of scoliosis than that after idiopathic curves. Lonstein and Akbarnia reported complications in 81% of their patients. Patients with cerebral palsy are believed to be at an increased risk for infection. Gersoff and Renshaw reported infections in 15% of their patients, which was comparable to the average of 19% for other studies. Patients with deep infections were treated by removal of all sutures down to the instrumentation and graft, irrigation and debridement, administration of systemic antibiotics, packing of the wound, frequent changes of dressing until granulation tissue covered the instrumentation and the graft, and delayed primary closure. All infections resolved without removal of the instrumentation.

Pulmonary complications often develop in these patients because they cannot cooperate in deep breathing and coughing exercises, and appropriate prophylactic pulmonary measures are needed. It should be noted that all three of Lonstein and

Akbarnia's patients who died after surgery succumbed to bronchial pneumonia 5 to 9 months after surgery.

If the upper limit of the fusion is not selected carefully (above T4), kyphosis cephalad to the upper limit of the fusion can occur. Pseudarthrosis is less frequent with newer instrumentation systems. Other possible complications are those inherent in any spinal operation, such as urinary tract infection, ileus, and blood loss.

Although the complications can be significant in these patients, the functional improvement or prevention of deterioration of function is well worth the effort and the risks of surgery. Complications should be expected and planned for; prompt treatment will lessen their severity.

FRIEDREICH ATAXIA

Friedreich ataxia is a recessively inherited condition characterized by spinocerebellar degeneration. The clinical onset takes place between the ages of 6 and 20 years. Primary symptoms include progressive ataxic gait, dysarthria, decreased proprioception or vibratory sense, muscle weakness, and a lack of deep tendon reflexes. Secondary symptoms include pes cavus, scoliosis, and cardiomyopathy. Affected children frequently are wheelchair-bound in the first or second decades of life. The cardiomyopathy often leads to death in the third or fourth decades of life.

The largest reported series of spinal deformity in patients with Friedreich ataxia is that of Labelle et al., who followed up on 56 patients in accordance with the criteria of Geoffrey et al. They found that all 56 patients had scoliosis. The most common pattern was double structural thoracic and lumbar curves (57%). The typical neuromuscular thoracolumbar curve with pelvic obliquity was found in only 14%. Similar findings were reported by Cady and Bobechko in 38 patients. Because no significant correlation could be established between overall muscle weakness and curve progression, as would be expected in neuromuscular scoliosis, they postulated that the pathogenesis of scoliosis in patients with Friedreich ataxia may be a disturbance of equilibrium and postural reflexes rather than muscle weakness. Labelle et al. also found that not all curves in patients with Friedreich ataxia were progressive; the onset of the disease at an early age and the presence of scoliosis before puberty were major factors in progression. They concluded that scoliosis appearing in the late teens or early twenties is less likely to be progressive.

Most authors have not found bracing to be useful for progressive curves in patients with Friedreich ataxia. The orthosis fails to control the curve, and by the time the patients develop scoliosis, they often have a significant degree of ataxia and the restriction of a spinal orthosis makes ambulation more difficult. Labelle et al. recommended that curves of less than 40 degrees be observed, curves of more than 60 degrees be treated surgically, and curves of between 40 and 60 degrees be observed or treated surgically, depending on the age of the patient, the onset of the disease, and such characteristics of the scoliosis as the patient's age when it is recognized and evidence of progression of the curve. If the curve is observed too long, cardiomyopathy may have progressed to the point that surgery is very risky, if not impossible; therefore early surgical treatment is recommended for progressive curves.

Cardiology evaluation is mandatory before any surgery is considered in these patients. Patients with Friedreich ataxia frequently are unable to walk with a postoperative cast or brace. Preoperative traction and prolonged bed rest postoperatively must be kept to a minimum, or weakness can increase rapidly. For these reasons, the ideal instrumentation for these patients is segmental spinal instrumentation, such as multihook devices, which do not require external support postoperatively. Generally, these patients require a long fusion with attention to sagittal contours to prevent later problems with thoracic kyphosis. The pelvis usually is not included in these fusions unless pelvic obliquity is significant.

CHARCOT-MARIE-TOOTH DISEASE

Classic Charcot-Marie-Tooth (CMT) disease is a demyelinating neuropathy. The condition is dominantly inherited, with considerable variation in severity. Hensinger and MacEwen studied 69 patients with CMT disease, of whom 7 (10%) had kyphoscoliosis; 2 patients had mild deformities and did not require treatment, 2 were successfully treated with Milwaukee braces, and 3 underwent posterior spine stabilization and fusion. Daher et al., in a study of 12 patients with CMT disease and scoliosis, also found that brace treatment was well tolerated. Both these reports emphasize that in patients with CMT disease and spinal deformity, the deformity can be managed with the same techniques used for idiopathic scoliosis, including bracing and surgery. The sagittal plane deformity accompanying this scoliosis most frequently is kyphosis, and fusion to the pelvis generally is not necessary unless pelvic obliquity exists.

SYRINGOMYELIA

Syringomyelia is a cystic, fluid-filled cavitation within the spinal cord. Scoliosis may be the first manifestation of a syringomyelia. Huebert and MacKinnon reported scoliosis in 63% of 43 children with syringomyelia. Scoliosis was found in 82% of children whose symptoms had been noted before the age of 16 years. Williams identified scoliosis in 73% of his 148 patients with syringomyelia. Physical findings that may indicate syringomyelia include neurological deficits and pain associated with the scoliosis, intrinsic muscle wasting of the hands, cavus deformity or, especially, loss of superficial abdominal reflexes. Roentgenographic features suggestive of syringomyelia include Charcot changes in joints and a left thoracic curvature. If the diagnosis of syringomyelia is suspected, MRI should be done (Fig. 38-141). When obtaining the MRI, care must be taken to include the craniocervical junction to rule out the presence of an Arnold-Chiari malformation.

The association of syringomyelia with scoliosis may have a

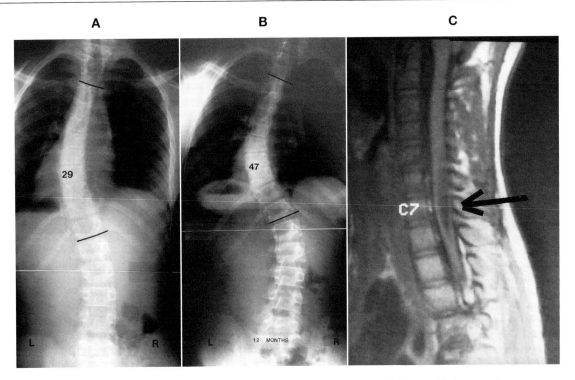

Fig. 38-141 Progressive curve in patient with syringomyelia. **A,** Initial curve. **B,** One year later. **C,** MRI shows syrinx at C7 *(arrow).*

significant influence on treatment. Heubert and MacKinnon reported one patient in whom spinal fusion after laminectomy was fatal when a large cyst in the cord ruptured. Nordwall and Wikkelso reported delayed onset of paraplegia in a patient with syringomyelia who was treated with Harrington rod instrumentation. Because of the possibility of these complications, surgery for scoliosis in patients with syringomyelia should be approached cautiously. The rate of progression of the neurological deficit and the prognosis of the curve should be considered carefully before any extensive surgery is considered. Bradford advocates initial treatment of this condition with drainage of the cyst, followed by observation to determine if the subsequent curve stabilizes. Gurr, Taylor and Stobo, in a series of 15 patients who had surgical drainage of the syrinx, noted that 3 had improvement of their curves, and in none of the remaining patients did the curves progress. Philips, Hensinger, and Kling found that drainage of the syrinx delayed but did not prevent curve progression in immature patients; however, drainage of the syrinx did allow use of distraction-type instrumentation without complications. If surgery becomes necessary for these patients, and the curve is suitable for anterior instrumentation and fusion, we believe this should be considered. Correction generally can be obtained without distraction when anterior instrumentation is used. Many patients have had posterior laminectomies that necessitate the use of anterior surgery. If posterior instrumentation is required, even if the cyst has been drained, only minimal distraction should be used and only moderate curve correction should be attempted.

SPINAL CORD INJURY

Several series in the literature have reported an incidence of spinal deformity in 99% of children with spinal cord injuries before the adolescent growth spurt. Spinal deformity is much more common and the rate of curve progression much greater in preadolescents than in older patients.

Increasing curvature with pelvic obliquity in a child with a spinal cord injury can lead to a loss of sitting balance that requires the use of the upper extremities for trunk support rather than for functional tasks. Pressure sores may occur on the downside of the ischium, and hip subluxation can occur on the high side of the pelvic obliquity.

Orthotic Treatment

Although Lancourt, Dickson, and Carter stated that alteration of the natural progression of scoliosis in these patients is impossible with devices such as braces or corsets, other authors, such as Mayfield et al., Bonnett, and Dearolf et al. indicated that orthotic treatment does have a place in the management of scoliosis in preadolescent patients with spinal cord injuries. Orthotic treatment is difficult because of potential skin problems, but Dearolf et al. noted effective slowing of progression in 7 of 12 patients in their series. The use of an orthosis may delay the need for surgery in preadolescent patients until longitudinal growth of the spine is more complete. Orthotic treatment requires close cooperation among the physician, the family, and the patient. A custom-fitted, well-padded, plastic total contact TLSO generally is used.

A   B   C

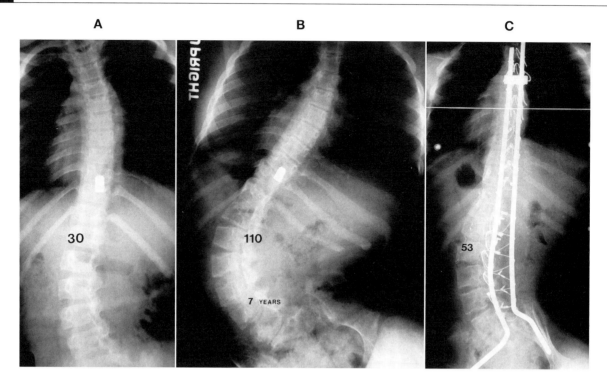

Fig. 38-142   Progressive paralytic scoliosis after gunshot wound. **A,** Initial curve of 30 degrees. **B,** Seven years later, curve is 110 degrees. **C,** After fusion and segmental instrumentation, correction to 53 degrees.

Close attention must be paid for any evidence of pressure changes on the skin. The brace can be removed at night and used only during sitting.

Operative Treatment

Most preadolescent children with spinal cord injuries ultimately require surgical stabilization of their scoliosis. In the series of Mayfield et al., 68% of preadolescent patients ultimately required stabilization and fusion of the spine. Dearolf et al. found that 61% of their patients injured before maturity required surgical stabilization, and Campbell and Bonnett reported surgery in 50%. If the curve progresses despite orthotic treatment, surgical intervention is indicated. If the curve is more than 60 degrees when the child is first seen, immediate surgery should be considered. Curves treated with an orthosis are considered for surgery if they progress beyond 40 degrees, and curves between 40 and 60 degrees are considered individually.

The prevalence of pseudarthrosis in these patients reported in the literature ranges from 27% to 53%. Dearolf et al. found pseudarthrosis in 26% of their patients, and they attributed the lower figure to the use of segmental fixation in recent years. Segmental instrumentation allows more rigid fixation, and postoperative casting can be avoided (Fig. 38-142). Complete urinary tract evaluation should be done before surgery because urinary tract infections are common in patients with spinal cord injuries. The urine should be cultured 2 weeks before surgery. If the culture is positive, the patient is treated with antibiotics

for 10 days, and the culture is repeated. If the organism is sensitive to a medication delivered orally, surgery is done when the culture is negative, and the antibiotic is continued through surgery. If the organism is sensitive only to intravenous antibiotics, surgery is delayed until the cultures are negative for 10 days after discontinuation of the antibiotics. Postoperatively, oral antibiotic prophylaxis should be continued for 3 months. Rapidly progressive curves in patients with spinal cord injury should be evaluated with MRI for the possibility of a posttraumatic syrinx.

Because of the frequency of pseudarthrosis, surgery should be delayed, if possible, until the patient weighs more than 100 pounds, so that ¼-inch L-rods or adult-size multihook segmental instrumentation systems can be used. If the curve does not bend to less than 60 degrees on bending films, combined anterior release and posterior fusion should be considered. For patients younger than 10 years of age with progressive curves of more than 50 degrees, a dilemma still exists. Luque instrumentation or subcutaneous Harrington rods without fusion failed in all four patients treated this way by Dearolf et al. If fusion is required in young children at risk for future crankshaft phenomenon, a first-stage anterior release and fusion should be done, followed by posterior segmental spinal instrumentation and fusion.

Dearolf et al. reported pseudarthroses in 3 of 10 preadolescent patients and in 1 mature patient who had fusion to the sacrum. They believed that if the residual pelvic obliquity would be slight, fusion to L4 or L5 is sufficient. If, on the other

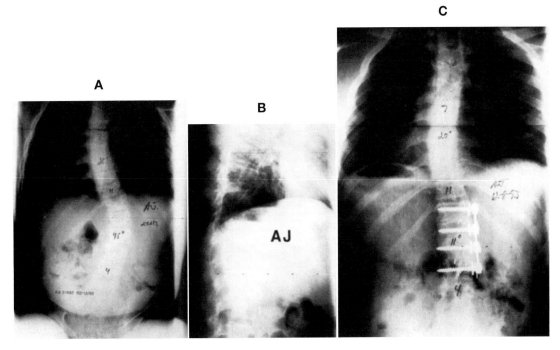

Fig. 38-143 Fourteen-year-old boy who was paraplegic as result of gunshot wound to spine. **A** and **B,** Anteroposterior and lateral sitting thoracolumbar spine view showing 45-degree right lumbar curve with minimal pelvic obliquity. Lateral view shows thoracolumbar junction to be fairly straight. Because patient wanted to continue walking with braces, preservation of as many mobile segments below fusion was thought advantageous. Because of behavior of lumbar curve on side bending, it was thought that anterior fusion alone with instrumentation would provide correction of scoliosis and maintain sagittal contour. **C,** Anteroposterior sitting thoracolumbar spine view postoperatively, showing excellent correction of scoliosis and preservation of sagittal contour. Anterior procedure was done using subperiosteal stripping of spine, and fusion healed rapidly within a few months. (From Shook JE, Lubicky JP: Paralytic scoliosis. In Bridwell KH, DeWald RL, eds: *The textbook of spinal surgery,* ed 2, Philadelphia, 1997, Lippincott-Raven.)

hand, the pelvis is significantly involved in the curve, fusion probably should include the sacrum. For patients who are ambulators and in whom adequate correction can be obtained without involving the pelvis, an effort should be made to end the instrumentation above the pelvis. In carefully selected patients, Lubicky used short anterior spinal fusion with instrumentation alone. He reported that this provided excellent curve correction over a short segment and allowed a number of open disc spaces below the fused segment (Fig. 38-143).

If laminectomy was used to treat the initial spinal cord injury, an increased incidence of kyphosis can be expected. A kyphosis that is rigid and cannot be corrected to less than 50 degrees on hyperextension views should be treated with a first-stage anterior release and spinal fusion, followed by a long posterior fusion with segmental instrumentation.

POLIOMYELITIS

Because the Salk and Sabin vaccines have made poliomyelitis in children rare in the United States, most recent experience in treating postpolio spinal deformities is in adult patients. The basic principles of treatment, however, are no different from those of treatment of spinal deformities resulting from other neuromuscular diseases. Bonnett et al. outlined the indications for correction and posterior spine fusion in patients with polio (Box 38-5).

As in any other neuromuscular curve, the length of fusion is much greater in patients with poliomyelitis than in those with idiopathic scoliosis. Segmental instrumentation is recommended. In evaluation of the distal extent of the fusion in a patient with poliomyelitis, it must be determined whether the pelvic obliquity is caused by the spinal curvature itself or by other factors, such as iliotibial band contractures.

SPINAL MUSCLE ATROPHY

Spinal muscle atrophy is an autosomal recessive condition in which the anterior horn cells of the spinal cord, and occasionally the bulbar nuclei, atrophy. Daher et al. proposed that this disorder is caused by one episode of neural destruction at different times in childhood. Children affected earlier in life are more severely involved than those affected later. Spinal muscle atrophy can be divided into three categories. Type I, or acute infantile Werdnig-Hoffman disease, manifests within the first 6 months of life. The course of the disease is progressive, with most of these children dying within the first 2 to 3 years of life. Children who have an acute period of deterioration followed by an arrest of the disease process and a relatively benign course are considered to have type II (chronic) infantile spinal muscle atrophy. Type III, or Kugelberg-Welander disease, usually is seen after 2 years of age. It is more slowly progressive, and most patients are able to ambulate independently.

Clinically, children with spinal muscle atrophy have severe weakness of the trunk and limb muscles. Fasciculations of the tongue and tremors of the extremities are frequent. Reflexes are diminished. Most patients have normal intelligence, and the heart is unaffected by the disease process. The cause of death usually is pulmonary insufficiency. Ninety percent of these patients have scoliosis, and it is the most severe problem in those who survive childhood. Granata et al. observed that once patients with spinal muscle atrophy were wheelchair bound, their scoliosis developed rapidly. Aprin et al. noted that scoliosis usually is diagnosed between 6 and 8 years of age, and the more severe the disease, the more likely the curve is to be progressive.

Orthotic Treatment

Schwentker and Gibson and Riddick et al. reported that bracing slowed progression of the curve in their patients and also allowed sitting for longer periods of time. Furumasu, Swank, and Brown, however, found that patients treated in braces were less functional because of decreased flexibility of the spine, and this resulted in noncompliance. As recommended by Shapiro et al., we believe that when the scoliosis in a skeletally immature patient reaches 20 degrees in the sitting position, orthotic treatment should be considered, usually a total contact TLSO. This is used only during sitting to minimize progression of the curve and to provide an extremely weak

child with a stable sitting support. As reported by Aprin et al. and Riddick et al., severe chest wall deformities can occur from bracing, and developing chest wall deformities are a contraindication to brace treatment. Although bracing may not eliminate the need for surgical stabilization, it may delay surgery until closer to the end of growth. Surgery at a young age would require anterior and posterior approaches to prevent the crankshaft phenomenon, and the anterior fusion adds considerably to the risk of the procedure in these patients. The anterior approach almost invariably involves "taking down" the diaphragm, which is the main respiratory muscle in patients with spinal muscle atrophy. Thoracoscopic anterior release and fusion (p. 1825) may be a satisfactory alternative in these patients at great risk of crankshaft development.

Operative Treatment

Surgical treatment of the spinal deformity is posterior spinal fusion with posterior segmental instrumentation and adequate bone grafting. Because fusion to the sacrum is needed for many of these patients, cross linked, L-rod fixation with hooks, sublaminar wires, and fixation to the pelvis by the Galveston technique provides optimal internal fixation. Augmentation of the fusion with bone-bank allograft bone usually is necessary. If the vertebrae are extremely osteoporotic, external support, such as a bivalved body jacket, can be used. For a severe fixed lumbar curve with pelvic obliquity, anterior release and fusion may be needed in addition to posterior instrumentation. It should be understood, however, that anterior surgery in patients with severe pulmonary compromise carries a great risk, and this risk must be evaluated carefully before surgery. If possible, endoscopic techniques of anterior release and fusion should be considered.

Complications should be expected in this group of patients. Daher et al. reported that 45% of their patients had complications, most of which were minor and did not require further surgery. Hensinger and MacEwen reported 2 postoperative deaths in 20 patients, and 3 patients required grafting for pseudarthroses. Aprin et al. reported that 10 of their 22 patients developed atelectasis or pneumonitis postoperatively. Brown et al. reduced their complication rate from 35% to 15% with the use of Luque segmental instrumentation and the elimination of postoperative immobilization.

Frequent pulmonary complications in patients with spinal muscle atrophy require respiratory support for longer than normal after surgery and rapid mobilization when possible. As indicated by Kepes et al., patients with spinal muscle atrophy may be especially sensitive to medications that depress the respiratory centers, and the use of these drugs in the postoperative period should be minimal. Lonstein and Renshaw found that patients with forced vital capacity of less than 20% of that predicted are at great risk for postoperative death. A vigorous preoperative and postoperative physical therapy program is mandatory.

The patient and the family should be warned of the possibility of some loss of function after spinal instrumentation and fusion in these patients. A flexible spine allows a weak trunk to collapse forward to increase the reach of the upper extremity. Also, flexibility of the spine and extremities allows the center of gravity to be placed where weak muscles have the best mechanical advantage. Spinal fusion creates a longer lever arm that weak hip muscles are unable to control. Brown et al. noted that gross motor activities such as transfers, rolling, bathing, dressing, and toileting declined after spinal fusion. This loss of function, however, must be weighed against the predicted functional loss and pulmonary compromise from severe, untreated spinal deformity. Over the long, progressive course of this disease, the advantages of a stable trunk far outweigh the disadvantages.

FAMILIAL DYSAUTONOMIA

Familial dysautonomia (Riley-Day syndrome), first described in 1949, is a rare autosomal recessive disorder found mostly in Jewish children of Eastern European extraction. Its clinical features include absence of overflow tears and sweating, vasomotor instability that often leads to hyperthermia, and relative indifference to pain. Other frequent findings include episodic hypertension, postural hypotension, transient blotching of the skin, hyperhidrosis, episodic vomiting, disordered swallowing, dysarthria, and motor incoordination. Death is caused most often by pulmonary disease. Yoslow et al. found scoliosis in 39 of 65 patients and indicated that it is the major orthopaedic problem in patients with this disease. The scoliosis may be progressive and may be large enough to contribute to early death because of kyphoscoliotic cardiopulmonary decompensation. Kyphosis also is a frequent sagittal plane deformity in these patients. If surgery for the scoliosis is considered, however, features of the syndrome such as vasomotor and thermal instability can cause troublesome and sometimes fatal operative or postoperative complications. Milwaukee brace treatment is complicated by the tendency for pressure ulcers to develop. Albanese and Bobechko and Kaplan et al. found brace treatment to be successful in their patients.

Posterior spinal fusion with instrumentation was required in 13 of 51 patients in the Israeli series of Kaplan et al. All children undergoing surgery had severe pulmonary problems. Intraoperative and postoperative respiratory and dysautonomic complications were frequent. Because of osteopenic bone, only minor improvement of the spinal deformity was possible and a small loss of correction was common; however, those surviving noted a marked decrease in the frequency of pneumonia and, for some reason, an improvement in the degree of ataxia. Albanese and Bobechko reported surgical stabilization of kyphoscoliosis in seven patients. Intraoperative complications included transient hypertension, failure of the lamina because of osteopenia, and an endotracheal tube that was plugged by thick secretions after the lung was collapsed for an anterior approach. All patients had at least one complication, although there were no intraoperative or immediate postoperative deaths.

One technical problem in instrumenting these curves is the frequent occurrence of severe kyphosis combined with weak bone. Anterior procedures should be approached with caution because of the frequency of respiratory problems. Despite the significant dangers and high complication rates in patients with familial dysautonomia, with proper precautions surgery can be done successfully and can improve the quality of life.

ARTHROGRYPOSIS MULTIPLEX CONGENITA

Arthrogryposis multiplex congenita is a syndrome of persistent joint contractures that are present at birth. A myopathic subtype is characterized by muscle changes similar to those found in progressive muscular dystrophy. In the neuropathic subtype, anterior horn cells are reduced or absent in the cervical, thoracic, and lumbosacral segments of the spinal cord. In the third subtype, joint fibrosis and contractures alone are the main problems.

Scoliosis is common in patients with arthrogryposis multiplex congenita. Herron, Westin, and Dawson found a 20% incidence, and Drummond and MacKenzie found a 28% incidence. The scoliosis usually is detected at birth or within the first few years of life. If after that time no scoliosis is present, deformity usually does not develop. Most curves are progressive and become rigid and fixed at an early age. Brace treatment rarely is successful and should be used only in patients with small, flexible curves. The onset of pelvic obliquity is a serious problem. If treatment of the pelvic obliquity by release of the contractures in the hip area does not halt progression of the curve, spinal fusion to the sacrum is necessary. As indicated by Daher et al., the onset of thoracic lordosis also requires prompt treatment. Because of the severity and rigidity of the curves, postoperative complications are frequent. The connective tissue is tough, and the bones are osteoporotic. Daher et al. reported an average blood loss of 2000 ml, and Herron et al. obtained a maximal correction of only about 25% with the use of Harrington instrumentation and posterior fusion. Segmental fixation with L-rod instrumentation and sublaminar wires or cables has significant advantages for these patients, with its improved fixation and ability to instrument to the pelvis. If a significant pelvic obliquity is present that does not correct to acceptable levels on preoperative bending films, a first-stage anterior release and fusion are indicated. This is then followed by posterior instrumentation and fusion to the pelvis.

DUCHENNE MUSCULAR DYSTROPHY

Scoliosis develops in almost all patients with Duchenne muscular dystrophy (Fig. 38-144). Smith et al. examined 51 males with Duchenne muscular dystrophy, and all had scoliosis despite preventive measures such as braces or wheelchair seating systems. Spinal deformity usually occurs after the patient becomes confined to a wheelchair, although very early scoliosis has been detected in some ambulatory patients. The curves are predominantly long thoracolumbar curves with pelvic obliquity, the collapse of which is caused by absence of muscles and not by asymmetrical muscle activity or contracture. Once a curve develops, it generally is progressive and

A   B   C

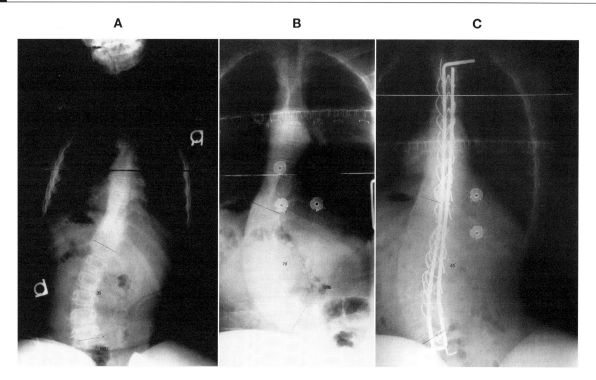

Fig. 38-144   **A** and **B,** Progressive scoliosis in patient with Duchenne muscular dystrophy. **C,** After fusion with Luque rod instrumentation.

cannot be controlled by braces or wheelchair seating systems. In patients with Duchenne muscular dystrophy, pulmonary function deteriorates approximately 4% each year after the age of 12 years. If orthotic treatment is continued while pulmonary function deteriorates significantly, surgical stabilization may become impossible. Diminution in pulmonary function is believed to be related to muscle weakness and not to the spinal deformity itself. If the forced vital capacity decreases to less than 40% of normal, surgery probably is not advisable because of the potential pulmonary problems postoperatively.

Lonstein and Renshaw's indications for spinal fusion in patients with Duchenne muscular dystrophy are curves of more than 30 degrees, a forced vital capacity of more than 30% of normal, and prognosis of at least 2 years of life remaining. Because the scoliosis invariably worsens, many authors, such as Shapiro and Specht, Galasko et al., and Smith et al., recommended spinal fusion at the onset of the deformity in patients who use a wheelchair full-time even when the curves are as small as 20 degrees or less. The patient's pulmonary function probably is more important in decision making than the size of the curve. The vital capacity should be more than 40% to 50% of normal. If the curve is allowed to progress beyond 30 to 40 degrees, the forced vital capacity can be less than 40% of predicted normal. Shapiro et al. stated that most patients with Duchenne muscular dystrophy generally have a forced vital capacity of 50% to 70% of normal when they begin to use a wheelchair full-time. They recommended surgery during the first few years of full-time wheelchair use, when the patient almost always has a small, flexible curve and little or

no pelvic obliquity but still has a forced vital capacity of 40% or more.

L-rod instrumentation with sublaminar wires and cross-link plates or the unit rod is the ideal instrumentation for these patients. In patients with smaller curves and no fixed pelvic obliquity, the fusion and instrumentation can end at L5. If fixed pelvic obliquity is more than 15 degrees, fusion to the pelvis with Galveston or S-rod pelvic fixation is indicated. Bronson et al. found that correction of pelvic obliquity was more certain with instrumentation and fusion to the sacrum in larger curves (average, 61 degrees). The fusion should extend to the high upper thoracic spine, to T2 or T3. The sagittal contours of the spine, especially lumbar lordosis, should be maintained for sitting balance and pressure distribution. As in patients with other neuromuscular conditions, adequate preoperative consultations and tests should be obtained. Preoperative cardiac assessment is necessary to help define subclinical cardiomyopathies. Large amounts of blood loss should be expected, and bone-bank allograft is needed because a massive amount of bone graft will be necessary. Because of the pulmonary compromise in these patients, rapid postoperative mobilization is important. We generally use no orthoses after surgery, although Shapiro and Specht recommended a bivalved plastic orthosis when the patient is sitting to minimize discomfort for 6 weeks postoperatively.

The use of multihook segmental fixation for patients with Duchenne muscular dystrophy has not been reported in the literature. If these curves are treated early, rotatory deformity usually is minimal. The bones often are extremely osteopenic, and rotational maneuvers are likely to cause hook cut-out. We have had no instrumentation failures in our patients treated with L-rods and sublaminar wire fixation. Lonstein and Renshaw listed the following benefits of spinal fusion in patients with Duchenne muscular dystrophy:

Preserves sitting balance

Prevents back pain

Improves spinal decompensation

Frees the arms of the necessity of trunk support

Improves body image

Possibly slows the deterioration of pulmonary function

Miller et al., however, found that the rate of decline of forced vital capacity was not changed by preventing scoliosis with spinal fusion. Shapiro et al. also found diminution of forced vital capacity at the same rate as before surgery in most of their patients.

VARIANTS OF MUSCULAR DYSTROPHY OTHER THAN DUCHENNE TYPE

In their report of 11 patients who had surgery for spinal deformity in association with non-Duchenne muscular dystrophy, Daher et al. concluded that spinal curvature in association with non-Duchenne muscular dystrophy is uncommon. The occurrence of scoliosis in patients with non-Duchenne muscular dystrophy depends on the specific type of dystrophic disease, and the prognosis is related to the severity of the primary problem. For instance, Siegel found that childhood dystrophia myotonica is not associated with spinal curvature. Facioscapulohumeral dystrophy is more rapidly progressive when the onset occurs in childhood. Frequently, it also is asymmetrical in distribution, and structural scoliosis can occur. None of the 11 patients reported by Daher et al. had pelvic obliquity. Thoracic lordosis was present in 36% of their patients, all of whom developed poor vital capacity and shortness of breath. The use of an orthosis during the juvenile years controlled the curve until the pubertal growth spurt, when progression occurred. The Milwaukee brace should not be used, however, when a thoracic lordosis exists. Spinal fusion is effective in maintaining correction and preventing curve progression in these patients.

Congenital Scoliosis

Congenital scoliosis is a lateral curvature of the spine caused by the presence of vertebral anomalies that result in an imbalance of the longitudinal growth of the spine. The critical time in the development of the spine embryologically is the fifth to sixth week—the time of segmentation processes—and congenital anomalies of the spine develop during the first 6 weeks of intrauterine life. Some type of anomaly must be visible on the roentgenograms of the spine before a diagnosis of congenital scoliosis can be made. Because congenital scoliosis often is rigid and correction can be difficult, it is important to detect these curves early and to institute appropriate treatment while

BOX 38-6 • Classification of Congenital Scoliosis

Failure of formation (Fig. 38-145)
Partial failure of formation (wedge vertebra)
Complete failure of formation (hemivertebra)
Failure of segmentation
Unilateral failure of segmentation (unilateral unsegmented bar)
Bilateral failure of segmentation (block vertebra) (Fig. 38-146)
Miscellaneous

the curve is small rather than to attempt salvage-type procedures that are necessary when the deformity is severe.

Wynne-Davies found no genetic etiology for isolated congenital abnormalities of the spine such as hemivertebrae. Winter reviewed the family histories of 1250 patients with congenital scoliosis and found only 13 who had first- or second-degree relatives with congenital spinal deformity. Most congenital scoliosis is believed to be caused by nongenetic, fetal environmental factors, but usually these factors cannot be determined by history.

CLASSIFICATION

The classification proposed by MacEwen et al. and later modified by Winter, Moe, and Eilers is the one most uniformly accepted (Box 38-6; Figs. 38-145 and 38-146). The congenital curve also should be classified according to the area of the spine involved because this is indicative of the prognosis of the specific deformity. The areas generally distinguished are the cervicothoracic spine, thoracic spine, thoracolumbar spine, and lumbosacral spine.

PATIENT EVALUATION

In addition to the routine spinal evaluation, some specific physical findings should be sought in patients with congenital scoliosis. The skin of the back should be carefully examined for signs such as hair patches, lipomata, dimples, and scars (Fig. 38-147), which may indicate an underlying anomalous vertebra. The neurological evaluation should be very thorough. Evidence of neurological involvement, such as a clubfoot, calf atrophy, absent reflexes, and atrophy of one lower extremity compared with the other, should be noted carefully. Many children with congenital scoliosis have other anomalies. MacEwen, Winter, and Hardy emphasized the importance of a complete evaluation of the genitourinary system: 18% of their patients had urological anomalies, including 2.5% who had obstructive disease that could be life threatening. Winter et al. found congenital heart disease in 7% of his patients. Diastematomyelia occurs in approximately 5% of patients (Fig. 38-148).

A high-quality series of routine roentgenograms is essential to evaluate the deformity. To obtain films of this quality, it often is necessary to take supine films at a 40-inch distance rather

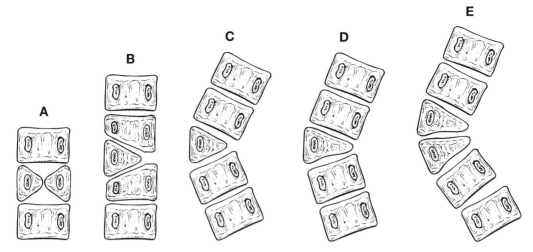

Fig. 38-145 Defects of formation. **A,** Anterior central defect. **B,** Incarcerated hemivertebra. **C,** Free hemivertebra. **D,** Wedge vertebra. **E,** Multiple hemivertebrae. (Redrawn from Bradford DS, Hensinger RM: *The pediatric spine*, New York, 1985, Thieme.)

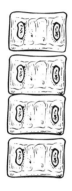

Fig. 38-146 Block vertebra. (Redrawn from Bradford DS, Hensinger RM: *The pediatric spine*, New York, 1985, Thieme.)

than the routine standing films, which are taken at a 72-inch distance. The use of relatively slow-speed film also improves the details of the roentgenograms. Once the anomalies have been identified, routine follow-up roentgenograms for curve measurements can then be made with the higher-speed films. The congenital curve should be classified as a failure of segmentation or a failure of formation, and the roentgenograms should be examined carefully for any evidence of widening of the pedicles or midline bony defects that may indicate an underlying cord anomaly.

Probably more important than classification of the curve is an analysis of the growth potential of the curve to better determine the possibility of curve progression. All congenital curves should be carefully measured with the Cobb technique, including compensatory or secondary curves in seemingly normal parts of the spine. Measurements should include each end of the anomalous area, as well as each end of the entire curve generally considered for treatment. Tomograms are sometimes helpful to further delineate the type of congenital curve, and myelography or MRI should be considered if

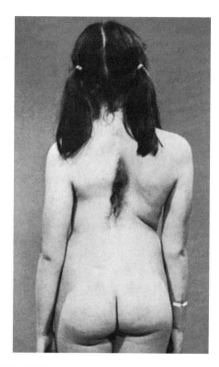

Fig. 38-147 Hair patch associated with diastematomyelia and congenital scoliosis. (From Winter RB et al: *J Bone Joint Surg* 56A:27, 1974.)

diastematomyelia or a neurological abnormality is suspected (Fig. 38-149). Gillespie et al. emphasized the high risk of congenital intraspinal anomalies in patients with congenital scoliosis and the lack of cutaneous manifestations in a significant number of patients. Winter et al. found the incidence of spinal dysraphism to be 10%. MRI scanning during infancy may help delineate the anatomical deformity, which may not be visible on plain roentgenograms, and also better delineates the

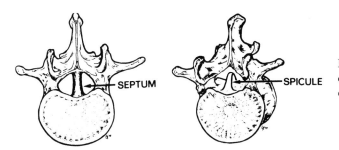

Fig. 38-148   Diastematomyelia spicule invaginates dura and divides spinal cord, either partially or completely. (From Hood RW et al: *J Bone Joint Surg* 62A:520, 1980.)

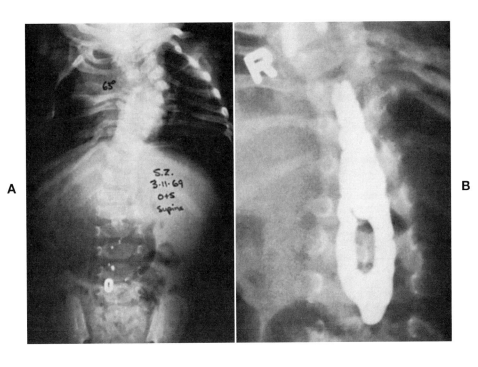

A

B

Fig. 38-149   **A,** Widening of spinal canal from T12 to L5. **B,** Myelogram shows classic midline defect at L2 of diastematomyelia. (From Winter RB et al: *J Bone Joint Surg* 56A:27, 1974.)

physis. MRI is helpful in evaluating patients whose curves are not too large, but the scans are difficult to interpret in patients with major scoliosis, in whom a water-soluble myelogram may be more useful. Drvaric et al. found urological abnormalities in 40% of 100 patients with congenital scoliosis, and they recommended urological evaluation of all patients with congenital scoliosis. They found diagnostic ultrasound evaluations of the urinary tract to be an acceptable alternative as an initial screening method, with excretory urography reserved for confirmation in patients in whom an abnormality is identified ultrasonographically or in whom the ultrasound is inconclusive.

NATURAL HISTORY

Several excellent studies have outlined the natural history of congenital scoliosis. McMaster and Ohtsuka followed 216 untreated patients for 5 years and found that the rate of deterioration and the ultimate severity of the curve depended on both the type of anomaly and the site at which it occurred. The most progressive of all anomalies was a concave, unilateral unsegmented bar with a convex hemivertebra (Fig. 38-150).

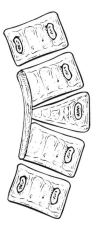

Fig. 38-150   Unilateral and unsegmented bar with a contralateral hemivertebra. (Redrawn from Lubicky JP: Congenital scoliosis. In Bridwell KH, DeWald RL, eds: *The textbook of spinal surgery,* ed 2, Philadelphia, 1997, Lippincott-Raven.)

Site of curvature	Block vertebra	Wedged vertebra	Hemivertebrae		Unilateral unsegmented bar	Unilateral unsegmented bar and contralateral hemivertebrae
			Single	Double		
Upper thoracic	< 1° – 1°	★ – 2°	1° – 2°	2° – 2.5°	2° – 4°	5° – 6°
Lower thoracic	< 1° – 1°	1° – 2°	2° – 2.5°	2° – 3°	5° – 6.5°	6° – 7°
Thoracolumbar	< 1° – 1°	1.5° – 2°	2° – 3.5°	5° – ★	6° – 9°	> 10° – ★
Lumbar	< 1° – ★	< 1° – ★	< 1° – 1°	★	> 5° – ★	★
Lumbosacral	★	★	< 1° – 1.5°	★	★	★

☐ No treatment required   ▨ May require spinal fusion   ☐ Require spinal fusion

★ Too few or no curves

Fig. 38-151   Median yearly rate of deterioration without treatment for each type of single congenital scoliosis in each region of spine. Numbers on left in each column refer to patients seen before 10 years of age; numbers on right refer to patients seen at age 10 years or older. (From McMaster MJ, Ohtsuka K: *J Bone Joint Surg* 64A:1128, 1982.)

Second in severity was a unilateral unsegmented bar, and next was a double-convex hemivertebra. For each type of anomaly, the rate of deterioration usually was less severe if the abnormality was in the upper thoracic region, more severe in the thoracic region, and most severe in the thoracolumbar region (Fig. 38-151). Other natural history studies from Nasca et al. and Winter et al. confirmed these findings. The rate of deterioration of the curve is not constant, but if the curve is present before the patient is 10 years of age, it usually increases, especially during the adolescent growth spurt. The least severe scoliosis is caused by a block vertebra.

The deformity produced by a failure of formation is much more difficult to predict than that caused by failure of segmentation. A hemivertebra produces scoliosis through an enlarging wedge on the affected side of the spine, whereas a unilateral unsegmented bar retards growth on the affected side. The growth imbalance in patients with hemivertebrae is not as severe as in those with unilateral unsegmented bars. Winter reported that a hemivertebra can exist tucked into the spine between adjacent normal vertebrae without causing a corresponding deformity. He called this an "incarcerated hemivertebra." If, however, the hemivertebra is separated from either of the adjacent vertebrae by a disc, it is a segmented hemivertebra with two functioning physes on either side and is likely to cause a slowly progressive curve (Fig. 38-152). Analysis of the growth status is the most important factor in predicting the possibility of progression of these congenital deformities. Dubousset et al. emphasized the importance of considering growth of the spinal canal in three dimensions (Fig. 38-153). Analysis of the potential growth on both sides of the curve will help with the prognosis. For example, if normal convex growth is expected and deficient concave growth is likely, major deformity will occur (Fig. 38-154); however, if growth is deficient on both the convex and concave sides, progressive lateral deformity may not occur. If both sides are deficient in growth potential over many levels, shortening of the trunk may occur without lateral curvature.

NONOPERATIVE TREATMENT

Nonoperative treatment is of limited value in patients with congenital scoliosis. Nonprogressive curves require regular

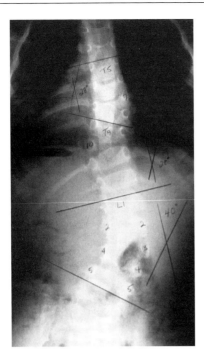

Fig. 38-152   Segmented hemivertebra with two functioning physes is likely to cause slowly progressive curve.

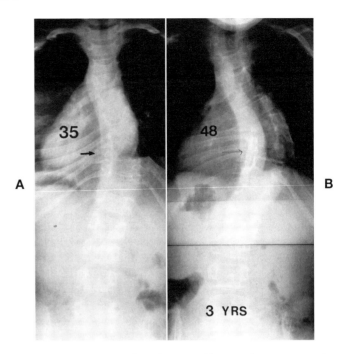

Fig. 38-154   Progression of curve with normal convex growth and deficient concave growth due to unsegmented bar. **A,** Initial curve of 35 degrees. **B,** Three years later, curve is 48 degrees.

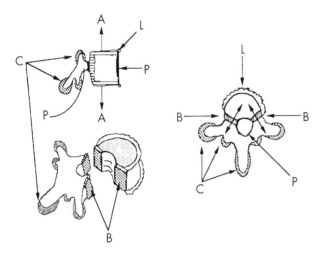

Fig. 38-153   Vertebral growth. *A,* Body endplates (superior and inferior). *B,* Neurocentral cartilage (bipolar) fusion at age 7 or 8 years. *C,* Posterior elements cartilage. *P,* Periosteum; *L,* ring apophysis (begins age 7 to 9 years, closed at age 14 to 24 years). (From Dubousset J, Katti E, Seringe R: *J Pediatr Orthop* 13:123, 1993.)

observation with quality roentgenograms twice a year. Observation also is helpful in patients with multiple anomalies in whom the prognosis is difficult to determine.

A few congenital curves can be managed orthotically. Winter et al. reported 63 patients with congenital scoliosis who were treated with a Milwaukee brace. They observed that three types of curves responded to brace management: (1) longer and flexible curves, (2) curves that could be corrected either in traction or on side bending, and (3) curves with a mixture of anomalous and nonanomalous vertebrae. Short, sharp, and rigid curves did not respond to brace treatment. Bracing usually works on the vertebrae outside the actual congenital deformity, and compensatory curves also can be successfully managed for several years with orthotic treatment. Lumbar curves can be treated in a TLSO, but thoracic curves require a Milwaukee brace. When using a TLSO, its effect on the child's developing thorax must be considered. If orthotic treatment is elected, careful measurement and comparison of spine roentgenograms at 6-month intervals must be made. Because of the slow progression of some curves, it is important to compare current roentgenograms with all previous films, including the original films, to detect curve progression.

OPERATIVE TREATMENT

Because 75% of congenital curves are progressive and only 5% to 10% can be treated with bracing, surgery remains the fundamental treatment. Winter delineated the several types of surgery available for this condition (Box 38-7).

Posterior Fusion Without Instrumentation

Winter et al. analyzed 290 patients ranging in age from 5 to 19 years who had congenital scoliosis and who were treated with posterior spinal fusion with or without Harrington instrumentation. They concluded that posterior fusion is satisfactory for most patients with congenital scoliosis. The most common problem was bending of the fusion mass in growing children, which occurred in 14% of patients. Use of instrumentation allowed slightly better correction but was associated with the only incidences of paraplegia and infection in the series. The advantages of posterior fusion without instrumentation are its simplicity, safety, and reliability. Difficulties include cast correction, an increased pseudarthrosis rate, the possibility of late bending, the possibility of crankshaft phenomenon, and the smaller amount of correction possible. Posterior fusion alone generally is used for smaller curves that are expected to progress slowly and curves in which anterior spinal fusion would be quite difficult, such as the cervicothoracic junction.

The basic posterior spinal fusion technique is described in Technique 38-3. Correction is achieved postoperatively by a corrective cast or brace. The most common errors are (1) failure to apply abundant bone graft, (2) failure to apply a tight-fitting cast or brace, (3) premature removal of the cast or brace, and (4) failure to recognize and repair pseudarthroses promptly. Many surgeons routinely explore all fusions for congenital scoliosis at 6 months after surgery to identify any pseudarthroses. For posterior fusion without instrumentation, the entire curve must be fused, and the fusion must be bilateral.

Winter et al. showed that most large posterior fusion masses do not bend. Bending, however, can occur despite the best of posterior fusions, especially in curves with significant potential for progression, such as a unilateral bar or a unilateral bar with an opposite side hemivertebra. Both posterior and anterior fusions should be done for these curves.

Posterior Fusion with Instrumentation

The advantages of instrumentation in congenital scoliosis are (1) slightly more correction can be obtained; (2) the rate of pseudarthrosis can be reduced somewhat; and (3) the postoperative cast or brace is less unpleasant. These advantages must be weighed against the risks of paralysis and infection, as indicated by Winter et al. Letts and Hollenberg reported that congenital scoliosis is the condition in which paraplegia occurs most often after Harrington instrumentation. The risk of neurological injury can be lowered but not eliminated with careful preoperative evaluation by myelography or MRI, by intraoperative spinal cord monitoring, and by the routine use of the wake-up test. Instrumentation does not alter the length of the fusion or the necessity for facet fusion, decortica-

tion, abundant bone graft, and postoperative external support (Box 38-8). Instrumentation usually should be reserved for larger curves in older children in whom obtaining and maintaining correction of the curves would be difficult in a plaster cast alone. The curves should be flexible, and no intraspinal abnormalities should be present. Ideally, kyphosis should not be significant. The goal of this surgery is modest correction and curve control. A wake-up test is mandatory in these patients. The instrumentation is used to increase the fusion rate and as a stabilizing strut, rather than to obtain significant correction.

♦ Combined Anterior and Posterior Fusions

The main indications for anterior and posterior fusions instead of isolated posterior fusion are (1) to treat sagittal plane problems, (2) to increase the flexibility of the scoliosis by discectomy, (3) to eliminate the anterior physis to prevent bending or torsion of the fusion mass with further growth (crankshaft phenomenon), and (4) to treat curves with a significant potential for progression. The anterior procedure consists of removal of the disc, cartilage endplates, and bony endplates. Bone graft in the form of bone chips is placed into the disc space for fusion. No anterior instrumentation is used. The spine is exposed on the convex side, but the approach is dictated by the level of the curve. After the anterior fusion, a posterior procedure is done. Instrumentation may or may not be used, depending on factors such as the severity of the curve. The postoperative management is the same as after posterior fusion with or without instrumentation. Dubousset et al. recommended anterior and posterior fusions in young patients who are fused at the lumbar level before Risser 0 and who have significant residual deformity of 30 degrees and 10 degrees of rotation. For thoracic curves the amount of crankshaft effect that can be tolerated is weighed against the inconveniences and risks of the thoracotomy necessary to perform the anterior epiphysiodesis.

King et al. described a technique of transpedicular convex anterior hemiepiphysiodesis combined with posterior arthrodesis for treatment of progressive congenital scoliosis. In effect,

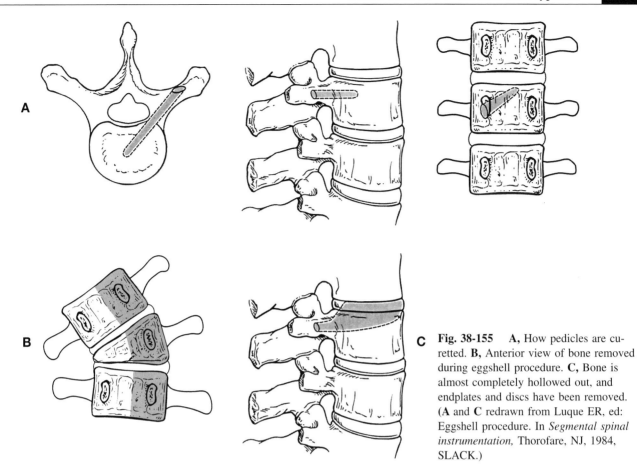

Fig. 38-155   **A,** How pedicles are curetted. **B,** Anterior view of bone removed during eggshell procedure. **C,** Bone is almost completely hollowed out, and endplates and discs have been removed. (**A** and **C** redrawn from Luque ER, ed: Eggshell procedure. In *Segmental spinal instrumentation,* Thorofare, NJ, 1984, SLACK.)

a combined anterior and posterior fusion can be done through a single posterior approach. These authors reported arrest of curve progression in all nine of their patients after this procedure. The average age of patients at surgery was 9 years. Their technique is based on the work of Michele and Krueger, who described a transpedicular approach to the vertebral body, and Heinig, who described the "eggshell" procedure, so-called because the vertebral body is hollowed out until it is "eggshell" thin before it is collapsed. King et al. found the pedicle dimensions to be adequate for this technique even in infants; however, they recommended preoperative CT through the center of each pedicle to be included in the epiphysiodesis.

TECHNIQUE 38-37 (King)

Position the patient prone on a radiolucent operating table, using a frame or chest rolls. After preparing and draping, obtain a roentgenogram over a skin marker to identify the appropriate level for the incision. Make a single midline posterior incision and retract the paraspinous muscles on both sides of the curve as far as the tips of the costotransverse processes in the thoracic spine and lateral to the facet joints in the lumbar spine. Remove the cortical bone in the area of the pedicle to be mined caudad to the facet joint and at the base of the costotransverse process in the thoracic spine. Use the curet to remove the cancellous

bone. The medullary cavity of the pedicle can now be seen. The cortex medially indicates the boundary of the spinal canal and caudally and cranially indicates the margins of the intervertebral neural foraminae. Use progressively larger curets until only the cortical rim of the pedicle remains (Fig. 38-155, *A*). The pedicle margins then expand into the vertebral body. Remove cancellous bone, creating a hole in the lateral half of the vertebral body. Use curved curets to remove cancellous bone from the vertebral body in the cephalad and caudad directions until the endplate bone, the physis, and intervertebral disc are encountered. Brisk bleeding may occur, and the surgeon should be prepared for it. For a single hemivertebra, mine the pedicle of the hemivertebra itself, along with that of the adjacent vertebra in the cephalad and caudad directions (Fig. 38-155, *B*). Communication with each pedicle hole across the physis and disc space is readily achieved (Fig. 38-155, *C*). Pack autogenous bone from the iliac crest down the pedicles and across the vertebral endplates and discs. Posteriorly, excise the convex and concave facet joints and pack with cancellous bone. Carry out decortication bilaterally. Use autologous iliac crest bone graft in all patients and augment with allograft bone if necessary. If internal fixation is needed, a wire or a compression device can be used.

AFTERTREATMENT. The patient is placed in a thoracolumbosacral orthosis for 4 to 6 months. Following that, no further immobilization is used.

Combined Anterior and Posterior Convex Hemiepiphysiodesis (Growth Arrest)

In 1981 Winter reported 10 patients with progressive congenital scoliosis treated by convex anterior and posterior epiphysiodeses and fusions. Roaf, in 1963, reported 188 patients treated by epiphysiodesis and posterior intraarticular fusion on the convex side. Many of his patients were older children with little residual growth potential, and his approach allowed only limited exposure. Andrew and Piggott reported 13 patients treated by anterior and posterior epiphysiodeses. These authors emphasized that this technique is appropriate in children younger than 5 years of age who meet certain criteria: (1) a documented progressive curve, (2) a curve of less than 60 degrees, (3) a curve of six segments or less, (4) concave growth potential, and (5) no pathological congenital kyphosis or lordosis. Even if the concave side ceases to grow, the anterior and posterior fusions obtain a good result. Epiphysiodesis of the entire curve, not merely the apical segment, should be done. Rigid spinal immobilization is used until the fusions are solid, usually at least 6 months after surgery.

Dubousset et al. emphasized the importance of preoperative planning. Each vertebra should be considered a cube divided into four quadrants, with each quadrant growing symmetrically around the spinal canal (Fig. 38-156). When growth is unbalanced, the zones that must be fused to reestablish balanced growth are determined preoperatively. King et al. noted a true epiphysiodesis effect after transpedicular convex anterior hemiepiphysiodesis (Technique 38-37) in four of their nine patients, all four of whom had single hemivertebrae. Based on these results, they recommended transpedicular hemiepiphysiodesis with posterior hemiarthrodesis in selected patients with single hemivertebrae.

◆ **Convex Anterior and Posterior Hemiepiphysiodeses and Fusion**

TECHNIQUE 38-38 *(Winter)*

Position the patient in a straight lateral position with the convexity of the curve upward. Prepare and drape the back and side in the same field. The anterior approach technique varies according to the level to be fused (p. 1820). The posterior approach is a standard subperiosteal exposure but always only on the convex side of the curve. Once the curve has been exposed, insert needles or other markers both anteriorly and posteriorly so that both are visible on one cross-table roentgenogram. Failure to place the fusion precisely in the proper area can lead to a poor result.

Once the proper area has been identified, incise the periosteum of the anterior vertebral bodies and peel it forward to the lateral edge of the anterior longitudinal ligament and backward to the base of the pedicle (Fig. 38-157, *A*).

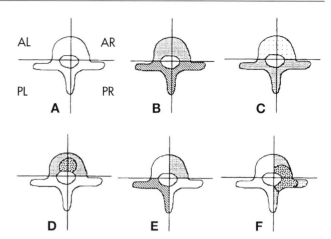

Fig. 38-156   A, Vertebral growth on horizontal plane, four segments: *AL,* Anterior left; *AR,* anterior right; *PL,* posterior left; and *PR,* posterior right. **B,** Congenital posterior bar involving PL and PR; level of epiphysiodesis must be AL and AR. **C,** Anterior defect involving AL and AR; epiphysiodesis must involve PL and PR. **D,** Anterior excess of growth potential involving both AR and AL; epiphysiodesis must involve both AR and AL above and below. **E,** Congenital posterolateral bar involving PL only; epiphysiodesis must involve only AR. **F,** Excess (hemivertebra) growth involving only AR and part of PR; hemiepiphysiodesis must involve AR and PR. (From Dubousset J, Katti E, Seringe R: *J Pediatr Orthop* 13:123, 1993.)

Incise the annulus of the disc at its superior and inferior margins and remove the superficial portion of the nucleus pulposus. Carefully remove the cartilaginous endplates, which are quite thick in children, taking at least one third of the physes but never more than half. Once the cartilaginous endplates have been removed, remove the cortical bony endplate with a curet. Make a trough in the lateral side of the vertebral bodies (Fig. 38-157, *B*) and lay the autogenous rib graft in the trough. Use cancellous bone to augment the autogenous rib graft. If autogenous rib is not available, use iliac or bone-bank bone.

The posterior procedure consists of a standard, unilateral, subperiosteal exposure of the area to be fused (Fig. 38-157, *C*). Excise the facet joints, remove any facet cartilage, decorticate the entire area, and apply a bone graft. Apply a corrective Risser cast while the child is still under anesthesia to avoid having to use a second anesthetic.

AFTERTREATMENT. Casting is continued for 6 months, and the cast is changed as frequently as necessary. Follow-up must be continued until the end of growth. Results may appear excellent for years but can deteriorate during the adolescent growth spurt.

Hemivertebra Excision

Hemivertebra excision usually is reserved for patients with pelvic obliquity (Fig. 38-158) or with fixed, lateral translation

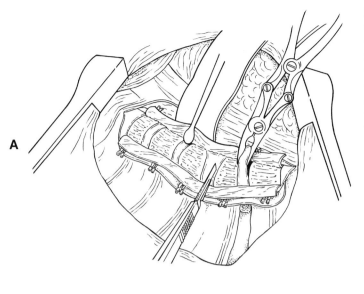

Fig. 38-157 Combined anterior and posterior convex hemiepiphysiodesis. **A,** Periosteum of anterior vertebral bodies is incised and peeled forward and backward. **B,** Trough is created in lateral side of vertebral bodies. Autogenous rib graft is placed in trough. **C,** Area to be fused is exposed through standard, unilateral, subperiosteal exposure. Area is decorticated, and bone graft is applied. (Redrawn from Winter RB, Lonstein JE, Denis F, et al: *J Pediatr Orthop* 8:633, 1988.)

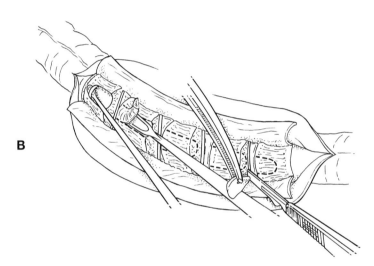

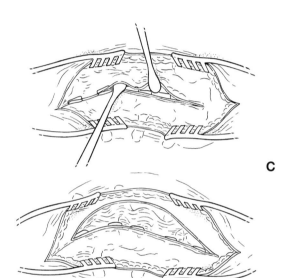

of the thorax that cannot be corrected by other means. Hemivertebra excision and fusion should be limited to very few patients. Preventive early fusion is preferable to allowing a curve to progress to the point where hemivertebra excision is indicated. At the lumbosacral area, however, excision of the hemivertebra can improve trunk imbalance. The L3, L4, or lumbosacral level, below the level of the conus medularis, is the safest level at which to excise a hemivertebra. Hemivertebra excision in the thoracic area is most dangerous because this area of the spinal canal is the narrowest and has the least blood supply.

The curves best managed by hemivertebra excision are angular curves in which the hemivertebra is the apex. This technique has been reported mostly in lumbosacral hemivertebrae that produce lateral spinal decompensation in patients for whom no other technique can achieve adequate alignment.

Winter emphasized that hemivertebra excision should be considered a convex osteotomy at the apex of the curve. The entire curve front and back must be fused. Neurological risk is inherent in hemivertebra excision because the spinal canal is entered both anteriorly and posteriorly. Winter reported two patients with lumbar root problems after hemivertebra excision.

Leatherman and Dickson reported serious complications when anterior hemivertebra excision was combined with posterior fusion in one operation. They recommended a two-stage procedure in which the vertebral body is removed through an anterior exposure; then in a second stage the posterior elements are removed and fusion is done. More recently, Bradford and Boachie-Adjei, Bergoin et al., Bollini et al., and Ulrich and Moushkin reported acceptable results with one-stage anterior and posterior hemivertebra resections. Generally, postoperative cast or brace immobilization is used for 6 months; the use of instrumentation may allow use of a brace rather than a cast, but the bone stock must be adequate to accept the instrumentation. Posterior instrumentation alone may cause more lordosis than compressing the convexity of the curve. A combination of anterior and posterior instrumentation can be used on the convex side.

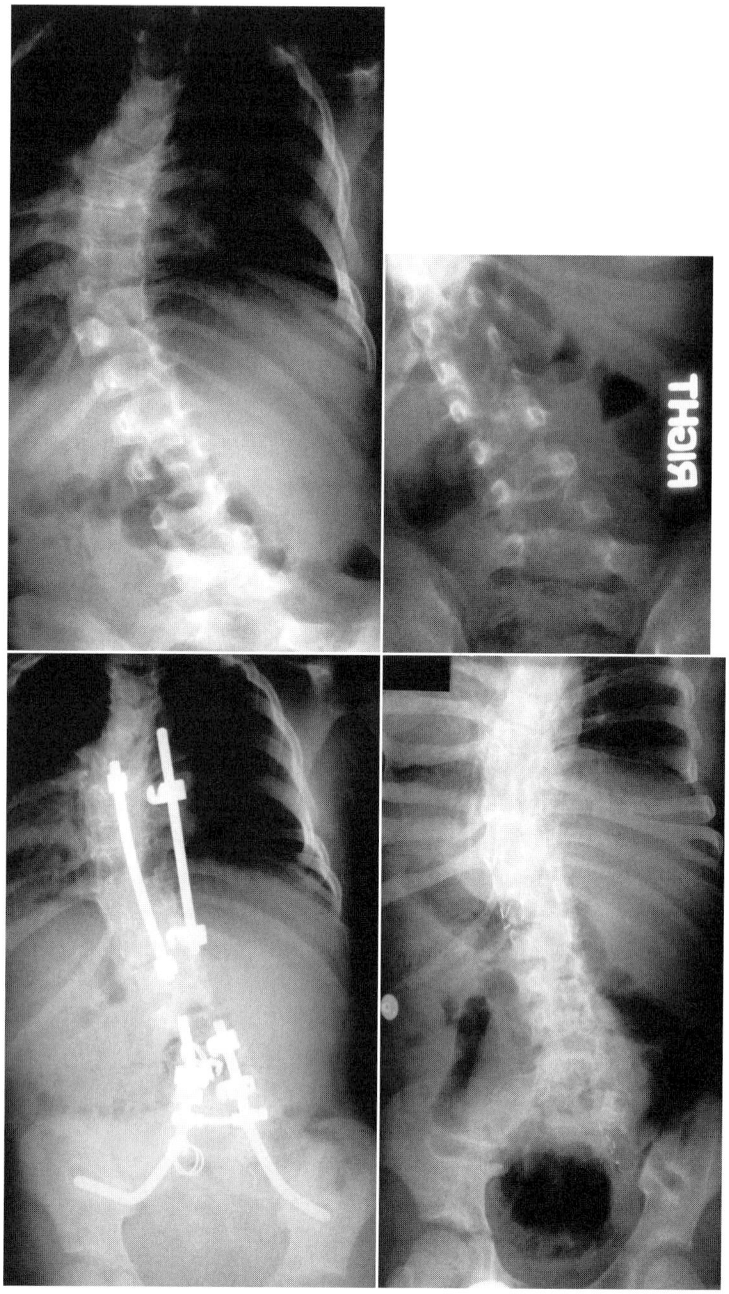

Fig. 38-158 **A** and **B**, Hemivertebra. **C**, After hemivertebral excision and fusion with short segment rods and cross links. **D**, After rod removal.

Heinig described a decancellation procedure done with curets through the pedicle. Lubicky recommended the use of both internal fixation and external immobilization with this technique. He found that the amount of immediate correction from this technique was unpredictable, but it did generally lead to a hemiepiphysiodesis when combined with a convex posterior fusion at the same level. He recommended that the technique be done with C-arm control (Figs. 38-159 to 38-161). Heinig and Lubicky advised leaving the hemilamina in place until the vertebral body resection is complete to protect the neural tube while the curet is used. This technique can be useful if the hemivertebra is located posteriorly next to the spinal canal, where seeing the hemivertebra from anteriorly can be difficult.

THORACIC INSUFFICIENCY SYNDROME

Campbell defined thoracic insufficiency syndrome as the inability of the thorax to support normal respiration or lung growth. This condition occurs in patients with hypoplastic thorax syndromes, such as Jarcho-Levin syndrome, progressive infantile scoliosis with reductive distortion of the thoracic volume from spinal rotation, and congenital scoliosis associated with fused ribs on the concave side of the curve. In a hypoplastic thorax associated with congenital scoliosis, "extrinsic" restrictive lung disease can be caused by volume restriction of the underlying growing lungs and motion restriction of the ribs with reduction of the secondary breathing mechanism.

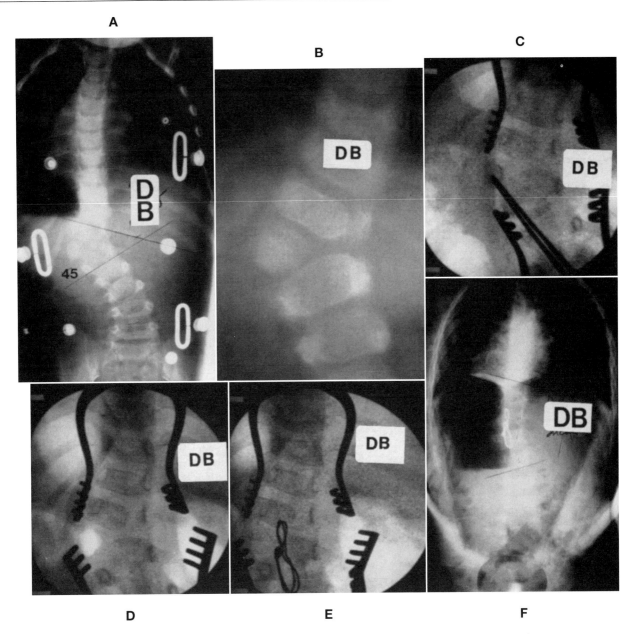

Fig. 38-159 Type I progressive congenital scoliosis in boy approximately 2½ years of age. **A,** Standing roentgenogram shows significant thoracolumbar curve with marked trunk decompensation. **B,** Anteroposterior tomogram demonstrates nature of congenital anomaly. Note healthy disc spaces on either side. **C,** Intraoperative posteroanterior view taken with C-arm, identifying pedicle of hemivertebra. Hemivertebra was removed using eggshell technique. **D,** Posteroanterior C-arm image demonstrating that hemivertebra has been excised. Space was filled with bone graft, sublaminar wire between two adjacent laminae was inserted and tightened, and bone graft was applied to lamina on convex side. **E,** C-arm image of completed construct and correction. **F,** Standing posteroanterior roentgenogram taken with patient in cast. Note tremendous correction of curvature and centering of trunk over pelvis. (From Lubicky JP: Congenital scoliosis. In Bridwell KH, DeWald RL, eds: *The textbook of spinal surgery,* ed 2, Philadelphia, 1997, Lippincott-Raven.)

Little is known about the natural history of global deformity of the thorax in patients with congenital scoliosis or how spinal surgery in very young children affects the general thoracic deformity and rib cage growth. Lung growth is limited to the anatomical boundaries of the thorax, so any spine or rib cage malformation that reduces the thoracic volume early in life may adversely affect the size of the lungs at skeletal maturity (Fig. 38-162). Campbell compared the thorax to a room with the spine as a corner. The shape of the room and its volume cannot be affected significantly by changing a single corner. He

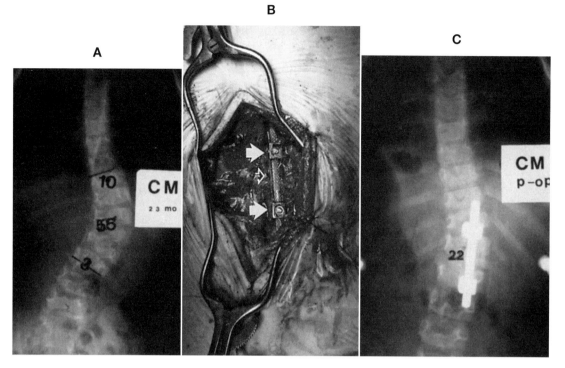

Fig. 38-160   Progressive type I congenital scoliosis in 23-month-old girl. **A,** Posteroanterior standing view shows significant curve with trunk shift to right. Child underwent eggshell verte-brectomy and hemiarthrodesis and hemiepiphysiodesis with acute correction provided by pediatric CD compression system. **B,** Intraoperative view of compression system in place. Closed arrows indicate hook position, upper one being two levels above hemivertebra and lower arrow one level below hemivertebra. Open arrow indicates where hemivertebra had been located before eggshell vertebrectomy. Construct is on convex side of curve. **C,** Posteroanterior standing view taken in brace postoperatively showing significant correction of curve and better centering of trunk over pelvis. (From Lubicky JP: Congenital scoliosis. In Bridwell KH, DeWald RL, eds: *The textbook of spinal surgery,* ed 2, Philadelphia, 1997, Lippincott-Raven.)

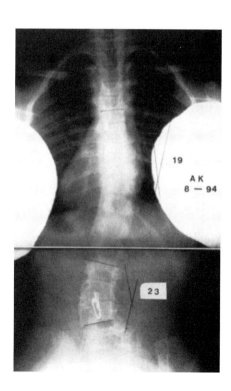

Fig. 38-161   Posteroanterior standing view of spine in 8-year, 6-month-old girl shows nicely balanced spine and solid hemiepiphysiodesis on left in lumbar spine 7 years after procedure similar to eggshell technique. (From Lubicky JP: Congenital scoliosis. In Bridwell KH, DeWald RL, eds: *The textbook of spinal surgery,* ed 2, Philadelphia, 1997, Lippincott-Raven.)

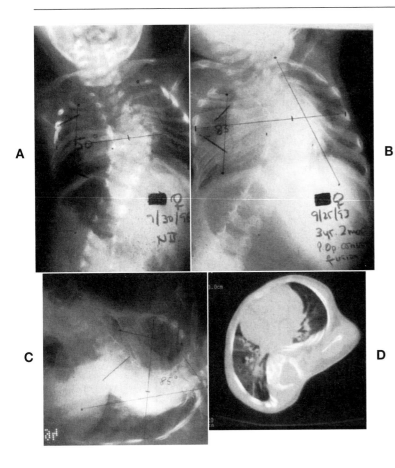

recommended not only evaluating the spinal deformity, but also analyzing global thoracic deformity and its effect on thoracic volume, symmetry, function, and growth.

For younger patients with progressive thoracic insufficiency syndrome associated with spinal deformity, Campbell listed as aims of treatment (1) to correct and stabilize spinal deformity, (2) to correct clinical deformity, (3) to preserve the growth potential of the spine as the posterior pillar of the thorax, (4) to improve volume, symmetry, and function of the thorax, and (5) to maintain improvements in volume, symmetry, and function of the thorax during growth. The volume of the thorax ultimately determines the volume of the lungs, and their function determines the adequacy of the secondary breathing mechanism. From birth to age 8, the lungs grow by alveolar cell multiplication, and during this golden period surgical treatment should, if possible, nurture the growth of all components of the thorax, including the spine, to facilitate the development of the underlying lungs. Because of the inability of traditional spinal correction techniques to effect changes in the dimensions of the thorax, Campbell developed a technique to directly treat chest wall deformity with indirect correction of the congenital scoliosis. This procedure treats the total global deformity of the thorax, allowing the spine to grow undisturbed by surgical intervention, with increased height of the thoracic spine and the thorax.

Gruca described a technique of surgical compression of the ribs to obtain correction of idiopathic scoliosis on the convex side of the curve. Campbell developed rib distraction instrumentation techniques for treating primary hemithorax constriction in severe spinal deformity in young children. He postulated that indirect correction of scoliosis could be obtained by surgical expansion of the chest through rib distraction on the concave side of the curve. He compared this technique to an opening wedge osteotomy of a malunion of a long bone. In this technique, the thoracic deformity is corrected by an "opening wedge thoracostomy" in the center of the deformity of the concave constricted hemithorax. Once the constricted hemithorax is lengthened, the thorax is equilibrated, with indirect correction of the scoliosis. Correction is maintained with an expandable titanium rib prosthesis. This technique is currently in phase III FDA clinical trials. A substantial correction of the hemithorax deformity, an average curve correction of approximately 20 degrees, and continued growth of the spine were noted as well. Elongation of unilateral unsegmented bars over time in patients treated with chest wall distraction techniques also has been noted (Fig. 38-163). According to Campbell, the advantages of this technique are that it directly treats the anatomical causes of thoracic insufficiency syndrome and does not interfere with any subsequent spinal procedures that may be needed later in life.

Campbell treated 34 patients who had progressive congenital scoliosis associated with fused ribs of the concave hemithorax with expansion thoracoplasty and a titanium rib prosthesis. He recommended consideration of spinal-growth-

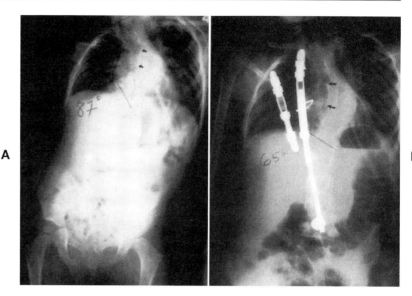

Fig. 38-163   **A,** Multiple congenital anomalies of thoracic spine, including hemivertebra on convex side of curve and long unilateral unsegmented bar on concave side *(arrows),* in a 2½-year old girl with 87-degree scoliosis. **B,** At 6-year follow-up, curve is corrected to 65 degrees. Length of large central, unilateral segmented bar from T5 to T11 on concave side of curve *(arrows)* when compared preoperatively and postoperatively suggests growth on concave side of curve. (From Campbell RM: Congenital scoliosis due to multiple vertebral anomalies associated with thoracic insufficiency syndrome, *Spine: State of the Art Reviews* 11: 210, 2000.)

sparing techniques, such as growth rods and expansion thoracoplasty, for patients with multiple levels of malformation in the thoracic spine ("jumbled spine") with associated areas of either rib deletion or fusion ("jumbled thorax"). Severe thoracic deformity in patients with thoracic insufficiency syndrome is best treated with expansion thoracoplasty.

◆ Expansion Thoracoplasty

The expandable prosthetic titanium rib device comes in two forms. The device with a radius of 220 mm is most commonly used in the treatment of fused ribs and scoliosis. The titanium alloy allows the use of MRI postoperatively. The upper end of the device is attached to the ribs by the superior rib cradle and a rib cradle cap that form a loose encirclement around the rib to avoid vascular compromise of the underlying rib. Lateral stability is provided by the surrounding soft tissues. The central portion of the device consists of the rib sleeve, which is a hollow component that attaches to the superior cradle. The inferior rib cradle is inserted into this rib sleeve, allowing the construct to later telescope for more correction. The rib cradle inferiorly is identical to the superior rib cradle except for a longer post that is sized to completely fill the rib sleeve to provide maximal expandability. The device is locked inferiorly by a peg-type lock through one of two holes, 5 mm apart in the distal rib sleeve, into partial-thickness holes in the inferior rib cradle post. This provides variable expandability for the device in increments of 5 mm. If the curves extend into the lumbar spine, a hybrid device is used. The inferior rib cradle is replaced with a modified spinal rod that has an expansion shaft proximally that can be inserted into the rib sleeve. A low profile laminar hook is connected to the rod distally, and the laminar hook is attached to one of the proximal lumbar vertebrae (Fig. 38-164). At the time of this writing, the device is available for investigative use under FDA investigational device exemption.

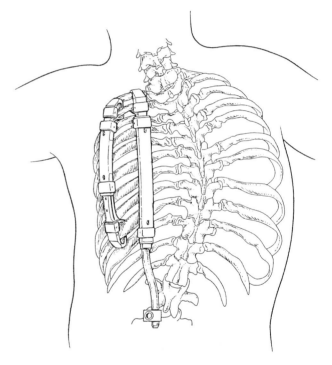

Fig. 38-164   Expandable prosthetic rib device. (Redrawn from Campbell RM, personal communication).

TECHNIQUE 38-39 *(Campbell)*

Place the patient in a lateral decubitus position with the concave side of the hemithorax upward. Intraoperative spinal monitoring is used. Pulse oximeters are attached to both hands to monitor vascularity. Administer prophylactic intravenous antibiotics. Make a thoracotomy incision around the tip of the scapula and carry it anteriorly. Often in patients with fused ribs, the scapula is both hypoplastic and elevated proximally. In these patients, the skin incision may need to be brought more distal as it courses around the scapula. If a hybrid device is to be used, make a second incision 1 cm lateral to the midline over the proximal lumbar spine (Fig. 38-165, *A*). Through the thoracotomy incision elevate the muscle flaps and proximally identify the middle scalene muscle. Place devices on the second rib posterior to the scalene muscle. Anterior to the middle scalene muscle device, attachment is not done proximally because of the risk of impingement on the neurovascular bundle (Fig. 38-165, *B*). Once exposure has been completed, identify the central rib fusion mass by the absence of intercostal muscles. This is the center of the apex of thoracic deformity where the concave hemithorax is most tightly constricted by rib fusion and is best seen on preoperative bending roentgenograms. Before performing the opening wedge thoracostomy, prepare the rib prosthesis cradle sites proximally and distally. Make 1-cm incisions using an electrocautery in the intercostal muscles under the second rib with a second 5-mm incision above it in the muscle. Use an elevator to carefully strip off only the anterior portion of the rib periosteum without violating the pleura (Fig. 38-165, *C*). Insert a second elevator into the proximal intercostal muscle incision to encircle the rib. Prepare the inferior rib cradle site in the same fashion. Insert the rib cradle cap into the proximal intercostal muscle incision sideways, then turn it distally to encircle the rib, similar to insertion of a spinal laminar hook. Pass the superior rib cradle into the inferior intercostal muscle incision (Fig. 38-165, *D*), mate it with the cradle cap, and lock it into place with pliers (Fig. 38-165, *E*).

The sites for the cradles should be just lateral to the transverse processes of the spine. The superior cradle site should be at the top of the area of the constricted hemithorax. If that site does not allow enough distance between the cradle sites for a device of sufficient length to have reasonable expansion capability, the site can be moved superiorly. In very flexible spines, however, care must be taken not to induce a large compensatory curve in the spine above the primary hemithorax constriction by placing the rib cradle too far superiorly. The inferior cradle site should be in a stable base of the area of the constricted hemithorax, below the line of the opening wedge thoracostomy, and usually encircling two fused ribs.

Select the inferior rib cradle site by picking a rib of attachment that is clinically stable, as horizontal as possible, and at the inferior edge of the thoracic constriction. Avoid unstable rib attachments distally (vestigial rib) because of the high loads placed on the device in the expansion of a fused chest wall. Insert the superior cradle before the opening wedge thoracostomy is made. The inferior cradle is not placed at this point because the size of the device required to hold acute hemithorax correction is not known until the hemithorax is lengthened by the opening wedge thoracostomy.

The deformity of the concave hemithorax is corrected by an opening wedge thoracostomy (Fig. 38-165, *F*). This corrects the "angulated thorax," similar to the use of an opening wedge osteotomy to correct malunion of a long bone. Place the thoracostomy in the apex of the thoracic constriction where it can best correct the concave hemithorax, lengthen the constricted segment, and flare out the superior ribs laterally to increase thoracic volume. In most patients, this line of correction passes not through the apex of the scoliosis but above it. To confirm the correct position, place metal markers on the chest wall and verify the location with C-arm roentgenograms and then compare with the preoperative plan. The line of cleavage for the primary opening wedge thoracostomy may be through a mass of fused ribs, an area of fibrous adhesions between two ribs, or vestigial intercostal muscle. If the chosen interval is osseous, use a rongeur and Kerrison punches to make the thoracostomy. Be careful not to reflect periosteum from the rib incision site, which will devascularize the rib. Strip away the underlying periosteum with a no. 4 Penfield elevator. The line of the thoracostomy extends from the sternum, along the contours of the ribs, to the transverse processes of the spine posteriorly.

Reflect the paraspinous muscles from lateral to medial. Take care not to expose the spine to minimize the risk of inadvertent fusion. Once exposure is completed, gently spread the thoracostomy interval apart with two vein retractors to allow a lamina spreader to be inserted between the ribs in the midaxillary line of the thorax. Then complete the opening wedge thoracostomy by gradually widening the lamina spreader about 5 mm every 3 minutes (Fig. 38-165, *G*) until the thoracic interval is widened to approximately 1 cm. If the ribs are easily distracted and there is at least 0.5 cm of soft tissue between the ribs as they articulate with the spine medially, no further resection is necessary. If rib distraction is difficult, additional rib fusion mass probably requires resection medially. If further resection is needed, cut a 1-cm wide channel medially at the posterior apex of the opening wedge thoracostomy, resecting the remaining fused rib anterior to the transverse process and following it down to the vertebral body for complete removal. Expose the bone to be removed a few millimeters at a time by subperiosteal dissection with a Freer elevator. Use a rongeur to remove the exposed bone. Take care to resect only visible bone, avoiding the spinal canal posteriorly and the esophagus and great vessels anteriorly. Preserve anomalous segmental vessels. Disarticulate the last 5 mm of fused rib from the spine with an angled curet, avoiding the neuroforamen, until the cartilage articular disc is visible. Secure hemostasis with bipolar cautery. Place bone wax over any raw bone surfaces.

If the maximal thoracostomy interval distraction is 2 cm or less, the underlying pleura generally stretches and remains intact. If distraction is more than 2 cm, the pleura

continued

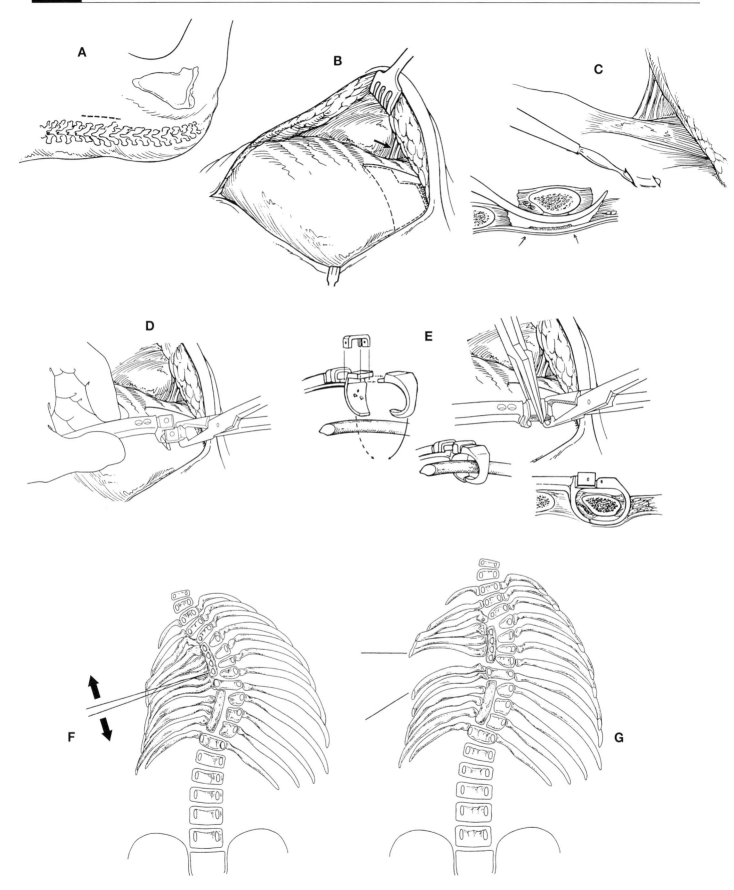

Fig. 38-165   **A** to **J,** Campbell technique of expansion thoracoplasty. See text for description. (Redrawn from Campbell RM, personal communication.)   *Continued*

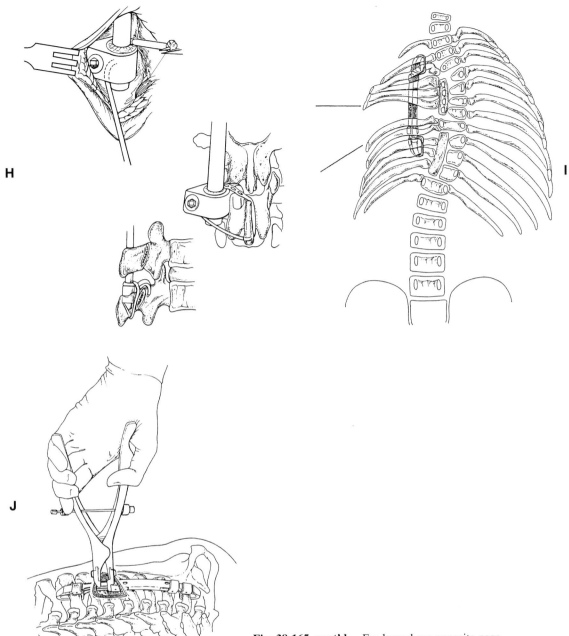

Fig. 38-165, cont'd   For legend see opposite page.

may begin to tear. Small tears in the pleura require no treatment, but substantial defects are treated with a Gore-Tex sheet sutured to the edges of the intact pleura. Avoid attaching it to rib, muscle, or periosteum because it will become a tether. A Gore-Tex sheet of 0.6-mm thickness is used for small defects, and a 2-mm sheet is used for larger defects. Usually the Gore-Tex sheet is placed after the device has been implanted to allow accurate sizing of the sheet needed for maximal thoracic volume. The surface of the sheet is brought outward to maximize volume.

After the chest is expanded by the laminar spreader,

measure the distance between the superior and inferior cradle sites to determine the size of the device needed. The inferior rib cradle and the rib sleeve should be of compatible sizes. An inferior rib cradle that is substantially shorter than the rib sleeve will reduce the device's ability for later expansion and require more frequent change-outs.

Assess the orientation of the device and cradle after acute thoracostomy expansion so that they conform best to the corrected anatomy. After the device is sized and the orientation for the inferior cradle is chosen, relax the laminar spreader to ease access to the cradle sites. Insert

continued

the cradle cap inferiorly, implant the inferior cradle, and lock the components together with a cradle lock. If a hybrid device is used to span down to the lumbar spine, secure the low-profile laminar hook with a loop of Secure Strand (Smith & Nephew Richards, Memphis) looped around the posterior spinous process (Fig. 38-165, *H*). Place a bone graft on the lamina down to the hook to further stabilize a construct with a one-level fusion. If the superior cradle has not been previously inserted, implant it now. Reinsert the laminar spreader between medial ribs at the apex of the opening wedge thoracostomy. Reexpand the interval, expanding the thorax by bringing the device components out to length. Assemble the device by threading the rib sleeve over the inferior cradle and levering the rib sleeve in line with the superior rib cradle by the device wrenches. The acute correction obtained by the opening wedge thoracostomy is now stabilized by the rib device (Fig. 38-165, *I*).

For primary thoracic scoliosis in children younger than 18 months, only a single thoracic device is placed posteriorly, adjacent to the transverse processes of the spine. If a patient is older than 18 months of age and has adequate lumbar canal size and laminae, more support of the thoracostomy can be provided by a hybrid device and a second thoracic prosthesis added posterolaterally. Place the thoracic prosthesis in the posterior axillary line to further expand the constricted hemithorax with proximal attachment just posterior to the middle scalene muscle with at least 0.5 cm between the superior rib cradles. Once assembled, tension both devices by expanding them 0.5 cm to fit snugly without excessive distraction pressure and then place two distraction locks on the rib sleeve. If the chest wall defect created by the opening wedge thoracostomy is larger than 2 cm, potential chest wall instability will need to be considered. A chest wall defect up to 3 cm wide is well tolerated proximally because of the splinting effect of the scapula posteriorly and the pectoralis muscle anteriorly. A distal chest wall defect of more than 2 cm and a proximal defect of more than 3 cm may need augmentation to provide chest wall stability, either by centralization of surgically created "pseudo-ribs" in the defect, addition of more devices, or implantation of a Gore-Tex sheet, 2 mm thick, over the defect.

In the first technique, called *transport centralization,* separate a single rib or "pseudo-rib" of two or three fused ribs away from the superior border of the opening wedge thoracostomy and rotate it downward, like a "bucket handle," to lie centrally in the chest wall defect. The goal of this technique is to divide the chest wall defect into a series of smaller defects, none larger than 2 cm. If the defect is too large for a single rib, separate another rib, or "pseudo-rib," from the inferior border of the open wedge thoracostomy and bring it into the defect, dividing the larger defect into three smaller ones. Take care to preserve all soft tissue attachments to avoid devascularization of the rib.

The second method of augmentation is to add additional devices if transport centralization is not feasible or bone stock is inadequate. This method is practical only in larger patients with adequate soft tissue for device coverage, and usually three devices are the maximum that can be used safely.

Finally, a 2-mm Gore-Tex sheet can be used to supplement either of the other two methods. When the scoliosis extends from the thorax into the lumbar spine, use a lumbar hybrid rod extension (see Fig. 38-165, *H*). This lumbar extension can be used only in patients with adequate lumbar spinal canal size for hook placement, and generally the patient should be at least 18 months of age. Preoperatively assess the width of the canal by CT. The usual site of distal insertion is at either L1 or L2, but if the scoliosis extends well distally into the lumbar spine, then L3 can be used. Avoid more distal insertion sites on the spine if possible.

Spinal dysraphism of the proximal lumbar spine may require that the laminar hook be placed in the distal lumbar spine or that a modified McCarthy hook for the pelvis be coupled to the hybrid lumbar extension. Through a separate skin incision over the lumbar spine, insert the hybrid distraction device and pass it percutaneously from proximal to distal through the paraspinal muscles. Because of the kyphosis of the thorax, if the device is passed in a proximal direction, it may inadvertently penetrate the chest. Size the device similar to the all-thoracic technique and complete the opening wedge thoracostomy. Implant the superior cradle with an empty rib sleeve sized to extend to the inferior border of the thorax at the twelfth rib. Size a hybrid rod lumbar extension to match the rib sleeve and select for implantation. Insert the inferior hook sublaminar. Size a hybrid rod lumbar extension to match the rib sleeve. With a lamina spreader in place to maintain the correction obtained with the opening wedge thoracostomy, use in situ benders to bend the hybrid rod into a slight kyphosis proximally and slight valgus and lordosis distally to best fit the laminar hook. The length of the rod should allow it to extend 1 cm distal to the hook. With a Kelly clamp, create a tunnel from the proximal incision through the paraspinal muscles, moving proximally to distally, with a finger in the lumbar incision to palpate the tip of the clamp as it exits the muscle. Use the Kelly clamp to grasp a small chest tube and pull it into the proximal incision. Attach the hybrid device to the tube and using the tube thread it proximally to engage the rib cradle and then into the hook. Distract the rib and tighten the hook. Wrap the hook with Secure Strand (Smith & Nephew Richards, Memphis) looped under the posterior spinous process and place bone graft over the laminae.

A large amount of correction may push the anterior portion of the proximal fused ribs proximally into the brachial plexus. To check for acute thoracic outlet syndrome, bring the scapula back into position while the anesthesiologist monitors pulses and ulnar nerve function is monitored by somatosensory potentials. If both are normal, close the muscle flaps with absorbable suture and close the skin in standard fashion with absorbable subcutaneous sutures. If either the pulse or ulnar nerve function is abnormal, retract the scapula and subperiosteally resect 2 cm of the proximal two ribs that are anterior under the brachial plexus. Bring the scapula back into position and check somatosensory potentials again. If normal, close the incision.

AFTERTREATMENT. The patient is placed in the intensive care unit until extubated. Generally, a patient may require several days of ventilator support. No bracing is used postoperatively to avoid constricting chest wall growth. At intervals of 4 to 6 months after the initial implantation, the device is expanded in an outpatient procedure. Prophylactic intravenous antibiotics are used, and the distal end of the device is exposed with an incision through the thoracostomy incision if possible. Once the underlying muscle is exposed, it is split along its fibers or cut vertically either on the medial or lateral side of the device to form a thick muscle flap. The distraction lock over the device is removed, and distractor pliers are inserted to lengthen the device (Fig. 38-165, *J*). The prosthesis is lengthened slowly, approximately 2 mm every 3 minutes to avoid fracture. Once maximal reactive pressure is reached, the device is locked in place with a new distraction rod block. Lengthening usually is a minimum of 0.5 cm and up to 1.5 cm. Once the device has exhausted its expandability, a "change-out" surgical procedure is done through small proximal and distal transverse incisions. The central rib sleeve and the inferior rib shaft are removed and replaced with larger components (implants). Devices that extend well under the scapula may require opening a large portion of the old thoracotomy incision to change out the components.

KYPHOSIS

Anatomy

In the sagittal plane the normal spine has four balanced curves: the cervical spine is lordotic; the thoracic spine is kyphotic (20 to 45 degrees), with the curvature extending from T2 to T12 and with T7 the most dorsal vertebra; the lumbar region is lordotic (40 to 60 degrees) with L3 the most ventral vertebra; and the sacral curve is kyphotic. When standing, the thoracic kyphosis and lumbar lordosis are balanced. The weight-bearing line, or sagittal vertical axis, falls from the craniovertebral articulation through the bodies of the cervical vertebrae and anterior to the thoracic spine (Fig. 38-166). The axis then crosses the spinal column at T12 and lies posterior to the lumbar spine. The anterior elements of the spinal column resist

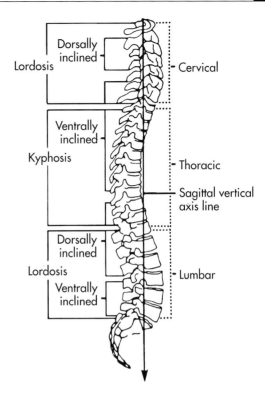

Fig. 38-166   Balance of sagittal contour depends on sagittal vertical axis. Each vertebra has unique orientation and spatial relationship to apical vertebra. (From Hammerberg KW: Kyphosis. In Bridwell KH, DeWald RL, eds: *The textbook of spinal surgery,* Philadelphia, 1991, JB Lippincott.)

compressive forces, and the posterior ligamentous structures resist tensile forces.

Kyphosis of 50 degrees or more in the thoracic spine usually is considered abnormal. Kyphotic deformity may occur if the anterior spinal column is unable to withstand compression, causing shortening of the anterior column. Disruption of the posterior column and inability to resist tension can lead to relative lengthening of the posterior column. Abnormal kyphosis is corrected by surgically shortening the posterior column or lengthening the anterior column or both.

Scheuermann Disease

Scheuermann disease is a structural kyphosis of the thoracic or thoracolumbar spine that occurs in 0.4% to 8.3% of the general population. It occurs slightly more often males. An increased frequency of the condition has been demonstrated in some families; however, no specific form of inheritance has been confirmed.

ETIOLOGY

The cause of Scheuermann disease is probably multifactorial. Scheuermann proposed that the kyphosis resulted from avascular necrosis of the ring apophysis of the vertebral body. Bick and Copel, however, demonstrated that the ring apophysis lies outside the true cartilaginous physis and contributes nothing to the longitudinal growth of the body; therefore a disturbance in the ring apophysis should not affect growth of the vertebra or cause vertebral wedging. In 1930 Schmorl suggested that the vertebral wedging was caused by herniation of disc material into the vertebral body; these herniations now are known as *Schmorl nodes*. Schmorl theorized that as the disc material is extruded into the vertebral body, the height of the intervertebral disc is diminished, which causes increased pressure anteriorly and disturbances of enchondral growth of the vertebral body and subsequent wedging. However, Schmorl nodes are relatively common and frequently occur in patients with no evidence of Scheuermann disease. Ferguson implicated the persistence of anterior vascular grooves in the vertebral bodies during preadolescence and adolescence. He suggested that these vascular defects create a point of structural weakness in the vertebral body, which leads to wedging and kyphosis.

Bradford and Moe investigated the gross and histological changes in two patients with Scheuermann kyphosis and found that the anterior longitudinal ligament was thickened and created a bowstring across the apex of the kyphosis. Disc material had been pushed out under this ligament, the bodies had become severely compressed, and the disc space was narrowed. Histological and electron microscopic examination showed normal bone, cartilage, and disc. The ring apophysis showed no definite avascular necrosis. Protrusion of disc material into the bony spongiosa of the vertebral body was noted. Based on the observations, with data obtained with the indices of Singh et al., Bradford et al. suggested that osteoporosis may be responsible for the development of Scheuermann disease. Lopez et al. noted a similar association between osteoporosis and Scheuermann disease on dual photon absorptiometry. Using quantitative CT Gilsanz et al. found no difference in vertebral bone density in a group of trauma patients and teenagers with Scheuermann disease. In a study of cadaver vertebrae, Scoles, Latimer, and Digiovanni also found no evidence of osteoporosis with single photon absorptiometric analysis.

Mechanical factors are a likely cause of Scheuermann disease. Lambrinudi and others suggested that the upright posture and the tightness of the anterior longitudinal ligament of the spine contribute to the deformity. Scheuermann kyphosis is more common in patients who do heavy lifting or manual labor. The fact that some correction of the kyphosis can be obtained by bracing that relieves pressure on the anterior vertebral regions also indicates that mechanical factors are important. The kyphosis probably causes increased pressure on the vertebral endplates anteriorly, causing uneven growth of the vertebral bodies as a response to the law of Wolff.

Aufdermaur and Spycher and Ippolito and Ponseti suggested that a biochemical abnormality of the collagen and matrix of the vertebral endplate cartilage may be important in the etiology. They found abnormal collagen fibers and a decrease in the ratio between collagen and proteoglycan in the matrix of the endplate cartilage in patients with Scheuermann disease.

In summary, no definitive cause of Scheuermann disease has been proved. The evidence suggests that it is unlikely to be caused solely by osteochondritis, avascular necrosis, hormonal abnormalities, osteoporosis, or growth aberrations. Likewise, conclusions regarding the genetic tendency of the condition cannot be made on the basis of current studies. Further research is required to better investigate the ultimate causes of Scheuermann disease.

CLINICAL FINDINGS

Scheuermann disease usually appears around the adolescent growth spurt. The presenting complaints are either pain in the middle or lower back or concern over posture. Frequently the parents believe that the kyphosis is postural, so diagnosis and treatment are delayed. Pain usually is located in the area of the deformity or in the lower back, is made worse by activity, and typically subsides with the cessation of growth. If pain is present in the lumbar area and the deformity is in the thoracic region, the possibility of spondylolysis should be considered.

Physical examination shows an angular thoracic or thoracolumbar kyphosis with compensatory hyperlordosis of the lumbar spine. The kyphosis is sharply angular and does not correct with the prone extension test (Fig. 38-167). The lumbar lordosis below the kyphosis usually is flexible and corrects with forward bending. Tight hamstrings and pectoral muscles are common. On forward bending, minimal structural scoliosis is present in as many as 30% of patients.

Physical findings in patients with lumbar Scheuermann disease may differ from those in patients with thoracic deformity. These patients usually have low back pain but, unlike patients with the more common form of Scheuermann disease, they do not have a noticeable deformity. Pain with spinal movement is the primary symptom. The condition is especially common in males involved in competitive athletics and in farm laborers, suggesting that it represents an injury to the vertebral physes from repeated trauma rather than true Scheuermann disease.

Neurological abnormalities usually are not present, but spinal cord compression from kyphosis, thoracic disc herniation, and epidural cysts have been reported occasionally. If lower extremity weakness, hyperreflexia, sensory changes, or other neurological findings are detected, MRI of the kyphotic area should be done.

ROENTGENOGRAPHIC FINDINGS

The criteria for the diagnosis of Scheuermann disease are more than 5 degrees of wedging of at least three adjacent vertebrae at the apex of the kyphosis and vertebral endplate irregularities with a thoracic kyphosis of more than 45 degrees (Fig. 38-168). On a lateral roentgenogram made with the patient standing, the degree of wedging is measured by drawing a line along the superior and inferior endplates of each vertebral body and

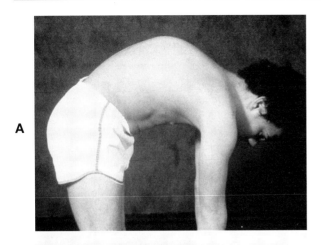

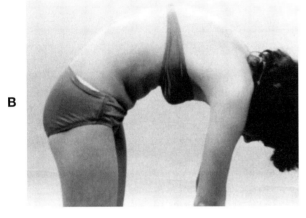

Fig. 38-167 **A,** Scheuermann kyphosis. **B,** Postural kyphosis.

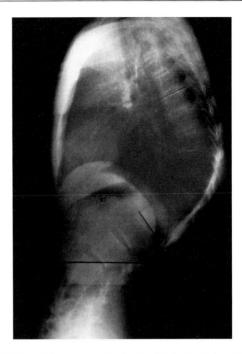

Fig. 38-168 Scheuermann kyphosis. Kyphotic deformity of 81 degrees and Schmorl nodes.

measuring the angle of intersection. Because the upper thoracic spine (T1 to T5) cannot always be seen on a routine lateral roentgenogram, abnormal kyphosis should be considered in a curve measuring more than 35 degrees from T5 to T12, and additional, better quality, lateral thoracic roentgenograms should be obtained.

Scoliosis is evident on posteroanterior roentgenograms in approximately a third of patients. A lateral roentgenogram should be made with the patient in the hyperextended position over a bolster to determine the structural nature of the deformity.

Two curve patterns occur in patients with thoracic Scheuermann disease. The most common type extends from T1 or T2 to T12 or L1 with the apex of the curve between T6 and T8. The second type extends from T4 or T5 to L2 or L3, with the apex of this curve at or near the thoracolumbar junction. The thoracolumbar pattern generally is more flexible because of a lack of support of the thoracic rib cage. Lowe noted that this type is more likely to be progressive and become painful in adult life.

Scheuermann disease of the lumbar spine is characterized by irregularity of the vertebral endplates, the presence of Schmorl nodes, and narrowing of the intervertebral discs,

without wedging of the vertebral bodies or kyphosis. Late degenerative changes such as disc space narrowing and Schmorl's nodes occur as in Scheuermann disease of the thoracic spine.

NATURAL HISTORY

In most cases, Scheuermann disease results in minimal deformity and few symptoms. Several investigators believe that untreated Scheuermann disease continues to progress throughout the adolescent growth period. Bradford et al. noted progression in 96 of 168 patients before brace treatment was instituted. Back pain and fatigue are common complaints during adolescence but usually disappear with skeletal maturity. Factors that contribute to the risk of continued progression of kyphosis include the number of years of growth remaining and the number of wedged vertebrae. Neurological injury occasionally has been reported in adolescents because of herniation of a thoracic disc, an epidural cyst, or the severe kyphotic deformity alone with subsequent compression of the cord.

The true natural history of untreated Scheuermann disease in adulthood is not well established. Travaglini and Conte found that the kyphosis increased during adulthood in 80% of their patients, although few developed severe deformity. During middle-age, degenerative spondylosis is common, but roentgenographic findings do not always correlate with the presence or absence of back pain. If the kyphosis is less than 60 degrees, these changes usually do not occur in adulthood.

Murray, Weinstein, and Sprall evaluated 67 patients with Scheuermann kyphosis and a mean angle of kyphosis of 71 degrees at an average follow-up of 32 years. They were compared with a control group of 34 subjects who were matched for age and sex. The group with Scheuermann kyphosis had more intense back pain, jobs that tended to have lower requirements for activity, loss of extension of the trunk, and different localization of pain. No significant differences between the patients and the control subjects were seen in level of education, number of days absent from work because of back pain, pain that interfered with activities of daily living, self-esteem, social limitations, use of medication for back pain, or level of recreational activities. The patients reported little preoccupation with their physical appearances. Normal or above-normal averages of pulmonary function were found in patients in whom the kyphosis was less than 100 degrees. Murray et al. concluded that patients who have Scheuermann kyphosis may have some functional limitations that do not significantly affect their lives. Patients who did not have surgery for the kyphosis adapted reasonably well to their condition.

Lumbar Scheuermann disease, which usually is associated with strenuous physical activity, generally becomes asymptomatic within several months after restriction of activities. It has not been shown to have any long-term sequelae in adult life, as long as those affected avoid strenuous jobs.

DIFFERENTIAL DIAGNOSIS

The most common entity to be differentiated from Scheuermann disease is postural round-back deformity. This deformity characteristically produces a slight increase in thoracic kyphosis, which is mobile clinically and is easily correctable on the prone-extension test. Roentgenograms show normal vertebral body contours without vertebral wedging. The kyphosis is more gradual than the angular kyphosis commonly seen in Scheuermann disease. The presence of a normal roentgenogram, however, may not rule out the presence of Scheuermann disease because roentgenographic changes may not be apparent until a child is 10 to 12 years of age.

If pain is a presenting symptom, infectious spondylitis must be considered. This usually can be excluded, however, by clinical and laboratory studies and tomograms or bone scans of the spine. Occasionally, traumatic injuries can confuse the differential diagnosis, but usually the wedging caused by a compression fracture involves only a single vertebra rather than the three or more vertebrae involved in true Scheuermann kyphosis. Osteochondrodystrophies, such as Morquio and Hurler syndromes, as well as tumors and congenital deformities, especially congenital kyphosis, also must be considered. In young men, ankylosing spondylitis must be ruled out, and this may require an HLA B-27 blood test.

The treatment of adolescents with Scheuermann disease generally consists of observation (with or without an exercise program), bracing, or surgery.

NONOPERATIVE TREATMENT

Observation

Adolescents with mildly increased kyphosis of less than 50 degrees without evidence of progression can be followed up with repeat standing lateral roentgenograms every 4 to 6 months. When growth is complete, further follow-up is not needed. Exercises alone have not been shown to provide any correction of the deformity in patients with Scheuermann disease. An exercise program, however, can help to maintain flexibility, correct lumbar lordosis, and strengthen the extensor muscles of the spine. Stretching exercises should be prescribed for patients with associated tightness of the hamstring or pectoralis muscles. Patients with lumbar Scheuermann disease and back pain should avoid heavy lifting and should be placed on an exercise program for the lower back.

Orthotic Treatment

Thoracic type Scheuermann kyphosis (apex T6 to T8) of more than 50 degrees in skeletally immature patients is managed with a Milwaukee brace. If the treatment is instituted before skeletal maturity, the kyphosis usually can be corrected. Bradford et al. reported 35% improvement in lumbar lordosis and 49% improvement in thoracic kyphosis in teenagers with Scheuermann kyphosis who were treated with full-time Milwaukee bracing for an average of 14 months, followed by an average of 18 months of part-time bracing. At long-term follow-up some loss of correction had occurred, but 69% of patients had improvement from the initial kyphosis. If the kyphosis exceeded 75 degrees, the wedging of the vertebral bodies was more than 10 degrees, and the patient was near or past skeletal maturity, the results were much poorer. Montgomery and Erwin reported long-term results in 21 patients who were treated with full-time Milwaukee bracing for an average of 18 months, followed by part-time bracing for an average of 6 months. The initial kyphosis improved about 30%, but final kyphosis correction averaged only 10%.

The Milwaukee brace functions as a dynamic three-point orthosis that promotes extension of the thoracic spine. The neck ring maintains proper alignment of the upper thoracic spine, and the padded posterior uprights apply pressure over the apex of the kyphosis. The pelvic girdle stabilizes the lumbar spine by flattening the lumbar lordosis. The occipital pads serve as a fulcrum to provide active extension of the spine at night as the neck is extended during sleep.

Although the Milwaukee brace has been shown to effectively prevent kyphosis progression and offers some modest permanent correction, full-time brace wear often is resisted by the adolescent. Gutowski and Renshaw found that the Boston lumbar kyphosis orthosis was satisfactory for correction of curves of less than 70 degrees and had better compliance. They recommended the Boston lumbar orthosis as an acceptable alternative to the Milwaukee brace in patients with flexible kyphotic curves of less than 70 degrees and in whom compliance may be a problem. The Milwaukee brace should be used in patients with larger curves or in patients who do not achieve satisfactory correction with the Boston lumbar orthosis. The rationale for the Boston lumbar orthosis is that reduction of the lumbar lordosis will cause the patient to dynamically straighten the thoracic kyphosis to maintain an upright posture. This presupposes a flexible kyphosis, a normal neurovestibular axis, and the absence of hip flexion contractures.

Lowe used a modified underarm, thoracolumbosacral orthosis with padded anterior, infraclavicular outriggers for patients with thoracolumbar-pattern Scheuermann disease (apex T9 and below) and found that it was as effective as the Milwaukee brace and was cosmetically more acceptable to patients.

Hyperextension casting has been used with excellent results in Europe but has not been popular in the United States because of problems with the skin, restrictions of physical activity, and the need for frequent cast changes.

OPERATIVE TREATMENT

Operative treatment occasionally is necessary for patients with Scheuermann kyphosis. Because of reported sequelae in adulthood, including backache, embarrassment about physical appearance, interruption of work or disability, severe progressive deformity, cardiopulmonary failure, spondylolisthesis, disc degeneration, and interference with recreational activities, many authors have recommended operative treatment in adolescents in whom the deformity cannot be controlled by bracing, which generally includes patients with a very rigid kyphosis of more than 80 degrees. Lowe recommends consideration of operative treatment in adults with a kyphosis of 75 degrees or more and persistent disabling pain despite conservative management and in those who have an unacceptable cosmetic appearance. Our experience with Scheuermann kyphosis in adults is similar to that of Murray et al., and we usually reserve operative treatment for patients with pain and unacceptable deformity from excessive thoracic or thoracolumbar kyphosis. We strongly recommend the use of a Milwaukee brace in growing children. If the curve progresses beyond 80 degrees despite brace treatment, surgery is considered. In skeletally mature adolescents, the presence of back pain, the size of the kyphosis, and the cosmetic appearance are considered in the decision-making process. The patient must then weigh the potential risks of surgery against the expected results of nonoperative treatment.

Surgical treatment for Scheuermann disease generally combines anterior release with posterior instrumentation and fusion. If the patient is skeletally immature with anterior spinal growth remaining and the kyphosis corrects to less than 50 degrees on hyperextension lateral roentgenograms, a posterior instrumented fusion with the newer segmental instrumentation systems can be considered. Otherwise, a combined anterior and posterior procedure is done to provide anterior and posterior column load sharing. Bradford et al. reported loss of correction in 16 of 22 patients treated with posterior Harrington

instrumentation and fusion. Loss of correction was caused by the presence of a severe initial deformity, inadequate length of the fusion, severe wedging of the vertebral bodies, and contraction of the anterior longitudinal ligament.

In a later report of 24 patients with combined anterior release and posterior instrumentation and fusion, Bradford et al. listed as indications for combined anterior and posterior fusion kyphosis of more than 70 degrees in patients who are skeletally mature and who have pain that cannot be controlled by conservative methods.

Speck and Chopin also emphasized the importance of fusing the entire length of the kyphosis. The end vertebra should be the last vertebra from the apex that is tilted maximally into the concavity of the curve. Ideally, at least one vertebra above and one vertebra below should be added to the fusion. Anteriorly the fusion should include the most rigid apical segment of the curve as identified by comparison of the standing lateral roentgenogram and the hyperextension lateral roentgenogram.

Other instrumentation techniques have been used for correction of Scheuermann kyphosis. Sturm, Dobson, and Armstrong reported good results with posterior fusion alone using large, threaded Harrington compression rods rather than small ones. Coscia et al. reported an average 23-degree improvement with a combined anterior and posterior approach with Luque sublaminar wires and rods used posteriorly for internal fixation. However, junctional kyphosis above the instrumented area developed in 13 of their 19 patients, probably because the interspinous ligament and ligamentum flavum must be removed to allow wire passage. The Luque rods can translate the kyphosis posteriorly, but they cannot shorten the posterior column, which is an important aspect in treating kyphotic deformity.

Currently, posterior double-rod, multihook segmental instrumentation systems are the most commonly used systems for the operative treatment of Scheuermann disease. Clark and Shufflebarger and Lowe reported excellent correction with combined anterior and posterior operative approaches using Cotrel-Dubousset posterior instrumentation. The versatility of these newer instrumentation systems allows for variation in hook placement, rod contouring (which allows both frontal and sagittal balance to be achieved), and no postoperative mobilization. For an average patient with a flexible deformity, the basic construct should include a minimum of eight hooks above the apex and six hooks or fixation sites below the apex. Above the apex there normally are two double-level pediculotransverse process claws on each side, for a total of eight fixation points above the apex of the kyphosis. Laminar hooks are avoided if possible to avoid intrusion into the neural canal. In patients with significant osteopenia, however, laminar hooks may be required because of the inferior strength of the transverse processes. A pedicle hook is used on each side, one or two levels below the apex of the deformity. This hook is placed below the kyphosis so that when the rod is attached to the upper hooks and manipulated into this pedicle hook, the rod is levered on the apical lamina rather than the pedicle hook. In

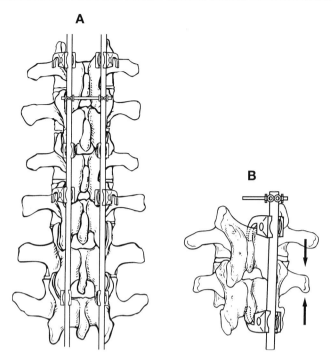

A

B

Fig. 38-169   **A,** Basic hook configuration above level of kyphosis in flexible kyphosis indicating two-level pedicle-transverse process claws on each side, for total of eight points of fixation above apex of kyphosis. **B,** Two-level laminar claw used at caudal end of instrumentation for Scheuermann's disease. These two hooks are combined with upgoing pedicle hooks, one or two levels below apex of deformity; consequently, total of six fixation points are used distally. (Redrawn from Sutterlin CE III: Occipitocervical and upper cervical methods of fusion and fixation. In Bridwell KH, DeWald RL, eds: *The textbook of spinal surgery,* ed 2, Philadelphia, 1997, Lippincott-Raven.)

adolescents, the distal end of the construct usually has a two-level laminar claw on each side. This then gives three hooks below the apex on each side of the spine. If a patient is osteopenic, pedicle screws can be substituted for the two distal hooks. Infralaminar hooks are added distally on each side to protect the most distal screws (Fig. 38-169).

◆ **Anterior Release and Fusion**

TECHNIQUE 38-40

The levels of the anterior release are those with the most wedging and the least flexibility on hyperextension lateral views. This region generally includes seven or eight interspaces centered on the apex of the kyphosis.

Select the appropriate anterior approach for the levels to be fused. If there is no associated scoliosis, make the approach through the left side. If there is a concomitant scoliosis, approach the spine on the convexity of the scoliosis; use the resected rib later for a bone graft. Release

the anterior longitudinal ligament and excise the entire disc and cartilaginous endplate, leaving only the posterior portion of the annulus and the posterior longitudinal ligament. Curet the bony endplates but do not remove them completely. Use a laminar spreader to loosen or mobilize each joint. Pack each disc space temporarily with Gelfoam or Surgicel to minimize blood loss. Perform an interbody fusion using the morselized rib graft.

◆ **Posterior Multihook Segmental Instrumentation**

TECHNIQUE 38-41

Place the patient prone on a Hall frame and make a posterior approach to the spine. (The instrumentation frequently extends proximally to T2 or T3.) Determine the apex of the kyphosis on preoperative roentgenograms. Use at least two sets of pediculotransverse process claws above the apex if the curve is flexible.

In very large patients with rigid curves, extra fixation sites may be needed, and a third set of pediculotransverse process claws can be used. If it is necessary to have three sets of hooks above the apex, use three single-level pediculotransverse process claws rather than double-level claws. Distal to the apex, use at least three hooks on each side (see Fig. 38-169). At the distal end of the instrumentation include not only the distal vertebra in the measured kyphosis but also the first lordotic vertebra. This vertebra is just caudad to the lordotic disc below the kyphotic deformity. Place the pediculotransverse claws proximally. Hammerberg recommended staggering the intermediate two pediculotransverse claws on either side of the spine above the apex to distribute the force at each level and increase segmental fixation. Staggering of the hooks allows easier access to at least one side of each vertebral body to apply bone graft for ultimate fusion. Below the apex, use pedicle hooks in the lower thoracic spine. In the lumbar spine, use laminar hooks of appropriate size.

Proper rod contouring is important. The amount of kyphosis placed in the rods is based on the hyperextension lateral roentgenogram. Do not correct the kyphosis more than 50% of the preoperative kyphosis, otherwise a proximal junctional kyphosis may occur. The upper end of the rod should have an additional kyphotic bend for insertion into the most superior transverse process hook. Contour lordosis, beginning at the thoracolumbar junction.

Insert the upper end of the rod into the proximal hooks. Then compress each claw to ensure that each hook remains seated. Tighten the threaded plugs to hold the upper hooks securely into the rod and secure the claw. In compression of each level, start at the uppermost claw and continue toward the apex of the deformity. Insert the rod into the pedicle hook below the apex of the deformity and use the appropriate plug to hold the rod in the open hook (Fig. 38-170).

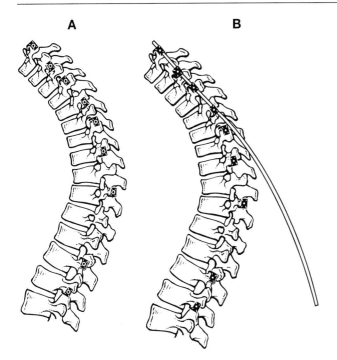

Fig. 38-170   Reduction of kyphosis, standard method. **A,** Insertion of hooks. Note three sets of pedicle–transverse claws above apex of kyphosis. **B,** Rod passed through hooks of proximal segment and distal end of rod is pushed to lower spine with rod pusher. Note that lower tip bend in rod facilitates hook insertion under distal lamina. (Redrawn from Sutterlin CE III: Occipitocervical and upper cervical methods of fusion and fixation. In Bridwell KH, DeWald RL, eds: *The textbook of spinal surgery,* ed 2, Philadelphia, 1997, Lippincott-Raven.)

Using a rod holder and spreader distal to the hook, apply compression toward the apex through this pedicle hook. Push the caudal end of the rod down to the spine and place it into the distal hooks. Apply compression to the distal hook with the rod holder and laminar spreader. Compress the downgoing laminar hook by spreading it distally. By seating the distal hook first, the posterior column is shortened and held fixed in the shortened position before the downgoing superior laminar hook is compressed.

Perform careful facet fusion and decortication and add abundant autogenous bone graft (Fig. 38-171).

AFTERTREATMENT. Unless the bone quality is poor and fixation is tenuous, postoperative bracing is not required. If there is any concern about fixation, an extension orthosis, such as a Jewett brace, is used until the fusion begins to consolidate, usually in 3 to 6 months. Ambulation is started as soon as possible. All patients are started on isometric and isotonic back exercise programs when the fusion appears solid. In adolescents, the fusion generally is solid in approximately 6 months. The patient generally is allowed to sit up on the second or third day after surgery.

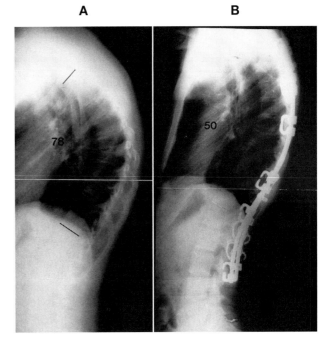

Fig. 38-171   **A,** Kyphosis of 78 degrees. **B,** After posterior fusion and multihook segmental instrumentation.

◆ ◆ ◆

Bradford described the use of four short rods to correct the kyphotic deformity by posterior compression and shortening rather than by three-point bending as produced by two long rods (Fig. 38-172). Cotrel-Dubousset or similar instrumentation is used.

◆ Four-Rod Instrumentation

TECHNIQUE 38-42 *(Bradford)*
The same proximal and distal hook patterns are used as in the single-rod technique (see Fig. 38-169). Place the proximal hooks above the apex of the deformity, beginning at the most proximal vertebra in the kyphosis. Insert the distal hook(s) and pedicle screws. Contour the upper rod to the corrected upper half of the kyphotic curve and pass through all of the hooks above the apex of the deformity. Contour the lower rod to fit the lower half of the corrected kyphosis, as well as the lumbar lordosis, and place in the hook(s) and screws below the apex. Cut the rods to length so that they overlap approximately 1 inch near the apex of the deformity. Bring the overlapping ends of the rods together and secure with wide CD domino-type connectors. Using a rod holder and spreader, apply compression alternately to each side of the deformity, causing the rods to overlap progressively until the deformity is corrected. After the wake-up test is done, finish tightening the hook plugs. If necessary, add additional cross links for support.

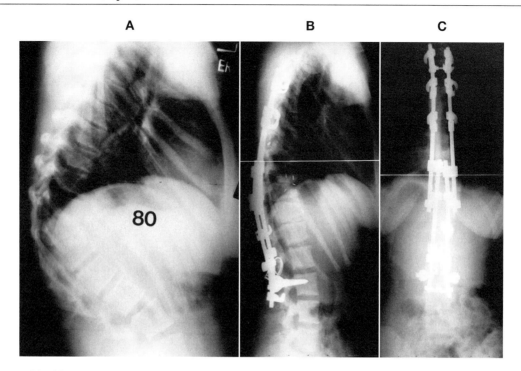

Fig. 38-172 **A,** Kyphosis of 80 degrees. **B** and **C,** After posterior fusion and instrumentation with four rods connected by domino cross links.

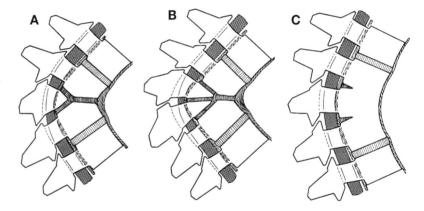

Fig. 38-173 Classification of congenital kyphosis. **A** and **B,** Type I, **C,** Type II. (Type III not shown.) (From Winter RB, Moe JH, Wang JF: *J Bone Joint Surg* 55A:223, 1973.)

Congenital Kyphosis

Kyphosis of the spine caused by congenital vertebral anomalies is uncommon, although it can cause significant deformities and disabilities. Winter et al. reported 130 patients with congenital kyphosis and described three types. Type I is congenital failure of vertebral body formation. Type II is failure of vertebral body segmentation (Fig. 38-173). Type III is a combination of both of these conditions. McMaster and Singh further subdivided type I congenital kyphosis into posterolateral quadrant vertebrae, posterior hemivertebrae, butterfly (sagittal cleft) vertebrae, and anterior or anterolateral wedged vertebrae (Fig. 38-174). This classification is important in predicting the natural history of these congenital kyphotic deformities.

Type I deformities are more common than type II deformities and occur more commonly in the thoracic spine and at the thoracolumbar junction. They are extremely rare in the cervical spine. In the series of McMaster and Singh, progression was most rapid in type III kyphosis, followed by type I. Kyphosis caused by two adjacent type I vertebral anomalies progressed more rapidly and produced a more severe deformity than did a single anomaly. Approximately 25% of patients with type I deformities had neurological deficits, and deformities in the upper thoracic spine were more likely to be associated with neurological problems. No patient in whom the apex of the kyphosis was at or caudad to the twelfth thoracic vertebra had neurological abnormalities. However, McMaster and Singh found that type I kyphosis progressed relentlessly during growth and usually accelerated during the adolescent growth

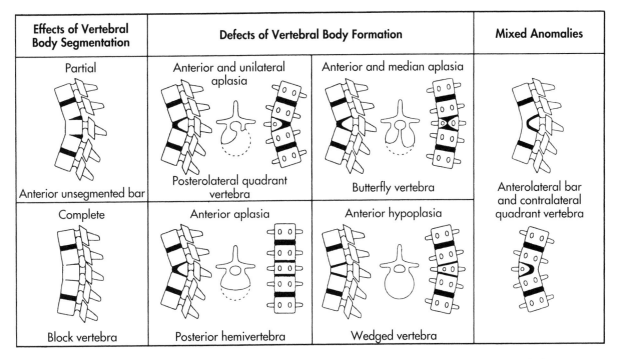

Effects of Vertebral Body Segmentation	Defects of Vertebral Body Formation		Mixed Anomalies
Partial	Anterior and unilateral aplasia	Anterior and median aplasia	
	Posterolateral quadrant vertebra	Butterfly vertebra	Anterolateral bar and contralateral quadrant vertebra
Anterior unsegmented bar			
Complete	Anterior aplasia	Anterior hypoplasia	
Block vertebra	Posterior hemivertebra	Wedged vertebra	

Fig. 38-174 Drawing showing different types of vertebral anomalies that produce a congenital kyphosis or kyphoscoliosis. (From McMaster MJ, Singh H: *J Bone Joint Surg* 81A:1369, 1999).

spurt before stabilizing at skeletal maturity. An anterior failure of vertebral body formation produces a sharply angular kyphosis that is much more deforming and potentially dangerous neurologically than a curve with a similar Cobb measurement owing to an anterior failure of segmentation that affects several adjacent vertebrae and produces a smooth, less obvious deformity.

Type II deformities (failure of segmentation) are less common. An absence of physes and discs anteriorly in one or more vertebrae results in the development of an anterior unsegmented bar. The amount of kyphosis produced is proportional to the discrepancy between the amounts of growth in the anterior and posterior portions of the defective vertebral segments. Mayfield et al. reported that these deformities progress at an average rate of 5 degrees a year and are not as severe as type I deformities. Paraplegia did not occur in any of their patients with type II kyphosis. This also was true in studies by Winter and McMaster. Low back pain and cosmetic deformities were, however, significant problems in Mayfield et al.'s report, and early treatment was warranted.

CLINICAL AND ROENTGENOGRAPHIC EVALUATION

An evaluation similar to that for congenital scoliosis should be done for every patient with congenital kyphosis, with special attention to the neurological evaluation. Genitourinary abnormalities, cardiac anomalies, Klippel-Feil syndrome, and intraspinal abnormalities are frequent in these patients. Cardiac evaluation and renal ultrasonography should be done, as well as evaluation of the spinal canal with MRI and an occasional myelogram in patients with neurological abnormalities or for whom operative correction is considered. Winter et al. emphasized that the patient should be placed supine for the myelogram evaluation so that the contrast medium pools at the apex of the kyphosis. If scoliosis is present, the patient must be turned to a semilateral position to place the convexity of the kyphoscoliosis in a dependent position.

In the series of McMaster and Singh, only 1 patient of 51 with congenital kyphosis was found to have an occult, congenital intraspinal anomaly on myelogram or MRI. In contrast, incidence rates of intraspinal anomalies in congenital scoliosis have been reported to be from 6% to as high as 58%. These authors postulated that the disparity is due to the fact that vertebral anomalies responsible for congenital scoliosis appear during the mesenchymal period, when the spinal cord is also developing, whereas vertebral anomalies responsible for congenital kyphosis occur during the late chondrification and ossification periods, when the basic anatomy of the neural structures already has been established.

OPERATIVE TREATMENT

As shown by Winter et al., treatment of congenital kyphosis with an orthosis is ineffective. The operative procedure depends on the type of deformity, the severity of the deformity, the age of the patient, and the presence or absence of neurological symptoms.

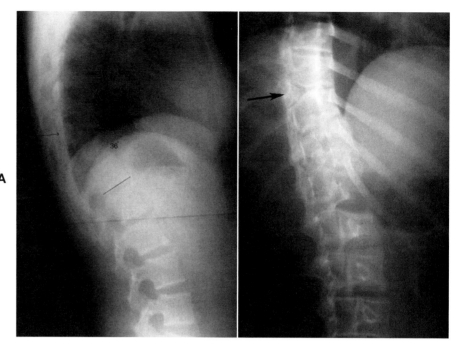

Fig. 38-175 **A** and **B,** Type I congenital kyphosis (defect of formation). **A**

B

Early detection and prompt treatment of type I deformities are essential (Fig. 38-175). For type I deformities, a Moe-type posterior fusion is appropriate in patients younger than 5 years of age with a supine lateral deformity of less than 50 degrees. In this patient population a solid posterior arthrodesis allows any remaining anterior physes to continue to grow, which may result in some degree of spontaneous reduction of the kyphosis over the growing years (Fig. 38-176). Only the vertebrae to be fused should be exposed, including pathological vertebrae plus one healthy vertebra proximal and distal. If available, autogenous bone is preferable, but allograft bone can be used. Postoperatively, the patient is placed in a corrective cast. Winter recommended that the patient remain at bed rest for 4 months, after which ambulation is allowed in a Risser cast. If at 6 months the solidity of the fusion is uncertain, the area is inspected surgically and bone graft is added after decortication of the fusion mass. The child may require casting for up to 12 months.

For children older than 5 years of age with type I deformity, combined anterior and posterior fusion generally is required. Winter et al. reported 94 patients 5 years of age or older with type I kyphosis and found that thoracic or thoracolumbar kyphosis of 55 degrees or less could be stabilized successfully by posterior fusion alone. If the kyphosis was more than 55 degrees or the patient was skeletally mature, both anterior and posterior fusions were required. We have found that, because of the progressive nature of type I kyphotic deformities, most children over the age of 5 years have curves that require anterior and posterior fusions. In these procedures, the spine is approached anteriorly, and the shortened ligaments, fibrous tissue, and cartilaginous remnants are removed. Autogenous bone graft is then positioned to support the anterior column. Vertebrectomy is unnecessary unless there are problems of

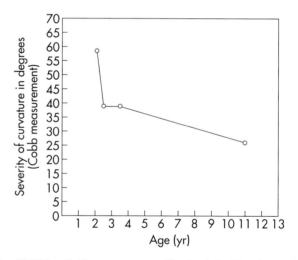

Fig. 38-176 Cobb measurement of kyphosis in 17 patients with congenital kyphosis having only posterior fusion before age 5 years. After initial significant improvement resulting from hyperextension cast, improvement was slow and steady as a result of posterior growth arrest combined with continued anterior growth. (From Winter RB, Moe JH: *J Bone Joint Surg* 64A:419, 1982.)

spinal cord compression. Once the discectomy is completed, the spine becomes much more flexible, and an anterior strut can be inserted while the assistant manually applies correction over the apex of the deformity (Fig. 38-177). Autogenous bone is then packed into all the spaces around the strut graft. The posterior procedure must encompass the entire length of the affected vertebrae and at least one normal vertebra above and one below. The posterior fusion is always slightly longer than the anterior fusion. Autogenous bone graft is recommended as

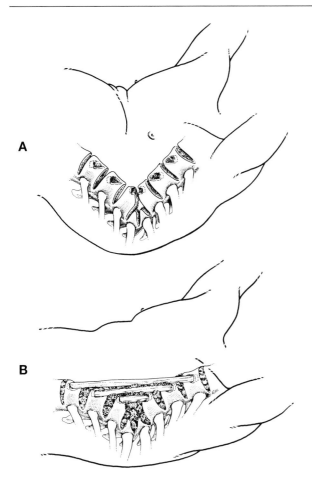

Fig. 38-177 **A,** Preparation of tunnels for strut grafts. **B,** Insertion of strut grafts into pre-prepared tunnels with cancellous bone graft in disc spaces. (Redrawn from Bradford DS et al: *Moe's textbook of scoliosis and other spinal deformities,* ed 2, Philadelphia, 1987, WB Saunders.)

graft material. If possible, internal fixation is used posteriorly. Only compression-type instrumentation is used; distraction should never be used. Traction also should not be used in patients with type I deformities because it is associated with a high incidence of paraplegia. If pediatric-size posterior instrumentation is used, generally it is supplemented with a Milwaukee brace and bed rest. If larger-size, more stable, multihook segmental instrumentation systems can be used, external support may not be needed. Patients with major neurological deficits require anterior spinal cord decompression with anterior and posterior fusions (Technique 38-44). Laminectomy is contraindicated in patients with type I kyphosis. If a patient has minor spinal cord compression with hyperactive reflexes and clonus only, the anterior release and correction often realigns the spinal canal enough to relieve the cord pressure.

Mayfield et al. outlined a treatment plan for congenital kyphosis caused by defects of anterior segmentation (type II) (Fig. 38-178). In younger children, progression of the deformity can be halted by posterior fusion extending from one

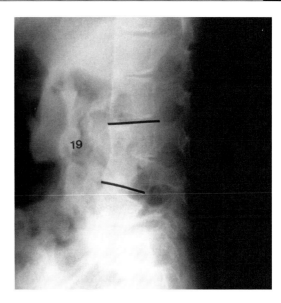

Fig. 38-178 Congenital kyphosis caused by anterior unsegmented bar.

vertebral segment above to one below the measured curve. In adolescents, mild to moderate thoracic deformities (up to 50 degrees) usually can be stabilized by posterior fusion with instrumentation that applies compression and shortens the posterior spinal column. In juveniles in whom instrumentation cannot be used, rigid immobilization in a cast for at least 1 year is recommended. Patients with severe kyphotic deformities require a combined anterior and posterior approach, including osteotomies of all levels of the anterior bar and anterior and posterior arthrodeses. The anterior osteotomies and interbody fusions extend the length of the kyphotic curve. In a second stage, posterior fusion is done with compression-type instrumentation to allow shortening of the posterior column. The posterior fusion should extend one to two levels beyond the ends of the kyphotic curve. With this technique, the anterior column is lengthened, the posterior column is shortened, and the middle column acts as a hinge.

◆ Anterior Osteotomy and Fusion

TECHNIQUE 38-43 *(Winter et al.)*

Expose the spine through an appropriate anterior approach (Chapter 34). Ligate the segmental vessels and expose the spine by subperiosteal stripping (Fig. 38-179, *A*). The anterior longitudinal ligament usually is thickened and must be divided at one or more levels. Make sure that a circumferential exposure is made all the way to the opposite foramen before beginning the osteotomy. Divide the bony bar with a sharp osteotome or high-speed burr. Start the division anteriorly and work posteriorly until the remaining disc material is entered. Once the remaining disc material is seen, use a laminar spreader and excise the disc material

continued

back to the level of the posterior longitudinal ligament (Fig. 38-179, *B*). If the bony bar is complete, make the osteotomy all the way through the posterior cortex at the level of the foramina. Take care in the area of the posterior longitudinal ligament because the ligament may be absent. Once the osteotomies have been completed, insert strut grafts, slotting them into bodies above and below the area of the kyphos. Hollow out the cancellous bone of each body with a curet. Using rib, fibula, or iliac crest grafts of sufficient length, insert the upper end of the graft into the slot first. As manual pressure is applied posteriorly against the kyphos, use an impactor to tap the lower end of the graft into place. Place additional grafts in the disc space defects and close the pleura over them if possible. More than one strut graft may be necessary, depending on the severity of the curve. The grafts should be placed as far anterior to the axis of the flexion deformity as possible.

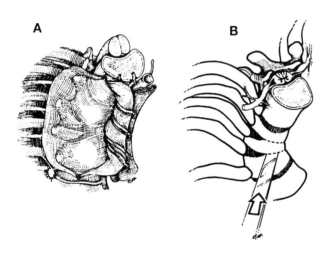

Fig. 38-179 **A,** Anterolateral exposure of spine in preparation for anterior osteotomy. **B,** Completion of osteotomy with osteotome. (Redrawn from Bradford DS et al: *Moe's textbook of scoliosis and other spinal deformities,* ed 2, Philadelphia, 1987, WB Saunders.)

Winter et al. found that failures of anterior fusion in their patients generally were associated with strut grafts that were too short or were placed too close to the apex of the kyphosis or with inadequate removal of the intervertebral discs in the fusion area.

In 42 patients with kyphosis and neurological deficits, Lonstein et al. found that except for a few flexible (and noncongenital) kyphoses, anterior decompression and fusion followed by a second-stage posterior fusion gave the best results. They recommended hyperextension roentgenograms in patients with paraparesis or paraplegia to differentiate a flexible from a rigid kyphosis. If the kyphosis is flexible, the patient may be placed in skeletal traction, with careful neurological monitoring. It should be noted, however, that in the series of Lonstein et al. most patients in this category had neurofibromatosis and not a type I congenital kyphosis. If the kyphosis is rigid, as is usually the case in type I kyphosis, and the patient's neurological deficit is significant, the best approach is anterior spinal cord decompression and fusion followed by a posterior fusion.

◆ Anterior Cord Decompression and Fusion

TECHNIQUE 38-44 *(Winter and Lonstein)*
Expose the spine through an appropriate anterior approach. Identify the apical vertebra and the site of compression and remove the intervertebral disc completely on each side of the vertebral body or bodies. Remove the vertebral body laterally at the apex of the kyphosis, using curets, rongeurs, or high-speed burrs. Remove the cancellous bone back to the posterior cortex of the vertebral body from pedicle to pedicle, removing a wedge-shaped area of bone (Fig. 38-180, *A*). Beginning on the side away from the surgeon, use angled curets to remove the posterior cortical shell. Removing the bone farthest away first prevents the spinal cord from falling into the defect and blocking vision on the far side (Fig. 38-180, *B*). Next, remove the closest

Fig. 38-180 **A,** Anterolateral exposure of spine and partial removal of apex of kyphosis. **B,** Posterior cortex is removed, allowing decompression of spinal cord. **C,** Cord is decompressed and strut grafts are in place. (Redrawn from Bradford DS et al: *Moe's textbook of scoliosis and other spinal deformities,* ed 2, Philadelphia, 1987, WB Saunders.)

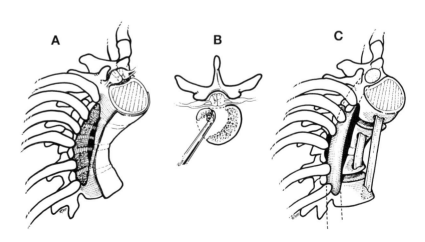

bony shell, working toward the apex. Control epidural bleeding with thrombin-soaked Gelfoam. Once the cord has been decompressed, perform an anterior strut graft fusion (Fig. 38-180, *C*). Close and drain the incision in the routine manner.

At a second stage, a posterior fusion with or without instrumentation is done. Before surgery a myelogram is necessary to rule out conditions such as tethered cord and diastematomyelia. In patients with congenital kyphosis and neurological deficits, definitely localizing the area of compression before surgery is helpful (Fig. 38-181).

◆ ◆ ◆

Bradford et al. noted frequent fracture of strut grafts when the grafts were not in contact with the vertebral bodies and simply spanned an open area between vertebrae. A rib or fibular graft may take up to 2 years for replacement, and it is weakest approximately 6 months after surgery. To prevent graft fracture,

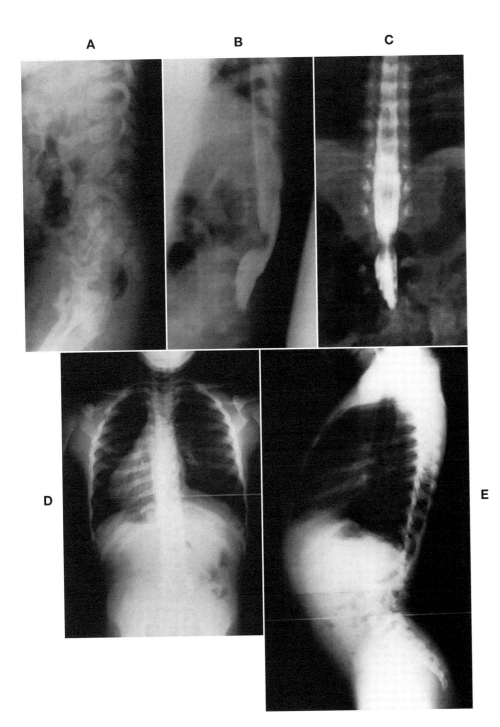

A   **B**   **C**

D   **E**

Fig. 38-181 **A** to **C,** Preoperative lateral roentgenogram and myelogram of young child with type I congenital kyphosis with neurological involvement of the lower extremities; myelogram indicates area of compression of cauda equina. **D** and **E,** Solid anterior fusion 8 years after excision of hemivertebra and anterior strut grafting.

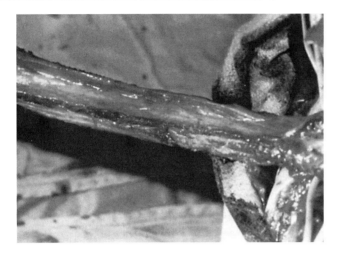

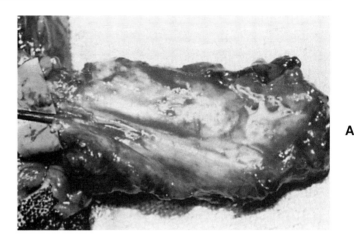

A

Fig. 38-182 Intraoperative photograph of harvest of vascularized rib. Caudal intercostal muscle is retained with rib. Towel clip anchors most distal aspect of graft. (From Shaffer JW, Bradford DS: The use of and techniques for vascularized rib pedicle grafts. In Bridwell KH, DeWald RL, eds: *The textbook of spinal surgery,* ed 2, Philadelphia, 1997, Lippincott-Raven.)

Bradford developed a technique of vascular pedicle bone graft for the treatment of severe kyphosis when the strut must be placed more than 4 cm from the spine. He credits Rose et al. with first describing the technique in 1975.

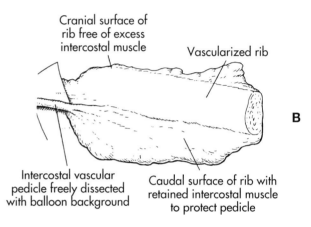

B

Cranial surface of rib free of excess intercostal muscle

Vascularized rib

Intercostal vascular pedicle freely dissected with balloon background

Caudal surface of rib with retained intercostal muscle to protect pedicle

Fig. 38-183 Intraoperative photographs of harvest of vascularized rib. **A** and **B,** Background balloon placed behind intercostal vascular pedicle. Ordinarily, it is not necessary to dissect out vascular pedicle. *Continued*

◆ Anterior Vascular Rib Bone Grafting

TECHNIQUE 38-45 *(Bradford)*

Plan the thoracotomy to remove enough rib to bridge the kyphosis. For a severe kyphotic deformity from T6 to T12, a vascularized fifth rib would be used to strut the deformity. Make a skin incision as in the routine transthoracic exposure. Take care to identify the appropriate rib and avoid the use of electrocautery over the rib periosteum. Divide the intercostal muscles sharply off the cranial portion of the rib. This rib dissection is always extraperiosteal. Divide the rib distally to provide enough length to span the area of deformity. At the level of the distal rib osteotomy, ligate the intercostal vessels and sharply cut the intercostal nerve and allow it to retract. The intercostal muscles attached to the caudal portion of the rib should remain attached to provide protection for the intercostal vessels that will perfuse the rib (Fig. 38-182). At the level for the proximal rib osteotomy, mobilize the periosteum away from the rib. Once the osteotomy is completed, the rib is connected only to the caudal intercostal muscle and its intercostal vascular pedicle. Carefully divide the intercostal vessels below the rib in the direction of the costovertebral joint, retaining the

muscle around the intercostal pedicle. Do not dissect out the intercostal artery and vein. If the rib and muscle are poorly perfused, dissect the vascular pedicle away from the intercostal vessels (Fig. 38-183). Mobilize the rib with its intact intercostal musculature and artery and vein complex (Fig. 38-184, *A*). Carefully peel back the periosteum on the rib graft for 2 or 3 mm on each end to provide bone-to-bone contact without soft tissue intervention when the graft is rotated into position. Identify the vertebral bodies proximally and distally to be included in the fusion. Make a hole in the anterior aspect of the vertebral body above and below to accept the ends of the rib graft. Trim the rib so that the ends will match the length of the spine to be fused. Rotate the rib on its axis approximately 90 degrees and wedge it into the vertebrae above and below (Fig. 38-184, *B*). Close the chest in a routine fashion over chest tubes. Immobilization of the spine after vascular grafting is the same as after nonvascular graft procedures.

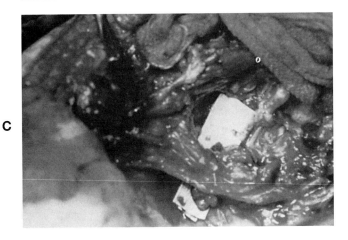

C

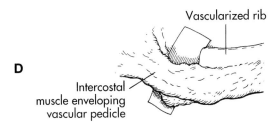

D

Vascularized rib

Intercostal muscle enveloping vascular pedicle

Fig. 38-183, cont'd   **C** and **D,** Retaining a portion of intercostal muscle with vessel as shown here reduces likelihood of pedicle injury during harvest. (From Shaffer JW, Bradford DS: The use of and techniques for vascularized rib pedicle grafts. In Bridwell KH, DeWald RL, eds: *The textbook of spinal surgery,* ed 2, Philadelphia, 1997, Lippincott-Raven.)

Spondylolysis and Spondylolisthesis

Herbiniaux, a Belgian obstetrician, noted a bony prominence in front of the sacrum that caused problems in delivery. He generally is credited with having first described spondylolisthesis. The term *spondylolisthesis* was used by Kilian in 1854 and is derived from the Greek *spondylos*, meaning vertebra, and *olisthesis*, meaning to slip or slide down a slippery path. Spondylolisthesis is defined as anterior or posterior slipping or displacement of one vertebra on another.

CLASSIFICATION

Wiltse, Newman, and Macnab's classification of spondylolisthesis (Fig. 38-185), based on the work of Neugebauer and Newman, is the most generally accepted (Box 38-9). Marchetti and Bartolozzi suggested that the Wiltse et al. classification is based on a mixture of etiological and topographical criteria, that it is difficult to predict progression or response to surgery with this classification, and that it also is difficult to identify the type of spondylolisthesis precisely. Therefore they have attempted to further classify spondylolisthesis, dividing the condition into developmental and acquired forms (Box 38-10). Their classification removes the isthmic or lysis part of spondylolisthesis from the primary role in causation and

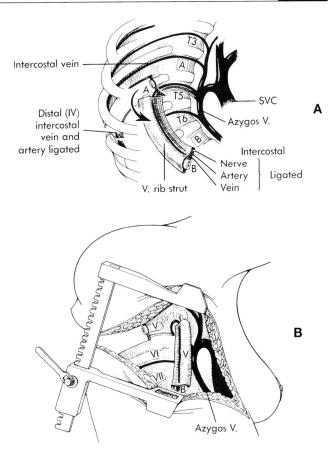

Fig. 38-184   Thoracotomy. **A,** Wide margin of intercostal muscle left attached to rib to ensure intact blood supply. **B,** Rib graft rotated 90 degrees on its axis and keyed into vertebral bodies over length of kyphosis to be fused. (Redrawn from Bradford DS: *Spine* 5:318, 1980.)

emphasizes the developmental and dysplastic aspects. When analyzing the spondylolisthesis, the surgeon must first decide if the condition is developmental or acquired. If it is developmental, the degree of dysplasia must be determined as high (severe) or low (mild) by evaluation of the quality of the posterior bony hook (Fig. 38-186). The degree of lordosis and the position of the gravity line also are important; the farther anterior the gravity line is, the more likely the spondylolisthesis is to increase. The competency of the disc at the level of the spondylolisthesis also is important; this may require an MRI to determine. Indications of an unstable situation include a significant localized kyphosis (high slip angle) of the slip. Bony changes such as a trapezoid-shaped L5 vertebral body and a dome-shaped sacrum also are indicative of instability and significant dysplasia. The implications of the classification system are that the more dysplastic and unstable the situation is, the more aggressive the surgical procedure should be to solve the problem.

Most spondylolistheses in children and adolescents are developmental. The child is born with a dysplastic bony hook. Once the child begins to ambulate, various mechanical forces take over. The pars is under increased stress and may stretch or

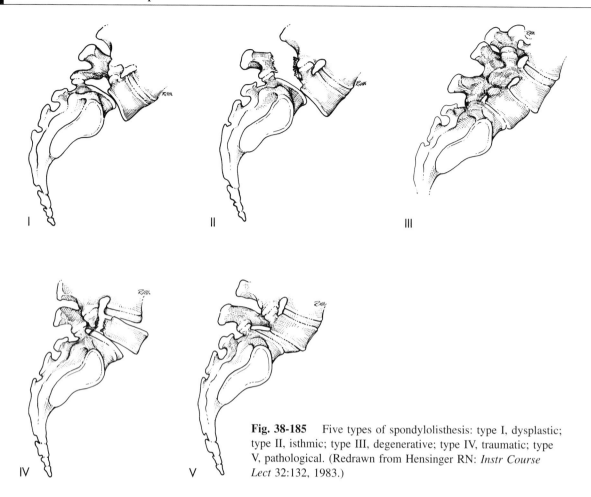

Fig. 38-185   Five types of spondylolisthesis: type I, dysplastic; type II, isthmic; type III, degenerative; type IV, traumatic; type V, pathological. (Redrawn from Hensinger RN: *Instr Course Lect* 32:132, 1983.)

BOX 38-9 • Classification of Spondylolisthesis

Type I. Dysplastic: Congenital abnormalities of the upper sacral facets or inferior facets of the fifth lumbar vertebra that allow slipping of L5 on S1. No pars interarticularis defect is present in this type.

Type II. Isthmic: Defect in the pars interarticularis that allows forward slipping of L5 on S1. Three types of isthmic spondylolistheses are recognized:

    Lytic—a stress fracture of the pars interarticularis

    An elongated but intact pars interarticularis

    An acute fracture of the pars interarticularis

Type III. Degenerative: This lesion results from intersegmental instability of a long duration with subsequent remodeling of the articular processes at the level of involvement.

Type IV. Traumatic: This type results from fractures in the area of the bony hook other than the pars interarticularis, such as the pedicle, lamina, or facet.

Type V. Pathological: This type results from generalized or localized bone disease and structural weakness of the bone such as osteogenesis imperfecta.

---

fracture. The disc is subsequently placed under increased stress, and early disc failure can occur. As these events occur, the situation becomes more unstable and progression results. If this unstable condition can be recognized early in children, early stabilization may prevent severe spondylolisthesis or spondyloptosis and avoid more extensive and riskier surgical interventions.

Developmental spondylolisthesis is the focus of this section. Acquired stress fracture–type spondylosis also is discussed. Acquired degenerative spondylolisthesis is discussed in Chapter 41.

ETIOLOGY AND NATURAL HISTORY

The prevalence of spondylolisthesis in the general population is approximately 5% and is about equal in men and women. Developmental spondylolisthesis with lysis seems to result from a stress fracture that occurs in children with a genetic predisposition for the defect. The defect has not been noted at birth or in chronically bedridden patients. Wiltse et al. postulated that lumbar lordosis is accentuated by the normal flexion contractures of the hip in childhood and that this posture places the weight-bearing forces on the pars interarticularis.

BOX 38-10 • Classification of Marchetti-Bartolozzi

DEVELOPMENTAL
High Dysplastic
With lysis
With elongation

Low Dysplastic
With lysis
With elongation

ACQUIRED
Traumatic
Acute fracture
Stress fracture

Postsurgery
Direct surgery
Indirect surgery

Pathological
Local pathology
Systemic path

Degenerative
Primary
Secondary

From DeWald RL: Spondylolisthesis. In Bridwell KH, DeWald RL, eds: *The textbook of spinal surgery,* ed 2, Philadelphia, 1997, JB Lippincott.

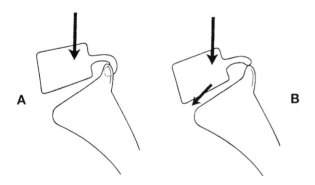

Fig. 38-186 **A,** Pedicle, pars interarticularis, inferior facets of L5, and sacral facets all form bony hook that prevents L5 vertebra from sliding forward along slope of sacral endplate. **B,** Figure demonstrates difference between normal bony hook and dysplastic bony hook that is incapable of providing resistance to forward slippage of the L5 vertebra under weight-bearing stresses in upright spine. (From DeWald RL: Spondylolisthesis. In Bridwell KH, DeWald RL, eds: *The textbook of spinal surgery,* ed 2, Philadelphia, 1997, Lippincott-Raven.)

Letts et al. suggested that shear stresses are greater on the pars interarticularis when the lumbar spine is extended. Cyron and Hutton found that the pars interarticularis is thinner and the vertebral disc is less resistant to shear in children and adolescents than in adults. It also is more common in certain types of athletes, such as female gymnasts. These observations indicate that the condition is acquired rather than congenital. However, as many as 50% of Eskimos are reported to have spondylolisthesis, whereas only 6% to 7% of white males and 1.1% of adult black females have the condition, indicating a definite genetic predisposition.

If increased slipping occurs, it usually occurs between the ages of 9 and 15 years and seldom after the age of 20 years. Fredrickson et al. studied 500 unselected first-grade children for approximately 20 years. They found a definite hereditary predisposition for the defect and a strong association with spina bifida occulta. Progression of the slip was unlikely after adolescence, and the slip was never symptomatic in their study population. Harris and Weinstein, in a long-term follow-up of untreated patients with grade III and grade IV spondylolistheses, found that 36% of patients were asymptomatic, 55% had mild symptoms, and only one patient had significant symptoms. All patients led active lives, and all had required only minor adjustments in their lifestyles. None were dissatisfied with their cosmetic appearance, and none stated that it had interfered with social or business relationships. In a similar group of patients treated with in situ posterior interlaminar arthrodeses, 57% were asymptomatic and 38% had mild symptoms.

CLINICAL FINDINGS

Spondylolysis and spondylolisthesis usually cause no symptoms in children, and many seek medical evaluation because of a postural deformity or gait abnormality. Pain most often occurs during the adolescent growth spurt and is predominantly backache, with only occasional leg pain. Symptoms are aggravated by high activity levels or competitive sports and are diminished by activity restriction and rest. The back pain probably results from instability of the affected segment, and the leg pain usually is related to irritation of the L5 nerve root.

The physical findings vary with the severity of the slip. With a significant slip, a step-off at the lumbosacral junction is palpable, motion of the lumbar spine is restricted, and hamstring tightness is evident on straight leg raising. As the vertebral body displaces anteriorly, the patient assumes a lordotic posture above the level of the slip to compensate for the displacement. The sacrum becomes more vertical, and the buttocks appear heart-shaped because of the sacral prominence (Fig. 38-187). With more severe slips the trunk becomes shortened and often leads to complete absence of the waistline. These children walk with a peculiar spastic gait, described as a "pelvic waddle" by Newman, because of the hamstring tightness and the lumbosacral kyphosis. Children, unlike adults, seldom have objective signs of nerve root compression, such as motor weakness, reflex change, or sensory deficit. Tight hamstrings often are the only positive physical finding.

Scoliosis is relatively common in younger patients with spondylolisthesis and is of three types: (1) sciatic, (2) olisthetic, or (3) idiopathic. Sciatic scoliosis is a lumbar curve caused by muscle spasm. Usually, this is not a structural curve, and it

A   **B**

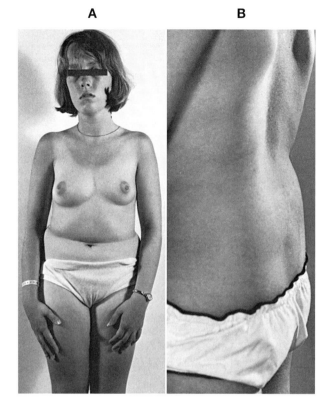

Fig. 38-187   Typical posture **(A)** and back contours **(B)** in adolescent with type III or IV spondylolisthesis. (From Hensinger RN: *Instr Course Lect* 32:132, 1983.)

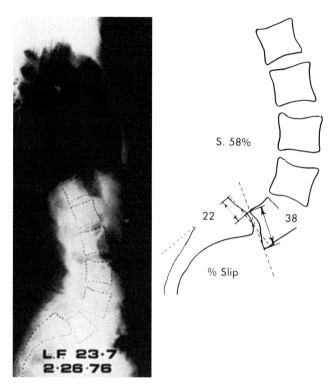

Fig. 38-188   Percentage of slipping calculated by measuring distance from line parallel to posterior portion of first sacral vertebral body to line parallel to posterior portion of body of L5; anteroposterior dimension of L5 inferiorly is used to calculate percentage of slipping. (From Boxall D et al: *J Bone Joint Surg* 61A:479, 1979.)

resolves with recumbency or relief of symptoms. Olisthetic scoliosis is a torsional lumbar curve with rotation that blends with the spondylolytic defect and results from asymmetrical slipping of the vertebra. These lumbar curves generally resolve after treatment of the spondylolisthesis. Severe curves, however, may become structural, and treatment is more complicated. Seitsalo et al. found that fusion of the lumbosacral area had no corrective effect on thoracic or thoracolumbar curves. When idiopathic scoliosis and spondylolisthesis occur together, they should be treated as separate problems.

ROENTGENOGRAPHIC FINDINGS

The key to diagnosis of spondylolysis and spondylolisthesis lies in routine roentgenograms. The initial evaluation should include anteroposterior and standing lateral views. The lateral view should be taken with the patient standing. Lowe et al. found a 26% increase in slipping on standing films compared with recumbent films. In spondylolysis without slippage, the pars interarticularis defect often is difficult to see. Oblique views of the lumbar spine can put the pars area in relief apart from the underlying bony elements, making viewing of the defect easier. A bone scan may be indicated in children in whom it is believed that an acquired pars defect is present but cannot be confirmed by plain films. The bone scan may detect the stress reaction stage before the fracture occurs. A single

photon emission computed tomography (SPECT) bone scan is necessary to show whether uptake is increased in the pars. If increased uptake is confirmed, a CT scan can be obtained to evaluate whether there are thickened cortices consistent with a stress reaction or whether there is an acute stress fracture.

The most commonly used roentgenographic grading system for spondylolisthesis is that of Meyerding. In this system, the slip grade is calculated by determining the ratio between the anteroposterior diameter of the top of the first sacral vertebra and the distance the L5 vertebra has slipped anteriorly (Fig. 38-188). Grade I spondylolisthesis is displacement of 25% or less, grade II between 25% and 50%, grade III between 50% and 75%, and grade IV more than 75%.

DeWald recommended a modification of the Newman system to better define the amount of anterior roll of L5 (Fig. 38-189). The dome and the anterior surface of the sacrum are divided into 10 equal parts. The scoring is based on the position of the posteroinferior corner of the body of the fifth lumbar vertebra with respect to the dome of the sacrum. The second number indicates the position of the anteroinferior corner of the body of the L5 vertebra with respect to the anterior surface of the first sacral segment.

According to Boxall et al., the angular relationships are the

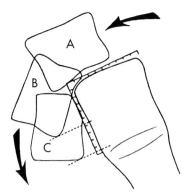

Fig. 38-189 Modified Newman spondylolisthesis grading system. Degree of slip is measured using two numbers—one along sacral endplate and second along anterior portion of sacrum: *A* = 3 + 0; *B* = 8 + 6; and *C* = 10 + 10. (From DeWald RL: Spondylolisthesis. In Bridwell KH, DeWald RL, eds: *The textbook of spinal surgery,* ed 2, Philadelphia, 1997, Lippincott-Raven.)

best predictors of instability or progression of the spondylolisthesis deformity. These relationships are expressed as the slip angle, which is formed by the intersection of a line drawn parallel to the inferior aspect of the L5 vertebra and a line drawn perpendicular to the posterior aspect of the body of the S1 vertebra (Fig. 38-190). Lateral roentgenograms should be made in the standing position. Boxall et al. found an association between a high slip angle (over 55 degrees) and progression of the deformity, even after a solid posterior arthrodesis. Further studies, such as MRI, can be useful in determining the extent of injury to the disc at the level of the spondylolisthesis. Herniation of the nucleus pulposus is rare in children, but the status of the disc can be predictive of the instability of the situation. Nerve root compression also can be evaluated. Objective signs of specific nerve root compression usually are absent in children, although hamstring spasm or tightness usually is present.

TREATMENT OF ACQUIRED SPONDYLOLYSIS

Treatment of acquired spondylolysis from a stress fracture in children and adolescents depends on whether the spondylolysis is acute or chronic. Micheli, Jackson et al., and Rabushka et al. reported children and adolescents in whom acute spondylolytic defects healed with cast or brace immobilization. Typically, these children have an acute onset of symptoms, and the episode of injury is clearly documented. Often they are participating in sports, such as gymnastics, that cause repetitive hyperextension of the spine. A SPECT scan is helpful in determining whether the process is acute or chronic. If the SPECT scan is positive, a CT scan of the suspected area can be obtained. If the SPECT scan reveals metabolic activity and a CT scan shows thickening of the pars, avoidance of aggravating activity or the use of a brace can be effective treatment methods. If the SPECT scan is metabolically active and CT indicates an acute stress fracture, a 3- to 6-month trial of

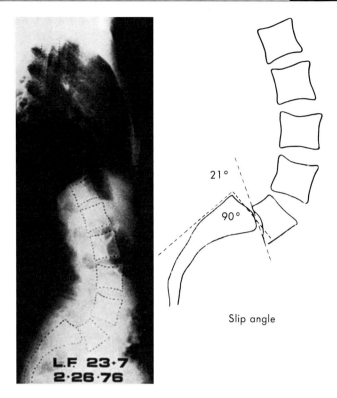

Fig. 38-190 Angle of slipping, formed by intersection of line drawn parallel to inferior aspect of L5 body and line drawn perpendicular to posterior aspect of body of S1. (From Boxall D et al: *J Bone Joint Surg* 61A:479, 1979.)

orthotic treatment is warranted. If the defect has not healed in 6 months, continued bracing is not indicated. CT probably is the most helpful roentgenographic technique to determine the presence or absence of healing.

Children and adolescents in whom the spondylolysis is of long duration are treated with routine nonoperative measures. Vigorous activities are restricted, and back-, abdominal-, and trunk-strengthening exercises are prescribed. If the symptoms are more severe, a brief period of bed rest or brace immobilization may be required. Once the pain has improved and the hamstring tightness has lessened, the child is allowed progressive activities. Yearly examinations with standing spot lateral roentgenograms of the lumbosacral spine are advised to rule out the development of spondylolisthesis. If the patient remains asymptomatic, limitation of activities or contact sports is not necessary. Most children with spondylolysis have excellent relief of symptoms or only minimal discomfort at long-term follow-up. If a child does not respond to conservative measures, other causes of back pain, such as infection, tumor, osteoid osteoma, or herniated disc, should be ruled out. Special attention should be paid to children whose symptoms do not respond to bed rest or who have objective neurological findings. A very small percentage of children with spondylolysis who do not respond to conservative measures and in whom the other possible causes of back pain have been eliminated may require operative treatment.

◆ Repair of Spondylolytic Defect

In symptomatic patients with an established pars intraarticularis defect, the possibility of direct repair can be considered. The principles of this pseudarthrosis repair are the same as for any long bone: debridement, grafting of the site with autogenous bone graft, and compression across the fracture. If a direct repair of the spondylolysis is considered, the disc status should be evaluated with MRI. If disc degeneration is significant, an arthrodesis at that level may be a better choice.

Several techniques for repair of the spondylolytic defect have been described. Buck described a technique in which screws are used for repair, but this technique is difficult, and neurological and mechanical problems are possible with screw fixation across the defect. Bradford reported 22 patients with repair of the defect by segmental wire fixation and bone grafting; 80% of patients obtained good or excellent results, and 90% obtained a solid fusion of the pars defect. Better clinical results were obtained in patients younger than 30 years of age, possibly because chronic instability leads to degenerative disc pathology in older patients, which causes continued symptoms despite fusion of the defect. Van Dam reported success in 16 patients using a modification of the Scott repair technique. In 26 direct pars repairs, union was achieved in 22.

TECHNIQUE 38-46 *(van Dam, Modified Scott Technique)*

Approach the lumbar spine posteriorly. Identify and debride the area of the pars pseudarthrosis. Place a 6.5-mm cancellous screw approximately two thirds of the way into the ipsilateral pedicle. Loop an 18-gauge wire around the screw head and pass the wire through a hole at the base of the spinous process (Fig. 38-191, *A*). Pass the ends of the wire through a metal button and tighten the wire loop around the screw head. Twist the wire ends tightly against the metal button. Cut the excess wire away (Fig. 38-191, *B*). Place autogenous cancellous bone in and around the debrided pars defect. Fully seat the screw to accomplish final tightening of the wire.

Taddonio described the use of pedicle screws attached to CD rods and offset laminar hooks to accomplish the same mechanical stability (Fig. 38-192) as in the Buck technique and Bradford technique.

AFTERTREATMENT. The patient should use a lumbosacral orthosis for a minimum of 3 months and up to 6 months after surgery. Healing of the pars is ascertained by follow-up CT.

Posterolateral Fusion

Posterolateral fusion is the conventional operative treatment for symptomatic spondylolysis unresponsive to conservative treatment. Postoperative immobilization is optional, but we generally immobilize the patient in a TLSO. A pantaloon cast generally is not necessary. Turner and Bianco and Rombold reported fusion rates of approximately 90% and similar percentages of relief of symptoms after fusion of L5 to the

sacrum. Extension of the fusion to L4 is not necessary. The Gill procedure or a wide laminectomy in a child is not necessary and may lead to spondylolisthesis.

TREATMENT OF DEVELOPMENTAL SPONDYLOLISTHESIS

Nonoperative Treatment

Surgery is not always necessary for spondylolisthesis. Restriction of the patient's activities, spinal, abdominal, and trunk muscular rehabilitation, and other nonoperative measures, including the intermittent use of a rigid back brace, often are sufficient if the symptoms are minimal and the slippage is mild. If symptoms improve, progressive increases in activity are permitted. Activity restrictions are unnecessary for patients with mild degrees of spondylolisthesis. For symptom-free patients with slips of more than 25% but less than 50%, Wiltse recommended avoiding contact sports and activities that carry a high probability of back injury. Standing spot lateral roentgenograms of the lumbosacral junction are made every 6 to 12 months until the completion of growth. This is especially important in females and in patients who have high-risk characteristics for progression of the slip.

Operative Treatment

Indications for surgery include persistent symptoms despite 9 months to 1 year of conservative treatment, persistent tight hamstrings, abnormal gait, and pelvic-trunk deformity. Development of a neurological deficit is an indication for surgical intervention, as is progression of the slip, which is indicative of a severe dysplasia. Early surgery may prevent more difficult or risky surgeries at a later time. If a patient is asymptomatic and has a slip of more than 50%, severe dysplasia (high dysplastic spondylolisthesis) is likely and surgery is indicated. Harris and Weinstein reported 12 patients with slips of more than 50% who were followed for as long as 25 years. They concluded that, although many of these patients function well, those with spinal fusion did slightly better.

A posterolateral fusion between L5 and the sacrum is recommended for slips of less than 50% in children and adolescents whose symptoms persist despite conservative treatment. This degree of slippage is a mild dysplasia (low dysplastic type) usually without a significant slip angle. In our experience these children do quite well with a posterolateral in situ fusion. Wiltse suggested that extremely tight hamstrings, decreased tendo calcaneal reflexes, and even a foot drop would improve after a solid arthrodesis. Laminectomy as an isolated technique in a growing child is contraindicated because further slipping will occur. Hensinger et al. and Boxall et al. expressed doubt as to whether decompression with removal of the posterior element of L5 should ever be done in children with slips of less than 50%, no matter what the signs and symptoms of neurological compromise. Lenke et al. emphasized the importance of obtaining a true anteroposterior (Ferguson) view of the lumbosacral junction to evaluate the success of arthrodesis. This view provides a true coronal profile of the L5 sacral ala region.

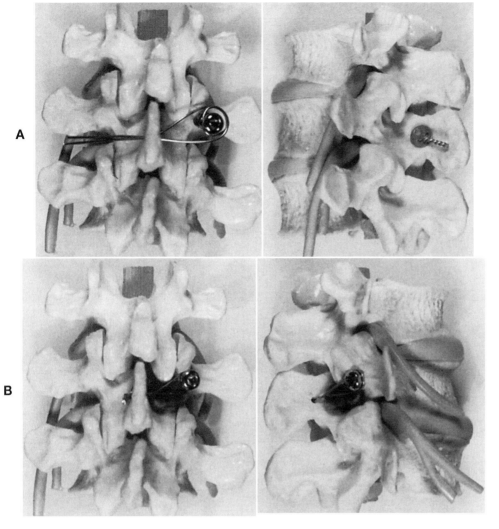

A

B

Fig. 38-191 **A,** Posterior view of lumbar spine model demonstrating 6.5 × 25 mm cancellous screw placed approximately two thirds into ipsilateral pedicle; 18-gauge wire has been looped around screw head and passed through hole in base of spinous process. **B,** Oblique view of lumbar model with wire ends passed through metal button and twisted tightly against metal button. (From van Dam BE: Nonoperative treatment and surgical repair of lumbar spondylolysis. In Bridwell KH, DeWald RL, eds: *The textbook of spinal surgery,* ed 2, Philadelphia, 1997, Lippincott-Raven.)

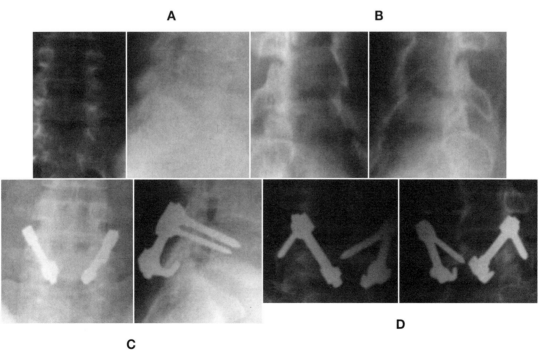

A   B

C   D

Fig. 38-192 **A** and **B,** Isthmic spondylolysis at L5-S1. **C** and **D,** Repair of the pars defect with Cotrel-Dubousset rods anchored to bilateral L5 pedicle screws and L5 offset laminar hooks. (From Taddonio RF: Isthmic spondylolisthesis. In Bridwell KH, DeWald RL, eds: *The textbook of spinal surgery*, Philadelphia, 1991, JB Lippincott.)

◆ **Bilateral Lateral Fusion**

TECHNIQUE 38-47 *(Wiltse)*

Place the patient prone on a Hall frame. Make curved incisions through the skin and subcutaneous tissue, about three fingerbreadths lateral to the midline and just medial to the posterosuperior iliac spine (Fig. 38-193, *A*); curve both incisions slightly inward at their caudal ends. Alternatively, make one midline incision and retract the skin to either side to allow the fascial incisions. Make similar incisions in the fascia at about the same distance lateral to the spinous processes, also curving these fascial incisions toward the midline on their distal ends. This transverse portion of the fascial incision allows adequate retraction. Use the index finger to dissect through the sacrospinalis muscle mass down to the sacrum and forward on the back of the sacrum to the articular processes of L5 and S1, as well as to the space between the transverse process of L5 and the ala of the sacrum. If the spondylolisthesis is more than 50%, it may be necessary also to expose the L4-L5 facet and the transverse process and the lamina of the L4 vertebral body. Two long Gelpi retractors are good instruments for retracting the muscle (Fig. 38-193, *B*). Expose the lamina of the vertebra to be fused to the bases of the spinous processes (Fig. 38-193, *C*). Denude the lumbar transverse processes of soft tissue all the way to their tips. If dissection is not carried anterior to the transverse processes, the spinal nerve roots will not be injured. Denude only the lateral surface of the superior articular process of the topmost vertebra to be included to prevent damage to the facet joint above the level of the fusion. Within the fusion area, denude of soft tissue the lateral surface of the superior articular process, the lamina as far medially as the base of the spinous processes, and the pars interarticularis. To preserve their ligamentous attachments and blood supply, do not expose the spinous processes. Carefully expose the facet joints within the fusion area and remove the articular cartilage in the posterior two thirds of each joint.

Prepare the graft bed as for a classic Hibbs fusion (Chapter 36). Turn an anteriorly based flap of bone from the top of the ala of the sacrum forward and cephalad to form a bridge to the transverse process of L4 or L5. Obtain iliac grafts from one or both sides of the pelvis through the ipsilateral skin incision. Ordinarily, one iliac crest supplies sufficient graft. Take the bone graft from the outer part of the ilium, leaving the inner cortex intact. Tamp cancellous bone between the denuded articular processes and tamp strips of iliac cancellous and cortical bone into place over the area to be fused (Fig. 38-193, *D*). Close the deep fascia with an absorbable stitch and close the wound over drains.

AFTERTREATMENT. Postoperative management varies, depending on the preference of the surgeon. In most patients with grade I, II, or III slips, an underarm Risser cast or a TLSO is used. For patients with more severe slips, or those with

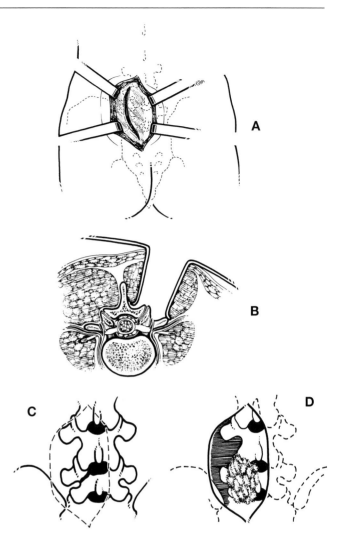

Fig. 38-193   Wiltse technique of bilateral lateral fusion. **A,** Skin incision and fascial incision. **B,** Axial view of paraspinal sacrospinalis-splitting approach to lumbar spine. **C,** Lateral portion of lamina of L4, L5, and ala of sacrum exposed. **D,** Bone graft applied in lateral position after decortication of lamina and transverse processes. (Redrawn from Wiltse LL et al: *J Bone Joint Surg* 50A:921, 1968.)

significantly high slip angles that are considered unstable, an underarm cast is used, with extension down the thigh on one side to better immobilize the lumbosacral joint. This pantaloon-type cast is worn for 3 months, followed by another 3 months in an underarm Risser cast or a TLSO. After 6 months in a cast or brace, a lumbosacral corset is worn for another 6 months. All immobilization is discontinued at the end of 12 months.

TREATMENT OF SEVERE (HIGH-DYSPLASTIC) SPONDYLOLISTHESIS

Operative treatment of high-dysplastic spondylolisthesis is more controversial. Most authors agree that slippage of over 50% requires fusion. The operative options, however, are many, including bilateral lateral fusion, anterior fusion and release

A   B   C

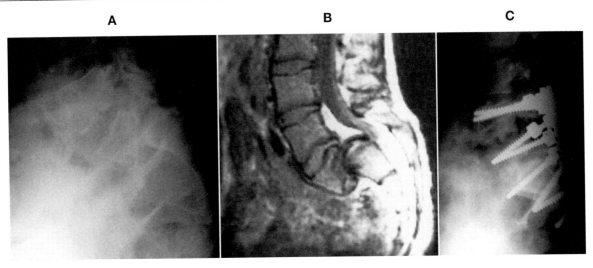

Fig. 38-194   **A,** Severe spondylolisthesis. **B,** MRI shows slip. **C,** After anterior and posterior reduction and fusion with posterior instrumentation.

A   B   C

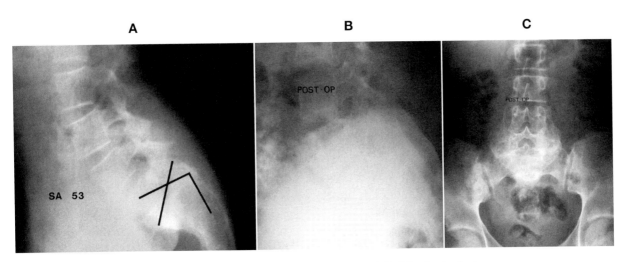

Fig. 38-195   **A,** Severe spondylolisthesis. **B** and **C,** After in situ fusion.

with posterior fusion, posterior interbody fusion, cast reduction and fusion, and posterior instrumentation with reduction and fusion.

Lenke et al. found that 21% of 56 in situ bilateral transverse process fusions for spondylolisthesis were definitely not fused. Despite this low fusion rate, overall clinical improvement was noted in over 80% of patients. Other authors, such as Bradford and DeWald et al., recommended combined anterior fusion and reduction with posterior spinal instrumentation for high-dysplastic slips because of problems with the healing of a posterior arthrodesis alone. In addition to improving appearance, the reduction of spondylolisthesis with instrumentation improves the chance of fusion, but these procedures have many risks and potential complications (Fig. 38-194). Johnson and Kirwan and Wiltse reported excellent results in patients with slips of more than 50% treated with bilateral lateral fusions. Freeman and Donati found similar results after in situ fusion in

patients followed for an average of 12 years (Fig. 38-195). Poussa et al. compared the results of in situ fusion of spondylolisthesis of more than 50% with results of newer techniques of reduction using a transpedicular system. They found no differences between the groups in functional improvement or pain relief. Fusion in situ gave a satisfactory cosmetic appearance. Reduction procedures were associated with increased operative time, complications, and reoperations. In immature patients with grade III or IV spondylolisthesis that can be partially reduced on flexion and extension roentgenograms, a posterolateral fusion can be done in conjunction with cast reduction. The reduction reduces the slip angle and places the fusion under less tensile stress. It also decompresses the anterior portion of the sacrum, allowing sacral remodeling. Burkus et al. compared the long-term results of in situ arthrodesis with and without cast reduction. Adolescents treated postoperatively with reduction and cast immobilization had less evidence of late progression of deformity and more improvement in the amount of sagittal translation and lumbosacral kyphosis. They also had a lower incidence of pseudarthrosis, but the sample was too small to be statistically significant.

Cauda equina injuries may occur after in situ fusions; Maurice and Morley reported four patients with immediate postoperative injuries. Schoenecker et al. reported the development of cauda equina syndromes after in situ fusion in 12 adolescent patients with grade III or IV spondylolisthesis. Posterolateral fusion was done through a bilateral paraspinous muscle–splitting technique in 4 of these patients. In severe spondylolisthesis, the sacral roots are stretched over the back of the body of S1 and are very sensitive to any movement of L5 on S1. Schoenecker et al. postulated that muscle relaxation after general anesthesia and the surgical dissection may have led to additional slippage that further stretched these sacral roots. Patients most at risk had an initial slip angle of more than 45 degrees. We also have seen cauda equina syndrome develop in one patient after in situ bilateral lateral fusion. Schoenecker et al. recommended thorough neurological evaluations before and after in situ arthrodesis in all patients with grade III or IV spondylolisthesis. Examination should include clinical assessment of perineal sensation, function of the bladder, and rectal tone. If a patient has a detectable neurological deficit preoperatively, decompression of the cauda equina at the time of the arthrodesis with removal of the posterior superior lip of the sacrum (Fig. 38-196) can be done. Because this decompression may cause additional instability, postoperative immobilization in a plaster cast with the patient recumbent is mandatory. Alternatively, decompression of the cauda equina can be combined with reduction of the forward slip with posterior pedicular instrumentation. However, this procedure lengthens the trunk and may lead to L5 nerve root deficits or sometimes to injury of the entire lumbosacral plexus. If injury to the cauda equina is evident after an otherwise uneventful in situ arthrodesis, prompt decompression with removal of the posterior aspect of S1 is recommended, with recumbent postoperative immobilization until fusion occurs. Partial reduction of the spondylolisthesis also should be considered.

There are no definite guidelines regarding the appropriate surgical treatment of children and adolescents with high-dysplastic spondylolisthesis. Intuitively it seems that the more dysplastic and unstable the spine is, the more justifiable is some

type of reduction and instrumentation. On the other hand, if a child is young and flexion and extension views show significant movement at the L5-S1 junction, fusion with cast reduction or fusion with instrumentation and limited reduction certainly is a reasonable option. The older the adolescent, the more unstable the deformity, and the more significant the deformity, the greater the need for aggressive surgery.

◆ Posterolateral Fusion and Cast Reduction

TECHNIQUE 38-48
Expose the spine and perform a posterolateral fusion from L4 to the sacrum. Make no attempt at reduction at the time of surgery. At approximately 7 days after surgery, place the patient on a Cotrel traction table without the use of analgesics. Use head-halter and pelvic straps to provide longitudinal traction and reduce the spondylolisthesis by the method of Scaglietti, Frontino, and Bartolozzi. Support the limbs and slowly lower them toward the floor to allow the hips to extend gradually while the sacrum is rotated anteriorly (Fig. 38-197). Apply a spica cast incorporating one or both lower extremities, depending on whether the patient will be allowed to walk. A single spica cast is adequate for most patients.

AFTERTREATMENT. If a single spica cast is used, the patient is allowed to walk immediately. If the cast needs to be changed for any reason (such as loosening or soiling), no further attempt at reduction is made. The cast is worn until there is roentgenographic evidence of fusion, generally 4 to 9 months. Follow-up evaluations are made at 4- to 6-week intervals until the fusion is solid, and then the cast is removed (Fig. 38-198).

Instrumented Reduction
Reduction and fusion in high-dysplastic spondylolisthesis with internal fixation and a sagittally aligned spine can eliminate the complication of progression of the deformity that can occur after in situ fusion. Lumbar root pain or deficit may require decompression of the L5 symptomatic roots and internal fixation. Internal fixation makes it possible to decompress these roots fully without fear of residual instability

Fig. 38-196   A, Severe spondylolisthesis. **B,** Increase that may occur intraoperatively. **C,** Operative decompression of cauda equina with sacroplasty. **D,** Appearance of sacrum after excision of posterosuperior aspect. (From Schoenecker PL, Cole HO, Herring JA, et al: Cauda equina syndrome after in situ arthrodesis for severe spondylolisthesis at the lumbosacral junction, *J Bone Joint Surg* 72A:369, 1990.)

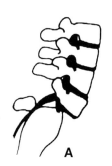

A

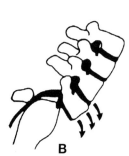

B

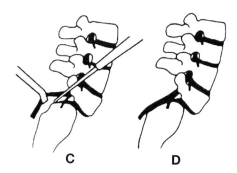

C   **D**

or progressive slipping (Fig. 38-199). Sacral radiculopathy caused by stretching of the sacral roots over the posterosuperior corner of the sacrum theoretically can be relieved by restoring the lumbar spine to its proper position over the sacrum. This relieves the anterior pressure from the sacral roots, shortens

their course, and relaxes the cauda equina. Correction of the slip angle (kyphosis) greatly reduces the bending moment and tensile stress that works against the posterior lumbosacral graft. When normal biomechanics are restored by correction of the deformity, it may be possible to fuse fewer lumbosacral segments. Theoretically, restoring body posture and mechanics to normal may lessen future problems in the proximal areas of the spine. Physical appearance is a concern of adolescents with high-grade spondylolisthesis, and this can be improved with reduction of the deformity.

These theoretical advantages, however, should be weighed carefully against the potential risks of the surgery. These procedures are technically demanding and carry with them significant risk of nerve root injury. As techniques are evolving, these risks are decreasing but are undeniably still present. Results of newer techniques should be compared with long-term studies of untreated high-dysplastic spondylolisthesis and those of in situ fusion.

Harms found that reduction could be accomplished by applying distraction between the middle lumbar spine and the sacrum and combining this with a dorsal extension moment at the vertebral body adjacent to the slipped vertebra (Fig. 38-200). This reduction technique was combined with restoration of the anterior column by a posterior interbody lumbar fusion or anterior interbody lumbar fusion. Harms reported that the use of a titanium cage with autologous bone material inserted from a posterolateral interbody fusion technique provided anterior column support (Fig. 38-201).

TREATMENT OF SPONDYLOPTOSIS

L5 Vertebrectomy

Spondyloptosis exists when the entire body of L5 on a lateral standing roentgenogram is totally below the top of S1. Gaines popularized a two-stage L5 vertebrectomy technique

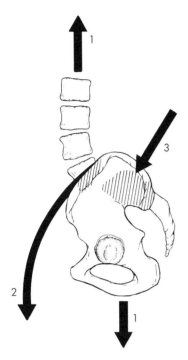

Fig. 38-197 Corrective forces applied to lumbosacral area to obtain reduction of spondylolisthesis. *1,* Elongation force applied to vertebral column including neck and pelvis. *2,* Pelvis rotated, bringing lumbosacral angle to normal value. Olisthesis reduced at same time. *3,* Direct pressure applied to proximal part of sacrum. (From Scaglietti O, Grontino G, Bartolozzi P: *Clin Orthop* 117:164, 1976.)

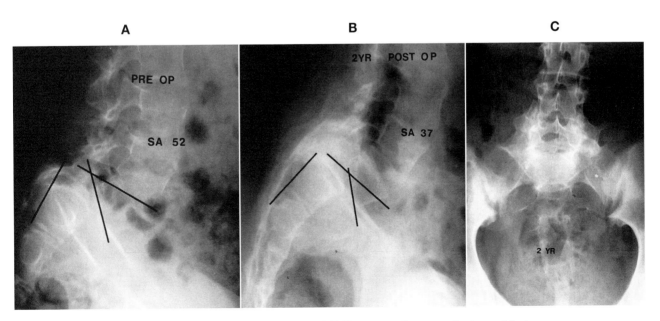

Fig. 38-198 **A,** Spondylolisthesis. **B** and **C,** Two years after cast reduction and fusion.

A   B   C

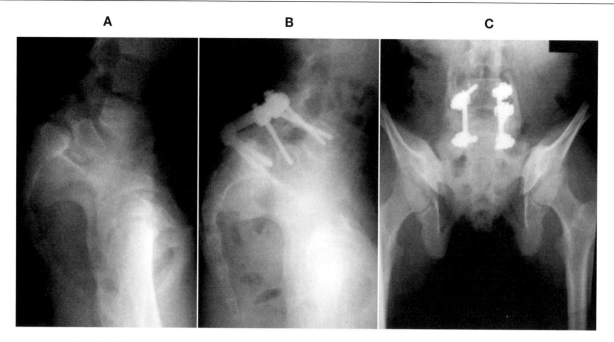

Fig. 38-199   **A,** Standing lateral roentgenogram of high dysplastic spondylolisthesis, L5 on S1, in 12-year-old patient who had significant leg pain. It was thought that decompression of L5 nerve roots was important part of surgical procedure. **B** and **C,** Postoperative Ferguson and lateral views of lumbosacral junction after decompression of L5 nerve roots with limited reduction and internal fixation L4 to S1. Postoperatively, patient's back and leg symptoms were completely relieved.

Fig. 38-200   Schematic illustration of reduction and fusion in spondylolisthesis. **A,** Distraction and dorsal extension forces. **B,** Reduction maintained by pedicle-screw-rod system. Screws are loaded in distraction, and L5-S1 interspace is still kyphotic. **C,** After anterior support, posterior compression is applied. (From Harms J, Jeszenszky D, Stoltze D, Böhm H: True spondylolisthesis reduction and monosegmental fusion in spondylolisthesis. In Bridwell KH, DeWald RL, eds: *The textbook of spinal surgery,* ed 2, Philadelphia, 1997, Lippincott-Raven.)

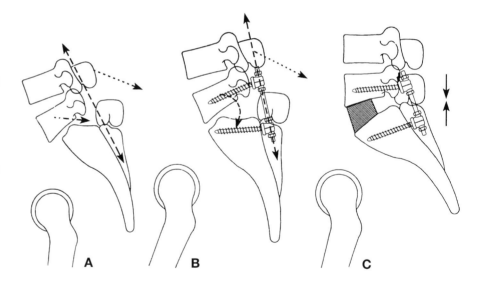

A   B   C

for this difficult problem. The objective is to restore sagittal plane balance and avoid nerve root damage from cauda equina and nerve root stretching during reduction. In the first stage, an L5 vertebrectomy with total removal of the L4-5 and L5-S1 discs is done through a transverse abdominal incision (Fig. 38-202, *A*). The L5 body is excised back to the base of the pedicles, and epidural bleeding is controlled with Gelfoam. No reduction of the deformity is attempted at this time. The caudal cartilage endplate of L4 is removed after the L5 vertebrectomy is completed. At a second stage, L4 is reduced onto S1 from a posterior approach. Harrington hooks and outriggers are placed

between L1 and the sacral ala. The L4-S1 interval is gently distracted to bring the transverse process and pedicle of L5 into direct view. The loose posterior element and pedicles and the transverse processes of L5 are excised. The L5 roots are identified and pedicle screws are placed into L4 and S1. The cartilage endplate of S1 is excised, leaving the bony endplate. The Harrington outriggers are removed, and L4-S1 pedicle screws are used to approximate the body of L4 onto S1. The cancellous bone from the L5 vertebrectomy is placed in the lateral gutter to produce an intertransverse process fusion (Fig. 38-202, *B* and *C*).

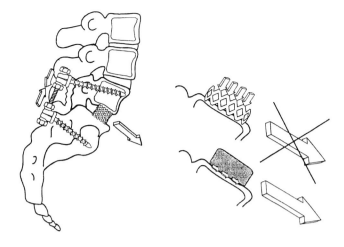

Fig. 38-201 Use of titanium 1 cages as anterior support together with posterior compression-instrumentation resulting in decrease of shear forces. (From Harms J, Jeszenszky D, Stoltze D, Böhm H: True spondylolisthesis reduction and monosegmental fusion in spondylolisthesis. In Bridwell KH, DeWald RL, eds: *The textbook of spinal surgery,* ed 2, Philadelphia, 1997, Lippincott-Raven.)

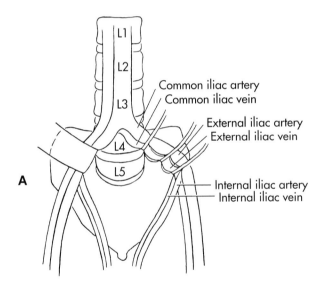

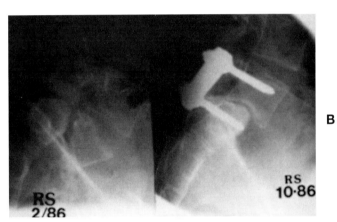

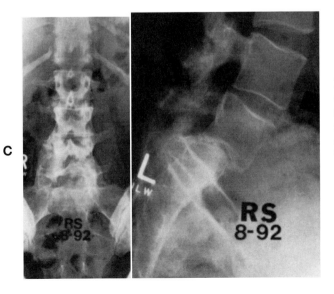

Fig. 38-202 **A,** Anterior approach for resection of L4-L5 disc, vertebral body of L5, and L5-S1 disc is made through incision extending transversely across both rectus abdominus muscles. Great vessels are mobilized laterally after being carefully identified, and structures to be resected are seen between bifurcation of vena cava and aorta. **B,** Preoperative and postoperative lateral roentgenogram. **C,** Roentgenograms of same patient 7 years later. Solid intertransverse fusion and interbody fusion are demonstrated. Reconstructed L4-S1 intervertebral foramen is wide open on lateral roentgenogram. (**A** redrawn from and **B** and **C** from Gaines RW, Jr: The L5 vertebrectomy approach for the treatment of spondyloptosis. In Bridwell KH, DeWald RL, eds: *The textbook of spinal surgery,* ed 2, Philadelphia, 1997, Lippincott-Raven.)

Kyphoscoliosis

MYELOMENINGOCELE

Treatment of patients with myelomeningocele spinal deformities is the most challenging in spine surgery. It requires a team effort, with cooperation of consultants in several subspecialties. These children often have multiple system dysfunctions that influence the treatment of their spinal deformity.

Incidence and Natural History

Scoliosis in children with myelomeningocele often is associated with lordotic or kyphotic deformities (Box 38-11). These deformities often are progressive and can lead to significant disabilities. Banta et al. found that the incidence of scoliosis increased with increasing age and neurological level.

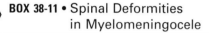

BOX 38-11 • Spinal Deformities
in Myelomeningocele

SCOLIOSIS
Congenital
Developmental (paralytic)
Combination

KYPHOSIS
Congenital
Developmental (paralytic)

LORDOSIS
Usually found in combination with scoliosis or kyphosis

From Brown HP: *Orthop Clin North Am* 9:392, 1978.

Almost all patients with a thoracolumbar level spina bifida have spinal deformity by the age of 14 years. Raycroft and Curtis differentiated two types of deformity: congenital and paralytic. Congenital scoliosis in myelomeningocele is associated with structural disorganization of the vertebrae with asymmetrical growth and includes all of the congenital anomalies associated with scoliosis, hemivertebrae, unilateral unsegmented bars, and various combinations of the two. Congenital scoliosis occurs in about 15% to 20% of myelomeningocele patients with scoliosis. Most scoliotic curves in myelomeningocele patients are paralytic curves. In these patients, the spine is straight at birth and gradually develops progressive curvature because of the neuromuscular problems. These generally are long, C-shaped curves with the apex in the thoracolumbar or lumbar spine (Fig. 38-203). These paralytic curves often extend into the lumbosacral junction and often are associated with pelvic obliquity. In these children, spinal curvatures often develop at a younger age than in children with idiopathic scoliosis, beginning at 3 to 4 years of age, and can become quite severe before the patient is 10 years old. Future trunk growth and final trunk height are considerations in treatment, although Lindseth noted that children with myelomeningocele have slow growth because of growth hormone deficiency and mature earlier than usual, often by 9 to 10 years in girls and 11 to 12 years in boys.

Clinical Evaluation

Thorough evaluation is critical for determining the appropriate management of patients with myelomeningocele and spinal deformity. The following areas are closely investigated: the presence of hydrocephalus, any operative procedures for shunting, bowel and bladder function, frequency of urinary tract infections, the use of an indwelling catheter or intermittent catheterization, current medications, mental status, method of

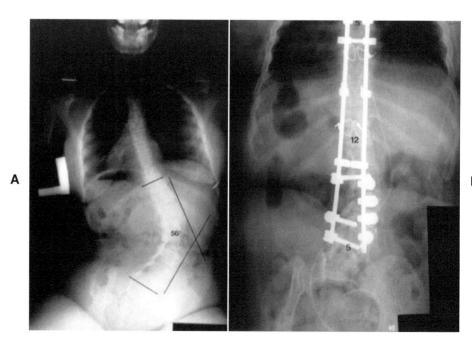

Fig. 38-203 **A,** Scoliotic deformity in patient with myelomeningocele. **B,** After anterior and posterior fusions and posterior instrumentation. (From Warner WC: Scoliosis in myelomeningocele. In Sarwark JF, Lubicky JP, eds: *Caring for the child with spina bifida,* Chicago, 2001, American Academy of Orthopaedic Surgeons.)

ambulation, the level of the defect, any noticeable progression of the curve, and any lower extremity contractures. The spine is examined to determine the type and flexibility of the deformity and to detect any evidence of pressure sores or lack of sitting balance. In patients with progressive paralytic scoliosis, hydromyelia, disturbed ventricular shunts, syringomyelia, tethered cord, or compression from an Arnold-Chiari syndrome may contribute to the progression of scoliosis. Lubicky noted that most patients with myelomeningocele have roentgenographic tethering of the spinal cord at the site of the sac closure. The mere presence of roentgenographic tethering does not necessarily imply traction on the cord. Other clinical signs and symptoms of cord tethering should be observed, including back pain, new or increased spasticity, changes in muscle strength, difficulty with gait, changes in bowel or bladder function, and the appearance of lower extremity deformities.

Careful evaluation of any pelvic obliquity is necessary. Winter and Pinto emphasized the importance of determining the precise cause of pelvic obliquity. Because patients with myelomeningocele are prone to develop contractures about the hips, careful physical examination of the hip adductors, extensors, and flexors is important in evaluating the cause of pelvic obliquity. Lubicky noted a difficult but unusual problem in some patients with myelomeningocele and extension contractures of the hips. In these patients, flexion through the thoracolumbar spine was needed for them to sit upright. Spinal fusion would make sitting impossible and would place significant mechanical stresses on the instrumentation (Fig. 38-204). Physiological hip flexion should be restored in these patients before undertaking spinal instrumentation and fusion.

Roentgenographic Findings

Roentgenograms should be taken with the patient upright and supine. If the patient can ambulate, standing films should be made. If the patient is nonambulatory, sitting films should be made. The upright films allow better evaluation of the actual deformity of the spine when the patient is functioning. The supine films show better detail of various associated spinal deformities. The flexibility of the curves is determined with traction or bending films.

Roentgenographic evaluation of the pelvic obliquity should include a supine view obtained with the hips in the "relaxed" position. In this view, the hips are flexed and abducted or adducted as dictated by the contractures. Alternatively, roentgenograms can be made with the patient prone and the hips off the edge of the roentgenographic table and placed in abduction or adduction (see Fig. 38-127).

Various specialized roentgenograms are helpful. Myelography and MRI are useful for evaluating such conditions as hydromyelia, tethered cord (Fig. 38-205), diastematomyelia, and Arnold-Chiari malformation. Intravenous pyelography should be done at regular intervals, according to the urologist's recommendation.

Scoliosis and Lordosis

Orthotic Treatment. Although the natural history of paralytic curves in patients with myelomeningocele is not changed by orthotic treatment, bracing can be useful to delay spinal fusion until adequate spinal growth has occurred. Bracing may accomplish this in paralytic curves but does not affect congenital curves. The brace also can improve sitting balance and free the hands for other activities. Custom-fitted body jackets, usually bivalved, are used but require very close and frequent observation by the parents. The skin must be examined frequently for pressure areas; any sign of pressure requires immediate brace adjustment. Bracing usually is not instituted until the curve is beginning to cause clinical problems, and generally it is worn only when the patient is upright. If the curve fails to respond to bracing or if bracing becomes impossible because of pressure sores or noncompliance, surgery is indicated. The patient and the parents need to understand that the brace is not the definitive treatment for these curves.

Operative Treatment. Hull et al., Mackel and Lindseth, Mayfield, and Sriram et al. have all indicated that surgery on the myelomeningocele spine is accompanied by potential serious complications. Although the operative procedures varied considerably in these reports, some observations could be made. Because of densely scarred and adherent soft tissue, spinal exposure often is lengthy and hemorrhagic. The deformity often is rigid, and proper correction is impossible. The quality of the bone often provides poor seating for instrumentation systems, and the inadequacy of the posterior bone mass provides a poor bed for bone grafting. The lack of normal posterior vertebral elements makes instrumentation and achieving a solid fusion difficult. The abnormal placement of the paraspinal muscles results in the lack of usual soft tissue coverage of the spine and instrumentation systems. Newer techniques of surgery and instrumentation, bank bone, and prophylactic antibiotics have lessened but not eliminated these problems. The parents must be aware of these potential problems before surgery and must accept these as inherent in the operative treatment.

Emans et al. called attention to the problem of latex allergy in patients with myelomeningocele. Repeated exposure to latex during daily catheterization and multiple operations most likely accounts for sensitization of these patients to natural latex. The allergy is to the residual plant proteins in natural latex products and is an IgE-mediated, immediate type of hypersensitivity. Anaphylaxis may occur intraoperatively and easily can be confused with other intraoperative emergencies. Patients with myelomeningocele should be closely questioned about any preoperative reactions to latex. If there is any question, strict avoidance of latex products during surgery appears to satisfactorily manage the problem.

Congenital abnormalities that cause scoliosis in patients with myelomeningocele are treated in the same manner as in other patients with congenital scoliosis—early operative intervention. Paralytic scoliosis is a more common cause of

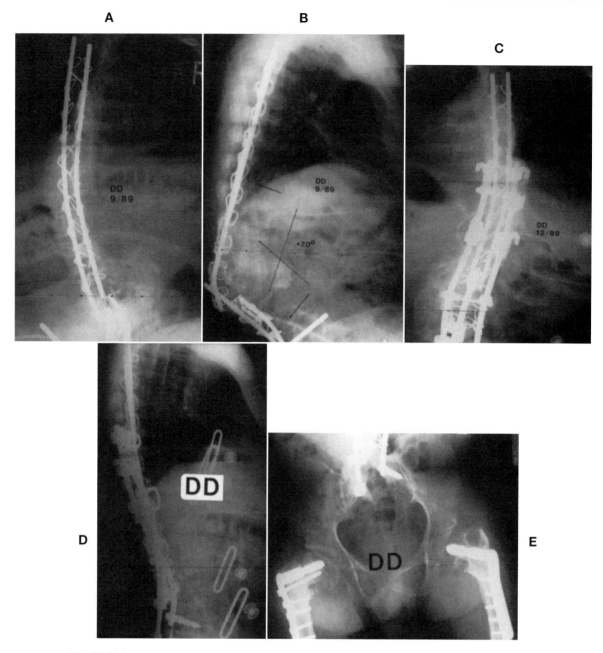

Fig. 38-204   Thoracic-level myelomeningocele in 16-year-old boy who had progressive scoliosis and underwent anterior interbody fusion and posterior Luque instrumentation. Unfortunately, he had extremely poor hip flexion. Three years later he had increasing deformity. Anteroposterior **(A)** and lateral **(B)** roentgenograms at time of presentation showing broken rods and severe kyphotic deformity. Pseudarthrosis provided flexion for sitting because hips could not. Anteroposterior **(C)** and lateral **(D)** roentgenograms after revision of pseudarthrosis anteriorly and posteriorly. After these procedures and during same hospitalization, patient underwent femoral shortening osteotomies, which allowed him to sit properly and prevented stress on instrumentation **(E)**. (From Lubicky JP: Spinal deformity in myelomeningocele. In Bridwell KH, DeWald RL, eds: *The textbook of spinal surgery,* ed 2, Philadelphia, 1997, Lippincott-Raven.)

scoliosis, and lordoscoliosis is the most common type. Osebold et al. reported that, in 40 patients with myelomeningocele and paralytic scoliosis, posterior spinal arthrodesis and Harrington instrumentation extending to the sacrum, combined with anterior fusion and either Dwyer or Zielke instrumentation,

gave the best results. The combined fusion method reduced the incidence of pseudarthrosis to 23%, compared with 45% when only posterior fusion and instrumentation were used. Prophylactic antibiotics were an important part of their regimen and reduced the infection rate to 8%. Posterior fusion or anterior

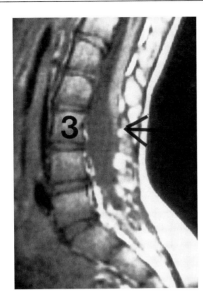

Fig. 38-205 MRI shows tethered cord at L3 in patient with kyphoscoliosis.

fusion alone was inadequate even with instrumentation. Early mobilization was allowed with the use of a bivalved TLSO. Other studies, such as those of McMaster, Banta, and Stark and Saraste, confirm the importance of combining anterior and posterior arthrodeses.

Selection of Fusion Levels. The levels of fusion depend on the age of the child, location of the curve, level of paralysis, ambulatory status, and presence or absence of pelvic obliquity. Spinal fusion generally should extend from neutral vertebra to neutral vertebra, with the end vertebra of the scoliotic curve located within the stable zone. Paralytic curves often tend to be fused too short, especially proximally. When deciding whether to stop the fusion short or long, the longer fusion usually is safer. In the past, instrumentation was extended to the pelvis because deficient posterior elements of the lumbar spine made adequate fixation impossible. With pedicle screw fixation, fusion and instrumentation sometimes can be stopped short of the pelvis. Mazur and Müller demonstrated that spinal fusion to the pelvis in ambulatory patients diminished their ambulatory status. They therefore recommended fusion short of the pelvis if possible in ambulatory patients. Ending the fusion above the pelvis eliminates the stresses on the instrumentation and fusion areas at the lumbosacral junction and allows some motion for adjustment of lordosis in those who have mild hip flexion contractures. In nonambulatory patients, unless the lumbar curve can be corrected to less than 20 degrees and the pelvic obliquity to less than 15 degrees, the scoliosis will continue to progress if the lumbosacral junction is not fused.

Attention to sagittal contour is extremely important. Even in a nonambulatory patient, maintenance of lumbar lordosis is important. If the lumbar lordosis is flattened, the pelvis rotates and much of the sitting weight is placed directly on the ischial tuberosities, which can result in the development of pressure sores.

Anterior-Only Fusion. Sponseller et al. recommended anterior fusion and instrumentation alone in selected patients with myelomeningocele and paralytic scoliosis. Their indications for this procedure include (1) thoracolumbar curves of less than 75 degrees, (2) compensatory proximal curves of less than 40 degrees, (3) no significant kyphosis in the primary curve, and (4) no evidence of syrinx. Fourteen patients were treated with this technique. A ³⁄₁₆-inch TSRH rod was used most frequently anteriorly. They noticed a decrease in quadriceps strength immediately after surgery in two patients and hypothesized that the amount of correction achieved with the anterior instrumentation systems was so great that traction was placed on the cord. They now have recognized that intraoperative monitoring of quadriceps function is essential in these patients.

◆ Posterior Instrumentation and Fusion

Posterior instrumentation and fusion alone have been reserved for flexible curves with most of the posterior elements intact so that adequate fixation can be obtained with pedicle screws. However, the curve must be flexible, and correction must allow for almost normal coronal and sagittal balance.

TECHNIQUE 38-49

Place the patient prone on a Hall frame. Prepare and drape the back in a sterile manner. Make a midline incision from the area of the superior vertebra to be instrumented down to the sacrum. In the area of the normal spine, carry out subperiosteal dissection. An inverted Y incision has been described to prevent exposure of the sac in the midline, but we have had difficulty with skin necrosis using this technique and have had better results with a midline incision that follows the scarred area of the skin posteriorly and careful dissection around the sac in the midline area. Make the skin incision carefully because the dural sac is just beneath the skin. If a dural leak is noted, repair it immediately. Carry the dissection laterally over the convex and concave facet areas and down to the ala of the sacrum (Fig. 38-206, *A*). Expose the area of normal spine to be fused and the bony elements in the region of the abnormal sac area. Pass sublaminar wires beneath the lamina of the normal vertebra above the sac area. In the area of the defect, attempt to achieve segmental fixation. Pass a wire around a pedicle and twist it on itself to secure fixation (Fig. 38-206, *B*). Pass wires on both the concave and the convex sides of the curve. Because these pedicles often are osteoporotic, take care in tightening the wires so that they do not "cut through." On the concave side of the curve, if distraction would help correct pelvic obliquity, a hook site for a pedicle hook can be prepared in the thoracic area. If the iliac wing is large enough to accept the Galveston fixation, make a Galveston bend in a short rod. Insert the short rods in the iliac crests. Connect two longer rods to the spine with the segmental wires and connect the long rods to the

continued

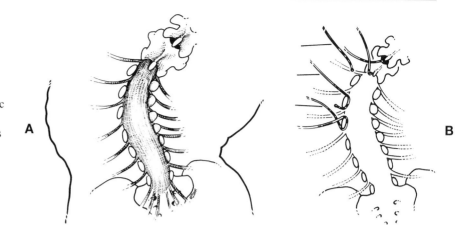

Fig. 38-206   Correction of scoliosis in myelomeningocele. **A,** Spinal exposure; dural sac is not dissected. **B,** Sublaminar wires placed in normal spine; in area of spina bifida, wires encircle pedicle for segmental fixation.

Galveston-type rods with domino-type cross links (Technique 38-35). Alternatively, contour the rods. Take care to preserve normal lumbar lordosis and secure them in place by tightening the segmental wires. Apply copious bone-bank allograft to any areas of bony structures posteriorly. It is important to link the two rods with a cross-link system.

Combined Anterior and Posterior Fusion. The most commonly required procedure for progressive scoliosis in patients with myelomeningocele combines anterior and posterior fusions with posterior instrumentation. Posterior instrumentation consists of a standard rod with hooks or sublaminar wires, cables, or a combination of these in the areas of normal posterior elements. The hooks allow distraction or compressive forces to be applied, and the wires or cables allow a translational force to be applied. The wires or cables also have the advantage of distributing the corrective forces over multiple vertebral levels and providing secure fixation of all instrumented levels. Although normally shaped, the vertebrae may be small, necessitating the use of pediatric-size hooks.

The absence of posterior elements in the dysraphic portion of the spine makes fixation more problematic, so various instrumentation systems need to be available (Fig. 38-207). Rodgers et al. noted that pedicle screws greatly improved fixation and correction of the dysraphic portion of the spine. In widely dysraphic vertebrae, the orientation and landmarks of the pedicle are altered (Fig. 38-208), and direct view of the pedicle is necessary to insert pedicle screws in these areas. The pedicle is exposed by either resection of a sufficient amount of facet or dissection along the medial wall of the spinal canal and retraction of the meningocele sac to identify the medial wall of the pedicle. During probing of the pedicle, remaining within the cortices of the pedicle is imperative. Rogers et al. emphasized that the pedicle screws do not necessarily need to penetrate the anterior vertebral cortex. Because of the small pedicles in these

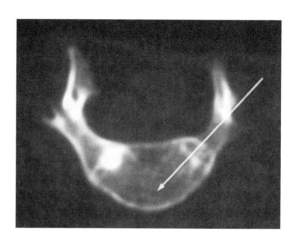

Fig. 38-207   CT scan showing abnormal pedicle orientation in dysraphic vertebra. (From Rodgers WB, Frim DM, Emans JB: *Clin Orthop* 338:19, 1997.)

patients, solid pedicle screws generally are necessary rather than cannulated screws. In the dysraphic spine, the pedicle screws often have to be inserted at an angle from lateral to medial (Fig. 38-209). This requires special attention to rod contouring to attach the rod to the screw because of the lateral position of the screw head.

Two other techniques for fixation of the dysraphic spine have been described but probably are not as secure as those using pedicle screws. Drummond spinous process button wires can be passed through laminar remnants (Fig. 38-210), or segmental wires can be looped around each pedicle. When Drummond button wires are used, the dysraphic laminae are exposed, and dissection is done between the sac and the adjacent laminae while the sac is carefully retracted medially. A hole is placed through the strongest available portion of the laminar remnant, and the wire is passed from medial to lateral, leaving the button on the inner surface of the lamina. Segmental wires can be looped around each pedicle by passing

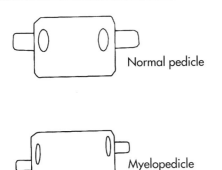

Fig. 38-208 Diagram showing alteration in anatomical relationship of pedicle–transverse process. (From Rodgers WB, Frim DM, Emans JB: *Clin Orthop* 338:19, 1997.)

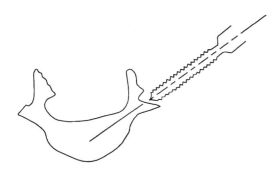

Fig. 38-209 Pedicle screw insertion. (From Rodgers WB, Frim DM, Emans JB: *Clin Orthop* 338:19, 1997.)

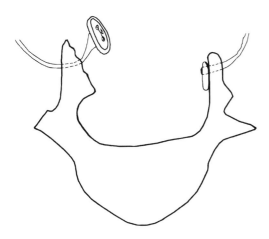

Fig. 38-210 Diagram of Wisconsin button wire fixation of a dysraphic vertebra. (Redrawn from Rodgers WB, Frim DM, Emans JB: *Clin Orthop* 338:19, 1997.)

from one foramen around the pedicle and other posterior remnants medial to the pedicle and then back through the next foramen and back to the original wire. The passage of these wires usually is blind. The wires then attach to the rod. The wire also can be looped around a pedicle bone screw if it is

difficult to contour the rod to easily fit in the screw (see Fig. 38-206, *A* and *B*).

Instrumentation to the pelvis frequently is necessary to correct associated pelvic obliquity in nonambulatory children. Fixation to the pelvis and sacrum is especially difficult in children with myelomeningocele because the bone often is osteoporotic and the pelvis is small, making secure instrumentation difficult. The stresses placed on distal fixation in scoliosis tend to displace sacral or sacropelvic instrumentation laterally. If there is associated kyphosis, these forces tend to displace sacral or pelvic instrumentation dorsally.

Several techniques have been described for extending fixation to the pelvis, including Galveston, Dunn-McCarthy, Jackson, Fackler, sacral bar, and pedicle screws. Our preferred technique for pelvic fixation in patients with myelomeningocele and paralytic scoliosis is the Galveston technique (Technique 38-35). We believe this provides the most secure pelvic fixation for scoliotic curves. However, many patients with myelomeningocele have hypoplastic iliac crests, and in these patients, L-rods are fixed to the sacrum using the technique described by McCarthy (Technique 38-34). Their technique does not restrict lateral displacement as well as the Galveston intrapelvic fixation, but cross linking of the two rods may help to decrease lateral displacement. Once the two rods are cross linked, pelvic obliquity can be corrected by cantilevering the cross-linked rods. The Jackson intrasacral rod technique consists of inserting the rods through the lateral sacral mass and into the sacrum. The rod then penetrates the anterolateral cortex and usually is attached to a sacral screw, providing fixation in flexion and extension. The anatomy of the sacrum in patients with myelomeningocele makes this technique quite difficult. Widmann, Hresko, and Hall described a technique using a sacral bar connected to standard CD-like rods in 10 patients and found it to be effective (Fig. 38-211). Pelvic fixation by sacral pedicle screws is not reliable in these small osteopenic patients.

In patients who are treated with combined anterior and posterior fusion, the necessity for anterior instrumentation is controversial. Ward, Wenger, and Roach found no statistical differences in fusion rate, curve correction, or change in pelvic obliquity with anterior and posterior instrumentation and fusion when compared with anterior arthrodesis with only posterior instrumentation and fusion. If anterior instrumentation is used, great care must be taken to not cause a kyphotic deformity in the spine. If the patient requires posterior fusion and instrumentation, especially to the pelvis, it is difficult to instrument the sacrum anteriorly. This would then leave the anterior instrumentation ending two or three levels above the distal extent of the posterior instrumentation. It has been our experience that combined anterior and posterior fusion generally requires an anterior release and fusion and posterior instrumentation. We have not found the need to use anterior and posterior instrumentation in these patients.

Fig. 38-211　**A,** Correct passage of sacral bar through body of sacrum, posterior to great vessels and anterior to spinal canal. **B,** Connection between sacral bar and vertical rods. (Redrawn from Torode IP, Dickens DRV: The spine. In Broughton NS, Menelaus MB, eds: *Menelaus' orthopaedic management of spina bifida cystica,* ed 3, London, Harcourt Brace, 1998.)

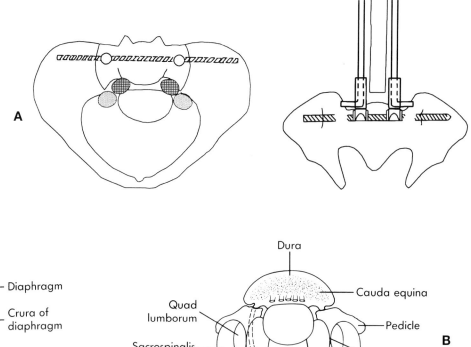

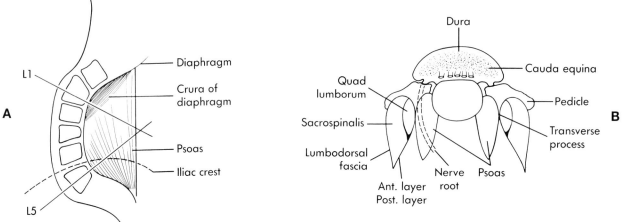

Fig. 38-212　**A,** Sagittal diagram showing deforming effect of psoas muscle on kyphosis. **B,** Transverse section of lumbar spine and attached muscles in region of kyphosis. Pedicles and laminae of vertebrae are splayed laterally; erector spinae muscles enclosed in thoracolumbar fascia lie lateral to vertebral bodies and act as flexors. (Redrawn from Sharrard WJW, Drennan JC: *J Bone Joint Surg* 54B:50, 1972.)

Kyphosis

Incidence and Natural History. Kyphosis in patients with myelomeningocele may be either developmental or congenital. Developmental kyphosis is not present at birth and progresses slowly. It is a paralytic kyphosis that is aggravated by the lack of posterior stability. Congenital kyphosis, which is a much more difficult problem, usually measures 80 degrees or more at birth. The level of the lesion usually is T12 with total paraplegia. The kyphosis is rigid and progresses rapidly during infancy. Children with severe kyphosis are unable to wear braces and often have difficulty sitting in wheelchairs because the center of gravity is displaced forward. An ulceration may develop over the prominent kyphos and make skin coverage quite difficult. Progression of the kyphosis may lead to respiratory difficulty because of incompetence of the inspiratory muscles, crowding of the abdominal contents, and upward pressure on the diaphragm. Increased flexion of the trunk can interfere with urinary drainage and also may cause problems if urinary diversion or ileostomy become necessary.

Hoppenfeld described the anatomy of this condition and noted that the pedicles are widely spread and the rudimentary laminae actually are everted. The anterior longitudinal ligament is short and thick. The paraspinal muscles are present but are displaced far anterolaterally (Fig. 38-212). All muscles therefore act anteriorly to the axis of rotation, which tends to worsen the kyphosis.

Operative Treatment. Apical vertebral ostectomy, as proposed by Sharrard, makes closure of the skin easier in neonates but provides only short-term improvement, and the kyphotic deformity invariably recurs. Lindseth and Selzer reported 23 children with myelomeningocele whose kyphosis was treated with vertebral excision. Their most consistent results were obtained with partial resection of the apical vertebra and the proximal lordotic curve, which was done in 12 patients. If only the apical vertebra and other vertebrae on either side were excised, correction of the kyphotic prominence was lost.

Although all severe congenital kyphoses in patients with myelomeningocele progresses, not all patients require surgery.

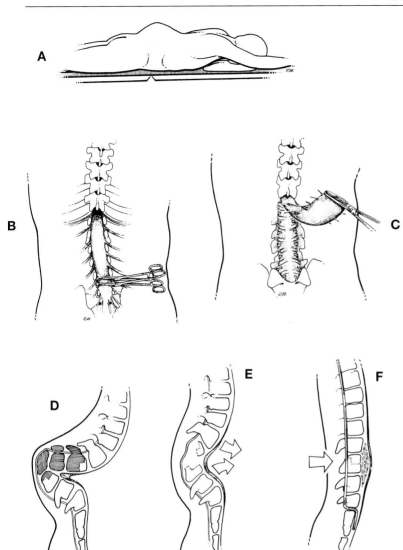

Fig. 38-213 Technique of vertebral excision (Lindseth and Selzer). **A,** Skin incision. **B,** Exposure of area of kyphosis and dural sac. **C,** Sac is divided distally and dissected proximally. **D,** Vertebrae between apex of lordosis and apex of kyphosis are removed. **E,** Kyphosis is reduced. **F,** Reduction is maintained with stable internal fixation (in this instance with Luque rods and segmental wires).

Kyphectomy is indicated to improve sitting balance or when skin problems occur over the apex. Surgery should be delayed until the patient is 7 or 8 years of age but should be done before skeletal maturity. Delaying the surgery, if possible, allows more secure internal fixation with less postoperative loss of correction.

◆ *Vertebral Excision and Reduction of Kyphosis*

TECHNIQUE 38-50 *(Lindseth and Selzer)*

Use a midline posterior incision (Fig. 38-213, *A*), which can be varied somewhat depending on local skin conditions. Expose subperiosteally the more normal vertebrae superiorly and the area of the abnormality, continuing the exposure past the lateral bony ridges.

At this point, remove the sac. Dissect inside the lamina until the foramina are exposed on each side of the spine. Expose, divide, and coagulate the nerve, artery, and vein within each foramen, exposing the sac distally where it is scarred down and thin. At its distal level, cross-clamp the sac with Kelly clamps and divide it between the clamps (Fig. 38-213, *B*). Close the scarred ends with a running stitch. Dissect the sac proximally. As this proximal dissection is done, large venous channels connecting the sac to the posterior vertebral body will be encountered; control the bleeding from the bone with bone wax and from the soft tissue with electrocautery. Dissect the sac up to the level of the more normal-appearing dura (Fig. 38-213, *C*).

The sac can be transected at this point. If this is done, close the dura with a purse-string suture. Do not suture the cord itself shut, but leave it open so that the spinal fluid can escape from the central canal of the cord into the arachnoid

continued

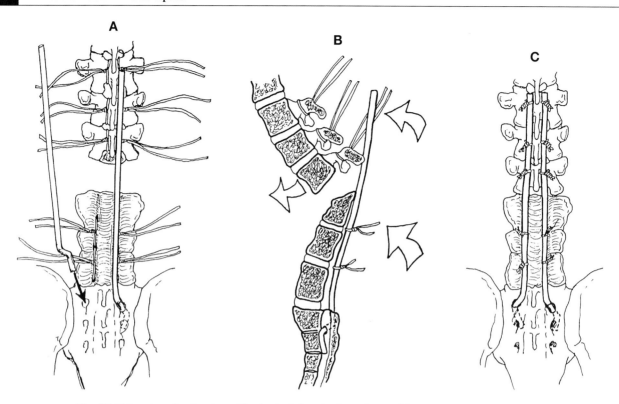

Fig. 38-214   Anterior fixation of kyphotic deformity in patients with myelomeningocele. (From Warner WC, Fackler CD: *J Pediatr Orthop* 13:704, 1993.)   *Continued*

space. If the sac is not removed, it can be used at the completion of the procedure to further cover the area of the resected vertebra.

Once the sac has been reflected proximally, continue dissection around the vertebral bodies, exposing only the area to be removed. If the entire kyphotic area of the spine is exposed subperiosteally, avascular necrosis of these vertebral bodies may occur. Remove the vertebrae between the apex of the lordosis and the apex of the kyphosis (Fig. 38-213, *D*). Remove the vertebra at the apex of the kyphosis first by removing the intervertebral disc with a Cobb elevator and curets. Take care to leave the anterior longitudinal ligament intact to act as a stabilizing hinge. Once this vertebra has been removed, temporarily correct the spine to determine how many cephalad vertebrae should be removed. Remove enough vertebrae to correct the kyphosis as much as possible but not so many that approximation is impossible (Fig. 38-213, *E*). Morselization of these vertebral bodies provides additional bone graft.

Many techniques have been described for fixation of the kyphotic deformity, but L-rod instrumentation to the pelvis with segmental wires is recommended (Fig. 38-213, *F*). The distal end of the rod can be contoured. We prefer to make a right-angled bend in the rod and pass the bend through the S1 foramen rather than around the ala of the sacrum, as described by Warner and Fackler (Fig. 38-214). Move the

distal segment to the proximal segment and tighten the segmental wires.

Gurr described an intramedullary technique for fixation of the distal vertebrae (personal communication). After the kyphectomy has been completed, place a single guide wire in the center of the distal remaining vertebrae into the sacrum. Confirm the position of the guide wire on anteroposterior and lateral roentgenograms (Fig. 38-215). Place the distal ends of the instrumentation rods parallel to the guide wire through the vertebrae and into the sacrum and check their position roentgenographically (Fig. 38-216). Contour the cephalad ends to the expected correction of the deformity or cut them short and link them with domino or side-to-side cross links to the upper construct. Apply additional allograft bone graft, irrigate the wound, and close it over suction drains. Antibiotics are given intravenously for several days before and after surgery.

AFTERTREATMENT. When the patient is stable after surgery, a plaster model is taken for a bivalved, plastic body jacket; it is not necessary to immobilize the hips. The patient is returned to the sitting position as soon as the jacket is available. Some patients in whom the bone is too osteoporotic and the stability of the internal fixation is in doubt may be kept on bed rest for several months or allowed to sit only in an inclined chair. The fusion usually is solid in 6 to 9 months.

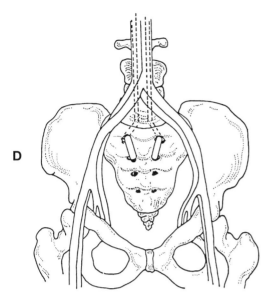

Fig. 38-214, cont'd   For legend see opposite page.

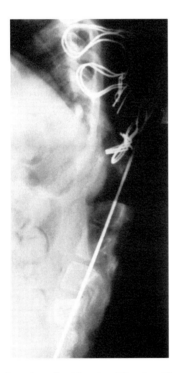

Fig. 38-215   Insertion of guide wire. (Courtesy Kevin Gurr, MD.)

The postoperative care of these patients requires close observation by all subspecialty consultants involved. Postoperative infections, urinary tract problems, skin problems, and pseudarthrosis are frequent. The improved function, however, and the prevention of progression of the kyphosis make surgery worth the risks (Fig. 38-217).

Paralytic kyphosis is treated with more standard techniques. When surgery becomes necessary, anterior fusion over the area of the apex and all levels of deficient posterior elements is done

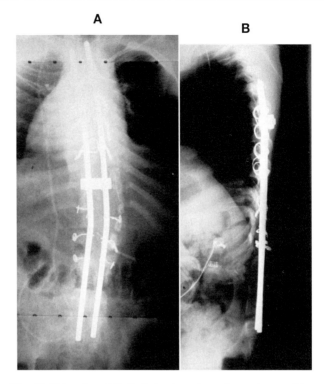

A   **B**

Fig. 38-216   A and B, Rods in place through vertebrae and into sacrum. (Courtesy Kevin Gurr, MD.)

with strut grafting (Technique 38-45). This is followed by posterior arthrodesis and instrumentation (Technique 38-41).

SACRAL AGENESIS

Sacral agenesis is a rare lesion that often is associated with maternal diabetes mellitus. Renshaw postulated that the condition is teratogenically induced or is a spontaneous genetic mutation that predisposes to or causes failure of embryonic induction of the caudal notocord sheath and ventral spinal cord. The dorsal ganglia and the dorsal (sensory) portion of the spinal cord continue to develop. The vertebrae and motor nerves are not subsequently induced, and the sacral agenesis results. Sensation remains intact because the dorsal ganglia and the dorsal portion of the spinal cord have been derived from the neural crest tissue. This disturbance in the normal sequence of development explains the observation that the lowest vertebral body with pedicles corresponds closely to the motor level, whereas the sensory level is distal to the motor level.

Renshaw studied 23 patients with sacral agenesis and proposed the following classification: type I, either total or partial unilateral sacral agenesis (Fig. 38-218, A); type II, partial sacral agenesis with partial but bilaterally symmetrical defects and a stable articulation between the ilia and a normal or hypoplastic S1 vertebra (Fig. 38-218, B); type III, variable lumbar and total sacral agenesis with the ilia articulating with the sides of the lowest vertebra present (Fig. 38-218, C); type IV, variable lumbar and total sacral agenesis with the caudal

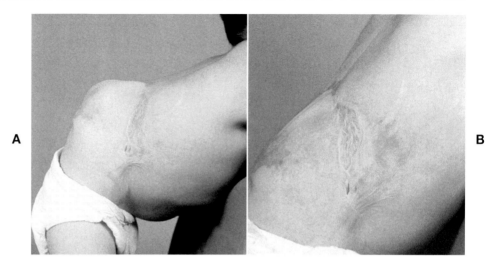

Fig. 38-217 Clinical appearance before (**A**) and after (**B**) surgery. (Courtesy Kevin Gurr, MD.)

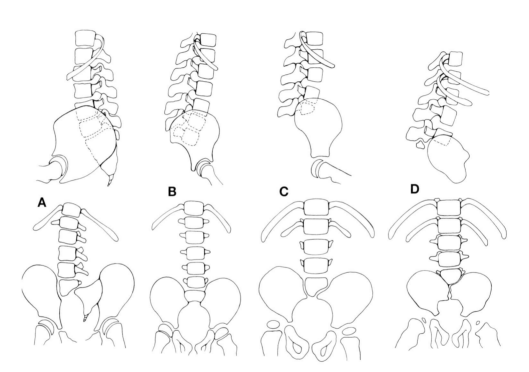

Fig. 38-218 Types of sacral agenesis. **A,** Type I, total or partial unilateral sacral agenesis. **B,** Type II, partial sacral agenesis with partial, bilateral symmetrical defects in stable articulation between ilia and normal or hypoplastic S1 vertebra. **C,** Type III, variable lumbar and total sacral agenesis; ilia articulate with lowest vertebra. **D,** Type IV, variable lumbar and total sacral agenesis; caudal endplate of lowest vertebra rests above fused ilia or iliac amphiarthrosis. (From Renshaw TS: *J Bone Joint Surg*: 60A:373, 1978.)

endplate of the lowest vertebra resting above either fused or an iliac amphiarthrosis (Fig. 38-218, *D*).

Type II defects are most common, and type I are least common. Types I and II usually have a stable vertebral-pelvic articulation, whereas types III and IV produce instability and possibly a progressive kyphosis.

The clinical appearance of a child with sacral agenesis ranges from one of severe deformities of the pelvis and lower extremities to no deformity or weakness whatsoever. Those

with partial sacral or coccygeal agenesis may have no symptoms. Those with lumbar or complete sacral agenesis may be severely deformed, with multiple musculoskeletal abnormalities, including foot deformities, knee flexion contractures with popliteal wedging, hip flexion contractures, dislocated hips, spinal-pelvic instability, and scoliosis. The posture of the lower extremities has been compared with a "sitting Buddha" (Fig. 38-219). Anomalies of the viscera, especially in the genitourinary system and the rectal area, are common.

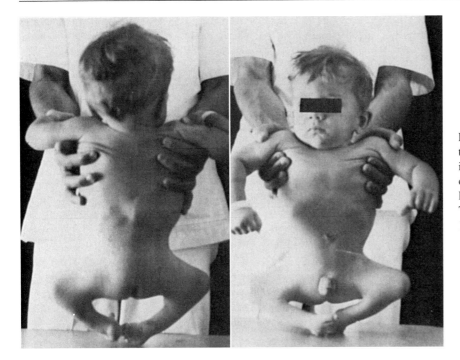

Fig. 38-219   Severe knee flexion contractures with popliteal wedging and hip flexion deformities or contractures as result of lumbosacral agenesis at T12 level. (From Phillips WA, Cooperman DR, Lindquist TC, et al: *J Bone Joint Surg* 64A:1282, 1982.)

Inspection of the back reveals a bony prominence representing the last vertebral segment, often with gross motion between this vertebral prominence and the pelvis. Flexion and extension may occur at the junction of the spine and pelvis rather than the hips.

Neurological examination usually reveals intact motor power down to the level of the lowest vertebral body that has pedicles. Sensation, however, is present down to more caudal levels. Even patients with the most severe involvement may have sensation to the knees and spotty hypesthesia distally. Bladder and bowel control often is impaired.

Treatment

In 1982 Phillips et al. reviewed the orthopaedic management of lumbosacral agenesis and concluded that patients with partial or complete absence of the sacrum only (types I and II) have an excellent chance of becoming community ambulators. Management of more severe deformities (types III and IV) is more controversial.

Scoliosis is the most common spinal anomaly associated with sacral agenesis. No correlation has been found between the type of defect and the likelihood of scoliosis. Scoliosis may be associated with congenital anomalies, such as hemivertebra, or with no obvious spinal abnormality above the level of the vertebral agenesis. Progressive scoliosis or kyphosis requires operative stabilization as for similar scoliosis without sacral agenesis.

The treatment of spinal-pelvic instability is more controversial. Perry et al. believe the key to rehabilitation of a patient with an unstable spinal-pelvic junction is establishment of a stable vertebral-pelvic complex about which lower extremity contractures can be stretched or operatively released. Renshaw also believes that patients with type III or type IV defects must

be observed closely for signs of progressive kyphosis. If progressive deformity is noted, he recommended lumbopelvic arthrodesis as early as is consistent with successful fusion. In his series, fusion was done in patients 4 years of age or older. Phillips et al., however, found that spinal-pelvic instability was not a problem in 18 of the 20 surviving patients at long-term follow-up. Others noted an actual decrease in the ability to sit after stabilization of the lumbopelvic area. Proper care of patients with sacral agenesis is best provided by a treatment team, including an orthopaedic surgeon, urologist, neurosurgeon, pediatrician, physical therapist, and orthotist-prosthetist.

Unusual Causes of Scoliosis

NEUROFIBROMATOSIS

Neurofibromatosis is a hereditary hamartomatous disorder of neural crest derivation. These hamartomatous tissues may appear in any organ system of the body. The most widely described clinical forms of neurofibromatosis are the peripheral (NF-1) and central (NF-2) types.

The classic neurofibromatosis (NF-1) described by von Recklinghausen is an autosomal dominant disorder that affects approximately 1 in 4000 people. Patients with NF-1 develop Schwann cell tumors and pigmentation abnormalities. Orthopaedic problems are frequent in patients with this type of neurofibromatosis, with spinal deformity being the most common.

Central (NF-2) neurofibromatosis also is an autosomal dominant disorder; however, it is much less common. It is characterized by bilateral acoustic neuromas. NF-2 neurofibromatosis does not have any bony involvement or orthopaedic manifestations. The diagnosis of NF-1 neurofibromatosis is based on clinical criteria (Box 38-12).

Scoliosis is the most common osseous defect associated with neurofibromatosis. In a group of patients with scoliosis, Crawford and Bagamery found that 3% had neurofibromatosis; in patients with neurofibromatosis, 60% had some disorder of the spine. Akbarnia et al. found spinal deformities in 10% of 220 patients with neurofibromatosis and believe that this is representative of the true prevalence of spinal deformity in an otherwise unselected cross section of neurofibromatosis patients.

The spinal deformities of neurofibromatosis are of two basic forms: nondystrophic and dystrophic. Nondystrophic deformities mimic idiopathic scoliosis. Dystrophic scoliosis characteristically is a short-segment, sharply angulated curve with severe wedging of the vertebral bodies, severe rotation of the vertebrae, scalloping of the vertebral bodies, spindling of the transverse processes, foraminal enlargement, and rotation of the ribs 90 degrees in the anteroposterior direction, making them appear abnormally thin. Curves with significant sagittal plane deformity are common in dystrophic scoliosis. Neurofibromatosis kyphoscoliosis is characterized by acute angulation in the sagittal plane and striking deformity of the vertebral bodies near the apex. Winter also described severe thoracic lordoscoliosis in patients with neurofibromatosis. Functional scoliosis may be caused by leg length discrepancy resulting from lower extremity hypertrophy or dysplasia of the long bones.

In a review of 102 patients with neurofibromatosis, Winter et al. found that 80 patients had curvatures associated with dystrophic changes in the vertebrae and ribs. Nondystrophic curves behaved according to their causative factors (idiopathic, congenital, and Scheuermann disease), and the neurofibromatosis appeared to have no influence on the curve or its treatment. Because only a few of the dystrophic curves remained small, Winter et al. emphasized that observation of progression of a dystrophic spinal deformity is unjustified in patients with neurofibromatosis. Spinal deformity caused

paraplegia only in patients with dystrophic kyphoscoliosis; paraplegia did not occur in those with dystrophic scoliosis alone. Laminectomy alone worsened spinal cord compression caused by kyphoscoliosis.

Management of Nondystrophic Curves

Nondystrophic curves have the same prognosis and evolution as do idiopathic curves, except for a higher risk of pseudarthrosis after operative fusion. Crawford reported that some nondystrophic curves developed dystrophic changes. The general guidelines for treating these curves are the same as for idiopathic curves. Curves of less than 20 to 25 degrees are observed; if no dystrophic changes occur, a brace is prescribed when the deformity progresses to 30 degrees. If the deformity exceeds 40 to 45 degrees, a posterior spinal fusion with multihook segmental instrumentation is recommended. Shufflebarger reported 10 patients with neurofibromatosis and nondystrophic curves treated with posterior spinal fusion, Cotrel-Dubousset instrumentation, and conventional hook patterns without postoperative immobilization. Although follow-up is short, results were similar to those after instrumentation of idiopathic curves. Also common in these patients are spinal canal neurofibromas, which may grow and cause pressure-induced dysplasia of the canal. CT myelography or MRI should be done before surgery to rule out the presence of any intraspinal canal neurofibroma.

Management of Dystrophic Scoliosis

Winter et al. reported an average progression of 27 degrees during brace treatment of 10 patients with dystrophic curves; none improved. They believe that brace treatment is not indicated for the typical dystrophic curve of neurofibromatosis.

Appropriate operative treatment is determined by the presence or absence of a kyphotic deformity and by the presence or absence of neurological deficits.

Before operative treatment of dystrophic curves in patients with neurofibromatosis, the presence of an intraspinal lesion, such as a pseudomeningocele, dural ectasia, or an intraspinal neurofibroma (dumbbell tumor) should be ruled out. Impingement of these lesions against the spinal cord has been reported to cause paraplegia after instrumentation of these curves. MRI or complete high-volume CT myelogram in the prone, lateral, and supine positions should be done before operative treatment. Although myelography is adequate to evaluate the presence of intraspinal tumors or dural ectasia, MRI is better to evaluate displacement of the cord, subarachnoid extent of neurofibroma, or anterior abnormalities; however, MRI may be inadequate for the severe kyphoscoliotic deformity associated with dystrophic kyphoscoliosis, and high-volume computed myelography often is necessary.

Scoliosis Without Kyphosis

Patients with dystrophic scoliosis without kyphosis should be followed at 6-month intervals if the curve is less than 20 degrees. As soon as the progression of the curve is noted, a posterior spinal fusion should be done. If this fusion is done

A   B   C   D

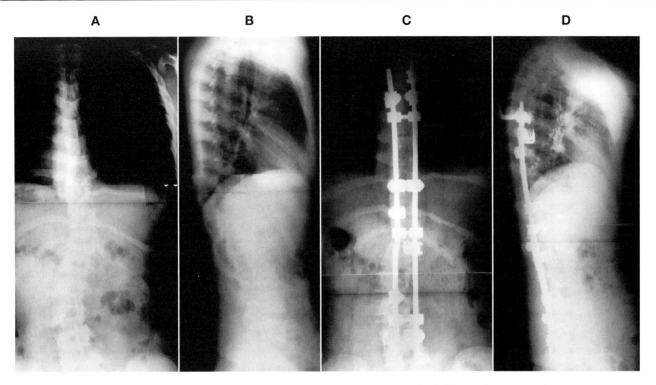

Fig. 38-220   **A** and **B**, Dystrophic scoliosis. **C** and **D**, After posterior fusion and instrumentation.

before the curve becomes too large, anterior fusion will not be necessary (Fig. 38-220). For curves larger than 80 degrees, Betz et al. recommended combined anterior and posterior arthrodesis unless there are contraindications to the anterior approach (e.g., patients with anterior neurofibromas, excessive venous channels, poor medical condition, or thrombocytopenia caused by splenic obstruction by a fibroma). Crawford and Gabriel recommended primary anterior and posterior fusion for dystrophic curves with scoliosis of more than 40 degrees, unless contraindicated (e.g., by young age, osteoporotic bone, or peculiar anatomical configurations). Multihook segmental instrumentation systems provide correction and permit ambulation with or without postoperative bracing. If instrumentation is tenuous, bracing should be used. The fusion mass must be followed carefully. If there is any question as to the status of the fusion mass, the surgical area is explored 1 year after surgery, and additional autogenous bone grafting is done. Similarly, if progression of more than 10 degrees occurs, the fusion mass is explored and reinforced.

Kyphoscoliosis

Winter et al. and Hsu et al. emphasized that patients with dystrophic scoliosis and angular kyphosis respond poorly to posterior fusion alone. Good results were consistently obtained only by combined anterior and posterior fusions. They also emphasized that not all patients had solid fusions initially, even with both anterior and posterior procedures. Winter et al. believe that the reasons for failure are too little bone and too limited a fusion area. They emphasized that the entire structural

area of the deformity must be fused anteriorly, with complete disc excision and strong strut grafts, preferably from the fibula, as well as rib and iliac crest grafts. Ideally, all anterior grafts should be in contact throughout with other grafts or with the spine. Those grafts surrounded by soft tissue tend to be resorbed in the midportion. Hsu et al., however, noted that an "adequate" anterior procedure can be difficult in severely angulated dystrophic curves. They emphasized the importance of early diagnosis and treatment by combined anterior and posterior fusions with internal fixation, if possible. Betz et al. and Calvert, Edgar, and Webb questioned the necessity of an anterior approach in all dystrophic kyphoscoliotic curves.

For smaller dystrophic scoliosis with kyphosis of less than 40 degrees, posterior spinal instrumentation with arthrodesis is considered as soon as possible. The fusion mass should be explored at 1 year after surgery or sooner if progression of more than 10 degrees occurs. If the kyphosis is larger than 50 degrees, anterior disc excision with fibular strut bone grafting should be done, followed by posterior arthrodesis and instrumentation. The anterior fusion should extend one or two levels past both end vertebrae. The fusion mass should be reexplored at 6 months after surgery with augmentation of the fusion mass if necessary. The bone structure and severity of the curvature may be such that conventional instrumentation cannot be used and halo casting may be necessary in these patients. Betz et al. recommended that if anterior fusion is necessary for kyphoscoliotic deformities, vascularized rib graft augmentation as described by Bradford (Fig. 38-221), should be considered.

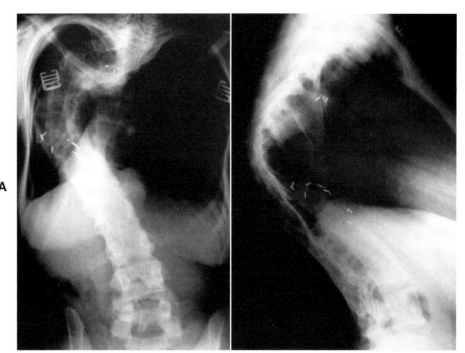

Fig. 38-221   **A** and **B,** After anterior fusion with vascularized rib graft in patient with dystrophic kyphoscoliosis.

Kyphoscoliosis with Spinal Cord Compression

Winter et al. reported 16 patients with spinal cord or cauda equina compression: 8 had cord compression from spinal angulation, 5 had neural signs caused by tumors, and 3 had problems caused both by tumors and by angulation. Cord compression caused by an intraspinal lesion must be distinguished from kyphotic angular cord compression by MRI or high-volume CT myelography in the prone, lateral, and supine positions. Patients with severe scoliosis without significant kyphosis and with evidence of paraplegia should be assumed to have an intraspinal lesion until proved otherwise. If cord compression is caused by kyphoscoliotic deformity, laminectomy is absolutely contraindicated. Removal of the posterior elements adds to the kyphosis and also removes valuable bone surface for a posterior fusion. If spinal cord compression is minor and no intraspinal tumor is present, halo gravity traction can be used (p. 1773). The patient's neurological status must be monitored carefully even if the kyphosis is mobile. As the alignment of the spinal canal improves and the compression is eliminated, anterior and posterior fusions can be done without direct observation of the cord. However, significant cord compression in patients with severe structural kyphoscoliosis requires anterior cord decompression. Anterior strut graft fusion must be done with this decompression, and posterior fusion is done as a second stage. If a tumor causes spinal cord compression anteriorly, anterior excision, spinal cord decompression, and fusion are indicated. If the lesion is posterior, a hemilaminectomy with tumor excision may be necessary. Instrumentation and fusion should be done at the time of decompression to prevent a rapidly increasing kyphotic deformity and neurological injury.

Thoracic Lordoscoliosis

Winter reported two patients with thoracic lordoscoliosis and neurofibromatosis who were treated with Harrington rod instrumentation and sublaminar wiring. Although fragility of the dystrophic laminae and the risk of injury to a fragile dural ectasia are reasons for concern, they do not exclude the possibility of correcting the thoracic lordosis. Both of his patients obtained solid arthrodeses with only posterior fusions. More severe lordosis may require anterior discectomy before the posterior procedure.

Postoperative Management

Patients with nondystrophic curves are managed the same as those with idiopathic curves. If, however, the instrumentation is tenuous, casting or bracing is used. All patients with dystrophic neurofibromatosis probably should be immobilized in a cast or brace until fusion is evident on anteroposterior, lateral, and oblique roentgenograms. Exploration of the fusion mass at 6 to 12 months after surgery generally is necessary in dystrophic curves, and prolonged immobilization often is needed. Even after the fusion is solid, the patient should be followed annually to be certain that no erosion of the fusion mass is occurring.

Complications of Surgery

In addition to the complications inherent in any major spinal surgery, several complications are related to the neurofibromatosis. McCarroll pointed out that a plexiform venous anomaly may be encountered in the soft tissues surrounding the spine that can impede the operative approach to the vertebral bodies and lead to excessive bleeding. The increased vascularity of the neurofibromatous tissue itself also may increase blood loss.

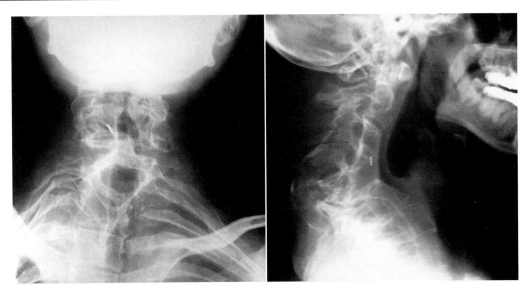

Fig. 38-222   Cervical spine deformity in patient with neurofibromatosis.

Hsu et al. noted that pheochromocytoma, a tumor arising from chromaffin cells, can be associated with neurofibromatosis. The angular deformity of the neurofibromatosis may cause significant mechanical problems with anterior strut grafting. The apical bodies may have subluxed into bayonet apposition or be so rotated that they no longer are in alignment with the rest of the spine. This malalignment does not allow the anterior strut grafts to be placed in the concavity of the kyphosis and makes them mechanically less effective in preventing its progression. Winter et al. and Hsu et al. emphasized the difficulty, as well as the necessity, of an adequate anterior fusion. Shufflebarger recommended performing the anterior procedure from the concave side, using multiple strut grafts. Convex discectomies further destabilize the spine, and placing struts from the convex approach is technically difficult.

Many patients with neurofibromatosis and scoliosis have cervical spine abnormalities (Fig. 38-222). Curtis et al. reported deformities in the cervical spine that caused cord compression in four of their eight patients who had neurofibromatosis with paraplegia. Yong-Hing, Kalamachi, and MacEwen found that 44% of their patients with scoliosis or kyphoscoliosis had associated cervical lesions, which they classified into two groups: abnormalities of bone structure and abnormalities of vertebral alignment. Cervical anomalies were most common in patients with short kyphotic curves or thoracic or lumbar curves that measured more than 65 degrees. This also is the group of patients more apt to require anesthesia, traction, and operative stabilization of the spine. They therefore recommended routine roentgenographic evaluation of the cervical spine in all patients with neurofibromatosis before anesthesia for any reason and before traction for treatment of the scoliosis.

Winter et al. reported postoperative paralysis in two patients caused by contusion of the spinal cord by the periosteal elevator during exposure. Both patients had unsuspected areas of laminar erosion because of dural ectasia. A complete, high-volume myelogram series in the prone, lateral, and supine positions would have alerted the surgeon to this before surgery. The most dangerous situation for neurologically intact patients with neurofibromatosis is instrumentation and distraction of the spine in the presence of unrecognized intraspinal lesions.

MARFAN SYNDROME

Marfan syndrome is a hereditary disorder of connective tissue inherited as an autosomal dominant trait. Sporadic occurrences reportedly account for 15% of patients. Studies by Boucek et al. have implicated a possible defect in collagen cross links.

Diagnosis

Pyeritz and McKusick divided the physical findings in Marfan syndrome into major signs and minor signs. Major signs include ectopia lentis, aortic dilation, severe kyphoscoliosis, and thoracic deformity. Minor signs include myopia, tall stature, mitral valve prolapse, ligamentous laxity, and arachnodactyly. Screening tests for the Marfan phenotype include the thumb sign (the thumb extends well beyond the ulnar border of the hand when overlapped by the fingers), the wrist sign (the thumb overlaps the fifth finger as the patient grasps the opposite wrist), and the knee sign (the patient has the ability to touch his toes on the floor when sitting with the knees crossed). The diagnosis of Marfan syndrome frequently is delayed because cardiovascular involvement is a major diagnostic criterion and may not be evident until adolescence or adulthood. No specific "test" exists to identify Marfan syndrome.

Joseph et al. divided patients with the Marfan phenotype into three groups: group I included patients with a definite diagnosis of Marfan syndrome (two or more major signs with additional minor signs); group II patients represented probable

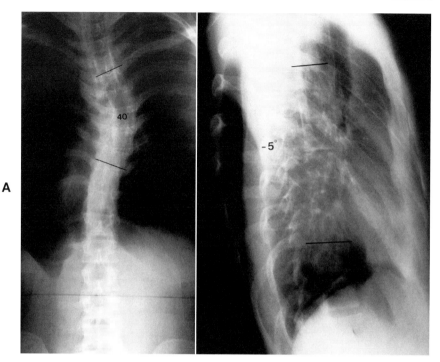

Fig. 38-223 **A** and **B,** Thoracic lordosis in patient with Marfan syndrome.

A

B

Marfan syndrome (patients with one major sign and multiple minor signs); and group III patients represented the Marfan phenotype (patients with multiple minor signs only). They concluded that even patients with the Marfan phenotype have a high incidence of severe progressive scoliosis. Scoliosis is reported to occur in 40% to 60% of patients with Marfan syndrome. Joseph et al. found scoliosis in 100% of patients with definite Marfan syndrome and in 89% of patients with probable Marfan syndrome or the Marfan phenotype. Sponseller et al. found that 62% of patients had curves of more than 10 degrees. In adulthood curves of less than 40 degrees tended not to progress, whereas curves over 40 degrees progressed an average of 2.8 degrees a year. The curve patterns of scoliosis in Marfan syndrome were similar to those in idiopathic scoliosis. Double major curves were the most frequent, and the scoliosis progressed more frequently in the infantile age group. Disabling back pain was more frequently a presenting complaint in patients with scoliosis associated with Marfan syndrome than in patients with idiopathic scoliosis. Sagittal plane deformities were common (Fig. 38-223), although only three patients had thoracic lordosis. Spondylolisthesis was found in 5%; the percentage of slip was more than that in the normal population.

Nonoperative Treatment

Observation. For young patients with small curves of less than 25 degrees, observation every 3 to 4 months is indicated. The family should be made aware, however, that many of these curves progress.

Orthotic Treatment. Robins, Moe, and Winter treated 14 patients with Milwaukee bracing and found that 3 curves were improved and 3 did not increase. They concluded that the use of the Milwaukee brace should be limited to mild flexible curves. Birch and Herring found orthotic treatment successful in only one of nine patients. Joseph et al. found orthotic management moderately successful but noted that an underarm TLSO in a patient with this syndrome often leads to chest wall deformity, with narrowing of the inferior portion of the thoracic cage, which serves to accentuate the slender trunk already present. They recommended the use of the Milwaukee brace, which is less restricting. Milwaukee bracing is indicated for patients with flexible progressive curves between 25 and 40 degrees that have no associated thoracic lordosis or lumbar kyphosis. Bracing is not indicated for rigid, large curves or curves associated with thoracic lordosis.

Operative Treatment

If progression occurs despite bracing or if the curve exceeds 40 degrees, spinal fusion is recommended. If nonoperative treatment is continued too long, cardiovascular involvement may progress to the point of making surgery dangerous, if not impossible. Before operative intervention is considered, a complete cardiovascular evaluation is mandatory. Aortic dilation can develop in these patients at any time from childhood to late adolescence or adulthood. Echocardiography is recommended because its sensitivity for aortic root dilation greatly exceeds that of auscultation. Any evidence of aortic dilation should be treated medically or operatively before treatment of the spinal deformity.

Robins et al. concluded that scoliosis in patients with Marfan syndrome can be corrected with no more morbidity than in patients with idiopathic scoliosis and that solid fusion and maintenance of correction can be anticipated. Birch and Herring reported frequent complications in these patients, including pseudarthroses in 44% and postoperative loss of correction. They emphasized that these patients require massive bone grafts, secure segmental internal fixation, and careful postoperative observation for pseudarthrosis. Generally the technique of instrumentation and selection of hook levels are the same as for idiopathic scoliosis (p. 1795). Donaldson and Brown emphasized that care must be taken in determining the distal extent of the fusion to avoid junctional kyphosis. The lumbar extent of the fusion must go to the intersection of the sagittal vertical line dropped from C7. They noted that this generally is at L2 or below.

Winter reported that thoracic lordosis is relatively common in patients with Marfan syndrome and spinal deformity, and sagittal plane balance must be obtained in addition to improvement of the coronal plane deformity. Multihook segmental instrumentation systems are effective in correcting this problem. Surgical treatment should provide a more normal anteroposterior diameter of the chest, since this frequently is quite narrow.

Birch and Herring emphasized the importance of kyphotic deformity in the sagittal plane. Not all adolescents with kyphosis required surgery, but those who did required anterior fusion and posterior instrumentation and fusion. Typically kyphosis has a low thoracic or thoracolumbar apex and involvement of the lumbar spine.

Severe spondylolisthesis associated with Marfan syndrome has been reported by Winter, Taylor, and Sponseller et al. It has been postulated that the spondylolisthesis may be more likely to progress because of poor musculoligamentous tissues. Taylor reported successful treatment of grade IV spondylolisthesis with in situ fusion.

VERTEBRAL COLUMN TUMORS

Because of their variable presentation, tumors of the vertebral column often present diagnostic problems. A team composed of a surgeon, diagnostic radiologist, pathologist, and often a medical oncologist and radiotherapist is necessary for treatment of the spectrum of tumors that involve the spine. This section discusses the most common primary tumors of the vertebral column in children.

Clinical Findings

A complete history is the first step in the evaluation of any patient with a tumor. The initial complaint of patients with tumors involving the spine generally is pain. The exact type and distribution of pain vary with the anatomical location of the pathological process. In general, pain caused by a neoplasm is not relieved by rest and often is worse at night. Occasionally, constitutional symptoms such as anorexia, weight loss, or fever may be present. The age and sex of the patient may be important in the differential diagnosis.

Physical examination should include a general evaluation in addition to careful examination of the spine. The tumor may produce local tenderness, muscle spasm, scoliosis, and limited spine motion. A careful neurological examination is essential.

Laboratory studies should include a complete blood count, urinalysis, and sedimentation rate, as well as serum calcium, phosphorus, and alkaline phosphatase concentrations. As the evaluation continues, further laboratory studies may be indicated.

Roentgenographic Evaluation and Treatment

Standing roentgenograms of the spine should be made in at least two planes at 90-degree angles. If a scoliotic curve is present, the curve usually shows significant coronal decompensation. There is an absence of the usual compensatory balancing curve above or below the curve containing the lesion. The scoliosis lacks the usual structural characteristics associated with idiopathic scoliosis, such as vertebral rotation and wedging. Curves with these characteristics should raise the index of suspicion for an underlying cause of the scoliosis.

Bone scanning is helpful in certain tumors of the spine, especially osteoid osteoma. CT has greatly improved evaluation of the extent of the lesion and the presence of any spinal canal compromise; sagittal and coronal reformatted images are necessary to define the exact anatomical location and extent of the lesion. MRI is useful in evaluating the extent of soft tissue involvement of the tumor and for determining the level and extent of neurological compromise in patients with a neurological deficit.

Arteriography may be indicated to evaluate the extent of the tumor and to localize major feeder vessels. Dick et al. reported the use of adjuvant arterial embolization in the treatment of benign primary bone tumors in children. Their indications for embolization are benign vascular tumors in central locations. Three of the four tumors they embolized were aneurysmal bone cysts. Contraindications include avascular tumors and tumors supplied by vessels that also supply important segments of the spinal cord, because embolization of these vessels may infarct the spinal cord. Dick et al. suggested that malignant tumors that are to be treated with radiation should not be embolized, since effective radiation requires high oxygenation of the cells.

Biopsy

Certain tumors such as osteochondroma and osteoid osteoma generally can be diagnosed by their clinical presentation and roentgenographic appearance. Other benign tumors such as osteoblastoma, aneurysmal bone cyst, and giant cell tumors often are difficult to diagnose preoperatively. Biopsy is the ultimate diagnostic technique for evaluating neoplasms. The biopsy may be incisional (removal of a small portion of the tumor) or excisional (removal of the entire tumor).

Percutaneous CT-guided needle biopsy is an excellent diagnostic tool. Ghelman et al. obtained histological diagnoses in 85% of 76 biopsies, and Kattapuram, Khurana, and Rosenthal obtained accurate diagnoses in 92%. Metastatic diseases were most often diagnosed accurately (95%), and benign primary tumors were diagnosed least often (82%). Fine-needle cytological aspirates are satisfactory for diagnosing metastatic disease and most infections, but large-core biopsy specimens are preferable for primary bone tumors. If the needle biopsy is not diagnostic, an open biopsy or transpedicular biopsy will yield more tissue. Care must be taken that the open biopsy does not interfere with the definitive surgery if total resection is anticipated.

◆ Open Biopsy of Thoracic Vertebra

TECHNIQUE 38-51 *(Michele and Krueger)*

With the patient prone, make an incision over the side of the spinous process of the involved vertebra. Retract the muscles and expose the transverse process. Perform an osteotomy at the base of the transverse process at its junction with the lamina (Fig. 38-224, *A*). By depressing or retracting the transverse process, expose the isthmus of the vertebra, revealing the cancellous nature of its bone structure. Roentgenographic verification of the level is very important. Insert a $^3/_{16}$-inch trephine with $^1/_4$-inch markings through the fenestra and guide it downward with slight pressure so that a mere twisting action leads the trephine into the pedicle and finally into the body (Fig. 38-224, *B*). Remove the trephine repeatedly, and in each instance check that the contents consist of cancellous bone, which indicates that the trephine is in the medullary substance of the pedicle and has created a channel from the posterior elements directly into the vertebral body. Remove the pathological tissue with a small blunt curet.

Alternatively, after the osteotomy of the base of the transverse process, expose the vertebral body by retracting the transverse process and depressing the adjacent rib to expose the junction of the pedicle and the body. Use the trephine to penetrate this junction at an angle of 45 degrees toward the midline and remove the material with a curet (Fig. 38-224, *C*).

Benign Tumors of Vertebral Column

The most common benign tumors of the vertebral column in children are osteoid osteoma, osteoblastoma, aneurysmal bone cyst, eosinophilic granuloma, and hemangioma.

Osteoid Osteoma. Osteoid osteoma is a benign growth that consists of a discrete osteoid nidus and reactive sclerotic bone thickening around the nidus. No malignant change of these tumors ever has been documented. The lesion occurs more frequently in males than females. Spinal lesions occur predominantly in the posterior elements of the spine, especially the lamina and the pedicles. Osteoid osteoma of the vertebral body has been reported but is quite rare. The lumbar spine is the most frequently involved area.

Typically, patients with spinal osteoid osteoma have pain that is worse at night and is relieved by aspirin. The pain increases with activity and often is localized to the site of the lesion. Radicular symptoms are especially common with lesions of the lumbar spine. Lesions in the cervical spine can produce radicular-type symptoms in the shoulders and arms, but the results of the neurological examination usually are normal.

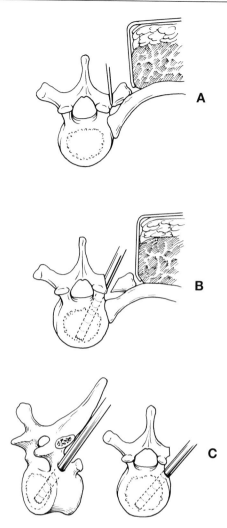

Fig. 38-224   **A,** Transverse osteotomy at base of thoracic transverse process. **B,** Trephine through fenestra of isthmus, into pedicle and body. **C,** Trephine inserted into body at junction of pedicle. (Redrawn from Michele AA, Krueger FJ: *J Bone Joint Surg* 31A:873, 1949.)

Physical examination reveals muscle spasm in the involved area of the spine. The patient's gait may be abnormal because of pain, and localized tenderness over the tumor may be moderate to severe.

Osteoid osteoma is the most common cause of painful scoliosis in adolescents. Marsh et al., Mehta, and Pettine and Klassen reported that scoliosis is common when the vertebral column is involved. The scoliosis associated with osteoid osteoma usually is described as a C-shaped curve, but Pettine and Klassen found that only 23% of the scoliotic curves in their patients had this classic curve pattern, and Keim and Reina noted that only three of their nine patients had typical C-shaped curves. The osteoid osteoma usually is located on the concave side of the curve and in the area of the apical vertebra.

When the osteoid osteoma is visible on plain roentgenograms, its appearance is diagnostic: a central radiolucency with surrounding sclerotic bony reaction; however, the lesion often is not visible on plain films. Technetium bone scanning should

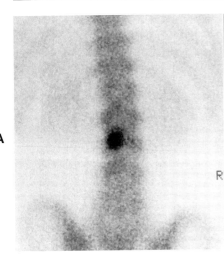 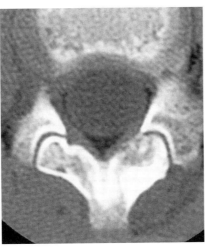

A   **B**

Fig. 38-225   Bone scan (**A**) and CT scan (**B**) of patient with spinal osteoid osteoma.

be considered in any adolescent with painful scoliosis (Fig. 38-225, *A*). False-negative bone scans have not been reported in patients with osteoid osteoma of the spine. CT using very narrow cuts will precisely define the location of the tumor and the extent of the osseous involvement (Fig. 38-225, *B*).

Mehta and Murray suggested that patients with spinal tumors and scoliosis reach a critical point after which the continuation of a painful stimulus results in structural changes in the spine. Pettine and Klassen found that 15 months is the critical duration of symptoms if antalgic scoliosis is to undergo spontaneous correction after excision of the tumor. They noted improvement or complete correction of the scoliosis in 11 of 12 patients in whom the lesion was removed before 15 months of symptoms. In 10 of 11 patients with symptoms for more than 15 months, no improvement in the scoliosis occurred after removal of the lesion. Although the natural course of many osteoid osteomas is spontaneous remission, spinal lesions in children or adolescents should be removed when diagnosed to prevent the development of structural scoliosis. The operative treatment of an osteoid osteoma is complete removal; recurrence is likely after incomplete removal. If pain and deformity persist after removal of the lesion, incomplete removal or perhaps a multifocal lesion should be suspected. Exact localization of the tumor is imperative; in the series of Pettine and Klassen, five patients had the initial operative procedure on the wrong locations. Rinsky et al. reported the use of intraoperative localization of the lesion by radionuclide imaging and the use of a gamma camera. In our experience the camera is rather bulky, and we have been unable to accurately pinpoint the location of the nidus of the osteoid osteoma in this manner. The best way to determine the exact location of the nidus preoperatively is with high-resolution CT scanning. Technetium can be injected 2 to 3 hours before surgery, and the specimen can be sent for in vitro radionuclide evaluation, as described by Israeli et al. If the specimen can be excised en bloc, a CT scan of the specimen may show the nidus.

Excision of these lesions usually does not require spinal fusion, but if removal of a significant portion of the facet joints

and pedicles makes the spine unstable, spinal fusion can be done at the time of tumor removal.

Osteoblastoma. Most authors believe that osteoid osteoma and osteoblastoma are variant manifestations of a benign osteoblastic process, resulting in an osteoid nidus surrounded by sclerotic bone. Histologically the lesions are similar. The primary difference is the tendency of the osteoblastoma to form a less sclerotic but more expansile mass. McLeod, Dahlin, and Beabout define lesions larger than 1.5 cm in diameter as osteoblastomas and those less than 1.5 cm as osteoid osteomas.

Benign osteoblastoma is an uncommon primary bone tumor that accounts for fewer than 1% of all bone tumors. Of these reported tumors, however, 40% have been located in the spine, and more than half were associated with scoliosis. Marsh et al. reported 197 osteoblastomas, 41 of which were in the spine. Nemoto et al., in a review of 75 spinal osteoblastomas, found that presenting symptoms for most patients included pain. The nonspecificity of symptoms often contributed to a delay in the diagnosis. Pain was present for an average of 16 months before the diagnosis was made. Scoliosis was present in 50% of patients with osteoblastomas involving the thoracic or lumbar spine. The osteoblastomas were always located in the concavity of the curve, near its apex.

In contrast to osteoid osteoma, plain roentgenograms often are sufficient to confirm the diagnosis of osteoblastoma. CT scans and bone scans (Fig. 38-226), however, can be helpful for a cross-sectional evaluation and localization of the tumor before operative excision. Osteoblastoma of the spine involves predominantly the posterior elements. Because 66% of their patients had lesions confined to the posterior elements and 31% had lesions that involved both the posterior elements and the vertebral bodies, Nemoto et al. concluded that a neoplasm involving only a vertebral body is unlikely to be an osteoblastoma. Spinal osteoblastomas are typically expansile with a scalloped or lobulated contour, well-defined margins, and frequently a sclerotic rim.

The treatment of osteoblastoma of the spine is complete operative excision. Marsh et al. reported a high cure rate even

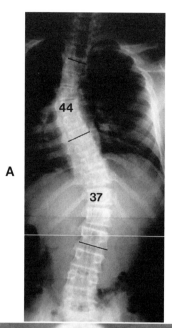

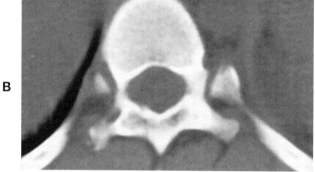

Fig. 38-226   Roentgenogram (**A**) and CT scan (**B**) of patient with osteoblastoma on right side of spine that caused left thoracic curve.

if curettage was incomplete because of the location of the tumor. Recurrences after incomplete curettage, however, are not rare, and malignant change has been reported after incomplete curettage; therefore complete excision is advised whenever possible. Because of the possibility of late sarcomatous changes, irradiation of this lesion is not recommended. The scoliosis associated with vertebral column osteoblastoma usually is reversible after excision if the diagnosis is made early and treatment is undertaken at that time. Akbarnia and Rooholamini found that the scoliosis improved in three patients who had symptoms for 9 months or less before excision of the tumor; the scoliosis did not improve in two patients whose symptoms had been present for longer periods of time.

Aneurysmal Bone Cysts. An aneurysmal bone cyst is a nonneoplastic, vasocystic tumor originating on either a previously normal bone or a preexisting lesion. It is most common in children and young adults, and vertebral involvement is common. Its roentgenographic appearance is characteristic: an expansile lesion confined by a thin rim of reactive bone. The

lesion occurs in both the vertebral body and in the posterior elements of the spine. Unlike other vertebral tumors, aneurysmal bone cysts may involve adjacent vertebrae. Pain is the most common symptom, and radicular symptoms may be caused by cord compression.

Treatment is operative excision whenever possible. The tumors can be quite vascular, and if operative resection is contemplated, preoperative embolization should be considered. Dick et al. emphasized that embolization should be done in addition to the operative excision and that vessels supplying important segments of the spinal cord or brain should not be embolized. DeCristofaro reported 19 aneurysmal bone cysts treated by selected arterial embolization alone, two of which involved the L2 vertebra. One of the lesions was treated with one embolization and one required a second embolization. Good clinical results were noted. They recommended selective arterial embolization as an excellent treatment choice for aneurysmal bone cysts. The major disadvantage is the need for repeat procedures and repeat CT scans and angiography. The diagnosis of the lesions in their patients was confirmed with incision or needle biopsies. Radiation therapy should be used only in those lesions that cannot be operatively excised.

Many patients with aneurysmal bone cysts of the vertebral column have neurological symptoms. Hay et al. reported that 21 of 71 patients with aneurysmal bone cysts of the vertebral column had significant neurological symptoms, including complete or incomplete paraplegia. An additional 18% had some root symptoms and signs. When these neurological symptoms occur, complete excision of the aneurysmal bone cyst with decompression of the spinal canal is indicated. The approach, whether anterior, posterior, or combined anterior and posterior, is dictated by the location of the lesion.

Eosinophilic Granuloma. Eosinophilic granuloma in childhood usually is a solitary lesion. The cause of this lesion, which may not represent a true neoplasm, is unknown. Approximately 10% involve the spine. Eosinophilic granuloma may produce varying degrees of vertebral collapse, including the classic picture of a vertebra plana. Considerable collapse of the vertebral body may occur without neurological compromise, and significant reconstitution in height may occur after treatment (Fig. 38-227). Villas et al. noted that bone scan demonstrated increased uptake in only one of six biopsy-confirmed eosinophilic granulomas. They suggested that a lytic roentgenographic image without vertebral plana with normal bone scan uptake probably is a benign lesion, but biopsy must still be done. The differential diagnoses include an aneurysmal bone cyst, acute leukemia, metastatic neuroblastoma, and Ewing sarcoma. Yu, Kasser, and O'Rourke reported vertebra plana in association with chronic recurrent multifocal osteomyelitis. If the lesion does not have the characteristic roentgenographic appearance, biopsy may be necessary. The treatment of vertebra plana generally focuses on relief of symptoms, and spontaneous healing of the lesion usually can be expected. Spinal deformity may be minimized by the use of an appropriate orthosis. Other treatment alternatives, including curettage and bone grafting, radiotherapy, and interlesional

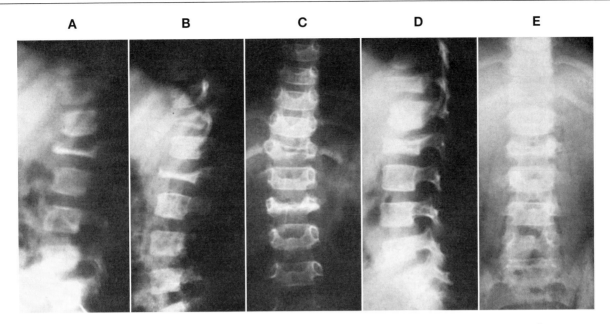

Fig. 38-227   **A,** Eosinophilic granuloma of spine in 3½-year-old patient. **B,** Sudden collapse of T12 3 weeks later, in addition to vertebra plana at L2. **C,** Collapse of T12 and L2. **D** and **E,** Considerable reconstitution of the vertebral height of T12 and L2 16 months later. (From Seimon LP: *J Pediatr Orthop* 1:371, 1981.)

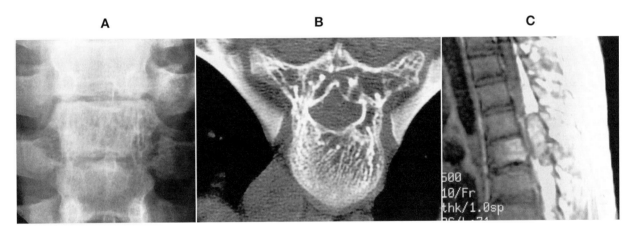

Fig. 38-228   Roentgenogram **(A),** CT scan **(B),** and MRI **(C)** of patient with spinal hemangioma with canal compromise.

installation of corticosteroids, also have been reported, but they rarely are needed.

Hemangioma. Hemangioma is the most common benign vascular tumor of bone. Most hemangiomas involve the vertebral bodies or skull, and involvement of other bones is rare. Vertebral involvement usually is an incidental finding and requires surgery only when neurological function is compromised (Fig. 38-228, *C*). Hemangioma has been reported in as many as 12% of spines studied by autopsy. The lesion usually produces a characteristic, vertical, striated appearance (Fig. 38-228, *A* and *B*). Laredo et al. subdivided vertebral hemangiomas into three subcategories. The most common is the asymptomatic vertebral hemangioma; the second is a compressive vertebral hemangioma that compresses the cord or

cauda equina; and the third is the rare vertebral hemangioma that causes clinical symptoms (symptomatic vertebral hemangioma). They noted six roentgenographic criteria that were indicative of vertebral hemangioma leading to compressive problems: thoracic location (from T3 to T9), entire vertebral body involvement, neural arch (particularly pedicles) involvement, irregular, honeycomb appearance, expanded and poorly defined cortex, and swelling of the soft tissue. They suggested that in patients with vertebral hemangioma and back pain of uncertain origin, the presence of three or more of these signs may indicate a potentially symptomatic vertebral hemangioma. Laredo et al. also compared MRI findings in asymptomatic and symptomatic vertebral hemangiomas. They found that vertebral hemangiomas with a low-signal intensity on T1-weighted images had a significant vascular component and might have been a major contributing factor to the patient's symptoms. Most vertebral hemangiomas contained predominant fat attenuation values on CT and showed high-signal intensity on T1-weighted imaging, indicating a predominantly fatty content. They emphasized, however, as has been our experience, that most vertebral hemangiomas are not symptomatic and are an incidental finding. If neurological dysfunction and anterior collapse occur, operative excision of the lesion, perhaps with adjuvant embolization, as described by Dick et al., is recommended.

Primary Malignant Tumors of Vertebral Column

Primary malignant tumors of the vertebral column are uncommon. In children, the most common are Ewing sarcoma and osteogenic sarcoma.

Ewing Sarcoma. Ewing sarcoma is a relatively rare, primary malignant tumor of bone of uncertain histogenesis. The tumor occurs most frequently in males in the second decade of life. All bones, including the spine, may be affected. The tumor most commonly begins in the pelvis or long bones and rapidly metastasizes to other skeletal sites, including the spine, especially the vertebral bodies and pedicles.

The currently recommended treatment for Ewing sarcoma is radiotherapy and adjuvant chemotherapy. Occasionally, surgery may be necessary to stabilize the spine because of compression of the neural elements and bony instability. If decompression of the neural elements is necessary, stabilization may be needed at the same time.

Osteogenic Sarcoma. Osteogenic sarcoma is the most common primary malignant bone tumor, excluding multiple myeloma, but fewer than 2% originate in the spine. It is a malignant tumor of bone in which tumor cells form neoplastic osteoid or bone, or both. Classic osteogenic sarcoma is more common in boys 10 to 15 years of age. This is a rapidly progressive malignancy, and multiple metastatic lesions to the vertebral column are more common than primary involvement. The role of surgery for vertebral involvement is based on whether the spinal lesion is solitary, primary, or metastatic. If decompression of the spinal cord becomes necessary or if structural integrity of the vertebral column is compromised, stabilizing procedures usually are required. If aggressive operative debridement is required, the neural structures limit the margin of the resection, making it impossible to achieve as wide a margin of resection as in the extremities.

POSTIRRADIATION SPINAL DEFORMITY

Perthes in 1903 first demonstrated inhibition of osseous development by irradiation. Later studies by Hinkel, Barr et al., and Reidy et al. indicated that the physis is particularly sensitive to radiation. A physis exposed to 600 rad or more showed some growth retardation, and complete inhibition of growth was produced by doses of more than 1200 rad. Bick and Copel reviewed histological sections of fresh autopsy material of vertebral bodies taken from subjects varying in age from 14

weeks of fetal development to 23 years of age. They demonstrated that the longitudinal growth of a vertebral body takes place by means of true physeal cartilage, similar to the longitudinal growth of the metaphysis of the long bones. Engel and Arkin et al. produced experimental scoliosis by asymmetrical irradiation, either internal or external.

Incidence

Mayfield et al. studied spinal deformity in children treated for neuroblastoma, and Riseborough et al. studied spinal deformity in children treated for Wilms tumor. Several principles can be summarized from these studies. A direct relationship seems to exist between the amount of radiation and the severity of the spinal deformity. In general, a dose of less than 2000 rad is not associated with significant deformity, a dose between 2000 and 3000 rad is associated with mild scoliosis, and a dose of more than 3000 rad is associated with more severe scoliosis. Irradiation in younger children, especially those 2 years of age or younger, produces the most serious disturbance in vertebral growth. Radiation treatment in children older than 4 years of age is less frequently associated with spinal deformity. Asymmetrical irradiation is associated with more frequent and also more severe deformities. In most patients the scoliosis remains slight until the adolescent growth spurt, at which time progression may occur. Scoliosis is the most frequent deformity, and the direction of the curve usually is concave toward the side of the irradiation. Kyphosis may occur in association with the scoliosis, or kyphosis alone may be present, most frequently at the thoracolumbar junction. Children who require a laminectomy because of epidural spread of tumor are especially prone to the development of moderate to severe spinal deformity. Similarly, those children whose disease causes paraplegia also are prone to rapid progression of the deformity. Without these two complicating features, most radiation-induced scoliotic deformities remain small and do not require treatment. Since progression of these curves generally occurs during the adolescent growth spurt, any child undergoing radiation therapy to the spine should have orthopaedic consultation and regular follow-up until skeletal maturity.

Roentgenographic Findings

Neuhauser et al. described the roentgenographic changes in previously irradiated spines, and Riseborough et al. divided the roentgenographic findings into four groups. The earliest noted changes were alterations in the vertebral bodies within the irradiated section of the spine, which are expressions of irradiation impairment of physeal enchondral growth at the vertebral endplates. The most obvious features of these lesions were growth arrest lines that subsequently led to the bone-in-bone picture (28%) (Fig. 38-229). Endplate irregularity with altered trabecular pattern and decreased vertebral body height were seen most frequently (83% of patients). Contour abnormalities, causing anterior narrowing and beaking of the vertebral bodies, such as in Morquio disease (Fig. 38-230), were present in 20% of patients. Asymmetrical or symmetrical

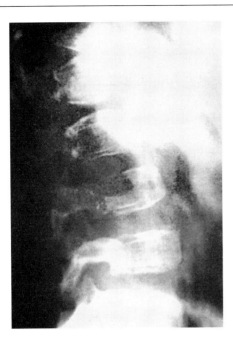

Fig. 38-229 "Bone-in-bone" appearance of irradiated spine, equivalent of growth arrest line in long bone. (From Katzman H et al: *J Bone Joint Surg* 51A:825, 1969.)

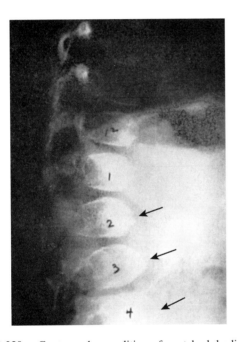

Fig. 38-230 Contour abnormalities of vertebral bodies after radiotherapy for Wilms tumor in 8-month-old patient. (From Katzman H et al: *J Bone Joint Surg* 51A:825, 1969.)

failure of vertebral body development was apparent on the anteroposterior roentgenograms of all 81 patients studied. The second group of roentgenographic changes included alterations in spinal alignment. Scoliosis was present in 70% of patients and kyphosis in 25%. The third group of roentgenographic findings included skeletal alterations in bones other than the

vertebral column, the most common of which were iliac wing hypoplasia (68%) and osteochondroma (6%). The fourth group consisted of patients with no evidence of deformity of the axial skeleton (27%).

Treatment

Most studies indicate that the curves usually remain slight until the adolescent growth spurt, when progression can be severe and rapid. Mayfield found that curves in 50% of patients treated with orthoses improved or did not progress; the other 50% progressed and required surgery. Riseborough et al. found that all three of their patients treated with Milwaukee braces required operative treatment. They concluded that the Milwaukee brace is ineffective in the treatment of postirradiation spinal deformity because of the severity of the changes in the architecture of the vertebrae and the excessive soft tissue scarring.

The indications for operative treatment include a scoliosis of more than 40 degrees or a thoracolumbar kyphosis of more than 50 degrees. Patients with progression despite brace treatment also are considered candidates for operative intervention. Riseborough et al. outlined the difficulties in obtaining adequate correction and fusion of these curves, which frequently are very rigid. Extensive soft tissue scarring may further complicate the surgery. Many patients requiring operative treatment have a kyphoscoliotic deformity, and many also have had previous laminectomies, which will inhibit solid fusion. Healing can be prolonged, and pseudarthrosis is common. Riseborough noted pseudarthroses in three of eight patients operatively treated, and King and Stowe found 10 pseudarthroses in 13 patients.

Combined anterior and posterior fusions with an anterior strut graft or anterior interbody fusion and posterior instrumentation should be considered for all patients with kyphotic deformities of more than 40 degrees. Anterior instrumentation rarely is used because of the unpredictable nature of the irradiated anterior bone stock. Multihook segmental instrumentation systems, with their ability to apply both compression and distraction, are ideal for posterior instrumentation in these patients. The fusion area is selected by the same criteria as for idiopathic curves (p. 1795). A large quantity of bone from the nonirradiated iliac crest should be used. Ogilvie suggested exploration of the fusion 6 months after surgery for repeated bone grafting of any developing pseudarthrosis. Because of problems with bone stock, postoperative immobilization in a TLSO is indicated until complete fusion is obtained.

Complications and Pitfalls

Pseudarthrosis, infection, and neurological injury are more frequent after spinal fusion for radiation-induced deformity than for other spinal deformities. The increase in pseudarthrosis is attributed to poor bone quality, decreased bone vascularity, skeletal immaturity, a kyphotic deformity, and the absence of posterior bone elements after laminectomy. Poor vascularity and skin quality have been associated with an increased infection rate. Severe scarring sometimes is present in the retroperitoneal space, making the anterior exposure more difficult.

OSTEOCHONDRODYSTROPHY

Diastrophic Dwarfism

Diastrophic dwarfism is inherited as an autosomal recessive disease. The dwarfing is severe, and almost all patients have scoliosis. Bethem, Winter, and Lutter found that the Milwaukee brace was useful only for small curves in these patients. If the curve cannot be braced successfully, fusion is indicated. In very young children, growth rod–type instrumentation can be considered. However, because growth is limited, repeat surgeries to lengthen the rods are done at 15- to 18-month intervals instead of the usual 6-month interval. By age 10, most of the spinal growth in a diastrophic dysplastic patient is complete and, definitive fusion is then done.

Cervical kyphosis occurs commonly, and although it usually resolves with age, it can cause quadriplegia if untreated. Roentgenographic evaluation of the cervical spine is mandatory in these patients. If the cervical kyphosis worsens, surgical treatment is necessary. If the kyphosis is mild, posterior fusion alone, combined with a halo brace should be considered. In an older child with a more severe kyphosis, combined anterior and posterior fusion should be considered. If the kyphosis is causing neurological problems, decompression anteriorly at the apex of the kyphosis is needed along with anterior and posterior fusion.

Spondyloepiphyseal Dysplasia

Orthopaedic aspects of spondyloepiphyseal dysplasia are discussed in Chapter 29.

The spinal problems most commonly associated with this condition are scoliosis, kyphoscoliosis, and odontoid hypoplasia with atlantoaxial instability (Fig. 38-231). If the scoliosis and kyphoscoliosis are progressive, orthotic treatment sometimes is useful for delaying the fusion until the patient is older. Bethem et al. found that the Milwaukee brace was more successful in managing the kyphotic deformity than the scoliotic deformity. Kopits found a 30% to 40% incidence of spondyloepiphyseal dysplasia in patients who had atlantoaxial instability. In children with this condition who are not walking by 2 to 3 years of age, the most likely explanation is spinal cord compression at the upper cervical region. Flexion-extension lateral cervical spine roentgenograms should be obtained. If ossification delay in vertebral bodies makes accurate determination of movement at this level impossible, a flexion-extension lateral MRI study is indicated. Once the instability is diagnosed, the treatment is surgical fusion.

If the scoliotic curve continues to progress despite bracing, surgical fusion is considered. Unlike achondroplasia, spinal stenosis generally is not present in patients with spondyloepiphyseal dysplasia, and standard-size instrumentation systems can be used.

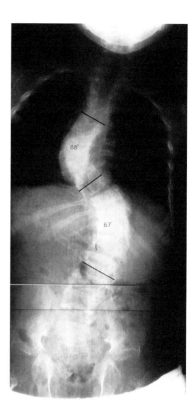

Fig. 38-231 Spinal deformity in patient with spondyloepiphyseal dysplasia.

OSTEOGENESIS IMPERFECTA

Patients with osteogenesis imperfecta have abnormal collagen production that results in defective bone (Fig. 38-232) and connective tissue. Other orthopaedic aspects of osteogenesis imperfecta are described in Chapter 29.

The reported incidence of spinal deformity in patients with osteogenesis imperfecta ranges from 40% to 90%. Hanscom et al. developed a classification system based on the degree of bony involvement and the likelihood of a spinal deformity developing. Patients with type A disease have mild bony abnormalities with normal vertebral contours. Patients with type B disease have bowed long bones and wide cortices with bioconcave vertebral bodies and normal pelvic contour. Patients with type C disease have thin, bowed long bones and protrusio acetabuli, which develop around the age of 10 years. Patients with type D disease have similar deformities as type C, with the addition of cystic changes around the knee by the age of 5 years. Patients with type E disease are totally dependent functionally. Scoliosis occurred in 46% of their patients with type A disease and in all patients with types C and D. Benson et al., in a review of 100 patients with osteogenesis imperfecta, came to the same conclusion that the severity of the disease correlates with the risk of development and severity of the scoliosis.

The natural history of scoliosis in patients with osteogenesis

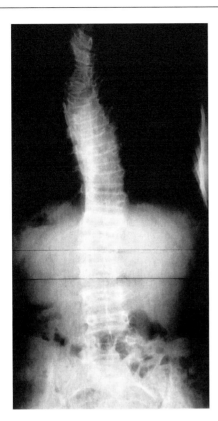

Fig. 38-232   Spinal deformity in patient with osteogenesis imperfecta.

imperfecta is continued progression. Benson et al. found that scoliosis present at a young age was almost always progressive, and Moorefield and Miller reported that progression may continue into adulthood. King and Bobechko found severe and disabling spinal deformities in many adults with osteogenesis imperfecta.

Anesthesia Problems

Libman emphasized several areas of concern in the administration of anesthesia for a patient with osteogenesis imperfecta. The primary concern is the risk of fractures. Extreme care must be taken in handling these patients, including positioning on the operating table with adequate padding and care in transfer. Care also should be taken in establishing the intravenous line or application of a blood pressure cuff, because both can result in fracture. Intubation and airway control also can be problematic because these patients have large heads and short necks, as well as tongues that often are disproportionately large. Extension of the head to facilitate intubation could cause a cervical spine fracture or a mandibular fracture. Because many patients with osteogenesis imperfecta have thoracic deformities, poor respiratory function should be expected. Libman also noted a tendency for hyperthermia to develop in patients with osteogenesis imperfecta. This does not appear to be a malignant type, however,

and may be related to elevated thyroid hormone levels, which are found in at least half of the patients with osteogenesis imperfecta. He found that hyperthermia can be induced by various anesthetic agents, as well as atropine, and suggested avoiding the use of atropine in these patients. If hyperthermia occurs, it is controlled with cooling, supplemental oxygen, sodium bicarbonate, cardiovascular stimulants, and dantrolene sodium. Libman suggested preoperative treatment with dantrolene sodium to perhaps prevent hyperthermia. He also recommended minimizing fasciculations associated with succinylchloride. If possible, other agents should be used. If succinylcholine is necessary, the fasciculations may be minimized by prior administration of a nondepolarizing muscle relaxant.

Orthotic Treatment

Most authors agree that bracing does not control progressive scoliosis in patients with severe osteogenesis imperfecta. Yong-Hing and MacEwen reviewed 121 patients treated by 51 different orthopaedic surgeons. They found that brace treatment was ineffective in stopping progression of scoliosis in patients with osteogenesis imperfecta even if the curves were small. Benson et al. reported Milwaukee brace treatment of nine patients with osteogenesis imperfecta and noted that eight curves progressed, and deformities of the chest wall developed in six patients. Hanscom et al. believe that orthotic treatment under carefully controlled circumstances may be a reasonable alternative to operative intervention in patients with type A or type B osteogenesis imperfecta. It is doubtful whether any effective forces from an orthosis can be transmitted to the spine of a patient with preexisting deformity of the chest wall, fragile ribs, and deformed vertebral bodies.

Operative Treatment

Yong-Hing and MacEwen recommended spinal fusion for curves of more than 50 degrees in patients with osteogenesis imperfecta, regardless of the age of the patient, provided there are no medical contraindications. They agreed with Benson et al. that the decision to fuse the spine should depend on the extent of the curvature and the presence of progression rather than on the age of the patient. In the series of Yong-Hing and MacEwen one third of patients had some complication; 5 of 60 patients developed pseudarthroses, 9 lost more than 2.5 liters of blood, and 14 had problems related to instrumentation. In the absence of a pseudarthrosis or kyphosis, late bending of the fused spine did not occur. Hanscom et al. recommended fusion for prevention of progression of the spinal deformity and cardiopulmonary problems in patients with types B, C, or E osteogenesis imperfecta.

Some type of multihook segmental instrumentation often can be used in patients with type A osteogenesis imperfecta. Patients with the milder form of the disease can be treated in the same manner as patients with idiopathic scoliosis, although significant correction of the curve should not be attempted. Bone graft should be obtained from the iliac crest, but often the

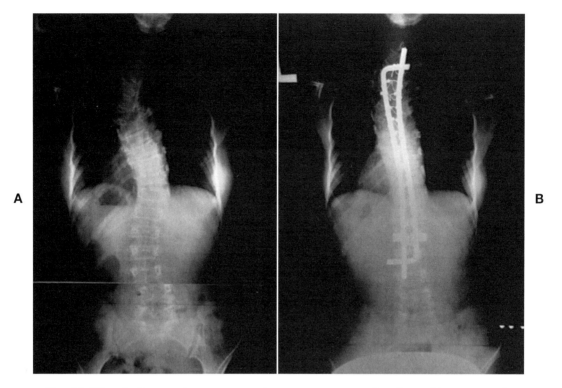

Fig. 38-233 **A,** Preoperative posteroanterior roentgenograms of patient with osteogenesis imperfecta with progressing curvature. **B,** Postoperative roentgenograms after instrumentation with sublaminar cables and Luque rods.

amount of bone available is inadequate and allograft is required for supplement. If the patient is small, pediatric-size hooks and instrumentation may be needed. The rod must be bent carefully to conform to the contours of the spine in both the coronal and sagittal planes to prevent excessive pull-out forces on the hooks. Methylmethacrylate has been used to supplement hook placement in these patients.

In patients with more severe disease (type C or type D), Hanscom et al. recommended the use of L-rods with segmental wires (Fig. 38-233). Great care in tightening these wires should be taken to prevent the wire from pulling through the lamina posteriorly. An alternative is to use Mersilene tapes. Anterior procedures should not be necessary if spinal deformities are stabilized before they become too severe.

Because of poor bone quality, immobilization in a two-piece TLSO is necessary for 6 to 9 months after surgery until the fusion is solid.

Unusual Causes of Kyphosis

POSTLAMINECTOMY SPINAL DEFORMITY

Laminectomies most often are done in children for the diagnosis and treatment of spinal cord tumors, although they also may be needed in other conditions such as neurofibromatosis and syringomyelia. Several authors, including Haft et al.,

Tachdjian and Matson, and Lonstein et al., reported the frequency of spinal deformities after laminectomy in children. The incidence of spinal deformity ranged from 33% in the series of Haft et al. to 100% of the 32 patients studied by Lonstein et al.

Kyphosis is the most common deformity that occurs after multiple level laminectomies. Yasuoka et al. found spinal deformity after laminectomy more frequent in children younger than 15 years of age. Both Yasuoka et al. and Fraser et al. found that the higher the level of the laminectomy, the greater the likelihood of spinal deformity or instability. They also found that all cervical or cervicothoracic laminectomies were followed by deformity. Lonstein et al. described two basic types of kyphosis, depending on the status of the facet joints posteriorly: sharp and angular or long and gradually rounding.

Scoliosis also may occur after laminectomy and generally is in the area of the laminectomy and associated with the kyphotic deformity. Scoliosis may occur at levels below the laminectomy, but this is caused by the paralysis from the cord tumor or its treatment rather than by the laminectomy.

The causes of instability of the spine after multiple laminectomies include skeletal and ligamentous deficiencies, neuromuscular imbalance, progressive osseous deformity, and radiation therapy. Yasuoka et al. noted increased wedging or excessive motion in children rather than subluxation as occurs in adults. They postulated that after laminectomy, pressure is increased on the cartilaginous endplates of the vertebral bodies

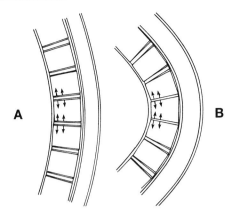

Fig. 38-234 Increased pressure on cartilaginous endplate of vertebra anteriorly after laminectomy (**A**) causes wedging of the vertebra (**B**). (Redrawn from Yasuoka S, Peterson H, Laws ER Jr, et al: *Neurosurgery* 9:145, 1981.)

anteriorly, and with time cartilage growth is decreased and vertebral wedging occurs (Fig. 38-234). Panjabi et al. showed that the loss of posterior stability caused by removal of interspinous ligaments, spinous processes, and laminae allows the normal flexion forces to produce a kyphosis. Lonstein et al. emphasized the importance of the facet joints posteriorly in these deformities. They showed that when the facet joints are completely removed at one level, gross instability results, with maximal angulation at that level causing a sharp, angular kyphos, enlargement of the intervertebral foramen, and opening of the disc space posteriorly. If complete removal is on one side only, the angular kyphosis is accompanied by a sharp scoliosis with the apex at the same level. If all the facets are preserved, a gradual rounding kyphos results in the area of the laminectomy. Many authors, including Kilfoyle et al. and Brown and Bonnett, reported extremely high incidences of spinal deformity in children younger than 10 years of age with complete paralysis. Children with extensive laminectomies and paralysis as a result of spinal cord tumors or their treatment are likely to have increasing spinal deformities. Radiation therapy, used to treat many spinal tumors, has been associated with injury to the vertebral physis and subsequent spinal deformity (see p. 1926). The cause of postlaminectomy spinal deformity is therefore multifactorial.

Treatment

When laminectomy is necessary, the facet joints should be preserved whenever possible. After surgery, the child should be examined regularly by an orthopaedic surgeon. If a spinal deformity is detected, Milwaukee brace treatment is begun immediately. Lonstein et al. found that the results of nonoperative treatment usually are temporary and provide lasting control in only a few patients. The goal of orthotic treatment should be to control the deformity until the patient is older, at which time fusion can be done.

If the deformity progresses despite orthotic treatment or if the deformity is severe, spinal fusion should be done. Of

course, if the patient has a very limited lifespan because of a highly malignant tumor, there is no reason to subject this child to an extensive operative procedure.

Most authors recommend combined anterior and posterior fusions for this condition because of the very small amount of bone surface posteriorly after a wide laminectomy. Also, many of these deformities have a kyphotic component, and anterior spinal fusion is more successful biomechanically than posterior fusion. Anteriorly the fusion mass is under compression rather than distraction forces. Of 45 patients treated for postlaminectomy scoliosis, Lonstein reported pseudarthroses in 33% with posterior fusion alone, in 22% with anterior fusion alone, and in 9.5% with combined anterior and posterior fusion. At the first stage, anterior fusion is done by removing all of the disc material, taking special care to remove the entire disc back to the posterior longitudinal ligament to prevent growth in the posterior aspect of the vertebral endplate with increasing kyphotic deformity. Strut grafting, using the rib graft obtained during the approach, or a fibular graft can be used to provide correction in addition to the fusion. Additional bone obtained locally from the vertebral bodies or ilium or remaining rib should be packed into the open disc spaces. Posterior fusion and instrumentation are done either immediately after anterior fusion or 1 to 2 weeks later. If the laminectomy is extensive, the defect may be crossed with posterior instrumentation (Fig. 38-235). If transverse processes or laminae remain, they can be used for segmental fixation with wire loops. In the lumbar spine, pedicle fixation can be useful. Often, the extent of the deformity and the absence of the posterior elements make instrumentation impossible, and in these patients a halo cast or vest may be necessary after surgery.

SKELETAL DYSPLASIAS

Achondroplasia

Achondroplasia is the most common of the bony dysplasias. The most frequent spinal deformity associated with this condition is thoracolumbar kyphosis that is present at birth. As muscle tone develops and walking begins, the kyphotic deformity usually resolves. Bailey found that approximately 30% of patients have a persistent kyphosis and that 35% of these curves become severe. This kyphosis is poorly tolerated by the patient with achondroplasia because of the decreased size of the spinal canal related to a marked decrease in the interpedicular distance in the lower lumbar region and to shortened pedicles, which cause a reduction in the anteroposterior dimensions of the spinal canal.

Hensinger and Bethem et al. emphasized awareness of the possibility of persistent or progressive thoracolumbar kyphosis in these patients. Early bracing to prevent progression and correction of any associated hip flexion contractures to prevent hyperlordosis below the kyphosis is recommended. If the kyphosis is progressive despite brace treatment, operative stabilization is indicated. Tolo recommended surgical treatment for any child with achondroplasia who is 5 or 6 years of age and has more than 40 degrees of localized thoracolumbar kyphosis with anterior vertebral wedging of the apical vertebrae. The spinal canal size reaches adult proportions by the age of 5 years and he suggested that circumferential fusion after this age should not lead to iatrogenic spinal stenosis and that surgery at this stage allows more correction than would be possible later with a more rigid kyphosis, which may decrease the need for

later decompressive laminectomies. Surgery must be done both anteriorly, with soft tissue release and strut grafting, and posteriorly with spinal fusion. Tolo used spinous process wires with Drummond buttons at all levels to be fused. Manual pressure was used to correct the kyphosis while the wires were tightened. Posterior instrumentation that invades the spinal

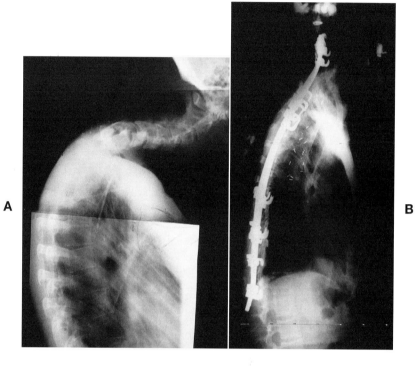

Fig. 38-235   **A,** Postlaminectomy kyphosis after removal of spinal cord tumor. **B,** After anterior and posterior fusions and posterior instrumentation crossing defect.

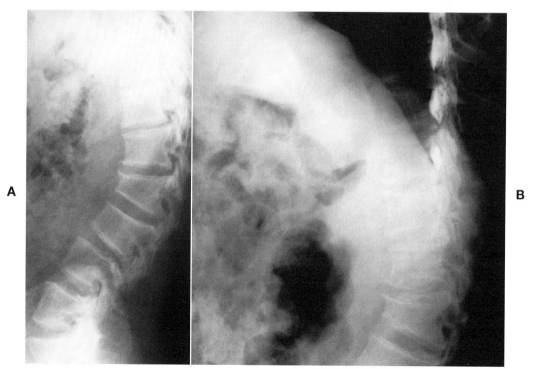

Fig. 38-236   **A** and **B,** Achondroplasia with complete block on myelogram.

canal poses a significant risk of neurological compromise because of the small size of the spinal canal and should be avoided. Since rigid instrumentation is impossible, postoperative casting or bracing is necessary. If the kyphosis is associated with paraparesis, anterior cord decompression followed by posterior spinal arthrodesis is indicated. However, patients with achondroplasia usually are free of any spine-related neurological problems during childhood and adolescence. Generally the symptoms of neurological compression and spinal stenosis develop in adulthood (Fig. 38-236).

Neurological deficits in infants with achondroplasia may indicate narrowing of the foramen magnum and basilar impression. This stenosis of the foramen magnum has been associated with ventilatory insufficiency, such as sleep apnea, and has caused sudden death in infants with achondroplasia. Evaluation of neurological deficits should include appropriate imaging studies of the foramen magnum and the occipitocervical junction.

Mucopolysaccharidoses

Of the many types of mucopolysaccharidoses, Morquio, Hurler, and Maroteaux-Lamy syndromes are the types most commonly associated with structural changes of the spine. The spinal deformity commonly seen in children with these conditions is kyphosis, usually in the thoracolumbar junction (Fig. 38-237). Treatment of the condition depends on the degree of the deformity, as well as the child's prognosis. Hurler syndrome usually is rapidly progressive, and affected children usually die before the age of 10 years.

Morquio syndrome is the most common of the muco-polysaccharidoses (Fig. 38-238). Children with this condition may well live into adult life and have normal mentality. Many authors, including Blaw and Langer, Kopits, Langer, and Lipson, have emphasized the frequent occurrence of atlanto-axial instability in patients with Morquio syndrome. The most common presenting symptom is reduced exercise tolerance, followed by progressive upper motor neuron deficits. Blaw and Langer stated that neurological problems in the first 2 decades

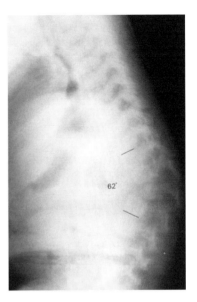

Fig. 38-237 Kyphosis at thoracolumbar junction in patient with Hurler syndrome.

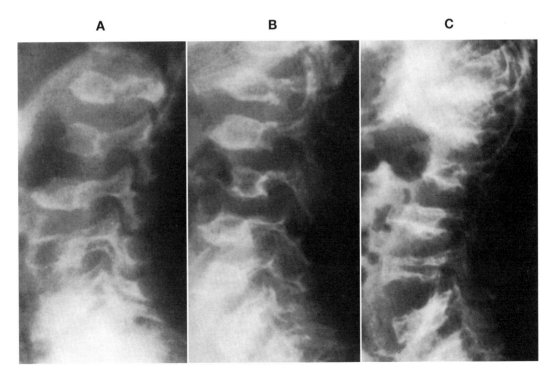

Fig. 38-238 **A,** Hook-shaped bodies in young child. **B,** Further anterior ossification in older child. **C,** Flattened, rectangular vertebral bodies in adult. (From Langer LO, Carey LS: *Am J Roentgenol* 97:1, 1966.)

of life usually are related to odontoid abnormalities or atlantoaxial instability; later, symptoms primarily are caused by the kyphosis or gibbus. Posterior fusion of C1 to C2 is the recommended treatment for atlantoaxial instability as soon as any signs of a myelopathy are identified. Blaw and Langer recommended that the developing gibbus during childhood be treated with an appropriate spinal orthosis to prevent neurological deficits.

References

INFANTILE AND JUVENILE IDIOPATHIC SCOLIOSIS

Branthwaite MA: Cardiorespiratory consequences of unfused idiopathic scoliosis, *Br J Chest Dis* 80:360, 1986.

Brown JK, Bell E, Fulford GE: Mechanism of deformity in children with cerebral palsy with special reference to postural deformity, *Pädiat Fortbidk Praxis* 53:78, 1982.

Ceballos T, Ferrer-Torrelles M, Costillo F, et al: Prognosis in infantile idiopathic scoliosis, *J Bone Joint Surg* 62A:863, 1980.

Conner AN: Early onset scoliosis: a call for awareness, *Br Med J* 289:962, 1994.

Davies G, Reid L: Effect of scoliosis on growth of alveoli, pulmonary arteries, and the right ventricle, *Arch Dis Child* 46:623, 1971.

Dickson RA: The etiology of spinal deformities, *Lancet* 1:1151, 1988.

Dickson RA, Lawton JO, Archer IA, Butt WP: The pathogenesis of idiopathic scoliosis: biplanar spinal asymmetry, *J Bone Joint Surg* 66B:8, 1984.

Dimeglio A: Growth of the spine before 5 years, *J Pediatr Orthop* 1B:102, 1993.

Dubousset J, Herring JA, Shufflebarger H: The crankshaft phenomenon, *J Pediatr Orthop* 9:541, 1989.

Emery JL, Mithal A: The number of alveoli in the terminal respiratory unit of man during late intrauterine life in childhood. *Arch Dis Child* 35:544, 1960.

Evans SC, Edgar MA, Hall-Craggs MA, et al: MRI of 'idiopathic' juvenile scoliosis, *J Bone Joint Surg* 78B:314, 1996.

Figueiredo UM, James JIP: Juvenile idiopathic scoliosis, *J Bone Joint Surg* 63B:61, 1981.

Gupta P, Lenke LG, Bridwell KH: Incidence of neural axis abnormalities in infantile and juvenile patients with spinal deformity. Is a magnetic resonance image screening necessary? *Spine* 23:206, 1998.

Hefti FL, McMaster MJ: The effect of the adolescent growth spurt on early posterior spinal fusion in infantile and juvenile idiopathic scoliosis, *J Bone Joint Surg* 65B:247, 1983.

James JIP: Infantile idiopathic scoliosis, *Clin Orthop* 21:106, 1961.

James JIP: The management of infants with scoliosis, *J Bone Joint Surg* 57B:422, 1975.

James JIP, Lloyd-Roberts GC, Pilcher MF: Infantile structural scoliosis, *J Bone Joint Surg* 41B:719, 1959.

Kahanovitz N, Levine DB, Lardone J: The part-time Milwaukee brace treatment of juvenile idiopathic scoliosis: long-term follow-up, *Clin Orthop* 167:145, 1982.

Koop SE: Infantile and juvenile idiopathic scoliosis, *Orthop Clin North Am* 19:331, 1988.

Krismundsdottir F, Burwell RG, James JIP: The rib-vertebra angles on the convexity and concavity of the spinal curve in infantile idiopathic scoliosis, *Clin Orthop* 201:205, 1985.

Lewonowski K, King JD, Nelson MD: Routine use of magnetic resonance imaging in idiopathic scoliosis patients less than 11 years of age, *Spine* 17(suppl):510, 1992.

Lloyd-Roberts GC, Pilcher MF: Structural idiopathic scoliosis in infancy, *J Bone Joint Surg* 47B:520, 1965.

Lonstein JE, Carlson JM: The prediction of curve progression in untreated idiopathic scoliosis during growth, *J Bone Joint Surg* 66A:1061, 1984.

Mannherz RE, Betz RR, Clancy M, et al: Juvenile idiopathic scoliosis followed to skeletal maturity, *Spine* 13:1087, 1988.

Mardjetko SM. In Bridwell KH, DeWald RL, eds: *The textbook of spinal surgery*, ed 2, Philadelphia, 1997, Lippincott-Raven.

Mardjetko SM, Hammerberg KW, Lubicky JP, et al: The Luque trolley revisited: review of 9 cases requiring revision, *Spine* 17:582, 1992.

Mau H: Etiology of idiopathic scoliosis, *Reconstr Surg Traumatol* 13:184, 1972.

McCarthy RE, McCullough FL: Growing instrumentation for scoliosis. Paper presented at the Twenty-eighth Annual Meeting of the Scoliosis Research Society, Dublin, Sept 1993.

McMaster MJ: Infantile idiopathic scoliosis: can it be prevented? *J Bone Joint Surg* 65B:612, 1983.

McMaster MJ, Macnicol MF: The management of progressive infantile idiopathic scoliosis, *J Bone Joint Surg* 61B:36, 1979.

Mehta MH: The rib-vertebra angle in the early diagnosis between resolving and progressive infantile scoliosis, *J Bone Joint Surg* 54B:230, 1972.

Moe JH, Kharrat K, Winter RB, et al: Harrington instrumentation without fusion plus external orthotic support for the treatment of difficult curvature problems in young children, *Clin Orthop* 185:35, 1984.

Morin MR: Pediatric Cotrel-Dubousset instrumentation system. In Bridwell KH, DeWald RL, eds: *Spinal surgery*, Philadelphia, 1991, JB Lippincott.

Patterson JF, Webb JK, Burwell RG: The operative treatment of progressive early onset scoliosis: a preliminary report, *Spine* 15: 809, 1990.

Pehrsson K, Nachemson A, Olofson J, Ström K, et al: Respiratory failure in scoliosis and other thoracic deformities, *Spine* 17:714, 1992.

Rinsky LA, Gamble JG, Bleck EE: Segmental instrumentation without fusion in children with progressive scoliosis, *J Pediatr Orthop* 5:687, 1985.

Roberts S, Menage J, Eisenstein SM: The cartilage end-plate and intervertebral disc in scoliosis: calcification and other sequelae, *J Orthop Res* 11:747, 1993.

Sanders JO, Herring JA, Browne RH: Behavior of the immature (Risser 0) spine in idiopathic scoliosis following posterior spinal instrumentation and fusion. Paper presented at the Twenty-eighth Annual Meeting of the Scoliosis Research Society, Dublin, Sept 1993.

Shufflebarger HL, Clark CE: Prevention of the crankshaft phenomenon, *Spine* 16:S409, 1991.

Thompson SK, Bentley G: Prognosis in infantile idiopathic scoliosis, *J Bone Joint Surg* 62B:151, 1980.

Tolo VT, Gillespie R: The characteristics of juvenile idiopathic scoliosis and results of its treatment, *J Bone Joint Surg* 60B:181, 1978.

Vanlommel E, Fabry G, Urlus M, et al: Harrington instrumentation without fusion for the treatment of scoliosis in young children, *J Pediatr Orthop* 11:116, 1992.

Winter RW: Scoliosis and spinal growth, *Orthop Rev* 7:17, 1977.

Wynne-Davies R: Infantile idiopathic scoliosis: causative factors, particularly in the first six months of life, *J Bone Joint Surg* 57B: 138, 1975.

NATURAL HISTORY OF ADOLESCENT IDIOPATHIC SCOLIOSIS

Aaro S, Ohlund C: Scoliosis and pulmonary function, *Spine* 9:220, 1984.

Arai S, Ohtsuka Y, Moriya H, et al: Scoliosis associated with syringomyelia, *Spine* 18:1591, 1993.

Apter A, Morein G, Munitz H, et al: The psychosocial sequelae of the Milwaukee brace in adolescent girls, *Clin Orthop* 131:156, 1978.

Archer IA, Dickson RA: Stature and idiopathic scoliosis: a prospective study, *J Bone Joint Surg* 67B:185, 1985.

Ascani E, Bartolozzi P, Logroscino CA, et al: Natural history of untreated idiopathic scoliosis after skeletal maturity, *Spine* 11:787, 1986.

Bagnall KM, Raso VJ, Hill DL, et al: Melatonin levels in idiopathic scoliosis: diurnal and nocturnal serum melatonin levels in girls with adolescent idiopathic scoliosis, *Spine* 21:1974, 1996.

Beals RK: Nosologic and genetic aspects of scoliosis, *Clin Orthop* 93:23, 1973.

Bergofsky GH, Turino GM, Fishman AP: Cardiorespiratory failure in kyphoscoliosis, *Medicine* 38:263, 1959.

Berman AT, Cohen DL, Schwentker EP, The effects of pregnancy on idiopathic scoliosis: a preliminary report on eight cases and review of the literature, *Spine* 7:76, 1982.

Betz RR, Bunnell WP, Lambrecht-Mulier E, et al: Scoliosis and pregnancy, *J Bone Joint Surg* 69A:90, 1987.

Biondi J, Weiner DS, Bethem D, Reed JR III: Correlation of Risser sign and bone age determination in adolescent idiopathic scoliosis, *J Pediatr Orthop* 5:697, 1985.

Bjerkreim I, Hassan I: Progression in untreated idiopathic scoliosis after end of growth, *Acta Orthop Scand* 53:897, 1982.

Bjure J, Nachemson A: Nontreated scoliosis, *Clin Orthop* 93:44, 1973.

Blount WP, Mellencamp DD: The effect of pregnancy on idiopathic scoliosis, *J Bone Joint Surg* 62A:1083, 1980.

Branthwaite MA: Cardiorespiratory consequence of unfused idiopathic scoliosis patients, *Br J Dis Chest* 80:360, 1986.

Bremberg S, Nilsson-Berggren B: School screening for adolescent idiopathic scoliosis, *J Pediatr Orthop* 6:564, 1986.

Bunnell WP: A study of the natural history of idiopathic scoliosis. Paper presented at the Nineteenth Annual Meeting of the Scoliosis Research Society, Orlando, Fla, 1984.

Bunnell WP: The natural history of idiopathic scoliosis before skeletal maturity, *Spine* 11:773, 1986.

Bunnell WP: The natural history of idiopathic scoliosis, *Clin Orthop* 229:20, 1988.

Burwell RG, James JN, Johnson F, et al: The rib hump score: a guide to referral and prognosis? *J Bone Joint Surg* 64B:248, 1982.

Burwell RG, James NH, Johnson F, et al: Standardized trunk asymmetry scores: a study of back contours in healthy school children, *J Bone Joint Surg* 65B:453, 1983.

Byl NN, Gray JM: Complex balance reactions in different sensory conditions: adolescents with and without idiopathic scoliosis. *J Orthop Res* 11:215, 1993.

Bylund P, Jansson E, Dahlberg E, Eriksson E: muscle fiber types in thoracic erector spinae muscles: fiber types in idiopathic and other forms of scoliosis, *Clin Orthop* 274:305, 1992.

Carpintero P, Mesa M, Garcia J, Carpintero A: Scoliosis induced by asymmetric lordosis and rotation: an experimental study, *Spine* 22:2202, 1987.

Carr AJ, Jefferson RJ, Turner-Smith AR: Family stature in idiopathic scoliosis, *Spine* 18;20, 1993.

Carr AJ, Ogilvie DJ, Wordsworth BP, et al: Segregation of structural collagen genes in adolescent idiopathic scoliosis, *Clin Orthop* 247:305, 1992.

Clayson D, Levine DB: Adolescent scoliosis patients: personality patterns and effects of corrective surgery, *Clin Orthop* 116:99, 1967.

Clayson D, Luz-Alterman S, Cataletto MM, Levine DB: Long-term psychological sequelae of surgically versus nonsurgically treated scoliosis, *Spine* 12:983, 1987.

Collis DK, Ponseti IV: Long-term follow-up of patients with idiopathic scoliosis, *J Bone Joint Surg* 51A:425, 1969.

Cowell HR, Hall JN, MacEwen GD: Genetic aspects of idiopathic scoliosis, *Clin Orthop* 86:121, 1972.

Cruickshank JL, Koike M, Dickson RA: Curve patterns in idiopathic scoliosis, *J Bone Joint Surg* 71B:259, 1989.

Cummings RJ, Loveless EA, Campbell J, et al: Interobserver reliability and intraobserver reproducibility of the system of King et al. for the classification of adolescent idiopathic scoliosis, *J Bone Joint Surg* 81A:743, 1999.

Czeizel A, Bellyei A, Barta O, et al: Genetics of adolescent idiopathic scoliosis, *J Med Genet* 15:424, 1978.

Davies G, Reid L: Effect of scoliosis on growth of alveoli and pulmonary arteries and on right ventricle, *Arch Dis Child* 46:623, 1971.

Deacon P, Archer IA, Dickson RA: The anatomy of spinal deformity: a biomechanical analysis, *Orthopedics* 10:897, 1987.

Deacon P, Flood BM, Dickson RA: Idiopathic scoliosis in three dimensions: a radiographic and morphometric analysis, *J Bone Joint Surg* 66B:509, 1984.

DeGeorge FV, Fisher RL: Idiopathic scoliosis: genetic and environmental aspects, *J Med Genet* 4:251, 1967.

Dickson RA: Scoliosis in the community, *Br Med J* 286:615, 1983.

Dickson RA: The etiology and pathogenesis of idiopathic scoliosis, *Acta Orthop Belgica* 58(suppl): 21, 1992.

Dickson R, Deacon P: Spinal growth, *J Bone Joint Surg* 69B:690, 1987.

Dickson RA, Lawton JO, Archer IA, Butt WP: The pathogenesis of idiopathic scoliosis: biplanar spinal asymmetry, *J Bone Joint Surg* 66B:8, 1984.

Dickson JH, Mirkovic S, Noble MS, et al: Results of operative treatment of idiopathic scoliosis in adults, *J Bone Joint Surg* 77A:513, 1995.

Dickson RA, Stamper P, Sharp AM, et al: School screening for scoliosis: cohort study of clinical course, *Br Med J* 281:265, 1980.

Dubousset J, Machida M: Melatonin: a possible role in the pathogenesis of human idiopathic scoliosis. In Proceedings of the Tenth International Philip Zorab Symposium on Scoliosis, abstract 3.19, Oxford, 1998, Oxford University Press.

Duval-Beupere G: Rib hump and supine angle as prognostic factors for mild scoliosis, *Spine* 17:103, 1992.

Duval-Beaupere G, Lamireau TH: Scoliosis of less than 30 degrees: properties of the evolutivity (risk of progression), *Spine* 10:421, 1985.

Echenne B, Barneon G, Pages M, et al: Skin elastic fiber pathology and idiopathic scoliosis, *J Pediatr Orthop* 8:522, 1988.

Edgar MA: The natural history of unfused scoliosis, *Clin Orthop* 10:931, 1987.

Edgar MA, Mehta M: Long-term follow-up of fused and unfused idiopathic scoliosis, *J Bone Joint Surg* 70B:712:1988.

Eliason JM, Richman LC: Psychological effects of idiopathic adolescent scoliosis, *Dev Behav Pediatr* 5:169, 1984.

Fallstrom K, Nachemson AL, Cochran TP: Psychologic effect of treatment for adolescent idiopathic scoliosis, *Orthop Trans* 8:150, 1984.

Ford DM, Bagnall KM, Clements CA, McFadden KD: Muscle spindles in the paraspinal musculature of patients with adolescent idiopathic scoliosis, *Spine* 13:461, 1988.

Fowles JV, Drummond DS, I'Ecuyer S, et al: Untreated scoliosis in the adult, *Clin Orthop* 134:212, 1978.

Gazioglu K, Goldstein LA, Femi-Pearse D, et al: Pulmonary function in idiopathic scoliosis: comparative evaluation before and after orthopaedic correction, *J Bone Joint Surg* 50A:1391, 1968.

Gibson JN, McMaster MJ, Scrimgeour CM, et al: Rates of muscle protein synthesis in paraspinal muscles: literal disparity in children with idiopathic scoliosis, *Clin Sci* 75:79, 1988.

Goldberg CJ, Dowling FE, Fogarty EE: Adolescent idiopathic scoliosis— early menarche, normal growth, *Spine* 18:529, 1993.

Goldberg MS, Mayo NE, Poitras B, et al: The Ste-Justine adolescent idiopathic scoliosis cohort study. II. Perception of health, self, and body image and participation in physical activities, *Spine* 19:1562, 1994.

Gucker T: Changes in vital capacity in scoliosis: preliminary report on effect of treatment, *J Bone Joint Surg* 44A:469, 1962.

Hadley-Miller N, Mims B, Milewicz DM: The potential role of the elastic fiber system in adolescent idiopathic scoliosis, *J Bone Joint Surg* 76A:1193, 1994.

Hamanishi C, Tanaka S, Kasahara Y, Shikata J: Progressive scoliosis associated with lateral gaze palsy, *Spine* 18:2545, 1993.

Harrington PR: The etiology of idiopathic scoliosis, *Clin Orthop* 126:17, 1977.

Hassan I, Bjerkreim I: Progression in idiopathic scoliosis after conservative treatment, *Acta Orthop Scand* 54:88, 1983.

Henderson MH, Rieger MA, Miller F, et al: Influence of parental age on degree of curvature in idiopathic scoliosis, *J Bone Joint Surg* 72A:910, 1990.

Herman R, Mixon J, Fisher A, et al: Idiopathic scoliosis and the central nervous system: a motor control problem, *Spine* 10:1, 1985.

Horal J: The clinical appearance of low back disorders in the city of Göteberg, Sweden, *Acta Orthop Scand Suppl* 118, 1969.

Howell FR, Mahood JK, Dickson RA: Growth beyond skeletal maturity, *Spine* 17:437, 1992.

James JIP: Idiopathic scoliosis: the prognosis, diagnosis, and operative indications related to curve pattern and age at onset, *J Bone Joint Surg* 36B:36, 1954.

Kane WJ, Moe JH: A scoliosis prevalence survey in Minnesota, *Clin Orthop* 69:216, 1970.

Keessen W, Crowe A, Hearn M: Proprioceptive accuracy in idiopathic scoliosis, *Spine* 17:149, 1992.

Kesling KL, Reinker KA: Scoliosis in twins: a meta-analysis of the literature and report of six cases, *Spine* 22:2009, 1997.

Kindsfater K, Lowe T, Lawellin D, et al: Levels of platelet calmodulin for the prediction of progression and severity of adolescent idiopathic scoliosis, *J Bone Joint Surg* 76A:1186, 1994.

Kolind-Sörensen V: A follow-up study of patients with idiopathic scoliosis, *Acta Orthop Scand* 44:98, 1973.

Kostuik JP, Bentivoglio J: The incidence of low-back pain in adult scoliosis, *Spine* 6:268, 1981.

Lenke LG, Betz RR, Bridwell KH, et al: Intraobserver and interobserver reliability of the classification of thoracic adolescent idiopathic scoliosis, *J Bone Joint Surg* 80A:1097, 1998.

Lindh M, Bjure J: Lung volumes in scoliosis before and after correction by Harrington instrumentation method, *Acta Orthop Scand* 46:934, 1975.

Little DG, Song KM, Katz D, Herring JA: The use of peak growth age in idiopathic scoliosis, *SRS*, 1995.

Little DG, Sussman MD: The Risser sign: a critical analysis, *J Pediatr Orthop* 14:569, 1994.

Lonstein JE: Natural history and school screening for scoliosis, *Orthop Clin North Am* 19:227, 1988.

Lonstein JE, Bjorklund S, Wanninger MH, et al: Voluntary school screening for scoliosis in Minnesota, *J Bone Joint Surg* 64A:481, 1982.

Lonstein JE, Carlson JM: The prediction of curve progression in untreated idiopathic scoliosis during growth, *J Bone Joint Surg* 66A:1061, 1984.

Low, WD, Chew EC, Kung LS, et al: Ultrastructures of nerve fibers and muscle spindles in adolescent idiopathic scoliosis, *Clin Orthop* 174:217, 1983.

Machida M, Dubousset J, Imamura Y, et al: Pathogenesis of idiopathic scoliosis: SEPs in chicken with experimentally induced scoliosis in patients with idiopathic scoliosis, *J Pediatr Orthop* 14:329, 1994.

Maguire J, Madigan R, Wallace S, et al: Intraoperative long-latency reflex activity in idiopathic scoliosis demonstrates abnormal central processing: a possible cause for idiopathic scoliosis, *Spine* 18:1621, 1993.

Makley JT, Herndon CH, Inkley S, et al: Pulmonary function in paralytic and nonparalytic scoliosis before and after treatment: a study of sixty-three cases, *J Bone Joint Surg* 50A:i379, 1968.

Mankin HJ, Graham JJ, Schack J: Cardiopulmonary function in mild and moderate idiopathic scoliosis, *J Bone Joint Surg* 46A:53, 1964.

Mayo NE, Goldberg MS, Poitras B, et al: The Ste-Justine adolescent idiopathic scoliosis cohort study. III. Back pain, *Spine* 19:1573, 1994.

McInnes E, Hill DL, Raso VJ et al: Vibratory response in adolescents who have idiopathic scoliosis, *J Bone Joint Surg* 73A:1208, 1991.

Miller NH, Mims B, Child A, et al: Genetic analysis of structural elastic fiber and collagen genes in familial adolescent idiopathic scoliosis, *J Orthop Res* 14:994, 1996.

Montgomery F, Willner S: A natural history of idiopathic scoliosis: a study of the incidence of treatment, *Spine* 13:401, 1988.

Muhlrad A, Yarom R: Contractile protein on platelets from patients with idiopathic scoliosis, *Haemostasis* 11:154, 1982.

Muirhead A, Conner AN: The assessment of lung function in children with scoliosis, *J Bone Joint Surg* 67B:699, 1985.

Nachemson A: A long-term follow-up study of nontreated scoliosis, *Acta Orthop Scand* 39:466, 1968.

Nachemson A long-term follow-up study of nontreated scoliosis, *J Bone Joint Surg* 50A:203, 1969.

Nachemson A: Adult scoliosis and back pain, *Spine* 4:513, 1979.

Nagi SJ, Riley LE, Newby LG: Social epidemiology of back pain in general population, *J Chronic Dis* 26:769, 1973.

Nash CL Jr, Lorig RA, Schatzinger LA, Brown RH: Spinal cord monitoring during operative treatment of the spine, *Clin Orthop* 126:100, 1977.

Nathan SW: Body image of scoliotic female adolescents before and after surgery, *Matern Child Nurs J* 6:139, 1977.

Nilsonne U, Lundgren KD: Long-term prognosis in idiopathic scoliosis, *Acta Orthop Scand* 39:456, 1968.

O'Beirne J, Goldberg C, Dowling FE, Fogarty EE: Equilibrial dysfunction in scoliosis—cause or effect? *J Spinal Disord* 2:184, 1989.

Oegema TR, Jr., Bradford DS, Cooper KM, Hunter RE: Comparison of biochemistry of proteoglycans isolated from normal, idiopathic scoliotic and cerebral palsy spine, *Spine* 8:378, 1983.

Ogilvie JW, Schendel MJ: Calculated thoracic volume as related to parameters of scoliosis correction, *Spine* 13:39, 1988.

Pedrini VA, Ponseti IV, Dohrman SC: Glycosaminoglycans of intervertebral disc in idiopathic scoliosis, *J Lab Clin Med* 82:938, 1973.

Pehrsson K, Bake B, Larsson S, Nachemson A: Lung function in adult idiopathic scoliosis: a 20-year follow-up, *Thorax* 46:474, 1991.

Pehrsson K, Larsson S, Oden A, et al: Long-term follow-up of patients with untreated scoliosis: a study of mortality, causes of death, and symptoms, *Spine* 17:191, 1992.

Picault C, deMauroy JC, Mouilleseaux B: Natural history of idiopathic scoliosis in girls and boys, *Spine* 11:777, 1986.

Perdriolle R, Vidal J: Thoracic idiopathic scoliosis curve evolution and prognosis, *Spine* 10:785, 1985.

Poitras B, Mayo NE, Goldberg MS, et al: The Ste-Justine adolescent idiopathic scoliosis cohort study. IV. Surgical correction and back pain, *Spine* 19:1582, 1994.

Ponseti IV, Friedman B: Prognosis in idiopathic scoliosis, *J Bone Joint Surg* 32A:381, 1950.

Renshaw TS: Screening school children for scoliosis, *Clin Orthop* 229:26, 1988.

Riseborough EJ, Wynne-Davies R: A genetic survey of idiopathic scoliosis in Boston, Massachusetts, *J Bone Joint Surg* 55A:974, 1973.

Robin GC, Span Y, Steinberg R, et al: Scoliosis in the elderly: a follow-up study, *Spine* 7:355, 1982.

Saunders JO, Little DG, Richard S: Prediction of the crankshaft phenomenon by peak height velocities, *Spine* 22:1352, 1997.

Scoles PV, Salvagno R, Villalba K, Riew D: Relationship of iliac crest maturation to skeletal and chronologic age, *J Pediatr Orthop* 8:639, 1988.

Shands AR, Eisberg HBL: The incidence of scoliosis in the state of Delaware: a study of 50,000 minifilms of the chest made during a survey for tuberculosis, *J Bone Joint Surg* 37A:1243, 1955.

Shannon DC, Roseborough EJ, Valenca LM, et al: The distribution of abnormal lung function in kyphoscoliosis, *J Bone Joint Surg* 52A:131, 1979.

Shuren N, Kasser JR, Emans JB, et al: Reevaluation of the use of the Risser sign in idiopathic scoliosis, *Spine* 17:359, 1992.

Smyrnis T, Antoniou D, Valavanis J, et al: Idiopathic scoliosis: characteristics and epidemiology, *Clin Orthop* 10:921, 1987.

Sponseller PD, Cohen MS, Nachemson AL, et al: Results of surgical treatment of adults with scoliosis, *J Bone Joint Surg* 69A:667, 1987.

Suh PB, MacEwen GD: Idiopathic scoliosis in males: a natural history study, *Spine* 13:1091, 1988.

Suk SI, Song HS, Lee CK: Scoliosis induced by anterior and poster rhizotomy, *Spine* 14:692, 1989.

Taylor TKF, Ghosh P, Bushnell GR: The contribution of the intervertebral disk to the scoliotic deformity, *Clin Orthop* 156:79, 1981.

Torell G, Nordwall A, Nachemson A: The changing pattern of scoliosis treatment due to effective screening, *J Bone Joint Surg* 63A:337, 1981.

Veraart BEEMJ, Jansen BJ: Changes in lung function associated with idiopathic thoracic scoliosis, *Acta Orthop Scand* 61:235, 1990.

Visscher W, Lonstein JE, Hoffman DA, et al: Reproductive outcomes in scoliosis patients, *Spine* 13:1096, 1988.

Weinstein SL: Idiopathic scoliosis: natural history, *Spine* 11:780, 1986.

Weinstein SL: The natural history of scoliosis in the skeletally mature patient. In Dickson JH, ed: *Spinal deformities*, vol 1, no. 2. *State of the art reviews. Spine*, Philadelphia, 1987, Hanley & Belfus.

Weinstein SL: Adolescent idiopathic scoliosis: prevalence and natural history, *Instr Course Lect* 38:115, 1989.

Weinstein SL, Dolan LA, Spratt KF, et al: Natural history of adolescent idiopathic scoliosis: back pain at 50 years. Paper presented at the annual meeting of the Scoliosis Research Society, New York, Sept 1998.

Weinstein SL, Ponseti IV: Curve progression in idiopathic scoliosis, *J Bone Joint Surg* 65A:447, 1983.

Weinstein SL, Zavala DC, Ponseti IV: Idiopathic scoliosis: long-term follow-up and prognosis in untreated patients, *J Bone Joint Surg* 63A:702, 1981.

Westgate HD, Moe JH: Pulmonary function in kyphoscoliosis before and after correction by Harrington instrumentation method. *J Bone Joint Surg* 51A:935, 1967.

Willner S: Prospective prevalence study of scoliosis in southern Sweden, *Acta Orthop Scand* 53:233, 1982.

Willner S: Prevalence study of trunk asymmetries and structural scoliosis in 10-year-old school children, *Spine* 9:644, 1984.

Willner S, Nilsson KO, Kastrup K, Berstrand CG: Growth hormone and somatomedin A in girls with adolescent idiopathic scoliosis, *Acta Paediatr Scand* 65:547, 1976.

Wynne-Davies R: Familial (idiopathic) scoliosis: a family survey, *J Bone Joint Surg* 50B:24, 1968.

Xiong B, Sevastik J, Hedlund R, Sevastik B: Sagittal configuration of the spine and growth of the posterior elements in early scoliosis, *J Orthop Res* 12:113, 1994.

Yamauchi Y, Yamaguchi T, Asaka Y: Prediction of curve progression in idiopathic scoliosis based on initial roentgenograms: a proposal of an equation, *Spine* 13:1258, 1988.

Yarom R, Blatt J, Gorodetsky R, Robin GC: Microanalysis and x-ray fluorescence spectrometry of platelets in diseases with elevated muscle calcium, *Eur J Clin Invest* 10:143, 1980.

Yarom R, Robin GC: Studies on spinal and peripheral muscles from patients with scoliosis, *Spine* 4:12, 1979.

Yarom R, Robin GC, Gorodetsky R: X-ray fluorescence analysis of muscles in scoliosis, *Spine* 3:142, 1978.

Yekutiel M, Robin GC, Yarom: Proprioceptive function in children with adolescent idiopathic scoliosis, *Spine* 6:560, 1981.

Zaoussis AL, James JIP: The iliac apophysis and the evolution of curves in scoliosis, *J Bone Joint Surg* 40B:442, 1958.

PATIENT EVALUATION IN ADOLESCENT IDIOPATHIC SCOLIOSIS

Aaro S, Dahlborn M: Vertebral rotation: estimation of vertebral rotation and spinal and rib cage deformity in scoliosis by computerized tomography, *Spine* 6:460, 1981.

Asher MA: Scoliosis evaluation, *Orthop Clin North Am* 19:805, 1988.

Barsanti CM, deBari A, Covino BM: The torsion meter: a critical review, *J Pediatr Orthop* 10:527, 1990.

Bernhardt M: Normal spinal anatomy: normal sagittal plane alignment. In Bridwell KH, DeWald RL, eds: *The textbook of spinal surgery*, ed 2, Philadelphia, 1997, Lippincott-Raven.

Bernhardt M, Bridwell KH: Segmental analysis of the sagittal plane alignment of the normal thoracic lumbar spines and thoracolumbar junction, *Spine* 14:717, 1989.

Bunnell WP: Vertebral rotation: a simple method of measurement in routine radiographs, *Orthop Trans* 9:114, 1985.

Carman DL, Browne RH, Birch JG: Measurement of scoliosis and kyphosis radiographs: intraobserver and interobserver variation, *J Bone Joint Surg* 72A:328, 1990.

Cobb JR: Outline for the study of scoliosis in instructional course lectures. In The American Academy of Orthopaedic Surgeons: *Instructional course lectures*, vol 5, Ann Arbor, Mich, 1948, JW Edwards.

Deacon P, Flood BM, Dickson RA: Idiopathic scoliosis in three dimension: a radiographic and morphometric analysis, *J Bone Joint Surg* 66B:509, 1984.

DeSmet A, Fritz SL, Asher MA: A method for minimizing the radiation exposure from scoliosis radiographs, *J Bone Joint Surg* 63A:156, 1981.

DeSmet A, Goin JE, Asher MA, et al: A clinical study of the differences between the scoliotic angles measured on the PA versus the AP radiographs, *J Bone Joint Surg* 64A:489, 1982.

Drummond D, Ranallo F, Lonstein J, et al: Radiation hazards and scoliosis management, *Spine* 8:741, 1983.

Farren J: Routine radiographic assessment of the scoliotic spine, *Radiography* 47:92, 1981.

Ferguson AB: Roentgen interpretations and decisions in scoliosis. In The American Academy of Orthopaedic Surgeons: *Instructional course lectures*, vol 7, Ann Arbor, Mich, 1950, JW Edwards.

Gelb DE, Lenke LB, Bridwell KH, et al: An analysis of sagittal spinal alignment in 100 asymptomatic middle and older age volunteers, *Spine* 20:1351, 1995.

Gray JE, Hoffman AE, Peterson HA: Reduction of radiation exposure during radiography for scoliosis, *J Bone Joint Surg* 65A:5, 1983.

Gunzburg R, Ganzberg J, Wagner J, et al: Radiologic interpretation of lumbar vertebral rotation, *Spine* 16:660, 1991.

Hopkins R, Grundy M, Sherr-Mehl M: X-ray filters in scoliosis x-rays, *Orthop Trans* 8:148, 1984.

James JIP: Idiopathic scoliosis: the prognosis, diagnosis, and operative indication related to curve patterns and the age at onset, *J Bone Joint Surg* 36B:36, 1954.

Kleinman RE, Csongradi JJ, Rinsky LA, et al: A radiographic assessment of spinal flexibility in scoliosis, *Clin Orthop* 162:47, 1982.

Lenke LG, Linville DA, Bridwell KH: Sagittal balance considerations in adults. In Margulies JY, Aebi M, Farcy JPC, eds: *Revision spine surgery*, St Louis, 1999, Mosby.

Leuonowaski K, King JD, Nelson MD: Routine use of magnetic resonance imaging in idiopathic scoliosis patients less than 11 years of age, *Spine* 17:S109, 1992.

Lonstein JE, Carlson JM: The prediction of curve progression in untreated idiopathic scoliosis during growth, *J Bone Joint Surg* 66A:1061, 1984.

Mehta MH: Radiographic estimation of vertebral rotation in scoliosis, *J Bone Joint Surg* 55B:513, 1973.

Morrissy RT, Goldsmith GS, Hall EC, et al: Measurement of the Cobb angle on radiographs of patients who have scoliosis: evaluation of intrinsic error, *J Bone Joint Surg* 72A:320, 1990.

Nash C, Moe J: A study of vertebral rotation, *J Bone Joint Surg* 51A:223, 1969.

Perdriolle R, Vidal J: Morphology of scoliosis: three-dimension evolution, *Orthopedics* 10:909, 1987.

Ponseti IV, Friedman B: Prognosis in idiopathic scoliosis, *J Bone Joint Surg* 32A:381, 1950.

Probst-Proctor SL, Bleck EE: Radiographic determination of lordosis and kyphosis in normal and scoliotic children, *J Pediatr Orthop* 3:344, 1983.

Pun WK, Lak KDK, Lee W, et al: A simple method to estimate the rib hump in scoliosis, *Spine* 12:342, 1987.

Richards BS: Measurement error in assessment of vertebral rotation using the Perdriolle torsiometer, *Spine* 17:513, 1992.

Risser JC: Important practical facts in the treatment of scoliosis. In The American Academy of Orthopaedic Surgeons: *Instructional course lectures*, vol 5, Ann Arbor, Mich, 1948, JW Edwards.

Risser JC: The iliac apophysis: an invaluable sign in the management of scoliosis, *Clin Orthop* 11:111, 1958.

Russell GG, Raso VJ, Hill D, et al: A comparison of four computerized methods of measuring vertebral rotation, *Spine* 15:24, 1990.

Sahlstrand T: The clinical value of Moiré topography in the management of scoliosis, *Spine* 11:409, 1986.

Sanders JO, Herring JA, Brown RH: Behavior of the immature Risser 0 (spine) in idiopathic scoliosis following posterior spinal instrumentation and fusion. Paper presented at the Twenty-eighth Annual Meeting of the Scoliosis Research Society, Dublin, Sept 1993.

Stagnara P: Examen du scoliotique. In *Deviations laterales du rachis: scolioses, encyclopedie mediocochirurgicale*, vol 7, Paris, 1974, Appareil Locomoteur.

Stokes IAF, Moreland MS: Measurement of the shape of the surface of the back in patients with scoliosis: the standing and forward-bending positions, *J Bone Joint Surg* 69A:203, 1987.

Stokes IAF, Shuma-Hartswick D, Moreland MS: Spine and back-shaped changes in scoliosis, *Acta Orthop Scand* 59:128, 1988.

Vedantam R, Lenke LG, Keeney JA, Bridwell KH: Comparison of standing sagittal alignment in asymptomatic adolescents versus adults, *Spine* 23:211, 1998.

Wamboldt A, Spencer DL: A segmental analysis of the distribution of lumbar lordosis in the normal spine, *Orthop Trans* 11:92, 1987.

Weisz I, Jefferson RJ, Turner-Smith AR, et al: ISIS scanning: a useful assessment to technique in the management of scoliosis, *Spine* 13:405, 1988.

NONOPERATIVE MANAGEMENT OF IDIOPATHIC SCOLIOSIS

Aaro S, Burstrom R, Dahlborn M: The derotating effect of the Boston brace: a comparison between computer tomography and a conventional method, *Spine* 6:477, 1981.

Andrews G, MacEwen GD: Idiopathic scoliosis: an 11-year follow-up study of the role of the Milwaukee brace in curve control and trunco-pelvic alignment, *Orthopedics* 12:809, 1989.

Apter A, Morein G, Munitz H, et al: The psychological sequelae of the Milwaukee brace in adolescent girls, *Clin Orthop* 131:156, 1978.

Axelgaard J, Brown JC: Lateral electrode surface stimulation for the treatment of progressive idiopathic scoliosis, *Spine* 8:242, 1983.

Bancel P, Kaelin A, Hall J, et al: The Boston brace: results of a clinical and radiologic study of 401 patients, *Orthop Trans* 8:33, 1984.

Bassett GS, Bunnell WP: Effect of a thoracolumbar orthosis on lateral trunk shift in idiopathic scoliosis, *J Pediatr Orthop* 6:182, 1986.

Benson DR, Wolf AW, Shoji H: Can the Milwaukee patient participate in competitive athletics? *Am J Sports Med* 5:7, 1977.

Bjerkreim I, Carlsen B, Korsell E: Preoperative Cotrel traction in idiopathic scoliosis, *Acta Orthop Scand* 53:901, 1982.

Bradford DS, Tanguy A, Vanselow J: Surface electrical stimulation in the treatment of idiopathic scoliosis: preliminary results in 30 patients, *Spine* 8:757, 1983.

Bunnell WP: Treatment of idiopathic scoliosis, *Orthop Clin North Am* 10:813, 1979.

Bunnell WP: Nonoperative treatment of spinal deformity: the case for observation. In The American Academy of Orthopaedic Surgeons: *Instructional course lectures*, vol 34, St Louis, 1985, Mosby.

Bylund P, Aaro S, Gottfries B: Is lateral electric surface stimulation an effective treatment for scoliosis? *J Pediatr Orthop* 7:298, 1987.

Carr WA, Moe JH, Winter RB, et al: Treatment of idiopathic scoliosis in the Milwaukee brace, *J Bone Joint Surg* 62A:599, 1980.

Clayson D, Luz-Alterman S, Cataletto MM, et al: Long-term psychological sequelae of surgically versus nonsurgically treated scoliosis, *Spine* 12:983, 1987.

Cochran T, Nachemson A: Long-term anatomic and functional changes in patients with adolescent idiopathic scoliosis treated with the Milwaukee brace, *Spine* 10:27, 1985.

Dickson RA: Spinal deformity—adolescent idiopathic scoliosis: nonoperative treatment, *Spine* 24:2601, 1999.

DiRaimondo CV, Green NE: Brace-wear compliance in patients with adolescent idiopathic scoliosis, *J Pediatr Orthop* 8:143, 1988.

Dove J, Hsu LC, Yau AC: The cervical spine after halo-pelvic traction: an analysis of the complications of 83 patients, *J Bone Joint Surg* 62B:158, 1980.

Durham JW, Moskowitc A, Whitney J: Surface electrical stimulation versus brace in treatment of idiopathic scoliosis, *Spine* 15:888, 1990.

Edgar MA, Chapman RH, Glasgow MM: Preoperative correction in adolescent idiopathic scoliosis, *J Bone Joint Surg* 64A:530, 1982.

Edmonson AS, Morris JT: Follow-up study of Milwaukee brace treatment in patients with idiopathic scoliosis, *Clin Orthop* 126:58, 1977.

Edmonson AS, Smith GR: Long-term follow-up study of Milwaukee brace treatment in patients with idiopathic scoliosis. Proceedings of the Scoliosis Research Society, Denver, Sept 22, 1982.

Emans JB, Kaelin A, Bancel P, et al: The Boston bracing system for idiopathic scoliosis: follow-up results of 295 patients, *Spine* 11:792, 1986.

Fallstrom K, Cochran T, Nachemson A: Long-term effects on personality development in patient with adolescent idiopathic scoliosis: influence of type of treatment, *Spine* 11:756, 1986.

Federico DJ, Renshaw TS: Results of treatment of idiopathic scoliosis with the Charleston bending orthosis, *Spine* 15:886, 1990.

Focarile FA, Bonaldi A, Giarolo M, et al: Effectiveness of nonsurgical treatment for idiopathic scoliosis: overview of available evidence, *Spine* 16:395, 1991.

Goldberg C, Poitras B, Mayo NE: Electro-spinal stimulation in children with adolescent and juvenile scoliosis, *Spine* 13:482, 1988.

Goldberg CJ, Dowling FE, Hall JE, et al: A statistical comparison between natural history of idiopathic scoliosis and brace treatment in skeletally immature adolescent girls, *Spine* 18:902, 1993.

Green NE: Part-time bracing of idiopathic scoliosis, *J Bone Joint Surg* 68A:738, 1986.

Hanks GA, Zimmer B, Nogi J: TLSO treatment of idiopathic scoliosis: an analysis of the Wilmington jacket, *Spine* 13:626, 1988.

Hassan J, Bjerkreim I: Progression in idiopathic scoliosis after conservative treatment, *Acta Orthop Scand* 54:88, 1983.

Humbyrd DE, Latimer FR, Lonstein JE, et al: Brain abscess as a complication of halo traction, *Spine* 6:364, 1981.

Jonassen-Rajala E, Josefsson E, Lundberg B, et al: Boston thoracic brace in the treatment of idiopathic scoliosis, *Clin Orthop* 183:37, 1984.

Kahanovitz N, Levine DB, Lardone J: The part-time Milwaukee brace treatment of juvenile idiopathic scoliosis: long-term follow-up, *Clin Orthop* 167:145, 1982.

Kahanovitz N, Weiser S: LESS compliance in adolescent female scoliosis patients. Proceedings of the Scoliosis Research Society, Coronado, Calif, Sept 1985.

Kahanovitz N, Weiser S: The psychological impact of idiopathic scoliosis on the adolescent female, *Spine* 14:483, 1989.

Katz DE, Richards S, Browne RH, Herring JA: A comparison between the Boston brace and the Charleston bending brace in adolescent idiopathic scoliosis, *Spine* 22:1302, 1997.

Kehl OK, Morrissy RT: Brace treatment in adolescent idiopathic scoliosis: an update on concepts and technique, *Clin Orthop* 229:34, 1988.

Keller RB: Nonoperative treatment of adolescent idiopathic scoliosis, *Instr Course Lect* 38:129, 1989.

Laurnen EL, Tupper JW, Mullen MP: The Boston brace in thoracic scoliosis: a preliminary report, *Spine* 8:388, 1983.

Leslie IJ, Dorgan JC, Bentley G, et al: A prospective study of deep vein thrombosis of the leg in children on halo-femoral traction, *J Bone Joint Surg* 63B:168, 1981.

Lindh M: The effect of sagittal curve changes on brace correction of idiopathic scoliosis, *Spine* 5:26, 1980.

Lonstein JE: Cast techniques. In Bradford DS et al, eds: *Moe's textbook of scoliosis and other spinal deformities*, ed 2, Philadelphia, 1987, WB Sanders.

Lonstein JE, Winter RB: Adolescent idiopathic scoliosis: nonoperative treatment, *Orthop Clin North Am* 19:239, 1988.

Lonstein JE, Winter RB: The Milwaukee brace for the treatment of adolescent idiopathic scoliosis: review of 1020 patients, *J Bone Joint Surg* 76A:1207, 1994.

MacLean WE, Green NE, Pierre CB, et al: Stress and coping with scoliosis: psychological effects on adolescents and their families, *J Pediatr Orthop* 9:257, 1989.

McCollough NC III: Nonoperative treatment of idiopathic scoliosis using surface electrical stimulation, *Spine* 11:802, 1986.

McCollough NC, Schultz M, Javech N, et al: Miami TLSO in the management of scoliosis: preliminary results from 100 cases, *J Pediatr Orthop* 1:141, 1981.

Meade KP, Bunch WH, Vanderby R Jr, et al: Progression of unsupported curves in adolescent idiopathic scoliosis, *Spine* 12:520, 1987.

Miller JAA, Nachemson AL, Schultz AB: Effectiveness of braces in mild idiopathic scoliosis, *Spine* 9:632, 1984.

Moe JH: Methods of correction and surgical techniques in scoliosis, *Orthop Clin North Am* 3:17, 1972.

Montgomery F, Willner S: Prognosis of brace-treated scoliosis: comparison of the Boston and Milwaukee methods in 244 girls, *Acta Orthop Scand* 60:383, 1989.

Montgomery F, Willner S, Appelgren G: Long-term follow-up of patients with adolescent idiopathic scoliosis treated conservatively: an analysis of the clinical value of progression, *J Pediatr Orthop* 10:48, 1990.

Mubarak SJ, Camp JF, Valetich W, et al: Halo application in the infant, *J Pediatr Orthop* 9:612, 1989.

Nachemson AL, Nordwall A: Effectiveness of preoperative Cotrel traction for idiopathic scoliosis, *J Bone Joint Surg* 59A:504, 1977.

Nachemson AL, Peterson L: Scoliosis Research Society brace study report. Part 1. Effectiveness of brace treatment in moderate adolescent idiopathic scoliosis. Paper presented at the Twenty-eighth Annual Meeting of the Scoliosis Research Society, Dublin, Sept 1993.

Nachemson AL, Cochran TP, Fällström K, et al: Somatic, social, and psychologic effects of treatment for idiopathic scoliosis, *Orthop Trans* 7:508, 1983.

Nash CL: Current concepts review: scoliosis bracing, *J Bone Joint Surg* 62A:848, 1980.

Nickel VL, Perry J, Garrett A, et al: The halo: a spinal skeletal traction fixation device, *J Bone Joint Surg* 50A:1400, 1968.

O'Brien JP: The halo-pelvic apparatus: a clinical, bioengineering, and anatomical study, *Acta Orthop Scand* 163(suppl), 1975.

O'Brien JP, Yau AC, Hodgson AR: Halo-pelvic traction: a technic for severe spinal deformities, *Clin Orthop* 93:179, 1973.

O'Brien JP, Yau ACMC, Smith TK, et al: Halo-pelvic traction: a preliminary report on a method of external skeletal fixation for correcting deformities and maintaining fixation of the spine, *J Bone Joint Surg* 53B:217, 1971.

Perry J: The halo in spinal abnormalities: practical factors and avoidance of complications, *Orthop Clin North Am* 3:69, 1972.

Perry J, Nickel VL: Total cervical-spine fusion for neck paralysis, *J Bone Joint Surg* 41A:37, 1959.

Piazza MR, Bassett GS: Curve progression after treatment with the Wilmington brace for idiopathic scoliosis, *J Pediatr Orthop* 10:39, 1990.

Price CT, Scott DS, Reed FE Jr, et al: Nighttime bracing for idiopathic scoliosis with the Charleston bending brace: preliminary report, *Spine* 16:1294, 1990.

Refsum HE, Naess-Andreson CF, Lange JE: Pulmonary function and gas exchange at rest and exercise in adolescent girls with mild idiopathic scoliosis during treatment with Boston thoracic brace, *Spine* 15:420, 1990.

Renshaw TS: Orthotic treatment of idiopathic scoliosis and kyphosis. In The American Academy of Orthopaedic Surgeons: *Instructional course lectures*, vol 34, St Louis, 1985, Mosby.

Risser JC: The application of body casts for the correction of scoliosis. In The American Academy of Orthopaedic Surgeons: *Instructional course lectures*, vol 12, Ann Arbor, Mich, 1955, JW Edwards.

Risser JC: Plaster body-jackets, *Am J Orthop* 3:19, 1961.

Risser JC, Norquist DM, Lauder CH Jr, et al: Three types of body casts. In The American Academy of Orthopaedic Surgeons: *Instructional course lectures*, vol 10, Ann Arbor, Mich, 1953, JW Edwards.

Rowe DE, Berstein SM, Riddick MF, et al: A meta-analysis of the efficacy of nonoperative treatments for idiopathic scoliosis, *J Bone Joint Surg* 79A:664, 1997.

Rudicel S, Renshaw TS: The effect of the Milwaukee brace on spinal decompensation in idiopathic scoliosis, *Spine* 8:385, 1983.

Schultz A, Haderspeck K, Takashima S: Correction of scoliosis by muscle stimulation: biomechanical analyses, *Spine* 6:468, 1981.

Shufflebarger HL, Kaiser RP: Nonoperative treatment of idiopathic scoliosis: a 10-year study, *Orthop Trans* 7:11, 1983.

Sullivan JA, Davidson R, Renshaw TS, et al: Further evaluation of the Scolitron treatment of idiopathic adolescent scoliosis, *Spine* 11:903, 1986.

Swank SM, Brown JC, Jennings MV, et al: Lateral electrical surface stimulation in idiopathic scoliosis: experience in two private practices, *Spine* 14:1293, 1989.

Swank SM, Winter RB, Moe JH: Scoliosis and cor pulmonale, *Spine* 7:343, 1982.

Toledo LC, Toledo CH, MacEwen GD: Halo traction with the Circolectric bed in the treatment of severe spinal deformities: a preliminary report, *J Pediatr Orthop* 2:554, 1982.

Tolo VT: Treatment follow-up or discharge, *Spine* 13:1189, 1988.

Uden A, Willner S: The effect of lumbar flexion and Boston thoracic brace on the curves in idiopathic scoliosis, *Spine* 8:846, 1983.

Watts HG: Bracing spinal deformities, *Orthop Clin North Am* 10:769, 1979.

Wiley JW, Thomson JD, Mitchell TM, et al: The effectiveness of the Boston brace in treatment of large curves in adolescent idiopathic scoliosis, *Spine* 25:2326, 2000.

Willers U, Mormelli H, Aaro S, et al: Long-term results of Boston brace treatment on vertebral rotation in idiopathic scoliosis, *Spine* 18:432, 1993.

Willner S: Effect of the Boston thoracic brace on the frontal and sagittal curves of the spine, *Acta Orthop Scand* 55:457, 1984.

Winter RB, Lonstein JE: Brace or not to brace: the true value of school screening, *Spine* 22:1283, 1997 (editorial).

Winter RB, Lonstein JE, Drogt J, et al: The effectiveness of bracing in the nonoperative treatment of idiopathic scoliosis, *Spine* 11:790, 1986.

Wynarsky GT, Schultz AB: Trunk muscle activities in braced scoliosis patients, *Spine* 14:1283, 1989.

Ylikoski M, Peltonen J, Poussa M: Biological factors and predictability of bracing in adolescent idiopathic scoliosis, *J Pediatr Orthop* 9:680, 1989.

OPERATIVE TREATMENT OF IDIOPATHIC SCOLIOSIS

Aaro S, Ohlen G: The effect of Harrington instrumentation on the sagittal configuration and mobility of the spine in scoliosis, *Spine* 8:570, 1983.

Akbarnia BA: Selection of methodology in surgical treatment of adolescent idiopathic scoliosis, *Orthop Clin North Am* 19:319, 1988.

Apel DM, Marrero G, King J, et al: Avoiding paraplegia during anterior spinal surgery: the role of somatosensory-evoked potential monitoring with temporary occlusion of segmental spinal arteries, *Spine* 16:365, 1991.

Asher M, Heinig C, Carson W, and Strippgen W: ISOLA spinal implant system: principles, design, and applications. In An HS, Cotler JM, eds: *Spinal instrumentation*, Baltimore, 1992, Williams & Wilkins.

Asher MA, Strippgen WE, Heinig CF, et al: *ISOLA Spine implant system: principles and practice*, Cleveland, 1991, AcroMed.

Ashman RB, Herring JA, Johnston CE II: Texas Scottish Rite Hospital (TSRH) instrumentation system. In Bridwell KH, DeWald RL eds: *The textbook of spinal surgery*, Philadelphia, 1991, JB Lippincott.

Aurori BF, Weierman RJ, Lowell HA, et al: Pseudarthrosis after spinal fusion for scoliosis: a comparison of autogenic and allogenic bone grafts, *Clin Orthop* 199:153, 1985.

Bailey TE, Mahoney OM: The use of banked autologous blood in patients undergoing surgery for spinal deformity, *J Bone Joint Surg* 69A:329, 1987.

Balderston RA: Cotrel-Dubousset instrumentation. In An HS, Cotler JM, eds: *Spinal instrumentation*, Baltimore, 1992, Williams & Wilkins.

Banta CJ, King AG, Dabezies EG, et al: Measurement of effective pedicle diameter in the human spine, *Orthopedics* 12:939, 1989.

Barr SJ, Scutte AM, Emans JB: Screws versus hooks: results in double-major curves in adolescent idiopathic scoliosis, *Spine* 22:1369, 1997.

Bell GR, Gurd AR, Orlowski JP, et al: The syndrome of inappropriate antidiuretic-hormone secretion following spinal fusion, *J Bone Joint Surg* 68A:720, 1986.

Ben-David B: Spinal cord monitoring, *Orthop Clin North Am* 19:427, 1988.

Benson L, Ibrahim K, Goldberg B: Coronal balance in Cotrel-Dubousset instrumentation: compensation versus decompensation. Paper presented at the annual meeting of the Scoliosis Research Society, Honolulu, Sept 1990.

Bergoin M, Bollini G, Hornung H: Is the Cotrel-Dubousset really universal in the surgical treatment of idiopathic scoliosis? *J Pediatr Orthop* 8:45, 1988.

Bernhardt M, Bridwell KH: Segmental analysis of the sagittal plane alignment of the normal thoracic and lumbar spines and thoracolumbar junction, *Spine* 14:717, 1989.

Berry JL, Moran JM, Berg WS, et al: A morphometric study of human lumbar and selected thoracic vertebrae, *Spine* 12:362, 1987.

Beschetti GD, Moore JS, Smith JG, et al: Techniques for exposure of the anterior thoracic and lumbar spine, *Spine: State of the Art Reviews* 12:599, 1998.

Betz RR, Harms J, Clements DH, et al: Comparison of anterior and posterior instrumentation for correction of adolescent thoracic idiopathic scoliosis, *Spine* 24:225, 1999.

Bieber E, Tolo V, Uematsu S: Spinal cord monitoring during posterior spinal instrumentation and fusion, *Clin Orthop* 229:121, 1988.

Birch JG, Herring JA, Roach JW, et al: Cotrel-Dubousset instrumentation in idiopathic scoliosis: a preliminary report, *Clin Orthop* 227:24, 1988.

Blackman R: Multiple level anterior thoracic diskectomy using an endoscopic exposure. Paper presented at the Twenty-eighth Annual Meeting of the Scoliosis Research Society, Dublin, Sept 18-23, 1993.

Blackman RG, Picetti G, O'Neal K: Endoscopic thoracic spine surgery. In White AH, Schofferman JA, eds: *Spine care: operative treatment*, vol 2, St Louis, 1995, Mosby.

Bradford DS: Techniques of surgery. In Bradford DS et al, eds: *Moe's textbook of scoliosis and other spinal deformities*, ed 2, Philadelphia, 1987, WB Saunders.

Bradshaw K, Webb JK, Faser AM: Clinical evaluation of spinal cord monitoring in scoliosis surgery, *Spine* 9:636, 1984.

Bridwell KH: Idiopathic scoliosis. In Bridwell KH, DeWald RL, eds: *The textbook of spinal surgery*, Philadelphia, 1991, JB Lippincott.

Bridwell KH, Betz RR, Capelli AM, et al: Sagittal plane analysis in idiopathic scoliosis patients treated with Cotrel-Dubousset instrumentation, *Spine* 15:921, 1990.

Bridwell KH, McCallister JW, Betz RR, et al: Coronal decompensation produced by Cotrel-Dubousset "derotation" maneuver for idiopathic right thoracic scoliosis, *Spine* 16:769, 1991.

Brinker MR, Willis JK, Cook SD, et al: Neurologic testing with somatosensory-evoked potentials in idiopathic scoliosis, *Spine* 17:277, 1992.

Brodsky JW, Dickson JH, Erwin WD, et al: Hypotensive anesthesia for scoliosis surgery in Jehovah's Witnesses, *Spine* 16:304, 1991.

Broome G, Simpson AHRW, Catalan J, et al: The modified Schollner costoplasty, *J Bone Joint Surg* 72B:894, 1990.

Brown RH, Nash CL Jr: Current status of spinal cord monitoring, *Spine* 4:466, 1979.

Casey MP, Asher MA, Jacobs RR, et al: The effect of Harrington rod contouring on lumbar lordosis, *Spine* 12:750, 1987.

Chopin D, Morin C: Cotrel-Dubousset instrumentation (CDI) for adolescent and pediatric scoliosis. In Bridwell KH, DeWald RL, eds: *The textbook of spinal surgery*, Philadelphia, 1991, JB Lippincott.

Cobb JR: The treatment of scoliosis, *Conn Med J* 7:467, 1943.

Cobb JR: Technique, after-treatment, and results of spine fusion for scoliosis. In The American Academy of Orthopaedic Surgeons: *Instructional course lectures*, vol 9, Ann Arbor, Mich, 1952, JW Edwards.

Cobb JR: The problem of the primary curve, *J Bone Joint Surg* 42A:1413, 1960.

Cochran T, Irstam L, Nachemson A: Long-term anatomic and function changes in patients with adolescent idiopathic scoliosis treated by Harrington rod fusions, *Spine* 8:576, 1983.

Corovessis PG, Zielke K: Does the combined ventral derotation system (VDS) followed by Harrington instrumentation improve the vital capacity in patients with idiopathic double major curve pattern scoliosis? *Clin Orthop* 283:130, 1992.

Cotrel Y, Dubousset J: New segmental posterior instrumentation of the spine, *Orthop Trans* 9:118, 1985.

Cotrel Y, Dubousset J, Guillaumat M: New universal instrumentation and spinal surgery, *Clin Orthop* 227:10, 1988.

Coventry MB, Topper EM: Pelvic instability: a consequence of removing iliac bone for grafting, *J Bone Joint Surg* 54:83.

Crawford AH: Video-assisted thoracoscopy. Minimally invasive spine surgery. *Spine: State of the Art Reviews* 11:341, 1997.

Crawford AH, Wall EJ, Wolf R: Video-assisted thoracoscopy, *Orthop Clin North Am* 30:367, 1999.

Crawford AH, Wolf RK, Wall EJ, et al: Pediatric spinal deformity. In Regan JJ, McAfee PC, Mack MF, eds: *Atlas of endoscopic spine surgery*, St Louis, 1995, Quality Medical Publishing.

Cundy PJ, Paterson DC, Hillier TM, et al: Cotrel-Dubousset instrumentation and vertebral rotation in adolescent idiopathic scoliosis, *J Bone Joint Surg* 72B:670, 1990.

Cunningham BW, Kotani Y, McNulte PS, et al: Video-assisted thoracoscopic surgery versus open thoracotomy for anterior thoracic spinal fusion: a comparative radiographic biomechanical and histologic analysis in a sheep model, *Spine* 23:1333, 1998.

D'Andrea LP, Betz RR, Lenke LG, et al: The effect of continued posterior spinal growth on sagittal contour in patients treated by anterior instrumentation for idiopathic scoliosis, *Spine* 25:813, 2000.

Dawson EG, Sherman JE, Kanim LEA, et al: Spinal cord monitoring: results of the Scoliosis Research Society and the European Spinal Society survey, *Spine* 16:S361, 1991.

Denis F: Cotrel-Dubousset instrumentation in the treatment of idiopathic scoliosis, *Orthop Clin North Am* 19:291, 1988.

Dickman CA, Mican C: Thoracoscopic approaches for the treatment of anterior thoracic spinal pathology, *Barrow Neurological Institute Quarterly* 12:4, 1996.

Dickman CA, Rosenthal D, Karahalios DG, et al: Thoracic vertebrectomy and reconstruction using a microsurgical thoracoscopic approach, *Neurosurgery* 38: 279, 1996.

Dickson JH, Erwin WD, Rossi D: Harrington instrumentation and arthrodesis for idiopathic scoliosis: a 21-year follow-up, *J Bone Joint Surg* 72A:678, 1990.

Dodd CAF, Fergusson CM, Freedman L, et al: Allograft versus autograft bone in scoliosis surgery, *J Bone Joint Surg* 70B:431, 1988.

Dove J, Lin YT, Shen YS, et al: Aortic aneurysm complicating spinal fixation with Dwyer's apparatus: report of a case, *Spine* 6:524, 1981.

Dowell JK, Powell JM, Webb PJ, et al: Factors influencing the result of posterior spinal fusion in the treatment of adolescent idiopathic scoliosis, *Spine* 15:803, 1990.

Dunn HK: Spinal instrumentation. I. Principles of posterior and anterior instrumentation. In The American Academy of Orthopaedic Surgeons: *Instructional course lectures*, vol 32, St Louis, 1983, Mosby.

Dwyer AF, Newton NC, Sherwood AA: An anterior approach to scoliosis: a preliminary report, *Clin Orthop* 62:192, 1969.

Dwyer AP, O'Brien JP, Seal PP, et al: The late complications after the Dwyer anterior spinal instrumentation for scoliosis, *J Bone Joint Surg* 59B:117, 1977.

Edgar MA, Mehta MH: Long-term follow-up of fused and unfused idiopathic scoliosis, *J Bone Joint Surg* 70B:712, 1988.

Edmonds HL, Markku PJ, Backman MH, et al: Transcranial magnetic motor evoked potentials (tc MMEP) for functional monitoring of motor pathways during scoliosis surgery, *Spine* 14:683, 1989.

Eker ML, Betz RR, Trent PS, et al: Computer tomography evaluation of Cotrel-Dubousset instrumentation in idiopathic scoliosis, *Spine* 13:1141, 1988.

Engler G: Preoperative and intraoperative considerations in adolescent idiopathic scoliosis, *Instr Course Lect* 38:137, 1989.

Engler GL, Spielholz NI, Bernhard WN, et al: Somatosensory-evoked potentials during Harrington instrumentation for scoliosis, *J Bone Joint Surg* 60A:528, 1978.

Fabry G, Melkebeek JV, Bockx E: Back pain after Harrington rod instrumentation for idiopathic scoliosis, *Spine* 14:620, 1989.

Farcy J, Weidenbaum M, Roye DP Jr: Correction of thoracic scoliosis using the Cotrel-Dubousset technique, *Surg Rounds Orthop* 1:11, 1987.

Fernyhough JC, Schimandle JJ, Weigel MC, et al: Chronic donor site pain complicating bone graft harvesting from the posterior iliac crest for spinal fusion, *Spine* 17:1474, 1992.

Fitch RD, Turi M, Bowman BE, et al: Comparison of Cotrel-Dubousset and Harrington rod instrumentations in idiopathic scoliosis, *J Pediatr Orthop* 10:44, 1990.

Flinchum D: Rib resection in the treatment of scoliosis, *South Med J* 56:1378, 1963.

Flinchum D: Scoliosis trouble, *J Med Assoc Ga* 52:67, 1963.

Fraser RD: A wide muscle-splitting approach to the lumbosacral spine, *J Bone Joint Surg* 64B:44, 1982.

Fraser RD, Gogan WJ: A modified muscle-splitting approach to the lumbosacral spine, *Spine* 17:943, 1992.

Freeman BL, Betz RR: The pediatric spine. In Canale ST, Beaty JH, eds: *Operative pediatric orthopaedics*, St Louis, 1995, Mosby.

Gaines RW Jr, York DH, Watts C: Identification of spinal cord pathways responsible for the peroneal-evoked response in the dog, *Spine* 9:810, 1984.

Gertzbein SD, Robbins SE: Accuracy of pedicular screw placement in vivo, *Spine* 15:11, 1990.

Giehl JP, Zielke K: Zielke procedures in scoliosis correction. In Bridwell KH, DeWald RL, eds: *The textbook of spinal surgery*, Philadelphia, 1991, JB Lippincott.

Goldstein LA: Concave rib resection and ligament release for correction of idiopathic scoliosis. In American Academy of Orthopaedic Surgeons: *Symposium on the spine*, St Louis, 1969, Mosby.

Gollehon D, Kahanovitz N, Happel LT: Temperature effects on the feline cortical and spinal evoked potentials, *Spine* 8:443, 1983.

Goodnough LT, Marcus RE: Effect of autologous blood donation in patients undergoing elective spine surgery, *Spine* 17:172, 1992.

Gray JM, Smith BW, Ashley RK, et al: Derotational analysis of Cotrel-Dubousset instrumentation in idiopathic scoliosis, *Spine* 16:S391, 1991.

Guidera KJ, Hoote J, Weatherly W, et al: Cotrel-Dubousset instrumentation: results in 52 patients, *Spine* 18:427, 1993.

Hales DD, Dawson EG, Delamarter R: Late neurological complications of Harrington-rod instrumentation, *J Bone Joint Surg* 71A:1053, 1989.

Hall JE: The anterior approach to spinal deformities, *Orthop Clin North Am* 3:81, 1972.

Hall JE: Preoperative assessment of the patient with a spinal deformity. In The American Academy of Orthopaedic Surgeons: *Instructional course lectures*, vol 34, St Louis, 1985, Mosby.

Hall JE, Millis MB, Snyder BD: Short segment anterior instrumentation for thoracolumbar scoliosis. In Bridwell KH, DeWald RL, eds: *The textbook of spinal surgery*, ed 2, Philadelphia, 1997, Lippincott-Raven.

Halsall AP, James DF, Kostuik JP, et al: An experimental evaluation of spinal flexibility with respect to scoliosis surgery, *Spine* 8:482, 1983.

Hamill CL, Lenke LG, Bridwell KH: Use of pedicle screw fixation to improve correction in the lumbar spine in patients with idiopathic scoliosis. Is it warranted? *Spine* **21:1241, 1996.**

Hammerberg KW, Rodts MF, DeWald RL: Zielke instrumentation, *Orthopedics* 11:1365, 1988.

Harms J: Surgical treatment of spondylolisthesis: the Harms technique. In Bridwell KH, DeWald RL, eds: *Spinal surgery*, Philadelphia, 1991, JB Lippincott.

Harms J, Jaczienski D, Biel B: Ventral correction of thoracic scoliosis. In Bridwell KH, DeWald RL, eds: *The textbook of spinal surgery*, ed 2, Philadelphia, 1997, Lippincott-Raven.

Harrington PR: Surgical instrumentation for management of scoliosis, *J Bone Joint Surg* 42A:1448, 1960.

Harrington PR: Treatment of scoliosis: correction and internal fixation by spine instrumentation, *J Bone Joint Surg* 44A:591, 1962.

Harrington PR: The management of scoliosis by spine instrumentation: an evaluation of more than two hundred cases, *South Med J* 56:1367, 1963.

Harrington PR, Dickson JH: An eleven-year clinical investigation of Harrington instrumentation: a preliminary report of 578 cases, *Clin Orthop* 93:113, 1973.

Harvey CJ, Betz RR, Huss GK, et al: Are there indications for partial rib resection in adolescent patients treated with Cotrel-Dubousset instrumentation? Paper presented at annual meeting of the Scoliosis Research Society, Kansas City, Mo, Sept 1992.

Hayes MA, Tompkins SF, Herndon WA, et al: Clinical and radiological evaluation of lumbosacral motion below fusion levels in idiopathic scoliosis, *Spine* 13:1161, 1988.

Herron LD, Newman MH: The failure of ethylene oxide gas-sterilized freeze-dried bone graft for thoracic and lumbar spinal fusion, *Spine* 14:496, 1989.

Hibbs RA: An operation for progressive spinal deformities, *NY Med J* 93:1013, 1911.

Hibbs RA: A report of 59 cases of scoliosis treated by the fusion operation, *J Bone Joint Surg* 6:3, 1924.

Hibbs RA, Risser JC, Ferguson AB: Scoliosis treated by the fusion operation, *J Bone Joint Surg* 13:91, 1931.

Hodgson AR, Stock FE: Anterior spine fusion, *Br J Surg* 44:266, 1956.

Hodgson AR, Stock FE: Anterior spine fusion, *Br J Surg* 48:172, 1960.

Holcomb GW 3rd, Menzio GA, Green NE: Video-assisted thoracoscopic diskectomy and fusion. *J Ped Surg* 32:1120, 1997.

Horton WC: Eliminating the reversed orientation in endoscopic spinal surgery: the technique of camera-monitor inversion. Paper presented at Endoscopic Approaches to the Spine, Memphis, Feb 5, 2000.

Horton WC, Hoh RT, Johnson JR, et al: Zielke instrumentation in idiopathic scoliosis: late effects and minimizing complications, *Spine* 13:1145, 1988.

Hsu LCS, Zucherman J, Tang SC, et al: Dwyer instrumentation in the treatment of adolescent idiopathic scoliosis, *J Bone Joint Surg* 64B:536, 1982.

Huang TJ, Hsu RW, Sum CW, Liu HP: Complications in thoracoscopic spinal surgery: a study of 90 consecutive patients, *Surg Endosc* 13:346, 1999.

Huang TJ, Hsu RW, Sum CW, et al: Video-assisted thoracoscopic surgery to the upper thoracic spine, *Surg Endosc* 13:123, 1999.

Hur S, Huizenga BA, Major M: Acute normovolemic hemodilution combined with hypotensive anesthesia and other techniques to avoid homologous transfusion in spinal fusion surgery, *Spine* 17:867, 1992.

Hutchinson DT, Bassett GS: Superior mesenteric artery syndrome in pediatric orthopaedic patients, *Clin Orthop* 250:250, 1990.

Jefferson RJ, Weisz I, Turner-Smith AR, et al: Scoliosis and its effect on back shape, *J Bone Joint Surg* 70B:261, 1988.

Johnson RM, McGuire EJ: Urogenital complications of anterior approaches to the lumbar spine, *Clin Orthop* 154:114, 1981.

Johnston CE II, Ashman RB, Baird AM, et al: Effect of construct stiffness on early fusion mass incorporation: experimental study, *Spine* 15:908, 1990.

Johnston CE II, Herring JA, Ashman RB: Texas Scottish Rite Hospital (TSRH) universal spinal instrumentation system. In An HS, Cotler JM, eds: *Spinal instrumentation*, Baltimore, 1992, Williams & Wilkins.

Jones SJ, Edgar MA, Ransford AO, et al: A system for the electrophysiological monitoring of the spinal cord during operations for scoliosis, *J Bone Joint Surg* 65B:134, 1983.

Kaiser LR, Bavaria JE: Complications of thoracoscopy, *Ann Thorac Surg* 56:796, 1993.

Kalen V, Conklin M: The behavior of the unfused lumbar curve following selective thoracic fusion for idiopathic scoliosis, *Spine* 15:271, 1990.

Kaneda K, Fujiya N, Satoh S: Results with Zielke instrumentation for idiopathic thoracolumbar and lumbar scoliosis, *Clin Orthop* 205:195, 1986.

Kaneda K, Shona Y, Situ S, Abumi K: Anterior correction of thoracic scoliosis with Kaneda anterior spinal system, a preliminary report, *Spine* 22:1358, 1997.

King AG, Mills TE, Loe WA, et al: Video-assisted thoracoscopic surgery in the prone position, *Spine* 25:2403, 2000.

King HA: Selection of fusion levels for posterior instrumentation and fusion in idiopathic scoliosis, *Orthop Clin North Am* 19:247, 1988.

King HA, Moe JH, Bradford DS, et al: The selection of the fusion levels in thoracic idiopathic scoliosis, *J Bone Joint Surg* 65A:1302, 1983.

Knapp DR, Jones ET: Use of cortical allograft for posterior spinal fusion, *Clin Orthop* 229:99, 1988.

Knapp DR Jr, Price CT, Jones ET, et al: Choosing fusion levels in progressive thoracic idiopathic scoliosis, *Spine* 17:1159, 1992.

Kohler R, Galland O, Mechin H, et al: The Dwyer procedure in the treatment of idiopathic scoliosis: a 10-year follow-up review of 21 patients, *Spine* 15:75, 1990.

Korovessis P: Combined VDS and Harrington instrumentation for treatment of idiopathic double major curves, *Spine* 12:244, 1987.

Kostuik JP: Recent advances in the treatment of painful adult scoliosis, *Clin Orthop* 147:238, 1980.

Krag MH, Van Hal ME, Beynnon BD: Placement of transpedicular vertebral screws close to anterior vertebral cortex: description of methods, *Spine* 14:879, 1989.

Krag MH, Weaver DL, Beynnon BD, et al: Morphometry of the thoracic and lumbar spine related to transpedicular screw placement for surgical spine fixation, *Spine* 13:27, 1988.

Krasna MJ, Mack MJ, eds: *Atlas of thoracoscopic surgery,* St Louis, 1994, Quality Medical Publishing.

Kray MH: Biomechanics of thoracolumbar spinal fixation: a review, *Spine* 16:84, 1991.

Krismer M, Bauer R, Sterzinger W: Scoliosis correction by Cotrel-Dubousset instrumentation: the effect of derotation and three-dimensional correction, *Spine* 17:S263, 1992.

Kurz LT, Garfin SR, Booth RE Jr: Harvesting autogenous iliac bone grafts: a review of complications and techniques, *Spine* 14:1324, 1989.

Lagrone MO: Loss of lumbar lordosis: a complication of spinal fusion for scoliosis, *Orthop Clin North Am* 19:393, 1988.

Lagrone MO, Bradford DS, Moe JH, et al: Treatment of symptomatic flatback after spinal fusion, *J Bone Joint Surg* 70A:569, 1988.

Landin P, Nachemson A: Transfusion-related non-a, non-b hepatitis in elective spine deformity surgery patients in Gothenburg, Sweden, *Spine* 14:1033, 1989.

Landreneau RJ, Mack MJ, Hazelrig SR et al: Video-assisted thoracic surgery: basic technical concepts and intercostal approach strategies, *Ann Thorac Surg* 54:800, 1992.

Larson SJ, Walsh PR, Sances A, et al: Evoked potentials in experimental myelopathy, *Spine* 5:299, 1980.

Lenke LG: Basic techniques of posterior segmental spine internal fixation. In Bridwell KH, DeWald RL, eds: *The textbook of spinal surgery*, ed 2, Philadelphia, 1997, Lippincott-Raven.

Lenke LG, Betz RR, Bridwell KH, et al: Spontaneous lumbar curve coronal correction after selective anterior or posterior thoracic fusion in adolescent idiopathic scoliosis, *Spine* 24:1663, 1999.

Lenke LG, Bridwell KH, Baldus C, et al: Analysis of pulmonary function and axis rotation in adolescent and young adult idiopathic scoliosis patients treated with Cotrel-Dubousset instrumentation, *J Spinal Disord* 5:16, 1992.

Lenke LG, Bridwell KH, Baldus C, et al: Cotrel-Dubousset instrumentation for adolescent idiopathic scoliosis, *J Bone Joint Surg* 74A:1056, 1992.

Lenke LG, Bridwell KH, Baldus C, et al: Preventing decompensation in King type II curves treated with Cotrel-Dubousset instrumentation: strict guidelines for selective thoracic fusion, *Spine* 17:S274, 1992.

Levy WJ Jr: Clinical experience with motor and cerebellar-evoked potential monitoring, *Neurosurgery* 20:169, 1987.

Lichtblau S: Dislocation of the sacroiliac joint: a complication of bone grafting, *J Bone Joint Surg* 44:193, 1962.

Lilijenqvist R, Halm, Henry FH, Link TM: Pedicle screw instrumentation of the thoracic spine in idiopathic scoliosis, *Spine* 22:2239, 1997.

Longley MCH, Lonstein JE: Spinal decompensation after Cotrel-Dubousset instrumentation, *Orthop Consul* 13:1, 1992.

Lowe TG: Morbidity and mortality committee report. Paper presented at Twenty-second Annual Meeting of the Scoliosis Research Society, Vancouver, Sept 1987.

Lowe TG, Peters JD: Anterior spinal fusion with Zielke instrumentation for idiopathic scoliosis: a frontal and sagittal curve analysis in 36 patients, *Spine* 18:423, 1993.

Lueders H, Gurd A, Hahn J, et al: A new technique for intraoperative monitoring of spinal cord function: multichannel recording of spinal cord and subcortical-evoked potentials, *Spine* 7:110, 1982.

Luk KDK, Lee FB, Leong JCY, et al: The effect on the lumbosacral spine of long spinal fusion for idiopathic scoliosis: a minimum ten-year follow-up, *Spine* 12:996, 1987.

MacEwen GD, Bennett E, Guille JT: Autologous blood transfusions in children and young adults with low body weight undergoing spinal surgery, *J Pediatr Orthop* 10:750, 1990.

Machida M, Weinstein SL, Yamada T, et al: Spinal cord monitoring: electrophysiological measures of sensory and motor function during spinal surgery, *Spine* 10:407, 1985.

Mack MGJ Regan JJ, McAfee PC, et al: Video-assisted thoracic surgery for the anterior approach to the thoracic spine, *Ann Thorac Surg* 59:1100, 1995.

Madigan RR, Linton BS, Wallace SL, et al: A new technique to improve cortical-evoked potentials in spinal cord monitoring, *Spine* 12:330, 1987.

Majd ME, Castro FE, Holt RT: Anterior fusion for idiopathic scoliosis, *Spine* 25:696, 2000.

Mann DC, Nash CL, Wilham MR, et al: Evaluation of the role of concave rib osteotomies in the correction of thoracic scoliosis, *Spine* 14:491, 1989.

Mann DC, Wilham MR, Brower EM, et al: Decreasing homologous blood transfusion in spinal surgery by use of the cell saver and predeposited blood, *Spine* 14:1296, 1989.

Marsicano JG, Lenke LG, Bridwell KH, et al: The lordotic effect of the OSI frame on operative adolescent idiopathic scoliosis patients, *Spine* 23:1341, 1998.

Mason DE, Crango P: Spinal decompensation in Cotrel-Dubousset instrumentation, *Spine* 16:S394, 1991.

Mason RJ, Betz RR, Orlowski JP, et al: The syndrome of inappropriate antidiuretic hormone secretion and its effect on blood indices following spinal fusion, *Spine* 14:722, 1989.

McAfee P, Regan J, Zdeblick T, et al: The incidence of complications in endoscopic anterior thoracolumbar spinal reconstructive surgery, *Spine* 20:1624, 1995.

McCall RE, Bronson W: Criteria for selective fusion in idiopathic scoliosis using Cotrel-Dubousset instrumentation, *J Pediatr Orthop* 12:475, 1992.

McCarthy RE, Peak RD, Morissy RT, et al: Allograft bone and spinal fusion for paralytic scoliosis, *J Bone Joint Surg* 68A:370, 1986.

Mehlman CT, Crawford AH: Video-assisted thoracoscopic surgery: pediatric orthopaedic applications. In Zdeblick T, ed: *Anterior approaches in spine surgery*, St Louis, 1995, Quality Medical Publishing.

Mehlman CT, Crawford AH, Wolf RK: Video-assisted thoracic surgery. Endoscopic thoracoplasty technique, *Spine* 22:2178, 1997.

Michel CR, Lalain JJ: Late results of Harrington's operation: long-term evolution of the lumbar spine below the fused segments, *Spine* 10:414, 1985.

Mirkovic S, Abitbol JJ, Steinman J, et al: Anatomic considerations for sacral screw placement, *Spine* 16(suppl):289, 1991.

Moe JH: A critical analysis of methods of fusion for scoliosis: an evaluation in 266 patients, *J Bone Joint Surg* 40A:529, 1958.

Moe JH: Methods of correction and surgical techniques in scoliosis, *Orthop Clin North Am* 3:17, 1972.

Moe JH, Gustilo RB: Treatment of scoliosis: results in 196 patients treated by cast correction and fusion, *J Bone Joint Surg* 46A:293, 1964.

Moe JH, Purcel GA, Bradford DS: Zielke instrumentation (VDS) for the correction of spinal curvature, *Clin Orthop* 180:133, 1983.

Moore MR, Baynham GC, Brown CW, et al: Analysis of factors related to truncal decompensation following Cotrel-Dubousset instrumentation, *J Spinal Disord* 4:188, 1991.

Moore SV: Segmental spinal instrumentation: complications, correction, and indications, *Orthop Trans* 7:413, 1983.

Moskowitz A, Moe JH, Winter RB, et al: Long-term follow-up of scoliosis fusion, *J Bone Joint Surg* 62A:364, 1980.

Mubarak SJ, Wenger DR, Leach J: Evaluation of Cotrel-Dubousset instrumentation for treatment of idiopathic scoliosis, *Update Spinal Disord* 2:3, 1987.

Naito M, Owen JH, Bridwell KH, et al: Effects of distraction on physiologic integrity of the spinal cord, spinal cord bloodflow, and clinical status, *Spine* 17:1154, 1992.

Nasca RJ, Lemons JE, Montgomery R: Evaluation of cryopreserved bone and synthetic biomaterials in promoting spinal fusion, *Spine* 16:S330, 1991.

Nash C, Moe J: A study of vertebral rotation, *J Bone Joint Surg* 51A:223, 1969.

Newton PO, Cardelia JM, Farnsworth CL, et al: Biomechanical comparison of open and thoracoscopic anterior spinal release in a goat model. *Spine* 23:530, 1998.

Newton PO, Shea KG, Granlund KF: Defining the pediatric spinal thoracoscopy learning curve, 65 consecutive cases, *Spine* 25:1028, 2000.

Newton PO, Wenger DR, Mubarak SJ, Myer RS: Anterior release and fusion in pediatric spinal deformity: a comparison of early outcome and cost of thoracoscopic and open thoracotomy approaches, *Spine* 22:1398, 1997.

Nickel VL, Perry J, Affeldt JE, Dail CW: Elective surgery on patients with respiratory paralysis, *J Bone Joint Surg* 39A:989, 1957.

O'Brien MF, Lenke LG, Bridwell KH, et al: Recognition and treatment of the proximal thoracic curve in adolescent idiopathic scoliosis treated with Cotrel-Dubousset instrumentation. Paper presented at the Twenty-eighth Annual Meeting of the Scoliosis Research Society, Dublin, Sept 1993.

Oga M, Ikuta H, Sugioka Y: The use of autologous blood and the surgical treatment of spinal disorders, *Spine* 17:1381, 1992.

Ogiela DM, Chan PK: Ventral derotation spondylodesis: a review of 22 cases, *Spine* 11:18, 1986.

Ogilvie JW: Anterior spine fusion with Zielke instrumentation for idiopathic scoliosis in adolescents, *Orthop Clin North Am* 19:313, 1988.

Olsewski JM, Simmons EH, Kallen FC, et al: Morphometry of the lumbar spine: anatomical perspectives related to transpedicular fixation, *J Bone Joint Surg* 72A:541, 1990.

Owen JH, Laschinger J, Bridwell KH, et al: Sensitivity and specificity of somatosensory- and neurogenic motor–evoked potentials in animals and humans, *Spine* 13:1111, 1988.

Owen R, Turner DA, Bamforth JSG, et al: Costectomy as the first stage of surgery for scoliosis, *J Bone Joint Surg,* 68B:91, 1986.

Passuti N, Daculsi G, Rogez JM, et al: Macroporous calcium phosphate ceramic performance in human spine fusion, *Clin Orthop* 248:169, 1989.

Perry J: Surgical approaches to the spine. In Pierce DS, Nickel VH, eds: *The total care of spinal cord injuries*, Boston, 1977, Little, Brown.

Phillips WA, Hensinger RN: Control of blood loss during scoliosis surgery, *Clin Orthop* 229:88, 1988.

Picetti GD III: CD Horizon Eclipse Spinal System surgical technique manual, Memphis, 1999 Sofamor Danek.

Pinto MR: Complications of pedicle screw fixation, *Spine: State of the art reviews,* 6:45, 1992.

Polly Jr DW: Material presented at Spinal Deformity: Challenges and Solutions of Surgical Treatment, Puerto Rico, May 12-13, 2000.

Ponseti IV, Friedman B: Changes in the scoliotic spine after fusion, *J Bone Joint Surg* 32A:751, 1950.

Pullock FE, Pollock FE Jr: Idiopathic scoliosis: Correction of lateral and rotational deformities using the Cotrel-Dubousset spinal instrumentation system, *South Med J* 83:161, 1990.

Puno RM, Grossfeld SL, Johnson JR, et al: Cotrel-Dubousset instrumentation in idiopathic scoliosis, *Spine* 17:S258, 1992.

Puno RM, Johnson JR, Ostermann PA, et al: Analysis of the primary and compensatory curvatures following Zielke instrumentation for idiopathic scoliosis, *Spine* 14:738, 1989.

Rappaport M, Hall K, Hopkins K, et al: Effects of corrective scoliosis surgery on somatosensory-evoked potentials, *Spine* 7:404, 1982.

Regan JJ, Mack MJ, Picetti MG: Comparison of VAT to open thoracotomy in thoracic spinal surgery, *Orthop Trans* 18:112, 1994.

Regan JR, Mack MJ, Pecetti GD: A technical report on video-assisted thoracoscopy in thoracic spinal surgery, *Spine* 20:831, 1995.

Regan JJ, McAfee PC: Thoracoscopy and laparoscopy of the spine. In Bridwell KH, DeWald RL, eds: *The textbook of spinal surgery,* ed 2, Philadelphia, 1997, Lippincott-Raven.

Relton JES, Hall JE: An operation frame for spinal fusion: a new apparatus designed to reduce haemorrhage during operation, *J Bone Joint Surg* 49B:327, 1967.

Richards BS: Lumbar curve response in type II idiopathic scoliosis after posterior instrumentation of the thoracic curve, *Spine* 17: S282, 1992.

Richards BS, Johnston II CE: Cotrel-Dubousset instrumentation for adolescent idiopathic scoliosis, *Orthopedics* 10:649, 1987.

Richards BS, Birch JG, Herring JA, et al: Frontal plane and sagittal plane balance following Cotrel-Dubousset instrumentation for idiopathic scoliosis, *Spine* 14:733, 1989.

Riseborough EJ: The anterior approach to the spine for the correction of deformities of the axial skeleton, *Clin Orthop* 93:207, 1973.

Roaf R: The treatment of progressive scoliosis by unilateral growth arrest, *J Bone Joint Surg* 45B:637, 1963.

Roth A, Rosenthal A, Hall JE, Mizel M: Scoliosis and congenital heart disease, *Clin Orthop* 93:95, 1973.

Roye DP Jr, Farcy JP, Rickert JB, et al: Results of spinal instrumentation of adolescent idiopathic scoliosis by King type, *Spine* 17:S270, 1992.

Ryan TP, Britt RH: Spinal and cortical sematosensory-evoked potential monitoring during corrective spinal surgery with 108 patients, *Spine* 11:352, 1986.

Schram RA, Allen BL Jr, Ferguson RL: Rib regeneration area as an indicator of fusion area in adolescent idiopathic scoliosis, *Spine* 12:346, 1987.

Shono Y, Kaneda K, Yamamoto I: A biomechanical analysis of Zielke, Kanada, and Cotrel-Dubousset instrumentations in thoracolumbar scoliosis: a calf spine model, *Spine* 16:1305, 1991.

Shufflebarger HL: *Clinical issue: rod rotation in scoliosis surgery*, Warsaw, 1994, Depuy Motech.

Shufflebarger HL: *The theory of the segmental approach to spinal instrumentation: a definitive method of planning spinal instrumentation for every spinal pathology*, Warsaw, 1994, DePuy Motech.

Shufflebarger HL: Thoracoplasty anterior technique. In Bridwell KH, DeWald RL, eds: *The textbook of spinal surgery,* ed 2, Philadelphia, 1997, Lippincott-Raven.

Shufflebarger HL, Clark CE: Cotrel-Dubousset instrumentation, *Orthopedics* 11:1435, 1988.

Shufflebarger HL, Clark CE: Fusion levels and hook patterns in thoracic scoliosis with Cotrel-Dubousset instrumentation, *Spine* 15:916, 1990.

Shufflebarger HL, Harms J: *Moss Miami 3-dimensional spinal instrumentation: surgical technique*, Warsaw, 1994, DePuy Motech.

Shufflebarger HL, Harms J: *Moss Miami 3-dimensional spinal instrumentation: taking spinal instrumentation to a new dimension*, Warsaw, 1994, DePuy Motech.

Smith AD, von Lackum WH, Wylie R: An operation for stapling vertebral bodies in congenital scoliosis, *J Bone Joint Surg* 36A:342, 1954.

Smith RM, Pool RO, Butt WP, et al: The transverse plane deformity of structural scoliosis, *Spine* 16:1126, 1991.

Sorenson J, Asher M: Six degrees freedom of motion analysis of biplanar radiographs: comparison of two instrumentation techniques for treatment of thoracolumbar/lumbar adolescent idiopathic scoliosis. Paper presented at the Twenty-eighth Annual Meeting of the Scoliosis Research Society, Dublin, Sept 1993.

Steel HH: Rib resection and spine fusion and correction of convex deformity in scoliosis, *J Bone Joint Surg* 65A:920, 1983.

Suk SJ, Kim WJ, Kim JH, Lee SM: Restoration of thoracic kyphosis in the hypokyphotic spine. A comparison between multiple-hook and segmental pedicle screw fixation in adolescent idiopathic scoliosis, *J Spinal Disord* 12:489, 1999.

Suk CL, Lee CK: Segmental pedicle screw fixation in the treatment of thoracic idiopathic scoliosis, *Spine* 20:1399, 1995.

Swank SM, Mauri TM, Brown JC: The lumbar lordosis below Harrington instrumentation for scoliosis, *Spine* 15:181, 1990.

Szalay EA, Carollo JJ, Roach JW: Sensitivity of spinal cord monitoring to intraoperative events, *J Pediatr Orthop* 6:437, 1986.

Tate DE, Friedman RJ: Blood conservation in spinal surgery: review of current techniques, *Spine* 17:1450, 1992.

Thompson JD, Callaghan JJ, Savory CG, et al: Prior deposition of autologous blood in elective orthopaedic surgery, *J Bone Joint Surg* 69A:320, 1987.

Thompson JP, Transfeldt EE, Bradford DS, et al: Decompensation after Cotrel-Dubousset instrumentation of idiopathic scoliosis, *Spine* 15:927, 1990.

Tolo VT: Surgical treatment of adolescent idiopathic scoliosis, *Instr Course Lect* 38:143, 1989.

Trammell TR, Benedict F, Reed D: Anterior spine fusion using Zielke instrumentation for adult thoracolumbar and lumbar scoliosis, *Spine* 16:307, 1991.

Tredwell SJ, Sawatzky B: The use of fibrin sealant to reduce blood loss during Cotrel-Dubousset instrumentation for idiopathic scoliosis, *Spine* 15:913, 1990.

Turi M, Johnston CE, Richards BS: Anterior correction of idiopathic scoliosis using TSRH instrumentation, *Spine* 18:417, 1993.

Vauzelle C, Stagnara P, Jouvinroux P: Functional monitoring of spinal activity during spinal surgery, *J Bone Joint Surg* 55A:441, 1973.

Waisman M, Saute M: Thoracoscopy spine release before posterior instrumentation and scoliosis, *Clin Orthop* 336:130, 1997.

Wall EJ, Bylski-Austrow DI, Shelton FS, et al: Endoscopic discectomy increases thoracic spine flexibility as effectively as open discectomy: a mechanical study in a porcine model, *Spine* 23:9, 1998.

Weatherly CR, Draycott V, O'Brien JF, et al: The rib deformity in adolescent idiopathic scoliosis: a prospective study to evaluate changes after Harrington distraction and posterior fusion, *J Bone Joint Surg* 69B:179, 1987.

Weinstein JN, Rydevik BL, Rauschning W, et al: Anatomic and technical considerations of pedicle screw fixation, *Clin Orthop* 284:34, 1992.

Weinstein JN, Spratt KF, Spengler D, et al: Spinal pedicle fixation: reliability and validity of roentgenogram-based assessment and surgical factors on successful screw placement, *Spine* 13:1012, 1988.

Weis JC, Betz RR, Clements DH: The prevalence of perioperative complications following anterior spinal fusion in patients with idiopathic scoliosis. Paper presented at the Twenty-eighth Annual Meeting of the Scoliosis Research Society, Dublin, Sept 1993.

Wenger DR, Mubarak SJ, Leach J: Managing complications of posterior spinal instrumentation and fusion, *Clin Orthop* 284:24, 1992.

Westfall SH, Akbarnia BA, Merenda JT, et al: Exposure of the anterior spine: technique, complications, and results in 85 patients, *Am J Surg* 154:700, 1987.

Willers U, Hedlund R, Aaro S, et al: Long-term results of Harrington instrumentation in idiopathic scoliosis, *Spine* 18:713, 1993.

Winter RB: Posterior spinal fusion in scoliosis: indications, techniques, and results, *Orthop Clin North Am* 10:787, 1979.

Winter RB: The idiopathic double thoracic curve pattern: its recognition and surgical management, *Spine* 14:1287, 1989.

Winter RB, Lovell WW, Moe JH: Excessive thoracic lordosis and loss of pulmonary function in patients with idiopathic scoliosis, *J Bone Joint Surg* 57A:972, 1974.

Wojcik AS, Webb JK, Burwell RG: An analysis of the effect of the Zielke operation on S-shaped curves in idiopathic scoliosis, *Spine* 14:625, 1989.

Wojcik AS, Webb JK, Burwell RG: An analysis of the effect of the Zielke operation on S-shaped curves in idiopathic scoliosis: a follow-up study revealing some skeletal and soft tissue factors involved in curve progression, *Spine* 15:816, 1990.

Wojcik AS, Webb JK, Burwell RG: Harrington-Luque and Cotrel-Dubousset instrumentation for idiopathic scoliosis: a postoperative comparison using segmental radiologic analysis, *Spine* 15:424, 1990.

Wood KB, Dekutoski MB, Schendel MJ: Rotational changes of the vertebral-pelvic axis following Isola sublaminar instrumentation. Paper presented at the Twenty-eighth Annual Meeting of the Scoliosis Research Society, Dublin, Sept 1993.

Wood KB, Olsewski JM, Schendel MJ et al: Rotational changes of vertebral pelvic access after sublaminar instrumentation in adolescent idiopathic scoliosis, *Spine* 22:51, 1997.

Wood KB, Transfeldt EE, Ogilvie JW, et al: Rotational changes of the vertebral-pelvic axis following Cotrel-Dubousset instrumentation, *Spine* 16:S404, 1991.

Woodson ST, Marsh JS, Tanner JB: Transfusion of previously deposited autologous blood for patients undergoing hip-replacement surgery, *J Bone Joint Surg* 69A:325, 1987.

Wu Z: Posterior vertebral instrumentation for correction of scoliosis, *Clin Orthop* 215:40, 1987.

York DH, Cabot RJ, Gaines RW: Response variability of somatosensory-evoked potentials during scoliosis surgery, *Spine* 12:864, 1987.

Zagra A, Lamartina C, Pace A, et al: Posterior spinal fusion in scoliosis: computer-assisted tomography and biomechanics of the fusion mass, *Spine* 13:155, 1988.

Zielke K: Derotation and fusion-anterior spinal instrumentation, *Orthop Trans* 2:270, 1978.

Zielke K: Ventral derotation spondylodesis: preliminary report on 58 cases, *Beitr Orthop Traumatol* 25:85, 1978.

Zindrick MR: Clinical pedicle anatomy, *Spine: State of the Art Reviews* 6:11, 1992.

Zindrick MR, Wiltse LL, Doornik A, et al: Analysis of the morphometric characteristics of the thoracic and lumbar pedicles, *Spine* 12:160, 1987.

NEUROMUSCULAR SCOLIOSIS (GENERAL)

Allen BL Jr: The place for segmental instrumentation in the treatment of spine deformity, *Orthop Trans* 6:21, 1982.

Allen BL Jr: Segmental spinal instrumentation. In The American Academy of Orthopaedic Surgeons: *Instructional course lectures*, vol 32, St Louis, 1983, Mosby.

Allen BL, Ferguson RL: The Galveston technique for L-rod instrumentation of the scoliotic spine, *Spine* 7:119, 1982.

Allen BL, Ferguson RL: L-rod instrumentation (LRI) for scoliosis in cerebral palsy, *J Pediatr Orthop* 2:87, 1982.

Allen BL Jr, Ferguson RL: Neurologic injuries with the Galveston technique of L-rod instrumentation for scoliosis, *Spine* 11:14, 1986.

Allen BL Jr, Ferguson RL: A 1988 perspective on the Galveston technique of pelvic fixation, *Orthop Clin North Am* 19:409, 1988.

Allen BL Jr, Ferguson RL: The Galveston experience with L-rod instrumentation for adolescent idiopathic scoliosis, *Clin Orthop* 229:59, 1988.

Bell DF, Moseley CF, Koreska J: Unit rod segmental spinal instrumentation in the management of patients with progressive neuromuscular spinal deformity, *Spine* 14:1301, 1989.

Bernard TN, Johnson CE II: Late complications due to wire breakage in segmental spinal instrumentation, *J Bone Joint Surg* 65A:1339, 1983.

Boachie-Adjei O, Asher M: ISOLA instrumentation. In McCarthy R, ed: Spinal instrumentation technique manual, Scoliosis Research Society.

Boachie-Adjei O, Lonstein JE, Winter RB, et al: Luque segmental instrumentation in management of neuromuscular spinal deformities, *J Bone Joint Surg* 71A:548, 1989.

Bonnett C, Brown JC, Perry J, et al: The evolution of treatment of paralytic scoliosis at Rancho Los Amigos Hospital, *J Bone Joint Surg* 57A:206, 1975.

Broadstone T: Consider postoperative immobilization of double L-rod SSI patients, *Orthop Trans* 8:171, 1984.

Broom MJ, Banta JV, Renshaw TS: Spinal fusion augmented by Luque-rod segmental instrumentation for neuromuscular scoliosis, *J Bone Joint Surg* 71A:32, 1989.

Brown JC, Swank SM, Matta J, et al: Late spinal deformity in quadriplegic children and adolescents, *J Pediatr Orthop* 4:456, 1984.

Camp JF, Caudle R, Ashman RD, et al: Immediate complications of Cotrel-Dubousset instrumentation to the sacropelvis: a clinical and biomechanical study, *Spine* 15:932, 1990.

DeWald RL, Faut MM: Anterior and posterior spinal fusion for paralytic scoliosis, *Spine* 4:401, 1979.

Eberle CF: Failure of fixation after segmental spinal instrumentation without arthrodesis in the management of paralytic scoliosis, *J Bone Joint Surg* 70A:696, 1988.

Farcy JC, Rawlins BA, Glassman SD: Technique and results of fixation to the sacrum with iliosacral screws, *Spine* 17:S190, 1992.

Ferguson RL, Allen BL Jr: Segmental spinal instrumentation for routine scoliotic curve, *Contemp Orthop* 2:450, 1980.

Ferguson RL, Allen BL: Staged correction of neuromuscular scoliosis, *J Pediatr Orthop* 3:555, 1983.

Gaines RW Jr, Abernathie DL: Mersilene tapes as a substitute for wire in segmental spinal instrumentation for children, *Spine* 11:907, 1986.

Goll SR, Balderston RA, Stambough JL, et al: Depth of intraspinal wire penetration during passage of sublaminar wires, *Spine* 13:503, 1988.

Greene WB, Miles JD: A modified technique for insertion of unit rod into the pelvis. *Am J Orthop* 29:401, 2000.

Herndon WA, Sullivan JA, Yngve DA, et al: Segmental spinal instrumentation with sublaminar wires: a critical appraisal, *J Bone Joint Surg* 69A:851, 1987.

Herring JA, Wenger DR: Early complications of segmental spinal instrumentation, *Orthop Trans* 6:22, 1982.

Herring JA, Wenger DR: Segmental spinal instrumentation: a preliminary report of 40 consecutive cases, *Spine* 7:285, 1982.

Johnston CE, Ashman RB, Sherman MC: Mechanical consequences of rod contouring and residual scoliosis in sublaminar pelvic SSI, *Orthop Trans* 10:5, 1986.

Johnston CE, Happel LT, Randall N, et al: Delayed paraplegia complicating sublaminar segmental spinal instrumentation, *J Bone Joint Surg* 68A:556, 1986.

Kepes ER, Martinez LR, Andrews IC, et al: Anesthetic problems in hereditary muscular abnormalities, *N Y State J Med* 72:1051, 1972.

Letts M, Rathbone D, Yamashita T, et al: Soft Boston orthosis in management of neuromuscular scoliosis: a preliminary report, *J Pediatr Orthop* 12:470, 1992.

Lieponis JV, Bunch WH, Lonser RE, et al: Spinal cord injury during segmental sublamina spinal instrumentation: an animal model, *Orthop Trans* 8:173, 1984.

Lonstein JE, Renshaw TS: Neuromuscular spine deformities. In The American Academy of Orthopaedic Surgeons: *Instructional course lectures*, vol 36, St Louis, 1987, Mosby.

Luque ER: Anatomy of scoliosis and its correction, *Clin Orthop* 105:298, 1974.

Luque ER: Segmental spinal instrumentation: a method of rigid internal fixation of the spine to induce arthrodesis, *Orthop Trans* 4:391, 1980.

Luque ER: Paralytic scoliosis in growing children, *Clin Orthop* 163:202, 1982.

Luque ER: Segmental spinal instrumentation for correction of scoliosis, *Clin Orthop* 163:192, 1982.

Luque ER: The anatomic basis and development of segmental spinal instrumentation, *Spine* 7:256, 1982.

Luque ER, Cardoso A: Segmental correction of scoliosis with rigid internal fixation, *Orthop Trans* 1:136, 1977.

Maloney WJ, Rinsky LA, Gamble JG: Simultaneous correction of pelvis obliquity, frontal plane, and sagittal plane deformities and neuromuscular scoliosis using a unit rod with segmental sublaminar wires: a preliminary report, *J Pediatr Orthop* 10:742, 1990.

McCarthy RE: Neuromuscular scoliosis: the tide mark for surgery. Material presented at Spinal Deformity: Challenges and Solutions of Surgical Treatment, Puerto Rico, May 12-13, 2000.

McCarthy RE, Dunn H, McCullough FL: Luque fixation to the sacral ala using the Dunn-McCarthy modification, *Spine* 14:281, 1989.

McCarthy RE, Peek RD, Morrissy RT, et al: Allograft bone in spinal fusion for paralytic scoliosis, *J Bone Joint Surg* 68A:370, 1986.

McCarthy RE, Saer III EH: The treatment of flaccid neuromuscular scoliosis. In Bridwell KH, DeWald RL, eds: *The textbook of spinal surgery,* ed 2, Philadelphia, 1997, Lippincott-Raven.

McCord DH, Cunningham BN, Shono Y, et al: Biomechanical analysis of lumbosacral fixation, *Spine* 17:S235, 1992.

Miller F, Dabney KW: Unit rod segmental instrumentation. In McCarthy RE, ed: Spinal instrumentation technique manual, Scoliosis Research Society.

Moe JH: The management of paralytic scoliosis, *South Med J* 50:67, 1957.

Nasca RJ: Segmental spinal instrumentation, *South Med J* 78:303, 1985.

Nash CL: Current concepts review: scoliosis bracing, *J Bone Joint Surg* 62A:848, 1980.

Neustadt JB, Shufflebarger HL, Cammisa FP: Spinal fusions to the pelvis augmented by Cotrel-Dubousset instrumentation for neuromuscular scoliosis, *J Pediatr Orthop* 12:465, 1992.

Nicastro JF, Traina J, Lancaster M, et al: Sublaminar segmental wire fixation: anatomic pathways during their removal, *Orthop Trans* 8:172, 1984.

Nickel VL, Perry J, Affeldt JE, et al: Elective surgery on patient with respiratory paralysis, *J Bone Joint Surg* 39A:989, 1957.

O'Brien JP, Yau AC: Anterior and posterior correction and fusion for paralytic scoliosis, *Clin Orthop* 86:151, 1972.

O'Brien MF: Sacropelvic fixation in spinal deformity. Material presented at Spinal Deformity: Challenges and Solutions of Surgical Treatment, Puerto Rico, May 12-13, 2000.

Ogilvie JW, Millar EA: Comparison of segmental spinal instrumentation devices in the correction of scoliosis, *Spine,* 8:416, 1983.

Olson SA, Gaines RW: Removal of sublaminar wires after spinal fusion, *J Bone Joint Surg* 69A:1419, 1987.

Osebold WR, Yamamoto SK, Hurley JH: Variability of response of scoliotic spines to segmental spinal instrumentation, *Spine* 17:1174, 1992.

Pampliega T, Beguiristain JL, Artieda J: Neurologic complications after sublaminar wiring: an experimental study in lambs, *Spine* 17:441, 1992.

Renshaw TS: Spinal fusion with segmental instrumentation, *Contemp Orthop* 4:413, 1982.

Sanders JO, Evert M, Stanley EA, et al: Mechanisms of curve progression following sublaminar (Luque) spinal instrumentation, *Spine* 17:781, 1992.

Schrader WC, Bethem D, Scerbin V: The chronic local effects of sublaminar wires: an animal model, *Spine* 13:499, 1988.

Shook JE, Lubicky JP: Paralytic scoliosis. In Bridwell KH, DeWald RL, eds: *The textbook of spinal surgery,* ed 2, Philadelphia, 1997, Lippincott-Raven.

Shufflebarger HL, Kahn A III, Rinsky LA, et al: Segmental spinal instrumentation in idiopathic scoliosis: a retrospective analysis of 234 cases, *Orthop Trans* 9:124, 1985.

Songer MN, Spencer DL, Meyer PR, et al: The use of sublaminar cables to replace Luque wires, *Spine* 16:S418, 1991.

Stevens DB, Beard C: Segmental spinal instrumentation for neuromuscular spinal deformity, *Clin Orthop* 242:164, 1989.

Sullivan JA, Conner SB: Comparison of Harrington instrumentation and segmental spinal instrumentation in the management of neuromuscular spinal deformity, *Spine* 7:299, 1982.

Taddonio RF: Segmental spinal instrumentation in the management of neuromuscular spinal deformity, *Spine* 7:305, 1982.

Taddonio RF, Weller K, Appel M: A comparison of patients with idiopathic scoliosis managed with and without postoperative immobilization following segmental spinal instrumentation with Luque rods, *Orthop Trans* 8:172, 1984.

Thompson GH, Wilber G, Shaffer JW, et al: Segmental spinal instrumentation in idiopathic scoliosis: a preliminary report, *Spine* 10:623, 1985.

Weiler PJ, McNeice GM, Medley JB: An experimental study of the buckling behavior of L-rod implants used in the surgical treatment of scoliosis, *Spine* 11:992, 1986.

Weiler PJ, Medley JB, McNeice GN: Numeric analysis of the load capacity of the human spine fitted with L-rod instrumentation, *Spine* 15:1285, 1990.

Wenger DR, Carollo JJ, Wilkerson JA: Biomechanics of scoliosis correction by segmental spinal instrumentation, *Spine* 7:260, 1982.

Wenger DR, Carollo JJ, Wilkerson JA, et al: Laboratory testing of segmental spinal instrumentation versus traditional Harrington instrumentation for scoliosis treatment, *Spine* 7:265, 1982.

Wenger DR, Miller S, Wilkerson J: Evaluation of fixation sites for segmental instrumentation of the human vertebra, *Orthop Trans* 6:23, 1982.

Wilber RG, Thompson GH, Shaffer JW, et al: Postoperative neurologic deficits and segmental spinal instrumentation: a study using spinal cord monitoring, *J Bone Joint Surg* 66A:1178, 1984.

Winter RB: Posterior spinal arthrodesis with instrumentation and sublaminar wire: 100 consecutive cases, *Orthop Trans* 9:124, 1985.

Winter RB, Carlson JM: Modern orthotics for spinal deformities, *Clin Orthop* 23:74, 1977.

Winter RB, Pinto WC: Pelvic obliquity: its causes and its treatment, *Spine* 11:225, 1986.

CEREBRAL PALSY

Allen BL, Ferguson RL: L-rod instrumentation for scoliosis in cerebral palsy, *J Pediatr Orthop* 2:87, 1982.

Balmer GA, MacEwen GD: The incidence and treatment of scoliosis in cerebral palsy, *J Bone Joint Surg* 52B:134, 1970.

Bleck EE: Orthopaedic management in cerebral palsy. In *Clinics in developmental medicine*, Philadelphia, 1987, JB Lippincott.

Bonnett C, Brown J, Brooks HL: Anterior spine fusion with Dwyer instrumentation for lumbar scoliosis in cerebral palsy, *J Bone Joint Surg* 55A:425, 1973.

Bonnett CA, Brown JC, Grow T: Thoracolumbar scoliosis in cerebral palsy: results of surgical treatment, *J Bone Joint Surg* 58A:328, 1976.

Brown JC, Swank SM, Specht L: Combined anterior and posterior spine fusion in cerebral palsy, *Spine* 7:570, 1982.

Bunnell WP, MacEwen GD: Nonoperative treatment in scoliosis in cerebral palsy: preliminary report on the use of a plastic jacket, *Dev Med Child Neurol* 19:45, 1977.

Ferguson RL, Allen BL: Considerations in the treatment of cerebral palsy patients with spinal deformities, *Orthop Clin North Am* 19: 419, 1988.

Gersoff WK, Renshaw JS: The treatment of scoliosis in cerebral palsy by posterior spinal fusion with Luque-rod segmented instrumentation, *J Bone Joint Surg* 70A:41, 1988.

Hennrikus WL, Rosenthal RK, Kasser JR: Incidence of spondylolisthesis in ambulatory cerebral palsy patients, *J Pediatr Orthop* 13:37, 1993.

Kalen V, Conklin MM, Shermann FC: Untreated scoliosis in severe cerebral palsy, *J Pediatr Orthop* 12:337, 1992.

Lonstein JE, Akbarnia BA: Operative treatment of spinal deformities in patients with cerebral palsy or mental retardation: an analysis of 107 cases, *J Bone Joint Surg* 65A:43, 1983.

MacEwen GD: Operative treatment of scoliosis in cerebral palsy, *Reconstr Surg Traumatol* 13:58, 1972.

Madigan RR, Wallace SL: Scoliosis in the institutionalized cerebral palsy population, *Spine* 6:583, 1981.

Neustadt JB, Shufflebarger HL, Cammisa FP: Spinal fusions to the pelvis augmented by Cotrel-Dubousset instrumentation for neuromuscular scoliosis, *J Pediatr Orthop* 12:465, 1992.

Rinsky LA: Surgery of spinal deformity in cerebral palsy: twelve years in the evolution of scoliosis management, *Clin Orthop* 253:100, 1990.

Samilson RL: Orthopedic surgery of the hips and spine in retarded cerebral palsy, *Orthop Clin North Am* 12:83, 1981.

Sponseller PD, Whiffen JR, Drummond DS: Interspinous process segmental spinal instrumentation for scoliosis in cerebral palsy, *J Pediatr Orthop* 6:559, 1986.

Stanitski CL, Micheli LJ, Hall JE, et al: Surgical correction of spinal deformity in cerebral palsy, *Spine* 7:563, 1982.

Swank SM, Cohen DS, Brown JC: Spine fusion in cerebral palsy with L-rod segmental spinal instrumentation: a comparison of single and two-stage combined approach with Zielke instrumentation, *Spine* 14:750, 1989.

Taddonio RF: Segmental spinal instrumentation and the management of neuromuscular spinal deformity, *Spine* 7:305, 1982.

Thometz JG, Simon SR: Progression of scoliosis after skeletal maturity in institutionalized adults who have cerebral palsy, *J Bone Joint Surg* 70A:1290, 1988.

Winter RB, Carlson JM: Modern orthotics for spinal deformities, *Clin Orthop* 126:74, 1977.

Winter RB, Pinto WC: Pelvic obliquity: its causes and its treatment, *Spine* 11:225, 1986.

INHERITABLE NEUROLOGICAL DISORDERS

Albanese SA, Bobechko WP: Spine deformity in familial dysautonomia (Riley-Day syndrome), *J Pediatr Orthop* 7:179, 1987.

Aprin H, Bowen JR, MacEwen GD, et al: Spine fusion in patients with spinal muscle atrophy, *J Bone Joint Surg* 64A:1179, 1982.

Axelrod FB, Iyer K, Fish I: Progressive sensory loss and familial dysautonomia, *Pediatrics* 67:517, 1981.

Brown JC, Zeller JS, Swank SM, et al: Surgical and functional results of spine fusion in spinal muscle atrophy, *Spine* 14:763, 1989.

Cady RB, Bobechko WP: Incidence, natural history, and treatment of scoliosis in Friedreich's ataxia, *J Pediatr Orthop* 4:673, 1984.

Daher YH, Lonstein JE, Winter RB, et al: Spinal surgery in spinal muscle atrophy, *J Pediatr Orthop* 5:391, 1985.

Daher YH, Winter RB, Lonstein JE, et al: Spinal deformities in patients with Friedreich's ataxia: a review of 19 patients, *J Pediatr Orthop* 5:553, 1985.

Daher YH, Winter RB, Lonstein JE, et al: Spinal deformities in patients with Charcot-Marie-Tooth: a review of 12 patients, *Clin Orthop* 202:219, 1986.

Evans GA, Drennan JC, Russman BS: Functional classification and orthopaedic management of spinal muscle atrophy, *J Bone Joint Surg* 63B:516, 1981.

Furumasu J, Swank SM, Brown JC: Functional activities in spinal muscular atrophy patients after spinal fusion, *Spine* 14:771, 1989.

Geoffrey G, Barbeau A, Breton G, et al: Clinical description and roentgenologic evaluation of patients with Friedreich's ataxia, *Can J Neurol Sci* 3:279, 1976.

Goldstein LA, Fuller J, Haake P, et al: Surgical treatment of thoracic scoliosis in patients with familial dysautonomia, *J Bone Joint Surg* 51A:205, 1969.

Granata C, Merlini L, Magni E, et al: Spinal muscle atrophy: natural history and orthopaedic treatment of scoliosis, *Spine* 14:760, 1989.

Hensinger RN, MacEwen GD: Spinal deformity associated with heritable neurologic conditions: spinal muscle atrophy, Friedreich's ataxia, familial dysautonomia, and Charcot-Marie-Tooth disease, *J Bone Joint Surg* 58A:13, 1976.

Hsu JD, Grollman T, Hoffer M, et al: The orthopaedic management of spinal muscular atrophy, *J Bone Joint Surg* 55B:663, 1973.

Kaplan L, Marguiles JY, Kadari A, et al: Spinal deformity in familial dysautonomia: the Israeli experience. Paper presented at the Twenty-eighth Annual Meeting of the Scoliosis Research Society, Dublin, Sept 1993.

Kepes, Martinez LR, Andrews IC, et al: Anesthetic problems and hereditary muscular abnormalities, *NY State J Med* 72:1051, 1972.

Kugelberg E, Welander L: Heredofamilial juvenile muscular atrophy simulating muscular dystrophy, *Arch Neurol* 75:500, 1956.

Labelle H, Thome S, Duhaine M, et al: Natural history in scoliosis in Friedreich's ataxia, *J Bone Joint Surg* 68A:564, 1986.

Merlini L, Granata C, Bonfiglioli S, et al: Scoliosis in spinal muscular atrophy: natural history and management, *Dev Med Child Neurol* 31:501, 1989.

Phillips DP, Roye DP Jr, Farcy JC, et al: Surgical treatment of scoliosis in a spinal muscle atrophy population, *Spine* 15:942, 1990.

Piasecki JO, Mahinpour S, Levine DB: Long-term follow-up for spinal fusion in spinal muscular atrophy, *Clin Orthop* 207:44, 1986.

Riddick M, Winter RB, Lutter L: Spinal deformities in patients with spinal muscle atrophy, *Spine* 8:476, 1982.

Riley CM, Day RL, Greeley DM, et al: Central autonomic dysfunction with defective lachrymation: report of five cases, *Pediatrics* 3:468, 1949.

Robin GC: Scoliosis in familial dysautonomia, *Bull Hosp Jt Dis* 44:16, 1984.

Schwentker EP, Gibson DA: The orthopaedic aspects of spinal muscle atrophy, *J Bone Joint Surg* 58A:32, 1976.

Shapiro F, Bresnan MJ: Current concepts reviewed: management of childhood neuromuscular disease. I. Spinal muscle atrophy, *J Bone Joint Surg* 64A:785, 1982.

Shapiro F, Bresnan MJ: Current concepts reviewed: orthopaedic management of childhood neuromuscular disease. II. Peripheral neuropathies, Friedreich's ataxia, and arthrogryposis multiplex congenita, *J Bone Joint Surg* 64A:949, 1982.

Stenqvist O, Sigurdson J: The anaesthetic management of a patient with familial dysautonomia, *Anaesthesia* 37:929, 1982.

Yoslow W, Becker MH, Bartels J, et al: Orthopaedic defects in familial dysautonomia: a review of 65 cases, *J Bone Joint Surg* 53A:1541, 1971.

SYRINGOMYELIA

Baker AS, Dove J: Progressive scoliosis as the first presenting sign of syringomyelia: report of a case, *J Bone Joint Surg* 65B:472, 1983.

Bertrand SL, Drvaric DM, Roberts JM: Scoliosis in syringomyelia, *Orthopedics* 12:335, 1989.

Bradford DS: Neuromuscular spinal deformity. In Bradford DS et al, eds: *Moe's textbook of scoliosis and other spinal deformities*, ed 2, Philadelphia, 1987, WB Saunders.

Gurr KR, Taylor TKF, Stobo P: Syringomyelia in scoliosis in childhood and adolescents, *J Bone Joint Surg* 70B:159, 1988.

Huebert HT, MacKinnon WB: Syringomyelia and scoliosis, *J Bone Joint Surg* 51B:338, 1969.

Nordwall A, Wikkelso C: A late neurologic complication of scoliosis surgery in connection with syringomyelia, *Acta Orthop Scand* 50:407, 1979.

Philips WA, Hensinger RN, Kling TF: Management of scoliosis due to syringomyelia in childhood and adolescents, *J Pediatr Orthop* 10:351, 1990.

Shook JE, Lubicky JP: Paralytic scoliosis. In Bridwell KH, DeWald RL, eds: *The textbook of spinal surgery,* ed 2, Philadelphia, 1997, Lippincott-Raven.

Williams B: Orthopaedic features in the presentation of syringomyelia, *J Bone Joint Surg* 61B:314, 1979.

SPINAL CORD INJURIES

Bonnett CA: The cord-injured child. In Lovell WW, Winter RB, eds: *Children's orthopaedics,* Philadelphia, 1978, JB Lippincott.

Brown HP, Bonnett CC: Spine deformity subsequent to spinal cord injury. In Proceedings of the Scoliosis Research Society, *J Bone Joint Surg* 55A:441, 1973.

Campbell J, Bonnett C: Spinal cord injury in children, *Clin Orthop* 112:114, 1975.

Dearolf WW, Betz RR, Vogel LC, et al: Scoliosis in pediatric spinal cord-injured patients, *J Pediatr Orthop* 10:214, 1990.

Johnston CE II, Hakaka MW, Rosenberger R: Paralytic spine deformity: orthotic treatment in spinal discontinuity syndromes, *J Pediatr Orthop* 2:233, 1982.

Lancourt JC, Dickson JH, Carter RE: Paralytic spinal deformity following traumatic spinal cord injury in children and adolescents, *J Bone Joint Surg* 63A:47, 1981.

Luque ER: Paralytic scoliosis in growing children, *Clin Orthop* 163:202, 1982.

Mayfield JK, Erkkila JD, Winter RB: Spine deformity subsequent to acquired childhood spinal cord injury, *J Bone Joint Surg* 63A:1401, 1981.

Shook JE, Lubicky JP: Paralytic scoliosis. In Bridwell KH, DeWald RL, eds: *The textbook of spinal surgery,* ed 2, Philadelphia, 1997, Lippincott-Raven.

POLIOMYELITIS

Bonnett C, Brown J, Perry J, et al: The evolution of treatment of paralytic scoliosis at Rancho Los Amigos Hospital, *J Bone Joint Surg* 57A:206, 1975.

Colonna PC, Vom Saal F: A study of paralytic scoliosis based on 500 cases of poliomyelitis, *J Bone Joint Surg* 23:335, 1941.

Garrett AL, Perry J, Nickel VL: Paralytic scoliosis, *Clin Orthop* 21:117, 1961.

Garrett AL, Perry J, Nickel VL: Stabilization of the collapsing spine, *J Bone Joint Surg* 43A:474, 1961.

Gucker T: Experience in poliomyelitis scoliosis after correction and fusion, *J Bone Joint Surg* 38A:1281, 1956.

Gui L, Savini R, Vincenzi G, et al: Surgical treatment of poliomyelitic scoliosis, *Ital J Orthop Traumatol* 2:191, 1976.

Irwin CE: The iliotibial band: its role in producing deformity in poliomyelitis, *J Bone Joint Surg* 31A:141, 1949.

James JIP: Paralytic scoliosis, *J Bone Joint Surg* 38B:660, 1956.

Leong JCY, Wilding K, Mok CD, et al: Surgical treatment of scoliosis following poliomyelitis: a review of 100 cases, *J Bone Joint Surg* 63A:726, 1981.

Mayer L: Further studies of fixed paralytic pelvic obliquity, *J Bone Joint Surg* 18:87, 1936.

Mayer PJ, Dove J, Ditmanson M, et al: Postpoliomyelitis paralytic scoliosis, *Spine* 6:573, 1981.

O'Brien JP, Dwyer AP, Hodgson AR: Paralytic pelvic obliquity: its prognosis and management and the development of a technique for full correction of the deformity, *J Bone Joint Surg* 57A:626, 1975.

O'Brien JP, Yau AC, Gertzbern S, et al: Combined staged, anterior and posterior correction and fusion of the spine in scoliosis following poliomyelitis, *Clin Orthop* 110:81, 1975.

Pavon SJ, Manning C: Posterior spine fusion for scoliosis due to anterior poliomyelitis, *J Bone Joint Surg* 52A:420, 1970.

Roaf R: Paralytic scoliosis, *J Bone Joint Surg* 38B:640, 1956.

Yount CC: Role of the tensor fascia femoris in certain deformities of the lower extremities, *J Bone Joint Surg* 8:171, 1926.

ARTHROGRYPOSIS MULTIPLEX CONGENITA

Brown LM, Robson MJ: The pathophysiology of arthrogryposis multiplex congenita neurologica, *J Bone Joint Surg* 62B:291, 1980.

Daher YH, Lonstein JE, Winter RB, et al: Spinal deformities in patients with arthrogryposis: a review of 16 patients, *Spine* 10:609, 1985.

Drummond D, Mackenzie DA: Scoliosis in arthrogryposis multiplex congenita, *Spine* 3:146, 1978.

Herron LD, Westin GW, Dawson EG: Scoliosis in arthrogryposis multiplex congenita, *J Bone Joint Surg* 60A:293, 1978.

Shapiro F, Bresnan MJ: Current concepts review: orthopaedic management of childhood neuromuscular disease. II. Peripheral neuropathies, Friedreich's ataxia, and arthrogryposis multiplex congenita, *J Bone Joint Surg* 64A:949, 1982.

MUSCULAR DYSTROPHY

Aprin H, Bowen JR, McEwen JD, Hall JE: Spine fusion in patients with spinal muscle atrophy, *J Bone Joint Surg* 64A:1179, 1982.

Bronson W, Drummond DS, Setal L, et al: Treatment of scoliosis patients with Duchenne muscular dystrophy. Paper presented at the Twenty-eighth Annual Meeting of the Scoliosis Research Society, Dublin, Sept 1993.

Cambridge W, Drennan JC: Scoliosis associated with Duchenne muscular dystrophy, *J Pediatr Orthop* 7:436, 1987.

Colbert AP, Clifford C: Scoliosis management in Duchenne muscular dystrophy: prospective study of modified Jewett hyperextension brace, *Arch Phys Med Rehabil* 60A:302, 1987.

Daher YH, Lonstein JE, Winter RB: Spinal deformities in patients with muscular dystrophy other than Duchenne: review of 11 patients having surgical treatment, *Spine* 10:614, 1984.

Daher YH, Lonstein JE, Winter RB, Bradford DS: Spinal surgery in spinal muscle atrophy, *J Pediatr Orthop* 5:391, 1985.

Galasko CSB, Delaney C, Morris P: Spinal stabilization in Duchenne muscular dystrophy, *J Bone Joint Surg* 74B:210, 1992.

Gibson DA, Koreska J, Robertson D, et al: The management of spinal deformity in Duchenne's muscular dystrophy, *Orthop Clin North Am* 9:437, 1978.

Granata C, Merlina L, Magne E, et al: Spinal muscle atrophy, natural history in orthopaedic treatment of scoliosis, *Spine* 14:760, 1989.

Green NE: The orthopaedic care of children with muscular dystrophy, *Instr Course Lect* 36:267, 1987.

Hsu JD: The natural history of spine curvature progression in the nonambulator Duchenne muscular dystrophy patient, *Spine* 8:771, 1983.

Jenkins JG, Bohn D, Edmonds JF, et al: Evaluation of pulmonary function in muscular dystrophy patients requiring spinal surgery, *Crit Care Med* 10:645, 1982.

Kurz LT, Mubarak SJ, Schultz P, et al: Correlation of scoliosis and pulmonary function in Duchenne muscular dystrophy, *J Pediatr Orthop* 3:347, 1983.

LaPrade RF, Rowe DE: The operative treatment of scoliosis in Duchenne muscular dystrophy, *Orthop Rev* 21:39, 1992.

Lonstein JE, Renshaw TS: Neuromuscular spine deformities. In The American Academy of Orthopaedic Surgeons: *Instructional course lectures,* vol 36, St Louis, 1987, Mosby.

Lord J, Behrman B, Varzos N, et al: Scoliosis associated with Duchenne muscular dystrophy, *Arch Phys Med Rehabil* 71:13, 1990.

Luque ER: Segmental spinal instrumentation for correction of scoliosis, *Clin Orthop* 163:192, 1982.

Miller F, Moseley CF, Koreska J, et al: Pulmonary function and scoliosis in Duchenne dystrophy, *J Pediatr Orthop* 8:133, 1988.

Miller F, Moseley CF, Koreska J: Spinal fusion in Duchenne muscular dystrophy, *Dev Med Child Neurol* 34:775, 1992.

Milne B, Rosales JK: Anesthetic considerations in patients with muscular dystrophy undergoing spinal fusion and Harrington rod insertion, *Can Anaesth Soc J* 29:250, 1982.

Mubarak SJ, Morin WD, Leach J: Spinal fusion in Duchenne muscular dystrophy-fixation and fusion to the sacropelvis? *J Pediatr Orthop* 13:756, 1993.

Rideau Y, Glorion B, Delaubier A, et al: The treatment of scoliosis in Duchenne muscular dystrophy, *Muscle Nerve* 7:281, 1984.

Rideau Y, Jankowski LW, Grellet J: Respiratory function in muscular dystrophies, *Muscle Nerve* 4:155, 1981.

Seeger BR, Sutherland AD, Clark MS: Orthotic management of scoliosis in Duchenne muscular dystrophy, *Arch Phys Med Rehabil* 65:83, 1984.

Shapiro F, Bresnan MJ: Orthopaedic management of childhood neuromuscular disease. III. Diseases of muscle, *J Bone Joint Surg* 64A:1102, 1982.

Shapiro F, Navil S, Colan S, et al: Spinal fusion in Duchenne muscular dystrophy: a multidisciplinary approach, *Muscle Nerve* 15:604, 1992.

Shapiro F, Specht L: Current concepts review: the diagnosis and orthopaedic treatment of inherited muscular diseases in childhood, *J Bone Joint Surg* 75A:439, 1993.

Siegel IM: Scoliosis in muscular dystrophy, *Clin Orthop* 93:235, 1973.

Siegel IM: Spinal stabilization in Duchenne muscular dystrophy: rationale and method, *Muscle Nerve* 5:417, 1982.

Smith PEM, Calverley PMA, Edwards RHT, et al: Practical problems in the respiratory care of patients with muscular dystrophy, *N Engl J Med* 316:1197, 1987.

Smith AD, Koreska J, Moseley CF: Progression of scoliosis in Duchenne muscular dystrophy, *J Bone Joint Surg* 71A:1066, 1989.

Sullivan JA, Conner SB: Comparison of Harrington instrumentation and segmental spinal instrumentation in the management of neuromuscular spinal deformity, *Spine* 7:299, 1982.

Sussman MD: Advantage of early spinal stabilization and fusion in patients with Duchenne muscular dystrophy, *J Pediatr Orthop* 4:532, 1984.

Swank SM, Brown JC, Perry RE: Spinal fusion in Duchenne's muscular dystrophy, *Spine* 7:484, 1982.

Taddonio RF: Segmental spinal instrumentation in the management of neuromuscular spinal deformity, *Spine* 7:305, 1982.

Weimann RL, Gibson DA, Moseley CF, et al: Surgical stabilization of the spine in Duchenne muscular dystrophy, *Spine* 8:776, 1983.

CONGENITAL SCOLIOSIS

Akbarnia BA, Heydarian K, Ganjavian MS: Concordant congenital spine deformity in monozygotic twins, *J Pediatr Orthop* 3:502, 1983.

Albanese SA, Coren AB, Weinstein MP, et al: Ultrasonography for urinary tract evaluation in patients with congenital spine anomalies, *Clin Orthop* 22A:302, 1988.

Andrew T, Piggott H: Growth arrest for progressive scoliosis: combined anterior and posterior fusion of the convexity, *J Bone Joint Surg* 67B:193, 1985.

Bergoin M, Bollini G, Gennari JM: One-stage hemivertebral excision and arthrodesis on congenital oblique take-off in children aged less than 5 years, *J Pediatr Orthop* 1:108, 1993.

Bernard TN Jr, Burke SW, Johnston CE III, et al: Congenital spine deformities: a review of 47 cases, *Orthopedics* 8:777, 1985.

Bollini G, Bergoin M, Labriet C, et al: Hemivertebrae excision and fusion in children aged less than five years, *J Pediatr Orthop* Part B, 1:95, 1993.

Bradford DS: Partial epiphyseal arrest and supplemental fixation for progressive correction of congenital spine deformity, *J Bone Joint Surg* 64A:610, 1982.

Bradford DS, Boachie-Adjei O: One-stage anterior and posterior hemivertebral resection and arthrodesis for congenital scoliosis, *J Bone Joint Surg* 72A:536, 1990.

Bradford DS, Tribus CB: Current concepts in management of patients with fixed decompensated spinal deformity, *Clin Orthop* 306:64, 1994.

Campbell RM: Congenital scoliosis due to multiple vertebral anomalies associated with thoracic insufficiency syndrome, *Spine: State of the Art Reviews* 14:209, 2000.

Danisa OA, Turner D, Richardson WJ: Surgical correction of lumbar kyphotic deformity: posterior reduction "eggshell" osteotomy, *J Neurosurg* (Spine I) 92:50, 2000.

Dimeglio A: Growth of the spine before age 5 years, *J Pediatr Orthop* 1:102, 1993.

Drvaric DM, Ruderman RJ, Conrad RW, et al: Congenital scoliosis and urinary tract abnormalities: are intravenous pyelograms necessary? *J Pediatr Orthop* 7:441, 1987.

Dubousset J, Katti E, Seringe R: Epiphysiodesis of the spine in young children for congenital spinal deformations, *J Pediatr Orthop* 1:123, 1993.

Freedman L, Leong J, Luk K, et al: One-stage combined anterior and posterior excision of hemivertebrae in the lower lumbar spine, *J Bone Joint Surg* 69B:854, 1987.

Gillespie R, Faithful D, Roth A, et al: Intraspinal anomalies and congenital scoliosis, *Clin Orthop* 93:103, 1973.

Goldberg C, Fenlon G, Blacke NS: Diastematomyelia: a critical review of the natural history and treatment, *Spine* 9:367, 1984.

Gruca A: On the pathology and treatment of "idiopathic" scoliosis, *Acta Med Pol* 15:139, 1974.

Hall JE, Herndon WA, Levine CR: Surgical treatment of congenital scoliosis with or without Harrington instrumentation, *J Bone Joint Surg* 63A:608, 1981.

Heinig CF: The egg shell procedure. In Luque ER, ed: *Segmental spinal instrumentation*, Thorofare, NJ, 1984, SLACK.

Hood RW, Riseborough E, Nehme A, et al: Diastematomyelia and structural spinal deformities, *J Bone Joint Surg* 62A:520, 1980.

King AG, MacEwen GD, Bose WJ: Transpedicular convex anterior hemiepiphysiodesis and posterior arthrodesis for progressive congenital scoliosis, *Spine* 17(suppl):291, 1992.

King JD, Lowery GL: Results of lumbar hemivertebral excision for congenital scoliosis, *Spine* 16:778, 1991.

Leatherman KD, Dickson RA: Two-stage corrective surgery for congenital deformities of the spine, *J Bone Joint Surg* 61B:324, 1979.

Letts RM, Hollenberg C: Delayed paresis following spinal fusion with Harrington instrumentation, *Clin Orthop* 125:45, 1977.

Lhowe D, Ehrlich MG, Chapman PH, et al: Congenital intraspinal lipomas: clinical presentation and response to treatment, *J Pediatr Orthop* 7:531, 1987.

Lonstein JE, Winter RB, Moe JH, et al: Neurologic deficit secondary to spinal deformity: a review of the literature and report of 43 cases, *Spine* 5:331, 1980.

MacEwen GD, Winter RB, Hardy JH: Evaluation of kidney anomalies in congenital scoliosis, *J Bone Joint Surg* 54A:1341, 1972.

McCarthy RE, Campbell Jr RM, Hall JE: Infantile and juvenile idiopathic scoliosis, *Spine: State of the Art Reviews* 14:163, 2000.

McMaster MJ: Occult intraspinal anomalies and congenital scoliosis, *J Bone Joint Surg* 66A:588, 1984.

McMaster MJ, David CV: Hemivertebra as a cause of scoliosis: a study of 104 patients, *J Bone Joint Surg* 68B:588, 1986.

McMaster MJ, Ohtsuka K: The natural history of congenital scoliosis: a study of 251 patients, *J Bone Joint Surg* 64A:1128, 1982.

Nasca RJ, Stelling FH, Steel HH: Progression of congenital scoliosis due to hemivertebrae and hemivertebrae with bars, *J Bone Joint Surg* 57A:456, 1975.

Onimus M, Manzone P, Michel F, et al: Early operation and congenital scoliosis, *J Pediatr Orthop* 1:119, 1993.

Roaf R: The treatment of progressive scoliosis by unilateral growth arrest, *J Bone Joint Surg* 45B:637, 1963.

Shapiro F, Eyre D: Congenital scolioses: a histopathologic study, *Spine* 6:107, 1981.

Slabaugh P, Lonstein J, Winter RB, et al: Lumbosacral hemivertebra: a review of 24 patients with resection in eight, *Spine* 5:234, 1980.

Smith AD, von Lackum WH, Wylie R: An operation for stapling vertebral bodies in congenital scoliosis, *J Bone Joint Surg* 36A:342, 1954.

Stoll J, Bunch W: Segmental spinal instrumentation for congenital scoliosis: a report of two cases, *Spine* 8:43, 1983.

Ulrich EV, Moushkin AY: Surgical treatment of scoliosis and kyphoscoliosis caused by hemivertebrae in infants, *J Pediatr Orthop* 1:113, 1993.

Whitecloud TS III, Brinker MR, Barrack RL, et al: Vibratory response in congenital scoliosis, *J Pediatr Orthop* 9:422, 1989.

Winter RB: Congenital scoliosis, *Clin Orthop* 93:75, 1973.

Winter RB: Congenital spine deformity: natural history and treatment, *Isr J Med Sci* 9:719, 1973.

Winter RB: Scoliosis and spinal growth, *Orthop Rev* 6:17, 1977.

Winter RB: Convex anterior and posterior hemiarthrodesis and epiphysiodesis in young children with progressive congenital scoliosis, *J Pediatr Orthop* 1:361, 1981.

Winter RB: *Congenital deformities of the spine*, New York, 1983, Thieme-Stratton.

Winter RB: Posterior spinal arthrodesis with instrumentation and sublaminar wire: 100 consecutive cases, *Orthop Trans* 9:124, 1985.

Winter RB: Congenital spine deformity. In Bradford DS et al, eds: *Moe's textbook of scoliosis and other spinal anomalies*, ed 2, Philadelphia, 1987, WB Saunders.

Winter RB: Congenital scoliosis, *Orthop Clin North Am* 19:395, 1988.

Winter RB: Congenital spine deformity: what's the latest and what's the best? *Spine* 14:1406, 1989.

Winter RB, Haven JJ, Moe JH, et al: Diastematomyelia and congenital spine deformities, *J Bone Joint Surg* 56A:27, 1974.

Winter RB, Lonstein JE, Denis F, et al: Convex growth arrest for progressive congenital scoliosis due to hemivertebrae, *J Pediatr Orthop* 8:633, 1988.

Winter RB, Moe JH: The results of spinal arthrodesis for congenital spine deformity in patients younger than 5 years' old, *J Bone Joint Surg* 64A:419, 1982.

Winter RB, Moe JH, Bradford DS: Congenital thoracic lordosis, *J Bone Joint Surg* 60A:806, 1978.

Winter RB, Moe JH, Eilers VE: Congenital scoliosis: a study of 234 patients treated and untreated, *J Bone Joint Surg* 50A:1, 1968.

Winter RB, Moe JH, Lonstein JE: Posterior spinal arthrodesis for congenital scoliosis: an analysis of the cases of 290 patients, 5 to 19 years old, *J Bone Joint Surg* 66A:1188, 1984.

Winter RB, Moe JH, Lonstein JE: The incidence of Klippel-Feil syndrome in patients with congenital scoliosis and kyphosis, *Spine* 9:363, 1984.

Winter RB, Moe JH, MacEwen D, et al: The Milwaukee brace and the nonoperative treatment of congenital scoliosis, *Spine* 1:85, 1976.

Wynne-Davies R: Congenital vertebral anomalies: aetiology and relationship to spina bifida cystica, *J Med Genet* 12:280, 1975.

SCHEUERMANN DISEASE

Ascani E, Ippolito E, Montanaro A: Scheuermann's kyphosis: histological, histochemical, and ultrastructural studies, *Orthop Trans* 7:28, 1982.

Asher M, Heinig C, Carson W, Strippgen W: ISOLA spinal implant system: principles, design, and applications. In An HS, Cotler JM, eds: *Spinal instrumentation*, Baltimore, 1992, Williams & Wilkins.

Asher MA, Strippgen WE, Heinig CF, et al: *ISOLA spine implant system: principles and practice*, Cleveland, 1991, AcroMed.

Aufdermaur M: Juvenile kyphosis (Scheuermann's disease): radiography, histology, and pathogenesis, *Clin Orthop* 154:166, 1981.

Aufdermaur M, Spycher M: Pathogenesis of osteochondrosis juvenilis, Scheuermann, *J Orthop Res* 4:452, 1986.

Bick EM, Copel JW: Longitudinal growth of the human vertebra: contribution to human osteogeny, *J Bone Joint Surg* 33A:783, 1951.

Blumenthal SL, Roach J, Herring JA: Lumbar Scheuermann's: a clinical series in classification, *Spine* 12:929, 1987.

Bradford DS: Neurological complications in Scheuermann's disease, *J Bone Joint Surg* 51A:657, 1969.

Bradford DS: Juvenile kyphosis, *Clin Orthop* 128:45, 1977.

Bradford DS: Juvenile kyphosis. In Bradford DS et al, eds: *Moe's textbook of scoliosis and other spinal deformities*, ed 2, Philadelphia, 1987, WB Saunders.

Bradford DS, Ahmed KB, Moe JH, et al: The surgical management of patients with Scheuermann's disease: a review of 24 cases managed by combined anterior and posterior spine fusion, *J Bone Joint Surg* 62A:705, 1980.

Bradford DS, Brown DM, Moe JH, et al: Scheuermann's kyphosis: a form of juvenile osteoporosis? *Clin Orthop* 118:10, 1976.

Bradford DS, Moe JH: Scheuermann's juvenile kyphosis: a histologic study, *Clin Orthop* 110:45, 1975.

Bradford DS, Moe JH, Montalvo FJ, et al: Scheuermann's kyphosis and roundback deformity: results of Milwaukee brace treatment, *J Bone Joint Surg* 56A:749, 1974.

Bradford DS, Moe JH, Montalvo FJ, et al: Scheuermann's kyphosis: results of surgical treatment in 22 patients, *J Bone Joint Surg* 57A:439, 1975.

Bradford DS, Moe JH, Winter RB: Kyphosis and postural roundback deformity in children and adolescents, *Minn Med* 56:114, 1973.

Bradford DS, Winter RB, Lonstein JE, et al: Techniques of anterior spine surgery for the management of kyphosis, *Clin Orthop* 128:129, 1977.

Clark CE, Shufflebarger HL: Cotrel-Dubousset instrumentation for Scheuermann's kyphosis. Paper presented at the annual meeting of the American Academy of Orthopaedic Surgeons, New Orleans, Feb 1990.

Coscia MF, Bradford DS, Ogilvie JW: Scheuermann's kyphosis: treatment with Luque instrumentation-a review of 19 patients. Paper presented at the Fifty-fifth Annual Meeting of the American Academy of Orthopaedic Surgeons, Atlanta, Feb 4-9, 1988.

Digiovanni BF, Scoles PV, Latimer BH: Anterior extension of the thoracic vertebral bodies in Scheuermann's kyphosis: an anatomic study, *Spine* 14:712, 1989.

Ferguson AB Jr: Etiology of preadolescent kyphosis, *J Bone Joint Surg* 38A:149, 1956.

Fon GT, Pitt MJ, Thies AC: Thoracic kyphosis: range in normal subjects, *Am J Roentgenol* 134:979, 1980.

Gilsanz V, Gibbens DT, Carlson M, et al: Vertebral bone density in Scheuermann disease, *J Bone Joint Surg* 71A:894, 1989.

Gutowski WT, Renshaw TS: Orthotic results in adolescent kyphosis, *Spine* 13:485, 1988.

Hensinger RN, Greene TL, Hunter LY: Back pain and vertebral changes simulating Scheuermann's kyphosis, *Spine* 6:341, 1982.

Herndon WA, Emans JB, Micheli LJ, et al: Combined anterior and posterior fusion for Scheuermann's kyphosis, *Spine* 6:125, 1981.

Ippolito E, Ponseti I: Juvenile kyphosis: histological and histochemical studies, *J Bone Joint Surg* 63A:175, 1981.

Kehl D, Lovell WW, MacEwen GD: Scheuermann's disease of the lumbar spine, *Orthop Trans* 6:342, 1982.

Kostuik J, Lorenz M: Long-term follow-up of surgical management in adult Scheuermann's kyphosis, *Orthop Trans* 7:28, 1983.

Lambrinudi L: Adolescent and senile kyphosis, *Br Med J* 2:800, 1934.

Lopez RA, Burke SW, Levine DB, et al: Osteoporosis in Scheuermann's disease, *Spine* 13:1099, 1988.

Lowe TG: Double L-rod instrumentation in the treatment of severe kyphosis, secondary to Scheuermann disease, *Spine* 12:336, 1987.

Lowe TG: Combined anterior-posterior fusion with Cotrel-Dubousset instrumentation for severe Scheuermann's kyphosis. Paper presented at the annual meeting of the American Academy of Orthopaedic Surgeons, New Orleans, Feb 1990.

Lowe TG: Scheuermann disease, *J Bone Joint Surg* 72A:940, 1990.

Moe JH: Treatment of adolescent kyphosis by nonoperative and operative methods, *Manitoba Med Rev* 45:481, 1965.

Montgomery SP, Erwin WE: Scheuermann's kyphosis: long-term results of Milwaukee brace treatment, *Spine* 6:5, 1978.

Murray PM, Weinstein SL, Spratt KF: The natural history and long-term follow-up of Scheuermann kyphosis, *J Bone Joint Surg* 75A:236, 1993.

Neithard FV: Scheuermann's disease and spondylolysis, *Orthop Trans* 7:103, 1983.

Ogilvie JW, Sherman J: Spondylolysis in Scheuermann's disease, *Spine* 12:251, 1987.

Ponseti IV, Friedman B: Changes in the scoliotic spine after fusion, *J Bone Joint Surg* 32A:751, 1950.

Ponte A, Gebbia F, Eliseo F: Nonoperative treatment of adolescent hyperkyphosis, *Orthop Trans* 9:108, 1985.

Ryan MD, Taylor TKF: Acute spinal cord compression in Scheuermann's disease, *J Bone Joint Surg* 64B:409, 1982.

Sachs BL, Bradford DS, Winter RB, et al: Scheuermann's kyphosis follow-up of Milwaukee brace treatment, *J Bone Joint Surg* 69A:50, 1987.

Scheuermann H: Kyphosis dorsalis juvenile, *Ztschr Orthop Chir* 41: 305, 1921.

Schmorl G: Die Pathogenese der juvenilen Kyphose, *Fortschr Geb Roentgenstr Nuklearmed* 41:359, 1930.

Scoles PV, Latimer BM, Digiovanni BF: Vertebral alterations in Scheuermann's kyphosis, *Spine* 16:509, 1991.

Shufflebarger HL: *Clinical issue: rod rotation in scoliosis surgery*, Warsaw, 1994, Depuy Motech.

Shufflebarger HL: *The theory of the segmental approach to spinal instrumentation: a definitive method of planning spinal instrumentation for every spinal pathology*, Warsaw, 1994, DePuy Motech.

Shufflebarger HL, Harms J: *Moss Miami three-dimensional spinal instrumentation: surgical technique*, Warsaw, 1994, DePuy Motech.

Shufflebarger HL, Harms J: *Moss Miami three-dimensional spinal instrumentation: taking spinal instrumentation to a new dimension*, Warsaw, 1994, DePuy Motech.

Singh M, Nagrath AR, Maini PS: Changes in trabecular pattern of the upper end of the femur as an index of osteoporosis, *J Bone Joint Surg* 52A:457, 1970.

Speck GR, Chopin DC: The surgical treatment of Scheuermann's kyphosis, *J Bone Joint Surg* 68B:189, 1986.

Sturm PF, Dobson JC, Armstrong GWD: The surgical management of Scheuermann's disease. Paper presented at the Fifty-fifth Annual Meeting of The American Academy of Orthopaedic Surgeons, Atlanta, Feb 4-9, 1988.

Sturm PF, Dobson JC, Armstrong GWD: The surgical management of Scheuermann's disease, *Spine* 18:685, 1993.

Travaglini F, Conte M: Untreated kyphosis: 25 years later. In Gaggi A, ed: *Kyphosis*, Bologna, 1984, Italian Scoliosis Research Group.

Voutsinas SA, MacEwen GD: Sagittal profiles of the spine, *Clin Orthop* 210:235, 1986.

Winter RB: Congenital scoliosis. In Bridwell KH, DeWald RL, eds: *The textbook of spinal surgery*, ed 2, Philadelphia, 1997, Lippincott-Raven.

Yablon JS, Kasdon DL, Levine H: Thoracic cord compression in Scheuermann's disease, *Spine* 13:896, 1988.

CONGENITAL KYPHOSIS

Bernard TN, Burke SW, Johnston CE III, et al: Congenital spine deformities: a review of 47 cases, *Orthopedics* 8:777, 1985.

Bjekreim I, Magnaes B, Semb G: Surgical treatment of severe angular kyphosis, *Acta Orthop Scand* 53:913, 1982.

Bradford DS: Anterior vascular pedicle bone grafting for the treatment of kyphosis, *Spine* 5:318, 1980.

Bradford DS, Ganjavian S, Antonious D, et al: Anterior strut-grafting for the treatment of kyphosis: a review of experience with 48 patients, *J Bone Joint Surg* 64A:680, 1982.

Guille JT, Forlin E, Bowen JR: Congenital kyphosis, *Orthop Rev* Feb 1993, p 235.

James JIP: Paraplegia in congenital kyphoscoliosis, *J Bone Joint Surg* 57B:261, 1975.

Lonstein JE, Winter RB, Moe JH, et al: Neurologic deficit secondary to spinal deformity: a review of the literature and report of 43 cases, *Spine* 5:331, 1980.

Mayfield JK, Winter RB, Bradford DS, et al: Congenital kyphosis due to defects of anterior segmentation, *J Bone Joint Surg* 62A:1291, 1980.

McMaster MJ, Singh H: Natural history of congenital kyphosis in kyphoscoliosis: a study of 112 patients, *J Bone Joint Surg* 81A:1367, 1999.

Montgomery SP, Hall JE: Congenital kyphosis, *Spine* 7:360, 1982.

Morrin B, Poitras B, Duhaime M, et al: Congenital kyphosis by segmentation defect: etiologic and pathogenic studies, *J Pediatr Orthop* 5:309, 1985.

Rose GK, Owen R, Sanderson JM: Transposition of rib with blood supply for the stabilization of spinal kyphosis, *J Bone Joint Surg* 57B:112, 1975.

Shaffer JW, Bradford DS: The use in techniques for vascularized rib pedicle grafts. In Bridwell KH, DeWald RL, eds: *The textbook of spinal surgery,* ed 2, Philadelphia, 1997, Lippincott-Raven.

Singh M, Nagrath AR, Maini PS: Changes in trabecular pattern of the upper end of the femur as an index of osteoporosis, *J Bone Joint Surg* 52A:457, 1970.

Winter RB: Congenital kyphoscoliosis with paralysis following hemivertebra excision, *Clin Orthop* 119:116, 1976.

Winter RB: Congenital spinal deformity: "What's the latest and what's the best?" *Spine* 14:1406, 1989.

Winter RB, Moe JH: The results of spinal arthrodesis for congenital spinal deformity in patients younger than 5 years' old, *J Bone Joint Surg* 64A:419, 1982.

Winter RB, Moe JH, Lonstein JE: The surgical treatment of congenital kyphosis: a review of 94 patients age 5 years or older with 2 years or more follow-up in 77 patients, *Spine* 10:224, 1985.

Winter RB, Moe JH, Wang JF: Congenital kyphosis, *J Bone Joint Surg* 55A:223, 1973.

SPONDYLOLISTHESIS AND SPONDYLOLYSIS

Ani N, Keppler L, Biscup RS, et al: Reduction of high-grade slips (grades III through V) with VSP instrumentation: report of a series of 41 cases, *Spine* 16:302, 1991.

Balderston RA, Bradford DS: Technique for achievement and maintenance of reduction for severe spondylolisthesis using spinous process traction wiring and external fixation of the pelvis, *Spine* 10:376, 1985.

Bell DF, Ehrlich MG, Zaleske DJ: Brace treatment for symptomatic spondylolisthesis, *Clin Orthop* 236:192, 1988.

Bohlman HH, Cook SS: One-stage decompression and posterolateral and interbody fusion for lumbosacral spondyloptosis through a posterior approach: report of two cases, *J Bone Joint Surg* 64A:415, 1982.

Boxall D, Bradford DS, Winter RB, et al: Management of severe spondylolisthesis in children and adolescents, *J Bone Joint Surg* 61A:479, 1979.

Bradford DS: Spondylolysis and spondylolisthesis, *Curr Pract Orthop Surg* 8:12, 1979.

Bradford DS: Treatment of severe spondylolisthesis: a combined approach for reduction and stabilization, *Spine* 4:423, 1979.

Bradford DS: Repair of spondylolysis or minimal degrees of spondylolisthesis by segmental wire fixation and bone grafting, *Orthop Trans* 6:1, 1982.

Bradford DS: Management of spondylolysis and spondylolisthesis. In The American Academy of Orthopaedic Surgeons: *Instructional course lectures*, vol 32, St Louis, 1983, Mosby.

Bradford DS: Closed reduction of spondylolisthesis: an experience in 22 patients, *Spine* 13:580, 1988.

Bradford DS, Boachie-Adjei O: Treatment of severe spondylolisthesis by anterior and posterior reduction and stabilization, *J Bone Joint Surg* 72A:1060, 1990.

Bradford DS, Iza J: Repair of the defect in spondylolysis or minimal degrees of spondylolisthesis by segmental wire fixation and bone grafting, *Spine* 10:673, 1985.

Buck JE: Direct repair of the defect in spondylolisthesis, *J Bone Joint Surg* 61A:479, 1979.

Burkus JK, Lonstein JE, Winter RB, Denis F: Long-term evaluation of adolescents treated operatively for spondylolisthesis: a comparison for in situ arthrodesis and reduction followed by immobilization in a cast, *J Bone Joint Surg* 74A:693, 1992.

Cloward RB: Spondylolisthesis: treatment by laminectomy and posterior interbody fusion: review of 100 cases, *Clin Orthop* 154:74, 1981.

Cyron BM, Hutton C: Variations in the amount and distribution of cortical bone across the pars interarticularis of L5: a predisposing factor in spondylolysis? *Spine* 4:163, 1979.

Danielson BI, Frennered AK, Irstam LKH: Radiologic progression of isthmic lumbar spondylolisthesis in young patients, *Spine* 16:422, 1991.

Dawson EG, Lotysch M III, Urist MR: Intertransverse process lumbar arthrodesis with autogenous bone graft, *Clin Orthop* 154:90, 1981.

DeWald RL: Spondylolisthesis. In Bridwell KH, DeWald RL, eds: *The textbook of spinal surgery,* ed 2, Philadelphia, 1997, Lippincott-Raven.

DeWald RL, Faut M, Taddonio RF, et al: Severe lumbosacral spondylolisthesis in adolescents and children: reduction and staged circumferential fusion, *J Bone Joint Surg* 63A:619, 1981.

Dick WT, Schnebel B: Severe spondylolisthesis: reduction in internal fixation, *Clin Orthop* 232:70, 1988.

Edwards CC: Reduction of spondylolisthesis. In Bridwell KH, DeWald RL, eds: *The textbook of spinal surgery,* ed 2, Philadelphia, 1997, Lippincott-Raven.

Fredrickson BE, Baker D, Yuan H, et al: The natural history of spondylolysis and spondylolisthesis, *J Bone Joint Surg* 66A:699, 1984.

Freeman BL, Donati NL: Spinal arthrodesis for severe spondylolisthesis in children and adolescents: a long-term follow-up study, *J Bone Joint Surg* 71A:594, 1989.

Frennered AK, Danielson BI, Nachemson AL: Midterm follow-up of young patients fused in situ for spondylolisthesis, *Spine* 16:409, 1991.

Gaines RW, Nichols WK: Treatment of spondyloptosis by two-stage L5 vertebrectomy and reduction of L4 onto S1, *Spine* 10:680, 1985.

Gaines RW Jr: The L5 vertebrectomy approach for the treatment of spondyloptosis. In Bridwell KH, DeWald RL, eds: *The textbook of spinal surgery,* ed 2, Philadelphia, 1997, Lippincott-Raven.

Garfin SR, Amundson GM: Spondylolisthesis, *Update Spinal Dis* 1:3, 1986.

Gelfand MJ, Strife JL, Kereiakes SG: Radionuclide bone imaging in spondylolysis of the lumbar spine in children, *Radiology* 140:191, 1981.

Gill GG, Manning JG, White HL: Surgical treatment of spondylolisthesis without spine fusion, *J Bone Joint Surg* 37A:493, 1955.

Gill GG, White HL: Surgical treatment of spondylolisthesis without spine fusion: a long-term follow-up of operated cases. Paper presented at the Western Orthopaedic Association, San Francisco, Nov 1962.

Goldberg MJ: Gymnastic injuries, *Orthop Clin North Am* 11:717, 1980.

Hambly M, Lee CK, Gutteling E, et al: Tension band wiring–bone grafting for spondylolysis and spondylolisthesis: a clinical and biomechanical study, *Spine* 14:455, 1989.

Haraldsson S, Willner S: A comparative study of spondylolisthesis in operations on adolescents and adults, *Arch Orthop Trauma Surg* 101:101, 1983.

Harms J, Jeszenszky D, Stoltze D, Böhm H: True spondylolisthesis reduction and monosegmental fusion in spondylolisthesis. In Bridwell KH, DeWald RL, eds: *The textbook of spinal surgery,* ed 2, Philadelphia, 1997, Lippincott-Raven.

Harrington PR, Dickson JH: Spinal instrumentation in the treatment of severe progressive spondylolisthesis, *Clin Orthop* 117:157, 1976.

Harrington PR, Tullos HS: Spondylolisthesis in children: observations and surgical treatment, *Clin Orthop* 79:75, 1971.

Harris IE, Weinstein SL: Long-term follow-up of patients with grade III and IV spondylolisthesis: treatment with and without fusion, *J Bone Joint Surg* 69A:960, 1987.

Hensinger RN: Spondylolysis and spondylolisthesis in children. In The American Academy of Orthopaedic Surgeons: *Instructional course lectures*, vol 32, St Louis, 1983, Mosby.

Hensinger RN: Spondylolysis and spondylolisthesis in children and adolescents, *J Bone Joint Surg* 71A:1098, 1989.

Hensinger RN, Lang JR, MacEwen GD: Surgical management of the spondylolisthesis in children and adolescents, *Spine* 1:207, 1976.

Herbiniaux G: *Traite sur divers accouchemens laborieux et sur les polypes de la matrice,* Braxelles, 1782, JL DeBoubers.

Huizenga BA: Reduction of spondyloptosis with two-stage vertebrectomy, *Orthop Trans* 7:21, 1983.

Jackson DW, Wiltse LL, Cirincione RJ: Spondylolysis in the female gymnast, *Clin Orthop* 117:68, 1976.

Johnson JR, Kirwan EOG: The long-term results of fusion in situ for severe spondylolisthesis, *J Bone Joint Surg* 65B:43, 1983.

Johnson LP, Nasca RJ, Dunham WK, et al: Surgical management of isthmic spondylolisthesis, *Spine* 13:93, 1988.

Kaneda K, Satoh S, Nohara Y, et al: Distraction rod instrumentation with posterolateral fusion in isthmic spondylolisthesis: 53 cases followed for 18 to 89 months, *Spine* 10:383, 1985.

Kilian HF: *Schilderungen neuer eckenformen und ihres verhaltens in Leven,* Mannheim, 1854, Verlag von Bassermann & Mathy.

Kiviluoto O, Santavirta S, Salenius P, et al: Posterolateral spine fusion: a 1- to 4-year follow-up of 80 consecutive patients, *Acta Orthop Scand* 56:152, 1985.

Klinghoffer L, Murdock MG: Spondylolysis following trauma: a case report and review of the literature, *Clin Orthop* 166:72, 1982.

Lenke LG, Bridwell KH, Bullis D, et al: Results of in situ fusion for isthmic spondylolisthesis, *J Spinal Disord* 5:433, 1992.

Letts M, Smallmon T, Afanasiev R, et al: Fracture of the pars inter-articularis in adolescent athletes: a clinical biomechanical analysis, *J Pediatr Orthop* 6:40, 1986.

Lindholm TS, Ragni P, Ylikoski M, et al: Lumbar isthmic spondylolisthesis in children and adolescents: radiologic evaluation and results of operative treatment, *Spine* 15:1350, 1990.

Lowe RW, Hayes TD, Kaye J, et al: Standing roentgenograms in spondylolisthesis, *Clin Orthop* 117:80, 1976.

Marchetti PG, Bartolozzi P: Classification of spondylolisthesis as a guideline for treatment. In Bridwell KH, DeWald RL, eds: *The textbook of spinal surgery,* ed 2, Philadelphia, 1997, Lippincott-Raven.

Matthiass HH, Heine J: The surgical reduction of spondylolisthesis, *Clin Orthop* 203:34, 1986.

Maurice HD, Morley TR: Cauda equina lesions following fusion in situ and decompressive laminectomy for severe spondylolisthesis: four case reports, *Spine* 14:214, 1989.

McCarroll JR, Miller JM, Ritter MA: Lumbar spondylolysis and spondylolisthesis in college football players: a prospective study, *Am J Sports Med* 14:404, 1986.

McPhee IB, O'Brien JP: Scoliosis in symptomatic spondylolisthesis, *J Bone Joint Surg* 62B:155, 1980.

Meyerding HW: Spondylolisthesis, *Surg Gynecol Obstet* 54:371, 1932.

Micheli LJ: Low back pain in the adolescent: differential diagnosis, *Am J Sports Med* 7:361, 1979.

Nachemson A: Repair of the spondylolisthetic defect and intertransverse fusion for young patients, *Clin Orthop* 117:101, 1976.

Neugebauer FL: A new contribution to the history and etiology of spondylolisthesis, *New Syndenham Society Selected Monographs* 121:1, 1988.

Newman PH: A clinical syndrome associated with severe lumbosacral subluxation, *J Bone Joint Surg* 47B:472, 1965.

Newman PH: Stenosis of the lumbar spine in spondylolisthesis, *Clin Ortnop* 115:116, 1976.

Nicol RO, Scott JHS: Lytic spondylolysis: repair by wiring, *Spine* 11:1027, 1986.

Ohki I, Inoue S, Murata T, et al: Reduction and fusion of severe spondylolisthesis using halo-pelvic traction with a wire reduction device, *Inter Orthop (SICOT)* 4:107, 1980.

Osterman K, Snellman O, Poussa M, et al: Treatment of lumbar lytic spondylolisthesis using osteoperiosteal transplants in young patients, *J Pediatr Orthop* 1:289, 1981.

Pedersen AK, Hagen R: Spondylolysis and spondylolisthesis: treatment by internal fixation and bone grafting of the defect, *J Bone Joint Surg* 70A:15, 1988.

Pizzutillo PD, Hummer CD III: Nonoperative treatment for painful adolescent spondylolysis or spondylolisthesis, *J Pediatr Orthop* 9:538, 1989.

Pizzutillo PD, Mirenda W, MacEwen GD: Posterolateral fusion for spondylolisthesis in adolescence, *J Pediatr Orthop* 6:311, 1986.

Poussa M, Schlenzka S, Seitsalo M, et al: Surgical treatment of severe isthmic spondylolisthesis in adolescents: reduction of fusion in situ, *Spine* 18:894, 1993.

Rabushka SE, Apfelbach H, Love L: Spontaneous healing of spondylolysis of the fifth lumbar vertebra: a case report, *Clin Orthop* 93:259, 1973.

Riley P, Gillespie R: Severe spondylolisthesis: results of posterolateral fusion, *Orthop Trans* 9:119, 1985.

Roka J, Moretta D, Fuster S, et al: Direct repair of spondylolysis, *Clin Orthop* 246:86, 1989.

Rombold C: Treatment of spondylolisthesis by posterolateral fusion, resection of the pars interarticularis, and prompt mobilization of the patient: an end-result study of seventy-three patients, *J Bone Joint Surg* 48A:1282, 1966.

Rosenberg NJ, Bargar WL, Friedman B: The incidence of spondylolysis and spondylolisthesis in nonambulatory patients, *Spine* 6:35, 1981.

Rosomoff HL: Lumbar spondylolisthesis: etiology of radiculopathy and role of the neurosurgeon, *Clin Neurosurg* 27:577, 1980.

Salib RM, Pettine KA: Modified repair of a defect in spondylolysis or minimal spondylolisthesis by pedicle screw, segmental wire fixation, and bone grafting, *Spine* 18:440, 1993.

Saraste H: Long-term clinical and radiological follow-up of spondy-lolysis and spondylolisthesis, *J Pediatr Orthop* 7:631, 1987.

Scaglietti O, Frontino G, Bartolozzi P: Technique of anatomical reduction of lumbar spondylolisthesis and its surgical stabilization, *Clin Orthop* 117:164, 1976.

Schlegel K, Pon MA: The biomechanics of posterior lumbar interbody fusion (PLIF) in spondylolisthesis, *Clin Orthop* 193:115, 1985.

Schoenecker PL: Developmental spondylolisthesis without lysis. In Bridwell KH, DeWald RL, eds: *The textbook of spinal surgery,* ed 2, Philadelphia, 1997, Lippincott-Raven.

Schoenecker PL, Cole HO, Herring JA, et al: Cauda equina syndrome after in situ arthrodesis for severe spondylolisthesis at the lumbosacral junction, *J Bone Joint Surg* 72A:369, 1990.

Seitsalo S: Operative and conservative treatment of moderate spondylolis-thesis in young patients, *J Bone Joint Surg* 72B:908, 1990.

Seitsalo S, Osterman K, Hyvarinen H, et al: Severe spondylolisthesis in children and adolescents: a long-term review of fusion in situ, *J Bone Joint Surg* 72B:259, 1990.

Seitsalo S, Osterman K, Hyvarinen H, et al: Progression of spondylolis-thesis in children and adolescents: a long-term follow-up of 272 patients, *Spine* 16:417, 1991.

Seitsalo S, Osterman K, Poussa M: Scoliosis associated with lumbar spondylolisthesis: a clinical survey of 190 young patients, *Spine* 13:899, 1988.

Seitsalo S, Osterman K, Poussa M, et al: Spondylolisthesis in children under 12 years of age: long-term results of 56 patients treated conservatively or operatively, *J Pediatr Orthop* 8:516, 1988.

Sevastikoglou JA, Spangfort E, Aaro S: Operative treatment of spondy-lolisthesis in children and adolescents with tight hamstrings syndrome, *Clin Orthop* 147:192, 1980.

Sherman FC, Rosenthal RK, Hall JE: Spine fusion for spondylolysis and spondylolisthesis in children, *Spine* 4:59, 1979.

Sijbrandij S: A new technique for the reduction and stabilisation of severe spondylolisthesis: a report of two cases, *J Bone Joint Surg* 63B:266, 1981.

Sijbrandij S: Reduction and stabilisation of severe spondylolisthesis: a report of three cases, *J Bone Joint Surg* 65B:40, 1983.

Stanton RP, Meehan P, Lovell WW: Surgical fusion in childhood spondylolisthesis, *J Pediatr Orthop* 5:411, 1985.

Steffee AD, Sitkowski DJ: Reduction and stabilization of grade IV spondylolisthesis, *Clin Orthop* 227:82, 1988.

Szappanos L, Szepesi K, Thomezz V: Spondylolysis in osteopetrosis, *J Bone Joint Surg* 70B:428, 1988.

Taddonio RF: Isthmic spondylolisthesis. In Bridwell KH, DeWald RL, eds: *The textbook of spinal surgery,* Philadelphia, 1991, JB Lippincott.

Takeda M: A newly devised "three-one" method for the surgical treatment of spondylolysis and spondylolisthesis, *Clin Orthop* 147:228, 1980.

Tower SS, Prat WB: Spondylolysis and associated spondylolisthesis in Eskimo and Athabascan populations, *Clin Orthop* 250:171, 1990.

Transfelt EE, Dendrinos GK, Bradford DS: Paresis of proximal lumbar roots after reduction of L5-S1 spondylolisthesis, *Spine* 14:884, 1988.

Turner RH, Bianco AJ Jr: Spondylolysis and spondylolisthesis in children and teen-agers, *J Bone Joint Surg* 53A:1298, 1971.

Van Dam DE: Nonoperative treatment and surgical repair of lumbar spondylolysis. In Bridwell KH, DeWald RL, eds: *The textbook of spinal surgery,* ed 2, Philadelphia, 1997, Lippincott-Raven.

van den Oever M, Merrick MV, Scott JHS: Bone scintigraphy in symptomatic spondylolysis, *J Bone Joint Surg* 69B:453, 1987.

Velikas EP, Blackburne JS: Surgical treatment of spondylolisthesis in children and adolescents, *J Bone Joint Surg* 63B:67, 1981.

Vidal J, Fassio B, Buscauret C, et al: Surgical reduction of spondylolisthesis using a posterior approach, *Clin Orthop* 154:156, 1981.

Wertzberger KL, Peterson HA: Acquired spondylolysis and spondylolisthesis in the young child, *Spine* 5:437, 1980.

Wiltse LL, Bateman JG, Hutchinson RH, et al: The paraspinal sacrospinalis-splitting approach to the lumbar spine, *J Bone Joint Surg* 50A:919, 1968.

Wiltse LL, Jackson DW: Treatment of spondylolisthesis and spondylolysis in children, *Clin Orthop* 117:92, 1976.

Wiltse LL, Newman PH, Macnab I: Classification of spondylolysis and spondylolisthesis, *Clin Orthop* 117:23, 1976.

KYPHOSCOLIOSIS IN MYELOMENINGOCELE

Allen B, Ferguson R: Operative treatment of myelomeningocele spinal deformities, *Orthop Clin North Am* 10:845, 1979.

Archibeck MJ, Smith JT, Carol KL, et al: Surgical release of the tethered spinal cord: survivorship analysis and orthopaedic outcome, *J Pediatr Orthop* 17:773, 1997.

Banta JV: Combined anterior and posterior fusion for spinal deformity in myelomeningocele, *Spine* 15:946, 1990.

Banta JV, Park SM: Improvement in pulmonary function in patients having combined anterior and posterior spine fusion for myelomeningocele scoliosis, *Spine* 8:766, 1983.

Banta JV, Whiteman S, Dyck PM, et al: Fifteen-year review of myelodysplasia, *J Bone Joint Surg* 58A:726, 1976.

Benson ER, Thomson JD, Smith BG, Banta JV: Results and morbidity in a consecutive series of patients undergoing spinal fusion for neuromuscular scoliosis, *Spine* 23:2308, 1998.

Bodel JG, Stephane JP: Luque rods in the treatment of kyphosis in myelomeningocele, *J Bone Joint Surg* 65B:98, 1983.

Christofersen MR, Brooks AL: Excision and wire fixation of rigid myelomeningocele kyphosis, *J Pediatr Orthop* 5:691, 1985.

D'Astous J, Drouin MA, Rhine E: Intraoperative anaphylaxis secondary to allergy to latex in children who have spina bifida: report of two cases, *J Bone Joint Surg* 74A:1084, 1992.

Drennan JC, Banta JV, Bunch WH, et al: Symposium, current concepts in the management of myelomeningocele, *Contemp Orthop* 19:63, 1989.

Drummond DS, Morear M, Cruess RL: The results and complications of surgery for the paralytic hip and spine in myelomeningocele, *J Bone Joint Surg* 62B:49, 1980.

Dunn HK: Kyphosis of myelodysplasia: operative treatment based on pathophysiology, *Orthop Trans* 7:19, 1983.

Dunn HK, Bender NK: The management of kyphosis of myelodysplasia. Paper presented at the Twenty-eighth Annual Meeting of the Scoliosis Research Society, Dublin, Sept 1993.

Emans JB: Allergy to latex in patients who have myelodysplasia, *J Bone Joint Surg* 74A:1103, 1992.

Feiwell E: Selection of appropriate treatment for patients with myelomeningocele, *Orthop Clin North Am* 12:101, 1981.

Gillespie R, Torode I, van Olm RS Jr: Myelomeningocele kyphosis fixed by kyphectomy and segmental spinal instrumentation, *Orthop Trans* 8:162, 1984.

Heydemann JS, Gillespie R: Management of myelomeningocele kyphosis in the older child by kyphectomy and segmental spinal instrumentation, *Spine* 12:37, 1987.

Hoppenfeld S: Congenital kyphosis in myelomeningocele, *J Bone Joint Surg* 49B:276, 1967.

Hull WJ, Moe JH, Winter RB: Spinal deformity in myelomeningocele: natural history, evaluation, and treatment, *J Bone Joint Surg* 56A:1767, 1974.

Johnston CE, Hakala MW, Rosenberg R: Paralytic spinal deformity: orthotic treatment in spinal discontinuity syndromes, *J Pediatr Orthop* 2:233, 1982.

Jones ET: Kyphectomy in myelodysplasia, *Orthop Trans* 7:432, 1983.

Kahanovitz N, Duncan JW: The role of scoliosis and pelvic obliquity on functional disability in myelomeningocele, *Spine* 6:494, 1981.

Kilfoyle RM, Foley JJ, Norton PL: Spine and pelvic deformity in childhood and adolescent paraplegia: a study of 104 cases, *J Bone Joint Surg* 47A:659, 1976.

Leatherman KD, Dickson RA: Congenital kyphosis in myelomeningocele: vertebral body resection and posterior spinal fusion, *Spine* 3:222, 1978.

Lindseth RE: Myelomeningocele spine. In Weinstein SL, ed: *The pediatric spine,* New York, 1994, Raven Press.

Lindseth RE, Selzer L: Vertebral excision of kyphosis in myelomeningocele, *J Bone Joint Surg* 61A:699, 1979.

Lubicky JP: The myelomeningocele spine. In Bridwell KH, DeWald RL, eds: *The textbook of spinal surgery,* Philadelphia, 1991, JB Lippincott.

Lubicky JP: Spinal deformity in myelomeningocele. In Bridwell KH, DeWald RL, eds: *The textbook of spinal surgery,* ed 2, Philadelphia, 1997, Lippincott-Raven.

Mackel JL, Lindseth RE: Scoliosis in myelodysplasia, *J Bone Joint Surg* 57A:131, 1975.

Mayfield JK: Severe spine deformity and myelodysplasia and sacral agenesis: an aggressive surgical approach, *Spine* 6:498, 1981.

Mazur J, Menelaus MB, Dickens DRV, et al: Efficacy of surgical management for scoliosis in myelomeningocele: correction of deformity and alteration of functional status, *J Pediatr Orthop* 6:568, 1986.

McIvor J, Kraibech JI, Hoffman H: Orthopaedic complications of lumboperitoneal shunts, *J Pediatr Orthop* 8:687, 1988.

McLaughlin TP, Banta JV, Gahm NH, et al: Intraspinal rhizotomy and distal cordectomy in patients with myelomeningocele, *J Bone Joint Surg* 68A:88, 1986.

McMaster MJ: Anterior and posterior instrumentation and fusion of thoracolumbar scoliosis due to myelomeningocele, *J Bone Joint Surg* 69B:20, 1987.

McMaster MJ: The long-term results of kyphectomy and spinal stabilization in children with myelomeningocele, *Spine* 13:417, 1988.

Meehan PL, Galina MP, Daftari T: Intraoperative anaphylaxis due to allergy to latex: report of two cases, *J Bone Joint Surg* 74A:1087, 1992.

Mintz LJ, Sarwark JF, Dias LS, et al: The natural history of congenital kyphosis in myelomeningocele: a review of 51 children, *Spine* 16:S348, 1991.

Müller EB, Nordwall A: Brace treatment of scoliosis in children with myelomeningocele, *Spine* 19:151, 1994.

Müller EB, Nordwall A, Oden A: Progression of scoliosis in children with myelomeningocele, *Spine* 19:144, 1994.

Osebold W, Mayfield JK, Winter RB, et al: Surgical treatment of paralytic scoliosis in myelomeningocele, *J Bone Joint Surg* 64A:841, 1982.

Poitras B, Rivard C, Duhaime M, et al: Correction of the kyphosis in myelomeningocele patients by both anterior and posterior stabilization procedure, *Orthop Trans* 7:432, 1983.

Raycroft JF, Curtis BH: Spinal curvature in myelomeningocele. In The American Academy of Orthopaedic Surgeons: *Symposium on myelomeningocele,* St Louis, 1972, Mosby.

Rodgers WB, Frim DM, Emans JB: Surgery of the spine in myelodysplasia: an overview, *Clin Orthop* 338:19, 1997.

Rodgers WB, Williams MS, Schwend RM, Emans JD: Spinal deformity in myelodysplasia: correction with posterior pedicle screw instrumentation, *Spine* 22:2435, 1997.

Samuelsson L, Eklof O: Scoliosis in myelomeningocele, *Acta Orthop Scand* 59:122, 1988.

Sharrard WJW: Spinal osteotomy for congenital kyphosis in myelomeningocele, *J Bone Joint Surg* 50B:466, 1968.

Sharrard WJW, Drennan JC: Osteoexcision of the spine for lumbar kyphosis in older children with myelomeningocele, *J Bone Joint Surg* 54B:50, 1972.

Smith RM, Emans JB: Sitting balance in spinal deformity, *Spine* 17:1103, 1992.

Sponseller PD, Young AT, Sarwark JF, Lim R: Anterior-only fusion for scoliosis in patients with myelomeningocele, *Clin Orthop* 364:117, 1999.

Sriram K, Bobechko WP, Hall JE: Surgical management of spinal deformities in spina bifida, *J Bone Joint Surg* 54A:666, 1972.

Stark A, Saraste H: Anterior fusion insufficient for scoliosis in myelomeningocele: eight children, 2 to 6 years after the Zielke operation, *Acta Orthop Scand* 64:22, 1993.

Szalay EA, Roach JW, Smith H, et al: Magnetic resonance imaging of the spinal cord and spinal dysraphisms, *J Pediatr Orthop* 7:541, 1987.

Vogel LC, Schrader T, Lubicky JT: Latex allergy in children and adolescents with spinal cord injuries, *J Pediatr Orthop* 15:517, 1995.

Ward T, Wenger DR, Roch JW: Surgical correction of myelomeningocele scoliosis: critical appraisal of various spinal instrumentation systems, *J Pediatr Orthop* 9:262, 1989.

Warner WC Jr, Fackler CD: Comparison of two instrumentation techniques in treatment of lumbar kyphosis in myelodysplasia, *J Pediatr Orthop* 13:704, 1993.

Widmann RF, Hresko MT, Hall JE: Lumbosacral fusion in children and adolescents using the modified sacral bar technique, *Clin Orthop* 364:85, 1999.

Winston K, Hall JE, Johnson D, et al: Acute elevation of intracranial pressure following transection of nonfunctional spinal cord, *Clin Orthop* 128:41, 1977.

Winter RB, Carlson JM: Modern orthotics for spinal deformities, *Clin Orthop* 126:74, 1977.

Winter RB, Pinto WC: Pelvic obliquity: its causes and treatment, *Spine* 11:225, 1986.

Yamane T, Shinoto A, Kamegaya M, et al: Spinal dysraphism: a study of patients over the age of 10 years, *Spine* 16:1295, 1991.

SACRAL AGENESIS

Abraham E: Lumbosacral coccygeal agenesis: autopsy case report, *J Bone Joint Surg* 58A:1169, 1976.

Abraham E: Sacral agenesis with associated anomalies (caudal regression syndrome): autopsy case report, *Clin Orthop* 145:168, 1979.

Andrish J, Kalamchi A, MacEwen GD: Sacral agenesis: a clinical evaluation of its management, heredity, and associated anomalies, *Clin Orthop* 139:52, 1979.

Dumont C, Dansin J, Forin V, et al: Lumbosacral agenesis: three cases of reconstruction using Cotrel-Dubousset or L-rod instrumentation, *Spine* 18:1229, 1993.

Elting JJ, Allen JC: Management of the young child with bilateral anomalous and functionless lower extremities, *J Bone Joint Surg* 54A:1523, 1972.

Ignelzi RJ, Lehman RAW: Lumbosacral agenesis: management and embryological implications, *J Neurol Neurosurg Psychiatry* 37:1273, 1974.

Koff SA, Deridder PA: Patterns of neurogenic bladder dysfunction in sacral agenesis, *J Urol* 188:87, 1977.

Marsh HO, Tejano NA: Four cases of lumbosacral and sacral agenesis, *Clin Orthop* 92:214, 1973.

Mongeau M, LeClaire R: Complete agenesis of the lumbosacral spine: a case report, *J Bone Joint Surg* 54A:161, 1972.

Nicol WJ: Lumbosacral agenesis in a 60-year-old man, *Br J Surg* 59:577, 1972.

Perry J, Bonnett CA Hoffer MM: Vertebral pelvic fusions in the rehabilitation of patients with sacral agenesis, *J Bone Joint Surg* 52A:288, 1970.

Phillips WA, Cooperman DR, Lindquist TC, et al: Orthopaedic management of lumbosacral agenesis: long-term follow-up, *J Bone Joint Surg* 64A:1282, 1982.

Redman JF: Congenital absence of the lumbosacral spine, *South Med J* 66:770, 1973.

Reeve AW, Mortimer JG: Lumbosacral agenesis or rumplessness, *N Z Med J* 73:340, 1971.

Renshaw TS: Sacral agenesis: a classification in review of 23 cases, *J Bone Joint Surg* 60A:373, 1978.

Rieger MA, Hall JE, Dalury DF: Spinal fusion in a patient with lumbosacral agenesis, *Spine* 12:1382, 1990.

Ruderman RJ, Keats P, Goldner JL: Congenital absence of the lumbo-sacral spine: a report of an unusual case, *Clin Orthop* 124:177, 1977.

Stanley JK, Owen R, Koff S: Congenital sacral anomalies, *J Bone Joint Surg* 61B:401, 1979.

White RI, Klauber GT: Sacral agenesis: analysis of 22 cases, *Urology* 8:521, 1976.

NEUROFIBROMATOSIS

Akbarnia BA, Gabriel KR, Beckman E, et al: Prevalence of scoliosis in neurofibromatosis, *Spine* 17:S244, 1992.

Betz RR, Iorio R, Lombardi AV, et al: Scoliosis surgery in neurofibromatosis, *Clin Orthop* 245:53, 1989.

Bradford DS: Anterior vascular pedicle bone grafting for the treatment of kyphosis, *Spine* 5:318, 1980.

Brown CW: Spinal deformities in neurofibromatosis. In Bridwell KH, DeWald RL, eds: *The textbook of spinal surgery*, Philadelphia, 1991, JB Lippincott.

Calvert PT, Edgar MA, Webb PJ: Scoliosis in neurofibromatosis: the natural history with and without operation, *J Bone Joint Surg* 71B:246, 1989.

Chee CP: Lateral thoracic meningocele associated with neurofibromatosis: total excision by posterolateral extradural approach: a case report, *Spine* 14:129, 1989.

Crawford AH: Pitfalls of spinal deformities associated with neurofibromatosis in children, *Clin Orthop* 245:29, 1989.

Crawford AH Jr, Bagamery N: Osseous manifestations of neurofibromatosis in childhood, *J Pediatr Orthop* 6:72, 1986.

Crawford AH, Gabriel KR: Dysplastic scoliosis: neurofibromatosis. In Bridwell KH, DeWald RL, eds: *The textbook of spinal surgery*, ed 2, Philadelphia, 1997, Lippincott-Raven.

Curtis B, Fisher R, Butterfield W, et al: Neurofibromatosis with paraplegia, *J Bone Joint Surg* 51A:843, 1969.

DiSimone RE, Berman AT, Schwentker EP: The orthopaedic manifestation of neurofibromatosis: a clinical experience and review of the literature, *Clin Orthop* 230:277, 1988.

Flood BM, Butt WP, Dickson RA: Rib penetration of the intervertebral foraminae in neurofibromatosis, *Spine* 11:172, 1986.

Hensinger R: Kyphosis secondary to skeletal dysplasias and metabolic disease, *Clin Orthop* 128:113, 1977.

Holt RT, Johnson JR: Cotrel-Dubousset instrumentation in neurofibromatosis spine curves: a preliminary report, *Clin Orthop* 245:19, 1989.

Hsu L, Lee P, Leong J: Dystrophic spinal deformities in neurofibromatosis, *J Bone Joint Surg* 66B:495, 1984.

Lonstein J, Winter RB, Moe JH, et al: Neurologic deficits secondary to spinal deformity, *Spine* 5:331, 1980.

McCarroll H: Clinical manifestations of congenital neurofibromatosis, *J Bone Joint Surg* 32A:601, 1950.

Miller A: Neurofibromatosis: with reference to skeletal changes, compression myelitis, and malignant degeneration, *Arch Surg* 32:109, 1936.

Mitchell G, Lourie H, Berne A: The various causes of scalloped vertebrae with notes on their pathogenesis, *Radiology* 89:67, 1967.

Riccardi V: Von Recklinghausen neurofibromatosis, *N Engl J Med* 305:1617, 1981.

Savini R, Parisini P, Cervellati S, Gualdrini G: Surgical treatment of vertebral deformities in neurofibromatosis, *Ital J Orthop Traumatol* 9:13, 1983.

Shufflebarger HL: Cotrel-Dubousset instrumentation in neurofibromatosis spinal problem, *Clin Orthop* 245:24, 1989.

Stone JW, Bridwell KH, Shackelford GD, et al: Dural ectasia associated with spontaneous dislocation of the upper part of the thoracic spine in neurofibromatosis: a case report and review of the literature, *J Bone Joint Surg* 69A:1079, 1987.

Tolo VT: Spinal deformity in skeletal dysplasia conditions. In Bridwell KH, DeWald RL, eds: *The textbook of spinal surgery*, ed 2, Philadelphia, 1997, Lippincott-Raven.

von Recklinghausen F: *Uber die multiplen Fibrome der Haut und ihre Beziehung zu den multiplen Neuromen, Festschrift dur Rudolph Virchow*, Berlin, 1882, August Hirschwald.

Winter RB: Thoracic lordoscoliosis in neurofibromatosis: treatment by Harrington rod with sublaminar wiring: report of two cases, *J Bone Joint Surg* 62A:1102, 1984.

Winter RB, Edwards W: Neurofibromatosis with lumbosacral spondylolisthesis, *J Pediatr Orthop* 1:91, 1981.

Winter RB, Lonstein JE, Anderson M: Neurofibromatosis hyperkyphosis: a review of 33 patients with kyphosis of 80 degrees or greater, *J Spinal Disord* 1:39, 1988.

Winter RB, Lonstein JE, Anderson M: Neurofibromatosis kyphosis. Paper presented at the Fifty-fifth Annual Meeting of the American Academy of Orthopaedic Surgeons, Atlanta, Feb 4-9, 1988.

Winter RB, Moe J, Bradford D, et al: Spine deformity in neurofibromatosis, *J Bone Joint Surg* 61A:677, 1979.

Yong-Hing K, Kalamchi A, MacEwen GD: Cervical spine abnormalities in neurofibromatosis, *J Bone Joint Surg* 61A:695, 1979.

MARFAN SYNDROME

Amis J, Herring J: Iatrogenic kyphosis: complication of Harrington instrumentation in Marfan's syndrome, *J Bone Joint Surg* 66A:460, 1984.

Birch JG, Herring JA: Spinal deformity in Marfan's syndrome, *J Pediatr Orthop* 7:546, 1987.

Boucek RJ, Noble NL, Gunya-Smith Z, et al: The Marfan's syndrome: a deficiency in chemically stable collagen cross links, *N Engl J Med* 305:988, 1981.

Donaldson DH: Spinal deformity associated with Marfan's syndrome. In Bridwell KH, DeWald RL, eds: *The textbook of spinal surgery*, Philadelphia, 1991, JB Lippincott.

Donaldson DH and Brown CW: Marfan's spinal pathology. In Bridwell KH, DeWald RL, eds: *The textbook of spinal surgery*, ed 2, Philadelphia, 1997, Lippincott-Raven.

Joseph KN, Kane HA, Milner RS, et al: Orthopaedic aspects of the Marfan phenotype, *Clin Orthop* 277:251, 1992.

Pyeritz RE, McKusick VA: The Marfan syndrome: diagnosis and management, *N Engl J Med* 300:772, 1979.

Pyeritz RE, McKusick VA: Basic defects in the Marfan syndrome, *N Engl J Med* 305:1011, 1981.

Robins PR, Moe JH, Winter RB: Scoliosis in Marfan syndrome: its characteristics and results of treatment in 35 patients, *J Bone Joint Surg* 57A:358, 1975.

Savini R, Cerrellati S, Beroaldo E: Spinal deformities in Marfan's syndrome, *Ital J Orthop Traumatol* 6:19, 1980.

Sponseller PD, Hobbs W, Riley LH III, et al: Spinal deformity and Marfan syndrome: prevalence and natural history. Paper presented at the Twenty-eighth Annual Meeting of the Scoliosis Research Society, Dublin, Sept 1993.

Taylor LJ: Severe spondylolisthesis and scoliosis in association with Marfan's syndrome: case report and review of the literature, *Clin Orthop* 221:207, 1987.

Waters P, Welch K, Micheli LJ, et al: Scoliosis in children with pectus excavatum and pectus carnatum, *J Pediatr Orthop* 9:551, 1989.

Winter RB: Severe spondylolisthesis in Marfan's syndrome: report of two cases, *J Pediatr Orthop* 2:51, 1982.

Winter RB: Thoracic lordoscoliosis in Marfan's syndrome: report of two patients with surgical correction using rods and sublaminar wires, *Spine* 15:233, 1990.

VERTEBRAL COLUMN TUMORS

Akbarnia BA, Bradford DS, Winter RB: Osteoid osteoma of the spine: an analysis of 14 patients, *Orthop Trans* 6:4, 1982.

Akbarnia BA, Rooholamini SA: Scoliosis caused by benign osteoblastoma of the thoracic or lumbar spine, *J Bone Joint Surg* 63A:1146, 1981.

Allison DJ: Therapeutic embolization, *J Bone Joint Surg* 64B:151, 1982.

Barwick KW, Huvos AG, Smith J: Primary osteogenic sarcoma of the vertebral column, *Cancer* 46:595, 1980.

deCristofaro R, Biagini R, Boriani S, et al: Selective arterial embolization in the treatment of aneurysmal bone cyst in angioma of bone, *Skeletal Radiol* 21:523, 1992.

Dick HM, Bigliani LU, Michelsen WJ, et al: Adjuvant arterial embolization in the treatment of benign primary bone tumors in children, *Clin Orthop* 139:133, 1979.

Dunn HK: Tumors of the thoracic and lumbar spine. In Evarts CM, ed: *Surgery of the musculoskeletal system*, New York, 1983, Churchill Livingstone.

Gelb DE, Bridwell KH: Benign tumors of the spine. In Bridwell KH, DeWald RL, eds: *The textbook of spinal surgery*, ed 2, Philadelphia, 1997, Lippincott-Raven.

Ghelman B, Lospinuso MF, Levine DB, et al: Percutaneous computed tomography–guided biopsy of the thoracic and lumbar spine, *Spine* 16:736, 1991.

Hay MC, Paterson D, Taylor TKF: Aneurysmal bone cysts of the spine, *J Bone Joint Surg* 60B:406, 1978.

Israeli A, Zwas ST, Horoszowski H, et al: Use of radionuclide method in preoperative and intraoperative diagnosis of osteoid osteoma of the spine: case report, *Clin Orthop* 175:194, 1983.

Jelsma RK, Kirsch PT: The treatment of malignancy of a vertebral body, *Surg Neurol* 13:189, 1980.

Kattapuram SV, Khurana JS, Rosenthal DI: Percutaneous needle biopsy of the spine, *Spine* 17:561, 1992.

Keim HA, Reina EG: Osteoid osteoma as a cause of scoliosis, *J Bone Joint Surg* 57A:159, 1975.

Laredo J, Assouline E, Gelbert F, et al: Vertebral hemangiomas: fat content as a sign of aggressiveness, *Radiology* 177:467, 1990.

Laredo J, Reizine D, Bard M, Murland J: Vertebral hemangiomas: radiologic evaluation, *Radiology* 161:183, 1986.

Marsh BW, Bonfiglio M, Brady LP, et al: Benign osteoblastoma: range of manifestations, *J Bone Joint Surg* 57A:1, 1975.

McLeod RA, Dahlin DC, Beabout JW: The spectrum of osteoblastoma, *Am J Radiol* 126:321, 1976.

Mehta MH: Pain-provoked scoliosis: observations on the evolution of the deformity, *Clin Orthop* 135:58, 1978.

Mehta MH, Murray RO: Scoliosis provoked by painful vertebral lesions, *Skeletal Radiol* 1:223, 1977.

Merryweather R, Middlemiss JH, Sanerkin NG: Malignant transformation of osteoblastoma, *J Bone Joint Surg* 62B:381, 1980.

Michele A, Krueger FJ: A surgical approach to the vertebral body, *J Bone Joint Surg* 31A:873, 1949.

Moon KL, Genant HK, Holmes CA: Muscular skeletal applications of nuclear magnetic resonance imaging, *Radiology* 147:161, 1983.

Nelson OA, Greer RB III: Localization of osteoid osteoma of the spine using computerized tomography, *J Bone Joint Surg* 65A:263, 1983.

Nemoto O, Moser RP, Van Dam BE, et al: Osteoblastoma of the spine: a report of 75 cases, *Spine* 15:1272, 1990.

Pettine KA, Klassen RA: Osteoid osteoma and osteoblastoma of the spine, *J Bone Joint Surg* 68A:354, 1986.

Ransford AO, Pozo JL, Hutton PAN, et al: The behavior pattern of the scoliosis associated with osteoid osteoma or osteoblastoma of the spine, *J Bone Joint Surg* 66B:16, 1984.

Richardson FL: A report of 16 tumors of the spinal cord in children: the importance of spinal rigidity as an early sign of disease, *J Pediatr* 57:42, 1960.

Rinsky LA, Goris M, Bleck EE, et al: Intraoperative skeletal scintigraphy for localization of osteoid-osteoma in the spine, *J Bone Joint Surg* 62A:143, 1980.

Schacked I, Tarudor R, Wolpin G, et al: Aneurysmal bone cyst of a vertebral body with acute paraplegia, *Paraplegia* 19:294, 1981.

Seiman LP: Eosinophilic granuloma of the spine, *J Pediatr Orthop* 1:371, 1981.

Villas C, Martinez-Peric R, Barrios RH, Beguiristain JL: Eosinophilic granuloma of the spine with and without vertebra plana: long-term follow-up of six cases, *J Spinal Def* 6:260, 1993.

Wedge JH, Tchang S, MacFadyen DJ: Computed tomography and localization of spinal osteoid osteoma, *Spine* 6:423, 1981.

Yu L, Kasser JR, O'Rourke E: Chronic recurrent multifocal osteomyelitis: association with vertebra plana, *J Bone Joint Surg* 71A;105, 1989.

POSTIRRADIATION SPINE DEFORMITY

Arkin AM, Pack GT, Ransohoff NS, et al: Radiation-induced scoliosis: a case report, *J Bone Joint Surg* 32A:401, 1950.

Barr JS, Lingley JR, Gall EA: The effect of roentgen irradiation on epiphyseal growth, *Am J Roentgenol* 49:104, 1943.

Bick EM, Copel JW: Longitudinal growth of the human vertebra: a contribution to human osteogeny, *J Bone Joint Surg* 32A:803, 1950.

Donaldson DH: Scoliosis secondary to radiation. In Bridwell KH, DeWald RL, eds: *The textbook of spinal surgery*, Philadelphia, 1991, JB Lippincott.

Engel D: Experiments on the production of spinal deformities by radium, *Am J Roentgenol* 42:217, 1939.

Frantz CH: Extreme retardation of epiphyseal growth from roentgen irradiation, *Radiology* 55:720, 1950.

Hinkel CL: The effect of roentgen rays upon the growing long bones of albino rats. II. Histopathological changes involving inchondral growth centers, *Am J Roentgenol* 49:321, 1943.

Katzman H, Waugh T, Berdon W: Skeletal changes following irradiation of childhood tumors, *J Bone Joint Surg* 51A:825, 1969.

King J, Stowe S: Results of spinal fusion for radiation scoliosis, *Spine* 7:574, 1982.

Mayfield JK: Postirradiation spinal deformity, *Orthop Clin North Am* 10:829, 1979.

Mayfield JK, Riseborough EJ, Jaffe N, et al: Spinal deformity in children treated for neuroblastoma, *J Bone Joint Surg* 63A:183, 1981.

Neuhauser EBD, Wittenborg MH, Berman CZ, et al: Radiation effects of roentgen therapy on the growing spine, *Radiology* 59:637, 1952.

Ogilvie JW: Spinal deformity following radiation. In Bradford DS et al, eds: *Moe's textbook of scoliosis and other spinal deformities*, ed 2, Philadelphia, 1987, WB Saunders.

Reidy JA, Lingley JR, Gall EA, et al: The effect of roentgen irradiation on epiphyseal growth, *J Bone Joint Surg* 29:853, 1947.

Riseborough EJ: Irradiation-induced kyphosis, *Clin Orthop Rel Res* 128:101, 1977.

Riseborough EJ, Grabias SL, Burton RI, et al: Skeletal alterations following irradiation for Wilms' tumor, *J Bone Joint Surg* 58A:526, 1976.

OSTEOCHONDRODYSTROPHIES

Bethem D, Winter RB, Lutter L: Spinal disorders of dwarfism: review of the literature and report of 80 cases, *J Bone Joint Surg* **63A:1412, 1981.**

OSTEOGENESIS IMPERFECTA

Albright JA: Management overview of osteogenesis imperfecta, *Clin Orthop* 159:80, 1981.

Benson DR, Newman DC: The spine and surgical treatment in osteogenesis imperfecta, *Clin Orthop* 159:147, 1981.

Bradford DS: Osteogenesis imperfecta. In Bradford DS et al, eds: *Moe's textbook of scoliosis and other spinal deformities*, ed 2, Philadelphia, 1987, WB Saunders.

Donaldson DH: Spinal deformity associated with osteogenesis imperfecta. In Bridwell KH, DeWald RL, eds: *The textbook of spinal surgery*, Philadelphia, 1991, JB Lippincott.

Gitelis S, Whiffen J, DeWald RL: The treatment of severe scoliosis in osteogenesis imperfecta, *Clin Orthop* 175:56, 1983.

Hanscom DA, Bloom BA: The spine in osteogenesis imperfecta, *Orthop Clin North Am* 19:449, 1988.

Hanscom DA, Winter RB, Lutter L, et al: Osteogenesis imperfecta: radiographic classification, natural history, and treatment of spinal deformities, *J Bone Joint Surg* 74A:598, 1992.

King JD, Bobechko WP: Osteogenesis imperfecta, *J Bone Joint Surg* 53B:72, 1971.

Libman RH: Anesthetic considerations for the patient with osteogenesis imperfecta, *Clin Orthop* 159:123, 1981.

Lubicky JP: The spine and osteogenesis imperfecta. In Bridwell KH, DeWald RL, eds: *The textbook of spinal surgery*, ed 2, Philadelphia, 1997, Lippincott-Raven.

Moorefield WG, Miller GR: Aftermath of osteogenesis imperfecta: the disease of adulthood, *J Bone Joint Surg* 62A:113, 1980.

Norimatsu H, Mayuzumi T, Takahashi T: The development of the spinal deformities in osteogenesis imperfecta, *Clin Orthop* 162:20, 1982.

Versfeld GA: Costovertebral anomalies in osteogenesis imperfecta, *J Bone Joint Surg* 67B:602, 1985.

Yong-Hing K, MacEwen GD: Scoliosis associated with osteogenesis imperfecta: results of treatment, *J Bone Joint Surg* 64B:36, 1982.

Ziv I, Rang M, Hoffman JH: Paraplegia in osteogenesis imperfecta: a case report, *J Bone Joint Surg* 65B:184, 1983.

POSTLAMINECTOMY SPINAL DEFORMITY

Brown HP, Bonnett CC: Spine deformity subsequent to spinal cord injury, *J Bone Joint Surg* 55A:441, 1973.

Fraser RD, Patterson DC, Simpson DA: Orthopaedic aspects of spinal tumors in children, *J Bone Joint Surg* 59B:143, 1977.

Haft H, Ransohoff J, Carter S: Spinal cord tumors in children, *Pediatrics* 23:1152, 1959.

Johnston CE II: Postlaminectomy kyphoscoliosis following surgical treatment for spinal cord astrocytoma, *Orthopedics* 9:587, 1986.

Kilfoyle RM, Foley JJ, Norton PL: Spine and pelvic deformity in childhood and adolescent paraplegia: a study of 104 cases, *J Bone Joint Surg* 47A:659, 1965.

Lonstein JE: Postlaminectomy kyphosis, *Clin Orthop* 128:93, 1977.

Lonstein JE, Winter RB, Bradford DS, et al: Postlaminectomy spine deformity, *J Bone Joint Surg* 58A:727, 1976.

Panjabi MM, White AA, Johnson RM: Cervical spine mechanics as a function of transection on components, *J Biomech* 8:327, 1975.

Tachdjian MO, Matson DD: Orthopaedic aspects of intraspinal tumors in infants and children, *J Bone Joint Surg* 47A:223, 1965.

Winter RB, McBride GG: Severe postlaminectomy kyphosis: treatment by total vertebrectomy (plus late recurrence of childhood spinal cord astrocytoma), *Spine* 9:690, 1984.

Yasuoka S, Peterson HA, MacCarty CS: Incidence of spinal column deformity after multilevel laminectomy in children and adults, *J Neurosurg* 57:441, 1982.

Yasuoka S, Peterson H, Laws ER Jr, et al: Pathogenesis and prophylaxis of postlaminectomy deformity of the spine after multiple level laminectomy: difference between children and adults, *Neurosurgery* 9:145, 1981.

SKELETAL DYSPLASIAS

Bailey JA: Orthopaedic aspects of achondroplasia, *J Bone Joint Surg* 52A:1285, 1970.

Beals RK: Hypochondroplasia, *J Bone Joint Surg* 51A:728, 1969.

Beighton P: Orthopaedic problems in dwarfism, *J Bone Joint Surg* 62B:116, 1980.

Bethem D, Winter RB, Lutter L: Disorders of the spine in diastrophic dwarfism: a discussion of nine patients and review of the literature, *J Bone Joint Surg* 62A:529, 1980.

Bethem D, Winter RB, Lutter L: Spinal disorders of dwarfism: review of the literature and report of 80 cases, *J Bone Joint Surg* 63A:1412, 1981.

Blaw MD, Langer LO: Spinal cord compression in Morquio-Brailsford disease, *J Pediatr* 74:593, 1969.

Eulert J: Scoliosis and kyphosis in dwarfing conditions, *Arch Orthop Traum Surg* 102:45, 1983.

Hensinger RN: Kyphosis secondary to skeletal dysplasias and metabolic disease, *Clin Orthop* 128:113, 1977.

Herring JA, Winter RB: Kyphosis in an achondroplastic dwarf, *J Pediatr Orthop* 3:250, 1983.

Hurler G: Uber einen Typ multipler Abartungen, vorwiegend am Skelettsystem, *Z Kinderheilk* 24:220, 1919.

Johnston CE II: Scoliosis in metatrophic dwarfism, *Orthopedics* 6:491, 1983.

Kahanovitz N, Rimoin DL, Silence DO: The clinical spectrum of lumbar spine disease in achondroplasia, *Spine* 7:137, 1982.

Kopits SE: Orthopaedic complications of dwarfism, *Clin Orthop* 114:153, 1976.

Kopits SE: Cervical myelopathy and dwarfism, *Orthop Trans* 3:119, 1979.

Kozlowski K, Beighton P: Radiographic features of spondyloepimetaphyseal dysplasia with joint laxity and progressive kyphoscoliosis, *Fortschr Roentgenstr* 141:337, 1984.

Lamy M, Maroteaux P: Le nanisme diastrophique, *Presse Med* 68:1977, 1960.

Langer LO, Bauman PA, Gorlin RJ: Achondroplasia: clinical radiologic features with comment on genetic implications, *Clin Pediatr* 7:474, 1968.

Langer LO, Carey LS: The roentgenographic features of the KS mucopolysaccharidosis of Morquio, *Am J Roentgenol* 97:1, 1966.

Lipson SJ: Dysplasia of the odontoid process in Morquio's syndrome causing quadriparesis, *J Bone Joint Surg* 59A:340, 1977.

Morgan DF, Young RF: Spinal neurologica complications of achondroplasia: results of surgical treatment, *J Neurosurg* 52:463, 1980.

Morquio L: Sur une forme de dystrophie osseuse familiale, *Arch Med Enf* 32:129, 1929.

Ponseti IV: Skeletal growth in achondroplasia, *J Bone Joint Surg* 52A:701, 1970.

Stanescu V, Stanescu R, Maroteaux P: Pathogenic mechanisms in osteochondrodysplasias, *J Bone Joint Surg* 66A:817, 1984.

Tolo VT: Surgical treatment of thoracolumbar kyphosis in achondroplasia. Paper presented at the Fifty-fifth Annual Meeting of the American Academy of Orthopaedic Surgeons, Atlanta, Feb 4-9, 1988.

Yamada H, Nakamura S, Tajima M, et al: Neurological manifestations of pediatric achondroplasia, *J Neurosurg* 54:49, 1981.

CHAPTER 39

Lower Back Pain and Disorders of Intervertebral Discs

Keith D. Williams ◆ Ashley L. Park

Humans have been plagued by back and leg pain since the beginning of recorded history. Primitive cultures attributed such pain to the work of demons. The early Greeks recognized the symptoms as a disease and prescribed rest and massage for the ailment. The Edwin Smith papyrus, the oldest surgical text dating to 1500 BC, includes a case of back strain. Unfortunately, the text does not include the treatment rendered by the ancient Egyptians. In the fifth century AD, Aurelianus clearly described the symptoms of sciatica. He noted that sciatica arose from either hidden causes or observable causes, such as a fall, a violent blow, pulling, or straining. In the eighteenth century Cotugnio (Cotunnius) attributed the pain to the sciatic nerve. Gradually, as medicine advanced as a science, the number of specific diagnoses capable of causing back and leg pain increased dramatically.

Several physical maneuvers were devised to isolate the true problem in each patient. The most notable of these is the *Lasègue sign,* or *straight leg raising test,* described by Forst in 1881 but attributed to Lasègue, his teacher. This test was devised to distinguish hip disease from sciatica. Although sciatica was widespread as an ailment, little was known about it because only rarely did it result in death, allowing examination at autopsy. Virchow (1857), Kocher (1896), and Middleton and Teacher (1911) described acute traumatic ruptures of the intervertebral disc that resulted in death. The correlation between the disc rupture and sciatica was not appreciated by these examiners. Goldthwait in 1911 attributed back pain to posterior displacement of the disc. Oppenheim and Krause in 1909 performed the first successful surgical excision of a herniated intervertebral disc. Unfortunately, they did not recognize the excised tissue as disc material and interpreted it as an enchondroma. Oil-contrast myelography was serendipitously introduced when iodized poppy seed oil, injected to treat sciatica in 1922, was inadvertently injected intradurally and was noted to flow freely. Dandy in 1929 and Alajouanine in the same year reported removal of a "disc tumor," or chondroma, from patients with sciatica. The commonly held opinion of that time was that the disc hernia was a neoplasm. Mixter and Barr in their classic paper published in 1934 attributed sciatica to lumbar disc herniation. This report also included a series of four patients with thoracic disc herniations, and four patients with cervical disc herniations. They suggested surgical treatment. Myelography was not used for confirmation of disc disease because of toxicity of the agents used in the years that followed. Myelography was refined with the development of nonionic contrast media, and the test was combined with CT; however, even this appears to have been supplanted by MRI of the spine.

The standard procedure for disc removal was a total laminectomy followed by a transdural approach to the disc. In 1939 Semmes presented a new procedure to remove the ruptured intervertebral disc that included subtotal laminectomy and retraction of the dural sac to expose and remove the ruptured disc with the patient under local anesthesia. Love in the same year also described this same technique independently. This procedure, now the classic approach for the removal of an intervertebral disc, has been improved with the use of microscopic and video imaging. Kambin, Onik, and Helms and others have popularized minimally invasive techniques for selected disc hernias.

As more people were treated for herniated lumbar discs, it became obvious that surgery was not universally successful. Over the past several decades, studies of patients with back or leg pain have led to improved treatment of those in whom a specific diagnosis was possible. Unfortunately, this group remains the minority of patients who are evaluated for low back or leg pain. Complex psychosocial issues, depression, and secondary gain are but a few of the nonanatomical problems that must be considered when evaluating these patients. In addition, the number of anatomical causes for these symptoms has increased as our understanding and diagnostic capabilities have increased. In an attempt to identify other causes of back pain Mooney and Robertson popularized facet injections, thus resurrecting an idea proposed originally in 1911 by Goldthwait. Smith et al. in 1963 approached the problem by suggesting a radical departure in treatment—enzymatic dissolution of the disc by injection of chymopapain. Although this technique is still used in Europe, it rarely is used in the United States because of medicolegal concerns.

The anatomical dissections and clinical observations of Kirkaldy-Willis and associates identified pathological processes associated with or complicating the process of spinal aging as primary causes of disc disease. Additional information about this process and its treatment continues to be collected.

A thorough and complete history of all aspects of lumbar spinal surgery was compiled by Wiltse in 1987.

Epidemiology

Back pain, the ancient curse, is now an international health issue of major significance. Hult estimated that up to 80% of people are affected by this symptom at some time in their lives. Impairments of the back and spine are ranked as the most frequent cause of limitation of activity in people younger than 45 years by the National Center for Health Statistics. Physicians who treat patients with spinal disorders and spine-related complaints must distinguish the complaint of back pain, which several epidemiological studies reveal to be relatively constant, from disability attributed to back pain. In 1984, disability was noted by Waddell to be exponentially increasing in the United Kingdom (Fig. 39-1). Conversely, an insurance industry study revealed a trend toward decreasing claim rates for low back pain in the United States from 1987 to 1995.

Although back pain as a presenting complaint may account for only 2% of the patients seen by a general practitioner, Dillane, Fry, and Kalton reported that in 79% of men and 89% of women the specific cause was unknown. Svensson and Andersson noted the lifetime incidence of low back pain to be 61% and the prevalence to be 31% in a random sample of 40- to 47-year-old men. They noted that 40% of those reporting back pain also reported sciatica. In women 38 to 64 years of age the lifetime incidence of low back pain was 66% with a prevalence of 35%. Svensson and Anderson noted psychological variables associated with low back pain to be dissatisfaction with the work environment and a higher degree of worry and fatigue at the end of the workday. The cost to society and the patient in the form of lost work time, compensation, and treatment is staggering. Snook reported that Liberty Mutual Insurance Company paid $247 million for compensable back

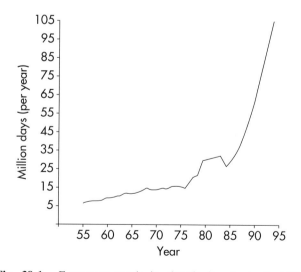

Fig. 39-1 Forty-year trends in chronic low back disability. United Kingdom statistics for sickness and invalidity benefits for back incapacities from 1953-1954 to 1993-1994 (based on statistics supplied by the Department of Social Security). (From Waddell G: *Spine* 21:2820, 1996.)

pain in 1980. Because this company represents only 9% of the insured workers' compensation market, Webster and Snook estimated the compensable costs of low back pain in the United States to be $11.1 billion in 1989. They reported that the mean cost of each reported claim of low back pain at Liberty Mutual had increased from $6807 in 1986 to $8321 in 1989, although they suggested that an increase in premiums sold, not an increase in low back pain claims, was the reason for this rise. More recent data from Liberty Mutual estimates that $8.8 billion was paid annually in the United States for claims related to low back pain. Of the billions of dollars spent annually in the United States because of back complaints, it was estimated that only about 39% was spent for medical treatment; the remaining costs were for disability payments. This did not include the losses from absenteeism. Although absenteeism because of back pain varies with the type of work, it rivals the common cold in total workdays lost.

Saal and Saal noted an 18% incidence of chronic back pain in 1135 adults; 80% of those reporting chronic pain did not report limitation of activity, and fewer than 4% reported significant limitation of activity. Females reported back pain more frequently than males. There were no racial differences, but the lower the educational level of those interviewed the greater the proportion of those reporting back pain. In 1992 Carey et al. interviewed 4437 North Carolinians by telephone and noted an incidence of 3.9% chronic low back pain. Of those who reported having chronic low back pain, 34% said that they were permanently disabled. These authors concluded that chronic back pain is common and associated with high costs. In the Netherlands van Doorn noted that the low back pain disability claims for self-employed dentists, veterinarians, physicians, and physical therapists increased 211% from 1977 to 1989, and the cost increased 13% over that same time period. Frymoyer and Cats-Baril noted an increase of 2500% in awards for back pain disability by the Social Security Disability Insurance from 1957 to 1976. They estimated that the total cost of low back pain was $25 billion to $100 billion per year, with 75% of those costs attributed to the 5% who became permanently disabled.

Multiple factors affect the development of back pain. Frymoyer et al. noted that risk factors associated with severe lower back pain include jobs requiring heavy and repetitive lifting, the use of jackhammers and machine tools, and the operation of motor vehicles. They also noted that patients with severe pain were more likely to be cigarette smokers and had a greater tobacco consumption. In an earlier study Frymoyer et al. noted that patients complaining of back pain reported more episodes of anxiety and depression; they also had more stressful occupations. Women with back pain had a greater number of pregnancies than those who did not. Jackson, Simmons, and Stripinis noted that adult patients with scoliosis are more likely to have back pain and that the pain persists and progresses. Deyo and Bass noted a strong relationship between smoking and back pain in patients younger than 45 years of age. They also noted a greater tendency for back pain in those patients who were the most obese. Other investigators, how-

ever, have found no relationship between obesity and back pain. Svensson and Anderson associated low back pain with cardiovascular risk factors, including calf pain on exertion, high physical activity at work, smoking, frequent worry, tension, and monotonous work.

The incidence of back pain appears to be constant. Efforts are being made to decrease the physical risk factors that may lead to low back pain. However, as shown by Boos et al., nonanatomical factors, specifically work perception and psychosocial factors, are intimately intertwined with physical complaints. Compounding diagnostic and treatment difficulties is the high incidence of significant abnormalities demonstrated by imaging studies, which in asymptomatic matched controls is as high as 76%.

General Disc and Spine Anatomy

The development of the spine begins in the third week of gestation and continues until the third decade of life. Formation of the primitive streak marks the beginning of spinal development, which is followed by the formation of the notochordal process. This process induces neurectodermal, ectodermal, and mesodermal differentiation.

Somites form in the mesodermal tissue adjacent to the neural tube (neurectoderm) and notochord. They number 42 to 44 in humans. The somites begin to migrate in preparation for the formation of skeletal structures. At the same time, the portion of the somites around the notochord separates into a sclerotome with loosely packed cells cephalad and densely packed cells caudally. Each sclerotome then separates at the junction of the loose and densely packed cells. The caudal dense cells migrate to the cephalad loose cells of the next more caudal sclerotome (Fig. 39-2).

The space where the sclerotome separates eventually forms the intervertebral disc. Vessels that originally were positioned between the somites now overlie the middle of the vertebral body. As the vertebral bodies form, the notochord that is in the center degenerates. The only remaining notochordal remnant forms the nucleus pulposus. Pazzaglia, Salisbury, and Byers reviewed the involution of the notochord in fetal and embryonic spines by several histological methods and concluded that all chordal cells disappear by early childhood. Notochordal remnants usually are not distinguishable in the adult nucleus pulposus.

The intervertebral disc in adults is composed of the annulus fibrosus and the nucleus pulposus. The annulus fibrosus is composed of numerous concentric rings or layers of fibrocartilaginous tissue. Fibers in each ring cross diagonally, and the rings attach to each other with additional radial fibers. The rings are thicker anteriorly (ventrally) than posteriorly (dorsally). The nucleus pulposus, a gelatinous material, forms the center of the disc. Because of the structural imbalance of the annulus, the nucleus is slightly posterior (dorsal) in relation to the disc as a whole. The discs vary in size and shape with their position in the spine. Discs also decrease in volume, resulting in a 16% to

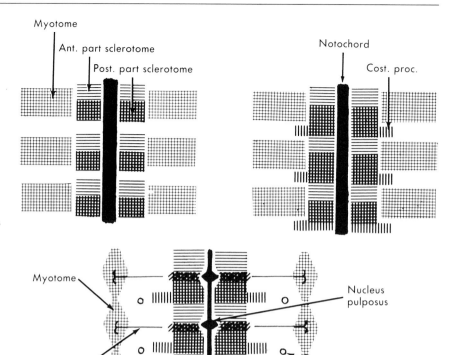

Fig. 39-2 Schematic representation of development of vertebrae and discs. (From Rothman RH, Simeone FA: *The spine*, vol 1, Philadelphia, 1982, WB Saunders.)

21% loss in disc height after 6 hours of standing or sitting. T2-weighted MRI signals increase as much as 25% after a night of bed rest. This diurnal variation has been substantiated by Botsford et al. and Paajanen et al.

The nucleus pulposus is composed of a loose, nonoriented, collagen fibril framework supporting a network of cells resembling fibrocytes and chondrocytes. This entire structure is embedded in a gelatinous matrix of various glucosaminoglycans, water, and salts. This material usually is under considerable pressure and is restrained by the crucible-like annulus. Inoue demonstrated that the cartilage endplate contains no fibrillar connection with the collagen of the subchondral bone of the vertebra. This lack of interconnection between the endplate and the vertebra may render the disc biomechanically weak against horizontal shearing forces. Inoue also demonstrated that the collagen fibrils in the outer two thirds of the annulus fibrosus are firmly anchored into the vertebral bodies (Fig. 39-3).

The intervertebral disc in the adult is avascular. Rudert and Tillmann were able to demonstrate blood vessels in the annulus until the age of 20 years and within the cartilage endplates until the age of 7 years. The cells within the disc are sustained by diffusion of nutrients into the disc through the porous central concavity of the vertebral endplate. Histological studies have shown regions where the marrow spaces are in direct contact with the cartilage and that the central portion of the endplate is permeable to dye. Motion and weight-bearing are believed to be helpful in maintaining this diffusion. The metabolic turnover

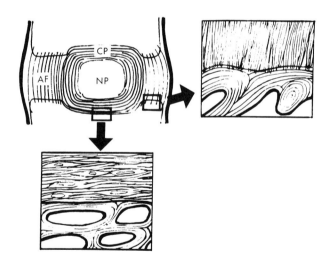

Fig. 39-3 Schematic representation of orientation of fibers in disc and endplate. *AF,* Annulus fibrosus; *NP,* nucleus pulposus; *CP,* cartilaginous plate. (From Inoue H: *Spine* 6:139, 1981.)

of the disc is relatively high when its avascularity is considered but slow compared with other tissues. The glycosaminoglycan turnover in the disc is quite slow, requiring 500 days. Inoue postulated that the degeneration of the disc may be prompted by decreased permeability of the cartilage endplate, which is normally dense.

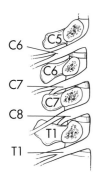
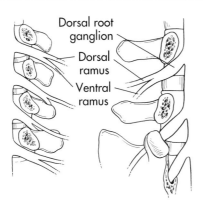
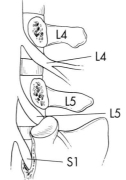

Fig. 39-4   Discs are named for vertebral level immediately cephalad. Pathology most commonly affects nerve root one segment caudal.

NEURAL ELEMENTS

The organization of the neural elements is strictly maintained throughout the entire neural system, even within the conus medullaris and cauda equina distally. Wall et al. noted that the orientation of the nerve roots in the dural sac and at the conus medullaris follows a highly organized pattern, with the most cephalad roots lying lateral and the most caudal lying centrally. The motor roots are ventral to the sensory roots at all levels. The arachnoid mater holds the roots in these positions.

The pedicle is the key to understanding surgical spinal anatomy. The relation of the pedicle to the neural elements varies by region within the spinal column. In the cervical region, there are seven vertebrae but eight cervical roots. Therefore, accepted nomenclature allows each cervical root to exit cephalad to the pedicle of the vertebra for which it is named (e.g., the C6 nerve root exits above or cephalad to the C6 pedicle). This relationship changes in the thoracic spine because the eighth cervical root exits between the C7 and T1 pedicles, requiring the T1 root to exit caudal or below the pedicle for which it is named. This relationship is maintained throughout the remaining more caudal segments. Of importance, the naming of the disc levels is different, in that all levels where discs are present are named for the vertebral level immediately cephalad (i.e., the C6 disc is immediately caudal to the C6 vertebra and disc pathology at that level typically would involve the C7 nerve root). In the lumbar spine classically a similar relationship exists in that disc pathology most commonly affects the nerve root one segment caudal (e.g., an L4 disc herniation would be expected to cause L5 root symptoms and findings) (Fig. 39-4).

At the level of the intervertebral foramen is the dorsal root ganglion. The ganglion lies within the outer confines of the foramen. Distal to the ganglion three distinct branches arise; the most prominent and important is the ventral ramus, which supplies all structures ventral to the neural canal. The second branch, the sinu-vertebral nerve, is a small filamentous nerve that originates from the ventral ramus and progresses medially over the posterior aspect of the disc and vertebral bodies, innervating these structures and the posterior longitudinal ligament. The third branch is the dorsal ramus. This branch courses dorsally, piercing the intertransverse ligament near the

pars interarticularis. Three branches from the dorsal ramus innervate the structures dorsal to the neural canal. The lateral and intermediate branches provide innervation to the posterior musculature and skin. The medial branch separates into three branches to innervate the facet joint at that level and the adjacent levels above and below (Fig. 39-5).

Pedersen, Blunck, and Gardner noted that the clinically significant function of the sinu-vertebral nerves and the posterior rami is the transmission of pain. The proprioceptive functions of these nerves are not known but assumed.

Studies by Bogduk and others demonstrated neural fibers in the outer layers of the annulus. These fibers are branches of the sinu-vertebral nerve dorsally. Ventral branches arise from the sympathetic chain that courses anterolaterally over the vertebral bodies. Rhalmi et al., using histological methods, demonstrated neural elements in all spinal ligaments. In the ligamentum flavum the nerve fibers are close to blood vessels and fat globules.

ANATOMICAL PROPORTIONS

Variation in the ratio of the cross-sectional area of the neural elements to the cross-sectional area of the spinal canal at various levels is relatively large. This is particularly true in patients with developmental stenosis in whom otherwise relatively minor intrusion into the spinal canal by pathological anatomy may cause compression of the neural structures. Many studies have documented that the changes in the foraminal dimensions increase with flexion and decrease with extension. Also, disc space narrowing causes significant volumetric decreases in the neural foramen at all levels.

Natural History of Disc Disease

The natural process of spinal aging has been studied by Kirkaldy-Willis and Hill and by others through observation of clinical and anatomical data. One theory of spinal degeneration assumes that all spines degenerate and that our current methods of treatment are for symptomatic relief, not for a cure.

The degenerative process has been divided into three separate stages with relatively distinct findings. The first stage

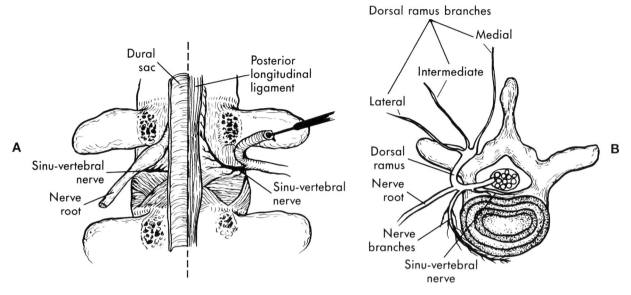

Fig. 39-5 **A,** Dorsal view of lumbar spinal segment with lamina and facets removed. On left side, dura and root exiting at that level remain. On right side, dura has been resected and root is elevated. Sinu-vertebral nerve with its course and innervation of posterior longitudinal ligament is usually obscured by nerve root and dura. **B,** Cross-sectional view of spine at level of endplate and disc. Note that sinu-vertebral nerve innervates dorsal surface of disc and posterior longitudinal ligament. Additional nerve branches from ventral ramus innervate more ventral surface of disc and anterior longitudinal ligament. Dorsal ramus arises from root immediately on leaving foramen. This ramus divides into lateral, intermediate, and medial branches. Medial branch supplies primary innervation to facet joints dorsally.

is dysfunction, which is seen in those 15 to 45 years of age. It is characterized by circumferential and radial tears in the disc annulus and localized synovitis of the facet joints. Varlotta et al. noted a familial predisposition to lumbar disc herniation in patients who had disc herniation before the age of 21 years. In this group the familial incidence was 32% compared with a matched control group of asymptomatic individuals in whom the rate was only 7%. A case control study of familial degenerative disc disease revealed a similar incidence of degenerative changes between first-order relatives of those with documented lumbar disc herniations and those without such a family history. However, the first-order relatives did have statistically significant more severe degenerative change.

The next stage is instability. This stage, found in 35- to 70-year-old patients, is characterized by internal disruption of the disc, progressive disc resorption, degeneration of the facet joints with capsular laxity, subluxation, and joint erosion. The final stage, present in patients older than 60 years, is stabilization. In this stage the progressive development of hypertrophic bone about the disc and facet joints leads to segmental stiffening or frank ankylosis (Table 39-1).

Each spinal segment degenerates at a different rate. As one level is in the dysfunction stage, another may be entering the stabilization stage. Disc herniation in this scheme is considered a complication of disc degeneration in the dysfunction and instability stages. Spinal stenosis from degenerative arthritis in this scheme is a complication of bony overgrowth compromis-

ing neural tissue in the late instability and early stabilization stages. Mayoux-Benhamou et al. noted that a 4-mm collapse of the disc produces sufficient narrowing of the foramen to threaten the nerve.

The stages and progression of degeneration have been confirmed by histological studies. Miller, Schmatz, and Schultz noted that disc degeneration progresses histologically as age increases. Males were found to have more degeneration than females. L4-5 and L3-4 disc levels showed the greatest degree of disc degeneration. Urban and McMullin noted that the hydration of disc material decreased with age. The relationship between the change in hydration and swelling pressure was dependent on the composition of the disc rather than on the age of the patient or the degree of degeneration. In their study L1-2 and L5-S1 discs had the lowest hydration. Yasuma et al. noted progressive histological changes in the prolapsed discs when compared with protruded discs. Urovitz and Fornasier were unable to detect any evidence of autoimmune reaction in human disc tissue, but they did detect evidence of the response to mechanical injury. Using postmyelogram CT scans, Takata et al. found that the cauda equina and affected nerve roots were swollen in 17 of 28 patients studied. The affected roots returned to normal size after disc excision. Ziv et al. reported coarsely fibrillated and ulcerated spinal facet joints in young patients, and this finding continued through progressive aging. The cartilage of the superior facets is thicker and has a higher water content than the inferior facets, indicating more frequent

Table 39-1 Spectrum of Pathological Changes in Facet Joints and Discs and the Interaction of These Changes

Phases of Spinal Degeneration	Facet Joints		Pathological Result		Intervertebral Disc
Dysfunction	Synovitis	→	Dysfunction	←	Circumferential tears
	Hypermobility		↓	↖	
	Continuing degeneration	↗	Herniation	←	Radial tears
Instability	Capsular laxity	→	Instability	←	Internal disruption
	Subluxation	→	Lateral nerve entrapment	←	Disc resorption
Stabilization	Enlargement of articular	→	One-level stenosis	←	Osteophytes
	processes	↘	Multilevel spondylosis and stenosis	↙	

Modified from Kirkaldy-Willis WH, ed: *Managing low back pain,* New York, 1983, Churchill Livingstone.

damage. Neumann et al. suggested that the amount of bone tissue in the spine may be functionally related to the structural properties of the spinal ligaments.

Long-term follow-up studies of lumbar disc herniations by Hakilius in 1970, Weber in 1983, and Seal in 1996 consistently documented several principles, the foremost being that generally symptomatic lumbar disc herniation (which is only one of the consequences of disc degeneration) has a favorable outcome in most patients. This was pointed out by Weber, who noted that the primary benefit of surgery was early on in the first year, but that with time the statistical significance of the improvement was lost. In addition, the review by Saal supported an active care approach, minimizing centrally acting medications. The judicious use of epidural steroids also is supported. Nonprogressive neurological deficits (except cauda equina syndrome) can be treated nonoperatively with expected improvement clinically. If surgery is necessary, it usually can be delayed 6 to 12 weeks to allow adequate opportunity for improvement. These principles are consistent with clinical findings and treatment practices at this clinic. Clearly, some patients are best treated surgically, and this is discussed in the section dealing specifically with lumbar disc herniation. Similar principles are valid regarding cervical disc herniations, which also generally can be treated nonoperatively. The important exceptions are patients with cervical myelopathy, who are best treated surgically.

The natural history of disc disease is one of recurrent episodes of pain followed by periods of significant or complete relief. Biering-Sørensen and Hilden noted that the memory of painful low back episodes was short. At initial evaluation and at 6 months' follow-up the question of ever having had low back pain was answered by patients with a *yes* or *no* and 84% answered consistently on the two occasions. However, in a questionnaire at 12 months only two fifths of those interviewed answered consistently. They questioned the long-term analysis of data from this standpoint and noted that the clinician should be aware of the potential vagueness and unreliability of a history of previous back injury.

Before a discussion of diagnostic studies, axial spine pain with radiation to one or more extremity must be considered.

Also, our understanding of certain pathophysiological entities must be juxtaposed to other entities of which we have only a rudimentary understanding. It is doubtful if there is any other area of orthopaedics in which accurate diagnosis is as difficult or the proper treatment as challenging as in patients with persistent neck and arm or low back and leg pain, despite appropriate evaluation and care. Although there are many patients with clear diagnoses properly arrived at by careful history and physical examination with confirmatory imaging studies, more patients with pain have absent neurological findings other than sensory changes and have normal imaging studies or studies that do not support the clinical complaints and findings. Inability to easily demonstrate an appropriate diagnosis in a patient does not relieve the physician of the obligation to recommend treatment or to direct the patient to a setting where such treatment is available. Careful assessment of these patients to determine if they have problems that can be orthopaedically treated (nonsurgically or surgically) is imperative to avoid overtreatment as well as undertreatment. Surgical treatment can benefit a patient if it corrects a deformity, corrects instability, or relieves neural compression, or treats a combination of these problems. Obtaining a history and completing a physical examination to determine a diagnosis that should be supported by other diagnostic studies is a very useful approach; conversely, matching the diagnosis and treatment to the results of diagnostic studies, as is done in other subspecialties of orthopaedics, is fraught with difficulty.

As pointed out by Waddell, most patients with nonspecific complaints and findings are best treated by their primary care physicians. For those with significant findings, evaluation and treatment by a specialist is appropriate. For a small minority of patients (although they are responsible for a much more significant portion of health care utilization) a multidisciplinary approach is best.

NONSPECIFIC LUMBAR PAIN

Nonspecific low back pain occurs at some point in the lives of most people. In Western societies a lifetime incidence of approximately 80% has been documented. A study of 1389

Table 39-2   Selective Indications for Roentgenography in Acute Low Back Pain

Age >50 years
Significant trauma
Neuromuscular deficits
Unexplained weight loss (10 pounds in 6 months)
Suspicion of ankylosing spondylitis
Drug or alcohol abuse
History of cancer
Use of corticosteroids
Temperature ≥37.8° C (100.0° F)
Recent visit (within 1 month) for same problem and no
    improvement
Patient seeking compensation for back pain

Adapted from Deyo RA, Diehl AK: *J Gen Intern Med* 1:20, 1986.

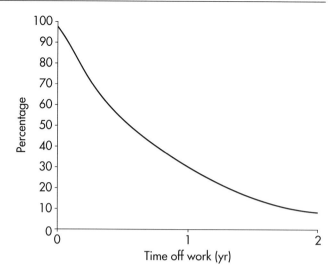

Fig. 39-6   Diminishing chance of return to work with increasing time out of work resulting from low back pain (based on data from Clinic Standards Advisory Group). (From Waddell G: *Spine* 21:2820, 1996.)

adolescents aged 13 to 16 years recorded low back pain in nearly 60%. The incidence and severity of this problem has remained fairly constant since the early 1980s. Appropriate treatment for what can be at times excruciating pain generally should begin with evaluation for significant spinal pathology. This being absent, a brief (1 to 3 days) period of bed rest with institution of an antiinflammatory regimen and rapid progression to an active exercise regimen with an anticipated return to full activity should be expected and encouraged. Generally, patients treated in this manner improve significantly in 4 to 8 weeks. Diagnostic studies, including roentgenograms, often are unnecessary because they add little information. More sophisticated imaging with CT scans and MRI or other studies have even less utility initially. An overdependence on the diagnosis of disc herniation occurred with early use of these diagnostic studies that show disc herniations in 20% to 36% of normal volunteers. This incidence increased to 76% of asymptomatic controls when they were matched to a population at risk for work-related lumbar pain complaints. Imaging guidelines have been set forth by Bigos et al. and Deyo and Diehl (Table 39-2).

Patients should understand that persistence of some pain is not indicative of treatment failure, necessitating further measures; however, it is important for treating physicians to recognize that the longer a person is limited by pain, the less likely is a return to full activity. Once a patient is out of work for 6 months, there is only a 50% chance that he will return to his previous job (Fig. 39-6).

For patients who do not respond to treatment regimens, early recognition that other issues may be involved is essential. Careful reassessment of complaints and reexamination for new information or findings as well as inconsistencies are necessary. Many studies of occupational back pain have revealed that depression, occupational mental stress, job satisfaction, intensity of concentration, anxiety, and marital status can be related to complaints of pain and disability. The role of these factors as causal or consequential of the symptoms remains an area of continued study; however, there is certainly some evidence that the psychological stresses occur before complaints of pain in

some patients. Another finding that is evident from the literature is the inability of physicians to detect psychosocial factors adequately without using specific instruments designed for this purpose in patients with back pain. In one particular study by Grevitt et al. experienced spinal surgeons were able to identify distressed patients only 26% of the time based on patient interviews. Given the difficulty of identifying patients with psychosocial distress, being aware of the high incidence of incidental abnormal findings on imaging studies underscores the need for critical individual review of these studies by treating physicians. Severe nerve compression demonstrated by MRI or CT correlates with symptoms of distal leg pain; however, mild to moderate nerve compression (Table 39-3), disc degeneration or bulging, and central stenosis do not significantly correlate with specific pain patterns.

A review of the pertinent literature reveals that similar psychological factors are important in patients with neck pain. As confounding as these psychological risk factors are, reasonable and logical measures are available that assist in evaluation and treatment.

Diagnostic Studies

ROENTGENOGRAPHY

The simplest and most readily available diagnostic tests for back or neck pain are anteroposterior and lateral roentgenograms of the involved spinal segment. These simple roentgenograms show a relatively high incidence of abnormal findings. Ford and Goodman reported only 7.3% normal spine roentgenograms in a group of 1614 patients evaluated for back pain. Scavone, Latshaw, and Rohrer reported a 46% incidence of abnormal incidental findings in lumbar spine films taken over

Table 39-3 Classification for Spinal Nerve and Thecal Sac Deformation

SPINAL NERVE DEFORMATION IN LATERAL RECESS OR INTERVERTEBRAL FORAMEN

0—Absent	No visible disc material contacting or deforming nerve
I—Minimal	Contact with disc material deforming nerve but displacement less than 2 mm
II—Moderate	Contact with disc material displacing 2 or more mm. The nerve is still visible and not obscured by disc material
III—Severe	Contact with disc material completely obscuring the nerve

THECAL SAC DEFORMATION IN VERTEBRAL CANAL

0—Absent	No visible disc material contacting or deforming thecal sac
I—Minimal	Disc material in contact with thecal sac
II—Moderate	Disc material deforming thecal sac, anteroposterior distance of thecal sac ≥7 mm
III—Severe	Disc material deforming thecal sac, anteroposterior distance of thecal sac <7 mm

From Beattie PF, Meyers SP, Strafford P, et al: *Spine* 25:819, 2000.

1 year in a university hospital. Unfortunately, when these roentgenographic abnormalities are critically evaluated with respect to the patients' complaints and physical findings, the correlation is very low. Fullenlove and Williams clearly identified the lack of definition between roentgenographic findings in symptomatic, asymptomatic, and operated patients. Rockey et al. and Liang and Komaroff concluded that spinal roentgenograms on the initial visit for acute low back pain do not contribute to patient care and are not cost effective. They recommended that plain roentgenograms be taken only after the initial therapy fails, especially in patients younger than 45 years of age.

There is insignificant correlation between back pain and the roentgenographic findings of lumbar lordosis, transitional vertebra, disc space narrowing, disc vacuum sign, and claw spurs. In addition, the entity of disc space narrowing is extremely difficult to quantify in all but the operated backs or in obviously abnormal circumstances. Frymoyer et al. in a study of 321 patients found that only when traction spurs or obvious disc space narrowing or both were present did the incidence of severe back and leg pain, leg weakness, and numbness increase. These positive findings had no relationship to heavy lifting, vehicular exposure, or exposure to vibrating equipment. Other studies have shown some relationship between back pain and the findings of spondylolysis, spondylolisthesis, and adult scoliosis, but these findings also can be observed in spine roentgenograms of asymptomatic patients.

Special roentgenographic views can be helpful in further defining or disproving the initial clinical roentgenographic impression. Oblique views are useful in further defining spondylolisthesis and spondylolysis but are of limited use in facet syndrome and hypertrophic arthritis of the lumbar spine. Conversely, in the cervical spine hypertrophic changes about the foramina are easily outlined. Lateral flexion and extension roentgenograms may reveal segmental instability. Hayes et al. attempted to identify the pathological level of abnormal lumbar spine flexion, but they found a wide range of motion in asymptomatic patients. They also found that translational movements of 2 to 3 mm were frequent, which means that there is little correlation between abnormal motion and pathological instability. No standards are available to make this distinction. Unfortunately, the interpretation of these views depends on patient cooperation, patient positioning, and reproducible technique. Knutsson, Farfan, Kirkaldy-Willis, Stokes et al., Macnab, and Bigos are excellent references on this topic. The Ferguson view (20-degree caudocephalic anteroposterior roentgenogram) has been shown by Wiltse et al. to be of value in the diagnosis of the "far out syndrome," that is, fifth root compression produced by a large transverse process of the fifth lumbar vertebra against the ala of the sacrum. Abel, Smith, and Allen note that angled caudal views localized to areas of concern may show evidence of facet or laminar pathological conditions.

◆ MYELOGRAPHY

The value of myelography is the ability to check all disc levels for abnormality and to define intraspinal lesions; it may be unnecessary if clinical and CT findings are in complete agreement. The primary indications for myelography are suspicion of an intraspinal lesion or questionable diagnosis resulting from conflicting clinical findings and other studies. In addition, myelography is of value in a previously operated spine and in patients with marked bony degenerative change that may be underestimated on MRI. Myelography is improved by the use of postmyelography CT scanning in this setting, as well as in evaluating spinal stenosis. Bell et al. found myelography more accurate than CT scanning for identifying herniated nucleus pulposus and only slightly more accurate than CT scanning in the detection of spinal stenosis. Szypryt et al. found myelography slightly less accurate than MRI in detecting spinal abnormalities.

Several contrast agents have been used for myelography: air, oil contrast, and water-soluble (absorbable) contrast including metrizamide (Amipaque), iohexol (Omnipaque), and iopamidol (Isovue-M). Since these nonionic agents are absorbable, the discomfort of removing them and the severity of the post-myelographic headache have been decreased.

Isophendylate (Pantopaque) was the contrast agent of choice from 1944 to the late 1970s (Fig. 39-7). This agent required aspiration at the conclusion of the study and was more of a meningeal irritant than the nonionic materials currently available. Occasionally, older patients are seen with small amounts of residual Pantopaque within the subarachnoid space. Rarely, patients have severe reactions such as transient paralysis, cauda equina syndrome, or focal neurological deficits.

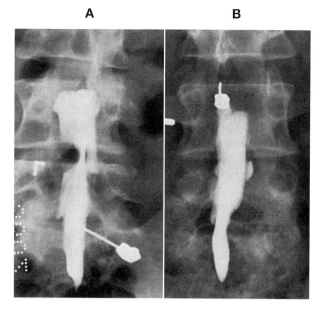

Fig. 39-7   A, Posteroanterior roentgenogram of iophendylate (Pantopaque) myelogram showing lumbar disc herniation. **B,** Oblique roentgenogram showing large L4-5 disc herniation.

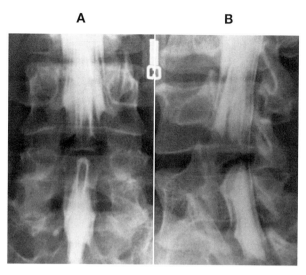

Fig. 39-8   A, Posteroanterior roentgenogram of metrizamide lumbar myelogram showing lumbar disc herniation. **B,** Oblique roentgenogram showing large L4-5 disc herniation.

Arachnoiditis is a severe complication that has been attributed on occasion to the combination of isophendylate and blood in the cerebrospinal fluid (CSF). Unfortunately, this diagnosis usually is confirmed only by repeat myelography. Attempts at surgical neurolysis have resulted in only short-term relief and a return of symptoms within 6 to 12 months after the procedure. Fortunately, time may decrease the effects of this serious problem in some patients, but progressive paralysis has been reported in rare instances. Arachnoiditis also can be caused by tuberculosis and other types of meningitis. Arachnoiditis has not been noted to be related to the use of water-soluble contrast, with or without injection, in the presence of a bloody tap. Myelography remains the best diagnostic study to evaluate arachnoiditis.

Water-soluble contrast media are now the standard agents for myelography (Fig. 39-8). Their advantages include absorption by the body, enhanced definition of structures, tolerance, absorption from other soft tissues, and the ability to vary the dosage for different contrasts. Like isophendylate they are meningeal irritants, but they have not been associated with arachnoiditis. The complications of these agents include nausea, vomiting, confusion, and seizures. Rare complications include stroke, paralysis, and death. Iohexol and iopamidol have significantly lower complication rates than metrizamide. The more common complications appear to be related to patient hydration, phenothiazines, tricyclics, and migration of contrast into the cranial vault. Many of the reported complications can be prevented or minimized by using the lowest possible dose to achieve the desired degree of contrast. Adequate hydration and discontinuation of phenothiazines and tricyclic drugs before, during, and after the procedure should also minimize the

incidence of the more common reactions. Likewise, maintenance of at least a 30-degree elevation of the patient's head until the contrast is absorbed also should help prevent reactions. Complete information about these agents and the dosages required is found in their package inserts.

Iohexol (Omnipaque) is a nonionic contrast medium approved for thoracic and lumbar myelography. The incidence of reactions to this medium is low. The most common reactions are headache (less than 20%), pain (8%), nausea (6%), and vomiting (3%). Serious reactions are very rare and include mental disturbances and aseptic meningitis (0.01%). Good hydration is essential to minimize the common reactions. The use of phenothiazine antinauseants is contraindicated when this medium is employed. Management before and after the procedure is the same as for metrizamide.

Air contrast is used rarely and probably should be used only in situations in which myelography is mandatory and the patient is extremely allergic to iodized materials. The resolution from such a procedure is poor. Air epidurography in conjunction with CT has been suggested in patients in whom further definition between postoperative scar and recurrent disc material is required.

Myelographic technique begins with a careful explanation of the procedure to the patient before its initiation. Hydration of the patient before the procedure may minimize postmyelographic complaints. Heavy sedation rarely is needed. Proper equipment, including a fluoroscopic unit with a spot film device, image intensification, tiltable table, and television monitoring, is useful. The type of needle selected also influences the risk of postdural puncture headaches (PDPH), which can be severe. Smaller gauge needles (22 or 25 gauge) have been found to result in a lower incidence of PDPH. Also, use of a Whitacre-type needle with a more blunt tip and side port opening results in fewer PDPH complaints.

The most common technical complications of myelography are significant retention of contrast medium (oil contrast only), persistent headache from a dural leak, and epidural injection. These problems usually are minor. Persistent dural leaks usually are responsive to a blood patch. With the use of a water-soluble contrast medium, the persistent abnormalities caused by retained medium and epidural injection are eliminated.

TECHNIQUE 39-1

Place the patient prone on the fluoroscopic table. Use of an abdominal pillow is optional. Prepare the back in the usual surgical fashion. Determine needle placement by the suspected pathological level. Placement of the needle cephalad to L2-3 is more dangerous because of the risk of damaging the conus medullaris.

Infiltrate the selected area of injection with a local anesthetic. Use the smallest-gauge needle that can be well placed. If a Whitacre-type needle is used, a 19-gauge needle may be placed through the skin, subcutaneous tissue, and fascia to form a track, since this relatively blunt needle may not penetrate these structures well. Midline needle placement usually minimizes lateral nerve root irritation and epidural injection. Advance the needle with the bevel parallel to the long axis of the body. Subarachnoid placement can be enhanced by tilting the patient up to increase intraspinal pressure and minimize the epidural space.

Once the dura and arachnoid have been punctured, turn the bevel of the needle cephalad. A clear continuous flow of CSF should continue with the patient prone. Manometric studies can be performed at this time if desired or indicated. Remove a volume of CSF equal to the planned injection volume for laboratory evaluation as indicated by the clinical suspicions. In most patients a cell count, differential white cell count, and protein analysis are performed.

Inject a test dose of the contrast material under fluoroscopic control to confirm a subarachnoid injection. If a mixed subdural-subarachnoid injection is suspected, change the needle depth; occasionally a lateral roentgenogram may be required to confirm the proper depth. If flow is good, inject the contrast material slowly.

Be certain of continued subarachnoid injection by occasionally aspirating as the injection continues. The usual dose of iohexol for lumbar myelography in an adult is 10 to 15 ml with a concentration of 170 to 190 mg/ml. Higher concentrations of water-soluble contrast are required if higher areas of the spine are to be demonstrated. Consult the package insert of the contrast used. The needle can be removed if a water-soluble contrast (iohexol) is used. The needle must remain in place and be covered with a sterile towel if isophendylate is used.

Allow the contrast material to flow caudally for the best views of the lumbar roots and distal sac. Make spot films in the anteroposterior, lateral, and oblique projections. A full lumbar examination should include thoracic evaluation to about the level of T7 because lesions at the thoracic level may mimic lumbar disc disease. Take additional spot films as the contrast proceeds cranially.

If a total or cervical myelogram is desired, allow the contrast to proceed cranially. Extend the neck and head maximally to prevent or minimize intracranial migration of the contrast medium.

If isophendylate (oil contrast) was used, remove the contrast medium by extracting through the original needle or a multiholed stylet inserted through the original needle or by inserting another needle if extraction through the first needle is difficult. A small amount of medium occasionally is retained, but remove as much as possible.

If blood is present in the initial tap, abandon the procedure if oil contrast is to be used. It can be attempted again in several days if the patient has no symptoms related to the first tap and is well hydrated. If the proper needle position is confirmed in the anteroposterior and lateral views and CSF flow is minimal or absent, suspect a neoplastic process. Then place the needle at a higher or lower level as indicated by the circumstances. If attempts to obtain CSF continue to fail, abandon the procedure and reevaluate the clinical situation.

COMPUTED TOMOGRAPHY

Computed tomography revolutionized the diagnosis of spinal disease (Fig. 39-9). Most clinicians now agree that CT is an extremely useful diagnostic tool in the evaluation of spinal disease.

The current technology and computer software have made possible the ability to reformat the standard axial cuts in almost any direction and magnify the images so that exact measurements of various structures can be made. Software is available to evaluate the density of a selected vertebra and compare it with vertebrae of the normal population to give a numerically reproducible estimate of vertebral density to quantitate osteopenia.

Numerous types of CT studies for the spine are available. These studies vary from institution to institution and even within institutions. One must be careful in ordering the study to be certain that the areas of clinical concern are included.

Several basic routines are used in most institutions. The most common routine for lumbar disc consists of making serial cuts through the last three lumbar intervertebral discs. If the equipment has a tilting gantry, an attempt is made to keep the axis of the cuts parallel with the disc. However, frequently the gantry cannot tilt enough to allow a parallel beam through the lowest disc space. This technique does not allow demon-

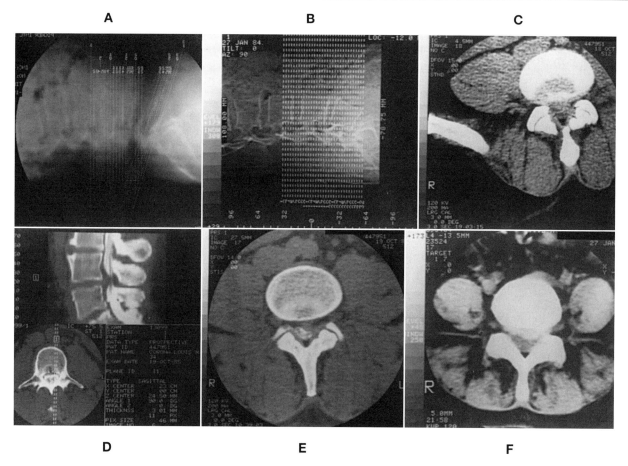

Fig. 39-9 **A,** CT scan "scout view" of lumbar disc herniation at lumbar disc level showing angled gantry technique. **B,** CT scan "scout view" of straight gantry technique. **C,** CT scan of lumbar disc herniation at L4-5 disc level showing cross-sectional anatomy with gantry straight. **D,** CT scan of L4-5 disc herniation at lumbar disc level showing cross-sectional, sagittal, and coronal anatomy using computerized reformatted technique. **E,** CT scan of L4-5 disc herniation at lumbar disc level showing cross-sectional anatomy 2 hours after metrizamide myelography. **F,** CT scan of lumbar disc herniation at L4-5 disc level showing cross-sectional anatomy after intravenous injection for greater soft tissue contrast.

stration of the canal at the pedicles. Another method involves making cuts through the discs without tilting the gantry. Once again, the entire canal is not demonstrated, and the lower cuts frequently have the lower and upper endplates of adjacent vertebrae superimposed in the same view.

The final and most complex method consists of making multiple parallel cuts at equal intervals. This allows computer reconstruction of the images in different planes—usually sagittal and coronal. These reformatted views allow an almost three-dimensional view of the spine and most of its structures. The greatest benefit of this technique is the ability to see beyond the limits of the dural sac and root sleeves. Thus the diagnosis of foraminal encroachment by bone or disc material can now be made in the face of a normal myelogram. The proper procedure can be chosen that fits all the pathological conditions involved.

Optimal reformatted CT should include enlarged axial and sagittal views with clear notation as to laterality and sequence of cuts. Several sections of the axial cuts should include the local soft tissue and contiguous abdominal contents. Finally, a set of images adjusted for improved bony detail should be included for evaluation of the facet joints as well as the lateral recesses. Naturally this study should be centered on the level of greatest clinical concern. The study can be enhanced further if done after water contrast myelography or with intravenous contrast medium. Enhancement techniques are especially useful if the spine being evaluated has been operated on previously.

This noninvasive, painless, outpatient procedure can supply more information about spinal disease than was previously available with a battery of invasive and noninvasive tests usually requiring hospitalization. Unfortunately, CT does not demonstrate intraspinal tumors or arachnoiditis and is unable to differentiate scar from recurrent disc herniation. Bell et al. compared myelography with CT scanning and noted that myelography was more accurate. They did not compare the

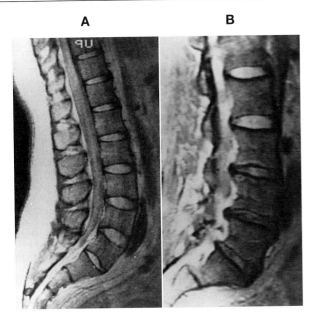

A   **B**

Fig. 39-10 Magnetic resonance imaging of lumbar spine. **A,** Normal T2-weighted image. **B,** T2-weighted image showing degenerative bulging and/or herniated discs at L3-4, L4-5, and L5-S1.

results of postmyelogram CT scanning. Weiss et al. and Teplick and Haskin in separate reports suggested that the use of intravenous contrast medium (Fig. 39-9, *E*) followed by CT can improve the definition between scar and disc herniation. Myelography is still required to demonstrate intraspinal tumors and to "run" the spine to detect occult or unsuspected lesions. The development of low-dose metrizamide or iohexol myelography with reformatted CT done as an outpatient procedure allows a maximum of information to be obtained with a minimum of time, risk, discomfort, and cost.

MAGNETIC RESONANCE IMAGING

Magnetic resonance imaging (MRI) is the newest technological advance in spinal imaging. This technique uses the interaction of an unpaired electron with an external oscillating electromagnetic field that is changing as a function of time at a particular frequency. Energy is absorbed and subsequently released by selected nuclei at particular frequencies after excitation with radiofrequency electromagnetic energy. The released energy is recorded and formatted by computer in a pattern similar to CT. Current MRI techniques concentrate on imaging the proton (hydrogen) distribution present as H_2O primarily. The advantages of this technique include the ability to demonstrate intraspinal tumors, examine the entire spine, and identify degenerative discs based on decreased H_2O content (Fig. 39-10). Unfortunately, the equipment required for this procedure is costly and requires specially constructed facilities.

Szypryt et al. found MRI slightly better than myelography in the identification of spinal lesions. The accuracy of MRI in their study was 88% and that of myelography was 75%;

combined accuracy was 94%. MRI is clearly superior in the detection of disc degeneration, tumors, and infections. Most MRI scans allow evaluation of a complete spinal region (such as cervical, thoracic, or lumbar) rather than three segments. They also can clearly view areas in the foramen and the paraspinal soft tissues.

MRI is so accurate that a significant number of lesions can be identified in asymptomatic patients. Gibson et al. found disc degeneration in all symptomatic adolescent patients and in 4 of 20 asymptomatic adolescents. Boden et al. found cervical spinal abnormalities in 14% of asymptomatic patients younger than 40 years of age and in 28% of asymptomatic patients over the age of 40 years. Cervical disc degeneration was found in 25% of those younger than 40 years of age and in 60% of those 60 years and older. They studied lumbar MRI scans of 67 asymptomatic patients and found that 20% of those younger than 60 years of age had herniated nuclei pulposi, which were also present in 36% of those over the age of 60 years. Asymptomatic abnormalities were found in 57% of those 60 years of age or older. Lumbar disc degeneration was found in 35% of those from 20 to 39 years of age and in 100% of those over 50 years of age. Therefore the demonstrated findings must be carefully correlated with the clinical impression.

POSITRON EMISSION TOMOGRAPHY

Positron emission tomography (PET) and single photon emission CT (SPECT) are other similar techniques that may offer additional diagnostic information. Collier et al. and others reported that SPECT is more sensitive than planar bone scintigraphy in the identification of symptomatic sites in spondylolysis. PET scanners are considered experimental by most third-party payers at this time. Their use currently is limited to relatively few centers.

Currently, imaging capabilities exceed clinical abilities to identify the source of pain. However, some patients may have nonanatomical causes for their pain and there is no imaginable explanation for their symptoms. In these patients, imaging studies are useful to rule out significant pathology that may explain their symptoms, such as with spinal cord tumors, infections, polyradiculopathies, or myeloradiculopathies.

OTHER DIAGNOSTIC TESTS

Numerous diagnostic tests have been used in the diagnosis of intervertebral disc disease in addition to roentgenography, myelography, and CT. The primary advantage of these tests is to rule out diseases other than primary disc herniation, spinal stenosis, and spinal arthritis.

Electromyography is the most notable of these tests. One advantage of electromyography is in the identification of peripheral neuropathy and diffuse neurological involvement indicative of higher or lower lesions. Electromyography and nerve conduction velocity can be helpful if a patient has a history and physical examination suggestive of radiculopathy at either the cervical or lumbar level with inconclusive imaging studies. Macnab et al. reported that denervation of the paraspinal muscles is found in 97% of previously operated lumbar spines as a result of the surgery. Therefore paraspinal muscles in a patient with a previous posterior operation usually are abnormal and are not a reliable diagnostic finding.

The somatosensory evoked potentials (SSEP) test is another diagnostic tool that can identify the level of root involvement. Unlike electromyography this test can only indicate a problem between the cerebral cortex and the end organs; the test cannot pinpoint the level of the lesion. This procedure is of benefit during surgery to avoid neurological damage. Both electromyography and SSEP depend on the skill of the technician and interpreter. Delamarter et al. used cortical evoked potentials to monitor experimentally induced spinal stenosis. They noted changes in the cortical response at 25% constriction. This was the only change noted in this group. Higher degrees of constriction were accompanied by much more significant changes. The SSEP is an extremely sensitive monitoring technique.

Bone scans are another procedure in which positive findings usually are not indicative of intervertebral disc disease, but they can confirm neoplastic, traumatic, and arthritic problems in the spine. Various laboratory tests such as a complete blood count, differential white cell count, biochemical profile, urinalysis, and sedimentation rate are extremely good screening procedures for other causes of pain in the spine. Rheumatoid screening studies such as rheumatoid arthritis latex, antinuclear antibody, lupus erythematosus cell preparation, and HLA-B27 also are useful when indicated by the clinical picture.

Some tests that were developed to enhance the diagnosis of intervertebral disc disease have been surpassed by the more advanced technology. Lumbar venography and sonographic measurement of the intervertebral canal are two examples.

Injection Studies

Whenever a diagnosis is in doubt and the complaints appear real or the pathological condition is diffuse, identification of the source of pain is problematic. The use of local anesthetics or contrast media in various specific anatomical areas can be useful. These agents are relatively simple, safe, and minimally painful. Contrast media such as diatrizoate meglamine (Hypaque), iothalamate meglumine (Conray), iohexol (Omnipaque), iopamidol, and metrizamide (Amipaque) have been used for discography and blocks with no reported ill effects. Reports of neurological complications with contrast media used for discography and subsequent chymopapain injection are well documented. The best choice of a contrast medium for documenting structures outside the subarachnoid space is an absorbable medium with low reactivity because it might be injected inadvertently into the subarachnoid space. Iohexol and metrizamide are the least reactive, most widely accepted, and best tolerated of the currently available contrast media. Local anesthetics such as lidocaine (Xylocaine), tetracaine (Pontocaine), and bupivacaine (Marcaine) are used frequently both epidurally and intradurally. The use of bupivacaine should be limited to low concentrations and low volumes because of reports of death after epidural anesthesia using concentrations of 0.75% or higher.

Steroids prepared for intramuscular injection also have been used frequently in the epidural space with few and usually transient complications. Spinal arachnoiditis in years past was associated with the use of epidural methylprednisolone acetate (Depo-Medrol). This complication was thought to be caused by the use of the suspending agent, polyethylene glycol, which has since been eliminated from the Depo-Medrol preparation. For epidural injections, we prefer the use of Celestone Soluspan, which is a mixture of betamethasone sodium phosphate and betamethasone acetate. Celestone Soluspan provides both immediate and long-term duration of action, is highly soluble, and contains no harmful preservatives. Isotonic saline is the only other injectable medium used frequently about the spine with no reported adverse reactions.

When discrete, well-controlled injection techniques directed at specific targets in and around the spine are used, grading the degree of pain before and after selective spinal injection is helpful in determining the location of the pain generator. The patient is asked to grade the degree of pain on a 0 to 10 scale before and at various intervals after the selective spinal injection (Box 39-1). If a selective spinal injection done under fluoroscopic control results in a 50% or more decrease in the level of pain, which corresponds to the duration of action of the anesthetic agent used, then the target area injected is presumed to be the pain generator.

EPIDURAL CORTISONE INJECTIONS

Epidural injections in the cervical, thoracic, and lumbosacral spine were developed to diagnose and treat spinal pain. Information obtained from epidural injections can be helpful in confirming pain generators that are responsible for a patient's discomfort. Structural abnormalities do not always cause pain and diagnostic injections can help to correlate abnormalities seen on imaging studies with associated pain complaints. In addition, epidural injections can provide pain relief during the recovery of disc or nerve root injuries and allow patients to increase their level of physical activity. Because severe pain from an acute disc injury with or without radiculopathy often is time-limited, therapeutic injections help to manage pain and may alleviate or decrease the need for oral analgesics.

Epidural injections were first done in the lumbar region. In 1901 the first reports were published of epidural injections of cocaine for low back pain and sciatica. In 1930 Evans reported good results in 22 of 40 patients treated with procaine and saline injection into the sacral epidural space for unilateral sciatica, and in the early 1950s Robecchi and Capral were the first to report epidural injection of cortisone into the first sacral neuroforamen for the treatment of low back pain. The earliest references for cervical epidural injections were published by Catchlove and Braha and Shulman et al. No historical information on thoracic epidural injections has been published.

BOX 39-1 • Pain Scale and Diary

0   No pain
1   Mild pain that you are aware of but not bothered by
2   Moderate pain that you can tolerate without medication
3   Moderate pain that is discomforting and requires medication
4-5   More severe and you begin to feel antisocial
6   Severe pain
7-9   Intensely severe pain
10   Most severe pain; you might contemplate suicide over it

Activity	Comments	Location of Pain	Time	Severity of Pain (0 to 10)

From White AH: *Back school and other conservative approaches to low back pain,* St Louis, 1983, Mosby.

The efficacy of epidural injections is not reliably known because of the lack of well-controlled studies. Inconsistencies in indications and protocols are striking among reports, and many epidural steroid injection studies were done without fluoroscopic-guided needle placement to confirm correct positioning, adding another variable to the interpretation of the results. Nevertheless, more than 40, mostly uncontrolled, studies on more than 4000 patients have been published on the efficacy of lumbar and caudal epidural corticosteroid injections, and according to Bogduk, only 4 recommended against the use of lumbosacral epidural corticosteroids in the management of radicular pain in the lumbosacral spine. Kepes and Duncalf calculated the average favorable response rate obtained with lumbar epidural steroid injections to be 60%, whereas White calculated the favorable response rate to be 75%. Several studies reported the usefulness of transforaminal epidural corticosteroid injections (selective epidural or selective nerve root block) to identify or confirm a specific nerve root as a pain generator when the diagnosis is not clear based on clinical evidence.

Few serious complications occur in patients receiving epidural corticosteroid injections; however, epidural abscess, epidural hematoma, durocutaneous fistula, and Cushing syndrome have been reported as individual case reports. The most adverse immediate reaction during an epidural injection is a vasovagal reaction. Dural puncture has been estimated to occur in 0.5% to 5% of patients having cervical or lumbar epidural steroid injections. The anesthesiology literature reported a 7.5% to 75% incidence of postdural puncture (positional) headaches, with the highest estimates associated with the use of 16- and 18-gauge needles. Headache without dural puncture has been estimated to occur in 2% and is attributed to air injected into the epidural space, increased intrathecal pressure from fluid around the dural sac, and possibly an undetected dural puncture. Some of the minor, more common complaints caused by corticosteroid injected into the epidural space include nonpositional headaches, fascial flushing, insomnia, low-grade fever, and transient increased back or lower extremity pain. Epidural corticosteroid injections are contraindicated in the presence of infection at the injection site, systemic infection, bleeding diathesis, uncontrolled diabetes mellitus, and congestive heart failure.

We do epidural corticosteroid injections in a fluoroscopy suite equipped with resuscitative and monitoring equipment. Intravenous access is established in all patients with a 20-gauge angiocatheter placed in the upper extremity. Mild sedation is achieved through intravenous access. We recommend the use of fluoroscopy for diagnostic and therapeutic epidural injections for several reasons. Epidural injections performed without fluoroscopic guidance are not always made into the epidural space or the intended interspace. Even in experienced hands, needle misplacement occurs in up to 40% of caudal and 30% of lumbar epidural injections when done without fluoroscopic guidance. Accidental intravascular injections also can occur, and the absence of blood return with needle aspiration before injection is not a reliable indicator of this complication. In the presence of anatomical anomalies, such as a midline epidural septum or multiple separate epidural compartments, the desired flow of epidural injectants to the presumed pain generator will be restricted and remain undetected without fluoroscopy. In addition, if an injection fails to relieve pain, it would be impossible without fluoroscopy to determine whether the failure was caused by a genuine poor response or by improper needle placement.

Cervical Epidural Injection

Cervical epidural steroid injections have been used with some success to treat cervical spondylosis associated with acute disc disruption and radiculopathies, cervical strain syndromes with associated myofascial pain, postlaminectomy cervical pain, reflex sympathetic dystrophy, postherpetic neuralgia, acute viral brachial plexitis, and muscle contraction headaches.

The best results with cervical epidural steroid injections have been in patients with acute disc herniations or well-defined radicular symptoms and in patients with limited myofascial pain.

◆ Interlaminar Approach

TECHNIQUE 39-2

Place the patient prone on a pain management table. We use a low-attenuated carbon fiber table top that allows better imaging and permits unobstructed C-arm viewing. For optimal placement and comfort, place the patient's face in a cervical prone cutout cushion. Cervical epidural injections using a paramedian approach should be done routinely at the C7-T1 interspace unless previous surgery of the posterior cervical spine has been done at that level, in which case the C6-C7 or T1-T2 level is injected. Aseptically prepare the skin area with isopropyl alcohol and povidone-iodine several segments above and below the laminar interspace to be injected. If the patient is allergic to povidone-iodine, then substitute with chlorhexidine gluconate (Hibiclens). Drape the patient in sterile fashion. Using anteroposterior fluoroscopic imaging, identify the target laminar interspace. With the use of a 27¼-gauge needle, anesthetize the skin so that a skin wheal is raised over the target interspace on the side of the patient's pain with 1 to 2 ml of 1% preservative-free Xylocaine without epinephrine. To diminish the burning discomfort of the anesthetic, mix 3 ml of 8.4% sodium bicarbonate in a 30-ml bottle of 1% preservative-free Xylocaine without epinephrine. Nick the skin with an 18-gauge hypodermic needle. Under fluoroscopic control insert and advance a 3½-inch, 22-gauge spinal needle in a vertical fashion until contact is made with the upper edge of the T1 lamina 1 to 2 mm lateral to the midline.

Anesthetize the lamina with 1 to 2 ml of 1% preservative-free Xylocaine without epinephrine. Then anesthetize the soft tissues with 2 ml of 1% preservative-free Xylocaine without epinephrine as the spinal needle is withdrawn. Insert a 3½-inch, 18-gauge Tuohy epidural needle and advance it vertically within the anesthetized soft tissue track until contact is made with the T1 lamina under fluoroscopy. "Walk off" the lamina with the Tuohy needle onto the ligamentum flavum. Remove the stylet from the Tuohy needle and attach a 10-ml syringe filled halfway with air and sterile saline. Advance the Tuohy needle into the epidural space using the loss of resistance technique. Once loss of resistance has been achieved, aspirate to check for blood or spinal fluid. If neither is evident, remove the syringe from the Tuohy needle and attach a 5-ml syringe containing 1.5 ml of nonionic contrast dye. Confirm epidural placement by producing an epidurogram with the nonionic contrast agent (Fig. 39-11). To further confirm proper placement adjust the C-arm to view the area from a lateral perspective. A spot roentgenogram can be obtained to document placement. Inject a test dose of 1 to 2 ml of 1% preservative-free Xylocaine without epinephrine and wait 3 minutes. If the patient is without complaints of warmth, burning, significant paresthesias, or signs of apnea, place a 10-ml syringe on the Tuohy needle and slowly inject 2 ml of 1% preservative-free Xylocaine without epinephrine and 2 ml of 6 mg/ml Celestone Soluspan slowly into the epidural space. If Celestone Soluspan cannot be obtained, 40 mg/ml of triamcinolone is a good substitute.

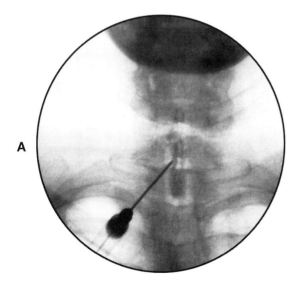 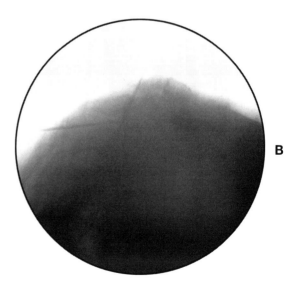

Fig. 39-11 **A,** Posteroanterior view of cervical interlaminar epidurogram demonstrating characteristic C7 to T1 epidural contrast flow pattern. **B,** Lateral roentgenogram of cervical epidurogram.

◆ Transforaminal Approach

TECHNIQUE 39-3

Place the patient in a modified lateral decubitus position with the painful side up on a pain management table. Aseptically prepare the skin area with isopropyl alcohol and povidone-iodine several segments above and below the neuroforamen to be injected. Drape the patient in sterile fashion. Identify the foramen level to be injected under fluoroscopy, orienting the beam so that it is slightly tilted caudal to cephalad and anterior to posterior to maximize the view of the neuroforamen. Insert and slowly advance a 3½-inch 25-gauge spinal needle until contact is made with the lower aspect of the superior articular process under fluoroscopy. Stay posterior to the foramen to avoid the vertebral artery. To maximize posterior positioning of the spinal needle bevel, orient the needle notch anteriorly. Orient the C-arm so that the fluoroscopy beam is in an anteroposterior projection. Redirect the spinal needle and "walk off" bone into the foramen 3 to 4 mm but no farther medially than the midpoint of the articular pillar on anteroposterior imaging. Remove the stylet. After a negative aspiration, inject 0.5 ml of nonionic contrast dye under fluoroscopy. Once an acceptable dye pattern is seen (filling of the oval neuroforamen and flow of contrast along the exiting nerve root), inject slowly a 1-ml volume, containing 0.5 ml of 2% to 4% preservative-free Xylocaine without epinephrine and 0.5 ml of 6 mg/ml Celestone Soluspan.

Thoracic Epidural Injection

Epidural steroid injections in the thoracic spine have been shown to provide relief from thoracic radicular pain secondary to disc herniations, trauma, diabetic neuropathy, herpes zoster, and idiopathic thoracic neuralgia, although reports in the literature are few.

◆ Interlaminar Approach

TECHNIQUE 39-4

A paramedian rather than a midline approach is used because of the angulation of the spinous processes. Place the patient prone on a pain management table. The preparation of the patient and equipment is identical to that used for interlaminar cervical epidural injections. Aseptically prepare the skin area several segments above and below the interspace to be injected. Drape the patient in sterile fashion. Identify the target laminar interspace using anteroposterior visualization under fluoroscopic guidance. Anesthetize the skin over the target interspace on the side of the patient's pain. Under fluoroscopic control, insert and advance a 3½-inch, 22-gauge spinal needle to the superior edge of the target lamina. Anesthetize the lamina and the soft tissues as the spinal needle is withdrawn. Mark the skin with an 18-gauge hypodermic needle and then insert a 3½-inch, 18-gauge Tuohy epidural needle and advance it at a 50- to 60-degree angle to the axis of the spine and a 15- to 30-degree angle toward the midline until contact with the lamina is made. To better view the thoracic interspace, position the C-arm so that the fluoroscopy beam is in the same plane as the Tuohy epidural needle. "Walk off" the lamina with the Tuohy needle into the ligamentum flavum. Remove the stylet from the Tuohy needle and, using the loss of resistance technique, advance it into the epidural space. Once loss of resistance has been achieved, aspirate to check for blood or spinal fluid. If neither is evident, inject 1.5 ml of nonionic contrast dye to confirm epidural placement. To further confirm proper placement, adjust the C-arm to view the area from a lateral projection (Fig. 39-12). A spot roentgenogram or epidurogram can be obtained. Inject 2 ml of 1% preservative-free Xylocaine without epinephrine and 2 ml of 6 mg/ml Celestone Soluspan slowly into the epidural space.

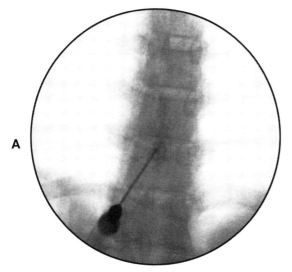
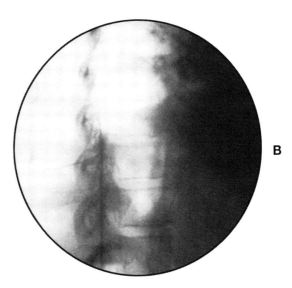

Fig. 39-12 **A,** Posteroanterior view of thoracic interlaminar epidurogram demonstrating characteristic contrast flow pattern. **B,** Lateral roentgenogram of thoracic epidurogram.

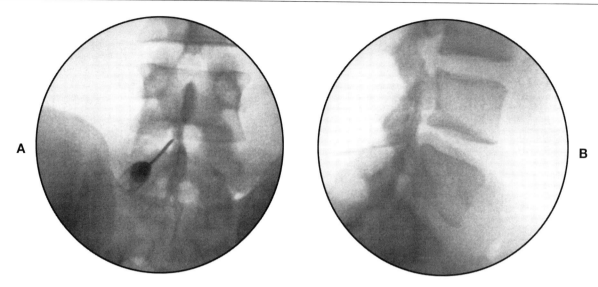

Fig. 39-13 **A,** Posteroanterior lateral view of lumbar epidurogram demonstrating characteristic contrast flow pattern. **B,** Lateral roentgenogram of lumbar epidurogram.

Lumbar Epidural Injection

Certain clinical trends are apparent with lumbar epidural steroid injections. When nerve root injury is associated with a disc herniation or lateral bony stenosis, most patients who received substantial leg pain relief from a well-placed transforaminal injection, even if temporary, will benefit from surgery for the radicular pain. Patients who do not respond and who have had radicular pain for at least 12 months are unlikely to benefit from surgery. Patients with back and leg pain of an acute nature (less than 3 months) respond better to epidural corticosteroids. Unless a significant reinjury results in an acute disc or nerve root injury, postsurgical patients tend to respond poorly to epidural corticosteroids.

◆ Interlaminar Approach

TECHNIQUE 39-5

Place the patient prone on a pain management table. Aseptically prepare the skin area with isopropyl alcohol and povidone-iodine several segments above and below the laminar interspace to be injected. Drape the patient in a sterile fashion. Under anteroposterior fluoroscopy guidance, identify the target laminar interspace. Using a 27¼-gauge needle, anesthetize the skin over the target interspace on the side of the patient's pain with 1 to 2 ml of 1% preservative-free Xylocaine without epinephrine. Insert a 3½-inch, 22-gauge spinal needle vertically until contact is made with the upper edge of the inferior lamina at the target interspace, 1 to 2 cm lateral to the caudal tip of the inferior spinous process under fluoroscopy. Anesthetize the lamina with 2 ml of 1% preservative-free Xylocaine without epinephrine. Then anesthetize the soft tissue with 2 ml of

1% Xylocaine as the spinal needle is withdrawn. Nick the skin with an 18-gauge hypodermic needle and then insert a 3½-inch, 17-gauge Tuohy epidural needle and advance it vertically within the anesthetized soft tissue track until contact with the lamina has been made under fluoroscopy. "Walk off" the lamina with the Tuohy needle onto the ligamentum flavum. Remove the stylet from the Tuohy needle and attach a 10-ml syringe filled halfway with air and sterile saline to the Tuohy needle. Advance the Tuohy needle into the epidural space using the loss of resistance technique. Avoid lateral needle placement to decrease the likelihood of encountering an epidural vein or adjacent nerve root. Remove the stylet once loss of resistance has been achieved. Aspirate to check for blood or spinal fluid. If neither is present, remove the syringe from the Tuohy needle and attach a 5-ml syringe containing 2 ml of nonionic contrast dye. Confirm epidural placement by producing an epidurogram with the nonionic contrast agent (Fig. 39-13). A spot roentgenogram can be taken to document placement. Remove the 5-ml syringe and place on the Tuohy needle a 10-ml syringe containing 2 ml of 1% preservative-free Xylocaine and 2 ml of 6 mg/ml Celestone Soluspan. Inject the corticosteroid preparation slowly into the epidural space.

◆ Transforaminal Approach

TECHNIQUE 39-6

Place the patient prone on a pain management table. Aseptically prepare the skin area with isopropyl alcohol and povidone-iodine several segments above and below the

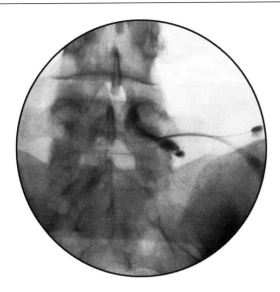

Fig. 39-14   Right L5 selective nerve root injection contrast pattern.

interspace to the injected. Drape the patient in sterile fashion. Under anteroposterior fluoroscopic guidance, identify the target interspace. Anesthetize the soft tissues over the lateral border and midway between the two adjacent transverse processes at the target interspace. Insert a 4¾-inch, 22-gauge spinal needle and advance it within the anesthetized soft tissue track under fluoroscopy until contact is made with the lower edge of the superior transverse process near its junction with the superior articular process. Retract the spinal needle 2 to 3 mm and redirect it toward the base of the appropriate pedicle and advance it slowly to the 6-o'clock position of the pedicle under fluoroscopy. Adjust the C-arm to a lateral projection to confirm the position then return the C-arm to the anteroposterior view. Remove the stylet. Inject 1 ml of nonionic contrast slowly to produce a perioneurosheathogram (Fig. 39-14). After an adequate dye pattern is observed, inject slowly a 2-ml volume containing 1 ml of 0.75% preservative-free bupivacaine and 1 ml of 6 mg/ml Celestone Soluspan.

The S1 nerve root also can be injected using the transforaminal approach. Place the patient prone on the pain management table. After appropriate aseptic preparation, direct the C-arm so that the fluoroscopy beam is in a cephalocaudad and lateral-to-medial direction so that the anterior and posterior S1 foramina are aligned. Anesthetize the soft tissues and the dorsal aspect of the sacrum with 2 to 3 ml of 1% preservative-free Xylocaine without epinephrine. Insert a 3½-inch, 22-gauge spinal needle and advance it within the anesthetized soft tissue track under fluoroscopy until contact is made with posterior sacral bone slightly lateral and inferior to the S1 pedicle. "Walk" the spinal needle off the sacrum into the posterior S1 foramen to the

medial edge of the pedicle. Adjust the C-arm to a lateral projection to confirm the position and then return it to the anteroposterior view. Remove the stylet. Inject 1 ml of nonionic contrast slowly to produce a perineurosheathogram. After an adequate dye pattern of the S1 nerve root is obtained, insert a 2-ml volume containing 1 ml of 0.75% preservative-free Marcaine and 1 ml of 6 mg/ml Celestone Soluspan.

◆ **Caudal Approach**

TECHNIQUE 39-7

Place the patient prone on a pain management table. Aseptically prepare the skin area from the lumbosacral junction to the coccyx with isopropyl alcohol and povidone-iodine. Drape the patient in sterile fashion. Try to identify by palpation the sacral hiatus, which is located between the two horns of the sacral cornu. The sacral hiatus can best be observed by directing the fluoroscopic beam laterally. Anesthetize the soft tissues and the dorsal aspect of the sacrum with 2 to 3 ml of 1% preservative-free Xylocaine without epinephrine. Keep the C-arm positioned so that the fluoroscopic beam remains lateral. Insert a 3½-inch, 22-gauge spinal needle between the sacral cornu at about 45 degrees, with the bevel of the spinal needle facing ventrally until contact with the sacrum is made. Using fluoroscopic guidance, redirect the spinal needle more cephalad, horizontal and parallel to the table, advancing it into the sacral canal through the sacrococcygeal ligament and into the epidural space. Remove the stylet. Aspirate to check for blood or spinal fluid. If neither is evident, inject 2 ml of nonionic contrast dye to confirm placement. Move the C-arm into the anteroposterior position and look for the characteristic "Christmas tree" pattern of epidural flow (Fig. 39-15). If a vascular pattern is seen, reposition the spinal needle and again confirm epidural placement with nonionic contrast dye. Once the correct contrast pattern is obtained, inject slowly a 10-ml volume containing 3 ml of 1% preservative-free Xylocaine without epinephrine, 3 ml of 6 mg/ml Celestone Soluspan, and 4 ml of sterile normal saline.

ZYGAPOPHYSEAL (FACET) JOINT INJECTIONS

The facet joint can be a source of back pain; the exact cause of the pain remains unknown. Theories include meniscoid entrapment and extrapment, synovial impingement, chondromalacia facetae, capsular and synovial inflammation, and mechanical injury to the joint capsule. Osteoarthritis is another cause of facet joint pain; however, the incidence of facet joint arthropathy is equal in both symptomatic and asymptomatic patients. As with other osteoarthritic joints, roentgenographic changes correlate poorly with pain.

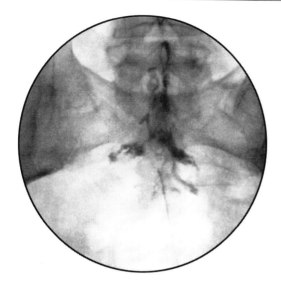

Fig. 39-15   Posteroanterior view of caudal epidurogram demonstrating characteristic contrast flow pattern.

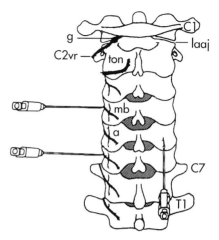

Fig. 39-16   Proper needle placement for posterior approach to C4 and C6 medial branch blocks. Second cervical ganglion *(g)*, third occipital nerve *(ton)*, C2 ventral ramus *(C2vr)* and lateral atlantoaxial joint *(laaj)* are noted. *a,* Articular facet; *mb,* medial branch. (Redrawn from Boduk N: Back pain: Zygapophyseal blocks and epidural steroids. In Cousins MJ, Bridenbaugh PO, eds: *Neural blockade in clinical anesthesia and management of pain,* ed 2, Philadelphia, 1988, JB Lippincott.)

Although the history and physical examination may suggest that the facet joint is the cause of spine pain, no noninvasive pathognomonic findings distinguish facet joint–mediated pain from other sources of spine pain. Fluoroscopically guided facet joint injections therefore are commonly considered the gold standard for isolating or excluding the facet joint as a source of spine or extremity pain.

Clinical suspicion of facet joint pain by a spine specialist remains the major indicator for diagnostic injection, which should be done only in patients who have had pain for more than 4 weeks and only after appropriate conservative measures have failed to provide relief. Facet joint injection procedures may help to focus treatment on a specific spinal segment and provide adequate pain relief to allow progression in therapy. Either intraarticular or medial branch blocks can be used for diagnostic purposes. Although injection of cortisone into the facet joint was a popular procedure through most of the 1970s and 1980s, many investigators have found no evidence that this effectively treats low back pain caused by a facet joint. The only controlled study on the use of intraarticular corticosteroids in the cervical spine found no added benefit from intraarticular betamethasone over bupivacaine.

directed fluoroscopy. Each cervical facet joint from C3-4 to C7-T1 is supplied from the medial nerve branch above and below that joint which curves consistently around the "waist" of the articular pillar of the same numbered vertebrae (Fig. 39-16). For example, to block the C6 facet joint nerve supply, anesthetize the C6 and C7 medial branches. Insert a 22- or 25-gauge, 3½-inch spinal needle perpendicular to the pain management table and advance it under fluoroscopic control ventrally and medially until contact is made with periosteum. Direct the spinal needle laterally until the needle tip reaches the lateral margin of the waist of the articular pillar and then direct the needle until it rests at the deepest point of the articular pillar's concavity under fluoroscopy. Remove the stylet. If there is a negative aspirate, inject 0.5 ml of 0.75% preservative Marcaine.

Cervical Facet Joint
◆ Medial Branch Block Injection

TECHNIQUE 39-8
Place the patient prone on the pain management table. Rotate the patient's neck so that the symptomatic side is down. This allows the vertebral artery to be positioned farther beneath the articular pillar, creates greater accentuation of the cervical waists, and prevents the jaw from being superimposed. Aseptically prepare and drape the side to be injected. Identify the target location using anteroposterior-

Lumbar Facet Joint
◆ Intraarticular Injection

TECHNIQUE 39-9
Place the patient prone on a pain management table. Aseptically prepare and drape the patient. Under fluoroscopic guidance, identify the target segment to be injected. Upper lumbar facet joints are oriented in the sagittal (vertical) plane and often can be seen on direct anteroposterior views, whereas the lower lumbar facet joints, especially at L5-S1, are obliquely oriented and require an

ipsilateral oblique rotation of the C-arm to be seen. Position the C-arm under fluoroscopy until the joint silhouette first appears. Insert and advance a 22- or 25-gauge, 3½-inch spinal needle toward the target joint along the axis of the fluoroscopy beam until contact is made with the articular processes of the joint. Enter the joint cavity through the softer capsule and advance the needle only a few millimeters. Capsular penetration is perceived as a subtle change of resistance. If midpoint needle entry is difficult, redirect the spinal needle to the superior or inferior joint recesses. Confirm placement with less than 0.1 ml of nonionic contrast dye with a 3-ml syringe to minimize injection pressure under fluoroscopic guidance. Once intraarticular placement has been verified, inject a total volume of 1 ml of injectant (local anesthetic with or without corticosteroids) into the joint.

◆ Medial Branch Block Injection

TECHNIQUE 39-10

Place the patient prone on a pain management table. Aseptically prepare and drape the patient. Because there is dual innervation of each lumbar facet joint, two medial branch blocks are required. It is important to remember that the medial branches cross the transverse processes below their origin (Fig. 39-17). For example, the L4-5 facet joint is anesthetized by blocking the L3 medial branch at the transverse process of L4, and the L4 medial branch at the transverse process of L5. In the case of the L5-S1 facet joint, anesthetize the L4 medial branch as it passes over the L5 transverse process and the L5 medial branch as it passes across the sacral ala. Using anteroposterior fluoroscopic imaging, identify the target transverse process. For L1 through L4 medial branch blocks, penetrate the skin using a 22- or 25-gauge, 3½-inch spinal needle lateral and superior to the target location. Under fluoroscopic guidance, advance the spinal needle until contact is made with the dorsal superior and medial aspects of the base of the transverse process so that the needle top rests against the periosteum. To ensure optimal spinal needle placement, reposition the C-arm so that the fluoroscopy beam is ipsilateral oblique and the "Scotty dog" is seen. Position the spinal needle in the middle of the "eye" of the "Scotty dog." Slowly inject (over 30 seconds) 0.5 ml of 0.75% Marcaine.

To inject the L5 medial branch (more correctly, the L5 dorsal ramus), position the patient prone on the pain management table with the fluoroscopic beam in the anteroposterior projection. Identify the sacral ala. Rotate the C-arm 15 to 20 degrees ipsilateral obliquely to maximize exposure between the junction of the sacral ala and the superior process of S1. Insert a 22- or 25-gauge, 3½-inch spinal needle directly into the osseous landmarks approxi-

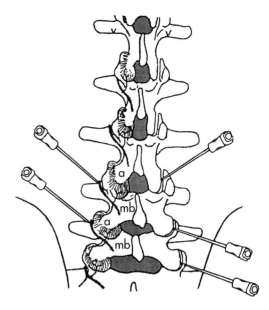

Fig. 39-17 Posterior view of lumbar spine demonstrating location of medial branches of dorsal rami, which innervate lumbar facet joints *(a)*. Needle position for L3 and L4 medial branch blocks shown on left half of diagram would be used to anesthetize the L4-5 facet joint. Right half of diagram demonstrates L3-4, L4-5, and L5-S1 intraarticular facet joint injection positions. *a,* Articular facet; *mb,* medial branch. (Redrawn from Boduk N: Back pain: zygapophyseal blocks and epidural steroids. In Cousins MJ, Bridenbaugh PO, eds: *Neural blockade in clinical anesthesia and management of pain,* ed 2, Philadelphia, 1988, JB Lippincott.)

mately 5 mm below the superior junction of the sacral ala with the superior articular process of the sacrum under fluoroscopy. Rest the spinal needle on the periosteum and position the bevel of the spinal needle medial and away from the foramen to minimize flow through the L5 or S1 foramen. Slowly inject 0.5 ml of 0.75% Marcaine.

◆ Sacroiliac Joint

The sacroiliac joint remains a controversial source of primary low back pain despite validated scientific studies. It often is overlooked as a source of low back pain because its anatomical location makes it difficult to examine in isolation and many provocative tests place mechanical stresses on contiguous structures. In addition, several other structures may refer pain to the sacroiliac joint.

The sacroiliac joint, like other synovial joints, moves; however, sacroiliac joint movement is involuntary and is caused by shear, compression, and other indirect forces. Muscles involved with secondary sacroiliac joint motion include the erectae spinae, quadratus lumborum, psoas major and minor, piriformis, latissimus dorsi, obliquus abdominis, and gluteal. Imbalances in any of these muscles as a result of central facilitation may cause them to function in a shortened state that tends to inhibit their antagonists reflexively.

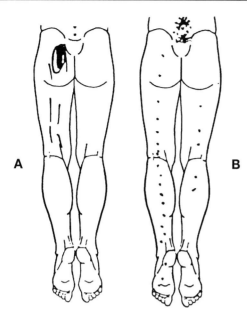

Fig. 39-18   Pain diagram. **A,** Patient reported pain diagram consistent with sacroiliac joint dysfunction. **B,** Patient reported diagram inconsistent with sacroiliac joint dysfunction. (From Fortin JD, Dwyer AP, West S, Pier J: *Spine* 19:1475, 1994.)

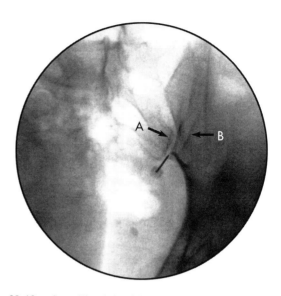

Fig. 39-19   Sacroiliac joint injection showing medial *(A)* and lateral *(B)* joint planes (silhouettes). Entry into joint is achieved above most posteroinferior aspect of joint.

Theoretically, dysfunctional movement patterns may result. Postural changes and body weight also can create motion through the sacroiliac joint.

Because of the wide range of segmental innervation (L2-S2) of the sacroiliac joint, there is a myriad of referral zone patterns. In studies of asymptomatic subjects, the most constant referral zone was localized to a 3 × 10 cm area just inferior to the ipsilateral posterior superior iliac spine (Fig. 39-18); however, pain may be referred to the buttocks, groin, posterior thigh, calf, and foot.

Sacroiliac dysfunction, also called *sacroiliac joint mechanical pain* or *sacroiliac joint syndrome,* is the most common painful condition of this joint. The true prevalence of mediated pain from sacroiliac joint dysfunction is unknown; however, several studies indicated that it is more common than expected. Because no specific or pathognomonic historical facts or physical examination tests accurately identify the sacroiliac joint as a source of pain, diagnosis is one of exclusion. However, sacroiliac joint dysfunction should be considered if an injury was caused by a direct fall on the buttocks, a rear-end motor vehicle accident with the ipsilateral foot on the brake at the moment of impact, a broadside motor vehicle accident with a blow to the lateral aspect of the pelvic ring, or a fall in a hole with one leg in the hole and the other extended outside. Lumbar rotation and axial loading that can occur during ballet or ice skating is another common mechanism of injury. Although somewhat controversial, the risk of sacroiliac joint dysfunction may be increased in individuals with lumbar fusion or hip pathology. Other causes include insufficiency stress fractures, fatigue stress fractures, metabolic processes, such as deposition diseases, degenerative joint disease, infection, and inflamma-

tory conditions, such as ankylosing spondylitis, psoriatic arthritis, and Reiter's disease. The diagnosis of sacroiliac joint pain can be confirmed if symptoms are reproduced upon distention of the joint capsule by provocative injection and subsequently abated with an analgesic block.

TECHNIQUE 39-11

Place the patient prone on a pain management table. Aseptically prepare and drape the side to be injected. Rotate the C-arm until the medial (posterior) joint line is seen. Use a 27¼-gauge needle to anesthetize the skin of the buttock 1 to 3 cm inferior to the lowest aspect of the joint. Using fluoroscopy insert a 3½-inch, 22-gauge spinal needle until the needle rests 1 cm above the most posteroinferior aspect of the joint (Fig. 39-19). Rarely, a larger spinal needle is required in obese patients. Advance the spinal needle into the sacroiliac joint until capsular penetration occurs. Confirm intraarticular placement under fluoroscopy with 0.5 ml of nonionic contrast dye. A spot roentgenogram can be taken to document placement. Inject a 2-ml volume containing 1 ml of 0.75% preservative-free Marcaine and 1 ml of 6 mg/ml Celestone into the joint.

DISCOGRAPHY

Discography has been used since the late 1940s for the experimental and clinical evaluation of disc disease in both the cervical and lumbar regions of the spine. Since that time discography has had a limited but important role in the evaluation of suspected disc pathology.

The clinical usefulness of the data obtained from discography remains controversial. In 1968 Holt published a landmark study that showed a 37% false-positive rate. He concluded that lumbar discography was an unreliable diagnostic tool. However, Holt's studies had numerous design flaws, including suboptimal imaging equipment, neurotoxic contrast agents, inadequate needle placement, and failure to determine if pain responses were concordant or discordant with patients' typical pain patterns. Using modern techniques, Walsh et al. in 1990 published a well-controlled prospective study that, unlike Holt's study, required an abnormal nucleogram and a concordant pain response to indicate a positive provocative discogram. The investigators of this study found a 0% false-positive rate for discography compared with 37% reported by Holt. These authors concluded that, with current technique and standardized protocol, discography was a highly reliable test.

In independent studies, Cloward and Smith emphasized that reproduction of a patient's pain was the key feature of cervical discography. In 1964 Holt reported that cervical discography had no diagnostic value because pain reproduction and fissuring were features of cervical discs in normal volunteers. Later investigative work by Simmons and Segil demonstrated the importance of discriminating between painful and nonpainful discs, while avoiding pain reproduction and disc morphology as absolute entities. Carrying this idea further, Roth in 1976 introduced analgesic cervical discography with the rationale that once a painful disc is identified, pain relief should occur by injecting a local anesthetic into the disc. He reported a high success rate for anterior disc excision and fusion using this form of precision diagnostic testing.

The most important aspect of discography is provocative testing for concordant pain (that which corresponds to a patient's usual pain) to provide information regarding the clinical significance of the disc abnormality. Although difficult to standardize, this distinguishes discography from other anatomical imaging techniques. If the patient is unable to distinguish customary pain from any other pain, the procedure is of no value. In patients who have a concordant response without evidence of a radial annular fissure on discography, CT should be considered because some discs that appear normal on discography show disruption on CT scan.

Indications for lumbar discography include surgical planning of spinal fusion, testing of the structural integrity of an adjacent disc to a known abnormality such as spondylolisthesis or fusion, identifying a painful disc among multiple degenerative discs, ruling out secondary internal disc disruption or suspected lateral or recurrent disc herniation, and determining the primary symptom-producing level when chemonucleolysis is being considered. Thoracic discography is a useful tool in the investigation of thoracic, chest, and upper abdominal pain. Degenerative thoracic disc disease, with or without herniation, has a highly variable clinical presentation, frequently mimicking visceral conditions, as well as causing back or musculoskeletal pain. In the cervical spine, discography is an important adjunct for diagnosing primary discogenic pain and determin-

ing which disc is affected and will require surgery. Discography also may be justified in medicolegal situations to establish a definitive diagnosis even though treatment may not be planned on that disc.

Compression of the spinal cord, stenosis of the roots, bleeding disorders, allergy to the injectable material, and active infection are contraindications to diagnostic discography procedures. Although the risk of complications from discography is low, potential problems include discitis, nerve root injury, subarachnoid puncture, chemical meningitis, bleeding, and allergic reactions. In addition, in the cervical region, retropharyngeal and epidural abscess can occur. Pneumothorax is a risk in both the cervical and thoracic regions.

◆ Lumbar Discography

Lumbar discography originally was done using a transdural technique in a manner similar to myelography with a lumbar puncture. The difference between lumbar myelography and discography was that the needle used for the latter was advanced through the thecal sac. The technique later was modified, consisting of an extradural, extralaminar approach that avoided the thecal sac, and it was refined further to enable entry into the L5-S1 disc using a two-needle technique to maneuver around the iliac crest.

A patient's response during the procedure is the most important aspect of the study. Pain alone does not determine if a disc is the cause of the back pain. The concordance of the pain in regard to the quality and location are paramount in determining whether the disc is a true pain generator. A control disc is necessary to validate a positive finding on discography.

TECHNIQUE 39-12 *(Falco)*

Place the patient on a procedure or fluoroscopic table. Insert an angiocatheter into the upper extremity and infuse intravenous antibiotics to prevent discitis. Some physicians prefer to give antibiotics intradiscally during the procedure in lieu of the intravenous route. Place the patient in a modified lateral decubitus position with the symptomatic side down to avoid having the patient confuse the pain caused by the needle with the actual pain on that same side. This position also allows for easier fluoroscopic imaging of the intervertebral discs and mobilizes the bowel away from the needle path. Lightly sedate the patient with an intravenous opioid and short-acting benzodiazepine. Prepare and drape the skin sterilely, including the lumbosacral region.

Under fluoroscopic control, identify the intervertebral discs. Adjust the patient's position or the C-arm so that the lumbar spine is in an oblique position with the superior articular process, dividing the intervertebral space in half (Fig. 39-20). Anesthetize the skin overlying the superior articular process with 1 to 2 ml of 1% lidocaine if necessary. Advance a single 6-inch spinal needle (or longer, depending on the patient's size) through the skin and deeper soft tissues to the outer annulus of the disc. The disc entry point is just

continued

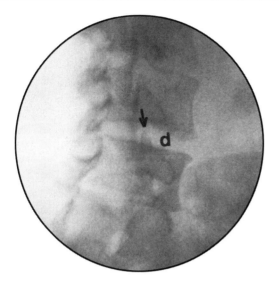

Fig. 39-20 Lumbar spine in an oblique position with superior articular process *(arrow)* dividing disc space *(d)* in half. (Courtesy Frank JE Falco, MD.)

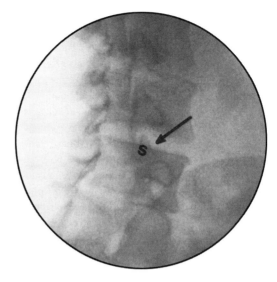

Fig. 39-21 Disc entry point is just anterior *(arrow)* to base of superior articular process *(s)* and just above superior endplate of vertebral body. (Courtesy Frank JE Falco, MD.)

anterior to the base of the superior articular process and just above the superior endplate of the vertebral body, which allows the needle to safely pass by the exiting nerve root (Fig. 39-21). Advance the needle into the central third of the disc, using anteroposterior and lateral fluoroscopic imaging. Confirm the position of the needle tip within the central third of the disc with anteroposterior and lateral fluoroscopic imaging. Inject either saline or nonionic contrast dye into each disc. Record any pain that the patient experiences during the injection as *none, dissimilar, similar,* or *exact* in relationship to the patient's typical low back pain. Record intradiscal pressures to assist in determining if the disc is the cause of the pain. Obtain roentgenograms of the lumbar spine upon completion of the study, paying particular attention to the contrast-enhanced disc. Obtain a CT scan if necessary to assess disc anatomy further.

An alternative method is a two-needle technique in which a 6- or 8-inch spinal needle is passed through a shorter introducer needle (typically 3½ inches in length) into the disc in the same manner as a single needle. This approach may reduce the incidence of infection by allowing the procedure needle to pass into the disc space without ever penetrating the skin. The introducer needle also may assist in more accurate needle placement, reducing the risk of injuring the exiting nerve root. The two-needle approach may require more time than the single-needle technique, and the larger introducer needle could cause more pain to the patient.

The two-needle technique often is used to enter the L5-S1 disc space with one modification. The procedure needle typically is curved (Fig. 39-22). To bypass the iliac crest, the introducer needle is advanced at an angle that

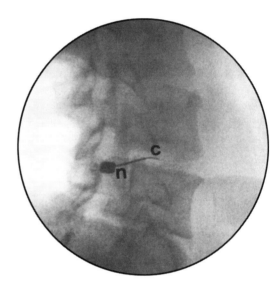

Fig. 39-22 Curved procedure needle *(c)* passing through straight introducer needle *(n)*. (Courtesy Frank JE Falco, MD.)

places the needle tip in a position that does not line up with the L5-S1 disc space, which makes it difficult if not impossible for a straight procedure needle to advance into the L5-S1 disc. A curved procedure needle, on the other hand, allows the needle tip to align with the L5-S1 disc as it is advanced towards and into the disc adjusting for malalignment.

◆ Thoracic Discography

Thoracic discography has been refined to provide a technique that is reproducible and safe. A posterolateral extralaminar

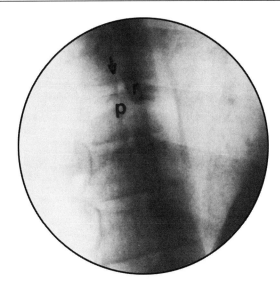

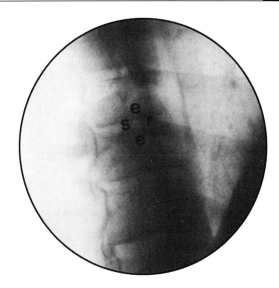

Fig. 39-23   Oblique position with superior articular process *(arrow)* dividing thoracic intervertebral space in half. *p*, Pedicle; *r*, rib head. (Courtesy Frank JE Falco, MD.)

Fig. 39-24   Thoracic endplates *(e)*, superior articular process *(s)*, and rib head *(r)* form "box." (Courtesy Frank JE Falco, MD.)

approach similar to lumbar discography is used with a single-needle technique. The significant difference between thoracic and lumbar discography is the potential for complications because of the surrounding anatomy of the thoracic spine. In contrast to lumbar discography, which typically is performed in the mid to lower lumbar spine below the spinal cord and lungs, thoracic discography has the inherent risk of pneumothorax and direct spinal cord trauma; other complications include discitis and bleeding.

Essentially the same protocol is used for thoracic discography as for lumbar discography.

TECHNIQUE 39-13 *(Falco)*

Place the patient in a modified lateral decubitus position on the procedure table with the symptomatic side down. Begin antibiotics through the intravenous catheter. Alternatively, intradiscal antibiotics may be given during the procedure. Lightly sedate the patient and prepare and drape the skin in a sterile manner.

Using fluoroscopic imaging, identify the intervertebral thoracic discs. Move the patient or adjust the C-arm obliquely to position the superior articular process so that it divides the intervertebral space in half (Fig. 39-23). At this point, the intervertebral discs and endplates, subjacent superior articular process, and adjacent rib head should be in clear view. The endplates, the superior articular process, and the rib head form a "box" (Fig. 39-24) that delineates a safe pathway into the disc, avoiding the spinal cord and lung. Keep the needle tip within the confines of this "box" while advancing it into the annulus.

After proper positioning and exposure, anesthetize the skin overlying the superior articular process with 1 to 2 ml of 1% lidocaine if necessary. Advance a single 6-inch spinal needle (a shorter or longer needle can be used, depending on the patient's size) through the skin and the deeper soft tissues into the outer annulus within the "box" just anterior to the base of the superior articular process and just above the superior endplate. Continue into the central third of the disc, using anteroposterior and lateral fluoroscopic guidance.

Inject either saline or a nonionic contrast dye into each disc in the same manner as for lumbar discography. Record any pain response and analyze for reproduction of concordant pain using the same protocol as for lumbar discography. Obtain roentgenograms and CT imaging of the thoracic spine upon completion of the study.

◆ Cervical Discography

The approach to the cervical spine is distinctly different from the approaches used for discography of the lumbar and thoracic spine. The cervical spine is approached anteriorly rather than posteriorly. Complications associated with cervical discography because of the surrounding anatomy include injury to the trachea, esophagus, carotid artery, and jugular veins, as well as spinal cord injury and pneumothorax. As with lumbar and thoracic discography, discitis also is a concern in the cervical spine, although the disc infection often originates from the gram-negative and anaerobic flora of the esophagus as opposed to the gram-positive skin flora seen in lumbar discography.

Traditionally, the approach to the cervical intervertebral discs has been via a paralaryngeal route that requires displacement of the trachea and esophagus away from the site of entry. A more lateral approach that is gaining popularity bypasses these structures and does not require such displacement.

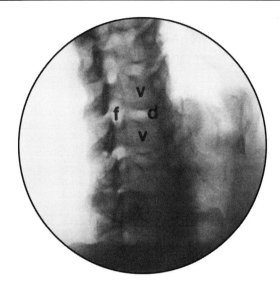

Fig. 39-25 Foraminal position for performing cervical discography with anterolateral approach. *f,* Foramen; *v,* vertebral body; *d,* intervertebral disc. (Courtesy Frank JE Falco, MD.)

The same protocol for lumbar and thoracic discography is used in cervical discography.

TECHNIQUE 39-14 *(Falco)*

Place the patient supine on the procedure table. Insert an angiocatheter into the upper extremity and begin intravenous antibiotic infusion. Alternatively, intradiscal antibiotics can be given during surgery. Sedate the patient and prepare and drape the skin sterilely, including the anterolateral aspect of the neck.

Under fluoroscopic imaging, identify the intervertebral discs with aligned endplates and sharp margins of the intervertebral discs. Approach the paralaryngeal area from the right, using a finger to displace the esophagus and trachea to the left and the carotid artery to the right side. With the other hand, insert a 2- or 3½-inch spinal needle over the finger through the skin and into the outer annulus of the disc. Advance the needle into the center of the disc, using anteroposterior and lateral fluoroscopic guidance.

An alternative method is a more lateral approach to the cervical spine using a single needle. This approach may reduce the incidence of infection by passing the needle posterior to the trachea and esophagus en route to the disc space. Position the patient or the C-arm to place the cervical spine in an oblique position for optimal foraminal exposure and continue adjusting until the endplates, disc space, and uncovertebral process are in sharp focus (Fig. 39-25). Insert a 2- or 3½-inch needle into the skin and advance it until the tip makes contact with the subjacent uncovertebral process. "Walk off" the needle just anterior to the uncovertebral process. Advance the needle into the center of the disc, using anteroposterior and lateral fluoroscopic guidance.

After needle placement with either technique, the rest of the procedure is essentially the same as that described for thoracic or lumbar discography. Inject either saline or a nonionic contrast dye into each disc. Record any pain response and analyze for concordance using the same protocol employed for lumbar and thoracic discography. Obtain roentgenograms and CT imaging of the cervical spine upon completion of the study.

Psychological Testing

As discussed previously in this section, pain in some patients is the result of nonanatomical causes. Many, but not all, patients report the onset of their symptoms after a work-related incident, which may have been relatively minor. Some patients present acutely, and for these patients treatment as outlined for nonspecific back pain should be followed. It is known that patients who do not return to work in 6 months are at increased risk for long-term disability. Patients with acute injuries or with history of chronic pain require closer evaluation. Increasing evidence suggests that the preeminence of psychosocial factors over physical variables is responsible for prolonged disability.

Over the past several decades extensive studies have been done on various evaluation tools for patients with "abnormal illness behavior." Waddell et al. defined this as "maladaptive overt illness-related behavior which is out of proportion to the underlying physical disease and more readily attributable to associated cognitive and affective disturbances." Waddell et al. also developed clinical tools designed to detect the presence of "abnormal illness behavior" by identifying physical signs or symptoms and descriptions that are nonorganic in nature. Five nonorganic signs and seven nonorganic symptom descriptions (Table 39-4) have been identified. Waddell initially described these for use in patients with chronic pain and suggested that the presence of three signs was required to determine "abnormal illness behavior." Several studies evaluated the ability of these signs and symptom descriptions to predict return to work but have proved inconclusive; nevertheless, they appear to be useful in detecting patients at increased risk for poor outcome with surgical intervention.

The Minnesota Multiphasic Personality Inventory (MMPI) has been used for psychological assessment in many previous studies and has been demonstrated to be a reasonable predictor of surgical and conservative treatment results regardless of the spinal pathological condition. Unfortunately, the MMPI is lengthy and difficult to administer in an orthopaedic clinical setting and probably is best given by a psychiatrist or psychologist. By comparison, the Distress and Risk Assessment Method (DRAM) is relatively easily administered and scored and has been validated in clinical settings with regard to patients with back pain. The DRAM consists of the Modified Somatic Perception Questionnaire (MSPQ) and the Zung Depression Index (ZDI). With this simplified method, patients

Table 39-4 Signs and Symptoms for Diagnosis of "Abnormal Illness Behavior"

Nonorganic Signs	Organic Signs
Regional disturbances	A widespread region of sensory changes or weakness that is divergent from accepted neuroanatomy
Superficial/nonanatomical tenderness	Tenderness of the skin to light touch (superficial) or deep tenderness felt over a widespread area not localized to one structure (nonanatomical)
Simulation	
Axial loading	Low back pain reported with pressure on the patient's head while standing
Rotation	Low back pain reported when the shoulders and pelvis are rotated in the same plane as the patient stands
Distraction	
Straight leg raising	Inconsistent limitation of straight leg raising in supine and seated positions
Overreaction	Disproportionate verbalization, facial expression, muscle tension, collapsing, sweating, and so forth during examination

Nonorganic Symptom Descriptors

1. Do you get pain in your tailbone?
2. Do you have numbness in your entire leg (front, side, and back of leg at the same time?)
3. Do you have pain in your entire leg (front, side, and back of the leg at the same time?)
4. Does your whole leg ever give way?
5. Have you had any time during this episode when you have had very little back pain?
6. Have you had to go to the emergency room because of back pain?
7. Has all treatment for your back made your pain worse?

From Fritz JM, Wainner RS, Hicks GE: *Spine* 25:1925, 2000.

Table 39-5 Result Expectancy Related to Hs and Hy T Scores on the MMPI Test

Hs and Hy T Scores	Number of Patients	Chances of Good or Excellent Functional Recovery (%)
85 and above	10	10
75 to 84	32	16
65 to 74	31	39
55 to 64	36	72
54 and below	21	90
Prediction from base rate	63	48

From Wiltse LL, Rocchio PD: *J Bone Joint Surg* 57A:478, 1975.

and well-documented tests used for this purpose. This test is predictive of preinjury susceptibility to back injury and the potential for failure of conservative and surgical treatment. Wiltse and Rocchio demonstrated that elevations of the hysteria (Hs) and hypochondriasis (Hy) T scores above 75 are indicative of a poor postoperative response (16% good results). Their study evaluated patients treated with chymopapain, and their clinical results are illustrated in Tables 39-5 and 39-6.

Table 39-5 indicates the rate of good or excellent results using the MMPI test Hs and Hy scores alone in the study by Wiltse and Rocchio. Table 39-6 illustrates the lack of statistical significance between the MMPI scores and the presence of the following objective findings: reflex changes, motor weakness, sensory deficits, positive myelogram, positive electromyogram, and elevated CSF protein.

Similar studies of surgically and conservatively treated patients have had similar findings. Written reports are helpful, but the raw T score read on the far right or left side of the standard test result sheet is the simplest guide to postoperative outcome. If surgery is necessary in a patient with an elevated Hs or Hy score, then psychiatric or psychological assistance before and after the procedure can be helpful, but a poor result should be anticipated. Gentry observed a group of patients with objective evidence of psychological disturbance as indicated by the MMPI. Those patients who had surgery were less likely to return to work, less likely to have a reduction in their pain, and more likely to have greater disability than similar patients who did not have surgery. Wiltse and Rocchio recommended restraint and conservative treatment in these patients. Elevation of the Hs and Hy scores on the MMPI should be a relative contraindication to elective spinal surgery.

Additional material on this test can be found in the excellent articles by Dennis et al., Wiltse and Rocchio, and Southwick and White. Numerous other tests are available, but none has been shown to be as predictive of surgical outcome as the Hs and Hy scores on the MMPI. Riley et al. investigated a MMPI-2 and found that the results replicated those of the older MMPI.

identified as psychologically distressed are three to four times more likely to have a poor outcome after any form of treatment. It is our recommendation that some type of formal psychological evaluation be used preoperatively in patients who have chronic pain but no clear cause of their symptoms; whether the MMPI or the DRAM is used is less important.

The experience at this clinic has been primarily with the MMPI, which we routinely use for assessment of patients who have symptoms seemingly out of proportion to their anatomical abnormalities and are being evaluated for surgical treatment, especially spinal fusion. The MMPI is one of the most reliable

Table 39-6 Hs and Hy T Scores of Patients with Good or Excellent Results Versus Number of Preexisting Objective Deficits

Hs and Hy T scores	Number of Patients	Percentage Good or Excellent Results	Percentage with the No. of Preinjection Objective Deficits Indicated*				
			1+	2+	3+	4+	5+
75 and over	42	25	95.0	57.5	30.0	7.5	2.5
64 and below	57	87	95.2	64.4	32.6	8.7	2.2

From Wiltse LL, Rocchio PD: *J Bone Joint Surg* 57A:478, 1975.
*X^2 <0.001.

Patients with MMPI and MMPI-2 findings of depressed-pathological profile and a conversion V profile reported greater dissatisfaction with surgical outcome.

Similar outcomes have been noted for nonoperative treatment of these patients. Gatchel et al. noted similar problems in patients with acute back pain who were questioned 6 months later.

The main problem with the MMPI is that it requires the ability to read and comprehend the material. Pincus et al. also noted that the MMPI questions may be in line with natural disease processes such as rheumatoid arthritis. Patients with chronic diseases may, by the nature of their disease symptoms, have MMPI elevations. Chronic back pain without a specific disease association should not be considered as similar to chronic disease such as rheumatoid arthritis. Chapman and Pemberton noted that the MMPI failed to predict the subjective outcome as reported by patients with chronic back pain who were in an interdisciplinary pain-management program.

A simple test that is a good screening aid is the pain drawing. The pain drawing correlates well with the Hs and Hy scores. This test also requires some ability to follow simple directions (Fig. 39-26). Additional information can be found in the articles by Rainsford, Cairns, and Mooney and by Dennis et al. Udén and Landin found that the pain drawing correlated well with clinical results. Ohnmeiss reported that the pain drawing remained consistent over 8 months in patients who reported no change in their symptoms. Also, the intraevaluator repeatability was found to be high in this as in other studies. Patients with low Rainsford scores were most likely to have definite pathological conditions and those with high Rainsford scores were least likely to have a demonstrable pathological condition. Cummings and Routan warned that the pain drawing should not be used to identify areas of somatic disturbance in chronic pain patients.

Cervical Disc Disease

Herniation of the cervical intervertebral disc with spinal cord compression has been identified since Key detailed the pathological findings of two cases of cord compression by "intervertebral substance" in 1838. During the late 1800s and early 1900s there were many reports of chondromas of the cervical spine. Stookey described the clinical findings and anatomical location of cervical disc herniation in 1928 but attributed the lesion to a cervical chondroma. Mixter and Barr reported lumbar disc herniation in 1934 and included four cervical disc protrusions.

The classic approach to discs in this region has been posteriorly with laminectomy. This approach had been used as a standard exposure for extradural tumors. In 1943 Semmes and Murphey reported four patients in whom cervical disc rupture simulated coronary disease and introduced the concept that cervical disc disease usually manifested itself in root symptoms and not cord compression symptoms. Bailey and Badgley, Cloward, and Smith and Robinson in the 1950s popularized the anterior approach coupled with interbody fusion. Robertson in 1973, after the initial report by Hirsch in 1960, reported anterior cervical discectomy without fusion. He showed that simple anterior disc excision without fusion can give results similar to anterior cervical disc excision with anterior interbody fusion. More recently, Yamamoto et al. reported the long-term (2 to 13 year) results of anterior cervical disc excision without fusion. They noted 81% improvement in patients with soft disc hernias but only 47% improvement in patients with spondylosis; 49% had neck and scapular pain as new postoperative symptoms for the first 4 weeks after surgery (Table 39-7). Spontaneous fusion was noted in 79% at 29 months. Currently, anterior cervical discectomy with fusion is the procedure of choice when the disc is removed anteriorly to avoid disc space collapse, prevent painful and abnormal cervical motion, and to speed intervertebral fusion. Foraminotomy is the procedure of choice when the disc fragment is removed posteriorly.

In an epidemiological study of acute cervical disc prolapse, Kelsey et al. indicated that cervical disc rupture was more common in men by a ratio of 1.4 to 1. Factors associated with the injury were frequent heavy lifting on the job, cigarette smoking, and frequent diving from a board. The use of vibrating equipment and time spent in motor vehicles were not positively associated with this problem. Participation in sports other than diving, frequent wearing of shoes with high heels, frequent twisting of the neck on the job, time spent sitting on the job, and smoking of cigars and pipes were not associated with cervical intervertebral disc collapse. Horal reported that 40% of the population in Sweden were sometimes affected by neck pain during their lives. Patients with cervical disc disease are also likely to have lumbar disc disease. MRI studies have shown increasing cervical disc degeneration with age.

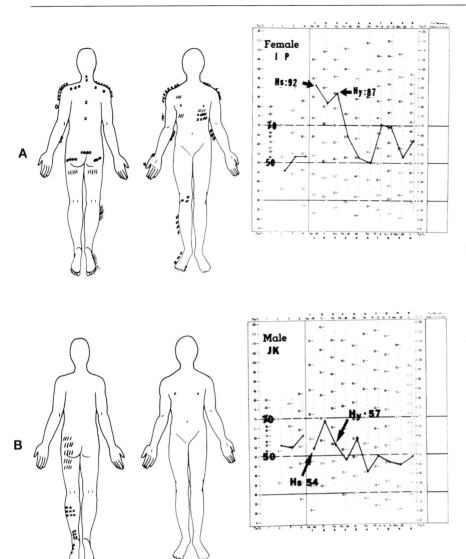

Fig. 39-26 **A,** Pain drawing and corresponding MMPI raw score sheet of patient with "conversion V" who was unrelieved of pain after disc surgery. **B,** Pain drawing and corresponding MMPI raw score sheet of patient with normal findings who was relieved of pain after disc surgery.

Table 39-7 Postoperative Neck or Scapular Pain

Follow-up Period	Soft Disc	Percentage	Spondy-losis	Percentage
1 month	4/11	36	8/34	53
1 year	1/11	9	10/29	34
2 years	0/10	0	6/24	25
4 years	0/5	0	4/21	19

From Yamamoto I, Ikeda A, Shibuya N, et al: *Spine* 16:272, 1991.

The pathophysiology of cervical disc disease is the same as degenerative disc disease in other areas of the spine. Disc swelling is followed by progressive annular degeneration. Frank extrusion of nuclear material can occur as a complication of this normal degenerative process. Kramer postulated that hydraulic pressure on the disc rather than excessive motion produces traumatic disc herniation. As the disc degeneration proceeds, hypermobility of the segment can result in instability or degenerative arthritic changes or both. Unlike in the lumbar spine, these hypertrophic changes are predominantly at the uncovertebral joint (uncinate process) (Fig. 39-27). Hypertrophic changes eventually develop about the facet joints and vertebral bodies. As in lumbar disease, progressive stiffening of the cervical spine and loss of motion are the usual result in the end stages. Hypertrophic spurring anteriorly occasionally results in dysphagia. Kang et al. identified the production of increased amounts of matrix metalloproteinases, nitric oxide, prostaglandin E2, and interleukin-6 in disc material removed from cervical disc hernias. They suggested that these products are involved in the biochemistry of disc degeneration. These substances also are implicated in pain production. These findings are similar to those in the lumbar spine. Kauppila and Penttila reported the presence of degenerative changes in the common arteries that supply the cervicobrachial area, and they suggested that impaired blood flow may play a part in cervicobrachial disorders.

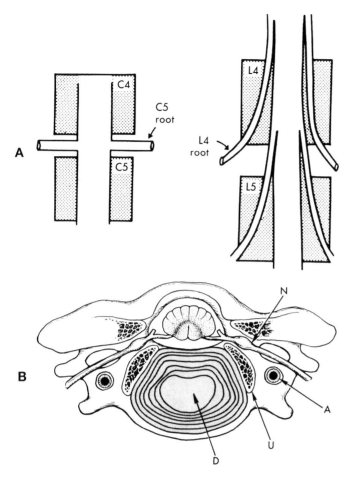

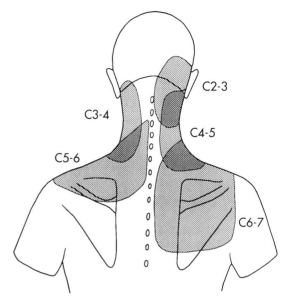

Fig. 39-28 Composite map of the results in all volunteers depicting characteristic distribution of pain from facet joints at segments C2-3 to C6-7. (Redrawn from Dwyer A, Aprill C, Bogduk N: *Spine* 15:456, 1990.)

Fig. 39-27 **A,** Comparison of points at which nerve roots emerge from cervical and lumbar spine. **B,** Cross-sectional view of cervical spine at level of disc *(D).* Uncinate process *(U)* forms ventral wall of foramen. Root *(N)* exits dorsal to vertebral artery *(A).* **(A** from Kikuchi S, Macnab I, Moreau P: *J Bone Joint Surg* 63B:272, 1981.)

SIGNS AND SYMPTOMS

The signs and symptoms of intervertebral disc disease are best separated into symptoms related to the spine itself, symptoms related to nerve root compression, and symptoms of myelopathy. Several authors reported that, when the disc is punctured anteriorly for the purpose of discography, pain is noted in the neck and shoulder. Complaints of neck pain, medial scapular pain, and shoulder pain are therefore probably related to primary pain about the disc and spine. Anatomical studies have indicated cervical disc and ligamentous innervations. This has been inferred to be similar in the cervical spine to that of the lumbar spine with its sinu-vertebral nerve. Tamura noted cranial symptoms such as headache, vertigo, tinnitus, and ocular problems associated with C3-4 root sleeve defects on myelography. Dwyer, Aprill, and Bogduk completed a two-stage investigation of the facet joints of the cervical spine as possible sources of pain. By injecting contrast medium into the facet joints of normal volunteers under roentgenographic

control to the point of pain production, a topographical map was produced. Although the number of volunteers was small, the findings were consistent (Fig. 39-28). The second stage of the study included a small number of patients who had therapeutic injections based on the location of their pain, as it related to the previously constructed pain map. Pain relief occurred immediately and completely in 9 of 10 patients who had had prior evaluation and failed other treatments. These pain patterns are not predicted by accepted dermatomal maps.

Symptoms of root compression usually are associated with pain radiating into the arm or chest with numbness in the fingers and motor weakness. Cervical disc disease also can mimic cardiac disease with chest and arm pain. Usually the radicular symptoms are intermittent and combined with the more frequent neck and shoulder pain.

The signs of midline cervical spinal cord compression (myelopathy) are unique and varied. The pain is poorly localized and aching in nature; pain may be only a minor complaint. Occasional sharp pain or generalized tingling may be described with neck extension. This is not unlike the Lhermitte sign in multiple sclerosis. The pain can be in both the shoulder and pelvic girdles; it is occasionally associated with a generalized feeling of weakness in the lower extremities and a feeling of instability.

In patients with predominant cervical spondylosis, symptoms of vertebral artery compression also may be found. These symptoms consist of dizziness, tinnitus, intermittent blurring of vision, and occasional episodes of retroocular pain.

The signs of lateral root pressure from a disc or osteophytes are predominantly neurological (Boxes 39-2 to 39-6). By evaluating multiple motor groups, multiple levels of deep

BOX 39-2 • C5 Nerve Root Compression*

Sensory Deficit
Upper lateral arm and elbow

Motor Weakness
Deltoid
Biceps (variable)

Reflex Change
Biceps (variable)

*Indicative of C4-5 disc rupture or other pathological condition at that level.

BOX 39-3 • C6 Nerve Root Compression*

Sensory Deficit
Lateral forearm, thumb, and index finger

Motor Weakness
Biceps
Extensor carpi radialis longus and brevis

Reflex Change
Biceps
Brachioradialis

*Indicative of C5-6 disc herniation or other local pathological condition at that level.

BOX 39-4 • C7 Nerve Root Compression*

Sensory Deficit
Middle finger (variable because of overlap)

Motor Weakness
Triceps
Wrist flexors (flexor carpi radialis)
Finger flexors (variable)

Reflex Change
Triceps

*Indicative of C6-7 disc rupture or other pathological condition at that level.

BOX 39-5 • C8 Nerve Root Compression*

Sensory Deficit
Ring finger, little finger, and ulnar border of palm

Motor Weakness
Interossei
Finger flexors (variable)
Flexor carpi ulnaris (variable)

Reflex Change
None

*Indicative of C7-T1 disc rupture or other pathological condition at that level.

BOX 39-6 • T1 Nerve Root Compression*

Sensory Deficit
Medial aspect of elbow

Motor Weakness
Interossei

Reflex Change
None

*Indicative of T1-2 disc rupture or other pathological condition at that level.

tendon reflexes, and sensory abnormalities, the level of the lesion can be localized as accurately as any other lesion in the nervous system. The multiple innervation of muscles can sometimes lead to confusion in determining the exact root involved. For this reason, myelography or other studies done for roentgenographic confirmation of the clinical impression usually are helpful.

Rupture of the C4-5 disc with compression of the C5 nerve root should result in weakness in the deltoid and biceps muscles. The deltoid is almost entirely innervated by C5, but the biceps has dual innervation. The biceps reflex may be diminished with injury to this nerve root, although it also has a C6 component, and this must be considered. Sensory testing should show a patch on the lateral aspect of the proximal arm to be diminished (Fig. 39-29).

Rupture of the C5-6 disc with compression of the C6 root can be confused with other root levels because of dual innervation of structures. Weakness may be noted in the biceps and extensor carpi radialis longus and brevis. As mentioned above, the biceps is dually innervated by C5 and C6, whereas the long extensors are dually innervated by C6 and C7. The brachioradialis and biceps reflexes also may be diminished at this level. Sensory testing usually indicates a decreased sensibility over the lateral proximal forearm, thumb, and index finger.

Rupture of the C6-7 disc with compression of the C7 root frequently results in weakness of the triceps. Weakness of the wrist flexors, especially the flexor carpi radialis, also is more indicative of C7 root problems. Extensor digitorum communis weakness also can indicate C7 root involvement and may be more readily apparent because of the normal relative weakness of this muscle compared to the triceps. Weakness of the flexor carpi ulnaris usually is caused more by C8 lesions. As mentioned above, finger extensors also may be weakened in that they have both C7 and C8 innervation. The triceps reflex may be diminished. Sensation is lost in the middle finger. C7 sensibility is variable because it is so narrow and overlap is prominent. Strong sensibility change can be difficult to document.

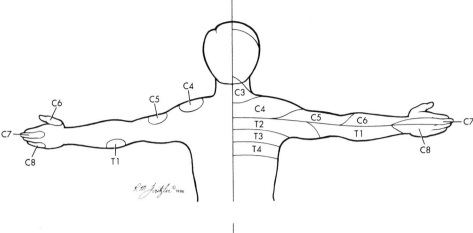

Fig. 39-29 C5 neurological level. (After Hoppenfeld S: *Physical examination of the spine and extremities*, Norwalk, Conn, 1976, Appleton-Century-Crofts.)

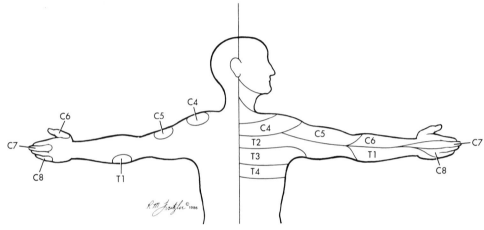

Rupture between C7 and T1 with compression of the C8 nerve root results in no reflex changes. Weakness may be noted in the finger flexors and in the interossei of the hand. Sensibility is lost on the ulnar border of the palm, including the ring and little fingers. Compression of T1 produces weakness of the interosseus muscles, decreased sensibility about the medial aspect of the elbow, and no reflex changes.

The clinical series of Odom, Finney, and Woodhall noted considerable variability in the level of compression and the neurological findings. Change in the triceps reflex was the predominant reflex change with compression of the sixth cervical root (56%). It also was the predominant reflex change in seventh root compression (64%). Similarly the index finger was the predominant digit with sensory change, with evidence of hypalgesia in both sixth (68%) and seventh (70%) cervical root compression.

Care should be taken in the examination of the extremity when radicular problems are encountered to rule out more distal compression syndromes in the upper extremities such as thoracic outlet syndrome, carpal tunnel syndrome, and cubital tunnel syndrome. The lower extremities should be examined with special attention to long tract signs indicative of myelopathy.

No tests for the upper extremity correspond with straight leg raising tests in the lower extremity. Davidson, Dunn, and

Metzmaker described the shoulder abduction relief sign. This can be helpful in the diagnosis of cervical root compression syndromes. The test consists of shoulder abduction and elbow flexion with placement of the hand on the top of the head. This should relieve the arm pain caused by radicular compression. It is interesting to note that if this position is allowed to persist for a minute or two and pain is increased, then more distal compressive neuropathies such as a tardy ulnar nerve syndrome (cubital tunnel syndrome) or primary shoulder pathological conditions often are the cause. Viikari-Juntura, Porras, and Laasonen noted that the shoulder abduction, axial compression, and manual axial traction tests are related to disc disease, but the sensitivity of these tests is low.

Cervical paraspinal spasm and limitation of neck motion are frequent findings of cervical spine disease but are not indicative of a specific pathological process. Special maneuvers involving neck motion can be helpful in the selection of conservative treatment and identification of pathological processes. The distraction test, which involves the examiner placing his hands on the occiput and jaw and distracting the cervical spine in the neutral position, can relieve root compression pain but also can increase pain caused by ligamentous injury. Neck extension and flexion with or without traction can be helpful in selecting conservative therapies.

Patients relieved of pain with the neck extended, with or

without traction, usually have hyperextension syndromes with ligamentous injury posteriorly, whereas patients relieved of pain with distraction and neck flexion are more likely to have nerve root compression caused by either a soft ruptured disc or most likely hypertrophic spurs in the neural foramina. Pain usually is increased in any condition with compression. One must be careful before applying compression or distraction to be sure no cervical instability or fracture is present. One must also be careful in interpreting the distraction test to be certain the temporomandibular joint is not diseased or injured because distraction also will increase the pain in this area.

The signs of midline disc herniation are those of spinal cord compression. If the lesion is high in the cervical region, paresthesias, weakness, atrophy, and occasionally fasciculations may occur in the hands. Also present may be a Hoffman's sign (upper cervical spinal cord) or the inverted radial reflex (typically indicating C5-6 pathology). Most commonly, however, the first and most prominent symptoms are those of involvement of the corticospinal tract; less commonly the posterior columns are affected. The primary signs are sustained clonus, hyperactive reflexes, and the Babinski reflex. Lesser findings are varying degrees of spasticity, weakness in the legs, and impairment of proprioception. Equilibrium may be grossly disturbed, but sense of pain and temperature sense rarely are lost and usually are of little localizing value.

DIFFERENTIAL DIAGNOSIS

The differential diagnosis of cervical disc disease is best separated into extrinsic and intrinsic factors. Extrinsic factors generally include disease processes extrinsic to the neck resulting in symptoms similar to primary neck problems. Included in this group are tumors of the chest, nerve compression syndromes distal to the neck, degenerative processes such as shoulder and upper extremity arthritis, temporomandibular joint syndrome, and lesions about the shoulder such as acute and chronic rotator cuff tears and impingement syndromes. Intrinsic problems primarily consist of lesions directly associated with the cervical spine, the most common being cervical disc degeneration with a concomitant complication of disc herniation and later development of hypertrophic arthritis. Congenital factors such as spinal stenosis in the cervical region also may produce symptoms. Primary and secondary tumors of the cervical spine and fractures of the cervical vertebrae also should be considered as intrinsic lesions.

Cervical disc disease has been categorized by Odom et al. into four groups: (1) unilateral soft disc protrusion with nerve root compression, (2) foraminal spur, or hard disc, with nerve root compression, (3) medial soft disc protrusion with spinal cord compression, and (4) transverse ridge or cervical spondylosis with spinal cord compression. Soft disc herniations usually affect one level, whereas hard disc herniations can affect multiple levels. Central lesions usually result in cord compression symptoms, and lateral lesions usually result in radicular symptoms.

Odom et al. reported that most of the soft disc herniations in their series occurred at the sixth cervical interspace (70%) and fifth cervical interspace (24%). Only six occurred at the seventh interspace. Foraminal spurs also were found predominantly at the sixth interspace (48%). The fifth interspace (39%) and seventh interspace (13%) accounted for the remaining levels where foraminal spurs were found. They also noted the incidence of medial soft disc protrusion with myelopathy to be rare (14 of 246 patients).

Disc material sometimes is extruded into the midline of the spinal canal anteriorly, with compression of the spinal cord and without nerve root involvement. Occasionally this is caused by a violent injury to the cervical spine, with or without fracture-dislocation, and at times it is associated with immediate quadriplegia. However, in some instances the symptoms are progressive and may be suggestive of spinal cord tumor or degenerative diseases of the spinal cord, such as amyotrophic lateral sclerosis, posterolateral sclerosis, and multiple sclerosis. In most of these ailments no block of the spinal canal has been reported, and for many years the mechanism causing the cervical cord compression was not understood. However, in the rare patients whom we have observed, spinal fluid block could be produced by hyperextending the neck, although with the neck in the neutral or flexed position the canal was completely open. This finding has been previously reported. It has since been observed that during operation on such patients when the neck is hyperextended, the superior edge of the lamina compresses the cord against the herniated disc, and it is therefore probable that repeated hyperextension of the neck over a period of weeks, months, or years gradually damages the spinal cord.

In view of the disturbances of the spinal fluid dynamics just mentioned, jugular compression should be carried out during lumbar puncture with the neck in the flexed, neutral, and hyperextended positions. Roentgenographically there is more often than not little or no alteration in the cervical curve. MRI usually demonstrates the abnormality without the need for myelography.

CONFIRMATORY TESTING

Roentgenographic evaluation of the cervical spine frequently shows loss of normal cervical lordosis. Disc space narrowing and hypertrophic changes frequent increase with age but are not indicative of cervical disc rupture. Usually roentgenograms are most helpful to rule out other problems. Oblique roentgenograms of the cervical spine may reveal foraminal encroachment.

MRI of the cervical spine has rapidly become the major diagnostic procedure for neck, arm, and shoulder symptoms. Maruyama evaluated the cervical discs in 36 cadavers using MRI and anatomical dissection and concluded that degeneration appeared to parallel T2 low intensity, but the incidence of false-positive posterior protrusion on MRI was remarkably high. MRI should confirm the objective clinical findings. Asymptomatic findings should be expected to increase with the age of the patient. Cervical myelography usually is indicated only after noninvasive evaluation by MRI fails to reveal the cause or level of the lesion. If MRI is inconclusive, electromyography or nerve conduction velocity may be indicated to demonstrate active radiculopathy before proceeding with myelography, especially if the history and physical examination are not strongly supportive of the presence of radiculopathy. Cervical myelography usually is more precise than lumbar myelography, regardless of the contrast medium used. Postmyelogram CT scanning with block imaging and thin cuts is very helpful.

Cervical discography is a highly controversial technique with limited benefits. It is not indicated in frank disc rupture, spondylosis, or spinal stenosis. The primary use is in patients with persistent neck pain without localized neurological findings in whom standard MRI, myelographic, and CT scan studies are negative. Some investigators maintain that isolated painful discs can be identified in some patients by discography. Certainly a degenerative disc without pain on injection is not the source of the patient's complaint. Cervical discography requires considerable care and caution. It should be considered a preoperative test in those patients in whom an anterior disc excision and interbody fusion are considered for primary neck and shoulder pain. Assessing the psychosocial well-being of a patient is recommended before proceeding with surgical treatment. Great care is required both in the technique and interpretation if reproducible results are desired. Cervical root blocks also have been suggested for the localization and confirmation of symptomatic root compression when used in conjunction with cervical discography. Facet joint injections also should be considered before fusion as a therapeutic as well as diagnostic procedure.

Myelography

When a component of dynamic cord compression is present, myelography remains a valuable tool, although dynamic MRI has reduced the role of myelography. Myelography is performed in the same way as for ruptured lumbar discs except that considerable attention must be paid to the flow of the column of contrast medium with the neck in hyperextended, neutral, and flexed positions. One cannot conclude that spinal cord compression is not present until one is certain that the cephalad flow of the medium is not obstructed with the neck acutely hyperextended. The neck should be hyperextended carefully because of the danger of further damage to the spinal cord.

NONOPERATIVE TREATMENT

As discussed earlier, most patients with symptomatic cervical disc herniations respond well to nonoperative treatment, including some patients with nonprogressive radicular weakness. Reasonably good evidence shows that acute disc herniations actually decrease in size over time in the cervical region. Many conservative treatment methods for neck pain are used for multiple diagnoses. The primary purpose of the cervical spine and associated musculature is to support and mobilize the head while providing a conduit for the nervous system. The forces on the cervical spine are therefore much smaller than on the lower spinal levels. The cervical spine is vulnerable to muscular tension forces, postural fatigue, and excessive motion. Most nonoperative treatments focus on one or more of these factors. The best primary treatment is short periods of rest, massage, ice, and antiinflammatory agents with active mobilization as soon as possible. The position of the neck for comfort is essential for relief of pain. The position of greatest relief may suggest the offending pathological process or mechanism of injury. Patients with hyperflexion injuries usually are more comfortable with the neck in extension over a small roll under the neck. No specific position is indicative of lateral disc herniation, although most tolerate the neutral position best. Patients with spondylosis (hard disc) are most comfortable with the neck in flexion.

Cervical traction can be helpful in selected patients. Care must be exercised in instructing the patient in the proper use of the traction. It should be applied to the head in the position of maximal pain relief. Traction never should be continued if it increases pain. The weights should rarely exceed 10 pounds (weight of the head). The proper head halter and duration of traction sessions should be chosen to prevent irritation of the temporomandibular joint. Traction applied by a patient-controlled pneumatic force, which is more mobile than halter-type units, avoids irritation of temporomandibular joint. Traction also should allow general relaxation of the patient. "Poor man's" traction is a simple method of evaluating the efficacy of cervical traction. It uses the weight of the unsupported head for the traction weight (about 10 pounds). For extension traction, the patient is supine and the head is allowed to gently extend off the examining table or bed. For flexion the same procedure is repeated in the prone position. The patient continues the exercise in the position that is most comfortable for 5 to 10 minutes several times daily.

The postural aspects of neck pain can be treated with more frequent changes in position and ergonomic changes in the work area to prevent fatigue and encourage good posture. Techniques to minimize or relieve tension also are helpful.

Cervical braces usually limit excessive motion. Like traction, they should be tailored to the most comfortable neck position. They may be most helpful for patients who are very active.

Neck and shoulder exercises are most beneficial as the acute pain subsides. Isometric exercises are helpful in the acute phase. Occasionally, shoulder problems such as adhesive capsulitis may be found concomitantly with cervical spondylosis; therefore complete immobilization of the painful extremity should be avoided.

OPERATIVE TREATMENT

The primary indications for operative treatment of cervical disc disease are (1) failure of nonoperative pain management, (2) increasing neurological deficit, and (3) cervical myelopathy that will predictably progress, based on natural history studies. In most patients the persistence of pain is the primary indication. Intuitively, the level of persistent pain should be severe enough to consistently interfere with the patient's desired activity and greater than would reasonably be expected after operative treatment. The choice of approach should be determined by the position and type of lesion. Soft lateral discs are easily removed from the posterior approach, whereas soft central or hard discs (central or lateral) probably are best treated with an anterior approach. Any controversy that existed relative to the need for fusion with anterior discectomy essentially has been resolved with long-term follow-up studies of patients without fusion, such as that by Yamamoto et al. mentioned previously. Osteophytes that were not removed at surgery have been shown frequently to be reabsorbed at the level of fusion. The use of a graft also prevents the collapse of the disc space and maintains adequate foraminal size.

◆ Removal of Posterolateral Herniations by Posterior Approach (Posterior Cervical Foraminotomy)

TECHNIQUE 39-15

With the patient under general endotracheal anesthesia in the prone position and the face in a Mayfield positioner, flex the neck to obliterate the cervical lordosis as much as possible. The upright position for surgery decreases venous bleeding, but concern regarding the possibility of air embolism and cerebral hypoxia in the event of a significant drop in blood pressure makes us reluctant to recommend its use. Usually a slight reverse Trendelenburg position works well in posterior cervical surgery coupled with careful dissection to minimize bleeding. The shoulders are retracted inferiorly with tape if roentgenograms of the lower cervical levels are contemplated.

Appropriately prepare and drape the operative field. Make a midline incision 2.5 cm lower than the interspace to be explored (Fig. 39-30). Retract the edges of this incision and the skin will withdraw in a cephalad direction so that the wound becomes properly placed. Divide the ligamentum nuchae longitudinally to expose the tips of the spinous processes above and below the designated area. The correct position is reasonably well ensured by palpation of the last bifid spine, which usually is the sixth cervical vertebra. However, it should be verified intraoperatively by a marker attached to the spinous process and documented on the lateral cervical spine roentgenogram. Dissect subperiosteally the paravertebral muscles from the laminae on the side of the lesion and retract them with a self-retaining retractor or with the help of an assistant using a Hibbs retractor.

With a small high-speed drill, grind away the caudal edge of the lateral portion of the lamina cephalad to the interspace. Usually minimal bone removal from the cephalad edge of the lateral portion of the caudal lamina is needed. Only a small amount of the medial portion of the facet needs to be removed in most patients. A small Kerrison rongeur (1 to 2 mm) can be used to enlarge this keyhole as needed. Sharply excise the ligamentum flavum with a small Kerrison rongeur and identify the nerve root, which is commonly displaced posteriorly and flattened by pressure from the underlying disc fragments. Removal of additional bone along the dorsal aspect of the foramen and immediately above and below the nerve root often is beneficial at this point. Once the bony removal has been completed, we prefer to use the operative microscope for the remainder of the procedure. This allows more delicate work around the neural elements while minimizing additional bone removal and allows better hemostasis.

The herniated nucleus pulposus most often lies slightly caudal to the center of the nerve root but occasionally cephalad. Gently retract the nerve root superiorly to expose the extruded nuclear fragments or a distended posterior longitudinal ligament. The nerve root should not be retracted in a caudal direction. If additional exposure is needed, remove more bone rather than risk nerve root or spinal cord injury from traction on the root. To control troublesome venous oozing at this point use bipolar cautery if possible. Otherwise, place tiny pledgets of cotton and thrombin-soaked Gelfoam above and below the nerve root. Take care not to pack the pledgets tightly around the nerve. The nerve root then can be retracted slightly in a cephalad direction to allow incision of the posterior longitudinal ligament over the herniated nucleus pulposus in a cruciate manner to permit the removal of the disc fragments.

After removal of all visible loose fragments, it is imperative to make a thorough search for additional fragments, both laterally and medially. It is equally important to be sure that the nerve root is thoroughly decompressed by inserting a probe in the intervertebral foramen. If the nerve root still seems to be tight, remove more bone from the articular facets until the nerve root is completely free. Since recurrence is so rare, do not curet the intervertebral space. Remove any cotton pledgets and Gelfoam after meticulous hemostasis has been achieved. Hemostasis must be complete because postoperative hemorrhage can produce cord compression and quadriplegia. Close the wound by suturing the fascia to the supraspinous ligament with interrupted sutures and then suturing the subcutaneous layers and skin.

AFTERTREATMENT. Neurological function is closely monitored after surgery. Discharge is permitted when the patient can walk and void. Pain should be controlled with oral medication. Currently most patients are discharged within 24 hours after surgery. Radicular pain relief usually is dramatic and prompt, although hypesthesia can persist for weeks or months. The patient is allowed to return to clerical work when comfortable

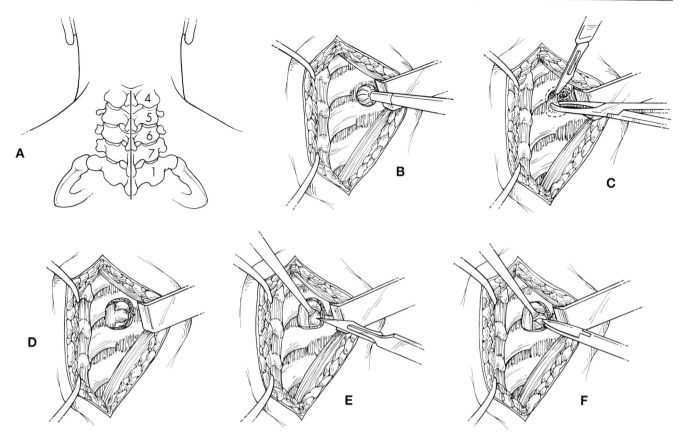

Fig. 39-30 Technique of removal of disc between fifth and sixth cervical vertebrae. **A,** Midline incision extending from spinous process of fourth cervical vertebra to that of first thoracic vertebra. **B,** Paraspinal muscles have been dissected from laminae and retracted laterally. Hole is to be drilled with Hudson burr (see text). **C,** Ligamentum flavum is being dissected. **D,** Defect measuring about 1.3 cm has been made (see text) to expose nerve root and lateral aspect of dura. **E,** Nerve root has been separated from nucleus and retracted superiorly to expose herniated disc. **F,** Longitudinal ligament has been incised, and loose fragment of nucleus is being removed.

and to manual labor after 6 weeks. As a rule, neither support nor physical therapy is necessary, and the patient's future activity is not restricted. Isometric neck exercises, upper extremity range-of-motion exercises, and posterior shoulder girdle exercises can be useful for patients in whom atrophy or inactivity has been considerable. A soft cervical collar can help relieve immediate postoperative pain.

Results. In few if any operations in orthopaedic surgery are the results better than after the removal of a lateral herniated cervical disc. In the series of 250 operations reported by Simmons there were no deaths or major complications involving the brain or spinal cord. Three patients had reflex sympathetic dystrophy postoperatively. Two of these completely recovered and one almost so. Two patients continued to have arm pain after operation and were reexplored during the initial hospital stay; in each, several more fragments of disc were found and removed. It is assumed that these fragments were overlooked at the initial operation. One patient had a recurrent extrusion at the same level. Two other patients had

soft extrusions on the opposite side at another level, also requiring a second operation.

Murphey, Simmons, and Brunson analyzed the results in a series of 150 patients who returned questionnaires concerning the success or failure of the operation. They were asked to state the percentage of benefit they derived from the procedure (Table 39-8), whether they were performing the same work as they had done preoperatively, and if not, whether the change of work had resulted from neck trouble. Approximately 90% had extremely good results, and there were none who were not significantly improved, as the data concerning work done confirm. Only 7 (6%) of the 125 patients who answered this part of the questionnaire found a change of work necessary because of neck trouble.

Anterior Approach to Cervical Disc

Smith and Robinson in 1955 were the first to recommend an anterior approach to the cervical spine in the treatment of cervical disc disease. They described an anterolateral discectomy with interbody fusion (Fig. 39-31). This pro-

Table 39-8 Results of Removal of Lateral Herniated Discs in Cervical Region (Patient's Estimate of Percent Improvement)

Relief (%)	Patients Improved (%)	Number of Patients
95-100	65.3	98
90-94	23.3	35
75-89	8.0	12
50-74	3.3	5
Total	100.0	150

Murphey F, Simmons JCH, Brunson B: *J Neurosurg* 38:679, 1973.

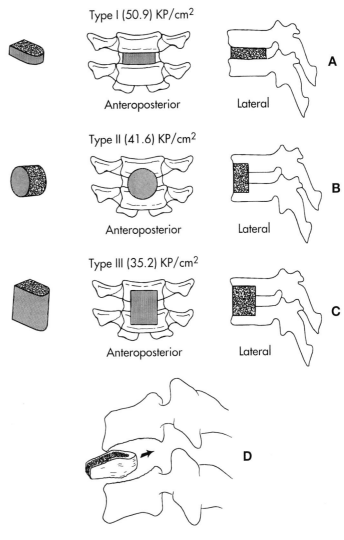

Fig. 39-31   Types of anterior cervical fusion. **A,** Smith-Robinson fusion. **B,** Cloward fusion. **C,** Bailey-Badgley fusion. **D,** Bloom-Raney modification of Smith-Robinson fusion. (**A** to **C** redrawn from White AA, Jupiter J, Southwick WO, Panjabi MM: *Clin Orthop* 91:21, 1973; **D** redrawn from Bloom MH, Raney FL: *J Bone Joint Surg* 63A:842, 1981.)

cedure attained widespread acceptance and application after Cloward in 1958 modified the procedure and introduced new instrumentation.

Three basic techniques are used for anterior cervical disc excision and fusion. The Cloward technique involves making a round hole centered at the disc space. A slightly larger, round iliac crest plug is then inserted into the disc space hole. The Smith-Robinson technique involves inserting a tricortical plug of iliac crest into the disc space after removing the disc and cartilaginous endplate. The graft is inserted with the cancellous side facing the cord (posterior). Bloom and Raney modified this technique by fashioning the tricortical graft to be thicker in its midportion and then inserting the graft with the cancellous portion facing anteriorly. The Bailey-Badgley technique involves the creation of a slot in the superior and inferior vertebral bodies. This technique is most applicable to reconstruction when one or more vertebral bodies are excised for tumor, stenosis, or other extensive pathological conditions. Simmons and Bhalla modified this technique by using a keystone graft that increases the surface area of the graft by 30% and allows more complete locking of the graft. Biomechanically, the Smith-Robinson technique provides the greatest stability and least risk of extrusion, compared to the Cloward or Bailey-Badgley type fusions.

White et al. reported relief of pain in 90% of 65 patients undergoing anterior cervical spine fusion for spondylosis with the technique of Smith and Robinson. Analysis of 90 patients with anterior cervical discectomies and fusion for cervical spondylosis with radiculopathy using the Cloward technique showed good or excellent results in 82% in the study by Jacobs, Krueger, and Levy. These investigators did not use discography. Others also have found that discography does not statistically improve the results. The Smith-Robinson technique is used almost exclusively at this clinic for anterior cervical discectomy procedures.

The choice of right- or left-sided approach to the cervical spine is somewhat controversial. The right side of the neck is preferred by some right-handed surgeons because of the ease of dissection. The reported increased risk of recurrent laryngeal nerve trauma when operating on the right is not judged by those who use it to be a significant deterrent to choosing this exposure. Exposure from the left is more inconvenient for a right-handed surgeon but decreases the risk of recurrent laryngeal nerve injury. This nerve on the left consistently descends with the carotid sheath and exits from the carotid sheath and vagus nerve intrathoracically. The nerve then courses under the arch of the aorta and ascends in the neck beside the trachea and esophagus. The course of the nerve on the right is not as consistent. The nerve usually descends with the carotid sheath and then loops around the subclavian artery and ascends between the trachea and esophagus. Occasionally the right recurrent laryngeal nerve exits the carotid sheath early and crosses anteriorly behind the thyroid. A large series of anterior cervical procedures implicated the endotracheal tube in combination with self-retaining retractors as the cause of recurrent laryngeal nerve injuries. The recommendation made was to deflate the cuff of the endotracheal tube after retractor placement to allow the tip of the tube to reposition itself. This significantly decreased the incidence of recurrent laryngeal nerve palsy in a series of 600 patients. See Chapter 36 for a complete description of anterior cervical discectomy and fusion.

Anterior Foraminotomy. Recently there have been several reports of microsurgical anterior foraminotomy to treat unilateral foraminal nerve compression from soft disc herniations or uncovertebral joint degenerative change. Verbiest first described this technique; Jho reported a modification, and Johnson reported a small clinical series. This technique appears to allow adequate decompression of the ventral aspect of the foramen unilaterally while removing the lateral portion of the disc, thus preserving the remaining disc. The long-term results are not yet available to compare this technique with anterior discectomy with fusion. We do not have any clinical experience with this technique.

◆ *Microsurgical Anterior Cervical Foraminotomy*

TECHNIQUE 39-16 *(Jho)*

After anesthesia has been administered by means of endotracheal intubation, place the patient supine, with a bolster placed behind both shoulders to maintain gentle extension of the cervical spine. Position the head with the midline upright. Gently pull both shoulders caudally and fix with tape for a good lateral view of the cervical spine on intraoperative roentgenogram. Do not use a cervical traction device. Prepare the anterior neck with antiseptic solution and drape.

Make a 3- to 5-cm long transverse incision in a skin crease ipsilateral to the radiculopathy. The first two thirds of the incision should be medial to the sternocleidomastoid muscle and the remainder should be lateral to the medial border of that muscle. Incise the subcutaneous tissue and platysma muscle along the line of the skin incision. Cleanly undermine the loose connective tissue layer under the platysma muscle to provide space in which to work. Use a combination of sharp and blunt dissection to access the anterior column of the cervical spine. Keep the carotid artery and the sternocleidomastoid muscle lateral and the strap muscle, trachea, and esophagus medial. Open the prevertebral fascia and expose the anterior column of the cervical spine. Confirm the correct level roentgenographically.

Use an anterior cervical discectomy retractor system to expose the ipsilateral longus colli muscle (Fig. 39-32, *A*). Use only smooth-tipped retractor blades to avoid injury to the trachea and esophagus medially and the carotid artery and vagus nerve laterally. Use the operating microscope at this stage and excise the medial portion of the longus colli muscle to expose the medial parts of the transverse

processes of the upper and lower vertebrae (Fig. 39-32, *B*). Expose the vertebral artery anterior to the C7 transverse process. When operating at C6-7 take care not to injure the vertebral artery while removing the medial portion of the longus colli muscle. For operations above C6-7, the vertebral artery is not exposed purposely at this point.

Once the medial parts of the transverse processes of the upper and lower vertebrae have been identified, the ipsilateral uncovertebral joint between them can be seen. The interface of the uncovertebral joint is angled approximately 30 degrees cephalad from the horizontal line of the intervertebral disc. Make a sharp vertical incision of the disc at the medial margin of the ipsilateral uncovertebral joint to prevent inadvertent internal disruption of the remaining disc. While drilling the bone, repeated sharp cutting of the deeper disc may be required. Remove the thin layer of disc material located at the uncovertebral joint.

Drill between the transverse processes of the uncovertebral joint using a high-speed microdrill attached to an angled handpiece (Fig. 39-32, *C*). To prevent injury to the vertebral artery, leave the thin cortical bone attached to the ligamentous tissue covering the medial portion of this artery. Continue drilling down to the posterior longitudinal ligament (see Fig. 39-32, *C*). While drilling posteriorly, gently incline medially. When the posterior longitudinal ligament is exposed, a piece of thin cortical bone remains attached lateral to the ligamentous tissue covering the vertebral artery. Dissect the lateral remnant of the uncinate process from the ligamentous tissue and fracture it at the base of the uncinate process (Fig. 39-32, *D*). Further dissect it from the surrounding soft tissue and remove it. The vertebral artery can be identified by its pulsation between the transverse processes of the vertebrae. Drilling at the base of the uncinate process must proceed cautiously because the nerve root lies just behind it. After the uncinate process becomes loosened at its base, remove the remaining thin bone of the uncinate process by fracturing it from its base rather than by continued drilling. Once the remaining piece of uncinate process is removed, the compressed nerve root will be distended forward by bone decompression (Fig. 39-32, *E*). The size of the hole that is made by drilling at the uncovertebral joint usually is approximately 5 to 8 mm wide transversely and 7 to 10 mm wide vertically. If there is no ruptured herniated disc fragment behind the posterior longitudinal ligament, this will end the nerve root decompression.

At this point the posterior longitudinal ligament still covers the nerve root and the lateral margin of the spinal cord. If the disc fragment has ruptured through the posterior longitudinal ligament, the tail of the disc material will be visible. Remove this disc fragment at this time. To avoid overlooking a hidden disc fragment, use a no. 15 blade knife or micro scissors to incise the ligament and remove any fragment with a 1- or 2-mm foot-plated bone punch. The

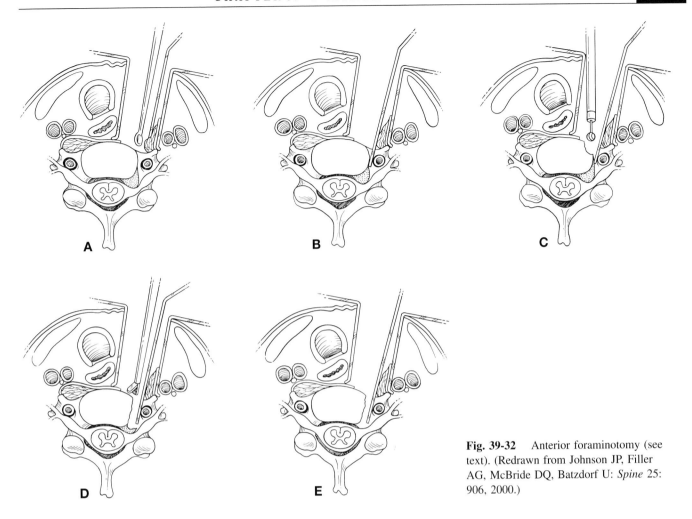

Fig. 39-32 Anterior foraminotomy (see text). (Redrawn from Johnson JP, Filler AG, McBride DQ, Batzdorf U: *Spine* 25: 906, 2000.)

ipsilateral one third to one half of the spinal cord is thus exposed and the nerve root can be seen laterally as it exits behind the vertebral artery.

Jho reported excision of the posterior longitudinal ligament in selected cases because it is unlikely that a hidden ruptured disc fragment could be present without disruption of this ligament. Removal of the ligament sometimes is complicated by epidural bleeding. If the ligament is not removed, the procedure is much simpler and the operating time is shorter. If epidural bleeding occurs during removal of the posterior longitudinal ligament, use bipolar coagulation. To avoid any potential compressive material coming into contact with the nerve root or spinal cord, do not use hemostatic agents. Although epidural bleeding usually is not a problem, removing the posterior longitudinal ligament is the most difficult part of this procedure. The disc within the intervertebral space remains untouched and preserved.

Close the platysma with interrupted 3-0 absorbable stitches and approximate the skin with subcuticular sutures. The operation can be performed at multiple levels. To minimize postoperative incisional pain, inject a few milliliters of local anesthetic subcutaneously.

Thoracic Disc Disease

The thoracic spine is the least common location for disc pathology. C.A. Key has been credited with the first report of a spinal cord injury caused by thoracic disc herniation, which appeared in 1838 in the Guy's Hospital Report. In the early twentieth century several reports of enchondromata, chondromata, or echondromata appeared. In their study in 1934 Mixter and Barr included four patients with a thoracic location of the herniated nucleus pulposus. Of the four patients in this series, three were treated operatively and one nonoperatively. The patient with nonoperative treatment died soon after diagnosis. Of the surgical group, two had complete paraplegia postoperatively. The third surgical patient died several months later for unknown reasons. These three were treated with posterior laminectomy. This initial report not only described the condition, but also revealed some of the difficulties of treatment.

Since the 1960s many other approaches have been described and validated through clinical experience. It is apparent that posterior laminectomy has no role in the surgical treatment of this problem. Other posterior approaches, such as costotransversectomy, have good indications. Fessler and Sturgill, as well as Vanichkachorn and Vaccaro, chronicled the history and treatment evolution for thoracic disc disease.

Symptomatic thoracic disc herniations remain relatively rare, with an estimated incidence of 1 in 1,000,000 persons per year. They represent 0.25% to 0.75% of the total incidence of symptomatic disc herniations. The most common age of onset is between the fourth and sixth decades. As with the other areas of the spine, the incidence of asymptomatic disc herniations is high. Wood et al. reviewed MRI studies in 90 asymptomatic patients and found thoracic disc abnormalities in 73%. Of these, 37% had frank herniations and 29% showed cord compression. At a mean follow-up of 26 months with repeat MRI of some of these patients none had become symptomatic. Also, Wood et al. noted that small herniations often increased, whereas the larger herniations often regressed. Operative treatment of thoracic disc herniations is indicated in the rare patient with acute disc herniation with myelopathic findings attributable to the lesion, especially progressive neurological symptoms.

SIGNS AND SYMPTOMS

Fortunately, the natural history of symptomatic thoracic disc disease is similar to that in other areas, in that symptoms and function typically improve with conservative treatment and time. However, the clinical course can be quite variable, and a high index of suspicion must be maintained to make the correct diagnosis. The differential diagnosis for the symptoms of thoracic disc herniations is fairly extensive and includes nonspinal causes occurring with the cardiopulmonary, gastrointestinal, and musculoskeletal systems. Spinal causes of similar symptoms can occur with infectious, neoplastic, degenerative, and metabolic problems within the spinal column as well as the spinal cord.

Two general patient populations have been documented in the literature. The smaller group of patients is younger and has a relatively short history of symptoms, often with a history of trauma. Typically, an acute soft disc herniation with either acute spinal cord compression or radiculopathy is present. Outcome generally is favorable with operative or nonoperative treatment. The larger group of patients has a longer history, often more than 6 to 12 months of symptoms, which result from chronic spinal cord or root compression. Disc degeneration, often with calcification of the disc, is the underlying process.

Pain is clearly the most common presenting feature of thoracic disc herniations. There appear to be two patterns of pain: one is axial and the other is bandlike radicular pain along the course of the intercostal nerve. The T10 dermatomal level is the most commonly reported distribution, regardless of the level of involvement. This is a band extending around the lower lateral thorax and caudally to the level of the umbilicus. This

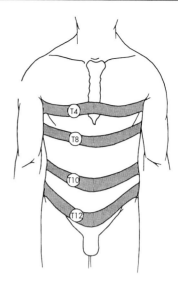

Fig. 39-33 Sensory dermatomes of trunk region. (Redrawn from Klein JD, Garfin SR: History and physical examination. In Weinstein JN, Rydevik BL, Somtag VKH, eds: *Essentials of the spine,* New York, 1995, Raven.)

radicular pattern is more common with upper thoracic and lateral disc herniations. Some axial pain often occurs with this pattern as well. Associated sensory changes of paresthesias and dysesthesia in a dermatomal distribution also occur. (Fig. 39-33). High thoracic discs (T2 to T5) can present similarly to cervical disc disease with upper arm pain, paresthesias, radiculopathy, and even Horner's syndrome. Myelopathy also may occur. Complaints of weakness, which may be generalized by the patient, typically involving both lower extremities present in the form of mild paraparesis. The presence of sustained clonus, a positive Babinski sign, and wide-based and spastic gait are all signs of myelopathy. Bowel and bladder dysfunction occur in only about 15% to 20% of these patients. The neurological evaluation of patients with thoracic disc herniations must be meticulous because there are few localizing findings. Abdominal reflexes, cremasteric reflex, dermatomal sensory evaluation, rectus abdominis contraction symmetry, lower extremity reflex, strength, and sensory examinations, as well as determination of long tract findings, are all important.

CONFIRMATORY TESTING

Plain roentgenograms are of some help to evaluate traumatic injuries and to determine potential osseous morphological variations that may help to localize findings, especially on intraoperative films, if these become necessary. MRI is the most important and useful imaging method to demonstrate thoracic disc herniations. In addition to the disc herniation, neoplastic or infectious pathology can be seen. The presence of intradural pathology, including disc fragments, also usually is demonstrated on MRI. The spinal cord signal may indicate the presence of inflammation or myelomalacia as well. Despite all these advantages, MRI may underestimate the thoracic disc herniation, which often is calcified and thus has low signal intensity on T1 and T2 sequences.

Myelography followed by CT scanning also can be useful in evaluating the bony anatomy, as well as more accurately assessing the calcified portion of the herniated thoracic disc. Regardless of the imaging methods used, the appearance and presence of a thoracic disc herniation must be carefully considered and correlated with the patient's complaints and detailed examination findings.

TREATMENT RESULTS

As mentioned previously, nonoperative treatment usually is effective. Brown reported that 63% of patients improved using a combination of nonoperative treatments. A specific regimen cannot be recommended for all patients; however, the principles of short-term rest, pain relief, antiinflammatory agents, and progressive directed activity restoration appear most appropriate. These measures generally should be continued at least 6 to 12 weeks if feasible. If neurological deficits progress or present as myelopathy, or if pain remains at an intolerable level, surgery should be recommended. The initial procedure recommended for this lesion was posterior thoracic laminectomy and disc excision. At least half of the lesions have been identified as being central, making the excision from this approach extremely difficult, and the results were somewhat disheartening. Most series reported fewer than half of the patients improving, with some becoming worse after posterior laminectomy and discectomy. Most recent studies suggest that lateral rachiotomy (modified costotransversectomy) or an anterior transthoracic approach for discectomy produces considerably better results with no evidence of worsening after the procedure. Video-assisted thoracic surgery (VATS) has been used in several series to successfully remove central thoracic disc herniations without the need for a thoracotomy or fusion. Bohlman and Zdeblick reported the results of anterior thoracic disc excision in 19 patients: 16 patients had excellent or good results, and 3 had fair or poor results. Pain was relieved in 10, decreased in 8, and unchanged in 1. None had worsening of neurological symptoms. Regan, BinYashay, and Mack reported a series of 29 thoracoscopic disc excisions with 76% satisfactory results.

OPERATIVE TREATMENT

The best surgical approach for these lesions depends on the specific characteristics of the disc herniation, as well as on the particular experience of the surgeon. Simple laminectomy really has no role in the treatment of thoracic disc herniations. Posterior approaches, including costotransversectomy, transpedicular approach, and the lateral extracavitary approach, have all been used successfully. Anterior approaches via thoracotomy, a transsternal approach, or VATS also have been used successfully (Fig. 39-34).

◆ Costotransversectomy

Costotransversectomy is probably best suited for thoracic disc herniations that are predominantly lateral or herniations that are suspected to be extruded or sequestered. Central disc herniations are probably best approached transthoracically. Some surgeons have recommended subsequent fusion after disc removal anteriorly or laterally.

TECHNIQUE 39-17

The operation usually is done with the patient under general anesthesia with a cuffed endotracheal tube or a Carlen tube to allow lung deflation on the side of approach. Place the patient prone and make a long midline incision or a curved incision convex to the midline centered over the side of involvement. Expose the spine in the usual manner out to the ribs. Remove a section of rib 5 to 7.5 cm long at the level of involvement, taking care to avoid damage to the intercostal nerve and artery. Carry the resection into the lateral side of the disc, exposing it for removal. Additional exposure can be made by laminectomy and excision of the pedicle and facet joint. Fusion is unnecessary unless more than one facet joint is removed. Close the wound in layers.

AFTERTREATMENT. The aftertreatment is similar to that for lumbar disc excision without fusion (Technique 39-21).

◆ Anterior Approach for Thoracic Disc Excision

Because of the relative age of patients with thoracic disc ruptures, special care must be taken to identify those with pulmonary problems. In these patients the anterior approach can be detrimental medically, making a posterolateral approach safer. Patients with midline protrusions probably are best treated with the transthoracic approach to ensure complete disc removal.

TECHNIQUE 39-18

The operation is done with the patient under general anesthesia, using a cuffed endotracheal tube or Carlen tube for lung deflation on the side of the approach. Place the patient in a lateral recumbent position. A left-sided anterior approach usually is preferred, making the operative procedure easier. Make a skin incision along the line of the rib that corresponds to the second thoracic vertebra above the involved intervertebral disc except for approaches to the upper five thoracic segments, where the approach is through the third rib. Choose the skin incision by inspection of the anteroposterior roentgenogram. Cut the rib subperiosteally at its posterior and anterior ends and then insert a rib retractor. Save the rib for grafting later in the procedure. One can then decide on an extrapleural or transpleural approach depending on familiarity and ease. Exposure of the thoracic vertebrae should give adequate access to the front and opposite side. Dissect the great vessels free of the spine.

continued

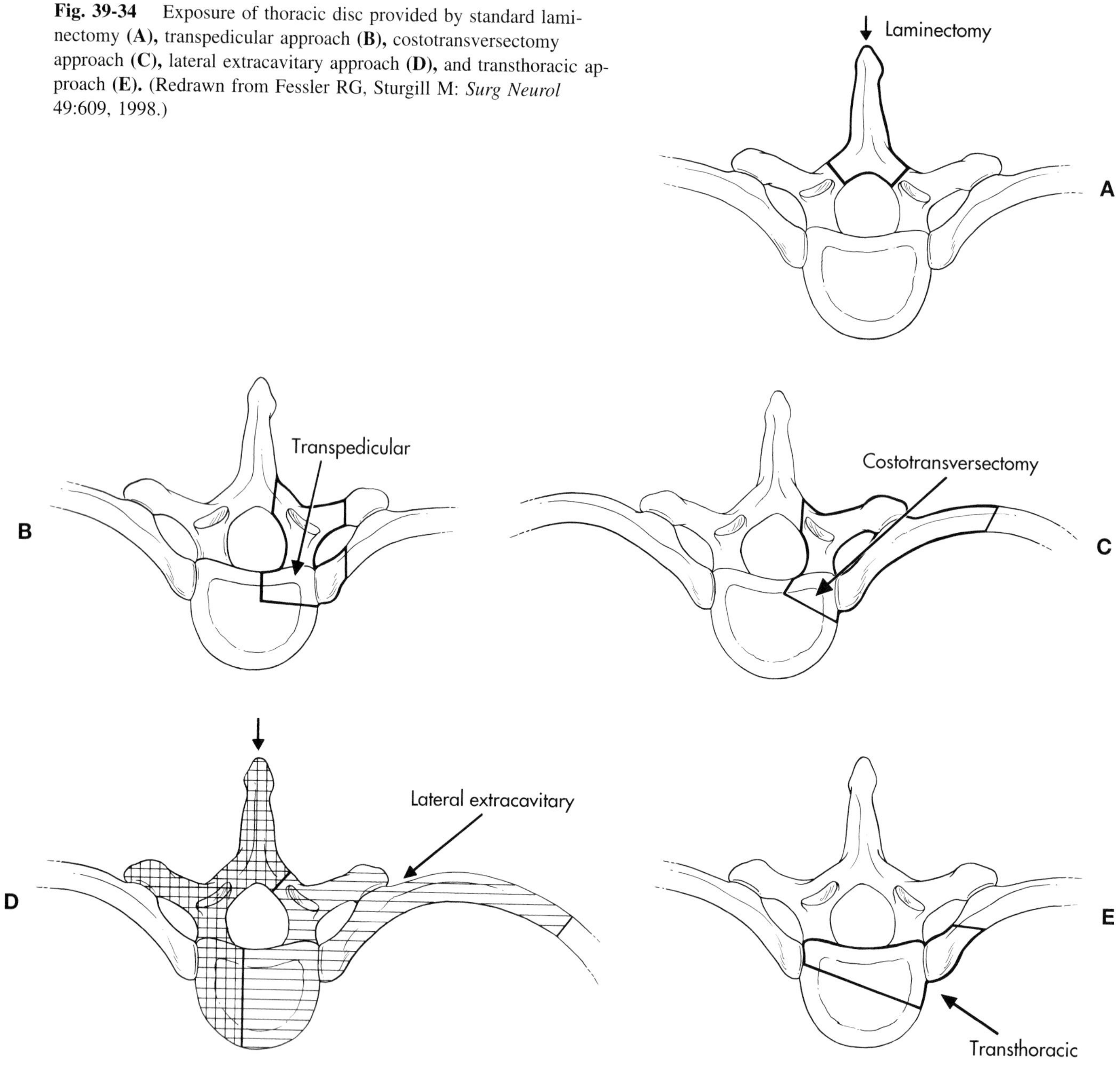

Fig. 39-34 Exposure of thoracic disc provided by standard laminectomy (**A**), transpedicular approach (**B**), costotransversectomy approach (**C**), lateral extracavitary approach (**D**), and transthoracic approach (**E**). (Redrawn from Fessler RG, Sturgill M: *Surg Neurol* 49:609, 1998.)

Laminectomy

A

Transpedicular

B

Costotransversectomy

C

Lateral extracavitary

D

E

Transthoracic

Ligate the intersegmental vessels near the great vessels and not near the foramen. One should be able to insert the tip of a finger against the opposite side of the disc when the vascular mobilization is complete. Exposure of the intervertebral disc without disturbing more than three segmental vessels is preferable to avoid ischemic problems in the spinal cord. In the thoracolumbar region strip the diaphragm from the eleventh and twelfth ribs. The anterior longitudinal ligament usually is sectioned to allow spreading of the intervertebral disc space. Remove the disc as completely as possible if fusion is planned. The use of the operating microscope or loupe magnification eases the removal of the disc near the posterior longitudinal ligament. Use curets and nibbling instruments to remove the disc up to the posterior longitudinal ligament. Then place a finger on the opposite side of the disc to avoid penetration when removing disc material on the more distant side. Carefully inspect the posterior longitudinal ligament for tears and extruded fragments. Remove the posterior longitudinal ligament only if necessary. Significant bleeding can occur if the venous plexus near the dura is torn. After removal of the disc, strip the endplates of their cartilage. Make a slot in one vertebral

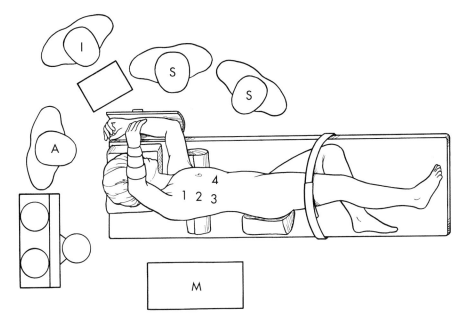

Fig. 39-35   Position on operating table and operating room setup. Surgeons *(S)* and nurse with instruments *(I)* stand in front of patient. Monitor *(M)* placed at back. "Working channels" *(1,2,3)* converge toward spine. Channel for optical system *(4)* situated ventrally. (From Rosenthal D, Rosenthal R, de Simone A: *Spine* 19:1087, 1994.)

body and a hole in the body on the opposite side of the disc space to accept the graft material. Make the hole large enough to accept several sections of rib, but make the slot large enough to accept only one rib graft at a time. Then insert iliac, tibial, or rib grafts into the disc space. Tie the grafts together with heavy suture material when the maximal number of grafts have been inserted. Close the wound in the usual manner and employ standard chest drainage. As an alternative, if fusion is not desired a more limited resection using the operating microscope can be done. After the vascular mobilization, resect the rib head to allow observation of the pedicle and foramen caudal to the disc space. The pedicle can be removed with a high-speed burr and Kerrison rongeurs, thus exposing the posterolateral aspect of the disc. This allows careful, blunt development of the plane ventral to the dura with removal of the disc herniation and preservation of the anterior majority of the disc, as well as limiting the need for fusion. A similar technique using VATS is described in Technique 39-19.

The transthoracic approach removing a rib two levels above the level of the lesion can be used up to T5. The transthoracic approach from T2 to T5 is best made by excision of the third or fourth rib and elevation of the scapula by sectioning of attachments of the serratus anterior and trapezius from the scapula. The approach to the T1-2 disc is best made from the neck with a sternal splitting incision.

AFTERTREATMENT. Postoperative care is the same as for a thoracotomy. The patient is allowed to walk after the chest tubes are removed. Extension in any position is prohibited. A brace or body cast that limits extension should be used if the

stability of the graft is questionable. The graft usually is stable without support if only one disc space is removed. Postoperative care is the same as for anterior corpectomy and fusion if more than one disc level is removed. If no fusion is done, the patient is mobilized as pain permits without a brace.

◆ Thoracic Endoscopic Disc Excision

Microsurgical and endoscopic surgical techniques are being applied to the anterior excision of thoracic disc herniation. Rosenthal et al. and Horowitz et al. first performed these procedures on cadavers to perfect the technique. Because these methods are highly technical, they should be performed by a surgeon who is proficient in this technique and in the use of endoscopic equipment and with the assistance of an experienced thoracic surgeon. Ideally the procedure should be done on cadavers or live animals first. Regan et al. also described this technique, with different portal positions.

TECHNIQUE 39-19 *(Rosenthal et al.)*
(Figs. 39-35 and 39-36)
Place the patient in the left lateral decubitus position to allow a right-sided approach and displacement of the aorta and heart to the left. Insert four trocars in a triangular fashion along the middle axillary line converging on the disc space. Introduce a rigid endoscope with a 30-degree optic angle attached to a video camera into one of the trocars, leaving the other three as working channels. Deflate the lung using a Carlin tube or similar method. Split the parietal pleura starting at the medial part of the intervertebral space and extending up to the costovertebral process. Preserve and mobilize the segmental arteries and sympathetic nerve out of the operating field. Drill away the rib head and lateral

continued

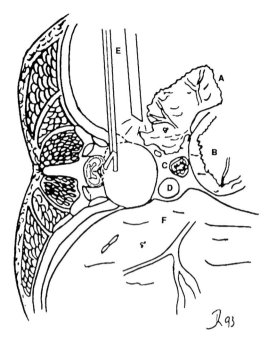

Fig. 39-36 Endoscopic removal of thoracic disc. Horizontal view at T6 level. Patient is in left lateral decubitus position. *A,* Right lung (collapsed). *B,* Heart and pericardium. *C,* Esophagus. *D,* Aorta. *E,* Forceps and endoscope. *F,* Left lung. (From Rosenthal D, Rosenthal R, de Simone A: *Spine* 19:1087, 1994.)

portion of the pedicle. Remove the remaining pedicle with Kerrison rongeurs to improve exposure to the spinal canal. Removing the superior posterior portion of the vertebra caudal to the disc space allows safer removal of the disc material, which then can be pulled anteriorly and inferiorly away from the spinal canal to be removed. Use endoscopic instruments for surgery in the portals. Remove the disc posteriorly and the posterior longitudinal ligament, restricting bone and disc removal to the posterior third of the intervertebral space and costovertebral area to maintain stability. Insert chest tubes in the standard fashion and set them to water suction; close the portals.

AFTERTREATMENT. The patient is rapidly mobilized as tolerated by the chest tubes. Discharge is possible once the chest tubes have been removed and the patient is ambulating well.

Lumbar Disc Disease

SIGNS AND SYMPTOMS

Although back pain is common from the second decade of life on, intervertebral disc disease and disc herniation are most prominent in otherwise healthy people in the third and fourth decades of life. Most people relate their back and leg pain to a traumatic incident, but close questioning frequently reveals that the patient has had intermittent episodes of back pain for many months or even years before the onset of severe leg pain. In many instances the back pain is relatively fleeting and is relieved by rest. This pain often is brought on by heavy exertion, repetitive bending, twisting, or heavy lifting. In other instances an exacerbating incident cannot be elicited. The pain usually begins in the lower back, radiating to the sacroiliac region and buttocks. The pain can radiate down the posterior thigh. Back and posterior thigh pain of this type can be elicited from many areas of the spine, including the facet joints, longitudinal ligaments, and the periosteum of the vertebra. Radicular pain, on the other hand, usually extends below the knee and follows the dermatome of the involved nerve root.

The usual history of lumbar disc herniation is of repetitive lower back and buttock pain, relieved by a short period of rest. This pain is then suddenly exacerbated by a flexion episode, with the sudden appearance of leg pain much greater than back pain. Most radicular pain from nerve root compression caused by a herniated nucleus pulposus is evidenced by leg pain equal to, or in many cases much greater than, the degree of back pain. Whenever leg pain is minimal and back pain is predominant, great care should be taken before making the diagnosis of a symptomatic herniated intervertebral disc. The pain from disc herniation usually is intermittent, increasing with activity, especially sitting. The pain can be relieved by rest, especially in the semi-Fowler position, and can be exacerbated by straining, sneezing, or coughing. Whenever the pattern of pain is bizarre or the pain itself is constant, a diagnosis of symptomatic herniated disc should be viewed with some skepticism.

Other symptoms of disc herniation include weakness and paresthesias. In most patients the weakness is intermittent, variable with activity, and localized to the neurological level of involvement. Paresthesias also are variable and limited to the dermatome of the involved nerve root. Whenever these complaints are generalized, the diagnosis of a simple unilateral disc herniation should be questioned.

Numbness and weakness in the involved leg and occasionally pain in the groin or testicle can be associated with a high or midline lumbar disc herniation. If a fragment is large or the herniation is high, symptoms of pressure on the entire cauda equina can be elicited. These include numbness and weakness in both legs, rectal pain, numbness in the perineum, and paralysis of the sphincters. This diagnosis should be the primary consideration in patients who complain of sudden loss of bowel or bladder control. Whenever the diagnosis of a cauda equina syndrome or acute midline herniation is suspected, evaluation and treatment should be aggressive.

PHYSICAL FINDINGS

The physical findings in back pain with disc disease are variable because of the time intervals involved. Usually patients with acute pain show evidence of marked paraspinal spasm that is sustained during walking or motion. A scoliosis or

---

BOX 39-7 • L4 Root Compression*

Sensory Deficit
Posterolateral thigh, anterior knee, and medial leg

Motor Weakness
Quadriceps (variable)
Hip adductors (variable)

Reflex Change
Patellar tendon
Tibialis anterior tendon (variable)

*Indicative of L3-4 disc herniation or pathological condition localized to the L4 foramen.

BOX 39-8 • L5 Root Compression*

Sensory Deficit
Anterolateral leg, dorsum of the foot, and great toe

Motor Weakness
Extensor hallucis longus
Gluteus medius
Extensor digitorum longus and brevis

Reflex Change
Usually none
Tibialis posterior (difficult to elicit)

*Indicative of L4-5 disc herniation or pathological condition localized to the L5 foramen.

BOX 39-9 • S1 Root Compression*

Sensory Deficit
Lateral malleolus, lateral foot, heel, and web of fourth and fifth toes

Motor Weakness
Peroneus longus and brevis
Gastrocnemius-soleus complex
Gluteus maximus

Reflex Change
Tendo calcaneus (gastrocnemius-soleus complex)

*Indicative of L5-S1 disc herniation or pathological condition localized to the S1 foramen.

---

a list in the lumbar spine may be present, and in many patients the normal lumbar lordosis is lost. As the acute episode subsides, the degree of spasm diminishes remarkably, and the loss of normal lumbar lordosis may be the only telltale sign. Point tenderness may be present over the spinous process at the level of the disc involved, and in some patients pain may extend laterally.

If there is nerve root irritation, it centers over the length of the sciatic nerve, both in the sciatic notch and more distally in the popliteal space. In addition, stretch of the sciatic nerve at the knee should reproduce buttock, thigh, and leg pain (i.e., pain distal to the knee). A Lasègue sign usually is positive on the involved side. A positive Lasègue sign or straight leg raising should elicit buttock or leg pain distal to the knee or both on the side tested. Occasionally if leg pain is significant the patient will lean back from an upright sitting position and assume the tripod stance to relieve the pain. Contralateral leg pain produced by straight leg raising should be regarded as pathognomonic of a herniated intervertebral disc. The absence of a positive Lasègue sign should make one skeptical of the diagnosis, although older individuals may not have a positive Lasègue sign. Likewise, inappropriate findings and inconsistencies in the examination usually are nonorganic in origin (see discussion of nonspecific back pain). If the leg pain has persisted for any length of time, atrophy of the involved limb may be present, as demonstrated by asymmetrical girth of the thigh or calf. The neurological examination will vary as determined by the level of root involvement (Boxes 39-7 to 39-9). Smith et al. examined the motion of the spinal roots in cadavers. They observed 0.5 to 5 mm of linear motion and 2% to 4% strain on the nerves at L4, L5, and S1. With increased strain, the roots moved lateral to the pedicle.

Unilateral disc herniation between L3 and L4 usually compresses the fourth lumbar root as it crosses the disc before exiting at the L4 intervertebral foramen. Pain may be localized around the medial side of the leg. Numbness may be present over the anteromedial aspect of the leg. The tibialis anterior may be weak as evidenced by inability to heel walk. The quadriceps and hip adductor group, both innervated from L2, L3, and L4, also may be weak and, in extended ruptures, atrophic. Reflex testing may reveal a diminished or absent patellar tendon reflex (L2, L3, and L4) or tibialis anterior tendon reflex (L4). Sensory testing may show diminished sensibility over the L4 dermatome, the isolated portion of which is the medial leg (Fig. 39-37), and the autonomous zone of which is at the level of the medial malleolus.

Unilateral disc herniation between L4 and L5 results in compression of the fifth lumbar root. Fifth lumbar root radiculopathy should produce pain in the dermatomal pattern. Numbness, when present, follows the L5 dermatome along the anterolateral aspect of the leg and the dorsum of the foot, including the great toe. The autonomous zone for this nerve is the dorsal first web of the foot and the dorsum of the third toe. Weakness may involve the extensor hallucis longus (L5), gluteus medius (L5), or extensor digitorum longus and brevis (L5). Reflex change usually is not found. A diminished tibialis posterior reflex is possible but difficult to elicit.

With unilateral rupture of the disc between L5 and S1 the findings of an S1 radiculopathy are noted. Pain and numbness involve the dermatome of S1. The S1 dermatome includes the lateral malleolus and the lateral and plantar surface of the foot, occasionally including the heel. There is numbness over the lateral aspect of the leg and, more important, over the lateral aspect of the foot, including the lateral three toes. The

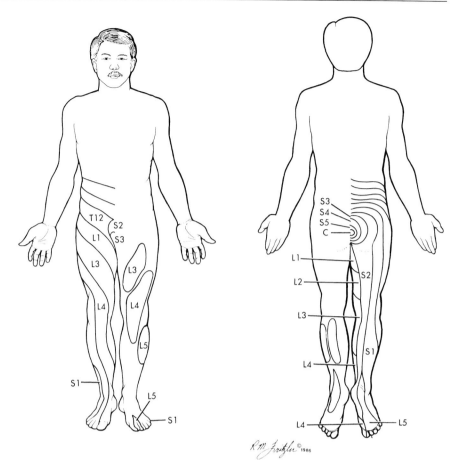

Fig. 39-37   L4 neurological level. (After Hoppenfeld S: *Physical examination of the spine and extremities*, Norwalk, Conn, 1976, Appleton-Century-Crofts.)

autonomous zone for this root is the dorsum of the fifth toe. Weakness may be demonstrated in the peroneus longus and brevis (S1), gastrocnemius-soleus (S1), or gluteus maximus (S1). In general, weakness is not a usual finding in S1 radiculopathy. Occasionally, mild weakness may be demonstrated by asymmetrical fatigue with exercise of these motor groups. The ankle jerk usually is reduced or absent.

Massive extrusion of a disc involving the entire diameter of the lumbar canal or a large midline extrusion can produce pain in the back, legs, and occasionally perineum. Both legs may be paralyzed, the sphincters may be incontinent, and the ankle jerks may be absent. Tay and Chacha in 1979 reported that the combination of saddle anesthesia, bilateral ankle areflexia, and bladder symptoms constituted the most consistent symptoms of cauda equina syndrome caused by massive intervertebral disc extrusion at any lumbar level. In these instances a cystometrogram may show bladder denervation.

More than 95% of the ruptures of the lumbar intervertebral discs occur at L4 or L5. Ruptures at higher levels in many patients are not associated with a positive straight leg raising test. In these instances, a positive femoral stretch test can be helpful. This test is carried out by placing the patient prone and acutely flexing the knee while placing the hand in the popliteal fossa. When this procedure results in anterior thigh pain, the result is positive and a high lesion should be suspected. In addition, these lesions may occur with a more diffuse neurological complaint without significant localizing neurological signs.

Often the neurological signs associated with disc disease vary over time. If the patient has been up and walking for a period of time, the neurological findings may be much more pronounced than if he has been at bed rest for several days, thus decreasing the pressure on the nerve root and allowing the nerve to resume its normal function. In addition, various conservative treatments can change the physical signs of disc disease.

Comparative bilateral examination of a patient with back and leg pain is essential in finding a clear-cut pattern of signs and symptoms. It is not uncommon for the evaluation to change. Adverse changes in the examination may warrant more aggressive therapy, whereas improvement of the symptoms or signs should signal a resolution of the problem. Early symptoms or signs suggestive of cauda equina syndrome or severe or progressive neurological deficit should be treated aggressively from the onset. McLaren and Bailey warn that the cauda equina syndrome is more frequent when disc excision is performed in the presence of an untreated spinal stenosis at the same level.

DIFFERENTIAL DIAGNOSIS

The differential diagnosis of back and leg pain is extremely lengthy and complex. It includes diseases intrinsic to the spine and those involving adjacent organs but causing pain referred to the back or leg. For simplicity, lesions can be categorized as being extrinsic or intrinsic to the spine. Extrinsic lesions include diseases of the urogenital system, gastrointestinal system, vascular system, endocrine system, nervous system not localized to the spine, and the extrinsic musculoskeletal system. These lesions include infections, tumors, metabolic disturbances, congenital abnormalities, and the associated diseases of aging. Intrinsic lesions involve those diseases that arise primarily in the spine. They include diseases of the spinal musculoskeletal system, the local hematopoietic system, and the local neurological system. These conditions include trauma, tumors, infections, diseases of aging, and immune diseases affecting the spine or spinal nerves.

Although the predominant cause of back and leg pain in healthy people usually is lumbar disc disease, one must be extremely cautious to avoid a misdiagnosis, particularly given the high incidence of disc herniations present in asymptomatic patients as discussed previously. Therefore a full physical examination must be completed before making a presumptive diagnosis of herniated disc disease. Common diseases that can mimic disc disease include ankylosing spondylitis, multiple myeloma, vascular insufficiency, arthritis of the hip, osteoporosis with stress fractures, extradural tumors, peripheral neuropathy, and herpes zoster. Infrequent but reported causes of sciatica not related to disc hernia include synovial cysts, rupture of the medial head of the gastrocnemius, sacroiliac joint dysfunction, lesions in the sacrum and pelvis, and fracture of the ischial tuberosity.

CONFIRMATORY IMAGING

Although the diagnosis of a herniated lumbar disc can be suspected from the history and physical examination, imaging studies are necessary to rule out other causes, such as a tumor or infection. Plain roentgenograms are of limited use in the diagnosis because they do not show disc herniations or other intraspinal lesions, but they can demonstrate infection, tumors, or other anomalies and should be obtained, especially if surgery is planned. Currently, the most useful test for diagnosing a herniated lumbar disc is MRI. Since the advent of MRI, myelography is used much less frequently, although in some situations it may help to demonstrate subtle lesions. When myelography is used, it should be followed with a CT scan.

NONOPERATIVE TREATMENT

The number and variety of nonoperative therapies for back and leg pain are overwhelming. Treatments range from simple rest to expensive traction apparatus. All these therapies are reported with glowing accounts of miraculous "cures"; unfortunately, few have been evaluated scientifically. In addition, the natural history of disc disease is characterized by exacerbations and remissions with eventual improvement regardless of treatment. Finally, several distinct symptom complexes appear to be associated with disc disease. Few if any studies have isolated the response to specific and anatomically distinct diagnoses.

The simplest treatment for acute back pain is rest. Deyo, Diehl, and Rosenthal reported that 2 days of bed rest were better than a longer period. Biomechanical studies indicate that lying in a semi-Fowler position (i.e., on the side with the hips and knees flexed) with a pillow between the legs should relieve most pressure on the disc and nerve roots. Muscle spasm can be controlled by the application of ice, preferably with a massage over the muscles in spasm. Pain relief and antiinflammatory effect can be achieved with nonsteroidal antiinflammatory drugs (NSAIDs). Most acute exacerbations of back pain respond quickly to this therapy. As the pain diminishes, the patient should be encouraged to begin isometric abdominal and lower extremity exercises. Walking within the limits of comfort also is encouraged. Sitting, especially riding in a car, is discouraged. Malmivaara et al. compared the efficacy of bed rest alone, back extension exercises, and continuation of ordinary activities as tolerated in the treatment of acute back pain. They concluded that continuation of ordinary activities within the limits permitted by pain led to a more rapid recovery.

Education in proper posture and body mechanics is helpful in returning the patient to the usual level of activity after the acute exacerbation is eased or relieved. This education can take many forms, from individual instruction to group instruction. Back education of this type is now usually referred to as "back school." Although the concept is excellent, the quality and quantity of information provided may vary widely. The work of Bergquist-Ullman and Larsson and others indicates that patient education of this type is extremely beneficial in decreasing the amount of time lost from work initially but does little to decrease the incidence of recurrence of symptoms or length of time lost from work during recurrences. Certainly the combination of back education and combined physical therapy is superior to placebo treatment. Cohen et al. reviewed 13 studies on group back education and concluded that the evidence was insufficient to recommend group education. A study by Galm et al. regarding sacroiliac joint dysfunction in patients with image-proven herniated nucleus pulposus and sciatica but without motor or sensory deficits found that 75% improved with respect to sciatic and back pain with intensive physiotherapy.

Numerous medications have been used with varied results in subacute and chronic back and leg pain syndromes. The current trend appears to be moving away from the use of strong narcotics and muscle relaxants in the outpatient treatment of these syndromes. This is especially true in the instances of chronic back and leg pain where drug habituation and increased depression are frequent. Oral steroids used briefly can be beneficial as potent antiinflammatory agents. The many types of NSAIDs also are helpful when aspirin is not tolerated or is of little help. Numerous NSAIDs are available for the treatment of low back pain. When depression is prominent, mood elevators such as amitriptyline can be beneficial in reducing sleep disturbance and anxiety without increasing depression. In addition, amitriptyline also decreases the need for narcotic medication.

Physical therapy should be used judiciously. The exercises should be fitted to the symptoms and not forced as an absolute group of activities. Patients with acute back and thigh pain eased by passive extension of the spine in the prone position can benefit from extension exercises rather than flexion exercises. Improvement in symptoms with extension is indicative of a good prognosis with conservative care. On the other hand, patients whose pain is increased by passive extension may be improved by flexion exercises. These exercises should not be forced in the face of increased pain. This may avoid further disc extrusion. Any exercise that increases pain should be discontinued. Lower extremity exercises can increase strength and relieve stress on the back, but they also can exacerbate lower extremity arthritis. The true benefit of such treatments may be in the promotion of good posture and body mechanics rather than of strength. Hansen et al. compared intensive, dynamic back muscle exercises, conventional physiotherapy (manual traction, flexibility, isometric and coordination exercises, and ergonomics counseling), and placebo-control treatment in a randomized, observer blind trial. Regardless of the method used, patients who completed therapy reported a decrease in pain. However, physiotherapy appeared to have better results in men, and intensive back exercises gave better results in women. Patients with hard physical occupations responded better to physiotherapy, whereas patients with sedentary occupations responded better to intensive back exercises.

Numerous treatment methods have been advanced for the treatment of back pain. Some patients respond to the use of transcutaneous electrical nerve stimulation (TENS). Others do well with traction varying from skin traction in bed with 5 to 8 pounds to body inversion with forces of over 100 pounds. Back braces or corsets may be helpful to other patients. Ultrasound and diathermy are other treatments used in back pain. The scientific efficacy of many of these treatments has not been proved. In addition, all therapy for disc disease is only symptomatic.

◆ EPIDURAL STEROIDS

The epidural injection of a combination of a long-acting steroid with an epidural anesthetic is an excellent method of symptomatic treatment of back and leg pain from discogenic disease and other sources. Most studies show a 60% to 85% short-term success rate that falls to a 30% to 40% long-term (6-month) good result rate. The local effect of the steroids has been shown to last at least 3 weeks at a therapeutic level. In a well-controlled study Berman et al. found that the best results were obtained in patients with subacute or chronic leg pain with no prior surgery. They also found that the worst results were in

patients with motor or reflex abnormalities (12% to 14% good results). A negative myelogram also was associated with a better result. Cuckler et al. in a double-blind, randomized study of epidural steroid treatment of disc herniation and spinal stenosis found no difference in the results at 6 months between placebo and a single epidural injection. Our experience parallels that of Berman et al. We agree that epidural steroids are not a cure for disc disease, but they do offer relatively prolonged pain relief without excessive narcotic intake if conservative care is elected. Hopwood and Abram observed that factors associated with poor surgical outcome also were associated with a poor outcome from epidural steroid injection. These factors included lower educational levels, smoking, lack of employment, constant pain, sleep disruption, nonradicular diagnosis, prolonged duration of pain, change in recreational activities, and extreme values on psychological scales.

In experienced hands the complication rate from this procedure should be small. White, Derby, and Wynne reported that the most common problem is a 25% rate of failure to place the material in the epidural space. Renfrew et al. and el-Khoury et al. observed that the use of fluoroscopic control dramatically decreased the failure rate. Another technique-related problem is intrathecal injection with inadvertent spinal anesthesia. Other reported complications include transient hypotension, difficulty in voiding, severe paresthesias, cardiac angina, headache, and transient hypercorticoidism. Kushner and Olson reported retinal hemorrhage in several patients who had epidural steroid injection for chronic back pain. They recommended careful consideration of this procedure in patients who have bleeding problems and in patients who have only one eye. DeSio et al. reported facial flushing and generalized erythema in patients after epidural steroid injection. The most serious complication reported was bacterial meningitis. The total complication rate in most series is about 5%, and the complications are almost always transient.

This procedure is contraindicated in the presence of infection, neurological disease (such as multiple sclerosis), hemorrhagic or bleeding diathesis, cauda equina syndrome, and a rapidly progressive neural deficit. Rapid injections of large volumes or the use of large doses of steroid also can increase the complication rate. The exact effects of intrathecal injection of steroids are not known. This technique must be used only in the low lumbar region. We prefer to abort the procedure if a bloody tap is obtained or if CSF is encountered.

We prefer to do the procedure in a room equipped for resuscitation and with the capability to monitor the patient. This procedure lends itself well to outpatient use, but the patient must be prepared to spend several hours to recover from the block. Methylprednisolone (Depo-Medrol) is the usual steroid injected. The dosage may vary from 80 to 120 mg. The anesthetics used may include lidocaine, bupivacaine, or procaine. Our current protocol is to inject the patient three times. These injections are made at 7- to 10-day intervals. This ensures at least one good epidural injection and decreases the volume of material injected at each procedure.

TECHNIQUE 39-20 *(Brown)*

The equipment needed includes material for an appropriate skin preparation, sterile rubber gloves, a 3½-inch, 20-gauge or 22-gauge disposable spinal needle (45-degree blunt- or curve-tipped epidural needles are preferred), several disposable syringes, bacteriostatic lidocaine, and methylprednisolone acetate, 40 mg/ml. The injection may be done with the patient in the sitting or lateral decubitus position. Anesthetize the skin near the midline. Advance the needle until the resistance of the ligamentum flavum is encountered. Then attach a syringe and slowly advance the needle while applying light pressure on the syringe. When the epidural space is encountered, the resistance is suddenly lost and the epidural space will accommodate the air. Remove the syringe and inspect the needle opening for blood or spinal fluid. If there is no flow out of the needle, then inject 3 ml of 1% lidocaine or other appropriate anesthetic. This may be preceded or followed by the chosen dosage of methylprednisolone.

Several variations also can be used. Some physicians use a sterile balloon to indicate the proper space. Others use the "disappearing drop" technique, which involves placing a drop of sterile saline over the hub of the needle. When the epidural space is entered, the drop disappears. Caudal injection also is used, but this may require larger volumes to wash the steroid up to the involved level. This method is safer but less reliable than an injection at L4-5.

OPERATIVE TREATMENT

If nonoperative treatment for lumbar disc disease fails, the next consideration is operative treatment. Before this step is taken, the surgeon must be sure of the diagnosis. The patient must be certain that the degree of pain and impairment warrants such a step. Both the surgeon and the patient must realize that disc surgery is not a cure but may provide symptomatic relief. It neither stops the pathological processes that allowed the herniation to occur nor restores the back to a normal state. The patient must still practice good posture and body mechanics after surgery. Activities involving repetitive bending, twisting, and lifting with the spine in flexion may have to be curtailed or eliminated. If prolonged relief is to be expected, then some permanent modification in the patient's lifestyle may be necessary.

The key to good results in disc surgery is appropriate patient selection. The optimal patient is one with predominant, if not only, unilateral leg pain extending below the knee that has been present for at least 6 weeks. The pain should have been decreased by rest, antiinflammatory medication, or even epidural steroids but should have returned to the initial levels after a minimum of 6 to 8 weeks of conservative care. Some managed care plans now insist on a trial of physiotherapy. The work of Hansen et al. is indicative of the problems with such

requirements, not only because of gender and occupation variations in response to physiotherapy and intensive back exercises, but also because no therapy appeared to have the same or better results. Physical examination should reveal signs of sciatic irritation and possibly objective evidence of localizing neurological impairment. CT, lumbar MRI, or myelography should confirm the level of involvement consistent with the patient's examination.

Surgical disc removal is mandatory and urgent only in cauda equina syndrome with significant neurological deficit, especially bowel or bladder disturbance. All other disc excisions should be considered elective. This should allow a thorough evaluation to confirm the diagnosis, level of involvement, and the physical and psychological status of patient. Frequently, if there is a rush to the operating room to relieve pain without proper investigation, both the patient and physician later regret the decision.

Regardless of the method chosen to treat a disc rupture surgically, the patient should be aware that the procedure is predominantly for the symptomatic relief of leg pain. Patients with predominant back pain may not be relieved of their major complaint—back pain. Spangfort, in reviewing 2504 lumbar disc excisions, found that about 30% of the patients complained of back pain after disc surgery. Failure to relieve sciatica was proportional to the degree of herniation. The best results of 99.5% complete or partial pain relief were obtained when the disc was free in the canal or sequestered. Incomplete herniation or extrusion of disc material into the canal resulted in complete relief for 82% of patients. Excision of the bulging or protruding disc that had not ruptured through the annulus resulted in complete relief in 63%, and removal of the normal or minimally bulging disc resulted in complete relief in 38%, which is near the stated level for the placebo response. Likewise, the incidence of persistent back pain after surgery was inversely proportional to the degree of herniation. In patients with complete extrusions the incidence was about 25%, but with minimal bulges or negative explorations the incidence rose to over 55% (Figs. 39-38 and 39-39).

General Principles for Open Disc Surgery

Most disc surgery is performed with the patient under general endotracheal anesthesia, although local anesthesia has been used with minimal complications. Patient positioning varies with the operative technique and surgeon. To position the patient in a modified kneeling position, a specialized frame or custom frame modified from the design of Hastings is popular. Positioning the patient in this manner allows the abdomen to hang free, minimizing epidural venous dilation and bleeding (Fig. 39-40). A head lamp allows the surgeon to direct light into the lateral recesses where a large proportion of the surgery may be required. The addition of loupe magnification also greatly improves the identification and exposure of various structures. Some surgeons also use the operative microscope to further improve visibility. The primary benefit of the operating microscope compared with loupes is the view afforded the

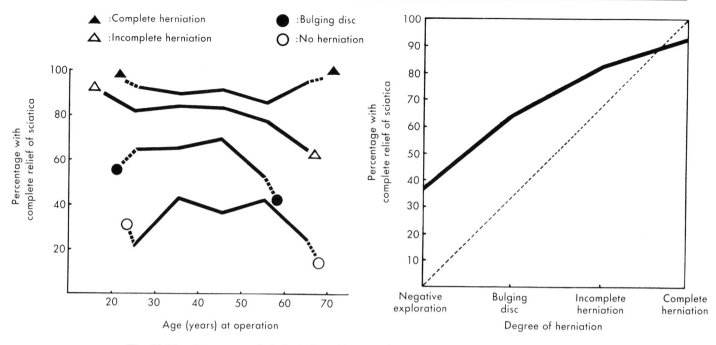

Fig. 39-38   Percentage relief of sciatica with type of disc herniation. (From Spangfort E: *Acta Orthop Scand Suppl* 142:1, 1972.)

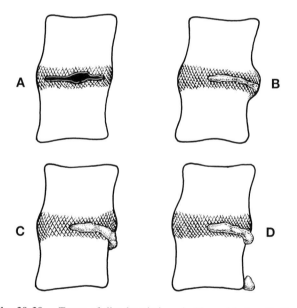

Fig. 39-39   Types of disc herniation. **A,** Normal bulge. **B,** Protrusion. **C,** Extrusion. **D,** Sequestration.

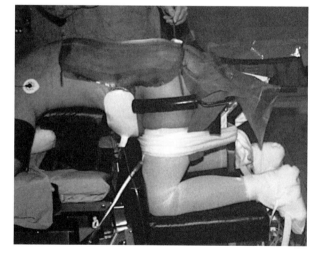

Fig. 39-40   Kneeling position for lumbar disc excision allows abdomen to be completely free of external pressure.

assistant. Roentgenographic confirmation of the proper level is necessary. Care should be taken to protect neural structures. Epidural bleeding should be controlled with bipolar electrocautery. Any sponge, pack, or cottonoid patty placed in the wound should extend to the outside. Pituitary rongeurs should be marked at a point equal to the maximal allowable disc depth to prevent accidental biopsy of viscera or aorta. Considerable

research has gone into techniques to prevent epidural fibrosis. Hoyland et al. noted dense fibrous connective tissue about previously operated nerve roots. They also found fibrillar foreign material within the scar in 55% of patients. This finding should remind the surgeon to minimize the use of cotton patties. The placement of autogenous fat appears to be a reasonable although not foolproof or complication-free tech-

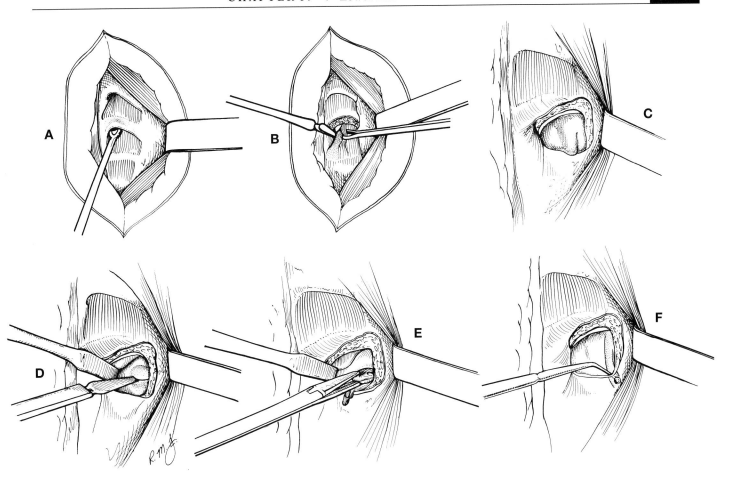

Fig. 39-41 Technique of lumbar disc excision. **A,** With lamina and ligamentum flavum exposed, use curet to remove the ligamentum flavum from inferior surface of lamina. Kerrison rongeur is used to remove bone. **B,** Elevate ligamentum flavum at upper corner and carefully dissect it back to expose dura and epidural fat below. Patties should be used to protect dura during this procedure. **C,** Expose dura and root. Remove additional bone if there is any question about adequacy of exposure. **D,** Retract nerve root and dural sac to expose disc. Inspect capsule for rent and extruded nuclear material. If obvious ligamentous defect is not visible, then carefully incise capsule of disc. If disc material does not bulge out, press on disc to try to dislodge herniated fragment. **E,** Carefully remove disc fragments. It is safest to avoid opening pituitary rongeur until it is inserted into disc space. **F,** After removing disc, carefully explore foramen, subligamentous region, and beneath dura for additional fragments of disc. Obtain meticulous hemostasis using bipolar cauterization.

nique of minimizing postoperative epidural fibrosis. Commercially available products may reduce scar volume, but clinical benefit remains uncertain.

◆ Ruptured Lumbar Disc Excision (Open Technique)

TECHNIQUE 39-21
After thoroughly preparing the back, identify the spinous processes of L3, L4, L5, and S1 by palpation. Make a midline incision 5 to 8 cm long, centered over the interspace where the disc herniation is located. Incise the supraspinous ligament; then, by subperiosteal dissection, strip the muscles from the spinous processes and laminae of these vertebrae on the side of the lesion. Retract the muscles either with a self-retaining retractor or with the help of an assistant and expose one interspace at a time. Verify the location with a roentgenogram so that no mistake is made regarding the interspaces explored. Secure hemostasis with electrocautery, bone wax, and packs. Leave a portion of each pack completely outside the wound for ready identification.

Denude the laminae and ligamentum flavum with a curet (Fig. 39-41, *A*). Commonly the lumbosacral interspace is large enough to permit exposure and removal of a herniated nucleus pulposus without removal of any bone. If not,

continued

remove a small part of the inferior margin of the fifth lumbar lamina. Exposure of the disc at higher levels usually requires removal of a portion of the inferior lamina. Thin the ligamentum flavum using a pituitary rongeur to remove the superficial layer. Detach the ligamentum from its cephalad or caudad laminar attachment using a small curet. Use care to keep the cutting edges of the curet directed posteriorly to minimize the chance of dural laceration. Using an angled Kerrison rongeur, preferably one with a thin foot plate and appropriate width, remove the detached ligamentum laterally and preserve the more medial ligamentum. Keep the Kerrison rongeur oriented parallel to the direction of the nerve root to minimize the risk of root injury, and the root will be more posterior than is normal due to the displacement caused by the herniated disc fragment. An alternative technique that can be used with good lighting and magnified visual aid is to divide the ligamentum parallel with its fibers using a no. 11 blade knife. Once the full thickness of the ligamentum has been divided, bluntly extend the division across the interspace with a Penfield 4 dissector and remove the lateral portion of the ligamentum. The lateral shelving portion of the ligamentum should be excised, often with a portion of the medial inferior facet to gain access to the lateral aspect of the nerve root. Next, retract the dura medially and identify the nerve root (Fig. 39-41, *C*). If the root is compressed by a large extruded fragment, it commonly will be displaced posteriorly. Retract the nerve root, once identified, medially so that the underlying extruded fragment or bulging posterior longitudinal ligament can be seen (Fig. 39-41, *D*). Occasionally the nerve root adheres to the fragment or to the underlying ligamentous structures and requires blunt dissection from these structures. If the position of the root is not known for certain, remove the lamina posterior to the root and medial to the pedicle until the root is clearly identified. Bipolar cautery on a low setting can be used to coagulate the epidural veins and maintain hemostasis. Gelfoam and small cottonoids also are useful. Take care to minimize packing about the nerve root. Retract the root or dura, identify any bleeding vein, and cauterize it with a bipolar cautery. Earlier insertion of cotton patties may well displace fragments from view. The underlying disc should be clearly visible at this time.

Gently retract the nerve with a Love root retractor or a blunt dissector, thus exposing the herniated fragment or posterior longitudinal ligament and annulus. If an extruded fragment is not seen, carefully palpate the posterior longitudinal ligament and seek a defect or hole in the ligamentous structures. A microblunt hook can be used for this. If no obvious abnormality is detected, follow the root around the pedicle or even outside the canal in search of fragments that may have migrated far laterally. Additional searching in the root axilla helps ensure that fragments that have migrated inferiorly are not missed. If the expected pathology is not found, obtain another roentgenogram with a blunt dissector at the level of the disc to be certain of the

proper level and review preoperative imaging studies to confirm proper sidedness.

If the herniated fragment is especially large, it is much better to sacrifice a portion of the facet to obtain a more lateral exposure than to risk injury to the root or cauda equina by excessive medial retraction. With such a lateral exposure the nerve root usually can be elevated, and the herniated fragment can be teased from beneath the nerve root and cauda equina, even when the fragment is large enough to block the entire canal. If the fragment is very large as with cauda equina lesions typically, a bilateral laminectomy is preferred to allow safer removal. If the disc cannot be teased from under the root, make a cruciate incision in the disc laterally. Gently remove disc fragments until the bulge has been decompressed to allow gentle retraction of the root over the defect (Fig. 39-41, *E*).

If the herniation is upward or downward, further removal of bone from the lamina and facet edges may be required. The herniated nucleus pulposus may be covered by a layer of posterior longitudinal ligament or may have ruptured through this structure. In the latter event, carefully lift the loose fragments out by suction, blunt hook, or pituitary forceps. If the ligament is intact, incise it in a cruciate fashion and remove the loose fragments. The tear or hole in the annulus should then be identifiable in most instances. The cavity of the disc can be entered through this hole, or occasionally the hole may need to be enlarged to allow insertion of the pituitary forceps. Remember that the anterior part of the annulus is adjacent to the aorta, vena cava, or iliac arteries and veins and that one of these structures can be injured if one proceeds too deeply. Remove other loose fragments of nucleus pulposus with the pituitary forceps and remove additional nuclear material along with the central portion of the cartilaginous plates, both above and below as necessary.

When placing instruments into the disc space do not penetrate beyond a depth of 15 mm to avoid injury to the anterior viscera. Then carry out a complete search for additional fragments of nucleus pulposus, both inside and outside the disc space (Fig. 39-41, *F*). Additional fragments commonly migrate medially beneath the posterior longitudinal ligament but outside the annulus and can easily be missed. Then remove all cotton pledgets and control residual bleeding with Gelfoam and bipolar cautery. Forcefully irrigate any loose fragments from the disc space using a syringe with a spinal needle placed into the disc space under direct vision until no fragments are returned with the irrigating solution. Close the wound with absorbable sutures in the supraspinous ligament and subcutaneous tissue. Various absorbable sutures are most commonly used in routine skin closure. Staples are avoided for patient comfort.

AFTERTREATMENT. Neurological function is closely monitored after surgery. The patient is allowed to turn in bed at will and to select a position of comfort such as a semi-Fowler position. Pain should be controlled with oral medication. Muscle relaxants are used postoperatively as well. Bladder stimulants can be used to assist voiding. The patient is allowed to stand with assistance on the evening after surgery to go to the bathroom. Discharge is permitted when the patient is able to walk and void. Currently most patients are discharged within 24 hours after surgery. Isometric abdominal and lower extremity exercises are started. The patient is instructed to minimize sitting and riding in a vehicle. Increased walking on a daily basis is recommended. Lifting, bending, and stooping are prohibited for the first several weeks. As the patient's strength increases, gentle isotonic leg exercises are started.

Between the fourth and sixth postoperative week, back school instruction is resumed or started, provided that pain is minimal. Lifting, bending, and stooping are gradually restarted after the sixth week. Increased sitting is allowed as pain permits, but long trips are to be avoided for at least 4 to 6 weeks. Lower extremity strength is increased from the eighth to twelfth postoperative weeks. Patients with jobs requiring much walking without lifting are allowed to return to work within 2 to 3 weeks. Patients with jobs requiring prolonged sitting usually are allowed to return to work within 4 to 6 weeks provided minimal lifting is required. Patients with jobs requiring heavy labor or long periods of driving are not allowed to return to work until 6 to 8 weeks and then to a modified duty. Some patients with jobs requiring exceptionally heavy manual labor may have to permanently modify their occupation or seek a lighter occupation. Keeping the patient out of work beyond 3 months rarely improves recovery or pain relief.

◆ **Microlumbar Disc Excision**

Microlumbar disc excision has replaced the standard open laminectomy as the procedure of choice for herniated lumbar disc. This procedure can be done on an outpatient basis and allows better lighting, magnification, and angle of view with a much smaller exposure. Because of the limited dissection required there is less postoperative pain and a shorter hospital stay. Zahrawi reported 103 outpatient microdiscectomies, noting 88% excellent and good results in the 83 who responded. Newman reported 75 conventional laminectomies done on an outpatient basis and noted 2 complications unrelated to the procedure or the outpatient setting. Kelly et al. noted less pulmonary morbidity and temperature elevation in patients after microlumbar discectomy. Numerous other investigators such as Silvers, Zahrawi, Lowell et al., and Moore et al. reported excellent results with low morbidity and early return to activity using microlumbar disc excision. Williams, the originator of the term, questioned its current usage, since the concept of the technique has changed over the years.

Microlumbar discectomy requires an operating microscope with a 400-mm lens, special retractors, a variety of small-angled Kerrison rongeurs of appropriate length, micro instruments, and preferably a combination suction–nerve root retractor. The procedure is performed with the patient prone. A vacuum pack is molded around the patient, and an inflatable pillow is positioned under the abdomen and is removed after evacuation of the vacuum pack. Alternatively, the Andrew's type frame previously described can be used. The microscope can be used from skin incision to closure. However, the initial dissection can be done under direct vision. A lateral roentgenogram is taken to confirm the level.

TECHNIQUE 39-22 *(Williams, Modified)*

Make the incision from the spinous process of the upper vertebra to the spinous process of the lower vertebra at the involved level. This usually results in a 1-inch (2.5-cm) skin incision (Fig. 39-42, *A*). Maintain meticulous hemostasis with electrocautery as the dissection is carried to the fascia. Incise the fascia at the midline using electrocautery. Then insert a periosteal elevator in the midline incision. Using gentle lateral movements separate the deep fascia and muscle subperiosteally from the spinous processes and lamina. Obtain a lateral roentgenogram with a metal clamp attached to the spinous process to verify the level. Now, using a Cobb elevator gently sweep the remaining muscular attachments off in a lateral direction exposing the interlaminar space and the edge of each lamina. Meticulously cauterize all bleeding points. Insert the microlumbar retractor into the wound and adjust the microscope. Identify the ligamentum flavum and lamina. Use a pituitary rongeur to remove the superficial leaf of the ligamentum. Using a no. 15 blade with the microscope, carefully incise the thinned ligamentum flavum superficially. Then use a Penfield no. 4 dissector to perforate the ligamentum. Minimal force should be used in this maneuver to prevent penetration of the dura (Fig. 39-42, *B*). Once the ligamentum is open, use a 45-degree Kerrison rongeur to remove the ligamentum flavum laterally (Fig. 39-42, *C*). The lamina, facet, and facet capsule should remain intact. However, one must remove the ligamentum flavum and bone from the lamina as needed to clearly identify the nerve root. Once identified, carefully mobilize the root medially; this may require some bony removal. Gently dissect the nerve free from the disc fragment to avoid excessive traction on the root. Bipolar cautery for hemostasis is very helpful. Once mobilized, retract the root medially. Maintain the orientation of the Kerrison parallel to that of the nerve root at all times. Once identified, the nerve root can be gently mobilized and retracted medially. Then make an extradural exploration using a 90-degree hook. In large herniations the nerve root appears as a large, white, glistening structure and can easily be mistaken for a ruptured disc. Follow the root to the pedicle if necessary to be certain of its location. The small opening and magnification can make the edge of the dural sac appear as the nerve root. When using bipolar cautery make sure only one side is in contact with the nerve root to avoid thermal injury to the nerve. Also, when using a Kerrison rongeur for bone or ligamentum removal, orient it parallel to the course of the nerve root as much as possible to minimize the risk of nerve root or dural injury. Epidural fat is not removed in this procedure. Insert the suction–nerve root retractor, with its tip turned medially under the nerve

continued

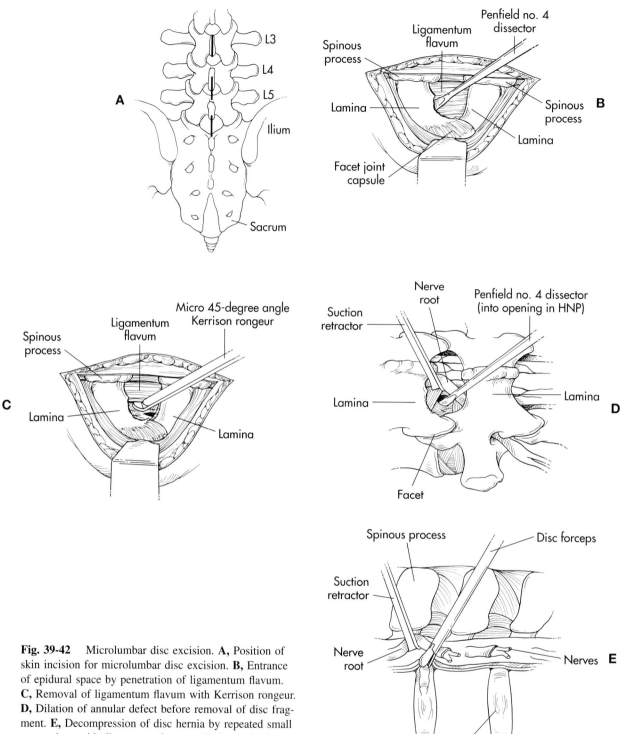

Fig. 39-42 Microlumbar disc excision. **A,** Position of skin incision for microlumbar disc excision. **B,** Entrance of epidural space by penetration of ligamentum flavum. **C,** Removal of ligamentum flavum with Kerrison rongeur. **D,** Dilation of annular defect before removal of disc fragment. **E,** Decompression of disc hernia by repeated small evacuations with discectomy forceps. (Redrawn from Cauthen JC: *Lumbar spine surgery*, Baltimore, 1983, Williams & Wilkins.)

root, and hold the manifold between the thumb and index finger. With the nerve root retracted, the disc will now be visible as a white, fibrous, avascular structure. Small tears may be visible in the annulus under the magnification. Now enlarge the annular tear with a Penfield no. 4 dissector and

remove the disc material with the microdisc forceps (Fig. 39-42, *D* and *E*). Do not insert the instrument into the disc space beyond the angle of the jaws, which usually is about 15 mm, to minimize the risk of anterior perforation and vascular injury. Remove the exposed disc material. Do not curet the disc space. Inspect the root and adjacent dura for disc fragments. Irrigate the disc space using a lock syringe and 18-gauge spinal needle inserted into the disc space. Obtain meticulous hemostasis. If the expected pathology is not found, review preoperative imaging studies for level and sidedness. Also obtain a repeat roentgenogram with a metallic marker at the disc level to verify the level. Be aware of bony anomalies that may alter the numbering of the vertebrae on imaging studies. Close the fascia and the skin in the usual fashion, using absorbable sutures.

AFTERTREATMENT. Postoperative care is similar to that after standard open disc surgery. Typically this procedure is done on an outpatient basis. Injecting the paraspinal muscles on the involved side with Bupivacaine 0.5% with epinephrine at the beginning of the procedure and additional Bupivacaine at the conclusion aids patient mobilization immediately postoperatively.

Endoscopic Techniques

Endoscopic techniques have been developed over the past several years with the purported advantage of shortened hospital stay and faster return to activity. These techniques generally are variations of the microdiscectomy technique using an endoscope rather than the microscope and different types of retractors. Thus far the purported advantages have not been demonstrated. This remains another alternative technique. Each system is somewhat unique, and the reader is referred to the technique guide of the various manufacturers for details. The basic principles remain the same as with microdiscectomy.

Additional Exposure Techniques

A large disc herniation or other pathological condition such as lateral recess stenosis or foraminal stenosis may require a greater exposure of the nerve root. Usually the additional pathological condition can be identified before surgery. If the extent of the lesion is known before surgery, the proper approach can be planned. Additional exposure includes hemilaminectomy, total laminectomy, and facetectomy. Hemilaminectomy usually is required when identifying the root is a problem. This may occur with a conjoined root. Total laminectomy usually is reserved for patients with spinal stenoses that are central in nature, which occurs typically in cauda equina syndrome. Facetectomy usually is reserved for foraminal stenosis or severe lateral recess stenosis. If more than one facet is removed, then a fusion should be considered in addition. This is especially true in the removal of both facets and the disc at the same interspace in a young, active person with a normal disc height at that level.

On rare occasions disc herniation has been reported to be intradural. An extremely large disc that cannot be dissected from the dura or the persistence of an intradural mass after dissection of the disc should alert one to this potential problem. Excision of an intradural disc requires a transdural approach,

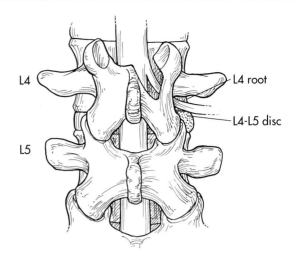

Fig. 39-43 Lateral approach for discectomy. L4 foraminotomy allows exposure of root. (Redrawn from Donaldson WF et al: *Spine* 18:1264, 1993; original by P Gretsky.)

which increases the risk of complications from CSF leak and intradural scarring.

A disc that is far lateral may require exposure outside the spinal canal. This area is approached by removing the intertransverse ligament between the superior and inferior transverse processes lateral to the spinal canal. The disc hernia usually is anterior to the nerve root that is found in a mass of fat below the ligament. A microsurgical approach or a percutaneous approach are good methods for dealing with this problem. Maroon et al. also recommended discography to confirm the lesion before surgery. Epstein noted little difference between lateral intertransverse exposure, facetectomy, and a more extensive hemilaminectomy with medial facetectomy. Donaldson et al. recommended the lateral approach after first finding the root medially and dissecting laterally down to a probe on top of the root (Fig. 39-43), and Strum et al. recommended an anterolateral approach.

Lumbar Root Anomalies

Lumbar nerve root anomalies (Figs. 39-44 to 39-47) are more common than may be expected, and they rarely are correctly identified with myelography. Kadish and Simmons identified lumbar nerve root anomalies in 14% of 100 cadaver examinations. They noted nerve root anomalies in only 4% of 100 consecutive metrizamide myelograms. They identified four types of anomalies. Type I is an intradural anastomosis between rootlets at different levels. Type II is an anomalous origin of the nerve roots. They separated this type into four subtypes: (1) cranial origin, (2) caudal origin, (3) combination of cranial and caudal origin, and (4) conjoined nerve roots. Type III is an extradural anastomosis between roots. Type IV is the extradural division of the nerve root. The surgeon must be aware of the possibility of anomalous roots hindering the disc excision. This may require a wider exposure. Sectioning of these roots results in irreversible neurological damage. Traction on anomalous nerve roots has been suggested as a cause of sciatic symptoms without disc herniation.

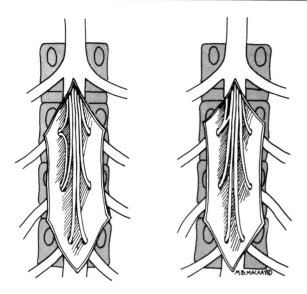

Fig. 39-44   Type I nerve root anomaly: intradural anastomosis. (From Kadish LJ, Simmons EH: *J Bone Joint Surg* 66B:411, 1984.)

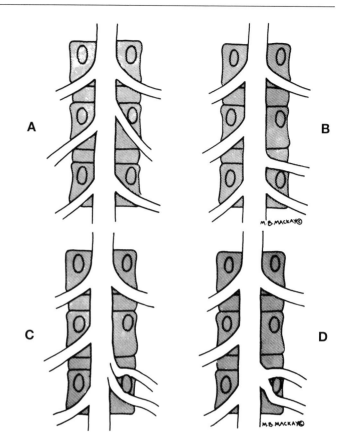

Fig. 39-45   Type II: anomalous origin of nerve roots. **A,** Cranial origin. **B,** Caudal origin. **C,** Closely adjacent nerve roots. **D,** Conjoined nerve roots. (From Kadish LJ, Simmons EH: *J Bone Joint Surg* 66B:411, 1984.)

Results of Open (Micro or Standard) Surgery for Disc Herniation

Numerous retrospective and some prospective reviews of open disc surgery are available. The results of these series vary greatly with respect to patient selection, treatment method, evaluation method, length of follow-up, and conclusions. Good results range from 46% to 97%. Complications range from none to over 10%. The reoperation rate ranges from 4% to over 20%. The detailed studies of Spangfort, Weir, and Rish are suggested for more detailed analysis. A comparison between techniques also reveals similar reports.

Several points do stand out in the analysis of the results of lumbar disc surgery. Patient selection appears to be extremely important. Several studies noted that a low educational level is significantly related to poor results of surgery. The works of Wiltse and Rocchio, and Gentry indicate that valid results of the MMPI (hysteria and hypochondriasis T scores) are very good indicators of surgical outcome regardless of the degree of the pathological condition. The extremely detailed work of Weir suggests that the duration of the current episode, the age of the patient, the presence or absence of predominant back pain, the number of previous hospitalizations, and the presence or absence of compensation for a work injury are factors affecting final outcome. Spangfort's work also indicates that the softer the findings for disc herniation clinically and at the time of surgery, the lower the chance for a good result.

Complications of Open Disc Excision

The complications associated with standard disc excision and microlumbar disc excision are similar. Spangfort's series (Table 39-9) of 2503 open disc excisions lists a postoperative mortality of 0.1%, a thromboembolism rate of 1.0%, a postoperative infection rate of 3.2%, and a deep disc space infection rate of 1.1%. Postoperative cauda equina lesions

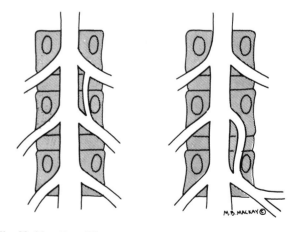

Fig. 39-46   Type III nerve root anomaly: extradural anastomosis. (From Kadish LJ, Simmons EH: *J Bone Joint Surg* 66B:411, 1984.)

developed in five patients. Laceration of the aorta or iliac artery also has been described as a rare complication of this operation. Rish, in a more recent report with a 5-year follow-up, noted a total complication rate of 4% in a series of 205 patients. The major complication in his series involved a worsening neuropathy postoperatively. There was one disc space infection

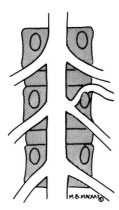

Fig. 39-47 Type IV nerve root anomaly: extradural division. (From Kadish LJ, Simmons EH: *J Bone Joint Surg* 66B:411, 1984.)

Table 39-9   Complications of Lumbar Disc Surgery

Complication	Incidence (%)
1. Cauda equina syndrome	0.2
2. Thrombophlebitis	1.0
3. Pulmonary embolism	0.4
4. Wound infection	2.2
5. Pyogenic spondylitis	0.07
6. Postoperative discitis	2.0 (1122 patients)
7. Dural tears	1.6
8. Nerve root injury	0.5
9. Cerebrospinal fluid fistula	*
10. Laceration of abdominal vessels	*
11. Injury to abdominal viscera	*

Modified from Spangfort EV: *Acta Orthop Scand Suppl* 142:65, 1972.
*Rare occurrence (numbers 10 and 11 not identified in Spangfort's study but reported elsewhere).

and one wound infection. Dural tears with CSF leaks, pseudomeningocele formation, CSF fistula formation, and meningitis also are possible but are more likely after reoperation. The complications of microlumbar disc excision appear to be lower than with standard laminectomy. Alexander reviewed patients who had sustained incidental durotomy at the time of disc surgery and found no perioperative morbidity or compromise of results if the dura was repaired. They noted a 4% incidence of this complication in 450 discectomies.

The presence of a dural tear or leak results in the potentially serious problems of pseudomeningocele, CSF leak, and meningitis. Eismont, Wiesel, and Rothman suggested five basic principles in the repair of these leaks (Fig. 39-48):

1. The operative field must be unobstructed, dry, and well exposed.
2. Dural suture of a 4-0 or 6-0 gauge with a tapered or reverse cutting needle is used in either a simple or running locking stitch. If the leak is large or inaccessible,

a free fat graft or fascial graft can be sutured to the dura. Fibrin glue applied to the repair also is helpful but will not seal a significant leak.

3. All repairs should be tested by using the reverse Trendelenburg position and Valsalva maneuvers.
4. Paraspinous muscles and overlying fascia should be closed in two layers with nonabsorbable suture used in a watertight fashion. Drains should not be used.
5. Bed rest in the supine position should be maintained for 4 to 7 days after the repair of lumbar dural defects. A lumbar drain should be placed if the integrity of the closure is questionable.

The development of headaches on standing and a stormy postoperative period should alert one to the possibility of an undetected CSF leak. This can be confirmed by MRI studies.

The presence of glucose in drainage fluid is not a reliable diagnostic test. On rare occasions a pseudomeningocele has been implicated as a cause of persistent pain from pressure on a nerve root by the cystic mass.

◆ Dural Repair Augmented with Fibrin Glue

Dural repair can be augmented with fibrin glue. Pressure testing of a dural repair without fibrin glue reveals that the dura is able to withstand 10 mm of pressure on day 1 and 28 mm on day 7. With fibrin glue the dura is able to withstand 28 mm on day 1 and 31 mm on day 7. Fibrin glue also can be used in areas of troublesome bleeding or difficult access for closure such as the ventral aspect of the dura.

TECHNIQUE 39-23

Mix 20,000 U of topical thrombin and 10 ml of 10 calcium chloride. Draw the mixture up into a syringe. In another syringe, draw 5 U of cryoprecipitate and inject equal quantities of each onto the dural repair or tear. Allow the glue to set to the consistency of "Jello" (Box 39-10). Commercially available kits also are available.

Free Fat Grafting

Fat grafting for the prevention of postoperative epidural scarring has been suggested by Kiviluoto; Jacobs, McClain, and Neff; and Bryant, Bremer, and Nguyen. The study by Jacobs et al. indicated that free fat grafts were superior to Gelfoam in the prevention of postoperative scarring. The current rationale for free fat grafting appears to be the possibility of making any reoperation easier. Unfortunately, the benefit of reduced scarring and its relationship to the prevention of postoperative pain have not been established, neither has the increased ease of reoperation in patients in whom fat grafting was performed. Caution should be taken in applying a fat graft to a large laminar defect because this has been reported to result in an acute cauda equina syndrome in the early postoperative period. We currently reserve the use of a fat graft (or fascial grafts) for dural repairs and small laminar defects where the graft is supported by the bone. A study by Jensen et al. found

Fig. 39-48   A, Illustration of dural repair using running-locking dural suture on taper or reverse-cutting, one-half-circle needle. A smaller-sized suture should be used. Use of suction with sucker and small cotton pledgets is essential to protect nerve roots while operative field is kept dry of CSF. **B,** Single dural stitches can be used to achieve closure, each suture end being left long. Second needle then is attached to free suture end, and ends of suture are passed through piece of muscle or fat, which is tied down over repaired tear to help to achieve watertight closure. Whenever dural material is inadequate to allow closure without placing excessive pressure on underlying neural tissues, free graft of fascia or fascia lata, or freeze-dried dural graft, should be secured to margins of dural tear using simple sutures of appropriate size. **C,** For small dural defects in relatively inaccessible areas, transdural approach can be used to pull small piece of muscle or fat into defect from inside out, thereby sealing CSF leak. Central durotomy should be large enough to expose defect from dural sac. Durotomy is then closed in standard watertight fashion. (From Eismont FJ, Wiesel SW, Rothman RH: *J Bone Joint Surg* 63A: 1132, 1981.)

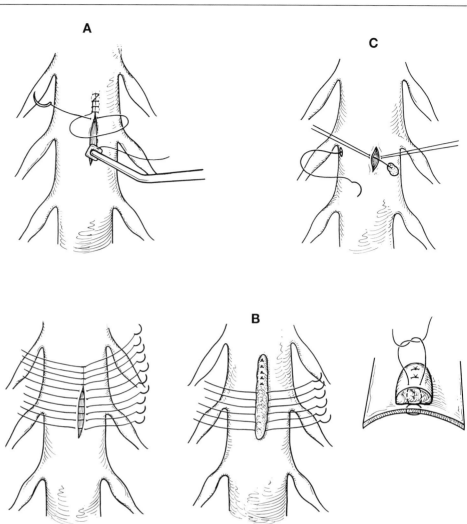

> **BOX 39-10 • Fibrin Glue**
>
> **INGREDIENTS**
> Two vials of topical thrombin, 10,000 U each
> 10 ml of calcium chloride
> 5 U of cryoprecipitate
> Two 5-ml syringes
> Two 22-gauge spinal needles
>
> **INSTRUCTIONS**
> Do not use saline that comes with thrombin
> Mix thrombin and calcium chloride
> Draw mixture into syringe
> Draw cryoprecipitate into second syringe
> Apply equal amounts to area of need
> Allow to set to a "Jello" consistency

that fat grafts decreased the dural scarring but not radicular scar formation. The clinical outcome was not improved.

The technique of free fat grafting is straightforward. At the end of the procedure, just before closing, take a large piece of subcutaneous fat and insert it over the laminectomy defect. If the patient is thin, a separate incision over the buttock may be required to get sufficient fat to fill the defect.

CHEMONUCLEOLYSIS

Chemonucleolysis has been used in the United States for more than 30 years. The enzyme was released for general use by the Food and Drug Administration (FDA) in December of 1982. Before its release in the United States it was used extensively in Europe and Canada. A wealth of experimental and clinical information exists concerning the technique and the enzyme. Specific guidelines have been suggested by the FDA regarding the use of the enzyme in the United States. The initial enthusiasm for the use of chymopapain has all but vanished in the United States; however, the use of this enzyme is still popular in Europe and elsewhere, with therapeutic results similar to surgery.

Because of the disclosure of neurological sequelae and other complications, the original guidelines issued in January of 1983 were radically changed. Those interested in performing the technique should contact the pharmaceutical companies that

Table 39-10 Results and Complications of Chemonucleolysis and Open Disc Excision

			Results (percent)						
Technique	Year	No. Performed	Excellent	Partial/ Good	None	Worse	Complications	Reoperation	Persistent Back Pain
Open Disc									
Semmes	1955	1440	53.6	43.3	1.7	1.4	NA	6.3	
Spangfort	1972	2503	76.9	17.0	5.0	0.5	8.0		31.5
Weir	1979	100	73.0	22.0	3.0	1.0	NA	NA	
Rish	1984	57	74.0	17.0	9.0		4.0	18.0	
Chemonucleolysis									
Illinois trial	1982	273	90.0		10.0		1.1		
Javid	1983	40	82.0		18.0				
Nordby	1983	641	55.0	25.0	20.0		NA	NA	

produce the drug for information regarding training and certification in the technique. Treating physicians also are encouraged to frequently check the package insert accompanying the drug and the information bulletins sent out by the FDA and the pharmaceutical companies regarding any new changes in the protocol or use of the enzyme. Careful patient selection and proficiency in performing this procedure are mandatory.

The indications for the use of chemonucleolysis are the same as for open surgery for disc herniation. Fraser reported the results of 60 patients treated for lumbar disc herniation in a 2-year double-blind study of chemonucleolysis. At 2 years 77% of the patients treated with chymopapain were improved, whereas only 47% of the saline injection group were improved. At 2 years from injection 57% of the chymopapain group were pain-free compared with 23% of the placebo group. Numerous other studies of the efficacy of the drug place the good or excellent results between 40% and 89%, which is comparable to the clinical reports for open surgery (Table 39-10). Tregonning et al. reviewed 145 patients who had received chymopapain injection and 91 patients who had laminectomy at 10-year follow-up and concluded that the surgically treated group had slightly better results than the chymopapain group. Javid compared 100 patients who had laminectomy with 100 patients who had chemonucleolysis and reported that patients who had received chymopapain had better results with respect to 6-month overall improvement, short-term improvement in numbness and motor strength, and longer improvement in sensory status. Also, chymopapain was significantly less expensive than laminectomy. Nordby and Wright reviewed 45 clinical studies of chymopapain and laminectomy. They concluded that chemonucleolysis was somewhat less effective than open disc excision, but it did avoid the trauma of surgery and postoperative fibrosis.

As with open disc surgery, this technique is not applicable in all lumbar disc herniations. The use of the drug is limited to the lumbar spine. The patient optimally has predominantly unilateral leg pain and localized neurological findings consistent with confirmatory testing with MRI, CT, or myelogra-

phy. Patients with moderate lateral recess or foraminal stenosis may worsen after the procedure because of collapse of the disc space and narrowing of the foraminal opening. Large disc herniations may not shrink sufficiently to result in relief of symptoms, and sequestered discs may be untouched by the enzyme. Smith et al. reported cauda equina syndromes in three patients after chymopapain was injected after a myelogram revealed a complete block.

Chymopapain injection is specifically contraindicated in patients with a known sensitivity to papaya, papaya derivatives, or food containing papaya, such as meat tenderizers. Other contraindications include severe spondylolisthesis, severe, progressive neurological deficit or paralysis, and evidence of spinal cord tumor or a cauda equina lesion. The enzyme cannot be injected in a patient who has been previously injected, regardless of the level injected. Use of chymopapain is limited to the lumbar intervertebral discs. Relative contraindications include allergy to iodine or iodine contrast material, use of the enzyme in a previously operated disc, patients with elevated allergy studies such as radioallergosorbent (RAST), Chymo-Fast, and skin testing with the drug, and patients with a severe allergic history, especially with a previous anaphylactic attack.

Spinal Instability from Degenerative Disc Disease

Farfan defined spinal instability (caused by degenerative disc disease) as a clinically symptomatic condition without new injury, in which a physiological load induces abnormally large deformations at the intervertebral joint. Biomechanical studies have revealed abnormal motion at vertebral segments with degenerative discs and the transmission of the load to the facet joints. Numerous attempts at roentgenographic definition of spinal instability with disc disease have resulted in more controversy than agreement as to a standard method of measurement. The method described by Knutsson is simple and relatively efficient in determining anteroposterior motion. The

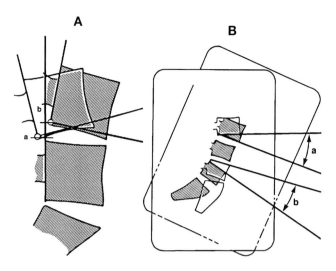

Fig. 39-49   Loss of motion segment integrity. **A,** Translation. **B,** Angular motion. (From American Medical Association: *Guide to the evaluation of permanent impairment*, ed 4, Chicago, 1993, AMA.)

fourth edition of the *American Medical Association Guide to the Evaluation of Permanent Impairment* defined instability as an anterior slip of 5 mm or more in the thoracic or lumbar spine (Fig. 39-49, *A*) or a difference in the angular motion of two adjacent motion segments more than 11 degrees from T1 to L5 and motion greater than 15 degrees at L5-1 compared with L4-5 (Fig. 39-49, *B*). There is little controversy as to the surgical treatment of lumbar spinal instability and spinal fusion of the unstable segments. The type of fusion performed and the indications for fusion are areas of controversy.

The major problem in spinal instability is the correlation of the patient's symptoms of giving way, catching, and predominant back pain to the roentgenographic identification of instability. Other factors such as concomitant spinal stenosis, disc herniation, and psychological problems only complicate any evaluation of spinal instability. Currently the decision for surgery for clinically significant lumbar spine instability caused by degenerative disc disease should be made on an individual patient basis with all the factors and risks weighed carefully.

DISC EXCISION AND FUSION

The necessity of lumbar fusion at the same time as disc excision was first suggested by Mixter and Barr. In the first 20 years after their discovery the combination of disc excision and lumbar fusion was common. More recent data comparing disc excision alone with the combination of disc excision and fusion by Frymoyer et al. and others indicate that there is little if any advantage to the addition of a spinal fusion to the treatment of simple disc herniation. These studies do indicate that spinal fusion increases the complication rate and lengthens recovery. The indications for lumbar fusion should be independent of the indications for disc excision for sciatica.

LUMBAR VERTEBRAL INTERBODY FUSION

Anterior lumbar intervertebral fusion (ALIF) and posterior lumbar intervertebral fusion (PLIF) have been suggested as definitive procedures for lumbar disc disease. Biomechanically the lumbar interbody fusion offers the greatest stability. It also eliminates the disc segment as a further source of pain. The primary problems are the more involved and potentially dangerous dissection, the risk of graft extrusion, and pseudarthrosis.

Most series of these fusions include a significant number of salvage procedures and complex pathological conditions, thus making direct comparison with primary disc surgery difficult. The routine use of such procedures for simple lumbar disc herniation with sciatica is not justified.

Most often, different types of grafts are taken from the iliac crest; however, hollow, perforated cylinders filled with autologous bone are now available for use in posterior and anterior lumbar intervertebral fusion. These cylinders are not indicated for spondylolisthesis greater than grade 1, osteopenia, malignancy, or gross obesity. Kuslich and Dowdle reported 98% fusion at one level anteriorly and 89% fusion at two levels with a slightly better functional improvement than the fusion rates using this device. This device also can be introduced by a percutaneous, laparoscopic anterior approach. The laparoscopic approach requires a team consisting of a laparoscopic general surgeon, spine surgeon, anesthesiologist, camera operator, scrub nurse, circulating nurse, and a radiology technician. It is strongly advised that the team attend a course on this technique or observe several cases before attempting such a procedure.

◆ Anterior Lumbar Interbody Fusion

TECHNIQUE 39-24

Place the patient supine on a radiolucent operating table. Support the lumbar spine with a rolled sheet or inflatable bag. Prepare and drape the patient's abdomen from upper chest to groin, leaving the iliac crests exposed for obtaining bone grafts. Expose the lumbar spine through a transabdominal or retroperitoneal approach as desired. Mobilize the great vessels over the segment to be excised. Ligate the median artery and vein at the bifurcation of the aorta to prevent tearing this structure when exposing the disc at L4-5 or L5-S1.

Identify and inspect all major structures before and after disc excision and fusion. Use anteroposterior fluoroscopy to confirm the proper disc level. Then incise the anterior longitudinal ligament superiorly or inferiorly over the edge of the vertebral body. Elevate the ligament as a flap if possible. Next remove the annular and nuclear material of the disc. The use of magnification can be beneficial as the dissection nears the posterior longitudinal ligament. Remove all nuclear material from the disc space.

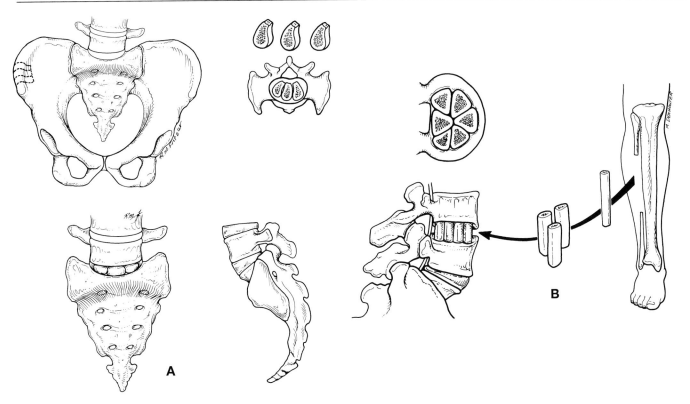

Fig. 39-50   Anterior lumbar intervertebral fusion (ALIF) can be performed using tricortical iliac crest graft **(A)** or fibular grafts **(B)**. **(A** from Ruge D, Wiltse LL: *Spinal disorders: diagnosis and treatment*, Philadelphia, 1977, Lea & Febiger; **B** from Wiltse LL: *Instr Course Lect* 28:207, 1979.)

Techniques for fusion vary. Some prefer to use dowel grafts to fill the space. Others prefer to use tricortical iliac grafts (Fig. 39-50). Obtain the grafts from the iliac crest as described for anterior cervical fusions (Chapter 36). Prepare the graft area for the desired grafting technique. We prefer tricortical grafts for this fusion. Good results using fibular grafts and banked bone also have been reported. Prepare the vertebrae by curetting the endplates to cancellous bone posteriorly. Then carefully make a slot in the vertebra to accommodate the grafts; use an osteotome slightly larger than the width of the disc space for this purpose and direct the cut toward the inferior vertebral body. Try to leave the upper and lower lips of the vertebral bodies intact. Remove enough tricortical iliac bone to allow insertion of at least three individual grafts. Fashion the grafts to fit snugly in the space with a laminar spreader in place. Insert the grafts so that the cancellous portions face the decorticated endplates. The grafts should be 3 to 4 mm shorter than the anteroposterior diameter of the vertebral body. Impact the grafts and seat them behind the anterior rim of the vertebral bodies. Usually three such grafts can be inserted. Add additional cancellous chips around the grafts. Suture the anterior longitudinal ligament. Close the retroperitoneum and abdomen in the usual manner.

AFTERTREATMENT. The patient is allowed to sit as soon as possible. Extension of the lumbar spine is prohibited for at least 6 weeks. Bracing or casting is left to the discretion of the surgeon after considering the stability of the grafts and reliability of the patient.

◆ Posterior Lumbar Interbody Fusion

TECHNIQUE 39-25 *(Cloward)*

Position the patient in the prone or kneeling position as desired. Expose the spine through a midline incision centered over the level of the pathological condition. Strip the muscle subperiosteally from the lamina bilaterally. Insert the laminar spreader between the spinous processes at the level of pathological findings. Open and remove the ligamentum flavum from the midline laterally. Enlarge the opening laterally by removing the lower one third of the inferior facet and the medial two thirds of the superior facet (Fig. 39-51, *A*). The upper lamina also can be thinned by undercutting to increase the anteroposterior diameter of the canal. Retract the lower nerve root and dura to the midline and protect it with the self-retaining nerve root retractor. Cauterize the epidural vessels with bipolar cautery. Cut out the disc and vessels over the annulus laterally. Remove as

continued

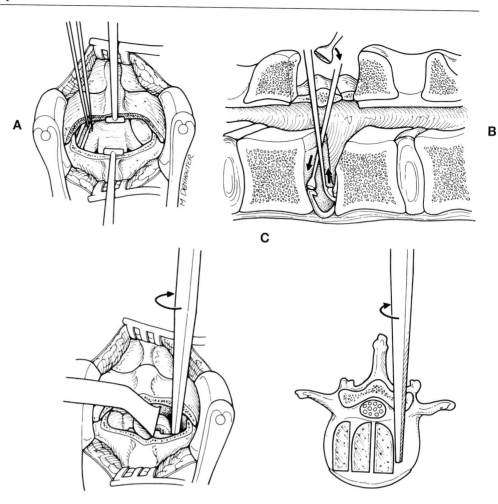

Fig. 39-51   Posterior lumbar interbody fusion technique. **A,** Bilateral laminotomy with preservation of facets. Control of epidural hemorrhage. Dipolar or insulated coagulation forceps are used on left side. On right side, epidural hemorrhage is controlled by impacted surgical tampons. Impacted surgical tampons also push nerve root medially and expose disc space without need for nerve root retractor. **B,** After intervertebral rims are removed, cleavage of disc attachment to cortical plate is identified. Curved, up-bite curet is used to remove concave centrum of lower cartilaginous plate. Then detached large chunks of disc material are removed with rongeur. **C,** Medial graft advancement with single chisel. (From Cauthen JC: *Lumbar spine surgery,* Baltimore, 1983, Williams & Wilkins.)

much disc material as possible (Fig. 39-51, *B*). Remove a thin layer of the endplates posteriorly. Repeat this process on the opposite side. Remove the remaining anterior edges of the endplates to the anterior longitudinal ligament. This must be done under direct vision to avoid injury to the great vessels. Prepare a surface of bleeding cancellous bone on both vertebral bodies. Obtain tricortical iliac crest grafts as previously noted from the posterior iliac crest. (Cloward used frozen human cadaver bone grafts.) Shape the grafts to be slightly shorter and the same height or slightly higher than the disc shape. Tamp the first graft in place and lever it medially to allow insertion of the remaining grafts. Repeat the procedure on the opposite side (Fig. 39-51, *C*). Remove the laminar spreader and check the graft for stability. Close the wound in the usual fashion.

AFTERTREATMENT. Aftertreatment is the same as for lumbar discectomy (p. 2006). Early walking is encouraged.

Failed Spine Surgery

One of the greatest problems in orthopaedic surgery and neurosurgery is the treatment of failed spine surgery. Numerous

reasons for the failures have been advanced. The best results from repeat surgery for disc problems appear to be related to the discovery of a new problem or identification of a previously undiagnosed or untreated problem. Waddell et al. suggested that the best results from repeat surgery occur when the patient had experienced 6 months or more of complete pain relief after the first procedure, when leg pain exceeded back pain, and when a definite recurrent disc could be identified. They identified adverse factors such as scarring, previous infection, repair of pseudarthrosis, and adverse psychological factors. Similar factors were identified by Lehmann and LaRocca and Finnegan et al. Satisfactory results from reoperation have been reported to be from 31% to 80%. Patients should expect improvement in the severity of symptoms rather than complete relief of pain. As the frequency of repeat back surgeries increases, the chance of a satisfactory result drops precipitously. Spengler et al. and Long et al. observed that the major cause of failure is improper patient selection.

The recurrence or intensification of pain after disc surgery should be treated with the usual conservative methods initially. If these methods fail to relieve the pain, the patient should be completely reevaluated. Frequently a repeat history and physical examination will give some indication of the problem. Additional testing should include psychological testing, myelography, MRI to check for tumors or a higher disc herniation, and reformatted CT scans to check for areas of foraminal stenosis or for lateral herniation. The use of the differential spinal, root blocks, facet blocks, and discograms also can help identify the source of pain. The presence of abnormal psychological test results or an abnormal differential spinal should serve as a modifier to any suggested treatment indicated by the other testing. Satisfactory nonoperative treatment of this problem should be attempted before additional surgery is performed, provided that this surgery is elective. A distinct, surgically correctable, anatomical problem should be identified before surgery is contemplated. The surgery should be tailored specifically to the anatomical problem(s) identified.

◆ REPEAT LUMBAR DISC SURGERY

The technique of repeat lumbar disc surgery at the same level and side as the previous procedure is nearly the same as for initial surgery. The procedure is longer and involves more meticulous dissection.

TECHNIQUE 39-26

Approach the spine using the method described previously. Identify normal tissue first. Use a curet to carefully remove scar from the edges of the lamina. Then remove additional bone as necessary to expose normal dura. Identify the pedicles superiorly and inferiorly if there is any question of position and status of the root. Carry the dissection from the pedicles to identify each root. This will allow the development of a normal plane between the dura and scar. Maintain meticulous hemostasis with bipolar cautery. Then remove disc material as indicated by the preoperative evaluation. Meticulously check the roots, dura, and posterior longitudinal ligament after removal of the offending disc herniation. Spinal fusion is not performed unless an unstable spine is created by the dissection or was identified preoperatively as a correctable and symptomatic problem.

AFTERTREATMENT. Aftertreatment is the same as for disc excision (p. 2006).

References

HISTORY

Alajouanine TH: From the presidential address for Professor Jean Cauchoix before the annual meeting of the International Society for the Study of the Lumbar Spine, San Francisco, June 1978.

Aurelianus C: *Acute diseases and chronic diseases*, Chicago, 1950, University of Chicago Press.

Barr JS, Hampton AO, Mixter WJ: Pain low in the back and "sciatica" due to lesions of the intervertebral discs, *JAMA* 109:1265, 1937.

Catchlove RF, Braha R: The use of cervical epidural nerve blocks in the management of chronic head and neck pain, *Can Anaesth Soc J* 31:188, 1984.

Cotugnio D: *Treatise on the nervous sciatica or nervous hip gout*, London, 1775, J Wilkie.

Dandy WE: Loose cartilage from the intervertebral disc simulating tumor of the spinal cord, *Orthop Surg* 19:1660, 1929.

de Sèze S: Sciatique "banale" et disques lombo-sacrés, *Presse Med* 51-52:570, 1940.

de Sèze S: Histoire de la sciatique, *Rev Neurol* 138:1019, 1982.

Dyck P: Lumbar nerve root: the enigmatic eponyms, *Spine* 9:3, 1984.

Elsberg CA: Experiences in spinal surgery: observations upon 60 laminectomies for spinal disease, *Surg Gynecol Obstet* 16:117, 1913.

Forst JJ: Contribution a l'etude clinique de la sciatique, thesis, Lyon, France, 1881.

Goldthwait JE: The lumbosacral articulations: an explanation of many cases of "lumbago," "sciatica," and paraplegia, *Bost Med Surg J* 164:365, 1911.

Hall GW: Neurologic signs and their discoverers, *JAMA* 95:703, 1930.

Kepes ER, Duncalf D: Treatment of backache with spinal injections of local anesthetics, spinal and systemic steroids: a review, *Pain* 22:33, 1985.

Kirkaldy-Willis WH, Hill RJ: A more precise diagnosis for low-back pain, *Spine* 4:102, 1979.

Kocher T: Die Verlitzungen der Wirbelsaule Zurleich Als Beitrag zur Physiologic des Menschichen Ruchenmarks, *Mitt Grenzgeb Med Chir* 1:415, 1896.

Lasègue C: Considerations sur la sciatique, *Arch Gen Med* 2:558, 1864.

Love JG: Removal of intervertebral discs without laminectomy, *Proc Staff Meet Mayo Clin* 14:800, 1939.

Middleton GS, Teacher JH: Extruded disc at T12-L1 level: microscopic exam showed it to be nucleus pulposus, *Glasgow Med J* 76:1, 1911.

Middleton GS, Teacher JH: Injury of the spinal cord due to rupture of an intervertebral disc during muscular effort, *Glasgow Med J* 76:1, 1911.

Mixter WJ, Barr JS: Rupture of the intervertebral disc with involvement of the spinal canal, *N Engl J Med* 211:210, 1934.

Murphy PL, Volinn E: Is occupational low back pain on the rise? *Spine* 24:691, 1999.

Oppenheim H, Krause F: Ueber Einklemmung bzw. Strangulation der Cauda equina, *Deutsche Med Wochenschr* 35:697, 1909.

Robinson JS: Sciatica and the lumbar disk syndrome: a historic perspective, *South Med J* 76:232, 1983.

Semmes RE: Diagnosis of ruptured intervertebral discs without contrast myelography and comment upon recent experience with modified hemilaminectomy for their removal, *Yale J Biol Med* 11:433, 1939.

Shulman M, Joseph NJ, Haller CA: Effect of epidural and subarachnoid injections of a 10% butamben suspension, *Reg Anesth* 15:142, 1990.

Sjöqvist O: The mechanism of origin of Lasègue's sign, *Acta Psych Neurol* 46(suppl):290, 1947.

Smith L, Garvin PJ, Gesler RM, et al: Enzyme dissolution of the nucleus pulposus, *Nature* 198:1131, 1963.

Sugar O: Charles Lasègue and his "Considerations on Sciatica," *JAMA* 253:1767, 1985.

Virchow R: *Untersuchunger uber die Enwickelung die Schadeigrunder*, Berlin, 1857, G Reimer.

Waddell G: Low back pain: a twentieth-century health care enigma, *Spine* 21:2820, 1996.

Wiltse LL: History of lumbar spine surgery. In White AA, ed: *Lumbar spine surgery: techniques and complications*, St Louis, 1987, Mosby.

EPIDEMIOLOGY

Andersson GBJ: Epidemiologic aspects of low-back pain in industry, *Spine* 6:53, 1981.

Andersson GBJ, Svensson HO, Oden A: The intensity of work recovery in low back pain, *Spine* 8:880, 1983.

Biering-Sorensen F, Hilden J: Reproducibility of the history of low-back trouble, *Spine* 9:280, 1984.

Buckle PW, Kember PA, Wood AD, Wood SN: Factors influencing occupational back pain in Bedfordshire, *Spine* 5:254, 1980.

Carey TS, Evans A, Haler N, et al: Care-seeking among individuals with chronic low back pain, *Spine* 20:312, 1995.

Damkot DK, Pope MH, Lord J, Frymoyer JW: The relationship between work history, work environment, and low-back pain in men, *Spine* 9:395, 1984.

Deyo RA, Bass JE: Lifestyle and low-back pain: the influence of smoking and obesity, *Spine* 14:501, 1989.

Dillane JB, Fry J, Kalton G: Acute back syndrome: a study from general practice, *Br Med J* 2:82, 1966.

Frymoyer JW, Cats-Baril WL: An overview of the incidences and costs of low back pain, *Orthop Clin North Am* 22:263, 1991.

Frymoyer JW, Newberg A, Pope MT, et al: Spine radiographs in patients with low-back pain: an epidemiological study in men, *J Bone Joint Surg* 66A:1048, 1984.

Frymoyer JW, Pope MT, Clements JH, et al: Risk factors in low-back pain: an epidemiological survey, *J Bone Joint Surg* 65A:213, 1983.

Grabias S: Current concepts review: the treatment of spinal stenosis, *J Bone Joint Surg* 62A:308, 1980.

Gyntelberg F: One-year incidence of low back pain among male residents of Copenhagen aged 40-59, *Dan Med Bull* 21:30, 1974.

Harreby M, Nygaard B, Jessen T, et al: Risk factors for low back pain in a cohort of 1389 Danish school children: an epidemiologic study, *Eur Spine J* 8:444, 1999.

Hult L: The Munkfors investigation, *Acta Orthop Scand Suppl* 16:1, 1954.

Jackson RP, Simmons EH, Stripinis D: Incidence and severity of back pain in adult idiopathic scoliosis, *Spine* 8:749, 1983.

Johnsson K, Willner S, Pettersson H: Analysis of operated cases with lumbar renal stenosis, *Acta Orthop Scand* 52:427, 1981.

Kelsey JL, White AA III: Epidemiology and impact of low-back pain, *Spine* 5:133, 1980.

Knutsson F: The instability associated with disk degeneration in the lumbar spine, *Acta Radiol* 25:593, 1944.

Kostuik JP, Bentivoglio J: The incidence of low-back pain in adult scoliosis, *Spine* 6:268, 1981.

Manning DP, Shannon HS: Slipping accidents causing low-back pain in a gearbox factory, *Spine* 6:70, 1981.

Middleton GS, Teacher JH: Injury of the spinal cord due to rupture of an intervertebral disc during muscular effort, *Glasgow Med J* 76:1, 1911.

Mooney V, Robertson J: The facet syndrome, *Clin Orthop* 115:149, 1976.

Nachemson AL: Prevention of chronic back pain: the orthopaedic challenge for the 80s, *Bull Hosp Jt Dis* 44:1, 1984.

Riihimaki H, Tola S, Videman T, Hanninen K: Low-back pain and occupation: a cross-sectional questionnaire study of men in machine operating, dynamic physical work and sedentary work, *Spine* 14:204, 1989.

Ryden LA, Molgaard CA, Bobbitt S, Conway J: Occupational low-back injury in a hospital employee population and epidemiologic analysis of multiple risk factors of a high-risk occupational group, *Spine* 14:315, 1989.

Sandover J: Dynamic loading as a possible source of low-back disorders, *Spine* 8:652, 1983.

Snook SH: The costs of back pain in industry, *Spine: State of the Art Reviews* 2:11, 1987.

Snook SH, Webster BS: The cost of disability, *Clin Orthop* 221:77, 1987.

Svensson HO, Andersson GBJ: Low back pain in 40- to 47-year-old men: work history and work environment factors, *Spine* 8:272, 1983.

Svensson HO, Andersson GBJ: The relationship of low-back pain, work history, work environment and stress: a retrospective cross-sectional study of 38- to 64-year-old women, *Spine* 14:517, 1989.

Svensson HO, Vedin A, Wilhelmsson C, Andersson GBJ: Low-back pain in relation to other diseases and cardiovascular risk factors, *Spine* 8:277, 1983.

Troup JDG, Martin JW, Lloyd DC: Back pain in industry: a prospective survey, *Spine* 6:61, 1981.

van-Doorn JW: Low back disability among self-employed dentists, veterinarians, physicians, and physical therapists in The Netherlands: a retrospective study over a 13-year period (N 1,119) and an early intervention program with 1-year follow-up (N 134), *Acta Orthop Scand Suppl* 263:1, 1995.

Waddell G, Main CJ, Morris EW, et al: Chronic low-back pain, psychological distress, and illness behavior, *Spine* 9:209, 1984.

Webster BS, Snook SH: The cost of compensable low back pain, *J Occup Med* 32:13, 1990.

Webster BS, Snook SH: The cost of 1989 workers' compensation low back pain claims, *Spine* 19:1111, 1994.

Weisz GM: Lumbar spinal canal stenosis in Paget's disease, *Spine* 8:192, 1983.

White AWM: Low back pain in men receiving workmen's compensation: a follow-up study, *Can Med Assoc J* 101:61, 1969.

Wilder DG, Woodworth BB, Frymoyer JW, Pope MH: Vibration and the human spine, *Spine* 7:243, 1982.

GENERAL DISC AND SPINE ANATOMY

Adams MA, Hutton WC: The mechanical function of the lumbar apophyseal joints, *Spine* 8:327, 1983.

Bogduk N: The clinical anatomy of the cervical dorsal rami, *Spine* 7:319, 1982.

Bogduk N: The innervation of the lumbar spine, *Spine* 8:286, 1983.

Bogduk N, Engel R: The menisci of the lumbar zygapophyseal joints: a review of their anatomy and clinical significance, *Spine* 9:454, 1984.

Bogduk N, Macintosh JE: The applied anatomy of the thoracolumbar fascia, *Spine* 9:164, 1984.

Bose K, Balasubramaniam P: Nerve root canals of the lumbar spine, *Spine* 9:16, 1984.

Botsford DJ, Esses SI, Ogilvie-Harris DJ: In vivo diurnal variation in intervertebral disc volume and morphology, *Spine* 15:935, 1994.

Crock HV: Normal and pathological anatomy of the lumbar spinal nerve root canals, *J Bone Joint Surg* 63B:487, 1981.

de Peretti F, Hovorka I, Ganansia P, et al: The vertebral foramen: a report concerning its contents, *Surg Radiol Anat* 15:287, 1993.

Hasue M, Kikuchi S, Sakuyama Y, Ito T: Anatomical study of the interrelation between lumbosacral nerve roots and their surrounding tissues, *Spine* 8:50, 1983.

Inoue H: Three-dimensional architecture of lumbar intervertebral discs, *Spine* 6:139, 1981.

Jayson MIV: Compression stresses in the posterior elements and pathologic consequences, *Spine* 8:338, 1983.

Kikuchi S, Hasue M, Nishiyama K, Ito T: Anatomical and clinical studies of radicular symptoms, *Spine* 9:23, 1982.

King AG: Functional anatomy of the lumbar spine, *Orthopedics* 6:1588, 1983.

Kirkaldy-Willis WH: The relationship of structural pathology to the nerve root, *Spine* 9:49, 1984.

Knutsson F: The instability associated with disc degeneration in the lumbar spine, *Acta Radiol* 25:593, 1944.

Mayoux-Benhamou MA, Revel M, Aaron C, et al: A morphometric study of the lumbar foramen: influence of flexion-extension movements and of isolated disc collapse, *Surg Radiol Anat* 11:97, 1989.

Miller JAA, Haderspeck KA, Schultz AB: Posterior element loads in lumbar motion segments, *Spine* 8:331, 1983.

Neumann P, Keller T, Ekstrom L, et al: Structural properties of the anterior longitudinal ligament: correlation with lumbar bone mineral content, *Spine* 18:637, 1993.

Paajanen H, Lehto I, Alanen A, et al: Diurnal fluid changes of lumbar discs measured indirectly by magnetic resonance imaging, *J Orthop Res* 12:509, 1994.

Pazzaglia UE, Salisbury JR, Byers PD: Development and involution of the notochord in the human spine, *J R Soc Med* 82:413, 1989.

Pedersen H, Blunck CFJ, Gardner E: The anatomy of lumbosacral posterior rami and meningeal branches of spinal nerves (sinu-vertebral nerves), *J Bone Joint Surg* 38A:2377, 1956.

Postacchini F, Urso S, Ferro L: Lumbosacral nerve-root anomalies, *J Bone Joint Surg* 64A:721, 1982.

Rhalmi S, Yahia LH, Newman N, Isler M: Immunohistochemical study of nerves in lumbar spine ligaments, *Spine* 18:264, 1993.

Rudert M, Tillman B: Lymph and blood supply of the human intervertebral disc: cadaver study of correlations to discitis, *Acta Orthop Scand* 64:37, 1993.

Rydevik B, Brown MD, Lundborg G: Pathoanatomy and pathophysiology of nerve root compression, *Spine* 9:7, 1984.

Spencer DL, Irwin GS, Miller JAA: Anatomy and significance of fixation of the lumbosacral nerve roots in sciatica, *Spine* 8:672, 1983.

Wall EJ, Cohen MS, Abitbol J, Garfin SR: Organization of intrathecal nerve roots at the level of the conus medullaris, *J Bone Joint Surg* 72A:1495, 1990.

Wilder DG, Pope MH, Frymoyer JW: The functional topography of the sacroiliac joint, *Spine* 5:575, 1980.

Young A, Getty J, Jackson A, et al: Variations in the pattern of muscle innervation by the L5 and S1 nerve roots, *Spine* 8:616, 1983.

Ziv I, Maroudas C, Robin G, Maroudas A: Human facet cartilage: swelling and some physiochemical characteristics as a function of age. II. Age changes in some biophysical parameters of human facet joint cartilage, *Spine* 18:136, 1993.

NATURAL HISTORY OF DISC DISEASE

Biering-Sørensen F, Hilden J: Reproducibility of the history of low-back trouble, *Spine* 9:280, 1984.

Gibson MJ, Szypryt EP, Buckley JH, et al: Magnetic resonance imaging of adolescent disc herniation, *J Bone Joint Surg* 69B:699, 1987.

Goldthwait E: Low-back lesions, *J Bone Joint Surg* 19:810, 1937.

Hakelius A: Prognosis in sciatica: a clinical follow-up of surgical and nonsurgical treatment, *Acta Orthop Scand* 129(suppl):1, 1970.

Jackson RP, Simmons EH, Stripinis D: Incidence and severity of back pain in adult idiopathic scoliosis, *Spine* 8:749, 1983.

Jayson MIV: Compression stresses in the posterior elements and pathologic consequences, *Spine* 8:338, 1983.

Kelsey JL, Githens PB, White AA III, et al: An epidemiologic study of lifting and twisting on the job and risk for acute prolapsed lumbar intervertebral disc, *J Orthop Res* 2:61, 1984.

Kirkaldy-Willis WH, Hill RJ: A more precise diagnosis for low-back pain, *Spine* 4:102, 1979.

Matsui H, Kanamori M, Ishihara H, et al: Familial predisposition for lumbar degenerative disc disease, *Spine* 23:1029, 1998.

Miller JAA, Schmatz C, Schultz AB: Lumbar disc degeneration: correlation with age, sex and spine level in 600 autopsy specimens, *Spine* 13:2173, 1988.

Pope MH, Bevins T, Wilder DG, Frymoyer JW: The relationship between anthropometric, postural, muscular, and mobility characteristics of males age 18-55, *Spine* 10:644, 1985.

Roland M, Morris R: A study of the natural history of back pain. I. Development of a reliable and sensitive measure of disability in low-back pain, *Spine* 8:141, 1983.

Rydevik B, Brown MD, Lundborg G: Pathoanatomy and pathophysiology of nerve root compression, *Spine* 9:7, 1984.

Saal JA: Natural history and nonoperative treatment of lumbar disc herniation, *Spine* 21:2S:1996.

Sandover J: Dynamic loading as a possible source of low-back disorders, *Spine* 8:652, 1983.

Takata K, Inoue S, Takahashi K, Ohtsuka Y: Swelling of the cauda equina in patients who have herniation of a lumbar disc: a possible pathogenesis of sciatica, *J Bone Joint Surg* 70A:3361, 1988.

Urban JPG, McMullin JF: Swelling pressure of the lumbar intervertebral discs: influence of age, spinal level, composition, and degeneration, *Spine* 13:2179, 1988.

Urovitz EP, Fornasier VL: Autoimmunity in degenerative disk disease: a histopathologic study *Clin Orthop* 142:215, 1979.

Varlotta GP, Brown MD, Kelsey JL, Golden AL: Familial predisposition for herniation of a lumbar disc in patients who are less than twenty-one years old, *J Bone Joint Surg* 73A:124, 1991.

Weber H: Lumbar disc herniation: a controlled, prospective study with ten years of observation, *Spine* 8:131, 1983.

Yasuma T, Koh S, Okamura T, Yamauchi Y: Histological changes in aging lumbar intervertebral discs, *J Bone Joint Surg* 72A:220, 1990.

DIAGNOSTIC STUDIES

Abel MS, Smith GR, Allen TNK: Refinements of the anteroposterior angled caudad view of the lumbar spine, *Skeletal Radiol* 7:113, 1981.

Abraham SR, Tedeschi AA, Partain CL, Blumenkopf B: Differential diagnosis of severe back pain using MRI, *South Med J* 81:487, 1988.

Alemohammad S, Bouzarth WF: Intracranial subdural hematoma following lumbar myelography: case report, *J Neurosurg* 52:256, 1980.

Amundsen P: Cervical myelography with Amipaque: seven years' experience, *Radiology* 21:282, 1981.

Angiari P, Crisi G, Merli GA: Aphasia and right hemiplegia after cervical myelography with metrizamide: a case report, *Neuroradiology* 26:61, 1984.

Asztely M, Kadziolka R, Nachemson A: A comparison of sonography and myelography in clinically suspected spinal stenosis, *Spine* 8:885, 1983.

Barrow DL, Wood JH, Hoffman JC Jr: Clinical indications for computer-assisted myelography, *Neurosurgery* 12:47, 1983.

Beattie PF, Meyers SP, Stratford P, et al: Associations between patient report of symptoms and anatomical impairment visible on lumbar magnetic resonance imaging, *Spine* 25:819, 2000.

Bell GR, Rothman RH, Booth RE, et al: A study of computer-assisted tomography. II. Comparison of metrizamide myelography and computed tomography in the diagnosis of herniated lumbar disc and spinal stenosis, *Spine* 9:552, 1984.

Birney TJ, White JJ, Berens D, Kuhn G: Comparison of MRI and discography in the diagnosis of lumbar degenerative disc disease, *J Spinal Disord* 5:417, 1992.

Bladé J, Gaston F, Montserrat E, et al: Spinal subarachnoid hematoma after lumbar puncture causing reversible paraplegia in acute leukemia: case report, *J Neurosurg* 58:438, 1983.

Bobest M, Furó I, Tompa K, et al: 1H nuclear magnetic resonance study of intervertebral discs: a preliminary report, *Spine* 11:709, 1986.

Boden SD, Davis DO, Dina TS, et al: Abnormal magnetic-resonance scans of the lumbar spine in asymptomatic subjects: a prospective investigation, *J Bone Joint Surg* 72A:403, 1990.

Boden SD, McCowin PR, Davis DO, et al: Abnormal magnetic-resonance scans of the cervical spine in asymptomatic subjects, *J Bone Joint Surg* 72A:1178, 1990.

Boos N, Rieder R, Schade V, et al: The diagnostic accuracy of magnetic resonance imaging, work perception, and psychosocial factors in identifying symptomatic disc herniations, *Spine* 20:2613, 1995.

Brem SS, Hafler DA, Van Uitert RL, et al: Spinal subarachnoid hematoma: a hazard of lumbar puncture resulting in reversible paraplegia, *N Engl J Med* 304:1020, 1981.

Charles MF, Byrd SE, Cohn ML, Huntington CT: Metrizamide computer tomography of the postoperative lumbar spine, *Orthop Rev* 11:49, 1982.

Coin CG: Cervical disk degeneration and herniation: diagnosis by computerized tomography, *South Med J* 77:979, 1984.

Collier BD, Johnson RP, Carrera GF, et al: Painful spondylolysis or spondylolisthesis studied by radiography and single-photon emission computed tomography, *Radiology* 154:207, 1985.

Deburge A, Benoist M, Boyer D: The diagnosis of disc sequestration, *Spine* 9:496, 1984.

Delamarter RB, Bohlman HH, Dodge LD, Biro C: Experimental lumbar spinal stenosis: analysis of the cortical evoked potentials, microvasculature, and histopathology, *J Bone Joint Surg* 72A:110, 1990.

Delamarter RB, Leventhal MR, Bohlman HH: Diagnosis of recurrent lumbar disc herniation vs postoperative scar by gadolinium-DTPA-enhanced magnetic resonance imaging (unpublished data).

Dvonch V, Scarff T, Bunch WH, et al: Dermatomal somatosensory evoked potentials: their use in lumbar radiculopathy, *Spine* 9:291, 1984.

Edelstein WA, Schenck JF, Hart HR, et al: Surface coil magnetic resonance imaging, *JAMA* 253:828, 1985.

Eisen A, Hoirch M: The electrodiagnostic evaluation of spinal root lesions, *Spine* 8:98, 1983.

Eldevik OP: Side effects and complications of myelography with water-soluble contrast agents, *J Oslo City Hosp* 32:121, 1982.

Esses SI, Moro JK: The value of facet joint blocks in patient selection for lumbar fusion, *Spine* 18:185, 1993.

Fager CA: Evaluation of cervical spine surgery by postoperative myelography, *Neurosurgery* 12:416, 1983.

Firooznia H, Benjamin V, Kricheff II, et al: CT of lumbar spine disc herniation: correlation with surgical findings, *Am J Roentgenol* 142:587, 1984.

Fitzgerald RH, Reines HD, Wise J: Diagnostic radiation exposure in trauma patients, *South Med J* 76:1511, 1983.

Ford LT, Goodman FG: X-ray studies of the lumbosacral spine, *South Med J* 10:1123, 1966.

Frymoyer JW, Newberg A, Pope MH, et al: Spine radiographs in patients with low-back pain: an epidemiological study in men, *J Bone Joint Surg* 66A:1048, 1984.

Fullenlove TM, Williams AJ: Comparative roentgen findings in symptomatic and asymptomatic backs, *Radiology* 63:572, 1957.

Gibson MJ, Buckley J, Mulholland RC, Worthington BS: The changes in the intervertebral disc after chemonucleolysis demonstrated by magnetic resonance imaging, *J Bone Joint Surg* 68B:719, 1986.

Gibson MJ, Szypryt EP, Buckley JH, et al: Magnetic resonance imaging of adolescent disc herniation, *J Bone Joint Surg* 69B:699, 1987.

Glasauer FE, Alker G: Metrizamide enhanced computed tomography: an adjunct to myelography in lumbar disc herniation, *Comput Radiol* 7:305, 1983.

Greenberg RP, Ducker TB: Evoked potentials in the clinical neurosciences, *J Neurosurg* 56:1, 1982.

Gulati AN, Guadognoli DA, Quigley JM: Relationship of side effects to patient position during and after metrizamide lumbar myelography, *Radiology* 141:113, 1981.

Haldeman S: The electrodiagnosis evaluation of nerve root function, *Spine* 9:42, 1984.

Harrington H, Tyler HR, Welch K: Surgical treatment of post-lumbar puncture dural CSF leak causing chronic headache: case report, *J Neurosurg* 57:703, 1982.

Haughton VM, Eldevik OP, Magnaes B, Amundsen P: A prospective comparison of computed tomography and myelography in the diagnosis of herniated lumbar disks, *Radiology* 142:103, 1982.

Hayes MA, Howard TC, Gruel CR, Kopta JA: Roentgenographic evaluation of lumbar spine flexion-extension in asymptomatic individuals, *Spine* 14:327, 1989.

Hemminghytt S, Daniels DL, Williams AL, Haughton VM: Intraspinal synovial cysts: natural history and diagnosis by CT, *Radiology* 145:375, 1982.

Herkowitz HN, Romeyn RL, Rothman RH: The indications for metrizamide myelography: relationship with complications after myelography, *J Bone Joint Surg* 65A:1144, 1983.

Herkowitz HN, Wiesel SW, Booth RE Jr, Rothman RH: Metrizamide myelography and epidural venography: their role in the diagnosis of lumbar disc herniation and spinal stenosis, *Spine* 7:55, 1982.

Hirschy JC, Leue WM, Berninger WH, et al: CT of the lumbosacral spine: importance of tomographic planes parallel to vertebral endplate, *Am J Roentgenol* 136:47, 1981.

Holt EP Jr: The question of lumbar discography, *J Bone Joint Surg* 50A:720, 1968.

Howie DW, Chatterton BE, Hone MR: Failure of ultrasound in the investigation of sciatica, *J Bone Joint Surg* 65B:144, 1983.

Hudgins WR: Computer-aided diagnosis of lumbar disc herniation, *Spine* 8:604, 1983.

James AE Jr, Partain CL, Patton JA, et al: Current status of magnetic resonance imaging, *South Med J* 78:580, 1985.

Jepson K, Nada A, Rymaszewski L: The role of radiculography in the management of lesions of the lumbar disc, *J Bone Joint Surg* 64B:405, 1982.

Johansen JP, Fossgreen J, Hansen HH: Bone scanning in lumbar disc herniation, *Acta Orthop Scand* 51:617, 1980.

Kambin P, Nixon JE, Chait A, Schaffer JL: Annular protrusion: pathophysiology and roentgenographic appearance, *Spine* 13:671, 1988.

Kapoor W, Hemmer K, Herbert D, Karpf M: Abdominal computed tomography: comparison of the usefulness of goal-directed vs non-goal-directed studies, *Arch Intern Med* 143:249, 1983.

Kelsey JL, Githens PB, Walter SD, et al: An epidemiological study of acute prolapsed cervical intervertebral disc, *J Bone Joint Surg* 66A:907, 1984.

Kieffer SA, Cacoyorin ED, Sherry RG: The radiological diagnosis of herniated lumbar intervertebral disk: a current controversy, *JAMA* 251:1192, 1984.

Kikuchi S, Macnab I, Moreau P: Localisation of the level of symptomatic cervical disc degeneration, *J Bone Joint Surg* 63B:272, 1981.

Killebrew K, Whaley RA, Hayward JN, Scatliff JH: Complications of metrizamide myelography, *Arch Neurol* 40:78, 1983.

Liang M, Komaroff AL: Roentgenograms in primary care patients with acute low back pain: a cost-effectiveness analysis, *Arch Intern Med* 142:1108, 1982.

MacGibbon B, Farfan HF: A radiologic survey of various configurations of the lumbar spine, *Spine* 4:258, 1979.

Macnab I: The traction spur: an indicator of segmental instability, *J Bone Joint Surg* 53A:663, 1971.

Macnab I, Cuthbert H, Godfrey CM: The incidence of denervation of the sacrospinales muscles following spinal surgery, *Spine* 2:294, 1977.

Macnab I, St Louis EL, Grabias SL, Jacob R: Selective ascending lumbosacral venography in the assessment of lumbar disc herniation, *J Bone Joint Surg* 58A:1093, 1976.

Macon JB, Poletti CE: Conducted somatosensory evoked potentials during spinal surgery. I. Control conduction velocity measurements, *J Neurosurg* 57:349, 1982.

Macon JB, Poletti CE, Sweet WH, et al: Conducted somatosensory evoked potentials during spinal surgery. II. Clinical applications, *J Neurosurg* 57:354, 1982.

MacPherson P, Teasdale E, MacPherson PY: Radiculography: is routine bed rest really necessary? *Clin Radiol* 34:325, 1983.

Meador K, Hamilton WJ, El Gammal TAM, et al: Irreversible neurologic complications of metrizamide myelography, *Neurology* 34:817, 1984.

Moufarrij NA, Hardy RW Jr, Weinstein MA: Computed tomographic, myelographic, and operative findings in patients with suspected herniated lumbar discs, *Neurosurgery* 12:184, 1983.

Paleari GL, Ballarati P, Gambrioli PL, Paleari M: Recent progress in vertebral body section roentgenography in the study of the pathology of the lumbar vertebrae, *Ital J Orthop Traumatol* 8:109, 1982.

Raskin SP, Keating JW: Recognition of lumbar disk disease: comparison of myelography and computed tomography, *Am J Roentgenol* 139:349, 1982.

Risius B, Modic MT, Hardy RW Jr, et al: Sector computed tomographic spine scanning in the diagnosis of lumbar nerve root entrapment, *Radiology* 143:109, 1982.

Rockey PH, Tompkins RK, Wood RW, Wolcott BW: The usefulness of x-ray examinations in the evaluation of patients with back pain, *J Fam Pract* 7:455, 1978.

Scavone JG, Latshaw RF, Rohrer GV: Use of lumbar spine films: statistical evaluation of a university teaching hospital, *JAMA* 246:1105, 1981.

Schelkun SR, Wagner KF, Blanks JA, Reinert CM: Bacterial meningitis following Pantopaque myelography: a case report and literature review, *Orthopedics* 8:74, 1985.

Schutte HE, Park WM: The diagnostic value of bone scintigraphy in patients with low back pain, *Skeletal Radiol* 10:1, 1983.

Schwarzer AC, Aprill CN, Derby R, et al: The relative contributions of the disc and zygapophyseal joint in chronic low back pain, *Spine* 19:801, 1994.

Shima F, Mihara K, Hachisuga S: Angioma in the paraspinal muscles complicated by spinal epidural hematoma: case report, *J Neurosurg* 57:274, 1982.

Siddiqi TS, Buchheit WA: Herniated nerve root as a complication of spinal tap: case report, *J Neurosurg* 56:565, 1982.

Siqueira EB, Kranzler LI, Schaffer L: Intraoperative myelography: technical note, *J Neurosurg* 58:786, 1983.

Smith GR: Nerve root cut-off on metrizamide-enhanced computerized tomography, *South Med J* 79:553, 1986.

Smith SE, Darden BV, Rhyne AL, Wood KE: Outcome of unoperated discogram-positive low back pain, *Spine* 20:1997, 1995.

Steiner RE: Nuclear magnetic resonance: its clinical application, *J Bone Joint Surg* 65B:533, 1983.

Stokes IAF, Wilder DG, Frymoyer JW, Pope MH: Assessment of patients with low-back pain by biplanar radiographic measurement of intervertebral motion, *Spine* 6:233, 1981.

Szypryt EP, Twining P, Wilde GP, et al: Diagnosis of lumbar disc protrusion, *J Bone Joint Surg* 70B:717, 1988.

Tchang SPK, Howie JL, Kirkaldy-Willis WH, et al: Computed tomography versus myelography in diagnosis of lumbar disc herniation, *J Can Assoc Radiol* 33:15, 1982.

Teplick JG, Haskin ME: Intravenous contrast-enhanced CT of the postoperative lumbar spine: improved identification of recurrent disk herniation, scar, arachnoiditis, and diskitis, *Am J Roentgenol* 143:845, 1984.

Tibrewal SB, Pearcy MJ: Lumbar intervertebral disc heights in normal subjects and patients with disc herniation, *Spine* 10:452, 1985.

Waddell G, McCulloch JA, Kummel E, Venner RM: Nonorganic physical signs in low-back pain, *Spine* 5:117, 1980.

Weiss T, Treisch J, Kazner E, et al: CT of the postoperative lumbar spine: the value of intravenous contrast, *Neuroradiology* 28:241, 1986.

Whelan MA, Gold RP: Computed tomography of the sacrum. I. Normal anatomy, *Am J Roentgenol* 139:1183, 1982.

Whelan MA, Hilal SK, Gold RP, et al: Computed tomography of the sacrum. II. Pathology, *Am J Roentgenol* 139:1191, 1982.

Wiesel S, Tsourmas N, Feffer HL, et al: A study of computer-assisted tomography. I. The incidence of positive CAT scans in an asymptomatic group of patients, *Spine* 9:549, 1984.

Wilberger JE Jr, Pang D: Syndrome of the incidental herniated lumbar disc, *J Neurosurg* 59:137, 1983.

Williams AL, Haughton VM, Daniels DL, Thornton RS: CT recognition of lateral lumbar disk herniation, *Am J Roentgenol* 139:345, 1982.

Williams PC: Reduced lumbosacral joint space: its relation to sciatic irritation, *JAMA* 99:1677, 1932.

Wiltse LL, Guyer RD, Spencer CW, et al: Alar transverse process impingement of the L5 spinal nerve: the far-out syndrome, *Spine* 9:31, 1984.

Winston K, Rumbaugh C, Colucci V: The vertebral canals in lumbar disc disease, *Spine* 9:414, 1984.

Witt I, Vestergaard A, Rosenklint A: A comparative analysis of x-ray findings of the lumbar spine in patients with and without lumbar pain, *Spine* 9:298, 1984.

Wood KB, Garvey TA, Gundry C, Heithoff KB: Magnetic resonance imaging of the thoracic spine: evaluation of asymptomatic individuals, *J Bone Joint Surg* 77A:1631, 1995.

INJECTION STUDIES

Ahlgren EW, Stephen R, Lloyd EAC, McCollum DE: Diagnosis of pain with a graduated spinal block technique, *JAMA* 195:125, 1966.

Angtuaco EJC, Holder JC, Boop WC, Binet EF: Computed tomographic discography in the evaluation of extreme lateral disc herniation, *Neurosurgery* 14:350, 1984.

Benoist M, Ficat C, Baraf P, Cauchoix J: Postoperative lumbar epiduro-arachnoiditis: diagnostic and therapeutic aspects, *Spine* 5:432, 1980.

Berman AT, Garbarino JL, Jr, Fisher SM, Bosacco SJ: The effects of epidural injection of local anesthetics and corticosteroids on patients with lumbosciatic pain, *Clin Orthop* 188:144, 1984.

Bogduk N, Long DM: The anatomy of the so-called "articular nerves" and their relationship to facet denervation in the treatment of low-back pain, *J Neurosurg* 51:172, 1979.

Bromley JW, Varma AO, Santoro AJ, et al: Double-blind evaluation of collagenase injections for herniated lumbar discs, *Spine* 9:486, 1984.

Brooks S, Dent AR, Thompson AG: Anterior rupture of the lumbosacral disc: report of a case, *J Bone Joint Surg* 65A:1186, 1983.

Brown FW: Management of discogenic pain using epidural and intrathecal steroids, *Clin Orthop* 129:72, 1977.

Colhoun E, McCall IW, Williams L, Pullicino VNC: Provocation discography as a guide to planning operations on the spine, *J Bone Joint Surg* 70B:267, 1988.

Cuckler JM, Bernini PA, Wiesel SW, et al: The use of epidural steroids in the treatment of lumbar radicular pain: a prospective, randomized, double-blind study, *J Bone Joint Surg* 67A:63, 1985.

Debaene A: Anatomo-radiological considerations about lumbar discography: an experimental study, *Neuroradiology* 17:77, 1979.

Deburge A, Benoist M, Rocolle J: La chirurgie dans les echecs de la nucleolyse des hernies discales lombaires, *Rev Chir Orthop* 70:637, 1984.

De La Porte C, Siegfried J: Lumbosacral spinal fibrosis (spinal arachnoiditis): its diagnosis and treatment by spinal cord stimulation, *Spine* 8:593, 1983.

Destouet JM, Bilula LA, Murphy WA, Monsees B: Lumbar facet joint injection: indication, technique, clinical correlation, and preliminary results, *Radiology* 145:321, 1982.

Dory MA: Arthrography of the lumbar facet joints, *Radiology* 140:23, 1981.

Eisenstein SM, Parry CR: The lumbar facet arthrosis syndrome, *J Bone Joint Surg* 69B:3, 1987.

Eng RHK, Seligman SJ: Lumbar puncture-induced meningitis, *JAMA* 245:1456, 1981.

Fortin JD, Dwyer AP, West S, Pier J: Sacroiliac joint: pain referral maps upon applying a new injection/arthrography technique. I. Asymptomatic volunteers, *Spine* 19:1475, 1994.

Fox AJ: Lumbar discography: a dissenting opinion letter, *J Can Assoc Radiol* 34:88, 1983.

Fraser RD, Osti OL, Vernon-Roberts B: Discitis after discography, *J Bone Joint Surg* 69B:26, 1987.

Ghia JN, Duncan GH, Teeple E: Differential spinal block for diagnosis of chronic pain, *Compr Ther* 8:55, 1982.

Ghormley RK: Low back pain with special reference to the articular facets with presentation of an operative procedure, *JAMA* 101:1773, 1933.

Goldthwait E: Low-back lesions, *J Bone Joint Surg* 19:810, 1937.

Green PWB, Burke AJ, Weiss CA, Langan P: The role of epidural cortisone injection in the treatment of diskogenic low back pain, *Clin Orthop* 153:121, 1980.

Hauelsen DC, Smith BS, Myers SR, Pryce RL: The diagnostic accuracy of spinal nerve injection studies, *Clin Orthop* 198:179, 1985.

Hodgkinson A: Neck pain localization by cervical disc stimulation and treatment by anterior interbody fusion, *J Bone Joint Surg* 52B:789, 1970.

Hoffman GS, Ellsworth CA, Wells EE, et al: Spinal arachnoiditis. What is the clinical spectrum? II. Arachnoiditis induced by Pantopaque/autologous blood in dogs, a possible model for human disease, *Spine* 8:541, 1983.

Holt EP: The fallacy of cervical discography, *JAMA* 188:799, 1964.

Jackson RP, Jacobs RR, Montesano PX: Facet joint injection in low-back pain: a prospective statistical study, *Spine* 13:966, 1988.

Johnson RG: Does discography injure normal discs? An analysis of repeat discograms, *Spine* 14:424, 1989.

Johnson RG, Macnab I: Localization of symptomatic lumbar pseudoarthroses by use of discography, *Clin Orthop* 197:164, 1985.

Kahanovitz N, Arnoczky SP, Sissons HA, et al: The effect of discography on the canine intervertebral disc, *Spine* 11:26, 1986.

Kikuchi S, Macnab I, Moreau P: Localisation of the level of symptomatic cervical disc degeneration, *J Bone Joint Surg* 63B:272, 1981.

Laun A, Lorenz R, Agnoli AL: Complications of cervical discography, *J Neurosurg Sci* 25:17, 1981.

Lownie SP, Ferguson GG: Spinal subdural empyema complicating cervical discography, *Spine* 14:1415, 1989.

Macnab I: Negative disc exploration: an analysis of the causes of nerve-root involvement in sixty-eight patients, *J Bone Joint Surg* 53A:891, 1971.

Macnab I, Grabias SL, Jacob R: Selective ascending lumbosacral venography in the assessment of lumbar-disc herniation: an anatomical study and clinical experience, *J Bone Joint Surg* 58A:1093, 1976.

Merriam WF, Stockdale HR: Is cervical discography of any value? *Eur J Radiol* 3:138, 1983.

Milette PC, Melanson D: A reappraisal of lumbar discography, *J Can Assoc Radiol* 33:176, 1982.

Murtagh FR: Computed tomography and fluoroscopy guided anesthesia and steroid injection in facet syndrome, *Spine* 13:6686, 1988.

Nachemson A: Lumbar discography: where are we today? *Spine* 14:555, 1989.

Quinnell RC, Stockdale HR: The significance of osteophytes on lumbar vertebral bodies in relation to discographic findings, *Clin Radiol* 33:197, 1982.

Quinell RC, Stockdale HR: Flexion and extension radiography of the lumbar spine: a comparison with lumbar discography, *Clin Radiol* 34:405, 1983.

Quinell RC, Stockdale HR, Harmon B: Pressure standardized lumbar discography, *Br J Radiol* 53:1031, 1980.

Roth DA: Cervical analgesic discography: a new test for the definitive diagnosis of the painful disk syndrome, *JAMA* 235:1713, 1976.

Sachs BL, Vanharanta M, Spirey MA et al: Dallas discogram description: a new classification of CT/discography in low back disorders, *Spine* 12:287, 1987.

Schellhas KP, Pollei SR, Dorwart RH: Thoracic discography: a safe and reliable technique, *Spine* 19:2103, 1994.

Shinomiya K, Nakao K, Shindoh S, et al: Evaluation of cervical diskography in pain origin and provocation, *J Spinal Disord* 6:422, 1993.

Simmons EH, Segil CM: An evaluation of discography in the localization of symptomatic levels in discogenic disease of the spine, *Clin Orthop* 108:57, 1975.

Simmons JW, April CN, Dwyer AP, Brodsky AE: A reassessment of Holt's data on: "The question of lumbar discography," *Clin Orthop* 237:120, 1988.

Skubic JN, Kostuik JP: Thoracic pain syndromes and thoracic disc herniation. In Frymoyer JN, ed: *The adult spine: principles and practice,* New York, 1991, Raven Press.

Smith GW: The normal cervical diskogram, *Am J Radiol* 81:1006, 1959.

Smith GW, Nichols P: The technic of cervical discography, *Radiology* 68:718, 1957.

Stambough JL, Booth RE Jr, Rothman RH: Transient hypercorticism after epidural steroid injection: a case report, *J Bone Joint Surg* 66A:1115, 1984.

Sussman BJ, Bromley JW, Gomez JC: Injection of collagenase for herniated lumbar disk: initial clinical report, *JAMA* 245:730, 1981.

Tajima T, Furukawa K, Kuramochi E: Selective lumbosacral radiculography and block, *Spine* 5:68, 1980.

Teeple E, Scott DL, Ghia JN: Intrathecal normal saline without preservative does not have a local anesthetic effect, *Pain* 14:3, 1982.

Walsh TR, Weinstein JN, Spratt KF, et al: Lumbar discography in normal subjects: a controlled, prospective study, *J Bone Joint Surg* 72A:1081, 1990.

White AH, Derby R, Wynne G: Epidural injections for the diagnosis and treatment of low-back pain, *Spine* 5:78, 1980.

Wilkinson HA: Field block anesthesia for lumbar puncture, *JAMA* 249:2177, 1983 (letter).

Yasuma T, Ohno R, Yamauchi Y: False-negative lumbar discograms: correlation of discographic and histological findings in postmortem and surgical specimens, *J Bone Joint Surg* 70A:1279, 1988.

PSYCHOLOGICAL TESTING

Barnes D, Smith D, Gatchel RJ, Mayer TG: Psychosocioeconomic predictors of treatment success/failure in chronic low-back pain patients, *Spine* 14:427, 1989.

Bigos SJ, Battié MC, Spengler DM, et al: A prospective study of work perceptions and psychosocial factors affecting the report of back injury, *Spine* 16:1, 1991.

Carron H, DeGood DE, Tait R: A comparison of low back pain patients in the United States and New Zealand: psychosocial and economic factors affecting severity of disability, *Pain* 21:77, 1985.

Chapman SL, Pemberton JS: Prediction of treatment outcome from clinically derived MMPI clusters in rehabilitation for chronic low back pain, *Clin J Pain* 10:267, 1994.

Cohen CA, Foster HM, Peck EA III: MMPI evaluation of patients with chronic pain, *South Med J* 76:316, 1983.

Colligan RC, Osborne D, Swenson WM, Offord KP: The aging MMPI: development of contemporary norms, *Mayo Clin Proc* 59:377, 1984.

Cummings GS, Routan JL: Accuracy of the unassisted pain drawings by patients with chronic pain, *J Orthop Sports Phys Ther* 8:391, 1987.

Dennis MD, Greene RL, Farr SP, Hartman JT: The Minnesota Multiphasic Personality Inventory: general guidelines to its use and interpretation of orthopedics, *Clin Orthop* 150:125, 1980.

Dennis MD, Rocchio PO, Wiltse LL: The topographical pain representation and its correlation with MMPI scores, *Orthopedics* 5:433, 1981.

Deyo RA, Diehl AK: Measuring physical and psychosocial function in patients with low-back pain, *Spine* 8:635, 1983.

Deyo RA, Walsh NE, Schoenfeld LS, Ramamurthy S: Studies of the Modified Somatic Perceptions Questionnaire (MSPQ) in patients with back pain: psychometric and predictive properties, *Spine* 14:507, 1989.

Feyer AM, Herbison P, Williamson AM, et al: The role of physical and psychological factors in occupational low back pain, *Occup Environ Med* 57:116, 2000.

Fritz JM, Wainner RS, Hicks GE: The use of nonorganic signs and symptoms as a screening tool for return-to-work in patients with acute low back pain, *Spine* 25:1925, 2000.

Gatchel RJ, Polatin PB, Kinney RK: Predicting outcome of chronic back pain using clinical predictors of psychopathology: a prospective analysis, *Health Psychol* 14:415, 1995.

Gentry WD: Chronic back pain: does elective surgery benefit patients with evidence of psychologic disturbance? *South Med J* 75:1169, 1982.

Gentry WD, Shows WD, Thomas M: Chronic low back pain: a psychological profile, *Psychosomatics* 15:174, 1974.

Grevitt M, Pande K, O'Dowd J, Webb J: Do first impressions count? A comparison of subjective and psychologic assessment of spinal patients, *Eur Spine J* 7:218, 1998.

Herron LD, Pheasant HC: Changes in MMPI profiles after low-back surgery, *Spine* 7:591, 1982.

Leavitt F, Garron DC, McNeill TW, Whisler WW: Organic status, psychological disturbance, and pain report characteristics in low-back-pain patients on compensation, *Spine* 7:398, 1982.

Linton SJ: A review of psychological risk factors in back and neck pain, *Spine* 25:1148, 2000.

Long CJ, Brown DA, Engelberg J: Intervertebral disc surgery: strategies for patient selection to improve surgical outcome, *J Neurosurg* 52:818, 1980.

Ohnmeiss DD: Repeatability of pain drawings in a low back pain population, *Spine* 25:980, 2000.

Pincus T, Callahan LF, Bradley LA, et al: Elevated MMPI scores for hypochondriasis, depression and hysteria in patients with rheumatoid arthritis reflect disease rather than psychological status, *Arthritis Rheum* 29:1456, 1986.

Rainsford AO, Cairns D, Mooney V: The pain drawing as an aid to the psychologic evaluation of patients with low-back pain, *Spine* 1:127, 1976.

Riley JL, Robinson ME, Geisser ME, Wittmer VT: Multivariate cluster analysis of the MMPI-2 in chronic low-back pain patients, *Clin J Pain* 9:248, 1993.

Riley JL, Robinson ME, Geisser ME, et al: Relationship between MMPI-2 cluster profiles and surgical outcome in low-back pain patients, *J Spinal Disord* 8:213, 1995.

Simmonds MJ, Kumar S, Lechelt E: Psychosocial factors in disabling low back pain: cause or consequences? *Dis Rehab* 18:161, 1996.

Southwick SM, White AA: The use of psychological tests in the evaluation of low-back pain, *J Bone Joint Surg* 65A:560, 1983.

Udén A, Landin LA: Pain drawing and myelography in sciatic pain, *Clin Orthop* 216:124, 1987.

Waddell G, McCulloch JA, Kummel E, et al: Nonorganic physical signs in low-back pain, *Spine* 5:117, 1980.

Wiltse LL, Rocchio P: Preoperative psychological tests as predictors of success of chemonucleolysis in the treatment of the low-back syndrome, *J Bone Joint Surg* 57A:478, 1975.

CERVICAL DISC DISEASE

Aldrich F: Posterolateral microdiscectomy for cervical monoradiculopathy caused by posterolateral soft cervical disc sequestration, *J Neurosurg* 72:370, 1990.

Aprill C, Dwyer A, Bogduk N: Cervical zygapophyseal joint pain patterns II: a clinical evaluation, *Spine* 15:458, 1990.

Bailey RW, Badgley CE: Stabilization of the cervical spine by anterior fusion, *J Bone Joint Surg* 42A:565, 1960.

Bernardo KL, Grubb RL, Coxe WS, Roper CL: Anterior cervical disc herniation: case report, *J Neurosurg* 69:134, 1988.

Bloom MH, Raney FL: Anterior intervertebral fusion of the cervical spine: a technical note, *J Bone Joint Surg* 63A:842, 1981.

Boden SD, McCowin PR, Davis DO, et al: Abnormal magnetic-resonance scans of the cervical spine in asymptomatic subjects, *J Bone Joint Surg* 72A:1178, 1990.

Braun IR, Pinto RS, De Fillip GJ, et al: Brain stem infarction due to chiropractic manipulation of the cervical spine, *South Med J* 76:1507, 1983.

Cloward RB: The treatment of ruptured lumbar intervertebral discs by vertebral body fusion. I. Indications, operative technique, after care, *J Neurosurg* 10:154, 1953.

Cloward RB: The anterior approach for removal of ruptured cervical discs, *J Neurosurg* 15:602, 1958.

Cosgrove GR, Théron J: Vertebral arteriovenous fistula following anterior cervical spine surgery: report of two cases, *J Neurosurg* 66:297, 1987.

Davidson RI, Dunn EJ, Metzmaker JN: The shoulder abduction test in the diagnosis of radicular pain in cervical extradural compressive monoradiculopathies, *Spine* 6:441, 1981.

Dwyer A, Aprill C, Bogduk N: Cervical zygapophyseal joint pain patterns. I. A study in normal volunteers, *Spine* 453, 1990.

Farley ID, McAfee PC, Davis RF, Long DM: Pseudarthrosis of the cervical spine after anterior arthrodesis, *J Bone Joint Surg* 72A:1171, 1990.

Garcia A: Cervical traction, an ancient modality, *Orthop Rev* 13:429, 1984.

Griffith SL, Zogbi SW, Guyer RD, et al: Biomechanical comparison of anterior instrumentation for the cervical spine, *J Spinal Disord* 8:429, 1995.

Hirsch D: Cervical disc rupture: diagnosis and therapy, *Acta Orthop Scand* 30:172, 1960.

Horal J: The clinical appearance of low back disorders in the city of Gothenburg, Sweden: comparisons of incapacitated probands with matched controls, *Acta Orthop Scand Suppl* 116:1, 1969.

Jacobs B, Krueger EG, Levy DM: Cervical spondylosis with radiculopathy: results of anterior diskectomy and interbody fusion, *JAMA* 211:2135, 1970.

Jenis L, Leclair WJ: Late vascular complication with anterior cervical discectomy and fusion, *Spine* 19:1291, 1994.

Jho: Microsurgical anterior cervical foraminotomy for radiculopathy: a new approach to cervical disc herniation, *J Neurosurg* 84:155, 1996.

Johnson JP, Filler AG, McBride DQ, Batzdorf U: Anterior cervical foraminotomy for unilateral radicular disease, *Spine* 25:905, 2000.

Kang JD, Georgescu HI, McIntryre LL, et al: Herniated cervical intervertebral discs spontaneously produce matrix metalloproteinases, nitric oxide, interleukin-6, and prostaglandin EW, *Spine* 20:2373, 1995.

Kauppila LI, Penttila A: Postmortem angiographic study of degenerative vascular changes in arteries supplying the cervicobrachial region, *Ann Rheum Dis* 53:94, 1994.

Kelly MF, Spiegel J, Rizzo KA, Zwillenberg D: Delayed pharyngoesophageal perforation: a complication of anterior spine surgery, *Ann Otol Rhinol Laryngol* 100:201, 1991.

Kelsey JL, Githens PB, Walter SD, et al: An epidemiological study of acute prolapsed cervical intervertebral disc, *J Bone Joint Surg* 66A:907, 1984.

Key CA: On paraplegia depending on the ligaments of the spine, *Guy's Hosp Rep* 7:1737, 1838.

Kikuchi S, Hasue M, Nishiyama K, Ito T: Anatomical and clinical studies of radicular symptoms, *Spine* 9:23, 1984.

Kikuchi S, Macnab I, Moreau P: Localisation of the level of symptomatic cervical disc degeneration, *J Bone Joint Surg* 63B:272, 1981.

Koop SE, Winter RB, Lonstein JE: The surgical treatment of instability of the upper part of the cervical spine in children and adolescents, *J Bone Joint Surg* 66A:403, 1984.

Kramer J: Pressure dependent fluid shift in the intervertebral disc, *Orthop Clin North Am* 8:211, 1977.

Lindsey RW, Newhouse KE, Leach J, Murphy MJ: Nonunion following two-level anterior cervical discectomy and fusion, *Clin Orthop* 223:155, 1987.

Lunsford LD, Bissonette DJ, Jannetta PJ, et al: Anterior surgery for cervical disc disease. I. Treatment of lateral cervical disc herniation in 253 cases, *J Neurosurg* 53:1, 1980.

Maruyama Y: Histological, magnetic resonance imaging, and discographic findings on cervical disc degeneration in cadaver spines: a comparative study, *Nippon Seikeigeka Gakkai Zasshi* 69:1102, 1995.

Murphey F, Simmons JCH, Brunson B: Surgical treatment of laterally ruptured cervical discs: a review of 648 cases, 1939 to 1972, *J Neurosurg* 38:679, 1973.

Naito M, Kurose S, Oyama M, Sugioka Y: Anterior cervical fusion with the Caspar instrumentation system, *Int Orthop* 17:73, 1993.

Odom GL, Finney W, Woodhall B: Cervical disk lesion, *JAMA* 166:23, 1958.

O'Laoire SA, Thomas DGT: Spinal cord compression due to prolapse of cervical intervertebral disc (herniation of nucleus pulposus), *J Neurosurg* 59:847, 1983.

Pennecot GF, Gouraud D, Hardy JR, Pouliquen JC: Roentgenographical study of the stability of the cervical spine in children, *J Pediatr Orthop* 4:346, 1984.

Rainer JK: Cervical disc surgery: a historical review, *J Tenn Med Assoc* 77:12, 1984.

Rath WW: Cervical traction: a clinical perspective, *Orthop Rev* 13:430, 1984.

Riley LH: Surgical approaches to the anterior structures of the cervical spine, *Clin Orthop* 91:16, 1973.

Robertson JT: Anterior removal of cervical disc without fusion, *Clin Neurosurg* 20:259, 1973.

Robinson JS: Sciatica and the lumbar disc syndrome: a historic perspective, *South Med J* 76:232, 1983.

Roda JM, Gonzalez C, Blazquez, MG, et al: Intradural herniated cervical disc: case report, *J Neurosurg* 57:278, 1982.

Rosenorn J, Hansen EB, Rosenorn MA: Anterior cervical discectomy with and without fusion, *J Neurosurg* 59:252, 1983.

Semmes RE, Murphey F: The syndrome of unilateral rupture of the sixth cervical intervertebral disk, with compression of the seventh nerve root: a report of four cases with symptoms simulating coronary disease, *JAMA* 121:1209, 1943.

Sherk HH, Watters WC III, Zeiger L: Evaluation and treatment of neck pain, *Orthop Clin North Am* 13:439, 1982.

Simmons EH, Bhalla SK: Anterior cervical discectomy and fusion: a clinical and biomechanical study with eight-year follow-up, with a note on discography: technique and interpretation of results by WP Butt, *J Bone Joint Surg* 51B:225, 1969.

Simmons JCH: Rupture of cervical intervertebral discs. In Edmonson AS, Crenshaw AH, eds: *Campbell's operative orthopaedics*, ed 6, St Louis, 1980, Mosby.

Smith GW, Robinson RA: Anterior lateral cervical disc removal and interbody fusion for cervical disc syndrome, *Bull Johns Hopkins Hosp* 96:223, 1955.

Stookey B: Cervical chrondroma, *Arch Neurol Psychol* 20:275, 1928.

Tamura T: Cranial symptoms after cervical injury: aetiology and treatment of the Barré-Lieou syndrome, *J Bone Joint Surg* 71B:282, 1989.

Verbeist H: A lateral approach to the cervical spine: technique and indications, *J Neurosurg* 28:191, 1968.

Viikari-Juntura E, Porras M, Laasonen EM: Validity of clinical tests in the diagnosis of root compression in cervical disc disease, *Spine* 14:253, 1989.

Welsh LW, Welsh JJ, Chinnici JC: Dysphagia due to cervical spine surgery, *Ann Otol Rhinol Laryngol* 96:112, 1987.

White AA, Jupiter J, Southwick WO, Panjabi MM: An experimental study of the immediate load-bearing capacity of three surgical constructions for anterior spine fusions, *Clin Orthop* 91:21, 1973.

White AA, Southwick WO, DePonte RJ, et al: Relief of pain by anterior cervical spine fusion for spondylosis: a report of sixty-five cases, *J Bone Joint Surg* 55A:525, 1973.

Whitecloud TS: *Management of radiculopathy and myelopathy by the anterior approach: the cervical spine*, Philadelphia, 1983, JB Lippincott.

Yamamoto I, Ikeda A, Shibuya N, et al: Clinical long-term results of anterior discectomy without interbody fusion for cervical disc disease, *Spine* 16:272, 1991.

THORACIC DISC DISEASE

Antoni N: Fall av kronisk rotkompression med ovanlig orsak, hernia nuclei pulposi disci intervertebralis, *Sv Lakartidn* 28:436, 1931.

Bohlman HH, Zdeblick TA: Anterior excision of herniated thoracic discs, *J Bone Joint Surg* 70A:1038, 1988.

de Looze MP, Toussaint HM, van Dieen JH, Kemper HC: Joint moments and muscle activity in the lower extremities and lower back in lifting and lowering tasks, *J Biomech* 26:1067, 1993.

Fessler RG, Sturgill M: Review: complications of surgery for thoracic disc disease, *Surg Neurol* 49:609, 1998.

Gajdosik RL, Albert CR, Mitman JJ: Influence of hamstring length on the standing position and flexion range of motion of the pelvic angle, lumbar angle, and thoracic angle, *J Orthop Sports Phys Ther* 20:213, 1994.

Hochman MS, Pena C, Ramirez R: Calcified herniated thoracic disc diagnosed by computerized tomography: case report, *J Neurosurg* 52:722, 1980.

Horowitz MB, Moossy JJ, Julian T, et al: Thoracic discectomy using video-assisted thoracoscopy, *Spine* 19:1082, 1994.

Love JG, Kiefer EJ: Root pain and paraplegia due to protrusions of thoracic intervertebral disks, *J Neurosurg* 15:62, 1950.

Maiman DJ, Larson SJ, Luck E, El-Ghatit A: Lateral extracavity approach to the spine for thoracic disc herniation: report of 23 cases, *Neurosurgery* 14:178, 1984.

Martucci E, Mele C, Martella P: Thoracic intervertebral disc protrusion, *Ital J Orthop Traumatol* 10:333, 1984.

Milgrom C, Finestone A, Lev B, et al: Overexertional lumbar and thoracic back pain among recruits: a prospective study of risk factors and treatment regimens, *J Spinal Disord* 6:187, 1993.

Naunheim KS, Barnett MG, Crandall DG, et al: Anterior exposure of the thoracic spine, *Ann Thorac Surg* 57:1436, 1994.

O'Leary PF, Camins MB, Polifroni NV, Floman Y: Thoracic disc disease: clinical manifestations and surgical treatment, *Bull Hosp Jt Dis* 44:27, 1984.

Omojola MF, Cardoso ER, Fox AJ, et al: Thoracic myelopathy secondary to ossified ligamentum flavum: case report, *J Neurosurg* 56:448, 1982.

Panjabi MM, Krag MH, Dimnet JC, et al: Thoracic spine centers of rotation in the sagittal plane, *J Orthop Res* 1:387, 1984.

Regan JJ, Ben-Yishay A, Mack MJ: Video-assisted thoracoscopic excision of herniated thoracic disc: description of technique and preliminary experience in the first 29 cases, *J Spinal Disord* 11:183, 1998.

Ridenour TR, Haddad SF, Hitchon PW, et al: Herniated thoracic disks: treatment and outcome, *J Spinal Disord* 6:218, 1993.

Rogers MA, Crockard HA: Surgical treatment of the symptomatic herniated thoracic disk, *Clin Orthop* 300:70, 1994.

Rosenthal D, Rosenthal R, de Simone A: Removal of a protruded thoracic disc using microsurgical endoscopy, a new technique, *Spine* 19:1087, 1994.

Sekhar LN, Jannetta PJ: Thoracic disc herniation: operative approaches and results, *Neurosurgery* 12:303, 1983.

Stone JL, Lichtor T, Banerjee S: Intradural thoracic disc herniation, *Spine* 19:1281, 1994.

Vaccaro AR, Rizzolo SJ, Allardyce TJ, et al: Placement of pedicle screws in the thoracic spine. I. Morphometric analysis of the thoracic vertebrae, *J Bone Joint Surg* 77A:1193, 1995.

Vaccaro AR, Rizzolo SJ, Balderston RA, et al: Placement of pedicle screws in the thoracic spine. II. An anatomical and radiographic assessment, *J Bone Joint Surg* 77A:1200, 1995.

Vanichkachorn JS, Vaccaro AR: Thoracic disk disease: diagnosis and treatment, *J Am Acad Orthop Surg* 8:159, 2000.

LUMBAR DISC DISEASE: ETIOLOGY, DIAGNOSIS, AND CONSERVATIVE TREATMENT

Alcoff J, Jones E, Rust P, Newman R: Controlled trial of imipramine for chronic low back pain, *J Fam Pract* 14:841, 1982.

American Medical Association: *Guides to the evaluation of permanent impairment*, ed 4, Chicago, 1993, American Medical Association.

Atkinson JH, Kremer EF, Garfin SR: Psychopharmacological agents in the treatment of pain, *J Bone Joint Surg* 67A:337, 1985.

Basmajian JV: Acute back pain and spasm: a controlled multicenter trial of combined analgesic and antispasm agents, *Spine* 14:438, 1989.

Bell GR, Rothman RH: The conservative treatment of sciatica, *Spine* 9:54, 1984.

Bergquist-Ullman M, Larsson U: Acute low back pain in industry: a controlled prospective study with special reference to therapy and confounding factors, *Acta Orthop Scand Suppl* 170:1, 1977.

Berman AT, Garbarino JL, Fisher ST, Bosacco SJ: The effects of epidural injection of local anesthetics and corticosteroids on patients with lumbosciatic pain, *Clin Orthop* 188:144, 1984.

Bernard TN, Kirkaldy-Willis WH: Recognizing specific characteristics of nonspecific low back pain, *Clin Orthop* 217:266, 1987.

Berwick DM, Budman S, Feldstein M: No clinical effects of back schools in an HMO: a randomized prospective trial, *Spine* 14:338, 1989.

Bigos SJ, Battié MC: Acute care to prevent back disability: ten years of progress, *Clin Orthop* 221:121, 1987.

Blower PW: Neurologic patterns in unilateral sciatica: a prospective study of 100 new cases, *Spine* 6:175, 1981.

Böstman OM: Body mass index and height in patients requiring surgery for lumbar intervertebral disc herniation, *Spine* 18:851, 1993.

Cauthen C: *Lumbar spine surgery*, Baltimore, 1983, Williams & Wilkins.

Christodoulides AN: Ipsilateral sciatica on femoral nerve stretch test is pathognomonic of an L4-5 disc protrusion, *J Bone Joint Surg* 71B:88, 1989.

Clarke NMP, Cleak DK: Intervertebral lumbar disc prolapse in children and adolescents, *J Pediatr Orthop* 3:202, 1983.

Cohen JE, Frank JW, Bombardier C, Guillemin F: Group education interventions for people with low back pain: an overview of the literature, *Spine* 19:1214, 1994.

Cuckler JM, Bernini PA, Wiesel SW, et al: The use of epidural steroids in the treatment of lumbar radicular pain, *J Bone Joint Surg* 67A:63, 1985.

de Sèze S: Sciatique "banale" et disques lombo-sacrés, *La Presse Medicale* 51-52:570, 1940.

de Sèze S: Histoire de la sciatique, *Rev Neurol* 138:1019, 1982.

DeSio JM, Kahn CH, Warfield CA: Facial flushing and/or generalized erythema after epidural steroid injection, *Anesth Analg* 80:617, 1995.

Deyo RA: Conservative therapy for low back pain: distinguishing useful from useless therapy, *JAMA* 250:1057, 1983.

Deyo RA, Diehl AK, Rosenthal M: How many days of bed rest for acute low back pain: a randomized clinical trial, *N Engl J Med* 315:1064, 1986.

Deyo RA, Walsh NE, Martin DC, et al: A controlled trial of transcutaneous electrical nerve stimulation (TENS) and exercise for chronic low back pain, *N Engl J Med* 322:1627, 1990.

el-Khoury GY, Ehara S, Weinstein JN, et al: Epidural steroid injection: a procedure ideally performed with fluoroscopic control, *Radiology* 168:554, 1988.

Estridge MN, Rouhe SA, Johnson NG: The femoral stretching test: a valuable sign in diagnosing upper lumbar disc herniations, *J Neurosurg* 57:813, 1982.

Fairbank JCT, O'Brien JP: The iliac crest syndrome: a treatable cause of low-back pain, *Spine* 8:220, 1983.

Farfan HF: The torsional injury of the lumbar spine, *Spine* 9:53, 1984.

Fisher RG, Saunders RL: Lumbar disc protrusion in children, *J Neurosurg* 54:480, 1981.

Friberg O: Clinical symptoms and biomechanics of lumbar spine and hip joint in leg length inequality, *Spine* 8:643, 1983.

Galm R, Frohling M, Rittmeister M, Schmitt E: Sacroiliac joint dysfunction in patients with imaging-proven lumbar disc herniation, *Eur Spine J* 7:450, 1998.

Giles LGF, Taylor JR: Low back pain associated with leg length inequality, *Spine* 6:510, 1981.

Grabel JD, Davis R, Zappulla R: Intervertebral disc space cyst simulating a recurrent herniated nucleus pulposus, *J Neurosurg* 69:137, 1988.

Hansen FR, Bendix T, Skov P, et al: Intensive, dynamic back-muscle exercises, conventional physiotherapy, or placebo-control treatment of low-back pain: a randomized, observer-blind trial, *Spine* 18:98, 1993.

Hazard RG, Fenwick JW, Kalisch SM, et al: Functional restoration with behavioral support: a one-year prospective study of patients with chronic low-back pain, *Spine* 14:157, 1989.

Herron LD, Pheasant HC: Prone knee-flexion provocative testing for lumbar disc protrusion, *Spine* 5:65, 1980.

Hopwood MB, Abram SE: Factors associated with failure of lumbar epidural steroids, *Reg Anesth* 18:238, 1993.

Kikuchi S, Hasue M, Nishiyama K, et al: Anatomical and clinical studies of radicular symptoms, *Spine* 9:23, 1984.

Kirkaldy-Willis WH, Hill RJ: A more precise diagnosis for low-back pain, *Spine* 4:102, 1979.

Klier I, Santo M: Low back pain as presenting symptoms of chronic granulocytic leukemia, *Orthop Rev* 11:111, 1982.

Kosteljanetz M, Bang F, Schmidt-Olsen S: The clinical significance of straight-leg raising (Lasègue's sign) in the diagnosis of prolapsed lumbar disc: interobserver variation and correlation with surgical findings, *Spine* 13:393, 1988.

Kostuik JP, Bentivoglio J: The incidence of low-back pain in adult scoliosis, *Spine* 6:268, 1981.

Kushner FH, Olson JC: Retinal hemorrhage as a consequence of epidural steroid injection, *Arch Ophthalmol* 113:309, 1995.

Macnab I, Cuthbert H, Godfrey CM: The incidence of denervation of the sacrospinales muscles following spinal surgery, *Spine* 2:294, 1977.

Malmivaara A, Hakkinen U, Aro T, et al: The treatment of acute low back pain—bed rest, exercises, or ordinary activity? *N Engl J Med* 332:1786, 1995.

Melleby A, Kraus H: Chronic back pain: use of a YMCA-developed exercise regimen, *J New Develop Clin Med* 5:75, 1987.

Miller A, Stedman GH, Beisaw NE, Gross PT: Sciatica caused by an avulsion fracture of the ischial tuberosity, *J Bone Joint Surg* 69A:143, 1987.

Nachemson AL: Prevention of chronic back pain: the orthopaedic challenge for the 80s, *Bull Hosp Jt Dis* 44:1, 1984.

Natchev E, Valentino V: Low back pain and disc hernia: observation during auto-traction treatment, *Manual Med* 1:39, 1984.

Offierski CM, Macnab I: Hip-spine syndrome, *Spine* 8:316, 1983.

Onel D, Tuzlaci M, Sari H, Demir K: Computed tomographic investigation of the effect of traction on lumbar disc herniations, *Spine* 14:82, 1989.

Pheasant H, Bursk A, Goldfarb J, et al: Amitriptyline and chronic low-back pain: a randomized double-blind crossover study, *Spine* 8:552, 1983.

Postacchini F, Urso S, Tovaglia V: Lumbosacral intradural tumours simulating disc disease, *Int Orthop* 5:283, 1981.

Ramamurthi B: Absence of limitation of straight leg raising in proved lumbar disc lesion: case report, *J Neurosurg* 52:852, 1980.

Renfrew DL, Moore TE, Kathol ME, et al: Correct placement of epidural steroid injections: fluoroscopic guidance and contrast administration, *Am J Neuroradiol* 12:1003, 1991.

Robinson JS: Sciatica and the lumbar disk syndrome: a historic perspective, *South Med J* 76:232, 1983.

Saag KG, Cowdery JS: Spine update: nonsteroid anti-inflammatory drugs: balancing benefits and risks, *Spine* 13:1530, 1994.

Saal JA, Saal JS: Nonoperative treatment of herniated lumbar intervertebral disc with radiculopathy and outcome study, *Spine* 14:431, 1989.

Sandover J: Dynamic loading as a possible source of low back disorders, *Spine* 8:652, 1983.

Shiqing X, Quanzhi Z, Dehao F: Significance of the straight leg raising test in the diagnosis and clinical evaluation of lower lumbar intervertebral disc protrusion, *J Bone Joint Surg* 69A:517, 1987.

Simmons JW, Dennis MD, Rath D: The back school: a total back management program, *Orthopedics* 7:1453, 1984.

Smith SA, Massie JB, Chesnut R, Garfin SR: Straight leg raising: anatomical effects on the spinal nerve root without and with fusion, *Spine* 18:992, 1993.

Solheim LF, Siewers P, Paus B: The piriformis muscle syndrome: sciatic nerve entrapment treated with section of the piriformis muscle, *Acta Orthop Scand* 52:73, 1981.

Sprangfort E: Lasegue's sign in patients with lumbar disc herniation, *Acta Orthop Scand* 42:459, 1971.

Tay EC, Chacha PB: Midline prolapse of a lumbar intervertebral disc with compression of the cauda equina, *J Bone Joint Surg* 61B:43, 1979.

Tonelli L, Falasca A, Argentieri C, et al: Influence of psychic distress on short-term outcome of lumbar disc surgery, *J Neurosurg Sci* 27:237, 1983.

Troup JDG: Straight leg raising (SLR) and the qualifying tests for increased root tension: their predictive value after back and sciatic pain, *Spine* 6:526, 1981.

Ueyoshi A, Shima Y: Studies on spinal braces with special reference to the effects of increased abdominal pressure, *Int Orthop* 9:255, 1985.

Verta MJ Jr, Vitello J, Fuller J: Adductor canal compression syndrome, *Arch Surg* 119:345, 1984.

Waddell G: A new clinical model for the treatment of low-back pain, *Spine* 12:632, 1987.

Waddell G, Main CJ, Morris EW, et al: Chronic low-back pain, psychologic distress, and illness behavior, *Spine* 9:209, 1984.

Waddell G, McCulloch JA, Kummel E, et al: Nonorganic physical signs of low-back pain, *Spine* 5:117, 1980.

Ward NG: Tricyclic antidepressants for chronic low-back pain: mechanisms of action and predictors of response, *Spine* 11:661, 1986.

Weber H: Lumbar disc herniation: a controlled, prospective study with ten years of observation, *Spine* 8:131, 1983.

Weise MD, Garfin SR, Gelberman RH, et al: Lower-extremity sensibility testing in patients with herniated lumbar intervertebral discs, *J Bone Joint Surg* 67A:1219, 1985.

Weitz EM: The lateral bending sign, *Spine* 6:388, 1981.

White AA III, Gordon SL: Synopsis: workshop on idiopathic low-back pain, *Spine* 7:141, 1982.

White AH, Derby R, Wynne G: Epidural injections for the diagnosis and treatment of low-back pain, *Spine* 5:78, 1980.

White AH, Taylor LW, Wynne G, Welch RB: Appendix: a diagnostic classification of low-back pain, *Spine* 5:83, 1980.

Willner S: Effect of a rigid brace on back pain, *Acta Orthop Scand* 56:40, 1985.

Yoganandan N, Maiman DJ, Pintar F, et al: Microtrauma in the lumbar spine: a cause of low back pain, *Neurosurgery* 23:162, 1988.

Zaleske DJ, Bode HH, Benz R, Krishnamoorthy KS: Association of sciatica-like pain and Addison's disease: a case report, *J Bone Joint Surg* 66A:297, 1984.

LUMBAR DISC DISEASE: SURGICAL TREATMENT AND RESULTS

Adams CB: "I've torn it: how to repair it," *Br J Neurosurg* 9:201, 1995.

Balderston RA, Gilyard GG, Jones AA, et al: The treatment of lumbar disc herniation: simple fragment excision versus disc space curettage, *J Spinal Disord* 4:22, 1991.

Blaauw G, Braakman R, Gelpke GJ, Singh R: Changes in radicular function following low-back surgery, *J Neurosurg* 69:649, 1988.

Blower PW: Neurologic patterns in unilateral sciatica: a prospective study of 100 new cases, *Spine* 6:175, 1981.

Bradford DS, Garcia A: Lumbar intervertebral disk herniations in children and adolescents, *Orthop Clin North Am* 2:583, 1971.

Bryant MS, Bremer AM, Nguyen TQ: Autogeneic fat transplants in the epidural space in routine lumbar spine surgery, *Neurosurgery* 13:367, 1983.

Capanna AH, Williams RW, Austin DC, et al: Lumbar discectomy—percentage of disc removal and detection of anterior annulus perforation, *Spine* 6:610, 1981.

Carruthers CC, Kousaie KN: Surgical treatment after chemonucleolysis failure, *Clin Orthop* 165:172, 1982.

Castellvi AE, Goldstein LA, Chan DPK: Lumbosacral transitional vertebrae and their relationship with lumbar extradural defects, *Spine* 9:493, 1984.

Cauthen C: *Lumbar spine surgery*, Baltimore, 1983, Williams & Wilkins.

Chow SP, Leong JCY, Yau AC: Anterior spinal fusion for deranged lumbar intervertebral disc: a review of 97 cases, *Spine* 5:452, 1980.

Clarke NMP, Cleak DK: Intervertebral lumbar disc prolapse in children and adolescents, *J Pediatr Orthop* 3:202, 1983.

Crawshaw C, Frazer AM, Merriam WF, et al: A comparison of surgery and chemonucleolysis in the treatment of sciatica: a prospective randomized trial, *Spine* 9:195, 1984.

Crock HV: Normal and pathological anatomy of the lumbar spinal nerve roots, *J Bone Joint Surg* 63B:487, 1981.

Delamarter RB, Leventhal MR, Bohlman HH: Diagnosis of recurrent lumbar disc herniation vs postoperative scar by gadolinium-DTPA enhanced magnetic resonance imaging (unpublished data).

Di Lauro L, Poli R, Bortoluzzi M, Marini G: Paresthesias after lumbar disc removal and their relationship to epidural hematoma, *J Neurosurg* 57:135, 1982.

Donaldson WF, Star MJ, Thorne RP: Surgical treatment for the far lateral herniated lumbar disc, *Spine* 18:1263, 1993.

Dvonch V, Scarff T, Bunch WT, et al: Dermatomal somatosensory evoked potentials: their use in lumbar radiculopathy, *Spine* 9:291, 1984.

Ebeling U, Kalbarcyk H, Reulen HJ: Microsurgical reoperation following lumbar disc surgery: timing, surgical findings, and outcome in 92 patients, *J Neurosurg* 70:397, 1989.

Ebersold MJ, Quast LM, Bianco AJ: Results of lumbar discectomy in the pediatric patient, *J Neurosurg* 67:643, 1987.

Eie N, Solgaard T, Kleppe H: The knee-elbow position in lumbar disc surgery: a review of complications, *Spine* 8:897, 1983.

Eismont FJ, Wiesel SW, Rothman RH: The treatment of dural tears associated with spinal surgery, *J Bone Joint Surg* 63A:1132, 1981.

Epstein JA, Carras R, Ferrar J, et al: Conjoined lumbosacral nerve roots, *J Neurosurg* 55:585, 1981.

Epstein NE: Different surgical approaches to far lateral lumbar disc herniations, *J Spinal Disord* 8:383, 1995.

Epstein NE: Evaluation of varied surgical approaches used in the management of 170 far-lateral lumbar disc herniations: indications and results, *J Neurosurg* 83:648, 1995.

Fisher RG, Saunders RL: Lumbar disc protrusion in children, *J Neurosurg* 54:480, 1981.

Floman Y, Wiesel SW, Rothman RH: Cauda equina syndrome presenting as a herniated lumbar disc, *Clin Orthop* 147:234, 1980.

Flynn JC, Price CT: Sexual complications of anterior fusion of the lumbar spine, *Spine* 9:489, 1984.

Frymoyer JW, Hanaley EN, Howe J: A comparison of radiographic findings in fusion and nonfusion patients ten or more years following lumbar disc surgery, *Spine* 5:435, 1979.

Garrido E, Rosenwasser RH: Painless footdrop secondary to lumbar disc herniation: report of two cases, *Neurosurgery* 8:484, 1981.

Getty CJM, Johnson JR, Kirwan E, Sullivan MF: Partial undercutting facetectomy for bony entrapment of the lumbar nerve root, *J Bone Joint Surg* 63B:330, 1981.

Greenberg RP, Ducker TB: Evoked potentials in the clinical neurosciences, *J Neurosurg* 56:1, 1982.

Hastings DE: A simple frame of operations of the lumbar spine, *Can J Surg* 12:251, 1969.

Hoyland JA, Freemont AJ, Denton J, et al: Retained surgical swab debris in post-laminectomy arachnoiditis and peridural fibrosis, *J Bone Joint Surg* 70B:659, 1988.

Hurme M, Torma AT, Einola S: Operated lumbar disc herniation: epidemiological aspects, *Ann Chir Gynaecol* 72:33, 1983.

Jacobs RR, McClain O, Neff J: Control of postlaminectomy scar formation: an experimental and clinical study, *Spine* 5:223, 1980.

Jane JA, Haworth CS, Broaddus WC, et al: A neurosurgical approach to far-lateral disc herniation, *J Neurosurg* 72:143, 1990.

Jensen TT, Asmussen K, Berg-Hansen E-M, et al: First-time operation for lumbar disc herniation with or without free fat transplantation, *Spine* 21:1072, 1996.

Kadish L, Simmons EH: Anomalies of the lumbosacral nerve roots and anatomical investigation and myelographic study, *J Bone Joint Surg* 66B:411, 1984.

Kahanovitz N, Viola K, Muculloch J: Limited surgical discectomy and microdiscectomy: a clinical comparison, *Spine* 14:79, 1989.

Kambin P: Lumbar discectomy, surgical technique. Paper presented at the American Academy of Orthopaedic Surgeons Course, St Louis, May 1996.

Kataoka O, Nishibayashi Y, Sho T: Intradural lumbar disc herniation: report of three cases with a review of the literature, *Spine* 14:529, 1989.

Kelly RE, Dinner MH, Lavyne MH, Andrews DW: The effect of lumbar disc surgery on postoperative pulmonary function and temperature: a comparison study of microsurgical lumbar discectomy with standard lumbar discectomy, *Spine* 18:287, 1993.

Key JA: Intervertebral-disk lesions in children and adolescents, *J Bone Joint Surg* 32A:97, 1950.

Kikuchi S, Hasue M, Nishiyama K, et al: Anatomical and clinical studies of radicular symptoms, *Spine* 9:23, 1984.

Kirkaldy-Willis WH, Hill RJ: A more precise diagnosis for low-back pain, *Spine* 4:102, 1979.

Kiviluoto O: Use of free fat transplants to prevent epidural scar formation: an experimental study, *Acta Orthop Scand Suppl* 164:1, 1976.

Kostuik JP, Harrington I, Alexander D, et al: Cauda equina syndrome and lumbar disc hernia, *J Bone Joint Surg* 68A:386, 1986.

Kuslich SD, Dowdle JA: Two-year follow-up results of the BAK interbody fusion device. Proceedings of the Ninth Annual Meeting of the North American Spine Society, Oct 1994.

Leavitt F, Garron DC, Whisler WW, D'Angelo CM: A comparison of patients treated by chymopapain and laminectomy for low back pain using a multidimensional pain scale, *Clin Orthop* 146:136, 1980.

Leong JCY, Chun SY, Grange WJ, Fang D: Long-term results of lumbar intervertebral disc prolapse, *Spine* 8:793, 1983.

Lewis PJ, Weir BKA, Broad RW, Grace MG: Long-term prospective study of lumbosacral discectomy, *J Neurosurg* 67:49, 1987.

Lindholm TS, Pylkkanen P: Discitis following removal of intervertebral disc, *Spine* 7:618, 1982.

Lowell TD, Errico TJ, Fehlings MG, et al: Microdiskectomy for lumbar disk herniation: a review of 100 cases, *Orthopedics* 18:985, 1995.

Macnab I: Management of low back pain. In Ahstrom JP Jr, ed: *Current practice in orthopaedic surgery*, St Louis, 1973, Mosby.

Macnab I, Cuthbert H, Godfrey CM: The incidence of denervation of the sacrospinales muscles following spinal surgery, *Spine* 2:294, 1977.

Macon JB, Poletti CE: Conducted somatosensory evoked potentials during spinal surgery. I. Control, conduction velocity measurements, *J Neurosurg* 57:349, 1982.

Macon JB, Poletti CE, Sweet WH, et al: Conducted somatosensory evoked potentials during spinal surgery. II. Clinical applications, *J Neurosurg* 57:354, 1982.

Maroon JC, Kopitnik TA, Schulhoff LA, et al: Diagnosis and microsurgical approach to far-lateral disc herniation in the lumbar spine, *J Neurosurg* 72:378, 1990.

Moore AJ, Chilton JD, Uttley D: Long-term results of microlumbar discectomy, *Br J Neurosurg* 8:319, 1994.

Mullen JB, Cook WA Jr: Reduction of postoperative lumbar hemilaminectomy pain with Marcaine, *J Neurosurg* 51:126, 1975.

Nachemson AL: Prevention of chronic back pain: the orthopaedic challenge for the 80s, *Bull Hosp Jt Dis Orthop* 44:1, 1984.

Nakano N, Tomita T: Results of surgical treatment of low back pain: a comparative study of the anterior and posterior approach, *Int Orthop* 4:101, 1980.

Neidre A, Macnab I: Anomalies of the lumbosacral nerve roots, *Spine* 8:294, 1983.

Newman MH: Outpatient conventional laminotomy and disc excision, *Spine* 20:353, 1995.

Nielsen B, deNully M, Schmidt K, Hansen RI: A urodynamic study of cauda equina syndrome due to lumbar disc herniation, *Urol Int* 35:167, 1980.

Onik G, Helms CA: Automated percutaneous lumbar diskectomy, *Am J Roentgenol* 156:531, 1991.

Pásztor E, Szarvas I: Herniation of the upper lumbar discs, *Neurosurg Rev* 4:151, 1981.

Pau A, Viale ES, Turtas S, Zirattu G: Redundant nerve roots of the cauda equina, *Ital J Orthop Traumatol* 4:95, 1984.

Posner I, White AA III, Edwards WT, Hayes WC: A biomechanical analysis of the clinical stability of the lumbar and lumbosacral spine, *Spine* 7:374, 1982.

Postacchini F, Urso S, Ferro L: Lumbosacral nerve-root anomalies, *J Bone Joint Surg* 64A:721, 1982.

Rechtine GR, Reinert CM, Bohlman HH: The use of epidural morphine to decrease postoperative pain in patients undergoing lumbar laminectomy, *J Bone Joint Surg* 66A:1, 1984.

Rish BL: A critique of the surgical management of lumbar disc disease in a private neurosurgical practice, *Spine* 9:500, 1984.

Ruggieri F, Specchia L, Sabalat S, et al: Lumbar disc herniation: diagnosis, surgical treatment, and recurrence: a review of 872 operated cases, *Ital J Orthop Traumatol* 14:15, 1988.

Semmes RE: Diagnosis of ruptured intervertebral discs without contrast myelography and comment upon recent experience with modified hemilaminectomy for their removal, *Yale J Biol Med* 11:433, 1939.

Silvers HR: Microsurgical versus standard lumbar discectomy, *Neurosurgery* 22:837, 1988.

Smith RV: Intradural disc rupture: report of two cases, *J Neurosurg* 55:117, 1981.

Solgaard T, Kleppe H: Long-term results of lumbar intervertebral disc prolapse, *Spine* 8:793, 1983.

Solheim LF, Siewers P, Paus B: The piriformis muscle syndrome: sciatic nerve entrapment treated with section of the piriformis muscle, *Acta Orthop Scand* 52:73, 1981.

Spangfort EV: The lumbar disc herniation: a computer-aided analysis of 2504 operations, *Acta Orthop Scand Suppl* 142:1, 1972.

Spencer DL, Irwin GS, Miller JA: Anatomy and significance of fixation of the lumbosacral nerve roots in sciatica, *Spine* 8:672, 1983.

Spengler DM: Lumbar discectomy: results with limited disc excision and selective foraminotomy, *Spine* 7:604, 1982.

Spengler DM, Freeman CW: Patient selection for lumbar discectomy: an objective approach, *Spine* 4:129, 1979.

Techakapuch S, Bangkok T: Rupture of the lumbar cartilage plate into the spinal canal in an adolescent, *J Bone Joint Surg* 63A:481, 1981.

Vaughan PA, Malcolm BW, Maistrelli GL: Results of L4-L5 disc excision alone versus disc excision and fusion, *Spine* 13:690, 1988.

Waddell G, Main CJ, Morris EW, et al: Chronic low-back pain, psychologic distress, and illness behavior, *Spine* 9:209, 1984.

Waddell G, Reilly S, Torsney B, et al: Assessment of the outcome of low back surgery, *J Bone Joint Surg* 70B:723, 1988.

Wayne SJ: A modification of the tuck position for lumbar spine surgery: a 15-year follow-up study, *Clin Orthop* 184:212, 1984.

Weber H: Lumbar disc herniation: a controlled, prospective study with ten years of observation, *Spine* 8:131, 1983.

Weinstein J, Spratt KF, Lehmann T, et al: Lumbar disc herniation: a comparison of the results of chemonucleolysis and open discectomy after ten years, *J Bone Joint Surg* 68A:43, 1986.

Weinstein JN, Scafuri RL, McNeill TW: The Rush-Presbyterian–St. Luke's lumbar spine analysis form: a prospective study of patients with "spinal stenosis," *Spine* 8:891, 1983.

Weir BKA: Prospective study of 100 lumbosacral discectomies, *J Neurosurg* 50:283, 1979.

Weise MD, Garfin SR, Gelberman RH, et al: Lower-extremity sensibility testing in patients with herniated lumbar intervertebral discs, *J Bone Joint Surg* 67A:1219, 1985.

Wilberger JE Jr, Pang D: Syndrome of the incidental herniated lumbar disc, *J Neurosurg* 59:137, 1983.

Wilkinson HA, Baker S, Rosenfeld S: Gelfoam paste in experimental laminectomy and cranial trephination: hemostasis and bone healing, *J Neurosurg* 54:664, 1981.

Williams RW: Microlumbar discectomy: a conservative surgical approach to the virgin herniated lumbar disc, *Spine* 3:175, 1978.

Williams RW: Microcervical foraminotomy: a surgical alternative for intractable radicular pain, *Spine* 8:708, 1983.

Williams RW: Microdiskectomy—myth, mania, or milestone? An 18-year surgical adventure, *Mt Sinai J Med* 58:139, 1991.

Yong-Hing K, Reilly J, de Korompay V, Kirkaldy-Willis WH: Prevention of nerve root adhesions after laminectomy, *Spine* 5:59, 1980.

Zahrawi F: Microlumbar discectomy (MLD), *Spine* 13:358, 1988.

Zahrawi F: Microlumbar discectomy: is it safe as an outpatient procedure? *Spine* 19:1070, 1994.

Zamani MH, MacEwen GD: Herniation of the lumbar disc in children and adolescents, *J Pediatr Orthop* 2:528, 1982.

CHEMONUCLEOLYSIS

Abdel-Salam A, Eyres KS, Cleary J: A new paradiscal injection technique for the relief of back spasm after chemonucleolysis, *Br J Rheumatol* 31:491, 1992.

Agre K, Wilson RR, Brim M, McDermott DJ: Chymodiactin postmarketing surveillance: demographic and adverse experience data in 29,075 patients, *Spine* 9:479, 1984.

Alexander AH: Debate: resolved—chemonucleolysis is the best treatment of the recalcitrant acute herniated nucleus pulposus: what's new and what's true in the Napa Valley. Paper presented March 14, 1985.

Apfelbach HW: Technique for chemonucleolysis, *Orthopedics* 6:1613, 1983.

Barach EM, Nowak RM, Lee TG, Tomlanovich MC: Epinephrine for treatment of anaphylactic shock, *JAMA* 251:2118, 1984.

Battit GE: Anaphylaxis associated with chymopapain injections, *JAMA* 253:977, 1985.

Benoist M, Bonneville JF, Lassale B, et al: A randomized, double-blind study to compare low-dose with standard-dose chymopapain in the treatment of herniated lumbar intervertebral discs, *Spine* 18:28, 1993.

Benoist M, Deburge A, Heripret G, et al: Treatment of lumbar disc herniation by chymopapain chemonucleolysis: a report on 120 patients, *Spine* 7:613, 1982.

Bernstein IL: Adverse effects of chemonucleolysis, *JAMA* 250:1167, 1983.

Boumphrey FRS, Bell GR, Modic M, et al: Computed tomography scanning after chymopapain injection for herniated nucleus pulposus: a prospective study, *Clin Orthop* 219:120, 1987.

Bradford DS, Cooper KM, Oegema TR, Jr: Chymopapain, chemonucleolysis, and nucleus pulposus regeneration, *J Bone Joint Surg* 65A:1220, 1983.

Brown MD, Tompkins JS: Pain response post-chemonucleolysis or disc excision, *Spine* 14:321, 1989.

Burkus JS, Alexander AH, Mitchell JB: Evaluation and treatment of chemonucleolysis failures, *Orthopedics* 11:1677, 1988.

Carruthers CC, Kousaie KN: Surgical treatment after chemonucleolysis failure, *Clin Orthop* 165:172, 1982.

Castro WH, Halm H, Jerosch J, et al: Long-term changes in the magnetic resonance image after chemonucleolysis, *Eur Spine J* 3:222, 1994.

Crawshaw C, Frazer AM, Merriam WF, et al: A comparison of surgery and chemonucleolysis in the treatment of sciatica: a prospective randomized trial, *Spine* 9:195, 1984.

Dolan P, Adams MA, Hutton WC: The short-term effects of chymopapain on intervertebral discs, *J Bone Joint Surg* 69B:422, 1987.

Eguro H: Transverse myelitis following chemonucleolysis: report of a case, *J Bone Joint Surg* 65A:1328, 1983.

Fraser RD: Chymopapain for the treatment of intervertebral disc herniation: the final report of a double-blind study, *Spine* 9:815, 1984.

Garreau C, Dessarts I, Lassale B, et al: Chemonucleolysis: correlation of results with the size of the herniation and the dimensions of the spinal canal, *Eur Spin J* 4:77, 1995.

Grammer LC, Ricketti AJ, Schafer MF, Patterson R: Chymopapain allergy: case reports and identification of patients at risk for chymopapain anaphylaxis, *Clin Orthop* 188:139, 1984.

Hall BB, McCulloch JA: Anaphylactic reactions following the intradiscal injection of chymopapain under local anesthesia, *J Bone Joint Surg* 65A:1215, 1983.

Hill GM, Ellis EA: Chemonucleolysis as an alternative to laminectomy for the herniated lumbar disc, *Clin Orthop* 225:229, 1987.

Hoogland T, Scheckenbach C: Low-dose chemonucleolysis combined with percutaneous nucleotomy in herniated cervical disks, *J Spinal Disord* 8:228, 1995.

Javid MJ: Chemonucleolysis versus laminectomy: a cohort comparison of effectiveness and charges, *Spine* 20:2016, 1995.

Kato F, Mimatsu K, Kawakami N, Miura T: Changes seen on magnetic resonance imaging in the intervertebral disc space after chemonucleolysis: a hypothesis concerning regeneration of the disc after chemonucleolysis, *Neuroradiology* 34:267, 1992.

Kato F, Mimatsu K, Kawakami N, et al: Serial changes observed by magnetic resonance imaging in the intervertebral disc after chemonucleolysis: a consideration of the mechanism of chemonucleolysis, *Spine* 17:934, 1992.

Leavitt F, Garron DC, Whisler WW, D'Angelo CM: A comparison of patients treated by chymopapain and laminectomy for low back pain using a multidimensional pain scale, *Clin Orthop* 146:136, 1980.

Maciunas RJ, Onofrio BM: The long-term results of chymopapain: ten-year follow-up of 268 patients after chemonucleolysis, *Clin Orthop* 206:37, 1986.

McCulloch JA: Chemonucleolysis: experience with 2000 cases, *Clin Orthop* 146:128, 1980.

McCulloch JA, Ferguson JM: Outpatient chemonucleolysis, *Spine* 6:606, 1981.

Moneret-Vautrin DA, Feldmann L, Kanny G, et al: Incidence and risk factors for latent sensitization to chymopapain: predictive skin-prick tests in 700 candidates for chemonucleolysis, *Clin Exp Allergy* 24:471, 1994.

Nachemson AL, Rydevik B: Chemonucleolysis for sciatica: a critical review, *Acta Orthop Scand* 59:56, 1988.

Naylor A, Earland C, Robinson J: The effect of diagnostic radiopaque fluids used in discography on chymopapain activity, *Spine* 8:875, 1983.

Nordby EJ, Wright PH: Efficacy of chymopapain in chemonucleolysis: a review, *Spine* 19:2578, 1994.

Nordby EJ, Wright PH, Schofield SR: Safety of chemonucleolysis: adverse effects reported in the United States, 1982-1991, *Clin Orthop* 293:122, 1993.

Oegema TR Jr, Swedenberg S, Johnson SL, et al: Residual chymopapain activity after chemonucleolysis in normal intervertebral discs in dogs, *J Bone Joint Surg* 74A:831, 1992.

Parkinson D: Late results of treatment of intervertebral disc disease with chymopapain, *J Neurosurg* 59:990, 1983.

Shields CB, Reiss SJ, Garretson HD: Chemonucleolysis with chymopapain: results in 150 patients, *J Neurosurg* 67:187, 1987.

Simmons JW, Stavinoha WB, Knodel LC: Update and review of chemonucleolysis, *Clin Orthop* 183:51, 1984.

Smith S, Leibrock LG, Gelber BR, Pierson EW: Acute herniated nucleus pulposus with cauda equina compression syndrome following chemonucleolysis: report of three cases, *J Neurosurg* 66:614, 1987.

Strum PF, Armstrong GW, O'Neil DJ, Belanger JM: Far lateral lumbar disc herniation treated with an anterolateral retroperitoneal approach: report of two cases, *Spine* 17:363, 1992.

Suguro T, Oegema TR, Bradford DS: Ultrastructural study of the short-term effects of chymopapain on the intervertebral disc, *J Orthop Res* 4:281, 1986.

Tregonning GD, Transfeldt EE, McCulloch JA, et al: Chymopapain versus conventional surgery for lumbar disc herniation: 10-year results of treatment, *J Bone Joint Surg* 73B:481, 1991.

Tsay YG, Jones R, Calenoff E, et al: A preoperative chymopapain sensitivity test for chemonucleolysis candidates, *Spine* 9:764, 1984.

van Leeuwen RB, Hoogland PH: CT examination of 91 patients after chemonucleolysis, *Acta Orthop Scand* 62:128, 1991.

Wakano K, Kasman R, Chao EY, et al: Biomechanical analysis of canine intervertebral discs after chymopapain injection: a preliminary report, *Spine* 8:59, 1983.

Weinstein J, Spratt KF, Lehmann T, et al: Lumbar disc herniation: a comparison of the results of chemonucleolysis and open discectomy after ten years, *J Bone Joint Surg* 68A:43, 1986.

Weitz EM: Paraplegia following chymopapain injection: a case report, *J Bone Joint Surg* 66A:1131, 1984.

Whisler WW: Anaphylaxis secondary to chymopapain, *Orthopedics* 6:1628, 1983.

Willis J, ed: Chymopapain administration procedures modified, *FDA Drug Bull* 14:14, 1984.

PERCUTANEOUS LUMBAR DISCECTOMY

Blankstein A, Rubinstein E, Ezra E, et al: Disc space infection and vertebral osteomyelitis as a complication of percutaneous lateral discectomy, *Clin Orthop* 225:234, 1987.

Davis GW, Onik G: Clinical experience with automated percutaneous lumbar discectomy, *Clin Orthop* 238:98, 1989.

Goldstein TB, Mink JH, Dawson EG: Early experience with automated percutaneous lumbar discectomy in the treatment of lumbar disc herniation, *Clin Orthop* 238:77, 1989.

Graham CE: Percutaneous posterolateral lumbar discectomy: an alternative to laminectomy in the treatment of backache and sciatica, *Clin Orthop* 238:104, 1989.

Hijikata S: Percutaneous nucleotomy: a new concept of technique and 12 years' experience, *Clin Orthop* 238:9, 1989.

Kahanovitz N, Viola K, Goldstein T, Dawson E: A multicenter analysis of percutaneous diskectomy, *Spine* 15:713, 1990.

Kahanovitz N, Viola K, McCullough J: Limited surgical diskectomy and microdiskectomy: a clinical comparison, *Spine* 14:79, 1989.

Kambin P, Brager MD: Percutaneous posterolateral discectomy: anatomy and mechanism, *Clin Orthop* 223:145, 1987.

Kambin P, Gellman H: Percutaneous lateral discectomy of the spine, *Clin Orthop* 174:127, 1983.

Kambin P, Schaffer JL: Percutaneous lumbar discectomy: review of 100 patients and current practice, *Clin Orthop* 238:24, 1989.

Maroon JC, Onik G, Sternau L: Percutaneous automated discectomy: a new approach to lumbar surgery, *Clin Orthop* 238:64, 1989.

Monteiro A, Lefevre R, Pieters G, Wilment E: Lateral decompression of a pathological disc in the treatment of lumbar pain and sciatica, *Clin Orthop* 238:56, 1989.

Morris J: Percutaneous discectomy, *Orthopedics* 11:1483, 1988.

Onik G, Helms CA, Ginsburg L: Percutaneous lumbar discectomy using a new aspiration probe, *Am J Radiol* 144:1137, 1985.

Onik G, Maroon J, Davis GW: Automated percutaneous discectomy at the L5-S1 level: use of a curved cannula, *Clin Orthop* 238:71, 1989.

Schreiber A, Suezawa Y, Leu H: Does percutaneous nucleotomy with discoscopy replace conventional discectomy? Eight years of experience and results in treatment of herniated lumbar disc, *Clin Orthop* 238:35, 1989.

Schweigel J: Automated percutaneous discectomy: comparison with chymopapain. In *Automated percutaneous discectomy*, San Francisco, 1988, University of California Press.

Shepperd JAN, James SE, Leach AB: Percutaneous disc surgery, *Clin Orthop* 238:43, 1989.

Stern MB: Early experience with percutaneous lateral discectomy, *Clin Orthop* 238:50, 1989.

Wilson D, Harbaugh R: Microsurgical and standard removal of protruded lumbar disc: a comparative study, *Neurosurgery* 8:422, 1986.

COMPLICATIONS OF LUMBAR SPINE SURGERY

Benoist M, Ficat C, Baraf P, Cauchoix J: Postoperative lumbar epiduroarachnoiditis: diagnostic and therapeutic aspects, *Spine* 5:432, 1980.

Bryant MS, Bremer AM, Nguyen TQ: Autogeneic fat transplants in the epidural space in routine lumbar spine surgery, *Neurosurgery* 13:367, 1983.

Caplan LR, Norohna AB, Amico LL: Syringomyelia and arachnoiditis, *J Neurol Neurosurg Psychiatr* 53:106, 1990.

Choudhury AR, Taylor JC: Cauda equina syndrome in lumbar disc disease, *Acta Orthop Scand* 51:493, 1980.

Di Lauro L, Poli R, Bortoluzzi M, Marini G: Paresthesias after lumbar disc removal and their relationship to epidural hematoma, *J Neurosurg* 57:135, 1982.

Eismont FJ, Wiesel SW, Rothman RH: The treatment of dural tears associated with spinal surgery, *J Bone Joint Surg* 63A:1132, 1981.

Floman Y, Wiesel SW, Rothman RH: Cauda equina syndrome presenting as a herniated lumbar disc, *Clin Orthop* 147:234, 1980.

Javid MJ, Nordby EJ, Ford LT, et al: Safety and efficacy of chymopapain (Chymodiactin) in herniated nucleus pulposus with sciatica: results of a randomized, double-blind study, *JAMA* 249:2489, 1983.

Jones AA, Stambough JL, Balderson RA, et al: Long-term results of lumbar spine surgery complicated by unintended incidental durotomy, *Spine* 14:443, 1989.

May ARL, Brewster DC, Darling RC, et al: Arteriovenous fistula following lumbar disc surgery, *Br J Surg* 68:41, 1981.

Mayer PJ, Jacobsen FS: Cauda equina syndrome after surgical treatment of lumbar spinal stenosis with application of free autogenous fat graft: a report of two cases, *J Bone Joint Surg* 71A:1090, 1989.

McLaren AC, Bailey SI: Cauda equina syndrome: a complication of lumbar discectomy, *Clin Orthop* 204:143, 1986.

Nielsen B, deNully M, Schmidt K, Hansen RI: A urodynamic study of cauda equina syndrome due to lumbar disc herniation, *Urol Int* 35:167, 1980.

Puranen J, Makela J, Lahde S: Postoperative intervertebral discitis, *Acta Orthop Scand* 55:461, 1984.

Salander JM, Youkey JR, Rich NM, et al: Vascular injury related to lumbar disc surgery, *J Trauma* 24:628, 1984.

Shaw ED, Scarborough JT, Beals RK: Bowel injury as a complication of lumbar discectomy: a case report and review of the literature, *J Bone Joint Surg* 63A:478, 1981.

Zide BM, Wisoff JH, Epstein FJ: Closure of extensive and complicated laminectomy wounds: operative technique, *J Neurosurg* 67:59, 1987.

FAILED SPINE SURGERY

Blaauw G, Braakman R, Gelpke GJ, Singh R: Changes in radicular function following low-back surgery, *J Neurosurg* 69:649, 1988.

Cauthen C: *Lumbar spine surgery*, Baltimore, 1983, Williams & Wilkins.

Ebeling U, Kalbarcyk H, Reulen HJ: Microsurgical reoperation following lumbar disc surgery: timing, surgical findings, and outcome in 92 patients, *J Neurosurg* 70:397, 1989.

Finnegan WJ, Fenlin JM, Marval JP, et al: Results of surgical intervention in the symptomatic multiply operated back patient, *J Bone Joint Surg* 61A:1077, 1979.

Frymoyer JW, Hanaley EN, Howe J: A comparison of radiographic findings in fusion and nonfusion patients ten or more years following lumbar disc surgery, *Spine* 5:435, 1979.

Lehmann TR, LaRocca AS: Repeat lumbar surgery: a review of patients with failure from previous lumbar surgery treated by spinal cord exploration and lumbar spinal fusion, *Spine* 6:615, 1981.

Long DM, Filtzer DL, BenDebba M, Hendler NH: Clinical features of the failed-back syndrome, *J Neurosurg* 69:61, 1988.

Nakano N, Tomita T: Results of surgical treatment of low back pain: a comparative study of the anterior and posterior approach, *Int Orthop* 4:101, 1980.

Quimjian JD, Matrka PJ: Decompression laminectomy and lateral spinal fusion in patients with previously failed lumbar spine surgery, *Orthopedics* 2:563, 1988.

Spengler DM, Freeman C, Westbrook R, Miller JW: Low-back pain following multiple lumbar spine procedures: failure of initial selection? *Spine* 5:356, 1980.

Tria AJ, Williams JM, Harwood D, Zawadsky JP: Laminectomy with and without spinal fusion, *Clin Orthop* 224:134, 1987.

C H A P T E R

40 Infections of Spine

George W. Wood II

Evidence of spinal infection in humans dates back to before the time of recorded history. Neolithic persons (c. 7000 to 300 BC) and Egyptian mummies (c. 3000 BC) have been found to have evidence of spinal deformity believed to be caused by tuberculosis. Hippocrates described the clinical condition of spinal infection and noted that the prognosis in this condition, believed to be tuberculosis, was better when the infection was below the diaphragm than when above it. In 1779 Percival Pott gave the first complete report of tuberculous infection of the spine. According to Wilensky, Nelaton coined the term *osteomyelitis* in 1854. The scientific understanding of osteomyelitis began in 1884 when Rodet described the development of osteomyelitis after injections of *Staphylococcus aureus* into the veins of animals. Early treatment for spinal infections was limited to abscess drainage, usually of tuberculosis infections; unfortunately, secondary bacterial infection frequently caused death.

Before the use of antibiotics, mortality in patients with infections of the spine and contiguous tissues was 40% to 70%. Advances in chemotherapy since the 1960s have dramatically altered the natural history of these diseases. Today spinal infections are relatively rare, accounting for only 2% to 4% of all osteomyelitis infections, and mortality is estimated to be 1% to 20%, depending on the patient group and the infecting agent.

Paralysis is reported to occur in up to 50% of patients with spinal infections, depending on the patient population and the spinal segment involved. The primary problems today are the delay in diagnosis (estimated to average 3 months), the long recovery period (averaging 12 months or more), and the great cost of treating such infections.

Reconstructive surgery for spinal infection required the development of safe surgical and anesthetic techniques. In 1911 Hibbs and Albee independently developed posterior spinal fusion techniques for treating tuberculous spinal disease; these procedures decreased the degree of kyphosis and shortened the course of the disease. Both Hibbs and Albee chose the posterior approach because it avoided involvement of the area of active infection. Posterior spinal fusion remained the mainstay of treatment of spinal tuberculous infection until the advent of antibiotics. With the development of chemotherapeutic agents, surgical approaches became more aggressive in the direct treatment of tuberculosis and other pyogenic infections. Hodgson and Stock in 1956 pioneered radical anterior decompression for Pott disease, and this procedure has been used with equal success in the treatment of other kinds of spinal infections.

Today, radical excision of infected bone is commonplace, provided that ancillary support for such procedures is adequate, and the use of bone graft in infected spaces is accepted by most authors. Govender et al. reported successful treatment of patients with spinal tuberculosis and HIV, using radical debridement, fresh frozen allografts, and 18 months of anti-tuberculous drugs without antiretroviral therapy.

Rigid internal fixation is being used more frequently in the treatment of pyogenic and nonpyogenic spinal infections. Caragee noted a 47% complication rate after instrumentation, including two instrumentation failures and one wound dehiscence, in 17 patients with pyogenic osteomyelitis. Wrobel, Chappell, and Taylor reported general success after instrumentation in 10 of 23 patients with coccidioidomycosis spinal infection. In a review of 31 patients with primary spinal infection treated with internal fixation, Faraj and Webb noted eradication of the infections. However, one patient died of infection, three had deep wound infections requiring further debridement, and one had an implant failure. Krodel et al. noted no additional risks when posterior instrumentation was used to augment anterior decompression and grafting for spinal tuberculosis. The use of autograft alone has a similar but less frequent complication rate. Allograft also has been used with fewer complications as noted by Schuster et al. and Govender and Parbhoo. Meticulous planning, proper implant choice, and appropriate long-term antibiotics are necessary when rigid internal fixation is used for infections of the spine. Nonpyogenic infections seem to be less reactive to instrumentation than pyogenic infections.

Biology of Spinal Infection

A knowledge of the structure and composition of the spinal elements is essential to an understanding of spinal infections. The intervertebral disc has been identified as the most commonly infected spinal element, but more recent evidence now points to the metaphyses and cartilaginous endplates as the starting areas for blood-borne infections. The disc space is now considered the primary starting area only for infections that result from direct inoculation.

Coventry, Ghormley, and Kernohan in 1945 described the microscopic anatomy of the intervertebral disc and its contiguous structures. They concluded that in adults older than 30 years the intervertebral disc receives its nutrition from tissue fluids rather than from direct blood supply. They noted multiple holes in the endplates of the vertebral bodies, which corresponded with the marrow cavities and were arranged in three distinct areas: (1) a central zone with numerous small holes, (2) a peripheral zone with a few large holes, and (3) an epiphyseal ring surrounding the endplate.

The epiphyseal ring overlaps the outer surface of the vertebral body and joins the more concave surface of the central and peripheral zones internally. Next to the bony endplate is the cartilaginous plate, which consists of hyaline cartilage and forms the inner base between the bone and the fibrous disc. Inoue in 1981 found that the disc was firmly adherent to the vertebral endplate: two thirds of its fibers were perpendicular to the endplate in this area. The central portion was less firmly

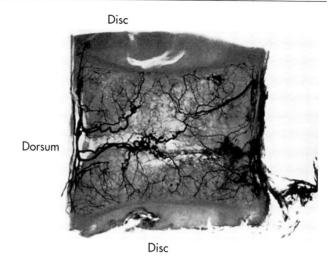

Fig. 40-1   Section through vertebral body after arterial injection. Nutrient vessels are visible on dorsal and ventral surfaces. (From Wiley AM, Trueta J: *J Bone Joint Surg* 41B:796, 1959.)

attached, with fibers parallel to the endplate. This composition most likely allows the transport of nutrients through the holes and into the central portion of the disc without disturbing the structural integrity.

The arterial and venous supply to the vertebrae has been studied by numerous investigators for more than 100 years. In 1959 Wiley and Trueta found marked similarities in the arterial and venous supply in humans and rabbits at the cervical, thoracic, and lumbar levels. At the level of each vertebra, the vertebral artery, intercostal artery, or lumbar arteries provide nutrient vessels that enter the vertebral body (Fig. 40-1). Posterior spinal branch arteries enter the spinal canal through each neural foramen. These arteries separate into ascending and descending branches that anastomose with similar branches at each level (Fig. 40-2). This posterior network joins centrally to enter a large posterior nutrient foramen.

Whalen et al. investigated the microvasculature of the vertebral endplates in fetal cadavers and young rabbits and described vessels oriented obliquely in the cartilage toward the intervertebral disc. These vessels were found to originate from the circumferential vessels fed from the arterial plexus outside the perichondrium or from nearby metaphyseal marrow vessels. They noted that venous drainage was by a similar route. They concluded that the intervertebral disc was avascular, even in infants. In contrast, the surrounding cartilaginous material was highly vascular. They found no change in this relationship with growth unless a pathological process was encountered (Fig. 40-3). The cartilaginous endplate therefore appears to be the anatomical area in which the arterial supply ends, regardless of age. The intervertebral disc is centrally avascular and dependent on diffusion for its nutrition.

The venous drainage of the pelvis and its relationship to spinal vasculature was first described by Breschet in 1819 and was later expanded by Batson in 1940 with the discovery that the pelvic veins drained into the spinal venous plexus. This

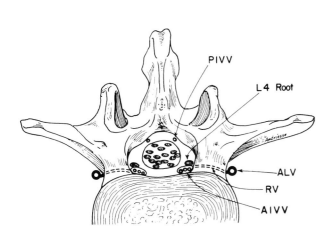

Fig. 40-2   Diagram of transverse section of lumbar vertebra. Anterior and internal vertebral arteries and veins are noted in canal. *PIVV*, Posterior internal vertebral vein; *ALV*, ascending lumbar vein; *RV*, radicular vein; *AIVV*, anterior internal vertebral vein. (From Macnab I, St Louis EL, Grabias SL, Jacob R: *J Bone Joint Surg* 58A:1093, 1976.)

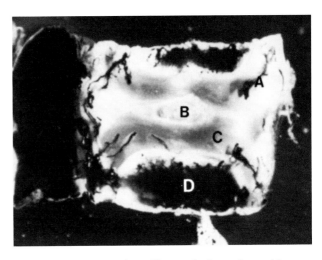

Fig. 40-3   Sagittal section of human fetal vertebra and intervertebral disc after arterial injection. Note oblique orientation of vessels to disc and absence of vessels penetrating disc. *A,* Neural canal. *B,* nucleus pulposus; *C,* hyaline cartilage endplate; *D,* ossified vertebral body. (From Whalen JL, Parke WW, Mazur JM, Stauffer ES: *J Pediatr Orthop* 5:403, 1985.)

explained the frequent metastasis of pelvic tumors and infections to the spine. In 1976 Crock and Yoshizawa described the microvascular circulation of the venous anatomy of the vertebral endplate.

The venous microcirculation begins in the vertebral endplate where the arterial circulation ends. The large subvenous or venous channels are oriented horizontally and parallel to the endplate. The horizontal system then drains through small vertical veins perforating the endplate and connecting with horizontal vessels in the cancellous bone adjacent to the endplate. Additional vertical veins drain to the basivertebral system and converge to form the anterior internal venous plexus as one or two major tributaries. These plexuses then drain externally into the external venous plexus. Externally these vessels join with the anterior internal vertebral, posterior internal vertebral, and posterior radicular veins. The internal vertebral veins course dorsal to the dural sac near the lamina. The anterior internal veins lie in the lateral aspect of the floor of the spinal canal bilaterally; these veins are sacrificed during disc excision. As the internal veins approach the midpoint of the body of the vertebra, they move centrally to drain the interosseous system through the nutrient foramen. The anterior internal veins also drain the articular vessels that course along the roots, joining the ascending lumbar veins outside the spinal canal. The series of interconnected veins continues from sacrum to skull (Figs. 40-2 to 40-4).

Spinal infection can occur by direct infection of the disc itself, usually through surgical manipulation directly or percutaneously, or by local spread from contiguous structures. Contiguous spread has been reported to occur from the colon via subphrenic abscesses and also from abdominal abscess extension from gunshot wounds without direct spinal injury. The most common method of spinal infection is through the

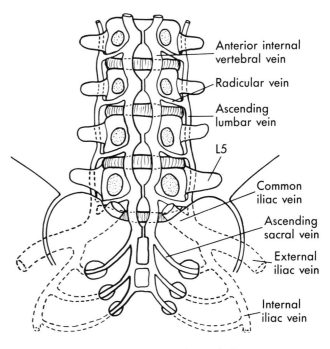

Fig. 40-4   Schematic diagram of vertebral venous system. (Modified from Macnab I, St Louis EL, Grabias SL, Jacob R: *J Bone Joint Surg* 58A:1093, 1976.)

arterial spread of pyogenic bacteria. This arterially spread infection originates in the endplate of the vertebra, probably in the venous channels, or in the vertebral body itself and spreads to the disc secondarily as the infection progresses.

On the other hand, because tuberculous spinal infection has been reproduced only by injecting the renal vein experimentally (Hodgson), it is believed that tuberculous infection results

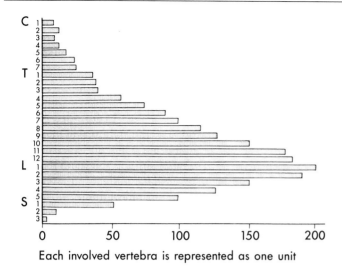

Fig. 40-5   Bar graph of 587 consecutive cases of spinal tuberculosis occurring in series of 1000 consecutive cases of bone and joint tuberculosis. (From Hodgson AR: Infectious disease of the spine. In Rothman RH, Simeone FA, eds: *The spine*, Philadelphia, 1975, WB Saunders.)

from venous spread, usually at the level of the renal veins. This is substantiated by the frequency of infection in tuberculous disease (Fig. 40-5). A similar frequency has not been noted with bacterial infection. Bacterial infections rapidly attack the intervertebral disc. Tuberculous and nonbacterial infections, on the other hand, usually preserve the intervertebral disc. This pathological characteristic may help identify the infecting organism at surgery.

Natural History

The natural history of pyogenic vertebral infections involves an infecting source or incident followed by a period of increased pain, with or without significant generalized sepsis. Generalized sepsis usually indicates a primary source of infection other than the spine. Blood-borne infection probably begins in the capillary loop or postcapillary venous channels in the endplate. Sludging in these channels results in suppurative inflammation, tissue necrosis, bony collapse, and spread of the infection into the adjacent intervertebral disc spaces. This eventually results in the endplate erosions that are the first roentgenographic findings. The infection can extend anteriorly to create a paravertebral abscess or posteriorly to cause an epidural abscess. Large paravertebral abscesses may extend down the psoas and into the groin. Likewise, epidural abscesses may cross the spinal epidural space and enter the meningeal space and spinal cord itself, although this occurs late in the course of pyogenic infections and rarely occludes the spinal arteries (Feldenzer et al.). As the bone becomes infected, it softens and may collapse under the body weight and stress. Neurological deficits are caused by (1) direct extension of the infection in the form of abscess or bacterial communication with the spinal

canal to the neural elements or (2) secondary compression from pathological fracture as a result of bone softening (Fig. 40-6). This progression of spinal infection is possible in both pyogenic and nonpyogenic infections. There are numerous reports of infection extending to the epidural space and even to the meninges. Doita et al. reported a patient who had contiguous spread to the aorta. The patient required prosthetic replacement of the aorta in addition to aggressive surgical debridement with strut grafting. Toxic shock syndrome also has been reported by Odom et al. after vertebral abscess drainage.

The course of the infection varies with the infecting organism and the patient's immune status. The infection itself may create a malnourished condition that compromises the immune system (Nichols). Hopkinson, Stevenson, and Benjamin noted that septic discitis was associated with invasive procedures, underlying cancer, and diabetes. According to Waldvogel and Vasey, death occurs in 10% of patients with overwhelming spinal infections.

Individuals with a good immune response may actually overcome the infection with no treatment. This has been proven experimentally by Fraser, Osti, and Vernon-Roberts. They injected *Staphylococcus epidermidis* into sheep discs and noted that 6 weeks later only those discs injected with bacteria showed evidence of discitis; however, bacteria could not be cultured from those discs. This finding indicates that there is an optimal period for bacteriological identification of disc space infections in otherwise healthy individuals. It also explains the widely varying clinical presentations of spinal infection and further compounds the difficulty of making an accurate and timely bacteriological diagnosis.

Paralysis from spinal infection may occur early or late. Early onset of paralysis frequently suggests epidural extension of an abscess. Late paralysis may be caused by the development of significant kyphosis, vertebral collapse with retropulsion of bone and debris, or late abscess formation in more indolent infections. Eismont et al. identified four factors that indicate an increased predisposition to paralysis in pyogenic and fungal vertebral osteomyelitis. They noted that the incidence of paralysis increased with (1) age, (2) a higher vertebral level of infection (cervical), (3) the presence of debilitating disease, such as diabetes mellitus, rheumatoid arthritis, or chronic steroid usage, and (4) *S. aureus* infections. Paralysis from tuberculosis is not related to those factors.

Epidemiology

The vertebral endplate is the most commonly reported focus of vertebral infection, followed by inoculation of the disc space itself, epidural abscess formation, and paraspinal abscess formation. Other spinal elements, including the articular processes, facet joints, and even the odontoid, also have been reported as primary areas of infection, but generally these are isolated case reports. According to Waldvogel and Vasey, the thoracic and lumbar spinal vertebrae are the most common areas of pyogenic infection, and according to Hodgson et al.,

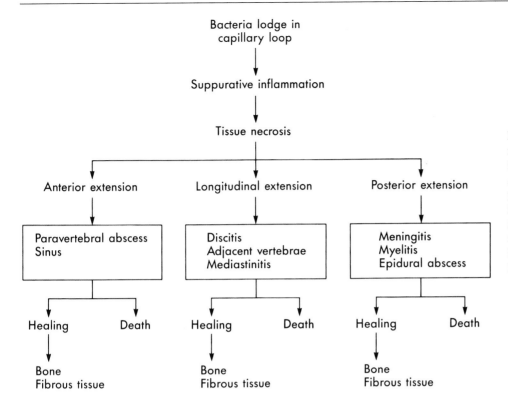

Fig. 40-6 Flow diagram of natural history of vertebral infection. (From Wood GW II: Anatomic, biologic, and pathophysiologic aspects of spinal infections. In Wood GW II, ed: *State of the art and review. Spine: spinal infections,* vol 3, no 3, Philadelphia, 1989, Hanley & Belfus.)

the thoracolumbar junction is the most common area of tuberculous infection.

Numerous organisms have been reported to infect the spine (Box 40-1). Waldvogel and Vasey noted that *S. aureus* was the most common organism in pyogenic infection: this organism, and to a lesser degree *S. epidermidis,* accounted for 60% of the infections in their review. The incidence of isolation of *S. aureus* varies from 40% to 90%. The current trend is a decrease in the frequency of *S. aureus* infections but an increase in the resistant strains of the organism. More recent reports indicate that more than half of the isolates of the organism are resistant to penicillin, and more than one third of that group are resistant to methicillin. Roca and Yoshikawa reported that intravenous drug users are more commonly infected with *Pseudomonas aeruginosa. Mycobacterium tuberculosis* is the most common nonpyogenic infecting agent.

Spinal surgery is the most common cause of iatrogenic disc infection, whereas genitourinary infection is the most common predisposing factor for blood-borne infection. Respiratory tract and dermal infections are implicated less frequently in blood-borne infection. Postabortal and postpartum infections also have been reported to cause spinal infections. According to Eismont et al., patients with chronic diseases that decrease the natural immune response, such as diabetes, alcoholism, rheumatoid arthritis, and chronic renal disease, are more likely to develop a spinal infection and its complications. Frazier et al. noted delayed diagnosis in 11 patients with primary fungal spinal infections; 9 of these patients were immunocompromised from diabetes, corticosteroids, chemotherapy, or malnutrition.

BOX 40-1 • Infecting Organisms in Spinal Osteomyelitis

Actinomyces
Aerobacter aerogenes
Bacteroides
Brucella
Corynebacterium
Clostridium perfringens
Enterobacter aerogenes
Escherichia coli
Gonococcus
Klebsiella
Micrococcus
Proteus
Pseudomonas
Pyocyaneus
Salmonella enteritidis
Salmonella oranienburg
Salmonella panama
Salmonella paratyphi A and B
Salmonella suipestifer
Salmonella typhimurium
Salmonella typhosa
Serratia marcescens
Staphylococcus aureus
Staphylococcus alba
Staphylococcus epidermidis
Streptococcus (microaerophilic)
Streptococcus (alpha)

From Wood GW III, Edmonson AS: Osteomyelitis of the spine. In Wood GW III, ed: *State of the art and review. Spine: spinal infections,* vol 3, no 3, Philadelphia, 1989, Hanley & Belfus.

Table 40-1 Sites of Tuberculous Involvement of Bones and Joints in 99 Cases,* British Columbia, 1967 Through 1976

Site	No. of Cases†	Site	No. of Cases†
Joint	59	Spine	37
Wrist	8	C4-5	1
Elbow	7	C5-6	3
Shoulder	5	C6-7	1
Costosternal	1	T5-6	1
Sternoclavicular	1	T6-7	2
Sacroiliac	4	T7-8	2
Hip	16	T8-9	4
Knee	12	T9-10	3
Ankle	2	T10-11	5
Foot	3	T11-12	4
Bone (osteomyelitis)	9	T12-L1	3
Finger	1	L1-2	6
Sternum	1	L2-3	8
Rib	1	L3-4	8
Pelvis	4	L4-5	5
Fibula	1	L5-S1	6
Calcaneus	1	Unknown	2

From Enarson DA et al: *Can Med Assoc J* 120:139, 1979.
*In six cases there was tuberculous disease at two sites.
†The numbers in the left-hand column indicate the frequency of involvement of an individual site; the numbers to the right are the total number of cases.

The incidence of tuberculous spondylitis has progressively declined since the advent of antituberculous medication but still accounts for more than one third of bone and joint infections (Table 40-1). Collert noted a marked decrease in tuberculous spondylitis since 1950, compared with a modest increase in pyogenic spondylitis. Other nonpyogenic infections are rare in healthy individuals but are much more common in immuno-compromised patients. The recent appearance of resistant strains of *Mycobacterium tuberculosis*, the continuing spread of HIV infection, the increased use of organ transplantation, and improvements in cancer chemotherapy may increase the potential for spinal infection. At this time, a rapid rise in spinal infection has not been reported.

Diagnosis

PHYSICAL EXAMINATION

The most common presenting symptom of spinal infection is pain. Ross and Fleming reported pain as the primary symptom in 85% of their patients with spinal infections. Pain occurs primarily with changes in position, ambulation, and other forms of activity. The intensity of the pain varies from mild to extreme. Constitutional symptoms include anorexia, malaise, night sweats, intermittent fever, and weight loss. Spinal deformity may be a late presentation of the disease. Paralysis is

a serious complication but rarely is the presenting complaint. A history of an immune-suppressing disease or a recent infection, or both, is not uncommon. Puig-Guri described four clinical syndromes that can be caused by the infection: (1) hip joint syndrome, with acute pain in the hip, flexion contracture, and limited motion, (2) abdominal syndrome, with symptoms and signs that may suggest acute appendicitis, (3) meningeal syndrome, with symptoms and signs that suggest acute suppurative or tuberculous meningitis, and (4) back pain syndrome, in which the onset of pain may be acute or insidious; pain may be mild or may be so severe that jarring the bed is agonizing.

Temperature elevation, if present, usually is minimal. Localized tenderness over the involved area is the most common physical sign. Sustained paraspinal spasm also is indicative of the acute process. Limitation of motion of the involved spinal segments because of pain is frequent. Torticollis may result from infection in the cervical spine, and bizarre posturing and physical positions that could be considered psychogenic in origin are not infrequent. Other possible findings include the Kernig sign, hamstring spasm, and generalized weakness. Clinical findings in elderly and immunosuppressed individuals may be minimal.

Because of the depth of the spine, abscess formation is difficult to identify unless it points superficially. Frequently these areas of abscess pointing are some distance from the primary process. A paraspinal abscess not uncommonly presents as a swelling in the groin below the Poupart ligament (inguinal ligament) because of extension along the psoas muscle. Straight leg raising examination usually is not helpful because it may be negative or may elicit back or rarely leg pain. Neurological findings rarely are radicular in nature and more frequently involve multiple nerve groups. Eismont et al. noted central cord syndrome in two thirds of patients with paralysis from cord compression, and anterior cord syndrome was found in one third. As might be expected, neurological symptoms become more frequent at higher spinal levels; neurological symptoms are most frequent with infections in the cervical and thoracic areas and are least common with infections in the thoracolumbar region.

Differentiation between pyogenic and caseating infections by physical examination is extremely difficult. The patient's history may suggest the etiological factor. The development of neurological signs should suggest the possibility of neural compression from abscess formation, bone collapse, or direct neural infection. Neurological symptoms from arterial thrombosis are rare (Feldenzer et al.). In our experience, once neurological symptoms appear, they progress rapidly unless active decompression or drainage is undertaken.

DIAGNOSTIC TECHNIQUES

The purpose of diagnostic techniques is confirmation of the clinical impression. In spinal infection, no single diagnostic technique is 100% effective as a confirmatory test. Culture of the organism from the infected tissue is the most definitive test,

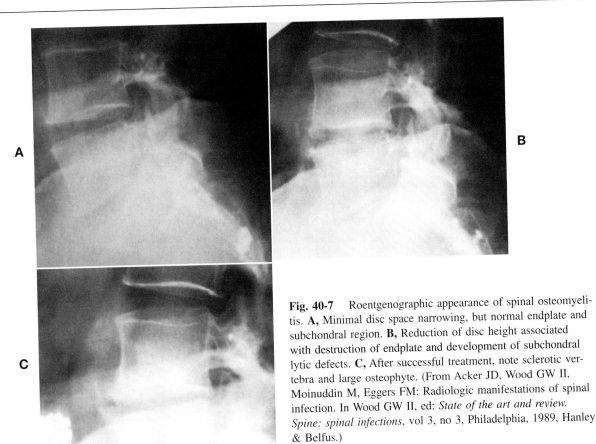

Fig. 40-7 Roentgenographic appearance of spinal osteomyelitis. **A,** Minimal disc space narrowing, but normal endplate and subchondral region. **B,** Reduction of disc height associated with destruction of endplate and development of subchondral lytic defects. **C,** After successful treatment, note sclerotic vertebra and large osteophyte. (From Acker JD, Wood GW II, Moinuddin M, Eggers FM: Radiologic manifestations of spinal infection. In Wood GW II, ed: *State of the art and review. Spine: spinal infections,* vol 3, no 3, Philadelphia, 1989, Hanley & Belfus.)

but results may be negative even under the most optimal conditions. Likewise, all imaging and laboratory studies may be inconclusive, depending on the time at which they are done relative to the onset of infection.

Roentgenograms

Plain roentgenograms of the involved area are the most common initial study in patients with spinal infection. According to Waldvogel and Vasey, roentgenographic findings appear 2 weeks to 3 months after the onset of the infection. Roentgenographic findings include disc space narrowing, vertebral endplate irregularity or loss of the normal contour of the endplate, defects in the subchondral portion of the endplate, and hypertrophic (sclerotic) bone formation (Fig. 40-7). Occasionally, paravertebral soft tissue masses may be noted with involvement of nearby areas of the spine. Late roentgenographic findings may include vertebral collapse, segmental kyphosis, and finally bony ankylosis. The sequence of events may range from 2 to 8 weeks for early findings to more than 2 years for later findings. The only definable abnormality on plain roentgenograms and computed tomographic scans related specifically to tuberculosis is fine calcification in the paravertebral soft tissue space.

Computed Tomography

Computed tomography (CT) adds another dimension to the plain roentgenograms. CT identifies paravertebral soft tissue

swelling and abscesses much more readily and also can monitor changes in the size of the spinal canal. Some clinicians prefer CT to roentgenography for determining clinical progress. Findings with CT scanning are similar to those with plain roentgenograms, including lytic defects in the subchondral bone, destruction of the endplate with irregularity or multiple holes visible in the cross-sectional views, sclerosis near the lytic irregularities, hypodensity of the disc, flattening of the disc itself, disruption of the circumferential bone near the periphery of the disc, and soft tissue density in the epidural and paraspinal regions. Postmyelogram CT more clearly defines compression of the neural elements by abscess or bone impingement and helps determine whether the infection extends to the neural structures themselves.

Magnetic Resonance Imaging

High-quality magnetic resonance imaging (MRI) is an accurate and rapid method for identifying spinal infection. It identifies infected and normal tissues and probably best determines the full extent of the infection. Unfortunately, MRI does not differentiate between pyogenic and nonpyogenic infections and cannot eliminate the need for diagnostic biopsy. Modic, Masaryk, and Plaushtek noted an MRI sensitivity of 96%, a specificity of 92%, and an accuracy of 94% in 37 patients with disc space infections. To detect infection, both T1 and T2 views in the sagittal plane should be obtained. These researchers described MRI findings in patients with vertebral osteomyelitis and noted that T1 images have a decreased signal intensity in the vertebral bodies and disc spaces. The margin between the disc and the adjacent vertebral body cannot be differentiated. In T2 images, the signal intensity is increased in the vertebral disc and is markedly decreased in the vertebral body. Abscesses in the paravertebral soft tissue about the thecal sac can be readily identified as areas of increased uptake. Frequently, the delineation of infection in the paravertebral tissues with extension to the thecal tissues eliminates the need for additional myelography. MRI also is useful to identify primary spinal cord infections (myelitis) without epidural or bone involvement. Kastenbauer et al. noted that in patients with bacterial myelitis, MRI demonstrated hyper-intensities on T2-weighted images that involved the gray matter and extended into the spinal cord. They noted one case of central cavitation of the cord in a follow-up MRI. Goebels, Helmchen, and Abele-Horn noted that MRI was useful in the identification of myelitis from *Mycoplasma pneumoniae* and that the improvement in follow-up MRI preceded clinical improvement. Gupta et al. noted that abscess formation and the presence of bone fragments were the only MRI findings that helped to distinguish spinal tuberculosis from neoplasia.

The addition of gadolinium-labeled diethylenetriaminepentaacetic acid (Gd-DTPA), which is being investigated for various pathological processes, appears to enhance the delineation of epidural abscesses and to further delineate the extent of spinal infection. Our experience has been that this delineation is confined more to involvement of infected soft tissues than to the identification of true liquefied abscess cavities. It is unclear at this time whether the added time, risk, and expense of this additional step yield significantly more information. This contrast material may be useful in older or questionable infections.

MRI is used to follow the progression of treatment. However, the clinical findings, such as decreased pain and improved neurological function, appear to be better indicators than an improvement seen on MRI. Veillard et al. noted that the presence of persisting lesions were of no significance in the face of improved clinical findings. Goebels et al., however, reported that MRI findings showed improvement of myelitis caused by *Mycoplasma pneumoniae* before clinical findings were evident.

Although MRI appears to be the best test for delineating spinal infection, it does have some significant drawbacks, the most important of which is degradation from motion. Motion artifact is common in patients with spinal infections because pain makes it difficult for them to remain still in the supine position for long periods. Additionally, they must lie in an enclosed container, and claustrophobia is a frequent problem. Finally, many of these patients are elderly, and if they have a pacemaker, MRI is contraindicated. The small calcifications seen in the paravertebral abscesses of tuberculosis, which make it so characteristic on plain roentgenograms, are not identifiable with MRI.

Radionuclide Scanning

Radionuclide studies are relatively effective in identifying spinal infection. These techniques include technetium 99 (Tc-99m) bone scan, gallium 67 (Ga-67) scan, and indium 111–labeled leukocyte (In-111 WBC) scan. The technetium bone scan has three basic phases: angiogram, blood pool images, and delayed static images. In infection, diffuse activity is seen on the blood pool images; the diffuse activity becomes focal on delayed views. This marked reactivity may persist for months. Bone scans are almost always positive in patients with infection, but they are not specifically diagnostic of infection. The gallium 67 scan is a good adjunct to bone scanning for the detection of osteomyelitis. Modic et al. reported a sensitivity of 90%, specificity of 100%, and accuracy of 94% in patients having combined Tc-99 and Ga-67 scanning for infection. Tzen et al. suggested the use of Ga-67 scans in patients with fever of unknown origin. They reported six patients in whom spinal infection was noted by Ga-67 scan and confirmed by MRI and biopsy. Gallium scans alone are not as accurate as the combination of bone scan and gallium scan for identifying infection. They also do not identify the type of organism involved. Because the gallium scan changes rapidly with the resolution of the acute active infection, it may be useful to document clinical improvement.

In-111 WBC scans are useful in detecting abscesses but do not differentiate between acute and chronic infections. False-negative indium scans have been reported in chronic infections because the radionuclide accumulates with any inflammatory, noninfectious lesion. Likewise, neoplastic noninfectious inflammatory lesions may lead to similar false-positive results with all scanning techniques. One major advantage of In-111 WBC scanning is that it differentiates between noninfectious lesions such as hematomas and seromas, which may appear as a mass or an abscess-like cavity on MRI or CT. Differentiation is important in the postoperative evaluation of potential infections.

Laboratory Studies

The erythrocyte sedimentation rate (ESR) is the best laboratory study to identify or to evaluate and clinically monitor osteomyelitic disc space infection. Unfortunately, the ESR is not diagnostic and indicates only an inflammatory process, as do most of the roentgenographic findings. The ESR is elevated in 71% to 97% of children with vertebral osteomyelitis. In 37% of adults with osteomyelitis, the rate exceeds 100 mm/hr, and in 67% rates greater than 50 mm/hr are noted. However, the ESR normally is elevated after surgery (approximately 25 mm/hr) but usually falls to a nearly normal level at 4 weeks after surgery. Therefore persistent elevation of the ESR 4 weeks after surgery, with associated clinical findings, indicates a persistent infection.

Elevation of C-reactive protein is an early indicator of infection, but the real value of the test is its rapid return to normal with resolution of the infection. Thelander and Larsson have compared this test with the ESR as an indicator of infection after spine surgery, including microscopic and conventional disc excision and anterior and posterior spinal fusion. They noted that in all patients both tests were elevated initially after the surgery, but in all the patients the C-reactive protein had returned to normal by 14 days, whereas ESR took much longer to return to normal. The major problem with this test is the longer time necessary to obtain the results compared with the ESR. Richards and Emara noted that both the sedimentation rate and C-reactive protein were elevated initially in instrumented spine surgeries. Without infection these values dropped within 4 to 6 days while postoperative infection was heralded by an increase in these values.

Leukocytosis is not especially helpful in diagnosing spinal infection. White cell counts may actually drop in infants and debilitated patients. High white cell counts may indicate areas of infection other than the spine. Blood cultures are helpful if positive, which usually occurs in times of active sepsis with a febrile illness, and may be adequate for the diagnosis and treatment of osteomyelitis, but this occurrence is rare. Skin testing for mycobacterial infections and organism-specific antibody testing may yield additional information while the surgeon awaits biopsy results.

CD4 counts are not helpful in determining the presence of infection in HIV patients. Frequently, these patients are engaging in activities, such as intravenous drug abuse, that predispose to spinal infection. Casado et al. compared musculoskeletal complaints in HIV-positive patients with their CD4 counts and found that spinal infection was present when the CD4 count was more that 200 while osteoarticular and soft tissue infection were present when the CD4 count was less than 200.

Diagnostic Biopsy

Needle biopsy of the suspected lesion is the best method of determining infection and identifying the etiological agent so that appropriate antibiotics can be administered; however, this technique is not foolproof. Administration of antibiotics before biopsy or the elapse of a long period between the onset of the disease and the biopsy may result in a negative biopsy; even open biopsy may not be positive in these situations. An inflammatory process can be confirmed pathologically, although the etiological agent cannot be isolated. Time, host resistance, bacterial virulence, prior antibiotic exposure, and culture of the proper anatomical part are all factors in successful isolation of the offending organism.

Needle biopsy for diagnosis should be and is the most common procedure performed for vertebral osteomyelitis. It frequently can be carried out with the patient under local anesthesia, with roentgenographic or CT control. Stoker and Kissin recommended general anesthesia only for biopsies in children. The reported success rates for percutaneous needle biopsy range from 71% to 96%; reported inadequate biopsy results range from 0% to 20%; and false-negative results range from 4% to 20%. Up to 25% of infections have been reported to have negative biopsy results when patients were treated with antibiotics before biopsy.

Needle biopsy is not without risks. In 1975 Evarts warned against percutaneous biopsy in the thoracic spine because of damage to the vascular structures and the possibility of pneumothorax. With the development of new techniques and the use of stronger and smaller needles, this is not as likely, but there is a definite risk of pneumothorax. Tube thoracostomy rarely is required to treat a pneumothorax, but chest roentgenograms and careful patient monitoring are mandatory after thoracic vertebral biopsy.

CT guidance has improved the success rate of biopsy in both the thoracic and cervical spines. Currently, closed biopsy with CT guidance appears to have the highest success rate and the lowest complication rate. However, even with this technique percutaneous biopsy is not safe in all areas of the spine.

Negative results from percutaneous biopsy should not preclude open biopsy if there is good clinical evidence of infection. Razak, Kamari, and Roohi reported only 22% positive results with percutaneous biopsy and 93% positive results with open biopsy. As in many other procedures results may vary widely. Confidence in a procedure must be determined by prior experience.

DIFFERENTIAL DIAGNOSIS

The differential diagnosis of spinal osteomyelitis should include primary and metastatic malignancies, metabolic bone diseases with pathological fractures, and infections in contiguous and related structures, including the psoas muscle, hip joint, abdominal cavity, and genitourinary system. Charcot spinal arthropathy has been reported by Kalen et al. to resemble spinal osteomyelitis. Rheumatoid arthritis and ankylosing spondylitis also may cause findings resembling osteomyelitis of the spine. Acquired immunodeficiency syndrome (AIDS) may be another underlying factor in these infections. Crawfurd, Baird, and Clark reported five HIV-positive patients with spinal osteomyelitis who presented with radicular symptoms. Myelitis from bacterial infection also has similar findings and distinctive MRI findings as reported by Kastenbauer et al. and Goebels et al.

Nonoperative Treatment

The traditional treatment of spinal infection has been bed rest and immobilization, and this is still the mainstay; however, the body cast now is often replaced with a removable body jacket in compliant patients. Antibiotic treatment for vertebral infection is the primary therapy. The antibiotic is chosen according to the positive stains, cultures, and sensitivities of the organism. Specific antibiotics, however, may not be adequate for spinal infections. Eismont et al. noted that 1 hour after injection, cephalothin was not detectable in the disc and penetrated to less than 4% of serum values. Clindamycin and tobramycin levels were present at better than 50% of serum levels 1 hour after injection. Gibson et al. confirmed these conclusions in their study of flucloxacillin and cephradine levels in the intravertebral discs of children during anterior spinal surgery. They found that neither antibiotic was identifiable in the discs even though high serum levels were present in other tissues.

The time for discontinuing antibiotic therapy also is variable. Collert suggested that antibiotic therapy should be continued until the ESR returns to normal. Intravenous antibiotics usually are continued for about 6 weeks and are followed by oral antibiotics as indicated by the ESR. Certainly a failure of improvement in the ESR or continued persistence of symptoms should prompt a reevaluation of the therapy and possibly a repeat biopsy or even open biopsy for cultures or to remove sequestered and infected material.

With an adequate biopsy and a reliable patient who responds rapidly to antibiotics, hospitalization and bed rest usually are required only for the primary symptoms. Home intravenous antibiotic therapy may allow the patient to complete treatment out of the hospital. A major risk with this technique is late pathological fracture of the infected bone. The exact incidence of this complication with current therapy is unknown. Eismont et al. reported that staphylococcal infections appear to be more prone to causing paralysis than other types of infection; their study did not include patients treated with ambulatory antibiotic therapy and immobilization. If ambulatory therapy is chosen, thorough education and close monitoring of the patient are mandatory. Long-term bed rest and cast immobilization are no longer necessary in most patients with spinal osteomyelitis or disc space infection, but they may be useful in recalcitrant infections that cannot be definitively diagnosed by standard techniques.

Muffoletto et al. reported successful conservative treatment using intravenous antibiotics in 85% of 27 patients with pyogenic facet infection; however, neurological deficit occurred in 25%. Infection is rare in this area.

Prognosis

Even if an absolute diagnosis is not made, most spinal infections resolve symptomatically and roentgenographically within 9 to 24 months of onset. Recurrence of the infection and periods of decreased immune response are always possible, as are delayed complications of kyphosis, paralysis, and myelopathy. These risks are greatest during the period when the infection is controlled but the bone is still soft, when the healing process has not advanced to the point where solid bone has formed around the infected tissue.

Specific Infections

PYOGENIC INFECTIONS

The vertebrae are involved in 0.15% to 3.9% of all osteomyelitic infections. Vertebral osteomyelitis has been reported by Digby and Kersley to occur in 1 of 250,000 inhabitants per year in a localized area of England. Males are affected more frequently than females, with a reported incidence from 55% to 75%. Adults are affected more frequently than children, with peak ages between 45 and 65 years. The most common organism reported is *S. aureus*. Drug abusers have been noted to be more likely to have *Pseudomonas aeruginosa* infections. Paralysis has been found by Eismont et al. to be the most common complication of *S. aureus* infection.

Infections in Children

The syndrome of discitis in children is characterized by fever and an elevated ESR, followed by disc space narrowing on plain roentgenograms at 4 to 6 weeks from onset. The syndrome frequently is associated with difficulty in walking, malaise, irritability, and the sudden inability to stand or walk comfortably. Most reports indicate that the cause is bacterial infection, although trauma also has been implicated. Most culture reports are positive for *S. aureus*. The average age of onset is between 6 and 7 years. Symptoms usually are present for 4 weeks before hospitalization. Physical findings are limited. The child may refuse to walk or may cry when walking, and spinal flexion may be limited and so painful that the child holds himself erect. Physical findings directly related to the spine are rare. Neurological findings are uncommon but are ominous when present. In older children, abdominal pain may be a presenting symptom. Other, less frequent symptoms include hamstring tightness and spinal tenderness.

Diagnosing disc space infection (vertebral osteomyelitis) in children is difficult initially, and plain roentgenograms usually are negative. There may be a mild febrile reaction, but patients do not appear systemically ill. Laboratory investigation reveals only an elevated ESR in most patients. The best test to identify the infection probably is either MRI scanning or a combination of bone scanning and gallium scanning. These should give the earliest indication of possible infection, but are not totally diagnostic, and other possibilities, including inflammatory processes and tumors, may give false-positive results. Blood cultures may be helpful if obtained during the initial febrile period of the illness.

The treatment of discitis in children varies considerably. Spiegel et al. and Boston, Bianco, and Rhodes did not recommend antibiotics and suggested bed rest and immobilization. On the other hand, Wenger, Bobechko, and Gilday recommended that the diagnosis be confirmed with blood cultures and that intravenous antibiotics be administered. They recommended placing the child at bed rest on intravenous antibiotics until he or she can walk and move about comfortably and then switching to oral antibiotics for an additional arbitrary 3 weeks. They did not recommend cast or brace immobilization unless pain or difficulty in walking persists. They found immobilization most frequently necessary in older children. Most patients are symptom free within several months. Spontaneous fusion occurs in about 25% of patients. Surgical procedures rarely are required, and persistent back pain rarely is a problem in children. Aggressive surgical treatment rarely is needed in children except in tuberculosis and other caseating diseases that have not responded well to antibiotics alone.

Special situations involving patients with immune suppression, suspected drug use, tumorous conditions, or poor response to conservative treatment require more vigorous evaluation by needle aspiration biopsy for culture and sensitivity. CT scan control during the percutaneous biopsy, with the patient under a light general anesthesia, makes this a relatively safe procedure with high rates of positive culture. Definitive diagnosis and organism-specific antibiotic treatment constitute a more efficient method of dealing with these difficult situations.

In children younger than 6 years of age, discitis may be viral in origin. Needle biopsy rarely is performed in these patients, and they may be the only group in whom careful monitoring without antibiotics is reasonable. Van Dalen and Heeg reported an epidural abscess in a 3-week old infant who presented with quadriplegia. The patient recovered full neurological function after treatment with aspiration and antibiotics.

The likelihood of paralysis depends on several factors. In the series of Eismont et al., no patient younger than 37 years of age developed paralysis. The higher the level of the infection in the spine, the greater the chance of paralysis.

Disc Space Infection in Adults

In adults the intervertebral disc appears to be avascular, making it impossible for primary disc space infection to occur by a blood-borne route without first infecting bone. Therefore a true disc space infection in adults most likely is caused by penetrating trauma, the most common form of which is surgical manipulation. The reported incidence of disc space infection after disc surgery ranges from 1% to 2.8%. The reported incidence of disc space infection after discography is 1% when the single-needle technique is used and 0.5% with the double-needle technique. Postoperative disc space infection rarely is associated with a frank wound infection and wound drainage. The usual infecting organism is *S. aureus*, but other bacterial and fungal organisms have been reported.

The diagnosis of postoperative disc space infection is difficult and almost always is delayed. Pain is the most common complaint; however, persistence of back pain is not uncommon after surgical disc procedures. The most common diagnostic studies, including the ESR, bone scan, and gallium scan, are positive shortly after a spinal surgical procedure. MRI may be the best way to identify this complication rapidly. The ESR should return to nearly normal within 4 weeks after surgery. The persistence of back pain, muscle spasm, and difficulty in walking, along with an elevated ESR, 4 to 6 weeks after surgery should be highly indicative of a potential disc space infection. Disc space biopsy by closed-needle techniques or open biopsy, preferably before the administration of antibiotics, should allow identification of the offending organism in more than 50% of patients.

Specific or empiric antibiotics have been suggested in most reports of postoperative disc space infection. Antibiotics should be continued until the ESR returns to normal. Immobilization in a body cast may be helpful to relieve pain, which usually lasts for 8 to 24 months. Spontaneous intervertebral fusion usually results in relief of pain. Occasionally spontaneous fusion does not occur. The indications for surgery are the same as for vertebral osteomyelitis.

Epidural Space Infection

Spinal epidural infections have a low reported incidence of 0.2 to 1.2 cases per 10,000 hospital admissions per year. The incidence of this infection is increased in immunosuppressed patients. Morbidity and mortality are high with epidural infections. The causes of infection are the same as those for osteomyelitis and discitis. Epidural space infection actually can complicate a primary disc space infection. Trauma has been implicated as a causative factor in 25% of reported cases, presumably from secondary infection of an epidural hematoma. Feldenzer et al. noted that experimental epidural infection created physical signs from compression rather than from vascular thrombosis.

No biological boundaries are present in the epidural space, and the infection frequently spans three to five vertebral segments, with the potential to cover the entire spinal canal. These infections occur more frequently in the thoracic and lumbar spine and are found more frequently on the dorsal and lateral portions of the epidural space. Ventral (anterior) infections are less frequent and are more likely to be related to a primary osteomyelitis or disc space infection; *S. aureus* is the most common infecting agent.

The clinical findings are similar to those of osteomyelitis but with several distinct differences: (1) a more rapid development of neurological symptoms (days instead of weeks), (2) a more acute febrile illness, and (3) signs of meningeal irritation, including radicular pain with a positive straight leg raising test and neck rigidity. The classic progression of the disease is generalized spinal ache, root pain, weakness, and finally paralysis, all occurring within 7 to 10 days. Confirmatory testing is similar to that for osteomyelitis. MRI is critical to the determination of associated osteomyelitis.

Heusner noted that, even before antibiotics and at the dawn of the antibiotic age, with early decompression (before the development of paralysis or within 36 hours of onset) the chance of complete recovery was better than 50%. He also noted that the progression of the process was slow enough to allow evaluation and preparation without endangering the patient. Nonetheless, failure to provide prompt drainage can result in serious paralysis and possibly death. Some authors have reported successful treatment without surgical drainage, but these are few. Nonoperative management demands close observation and more active intervention if necessary.

The primary methods of treatment are surgical drainage and appropriate antibiotic therapy. The method of surgical treatment requires an accurate assessment of the location of the abscess and the presence of an associated osteomyelitis. Acute or chronic isolated dorsal (posterior), lateral, and some ventral (anterior) infections are best treated with total laminectomy for drainage, with closure over drains or secondary closure at a later date. Epidural infections associated with osteomyelitis are best exposed by anterior or posterolateral exposures that allow treatment of both the osteomyelitis and the epidural infection. Laminectomy in patients with ventral (anterior) osteomyelitis results in late deformity and collapse.

Other intraspinal infections include subdural abscess and spinal cord abscess. These infections are rare. Subdural abscesses progress at a slower pace than epidural abscesses and can be confused with tumors. Treatment requires durotomy without opening the arachnoid, thorough debridement, and dural closure if possible. Spinal cord abscesses cause pronounced incontinence and long tract signs. They frequently are confused with intramedullary tumors and transverse myelitis. In both of these conditions, the bone scan will be normal but the gallium scan should be positive. MRI, preferably with gadolinium contrast, is extremely helpful in defining the extent of the abscess. Some spinal cord abscesses can be treated successfully with antibiotics alone.

MRI also may be useful in the determining the outcome of spinal epidural abscesses. Tung et al. noted that weakness at follow-up was associated with 50% or more narrowing of the central canal, peripheral contrast enhancement, and abnormal spinal cord signal intensity. Incomplete recovery was associated with abscess size and the severity of canal narrowing.

POSTOPERATIVE INFECTIONS

Postoperative infections are pyogenic and usually occur shortly after the operation. Takahashi et al. compared the erythrocyte sedimentation rate, C-reactive protein, white blood cell count, and body temperature in patients who had spinal procedures with and without spinal instrumentation. They noted that patients with instrumentation had a significantly higher sedimentation rate and C-reactive protein than patients without, but these parameters normally decreased after surgery unless infection was present. Patients with postoperative infection tended to have a renewed elevation of these parameters. Richards et al. found that low-virulence organisms, such as *Propionibacterium acnes,* were most likely to cause late postoperative infections. These infections were associated with spontaneous drainage and back pain occurring an average of 27 months after surgery. Treatment was removal of the instrumentation when the fusion was solid. Weinstein, McCabe, and Cammisa reported 46 wound infections in 2391 spinal surgeries. Prior surgery (37%) was a high risk factor in their series. These infections were for the most part acute. Wound drainage was very common and occurred at an average of 15 days after surgery; however, fever was not common. Surgical treatment consisted of initial drainage and debridement without primary closure followed by delayed closure. Instrumentation was removed only when the fusion was solid or when fixation was lost. Viable bone graft and instrumentation were left in situ. This is also our method of treatment of acute postoperative infections. Picada et al. reviewed 817 instrumented lumbosacral fusions with 26 postoperative infections treated with

retention of the instrumentation; only 2 failed to heal. Recalcitrant wounds may require local V-Y flaps or free flaps when bone or implants are exposed according to Chen et al.

BRUCELLOSIS

Brucellosis results in a noncaseating, acid-fast, negative granuloma caused by a gram-negative capnophilic coccobacillus. This infection occurs most frequently in individuals involved in animal husbandry and meat processing (abattoirs). Pasteurization of milk and antibiotic treatment of animals have led to a significant decrease in the incidence of this disease. Symptoms include polyarthralgia, fever, malaise, night sweats, anorexia, and headache. Psoas abscesses are found in 12% of patients. Bone involvement, most frequently the spine, occurs in 2% to 30% of patients. The lumbar spine is the most frequently involved spinal segment.

Roentgenographic changes of steplike erosions of the margin of the vertebral body require 2 months or more to develop. Disc space thinning and vertebral segment ankylosis by bridging are similar to changes in other forms of osteomyelitis (Fig. 40-8). CT scans and MRI may show soft tissue involvement. Moehring noted that gallium scanning is not helpful in sacroiliac infections. MRI may be helpful in the early identification of the disease but has not been reported for this specific infection. The diagnosis usually is indicated by brucella titers of 1:80 or greater; confirmatory cultures also should be done, if possible using special techniques. Treatment usually consists of antibiotic therapy for 4 months and close monitoring of the *Brucella* titers. Persistence of a titer of 1:160 or greater after 4 months of treatment may indicate recurrence or resistance of the infection. Indications for surgical treatment are the same as for tubercular spinal infections. Neurological improvement after radical decompression and fusion is frequent. Because of the indolent nature of this disease, it can be mistaken for a degenerative process. Nas et al. recommended 6 months of antibiotic therapy (rifampicin and doxycycline) with surgery for spinal cord compression, instability, or radiculopathy.

FUNGAL INFECTIONS

Fungal infections generally are noncaseating, acid-fast, negative infections. They usually occur as opportunistic infections in immunocompromised patients. The development of symptoms usually is slow. Pain is less prominent as a physical symptom than in other forms of spinal osteomyelitis. Laboratory and roentgenographic findings are similar to those of pyogenic infections. Tubercular infection and tumors are the primary differential diagnoses. Direct culture by biopsy is the only method of absolute determination of the infecting organism.

Aspergillus and cryptococcal infections are of special note with regard to spinal infections. *Aspergillus* is an opportunistic infecting agent in most reported cases. Barnwell, Jelsma, and Raff noted spinal involvement in 63% of 26 patients with

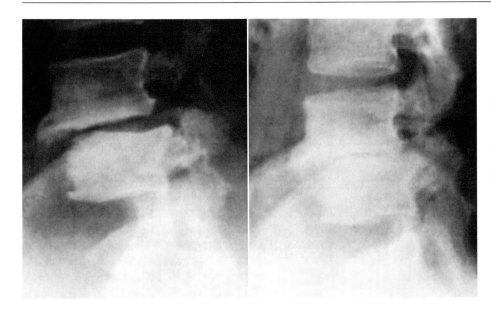

Fig. 40-8   Brucellosis of lumbar spine. Note vertebral sclerosis, spondylolisthesis, steplike irregularity in anterior vertebral body, and anterior osteophytes. (From Lifeso RM, Harder E, McCorkell SJ: *J Bone Joint Surg* 67B:345, 1985.)

Aspergillus infections. Vinas, King, and Diaz noted a predominant lumbar involvement, and neurological involvement occurred in 30%. Pain, tenderness, and an elevated ESR were the most common symptoms but white cell elevations are rare. The diagnosis requires biopsy. Most patients do not require further surgery, but Ferris and Jones reported 10 patients who required radical debridement. Their patients with paraplegia and epidural abscesses did not improve after surgery, but two patients did improve with medical therapy alone. More recent reports by Govender et al. and Assaad et al. are more encouraging with regard to neurological recovery after early, aggressive surgical debridement and stabilization and antibiotic therapy. In a literature review, Vinas et al. found a 27% mortality rate in 39 reported cases.

Cryptococcal infection is a less opportunistic but more prevalent fungal infection. These organisms are found in avian excreta and usually infect the human respiratory system. Spinal infection is rare and usually is associated with generalized cryptococcal dissemination. The primary findings are pain, weakness, and a mildly elevated ESR. Roentgenograms show lytic lesions that on biopsy reveal non-acid-fast, caseating granulomas without pus. The indications for radical surgery are the same as for tuberculosis.

TUBERCULOSIS

Tuberculosis was previously the primary cause of infectious spondylitis. Before the advent of effective chemotherapy, time and surgery for paralysis were the only treatment options. Laminectomy initially was performed for paralysis, but the results were disappointing until Menard accidentally opened an abscess and the patient improved. Unfortunately, many patients treated in this manner died of a secondary bacterial infection and the practice was abandoned. Posterior spinal fusion, as described by Hibbs and Albee, was the preferred operation to prevent deformity and promote healing by internal immobili-

Table 40-2   Mean Annual Incidence (per 100,000 Population) of Bone and Joint Tuberculosis According to Age and Sex, Canada, 1970 Through 1974

	Sex	
Age (yr)	Male	Female
0-14	0.14	0.12
15-24	0.18	0.20
25-34	0.25	0.43
35-44	0.63	0.43
45-54	1.00	0.75
55-64	1.30	1.02
65	1.60	1.40

From Enarson DA, Fujii M, Nakielna EM, Grzybowski S: *Can Med Assoc J* 120:139, 1979.

zation. Ito, Tsuchija, and Asami in 1934 reported the first radical debridement and bone-grafting procedure for abscess formation. After the development of satisfactory chemotherapeutic agents, more aggressive surgery was attempted, including costotransversectomy with bone grafting and radical debridement with bone grafting as popularized by Hodgson. Tubercular bone and joint infections currently account for 2% to 3% of all reported cases of *Mycobacterium tuberculosis*. Spinal tubercular infections account for one third to one half of the bone and joint infections. The thoracolumbar spine is the most commonly infected area. The incidence of infection appears to increase with age, but males and females are almost equally infected (Table 40-2).

Pathologically the infection is characterized by acid-fast, positive, caseating granulomas with or without pus. Tubercles composed of monocytes and epithelioid cells, forming minute masses with central caseation in the presence of Langerhans-type giant cells, are typical on microscopic examination. Abscesses expand, following the path of least resistance, and contain necrotic debris. Skin sinuses form, drain, and heal spontaneously. Bone reaction to the infection varies from intense reaction to no reaction. In the spine the infection spares the intervertebral discs and spreads beneath the anterior and posterior longitudinal ligaments. Epidural infection is more likely to result in permanent neurological damage.

Slowly progressive constitutional symptoms are predominant in the early stages of the disease, including weakness, malaise, night sweats, fever, and weight loss. Pain is a late symptom associated with bone collapse and paralysis. Cervical involvement can cause hoarseness because of recurrent laryngeal nerve paralysis, dysphagia, and respiratory stridor (known as *Milar asthma*). These symptoms may result from anterior abscess formation in the neck. Sudden death has been reported with cervical disease after erosion into the great vessels. Neurological signs usually occur late and may wax and wane. Motor function and rectal tone are good prognostic predictors. Jain et al. calculated that the spinal canal can accommodate 76% encroachment on CT scan without neurological abnormality. Seddon reported that 60% to 90% of patients with Pott paraplegia recovered with prolonged bed rest in an open-air hospital.

Laboratory studies suggest chronic disease. Findings include anemia, hypoproteinemia, and mild ESR elevation. Skin testing may be helpful but is not diagnostic. The test is contraindicated in patients with prior tuberculous infection because of the risk of skin slough from an intense reaction and therefore is not of use in patients with suspected reactivation of the disease.

Early roentgenographic findings include a subtle decrease in one or more disc spaces and localized osteopenia. Later findings include vertebral collapse, called "concertina collapse" by Seddon because of its resemblance to an accordion. Soft tissue swelling and its late calcification are highly predictable roentgenographic findings. CT scanning, with or without contrast, allows better evaluation of the pathological process and the degree of neural compromise. MRI permits further delineation of the pathological process. Gupta et al. noted that abscess formation and the presence of bone fragments were the only MRI findings that helped distinguish spinal tuberculosis from neoplasia. None of these tests, however, is confirmatory for tuberculosis. Gorse et al. noted that gallium scanning was most useful in patients with disseminated tuberculosis.

Definitive diagnosis is dependent on culture of the organism and requires biopsy of the lesion. Percutaneous techniques with roentgenographic or CT control usually are adequate. Francis et al. reported 29 patients with suspected spinal tuberculosis. Epithelioid granulomas were seen in 89%, positive AFB cultures in 83%, and positive AFB smears in 52%. Percutaneous thoracoscopic or laparoscopic biopsy is another reported option as noted by Dusmet, Halkic, and Corpataux. Open biopsy may be required if the needle biopsy is dangerous or nonproductive or if other open procedures are required.

Delayed diagnosis and missed diagnosis are common. Differential diagnoses include pyogenic and fungal infections, secondary metastatic disease, primary tumors of bone (such as osteosarcoma, chondrosarcoma, myeloma, eosinophilic granuloma, and aneurysmal bone cyst), sarcoidosis, giant cell tumors of bone, and bone deformities such as Scheuermann disease.

Treatment of Tubercular Spinal Infection

Definitive diagnosis by biopsy culture is important because of the toxicity of the chemotherapeutic agents and the length of treatment required. If open biopsy is required, Hodgson et al. suggested definitive debridement and grafting at the same time. In 1960 Hodgson et al. reported 412 patients treated by radical removal of the diseased area and anterior spinal arthrodesis. Their technique requires a more extensive excision of bone than that of Roaf, Kirkaldy-Willis, and Cathro, but their mortality was only 2.9%, and no deaths occurred in patients who had disease of limited extent or of short duration and who had no pulmonary involvement. No patient developed paraplegia after surgery. Hodgson et al. advised this method for all patients with early tuberculosis of the spine and proposed that it supplant conservative treatment in most patients. They operated on all patients, even those in whom the disease was far advanced, and of the first 100 patients observed for 2 to 4 years, 93 had solid arthrodeses consisting of an uninterrupted bridge of mature bone and healing of the tuberculous focus. Yilmaz et al. reported 22 patients with moderate to severe localized kyphosis from spinal tuberculosis successfully treated with anterior debridement, grafting, and anterior instrumentation alone. They concluded that this treatment was more effective than posterior instrumentation for stabilization and reduction of deformity.

Nonoperative and operative methods were extensively evaluated by the Medical Resource Council Working Party. Their reports indicated better results with regard to deformity, recurrence, development of paralysis, and resolution when radical surgery is performed with chemotherapeutic coverage. The resolution of paraplegia was not dependent on surgical intervention. Long-term bed rest, with or without cast immobilization, was ineffective. If the facilities for radical surgery are not available, ambulatory chemotherapy is the treatment of choice. Their most recent report identified the 6-month use of isoniazid with ethambutol or isoniazid with PAS to be inferior to isoniazid with rifampicin. They also stressed the use of adequate patient supervision for a successful result. Upadhyay et al. reported similar results. Leibert et al. had good results in 26 HIV patients with spinal tuberculosis after treatment with medication.

The indications for surgery in the absence of neurological symptoms vary widely. Involvement of more than one vertebra significantly increases the risk of kyphosis and collapse. Open biopsy for diagnosis, debridement, and grafting with or without anterior instrumentation may offer the most direct approach in

Table 40-3   Analysis of Results in Relation to Type of Graft

Type of Graft	No.	No. Follow-Up	Nonunion or Incomplete Fusion	Body Fusion	Average Time to Fusion (Mo)	Final Kyphosis		
						Decreased	Static	Increased (and Average)
Autologous rib	63	8	21	34 (62%)	24	1	30	24 (13 degrees)
Autologous ilium* (series I)	23	—	6	17 (74%)	14	1	21	1 (nil)
Autologous ilium (series II)	18	—	1	17 (94.5%)	10	2	11	5 (7 degrees)
Homologous rib	1	—	—	1	24	—	1	—
Homologous tibia	7	—	2	5 (71%)	28	—	5	2
Heterologous	5	—	1	4 (80%)	18.5	—	3	2
†Kiel bone	4							
Kiel bone ilium	1							

From Kemp HBS, Jackson JW, Jeremiah JD, Cook J: *J Bone Joint Surg* 55B:715, 1973.
*Autologous ilium: *Series I* denotes full-thickness ilium used as an inlay graft. *Series II* denotes full-thickness ilium crossing the coronal diameters of the affected vertebrae. The difference between the rate of fusion for autologous rib and autologous ilium was statistically significant ($P < 0.001$).
†Kiel bone = bovine bone.

these patients. Resistance to chemotherapy and recurrence of the disease are other indications for radical surgical treatment. Yau and Hodgson listed the indications for surgery in early or late disease as severe kyphosis with active disease, signs and symptoms of cord compression, progressive impairment of pulmonary function, and progression of the kyphotic deformity. Primary contraindications to surgery are cardiac and respiratory failure.

Posterior fusion, with or without spinal instrumentation, is indicated after anterior decompression and grafting to prevent late collapse and stress fracture of the graft if more than two vertebrae are involved and if anterior instrumentation is not used. Posterior fusion alone rarely is indicated at this time. High incidences of failure and late progression of kyphotic deformity, with or without fatigue fracture of the fusion, have followed posterior fusion alone. Tricortical iliac crest is the preferred bone graft material for all levels, provided it is long enough. If the ribs are strong, autogenous rib grafts can be used in the thoracic region, although Rajasekaran and Shanmugasundaram and others reported frequent failure with the use of ribs as grafts. Fibular grafts may be required if the area of debridement is extensive and the available iliac crest graft is too short or if the ribs are not strong enough. The incidence of late stress fracture increases with the use of fibular or rib grafts (Table 40-3). External immobilization is mandatory whenever debridement and grafting are performed. Halo (vest, cast, or pelvic) immobilization for up to 3 months is used after cervical and cervicothoracic procedures. Removable or nonremovable thoracolumbar immobilization is used after thoracic and thoracolumbar procedures until the grafts have completely healed (9 to 12 months or longer). Lumbosacropelvic immobilization is used after low lumbar procedures and should

be from the hip to the knee of at least one leg for 6 to 8 weeks, followed by thoracolumbosacral immobilization until the graft has healed and the infection has resolved.

Cervical tuberculosis is a rare disease with a high complication rate. Hsu and Leong reported a 42.5% spinal cord compression rate in 40 patients. Children younger than 10 years of age were more likely to develop abscesses, whereas older children were more likely to develop paraplegia. Drainage and chemotherapy were adequate for the younger children. For older patients these researchers recommended radical anterior debridement and strut grafting followed by chemotherapy. Cervical laminectomy resulted in increased kyphosis, subluxation, and neurological deficits. Posterior cervical fusion resulted in persistent pain, kyphosis, and neurological deficits that required anterior debridement and strut grafting. Subluxation was treated with skull traction for reduction, followed by anterior decompression and strut grafting.

Lifeso recommended various treatments for three different stages of C1-C2 tubercular infection. Stage 1 infections involve minimal bone and ligamentous destruction. Surgical treatment for this consists of transoral biopsy, decompression, and immobilization in an orthosis. Stage 2 infections involve ligamentous destruction, minimal bone loss, and anterior displacement of C1 on C2. The suggested treatment for this is transoral biopsy and decompression, followed by reduction with halo traction and later C1-C2 posterior fusion. Stage 3 infections exhibit marked ligamentous and bone destruction with C1-C2 displacement. The suggested treatment here is transoral biopsy and decompression, followed by reduction with halo traction and later occiput to C3 posterior fusion.

The thoracic and lumbar spines are more commonly involved with tubercular infection. Rajasekaran and Shanmu-

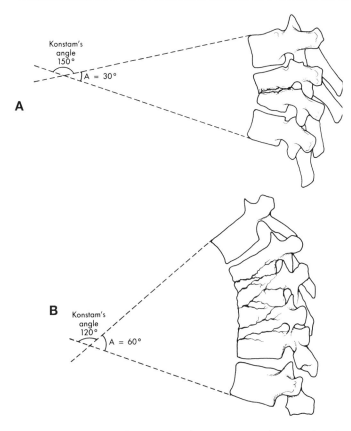

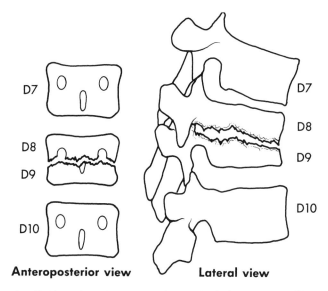

Fig. 40-9   Line diagrams showing Konstam angle *(K)* and angle A (see text). (Redrawn from Rajasekaran S, Shanmugasundaram K: *J Bone Joint Surg* 69A:503, 1987.)

Fig. 40-10   Line diagram showing method of assessment of loss of vertebral body. (Redrawn from Rajasekaran S, Shanmugasundaram K: *J Bone Joint Surg* 69A:503, 1987.)

gasundaram compared the development of kyphosis with the degree of collapse at the time of presentation of tubercular disease and the institution of antibiotic treatment. They developed a formula to predict the degree of final gibbus deformity that was 90% accurate: y = a + bx, where *y* is the measurement of the final angle of gibbus deformity, *x* is the initial loss of vertebral body, and *a* and *b* are constants 5.5 and 30.5, respectively. Initial vertebral loss was determined by dividing the vertebra into tenths for each involved vertebra (Figs. 40-9 and 40-10). These researchers suggested that this formula can be used to identify patients most likely to develop significant kyphosis.

Pott Paraplegia

The development of neurological deficit is a strong indication for surgical treatment. Seddon noted that 70% to 95% of patients with Pott paralysis recovered. He noted a poorer prognosis in paralysis caused by vascular embarrassment, penetration of the dura by the infection, and transection of the cord by a bony ridge. Paralysis persisting longer than 6 months was unlikely to improve.

Hodgson et al. (1964) described two basic groups: *group A, paraplegia with active disease,* which included subtypes 1

(external pressure on the cord) and 2 (penetration of the dura by infection) and *group B, paraplegia of healed disease,* which included subtypes 1 (transection of the cord by a bony ridge) and 2 (constriction of the cord by granulation and fibrous tissue). Hodgson et al. recommended early surgery to prevent the development of dural invasion by the infection, resulting in irreversible paralysis. A thorough preoperative examination, using MRI and CT scans of the involved segment, allows a complete evaluation of the extent of the disease and thus the development of a satisfactory approach for complete debridement and grafting. Late paralysis with inactive disease and significant kyphosis is much less responsive to treatment.

Atypical Tubercular Infections

Reports of atypical tubercular infections are limited to isolated case reports, usually in individuals who are elderly or immunocompromised by disease or medication. These atypical infections require much more aggressive surgical intervention because of the lack of antibiotic sensitivity and the risk of progression with standard tubercular therapy. The clinical manifestations and aggressive surgical treatment of atypical tubercular spinal infections and mycobacterial infections are similar.

Abscess Drainage by Anatomical Level

Any abscess cavity about the spine and pelvis can be drained as summarized in the following techniques.

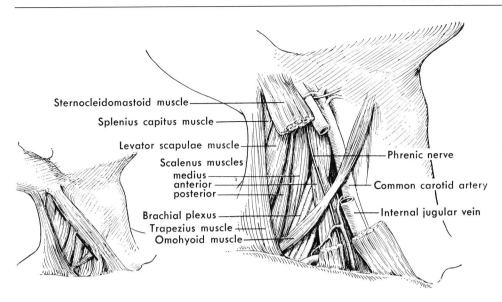

Fig. 40-11   Drainage of tuberculous abscess of cervical spine.

CERVICAL SPINE

If the cervical spine is involved, the abscess may be present retropharyngeally in the posterior triangle of the neck or supraclavicular area, or the tuberculous detritus may gravitate downward under the prevertebral fascia to form a mediastinal abscess.

◆ Drainage of Retropharyngeal Abscess

Drainage of a retropharyngeal abscess through an incision in the posterior wall of the pharynx is warranted only in an emergency, as indicated by cyanosis and respiratory difficulty. Usually drainage should be through an extraoral approach (Fig. 40-11).

TECHNIQUE 40-1

Make a 7.5-cm incision along the posterior border of the sternocleidomastoid muscle at the junction of its middle and upper thirds. Incise the superficial layer of cervical fascia and protect the spinal accessory nerve that pierces the sternocleidomastoid muscle and runs obliquely across the posterior triangle. Retract the sternocleidomastoid muscle medially or divide it transversely. Using blunt dissection, expose the levator scapulae and splenius muscles, displace the internal jugular vein anteriorly, and palpate the abscess in front of the transverse processes and bodies of the vertebrae. Puncture the abscess wall with a hemostat, enlarge the opening, and gently but thoroughly evacuate the abscess. If the abscess is unusually large and symptoms are severe, do not close the wound; if not, close the wound in layers. A tracheostomy set should be available should the patient develop respiratory difficulty from edema of the larynx or should the abscess rupture into the pharynx.

◆ Drainage of Abscess of Posterior Triangle of Neck

TECHNIQUE 40-2

Incise obliquely the skin and superficial fascia for 6.3 cm along the posterior border of the sternocleidomastoid muscle. Retract this muscle medially but carefully protect the superficial nerves and external jugular vein. Identify the scaleni muscles without injuring the phrenic nerve. Locate and divide the line of cleavage between the scalenus anterior and longus colli muscles by blunt dissection obliquely inward to the abscess beneath the paravertebral fascia. Evacuate the cavity and close the wound.

◆ Alternative Approach for Drainage of Retropharyngeal Abscess

Expose the anterior aspect of the cervical vertebrae as for standard anterior disc excision. This technique allows exposure from C2 to C7. A transverse incision is possible if only two or three vertebrae are involved. A longitudinal incision is made along the medial border of the sternocleidomastoid muscle if longer exposure is necessary.

TECHNIQUE 40-3

Place the patient supine on the operating table with endotracheal anesthesia administered through a noncollapsible tube. Place the head turned to the right 10 to 20 degrees. The insertion of a small nasogastric tube may facilitate the positive identification of the esophagus. Place a small roll between the scapulas; the shoulders can be pulled downward with tape to allow easy roentgen exposure. Slightly extend the neck over a small roll placed beneath it. Then place a head halter on the mandible and occiput and apply several pounds of traction. Prepare and drape the area from

continued

the mandible to the upper chest. It may be necessary to suture the initial drapes in place.

Undermine the subcutaneous tissue both above and below and divide the platysma muscle longitudinally in the direction of its fibers. Open the cervical fascia along the anteromedial border of the sternocleidomastoid muscle. Develop a plane between the sternocleidomastoid laterally and the omohyoid and sternohyoid medially. Palpate the carotid artery in this plane and gently retract it laterally with a finger. With combined blunt and sharp dissection develop a relatively avascular plane between the carotid sheath laterally and the thyroid, trachea, and esophagus medially. Insert hand-held retractors initially. Identify the esophagus by palpation of the nasogastric tube. Dissect free the filmy connective tissue on the posterolateral aspect of the esophagus along the entire exposed wound to prevent ballooning of the esophagus above and below the retractor. Expose the prevertebral fascia and open the abscess cavity. Insert a hypodermic needle into this material and obtain a lateral roentgenogram to confirm the proper level. Drain the wound in a standard fashion. Do not close the neck fascia but let it fall together. The skin can be loosely closed or left open for delayed closure.

DORSAL SPINE

◆ Costotransversectomy

Most abscesses caused by disease of the dorsal spine can be evacuated by costotransversectomy (Fig. 40-12). This procedure, originally performed by Haidenhaim, was described by Menard in 1894.

TECHNIQUE 40-4

Make a midline incision over three spinous processes. Reflect the periosteum and soft tissues laterally from the spinous processes and laminae on the side containing the abscess. Expose fully the middle transverse process and resect it at its base. After reflecting the periosteum from the contiguous rib, resect its medial end by division 5 cm from the tip of the transverse process. Bevel the end of the rib, taking care to avoid puncture of the pleura. Open the abscess by blunt dissection close to the vertebral body. The opening should be large enough to permit thorough exploration of the cavity and removal of all debris. If resection of more than one rib is necessary, enlarge the initial incision accordingly. After resecting the ribs, doubly ligate and divide the intervening neurovascular bundle. Close the wound in layers.

TECHNIQUE 40-5 *(Seddon)*

Begin a semicircular skin incision in the midline about 10 cm proximal to the apex of the kyphos, curve it distally

and laterally to a point 10 cm from the midline at this apex, and continue distally and medially to the midline at a point 10 cm distal to the apex (Fig. 40-13). If the infection is pyogenic without a kyphosis, a midline incision can be used. Elevate the skin flap and retract it medially. Cut the superficial muscles and turn them in whatever direction is appropriate for the particular level. Divide the erector spinae muscles transversely opposite the apex of the deformity. Using diathermy dissection, expose the medial 8.3 cm of not less than three ribs, the corresponding transverse processes, and the lateral third of the laminae (Fig. 40-14).

Resect the rib that roentgenograms show to be level with the widest bulge of the abscess as follows. After dividing the

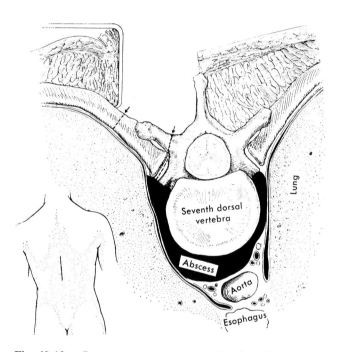

Fig. 40-12   Costotransversectomy to drain tuberculous abscess of dorsal spine.

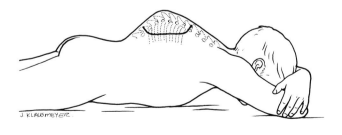

Fig. 40-13   Incision for costotransversectomy or anterolateral decompression. (From Seddon HJ: Pott's paraplegia. In Platt H, ed: *Modern trends in orthopedics*, second series, London, 1956, Butterworth.)

costotransverse ligaments, remove the transverse process in one piece with large bone-cutting forceps. Using subperiosteal dissection, expose the rib, being careful not to perforate the pleura. If such a perforation occurs, place a small swab over it and try to close it as soon as the rib has been removed. The use of a Carlen tube will allow deflation of the lung. Transect the rib at a point not less than 6.8 cm (in adults) lateral to the costotransverse joint. Use a curved gouge to free the medial end of the rib, pushing the gouge gently anteriorly and medially until it strikes the head of the rib or the vertebral column. Gently rotate the medial end of the rib and use the gouge to divide any remaining attachment. If the operation is successful, pus will pour out of the hole; remove it immediately with a sucker. Explore the abscess with a finger, reaching the vertebral

bodies, opening small cavities, and dislodging necrotic material. If the abscess is unusually large, remove a second transverse process and rib for more exposure. Remove the tuberculous material from the abscess cavity and superficial tissues. After dusting the wound and the cavity with streptomycin powder, close the muscles and skin without a drain.

LUMBAR SPINE AND PELVIC DRAINAGE

◆ Drainage of Paravertebral Abscess

TECHNIQUE 40-6
Make a 7.5- to 10-cm longitudinal incision 5 to 7.5 cm lateral to the midline parallel to the spinous processes. Divide the lumbodorsal fascia in line with the incision and pass a hemostat bluntly around the lateral and anterior borders of the erector spinae muscles to the transverse processes (Fig. 40-15). Usually the abscess is encountered immediately; if not, puncture the layer of lumbodorsal fascia that separates the quadratus lumborum muscle from the erector spinae group and force the hemostat along the anterior border of the transverse processes. After thorough evacuation of the abscess, close the incision in layers.

Drainage of Psoas Abscess
Psoas abscesses are entirely extraperitoneal and follow the course of the iliopsoas muscle. Drainage can be done posteriorly through the Petit triangle, by a lateral incision along the crest of the ilium, or anteriorly under the Poupart ligament, depending on the size of the abscess and the area in which it appears. Occasionally an abscess burrows beneath the Poupart ligament and is seen subcutaneously in the proximal third of the thigh in the adductor region (Fig. 40-16).

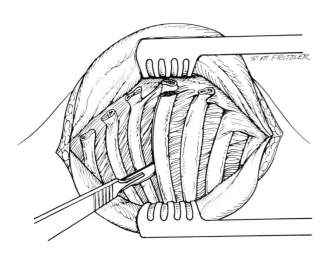

Fig. 40-14 Exposure of ribs and resection of transverse processes. (From Seddon HJ: Pott's paraplegia. In Platt H, ed: *Modern trends in orthopedics,* second series, London, 1956, Butterworth.)

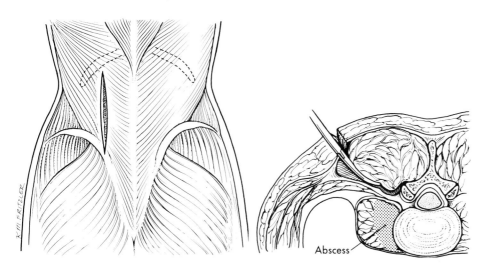

Fig. 40-15 Drainage of paravertebral abscess.

Abscess

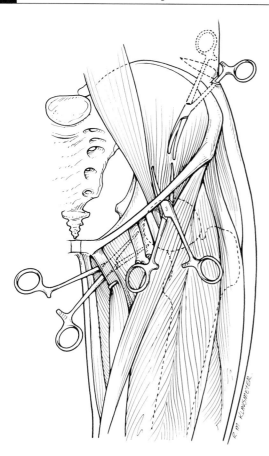

Fig. 40-16 Drainage of psoas abscess. Hemostat in adductor region is pointed toward inferior edge of acetabulum; abscess is usually located nearer junction of femoral head and neck. (Adapted from Freiberg JA, Perlman R: *J Bone Joint Surg* 18:417, 1936.)

◆ Drainage Through Petit Triangle

The sides of the Petit triangle are formed by the lateral margin of the latissimus dorsi muscle and the medial border of the obliquus externus abdominis muscle and its base by the crest of the ilium. The floor of the triangle is the obliquus internus abdominis muscle.

TECHNIQUE 40-7

Make a 7.5-cm incision 2.5 cm proximal to and parallel with the posterior crest of the ilium, beginning lateral to the erector spinae group of muscles (Fig. 40-17). After exposure of the Petit triangle, bluntly dissect through the obliquus internus abdominis muscle directly into the abscess. After thorough evacuation of the abscess, close the incision in layers.

AFTERTREATMENT. Since flexion contracture of the hip usually accompanies a psoas abscess, Buck traction should be used to correct the deformity and relax the spastic muscles until the hip is fully extended.

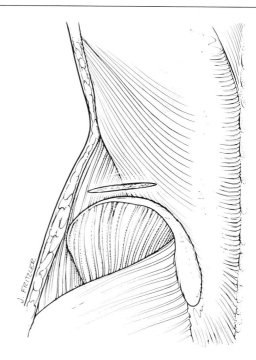

Fig. 40-17 Drainage of pelvic abscess through Petit triangle.

◆ Drainage by Lateral Incision

TECHNIQUE 40-8

Make a 10-cm incision along the middle third of the crest of the ilium and free the attachments of the internal and external obliquus abdominis muscles. With a hemostat, puncture the abscess, which can be palpated as a fluctuant extraperitoneal mass on the inner surface of the wing of the ilium. Avoid rupture of the peritoneum.

◆ Drainage by Anterior Incision

TECHNIQUE 40-9

Begin a longitudinal skin incision at the anterosuperior spine and continue it distally for 5 to 7.5 cm on the anterior aspect of the thigh. Identify the sartorius muscle and carry the dissection deep to its medial border to the level of the anteroinferior spine. Protect the femoral nerve, which lies just medial to this area. Now insert a long hemostat along the medial surface of the wing of the ilium under the Poupart ligament and puncture the abscess. Separate the blades of the hemostat to enlarge the opening and permit complete evacuation. Close the incision in layers.

Drainage by Ludloff Incision. When a psoas abscess points subcutaneously in the adductor region of the thigh, drainage is accomplished by a Ludloff incision, as described in Chapter 1.

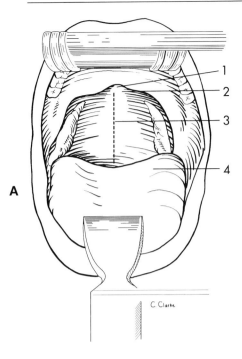
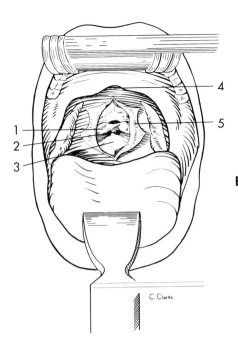

Fig. 40-18   Transoral approach to upper cervical area. **A,** Incision in posterior pharyngeal wall. *1*, Uvula; *2*, soft palate; *3*, incision in posterior pharyngeal wall; *4*, tongue. **B,** Atlas and axis exposed. *1*, Atlas; *2*, odontoid process; *3*, axis; *4*, uvula; *5*, edge of posterior pharyngeal wall retracted. (Redrawn from Fang HSY, Ong GB: *J Bone Joint Surg* 44A:1588, 1962.)

Weinberg described a method of excising a psoas abscess when simpler treatment has failed or is likely to fail because of the size of the abscess, its chronicity, or involvement with mixed bacterial infection. He removed the abscess and also any bony or cartilaginous sequestra lodged in the tract or in the diseased vertebrae. The reader is referred to his work for details of technique and aftertreatment.

Coccygectomy for Drainage of Pelvic Abscess

Lougheed and White noted that when tuberculosis involves the lower lumbar and lumbosacral areas, soft tissue abscesses may gravitate into the pelvis, forming a large abscess anterior to the sacrum. These soft tissue abscesses may point to the skin on the anterior surface of the thigh or above the iliac crest, but drainage at these sites alone is insufficient, resulting only in a chronically draining sinus despite antibacterial therapy. The pelvic abscess usually can be demonstrated roentgenographically by retrograde injection of an opaque medium. Lougheed and White devised a method of establishing dependent drainage posteriorly by coccygectomy. Their results in treatment of 10 patients by this method were uniformly good. The wound usually healed within 6 to 8 weeks, and the spinal lesions all became inactive.

TECHNIQUE 40-10 *(Lougheed and White)*

Make a 15-cm elliptical incision over the coccyx, removing a strip of skin. After freeing the coccyx from soft tissues, disarticulate it from the sacrum. With careful hemostasis carry the dissection upward, staying close to the sacrum until the resulting pyramidal tunnel communicates with the abscess cavity. After evacuating the purulent matter, insert

an irrigating catheter to the top of the cavity and pack the wound with iodoform gauze.

AFTERTREATMENT. For 2 to 3 weeks the wound is irrigated through the catheter several times daily with a solution of streptomycin. The packing is changed at intervals until the wound has healed by granulation tissue from within.

Surgical Treatment for Tuberculosis of Spine

◆ RADICAL DEBRIDEMENT AND ARTHRODESIS

TECHNIQUE 40-11 *(Hodgson et al.)*

Approach the upper cervical area (C1 and C2) through either the transoral or transthyrohyoid approach. In either approach perform a tracheostomy before operation. Have the anesthesia given through the tracheostomy opening, thus leaving the pharynx free of endotracheal tubing that would obstruct the view.

In the transoral approach, place the head in hyperextension and pack the hypopharynx. Turn back the soft palate on itself and anchor it with stay sutures, exposing the nasopharynx. Next, in the posterior pharyngeal wall make a midline incision 5 cm long with its center one fingerbreadth inferior to the anterior tubercle of the atlas that is palpable (Fig. 40-18, *A*). Carry the incision down to bone. Now strip

continued

Fig. 40-19 Transthyrohyoid approach to upper cervical area. **A,** Skin incision. *1,* Sternocleidomastoid muscle; *2,* hyoid bone; *3,* skin incision; *4,* thyroid cartilage. **B,** Incision in thyrohyoid membrane. *1,* Cut ends of sternohyoid and thyrohyoid muscles; *2,* omohyoid muscle; *3,* thyrohyoid membrane; *4,* incision in thyrohyoid membrane; *5,* epiglottis; *6,* internal laryngeal nerve and superior laryngeal artery; *7,* thyroid cartilage. **C,** Incision in posterior pharyngeal wall. *1,* Omohyoid muscle; *2,* cut ends of sternohyoid and thyrohyoid muscles; *3,* incision; *4,* posterior pharyngeal wall; *5,* cut edges of thyrohyoid membrane and hypopharyngeal mucosa. **D,** Vertebral bodies exposed. *1,* Cut edges of thyrohyoid membrane and hypopharyngeal mucosa; *2,* retracted edge of posterior pharyngeal wall; *3,* bodies of C2, C3, and C4 are exposed. (From Fang HSY, Ong GB, Hodgson AR: *Clin Orthop* 35:16, 1964.)

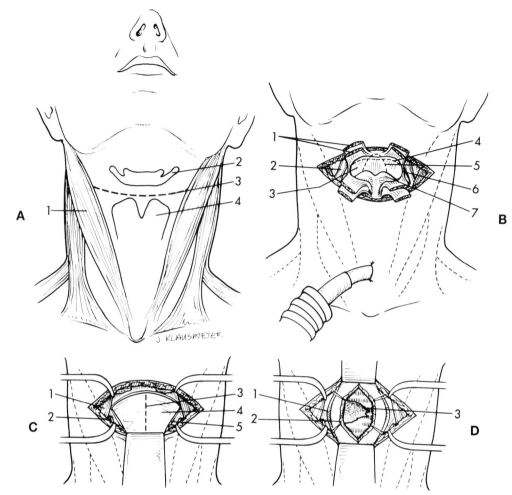

the posterior pharyngeal wall subperiosteally as far laterally as the lateral margin of the lateral masses of the atlas and the axis. Retract the raised soft tissue flaps with long stay sutures (Fig. 40-18, *B*) and control any oozing of blood by packing. The anterior arch of the atlas, the body of the axis, and the atlantoaxial joints on either side now are exposed.

For the transthyrohyoid approach, make a collar incision along the uppermost crease of the neck between the hyoid bone and the thyroid cartilage extending as far laterally as the carotid sheaths (Fig. 40-19, *A*). Divide the sternohyoid and thyrohyoid muscles, exposing the thyrohyoid membrane. Detach this membrane as near to the hyoid bone as possible to avoid damaging the internal laryngeal nerve and the superior laryngeal vessels that pierce it from the side nearer to its inferior attachment (Fig. 40-19, *B*). Next enter the hypopharynx by cutting into the exposed mucous membrane from the side to avoid damaging the epiglottis. Expose the posterior pharyngeal wall by retracting the hyoid bone and the epiglottis; make a midline incision in it down to bone (Fig. 40-19, *C*). Raise subperiosteally soft tissue flaps on either side and retract them to expose the bodies of

C2, C3, and C4 (Fig. 40-19, *D*). As an alternative, approach the upper cervical vertebrae (anterior base of the skull and C1 through C4) through a transmaxillary approach (Chapter 34).

Approach the lower cervical vertebrae (C3 through C7) through a collar incision or one along the anterior or posterior border of the sternocleidomastoid muscle (Chapter 34). Incise the abscess longitudinally, exposing the spine.

Approach the lower cervical and upper thoracic vertebrae (C7 through T3) on the side with the larger abscess through a periscapular incision similar to that used for a first-stage thoracoplasty. Elevate the scapula with a mechanical retractor and resect the third rib. The pleura usually is opened, but if it is adherent, or if for other reasons it is necessary, make an extrapleural approach. Divide the superior intercostal artery at its origin, along with the accompanying vein.

Approach the midthoracic vertebrae (T4 through T11) usually from the left side. Select the rib that in the midaxillary line lies opposite the maximal convexity of the kyphos. It usually is two ribs superior to the center of the

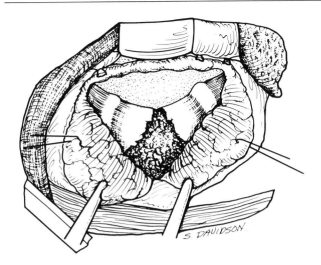

Fig. 40-20   Abscess opened with T-shaped incision through its wall. (From Hodgson AR, Stock FE: Anterior fusion. In Rob C, Smith R, eds: *Operative surgery service,* vol 9, London, 1960, Butterworth.)

vertebral focus. Make an incision along this rib, resect it, and do a standard thoracotomy. The abscess usually is seen immediately, or there may be adhesions between it and the adjacent lung. Mobilize the lung and push it anteriorly. Now make a longitudinal incision in the pleura close to the aorta in the groove between the aorta and the abscess. Displace the aorta anteriorly and medially, revealing the intercostal vessels; secure and divide these for the entire length of the abscess cavity. Divide also elements of the splanchnic nerves. Now displace the aorta anteriorly away from the spine and palpate the abscess across the anterior aspects of the vertebrae. Make a T-shaped incision through the abscess wall: the first incision is transverse and opposite the center of the disease process, and the second is longitudinal and medial to the distally placed ligatures on the intercostal vessels. Now raise the two triangular flaps, revealing the diseased area, including the inside of the abscess cavity (Fig. 40-20).

Approach the thoracolumbar area (T12 through L2) through an incision along the left eleventh rib. Keep the dissection extrapleural and retroperitoneal and separate the diaphragm from the spine. Divide the psoas muscle transversely and turn it distally. Ligate the lumbar arteries and veins, as just described for the intercostals, and proceed with the approach as for the middorsal area.

Expose the lower lumbar vertebrae (L3 and L4) through a renal approach, using a left twelfth rib incision. The psoas muscle usually is divided transversely at a more distal level, often going through an ill-defined abscess between the muscle fibers. Avoid the trunks of the lumbar plexus posterior to the muscle.

Expose the fifth lumbar and first sacral vertebrae through an extraperitoneal approach. Start the incision in the midline midway between the symphysis pubis and the umbilicus and carry it to the left in a lazy-S fashion to a point midway between the iliac crest and the lowest rib in the flank (Fig. 40-21, *A*). Divide the skin, superficial fascia, and deep fascia in line with the incision. Divide the obliquus internus abdominis muscle in the same line but across its fibers. Divide also the transversus abdominis muscle and fascia in the same line. Then expose and dissect the peritoneum from the lateral wall of the abdomen, the left psoas muscle, and the lower lumbar spine. If the bifurcation of the aorta is high, the easiest approach to the lumbosacral region is between the common iliac vessels. The only vessels encountered are the middle sacral artery and vein; cauterize and divide these (Fig. 40-21, *B*). Retract or divide any fibers of the presacral plexus as necessary. If the bifurcation of the aorta is low, make the approach lateral to the aorta, the vena cava, and the common iliac vessels. Ligate and divide the iliolumbar and ascending lumbar veins to mobilize adequately the left common iliac vein (Fig. 40-21, *C*). If necessary, ligate and divide the fifth lumbar artery and vein and, if a higher approach is required, the fourth lumbar artery and vein as well. Then displace the large vessels to the right side and protect them with retractors.

The technique of excision of the diseased tissue and of anterior arthrodesis is about the same at all levels of the spine. Remove debris, pus, and sequestrated bone or disc by suction or with a pituitary rongeur. If possible, pass the sucker anterior to or between diseased vertebrae into the abscess cavity on the opposite side, and evacuate all material. Remove with an osteotome, rongeur, or chisel all diseased bone, both soft and sclerotic, exposing the spinal canal for the whole length of the disease. Also remove with a knife or rongeur the posterior common ligament and tuberculous granulation and fibrous tissue, exposing the dura. Excise the entire vertebral body affected by the disease because collections of pus or sequestrated bone or disc material often are found in the spinal canal posterior to apparently normal posterior parts of diseased bodies. If there is a definite indication, open the dura for inspection of the cord.

Now remove the disc at each end of the cavity, exposing normal bleeding bone (Fig. 40-22, *A*). Partially correct the kyphosis by direct pressure posteriorly on the spine. After cutting a mortise in the vertebrae at each end, insert one or more strut grafts of the correct length, keeping the vertebrae sprung apart (Fig. 40-22, *B*). For the dorsal area, fashion the grafts from the rib removed during thoracotomy (Fig. 40-23); bone bank grafts may be added. For the cervical area obtain the grafts from the bone bank or from the iliac crest. For the lumbar area take a massive graft from the iliac crest (Figs. 40-24 and 40-25).

Put streptomycin and isoniazid into the cavity before closure. After thoracotomy, close the chest in the usual way

continued

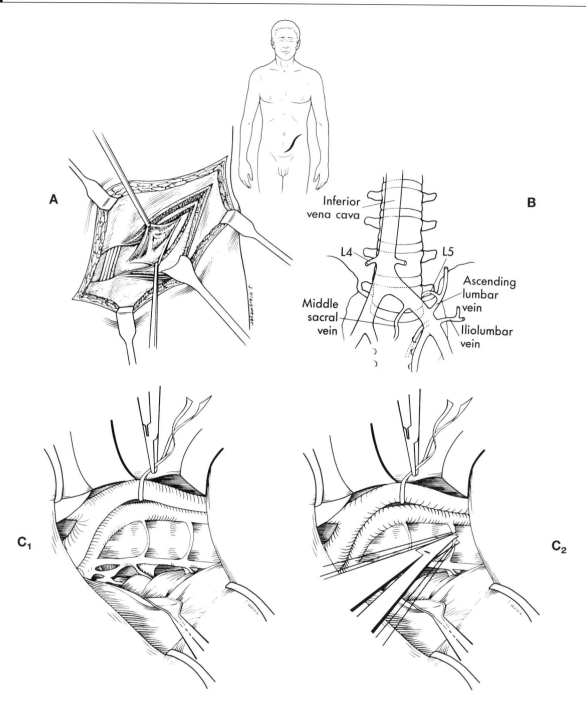

Fig. 40-21 **A,** Extraperitoneal approach to fifth lumbar and first sacral vertebrae (see text). *Inset,* Skin incision. **B,** In high bifurcation of aorta, middle sacral artery and vein are cauterized and divided. In low bifurcation of aorta, iliolumbar and ascending lumbar veins are cauterized and divided. **C1,** Exposed vertebrae are crossed by ascending lumbar vein. **C2,** Ascending lumbar vein is ligated and divided. (**A** and **B** from, **C₁** and **C₂** redrawn from Hoover NW: *J Bone Joint Surg* 50A:194, 1968.)

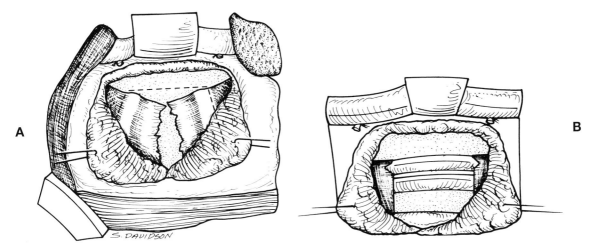

Fig. 40-22 **A,** Excision of diseased bone. **B,** Grafts inserted, keeping vertebrae sprung apart. (From Hodgson AR, Stock FE: Anterior fusion. In Rob C, Smith R, eds: *Operative surgery service*, vol 9, London, 1960, Butterworth.)

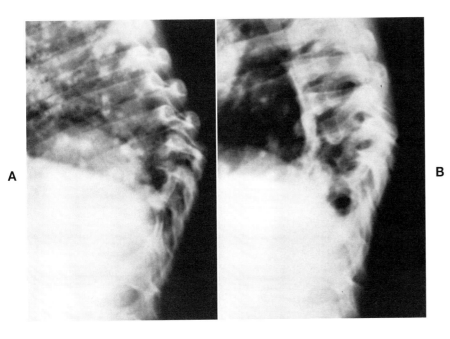

Fig. 40-23 Tuberculosis of spine without paraplegia in 4-year-old girl. **A,** Destruction of vertebral bodies before surgery. **B,** Six months after thoracotomy approach, excision of diseased bone, and anterior fusion from T6 to T11 using resected ribs for grafts; 4½ years later, pain and evidence of activity are absent.

and maintain suction drainage of the pleural space for 2 or 3 days.

AFTERTREATMENT. The patient is placed in a plaster cast consisting of anterior and posterior shells and remains there until the spine is judged to have united clinically. The time of immobilization after surgery averages about 3 months. Mobilization is then gradually started and is continued for 6 to 8 weeks, the patient being carefully watched for increasing kyphosis or other signs of disease activity.

◆ DORSOLATERAL APPROACH TO DORSAL SPINE

TECHNIQUE 40-12 *(Roaf, Kirkaldy-Willis, and Cathro)*

Expose the dorsal spine through a dorsolateral approach. Maintain careful hemostasis throughout. Select the side with the larger abscess shadow or, in the absence of an abscess, use the left side; make a curved incision. Begin posteriorly 3.8 cm from the midline, 7.5 cm proximal to the center of the lesion, and curve distally and laterally to a point 12.5 cm

continued

A B C

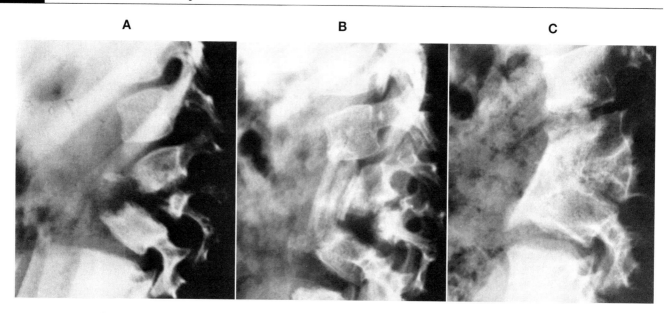

Fig. 40-24 Tuberculosis of spine in 13-year-old girl. **A,** L2, L3, and L4 are destroyed, with resulting kyphosis. **B,** One month after excision of diseased bone and grafting of bone between L1 and L4 from resected twelfth rib and from iliac crest. **C,** Three years after operation. Fusion is almost complete. (Courtesy Professor AR Hodgson.)

A B C

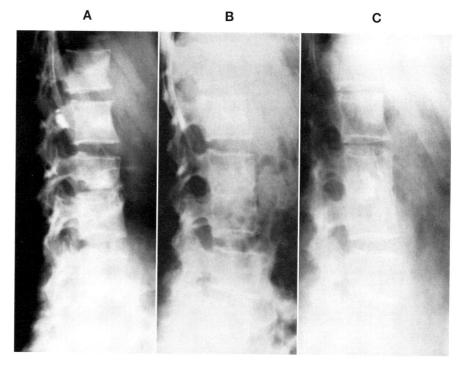

Fig. 40-25 Tuberculosis of bodies of L2 and L3 without paraplegia in 23-year-old woman. **A,** Before surgery. **B,** Six months after debridement and anterior arthrodesis through left extraperitoneal approach; grafts were from ilium. **C,** Four years after surgery; fusion is complete.

from the midline at the center of the lesion; continue medially and distally, ending 3.8 cm from the midline 7.5 cm distal to the center of the lesion (Fig. 40-26). Divide the superficial and deep fascia and the underlying muscles down to the ribs in the line of the incision. Retract the flap of the skin and muscle medially. Now locate the rib opposite the center of the focus and remove 7.5 to 10 cm of this rib and the one proximal and distal in the following manner. Free the ribs with a periosteal elevator and divide them with rib shears 7.5 to 10 cm from the tips of the transverse processes. Now resect each at the tip of the transverse process. Divide under direct vision the ligaments and

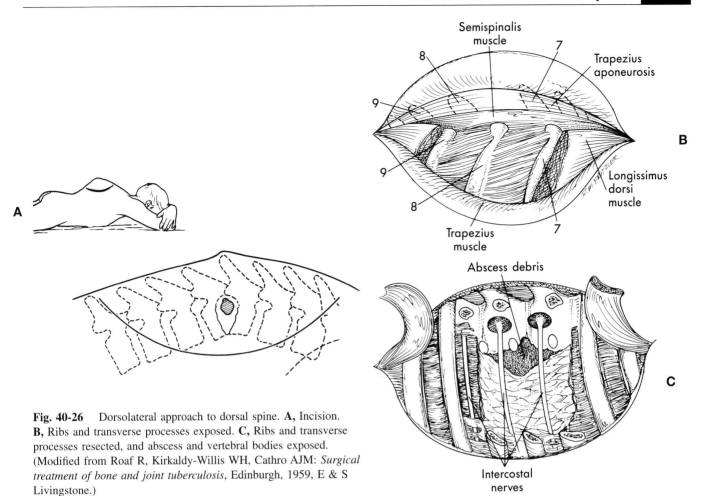

Fig. 40-26   Dorsolateral approach to dorsal spine. **A,** Incision. **B,** Ribs and transverse processes exposed. **C,** Ribs and transverse processes resected, and abscess and vertebral bodies exposed. (Modified from Roaf R, Kirkaldy-Willis WH, Cathro AJM: *Surgical treatment of bone and joint tuberculosis*, Edinburgh, 1959, E & S Livingstone.)

muscles attached to the rib heads and transverse processes and resect these bony parts. Identify two and preferably three intercostal nerves and trace them medially to the intervertebral foramina. These nerves, as they pass into the foramina, indicate the level of the cord in the spinal canal. Expose the intercostal vessels near the spinal column and cut them between clamps. Divide the intercostal muscles near the vertebral column. Separate the pleura from the spinal column by blunt dissection, exposing the lateral and anterolateral aspects of the vertebral bodies. Take care to avoid perforating the pleura, as it is often adherent and thickened; if a perforation should occur, suture it at once. Locate the center of the lesion by passing a finger into the wound anterior to the vertebral bodies. Remove all pus, granulation tissue, and necrotic matter. Occasionally one or more vertebral bodies may be sequestrated and lying free in the abscess cavity. Usually two or three small bony sequestra and pieces of necrotic disc material are found. If the paravertebral shadow, thought to be an abscess, is found to be mainly fibrous tissue, it is more difficult to find the lesion. Under these circumstances using roentgenographic

control, explore the bone with a fine gouge, burr, and rongeur. After thorough debridement decide whether bone grafts are advisable. The simplest method of grafting is to pack the cavity with bone chips. Or a more extensive procedure may be undertaken: with a chisel or gouge roughen the lateral and anterolateral aspects of the diseased vertebral bodies and, if possible, of one healthy vertebra above and below and cut a groove in them, passing from healthy bone above to healthy bone below. Wedge a full-thickness rib graft into the groove and sink it deeply within the vertebral bodies. Place cancellous bone chips obtained from the remaining portion of the resected ribs in the groove and laterally along the roughened surface of the vertebral bodies. If the pleura has been accidentally opened, drain the pleural cavity with a chest tube inserted through a small stab incision in the eighth intercostal space in the midaxillary line and connected to an underwater seal for 48 hours after surgery.

COSTOTRANSVERSECTOMY

Costotransversectomy is discussed on p. 2046.

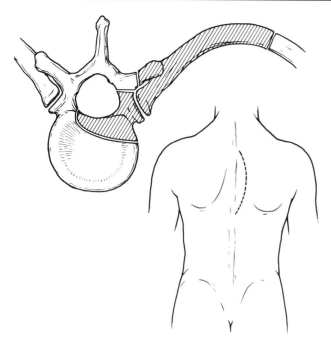

Fig. 40-27 Capener anterolateral decompression for tuberculous abscess of dorsal spine. *Stippled areas,* Extent of bone resection. *Inset,* Skin incision.

◆ ANTEROLATERAL DECOMPRESSION (LATERAL RHACHOTOMY)

In 1933 Capener originated a procedure that he called *lateral rhachotomy* and that is now popularly known as *anterolateral decompression,* in which the spine is opened from its lateral side. This affords access to the front and side of the cord, permitting decompression by the removal of bony spurs, granulation tissue, and sequestra or the evacuation of abscesses. Since the procedure entails resection of one or more pedicles, it is contraindicated if the spine is unstable. The operation at best is difficult, but is easiest when there is a sharp kyphos.

TECHNIQUE 40-13 *(Capener)*

If the disease is in the middorsal region, begin the incision in the midline at a point 10 cm proximal to the lesion, gently curve it laterally a distance of 7.5 cm, and return to the midline at a point 10 cm distal to the lesion (Fig. 40-27). Reflect the skin and superficial and deep fasciae as a thick flap. Now incise and retract laterally the origin of the trapezius muscle; divide the erector spinae muscles transversely over the rib leading to the affected intervertebral space and retract them proximally and distally. After exposing the rib subperiosteally, resect it from its angle to the transverse process; if necessary, resect the rib proximal and distal in the same manner. Now separate the intercostal nerve from its accompanying vessels and divide it, using the proximal end as a guide to further dissection and later for traction on the cord. Carefully retract the pleura along with

the intercostal vessels and remove the medial end of the rib and the transverse process and pedicle of the vertebra with a rongeur; a sphenoid punch and a motor-driven burr are of assistance at this stage. The dura and the posterolateral aspect of the vertebral body are seen after anterior depression of the pleura and the intercostal vessels and traction on the intercostal nerve. Now work from the more normal tissues in the vertebral canal toward the site of compression.

Gently remove diseased bone with a curet; also remove all impinging and encroaching tissues so carefully that the dura is not even momentarily dented. Thoroughly evacuate a paravertebral abscess if present. Close the wound in layers.

AFTERTREATMENT. Anterior and posterior plaster shells, prepared before surgery, are applied; when the lesion is in the cervical or upper dorsal region, skeletal traction should be employed. Alexander recommended that three or more ribs be widely resected to provide better exposure; Griffiths, Seddon, and Roaf, Kirkaldy-Willis, and Cathro also endorsed the more extensive approach.

TECHNIQUE 40-14 *(Seddon)*

The approach and the method of rib resection are as described for costotransversectomy on p. 2046. Resect not less than three and not more than four ribs. Isolate the intercostal nerves and trace them medially to the intervertebral foramina; now cut away the intervening intercostal muscles (Fig. 40-28, *A*). Gently push the pleura anteriorly with the fingers and determine by palpation the position of the two or three pedicles to be resected. To increase exposure, cut away small parts of the overhanging neural arches. Remove as little bone as possible dorsal to the pedicles, since anything in the least approaching hemilaminectomy is likely to be followed by a lateral subluxation of the spine. Now resect the pedicles by nibbling away from their lateral surfaces with a rongeur (Fig. 40-28, *B*). Use utmost care to avoid tearing the dura, which may be adherent to the inner surface of the pedicles. If a rent occurs, suture it as soon as possible.

Remove the offending material, such as a caseous mass, granulation tissue, a necrotic disc, or a nest of sequestra. This may be accomplished easily, but the removal of a ridge of living bone is difficult. Do not retract the cord; leave it untouched and approach the bony ridge from the side or from beneath. Drill the ridge in several places with a slowly rotating hand drill and then nibble away from the side and below with a small rongeur. The mass can be further broken up with an osteotome. The cord now rests on a shell of bone; gently push this bone anteriorly with a blunt instrument. Be sure to leave no offending ridges. Now pass a probe along the anterior surface of the cord both proximally and distally to locate any secondary cause of compression inside the

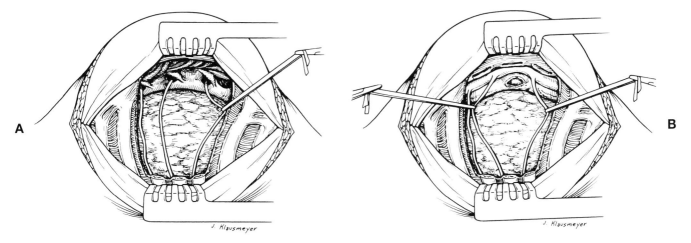

Fig. 40-28 **A,** Intercostal nerves isolated and pedicles exposed. **B,** Exposure of spinal cord after resection of three pedicles. Material anterior to cord now can be removed. Sequestrum is shown within abscess. (From Seddon HJ: Pott's paraplegia. In Platt H, ed: *Modern trends in orthopedics,* second series, London, 1956, Butterworth.)

spinal canal, such as an encapsulated caseous mass. Wash the wound with saline solution and dust it with streptomycin. Suture the muscles and skin without drainage.

AFTERTREATMENT. Aftertreatment is the same as for Technique 40-13.

References

BIOLOGY, DIAGNOSIS, AND TREATMENT OF SPINAL INFECTION

Abbey DM, Turner DM, Warson JS, et al: Treatment of postoperative wound infections following spinal fusion with instrumentation, *J Spinal Disord* 8:278, 1995.

Astagneau P, Desplaces N, Vincent V, et al: *Mycobacterium xenopi* spinal infections after discovertebral surgery: investigation and screening of a large outbreak, *Lancet* 358:747, 2001.

Batson OV: The function of the vertebral veins and their role in the spread of metastases, *Ann Surg* 112:138, 1940.

Boden SD, Davis DO, Dina TS, et al: Postoperative diskitis: distinguishing early MR imaging findings from normal postoperative disk space changes, *Radiology* 184:765, 1992.

Brant-Zawadzki M, Burke VD, Jeffrey RB: CT in the evaluation of spine infection, *Spine* 8:358, 1983.

Breschet G: *Essai sur les veines des rachis,* Paris, 1819, Méquigon-Morvith.

Casado E, Olive A, Holgado S, et al: Musculoskeletal manifestations in patients positive for human immunodeficiency virus: correlation with CD4 count, *J Rheumatol* 28:802, 2001.

Chen HC, Chen HH, Chen WJ, Tang YB: Chronic osteomyelitis of the spine managed with a free flap of latissimus dorsi: a case report, *Spine* 21:2016, 1996.

Collert S: Osteomyelitis of the spine, *Acta Orthop Scand* 48:283, 1977.

Corpataux JM, Halkic N, Wettstein M, Dusmet M: The role of laparoscopic biopsies in lumbar spondylodiscitis, *Surg Laparosc Endosc Percutan Tech* 10:417, 2000.

Coventry MB, Ghormley RK, Kernohan JW: The intervertebral disc: its microscopic anatomy and pathology. I. Anatomy, development, and physiology, *J Bone Joint Surg* 27:105, 1945.

Coventry MB, Ghormley RK, Kernohan JW: The intervertebral disc: its microscopic anatomy and physiology. III. Pathological changes in the intervertebral disc, *J Bone Joint Surg* 27:460, 1945.

Crawfurd EJ, Baird PR, Clark AL: Cauda equina and lumbar nerve root compression in patients with AIDS, *J Bone Joint Surg* 69B:36, 1987.

Croce MA, Fabian TC, Waddle-Smith L, Maxwell RA: Identification of early predictors for posttraumatic pneumonia, *Am Surg* 67:105, 2001.

Crock HV, Yoshizawa H: The blood supply of the lumbar vertebral column, *Clin Orthop* 115:6, 1976.

Darouiche RO, Hull RA: Bacterial interference for prevention of urinary tract infection: an overview, *J Spinal Cord Med* 23:136, 2000.

Digby JM, Kersley J: Pyogenic nontuberculous spinal infection, *J Bone Joint Surg* 61B:47, 1979.

Eismont FJ, Wiesel SW, Brighton CT, Rothman RH: Antibiotic penetration into rabbit nucleus pulposus, *Spine* 12:254, 1987.

Evarts CM: Diagnostic technique: closed needle biopsy, *Clin Orthop* 107:100, 1975.

Feldenzer JA, McKeever PE, Schaberg DR, et al: The pathogenesis of spinal epidural space abscess: microangiographic studies in an experimental model, *J Neurosurg* 69:110, 1988.

Fraser RD, Osti OL, Vernon-Roberts B: Discitis following chemonucleolysis: an experimental study, *Spine* 11:679, 1986.

Ghogawala Z, Mansfield FL, Borges LF: Spinal radiation before surgical decompression adversely affects outcomes of surgery for symptomatic metastatic spinal cord compression, *Spine* 26:818, 2001.

Gibson MJ, Karpinski MRK, Slack RCB, et al: The penetration of antibiotics into the normal intervertebral disc, *J Bone Joint Surg* 69B:784, 1987.

Goebels N, Helmchen C, Abele-Horn M: Extensive myelitis associated with *Mycoplasma pneumoniae* infection: magnetic resonance imaging and clinical long-term follow-up, *J Neurol* 248:204, 2001.

Golimbu C, Firooznia H, Rafii M: CT of osteomyelitis of the spine, *Am J Roentgenol* 142:159, 1984.

Hodgson AR: Infectious disease of the spine. In Rothman RH, Simeone FA, eds: *The spine,* Philadelphia, 1975, WB Saunders.

Hodgson AR, Stock FE: Anterior spinal fusion: a preliminary communication on the radical treatment of Pott's disease and Pott's paraplegia, *Br J Surg* 44:266, 1956.

Hopkinson N, Stevenson J, Benjamin S: A case ascertainment study of septic discitis: clinical, microbiological and radiological features, *QJM* 94:465, 2001.

Inoue H: Three-dimensional architecture of lumbar intervertebral discs, *Spine* 6:139, 1981.

Kalen V, Isono SS, Colin SC, Perkash I: Charcot arthropathy of the spine in long-standing paraplegia, *Spine* 12:480, 1987.

Kastenbauer S, Winkler F, Fesl G, et al: Acute severe spinal cord dysfunction in bacterial meningitis in adults: MRI findings suggest extensive myelitis, *Arch Neurol* 58:717, 2001.

Kattapuram SV, Phillips WC, Boyd R: Computed tomography in pyogenic osteomyelitis of the spine, *Am J Roentgenol* 140:1199, 1983.

Konnberg M: Erythrocyte sedimentation rate following lumbar discectomy, *Spine* 11:766, 1986.

Krodel A, Kruger A, Lohscheidt K, et al: Anterior debridement, fusion, and extrafocal stabilization in the treatment of osteomyelitis of the spine, *J Spinal Disord* 12:17, 1999.

Macnab I, St Louis EL, Grabias SL, Jacob R: Selective ascending lumbosacral venography in the assessment of lumbar-disc herniation, *J Bone Joint Surg* 58A:1093, 1976.

Modic T, Masaryk T, Plaushtek D: Magnetic resonance imaging of the spine, *Radiol Clin North Am* 14:229, 1986.

Nélaton A: *Éléments de pathologie chirurgicale*, Paris, 1844, Baillière.

Ogata K, Whiteside LA: Nutritional pathways of the intervertebral disc, *Spine* 6:211, 1981.

Picada R, Winter RB, Lonstein JE, et al: Postoperative deep wound infection in adults after posterior lumbosacral spine fusion with instrumentation: incidence and management, *J Spinal Disord* 13:42, 2000.

Pinner RW, Teutsch SM, Simonsen L, et al: Trends in infectious diseases mortality in the United States, *JAMA* 275:189, 1996.

Pott P: *Remarks on that kind of palsy of the lower limbs which is frequently found to accompany a curvature of the spine*, London, 1779, J Johnson.

Puig-Guri J: Pyogenic osteomyelitis of the spine: differential diagnosis through clinical and roentgenographic observations, *J Bone Joint Surg* 28:29, 1946.

Razak M, Kamari ZH, Roohi S: Spinal infection—an overview and the results of treatment, *Med J Malaysia* 55:C18, 2000.

Richards BR, Emara KM: Delayed infections after posterior TSRH spinal instrumentation for idiopathic scoliosis: revisited, *Spine* 26:1990, 2001.

Riley LH III, Banovac K, Martinez OV, Eismont FJ: Tissue distribution of antibiotics in the intervertebral disc, *Spine* 19:2619, 1994.

Roca RP, Yoshikawa TT: Primary skeletal infections in heroin users: a clinical characterization, diagnosis and therapy, *Clin Orthop* 144: 238, 1979.

Rodet A: Étude expérimentale sur l'ostéomyélite infectieuse, *Compt Rend Acad Sci*, pp 569-571, 1884.

Ross PM, Fleming JL: Vertebral body osteomyelitis: spectrum and natural history: a retrospective analysis of 37 cases, *Clin Orthop* 118:1890, 1976.

Ryan LM, Carrera GF, Lightfoot RW Jr, et al: The radiographic diagnosis of sacroiliitis: a comparison of different views with computed tomograms of the sacroiliac joint, *Arthritis Rheum* 26:760, 1983.

Sar C, Hamzaoglu A, Talu U, Domanic U: An anterior approach to the cervicothoracic junction of the spine (modified osteotomy of manubrium sterni and clavicle), *J Spinal Disord* 12:102, 1999.

Schellinger D: Patterns of anterior spinal canal involvement by neoplasms and infections, *Am J Neuroradiol* 17:953, 1996.

Schuster JM, Avellino AM, Mann FA, et al: Use of structural allografts in spinal osteomyelitis: a review of 47 cases, *J Neurosurg* 93:8, 2000.

Sharif HS: Role of MR imaging in the management of spinal infections, *Am J Roentgenol* 158:1333, 1992.

Stoker DJ, Kissin CM: Percutaneous vertebral biopsy: a review of 135 cases, *Clin Radiol* 36:569, 1985.

Suttner NJ, Adhami Z, Aspoas AR: *Mycobacterium chelonae* lumbar spinal infection, *Br J Neurosurg* 15:265, 2001.

Takahashi J, Ebara S, Kamimura M, et al: Early-phase enhanced inflammatory reaction after spinal instrumentation surgery, *Spine* 26:1698, 2001.

Thalgott JS, Cotler HB, Sasso RC, et al: Postoperative infections in spinal implants: classification and analysis—a multicenter study, *Spine* 16:981, 1991.

Thelander U, Larsson S: Quantitation of C-reactive protein levels and erythrocyte sedimentation rate after spinal surgery, *Spine* 17:400, 1992.

Waldvogel FA, Vasey H: Osteomyelitis: the past decade, *N Engl J Med* 303:360, 1980.

Weinstein MA, McCabe JP, Cammisa FP Jr: Postoperative spinal wound infection: a review of 2391 consecutive index procedures, *J Spinal Disord* 13:422, 2000.

Whalen JL, Parke WW, Mazur JM, Stauffer ES: The intrinsic vasculature of developing vertebral end plates and its nutritive significance to the intervertebral discs, *J Pediatr Orthop* 5:403, 1985.

Wheeler MD, Ikejema K, Enomoto N, et al: Glycine: a new antiinflammatory immunonutrient, *Cell Mol Life Sci* 56:843, 1999.

Whelan MA, Schonfeld S, Post JD, et al: Computed tomography of nontuberculous spinal infection, *J Comp Assist Tomogr* 9:280, 1985.

Wilensky AO: Osteomyelitis of the vertebra, *Ann Surg* 89:561, 1929.

Wiley AM, Trueta J: The vascular anatomy of the spine and its relationship to pyogenic vertebral osteomyelitis, *J Bone Joint Surg* 41B:796, 1959.

Wood GW II: Anatomic, biologic, and pathophysiologic aspects of spinal infections. In Wood GW II, ed: *State of the art and review, spine: spinal infections*, vol 3, no 3, Philadelphia, 1989, Hanley & Belfus.

PYOGENIC INFECTIONS

Caragee EJ: Instrumentation of the infected and unstable spine: a review of 17 cases from the thoracic and lumbar spine with pyogenic infections, *J Spinal Disord* 10:317, 1997.

Collert S: Osteomyelitis of the spine, *Acta Orthop Scand* 48:283, 1977.

Digby JM, Kersley JB: Pyogenic nontuberculous spinal infection, *J Bone Joint Surg* 61B:47, 1979.

Doita M, Marui T, Kurosaka M, et al: Contained rupture of the aneurysm of common iliac artery associated with pyogenic vertebral spondylitis, *Spine* 26:303, 2001.

Eismont FJ, Bohlman HH, Soni PL, et al: Pyogenic and fungal vertebral osteomyelitis with paralysis, *J Bone Joint Surg* 65A:19-29, 1983.

Emery SE, Chan DPK, Woodward HR: Treatment of hematogenous pyogenic vertebral osteomyelitis with anterior debridement and primary bone grafting, *Spine* 14:284, 1989.

Faraj AA, Webb JK: Spinal instrumentation for primary pyogenic infection: report of 31 patients, *Acta Orthop Belg* 66:242, 2000.

Gleckman R: Afebrile bacteremia: a phenomenon in geriatric patients, *JAMA* 248:1478, 1982.

Hadjipavlou AG, Mader JT, Necessary JT, Muffoletto AJ: Hematogenous pyogenic spinal infections and their surgical management, *Spine* 25:1668, 2000.

Kirkaldy-Willis WH, Thomas TG: Anterior approaches in the diagnosis and treatment of infections of the vertebral bodies, *J Bone Joint Surg* 47A:87, 1965.

Lindholm TS, Pylkkänen P: Discitis following removal of intervertebral disc, *Spine* 7:618, 1982.

Morrey BF, Kelly PJ, Nichols DR: Viridans streptococcal osteomyelitis of the spine, *J Bone Joint Surg* 62A:1009, 1980.

Muffolerro AJ, Ketonen LM, Mader JT, et al: Hematogenous pyogenic facet joint infection, *Spine* 26:1570, 2001.

Muffolerro AJ, Nader R, Westmark RM et al: Hematogenous pyogenic facet joint infection of the subaxial cervical spine: a report of two cases and review of the literature, *J Neurosurg* 95:135, 2001.

Nichols BL: Nutrition and infection, *South Med J* 71:705, 1978.

Przybylski GJ, Sharan AD: Single-stage autogenous bone grafting and internal fixation in the surgical management of pyogenic discitis and vertebral osteomyelitis, *J Neurosurg* 94:1, 2001.

Puranen J, Mäkelä J, Lähde S: Postoperative intervertebral discitis, *Acta Orthop Scand* 55:461, 1984.

Ray MJ, Bassett RL: Pyogenic vertebral osteomyelitis, *Orthopedics* 8:506, 1985.

Stone JL, Cybulski GR, Rodriguez J, Gryfinski ME: Anterior cervical debridement and strut-grafting for osteomyelitis of the cervical spine, *J Neurosurg* 70:879, 1989.

Velan GJ, Leitner J, Gepstein R: Pyogenic osteomyelitis of the spine in the elderly: three cases of a synchronous non-axial infection by a different pathogen, *Spinal Cord* 37:215, 1999.

Waldvogel FA, Medoff G, Swartz MN: Osteomyelitis: a review of clinical features, therapeutic considerations and unusual aspects. I, *N Engl J Med* 282:198, 1976.

Waldvogel FA, Vasey H: Osteomyelitis: the past decade, *N Engl J Med* 303:360, 1980.

Wilensky AO: Osteomyelitis of the vertebra, *Ann Surg* 89:561, 1929.

Wrobel CJ, Chappell ET, Taylor W: Clinical presentation, radiological findings, and treatment results of coccidioidomycosis involving the spine: report on 23 cases, *J Neurosurg* 95:33, 2001.

INFECTIONS IN CHILDREN

Boston HC Jr, Bianco AJ Jr, Rhodes KH: Disk space infections in children, *Orthop Clin North Am* 6:953, 1975.

Muffoletto AJ, Ketonen LM, Mader JT, et al: Hematogenous pyogenic facet joint infection, *Spine* 15:1570, 2001.

Nade S: Acute haematogenous osteomyelitis in infancy and childhood, *J Bone Joint Surg* 65B:109, 1983.

Scoles PV, Quinn TP: Intervertebral discitis in children and adolescents, *Clin Orthop* 162:31, 1982.

Spiegel PG, Kengla KW, Isaacson AS, Wilson JC Jr: Intervertebral disc space inflammation in children, *J Bone Joint Surg* 54A:284, 1972.

Van Dalen IV, Heeg M: Neonatal infectious spondylitis of the cervical spine presenting with quadriplegia: a case report, *Spine* 25:1450, 2000.

Wenger DR, Bobechko WP, Gilday DL: The spectrum of intervertebral disc-space infection in children, *J Bone Joint Surg* 60A:100, 1978.

EPIDURAL SPACE INFECTION

Chandnani VP, Beltran J, Morris CS, et al: Acute experimental osteomyelitis and abscesses: detection with MR imaging versus CT, *Radiology* 174:233, 1990.

Feldenzer JA, McKeever PE, Schaberg DR, et al: The pathogenesis of spinal epidural abscess: microangiographic studies in an experimental model, *J Neurosurg* 69:110, 1988.

Heusner AP: Nontuberculous spinal epidural infection, *N Engl J Med* 239:845, 1948.

Mampalam TJ, Rosegay H, Andrews BT, et al: Nonoperative treatment of spinal epidural infections, *J Neurosurg* 71:208, 1989.

Reihsaus E, Waldbaur H, Seeling W: Spinal epidural abscess: a meta-analysis of 915 patients, *Neurosurg Rev* 23:175, 2000.

Smith AS, Blaser SI: Infectious and inflammatory processes of the spine, *Radiol Clin North Am* 29:809, 1991.

Tung GA, Yim JW, Mermel LA, et al: Spinal epidural abscess: correlation between MRI findings and outcome, *Neuroradiology* 41:904, 1999.

Tzen KY, Yen TC, Yang RS, et al: The role of 67Ga in the early detection of spinal epidural abscesses, *Nucl Med Commun* 21:165, 2000.

Veillard E, Guggenbuhl P, Morcet N, et al: Prompt regression of paravertebral and epidural abscesses in patients with pyogenic discitis. Sixteen cases evaluated using magnetic resonance imaging, *Joint Bone Spine* 67:219, 2000.

Wang LP, Hauerberg J, Schmidt JF: Long-term outcome after neurosurgically treated spinal epidural abscess following epidural analgesia, *Acta Anaesthesiol Scand* 45:233, 2001.

BRUCELLOSIS

Goodhart GL, Zakem JF, Collins WC, Meyer JD: Brucellosis of the spine: report of a patient with bilateral paraspinal abscesses, *Spine* 12:414, 1987.

Lifeso RM, Harder E, McCorkell SJ: Spinal brucellosis, *J Bone Joint Surg* 67B:345, 1985.

Moehring HD: Brucella sacroiliitis: a case report, *Orthopedics* 8:499, 1985.

Nas K, Gur A, Kemaloglu MS, et al: Management of spinal brucellosis and outcome of rehabilitation, *Spinal Cord* 39:223, 2001.

Samra Y, Hertz M, Shaked Y, et al: Brucellosis of the spine: a report of three cases, *J Bone Joint Surg* 64B:429, 1982.

FUNGAL INFECTIONS

Assaad W, Cohen L, Esguerra JV, Whittier FC: *Aspergillus* discitis with acute disc abscess, *Spine* 19:2226, 1994.

Barnwell PA, Jelsma LF, Raff MJ: Aspergillus osteomyelitis: report of a case and review of the literature, *Diagn Microbiol Infect Dis* 3:515, 1985.

Eismont FJ, Bohlman HH, Soni PL, et al: Pyogenic and fungal vertebral osteomyelitis with paralysis, *J Bone Joint Surg* 65A:19, 1983.

Ferris B, Jones C: Paraplegia due to aspergillosis: successful conservative treatment of two cases, *J Bone Joint Surg* 67B:800, 1985.

Frazier DD, Campbell DR, Garvey TA, et al: Fungal infections of the spine: report of eleven patients with long-term follow-up, *J Bone Joint Surg* 83A:560, 2001.

Govender S, Rajoo R, Goga IE, Charles RW: *Aspergillus* osteomyelitis of the spine, *Spine* 16:746, 1991.

Halpern AA, Rinsky LA, Fountain S, Nagel DA: Coccidioidomycosis of the spine: unusual roentgenographic presentation, *Clin Orthop* 140:78, 1979.

Matsushita T, Suzuki K: Spastic paraparesis due to cryptococcal osteomyelitis: a case report, *Clin Orthop* 196:279, 1985.

Mawk JR, Erickson DL, Chou SN, Seljeskog EL: *Aspergillus* infections of the lumbar disc spaces: report of three cases, *J Neurosurg* 58:270, 1983.

Vinas FC, King PK, Diaz FG: Spinal Aspergillus osteomyelitis, *Clin Infect Dis* 28:1223, 1999.

Williams RL, Fukui MB, Meltzer CC, et al: Fungal spinal osteomyelitis in the immunocompromised patient: MR findings in three cases, *Am J Neuroradiol* 20:381, 1999.

TUBERCULOSIS

Acker JD, Wood GW II, Moinuddin M, Eggers FM: Radiologic manifestations of spinal infection. In Wood GW II, ed: *Spinal infections*, Philadelphia, 1989, Hanley & Belfus.

Albee FH: Transplantation of a portion of the tibia into the spine for Pott's disease: a preliminary report, *JAMA* 57:885, 1911.

Alexander GL: Neurological complications of spinal tuberculosis, *Proc R Soc Med* 39:730, 1945-1946.

Capener N: Personal communication to Girdlestone GR, 1934. Cited in Platt H, ed: *Modern trends in orthopaedics*, New York, 1950, Paul B Hoeber.

Capener N: The evolution of lateral rhachotomy, *J Bone Joint Surg* 36B:173, 1954.

Davies PDO, Humphries MJ, Byfield SP, et al: Bone and joint tuberculosis: a survey of notifications in England and Wales, *J Bone Joint Surg* 66B:326, 1984.

Dickson JA: Spinal tuberculosis in Nigerian children: a review of ambulant treatment, *J Bone Joint Surg* 49B:682, 1967.

Dove J, Hsu LCS, Yau ACMC: The cervical spine after halo-pelvic traction: an analysis of the complications in 83 patients, *J Bone Joint Surg* 62B:158, 1980.

Dusmet M, Halkic N, Corpataux JM: Video-assisted thoracic surgery diagnosis of thoracic spinal tuberculosis, *Chest* 116:1471, 1999.

Ehara S: Osteoarticular tuberculosis, *Semin Musculoskelet Radiol* 5:107, 2001.

Eighth report of the Medical Research Council Working Party on Tuberculosis of the Spine. A 10-year assessment of a controlled trial comparing debridement and anterior spinal fusion in the management of tuberculosis of the spine in patients on standard chemotherapy in Hong Kong, *J Bone Joint Surg* 64B:393, 1982.

Enarson DA, Fujii M, Nakielna EM, Grzybowski S: Bone and joint tuberculosis: a continuing problem, *Can Med Assoc J* 120:139, 1979.

Fang D, Leong JC, Fang HS: Tuberculosis of the upper cervical spine, *J Bone Joint Surg* 65B:47, 1983.

Fang HSY, Ong GB, Hodgson AR: Anterior spinal fusion, the operative approaches, *Clin Orthop* 35:16, 1964.

Fifth report of the Medical Research Council Working Party on Tuberculosis of the Spine, Brompton Hospital, London, England: A five-year assessment of controlled trials of in-patient and out-patient treatment and of plaster-of-Paris jackets for tuberculosis of the spine in children on standard chemotherapy: studies in Masan and Pusan, Korea, *J Bone Joint Surg* 58B:399, 1976.

First report of the Medical Research Council Working Party on Tuberculosis of the Spine: A controlled trial of ambulant out-patient treatment and in-patient rest in bed in management of tuberculosis of the spine in young Korean patients on standard chemotherapy: a study in Masan, Korea, *J Bone Joint Surg* 55B:678, 1973.

Fourteenth report of the Medical Research Council Working Party on Tuberculosis of the Spine: Five-year assessment of controlled trials of short-course chemotherapy regimens of 6, 9, or 18 months' duration for spinal tuberculosis in patients ambulatory from the start or undergoing radical surgery, *Int Orthop* 23:73, 1999.

Fourth report of the Medical Research Council Working Party on Tuberculosis of the Spine: A controlled trial of anterior spinal fusion and debridement in the surgical management of tuberculosis of the spine in patients on standard chemotherapy: a study in Hong Kong, *Br J Surg* 61:853, 1974.

Francis IM, Das DK, Luthra UK, et al: Value of radiologically guided fine needle aspiration cytology (FNAC) in the diagnosis of spinal tuberculosis: a study of 29 cases, *Cytopathology* 10:390, 1999.

Gorse GJ, Pais MP, Kusske JA, Cesario TC: Tuberculous spondylitis: a report of six cases and a review of the literature, *Medicine* 62:178, 1983.

Govender S, Parbhoo AH: Support of the anterior column with allografts in tuberculosis of the spine, *J Bone Joint Surg* 81:106, 1999.

Govender S, Parbhoo AH, Kumar KP, Annamalai K: Anterior spinal decompression in HIV-positive patients with tuberculosis: a prospective study, *J Bone Joint Surg* 83:864, 2001.

Griffiths DL: Pott's paraplegia and its operative treatment, *J Bone Joint Surg* 35B:487, 1953.

Gupta RK, Agarwal P, Rastogi H, et al: Problems in distinguishing spinal tuberculosis from neoplasia on MRI, *Neuroradiology* 38:S97, 1996.

Hibbs RA: An operation for progressive spinal deformities, *NY Med J* 93:1013, 1911.

Hodgson AR, Skinsnes OK, Leong CY: The pathogenesis of Pott's paraplegia, *J Bone Joint Surg* 49A:1147, 1967.

Hodgson AR, Stock FE: Anterior spinal fusion: a preliminary communication on the radical treatment of Pott's disease and Pott's paraplegia, *Br J Surg* 44:266, 1956.

Hodgson AR, Stock FE: Anterior fusion. In Rob C, Smith R, eds: *Operative surgery service*, vol 9, London, 1960, Butterworth.

Hodgson AR, Stock FE: Anterior spine fusion for the treatment of tuberculosis of the spine: the operative findings and results of treatment of the first one hundred cases, *J Bone Joint Surg* 42A:295, 1960.

Hodgson AR, Stock FE, Fang HSY, Ong GB: Anterior spinal fusion: the operative approach and pathological findings in 412 patients with Pott's disease of the spine, *Br J Surg* 48:172, 1960.

Hodgson AR, Yau A, Kwon JS, Kim D: A clinical study of 100 consecutive cases of Pott's paraplegia, *Clin Orthop* 36:128, 1964.

Hoover MJ Jr: The treatment of the tuberculous psoas abscess, *South Surg* 16:729, 1950.

Hoover NW: Methods of lumbar fusion, *J Bone Joint Surg* 50A:194, 1968.

Hsu LCS, Leong JCY: Tuberculosis of the lower cervical spine (C2 to C7): a report on 40 cases, *J Bone Joint Surg* 66B:1, 1984.

Hsu LCS, Cheng CL, Leong JCY: Pott's paraplegia of late onset: the cause of compression and results after anterior decompression, *J Bone Joint Surg* 70B:534, 1988.

Ito H, Tsuchija J, Asami G: A new radical operation for Pott's disease, *J Bone Joint Surg* 16:449, 1934.

Jain AK, Aggarwal A, Mehrotra G: Correlation of canal encroachment with neurological deficit in tuberculosis of the spine, *Int Orthop* 23:85, 1999.

Jain AK, Kumar S, Tuli SM: Tuberculosis of the spine (C1 to D4), *Spinal Cord* 37:362, 1999.

Jones AR: The influence of Hugh Owen Thomas on the evolution of treatment of skeletal tuberculosis, *J Bone Joint Surg* 35B:309, 1958.

Jones BS: Pott's paraplegia in the Nigerian, *J Bone Joint Surg* 40B:16, 1958.

Kemp HBS, Jackson JW, Jeremiah JD, Cook J: Anterior fusion of the spine for infective lesions in adults, *J Bone Joint Surg* 55B:715, 1973.

Leibert E, Schluger NW, Bonk S, Rom WN: Spinal tuberculosis in patients with human immunodeficiency virus infection: clinical presentation, therapy and outcome, *Tuber Lung Dis* 77:329, 1996.

Li JQ: Operative treatment of 183 cases of tuberculosis of the cervical spine, *Chinese J Orthop* 3:231, 1983.

Lifeso R: Atlanto-axial tuberculosis in adults, *J Bone Joint Surg* 69B:183, 1987.

Lonser RR, Brodke DS, Dailey AT: Vertebral osteomyelitis secondary to *Pseudallescheria boydii, J Spinal Disord* 14:361, 2001.

Lougheed JC, White WG: Anterior dependent drainage for tuberculous lumbosacral spinal lesions: coccygectomy and dependent drainage in treatment of tuberculous lesions of the lower spine with associated soft-tissue abscesses, *Arch Surg* 81:961, 1960.

Medical Resource Council Working Party on Tuberculosis of the Spine. Five-year assessments of controlled trials of ambulatory treatment, debridement and anterior spinal fusion in the management of tuberculosis of the spine: studies in Bulawayo (Rhodesia) and in Hong Kong, *J Bone Joint Surg* 60B:163, 1978.

Ménard V: *Étude pratique sur le mal du Pott*, Paris, 1900, Masson et Cie.

Naim-Ur-Rahman: Atypical forms of spinal tuberculosis, *J Bone Joint Surg* 62B:162, 1980.

Neal SL, Kearns MA, Seelig JM, Harris JP: Manifestations of Pott's disease in the head and neck, *Laryngoscope* 96:494, 1986.

Odom SR, Stallard JD, Pacheco HO, Ho H: Postoperative staphylococcal toxic shock syndrome due to preexisting staphylococcal infection: case report and review of the literature, *Am Surg* 67:745, 2001.

Rajasekaran S, Shanmugasundaram TK: Prediction of the angle of gibbus deformity in tuberculosis of the spine, *J Bone Joint Surg* 69A:503, 1987.

Roaf R, Kirkaldy-Willis WH, Cathro AJM: *Surgical treatment of bone and joint tuberculosis*, Edinburgh, 1959, E & S Livingstone.

Seddon HJ: Pott's paraplegia, *Br J Surg* 22:769, 1935.

Seddon HJ: The pathology of Pott's paraplegia, *Proc R Soc Med* 39:723, 1945-1946.

Seddon HJ: Anterolateral decompression of Pott's paraplegia, *J Bone Joint Surg* 33B:461, 1951.

Seddon HJ: Treatment of Pott's paraplegia by anterolateral decompression, *Mém Acad Chir* 79:281, 1952.

Seddon HJ: Pott's paraplegia and its operative treatment, *J Bone Joint Surg* 35B:487, 1953.

Seddon HJ: Pott's paraplegia. In Platt H, ed: *Modern trends in orthopaedics* (second series), London, 1956, Butterworth.

Seddon HJ, Alexander GL: Discussion of spinal caries with paraplegia, *Proc R Soc Med* 39:723, 1946.

Shanley DJ: Tuberculosis of the spine: imaging features, *Am J Roentgenol* 164:659, 1995.

Sixth report of the Medical Research Council Working Party on Tuberculosis of the Spine: Five-year assessments of controlled trials of ambulatory treatment, debridement and anterior spinal fusion in the management of tuberculosis of the spine studies in Bulawayo (Rhodesia) and in Hong Kong, *J Bone Joint Surg* 60B:163, 1978.

Smith TK, Livermore NB: Hoarseness accompanying Pott's paraplegia, *J Bone Joint Surg* 63A:159, 1981.

Upadhyay SS, Orth D, Saji MJ, et al: Longitudinal changes in spinal deformity after anterior spinal surgery for tuberculosis of the spine in adults: a comparative analysis between radical and debridement surgery, *Spine* 19:542, 1994.

Upadhyay SS, Saji MJ, Yau AC: Duration of antituberculosis chemotherapy in conjunction with radical surgery in the management of spinal tuberculosis, *Spine* 21:1898, 1996.

Weinberg JA: The surgical excision of psoas abscesses resulting from spinal tuberculosis, *J Bone Joint Surg* 39A:17, 1957.

Yau ACMC, Hodgson AR: Penetration of the lung by the paravertebral abscess in tuberculosis of the spine, *J Bone Joint Surg* 50A:243, 1968.

Yilmaz C, Selek HY, Gurkan I, et al: Anterior instrumentation for the treatment of spinal tuberculosis, *J Bone Joint Surg* 81A:1261, 1999.

C H A P T E R

41 Other Disorders of Spine

Douglas A. Linville

Spinal Stenosis

Before the development of roentgenograms, there were scattered reports of paralysis caused by narrowing of the spinal canal. The first verifiable report of lumbar spinal stenosis relieved by two-level laminectomy was that of Sachs and Fraenkel in 1900. Bailey and Casamajor in 1911 and Elsberg in

1913 wrote similar descriptions of the symptoms, pathological findings, and relief after surgery. The syndrome was not widely diagnosed until Verbiest in 1954 described the classic findings of middle-aged and older adults with back and lower extremity pain precipitated by standing and walking and aggravated by hyperextension. He delineated congenital narrowing of the spinal canal as a contributing factor in many and the secondary development of degenerative changes that further narrowed the lumbar canal and precipitated symptoms. Myelographic block in the midlumbar region with the characteristic degenerative hypertrophic changes about the discs, facets, and ligamentous structures was described in detail. A subsequent article by Verbiest on lumbar spondylosis documented detailed measurements of the spinal canal obtained during surgery. Since that time the syndrome has been well recognized, and numerous well-documented series have been reported. An excellent four-part review of the entire topic was published by Ehni et al. in 1969.

Dunlop, Adams, and Hutton in a cadaver study found a significant increase in pressure on the facet joints with disc space narrowing and increasing angles of extension. Degenerative spinal stenosis has been attributed to simple hypertrophic overgrowth of the superior articular facets that is the result of a progressive degeneration of the disc with resultant instability or hypermobility in the facet joints. As joint destruction progresses, the hypertrophic process finally results in local ankylosis. Calcification and hypertrophy of the ligamentum flavum and venous hypertension resulting in generalized bone overgrowth also may be contributing factors. Mild trauma and occupational activity do not appear to significantly affect the development of this disease, but they may exacerbate a preexisting condition.

ANATOMY

Spinal stenosis can be categorized according to the anatomical area of the spine affected, the region of each vertebral segment affected, and the specific pathological entity involved (Table 41-1). Stenosis can be generalized or localized to specific anatomical areas of the cervical, thoracic, or lumbar spine. It is most common in the lumbar region, but cervical stenosis also occurs frequently. It has been reported rarely in the thoracic spine. Spinal stenosis can be localized or diffuse, affecting multiple levels as in congenital stenosis. Degeneration of the disc occurs with disc narrowing and subsequent ligamentous redundancy, which compromises the spinal canal area. Instability may ensue, aggravating symptoms by the formation of facet overgrowth and ligamentous hypertrophy. The ligamentum flavum may be markedly thickened into the lateral recess where it attaches to the facet capsule, causing nerve root compression. These phenomena occur alone or in combination to create the symptomatic complex characteristic of spinal stenosis.

A description of spinal stenosis requires an understanding of the anatomy affected and the use of consistent terminology (Fig. 41-1). *Central spinal stenosis* denotes involvement of the area between the facet joints, which is occupied by the dura and its contents. Stenosis in this region usually is caused by protrusion of a disc, annulus, or osteophytes or by buckled or thickened ligamentum flavum. Symptomatic central spinal stenosis results in neurogenic claudication. Lateral to the dura is the lateral canal, which contains the nerve roots; compression in this region results in radiculopathy. The *lateral recess*, also

known as "Lee's entrance zone," begins at the lateral border of the dura and extends to the medial border of the pedicle. This is where the nerve root exits the dura and courses distally and laterally under the superior articular facet (Fig. 41-2, *A*). The borders of the lateral recess are the pedicle laterally, the superior articular facet dorsally, the disc and posterior ligamentous complex (PLC) ventrally, and the central canal medially. Ciric et al. reported that facet arthritis most frequently causes stenosis in this zone, along with vertebral body spurring and disc or annulus pathology. "Lee's mid-zone" describes the *foraminal region,* which lies ventral to the pars. Its borders are the lateral recess medially, the posterior vertebral body and disc ventrally, the pars distally, and the lateral border of the pedicle laterally. The dorsal root ganglion and ventral motor root occupy up to 30% of this space. This also is the point where the dura becomes confluent with the nerve root as epineurium. Causes of stenosis in this area are pars fracture with proliferative fibrocartilage or a lateral disc herniation (Fig. 41-2, *B*). Thickening of the ligamentum flavum sometimes persists into the foramen and can be associated with a spur from the undersurface of the pars, especially if foraminal height is less than 15 mm and posterior vertebral body height is less than 4 mm. The *exit zone* is identified as the area lateral to the facet

◤ **Table 41-1** Classification of Spinal Stenosis

Anatomical Area	Anatomical Region (Local Segment)
ANATOMICAL	
Cervical	Central
	Foraminal
Thoracic	Central
Lumbar	Central
	Lateral recess
	Foraminal
	Extraforaminal (far-out)

PATHOLOGICAL
Congenital
Achondroplastic (dwarfism)
   Congenital forms of spondylolisthesis
   Scoliosis
   Kyphosis
   Idiopathic

Degenerative and Inflammatory
Osteoarthritis
Inflammatory arthritis
Diffuse idiopathic skeletal hyperostosis (DISH)
Scoliosis
Kyphosis
Degenerative forms of spondylolisthesis

Metabolic
Paget disease
Fluorosis

joint. The nerve root is present in this location and can be compressed by a "far-lateral" disc, spondylolisthesis and associated subluxation, or facet arthritis.

The most common type of spinal stenosis is caused by degenerative arthritis of the spine, including Forestier syndrome, and is characterized by hyperostosis and spinal rigidity in elderly patients. Congenital forms caused by disorders such as achondroplasia and dysplastic spondylolisthesis are much less frequent. Finally, other processes such as Paget disease, fluorosis, kyphosis, scoliosis, and fracture with canal narrowing

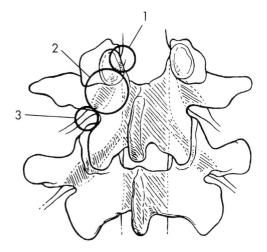

Fig. 41-1 Zones of lateral canal as described by Lee. *Entrance zone (1)* is cephalad and medial aspects of lateral recess that begins at lateral aspect of thecal sac and runs obliquely down and laterally toward intervertebral foramen. *Mid-zone (2)* is located beneath pars interarticularis and just inferior to pedicle and is bounded anteriorly by posterior aspect of vertebral body and posteriorly by pars; medial boundary is open to central spinal canal. *Exit zone (3)* is formed by intervertebral foramen. (From An HS, Butler JP: *Semin Spine Surg* 11:184, 1999.)

have been reported to result in spinal stenosis. Hypertrophy and ossification of the posterior longitudinal ligament in the cervical spine (diffuse idiopathic skeletal hyperostosis [DISH] syndrome) also may result in an acquired form of spinal stenosis. This disease usually is confined to the cervical spine.

Differentiation between the pathological processes causing spinal stenosis is relatively simple. Congenital spinal stenosis usually is central and evident on imaging studies. In achondroplasia the canal is narrowed in both the anteroposterior plane due to shortened pedicles and in lateral diameter because of diminished interpedicular distance. These findings occur in addition to the other characteristic features of achondroplasia. Idiopathic congenital narrowing usually involves one dimension of canal measurement, and the patient otherwise is normal.

Acquired forms of spinal stenosis usually are degenerative (Box 41-1) and are localized to the facet joints and ligamentum flavum, with additional arthritic changes in the joints visible on roentgenographic studies. Frequently these abnormalities are symmetrical. The L4-5 level is the most commonly involved, followed by L5-S1 and L3-4. Disc herniation and spondylolisthesis may further exacerbate the narrowing. Spondylolisthesis and spondylolysis rarely cause spinal stenosis in young patients. The combination of degenerative change, aging, and spondylolisthesis or spondylolysis in patients 50 years or older frequently results in lateral recess or foraminal stenosis. Paget disease and fluorosis have been reported to result in central or lateral spinal stenosis. Paget disease is one form of spinal stenosis that responds well to medical treatment with calcitonin.

NATURAL HISTORY

The natural course of all forms of spinal stenosis is the insidious development of symptoms occasionally exacerbated

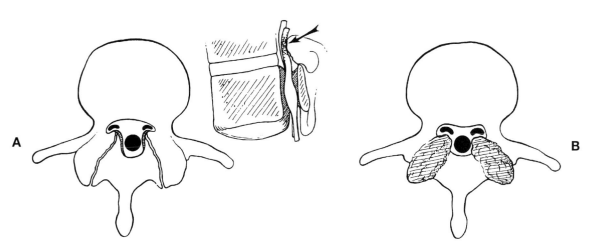

Fig. 41-2   A, Entrance zone stenosis. Hypertrophy of superior articular process narrows lateral recess and compresses nerve root. **B,** Mid-zone stenosis. Fibrocartilaginous mass associated with spondylolysis may impinge on nerve root at distal level and medial to pedicle level. (From An HS, Butler JP: *Semin Spine Surg* 11:184, 1999.)

BOX 41-1 • Classification of Spinal Stenosis

CONGENITAL
Idiopathic
Achondroplastic

ACQUIRED
Degenerative
  Central canal
  Lateral recess, foramen
  Degenerative spondylolisthesis
  Degenerative scoliosis
Combination of congenital and degenerative stenosis
Iatrogenic
  Postlaminectomy
  Postfusion
  Postchemonucleolysis
Spondylolytic
Posttraumatic
Miscellaneous
  Paget disease
  Fluorosis
  Diffuse idiopathic skeletal hyperostosis syndrome
  Hyperostotic lumbar spinal stenosis
  Oxalosis
  Pseudogout

---

by trauma or heavy activity. Many patients have significant roentgenographic findings with minimal complaints or physical findings. Johnsson, Rosén, and Udén reported that 19 (70%) of 27 patients with moderate, untreated spinal stenosis (11 mm or more anteroposterior canal diameter) remained unchanged after 4 years of observation; 4 (15%) improved, and 4 deteriorated without serious sequelae. In a separate study, Johnsson et al. found that 11 of 19 (58%) untreated patients were unchanged at 31-month follow-up, 6 were improved, and only 2 were worse.

In a prospective, randomized study by Amundsen et al. of 100 patients with symptomatic spinal stenosis, 19 patients with severe symptoms were treated operatively, 50 patients with moderate symptoms were treated conservatively, and 31 patients were randomized to receive operative (13) or conservative (18) treatment. Pain relief was noted after 3 months in most patients regardless of treatment but took as long as 12 months in a few patients. However, results in conservatively treated patients deteriorated over time, and at 4 years were excellent or fair in 50% of patients treated nonoperatively; 80% of those treated operatively still had good results. Results were not worse if surgery was done 3 years after failed conservative treatment, and significant deterioration did not occur during the 6 years of follow-up in any of the three groups of patients. Predictors of poor outcomes could not be identified. These authors concluded that conservative treatment is appropriate for patients with moderate pain, 50% of whom will have pain relief in less than 3 months, but operative treatment probably is indicated for patients with severe pain and those in whom conservative treatment fails.

Reported studies suggest that for most patients with spinal stenosis a stable course can predicted, with 15% to 50% showing some improvement with nonoperative treatment. Worsening of symptoms despite adequate conservative treatment is an indication for operative treatment.

CLINICAL EVALUATION

In a group of 100 patients, Amundsen et al. found back pain and sciatica present in 95% and claudication present in 91%. Sensory disturbance in the legs was present in 70%, with motor weakness in 33%, and voiding disturbance present in only 12% of patients. Despite the coexistent symptoms, back pain had been present for a median duration of 14 years and sciatica for a median duration of 2 years before presentation. Bilateral leg complaints were present in 42%, and unilateral leg symptoms were present in the other 58%. Distribution of symptoms was L5 in 91%, S1 in 63%, L1-4 in 28%, and S2-5 in 5%. Forty-seven patients (47%) had symptoms specific for two nerve roots, and 35% had monoradiculopathy. Three- and four-level radicular complaints were recorded in 17% and 1%, respectively. In patients with central spinal stenosis, symptoms usually are bilateral and involve the buttocks and posterior thighs in a nondermatomal distribution. With lateral recess stenosis, symptoms usually are dermatomal because they are related to a specific nerve being compressed. Patients with lateral recess stenosis may have more pain during rest and at night but more walking tolerance than patients with central stenosis.

Differentiation of symptoms of vascular claudication from those of neurogenic claudication is important (Table 41-2). Vascular symptoms typically are felt in the upper calf, are relieved after a short rest (5 minutes) while still standing, do not require sitting or bending, and worsen despite walking uphill or riding a stationary bicycle. Neurogenic claudication improves with trunk flexion, stooping, or lying but may require up to 20 minutes to improve. Patients often report better endurance walking uphill or up steps and tolerate riding a bicycle better than walking on a treadmill because of the flexed posture that occurs. Pushing a grocery cart also allows spinal flexion, which enhances endurance in most patients with neurogenic claudication.

Generally, physical findings with all forms of spinal stenosis are inconsistent. Distal pulses should be felt and confirmed to be strong, and internal and external rotation of the hips in extension should be full, symmetrical, and painless. Straight leg raising and sciatic tension tests usually are normal. The neurological examination usually is normal, but some abnormality may be detected if the patient is allowed to walk to the limit of pain and is then reexamined. The gait and posture after walking may reveal a positive "stoop test." This test is done by asking the patient to walk briskly. As the pain intensifies, the patient may complain of sensory symptoms followed by motor symptoms. If the patient is asked to continue to walk, he may assume a stooped posture, and the symptoms may be eased; or, if he sits in a chair bent forward, the same resolution of symptoms will occur.

Table 41-2 Differentiation of Symptoms of Vascular Claudication from Those of Neurogenic Claudication

Evaluation	Vascular	Neurogenic
Walking distance	Fixed	Variable
Palliative factors	Standing	Sitting/bending
Provocative factors	Walking	Walking/standing
Walking uphill	Painful	Painless
Bicycle test	Positive (painful)	Negative
Pulses	Absent	Present
Skin	Loss of hair; shiny	Normal
Weakness	Rarely	Occasionally
Back pain	Occasionally	Commonly
Back motion	Normal	Limited
Pain character	Cramping—distal to proximal	Numbness, aching—proximal to distal
Atrophy	Uncommon	Occasional

DIAGNOSTIC IMAGING

Roentgenography

Although plain roentgenography cannot confirm spinal stenosis, findings such as short pedicles on the lateral view, narrowing between the pedicles on the anteroposterior view, ligament ossification, narrowing of the foramen, and hypertrophy of the posterior articular facets can be helpful hints. Leroux et al. outlined hypertrophic roentgenographic changes associated with hyperostosis on plain and computed tomography (CT) (Box 41-2).

The roentgenographic identification and confirmation of lumbar spinal stenosis have improved with the development of new imaging techniques. Initially only central spinal stenosis was recognized, with canal narrowing to 10 mm considered absolute stenosis. This could be measured using roentgenograms or preferably myelography. In 1985 Schönström, Bolender, and Spengler compared the identification of central spinal stenosis with anteroposterior canal measurement by CT to identification by measurement of the dural sac with myelography in patients undergoing surgery for spinal stenosis. They found no correlation between the transverse area of the bony canal in normal patients and patients with spinal stenosis. A dural sac transverse area of 100 mm^2 or less did correlate with symptomatic spinal stenosis. This method allows the inclusion of soft tissue in the determination of spinal stenosis. The analysis of this area can be calculated relatively easily using standard CT scanning software.

Currently, axial imaging has supplanted standard roentgenograms in the diagnosis of spinal stenosis, although roentgenograms are important in the initial evaluation of patients with persistent pain of more than 6 weeks' duration or of those with "red flags" of other disease, including recent trauma, history of cancer, immunosuppression, age more than 50 or less than 20

BOX 41-2 • Hypertrophic Roentgenographic Changes Associated with Hyperostosis

PLAIN ROENTGENOGRAPHS
Dorsal level
    Intervertebral osseous bridge
    "Lobster claw"
Cervical level
    Exuberant osteophytosis
    Narrow cervical canal
Lumbar level
    Marginal somatic osseous proliferation
    "Candle flame"
    "Lobster claw"
    Intervertebral osseous bridge
    Discarthrosis
    Acquired vertebral block
    Hypertrophy of the posterior articular processes
    "Bulb" appearance of the posterior articular hypertrophy
    Anterior subluxation
    Posterior subluxation

LUMBAR CT SCAN
Herniated disc
Disc protrusion
Vacuum disc sign
Hypertrophy of the posterior articular processes
Osteoarthritis of apophyseal joints
Osseous proliferations of the nonarticular aspects of the superior apophyseal joint
Osseous proliferations of the nonarticular aspects of the inferior apophyseal joint
Calcification and/or ossification (C/O) of the posterior logitudinal ligament (PLL)
C/O of the yellow ligament (YL)
C/O of the supra-spinal ligament (SL)
Anterior C/O of the posterior articular capsule
Posterior C/O of the posterior articular capsule
Anteroposterior diameter of the spinal canal
Transverse diameters of the spinal canal

Modified from Leroux JL, Legeron P, Moulinier L, et al: *Spine* 17:1214, 1992.

years, neurological deficit, or previous surgery. Flexion and extension views are useful to identify preexisting instability before laminectomy and may be useful in determining the need for subsequent fusion. Translation of more than 4 to 5 mm or rotation of more than 10 degrees to 15 degrees is indicative of instability. A reversal of the normal trapezoidal disc geometry with widening posteriorly and narrowing anteriorly also may indicate instability.

MRI

Boden et al. noted abnormal findings in 67% of asymptomatic patients evaluated by MRI. In patients older than 60 years, 57% of MRI scans were abnormal, including 36% of patients with herniated nucleus pulposus and 21% with spinal stenosis. MRI is helpful in identifying other disease processes, such as tumors and infections, and is a good noninvasive study for patients with persistent lower extremity complaints after roentgenographic screening evaluation. MRI should be confirmatory in patients with a consistent history of neurogenic claudication or radiculopathy, but it should not be used as a screening examination because of the high rate of asymptomatic disease. Sagittal T2-weighted images are a good starting point because they give a myelogram-like image. Sagittal T1-weighted images are evaluated with particular attention focused on the foramen. An absence of normal fat around the root is indicative of foraminal stenosis. Axial images provide a good view of the central spinal canal and its contents on T1- and T2-weighted images. Far-lateral disc protrusions are identified on axial T1-weighted images by obliteration of the normal interval of fat between disc and root (Fig. 41-3). The foraminal zone is better evaluated with sagittal T1-weighted sequences, which confirm the presence of fat around the nerve root. Absolute anatomical measures also can be used, as previously discussed (p. 2065). Schnebel et al. noted a 96.6% agreement in pathological anatomy defined by postmyelogram CT and MRI. They noted the greatest disagreement in the MRI L5-S1 axial cuts because of the inability of the cut to be aligned parallel to the disc space. This can be a problem with spinal deformity, including scoliosis and significant spondylolisthesis, because true axial images are difficult to obtain. A disadvantage of MRI is the cost; nonetheless, MRI has become a useful, noninvasive diagnostic tool for the evaluation of patients with extremity complaints.

CT and Myelography

Despite the prevalence of MRI, myelography followed by CT scanning is still accepted and widely used for operative planning in patients with spinal stenosis; it has a diagnostic accuracy of 91%. The addition of CT scanning after a myelogram allows detection of as many as 30% more abnormalities than with myelography alone. Because of the dynamic nature of the study, stenosis not visible on MRI with the patient recumbent may be identified on standing flexion and extension lateral views. CT scanning after myelography characterizes the bony anatomy better than MRI, which helps the surgeon plan decompression surgery. However, imaging of the nerve roots in the foraminal region lateral to the pedicle is not possible because of the confluence of the dura with the epineurium at this point. Thus myelography followed by CT scanning is best suited for dynamic stenosis, postoperative leg pain, severe scoliosis or spondylolisthesis, around metallic implants, or in patients with lower extremity symptoms in the absence of findings on MRI.

Wiesel et al. evaluated 52 patients without low back symptoms or spinal disease and discovered that 50% over 40 years old had abnormal CT scans. They identified herniated nucleus pulposus in 29.2%, facet degeneration in 81.5%, and spinal stenosis in 48.1%. It must be reiterated that abnormal findings occur in as many as 24% to 34% of asymptomatic individuals evaluated with CT and myelography, just as with MRI, so clinical correlation is a must.

Ciric et al. and others used CT to further define lateral recess

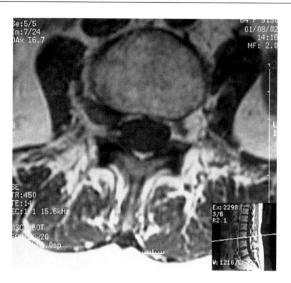

Fig. 41-3   T1-weighted MRI showing far lateral disc protrusion. Note obliteration of normal interval of fat between disc and root.

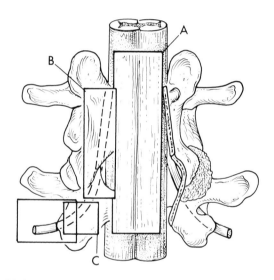

Fig. 41-4   Three-dimensional illustration of segmental stenoses. *A,* Anatomical; *B,* segmental; *C,* pathological. (Redrawn from Ciric I, Mikhael MA, Tarkington JA, Vic NA: *J Neurosurg* 53:433, 1980.)

stenosis and foraminal stenosis. These types of stenosis rarely are identified with myelography. The lateral recess is anatomically the area bordered laterally by the pedicle, posteriorly by the superior articular facet, and anteriorly by the posterolateral surface of the vertebral body and the adjacent intervertebral disc. The superior border of the corresponding pedicle is the narrowest portion of the lateral recess. Measurement of the recess in this area using the tomographic cross section usually is 5 mm or greater in normal patients, but in symptomatic patients the diagnosis is confirmed if the height is 2 mm or less (Fig. 41-4). The foramen is the area of the spine bordered by the inferior edge of the pedicle cephalad, the pars interarticularis with the associated inferior articular facet and the superior

A   B   C

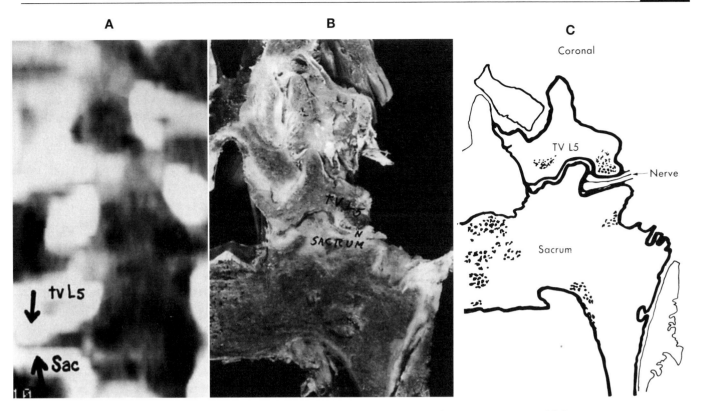

Fig. 41-5   **A,** Coronal view of CT scan showing impingement of transverse process of L5 on sacrum. **B,** Coronal section showing right transverse process. **C,** Drawing of coronal section. (From Wiltse LL, Guyer RD, Spencer CW, et al: *Spine* 9:31, 1984.)

articular facet from the lower segment posteriorly, the superior edge of the pedicle of the next lower vertebra caudally, and the vertebral body and disc anteriorly. This area rarely can be seen with myelography. A standard CT scan in the cross-sectional mode suggests narrowing if the foraminal space immediately after the pedicle cut is present for only one or two more cuts (provided the cuts are close together). The best way to appreciate foraminal narrowing is to reformat the lumbar scan, which can create sagittal views through the pedicles and structures situated laterally. Riew et al. reported that myelography influenced operative decision making more than MRI. When requested by the treating physician, CT myelography altered the operative plan in 74% of patients. Even when CT myelography was considered unnecessary, it altered the treatment plan in 49% of patients.

Wiltse et al. described a far-out compression of the root that occurs predominantly in spondylolisthesis when the root is compressed by a large L5 transverse process subluxed below the root and pressing the root against the ala of the sacrum. This diagnosis is best confirmed with a reformatted CT scan with coronal cuts (Fig. 41-5).

Some studies have attempted to correlate clinical outcomes with pathological findings on myelography and CT. In a retrospective review of 251 patients who underwent surgery for lumbar spinal stenosis, operative outcomes, as determined by Oswestry questionnaires, were evaluated and correlated with myelographic results. Patients who had a block on myelogram

had a better chance of obtaining a good outcome. A prospective study by Herno et al. confirmed postoperative stenosis in 64% of 191 patients at 4-year follow-up. Slight differences between those with and without stenosis were noted on the Oswestry questionnaire, but not in walking distances; instability was present in 21% without demonstrable clinical effect. In fact, the degree of decompression on CT myelography did not correlate at all with outcomes. Herno et al. reported similar results whether all stenotic levels were decompressed, only one level was decompressed leaving adjacent stenotic levels alone, or incomplete decompression of stenotic levels was done. Other studies by Paine and Surin et al. contradicted this, reporting worse results in patients with severe postoperative stenosis. Nonetheless, decompression of all symptomatic levels with evidence of compression is recommended to enhance neural circulation and function and to avoid reoperation for recurrent spinal stenosis.

Other Diagnostic Studies

Electrodiagnostic studies should be used if the diagnosis of neuropathy is uncertain, especially in patients with diabetes mellitus. The diagnostic use of such studies, including somatosensory evoked potentials, is limited by the lack of prospective studies to determine sensitivity or specificity. Vascular Doppler examinations are useful in identification of inflow problems into the lower extremities and should be accompanied by a vascular surgery consultation when indicated. Differential diagnosis also can be aided by the use of exercise testing. Tenhula et al. described a bicycle-treadmill test that stresses the patient in an upright position on an exercise treadmill and subsequently in a seated position on an exercise bicycle that allows spinal flexion. This study showed significant postoperative improvement in treadmill walking duration, lower visual analog pain scores, and a later onset of pain. Of the 32 patients evaluated preoperatively, 88% had symptoms during treadmill testing, and 41% had symptoms during bicycle testing. After decompression with or without fusion, only 9% had positive exercise treadmill findings, and 17% developed symptoms on the bicycle. Fritz et al. reported similar results with a two-stage exercise treadmill test. Earlier onset of leg symptoms with level walking and delayed onset of symptoms with inclined treadmill walking were significantly associated with stenosis. Exercise treadmill testing also is useful to help determine baseline function for quantitative evaluation of functional status after surgery.

NONOPERATIVE TREATMENT

Symptoms of spinal stenosis usually respond favorably to nonoperative management. Despite symptoms of back pain, radiculopathy, or neurogenic claudication, conservative management is successful in most patients. Conservative measures should include rest not exceeding 2 days, pain management with antiinflammatory medications or acetaminophen, and participation in a trunk-stabilization exercise program, along with good aerobic fitness. Other methods should be reserved for patients who are limited by pain and should be used to maximize participation in the exercise program. Traction has no proven benefit in the adult lumbar spine. For a patient with unremitting symptoms of radiculopathy or neurogenic claudication, epidural steroid injections may be useful in alleviating symptoms to allow better participation in physical therapy. Epidural steroids can give significant symptomatic relief, although no scientific study has documented long-term efficacy. If spinal stenosis is present with coexistent degenerative arthritis in the hips or knees, some permanent limitation in activity may be necessary regardless of treatment.

Simotas et al. treated 49 patients with an aggressive nonoperative protocol of therapeutic exercise, analgesics, and epidural steroid injection. All had spinal stenosis documented by CT or MRI and symptoms of disabling back, buttock, or leg pain. Except for a few patients with acute neurological changes who initially were prescribed 1 to 2 weeks of bed rest, patients were given one course of oral corticosteroids on a 7-day tapered schedule. An epidural steroid injection was given if symptoms persisted, with a repeat injection given if necessary by the transforaminal route at the point of most severe constriction. A third injection was administered only at the treating physician's discretion, usually for flare-ups during follow-up. For less severe symptoms, nonsteroidal antiinflammatory medications were used for 4 to 6 weeks, and this occasionally was repeated. All patients participated in physical therapy that included postural exercises, gentle lumbopelvic mobilization exercises,

and a daily flexion lumbar stabilization program. At 3-year follow-up, only 9 patients (18%) had required surgery after this treatment regimen. At final follow-up, 42% rated overall pain as none or mild, and 56% rated leg pain as none or mild. Sustained improvement was reported in 24% and mild improvement in 28%, with 13% definitely worse. Regarding walking, 40% reported improvement, 35% reported no change, and 25% reported worsening at final follow-up. This study documented the effectiveness of a structured nonoperative treatment regimen in patients with spinal stenosis, reporting satisfactory results in 69% at 3 years.

Epidural Steroid Injection

Although epidural steroid injections have been used in the treatment of spinal stenosis for a number of years, reports in the literature have not substantiated a positive effect, and most prospective reports show no statistically significant benefit. The technique of placement—caudal, translaminar, or transforaminal—also is debated, as is whether fluoroscopy should be used. Using anatomical landmarks for caudal injections, Stitz et al. reported accurate placement in 65% to 74% of patients, with intravascular placement in 4%. Accurate placement of translaminar injections appears to be equally difficult, with successful placement reported in 70%. Complications are infrequent but can occur and include hypercorticism, epidural hematoma, temporary paralysis, retinal hemorrhage, epidural abscess, chemical meningitis, and intracranial air. A 5% incidence of dural puncture has been reported, and, if it occurs, subarachnoid injection of steroids or local anesthetic should be avoided to prevent mechanical or chemical nerve root irritation. Headaches occur in 1% to 5% of patients and are related to dural puncture or the use of the caudal injection route. In patients with headaches associated with caudal injections, the cause has not been determined because dural puncture should not occur at this level, since the dural sleeve has terminated at midsacrum.

No scientifically validated long-term outcomes have been reported to substantiate the use of epidural steroid injections. A meta-analysis showed that epidural steroids have little short-term advantage over placebo for the treatment of leg pain. Unfortunately, studies are divided on the long-term results and the avoidance of surgery. The ideal candidate for epidural steroid injection appears to be a patient who has acute radicular symptoms or neurogenic claudication unresponsive to traditional analgesics and rest, with significant impairment in activities of daily living. We have used this technique successfully in our treatment algorithm for neurogenic claudication and radiculopathy.

OPERATIVE TREATMENT

The primary indication for surgery in patients with spinal stenosis is increasing pain that is resistant to conservative measures. Since the primary complaint is back pain and some leg pain, pain relief after surgery may not be complete. Most series report a 64% to 91% rate of improvement, 42% in patients with diabetes, but most patients still have some minor complaints, usually referable to the preexisting degenerative arthritis of the spine. Neurological findings, if present, improve inconsistently after surgery. In a series reported by Guigui et al., only 30% had complete improvement in motor symptoms after laminectomy, with 58% regaining grade 4 strength or better at a mean follow-up of 3 years. Reoperation rates vary from 6% to 23%. Prognostic factors include better results with a disc herniation, stenosis at a single level, weakness of less than 6 weeks' duration, age less than 65 years, and monoradiculopathy. Reversal of neurological consequences of spinal stenosis seems to be a relative indication for surgery unless the symptoms are acute.

Roentgenographic findings alone are never an indication for surgery, as clearly indicated in the studies by Wiesel et al. and Boden et al. Localized lesions without general involvement respond best. Ganz reported 86% good results in his series of 33 patients treated by decompressive surgery. In patients whose preoperative symptoms were relieved by postural change, the success rate was 96%, compared with only 50% in those not relieved by postural change. Factors predicting outcome are variable, and correlation of imaging with symptoms seems to be the best guarantee of improvement after surgery.

A patient's inability to tolerate the restricted lifestyle necessitated by the disease and the failure of a good conservative treatment regimen should be the primary determining factors for surgery in a well-informed patient. The patient should understand the potential for the operation to fail to relieve pain or to actually worsen it, especially back pain. In addition to the general risks of spinal surgery, the severity of symptoms and lifestyle modifications should be considered. Lumbar spinal stenosis does not result in paralysis, only decreased ambulatory capacity, and conservative management is warranted indefinitely in a patient with good function and manageable symptoms. Cervical and thoracic spinal stenoses, on the other hand, are associated with painless paralysis in the form of cervical and thoracic myelopathy and require closer attention and follow-up.

Principles of Spinal Stenosis Surgery

Decompression by laminectomy or a fenestration procedure is the treatment of choice for lumbar spinal stenosis (Fig. 41-6). Fusion is required if excessive bony resection compromises stability or if isthmic or degenerative spondylolisthesis, scoliosis, or kyphosis is present. Other important indications for fusion include adjacent segment degeneration after prior fusion and recurrent stenosis or herniated disc after decompression. Laminectomy may be preferable in older patients with severe, multilevel stenosis, whereas fenestration procedures, consisting of bilateral laminotomies and partial facetectomies that preserve the midline structures, are an alternative in younger patients with intact discs. Whenever possible, the source of pain should be localized with root blocks preoperatively to allow a more focal decompression. At surgery, specific attention should be directed to the symptomatic area, which may result in more extensive decompression than would normally be done with the pain source unconfirmed. If radical decompression of only one root is necessary, additional stabilization by fusion with or without instrumentation is unnecessary. The removal of more than one complete facet joint usually requires instrumented fusion unless the patient is elderly or has a narrow disc at that level. It is advisable to prepare the patient for fusion in case the findings at surgery require a more radical approach than anticipated. Positioning the patient with the abdomen hanging free minimizes bleeding. If fusion is likely, the hips should remain extended to prevent positional kyphosis. As in disc surgery, a microscope or magnifying loupes and a head lamp are helpful. When proceeding with the decompression, care should be taken to watch for adhesions that can result in dural tears, even if no previous surgery has been done. Frequently the narrowing in the lateral recess and foramen is so great that a Kerrison rongeur cannot be used without damaging the root. Dissection in the lateral recess and foramen usually requires a small, sharp osteotome or a high-speed burr, which allows the surgeon to thin the bone sufficiently to allow removal with angled curets. Unlike disc surgery, for decompression the lateral recess is best seen from the opposite side of the table. The operating surgeon may find it necessary to switch sides during the operation to better view the pathology and nerve roots. Blunt probes with increasing diameters also are useful for determining adequate foraminal enlargement. McLaren and Bailey reported that five of six patients with postoperative cauda equina syndrome had a disc removed from a stenotic spine without adequate decompression of the stenosis. Spinal stenosis should be treated at the same time as the disc herniation. A good approach is to start the decompression at a point of lesser stenosis and work toward the area of most severe stenosis. This often frees the neural structures enough to make the final decompression simpler and decreases the risk of damage to dura or nerve roots.

Adjacent Segment Degeneration

Adjacent disc degeneration and stenosis, or the transition syndrome, deserves special mention. It is known that disc degeneration occurs adjacent to a fusion in 35% to 45% of patients because of the ensuing hypermobility of the unfused joint. Lehmann et al. reported a 45% prevalence (15 of 33) of adjacent segment instability, defined as more than 3 mm of translation, and a 42% occurrence of spinal stenosis (14 of 33), usually above the fusion mass. Adjacent segment stenosis below the fusion mass, although less frequent, always occurred along with stenosis above the fusion.

Adjacent segment breakdown may cause symptoms that require surgery in 30% of patients. Pathology, including spinal stenosis, herniated nucleus pulposus, and instability, may require treatment years after successful surgery. Breakdown is possible one or two levels above lumbosacral fusions and above or below thoracolumbar and "floating" lumbar fusions. Schlegel et al. reported 58 patients who developed spinal stenosis, disc herniation, or instability at a segment adjacent to a previously asymptomatic fusion that was done an average of 13.1 years earlier. They found that floating lumbar fusions had

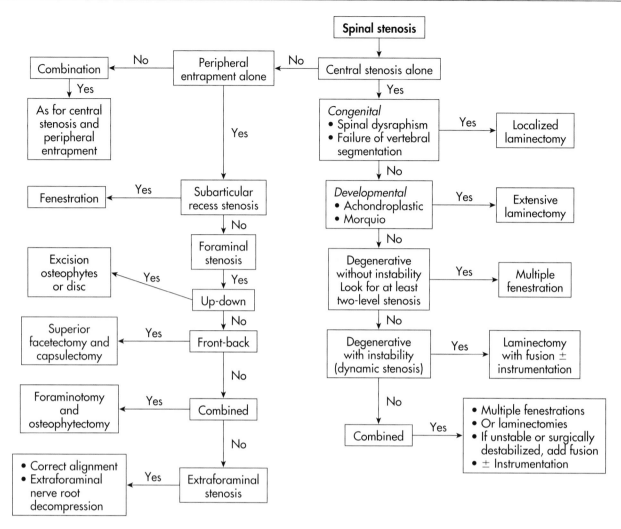

Fig. 41-6 Algorithm for treatment of spinal stenosis. (From Hadjipavlou AG, Simmons JW, Pope MH: *Semin Spine Surg* 10:193, 1998.)

a much shorter symptom-free interval (6.3 years) than did other fusions (range, 13 to 16.6 years). Of 37 patients followed for more than 2 years after identification of adjacent segment breakdown and subsequent surgery, 26 (70%) had good or excellent results, and 7 (19%) required additional operative procedures. Some contribution of postoperative loss of lordosis after index surgery was suggested but was not statistically significant in their data. These clinical findings have been substantiated by subsequent biomechanical studies that confirmed kinematic changes in segments adjacent to spinal fusions. Simple malalignment that occurs during patient positioning when the hips are not extended may result in hypolordosis and increase the load across implants, as well as increase posterior shear and laminar strain at adjacent levels. These changes may help to explain the cause of adjacent segment breakdown. Posterior lumbar interbody fusion (PLIF) also resulted in adjacent segment changes in all patients, but this did not affect results at 5 years in the series of Miyakoshi et al.

Rigidity of instrumentation has been hypothesized to correlate with motion at adjacent segments. A study by Even-Sapir et al. using single photon emission computed tomography (SPECT) revealed increased uptake in adjacent motion segments 4 years after surgery in 46% of patients with posterolateral fusions and in 67% of patients with circumferential fusions. However, Doeer et al. found little difference in adjacent segment motion between circumferential fusion and posterior fusion in a calf spine model. Motion at the adjacent segment increased by 29% after posterior fusion and by 21% after circumferential fusion. Thus it is undetermined whether more rigid fusion increases the likelihood of adjacent segment changes.

Fusion is more difficult as the number of levels fused increases, with L4-5 being the most frequent site of pseudarthrosis. Addition of a second level of fusion should be avoided if possible, and fusing a degenerative disc as a prophylactic measure does not seem to be supported by the data available. The actual source of transition syndromes cannot be determined from published studies; however, postoperative hypolordosis and rigidity of the fused segment probably both contribute to the problem. Surgery should attempt to maintain normal segmental lordosis and global sagittal balance, in addition to fusing the fewest segments possible.

Complications are relatively infrequent after decompression for spinal stenosis and occur more often in patients who are older than 80 years or age or who have diabetes. Complications are three times more likely after the age of 75 than before age 40 and are twice as likely in those older than 80 years as in patients younger than 70 years. The mortality rate is 2.3% after spinal stenosis in patients older than 80 years compared with 0.8% in those younger than 75 years. Comorbidities also contribute to poorer patient satisfaction and increased operative complications. Deep venous thrombosis also must be considered in patients after decompression. The incidence of this complication varies but is likely higher than reported. Pulmonary emboli, however, are exceedingly rare. Prophylaxis is best limited to pneumatic compression devices of the foot or calf and early ambulation, since the risk of epidural hematoma from pharmacological agents is greater than the risk of a significant pulmonary event or deep venous thrombosis. Reoperation is necessary in 9% to 23% of patients with spinal stenosis.

Decompression

There are no universal indicators of outcome after decompression. Outcome studies of lumbar decompression for spinal stenosis by Herron and Mangelsdorf and McCullen et al. identified subgroups associated with decreased rates of improvement. The factors they associated with poorer outcomes included questionable roentgenographic confirmation of stenosis, female sex, litigation, previous failed surgery, and the presence of spondylolisthesis. Katz et al. stated that for patients treated with laminectomy with or without fusion, the patient's self-assessment of health was the best predictor of satisfaction, with cardiac comorbidity also being predictive.

A 5-year follow-up study by Jönsson et al. described the "ideal patient" as one who has a pronounced constriction of the spinal canal, insignificant lower back pain, no concomitant disease affecting walking ability, and a symptom duration of less than 4 years. In their study, successful results were present in 63% to 67% of patients, deteriorating to 52% at 5 years, with reoperations necessary in 18%. Specifically, patients with 6 mm or less anteroposterior canal diameter preoperatively had better results. Similar results were reported by Airaksinen et al., with 62% good or excellent results at 4.3 years after surgery in 438 patients who had undergone decompression only. Results were worse in patients with hip arthritis, diabetes mellitus, previous surgery, vertebral fracture, or a postoperative complication. At an average 8.1-year follow-up, Katz et al. reported that 75% of patients were satisfied with the results of decompression despite severe back pain in 33% and inability to walk two blocks in 53%.

Prospective analysis of the Maine Lumbar Spine Group (Atlas et al.) identified a cohort of 67 patients with spinal stenosis studied 4 years after surgery and compared with a less severely affected group of 52 patients treated conservatively.

Better outcomes were noted in the operatively treated group despite their being more severely affected and worse functionally before surgery: 70% of the operatively treated group and 52% of the conservatively managed group reported improvement in back or leg pain. Some loss in functional improvement was noted in the operatively treated group over time, with no worsening in the conservative group. This also was confirmed in a later study by the same group. Of 148 patients with lumbar spinal stenosis followed for 4 years after treatment, 81 had been treated with surgery and 67 were treated without surgery. Those treated with surgery had more severe symptoms and worse function preoperatively but had better outcomes at 4-year follow-up. Back and leg pain were much improved or completely gone in 70% of the operatively treated group compared with 52% of those treated nonoperatively. Of those having surgery, 63% were satisfied with their current status, compared with 47% of those treated nonoperatively. Maximal benefit was noted 3 months after surgery. A modest decline in outcomes over the 4-year follow-up was noted in the operatively treated group, with no significant changes, either positive or negative, in those treated nonoperatively.

Progressive instability after decompression does not predict poor results. Poor ambulation has been correlated with roentgenographic signs of instability; however, Frazier et al. found that normal walking, sensory deficits, and ability to perform activities of daily living improved despite instability. Some further anterolisthesis is tolerated well after decompression, and it is appropriate to observe these patients for further symptoms before recommending fusion because as many as 30% of patients develop anterolisthesis after decompression.

◆ Midline Decompression (Neural Arch Resection)

TECHNIQUE 41-1

Perform the procedure with the patient under general endotracheal anesthesia. Position the patient prone using the frame of choice. Make the incision in the midline centered over the level of stenosis. Localizing roentgenograms should be taken if the level of dissection is uncertain. Carry the incision in the midline to the fascia. Strip the fascia and muscle subperiosteally from the spinous processes and laminae to the facet joints to expose the pars interarticularis. Take care to avoid damaging facet joints that are not involved in the bony dissection. Identify and remove the spinous processes of the levels to be decompressed. Then clear the soft tissue with a sharp curet. Dissect the lower edge of ligamentum flavum from the lamina with a curet and remove the lamina with a Kerrison rongeur. If the lamina is extremely thick, a high-speed drill with a diamond or side-cutting burr can be used to thin the outer cortex to allow easier removal of the inner portion with a Kerrison rongeur. Take special care in removal of the lamina and ligamentum flavum. The neural structures will be found compressed, and the usual space for instrument insertion may not be

continued

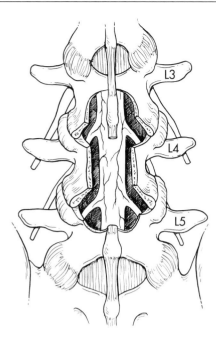

Fig. 41-7 Typical midline decompression for spinal stenosis. Note medial facetectomy and foraminotomy with preservation of the pars. Decompression is from inferior border of L3 pedicle to superior border of L5 pedicle, exposing both lateral borders of dura in lateral recess. (Redrawn from Whiffen JR, Neuwirth MG: Spinal stenosis. In Bridwell KH, DeWald RL, eds: *The textbook of spinal surgery,* ed 2, Philadelphia, 1997, Lippincott-Raven.)

available. Remove the lamina until the pedicles can be felt. Using the pedicle as a guide, identify the nerve root and trace it out to the foramen. With a chisel or rongeur, carefully remove the medial portion of the superior facet that forms the upper portion of the lateral recess (Fig. 41-7). Check the foramen for patency with an angled dural elevator or graduated probes. If there is further restriction, carry the dissection laterally and open the foramen, taking care not to remove more than half of the pars. Undercutting into the foramen is especially helpful in this regard. Inspect the disc and remove gross herniations unilaterally but try to avoid bilateral annulotomy because this compromises stability. Usually the disc is bulging, and the annulus is firm. Remove the annulus and bony ridge ventrally if it is kinking the nerve. This procedure involves some risk of nerve injury and requires a bloodless field. If safety is a concern, a complete facetectomy may be better. Complete the dissection at all symptomatic levels. Decompression should be from the caudal aspect of the most proximal pedicle to the cephalad aspect of the most distal pedicle, allowing observation of the lateral margins of the dura in the lateral recesses. This can be done with preservation of the proximal portion of the lamina and the intervening ligamentum flavum at the level above and below. Many failed decompressions are the result

of inadequate decompression of the foraminal region, so probing the foramen is mandatory to determine if the decompression is adequate. If no obstructions are noted and all areas have been decompressed adequately, close the incision. If desired, take a large fat graft from the incision or buttock and place it over the laminectomy defect and then close the incision.

Less-Invasive Decompression. The consequences of bone and ligament removal must be considered when performing decompression for spinal stenosis. Removal of the spinous processes, laminae, variable portions of the facets and pars, supraspinous and interspinous ligaments, ligamentum flavum, and portions of facet capsules is routine during these operative procedures. Denervation of the paraspinal musculature occurs with wide exposures, which results in altered muscle function. A minimally invasive technique allows decompression of the significant compressing anatomy while preserving paraspinal muscles, the spinous processes, and intervening supraspinous and interspinous ligaments.

◆ *Spinous Process Osteotomy (Weiner et al.)*

TECHNIQUE 41-2 (Fig. 41-8)
Patient positioning and localization of spinal levels are as described in the previous technique. Make a midline incision to expose the dorsolumbar fascia. Make a paramedian incision in the fascia, preserving the supraspinous and interspinous ligaments with subperiosteal dissection of the paraspinal muscles from the spinous process and laminae. Take care to avoid lifting the multifidus muscles beyond the medial aspect of the facet joint to preserve their innervation. With a curved osteotome, free each spinous process from the lamina at its base. Release only the levels shown to be affected on preoperative imaging. Once the spinous process is freed, retract it to one side with the paraspinal muscles beneath the retractor and the other blade of the retractor beneath the multifidus muscles to expose the midline (Fig. 41-8, *A*). Resect approximately half of the cephalad lamina and one fourth of the caudal lamina along with the underlying ligamentum flavum. Using a loupe or microscope for magnification, undercut the lateral recess and open the foraminal zone (Fig. 41-8, *B*). Complete laminectomy is recommended for severe stenosis or congenital stenosis involving all anatomical zones (central, lateral recess, and foraminal zones). Close the incision in routine fashion, allowing the spinous process to return to its normal position with suture of the fascia (Fig. 41-8, *C*).

Weiner et al. reported a 47% improvement in the Low Back Outcome Score and a 66% improvement in average pain level

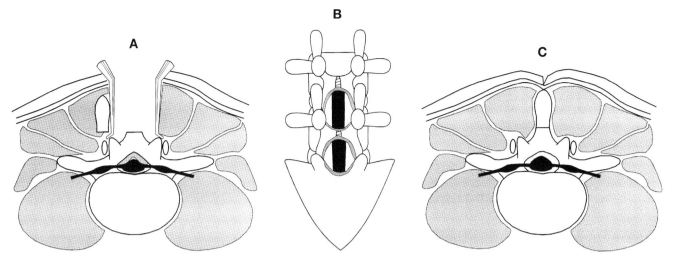

Fig. 41-8   Spinous process osteotomy. **A,** Muscle is taken down on only one side and only to medial facet border. **B,** Decompression is performed under microscopic magnification. **C,** After closure, spine returns to normal position. (Redrawn from Weiner BK, Brower RS, McCulloch JA: *Semin Spine Surg* 11:253, 1999.)

in 46 of 50 patients evaluated 9 months after surgery. Spinous process osteotomy was done at one to four levels; the only complications were dural tears in four patients. Although 3 patients died of unrelated causes, 38 of the 46 remaining patients were satisfied or very satisfied with their operative results. On reexploration or postoperative CT scans, spinous processes usually united with the remaining lamina in patients with short decompressions, although nonunion did not correlate with poor results. Complete laminectomy may be necessary if adequate decompression is not possible through the limited laminotomy in patients with severe involvement.

◆ Microdecompression

Microdecompression can be done in patients without disc herniations or instability including degenerative spondylolisthesis. This is a technically demanding procedure and is not recommended for patients with severe stenosis or congenital stenosis, which require complete laminectomy. McCulloch reported that decompressions were done at one to five levels without intraoperative complications in 30 patients treated for neurogenic claudication unresponsive to nonoperative measures. One superficial wound infection occurred. Of the 30 patients, 26 were very satisfied or fairly satisfied with their results; all but one stated that they would recommend the procedure to a friend with a similar problem.

TECHNIQUE 41-3 *(McCulloch)* (Fig. 41-9)
Place the patient in a kneeling position to increase interlaminar distance and identify the operative level on standard roentgenograms. Make a midline incision centered over the affected levels documented on preoperative imaging studies. Make a paramedian fascial incision on the most symptom-

atic side 1 cm from the midline. Elevate the multifidus muscles subperiosteally from the spinous process and laminae but do not retract them beyond the medial aspect of the facet joint. Obtain unilateral interlaminar exposure and maintain it with a discectomy retractor. Under microscopic magnification, perform laminotomy cephalad until the origin of the ligamentum flavum is encountered. Use undercutting to preserve as much dorsal bone as possible; angle the microscope to accomplish this. In a similar fashion, resect the proximal one fourth of the caudal lamina, thus completing removal of the ligamentum flavum from origin to insertion. Again, angling of the microscope into the lateral recess allows further decompression of the cephalad and caudad nerve roots and lateral dura. Once decompression is completed on one side, angle the microscope toward the midline for contralateral decompression (Fig. 41-9, *A*). Rotation of the operative table allows better viewing of the contralateral structures (Fig. 41-9, *B*). Use a no. 4 Penfield elevator or similar instrument to release adhesions between the dura and opposite ligamentum flavum, which is then resected in a similar fashion. Remove the bone at the base of the spinous processes of the cephalad and caudal levels to provide adequate vision of the opposite side (Fig. 41-9, *C*). Some removal of the deepest portions of the interspinous ligament also will be necessary to adequately view the structures across the midline.

AFTERTREATMENT. Special considerations are not necessary after a simple decompression. The patient should be examined carefully for the first few days for new neurological changes that may indicate the formation of an epidural hematoma. The patient is encouraged to walk on the first day.

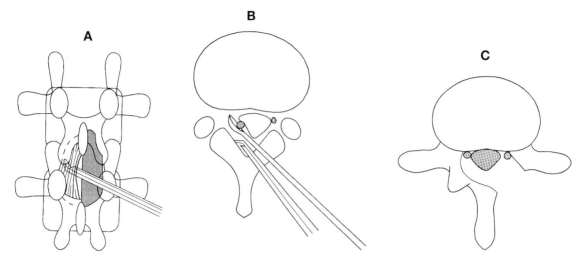

Fig. 41-9   Microdecompression. **A,** Muscle is taken down on only one side and ipsilateral decompressive hemilaminotomy is done (gray area); then contralateral side is accessed under midline structures. **B,** Sac and root are gently retracted for contralateral decompression. **C,** End result is complete decompression with preservation of paraspinal musculature and interspinous and supraspinous ligaments, limited dead space, and excellent cosmetic result. (Redrawn from Weiner BK, Brower RS, McCulloch JA: *Semin Spine Surg* 11:253, 1999.)

Sutures are removed at 14 days if nonabsorbable sutures have been used. The same limitations as after disc surgery (Chapter 39) apply to decompressions without fusion. For patients engaged in heavy manual labor, a permanent job change may be required. Return to work also is similar to return after disc surgery.

Decompression with Spinal Fusion. The indications for spinal fusion with decompression for spinal stenosis are becoming more clearly defined. The prevalence of postoperative problems related to instability is highly variable, possibly because of the great variations in the extent of the operative decompression. Shenkin and Hash noted a 6% occurrence of postoperative spondylolisthesis in patients with bilateral facetectomy and a 15% occurrence when three or more facets were removed. White and Wiltse noted subluxation after decompression in 66% of patients with degenerative spondylolisthesis. They suggested that a fusion be done in conjunction with decompression in (1) patients younger than 60 years of age with instability caused by the loss of an articular process on one side, (2) patients younger than 55 years of age with a midline decompression for degenerative spondylolisthesis that preserves the facets, and (3) patients younger than 50 years of age with isthmic spondylolisthesis. Others have suggested that patients with spinal stenosis and concomitant scoliosis should be treated with fusion because of the potential for instability and progression of deformity. The complete removal of one facet, or more than 50% resection of both facets, may result in instability. In addition, generalized spinal stenosis that requires extensive decompression with the loss of multiple articular processes may require fusion. When complete bilateral facetectomies are necessary, the addition of a lateral fusion may be difficult, and the bone graft may impinge on the exposed nerve roots. In this instance, an anterior interbody fusion is warranted to prevent postoperative instability. New posterior segmental fixation instrumentation for posterior spinal fusion has decreased the high incidence of pseudarthrosis after these long lumbar fusions.

The complications of this procedure are similar to those of disc surgery; however, the risk of nerve root damage and dural laceration is greater. The rates of infection, thrombophlebitis, and pulmonary embolism also are slightly higher. When a facet has been partially resected, later facet or pars fracture may account for a recurrence of symptoms. However, Getty et al. found that in their series the most important cause of failure to relieve symptoms was inadequate decompression. Postacchini and Cinotti noted bone regrowth at an average follow-up of 8.6 years in 88% of 40 patients who had total laminectomy for spinal stenosis. Bone regrowth was noted in all patients with associated spondylolisthesis.

Degenerative Spondylolisthesis and Scoliosis

Junghanns first described degenerative spondylolisthesis in 1930, separating the pathology from isthmic spondylolisthesis. He described this entity as "pseudospondylolisthesis," which was later renamed by Newman as *degenerative spondylolisthesis* because of the associated arthritic changes noted on roentgenograms. Degenerative spondylolisthesis often is accompanied by spinal stenosis, which usually is the cause of aggravation of symptoms and must be considered in patients with degenerative spondylolisthesis.

"Unstable stenosis," as described by Hanley, exists in two forms: unisegmental, which is manifested by degenerative spondylolisthesis, and multisegmental, which is represented by degenerative scoliosis. Thus treatment of either of these entities is really a continuum, and therefore they are considered together.

INCIDENCE

Degenerative spondylolisthesis occurs in patients older than 40 years and rarely is identified before that time. It is characterized by a posterior slip of one vertebra on another of less than 33%, with deformity occurring at L4-5 six times more often than at other lumbar levels and four times more often above a sacralized L5. Other levels may be similarly affected, with L3-4 affected more often than L5-S1. This disorder was found in approximately 4% of autopsy specimens and was identified in 10% of women older than 60 years. Women are affected by this condition four to six times more often than men, probably because of ligamentous laxity and abnormal facet morphology. Diabetes has been present in a disproportionate number of study patients, and Imada et al. found that oophorectomized patients had a three times greater rate of degenerative spondylolisthesis than did non-oophorectomized patients.

Degenerative scoliosis develops in patients with previously straight spines after the age of 40 years, typically affecting the lumbar spine with an associated lumbar hypolordosis, lateral olisthesis, and spinal stenosis. Men and women are affected more equally than patients with idiopathic curves, with about 60% to 70% of those affected being women. Degenerative scoliosis also affects fewer segments (2 to 5 segments) than does adult idiopathic scoliosis (7 to 11 segments), with an equal distribution of right and left lumbar curves. Symptoms of spinal stenosis occur most often in degenerative curves that have defects in both the convexity and concavity, possibly because significant degenerative changes preceded the development of the scoliosis. As a result, treatment for degenerative scoliosis often is necessary to relieve spinal stenosis by decompression, with instrumented fusion to prevent instability and further progression of deformity.

ANATOMY AND BIOMECHANICS

Degenerative spondylolisthesis is differentiated from isthmic spondylolisthesis by the presence of an intact pars. Because the arch is intact and moves forward with the L4 vertebral body, progressive spinal stenosis occurs in addition to facet degenerative changes. The true deformity of degenerative spondylolisthesis does not appear to be pure translation but rather a rotary deformity that may distort the dura and its contents and exaggerate the appearance of spinal stenosis. Existing theories to explain the development of degenerative spondylolisthesis include the primary occurrence of sagittal facets and disc degeneration, with secondary facet changes accounting for anterolisthesis. The sagittal facet theory suggests a predilection for slippage because of facet orientation that does not resist anterior translation forces and, over time, results in degenerative spondylolisthesis. The disc degenerative theory proposes that the disc narrows first, and subsequent overloading of the facets results in accelerated arthritic changes, secondary remodeling, and anterolisthesis.

It appears that facet arthritic changes are more severe than disc space narrowing, with the most advanced anterolisthesis present when disc narrowing is more pronounced. Thus a continuum seems to exist as degeneration progresses. In addition, facets that are aligned in a more sagittal orientation provide less stability at the involved level, but whether these changes result from chronic instability or from a primary anatomical variant is debatable. Boden et al. showed that sagittal facet angles of more than 45 degrees at L4-5 predicted a 25 times greater likelihood of degenerative spondylolisthesis. Despite the increased frequency of degenerative spondylolisthesis in women, there appears to be no gender-specific difference in facet orientation, which calls into question the theory that sagittal facet joints are a primary cause of degenerative spondylolisthesis. Sagittal facet orientation has been correlated with disc space narrowing, suggesting that disc narrowing increases loading of the facet, resulting in secondary facet changes. Regardless of the exact nature of the first inciting event, this instability causes facet arthritis, disc degeneration, and ligamentous hypertrophy, which all contribute to produce symptoms. Facet orientation therefore may be part of the consideration of potential instability when evaluating a patient for surgery, especially decompression alone.

In degenerative scoliosis, severe degenerative changes result in significant back pain. Mechanical insufficiency of the lumbar spine with a decrease in lordosis is caused by the degenerative changes. Curves usually are less than 60 degrees, with 81% developing a lateral olisthesis. Spinal stenosis occurs most commonly at the apex of the primary curvature (either concave or convex), with variable amounts of structural rotary deformity, although as many as 33% of patients develop symptoms because of stenosis within the distal compensatory curve. Characteristically, patients with neurogenic claudication and degenerative scoliosis do not obtain relief simply by bending forward or sitting. These patients require support of the torso by the upper extremities to obtain relief of their neurogenic claudication. Finally, osteoporosis is a significant consideration in the treatment of these patients. Although there is no cause-effect relationship between bone density and degenerative scoliosis, these patients usually are older and more predisposed to senile osteoporosis, and compression fractures may complicate the treatment.

NATURAL HISTORY

Most of the literature describing natural history concerns spinal stenosis rather than degenerative spondylolisthesis. Matsunaga, Ijiri, and Hayashi reported that in 145 patients examined annually for a minimum of 10 years progressive spondylolisthesis occurred in 34%, and further disc space narrowing continued in those without further slip. There was no correlation between roentgenographic findings and a patient's clinical picture. In fact, low back pain actually improved in those with continued disc space narrowing, which may imply autostabilization. Of the 145 patients, 76% remained without neurological deficits; however, 83% of patients with neurological symptoms, including claudication and vesicorectal disorder, deteriorated and had a poor prognosis. This is in agreement with an earlier study by Matsunaga et al, which showed that, over 60 to 176 months, progressive slipping occurred in 30% of patients without significant effect on clinical outcome.

Degenerative scoliosis occurs in 6% to 30% of the aged population, with most curves being minor. Rotary subluxation is variable and appears to be worse after decompression surgery without fusion. Men and women appear nearly equally affected, although a propensity for women has been noted. Curves can be progressive, but the natural history has not been elucidated conclusively. Grubb et al. reported progression of 1 to 6 degrees a year in 8 patients, but the small number of patients limits generalizations.

It appears from the literature that observation and nonoperative treatment are warranted initially in these patients. For those who develop neurological symptoms or who fail to improve despite nonoperative treatment, operative intervention should be considered.

CLINICAL EVALUATION

Symptoms of degenerative spondylolisthesis include back pain, neurogenic claudication, radiculopathy, and rarely bowel and bladder dysfunction. Although symptoms of spinal stenosis are more common, with leg pain and claudication in 68%, 32% have axial back pain only. Radiculopathy occurs in 32%, and cauda equina is rarely noted (3%). Overlap of symptoms of neurogenic claudication and vascular claudication requires a careful evaluation. Peripheral neuropathy also must be considered in the differential diagnosis.

Symptoms of neurogenic claudication are present in 71% to 90% of patients with degenerative scoliosis and usually cause patients to seek medical attention, with deformity incidentally noted. These symptoms usually do not improve with forward bending, and to obtain relief patients support the trunk with the arms or assume a supine position. This is in contrast to the usual patient with spinal stenosis and neurogenic claudication. Radiculopathy from facet overgrowth, foraminal stenosis within the concavity of curvature, or nerve root tension along the curve convexity can occur, although neurological deficits are rare and back pain is ubiquitous. Thus primary treatment is directed at decompression of spinal stenosis, with fusion or instrumentation indicated based on the potential for instability.

Physical findings are nonspecific in most patients. Motion usually is preserved, but patients guard against hyperextension. Symptoms may be reproduced by this maneuver in the presence of spinal stenosis. Neurological examination rarely identifies significant motor, sensory, or reflex deficits; however, any abnormal findings should be documented. Evaluation of distal pulses is necessary to help rule out peripheral vascular disease and vascular claudication. Bilateral absence of tendo calcaneus reflexes may be an indicator of peripheral neuropathy. Flattening of the lumbar spine is representative of degenerative change, and a lumbar prominence on forward bending accentuates the convexity of a coronal deformity, which is absent in those with degenerative spondylolisthesis. Sagittal and coronal balance should be estimated clinically.

DIAGNOSTIC IMAGING

Roentgenography

Roentgenographic imaging is straightforward in the diagnosis of degenerative spondylolisthesis and scoliosis. Anterolisthesis typically is seen at L4-5 without an associated pars defect. Standing roentgenograms are imperative because 15% of deformities spontaneously reduce on supine imaging. Variable disc space narrowing is indicative of degenerative changes. Flexion-extension lateral views may reveal instability, which is considered to be present when 4 to 5 mm of translation or more than 10 to 15 degrees of sagittal rotation is identified. Degenerative scoliosis is evident, with a solitary lumbar curve and associated degenerative disc changes. Flattening of the normal lumbar lordosis is present, and rotary subluxation may be evident in some patients, with lateral olisthesis of varying degrees.

Bending films add information for operative decision making. Flexion-extension views should be obtained with any spondylolisthesis or kyphosis, and lateral bending films should be obtained for coronal deformities. These studies are useful in determining whether supplemental anterior surgery is necessary or if all decompression and stabilization can be done from a posterior approach alone.

The Ferguson anteroposterior view shows any significant degenerative changes in the lumbosacral joint and allows better visualization of the transverse processes of L5. Hypoplastic transverse processes also should prompt the consideration of interbody fusion because of the paucity of bony substrate for fusion, especially for lumbosacral fusions.

CT Myelography and MRI

CT myelography and MRI are used as indicated for the evaluation of spinal stenosis (p. 2065) and may show facet overgrowth, hypertrophy of the ligamentum flavum, and rarely disc herniation. Because of the arthritic component affecting the facet joints, synovial cysts also have been documented. When identified, synovial cysts may alter the treatment plan, necessitating more extensive decompression into the foraminal zone.

Deformity, specifically scoliosis, is still a common indication for the use of CT scanning after myelography. Because of the difficulty of obtaining MR images parallel to the disc spaces in patients with scoliosis or spondylolisthesis and leg pain or claudication, myelography is better for evaluating the spinal canal and nerve roots. Flexion and extension myelography studies should be obtained with the patient standing and should be followed by CT scanning. Dynamic images may reveal nerve compression not apparent on supine images. The axial images show the bony deformities clearly, including the facet subluxations and bony spurring that often cause lower extremity complaints, lateral recess stenosis from ligamentum flavum hypertrophy, and pedicular kinking of the concave nerve roots. Pathology lateral to the dorsal root ganglion cannot be seen, however, because of the absence of subarachnoid space. MRI may supplement the information obtained by CT myelography, especially regarding the soft tissues, and often is helpful in decision making.

Although axial images are limited in larger deformities, with attention to the neural foramen and far-lateral regions, MRI can be very useful in preoperative evaluation. Disc hydration is a useful piece of information provided by T2-weighted sequences and may influence whether surgery stops at or includes a lower degenerative segment. Desiccation of the L5-S1 disc should prompt extra consideration to end at the adjacent disc above or include the degenerative segment. Adjacent segment pathology is common, and in older patients it may be prudent to include such diseased discs. Discography also may be warranted in such cases.

Discography

Kostuik advocated the use of discography to decide if instrumentation must include the lumbosacral disc or other discs not anticipated to be included in the fusion for adult idiopathic scoliosis. Although no prospective randomized study has proved the usefulness of discography for this purpose, Kostuik reported satisfying results with this testing protocol. Grubb and Lipscomb also used this protocol for determining fusion levels and reported good results, although they did not find discography necessary in patients with degenerative scoliosis. In fact, in their study, discography was abandoned for the evaluation and treatment of patients with degenerative scoliosis because fusion with instrumentation to the L5 or S1 levels was done in most patients, and all degenerative levels evident on plain roentgenograms were included in the fusion. Results were only slightly less satisfactory in patients with degenerative scoliosis than those in patients with idiopathic scoliosis.

Other Studies

EMG and nerve conduction velocity studies are useful in differentiating peripheral neuropathy from other abnormalities, especially in patients with diabetes mellitus. Nerve conduction studies should be used if the diagnosis is uncertain because the results of surgery are less predictable in patients with neuropathy. In addition, arterial Doppler studies, angiography, or vascular surgery consultation may be necessary in some patients. A noninvasive functional study using the bicycle-treadmill test (p. 2068) also may help to differentiate neurogenic from vascular claudication.

NONOPERATIVE TREATMENT

Conservative treatment is warranted for patients with neurogenic claudication from spinal stenosis caused by degenerative scoliosis and spondylolisthesis. Standard interventions should include short periods of rest, antiinflammatory medications, and, rarely, bracing. The use of specific exercise programs has not been evaluated; however, trunk-stabilization exercises and low-impact aerobic exercises seem to benefit this patient group.

Epidural Steroid Injection

Epidural steroid injections have been advocated, but randomized or placebo-controlled trials are lacking to determine their effectiveness in the treatment of spinal stenosis. The antiinflammatory effect of corticosteroids is the basis for their use. Long-term effects also may be a result of the local anesthetic agent administered with the steroid. Epidural steroid injections appear to be most beneficial in patients with radiculopathy; fluoroscopic guidance is helpful because a dorsal medium septum may be present, which can restrict injectate diffusion. No literature exists to support the use of a series of three epidural steroid injections unless symptoms improve partially after the first injection. If the first injection is done without fluoroscopy and is ineffective, a second injection can be done with fluoroscopy to ensure proper placement and diffusion. Further injections are not warranted if there is not a favorable response after a single well-placed injection. If epidural steroid injection is successful, physical therapy should be instituted.

OPERATIVE TREATMENT

For patients with unremitting back and leg pain after adequate nonoperative treatment, operative intervention is indicated. Only 10% to 15% of patients with degenerative spondylolisthesis require surgery. Caution should be exercised in proceeding with surgery for back pain alone because adjacent level pathology may account for symptoms.

Decompression

Degenerative Spondylolisthesis. Similar criteria for decompression alone are used for degenerative and isthmic spondylolisthesis. For patients with significant disc collapse and no pathological motion on dynamic roentgenograms and for young patients with multiple level congenital stenosis, decompression alone is indicated. Epstein reported the results of decompression in 290 patients. Laminectomy was done in 249 patients over an average of 3.4 levels, and limited decompression by fenestration, hemilaminectomy, or coronal hemilaminectomy was done over an average of 1.7 levels. Progressive slips required fusion in only 5 patients (1.7%), and secondary decompressions were necessary in 7 (2.8%). Roentgenographic findings did not correlate with clinical results, which were good or excellent in 82%. Several studies reported successful 5-year results in 90% of patients after fenestration procedures and in 71% to 81% after laminectomy.

Subsequent fusions were required in only 0.8% to 4%. Epstein reported a higher rate of reoperation for instability in patients with decompression and simultaneous disc excision. Of the eight patients undergoing reoperation for instability, five had discectomy at the time of the index decompression. The violation of the disc may have contributed to instability, which has been documented biomechanically in ligament-sectioning studies.

In the meta-analysis of Mardjetko, Connolly, and Shott, a review of 11 papers representing 216 patients showed that decompression without fusion was satisfactory in 69%, with progressive slips in 31% postoperatively. This occurrence is similar to the natural history of degenerative spondylolisthesis and did not compromise the operative results in most reports.

Degenerative Scoliosis. Decompression is a viable option for a patient with symptomatic spinal stenosis and minimal kyphosis, a neutral sagittal vertical axis, and no instability on dynamic imaging. Attempts should be made to avoid destabilizing the spine during decompression, and fusion should be done if more than 50% of both facets or an entire facet is resected. Degenerative scoliosis should be considered the coronal variant of spondylolisthesis; if the ligamentous structures are violated, facet and disc resection is necessary and fusion should be considered.

Decompression and Fusion

Degenerative Spondylolisthesis. Patients with preserved disc height are prone to instability after decompression, and fusion should be considered. Other indications for the addition of fusion include osteoporosis (which predisposes to pars fracture), absence of osteophytes on roentgenograms, and minor nonpathological motion on roentgenograms. After the report of Herkowitz and Kurz, the addition of fusion to decompression has become the standard in the treatment of degenerative spondylolisthesis and concomitant spinal stenosis. Outcomes are improved with the addition of in situ fusion regardless of whether there is a solid roentgenographic fusion. Most studies report that fusion rates are better with instrumentation, but clinical results are not different from those after uninstrumented fusion. Bridwell et al., however, reported better functional results, correction of sagittal alignment, and a fusion rate of 87% in patients with instrumented fusions compared with a 30% fusion rate in those with uninstrumented fusion. Similar findings were documented by Mardjetko et al. in their meta-analysis, with 90% satisfactory outcomes in instrumented fusions compared with 69% satisfactory results with decompression alone at 12- to 84-month follow-up. Booth et al. reported 6.5-year follow-up of 36 patients who had decompression, autogenous iliac crest bone grafting, intertransverse fusion, and pedicle screw instrumentation for degenerative spondylolisthesis. Stenosis at the level of previous decompression did not recur, but five patients developed symptomatic adjacent level "transition syndromes," with another seven having asymptomatic adjacent level degenerative changes. Sagittal alignment was maintained at the fused segments in all patients. Eighty-three percent were satisfied with their results,

86% reported that back and leg pain was better than before surgery, and 77% stated that they would have the surgery again. Dissatisfaction was associated with more than four medical comorbidities. Major complications were rare (2%) and involved screw breakage without symptoms. In Nork et al.'s report of 30 patients evaluated after decompression and instrumented posterior fusion, 93% were satisfied with their outcomes, based on SF-36 questionnaires, and showed improvement in abilities to perform heavy and light activities, participate in social activities, sit, and sleep. Pain, depression, and medication use also were decreased in this group. The fusion rate was 93% at an average of 128 days. Complications were rare, and poorer outcome was associated with more severe preoperative stenosis or the occurrence of a complication.

Pedicle screw implants appear to be better for maintaining anatomical alignment than distraction constructs and Luque rods or rectangles, which are reported to worsen anterolisthesis. Fusion rates with pedicle screws also are higher (86%) than with rod constructs (69%). Although fusion is not a necessity for successful results, it does appear to improve results when added to adequate decompression. Long-term results, however, are necessary to determine if adjacent segment "transition syndromes" are more likely in patients with more rigid instrumented fusions than in those with posterolateral in situ fusions. Therefore decompression and fusion, with or without instrumentation, are recommended for patients with degenerative spondylolisthesis and spinal stenosis in the absence of multiple medical comorbidities.

Degenerative Scoliosis. In a patient with a flexible spine and mild to moderate scoliosis, symptomatic spinal stenosis is treated with traditional decompression. Occasionally, facetectomy or partial pedicle resection is necessary to decompress symptomatic nerve roots. In this situation, posterior intertransverse fusion is recommended. If laxity is present, instrumentation should extend from neutral and stable vertebrae at each end of the construct. Ending the instrumented fusion at a level of kyphosis potentiates adjacent segment changes and may result in an adjacent compression fracture. This occurs at the thoracolumbar junction in as many as 15% of patients, which may be an indication for prophylactic polymethylmethacrylate augmentation. Rotary subluxation also can occur after decompression alone in the presence of unstable degenerative scoliosis. The fusion should end at a neutrally rotated, level, and stable end vertebra and should restore sagittal and coronal balance. Simmons and Simmons advocated avoiding fusion into the thoracic spine. Care should be taken to avoid stopping instrumentation and fusion at any apical segments or at the apex of a kyphosis or scoliosis because this creates deformity later.

Posterior Lumbar Interbody Fusion (PLIF) and Transforaminal Lumbar Interbody Fusion (TLIF)

Recent advances in instrumentation and techniques have resulted in an increased use of the PLIF technique with threaded interbody fusion cages. These cages may be allograft bone dowels or metal cylinders filled with bone graft. Biomechanically, bone dowels or metal cages appear equiva-

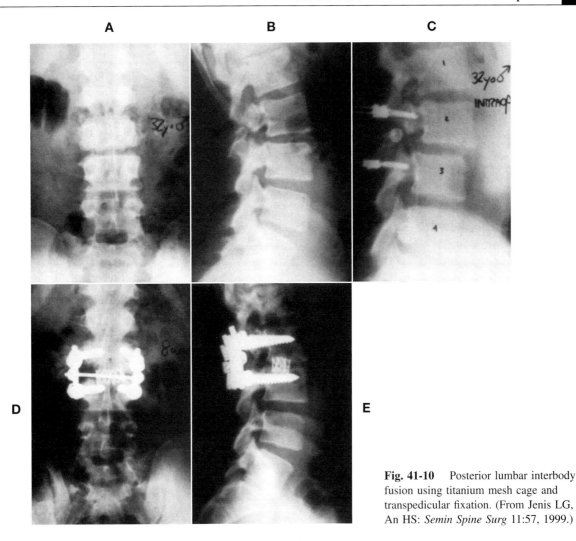

Fig. 41-10   Posterior lumbar interbody fusion using titanium mesh cage and transpedicular fixation. (From Jenis LG, An HS: *Semin Spine Surg* 11:57, 1999.)

lent. The use of these as stand-alone implants inserted through a posterior approach for grade I degenerative spondylolisthesis has provided only "moderate stability" in in vitro studies. Both implants appear to be susceptible to loosening with cyclic fatigue when used alone. This likely is a result of the posterior decompression and the resection of the disc for implant placement. It appears that significant disruption of the disc results in increased motion when loaded. If these implants are used posteriorly, further stabilization is necessary and is best provided by pedicle screw implants (Fig. 41-10). No reports have yet compared the outcomes of PLIF with traditional intertransverse fusion, with or without instrumentation, for degenerative spondylolisthesis. Ideal indications for interbody fusion in a patient with degenerative spondylolisthesis include discographically concordant single-level axial back pain with radiculopathy, minimal disc degenerative changes, and preserved disc height; it also is indicated for revision surgery with an inadequate posterior fusion mass. PLIF or TLIF also is appropriate for small or absent transverse processes at the levels to be fused, which would make intertransverse fusion impractical. The technique for PLIF is described on p. 2094.

Anterior Spinal Fusion

Anterior spinal fusion can be used for the treatment of degenerative spondylolisthesis if some indirect spinal decompression is provided by eradication of the disc, restoration of disc height, and ligamentotaxis by placement of structural bone graft or cage after distraction of the disc space and tensioning of the posterior ligamentous structures. Mardjetko et al. reported that the fusion rate with anterior procedures in pooled studies was 94%, with an 86% satisfaction rate, suggesting that there may be a place for anterior lumbar interbody fusion in this patient population because the results are similar to those obtained with decompression and instrumented fusion.

Decompression and Combined Fusion (360-Degree Fusion)

Any adult spinal deformity that requires fusion of L5-S1 also requires anterior fusion of the L5-S1 disc. This can be accomplished by an anterior procedure or a posterior interbody procedure. In patients with degenerative scoliosis, kyphosis, and a positive sagittal vertical axis, anterior interbody fusion usually is necessary to restore the height of L5-S1 and restore

A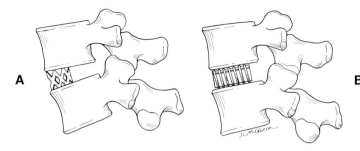

B

Fig. 41-11 Geometry of threaded interbody cylinder devices (**B**) does not allow replication of lordotic contour of intervertebral disc, as mesh cage does (**A**).

the normal segmental lordosis at this level. Because of the disproportionate amount of lumbar lordosis at this and the adjacent L4-5 level, the kyphosis that ensues often can be corrected with restoration of anterior disc height and without osteotomy. Posterior interbody procedures often do not allow safe excision of a contracted annulus and anterior longitudinal ligament for height restoration. Flexion and extension roentgenograms help with this aspect of the decision-making process by showing a narrow, immobile disc space.

For sagittally neutral or lordotic spines and an intact disc, posterior interbody fusion techniques can be considered. If disc height is maintained, it is easier to maintain normal lordotic disc anatomy during interbody fusion.

Regardless of the technique, restoration of normal segmental anatomy is of paramount importance at the L4-5 and L5-S1 levels. The objective of interbody grafts at these levels is to recreate the segmental lordosis of -20 to -28 degrees. This can be done with mesh cages, femoral ring allografts, iliac crest tricortical autograft wedges, fibular rings, or carbon fiber trapezoidal cages. Threaded interbody cylinder devices should be used cautiously in these applications, especially at the L4-5 and L5-S1 levels. Because of the geometry of the cylinder, the lordotic contour of the intervertebral disc cannot be replicated with this device (Fig. 41-11).

Adult Idiopathic Scoliosis

Treatment of adult scoliosis, both idiopathic and degenerative, requires a different approach from that used for typical adolescent idiopathic scoliosis. By definition, adult idiopathic curves are curves that are diagnosed in a patient older than 20 years of age. These curves have been present since adolescence but, for any number of reasons, the diagnosis was delayed. The prevalence of adult scoliosis is from 4% to 6%, with a similar female-to-male ratio as idiopathic adolescent scoliosis (Chapter 38).

In contrast, approximately 60% of patients with late-onset degenerative scoliosis are female. Degenerative curves are short segment, usually lumbar, and less severe than those in idiopathic scoliosis. Symptoms of spinal stenosis are more

common than in patients with degenerative scoliosis, and myelographic defects, if present, are within the primary curve. The goal of treatment of degenerative scoliosis is to relieve back pain and the symptoms of spinal stenosis, whereas the treatment goals for adult scoliosis usually are pain control and deformity correction.

SAGITTAL BALANCE

In the treatment of adult spinal deformities, it is important to understand the normal sagittal relationships. In a normal spine, the primary curvature is kyphosis of the thoracic spine, which develops first in infants. Subsequent to upright posture, the secondary lordotic curvatures in the cervical and lumbar spine develop between the ages of 5 and 15 years. Curves in males and females are similar at the cessation of growth, although the curves develop more quickly in females.

Sagittal balance is the alignment that is necessary to center the head over the pelvis or hips in both the sagittal and coronal planes. A plumb line dropped from the center of the C7 vertebral body is referred to as the sagittal vertical axis (SVA). On the lateral long-cassette view, the plumb line normally falls through or behind the sacrum. Normal values for the SVA are −3.2 ± 3.2 cm for adult populations, with negative values indicating a position behind the sacral promontory. The coronal vertical axis (CVA) is represented in a similar fashion with a plumb line on the posteroanterior roentgenogram, with a normal balance through the center of the sacrum. Any translation of the coronal vertical axis to either side of the midline is considered decompensation.

Sagittal and coronal vertical axes are used to evaluate and estimate global balance. Global balance is the result of segmental alignment of the functional spinal unit, and regional alignment of the cervical, thoracic, and lumbar segments. Bernhardt and Bridwell measured 102 roentgenograms of normal spines to determine normal sagittal plane alignment (Fig. 41-12). By convention, kyphosis is represented as a positive measurement, and lordosis as a negative value. In a normal adult spine, there is a small amount of kyphosis segmentally at each end of the thoracic kyphosis, reaching a maximum at the apical region (T6-7) of about +5 degrees. Apical discs or vertebrae are identified in the sagittal plane as those that are parallel to the floor. Considered independently, the thoracolumbar junction is a transition zone of force transmission and alignment. In this region a shift occurs from the thoracic kyphosis to lumbar lordosis. The first lordotic disc is typically at L1-2, and normal thoracolumbar alignment as measured from the cephalad T12 endplate to the caudal L2 endplate is 0 to −10 degrees. The lumbar spine is a region of lordosis, reaching a maximal segmental lordosis at L4-5 and L5-S1. The sagittal apex of the lumbar spine usually is L3. It is important to note that over 60% of lumbar lordosis is created by the discs at L4-5 and L5-S1, which contribute −20 degrees and −28 degrees, respectively, to the regional lordotic measurement.

Because most lordosis is present in the distal lumbar spine, it is important to maintain normal segmental and regional

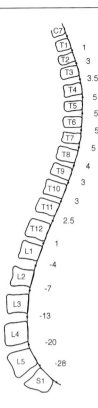

Fig. 41-12   Segmental sagittal measures of thoracic and lumbar spine. Note contribution of L4-5 and L5-S1 discs to overall lumbar lordosis (67%). (From Bernhardt M, Bridwell KH: *Spine* 14:717, 1989.)

interrelationships so that global balance is preserved. As a rule of thumb, on a lateral roentgenogram taken with the patient facing the surgeon's right, there is a "sagittal clock," as described by Bridwell. In a normal, standing patient, the apical L3 disc or endplate points at the 3-o'clock position, L4 points at the 4-o'clock position, and L5 points at the 5-o'clock position. If this regional alignment is maintained, then the likelihood of a postoperative flatback deformity is minimized.

Static normal values of kyphosis and lordosis probably are not useful in the treatment of spinal deformities. Because of the dynamic nature of the curves, normal is balanced. Hardacker et al. confirmed the dynamic nature of the spine in their study of cervical lordosis. They concluded that 75% of cervical lordosis occurs at C1-2, with only −10 degrees occurring in the rest of the subaxial cervical spine. Dynamic interrelationships also were confirmed. Increased cervical or lumbar lordosis correlated with increased thoracic kyphosis. Their study documented the dynamic nature of the spine and showed how compensatory changes occur to maintain global balance. Therefore normal kyphosis should be balanced by lordosis in the lumbar and cervical spines so that the plumb line falls through or behind the sacrum. A good rule of thumb is that lumbar lordosis should measure approximately 20 to 30 degrees more than the thoracic curve.

INCIDENCE

Adult idiopathic scoliosis is defined as a coronal deformity of more than 10 degrees with associated structural changes in a patient older than 20 years at time of diagnosis, most commonly in patients in their late thirties. Women are affected much more frequently than men, similar to the incidence of adolescent scoliosis. Studies have shown a prevalence of 2% to 4% for curves of more than 10 degrees. It is estimated that as many as 500,000 adults have coronal curves of more than 30 degrees. As noted by Weinstein and Ponseti in their classic description of the natural history of adult scoliosis, some of these curves are progressive. According to their report, thoracic curves of more than 50 degrees progress approximately 1 degree per year up to 75 degrees, when progression slows to about 0.3 degrees per year, finally stopping at about 90 degrees. Lumbar curves progress at a rate of 0.4 degrees per year after reaching only 30 degrees; thus a more aggressive approach is warranted for lumbar curves, especially after progression is documented. Predictors of lumbar curve progression include L5 above the intercristal line, apical rotation of more than 30%, an unbalanced or decompensated curve, a thoracic curve of more than 50 degrees, and a thoracolumbar or lumbar curve of more than 30 degrees. As many as 68% of adult curves progress more than 5 degrees over time.

Patients with idiopathic scoliosis rarely develop significant pulmonary complications, even with curves exceeding 100 degrees. Pehrsson et al. showed that over a 20-year period, diminished lung function in scoliosis patients paralleled that of the general aging population. In the absence of overt thoracic lordosis, surgery generally is not warranted to maintain or improve pulmonary function in adults.

CLINICAL EVALUATION

Back pain occurs in 60% to 80% of patients with scoliosis, which is similar to the occurrence in the general population. Despite this, 25% to 80% of patients with adult idiopathic curvatures present with the chief complaint of pain. Pain symptoms include mechanical back pain, buttock pain, and occasionally radiculopathy or neurogenic claudication. Neurogenic claudication occurs in 13% as a result of degenerative changes within or, more commonly, distal to the lumbar curve. Radiculopathy occurs in only 4%, with entrapment of nerve roots within the foramina of the concavity. In contrast to degenerative scoliosis, most adult patients with idiopathic scoliosis have more mechanical symptoms than neurological complaints. Patients may relate symptoms of curve progression: a progressive lean or list to one side, changes in waistline symmetry, hip prominence, protuberant or flaccid abdomen, hemline changes, or a loss in height in the absence of fracture. Neurological symptoms may include radiculopathy or neurogenic claudication, which usually is a result of degenerative changes in the distal fractional curve. Diminished pulmonary function in patients with curves of more than 60 degrees or cor pulmonale in patients with curves of more than 100 degrees occasionally is caused by the scoliosis and should be evaluated carefully to rule out other causes. Predictors of pain include curves of more than 45 degrees, lumbar curves, and thoracolumbar and lumbar curves of more than 45 degrees with apical rotation and coronal decompensation.

Physical examination findings usually are negative except for the spinal deformity. The skin should be examined for evidence of pathological lesions and hair patches that suggest underlying intraspinal anomalies. If spinal cord anomalies exist, atrophy may be evident in the lower extremities, or intrinsic atrophy of the foot may be present with pes cavus and clawing of the toes. Reflexes should be documented, as should the results of a comprehensive neurological examination.

The deformity should be evaluated by looking for structural features of the rib and lumbar paraspinal prominence on forward bending while also recording flexibility. This test also helps to determine which curve is primary, since more rotation and subsequent prominence is found in the more structural primary curve. If rib prominence exceeds 3 cm, thoracoplasty should be considered if surgery is performed. Trunk shift is identified by dropping an imaginary line perpendicular to the floor from the lateral ribs. These should symmetrically intersect the pelvis. Plumb lines should be dropped to evaluate for coronal decompensation and also to help in estimating sagittal balance. Special attention should be paid to the left shoulder because instrumentation of a curve with a structural upper thoracic curve must include this segment to avoid a high left shoulder postoperatively. Waistline asymmetry should be noted, and any limb length inequality must be considered. Equalizing limb length with ¼-inch blocks sometimes is helpful if limb length discrepancy is more than 1 inch.

ANATOMY AND BIOMECHANICS

Adult scoliosis shares most of the anatomical features of idiopathic adolescent scoliosis. There is a more structural and rigid primary curve and a compensatory secondary curve, and there also can be a structural upper thoracic curve similar to the King type V (see Fig. 38-29) or types 2 and 4 curves using the classification scheme of Lenke et al. (see Fig. 38-30). Unique to adult scoliosis patients are the diminished elasticity of the ligamentous structures and the narrowing of disc spaces, which combine to stiffen primary and secondary or compensatory curves. Osteopenia also must be considered in older patients, especially in those with risk factors for osteoporosis, such as glucocorticoid use and a significant family history.

The biomechanics of the bone-implant interface must be considered if long instrumentation constructs are used, especially when extended to the sacrum. Because of the long lever arm produced, the poor fixation obtained in the sacrum, even when bicortical screws are used, will fail if not protected. Of the different constructs used for instrumenting and fusing the lumbosacral joint, the most rigid fixation appears to be obtained with a modified Galveston technique and the use of iliac screws in addition to sacral bicortical screws. Fixation can be augmented with a structural interbody fusion device, but the

most significant biomechanical increase in strength is with the addition of the iliac screws. Other techniques that have been used include the Jackson intrasacral rod and a transiliac rod used to anchor the distal instrumentation as described by Kostuik. With the exception of the intrasacral rods, however, these techniques limit the amount of bone graft available for harvest. The superiority of any of these techniques has not been established, and the surgeon's experience and preference determine the choice.

DIAGNOSTIC IMAGING

Roentgenography

Standard roentgenograms on 36-inch cassettes must be obtained and scrutinized for coronal and, more important, sagittal balance. Depending on the level of proposed instrumentation, a Ferguson anteroposterior view (see p. 2089) may be helpful in determining the presence of significant degenerative changes at L5-S1, which would prompt its inclusion in the proposed fusion. Bending roentgenograms over a foam fulcrum are ideal for assessing flexibility, although standard maximal effort bending films often will suffice. For sagittal deformities, appropriate fulcrum bending films should be obtained to determine flexibility. Push prone views, as described by Kleinmann et al. and Vedantam et al., are useful in determining the response of the lowest instrumented vertebra to instrumentation.

Discography

Special imaging studies, including MRI and myelography supplemented with CT scanning, are discussed on p. 2076. Discography, although not yet validated by prospective data, may have a place in the evaluation of spinal deformity in adults. Grubb and Lipscomb reported that in patients with degenerative scoliosis, discographic findings were similar to those in other patients with spinal stenosis and added little to the diagnostic picture. However, in patients with idiopathic scoliosis and mechanical complaints, discography consistently identified abnormal, painful discs with reproduction of pain. These abnormal discs were most commonly, but not exclusively, in a compensatory lumbar or lumbosacral curve. Painful disc abnormalities frequently were identified in areas that would not have been included in the fusion area, according to accepted rules for fusion of idiopathic adolescent scoliosis. Therefore for operative decision making it is important to distinguish idiopathic scoliosis from degenerative scoliosis and to use discography as indicated clinically.

NONOPERATIVE TREATMENT

Traditional methods of nonoperative treatment of back and leg pain (p. 2068) are appropriate in patients with adult idiopathic scoliosis. Orthotics may be helpful for the relief of axial degenerative symptoms. Intermittent use of a soft thoracolumbosacral orthosis (TLSO) (Fig. 41-13) is better tolerated than a rigid TLSO by older, often endomorphic, patients. The orthosis

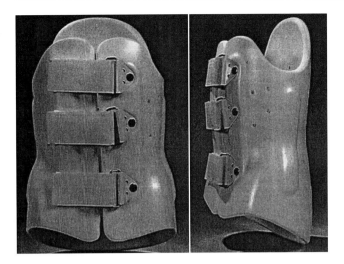

Fig. 41-13 Soft TLSO is better tolerated than rigid orthosis, especially by older patients. (Courtesy Boston Brace International, Avon, Mass.)

should be worn during symptomatic periods and kept to a minimum otherwise. Correction of deformity or prevention of progression of these curves is not possible, and an orthosis is used only for the management of symptoms; the patient should be aware of the treatment goals. Physical therapy should be continued in addition to bracing, with the ultimate goal of paraspinal strengthening and subsequent stabilization that allow the brace to be discarded.

OPERATIVE TREATMENT

Once adequate nonoperative treatment has failed in a patient with unremitting symptoms or roentgenographic progression, surgery should be considered. Curves of more than 50 degrees with documented progression, loss of pulmonary function believed to be caused by the scoliosis when curves exceed 60 degrees, progressive neurological changes, and significant coronal or sagittal decompensation are relative indications for surgery. Cosmetic considerations are a genuine concern for patients as well and may play a part in operative decision making.

A spinal implant should be used that allows segmental placement of hooks or screws and also allows iliac fixation. If fusion of the lumbosacral joint is anticipated, interbody fusion must be obtained with either allograft or fusion cages that are cut to maintain the normal segmental lordotic disc alignment. Autologous blood donation is encouraged, and a cell saver is useful in preserving blood lost intraoperatively. Spinal cord monitoring should include somatosensory and motor evoked potentials (SSEP and MEP). If useful data are obtained and maintained with SSEP and MEP, wake-up testing is unnecessary until the conclusion of the surgery. If pedicle screws are used below T8, pedicle screw stimulation also is useful to confirm proper placement. Fluoroscopy or computer-aided navigation enhances the use of anatomical landmarks and is

helpful for some surgeons. Regardless, this surgery is complex and has an extended recuperation period, with a significant risk of complications, which the patient must understand when operative treatment is chosen.

Posterior Instrumentation and Fusion

Patients with flexible curves of less than 70 degrees and no significant kyphosis or decompensation are candidates for posterior instrumentation and fusion alone. This can be done with a number of instrumentation systems and techniques (Chapter 38). The ideal candidate for a posterior procedure has a smaller, flexible curve, hypokyphosis, and a flexible compensatory lumbar curve. Posterior procedures also are an appropriate choice for a King type V or Lenke subclass 2 or 4 structural upper thoracic curve.

Standard posterior approaches are used (Chapter 34), and instrumentation may include hooks, wires, or screws for curve correction. The current trend involves the use of all pedicle screw constructs for deformity correction because of the segmental fixation that is obtained and the three-column control that is provided by a pedicle screw placed into the vertebral body. With this fixation, derotation may be possible to some extent during the correction maneuver. Another benefit of the use of pedicle screws is the extraspinal placement of implants, which avoids the space-occupying phenomenon created by hooks or wires placed within the spinal canal. Finally, the cortical fixation of a screw through the pedicle is superior biomechanically to hook fixation, which makes this technique appealing for an osteoporotic adult spine. These benefits are not without risks, however, and the primary concern is pedicle screw malposition that affects either the great vessels or the spinal cord, dura, or nerve roots. Thus far, when done by surgeons with proper training, pedicle screw placement has been safe and effective for the treatment of adult scoliosis; however, it is wise to discuss procedures in detail with patients before surgery and to explain the FDA status of devices used.

Selection of fusion levels is similar to that in adolescent scoliosis patients. The goal of surgery is a balanced spine with the head centered over the pelvis in the sagittal and coronal planes. Fusion should be from stable vertebra to stable vertebra unless pedicle screw instrumentation is used and fusion can safely be stopped short of the stable vertebra. For curves with features similar to King types II and V curves without severe kyphosis, pedicle screw fixation appears ideal. This technique allows fusion of the curve from end vertebra to end vertebra, which can save one to three fusion levels distally in some patients compared with typical hook constructs. In adults, flexibility of the compensatory curve must be considered more than in adolescents with scoliosis because overcorrection of the thoracic curve in a spine with a relatively inflexible lumbar curve results in decompensation and an unsatisfactory result. Therefore it is prudent to apply only a conservative amount of correction that can be accommodated by the compensatory curve so that normal balance is restored and further progression is halted. The amount of correction that can be obtained is estimated from preoperative bending films.

Avoiding a flatback deformity during posterior distraction is mandatory because this deformity is much easier to prevent than to treat. Nonetheless, because of pseudarthrosis, implant failure, transition syndromes, adjacent level fracture, patient positioning, and other technical reasons, flatback deformity can occur in some patients under the best of circumstances. Concave distraction of the lumbar spine, especially beyond L2, should be avoided because this maneuver is kyphogenic. Segmental instrumentation allows differential correction along the same rod, which is helpful in preventing flatback deformity and shoulder decompensation. Avoiding distraction, or even applying some convex compression, along with precontouring the rods into lordosis helps to maintain normal lumbar alignment.

Anterior Spinal Instrumentation and Fusion

Deformity correction through an anterior approach is described in Chapter 38 but deserves mention here because anterior instrumentation and fusion with third-generation implants have given excellent deformity correction in adults and have not caused significant problems with kyphosis as did the early Zielke and Dwyer implants. With single or double rod implant systems and structural grafts, anterior deformity correction is an excellent alternative for lumbar and thoracolumbar curves because it allows short segment correction of flexible curves. Primary thoracic curves with flexible and compensatory lumbar curves in adults also can be treated effectively with anterior fusion. However, correction must be appropriate for the ability of the lumbar curve to compensate; overcorrection in adults results in more decompensation than in the flexible spines of children with scoliosis. Also, as in pediatric deformities, strict attention must be paid to the upper thoracic spinal segment from T1 or T2 to T6 to prevent shoulder asymmetry due to a structural upper thoracic curve. An upper thoracic curve is a relative contraindication for anterior spinal instrumentation and fusion unless measures are taken to allow persistent tilt of the cephalad end vertebra, which will allow the upper thoracic curve to remain balanced.

Postoperative Management

Patients are monitored routinely in the intensive care unit with frequent neurological evaluations and observation to prevent complications associated with fluid shifts, which occur after such long procedures. Sitting is encouraged the day after surgery, and formal physical therapy is initiated. Walking as tolerated is encouraged with assistance until independent ambulation is achieved. A rigid TLSO is used in patients with osteoporosis but is not necessary except when patients are getting up from a supine position and ambulating. The Foley catheter is removed once the patient is able to get to a bedside commode with minimal assistance. Antibiotics are discontinued once drains are pulled, and oral narcotic analgesics usually are well tolerated by the third day after surgery. Pneumatic foot pulsation devices are used as prophylaxis against deep venous thrombosis because of the possible risk of epidural hematoma associated with pharmacological agents. These are discontin-

ued once the patient is fully independently ambulatory. Nonsteroidal antiinflammatory medications are avoided for 3 months postoperatively because of their inhibitory effect on fusion. The TLSO is discontinued at 4 to 6 months after surgery in most patients.

◆ Combined Anterior and Posterior Fusions

For a rigid curve of more than 70 degrees or a curve that is decompensated either sagittally or coronally, or for instrumentation that crosses the lumbosacral joint, a combined approach is necessary. For severe rigid thoracic deformities of more than 100 degrees, which often are associated with translation of the trunk of more than 4 to 6 cm anterior or lateral to the pelvis, Boachie-Adjei and Bradford showed that vertebrectomy, as a combined or staged procedure, was effective in achieving spinal balance. It is preferable to complete combined procedures, if possible, under a single anesthesia because this results in fewer complications and a shorter hospitalization; however, if any portion of the procedure is unexpectedly long, blood loss is excessive, or a patient is not able to tolerate continuation of the procedure, then it is prudent to postpone the second stage of the procedure. Parenteral nutrition between stages is recommended because patients often develop a postoperative ileus and do not tolerate enteral nutrition.

When a combined procedure is used, the first stage usually includes anterior release, discectomy, and fusion of the primary curve. If instrumentation is extended to the lumbosacral joint, anterior interbody fusion is necessary at L4-5 and L5-S1, with structural grafting of these discs to maintain lordosis, improve fusion rates, and decrease stresses on the posterior implants. Morselized bone graft is placed in the thoracic disc spaces and usually consists of the rib excised for the exposure. Supplemental bone graft can be obtained from the inner table of the anterior iliac crest if the rib is small or osteoporotic. Instrumentation may or may not be necessary during the anterior portion of the procedure and is placed at the surgeon's discretion.

After anterior release and fusion, posterior instrumentation and fusion are done, with segmental fixation from stable vertebra to stable vertebra. Care is taken to avoid ending an instrumentation construct at the apex of a curve in either the coronal or sagittal plane because of the risk of later decompensation. It also is prudent to include any disc level with severe degenerative changes, especially in degenerative deformities.

TECHNIQUE 41-4 *(Boachie-Adjei and Bradford)*
Approach the convex side of the curve. The specific exposure is dictated by the levels to be fused (p. 2083). Ligate the segmental vessels and elevate the outer cortex of the vertebral body as an osteoperiosteal flap. Resect the remaining vertebrae down to the dura at one or at multiple levels. For more severe deformities, resect multiple vertebrae. Excise the intervertebral discs completely to the

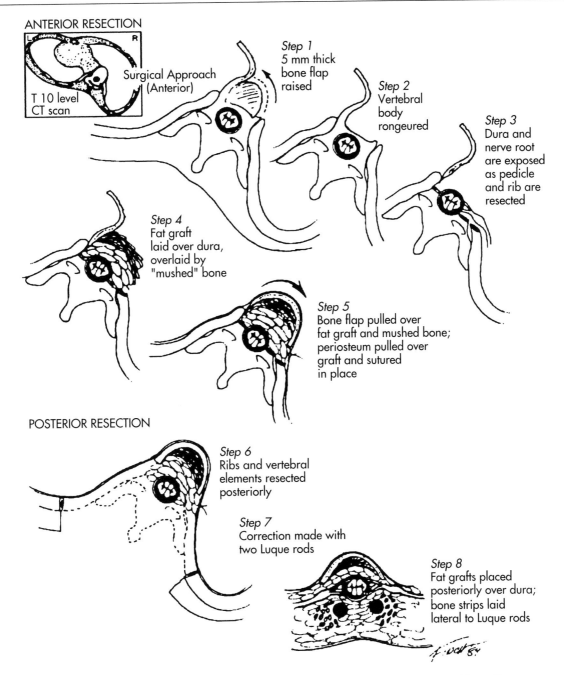

Fig. 41-14   Vertebral column resection and arthrodesis for complex deformities. (From Boachie-Adjei O, Dendrinos GK, Ogilvie JW, Bradford DS: *J Spinal Disord* 4:131, 1991.)

posterior longitudinal ligament at all levels encompassing the curve. Place the spongy cancellous bone removed from the resected vertebral bodies loosely over the dura, which is protected by fat or Gelfoam. Loosely reattach the outer cortex of the osteoperiosteal flap back over the spinal column. Remove the pedicles on the concave and the convex sides over the resected segments. The concave pedicle resection requires care and meticulous technique to resect the segment to its base. If this is not possible because of dural tube transposition, then most of it should be resected; whatever portion remains is removed during the second stage of the posterior procedure (Fig. 41-14).

The second stage of the procedure, done 1 to 2 weeks later, consists of concave rib osteotomies throughout the curvature and a thoracoplasty on the convex side. Remove the pedicles, laminae, and facets over the area and resect

continued

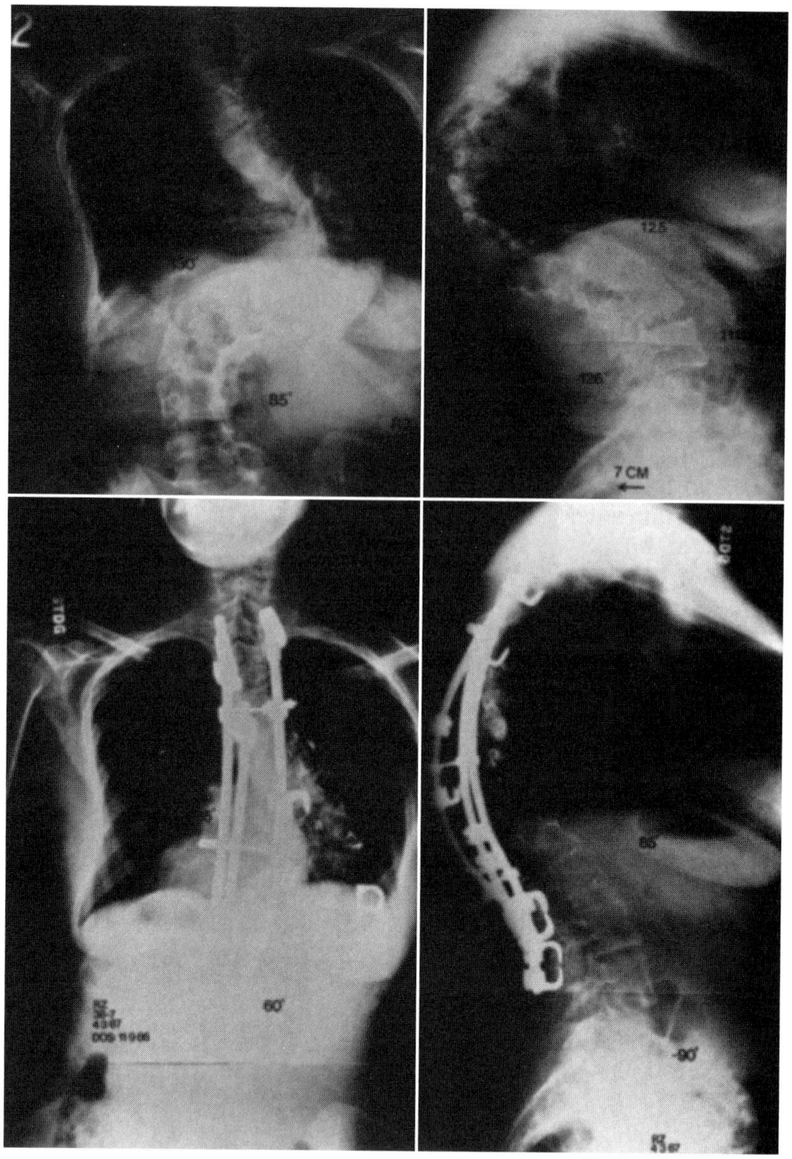

Fig. 41-15 **A** and **B**, Severe structural deformity with marked scoliosis, as well as kyphosis and sagittal plane imbalance. Correction was possible only by vertebral resection carried out over apical portion of curvature. Although Cotrel-Dubousset instrumentation was used, rods were placed so that correction without distraction was possible. Rods were positioned to allow cantilevered bending and coronal realignment without distraction, which would have run risk of producing paralysis. **C** and **D**, Postoperative appearance. (From Bradford DS: Adult scoliosis. In Lonstein JE, Bradford DS, Winter RB, Ogilvie JW, eds: *Moe's textbook of scoliosis and other spinal deformities*, ed 3, Philadelphia, 1995, WB Saunders.)

anteriorly. Examine the spinal cord over the entire resected area and continually monitor the dura to be certain that pulsation continues throughout the procedure. Perform segmental spinal instrumentation with L-rods or segmental instrumentation (Chapter 38). Insert iliac fixation in addition to sacral pedicle screws (Chapter 38) for fusion to the sacrum. Cut the ribs into match sticks and place over the fusion area lateral to the implants, taking care that no loose fragments lie against the spinal cord. Use fat or Gelfoam to protect the dura. Attempt to balance the spine in both the anteroposterior and sagittal planes. Total correction is not essential and therefore should not be attempted. Monitor somatosensory evoked potentials throughout the procedure. In addition, perform a wake-up test on all patients who do not have dependable somatosensory and motor evoked potentials.

AFTERTREATMENT. An underarm polypropylene body jacket is applied, and the patient is allowed to ambulate at will. The body jacket is worn for 4 to 6 months, depending on the quality of fusion mass (Fig. 41-15).

New Techniques

The newest generation of implants can be used to treat most deformities, allowing instrumentation of all thoracic levels down to the sacrum and pelvis. Approaches and techniques generally have remained the same, however. Pedicle screw instrumentation has been used in all levels in the treatment of spinal deformities, with excellent clinical and roentgenographic results. For lumbar curves, pedicle screw instrumentation is applied to the convexity and compressed to create lordosis; for typical thoracic curves, the pedicle screws are applied to the concavity of the deformity and distracted to restore kyphosis. Any compensatory curves must be treated appropriately with compression where lordosis is required and distraction where kyphosis is desired. Upper thoracic curves are controlled by compression of the convexity, since most of these curves also are kyphotic. Suk et al. achieved excellent correction and balance, while saving distal fusion levels, with the use of all-pedicle-screw constructs in the treatment of adolescent idiopathic scoliosis.

Computer navigation devices allow the placement of fiducials, or reference points, intraoperatively. Once computer reconstructions are calculated, video referencing creates a best-fit overlay over the known anatomy. This allows interpolation or animation of the placement and trajectories of proposed implants on preoperatively obtained images. This technique initially was used with CT and MRI studies but more recently has been used with fluoroscopy. Fluoroscopy has the advantage of "real-time" images that are not dependent on patient position and are not subject to as much error from motion as are CT and MRI. These technologies can confirm anatomical relationships and, although expensive, are being used more frequently.

Video-assisted thoracoscopic surgery (VATS) also has been gaining more widespread use. For skilled endoscopic spinal surgeons, VATS provides excellent visualization through relatively small incisions with the potential to decrease blood loss, postoperative pain, periscapular winging, and pulmonary dysfunction. However, the learning curve is very steep, with initial procedures taking a good deal longer than the typical thoracotomy. This technique requires double lumen intubation and places increased demands on the anesthesia staff. Although VATS continues to develop, the options for its use in anterior instrumentation are still limited. In adult patients with spinal deformity, in whom osteoporosis and osteopenia are prevalent, structural grafts may be more difficult to place endoscopically, thus limiting the application of VATS.

Adult Isthmic Spondylolisthesis

Spondylolisthesis is most commonly an acquired condition. Most progressive deformities occur in childhood, and deformities in adults usually are static and low grade. Two types of spondylolisthesis occur in adult patients: isthmic and degenerative. Each has its own characteristic etiology and pathoanatomy, and treatment varies slightly for each. Degenerative spondylolisthesis is discussed on p. 2074.

INCIDENCE

Isthmic spondylolisthesis is absent in newborns but occurs in juveniles and reaches the adult prevalence of 5% to 8% by the age of 18 years. Upright walking and its associated weight-bearing appear to be prerequisites for its development, since this disorder has not been reported in nonambulatory patients. Males are affected twice as often as females, and risk factors for isthmic spondylolisthesis include gymnastics, football, and pole-vaulting. Other at-risk avocations include weight-lifting, dancing, and volleyball, among other activities that cause

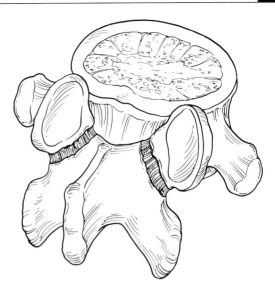

Fig. 41-16 Defect in isthmic spondylolysis, type IIA. (Redrawn from Wiltse LL, Rothman SLG: *Semin Spine Surg* 5:264, 1993.)

excessive lordosis or hyperflexion of the lumbar spine. People with active vocations, especially military recruits, may have a higher incidence of symptomatic or asymptomatic pars fractures (reported to occur in 9.7% of 1598 soldiers). Genetic transmission appears to occur and may be contributory.

ANATOMY

Generally, adult isthmic spondylolisthesis is nonprogressive, although symptoms of back pain and radiculopathy are common. Isthmic spondylolisthesis affects L5 in 89% of patients, L4 in 11%, and L3 in 3%. In adults, the slip usually is less than 50% and usually causes accelerated degeneration of the disc at the level of the pars defect. The slip occurs as the result of a defect in the pars interarticularis that interferes with the bony hook of the affected spinal motion segment (Fig. 41-16). The bony hook consists of the pedicle, pars, and inferior articular facet of the cephalad segment and the superior articular facet of the caudal segment. This structural linkage is weakened as a result of spondylolisthesis and can no longer resist translational instability. The posterior elements subsequently separate through the pars fracture, leaving the facet joints located, and the entire trunk translates anteriorly over the sacrum or caudal vertebral body. Severe slips can severely affect global sagittal balance because of the forward shift of the body's center of gravity. High-grade spondylolisthesis, however, is rare in adults.

Progression is rare in adult patients with L5 isthmic spondylolisthesis unless a previous decompression has been done to destabilize the posterior elements. The restraints to progression include the strong iliolumbar ligaments, large L5 transverse processes, disc, and annulus; further protection is provided by "deep seating" of L5 below the intercristal line. A stress riser necessarily exists at the level of the L4-5 disc at its junction with the immobile pelvis and stabilized L5, and this explains the increased progression and instability at the L4-5 level. Clinically, multiple factors likely contribute to stability and the resistance to spondylolisthesis. Increased instability should be suspected in the rare adult patient with isthmic spondylolisthesis at L4-5, and some degree of slip progression may occur.

In the presence of a pars fracture, shear stresses are placed across the disc, with 100% of the body weight creating an anteriorly directed force, compared with approximately 80% of the body weight when the intact facets share the load. This increased stress exacerbates disc space degeneration in adults and also may contribute to the formation of foraminal stenosis and subsequent radiculopathy. As callus formation occurs at the pars, a hook protrudes anteriorly from the bone itself and may be present simultaneously with superior articular facet overgrowth, both of which narrow the neural foramen. Fibrocartilaginous tissue also is present in the area of the pars fracture from failed attempts to heal the stress fracture. This pathoanatomy usually affects the L5 nerve root in patients with L5-S1 spondylolisthesis. Once the nerve is tethered within the neural foramen, further slipping mechanically stretches the nerve over the sacrum, contributing to radiculopathy.

Abnormal anatomy, such as dysplasia, also may predispose to progressive spondylolisthesis. Spina bifida occulta and dysplastic facet joints are defects in the bony hook that decrease the stability of the spondylolisthetic spinal segment, diminishing the normal resistance to shear forces and translation and allowing olisthesis. According to the classification of Marchetti and Bartolozzi, dysplasia can be divided into high and low dysplasia. Untreated high dysplasia is rare in adults and has a high incidence of progression. Low dysplasia is more common, with features consistent with spina bifida occulta, does not tend to progress, and is more commonly noted incidentally in adult patients.

BIOMECHANICS

Although pars fractures have been simulated in the laboratory, recreating spondylolisthesis has not been as straightforward. For instance, division of the pars in vitro resulted in significant motion in the axial and coronal planes, but translational instability did not occur. Biomechanical data also suggest that rotation and not a pure extension force may be the cause of pars fracture. In addition, the inability to recreate spondylolisthesis in biomechanical studies suggests that pars fracture is not the sole cause of translational instability. Further sectioning of the iliolumbar ligaments by Grobler et al. did not create any translation. In comparisons with a normal spine, Grobler et al. showed 12% more rotation, 33% more shear translation, and 43% more axial translation after creation of pars defects at L4-5 than after creation of pars defects at L5-S1. This difference was not attributable to the iliolumbar ligament because transection of the ligament alone did not result in a statistically significant increase in motion at the lumbosacral level. Thus it appears that instability is greater after pars fracture at the L4-5 level than at

the L5-S1 level. The iliolumbar ligaments may contribute some stability to the L5 level, but other mechanical or anatomical factors also must contribute to resistance of translational instability.

NATURAL HISTORY

Although not as likely as in adolescent patients, progression to a lesser degree may occur in adults, causing worsening of symptoms and progressive loss of function. Slips of 50% or more are rare in adults. Thus most adult patients are treated after pain develops and not prophylactically, as are children and adolescents. Postoperative progression of spondylolisthesis must be considered and prevented in patients with pars fractures who have decompressive procedures because of the possible disruption of the posterior ligamentous complex, facet capsules, or annulus. In a study by Haraldsson and Willner comparing adolescents and adults with spondylolisthesis, only 2 of 20 adults had progression of slips after age 25; both were after laminectomies. In contrast, 10 of 25 of those younger than 25 years of age had progressive slips. Thus laminectomy or combined bilateral resection of more than one facet must be considered a relative indication for fusion to prevent translational instability in the presence of a pars fracture.

Progressive disc degeneration occurs in most patients with isthmic spondylolisthesis and may be a contributing factor in the development of back pain. Floman documented progression of the slip from 9% to 30% (average, 14.6%) in 18 adult patients (32 to 55 years of age) with incapacitating lumbar back pain over a mean of 6.8 years. Progression began after the third decade and coincided with marked disc degeneration. A study of elite child and adolescent athletes by Muschik et al. and a study of 139 adults by Osterman et al. confirmed that in 80% to 90% most of the slipping had already occurred at the time of initial diagnostic studies and that competitive sports did not affect the progression of spondylolisthesis. The degree of slipping has been associated with same-level disc degeneration, but this was not associated with increased back symptoms. Excellent function can be maintained despite the presence of spondylolisthesis and disc degeneration and, accordingly, treatment should be directed at alleviating symptoms and not at preventing progression, since this rarely occurs.

CLINICAL EVALUATION

Patients often report distal lumbar pain; 11% of patients with distal back pain reported by Wiltse were found to have pars defects. Other authors have reported back pain of varying degrees in up to 91% of patients, occurring daily in about half and reported as severe and disabling in approximately 10% to 15%. However, spondylolysis and spondylolisthesis do not seem to predispose patients to more disability or pain than in the general population. However, pars fractures, with or without slipping, appear to be more common in symptomatic than asymptomatic patients. Antecedent trauma may be minimal, and the pars fracture may be an incidental finding. Disc

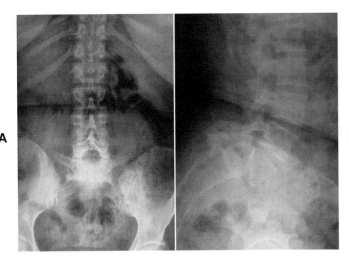

A

B

Fig. 41-17   Standing anteroposterior (**A**) and lateral (**B**) roentgenograms of patient with isthmic spondylolisthesis.

degeneration, facet arthritis, and pars fracture all may contribute to the back pain syndrome. Risk factors for back pain include grade II slip, increased wedging of L5 (low lumbar index), early disc degeneration, and spondylolisthesis at L4-5. L4-5 slips may be more symptomatic and more pronounced, probably because of increased biomechanical stresses and more inherent instability than at L5-S1.

Nerve compression may cause symptoms of radiculopathy or neurogenic claudication. Tension signs have been reported to be present in 19%, hamstring contractures in 27%, and a palpable step-off in 42% of patients. Sciatica is found more frequently in adults than in adolescents, is caused by foraminal stenosis, and usually affects the L5 root. Symptoms of neurogenic claudication caused by central spinal stenosis are not common in patients with isthmic spondylolisthesis because of the relative decompression of the spinal canal by the pars fractures. Symptoms of neurogenic claudication should prompt further evaluation of the spinal canal to identify the source of neural compression.

History and physical examination are important in determining the severity of symptoms and dysfunction. Special attention should be paid to aggravating and alleviating factors and the location of the pain. Pain in the distal lumbar spine that is worse with extension is characteristic of facet or pars pathology. Pain with flexion or sitting often is associated with discogenic causes. Radiculopathy may be aggravated with either maneuver. Pain that improves with walking uphill, resting on a grocery cart, or pushing a lawnmower indicates posterior element pathology. Tension signs may or may not be present but may be helpful in determining whether leg and buttock pain is radicular, referred, or muscular. Hamstring spasm, paraspinal muscle spasms that cause flattening of the back, and a spinous process step-off also can be identified. Claudication symptoms may signal the development of lateral recess stenosis, foraminal stenosis, or far-out compression of the L5 root by pressure between a large L5 transverse process and the sacrum. Bowel or bladder dysfunction is rare; however, if suspected, it can be identified with urological studies.

DIAGNOSTIC IMAGING
Roentgenography

Standing anteroposterior and lateral roentgenograms are diagnostic in most patients (Fig. 41-17). Standing films may show some slips that spontaneously reduce when the patient is supine. Supine films may be helpful in the evaluation of spinal tumors, for which better bone detail is necessary. Inspection of the pars region on the anteroposterior view usually identifies a lucency suggesting fracture, reactive sclerosis often contralateral to a spondylolysis—the "Napoleon's hat sign—or other indications of posterior element insufficiency, such as laminectomy or spina bifida occulta. The standing lateral view allows loading of the disc to translate any spondylolisthesis, making it and the pars fractures more visible. Lowe et al. showed that in 13 of 50 patients with spondylolisthesis translation was visible only on standing films. Occasionally, oblique views that show the traditional "Scotty dog" profile are necessary; oblique views identify as many as 19% of pars fractures that would be missed otherwise. A Ferguson anteroposterior view, which is a modified pelvic outlet view, may be useful as a preoperative study to evaluate the transverse processes of L5, the disc space between L5 and S1 for degeneration, and the posterior elements at L5 and S1. This image is acquired by focusing the roentgen beam on the L5-S1 disc with the beam parallel to the disc space (approximately a 30-degree cephalad tilt). Flexion-extension lateral images are useful for preoperative planning and for identifying hypermobility. In a patient with severe lumbosacral kyphosis, hyperlordosis, or sagittal decompensation, scoliosis films are warranted to assess global sagittal balance.

MRI

MRI is useful as a noninvasive screening tool for detection of compression on the neural elements and for early identification of disc desiccation. Sagittal images clearly delineate the discs and spinal canal, and parasagittal sequences give excellent detail of the neural foramen on T1-weighted images unless the patient has a concomitant scoliosis. Occasionally, horizontalization of the facet and diminished perineural fat obscure the nerve root, with an area of low signal intensity. This low-signal material identified on MRI has been found at surgery to correlate with fibrocartilaginous tissue and hypertrophic ligament within the neural foramen. T2-weighted images show disc hydration and edematous vertebral endplate changes, as described by Modic. A typical adult disc is white on T2-weighted images, with a slight cleft of decreased intensity. Asymmetry in disc attenuation is an indicator of desiccation and degeneration. In patients with adult isthmic spondylolisthesis, disc degeneration is present at the level of pars fracture. Of 40 patients studied with MRI by Szypryt et al., only 4 of 20 patients younger than 25 years had degeneration of the disc below the pars fracture; in contrast, 14 of 20 discs were degenerative in patients aged 25 to 45 years. At the adjacent level disc above the pars fracture, 4 of the 20 younger patients had disc desiccation, whereas half of those 25 to 45 years of age had degenerative changes. Osterman et al. confirmed disc degeneration in all 27 of their patients treated operatively. MRI also is helpful for the identification of fusion levels when surgery is planned and for guiding invasive diagnostic procedures such as discogram and myelogram. However caution must be exercised because of the large number of asymptomatic abnormalities on diagnostic studies even in young patients.

Bone Scintigraphy

Technetium bone scanning occasionally is helpful in adults to identify other causes of axial lumbar pain. Sacroiliac arthritis can mimic pars and facet pain syndromes because of sclerotomal referred pain. Facet arthritis, acute fractures, impending pars fractures, benign or malignant tumors, infection, pseudarthrosis, and metabolic bone diseases all may be identified by bone scanning. Bone scanning is more useful in younger patients to identify acute fractures of the pars, which may have healing potential, and to identify occult fractures of the pars. In a study by Lowe at al., 25% of a group of military recruits had increased uptake in the presence of a pars fracture documented on roentgenograms. Similarly, Van Den Oever et al. found that 74% of their patients with spondylolysis had normal bone scans. Both studies noted that increased activity was more common when symptoms were present for less than a year. Although bone scanning generally is not required for the diagnosis of adult isthmic spondylolisthesis, it may be helpful in excluding other conditions that can cause similar symptoms.

CT Myelography

Myelography followed by CT scanning is a dynamic study that allows observation of spinal fluid flow along the nerve roots and the conus medullaris. Because of its invasive nature, it should be used only as a preoperative study or if MRI is indeterminate or technically not feasible. Myelography is indicated for preoperative correlation with MRI studies in patients with (1) radicular complaints and multiple foci of pathology on the MRI, (2) continued radiculopathy in the absence of MRI findings, (3) radiculopathy and significant spinal deformity that precludes the use of MRI, and (4) contraindications to MRI. Standard myelogram images should be obtained, including anteroposterior, lateral, and oblique views, with the addition of flexion and extension lateral views in the upright position. Flexion and extension lateral images provide a dynamic picture of the bony structures and their relationship with the dural sac and neural elements and may identify nerve root compression that is missed by the static positioning of MRI or CT alone. After the myelogram, CT images are obtained to complete the study. For optimal reconstructions, 1.0- to 1.5-mm cuts should be obtained through the area in question. Alternatively, for helical CT scanners, 3.0-mm cuts can be used, with 1.0- to 1.5-mm reformatted images giving a similar high resolution.

Discography

Discography is a provocative procedure that seeks to elicit and reproduce exactly a patient's primary pain pattern. This can be done before surgery in a patient with adjacent level disc degeneration or multiple level degenerative disease that has been documented on MRI to determine if an adjacent level should be included in a fusion. Care must be taken in the interpretation of discograms because abnormal discographic findings may be present in as many as 17% of normal subjects. Discography may be useful in identifying symptomatic adjacent level degenerative disease, which was noted Henson, McCall, and O'Brien to be present in 27 (51%) of 52 patients with back pain and spondylolisthesis at L5-S1. Spondylolisthesis at L4-5 was noted in 14 of 27 patients with discographically confirmed disc degeneration; however, the extent of disc degeneration did not correlate with the amount of slippage. No prospective randomized trial has correlated operative outcome with preoperative discographic findings.

In clinical practice, discography may still be considered in the preoperative evaluation of patients with spondylolisthesis. In patients with multiple degenerated segments, if pain is elicited at all levels, elective fusion might be reconsidered because all levels may be affected or a significant psychosocial component may be present. Under these circumstances, a long fusion to the sacrum would likely be debilitating to the patient. If pain is identified at a single segment, or at most two segments, fusion can be done with more reassurance of improvement. At least one normal level should be identified and injected as a control, and, if possible, the patient should be lightly sedated and able to respond to questioning during the procedure. Concordance of pain response seems to be more important than morphology of the disc. Correlation between MRI and discography has been found to be high, and some authors reported equivalent results using MRI alone. Discography has yet to be proved as a diagnostic and predictive study, and its use must be carefully considered. Anecdotal reports have shown its usefulness in determining fusion levels if uncertainty exists after conventional imaging has been done.

NONOPERATIVE TREATMENT

Nonoperative management of isthmic spondylolisthesis is effective in most adult patients. Initial treatment includes a short period of rest and the use of acetaminophen or nonsteroidal antiinflammatories for pain control. The use of muscle relaxants and narcotics is minimized because of potential dependence and the lack of data to support their efficacy above over-the-counter medications. Manipulation and modalities, such as heat, cold, ultrasound, and transcutaneous electrical nerve stimulation, are short-term remedies and may be effective; however, a more preventive approach should be considered. Physical therapy should be initiated early for symptoms that do not improve. Trunk-stabilization exercises, avoiding hyperextension, are useful in improving posture and extensor muscle strength and may prevent later flare-ups. Proper instruction in isometric trunk stabilization has been reported by O'Sullivan et al. to result in sustained reduction of pain and disability compared with controls as confirmed by visual analog pain scores and the Oswestry functional disability scores at 30-month follow-up. At 3-year follow-up of an extension exercise program, pain described as moderate or severe was present in 62%, with 61% unable to work or limited in their vocation. In a demographically similar group of patients with spondylolisthesis treated with an abdominal flexion program and evaluated at 3 years, only 19% had moderate or severe pain, and only 24% were unable to work or were limited in their vocation. Thus it appears that pure extension exercise programs are not as effective as isometric stabilization programs or flexion programs. Aerobic fitness also has been shown to be effective in the treatment of back pain and should be considered early. Inactivity should be minimized because this produces debilitation and depression, both of which may contribute to the development of a chronic pain syndrome.

Bracing is an option for pain management in some patients, but without a thigh cuff no orthosis is particularly effective in immobilizing the lumbar spine below L3. Because pars fractures in adults do not heal, bracing provides only symptomatic treatment. An orthosis may have an indirect positive effect by limiting activity, but this restriction also may result in atrophy of the trunk muscles and more pain when unsupported, which leads to a patient's dependency on the orthosis. If bracing is used, it should be continued only until symptoms abate, and then trunk-stabilization exercises should be started as long as the patient remains pain free during extension maneuvers. If symptoms allow, isometric exercises while wearing the brace can be done until the brace is discontinued.

Epidural Steroid Injections

A corticosteroid and anesthetic solution can be used for pars injections, transforaminal, translaminar, or caudal epidural steroid injections, and facet injections, but no literature exists to guide the surgeon in the use of injections for spondylolisthesis. Radicular symptoms seem to respond better to steroid injection than does axial pain.

Nonoperative treatment can be effective for back pain and radiculopathy. In adult patients the actual diagnosis may be new to the patient, but the pathology likely has been present without symptoms for decades. Therefore every attempt should be made to control symptoms nonoperatively if possible.

OPERATIVE TREATMENT

For patients in whom nonoperative treatment is unsuccessful, who have a favorable psychological profile, and who are compliant and aware of surgical shortcomings, operative intervention should be considered. Patient selection is extremely important when decompression or fusion is done in adults with spondylolisthesis. Hanley and Levy noted that satisfactory results were significantly fewer in compensation cases, in patients with radicular symptoms, and in smokers. Franklin et al. reported that in compensation cases, back pain persisted in 66.7% of patients, and the quality of life was the same or worse in 55.8%. They also noted that the use of instrumentation increased the rate of failure in this population. Pseudarthrosis correlated with poor results. An educational level of less than the twelfth grade also was related to a poor prognosis for pain relief and return to work.

Back pain or radicular symptoms that have not improved with conservative treatment are the most common indications for surgery in adults with isthmic spondylolisthesis. Information obtained from a thorough history and physical examination and appropriate diagnostic imaging studies determines which operative procedure is best for an individual patient.

◆ Decompression

Lumbar decompression without fusion may be indicated in patients with symptoms of radiculopathy or neurogenic claudication. Although not recommended in children because of the risk of progressive spondylolisthesis, the Gill laminectomy has provided satisfactory long-term results in 75% to 90% of patients, regardless of postoperative slipping. In Gill's report, a maximum of 14% slip progression occurred in a group of 52 patients followed for an average of 71 months. Progression of spondylolisthesis may occur less frequently after Gill laminectomy if there is antecedent stabilizing disc degeneration. This procedure simply is a resection of all bone and fibrous tissue from the pars defect distally, including the lower portion of the pars interarticularis, lamina, spinous process, inferior articular facet, and all intervening ligamentous structures. Radiculopathy is relieved in most patients; however, significant back pain should be considered as an indication for fusion.

TECHNIQUE 41-5 *(Gill et al.)*

Place the patient prone on the operating table and through a midline incision expose subperiosteally the spinous processes of the fourth and fifth lumbar and the first sacral vertebrae (Fig. 41-18, *A*). Demonstrate the mobility of the fifth lumbar neural arch and with a rongeur resect the spinous processes of all three vertebrae (Fig. 41-18, *B*). Also with a rongeur resect the middle part of the loose fifth lumbar neural arch (Fig. 41-18, *C*). Then bite away the inferior aspect of the laminae of the fourth lumbar vertebra until the ligamentum flavum has been freed. By sharp dissection excise the ligamentum flavum from between the

continued

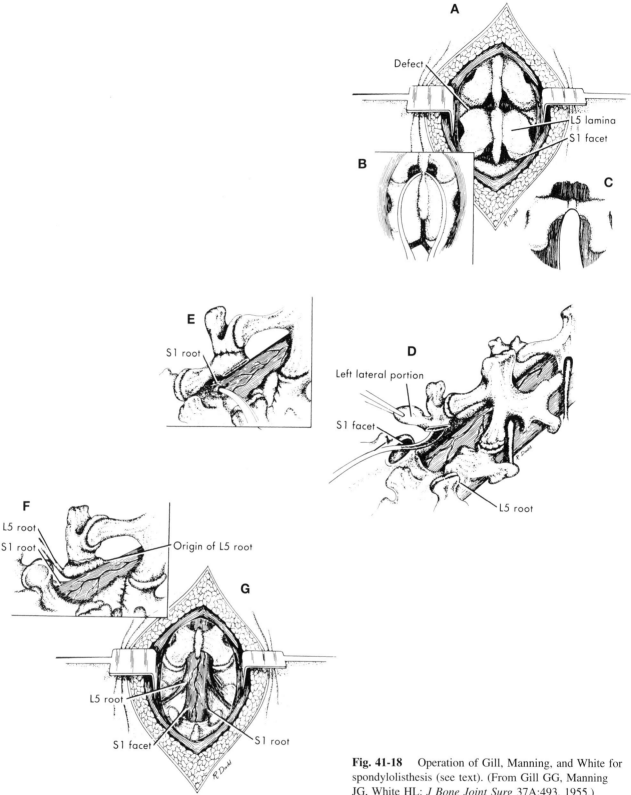

Fig. 41-18 Operation of Gill, Manning, and White for spondylolisthesis (see text). (From Gill GG, Manning JG, White HL: *J Bone Joint Surg* 37A:493, 1955.)

fourth and fifth vertebrae. Again by sharp dissection excise on one side the lateral part of the loose fifth lumbar arch, freeing it from its articulation with the sacrum and from the tissues in the defect in the pars interarticularis (Fig. 41-18, *D*); dissect close to bone to avoid damaging the fifth lumbar nerve root (Fig. 41-18, *E*). Next retract this root superiorly and medially. Carefully dissect it from the fibrocartilaginous tissue and free it laterally until it passes through the intervertebral foramen (Fig. 41-18, *F* and *G*). Resect bone from the pedicle as necessary to free the root. Then examine the exposed fourth and fifth lumbar discs and, if indicated, excise one or both. Carry out the same procedure on the opposite side.

AFTERTREATMENT. Postoperative care involves routine use of epidural or parenteral narcotics. Physical therapy is employed in the initial mobilization of the patient, which is started on the day after surgery. No anticoagulation is used if epidural anesthesia has been given. Pneumatic compression devices should be worn until the patient is ambulatory. A bladder catheter is retained until the patient can get to a bedside commode or to the bathroom with assistance, usually at 1 or 2 days. The epidural catheter is removed on the basis of patient analgesic requirements or by the third day after surgery. Diet is advanced as tolerated, walking is encouraged, and the patient is discharged when independent ambulation is possible and only oral pain medication is required.

◆ Posterolateral in Situ Fusion

Presently, standard treatment for adult patients with isthmic spondylolisthesis is in situ fusion from L5 to S1, with or without instrumentation, using autogenous cancellous bone graft. Fusion appears superior to decompression alone for resolution of symptoms. Single-level fusion is required in approximately 85% of patients, and good results are obtained in 89%. Although 30% of patients had progression of their slips after laminectomy and in situ fusion, Bosworth et al. found no difference in symptoms among these patients compared with those with in situ fusion alone. If slip progression does occur after posterolateral in situ fusion, observation is warranted.

TECHNIQUE 41-6 *(Wiltse, Modified)*
Induce anesthesia and insert an endotracheal tube, Foley catheter, and arterial intravenous line as indicated by the clinical status of the patient. Place the patient on a spinal frame that allows the abdomen to hang free. Make a midline skin incision extending one spinous process above and one below the levels to be fused. Elevate the subcutaneous tissue off the fascia for a distance of three or four fingerbreadths bilaterally; include exposure of the posterosuperior iliac crest on the side to be used for the bone graft donor site. Make a fascial incision two fingerbreadths lateral to the

midline, extending over the area to be fused. Bluntly dissect the paraspinal muscles down to the facet joint capsules. Carry the dissection down to the transverse processes to be fused. Clean the muscle subperiosteally to expose the transverse process and intertransverse ligament. Denude the facet joints by removing the fascia over them and then stripping them clean by subperiosteal dissection. Carry the dissection around the pars interarticularis. Prepare the opposite side in a similar manner. Do not denude the superior facets of the most cephalad level to be fused.

Obtain the bone graft from the donor site before denuding the recipient site. Incise the fascia over the iliac crest with sharp or electrocautery dissection. Carry the dissection from the posterosuperior iliac spine to about 3 to 4 cm lateral on the iliac crest. Strip the gluteal musculature from the crest laterally. Remove a corticocancellous bone graft from the exposed portions of the crest down to the inner table. Close the wound over closed suction drainage.

Prepare the recipient site for grafting by first placing corticocancellous strips beneath the transverse processes, bridging the transverse ligament. Place the grafts with the cortical side toward the ligament. Remove all cartilage from the facets to be fused. Place cancellous bone grafts in the facet defects. Denude all areas of exposed bone, including the ala of the sacrum, the transverse processes, and the exposed pars interarticularis. Carefully pack the remaining bone in the gutters bilaterally from the pars interarticularis to the tips of the transverse processes. Close the wound in layers. Place closed suction drains in the subcutaneous tissue bilaterally.

AFTERTREATMENT. The patient is allowed to be up the next day, wearing a rigid lumbosacral brace, but is strongly advised to refrain from smoking until the fusion is solid. Aspirin and nonsteroidal medication are discontinued, and bracing is continued until the fusion is solid.

Modifications of Bilateral Lateral Fusion
Spinal decompression can be done through a midline exposure of the spine over the areas to be decompressed. This incision is closed before the lateral approach is made. Decompression should always accompany a reduction attempt to help minimize the risk of injury to the cauda equina. This not only prevents impingement of nerve roots on bony or ligamentous structures during the reduction maneuver, but also allows the surgeon to assess tension directly by palpation. Reduction is indicated based on the pathology present and the patient's symptoms. For predominant symptoms of radiculopathy in a patient with spondylolisthesis, decompression should accompany posterolateral fusion. Pedicle screw instrumentation to improve the fusion rate is becoming increasingly popular. A prospective, randomized study of 77 patients treated with posterolateral fusion either with pedicle screw fixation (37) or without instrumentation (40) found no significant

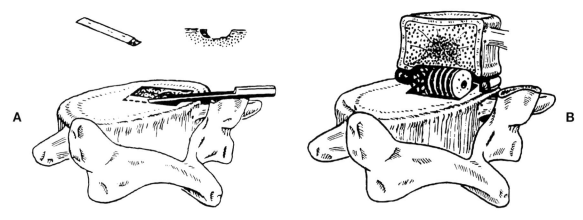

Fig. 41-19   Unilateral posterior lumbar interbody fusion (uPLIF or transforaminal lumbar interbody fusion). **A,** Decorticated vertebral body and preparation of osteotomy site. **B,** Bone chips and stacked dowels in place. (Redrawn from Blume HG: *Clin Orthop* 193:75, 1985.)

differences in level of pain, disability, or fusion rates between the two groups of patients. As in children and adolescents, fusion alone may relieve symptoms in adults with low-grade spondylolisthesis. In a retrospective study, Nooraie et al. compared 19 patients undergoing stabilization and fusion to 26 patients treated with decompression, stabilization, and fusion. Results showed no significant differences between the two groups. Instrumentation should be considered for high-risk groups (e.g., smokers). Instrumentation is especially important if a reduction has been done, even if unintentional. The pedicles usually are identified after the primary exposure is complete. They can be identified at the point formed by the intersection of an imaginary line bisecting the transverse process and another line bisecting the superior facet. This area is denuded, and the pedicle is probed with special instruments or guide wires. The pedicles can be tapped to receive the screws after the position of the probes or guide wires has been confirmed by roentgenograms, fluoroscopy, or computer-assisted navigation. Direct EMG stimulation of pedicle screws also is helpful to determine if pedicle cortical bone has been violated, especially medial and inferiorly. The placement of the screws and plates or rods varies with the type of instrumentation used.

◆ Posterior Lumbar Interbody Fusion

A technique for PLIF described by Cloward in 1943 has been used extensively by him and others for the treatment of spondylolisthesis. It is best suited for grade I or II displacement but is generally unsuited for displacements of grade III or higher unless reduction is done by posterior Harrington or similar instrumentation, as advocated by Vidal et al. Bohlman and Cook combined posterior interbody fusion with a posterolateral fusion, and Takeda combined it with a Bosworth H-graft fusion. Retraction of nerve roots and the dural sac is necessary to insert the grafts, and cauda equina deficits have been reported. Cloward reported a 4% incidence of footdrop in his series, all of which improved. This technique frequently requires internal fixation to prevent displacement of the graft

and further slip. Cloward used spinous process wiring. Steffee and Sitkowski and others suggested the use of pedicle screws and plates for this type of fixation. Cloward achieved fusion in 97% and complete resolution of pain in 83% of patients. Suk et al. reported the results of PLIF combined with pedicle screw instrumentation for patients with combinations of back pain, radiculopathy, and neurogenic claudication. In their retrospective review of 76 patients, claudication symptoms resolved in 96%, motor symptoms improved in 71%, and sensory changes were better in 55%. Success rates were equal in the PLF and PLIF groups, although the PLIF group had significantly more excellent results (75% compared with 45%). Reduction of approximately 50% was obtained in both groups; however, only 28% reduction was maintained with PLF with pedicle screws compared with 42% reduction maintained in the PLIF group.

A variation of PLIF is unilateral PLIF (uPLIF) or transforaminal lumbar interbody fusion (TLIF). Originally described by Blume, uPLIF produced successful results in 80% of patients treated for lumbar disc pathology. Unique to this procedure is the preservation of the ligamentum flavum by approaching the disc in the foraminal region after unilateral facetectomy (Fig. 41-19). This theoretically avoids epidural scarring and excessive postoperative instability because the spinal canal is not opened and the interspinous-supraspinous ligament complex, lamina, and contralateral facet are left intact. Harms et al. reported successful arthrodesis with TLIF in 97% of patients. Complications have been few, and in carefully selected patients this procedure has definite advantages over traditional PLIF.

TECHNIQUE 41-7 *(PLIF)*

Make a posterior approach to the spine to expose the transverse processes of L5 bilaterally as well as the sacral ala. Pedicle screws can be placed before laminectomy so that distraction can be applied through the screws to assist in providing tension. Once the posterior structures are on tension, removal of the loose posterior element of L5 is easier. Perform a Gill decompression (p. 2091) to expose the nerve roots and create a pedicle-to-pedicle working window. Carefully retract the S1 nerve root medially to expose the disc space, with periodic rest periods to allow blood flow to the root. Perform annulotomy sharply from each side of the dura and remove the disc with curets and pituitary rongeurs. A bone chisel also is helpful in removing the posterior endplate to a level flush with the central concavity of the endplate. This maneuver decorticates the endplate and also allows a better fit of the graft material. Further decorticate the anterior third of the disc under lateral fluoroscopy using an angled bone chisel or an angled curet under direct observation. Place cancellous autograft in the anterior third of the disc space and use tamps to compact it against the annulus and anterior longitudinal ligament (ALL). Place mesh or trapezoidal carbon fiber cages, allograft struts, or tricortical autograft into the disc space while distraction is maintained, first from one then the other side of the dura. After the structural graft or implant is placed, pack and tamp more cancellous autograft behind it. Take care not to overfill the disc space so that the graft is not retropulsed into the spinal canal.

This technique allows restoration of the normal lordotic disc configuration after the posterior instrumentation is compressed. Use of threaded cylindrical interbody fusion cages results in parallel endplates of adjacent discs and may contribute to loss of normal segmental lordosis, which is most important at L5-S1. If these implants are used, take care to maintain this normal alignment. Close the incision over drains and use an epidural catheter or parenteral narcotics for postoperative analgesia.

AFTERTREATMENT. Aftertreatment is similar to that after other fusion techniques, but the use of an orthosis is optional. The epidural catheter, if used, is removed the morning of the third postoperative day, and the patient usually is discharged 5 days after surgery.

Anterior Lumbar Interbody Fusion

Anterior lumbar interbody fusion (ALIF) can be used alone or as part of a combined procedure. For low-grade slips, ALIF alone allows removal of the disc, which is degenerative in most adult patients. This, theoretically, should alleviate discogenic pain. Removal of the disc and placement of a graft also can restore disc height significantly. The bone graft is under constant compression, which should improve fusion, paraspinal muscles are not disturbed, and in revisions the difficulty of reexploration can be avoided. For severe slips, in situ L5-S1 fibular peg grafting can be done with relative ease but requires posterior stabilization.

Disadvantages of ALIF are well known: retrograde ejaculation, vascular injury, visceral injury, and deep venous thrombosis. Herniated disc fragments are not visible from the anterior approach, nor are the nerve roots or pars fractures, to aid in determining whether decompression is adequate.

Satisfactory results after ALIF appear to be independent of the fusion rate and comparable to the results of decompression and PLF. Of 20 patients treated with ALIF for adult isthmic spondylolisthesis, Cheng et al. reported satisfactory results in 19, with definite fusions in 15 at an average of 10.5 years after surgery. Symptoms of back pain predominated and responded well to ALIF. Of the 9 patients in this study with sciatica, 6 had resolution of symptoms, 2 had occasional sciatica, and 1 had constant pain. The improvement in nerve root symptoms seems to be related to disc height restoration, ligamentotaxis, and increased volume of the neuroforamen. Using threaded interbody fusion cages in a human cadaver model, Chen et al. showed a 29% increase in neuroforaminal area at L4-5 and a 34% increase at L5-S1. Posterior disc height also increased 37% and correlated well with the neuroforaminal area increases. Thus by removing and fusing the degenerative disc, restoring disc height, and increasing neuroforaminal area, ALIF can be successful in the treatment of adult isthmic spondylolisthesis. The fusion rate, despite satisfactory results, has remained low in comparison to PLF.

◆ Spondylolisthesis Reduction

High-grade spondylolisthesis is rare in adults, and when it occurs, the slip usually is quite rigid. If a slip of more than 50% is identified in an adult patient, reduction should be considered. The goal should be reduction of the slip angle to neutral, or lordosis if possible, and the slip should be reduced to 50% or less but not necessarily to an anatomical position. Complete reduction of slips carries great morbidity in children and is likely more dangerous in adults, except in low-grade slips. For stiff, high-grade slips in adults, resection of L5 anteriorly followed by reduction of L4 onto the sacrum probably is the best option if in situ fusion will not suffice.

The technique described by Speed generally is used for high-grade slips after posterior instrumentation, fusion, and decompression.

TECHNIQUE 41-8 *(Speed)*

Make a midline incision from the umbilicus to the pubis and fully expose the sacral promontory. Then raise the foot of the table and pack the intestines out of the way. Palpate the relations of the fifth lumbar vertebra with the sacrum and confirm the roentgenographic findings. If the bifurcation of the aorta is low, retract it along with the left common iliac vein. Just to the right of the midline and avoiding the midsacral nerve and artery and the sympathetic ganglia, incise the peritoneum from the fourth lumbar interspace to the sacrum. Then determine the proper angle and depth for a drill to be inserted to pass obliquely through the body of the fifth lumbar vertebra and into the sacrum; with the patient supine, the direction is almost perpendicular to the floor. Then pass a large drill through the fifth lumbar

continued

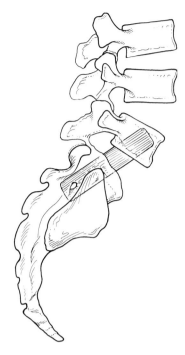

Fig. 41-20   Kellogg-Speed anterior fusion for spondylolisthesis. (Redrawn from Speed K: *Arch Surg* 37:715, 1983.)

vertebra and into the sacrum; as the drill passes from the body of the fifth lumbar vertebra and into the intervertebral space, advancing the drill is easier until the body of the sacrum is reached, when it becomes more difficult. From the tibia take a cortical graft and insert it into the hole, transfixing the fifth lumbar vertebra to the sacrum (Fig. 41-20).

AFTERTREATMENT. In patients with high-grade slips, a rigid TLSO with a hip spica cast is fitted, and the patient is non-weight-bearing for 6 weeks. Weight-bearing then is initiated, and the brace is discontinued at 3 months or once fusion is evident.

◆ Paramedian Retroperitoneal Approach

The retroperitoneal approach is useful for exposure of the lumbosacral joint and lumbar spine distal to the renal vessels. This approach is made with the patient supine, which allows a direct anterior approach to the discs. A left-sided longitudinal incision or a "bikini" incision can be used to allow access to the confluence of the fascia over the rectus abdominis muscle and the oblique abdominal muscles. The fascia is divided to expose the pre-peritoneal fat, and blunt dissection is used to expose the peritoneal contents, which are ligated anteriorly. The segmental vessels are ligated with special attention to ligating the presacral vessels and the iliolumbar vein at L5. This mobilizes the iliac vessels and allows exposure of the entire

L5-S1 disc. Care must be taken to avoid the use of electro-cautery near the superior hypogastric plexus because damage to this structure, which lies on the left iliac artery, can cause sexual dysfunction in women or retrograde ejaculation in men. Multiple ALIFs can be done using this approach, although thorough dissection of L5-S1 may be difficult if spondylolisthesis is significant.

TECHNIQUE 41-9 *(Lehmer)*

This procedure consists of two stages. The determination of when the second stage should be done depends on the stability after completion of the first stage. In the first stage, approach the anterior lumbosacral spine transperitoneally or retroperitoneally. Remove the body of L5 along with the L4-5 and L5-S1 discs to the bases of the pedicles. In the second stage, excise the loose neural arch and the pedicles of L5 through a midline posterior approach. Prepare the opposing L4 and S1 endplates for fusion. Reduce the body of L4 onto S1 (with or without an interbody fusion). Stabilize the L4 and S1 reduction and fusion with trans-pedicular instrumentation. Perform a routine bilateral posterolateral fusion.

AFTERTREATMENT. A lumbosacral orthosis is worn for 6 to 12 weeks. Ambulation is begun on the second postoperative day after the second stage.

Rheumatoid Arthritis of Spine

Rheumatoid arthritis is a systemic inflammatory disorder caused by lymphoproliferative disease within synovium, which results in cartilaginous destruction, periarticular erosions, and attenuation of ligaments and tendons. Pannus formation in the spine also may cause spinal cord compression. This entity occurs twice as often in young women, with the age at diagnosis typically between 30 to 50 years. Cervical instability is the most serious and potentially lethal manifestation of rheumatoid arthritis, with roentgenographic changes or instability present in 19% to 88% of patients. Lumbar or thoracic pathology rarely is present in patients with rheumatoid arthritis. Spinal disease is more common in patients severely affected by erosive peripheral disease and in patients with a longer disease history. Three basic types of cervical instability are present in this disease: atlantoaxial instability is most common, affecting 19% to 70% of patients, basilar impression or atlantoaxial impaction occurs in up to 38%, and subaxial subluxation occurs in 7% to 29%.

CLINICAL EVALUATION

Pain, neurological sequelae, or instability often are the presenting symptoms. Approximately 61% of individuals undergoing total joint replacement were reported to have instability in the cervical spine; 50% of these patients had no symptoms attributable to the neck preoperatively. From 40% to 88% of patients with rheumatoid arthritis of the spine have neck pain, and 7% to 58% have neurological findings. Axial neck pain usually is occipital and may be associated with headaches. Myelopathic symptoms include early weakness and gait disturbance, with frequent tripping or clumsiness. Hand function may be impaired, with coordination disturbances that cause difficulty differentiating coins or buttoning clothing. Sensory changes and bowel and bladder incontinence are late myelopathic symptoms. In patients with atlantoaxial instability, vertebrobasilar insufficiency due to kinking of the vertebral arteries can cause vertigo, tinnitus, or visual disturbances that lead to loss of equilibrium. Neurological evaluation often is difficult because of the peripheral disease. Tendon ruptures, severe joint disturbances, and previous surgery also make neurological examination difficult. Any findings consistent with myelopathy should stimulate further investigation.

DIAGNOSTIC IMAGING

Roentgenography

Roentgenograms should include anteroposterior, lateral, odontoid, and lateral flexion and extension views. Instability and potential for neurological sequelae are correlated best with the posterior atlantodens interval (PADI), which is determined by measuring the distance between the ventral surface of the lamina of C1 and the dorsal aspect of the odontoid; the interval should be more than 14 mm. This measurement is 97% sensitive for the presence of paralysis. In patients with preoperative paralysis caused by atlantoaxial subluxation, recovery is not expected if the spinal canal diameter is less than 10 mm. If basilar impression is coexistent, then significant recovery occurs only if the space available for the cord is at least 13 mm. If the space for the cord is 14 mm or less, decompression must be considered because of the risk of paralysis in patients with atlantoaxial instability. The PADI, however, does not represent the space available for the cord because the soft tissues are not included in the measurement. The atlantodens interval (ADI) is determined by measuring the distance between the posterior edge of the ring of C1 and the anterior edge of the odontoid and normally should be 3.5 mm or less in an adult. An ADI of more than 10 to 12 mm is clinically significant and suggests transverse ligament disruption; however, this measurement is not useful in predicting neurological sequelae caused by instability, possibly because of the natural history of atlantoaxial instability. As atlantoaxial instability progresses, subsequent vertical instability develops. As this superior migration occurs, the ADI actually decreases. Despite significant progression of instability and potential neurological deficit, the ADI will not increase further. Posterior subluxation is best determined by acute angulation of the cord and upper cervical spine as identified by sagittal reformatted CT scanning, lateral air contrast tomography, or preferably MRI. Lateral subluxation implies some rotation of the atlas and is present when the lateral masses of C1 lie 2 mm or more laterally than those of C2.

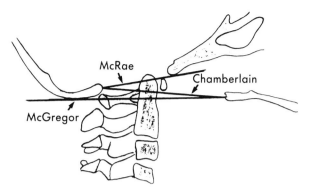

Fig. 41-21 Drawing of base of skull and upper spine showing McGregor's line, McRae's line, and Chamberlain's line. (From Hensinger RN: Section 23, Cervical Spine: pediatric. In American Academy of Orthopaedic Surgeons: *Orthopaedic knowledge update I: Home study syllabus*, 1984.)

Atlantoaxial impaction is measured using the McGregor line (Fig. 41-21). This line is constructed from the base of the hard palate to the outer cortical table of the occiput. The tip of the odontoid is then measured perpendicular to this line. Superior migration is considered present in men if the tip of the odontoid is 4.5 mm above this line. Ranawat et al. described a method of determining the degree of settling on the lateral roentgenogram using the minimal distance between a line drawn from the center of the anterior arch to the center of the posterior arch of the atlas, and a vertical line drawn along the posterior aspect of the odontoid from the center of the pedicles of C2. They reported that the normal value was 15 mm for women and 17 mm for men, with less than 13 mm considered abnormal (Fig. 41-22). To determine vertebral settling, Redlund-Johnell and Pettersson used the minimal distance between the McGregor line and the midpoint of the inferior margin of the body of the axis on the lateral roentgenogram in the neutral position (Fig. 41-23). They noted the normal value for men to be 34 mm or more and 29 mm or more for women (100 patients each). Kawaida, Sakou, and Morizono compared the predictive power of these screening methods and reported that they found the Redlund-Johnell method better for diagnosing basilar impression.

Subaxial subluxations produce a cascading, or "staircase," appearance of the spine. Any slippage of 4 mm or more, or 20% of the adjacent vertebral body, is considered significant. Measurement of sagittal spinal canal diameter is most useful and should be more than 13 mm. The risk of spinal cord compression and injury is higher in patients with smaller canal diameters.

CT Myelography and MRI

Three-dimensional imaging is useful in patients who have a neurological deficit or roentgenographic evidence of instability. MRI or CT myelography helps delineate the true space available for the cord. MRI is excellent for viewing soft tissues and the neural elements, but myelography followed by CT scanning gives similar information. In addition to bony

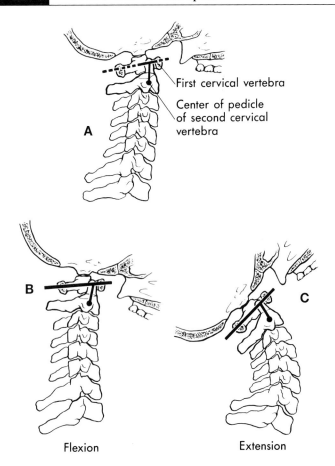

Fig. 41-22 Measurement of superior migration in rheumatoid arthritis. **A,** Diameter of ring of first cervical vertebra and distance from center of pedicle of second cervical vertebra to this diameter are measured. **B** and **C,** Measurement of superior migration is not changed in flexion or extension of spine. (Modified from Ranawat CS, O'Leary P, Pellicci P, et al: *J Bone Joint Surg* 61A:1003, 1979.)

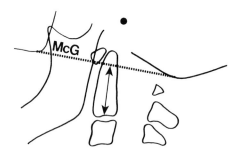

Fig. 41-23 Determination of vertebral settling in rheumatoid arthritis. Distance is measured between McGregor line *(McG)* and midpoint of base of C2. (From Redlund-Johnell I, Pettersson H: *Acta Radiol [Diagn]* 25:23, 1984.)

compression, pannus further decreases the space available for the cord by 3 mm or more in approximately 66% of patients. Determining the cervicomedullary angle is helpful in identifying vertical instability. A line drawn along the dorsal surface of the odontoid will intersect a line drawn ventral and parallel to the medulla. This angle normally should be 135 to 175 degrees,

with angles less than 135 suggesting atlantoaxial impaction and correlating with the presence of myelopathy. Kawaida et al. noted that MRI was 100% accurate in identifying vertical settling, and it is currently the most definitive, least invasive test for cord compression. Flexion and extension MRI scanning also has been used to determine dynamic compression of the spinal cord. Data from anatomical studies indicate that the space available for the cord should be 14 mm at the foramen magnum, 13 mm at the atlantoaxial articulation, and 12 mm in the subaxial cervical spine.

CERVICAL INSTABILITY

Cervical disease has an early onset and is correlated with appendicular disease activity. Other factors that predict more severe spinal involvement include longer duration of disease, positive rheumatoid factor, use of corticosteroids, and male sex. Once cervical myelopathy is established, mortality is common if this condition remains untreated. In fact, 100% of 21 patients refusing surgery for cervical instability died within 7 years of the onset of myelopathy. The incidence of sudden death from the combination of basilar impression and atlantoaxial instability is about 10%. Patients with rheumatoid arthritis have a shorter life expectancy than the normal population. Pellicci et al. reported a mortality rate significantly higher than the normal rate for comparable ages in patients with rheumatoid arthritis, even though none died as a result of cervical disease.

Atlantoaxial subluxation (AAS) is the most common instability, with a reported incidence of 11% to 46% of cases at necropsy. Atlantoaxial subluxation can be anterior, posterior, or lateral, with anterior instability predominating. Posterior instability may occur in 20% and lateral instability in 7% of patients. This instability results from erosive synovitis of the atlantoaxial, atlantoodontoid, and atlantooccipital joints. Basilar impression, vertical settling, or atlantoaxial impaction (AAI) is the settling of the skull onto the atlas and the atlas onto the axis as a result of erosive arthritis and bone loss. This settling can result in vertebral arterial thrombosis. According to Ranawat et al., atlantoaxial instability is present in as many as 38% of patients with rheumatoid arthritis; however, its frequency increases with disease severity. In the report of Oda et al., patients with mild disease did not develop this instability, but 52% of patients with moderate erosive disease developed vertical instability, as did 88% of those with severe erosive disease.

Subaxial subluxations (SAS) are more subtle and frequently multiple, affecting 10% to 20% of patients with rheumatoid arthritis. They are believed to result from synovitis of the facet joints and uncovertebral joints, accompanied by erosion of the ventral endplates. They may result in root compression from foraminal narrowing. Myelography, postmyelography reformatted CT scans, and MRI all show root cut off and partial or complete block. Postmyelography reformatted CT scans and MRI are clearly superior in identifying soft tissue obstructions and cord compression. Absolute subluxation distances of clinical significance are not known for this problem.

The signs and symptoms of these instability patterns include pain, stiffness, pyramidal tract involvement, vertebrobasilar insufficiency, root findings, and symptoms similar to the Lhermitte sign in multiple sclerosis. Early clinical manifestations include the Hoffman and Babinski signs and hyperreflexia.

Nonoperative Treatment

Goals of nonoperative treatment include preventing neurological injury, avoiding sudden death, minimizing pain, and maximizing function. Many patients, despite roentgenographic abnormalities, remain asymptomatic, and supportive treatment is all that is necessary. Medical management during disease flares is important for patient comfort and should be coordinated with a rheumatologist. A cervical orthosis is helpful in some patients if pain persists. Isometric exercises help stabilize the neck without excessive motion and also may help alleviate mechanical symptoms. Yearly follow-up with five-view roentgenograms is indicated to detect instability so that stabilization can be done before neurological deficits develop.

Operative Treatment

The indications for operative treatment are neurological impairment, instability, and pain. Boden et al. recommended arthrodesis for patients, with or without neurological deficits, who have atlantoaxial subluxation and a posterior atlanto-odontoid interval of 14 mm or less, atlantoaxial subluxation with at least 5 mm of basilar invagination, or subaxial subluxation with a sagittal spinal canal diameter of 14 mm or less. Axial imaging that shows compression of the spinal cord to a diameter of less than 6 mm also is an indication for surgery.

Atlantoaxial subluxation is best treated by posterior C1 and C2 fusion. This is accomplished with a posterior wiring technique using interlaminar autogenous iliac crest; transarticular screws can be added from C2 into C1, which obviates the need for a halo and allows the use of a Philadelphia collar or other similar postoperative orthosis. Preoperative planning must include axial CT scans with sagittal reconstructions to determine whether ample lateral mass is present for fixation and also to confirm that anomalies of the vertebral arteries do not put these structures at risk. Stabilization alone will result in some decrease of pannus, and odontoid excision is unnecessary unless anterior compression persists after fusion or if compression is purely bony.

In patients with basilar impression a trial of halo or tong traction for reduction is an option, if tolerated. If reduction is accomplished, a posterior occipitocervical fusion is done. If reduction is not possible, posterior fusion is done after anterior transoral decompression or posterior decompression that includes decompression of the foramen magnum. Posterior stabilization can be obtained with wiring and corticocancellous struts, Luque rods, lateral mass plates, Y-plates, and newer rod-screw or rod-hook systems. The prognosis is guarded in patients with preoperative neurological deficits, and basilar impression is associated with poorer recovery of function. As a result, aggressive treatment is indicated to prevent neurological deficits once progressive atlantoaxial impaction is identified.

Symptomatic subaxial subluxation probably is best treated by posterior fusion. Halo traction can be used to reduce subluxations preoperatively, especially in patients with myelopathy or paraplegia. Ranawat et al. reported that the results of anterior cervical decompression and fusion for subaxial subluxation were not satisfactory. Decompression occasionally is necessary if reduction is not possible and if narrowing of the space available for the cord is clinically significant. After reduction of the subluxation, posterior fusion is done using wires, plates, or rods and autogenous bone graft. If plates or rods are used, fixation is either into the lateral masses or transpedicular, with the latter more suited for C2 and C7 or T1, where the lateral masses are thin. Stability can be increased by the placement of polymethylmethacrylate around the wires. A bone graft is placed laterally to provide long-term stability. The mortality associated with surgery for these problems is 8% to 20%. The complication rate also is high, including a nonunion rate of 20% to 33%. Boden and Clark developed a treatment algorithm for atlantoaxial subluxation (Fig. 41-24).

The techniques for occipitocervical, atlantoaxial, and subaxial posterior cervical fusion are described in Chapter 36.

Pain is decreased after surgery in 90% to 97% of patients. Peppelman et al. reported that neurological function improved in 95% of their patients with atlantoaxial subluxations, in 76% of those with combined atlantoaxial subluxation and atlantoaxial impaction, and in 94% of those with subaxial subluxations. Atlantoaxial subluxations have a poor prognosis for neurological recovery, with several studies reporting improvement of function of one Ranawat class in only 40% to 50% of patients. The severity of the preoperative neurological deficit also influenced results. Casey et al. reported that, of 134 patients with Ranawat class III neurological deficits, 58% of ambulatory patients (IIIA) improved but only 20% of non-ambulatory patients (IIIB) did so.

Ankylosing Spondylitis

Ankylosing spondylitis is one of a variety of inflammatory spondyloarthropathies that affect the spine, sacroiliac joints, peripheral joints, and entheses, as well as possibly cause conjunctivitis and uveitis. Enteropathic spondyloarthropathies are associated with Crohn disease and ulcerative colitis, and reactive arthritis or Reiter syndrome also may affect the spine. Of these disorders, ankylosing spondylitis has a significantly more severe course once the spine is involved. There is a known association with the HLA-B27 antigen, which is present in 88% to 96% of patients who have ankylosing spondylitis.

Initially, morning stiffness is the primary symptom. Men are affected four times more frequently than women, usually in the second and third decades, with disease prevalence in white men estimated at 0.5 to 1 per 1000. As the disease progresses, ankylosis can cause various disfiguring and disabling spinal deformities. Ankylosis usually progresses from caudal to

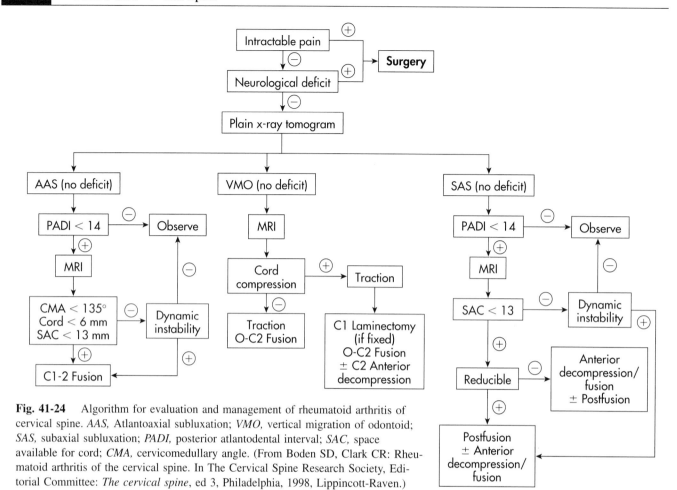

Fig. 41-24   Algorithm for evaluation and management of rheumatoid arthritis of cervical spine. *AAS,* Atlantoaxial subluxation; *VMO,* vertical migration of odontoid; *SAS,* subaxial subluxation; *PADI,* posterior atlantodental interval; *SAC,* space available for cord; *CMA,* cervicomedullary angle. (From Boden SD, Clark CR: Rheumatoid arthritis of the cervical spine. In The Cervical Spine Research Society, Editorial Committee: *The cervical spine,* ed 3, Philadelphia, 1998, Lippincott-Raven.)

cephalad. After ankylosis, however, pain symptoms often improve. Other symptoms may be related to hip arthritis, which occasionally progresses to spontaneous arthrodesis. Pulmonary cavitary lesions with fibrosis occur, as do aortic insufficiency and conduction defects. Amyloid deposition can cause renal failure. Uveitis requires special ophthalmological care and follow-up to prevent permanent vision changes. Breathing may be restricted because of fusion of the costochondral and costovertebral articulations.

Roentgenograms initially show fusion of the sacroiliac joints, which characteristically occurs bilaterally. In the vertebral bodies, inflammatory resorption of bone at the enthesis causes periarticular osteopenia. This resorption initially is seen as a "squaring off" of the corners of the vertebral bodies. Subsequent ossification occurs in the annulus fibrosis, sparing the anterior longitudinal ligament and disc and giving the "bamboo spine" appearance on roentgenograms. The posterior elements are similarly affected, with ossification of the facet joints, interspinous and supraspinous ligaments, and ligamentum flavum. Atlantoaxial instability must be identified, especially in any patient having surgery for conditions associated with ankylosing spondylitis. Because of the stiff subaxial spine, instability occurs in 25% to 90% of patients with ankylosing spondylitis.

Treatment is directed at maintaining flexibility with stretching of the hip flexors and hamstrings and maintaining spinal alignment with exercises. Antiinflammatory medications are useful in symptomatic management. All nonoperative measures essentially are supportive.

Spinal fractures in patients with ankylosing spondylitis are always serious and frequently are life-threatening injuries. Detwiler et al., Wade et al., Broom and Raycroft, and Graham and Van Peteghem noted that these fractures usually occur in the lower cervical spine, frequently are unstable, and usually are discovered late. Persistent pain may be the only finding until late neurological loss occurs. In patients with established kyphosis the deformity may suddenly improve. Unfortunately, the patient's previous deformity may not be known to those providing emergency care. Any perceived change in spinal alignment, even if the result of trivial trauma, should be considered a fracture in a patient with ankylosing spondylitis. The standard procedure is to immobilize the patient in the position in which he is found, since extension may result in sudden neurological loss. A widened anterior disc space, which may be the only obvious roentgenographic finding, creates a very unstable configuration that is prone to translation, late neurological loss, and very slow healing. Imaging with MRI or CT with sagittal reconstructions is helpful in making the diagnosis.

Graham and Van Peteghem, Rowed, and Broom and Raycroft advocated conservative treatment with traction and halo immobilization unless displacement and neurological compromise are present. They noted fewer complications with this approach. Detwiler et al. and Trent et al. advised early surgical stabilization by posterior fusion with posterior rods. Ho et al. recommended an anterior approach for stabilization. Surgical stabilization should be undertaken only with great care. Combined anterior and posterior stabilization with instrumentation may be required. It is important to note that the morbidity and mortality for these procedures in patients with ankylosing spondylitis are very high.

Traction should be carefully designed to reestablish the patient's previous deformity. This may require placing the patient in a kyphotic position that protects the spine but creates skin and mobility problems. Halo immobilization also can be difficult to institute and maintain without displacement.

Each patient with ankylosing spondylitis who has a fracture should be evaluated carefully to determine the best therapy for the specific injury. Nonoperative therapy appears to be more successful than surgery.

Pseudarthrosis is a frequent complication of a fracture in patients with ankylosing spondylitis. Wu et al. and Peh et al. noted late roentgenographic findings of disc space widening and discovertebral disruption. Collie et al. noted that the bone scan frequently is "hot" in these occult fractures, whereas the rest of the spine is no longer active on bone scan because of the disease process. Iplikcioglu et al. noted that MRI is superior to other imaging methods if the diagnosis is questionable.

OSTEOTOMY OF LUMBAR SPINE

Smith-Petersen, Larson, and Aufranc in 1945 described an osteotomy of the spine to correct the flexion deformity that often develops in ankylosing spondylitis and sometimes in rheumatoid arthritis. Since then, LaChapelle, Herbert, Wilson, Law, Simmons, and others have reported similar procedures. The technique described by Smith-Petersen et al. is carried out in one stage. Others have described surgery done in two stages, one consisting of division of the anterior longitudinal ligament under direct vision instead of allowing it to rupture when the deformity is corrected by gentle manipulation, as in the method of Smith-Petersen et al.

If the flexion deformity is severe, the patient's field of vision is limited to a small area near the feet, and walking is extremely difficult. This is evident by looking at the chin-brow to vertical angle (Fig. 41-25). Respiration becomes almost completely diaphragmatic, and gastrointestinal symptoms resulting from pressure of the costal margin on the contents of the upper abdomen are common; dysphagia or choking may occur. In addition to improvement in function, the improvement in appearance made by correcting the deformity is of great importance to the patient. If extreme, the deformity should be corrected in two or more stages because of contracture of soft tissues and the danger of damaging the aorta, the inferior vena cava, and the major nerves to the lower extremities. Lichtblau

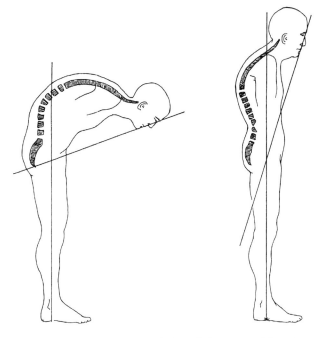

Fig. 41-25 Chin-brow to vertical angle is measured from brow to chin to vertical while patient stands with hips and knees extended and neck in its fixed or neutral position. (From Kostuik JP: Ankylosing spondylitis: surgical treatment. In Frymoyer JW: *The adult spine: principles and practice,* ed 2, Philadelphia, 1997, Lippincott-Raven.)

and Wilson reported one patient with transverse rupture of the aorta caused by manipulation of the spine for ankylosing spondylitis with severe flexion deformity. The patient had previously received 2000 units of roentgen therapy. These authors suggested that the roentgen therapy once used for this type of arthritis, not the arthritis itself, causes the aorta to adhere to the anterior longitudinal ligament and makes it subject to rupture during manipulation or osteotomy. They advocated a procedure in two stages in which the aorta is freed from the anterior longitudinal ligament in the first and the osteotomy is made in the second. They pointed out that in all their patients, regardless of the number of levels at which osteotomies were made, all correction took place at only one level. Law reported a series of 114 patients and Herbert one of 50 in which the patients were treated by osteotomy; in each series the mortality was about 10%, but in both reports most of the deaths occurred early in the series, and both surgeons predicted that the rate would be lower with more experience. Goel later reported a series of 15 patients in whom no deaths or serious complications occurred. According to Law, 25 to 45 degrees of correction usually can be obtained, resulting in marked improvement both functionally and cosmetically.

Adams suggested that the operation be carried out with the patient lying on his side. This lateral position has several advantages: (1) it is easier to place the grossly deformed patient on the table; (2) the danger of injuring the ankylosed cervical spine by pressure of the forehead against the table is eliminated; (3) the anesthesia is easier to manage because maintaining a

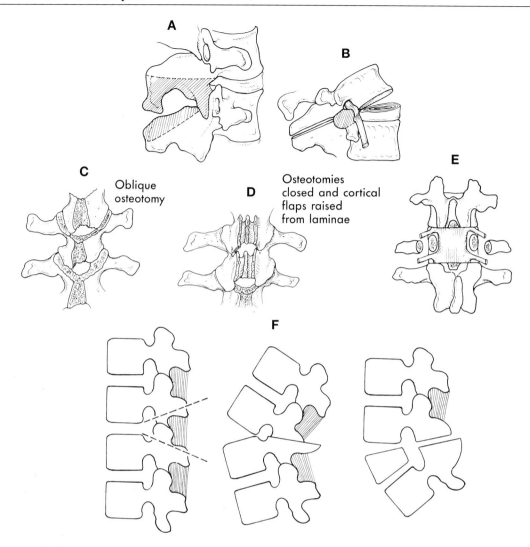

Fig. 41-26 Methods of high lumbar spinal osteotomy. **A** and **B,** Simple wedge resection of spinous processes into neural foramina. **C** and **D,** Chevron excision of laminae and spinous processes. **E,** Total laminectomy. **F,** Rather than osteotomy with opening of disc in front *(middle),* Thomasen used resection of posterior wedge and resection of pedicles *(right).* (**A, B, E,** and **F** redrawn from Thomasen E: *Clin Orthop* 194:142, 1984; **C** and **D** redrawn from Smith-Petersen MN, Larson CB, Aufranc OE: *J Bone Joint Surg* 27:1, 1945.)

clear airway and free respiratory exchange are less difficult; and (4) the operation is easier because any blood will flow out from the depth of the wound rather than into it. We agree that this is the safest and most efficient position for this procedure. Adams described hyperextending the spine with an ingenious three-point pressure apparatus, and Simmons described surgery with the patient on his side and under local anesthesia. When the osteotomy is complete, the patient is turned prone, carefully fracturing the anterior longitudinal ligament with the patient briefly under nitrous oxide and fentanyl anesthesia.

Osteotomy usually is made at the upper lumbar level because the spinal canal here is large and the osteotomy is distal to the end of the cord. A lumbar lordosis is created to compensate for the thoracic kyphosis; motion of the spine is not increased. Osteotomy methods include resection of the spinous processes from the laminae to the pedicles, simple wedge resection of the spinous processes into the neural foramina (Fig. 41-26, *A* and *B*), chevron excision of the laminae and spinous processes (Fig. 41-26, *C* and *D*), and combined anterior opening wedge osteotomy following posterior resection of the spinous processes and laminae (Fig. 41-26, *E* and *F*).

Styblo, Bossers, and Slot in 1985 reported an average correction from 80 degrees to 44 degrees after upper lumbar osteotomy; correction was maintained by internal fixation. Manual osteoclasis worked best in patients with calcified ligaments. They noted seven different types of spinal disruption caused by the manual osteoclasis. Complications from this procedure included hypertension, gastrointestinal problems, neurological defects, urinary tract infections, psychological problems, dural tears with leakage, and retrograde ejaculation. One rupture of the aorta was reported by Lichtblau and Wilson.

Spinal osteotomy is a demanding procedure for which

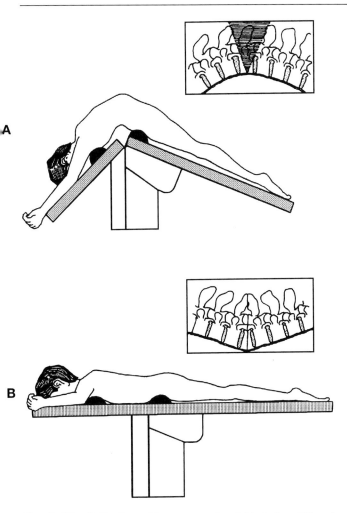

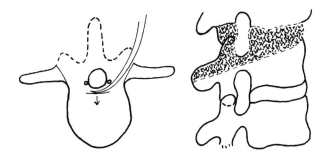

Fig. 41-28 Eggshell procedure. After posterior elements have been removed and pedicles have been collapsed outward, long, sharp curet is used to collapse "eggshell." (From Heinig CF: Eggshell procedure. In Luque ER, ed: *Segmental spinal instrumentation,* Thorofare, NJ, 1984, SLACK.)

Fig. 41-27 Patient's position on operating table before (**A**) and after (**B**) reduction of osteotomy. Osteotomy gap is closed when table is brought from flexed to straight position. (From Thiranont N, Netrawichien P: *Spine* 18:2517, 1993.)

proper training and experience are mandatory. The surgeon should be familiar with the several options available.

Smith-Peterson Osteotomy

The Smith-Peterson osteotomy is an excellent option for correction of smaller degrees of spinal deformity. Bone is removed through the pars and facet joints (Fig. 41-26, *C* and *D*). If a previous fusion has been done, care should be taken to thin the fusion mass gradually until the ligamentum flavum or dura is exposed. Symmetrical resection is necessary to prevent creating a coronal deformity. Removal of the underlying ligament also is helpful in preventing buckling of the dura or iatrogenic spinal stenosis. Approximately 10 degrees of correction can be obtained with each 10 mm of resection. Excessive resection should be avoided because it may result in foraminal stenosis. In patients with degenerative discs, decreased flexibility may limit the amount of correction that can be obtained. The osteotomy is closed with compression or with in situ rod contouring and bone graft is applied.

Pedicle Subtraction Osteotomy (Thomasen)

Pedicle subtraction osteotomy (Fig. 41-26, *A* and *B*) is best suited for patients who have significant sagittal imbalance of 4 cm or more and immobile or fused discs. Pedicle subtraction osteotomy is inherently safer than the Smith-Peterson osteotomy because it avoids multiple osteotomies. Typically, 30 degrees or more of correction can be obtained with a single posterior osteotomy, preferably at the level of the deformity. If the deformity is at the spinal cord level, pedicle subtraction osteotomy can be used, but care must be taken to avoid manipulation of the cord. Thomasen, and Thiranont and Netrawichien described the use of this osteotomy after laminectomy and pedicle resection. In their technique, compression instrumentation is used, along with simultaneous flexion of the head and foot of the operating table (Fig. 41-27). Care must be taken to avoid compression of the dura or creation of a coronal deformity. A wake-up test is done once correction and cancellous bone grafting have been completed.

Eggshell Osteotomy

The eggshell osteotomy requires both anterior and posterior approaches and usually is reserved for severe sagittal or coronal imbalance of more than 10 cm from the midline (Fig. 41-28). This is a spinal shortening procedure with anterior decancellization followed by removal of posterior elements, instrumentation, deformity correction, and fusion.

OSTEOTOMY OF CERVICAL SPINE

In patients with chin-on-chest deformity, often the mandible is so near the sternum that opening the mouth and chewing properly are difficult. Law reported a series of 14 patients treated by osteotomy of the cervical spine for this deformity. He pointed out that cervicodorsal kyphosis usually can be treated satisfactorily by lumbar osteotomy, which provides a compensatory lumbar lordosis and results in an erect posture. However, cervical osteotomy may be indicated (1) to elevate the chin from the sternum, thus improving the appearance, the ability to eat, and the ability to see ahead; (2) to prevent atlantoaxial and

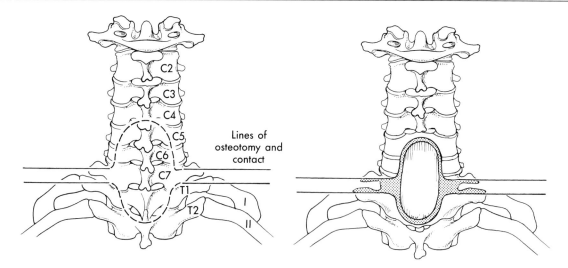

Fig. 41-29   Extent of resection of cervical laminae for safe osteotomy. Lateral resections are beveled toward each other so that opposing surfaces are parallel and in apposition after extension osteotomy. (Redrawn from Simmons EH: *Clin Orthop* 86:132, 1972.)

cervical subluxations and dislocations, which result from the weight of the head being carried forward by gravity; (3) to relieve tracheal and esophageal distortion, which causes dyspnea and dysphagia; and (4) to prevent irritation of the spinal cord tracts or excessive traction on the nerve roots, which causes neurological disturbances. The appropriate level for osteotomy is determined by the deformity and the degree of ossification of the anterior longitudinal ligament. Law successfully performed osteotomies at the levels of C3 and C4, C5 and C6, and C6 and C7. He fixed the spine internally with the plates devised by Wilson and Straub for use in lumbosacral arthrodesis. However, wiring of the spinal processes (Chapter 36), or use of a halo alone, also should be effective. In the osteotomy technique described by Simmons (Fig. 41-29), decompression is done first and is extended into the neural foramen. After decompression and resection of the inferior aspect of the pedicles, extension manipulation is done. The operation is carried out with the patient sitting in a dental chair and inclined forward with the arms resting on an operating table (Fig. 41-30). Overcorrection of the deformity must be avoided because otherwise the trachea and esophagus could be overstretched and become obstructed. If halo stabilization alone is used, postoperative neurological symptoms are treated by lessening correction; if internal fixation is used for more postoperative stability, reoperation is required for adjustment of correction. The halo is worn for 3 months, and a Philadelphia collar or similar orthosis is worn an additional 6 to 8 weeks.

Freeman reported using skeletal traction to treat a patient with severe cervicodorsal kyphosis who could not actively lift his chin from the sternum but in whom minimal passive motion of the cervical spine was demonstrated by skeletal traction. The traction reduced a subluxation of C4 on C5 but failed to restore acceptable alignment. The Crutchfield tongs were then

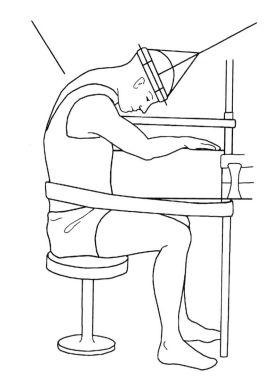

Fig. 41-30   Position of patient for cervical osteotomy: sitting on stool with head suspended by halo and traction. (Redrawn from Simmons EH: *Clin Orthop* 86:132, 1972.)

removed, and a plaster jacket with an attached halo was applied. The neck was extended gradually until some of the cervical lordosis had been restored. Then, with the halo still in place and the patient under a local anesthesia, an arthrodesis from the occiput to T3 was carried out successfully.

Tumors of Spine

BENIGN TUMORS

Of all primary benign bone tumors, 8% occur in the spine or sacrum. Although most spinal tumors are metastases and malignancies, 20% to 40% are primary benign spinal tumors. Benign lesions have a predilection for younger patients, with 60% of benign lesions identified in the second and third decades (Box 41-3). The exception to this is sacral tumors, which more often are malignant, even in the younger age groups. However, 70% of spinal tumors are malignant in patients over 21 years of age. Typically, benign lesions are in the posterior elements, with most anteriorly located lesions malignant (76%).

Kostas et al. reported 22 patients who had back pain and deformity caused by benign tumors or tumorlike lesions of the spine (15 lumbar, 7 thoracic); the duration of pain ranged from 1 to 6 years. Management included tumor excision and thorough debridement; spinal fusion with instrumentation was used to correct deformity and provide stability in five patients. Of five patients who had preoperative incomplete paraplegia, four recovered completely and one (who had a spinal cord hemangioma) improved two Frankel grades. They noted that because these lesions are rare in the thoracolumbar and lumbar spine, they are easily misdiagnosed in patients with persistent back pain.

During operative treatment of tumors, certain fundamentals must be followed to maintain function and anatomy and to minimize the risk of recurrence or instability. These principles are most important in the region of the spinal cord. For cervical and thoracic lesions, the spinal cord must be preserved. Roots vary in importance depending on anatomical location and can be resected if long-term benefit is to be gained. Some paired vascular structures, including the vertebral arteries, also can be singly resected. Adequate collateral circulation is identified by temporary occlusion during angiography if resection of the vertebral artery is anticipated.

In the thoracic spine, laminectomy alone does not provide safe access to the anterior column. The risk of paralysis is significant, and alternative approaches must be used. For patients who are unable to tolerate a thoracotomy, a costotransversectomy is a reasonable and safe approach to the anterior column. Unfortunately, with aggressive lesions, the spinal canal may be contaminated. Nerve roots serve only the intercostal muscles, so sacrifice of some of the thoracic roots does not severely affect function unless numerous roots are taken. As more thoracic roots are sacrificed, there is some effect on chest cage function and respiration due to interference with intercostal innervation.

Sacral tumors requiring wide excision are rare. Combined approaches often are necessary for wide excision and require complex reconstruction to stabilize the ilia to the distal lumbar spine. Resection of the sacrum and its associated nerve roots also affects continence. If both S1 nerve roots and a single S2

BOX 41-3 • Radiographic Diagnosis of Spine Tumors According to Age and Location

DIAGNOSIS ACCORDING TO AGE
10 to 30 Years of Age
Aneurysmal bone cyst (ABC)
Ewing
Giant cell
Histiocytosis X
Osteoblastoma
Osteoid osteoma
Osteochondroma
Osteosarcoma

30 to 50 Years of Age
Chondrosarcoma
Chordoma
Hodgkins
Hemangioma

50 + Years of Age
Metastatic
Myeloma

DIAGNOSIS ACCORDING TO LOCATION
Vertebral Body
Chordoma
Giant cell
Hemangioma
Histiocytosis X
Metastatic disease
Multiple myeloma

Posterior Elements
ABC
Osteoblastoma
Osteoid osteoma
Osteochondroma

Adjacent Vertebrae
ABC
Chondrosarcoma
Chordoma

Multiple Vertebrae
Histiocytosis X
Metastatic
Myeloma

From Parks P, Herkowitz HN: *Semin Spine Surg* 2:3, 1990.

nerve root are preserved, 50% of patients retain continence. If only a single S3 root is taken, with S1 and S2 undisturbed, bowel and bladder function are retained. The nature of the tumor to be resected, however, often dictates the anatomical level of resection.

Stability

Stability considerations after resection are different in adult and pediatric patients. In the cervical and thoracic regions,

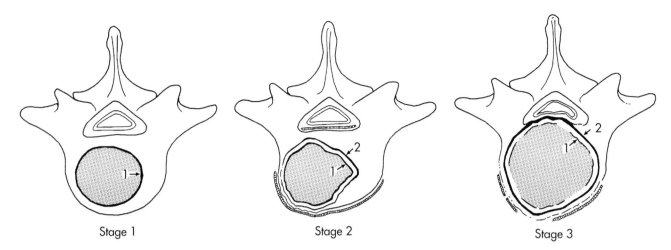

Stage 1   Stage 2   Stage 3

Fig. 41-31   Enneking staging of benign spinal tumors. Capsule of tumor is indicated by *1,* reactive pseudocapsule by *2.* Stage 3 aggressive benign tumors can expand through posterior vertebral wall and compress cord. Pseudocapsule is vascularized reactive tissue and can adhere to dura. (Redrawn from Boriani S, Biagini R, DeIure F: *Semin Spine Surg* 7:317, 1995.)

laminectomy creates instability in an immature spine, so arthrodesis should be done. The adult spine seems to tolerate laminectomy better, and some biomechanical considerations are useful when choosing instrumentation and fusion procedures. Instability created by anterior resection increases as more vertebral body is resected. As a rule of thumb, fusion should be done when any significant amount of vertebral body is resected. The exception to this is curettage: if adequate bone graft is placed after curettage, fusion usually is not necessary. After anterior fusion, with or without instrumentation, immobilization with a TLSO generally is recommended. Once incorporation of fusion bone is identified, usually 3 to 6 months postoperatively, the orthosis is discontinued.

Determination of instability after posterior spinal resections is not as straightforward as after anterior procedures. Important bony and ligamentous structures posteriorly individually contribute to overall stability in the intact spine. Soft tissue restraints include the supraspinous, interspinous, and posterior longitudinal ligaments, the ligamentum flavum, and the facet capsules. Bony stability is provided by the spinous processes, laminae, pars interarticularis, facet joints individually on the left and right, and the posterior vertebral wall. Point systems have been created to assist in the determination of stability. Bridwell assigned 25% of posterior vertebral stability for each stabilizing structure, including the midline osteoligamentous complex (laminae, spinous processes, and intervening ligaments), the two facet joint complexes (left and right), and the posterior vertebral wall, disc, and annulus. Violation of two of the four complexes, or disruption of 50% of the stabilizing structures, is an indication for instrumentation and fusion. Bony involvement of tumors also contributes to impending pathological fracture and instability. Considerations for impending instability or for determining stability after fracture include more than 50% collapse of the vertebral body, translation, segmental kyphosis of more than 20 degrees above normal, and involvement of both anterior and posterior columns.

Classification

As with tumors in other locations, the Enneking classification is useful in determining treatment of spinal tumors (Fig. 41-31). Stage 1 tumors (such as osteoid osteoma, eosinophilic granuloma, osteochondroma, and hemangioma) are latent and typically require no treatment. If surgery is necessary, often intralesional excision is all that is necessary, with or without adjuvants like liquid nitrogen, phenol, or PMMA. Stage 2 lesions are active, become symptomatic, and usually require only en bloc excision (i.e., removal of the tumor as a whole, as opposed to piecemeal). Intralesional excision, again, often suffices for these tumors. Examples of stage 2 lesions include osteoid osteoma, osteoblastoma, eosinophilic granuloma, more aggressive hemangiomas, osteochondroma, and aneurysmal bone cysts. Aggressive lesions are characterized as stage 3. Despite being classified as benign tumors, lesions such as giant cell tumors and osteoblastomas are locally aggressive and have a tendency to recur. Wide excision is indicated for these lesions and consists of removal of the tumor with a cuff of normal tissue if possible. A marginal excision would result in a biopsy specimen that includes the reactive zone around the tumor. The exact type of excisional biopsy often is dictated by the anatomy of the spine and the location of the tumor.

Posterior Element Tumors

Osteoid Osteoma.   Osteoid osteoma is a lesion of bony origin that was first described by Jaffe in 1935. These lesions are most common in the spine (42%), affect males more often than females, and are most common in the second decade. The lumbar spine is the most common location, the cervical next, and the thoracic last, and the lesion is almost invariably located in the posterior elements. Few osteoid osteomas of vertebral bodies have been reported. This lesion is not locally aggressive and is defined by a size of less than 2 cm; larger lesions are classified as osteoblastomas.

Pain is the primary complaint in 83% of patients, is worse at night with awakening in nearly 30%, and is relieved by aspirin in 27%. Because of the location in the posterior elements, radiculopathy occurs in up to 28% of patients. A painful scoliosis may result, with the lesion usually present at the apex of the curve in the concavity. Although various curve types may result, the usual structural features of vertebral rotation normally present in idiopathic scoliosis are absent. The resultant scoliosis is rigid and rapidly progressive. Saifuddin et al, in a meta-analysis of spinal osteoid osteoma and osteoblastoma, determined that (1) 63% of patients had scoliosis, (2) scoliosis was significantly more common with osteoid osteomas than with osteoblastomas, (3) lesions were more common in the thoracic and lumbar regions than in the cervical region and more common the lower cervical region than the upper cervical region, and (4) lesions were more commonly located to one side of the midline. They concluded that these findings support the concept that in patients with spinal osteoid osteoma or osteoblastoma scoliosis is secondary to asymmetrical muscle spasm.

Diagnosis can be difficult, since early roentgenograms may appear normal. Frequently, a sclerotic lesion of the pedicle is all that is apparent, and even this may be a subtle asymmetry. Later, the usual configuration of a central nidus with surrounding sclerosis may be found, but in only half of patients will it be typical in appearance. Oblique roentgenograms can be helpful when the pedicle, facet, and pars interarticularis are studied. A radioisotopic bone scan is most helpful in accurate localization, and CT scanning often shows the nidus.

Treatment should consist of surgical excision of the lesion if symptoms fail to improve or the scoliosis is progressive. Confirmation of nidus excision can be made by specimen CT. If the spine is considered unstable because of facet or pedicle removal, a single-level fusion is done simultaneously. Complete excision should result in improvement in the angular degree of the scoliosis, although resolution is less likely in patients aged 9 to 13.5 years. Scoliosis persists in 20% to 30% of patients after successful resection. Curves that persist for more than 18 months after resection may require treatment. Brace management may be necessary in immature patients, and regular follow-up is advised. Surgery for spinal deformity usually is deferred until after treatment and resection of the osteoid osteoma and follows the same principles as for idiopathic scoliosis. Prompt relief of pain is the best postoperative indicator of successful removal of the tumor.

More recently described treatment methods include high-frequency radio wave ablation (Osti and Sebben) and percutaneous CT-guided thermocoagulation (Cove et al.). Reports at present are anecdotal, and the effectiveness and safety of these minimally invasive techniques have yet to be proved.

Osteoblastoma. Osteoblastoma accounts for 10% of all spinal tumors and, of those reported, 32% appear in the spine. Like osteoid osteoma, it is most common in the second and third decades, with a male-to-female ratio of 2:1. These lesions almost always involve the pedicle or posterior elements, or both, although contiguous levels may be affected. The predominant spinal region affected is the cervical region (40%), followed by the lumbar (23%), thoracic (21%), and sacral regions (17%). Osteoblastoma may be misdiagnosed as an osteosarcoma, Ewing sarcoma, lymphoma, or aneurysmal bone cyst, which all are high on the list of differential diagnoses. Differentiation from osteoid osteoma is based on size, as these lesions exceed 2 cm.

Roentgenographic evaluation reveals a destructive, expansile lesion with a thin rim of cortical bone. Lytic features are predominant and occur in 50%, with purely blastic changes in 20%. Bone scanning always is positive and is helpful in identification. Although MRI is useful in identifying a soft tissue mass, it may confuse the picture. A "flare" reaction may occur, suggesting extracompartmental extension and confusing the diagnosis of a benign lesion. As with other bony lesions, CT is best for definition of the extent of the tumor and for identification of the nidus.

Wide excision, if possible, is the treatment of choice. The tumor recurs as late as 9 years after resection in as many as 10% to 20% of patients with intralesional excision. The best indication of successful removal is relief of preoperative pain. Ozaki et al. reported open resection of 13 osteoblastomas and 9 osteoid osteomas; 17 of the 22 patients had scoliosis before surgery, which improved in 16 after tumor resection. Two patients with osteoid osteomas had recurrences because of incomplete resection. Because of the possibility of recurrence and malignant transformation, however, long term CT follow-up is mandatory. Operative treatment is necessary for recurrences because these lesions are not radiosensitive.

Osteochondroma. Although rarely symptomatic, osteochondroma is the most common benign primary bone tumor. Half of patients with symptomatic tumors are younger than 20 years of age, which is consistent with the growing cartilaginous cap. Males are affected three times more often than females, with most lesions protruding eccentrically from the neural arch. Because the spinal canal is occupied by spinal cord in the thoracic and cervical spine, lesions here are more frequently symptomatic. As many as 91% of osteochondromas occur in the cervical and upper thoracic spine, although the lumbar spine and sacrum also are affected. The lack of symptoms may result in underdiagnosis of lesions in the lumbar and sacral regions.

Roentgenographic evaluation often is diagnostic, with the lesions found most often in the posterior elements. Because of the radiolucent cartilaginous cap, however, MRI or myelography may be necessary to determine if impingement of the neural structures is present. These lesions are slow growing and require excision only if symptomatic. Malignant transformation occurs in fewer than 1% of tumors and is suspected when symptoms are rapid in onset with growth of a previously stable osteochondroma. A cartilaginous cap larger than 1 cm also is suspect. En bloc excision to include all of the cartilaginous cap is done, with neurological recovery the rule and recurrence the exception.

Aneurysmal Bone Cyst. Aneurysmal bone cysts are relatively uncommon, accounting for only 1% to 2% of benign bone tumors. Although predominantly a posterior element lesion, an aneurysmal bone cyst may expand to include the pedicle and vertebral body. Of all aneurysmal bone cysts, 11% to 30% occur in the spine and are most frequent in patients younger than 20 years of age. There does not appear to be a gender preference. Back pain is the predominant symptom in 95% of patients, although muscle spasms causing spinal rigidity or scoliosis also may be present. The differential diagnosis includes giant cell tumors, tuberculosis, fibrous dysplasia, eosinophilic granuloma, Ewing sarcoma, and osteoblastoma.

The characteristic roentgenographic finding with aneurysmal bone cysts is an expansile lesion with a reactive rim of cortical bone outlining the lesion as it expands from the cortex, although this may be absent in 30%. Another characteristic feature is that these lesions may affect contiguous levels. Arteriography may show a lesion with multiple septa and blood-filled spaces. MRI with gadolinium enhancement also shows the fluid levels within the septations.

De Cristofaro et al. reported that embolization was successful in 79% of their patients (19 of 24), although some required repeated embolizations. Low-dose irradiation has had limited success, with few side effects when dosages are kept below 30 Gy. Radiation alone, however, is successful in only approximately 50%. Surgery therefore has remained the standard of care for aneurysmal bone cysts. After embolization to decrease intraoperative blood loss, curettage and bone grafting are done. Despite intralesional margins, the recurrence is only 13%. Any instability created must be treated at the time of surgery and often requires a single-level fusion in skeletally immature patients. Papagelopoulos et al. reported a recurrence rate of 10% within 10 years of treatment of 52 patients with aneurysmal bone cysts of the spine.

Vertebral Body Tumors

Typical benign lesions found in the vertebral bodies include eosinophilic granuloma, hemangioma, and giant cell tumors. Historically, lesions such as these were considered surgically inaccessible when in the vertebrae. The older literature recommended irradiation or chemotherapy. Although this still may be appropriate in special circumstances, such as in highly radiosensitive malignant tumors, angular deformity with potential paraplegia may result because of subsequent spinal instability. Benign tumors are best treated without irradiation to avoid secondary sarcomatous change. Optimal treatment of aggressive benign or solitary malignant tumors, however, may be anterior resection of the tumor to effect a cure or for tumor debulking.

Hemangioma. Hemangioma is a common lesion, present in as many as 10% to 12% of autopsy specimens. Most of these lesions are clinically silent and are detected only incidentally during evaluation for other problems. Occurrence may be single or multiple with contiguous levels affected, but the vertebral body is the most common location for hemangiomas, especially in the lumbar and lower thoracic regions. The posterior elements are involved in 10% to 15% of patients; however, this is atypical and indicative of an aggressive lesion. Patients with symptomatic hemangiomas most commonly have pain (60%), neurological compromise (30%), or symptomatic fracture (10%).

Epidural cavernous hemangiomas are extremely rare. Shin et al. reported five epidural cavernous hemangiomas (four thoracic and one lumbosacral), all of which showed paravertebral extension and partially encircled the spinal cord, and Zevgaridis et al. reported three such lesions that produced symptoms of spinal cord syndrome, thoracic radiculopathy, and lumbar radiculopathy. MRI findings included a homogeneous signal intensity similar to spinal cord and muscle on T1-weighted images and a high signal intensity, slightly less intense than that of cerebrospinal fluid, on T2-weighted images.

Roentgenograms detect larger lesions, which have vertical striations and coarse, thick trabeculae, described as a "corduroy" vertebra. Expansion may be noted in aggressive hemangiomas, with erosion of the vertebral body. Axial CT scanning shows a classic "polka dot" appearance. Bone scanning is not particularly helpful because lesions may be either hot or cold. MRI scanning has become the standard for diagnosing these lesions. Typical hemangioma is identified by increased intensity on both T1- and T2-weighted sequences and can be differentiated from Paget disease because Pagetic bone has more cortical thickening and affects the entire vertebral body. Aggressive hemangiomas can involve the entire vertebral body, may be expansile and have a soft tissue component, which is differentiated from typical hemangioma by hypointensity on T1-weighted images and hyperintensity on T2-weighted images.

Most hemangiomas do not require treatment, and other causes of pain must be excluded. For the rare symptomatic lesions, radiation is successful in 50% to 80%. Embolization also is useful, especially in patients with progressive neurological deficits, and may provide temporary relief of pain. Vertebroplasty has been successfully used for treatment of aggressive hemangiomas by stabilizing pathological bone with an injection of bone cement into the vertebral body. Recent use of inflatable bone tamps has had similarly good short-term results. Direct intralesional injection of ethanol has been reported to be effective in obliterating symptomatic vertebral hemangiomas. CT angiography is required before injection to identify functional vascular spaces of the hemangioma and to direct needle placement. Doppman, Oldfield, and Heiss reported complete obliteration of hemangiomas in 11 patients; 5 of 6 patients with paraplegia recovered completely, and 1 had improved at short-term follow-up. These authors cautioned that less than 15 ml of ethanol should be used because two patients who received 42 and 50 ml developed pathological fractures of the involved vertebrae 4 and 16 weeks after treatment. For progressive neurological deficit, radiation alone may be successful in arresting progression. With neurological deficit and fracture, however, surgery is necessary to remove an aggressive hemangioma, and embolization should be done preoperatively to minimize bleeding intraoperatively.

Eosinophilic Granuloma. Eosinophilic granuloma is most common in patients younger than 10 years of age. It typically is a solitary lesion of bone, with 7% to 15% occurring in the spine, and has a predilection for the thoracic region. Symptoms usually include pain, muscular rigidity, and neurological deficits; systemic symptoms may occur. The classic roentgenographic finding is vertebra plana seen as a complete collapse of the vertebral body on the lateral view. Bone scans are "cold," and MRI often reveals a "flare" reaction on T2-weighted images, which can be mistaken for a malignant lesion. Differential diagnosis includes Ewing sarcoma, aneurysmal bone cyst, infection, tuberculosis, leukemia, and neuroblastoma. Because roentgenographic findings are not pathognomonic, biopsy is necessary.

Once the diagnosis is made, immobilization and observation alone often are sufficient treatment. These lesions typically regress spontaneously over time with some, although incomplete, restoration of vertebral deformity. Raab et al. reported partial to nearly complete reconstitution of vertebral height (72% to 97%) in 14 patients between the ages of 1 and 11 years with eosinophilic granulomas treated with brace immobilization. Follow-up is important to detect instability. Operative intervention, including curettage and grafting, may speed healing. There presently is no role for radiation in the treatment of eosinophilic granuloma. Recurrence is unusual, and resolution of neurological deficits usually occurs as the tumor regresses.

Giant Cell Tumor. Giant cell tumor is the most prevalent benign tumor of the sacrum, rarely affecting other spinal sites, and is second only to hemangioma as the most common benign spinal neoplasm. Giant cell tumors account for 4% to 5% of all primary bone tumors, occurring most often between the third and fifth decades. Females are affected twice as frequently as males, and 1% to 18% of giant cell tumors occur in the spine. Because of its lytic appearance, differential diagnosis includes aneurysmal bone cysts, osteoblastoma, and metastasis.

Pain is the most common complaint and often is of long duration before diagnosis. Neurological deficits occur in 20% to 80% of patients with giant cell tumors of the spine. Roentgenograms show the lesions as lytic, septated, and expansile, often with cortical breakthrough and an associated soft tissue mass. More than 50% of these lesions involve the vertebral body only. When present in the sacrum, the lesion is in the proximal aspect and eccentrically located.

Because of the aggressive nature of these lesions, en bloc resection with wide margins is necessary. Despite aggressive operative treatment, a 10% to 50% recurrence rate has been reported. Preoperative embolization is recommended, and embolization and radiation are reserved for lesions that cannot be resected. Kahn et al. reported treatment of six patients with giant cell tumors of the spine treated with radiation and conservative surgery (biopsy or subtotal tumor resection). At an average follow-up of 13 years, five of the six patients had no evidence of disease, and one had disease that was not clinically apparent. These authors concluded that radiotherapy is a reasonable treatment alternative for tumors that cannot be excised completely or in which surgery would result in significant functional morbidity. Although the dose response in their patients was not clear, their review of the literature suggested that doses ranging from 3500 to 4500 cGy are safe and effective in controlling giant cell tumor. If intralesional excision is done, adjuvant cryotherapy should be considered. Metastases occur in 1% to 11% of patients, with a 10% incidence of sarcomatous change.

PRIMARY MALIGNANT TUMORS

Almost all patients with malignancies of the spine have pain. More than 95% seek medical care for pain, with radiculopathy occurring in around 20% of these patients.

Classification

The Enneking classification of malignant tumors also is useful for spinal tumors: stage I, low-grade; stage II, high-grade; and stage III, regional or distant metastases (Fig. 41-32). The site of the tumor is indicated by A, intracompartmental, or B, extracompartmental. This classification scheme is useful in determining if marginal or wide excision is best. Radical excision is not possible in the spine.

Osteosarcoma

Primary osteosarcoma of the spine is rare, accounting for only 3% of all osteosarcomas, and frequently is lethal. Pain is the most common presenting complaint, but neurological symptoms also are present in up to 70% of patients. These tumors are anterior column tumors, and 95% affect the vertebral body. Men and women are equally affected. Secondary osteosarcomas, which occur most commonly after irradiation or develop in patients with Paget disease, affect patients in the seventh decade. Soft tissue extension, or extracompartmental disease, is the rule at the time of diagnosis, which is evident on MRI scans or at surgery.

Roentgenograms may show a lytic, blastic, or a mixed picture affecting the vertebral body. Bone scanning is useful in identifying multicentric or metastatic disease, and axial CT scans are useful in delineating the bony anatomy. Intensive radiation therapy and chemotherapy are the primary treatments. Radical surgery has been suggested, including wide resection with adjuvant radiotherapy. In a series of 30 consecutive patients with primary spinal sarcomas, Talac et al. reported that the risk of local recurrence was five times greater in patients with positive resection margins than in patients with tumor-free resection margins. Ozaki et al. also noted that wide or marginal excision of the tumor improved survival and recommended treatment with chemotherapy and at least marginal excision if possible. In their series, patients with metastases, large tumors, and sacral tumors had a poor prognosis. Venkateswaran et al., however, found no association between the affected

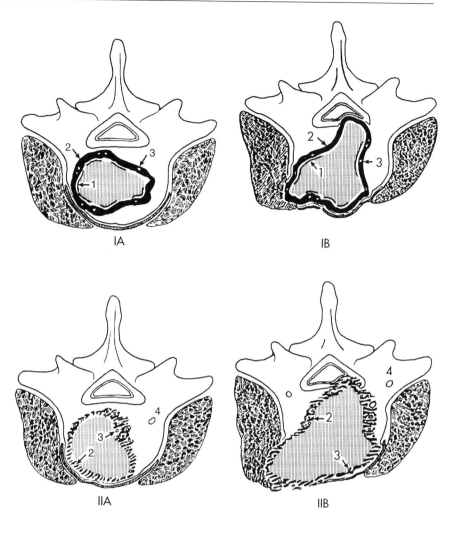

Fig. 41-32 Enneking staging of malignant spinal tumors. Capsule of tumor is indicated by *1*, pseudocapsule by *2*, island of tumor within pseudocapsule (satellites) or at distance (skip metastases) by *3*. Types I and IIB tumors can compress cord if expanding posteriorly. Pseudocapsule is more or less infiltrated by neoplastic tissue, which can have direct contact with dural sac. (Redrawn from Boriani S, Biagini R, DeIure F: *Semin Spine Surg* 7:317, 1995.)

spinal region and outcome in 33 children and adolescents with primary Ewing-family tumors of the vertebrae. Total sacrectomy and reconstruction with polymethylmethacrylate, plate-and-screw devices, and custom-made prostheses have been reported to be successful in the treatment of sacral osteosarcoma.

Ewing Sarcoma

Another anterior column primary bone tumor, Ewing sarcoma, is a permeative lesion that affects the spine only 3.5% to 8% of the time, with half of these tumors found in the sacrum. Neurological deficits are present in many patients because of soft tissue extension, and constitutional symptoms are common. Roentgenographic findings are confusing, with vertebra plana apparent in some patients, which may be confused with eosinophilic granuloma. Generally, these tumors are lytic, with a soft tissue mass identified on MRI. Treatment is similar to that for appendicular Ewing sarcoma: chemotherapy and radiation. Surgical decompression is indicated only for tumors causing neurological compromise and for potential instability to preserve neurological function. Long-term survival is possible with this tumor; 5-year survival using

chemotherapy and irradiation is between 20% and 44%. The frequency of cerebral and skeletal metastasis is higher than in appendicular disease, where pulmonary metastasis is most prevalent.

Chordoma

Primarily a tumor of adults, chordoma is an uncommon tumor that affects the sacrum and coccyx. It originates embryologically from the notochord remnants and, as such, usually is a midline tumor. It is relatively slow growing, but relentless in progression with high recurrence rates when a wide excision is not obtained. Symptoms usually are indolent with a palpable mass in the sacrum anteriorly on rectal examination. Men are affected twice as often as women, and the tumor affects an older population, with peak incidences during the fifth and seventh decades.

Roentgenograms reveal a lytic lesion in the midline of the sacrum with variable calcification. Bone scans often are negative because of the indolent biological behavior of these tumors. MRI provides excellent delineation of the anterior soft tissue extension that typically occurs with these tumors. Treatment involves a wide en bloc excision that may not be possible in the proximal sacrum without sacrifice of the S2 nerve roots. Recurrence rates approach 28% with sacrectomy, and bowel and bladder continence are retained only if both the S2 roots and one of the S3 roots are preserved. If for any reason the tumor is incised during excision, recurrence may be as great as 64%. As a result, great care is necessary in resection of these tumors, and radiation should be used for tumors with incisional margins. Long-term survival may approach 50% to 75% if marginal resection or better is achieved.

Multiple Myeloma

Plasmacytoma is the single-lesion variety of multiple myeloma and is rare, accounting for only 3% of plasma cell dyscrasias. This diagnosis carries a 60% 5-year survival rate. Thereafter, however, gradual progression to multiple myeloma occurs, although extended survival has been reported. Multiple myeloma, in contrast, accounts for 1% of newly diagnosed malignancies and is uniformly fatal within 4 years of diagnosis in all patients once spinal disease is diagnosed. Men and women are equally affected during the sixth to eighth decades. These tumors result from unregulated proliferation of plasma cells, causing systemic manifestations. Diagnosis is confirmed by the presence of at least 10% abnormal plasma cells, lytic bone lesions, and monoclonal gammopathy diagnosed on serum protein electrophoresis (SPEP) or urine protein electrophoresis (UPEP). Anemia and elevation of sedimentation rate also are characteristic on laboratory studies. Protein electrophoresis may be negative in as many as 3% of patients with myeloma, which requires a low threshold for bone marrow aspiration in patients at risk. Treatment of plasmacytoma and multiple myeloma is irradiation, with operative intervention reserved for patients with neurological deficits or progression despite maximal chemotherapy and irradiation.

METASTATIC TUMORS

Metastatic tumors are the most common malignant lesions found in bone, present 40 times more often than all other primary malignant bone tumors combined. Tumor types include breast, lung, prostate, kidney, gastrointestinal, and thyroid. Lymphoma is another tumor that commonly affects the spine and must be considered. Recent advances in chemotherapy, radiation therapy, and other cancer therapies have resulted in a significant improvement in survival for many of these types of cancer. With the improved survival, previously silent spinal metastases are becoming clinically apparent and significantly impairing quality of life. Metastatic disease involves the spine in 50% to 85% of patients, most often affecting the vertebral bodies of the lumbar spine, followed by the thoracic, cervical, and sacral regions.

The chief complaint in most patients is pain, although 36% of spinal metastases do not cause symptoms. Pain usually is progressive and unremitting, and often no relief occurs even with rest or at night. A previous history of cancer, regardless of how remote, must prompt a search for metastatic disease in patients with progressive pain. Neurological symptoms or signs may be present but are less frequent, occurring in 5% to 20% of patients with spinal metastases. For patients with thoracic metastasis, however, the rate of neurological symptoms increases to 37%, probably because of the more sensitive spinal cord with less space available at this level compared with compression of the nerve roots in the lumbar spine. In patients who develop neurological deterioration and paraparesis, only 25% to 35% regain lost motor function. Patients who are paraplegic or have complete bowel or bladder dysfunction are not likely to regain function regardless of treatment. Rapid onset of symptoms over a period of less than 24 hours also indicates a poor prognosis for neurological recovery in contrast to a lesion with a slower onset of symptoms. Fortunately, with aggressive treatment, 60% of patients who retain the ability to walk before treatment of spinal metastasis will maintain this function after treatment.

Imaging often is inconclusive and nondiagnostic in these patients. Plain roentgenograms of the spine are inconclusive in many with metastatic disease. The most sensitive study is bone scanning, which identifies most lesions larger than 2 mm, although false negatives occur in 5%. Multiple myeloma, breast, nasopharyngeal, lung, and renal tumors are the most likely neoplasms to appear falsely negative on bone scans. Use of CT scanning is helpful in delineating soft tissue extension from the bone or into the bone from extrinsic sources. Also, certain features of the CT scan are useful in determining whether a compression fracture is a result of osteoporosis or metastasis. Osteoporotic compression fractures reveal no evidence of cortical destruction, homogeneous involvement of the vertebral body, localized pathology, and the absence of a soft tissue mass. MRI is more useful in evaluating soft tissue masses, neural elements, and vertebral body lesions. Characteristic features of metastatic lesions are hypointensity on T1-weighted images, with enhancement on T2-weighted images and gadolinium-enhanced T1-weighted images. Myelography occasionally is necessary for tumors not well defined by other, less-invasive procedures but should be used cautiously because it can precipitate neurological deterioration in 16% to 24% of patients, necessitating immediate decompression.

The standard methods of treatment for benign tumors involving excision and grafting usually are insufficient for the early mobilization of patients with symptomatic metastatic disease. Siegal, Tiqva, and Siegal estimated that 5% of patients with metastatic cancer develop spinal cord compression. Kawabata et al. noted that 2 of 3880 autopsied patients with the diagnosis of metastatic cancer had previous clinical evidence of spinal metastasis but that at autopsy the rate of metastasis varied from 21% to 48%. Schaberg and Gainor analyzed 322 patients with metastatic cancer. The rate of spinal metastases varied from 2.2% to 31%. Breast and prostate tumors were the most frequent, followed by thyroid, lung, and renal cancer. Of patients with spinal metastases, 36% did not have back pain. Spinal cord compression was noted in 20% of the patients.

Prostatic tumors were the most common cause of epidural impingement. Hypernephroma was the most common malignancy to cause neurological impairment as the first sign of malignancy.

Pathoanatomy

The distal lumbar spine is interconnected with an extensive venous plexus that is valveless, allowing drainage of the brain, thorax, and pelvis. Batson's plexus allows retrograde blood flow within these systems, which interconnect the vertebral bodies, epidural veins, basivertebral, and paraarticular veins. As a result, metastases may follow these pathways, resulting in the characteristic pattern of bony spread. Interconnections of the epidural plexus with both the pelvic and mammary veins lends a relatively unimpeded pathway for the spread of prostate and breast cancer, which show the most affinity for spread to spinal sites.

Classification

DeWald et al. suggested a classification of spinal metastases. Class I is destruction without collapse but with pain. This class is divided further into (a) less than 50% vertebral body destruction, (b) greater than 50% vertebral body destruction, and (c) pedicle destruction. In this class they considered surgery only for grades Ib and Ic. Class II is the addition of moderate deformity and collapse with immune competence. This class is considered a good risk for surgery. Class III patients are immunocompromised with moderate deformity and collapse. This class carries greater risk for surgery. Class IV includes patients with paralysis, collapse, and deformity with immune competence. This class is considered a relative surgical emergency. Class V adds immune incompetence to paralysis, collapse, and deformity. This class is not considered a good operative risk. Further, surgical reconstruction is recommended when more than 50% vertebral body destruction is identified or in the presence of involvement of one or both pedicles due to the risk of later fracture and deformity. This classification allows consideration of the tumor, potential instability, and patient physiology, which is a sensible approach to a difficult problem.

Irradiation

For most metastatic tumors, irradiation is sufficient for the palliation of symptoms of pain and neurological deficit. Indications for irradiation include pain and mild, slowly progressive neurological symptoms in the presence of a radiosensitive tumor, spinal canal compromise that results from soft-tissue compression and not bony retropulsion, and multifocal lesions compressing the spinal canal. Instability is a relative contraindication for irradiation because of the potential collapse and progression of deformity that could occur with tissue necrosis. Use of irradiation causes initial necrosis of tumor bone, which later is converted to lamellar bone and normal bone marrow. This process results in remineralization of the lesion at 2 months, formation of woven bone at 4 months,

and reorganization into mature bone at 6 to 12 months. Initial necrosis after irradiation of large and potentially unstable lesions may result in acute instability and neurological deterioration.

Successful treatment has been documented in 62% of patients with pain and in 52% of patients with neurological impairment. Improvement in neurological symptoms was noted in 25%. Surgery has failed to show a benefit in survival rates over irradiation; therefore, if symptoms can be controlled, radiation therapy appears to be the logical choice. Acute neurological deterioration, however, is an indication for immediate surgical decompression.

Operative Treatment

Indications for surgical decompression include the requirement of tissue for diagnosis, treatment of an isolated lesion, treatment of a fracture causing instability, pain, or spinal canal compromise, radioresistant tumors, which usually include gastrointestinal and kidney metastases, recurrent tumor in a previously irradiated field, neurological symptoms that are progressive despite adjuvant measures, and potential instability. Operative procedures often are extensive and involve significant blood loss; therefore the patient must be in a physical state that allows for survival of the proposed procedure. Expected survival of more than 6 weeks is a relative condition for surgery in the presence of unremitting or progressive symptoms, although general physical condition also is important in operative decision making. In patients with a reasonable long-term survival, bone grafting is recommended rather than polymethylmethacrylate because of the likely failure of such materials. Adjunctive radiotherapy must be planned carefully, however, to allow for incorporation of grafts when used. This is best accomplished by performing radiotherapy preoperatively or delaying it until at least 3 weeks postoperatively if at all possible to improve fusion rates. Because of the hypercoagulable state of malignancy, especially in patients with paraplegia, the use of a preoperative inferior vena cava filter also should be considered.

Laminectomy has been shown to be of little value in the treatment of progressive paralysis caused by malignant spinal tumors in the anterior column. Successful results using this approach have been reported in only 30% to 40% of patients and are inferior to those obtained with radiation alone. Radical laminectomy for tumor resection is of value, however, and should be considered when compression is caused by lesions in the posterior elements compressing the dura. Careful evaluation of diagnostic images is necessary for appropriate preoperative planning of the operative approach and subsequent procedures.

Because of the predominant vertebral body location of malignant tumors, anterior decompression is most often necessary to remove the pathology responsible for neurological deterioration and pain. Other indications for anterior surgery include pathological kyphosis with an intact posterior osteoligamentous complex. Improvement in pain is possible in 80% to

95% of patients, with restoration of neurological function in 75%. Decompression often creates instability that requires reconstruction with instrumentation, allografts, and occasionally structural bone cement. Although circumferential instrumentation is definitely superior in stabilization, anterior instrumentation alone often will suffice if the posterior osteoligamentous complex is intact and resection is less than a complete spondylectomy. Additional posterior decompression and stabilization in a combined approach often are necessary if the spinal canal is compressed both anteriorly and posteriorly or if the posterior column is attenuated. If exposure of both anterior and posterior columns is necessary, a two-stage approach combined under one anesthesia or a simultaneous approach can be used. High-grade instability, contiguous vertebral involvement, destruction of both anterior and posterior columns, and need for en bloc resection are indications for these approaches. Solid fixation is possible with structural grafting anteriorly, and solid segmental instrumentation can be applied both anteriorly and posteriorly if necessary to provide the most rigid surgical constructs.

For patients with anterior column involvement who are unable to tolerate a thoracotomy, or those with circumferential spinal cord or neural constriction, a costotransversectomy is useful in the thoracic spine, and a posterolateral approach is useful in the lumbar and cervical spines. Admittedly, excision is intralesional, but decompression often is acceptable with the ability to restore stability using structural grafts or devices anteriorly with segmental instrumentation posteriorly. The morbidity of a thoracotomy is avoided, which is a necessity in some patients, especially those with symptomatic metastasis from lung cancer. By excising the rib head, intercostal neurovascular bundle, and transverse process on the side of the lesion, the anterior and middle columns are accessible to about the midline using special curets. If the pedicle is uninvolved, this medial wall is preserved to avoid contamination of the spinal canal or damage to the spinal cord. Bilateral approaches occasionally are necessary for extensive posterior vertebral body involvement to allow access to both sides of the middle column. Care must be taken with soft tissue extension to avoid inadvertent entry into the great vessels anteriorly. These procedures should be followed by instrumentation and fusion, and structural interbody grafting should be used if significant bony resection is done anteriorly to decrease tension stresses on the posterior implants.

Scoville et al. in 1967 were the first to use polymethylmethacrylate to fill defects in the vertebral bodies. Keggi, Southwick, and Keller reported the use of polymethylmethacrylate (PMMA) as an adjunct to internal fixation in situations in which bone fixation was questionable. There have been numerous reports on the efficacy of this material as an adjunct to internal fixation and bone grafting. Bone cement functions well in compression; however, results have been disappointing on the tension side of spinal reconstructions. Failure has been noted at a mean of 200 days after treatment, and therefore its use has been recommended for patients with a short life expectancy or in salvage cases. Generally, if life expectancy is more than 3 to 6 months, bone graft incorporation is possible. Fear of neural injury from the use of PMMA has been a frequent concern. Wang et al. showed that, although the temperature of the curing cement may reach 176° to 194° F, the temperature measured beneath an intact lamina and under Gelfoam covering the dura at a laminar defect was significantly less (45° F). Later examination of the spinal cord in test animals did not show evidence of neural injury. Clinically we have noted a fall in amplitude of somatosensory evoked potentials during the curing phase that returns to normal within 20 to 30 minutes of insertion of PMMA. Injury from the use of the material near the spinal cord has not been reported. PMMA can be used to augment existing internal fixation devices; however, loosening is to be expected. If long-term survival is expected, then provision for bone grafting and graft incorporation must be made.

Percutaneous vertebroplasty has been reported to be effective treatment for osteolytic spinal metastases and multiple myelomas. Cortet et al. reported decreased pain 48 hours after vertebroplasty in 36 (97%) of 37 patients. Beneficial effects were increased or unchanged in all after 1 month, in 89% after 3 months, and in 75% after 6 months. Although leakage of the cement outside the vertebral body occurred in 29, only 2 patients developed severe nerve root pain due to leakage into a neural foramen. They cautioned that vertebroplasty should be done only in centers with experienced neurosurgeons or orthopaedic surgeons because of the possibility of severe complications.

◆ Anterior Decompression

TECHNIQUE 41-10

Approach the diseased spine using the standard anterior approach for that spinal segment from the side of the most prominent tumor mass, but choose an approach that allows for more radical or extensive exposure if necessary. Identify normal bone and disc cranially and caudally. First ligate segmental vessels to allow discectomy, which is done to the posterior longitudinal ligament. Ligation of the segmental vessel at the level of vertebral body involvement may be difficult because of encasement by soft tissue extension. Decompression of the spinal canal or resection of tumor is possible if lesions are anteriorly situated. If decompression is necessary, create an access portal within the vertebral body anterior to the tumor and then use curets to pull tumoral tissue anteriorly away from the spinal canal into the void. This allows decompression without forcing material against the already compressed dura. Piecemeal resection commonly is done for metastatic lesions; however, for en bloc resection the tumor must not be violated. In these cases, osteotomize the pedicles after discectomy to allow en bloc resection. Be prepared for a spinal fluid leak, as adherence

continued

of the tumor to the dura is certainly a possibility. If any extension of tumor is present into the posterior elements, a staged posterior procedure for completion of vertebrectomy is done.

Once resection of tumor is complete, prepare for fixation. For patients with expected long-term survival of more than 1 to 2 years, place allograft or autograft for structural support. These grafts include allograft femur, humerus, fibula, or iliac crest. Autograft fibula or iliac crest are the only options unless a structural spacer, such as a mesh cage, is applied. Bone cement is a consideration in patients with a poor expected survival and allows for irradiation and immediate compressive strength when combined with anterior instrumentation. Cover the exposed dura or anterior longitudinal ligament or both with Gelfoam. Insert the polymethylmethacrylate in a semiliquid or doughy state. Use of a reinforcement device is recommended; this may include Harrington or other hook-rod implants used as a distraction device, Steinmann pins, or a mesh titanium cage that engages the vertebral bodies and is totally covered with polymethylmethacrylate to provide a smooth external surface. Remove excess cement, which is especially important in the cervical spine, where a large mass of cement can cause dysphagia. Take care to avoid pushing the cement against the dura and spinal cord. As soon as the cement has been trimmed, begin continuous irrigation of the wound with normal saline. This theoretically keeps perineural temperatures at a minimum, although due to CSF convection this may be unnecessary. Anterior instrumentation is added to provide maximal fixation. Numerous implants that are of low profile and provide at least four fixation points are available. For optimal fixation, place vertebral body screws in a bicortical fashion. If a later posterior instrumentation construct is planned, slight modification of screw placement is necessary to allow for placement of pedicle screws if these are to be used. Under these circumstances, identify the pedicle and simply keep the vertebral body screws just inferior to these structures. Once fixation is complete and compression of the interbody construct is maintained, test the construct for stability before closing. Remove and replace the cement and metal fixation if it is loose. Close the wound in the standard fashion. If corpectomy of more than a single level is done or if posterior column involvement is present, then a combined approach with posterior instrumentation is preferred.

AFTERTREATMENT. Rigid immobilization is preferable after these procedures, especially when the bone quality is in question due to osteoporosis or other metabolic causes. A TLSO is typically worn when getting out of bed and while up; however, it is not necessary for the patient to wear this during sleep. Once the graft incorporates over the next 3 to 6 months, the TLSO is discontinued. Radiation is deferred for 3 weeks if possible. Great attention is paid to nutrition during the perioperative period and may require parenteral or enteral supplementation.

◆ Costotransversectomy

TECHNIQUE 41-11

Using a standard posterior incision or a paramedian incision, expose the spinous processes and transverse processes bilaterally over the levels of anticipated instrumentation (Chapter 34). Once roentgenographic localization is complete, identify and expose the rib of the level and side of pathology. To perform corpectomy, it usually is necessary to subperiosteally expose three ribs and disarticulate them at the costotransverse articulation and also to excise the medial 8 to 10 cm of the ribs. Removal of the transverse processes aids in vertebral body exposure. Once the ribs are removed, use peanut dissectors to bluntly elevate the pleura from the vertebral bodies. Create working portals between the intercostal neurovascular bundles for placement of retractors and instruments. During this step of the procedure, headlight illumination is mandatory to see into the retropleural space. Laminectomy or facetectomy can be done if necessary for posterior decompression. Ligation of the segmental vessels is possible, if necessary, under direct observation. Retention of the intercostal nerves is preferable; however, these can be sacrificed if they interfere with proper decompression. The tradeoff is chest wall anesthesia, intercostal paralysis, and potentially upper abdominal muscle paralysis below T7. Perform discectomy above and below the affected vertebral body in the standard fashion. Remove the tumor with curets and rongeurs to the level of the posterior longitudinal ligament or dura as necessary. Brisk bleeding as the tumor is curetted is to be expected but is minimized by preoperative embolization. Intermittent packing of the tumor also helps to control bleeding, with continuation of the procedure after bleeding subsides. Once the tumor is excised, hemostasis usually occurs without much difficulty.

For curative resections, it is difficult to obtain en bloc or wide margins using this approach. Osteotomes can be safely directed to parallel the posterior vertebral body wall; however, obtaining margins beyond the opposite lateral cortical wall of the vertebral body is not possible because of the risk of injury to the opposite segmental vessels. Nonetheless, the approach is useful in patients unable to tolerate thoracotomy when anterior pathology is predominant and stabilization is necessary. Instrumentation is necessary for stabilization and can be used posteriorly at any time during the procedure, although we prefer to place implants before exposure of the spinal canal to minimize incidental dural tear while placing implants. Early placement of implants also can be helpful to distract the ligamentous structures and disc during the decompression. Pedicle fixation avoids the concerns of spinal canal compromise of hooks or wires and allows fixation of levels after laminectomy. Hook-rod or Luque-type constructs also are applicable, and the type used is determined by surgeon's experience. Before closure, maintain positive pressure ventilation momentarily while irrigation is allowed to cover the pleura. This is done to inspect the pleura for leaks that usually would necessitate placement of a chest tube. After bone grafting, standard closure is done over drains.

◆ Posterolateral Decompression

TECHNIQUE 41-12

This approach is indicated for patients with tumors that involve the anterior, middle, and posterior columns simultaneously. This is done without the risks or the extensive exposure required for a simultaneous approach. If a posterolateral approach is used, make a midline incision to expose the pathological level. Once identification of the correct level is confirmed, decompression can be done or posterior instrumentation can be placed. Regardless, because of the potential destabilization that occurs with laminectomy and pedicle resection, place posterior instrumentation before completion of the procedure.

Begin decompression as the pedicle that leads into the tumor is sounded, and use sequentially larger curets to remove bone through this access site. Hemilaminectomy is helpful to expose the medial border of the pedicle to avoid medial penetration, unless adequate decompression requires laminectomy, in which case this is done before the transpedicle decompression. Resect the lateral wall of the pedicle with a Leksell rongeur, which allows medialization of the curets. If the posterior vertebral body wall is retropulsed, resect the medial pedicle border as well. If compression is bilateral, a bilateral transpedicle approach is necessary. Once the pedicle is resected, a reverse-angle curet or even a PLIF tamp can be placed ventral to the dura, against the tumor or retropulsed posterior vertebral wall so that it is tamped or pushed back into the vertebral body. Decancellation of the middle column often is necessary before this maneuver to create a space for the bone that is reduced. Once the retropulsed material is pushed anteriorly, resect it with curets and pituitary rongeurs. Anterior column grafting depends on the procedure performed. Take care that morselized graft is not retropulsed into the spinal canal after placement, creating the same problem the procedure was intended to correct. Perform appropriate bone grafting and instrumentation. If a large anterior vertebral body was resected, a structural device should be placed in addition to posterior segmental spinal instrumentation.

AFTERTREATMENT. Patients are fitted for a TLSO, and immobilization is continued after the procedure for 3 to 6 months. Ambulation is started on the first postoperative day, unless neurological deficit was preexistent, in which case bed-to-chair transfers are started. Anticoagulants are not used in spinal surgery patients because of the inherent risk of epidural hematoma, so lower extremity antiembolism stockings and compression foot devices are used until the patient is ambulatory. A vena cava filter should be considered for high-risk patients. Radiation is deferred, if at all possible, for at least 3 weeks when autogenous or allograft bone is used.

References

SPINAL STENOSIS

Airaksinen O, Herno A, Turunen V, et al: Surgical outcome of 438 patients treated surgically for lumbar spinal stenosis, *Spine* 22:2278, 1997.

Amundsen T, Weber H, Nordal HJ, et al: Lumbar spinal stenosis: conservative or surgical management? A prospective 10-year study, *Spine* 25:1424, 2000.

An HS, Butler JP: Lumbar spinal stenosis: historical perspectives, classification, and pathoanatomy, *Semin Spine Surg* 11:184, 1999.

Arnoldi CC, Brodsky AE, Cauchoix J, et al: Lumbar spinal stenosis and nerve root entrapment syndromes: definition and classification, *Clin Orthop* 115:4, 1976.

Atlas SJ, Deyo RA, Keller RB, et al: The Maine Lumbar Spine Study. III. 1-year outcomes of surgical and nonsurgical management of lumbar spinal stenosis, *Spine* 21:1787, 1996.

Atlas SJ, Deyo RA, Patrick DL, et al: The Quebec Task Force classification for spinal disorders and the severity, treatment, and outcomes of sciatica and lumbar spinal stenosis, *Spine* 21:2885, 1996.

Atlas SJ, Keller RB, Robson D, et al: Surgical and nonsurgical management of lumbar spinal stenosis: four-year outcomes from the Maine Lumbar Spine Study, *Spine* 25:556, 2000.

Axelsson P, Johnsson R, Stromqvist B: The spondylolytic vertebra and its adjacent segment mobility measured before and after posterolateral fusion, *Spine* 22:414, 1997.

Bailey P, Casamajor L: Osteoarthritis of spine compressing cord, *J Nerv Ment Dis* 38:588, 1911.

Bassett G, Johnson C, Stanley P: Comparison of preoperative selective spinal angiography and somatosensory-evoked potential monitoring with temporary occlusion of segmental vessels during anterior spinal surgery, *Spine* 21:199, 1996.

Bell GR: Office evaluation of patients with spinal stenosis, *Semin Spine Surg* 11:191, 1999.

Bell GR, Rothman RH, Booth RE, et al: A study of computer-assisted tomography. II. Comparison of metrizamide myelography and computed tomography in the diagnosis of herniated lumbar disc and spinal stenosis, *Spine* 9:552, 1984.

Bell GR, Rothman RH: The conservative treatment of sciatica, *Spine* 9:54, 1984.

Boden SD: Point of view: 5-year reoperation rates after different types of lumbar spine surgery, *Spine* 23:820, 1998.

Boden SD, Davis DO, Dina TS, et al: Abnormal magnetic-resonance scans of the lumbar spine in asymptomatic subjects, *J Bone Joint Surg* 72A:403, 1990.

Bohl WR, Steffee AD: Lumbar spinal stenosis: a cause of continued pain and disability after total hip arthroplasty, *Spine* 4:168, 1979.

Bolender NF, Schönström N, Spengler DM: Role of computed tomography and myelography in the diagnosis of central spinal stenosis, *J Bone Joint Surg* 67A:240, 1985.

Butterman GR, Garvey TA, Hunt AF, et al: Lumbar fusion results related to diagnosis, *Spine* 23:116, 1998.

Choy DS, Ngeow J: Percutaneous laser disc decompression in spinal stenosis, *J Clin Laser Med Surg* 16:123, 1998.

Ciric I, Mikhael MA, Tarkington JA, Vick NA: The lateral recess syndrome: a variant of spinal stenosis, *J Neurosurg* 53:433, 1980.

Claussen CD, Lohkamp FW, v Bazan UB: The diagnosis of congenital spinal disorders in computed tomography (CT), *Neuropadiatrie* 8:405, 1977.

Cranston PE, Patel RB, Harrison RB: Computed tomography for metastatic lesions of the osseous pelvis, *South Med J* 76:1503, 1983.

Crawshaw C, Kean DM, Mulholland RC, et al: The use of nuclear magnetic resonance in the diagnosis of lateral canal entrapment, *J Bone Joint Surg* 66B:711, 1984.

Deen HG, Zimmerman RS, Lyons MK, et al: Use of the exercise treadmill to measure baseline functional status and surgical outcome in patients with severe lumbar spinal stenosis, *Spine* 23:244, 1998.

Dillin W: Spinal stenosis surgery outcome, *Semin Spine Surg* 11:297, 1999.

Dodge LD, Bohlman HH, Rhodes RS: Concurrent lumbar spinal stenosis and peripheral vascular disease, *Clin Orthop* 230:141, 1988.

Dorwart RH, Vogler JB, Helms CA: Spinal stenosis, *Radiol Clin North Am* 21:301, 1983.

Drew R, Bhandari M, Kulkarni AV, et al: Reliability in grading the severity of lumbar spinal stenosis, *J Spinal Disord* 13:253, 2000.

Dunlop RB, Adams MA, Hutton WC: Disc space narrowing and the lumbar facet joints, *J Bone Joint Surg* 66B:706, 1984.

Dyck P: The stoop-test in lumbar entrapment radiculopathy, *Spine* 4:89, 1979.

Ehni G, Clark K, Wilson CB, Alexander E Jr: Significance of the small lumbar spinal canal cauda equina compression syndromes due to spondylosis (parts 1 to 4), *Neurosurg* 31:490, 1969.

Eisenstein S: The morphometry and pathological anatomy of the lumbar spine in South African Negroes and Caucasoids with specific reference to spinal stenosis, *J Bone Joint Surg* 59B:173, 1977.

Elsberg CA: Experiences in spinal surgery, *Surg Gynecol Obstet* 16:117, 1913.

Etebar S, Cahill DW: Risk factors for adjacent-segment failure following lumbar fixation with rigid instrumentation for degenerative instability, *J Neurosurg* 90(suppl):163, 1999.

Farfan HF: The pathological anatomy of degenerative spondylolisthesis: a cadaver study, *Spine* 5:412, 1980.

Foley RK, Kirkaldy-Willis WH: Chronic venous hypertension in the tail of the wistar rat, *Spine* 4:251, 1979.

Forestier J, Rotes-Querol J: Senile ankylosing hyperostosis of the spine, *Ann Rheum Dis* 9:321, 1950.

Fox MW, Onofrio BM, Onofrio BM, Hanssen AD: Clinical outcomes and radiological instability following decompressive lumbar laminectomy for degenerative spinal stenosis: a comparison of patients undergoing concomitant arthrodesis versus decompression alone, *J Neurosurg* 85:793, 1996.

Frazier DD, Lipson SJ, Fossel AH, Katz JN: Associations between spinal deformity and outcomes after decompression for spinal stenosis, *Spine* 22:2025, 1997.

Fritz JM, Erhard RE, Delitto A, et al: Preliminary results of the use of a two-stage treadmill test as a clinical diagnostic tool in the differential diagnosis of lumbar spinal stenosis, *J Spinal Disord* 10:410, 1997.

Fritz JM, Erhard RE, Vignovic M: A nonsurgical treatment approach for patients with lumbar spinal stenosis, *Phys Ther* 77:962, 1997.

Fukusaki M, Kobayashi I, Hara T, Sumikawa K: Symptoms of spinal stenosis do not improve after epidural steroid injection, *Clin J Pain* 14:148, 1998.

Ganz JC: Lumbar spinal stenosis: postoperative results in terms of preoperative posture-related pain, *J Neurosurg* 72:71, 1990.

Garfin SR, Herkowtiz HN, Mirkovic S: Spinal stenosis, *Instr Course Lect* 49:361, 2000.

Gelalis ID, Kang JD: Thoracic and lumbar fusions for degenerative disorders: rationale for selecting the appropriate fusion techniques, *Orthop Clin North Am* 29:829, 1998.

Getty CJM: Lumbar spinal stenosis: the clinical spectrum and the results of operation, *J Bone Joint Surg* 62B:481, 1980.

Getty CJM, Johnson JR, Kirwan E, Sullivan MF: Partial undercutting facetectomy for bony entrapment of the lumbar nerve root, *J Bone Joint Surg* 63B:330, 1981.

Gill TJ, Mason MD: Assessment of neuroforaminal decompression in degenerative spinal stenosis, *Clin Orthop* 348:135, 1998.

Goel VK: Point of view: the effects of rigid spinal instrumentation and solid bony fusion on spinal kinematics: a posterolateral spinal arthrodesis model, *Spine* 23:773, 1998.

Gokalp HZ, Ozkai E: Intradural tuberculomas of the spinal cord: report of two cases, *J Neurosurg* 55:289, 1981.

Grabias S.: The treatment of spinal stenosis: current concepts review, *J Bone Joint Surg* 62A:308, 1980.

Grob D, Humke T, Dvorak J: Degenerative lumbar spinal stenosis: decompression with and without arthrodesis, *J Bone Joint Surg* 77A:1036, 1995.

Guigui P, Benoist M, Delecourt C, et al: Motor deficit in lumbar spinal stenosis: a retrospective study of a series of 50 patients. *J Spinal Disord* 11:283, 1998.

Hadjipavlou AG, Simmons JW, Pope MH: An algorithmic approach to the investigation, treatment, and complications of surgery for low back pain, *Semin Spine Surg* 10:193, 1998.

Hanley EN Jr: The indications for lumbar spinal fusion with and without instrumentation, *Spine* 20(suppl):143, 1995.

Hansraj KK, O'Leary PF, Cammisa FP Jr, et al: Decompression, fusion, and instrumentation surgery for complex lumbar spinal stenosis, *Clin Orthop* 384:18, 2001.

Hasegawa T, An HS, Haughton VM, et al: Lumbar foraminal stenosis: critical heights of the intervertebral discs and foramina: a cryomicrotone study in cadavers, *J Bone Joint Surg* 77A:32, 1995.

Herkowitz HN, Abraham DJ, Albert TJ: Controversy: management of degenerative disc disease above an L5-S1 segment requiring arthrodesis, *Spine* 24:1268, 1999.

Herkowitz HN, Garfin SR, Bell G, et al: The use of computerized tomography in evaluating nonvisualized vertebral levels caudad to a complete block on a lumbar myelogram, *J Bone Joint Surg* 69A:218, 1987.

Herno A, Airaksinen O, Saari T, Luukkonen M: Lumbar spinal stenosis: a matched-pair study of operated and nonoperated patients, *Br J Neurosurg* 10:461, 1996.

Herno A, Airaksinen O, Saari T, et al: The predictive value of preoperative myelography in lumbar spinal stenosis, *Spine* 19:1335, 1994.

Herno A, Airaksinen O, Saari T, Sihovonen T: Surgical results of lumbar spinal stenosis: a comparison of patients with or without previous back surgery, *Spine* 20:964, 1995.

Herno A, Airaksinen O, Saari T, et al: Computed tomography findings 4 years after surgical management of lumbar spinal stenosis: no correlation with clinical outcome, *Spine* 24:2234, 1999.

Herno A, Partanen K, Talaslahti T, et al: Long-term clinical and magnetic resonance imaging follow-up assessment of patients with lumbar spinal stenosis after laminectomy, *Spine* 24:1533, 1999.

Herno A, Saari T, Suomalainen O, Airaksinen O: The degree of decompressive relief and its relation to clinical outcome in patients undergoing surgery for lumbar spinal stenosis, *Spine* 24:1010, 1999.

Herron LD, Mangelsdorf C: Lumbar spinal stenosis: results of surgical treatment, *J Spinal Disord* 4:26, 1991.

Herron LD, Pheasant HC: Bilateral laminotomy and discectomy for segmental lumbar disc disease: decompression with stability, *Spine* 8:86, 1983.

Hiraizumi Y, Transfeldt EE, Fujimaki E, et al: Electrophysiologic evaluation of intermittent sacral nerve dysfunction in lumbar spinal canal stenosis, *Spine* 18:1355, 1993.

Hirsh LF, Finneson BE: Intradural sacral nerve root metastasis mimicking herniated disc: case report, *J Neurosurg* 49:764, 1978.

Hitselberger WE, Witten RM; Abnormal myelograms in asymptomatic patients, *J Neurosurg* 28:204, 1968.

Hurri H, Slatis P, Soini J, et al: Lumbar spinal stenosis: assessment of long-term outcome 12 years after operative and conservative treatment. *J Spinal Disord* 11:110, 1998.

Iguchi T, Kurihara A, Nakayama J, et al: Minimum 10-year outcome of decompressive laminectomy for degenerative lumbar spinal stenosis, *Spine* 25:1754, 2000.

Inufusa A, An H, Lim T, et al: Anatomic changes of the spinal canal and intervertebral foramen associated with flexion-extension movement, *Spine* 21:2412, 1996.

Jackson RP, Cain JE, Jacobs RR, et al: The neuroradiographic diagnosis of lumbar herniated nucleus pulposus (parts I and II), *Spine* 13:1352.

Jiang GX, Xu WD, Wang AH: Spinal stenosis with meralgia paraesthetica, *J Bone Joint Surg* 70B:272, 1988.

Johansson JE, Barington TW, Amelie M: Combined vascular and neurogenic claudication, *Spine* 7:150, 1992.

Johnsson K, Rosén I, Udén A: The natural course of lumbar spinal stenosis, *Clin Orthop* 279:82, 1992.

Johnsson K, Udén A, Rosén I: The effect of decompression on the natural course of spinal stenosis: a comparison of surgically treated and untreated patients, *Spine* 16:615, 1991.

Johnsson K, Willner S, Pettersson H: Analysis of operated cases with lumbar spinal stenosis, *Acta Orthop Scand* 52:427, 1981.

Jönsson B, Annertz M, Sjoberg C, Strömqvist B: A prospective and consecutive study of surgically treated lumbar spinal stenosis. I. Clinical features related to radiographic findings, *Spine* 22:2932, 1997.

Jönsson B, Annertz M, Sjoberg C, Strömqvist B: A prospective and consecutive study of surgically treated lumbar spinal stenosis. II. Five-year follow-up by an independent observer, *Spine* 22:2938, 1997.

Jönsson B, Strömqvist B: Symptoms and signs in degeneration of the lumbar spine: a prospective consecutive study of 300 operated patients, *J Bone Joint Surg* 75B:381, 1993.

Jönsson B, Strömqvist B: Decompression for lateral lumbar spinal stenosis: results and impact on sick leave and working conditions, *Spine* 19:2381, 1994.

Kanamori M, Matsue H, Hirano N, et al: Trumpet laminectomy for lumbar degenerative spinal stenosis, *J Spinal Disord* 6:232, 1993.

Karayannacos PE, Yashon D, Vasko JS: Narrow lumbar spinal canal with "vascular" syndromes, *Arch Surg* 111:803, 1976.

Katz JN, Lipson SJ, Change LC, et al: Seven- to 10-year outcome of decompressive surgery for degenerative lumbar spinal stenosis, *Spine* 21:92, 1996.

Katz JN, Lipson SJ, Lew RA, et al: Lumbar laminectomy alone or with instrumented or noninstrumented arthrodesis in degenerative lumbar spinal stenosis: patient selection, costs, and surgical outcomes, *Spine* 22:1123, 1997.

Katz JN, Stucki G, Lipson SJ, et al: Predictors of surgical outcome in degenerative lumbar spinal stenosis, *Spine* 24:2229, 1999.

Kauffman C, Garfin SR: Spinal stenosis: pathophysiology and symptom complex update 1999, *Semin Spine Surg* 11:209, 1999.

Keller RB, Atlas SJ, Soule DN, et al: Relationship between rates and outcomes of operative treatment for lumbar disc herniation and spinal stenosis, *J Bone Joint Surg* 81A:752, 1999.

Kimura I, Oh-Hama M, Shingu H: Cervical myelopathy treated by canal-expansive laminaplasty: computed tomographic and myelographic findings, *J Bone Joint Surg* 66A:914, 1984.

Kirkaldy-Willis WH: The relationship of structural pathology to the nerve root, *Spine* 9:49, 1984.

Kirkaldy-Willis WH, Wedge JH, Yong-Hing K, Reilly J: Pathology and pathogenesis of lumbar spondylosis and stenosis, *Spine* 4:319, 1978.

Kirkaldy-Willis WH, Wedge JH, Yong-Hing K, et al: Lumbar spinal nerve lateral entrapment, *Clin Orthop* 169:171, 1982.

Kostuik JP, Musha Y: Extension to the sacrum of previous adolescent scoliosis fusions in adult life, *Clin Orthop* 364:53, 1999.

Kuntz KM, Snider RK, Weinstein JN, et al: Cost-effectiveness of fusion with and without instrumentation of patients with degenerative spondylolisthesis and spinal stenosis, *Spine* 25:1132, 2000.

Lanes TC, Gauron EF, Spratt KF, et al: Long-term follow-up of patients with chronic back pain treated in a multidisciplinary rehabilitation program, *Spine* 20:801, 1995.

Larequi-Lauber T, Vader JP, Burnand B, et al: Appropriateness of indications for surgery of lumbar disc hernia and spinal stenosis, *Spine* 22:203, 1997.

Lee BCP, Kazam E, Newman AD: Computed tomography of the spine and spinal cord, *Radiology* 128:95, 1978.

Lehmann TR, Spratt KF, Tozzi JE, et al: Long-term follow-up of lower lumbar fusion patients, *Spine* 12:97, 1987.

Leroux JL, Legeron P, Moulinier L, et al: Stenosis of the lumbar spinal canal in vertebral ankylosing hyperostosis, *Spine* 17:1213, 1992.

Liew SM, Simmons ED Jr: Cervical deformity: rationale for selecting the appropriate fusion technique (anterior, posterior, and 360 degree), *Orthop Clin North Am* 29:779, 1998.

Lipson SJ: Spinal stenosis definitions, *Semin Spine Surg* 1:135, 1989.

Liyang D, Yinkan X, Wenming Z, Zhihua Z: The effect of flexion-extension motion of the lumbar spine on the capacity of the spinal canal: an experimental study, *Spine* 14:523, 1989.

Macnab I: Cervical spondylosis, *Clin Orthop* 109:69, 1975.

Mariconda M, Zanforlino G, Celestino GA, et al: Factors influencing the outcome of degenerative lumbar spinal stenosis, *J Spinal Disord* 13:131, 2000.

Matsui H, Kanamori M, Ishihara H, et al: Expansive lumbar laminoplasty for degenerative spinal stenosis in patients below 70 years of age, *Eur Spine J* 6:191, 1997.

Matsui H, Tsuji H, Sekido H et al: Results of expansive laminoplasty for lumbar spinal stenosis in active manual workers, *Spine* 17:S37, 1992.

McCullen GM, Bernini PM, Bernstein SH, Tosteson TD: Clinical and roentgenographic results of decompression for lumbar spinal stenosis, *J Spinal Disord* 7:380, 1994.

McGuire RA: Instrumentation of the stenotic spine with and without deformity, *Semin Spine Surg* 11:277, 1999.

McPhee IB, Swanson CE: The surgical management of degenerative lumbar scoliosis: posterior instrumentation alone versus two-stage surgery, *Bull Hosp Jt Dis* 57:16, 1998.

Messersmith RN, Cronan J, Esparza AR: Computed tomography–guided percutaneous biopsy: combined approach to the retroperitoneum, *Neurosurgery* 14:218, 1984.

Middlebrooks ES, Balderston RA: Decision making and operative treatment: decompression versus decompression and arthrodesis, *Semin Spine Surg* 11:234, 1999.

Miyakoshi N, Abe E, Shimada Y, et al: Outcome of one-level posterior lumbar interbody fusion for spondylolisthesis and postoperative intervertebral disc degeneration adjacent to the fusion, *Spine* 25:1837, 2000.

Mullin BB, Rea GL, Irsik R, et al: The effect of postlaminectomy spinal instability on the outcome of lumbar spinal stenosis patients, *J Spinal Disord* 9:107, 1996.

Nelson MA: Lumbar spinal stenosis, *J Bone Joint Surg* 55B:506, 1973.

Paine KWE: Clinical features of lumbar spinal stenosis, *Clin Orthop* 115:77, 1976.

Paine KWE: Results of decompression for lumbar spinal stenosis, *Clin Orthop* 115:96, 1976.

Phillips FM, Carlson GD, Bohlman HH, Hughes SS: Results of surgery for spinal stenosis adjacent to previous lumbar fusion, *J Spinal Disord* 13:432, 2000.

Porter RW, Hibbert C: Calcitonin treatment for neurogenic claudication, *Spine* 8:585, 1983.

Porter RW, Hibbert C, Evans C: The natural history of root entrapment syndrome, *Spine* 9:418, 1984.

Porter RW, Hibbert C, Wellman P: Backache and the lumbar spinal canal, *Spine* 5:99, 1980.

Porter RW, Miller CG: Neurogenic claudication and root claudication treated with calcitonin: a double-blind trial, *Spine* 13:1061, 1988.

Posner I, White AA III, Edwards WT, Hayes WC: A biomechanical analysis of the clinical stability of the lumbar and lumbosacral spine, *Spine* 7:374, 1982.

Postacchini F: Surgical management of lumbar spinal stenosis. *Spine* 24:1043, 1999.

Postacchini F, Cinotti G: Bone regrowth after surgical decompression for lumbar spinal stenosis, *J Bone Joint Surg* 74B:862, 1992.

Postacchini F, Pezzeri G, Montanaro A, Natali G: Computerized tomography in lumbar stenosis: a preliminary report, *J Bone Joint Surg* 62B:78, 1980.

Raskin SP: Degenerative changes of the lumbar spine: assessment by computed tomography, *Orthopedics* 4:186, 1981.

Rinaldi I, Mullins WJ, Delandy WF, et al: Computerized tomographic demonstration of rotational atlanto-axial fixation: case report, *J Neurosurg* 50:115, 1979.

Rivest C, Katz JN, Ferrante FM, Jamison RN: Effects of epidural steroid injection on pain due to lumbar spinal stenosis or herniated disks: a prospective study, *Arthritis Care Res* 11:291, 1998.

Rydevik B, Brown MD, Lundborg G: Pathoanatomy and pathophysiology of nerve root compression, *Spine* 9:7, 1984.

Saifuddin A: The imaging of lumbar spinal stenosis, *Clin Radiol* 55:581, 2000.

San Martino A, D'Andria FM, San Martino C: The surgical treatment of nerve root compression caused by scoliosis of the lumbar spine, *Spine* 8:261, 1983.

Schillberg B, Nystrom B: Quality of life before and after microsurgical decompression in lumbar spinal stenosis, *J Spinal Disord* 13:237, 2000.

Schmid G, Better S, Gottmann D, Strecker EP: CT-guided epidural/perineural injections in painful disorders of the lumbar spine: short- and extended-term results, *Cardiovasc Intervent Radiol* 22:493, 1999.

Schnebel B, Kingston S, Watkins R, Dillin W: Comparison of MRI to contrast CT in the diagnosis of spinal stenosis, *Spine* 14:332, 1989.

Schönström NSR, Bolender N, Spengler DM: The pathomorphology of spinal stenosis as seen on CT scans of the lumbar spine, *Spine* 10:806, 1985.

Shakil MS, Vaccaro AR, Albert TJ, Klein GR: Efficacy of conservative treatment of lumbar spinal stenosis, *Semin Spine Surg* 11:229, 1999.

Sheehan JM, Helm GA, Kallmes DFR, et al: Partial pediculectomy in the treatment of lumbar spinal stenosis: technical note, *Neurosurgery* 41:308, 1997.

Shenkin HA, Hash CJ: Spondylolisthesis after multiple bilateral laminectomies and facetectomies for lumbar spondylosis, *J Neurosurg* 50:45, 1979.

Simmons ED: Surgical treatment of patients with lumbar spinal stenosis with associated scoliosis, *Clin Orthop* 384:45, 2001.

Simmons ED Jr, Simmons EH: Spinal stenosis with scoliosis, *Spine* 17(suppl):117, 1992.

Simotas AC: Nonoperative treatment for lumbar spinal stenosis, *Clin Orthop* 384:153, 2001.

Simotas AC, Dorey FJ, Hansraj KK, Cammisa F Jr: Nonoperative treatment for lumbar spinal stenosis: clinical and outcome results and a 3-year survivorship analysis, *Spine* 15:197, 2000.

Spengler DM: Current concepts review: degenerative stenosis of the lumbar spine, *J Bone Joint Surg* 69A:305, 1987.

Spivak JM: Degenerative lumbar spinal stenosis, *J Bone Joint Surg* 80A:1053, 1998.

Stambough JL, Templin CR: Indirect decompression and reduction in the stenotic spine: is there a role for fusion? *Semin Spine Surg* 11:262, 1999.

Stambough JL: Principles of decompression for lumbar spinal stenosis, *Semin Spine Surg* 11:244, 1999.

Stitz MY, Sommer HM: Accuracy of blind versus fluoroscopically guided caudal epidural injection, *Spine* 24:1371, 1999.

Styblo K, Bossers GT, Slot GH: Osteotomy for kyphosis in ankylosing spondylitis, *Acta Orthop Scand* 56:294, 1985.

Surin V, Hedelin E, Smith L: Degenerative lumbar spinal stenosis: results of operative treatment, *Acta Orthop Scand* 53:79, 1982.

Templin CR, Stambough JL: Uncommon causes of spinal stenosis, *Semin Spine Surg* 11:215, 1999.

Tenhula J, Lenke LG, Bridwell KH, et al: Prospective functional evaluation of the surgical treatment of neurogenic claudication in patients with lumbar spinal stenosis, *J Spinal Disord* 13:276, 2000.

Tile M: The role of surgery in nerve root compression, *Spine* 9:57, 1984.

Tile M, McNeil SR, Zarins RK, et al: Spinal stenosis: results of treatment, *Clin Orthop* 115:104, 1976.

Truumees E, Fischgrund J, Herkowitz HN: Management of spinal stenosis adjacent to a previously treated segment, *Semin Spine Surg* 11:282, 1999.

Tsai RY, Yang RS, Bray RS Jr: Microscopic laminotomies for degenerative lumbar spinal stenosis, *J Spinal Disord* 11:389, 1998.

Turner JA, Ersek M, Herron L, Deyo R: Surgery for lumbar spinal stenosis: attempted meta-analysis of the literature, *Spine* 17:1, 1992.

Ullrich CG, Binet EF, Sanecki MG, Kieffer SA: Quantitative assessment of lumbar spinal canal by computed tomography, *Radiology* 134:137, 1980.

Umehara S, Zindrick MR, Patwardhan AG, et al: The biomechanical effect of postoperative hyperlordosis in instrumented lumbar fusion on instrumented and adjacent spinal segments, *Spine* 25:1617, 2000.

Vaccaro AR, Ball ST: Indications for instrumentation in degenerative lumbar spinal disorders, *Orthopedics* 23:260, 2000.

Velan GJ, Currier BL, Yaszemski MJ: Decision making in the evaluation and management of acquired spinal stenosis: an algorithmic approach, *Semin Spine Surg* 11:195, 1999.

Verbiest H: Pathological influence of developmental narrowness of bony lumbar vertebral canal, *J Bone Joint Surg* 37B:576, 1954.

Verbiest H: Results of surgical treatment of idiopathic developmental stenosis of the lumbar vertebral canal: a review of twenty-seven years' experience, *J Bone Joint Surg* 59B:181, 1977.

Verbiest H: The significance and principles of computerized axial tomography in idiopathic developmental stenosis of the bony lumbar vertebral canal, *Spine* 4:369, 1979.

Vitaz TW, Raque GH, Shileds CB, Glassman SD: Surgical treatment of lumbar spinal stenosis in patients older than 75 years of age. *J Neurosurg* 91(suppl):181, 1999.

Voelker JL, Mealey J, Eskridge J, et al: Metrizamide enhanced computed tomography as an adjunct to metrizamide myelography in the evaluation of lumbar disc herniation and spondylosis, *Neurosurgery* 20:379, 1987.

Walpin LA, Singer FR: Paget's disease: reversal of severe paraparesis using calcitonin, *Spine* 4:213, 1979.

Weiner BK, Brower RS, McCulloch JA: Minimally invasive alternatives in the treatment of lumbar stenosis, *Semin Spine Surg* 11:253, 1999.

Weiner BK, Fraser RD, Peterson M: Spinous process osteotomies to facilitate lumbar decompression surgery, *Spine* 24:62, 1999.

Weinstein JM, Scafuri RL, McNeill TW: The Rush-Presbyterian–St. Luke's lumbar spine analysis form: a prospective study of patients with "spinal stenosis," *Spine* 8:891, 1983.

Weisz M: Lumbar spinal canal stenosis in Paget's disease, *Spine* 8:192, 1983.

Whiffen JR, Neuwirth MG: Spinal stenosis. In Bridwell KH, DeWald RL, eds: *The textbook of spinal surgery,* ed 2, Philadelphia, 1997, Lippincott-Raven.

White AH, Wiltse LL: Postoperative spondylolisthesis. In Weinstein PR, Ehni G, Wilson CB, eds: *Lumbar spondylosis: diagnosis, management, and surgical treatment,* St Louis, 1977, Mosby.

Wiesel SW, Tsourmas N, Feffer HL, et al: A study of computer-assisted tomography. 1. The incidence of positive CAT scans in an asymptomatic group of patients, *Spine* 9:549, 1984.

Wiesz GM: Stenosis of the lumbar spinal canal in Forestier's disease, *Int Orthop* 7:61, 1983.

Williamson JB: Percutaneous stimulation of the cauda equina: a new diagnostic method in spinal stenosis, *Spine* 16:460, 1991.

Wilson PD, Straub LR: Operative indications in trauma to the low back, *Am J Surg* 74:270, 1947.

Wiltse LL: Common problems of the lumbar spine: degenerative spondylolisthesis and spinal stenosis, *J Cont Ed Orthop* 7:17,1979.

Wiltse LL, Guyer RD, Spencer CW, et al: Alar transverse process impingement of the L5 spinal nerve: the far-out syndrome, *Spine* 9:31, 1984.

Wiltse LL, Kirkaldy-Willis WH, McIvor GWD: The treatment of spinal stenosis, *Clin Orthop* 115:83, 1976.

Wolfe RM, Wiesel SW, Boden SD: Lumbar spinal stenosis: neurodiagnostic evaluation including myelography, *Semin Spine Surg* 11:219, 1999.

Yone K, Sakou T, Kawauchi Y, et al: Indication of fusion for lumbar spinal stenosis in elderly patients and its significance, *Spine* 21:242, 1996.

SPONDYLOLISTHESIS

Adkins EWO: Spondylolisthesis, *J Bone Joint Surg* 37B:148, 1955.

Antoniades SB, Hammerberg KW, DeWald RL: Sagittal plane configuration of the sacrum in spondylolisthesis, *Spine* 25:1085, 2000.

Apel DM, Lorenz MA, Zindrick MR: Symptomatic spondylolisthesis in adults: four decades later, *Spine* 14:345, 1989.

Balderston RA, Bradford DS: Technique for achievement and maintenance of reduction for severe spondylolisthesis using spinous process traction wiring and external fixation of the pelvis, *Spine* 10:376, 1985.

Bell DF, Ehrlich MG, Zaleske DJ: Brace treatment for symptomatic spondylolisthesis, *Clin Orthop* 236:192, 1988.

Berlemann U, Jeszenszky DJ, Buhler DW, Harms J: The role of lumbar lordosis, vertebral end-plate inclincation, disc height, and facet orientation in degenerative spondylolisthesis, *J Spinal Disord* 12:68, 1999.

Blackburne JS, Velikas EP: Spondylolisthesis in children and adolescents, *J Bone Joint Surg* 59B:490, 1977.

Blume HG: Unilateral posterior lumbar interbody fusion: simplified dowel technique, *Clin Orthop* 193:75, 1985.

Boccanera L, Pellicioni S, Laus M, Lelli A: Surgical treatment of isthmic spondylolisthesis in adults (review of 44 cases with long-term control), *Ital J Orthop Traumatol* 8:271, 1982.

Bohlman HH, Cook SS: One-stage decompression and posterolateral and interbody fusion for lumbosacral spondyloptosis through a posterior approach: report of two cases, *J Bone Joint Surg* 64A:415, 1982.

Boos N, Marchesi D, Aebi M: Treatment of spondylolysis and spondylolisthesis with Cotrel-Dubousset instrumentation: a preliminary report, *J Spinal Disord* 4:472, 1991.

Booth KC, Bridwell KH, Eisenberg BA, et al: Minimum 5-year results of degenerative spondylolisthesis treated with decompression and instrumented posterior fusion, *Spine* 24:1721, 1999.

Bosworth DM: Technique of spinal fusion in the lumbosacral region by the double clothespin graft (distraction graft; H graft) and results, *Instr Course Lect* 9:44, 1952.

Bosworth DM, Fielding JW, Demarest L, Bonaquist M: Spondylolisthesis: a critical review of a consecutive series of cases treated by arthrodesis, *J Bone Joint Surg* 37A:767, 1955.

Boxall D, Bradford DS, Winter RB, Moe JH: Management of severe spondylolisthesis in children and adolescents, *J Bone Joint Surg* 61A:479, 1979.

Bradford, DS: Treatment of severe spondylolisthesis: a combined approach for reduction and stabilization, *Spine* 4:423, 1979.

Bradford DS: Closed reduction of spondylolisthesis and experience in 22 patients, *Spine* 13:580, 1988.

Bradford DS, Gotfried Y: Staged salvage reconstruction of grade IV and V spondylolisthesis, *J Bone Joint Surg* 69A:191, 1987.

Bradford DS, Iza J: Repair of the defect in spondylolysis or minimal degrees of spondylolisthesis by segmental wire fixation and bone grafting, *Spine* 10:673, 1985.

Buck JE: Direct repair of the defect in spondylolisthesis preliminary report, *J Bone Joint Surg* 52B:432, 1970.

Cagli S, Crawford NR, Sonntag VK, Dickman CA: Biomechanics of grade I degenerative lumbar spondylolisthesis. 2. Treatment with threaded interbody cages/dowels and pedicle screws. *J Neurosurg* 94(suppl):51, 2001.

Capener N: Spondylolisthesis, *Br J Surg* 19:374, 1932.

Carragee EJ: Single-level posterolateral arthrodesis, with or without posterior decompression, for the treatment of isthmic spondylolisthesis in adults: a prospective, randomized study, *J Bone Joint Surg* 79A:1175, 1997.

Cauchoix J, Benoist M, Chassaing V: Degenerative spondylolisthesis, *Clin Orthop* 115:122, 1976.

Chen D, Fay L, Lok J, et al: Increasing neuroforaminal volume by anterior interbody distraction in degenerative lumbar spine, *Spine* 20:74, 1995.

Cheng CL, Fang F, Lee PC, Leong JCY: Anterior spinal fusion for spondylolysis and isthmic spondylolisthesis: long-term results in adults, *J Bone Joint Surg* 71B:264, 1989.

Cinotti G, Postacchini F, Fassari F, Urso S: Predisposing factors in degenerative spondylolisthesis: a radiographic and CT study, *Int Orthop* 21:337, 1997.

Cloward RB: Treatment of ruptured intervertebral discs by vertebral body fusion: indications, operative technique, and after care, *J Neurosurg* 10:154, 1953.

Cloward RB: Spondylolisthesis: treatment by laminectomy and posterior interbody fusion: review of 100 cases, *Clin Orthop* 154:74, 1981.

Crawford NR, Cagli S, Sonntag VK, Dickman CA: Biomechanics of grade I degenerative lumbar spondylolisthesis. I. In vitro model, *J Neurosurg* 94(suppl):45, 2001.

Csescei GI, Klekner AP, Dobai J, et al: Posterior interbody fusion using laminectomy bone and transpedicular screw fixation in the treatment of lumbar spondylolisthesis, *Surg Neurol* 53:2, 2000.

Cyron BM, Hutton WC, Troup JDG: Spondylolytic fractures, *J Bone Joint Surg* 58B:462, 1976.

Danielson BI, Frennered K, Irstam RK: Radiologic progression of isthmic lumbar spondylolisthesis in young patients, *Spine* 16:422, 1991.

Davis IS, Bailey RW: Spondylolisthesis: indications for lumbar nerve root decompression and operative technique, *Clin Orthop* 117:129, 1976.

Dawson EG, Lotysch M III, Urist MR: Intertransverse process lumbar arthrodesis with autogenous bone graft, *Clin Orthop* 154:90, 1981.

DeWald RL, Faut MM, Taddonio RF, Neuwirth MG: Severe lumbosacral spondylolisthesis in adolescents and children: reduction and staged circumferential fusion, *J Bone Joint Surg* 63A:619, 1981.

Dick WT, Schnebel B: Severe spondylolisthesis reduction and internal fixation, *Clin Orthop* 232:70, 1988.

Dreyzin V, Esses SI: A comparative analysis of spondylolysis repair, *Spine* 19:1909, 1994.

Eisenstein S: Spondylolysis: a skeletal investigation of two population groups, *J Bone Joint Surg* 60B:488, 1978.

Epstein NE: Decompression in the surgical management of degenerative spondylolisthesis: advantages of a conservative approach in 290 patients, *J Spinal Disord* 11:116, 1998.

Even-Sapir E, Martin RH, Mitchell MJ, et al: Assessment of painful late effects of lumbar spinal fusion with SPECT, *J Nucl Med* 35:416, 1994.

Farfan HF, Osteria V, Lamy C: The mechanical etiology of spondylolysis and spondylolisthesis, *Clin Orthop* 117:40, 1976.

Fischgrund JS, Mackay M, Herkowitz HN, et al: 1997 Volvo Award winner in clinical studies. Degenerative lumbar spondylolisthesis with spinal stenosis: a prospective, randomized study comparing decompressive laminectomy and arthrodesis with and without spinal instrumentation, *Spine* 22:2807, 1997.

Fitzgerald JAW, Newman PH: Degenerative spondylolisthesis, *J Bone Joint Surg* 58B:184, 1976.

Floman Y: Progression of lumbosacral isthmic spondylolisthesis in adults, *Spine* 25:342, 2000.

Flynn JC, Hoque MA: Anterior fusion of the lumbar spine: end-result study with long-term follow-up, *J Bone Joint Surg* 61A:1143, 1979.

Franklin GM, Haug J, Heyer NJ, et al: Outcome of lumbar fusion in Washington State workers' compensation, *Spine* 19:1897, 1994.

Fredrickson B, Baker D, McHolick W, et al: The natural history of spondylolysis and spondylolisthesis, *J Bone Joint Surg* 66A:699, 1984.

Freebody D, Bendall R, Taylor RD: Anterior transperitoneal lumbar fusion, *J Bone Joint Surg* 53B:617, 1971.

Freeman BL, Donati NL: Spinal arthrodesis for severe spondylolisthesis in children and adolescents, *J Bone Joint Surg* 71A:594, 1989.

Friberg O: Disc disease update: instability in spondylolisthesis, *Orthopedics* 14:463, 1991.

Gill GG: Treatment of spondylolisthesis and spina bifida. Exhibit displayed at the American Academy of Orthopaedic Surgeons meeting, Chicago, Jan 1952.

Gill GG, Manning JG, White HL: Surgical treatment of spondylolisthesis without spine fusion, *J Bone Joint Surg* 37A:493, 1955.

Gill GG, White HL: Surgical treatment of spondylolisthesis without spine fusion: a long-term follow-up of operated cases. Paper presented at the Western Orthopaedic Association, San Francisco, Nov 1962.

Goldstein LA, Haake PW, Devanney JR, Chan DPK: Guidelines for the management of lumbosacral spondylolisthesis associated with scoliosis, *Clin Orthop* 117:135, 1976.

Gramse RR, Sinaki M, Ilstrup DM: Lumbar spondylolisthesis—a rational approach to conservative treatment, *Mayo Clin Proc* 55:681, 1980.

Grobler LJ, Novotny JE, Wilder DG, et al: L4-L5 isthmic spondylolisthesis: a biomechanical analysis comparing stability in L4-L5 and L5-S1 isthmic spondylolisthesis, *Spine* 19:222, 1994.

Hambley M, Lee CK, Gutteling E, et al: Tension band wiring bone grafting for spondylolysis and spondylolisthesis: a clinical and biomechanical study, *Spine* 14:455, 1989.

Hanley EN, Levy JA: Surgical treatment of isthmic lumbosacral spondylolisthesis analysis of variables influencing results, *Spine* 14:148, 1989.

Haraldsson S, Willner S: A comparative study of spondylolisthesis in operations on adolescents and adults, *Arch Orthop Trauma Surg* 101:101, 1983.

Hardacker JW, Shuford RF, Capicotto PN, Pryor PW: Radiographic standing cervical segmental alignment in adult volunteers without neck symptoms, *Spine* 22:1472, 1997.

Harms J, Jeszenszky D, Stoltze D, et al: True spondylolisthesis reduction and monosegmental fusion in spondylolisthesis. In Bridwell KW, deWald RL, eds: *The textbook of spinal surgery*, ed 2, Philadelphia, 1997, Lippincott-Raven.

Harrington PR, Dickson JH: Spinal instrumentation in the treatment of severe progressive spondylolisthesis, *Clin Orthop* 117:157, 1976.

Harrington PR, Tullos HS: Spondylolisthesis in children: observations and surgical treatment, *Clin Orthop* 79:75, 1971.

Harris IE, Weinstein SL: Long-term follow-up of patients with grades III and IV spondylolisthesis, *J Bone Joint Surg* 69A:960, 1987.

Harris RI: Spondylolisthesis. In *Essays in surgery*, Toronto, 1950, University of Toronto.

Harris RI: Spondylolisthesis, *Ann R Coll Surg Engl* 8:259, 1951.

Haukipuro K, Keranen N, Koivisto E, et al: Familial occurrence of lumbar spondylolysis and spondylolisthesis, *Clin Genet* 13:471, 1978.

Henderson ED: Results of the surgical treatment of spondylolisthesis, *J Bone Joint Surg* 48A:619, 1966.

Henson J, McCall IW, O'Brien JP: Disc damage above a spondylolisthesis, *Br J Radiol* 60:69, 1987.

Herkowitz HN, Kurz LT: Degenerative lumbar spondylolisthesis with spinal stenosis: a prospective study comparing decompression with decompression and intertransverse process arthrodesis, *J Bone Joint Surg* 73A:802, 1991.

Herman S, Pouliquen JC: Spondylolisthesis with severe displacement in children and adolescents—results of posterior reduction and fixation in 12 cases, *Fr J Orthop Surg* 2:512, 1988.

Herron LD, Trippi AC: L4-5 degenerative spondylolisthesis: the results of treatment by decompressive laminectomy without fusion, *Spine* 14:534, 1989.

Hutton WC, Stott JR, Cyron BM: Is spondylolysis a fatigue fracture? *Spine* 2:202, 1977.

Imada K, Matsui H, Tsuji H: Oophorectomy predisposes to degenerative spondylolisthesis, *J Bone Joint Surg* 77B:126, 1995.

Inoue S, Wantanabe T, Goto S, et al: Degenerative spondylolisthesis: pathophysiology and results of anterior interbody fusion, *Clin Orthop* 227:90, 1988.

Jackson AM, Kirwan EO, Sullivan MF: Lytic spondylolisthesis above the lumbosacral level, *Spine* 3:260, 1978.

Jenis LG, An HS: Posterior lumbar interbody fusion for spondylolisthesis, *Semin Spine Surg* 11:57, 1999.

Jenkins JA: Spondylolisthesis, *Br J Surg* 24:80, 1936.

Johnson JR, Kirwan EO'G.: The long-term results of fusion in situ for severe spondylolisthesis, *J Bone Joint Surg* 65B:43, 1983.

Jones AA, McAfee PC, Robinson RA, et al: Failed arthrodesis of the spine for severe spondylolisthesis: salvage by interbody arthrodesis, *J Bone Joint Surg* 70A:25, 1988.

Kaneda K, Satoh S, Nohara Y, Oguma T: Distraction rod instrumentation with posterolateral fusion in isthmic spondylolisthesis: 53 cases followed for 18-89 months, *Spine* 10:383, 1985.

King AB, Baker DR, McHolick WJ: Another approach to the treatment of spondylolisthesis and spondyloschisis, *Clin Orthop* 10:257, 1957.

Kip PC, Esses SI, Doherty BI, et al: Biomechanical testing of pars defect repairs, *Spine* 19:2692, 1994.

Kirkaldy-Willis WH, Wedge JH, Yong-Hing K, Reilly J: Pathology and pathogenesis of lumbar spondylosis and stenosis, *Spine* 3:319, 1978.

Kiviluoto O, Santavirta S, Salenius P, et al: Postero-lateral spine fusion; a 1- to 4-year follow-up of 80 consecutive patients, *Acta Orthop Scand* 56:152, 1985.

Knox BD, Harvell JC Jr, Nelson PB, et al: Decompression and Luque rectangle fusion for degenerative spondylolisthesis, *J Spinal Disord* 2:223, 1989.

Kuntz KM, Snider RK, Weinstein JN, et al: Cost-effectiveness of fusion with and without instrumentation for patients with degenerative spondylolisthesis and spinal stenosis, *Spine* 25:2231, 2000.

Laurent LE: Spondylolisthesis: a study of 53 cases treated by spine fusion and 32 cases treated by laminectomy, *Acta Orthop Scand* 35(suppl):1, 1958.

Laurent LE, Einola S: Spondylolisthesis in children and adolescents, *Acta Orthop Scand* 31:45, 1961.

Laurent LE, Österman K: Operative treatment of spondylolisthesis in young patients, *Clin Orthop* 117:85, 1976.

Lehmer SM, Steffee AD, Gaines RW: Treatment of L5-S1 spondyloptosis by staged L5 resection with reduction and fusion of L4 onto S1 (Gaines procedure), *Spine* 19:1916, 1994.

Lenke LG, Bridwell KH, Bullis D, et al: Results of in situ fusion for isthmic spondylolisthesis, *J Spinal Disord* 5:433, 1992.

Lisai P, Rinonapoli G, Doria C, et al: The surgical treatment of spondylolisthesis with transpedicular stabilization: a review of 25 cases. *Chir Organi Mov* 83:369, 1998.

Lowe RW, Hayes TD, Kaye J, et al: Standing roentgenograms in spondylolisthesis, *Clin Orthop* 117:80, 1976.

Macnab I: Spondylolisthesis with an intact neural arch—the so-called pseudo-spondylolisthesis, *J Bone Joint Surg* 32B:325, 1950.

Macnab I, Dall D: The blood supply of the lumbar spine and its application to the technique of intertransverse lumbar fusion, *J Bone Joint Surg* 53B:628, 1971.

Magora A: Conservative treatment in spondylolisthesis. *Clin Orthop* 117:74, 1976.

Majd ME, Holt RT: Anterior fibular strut grafting for the treatment of pseudarthrosis in spondylolisthesis, *Am J Orthop* 29:99, 2000.

Marchetti P, Bartlozzi P: Classification of spondylolisthesis as a guideline for treatment. In Bridwell KW, deWald RL, eds: *The textbook of spinal surgery*, ed 2, Philadelphia, 1997, Lippincott-Raven.

Mardjetko SM, Connolly PJ, Shott S: Degenerative lumbar spondylolisthesis: a meta-analysis of the literature, *Spine* 19(suppl):2256, 1994.

Matsunaga S, Ijiri K, Hayashi K: Nonsurgically managed patients with degenerative spondylolisthesis: a 10- to 18-year follow-up study, *J Neurosurg* 93(suppl):194, 2000.

Matsunaga S, Sakou T, Morizono Y, et al: Natural history of degenerative spondylolisthesis: pathogenesis and natural course of the slippage, *Spine* 15:1204, 1990.

Mau H: Scoliosis and spondylolysis-spondylolisthesis, *Arch Orthop Trauma Surg* 99:129, 1981.

Maurice HD, Morley TR: Cauda equina lesions following fusion in situ and decompressive laminectomy for severe spondylolisthesis four case reports, *Spine* 14:214, 1989.

McAfee PC, Yuan HA: Computed tomography in spondylolisthesis, *Clin Orthop* 166:62, 1982.

McCulloch JA: Microdecompression and uninstrumented single-level fusion for spinal canal stenosis with degenerative spondylolisthesis. *Spine* 23:2243, 1998.

McPhee IB, O'Brien JP: Reduction of severe spondylolisthesis: a preliminary report, *Spine* 4:430, 1979.

McPhee IB, O'Brien JP: Scoliosis in symptomatic spondylolisthesis, *J Bone Joint Surg* 62B:155, 1980.

Mochida J, Suzuki K, Chiga M: How to stabilize a single level lesion of degenerative lumbar spondylolisthesis, *Clin Orthop* 368:126, 1999.

Modic MT: Degenerative disc disease and back pain, *Magn Reson Imaging Clin North Am* 7:481, 1999.

Moller H, Hedlund R: Instrumented and noninstrumented posterolateral fusion in adult spondylolisthesis—a prospective randomized study. 2, *Spine* 25:1716, 2000.

Moller H, Hedlund R: Surgery versus conservative management in adult isthmic spondylolisthesis—a prospective randomized study. 1, *Spine* 25:1711, 2000.

Muschik M, Hähnel H, Robinson PN, et al: Competitive sports and the progression of spondylolisthesis, *J Pediatr Orthop* 16:364, 1996.

Nachemson A: Repair of the spondylolisthetic defect and intertransverse fusion for young patients, *Clin Orthop* 117:101, 1976.

Nagaosa Y, Kikuchi S, Hasue M, Sato S: Pathoanatomic mechanisms of degenerative spondylolisthesis: a radiographic study, *Spine* 23:1447, 1998.

Newman PH: Stenosis of the lumbar spine in spondylolisthesis, *Clin Orthop* 115:116, 1976.

Newman PH: Surgical treatment for spondylolisthesis in the adult, *Clin Orthop* 117:106, 1976.

Newman PH, Stone KH: The etiology of spondylolisthesis, *J Bone Joint Surg* 45B:39, 1963.

Nooraie H, Ensafdaran A, Arasteh MM: Surgical management of low-grade lytic spondylolisthesis with C-D instrumentation in adult patients, *Arch Orthop Trauma Surg* 119:337, 1999.

Nork SE, Hu SS, Workman KL, et al: Patient outcomes after decompression and instrumented posterior spinal fusion for degenerative spondylolisthesis, *Spine* 24:561, 1999.

O'Brien JP, Mehdian H, Jaffray D: Reduction of severe lumbosacral spondylolisthesis, *Clin Orthop* 300:64, 1994.

Ohki I, Inoue S, Murata T, et al: Reduction and fusion of severe spondylolisthesis using halo-pelvic traction with a wire reduction device, *Int Orthop* 4:107, 1980.

Österman K, Lindholm TS, Laurent LE: Late results of removal of the loose posterior element (Gill's operation) in the treatment of lytic lumbar spondylolisthesis, *Clin Orthop* 117:121, 1976.

Österman K, Schlenzka D, Poussa M, et al: Isthmic spondylolisthesis in symptomatic and asymptomatic subjects: epidemiology and natural history with special reference to disk abnormality and mode of treatment, *Clin Orthop* 297:65, 1993.

O'Sullivan PB, Phyty GDM Twomey LT, Allison GT: Evaluation of specific stabilizing exercise in the treatment of chronic low back pain with radiologic diagnosis of spondylolysis or spondylolisthesis, *Spine* 22:2959, 1997.

Pedersen AK, Hagen R: Spondylolysis and spondylolisthesis: treatment by internal fixation and bone grafting of the defect, *J Bone Joint Surg* 70A:15, 1988.

Peek RD, Wiltse LL, Reynolds JB, et al: In situ arthrodesis without decompression for grade III or IV isthmic spondylolisthesis in adults who have severe sciatica, *J Bone Joint Surg* 71A:62, 1989.

Pellicci PM, Ranawat CS, Tsairis P, Beyan WJ: A prospective study of the progression of rheumatoid arthritis of the cervical spine, *J Bone Joint Surg* 63A:342, 1981.

Prothero SR, Parkes JC, Stinchfield FE: Complications after low-back fusion in 1000 patients, *J Bone Joint Surg* 48A:157, 1966.

Raugstad TS, Harbo K, Ogberg A, Skeie S: Anterior interbody fusion of the lumbar spine, *Acta Orthop Scand* 53:561, 1982.

Ravichandran G: Multiple lumbar spondylolyses, *Spine* 5:552, 1980.

Rechtine GR, Sutterline CE, Wood GW, et al: The efficacy of pedicle screw/plate fixation on lumbar/lumbosacral autogenous bone graft fusion in adult patients with degenerative spondylolisthesis, *J Spinal Disord* 9:382, 1996.

Ricciardi JE, Pflueger PC, Isaza JE, Whitecloud TS: Transpedicular fixation for the treatment of isthmic spondylolisthesis in adults, *Spine* 20:1917, 1995.

Riew KD, Hilibrand A, Bridwell KH, et al: MR versus CT myelography: surgical decision making for lumbar stenosis. Paper presented at the Scoliosis Research Society annual meeting, New York, Sept 16-20, 1998.

Rombold C: Treatment of spondylolisthesis by posterolateral fusion, resection of the pars interarticularis, and prompt mobilization of the patient: an end-result study of seventy-three patients, *J Bone Joint Surg* 48A:1282, 1966.

Rosenberg NJ, Bargar WL, Friedman B: The incidence of spondylolysis and spondylolisthesis in nonambulatory patients, *Spine* 6:135, 1981.

Rosomoff HL: Neural arch resection for lumbar spinal stenosis, *Clin Orthop* 154:83, 1981.

Scaglietti O, Frontino G, Bartolozzi P: Technique of anatomical reduction of lumbar spondylolisthesis and its surgical stabilization, *Clin Orthop* 117:164, 1976.

Schlegel JD, Smith JA, Schleusener RL: Lumbar motion segment pathology adjacent to thoracolumbar, lumbar, and lumbosacral fusions. *Spine* 21:970, 1996.

Schoenecker PL, Cole HO, Herring JA, et al: Cauda equina syndrome after in situ arthrodesis for severe spondylolisthesis at the lumbosacral junction, *J Bone Joint Surg* 72A:369, 1990.

Seitsalo S, Osterman K, Poussa M, Laurent L: Spondylolisthesis in children under 12 years of age: long-term results of 56 patients treated conservatively or operatively, *J Pediatr Orthop* 8:516, 1988.

Semon RL, Spengler D: Significance of lumbar spondylolysis in college football players, *Spine* 6:2172, 1981.

Sevastikoglou JA, Spangfort E, Aaro S: Operative treatment of spondylolisthesis in children and adolescents with tight hamstrings syndrome, *Clin Orthop* 147:192, 1980.

Sherman FC, Rosenthal RK, Hall JE: Spine fusion for spondylolysis and spondylolisthesis in children, *Spine* 4:59, 1979.

Shirado O, Zdeblick TA, McAfee PC, Warden KE: Biomechanical evaluation of methods of posterior stabilization of the spine and posterior lumbar interbody arthrodesis for lumbosacral isthmic spondylolisthesis, *J Bone Joint Surg* 73A:518, 1991.

Sienkiewicz PJ, Flatley TJ: Postoperative spondylolisthesis, *Clin Orthop* 221:172, 1987.

Sijbrandij S: A new technique for the reduction and stabilisation of severe spondylolisthesis: a report of two cases, *J Bone Joint Surg* 63B:266, 1981.

Sijbrandij S: Reduction and stabilisation of severe spondylolisthesis: a report of three cases, *J Bone Joint Surg* 65B:40, 1983.

Smith MD, Bohlman HH: Spondylolisthesis treated by a single-stage operation combining decompression with in situ posterolateral and anterior fusion: an analysis of eleven patients who had long-term follow-up, *J Bone Joint Surg* 72A:415, 1990.

Sørensen KH: Anterior interbody lumbar spine fusion for incapacitating disc degeneration and spondylolisthesis, *Acta Orthop Scand* 49:269, 1978.

Speed K: Spondylolisthesis: treatment by anterior bone graft, *Arch Surg* 37:175, 1938.

Stanton RP, Meehan P, Lovell WW: Surgical fusion in childhood spondylolisthesis, *J Pediatr Orthop* 5:411, 1985.

Steffee A, Sitkowski D: Reduction and stabilization of grade IV spondylolisthesis, *Clin Orthop* 227:82, 1988.

Suk S, Lee CK, Kim WJ, et al: Adding posterior lumbar interbody fusion to pedicle screw fixation and posterolateral fusion after decompression in spondylolytic spondylolisthesis. *Spine* 22:210, 1997.

Szypryt EP, Twinning P, Mulholland RC, Worthington BS: The prevalence of disc degeneration associated with neural arch defects of the lumbar spine assess by magnetic resonance imaging. *Spine* 14:977, 1989.

Taillard WF: Etiology of spondylolisthesis, *Clin Orthop* 117:30, 1976.

Tajima T, Furukawa K, Kuramochi E: Selective lumbosacral radiculography and block, *Spine* 5:168, 1980.

Takahashi K, Yamagata M, Takayanagi K, et al: Changes of the sacrum in severe spondylolisthesis: a possible key pathology of the disorder, *J Orthop Sci* 5:18, 2000.

Takeda M: A newly devised "three-one" method for the surgical treatment of spondylolysis and spondylolisthesis, *Clin Orthop* 147:228, 1980.

Thalgott JS, Sasso RC, Cotler HB, et al: Adult spondylolisthesis treated with posterolateral lumbar fusion and pedicular instrumentation with AO D-C plates, *J Spinal Disord* 10:204, 1997.

Todd EM Jr, Gardner WJ: Simple excision of the unattached lamina for spondylolysis, *Surg Gynecol Obstet* 106:724, 1958.

Troup JD: The etiology of spondylolysis, *Orthop Clin North Am* 8:157, 1977.

van den Oever M, Merrick MV, Scott JHS: Bone scintigraphy in symptomatic spondylolysis, *J Bone Joint Surg* 69B:453, 1987.

Velikas EP, Blackburne JS: Surgical treatment of spondylolisthesis in children and adolescents, *J Bone Joint Surg* 63B:67, 1981.

Verbiest H: The treatment of spondyloptosis or impending lumbar spondyloptosis accompanied by neurologic deficit and/or neurogenic intermittent claudication, *Spine* 4:68, 1979.

Vidal J, Fassio B, Fuscayret CH, Allieu Y: Surgical reduction of spondylolisthesis using a posterior approach, *Clin Orthop* 154:156, 1981.

Virta L, Rönnefaa T: The association of mild-moderate isthmic lumbar spondylolisthesis and low back pain in middle-aged patients is weak and only occurs in women, *Spine* 18:1496, 1993.

Walsh TR, Weinstein JN, Spratt KF, et al: Lumbar discography in normal subjects: a controlled, prospective study, *J Bone Joint Surg* 72A:1081, 1990.

Watkins MB: Posterolateral fusion in pseudarthrosis and posterior element defects of the lumbosacral spine, *Clin Orthop* 35:80, 1964.

Wiltse LL: Spondylolisthesis in children, *Clin Orthop* 21:156, 1961.

Wiltse LL: The etiology of spondylolisthesis, *J Bone Joint Surg* 44A:539, 1962.

Wiltse LL: Common problems of the lumbar spine: spondylolisthesis and its treatment, *J Cont Ed Orthop* 7:713, 1979.

Wiltse LL, Bateman JG, Hutchinson RH, Nelson WE: The paraspinal sacrospinalis-splitting approach to the lumbar spine, *J Bone Joint Surg* 50A:919, 1968.

Wiltse LL, Hutchinson RH: Surgical treatment of spondylolisthesis, *Clin Orthop* 35:116, 1964.

Wiltse LL, Jackson DW: Treatment of spondylolisthesis and spondylolysis in children, *Clin Orthop* 117:92, 1976.

Wiltse LL, Newman PH, Macnab I: Classification of spondylolysis and spondylolisthesis, *Clin Orthop* 117:23, 1976.

Wiltse LL, Rothman SLG: Spondylolisthesis: classification, diagnosis, and natural history, *Semin Spine Surg* 5:264, 1993.

Wiltse LL, Widell EH Jr, Jackson DW: Fatigue fracture: the basic lesion in isthmic spondylolisthesis, *J Bone Joint Surg* 57A:17, 1975.

Wiltse LL, Winter RB: Terminology and measurement of spondylolisthesis, *J Bone Joint Surg* 65A:768, 1983.

Wood KB, Popp CA, Transfeldt EE, Geissele AE: Radiographic evaluation of instability in spondylolisthesis, *Spine* 19:1697, 1994.

Wu SS, Lee CH, Chen PQ: Operative repair of symptomatic spondylolysis following a positive response to diagnostic pars injection. *J Spinal Disord* 12:10, 1999.

Wynne-Davies R, Scott JH: Inheritance and spondylolisthesis: a radiographic family survey, *J Bone Joint Surg* 61B:301,1979.

ADULT SCOLIOSIS

Abei M: Correction of degenerative scoliosis of the lumbar spine: a preliminary report, *Clin Orthop* 232:80, 1988.

Allen Jr BL, Ferguson RL: The Galveston technique of pelvic fixation with L-rod instrumentation of the spine, *Spine* 9:388, 1984.

Ascani E, Bartolozzi P, Logroscino CA, et al: Natural history of untreated idiopathic scoliosis after skeletal maturity, *Spine* 11:784, 1986.

Baki B, Bjure J, Kasalichy J, Nachemson A: Regional pulmonary ventilation and perfusion distribution in patients with untreated idiopathic scoliosis, *Thorax* 27:703, 1972.

Balderston RA: The surgical management of spinal deformity in adults—theoretical considerations, *Semin Spine Surg* 5:199, 1993.

Balderston RA, Winter RB, Moe JH, et al: Fusion to the sacrum for nonparalytic scoliosis in the adult, *Spine* 11:824, 1986.

Bengtsson G, Fallstrom K, Jansson B, Nachemson A: A psychological psychiatric investigation of the adjustment of female scoliosis patients, *Acta Psychiactrica Scand* 50:50, 1974.

Benner B, Ehni G: Degenerative lumbar scoliosis, *Spine* 4:548, 1979.

Bergofsky EH: Respiratory failure in disorders of the thoracic cage, *Am Rev Resp Dis* 119:643, 1979.

Bernhardt M, Bridwell KH: Segmental analysis of the sagittal plane alignment of the normal thoracic and lumbar spines and thoracolumbar junction, *Spine* 14:717, 1989.

Bjure J, Nachemson A: Non-treated scoliosis, *Clin Orthop* 93:44, 1973.

Boachie-Adjei O, Bradford DS: Vertebral column resection and arthrodesis for complex spinal deformities, *J Spinal Disord* 4:193, 1991.

Boachie-Adjei O, Dendrinos GK, Ogilvie JW, Bradford DS: Management of adult spinal deformity with combined anterior-posterior arthrodesis and Luque-Galveston instrumentation, *J Spinal Disord* 4:131, 1991.

Bradford DS: Adult scoliosis: current concepts of treatment, *Clin Orthop* 229:70, 1988.

Briard JL, Jegou D, Cauchoix J: Adult lumbar scoliosis, *Spine* 4:526, 1979.

Bridwell KH: Where to stop the fusion distally in adult scoliosis: L4, L5, or the sacrum? *Instr Course Lect* 45:101, 1996.

Bridwell KH: Osteotomies for fixed deformities in the thoracic and lumbar spine. In Bridwell KH, DeWald RL, eds: *The textbook of spinal surgery*, ed 2, Philadelphia, 1997, Lippincott-Raven.

Brodsky AE, Binder WF: Lumbar discography: its value and diagnosis and treatment of lumbar disc lesions, *Spine* 4:110, 1979.

Broom MJ, Price CT, Flynn JC: Adult scoliosis: current concepts, *J Fla Med Assoc* 77:21, 1990.

Brown CW, Orme TJ, Richardson HD: The rate of pseudarthrosis (surgical nonunion) in patients who are smokers and patients who are nonsmokers: a comparison study, *Spine* 11:942, 1986.

Byrd III JA, Scoles PV, Winter RB, et al: Adult idiopathic scoliosis treated by anterior and posterior spinal fusion, *J Bone Joint Surg* 69A:843, 1987.

Camp JF, Caudle R, Ashmun RD, Roach J: Immediate complications of Cotrel-Dubousset instrumentation to the sacro-pelvis: a clinical and biomechanical study, *Spine* 15:932, 1990.

Cochran T, Nachemson A: Long-term anatomic and functional changes in patients with adolescent idiopathic scoliosis treated with the Milwaukee brace, *Spine* 10:127, 1985.

Collis DK, Ponseti IV: Long-term follow-up of patients with idiopathic scoliosis not treated surgically, *J Bone Joint Surg* 51A:425, 1969.

Cooper DM, Rojas JV, Mellins RB, et al: Respiratory mechanics in adolescents with idiopathic scoliosis, *Am Rev Resp Dis* 130:22, 1984.

Dawson EG, Moe JH, Caron A: Surgical management of scoliosis in the adult, *J Bone Joint Surg* 55A:437, 1973.

Deckey JE, Court C, Bradford DS: Loss of sagittal plane correction after removal of spinal implants, *Spine* 25:2453, 2000.

Devlin VJ, Boachie-Adjei O, Bradford DS, et al: Treatment of adult spinal deformity with fusion to the sacrum using CD instrumentation, *J Spinal Disord* 4:1, 1991.

Dick J, Boachie-Adjei O, Wilson M: One-stage versus two-stage anterior and posterior spinal reconstruction in adults: comparison of outcomes, including nutritional status, complication rates, hospital costs, and other factors, *Spine* 17(suppl):310, 1992.

Donelson R., Aprill C, Medcalf R, Grant W: A prospective study of centralization of lumbar and referred pain: a predictor of symptomatic discs and annular competence, *Spine* 22:1115, 1997.

Drummond DS, Fowles JV, Ecuyer S, et al: Untreated scoliosis in the adult. Proceedings of the Scoliosis Research Society, *J Bone Joint Surg* 58A:156, 1976.

Epstein JA, Epstein BS, Jones MD: Symptomatic lumbar scoliosis and degenerative changes in the elderly, *Spine* 4:542, 1979.

Epstein JA, Epstein BS, Lavine LS: Surgical treatment of nerve root compression caused by scoliosis of the lumbar spine, *J Neurosurg* 14:449, 1974.

Erwin WD, Dickson JH, Harrington PR: Clinical review of patients with broken Harrington rods, *J Bone Joint Surg* 62A:1302, 1980.

Fowles JV, Drummond DS, L'Ecuyer S, et al: Untreated scoliosis in the adult, *Clin Orthop* 134:212, 1978.

Girardi FP, Boachie-Adjei O, Rawlins BA: Safety of sublaminar wires with Isola instrumentation for the treatment of idiopathic scoliosis, *Spine* 25:691, 2000.

Goldstein JM, Nash Jr CL, Wilham MR: Selection of lumbar fusion levels in adult idiopathic scoliosis, *Spine* 16:1150, 1991.

Grubb SA, Lipscomb HJ: Diagnostic findings in painful adult scoliosis, *Spine* 17:518, 1992.

Grubb SA, Lipscomb HJ, Coonrad RW: Degenerative adult onset scoliosis, *Spine* 13:241, 1988.

Grubb SA, Lipscomb HJ, Guilford WB: The relative value of lumbar roentgenograms, metrizamide myelography, and discography in the assessment of patients with chronic low back syndrome, *Spine* 12:282, 1987.

Grubb SA, Lipscomb HJ, Suh PB: Results of surgical treatment of painful adult scoliosis, *Spine* 19:1619, 1994.

Gurr KR, McAfee PC: Cotrel-Dubousset instrumentation in adults, *Spine* 13:510, 1988.

Horton WC, Holt RT, Muldowny DS: Controversy. Fusion of L5-S1 in adult scoliosis, *Spine* 21:2520, 1996.

Jackson RP, Simmons EH, Stripinis D: Instance and severity of back pain in adult idiopathic scoliosis, *Spine* 8:749, 1983.

Jackson RP, Simmons EH, Stripinis D: Coronal and sagittal plane spinal deformities correlating with back pain and pulmonary function in adult idiopathic scoliosis, *Spine* 14:1391, 1989.

Johnson JR, Holt RT: Combined use of anterior and posterior surgery for adult scoliosis, *Orthop Clin North Am* 19:361, 1988.

Kitahara H, Inoue S, Minami S, et al: Long-term results of spinal instrumentation surgery for scoliosis 5 years or more after surgery in patients over 20 to 23 years of age, *Spine* 14:744, 1989.

Kleinmann RG, Csongradi JJ, Rinsky LA, Bleck EE: The radiographic assessment of spinal flexibility in scoliosis: a study of the efficacy of the push prone film. *Clin Orthop* 162:47, 1989.

Kostuik JP: Decision making in adult scoliosis, *Spine* 4:521, 1979.

Kostuik JP: Recent advances in the treatment of painful adult scoliosis, *Clin Orthop* 147:238, 1980.

Kostuik JP: Treatment of scoliosis in the adult thoracolumbar spine with special reference to fusion to the sacrum, *Orthop Clin North Am* 19:371, 1988.

Kostuik JP: Operative treatment of idiopathic scoliosis: current concepts review, *J Bone Joint Surg* 72A:1108, 1990.

Kostuik JP, Israel J, Hall JE: Scoliosis surgery in adults, *Clin Orthop* 93:225, 1973.

Kostuik JP, Mauras GR, Richardson WJ, Okajima Y: Combined single-stage anterior and posterior osteotomy for correction of iatrogenic lumbar kyphosis, *Spine* 13:257, 1988.

Kostuik JP, Ventivoglio J: The incidence of low-back pain in adult scoliosis, *Spine* 6:268, 1981.

Lagrone MO, Bradford DS, Moe JH, et al: Treatment of symptomatic flatback after spinal fusion, *J Bone Joint Surg* 70A:569, 1988.

Lieberman IH, Salt PT, Orr RD, Draetschmer B: Prone position endoscopic transthoracic release with simultaneous posterior instrumentation for spinal deformity: a description of the technique, *Spine* 25:2251, 2000.

Lonstein JE: The Galveston technique using Luque or Cotrel-Dubousset rods, *Orthop Clin North Am* 25:311, 1994.

Luque ER: Segmental spinal instrumentation for correction of scoliosis, *Clin Orthop* 163:192, 1982.

Marchesi DG, Aebi M: Pedicle fixation devices in the treatment of adult lumbar scoliosis, *Spine* 17:304, 1992.

McClain RF: Revision and salvage in deformity surgery, *Semin Spine Surg* 5:214, 1993.

McCord DH, Cunningham BW, Shono Y, et al: Biomechanical analysis of lumbosacral fixation, *Spine* 17:S235, 1992.

McCutcheon ME, Thompson III WC: CT scanning of lumbar discography: a useful diagnostic adjunct, *Spine* 11:257, 1986.

Micheli L, Riseborough E, Hall J: Scoliosis in the adult, *Orthop Rev* 6:27, 1977.

Moskowitz A, Moe JH, Winter RB, Binner H: Long-term follow-up of scoliosis fusion, *J Bone Joint Surg* 62A:364, 1980.

Nachemson A: Adult scoliosis in back pain, *Spine* 4:513, 1979.

Nachemson A: A long-term follow-up study of nontreated scoliosis, *Acta Orthop Scand* 39:466, 1968.

Nilssone U, Lundgren KD: Long-term prognosis in idiopathic scoliosis, *Acta Orthop Scand* 39:456, 1968.

Nuber GW, Schafer MF: Surgical management of adult scoliosis, *Clin Orthop* 208:228, 1986.

Ogilvie JW: Adult scoliosis: evaluation and nonsurgical treatment, *Instr Course Lect* 42:251, 1992.

Ogon M, Haid C, Krismer M, et al: The possibility of creating lordosis and correcting scoliosis simultaneously after partial disc removal: balance lines of lumbar motion segments, *Spine* 21:2458, 1996.

Pehrsson K, Bake B, Larsson S, Nachemson A: Lung function in adult idiopathic scoliosis: a 20-year follow-up. *Thorax* 46:474, 1991.

Perennou D, Marcelli C, Herisson C, Simon L: Adult lumbar scoliosis: epidemiologic aspects in a low-back pain population, *Spine* 19:123, 1994.

Perra JH: Techniques of instrumentation and long fusions to the sacrum, *Orthop Clin North Am* 25:287, 1994.

Ponder RC, Dickson JH, Harrington PR, Erwin WD: Results of Harrington instrumentation in fusion in the adult idiopathic scoliosis patient, *J Bone Joint Surg* 57A:797, 1975.

Pritchett JW, Bortel DR: Degenerative symptomatic lumbar scoliosis, *Spine* 18:700, 1993.

Riseborough EJ: Scoliosis in adults, *Curr Pract Orthop Surg* 7:36, 1977.

Robin GS, Span Y, Steinberg RL et al: Scoliosis in the elderly: a follow-up study, *Spine* 7:355, 1982.

Saer III EH, Winter RB, Lonstein JE: Long scoliosis fusion to the sacrum in adults with nonparalytic scoliosis, an improved method, *Spine* 15:650, 1990.

Shufflebarger HL, Grimm JO, Bui V, Thomson JD: Anterior and posterior spinal fusion: staged versus same-day surgery, *Spine* 16:930, 1991.

Simmons ED Jr, Kowalski JM, Simmons EH: The results of surgical treatment for adult scoliosis, *Spine* 18:718, 1993.

Simmons EH, Jackson RP: The management of nerve root entrapment syndrome associated with the collapsing scoliosis of idiopathic lumbar and thoracolumbar curves, *Spine* 4:533, 1979.

Simmons EH, Segil CM: An evaluation of discography in the localization of symptomatic levels in discogenic disease of the spine, *Clin Orthop* 108:57, 1975.

Sponseller PD, Cohen MS, Nachemson AL, et al: Results of surgical treatment of adults with idiopathic scoliosis, *J Bone Joint Surg* 69A:667, 1987.

Swank S, Lonstein JE, Moe JH, et al: Surgical treatment of adult scoliosis: a review of 222 cases, *J Bone Joint Surg* 63A:268, 1981.

Swank S, Winter RB, Moe JH: Scoliosis and cor pulmonale, *Spine* 7:342, 1982.

Taylor BA, Webb PJ, Hetreed M, et al: Delayed postoperative paraplegia with hypotension in adult revision scoliosis surgery, *Spine* 19:470, 1994.

Trammell TR, Benedict F, Reed D: Anterior spine fusion using Zielke instrumentation for adult thoracolumbar and lumbar scoliosis, *Spine* 16:307, 1991.

Trammell TR, Schroeder RD, Reed DB: Rotatory olisthesis in idiopathic scoliosis, *Spine* 13:1378, 1988.

vanDam BE: Nonoperative treatment of adult scoliosis, *Orthop Clin North Am* 19:347, 1988.

vanDam BE, Bradford DS, Lonstein JE, et al: Adult scoliosis treated by posterior spinal fusion and Harrington instrumentation, *Spine* 12:32, 1987.

Vanderpool DW, James JIP, Wynne-Davies R: Scoliosis in the elderly, *J Bone Joint Surg* 51A:446, 1959.

Vedantam R, Lenke LG, Bridwell KH, Linville DL: Comparison of push-prone and lateral-bending radiographs for predicting postoperative coronal alignment in thoracolumbar and lumbar scoliotic curves, *Spine* 25:76, 2000.

Velis KP, Healey JH, Schneider R: Osteoporosis in unstable adult scoliosis, *Clin Orthop* 237:132, 1988.

Weinstein SL, Ponseti IV: Curve progression in idiopathic scoliosis, *J Bone Joint Surg* 65A:447, 1983.

West III JL, Anderson LD: Instance of deep vein thrombosis in major adult spinal surgery, *Spine* 17:S254, 1992.

Winter RB, Lonstein JE: Adult idiopathic scoliosis treated with Luque or Harrington rods and sublaminar wiring, *J Bone Joint Surg* 71A:1308, 1989.

Winter RB, Lonstein JE, Denis F: Pain patterns in adult scoliosis, *Orthop Clin North Am* 19:339, 1988.

Wong DA: Adult congenital scoliosis, *Semin Spine Surg* 5:226, 1993.

Zurbriggen C, Markwalder TM, Wyss S: Long-term results in patients treated with posterior instrumentation and fusion for degenerative scoliosis of the lumbar spine. *Acta Neurochir Wien* 141:21, 1999.

RHEUMATOID ARTHRITIS

Abe H, Tsuru M, Ito T, et al: Anterior decompression for ossification of the posterior longitudinal ligament of the cervical spine, *J Neurosurg* 55:108, 1981.

Adams JC: Technic, dangers and safeguards in osteotomy of the spine, *J Bone Joint Surg* 34B:226, 1952.

Alenghat JP, Hallett M, Kido DK: Spinal cord compression in diffuse idiopathic skeletal hyperostosis, *Radiology* 142:119, 1982.

Boden SD, Clark CR: Rheumatoid arthritis of the cervical spine. In The Cervical Spine Research Society, Editorial Committee: *The cervical spine*, ed 3, Philadelphia, 1998, Lippincott-Raven.

Boni M, Cherubino P, Denaro V, Benazzo F: Multiple subtotal somatectomy: technique and evaluation of a series of 39 cases, *Spine* 9:358, 1984.

Burkus JK, Denis F: Hyperextension injuries of the thoracic spine in diffuse idiopathic skeletal hyperostosis, *J Bone Joint Surg* 76A:237, 1994.

Casey AT, Crockard HA, Bland JM, et al: Surgery on the rheumatoid cervical spine for the non-ambulant myelopathic patient—too much, too late? *Lancet* 347:1004, 1996.

Chiba H, Annen S, Shimada T, Imura S: Atlantoaxial subluxation complicated by diffuse idiopathic skeletal hyperostosis, *Spine* 17:1414, 1992.

Clark CR: Occipitocervical fusion for the unstable rheumatoid neck, *Orthopedics* 12:469, 1989.

Clark CR, Goetz DD, Menezes AH: Arthrodesis of the cervical spine in rheumatoid arthritis, *J Bone Joint Surg* 71A:381, 1989.

Cocke EW, Robertson JH, Robertson JT, Crook JP Jr: The extended maxillotomy and subtotal maxillectomy for excision of skull base tumors, *Arch Otolaryngol Head Neck Surg* 116:92, 1990.

Conlon PW, Isdale IC, Rose BS: Rheumatoid arthritis of the cervical spine: an analysis of 333 cases, *Ann Rheum Dis* 25:120, 1966.

Crandall PH, Gregorius FK: Long-term follow-up of surgical treatment of cervical spondylotic myelopathy, *Spine* 2:139, 1977.

Crockard A, Grob D: Rheumatoid arthritis: upper cervical involvement. In The Cervical Spine Research Society, Editorial Committee: *The cervical spine*, ed 3, Philadelphia, 1998, Lippincott-Raven.

Crockard HA: Surgical management of cervical rheumatoid problems, *Spine* 20:2584, 1995.

de los Reyes RA, Malik GM, Wu KK, Ausman JI: A new surgical approach to stabilizing C1-2 subluxation in rheumatoid arthritis, *Henry Ford Hosp Med J* 29:127, 1981.

Dreyer SJ, Boden SD: Natural history of rheumatoid arthritis of the cervical spine, *Clin Orthop* 366:98, 1999.

Edwards WC, LaRocca H: The developmental segmental sagittal diameter of the cervical spinal canal in patients with cervical spondylosis, *Spine* 8:20, 1983.

Epstein JA, Carras R, Hyman RA, Costa S: Cervical myelopathy caused by developmental stenosis of the spinal canal, *J Neurosurg* 51:362, 1979.

Fehring TK, Brooks AL: Upper cervical instability in rheumatoid arthritis, *Clin Orthop* 221:137, 1987.

Floyd AS, Learmonth ID, Mody SAG, Meyers OL: Atlantoaxial instability and neurologic indicators in rheumatoid arthritis, *Clin Orthop* 241:177, 1989.

Freeman GE Jr: Correction of severe deformity of the cervical spine in ankylosing spondylitis with the halo device, *J Bone Joint Surg* 43A:547, 1961.

Fujiwara K, Jufimoto M, Owaki H, et al: Cervical lesions related to the systemic progression in rheumatoid arthritis, *Spine* 23:2052, 1998.

Fujiwara K, Owaki H, Fujimoto M, et al: A long-term follow-up study of cervical lesions in rheumatoid arthritis, *J Spinal Disord* 13:519, 2000.

Fujiwara K, Yonenobu K, Ochi T: Natural history of upper cervical lesions in rheumatoid arthritis, *J Spinal Disord* 10:275, 1997.

Goel MK: Vertebral osteotomy for correction of fixed flexion deformity of the spine, *J Bone Joint Surg* 50A:287, 1968.

Grob D, Schutz U, Poltz G: Occipitocervical fusion in patients with rheumatoid arthritis, *Clin Orthop* 366:46, 1999.

Gui L, Merlini L, Savini R, Davidovits P: Cervical myelopathy due to ossification of the posterior longitudinal ligament, *Ital J Orthop Traumatol* 9:269, 1983.

Hadley MN, Spetzler RT, Sonntag VKH: The transoral approach to the cervical spine: a review of 53 cases of extradural cervicomedullary compression, *J Neurosurg* 71:16, 1989.

Harta S, Tohno S, Kawagishi T: Osteoarthritis of the atlanto-axial joint, *Int Orthop* 5:277, 1981.

Herbert JJ: Vertebral osteotomy, technique, indications, and results, *J Bone Joint Surg* 30A:680, 1948.

Herbert JJ: Vertebral osteotomy for kyphosis, especially in Marie-Strümpell arthritis: a report on fifty cases, *J Bone Joint Surg* 41A:291, 1959.

Heywood AWB, Learmonth ID, Thomas M: Cervical spine instability in rheumatoid arthritis, *J Bone Joint Surg* 70B:702, 1988.

Hirabayashi K, Watanabe K, Wakano K, et al: Expansive open-door laminoplasty for cervical spinal stenotic myelopathy, *Spine* 8:693, 1983.

Hoff J, Nishimura M, Pitts L, et al: The role of ischemia in the pathogenesis of cervical spondylotic myelopathy: a review and new microangiographic evidence, *Spine* 2:100, 1977.

Hukuda S, Mochizuki T, Ogata M, Shichikawa K: The pattern of spinal and extraspinal hyperostosis in patients with ossification of the posterior longitudinal ligament and the ligamentum flavum causing myelopathy, *Skeletal Radiol* 10:79, 1983.

Jacobs B, Krueger EG, Leivy DM: Cervical spondylosis with radiculopathy, *JAMA* 211:2135, 1970.

Kandziora F, Mittlmeier T, Kerschbaumer F: Stage-related surgery for cervical spine instability in rheumatoid arthritis, *Eur Spine J* 8:371, 1999.

Karlins NL, Yagan R: Dyspnea and hoarseness: a complication of diffuse idiopathic skeletal hyperostosis, *Spine* 16:235, 1991.

Kawaida H, Sakou T, Morizono Y: Vertical settling in rheumatoid arthritis: diagnostic value of the Ranawat and Redlund-Jonell methods, *Clin Orthop* 239:128, 1989.

Kerschbaumer F, Kandzlora F, Klein C, et al: Transoral decompression, anterior plate fixation, and posterior wire fusion for irreducible atlantoaxial kyphosis in rheumatoid arthritis, *Spine* 25:2708, 2000.

Kimura I, Oh-Hama M, Shingu H: Cervical myelopathy treated by canal-expansive laminaplasty: computed tomographic and myelographic findings, *J Bone Joint Surg* 66A:914, 1984.

Kubota M, Baba I, Sumida T: Myelopathy due to ossification of the ligamentum flavum of the cervical spine: a report of two cases, *Spine* 6:553, 1981.

Kudo H, Iwano K, Yoshizawa H: Cervical cord compression due to extradural granulation tissue in rheumatoid arthritis, *J Bone Joint Surg* 66B:426, 1984.

LaChapelle EH: Osteotomy of the lumbar spine for correction of kyphosis in a case of ankylosing spondylarthritis, *J Bone Joint Surg* 28:851, 1946.

Law WA: Osteotomy of the spine and the treatment of severe dorsal kyphosis: four cases, *Proc R Soc Med* 42:594, 1949.

Law WA: Arthritis: surgical treatment of chronic arthritis. In Carling ER, Ross JP, eds: *British surgical practice, surgical progress*, London, 1952, Butterworth.

Law WA: Surgical treatment of the rheumatic diseases, *J Bone Joint Surg* 34B:215, 1952.

Law WA: Lumbar spinal osteotomy, *J Bone Joint Surg* 41B:270, 1959.

Law WA: Osteotomy of the spine, *J Bone Joint Surg* 44A:1199, 1962.

Law WA: The spine in rheumatoid spondylitis, *Clin Orthop* 36:35, 1964.

Lichtblau PO, Wilson PD: Possible mechanism of aortic rupture in orthopaedic correction of rheumatoid spondylitis, *J Bone Joint Surg* 38A:123, 1956.

Lipson SJ: Rheumatoid arthritis of the cervical spine, *Clin Orthop* 182:143, 1984.

Lipson SJ: Rheumatoid arthritis in the cervical spine, *Clin Orthop* 239:121, 1989.

Lipson SJ: Subaxial cervical involvement in rheumatoid arthritis. In The Cervical Spine Research Society, Editorial Committee: *The cervical spine*, ed 3, Philadelphia, 1998, Lippincott-Raven.

Lourie H, Stewart WA: Spontaneous atlantoaxial dislocation: a complication of rheumatoid disease, *N Engl J Med* 265:677, 1961.

Lunsford LD, Bissonette DJ, Zorub DS: Anterior surgery for cervical disc disease. II. Treatment of cervical spondylotic myelopathy in 32 cases, *J Neurosurg* 53:12, 1980.

Martel W, Page JW: Cervical vertebral erosions and subluxations in rheumatoid arthritis and ankylosing spondylitis, *Arthritis Rheum* 3:546, 1960.

Matsunaga S, Ijiri K, Koga H: Results of a longer than 10-year follow-up of patients with rheumatoid arthritis treated by occipitocervical fusion. *Spine* 25:1749, 2000.

Matthews JA: Atlanto-axial subluxation in rheumatoid arthritis: a five-year follow-up study, *Ann Rheum Dis* 33:526, 1974.

Mayfield FH: Cervical spondylosis: a comparison of the anterior and posterior approaches, *Clin Neurosurg* 13:181, 1966.

McCarron RF, Robertson WW: Brooks fusion for atlantoaxial instability in rheumatoid arthritis, *South Med J* 81:474, 1988.

McKenzie MK, Bartal E, Pay NT: A hyperextension injury of the thoracic spine in association with diffuse idiopathic skeletal hyperostosis, *Orthopedics* 14:895, 1991.

McLaren AC, Bailey SI: Cauda equina syndrome: a complication of lumbar discectomy, *Clin Orthop* 204:143, 1986.

McMaster MJ: Osteotomy of the cervical spine in ankylosing spondylitis, *J Bone Joint Surg* 79B:197, 1997.

McMaster PE: Osteotomy of the spine for fixed flexion deformity, *J Bone Joint Surg* 44A:1207, 1962.

Menezes AH, Van Gilder JC, Graf CJ, McDonnell DE: Craniocervical abnormalities: a comprehensive surgical approach, *J Neurosurg* 53:444, 1980.

Moskovich R, Crockard HA, Shott S, Ransford AO: Occipitocervical stabilization for myelopathy in patients with rheumatoid arthritis: implications of not bone-grafting, *J Bone Joint Surg* 82A:349, 2000.

Moskowitz RW, Ziv I, Denko CW, et al: Spondylosis in sand rats: a model of intervertebral disc degeneration and hyperostosis, *J Orthop Res* 8:401, 1990.

Neva MN, Kaarela K, Kauppi M: Prevalence of radiological changes in the cervical spine—a cross-sectional study after 20 years from presentation of rheumatoid arthritis, *J Rheumatol* 27:90, 2000.

Oda T, Fujiwara K, Yonenobu K, et al: Natural course of cervical spine lesions in rheumatoid arthritis, *Spine* 20:1128, 1995.

Olerud C, Larsson BE, Rodriguez M: Subaxial cervical spine subluxation in rheumatoid arthritis: a retrospective analysis of 16 operated patients after 1-5 years, *Acta Orthop Scand* 68:109, 1997.

Ono K, Ota H, Tada K, Yamamoto T: Cervical myelopathy secondary to multiple spondylotic protrusions: a clinicopathologic study, *Spine* 2:109, 1977.

Oostveen JC, Roozeboom AR, van de Laar MA, et al: Functional turbo spin echo magnetic resonance imaging versus tomography for evaluating cervical spine involvement in rheumatoid arthritis, *Spine* 23:1237, 1998.

Paley D, Schwartz M, Cooper P, et al: Fractures of the spine in diffuse idiopathic skeletal hyperostosis, *Clin Orthop* 267, 1991.

Peppelman WC, Kraus DR, Donaldson WF III, Agarwal A: Cervical spine surgery in rheumatoid arthritis: improvement of neurologic deficit after cervical spine fusion, *Spine* 18:2375, 1993.

Puttlitz CM, Goel VK, Clark CR, et al: Biomechanical rationale for the pathology of rheumatoid arthritis in the craniovertebral junction. *Spine* 25:1607, 2000.

Ranawat CS, O'Leary P, Pellicci P, et al: Cervical spine fusion in rheumatoid arthritis, *J Bone Joint Surg* 61A:1003, 1979.

Rawlins BA, Girardi FP, Boachie-Adjei O: Rheumatoid arthritis of the cervical spine, *Rheum Dis Clin North Am* 24:55, 1998.

Redlund-Johnell I, Pettersson H: Radiographic measurements of the cranio-vertebral region, designed for evaluation of abnormalities in rheumatoid arthritis, *Acta Radiol Diagn Stockh* 25:23, 1984.

Reijnierse M, Breedveld FC, Kroon HM, et al: Are magnetic resonance flexion views useful in evaluating the cervical spine of patients with rheumatoid arthritis? *Skeletal Radiol* 29:85, 2000.

Reiter MF, Boden SD: Inflammatory disorders of the cervical spine, *Spine* 23:2755, 1998.

Robinson RA, Afeiche N, Dunn EJ, Northrup BE: Cervical spondylotic myelopathy: etiology and treatment concepts, *Spine* 2:89, 1977.

Sachs B, Fraenkel J: Progressive ankylotic rigidity of the spine (spondylose rhizomélique), *J Nerv Ment Dis* 27:1, 1900.

Santavirta S, Sandelin J, Slatis P: Posterior atlanto-axial subluxation in rheumatoid arthritis, *Acta Orthop Scand* 56:298, 1985.

Santavirta S, Slatis P, Kankaanpaa U, et al: Treatment of the cervical spine in rheumatoid arthritis, *J Bone Joint Surg* 70A:658, 1988.

Slatis P, Santavirta S, Sandelin J, Konttinen YT: Cranial subluxation of the odontoid process in rheumatoid arthritis, *J Bone Joint Surg* 71A:189, 1989.

Smith HP, Challa VR, Alexander E Jr: Odontoid compression of the brain stem in a patient with rheumatoid arthritis: case report, *J Neurosurg* 53:841, 1980.

Smith-Petersen MN, Larson CB, Aufranc OE: Osteotomy of the spine for correction of flexion deformity in rheumatoid spondylitis, *J Bone Joint Surg* 27:1, 1945.

Styblo K, Bossers GT, Slot GH: Osteotomy for kyphosis in ankylosing spondylitis, *Acta Orthop Scand* 56:294, 1985.

Sunahara N, Matsunaga S, Mori T, et al: Clinical course of conservatively managed rheumatoid arthritis patients with myelopathy, *Spine* 22:2603, 1997.

Thomas WH: Surgical management of the rheumatoid cervical spine, *Orthop Clin North Am* 6:793, 1975.

Thomasen E: Vertebral osteotomy for correction of kyphosis in ankylosing spondylitis, *Clin Orthop* 194:142, 1985.

Tsuji H: Laminoplasty for patients with compressive myelopathy due to so-called spinal canal stenosis in cervical and thoracic regions, *Spine* 7:28, 1982.

Veidlinger OF, Colwill JC, Smyth HS, Turner D: Cervical myelopathy and its relationship to cervical stenosis, *Spine* 6:550, 1981.

Weinstein PR, Karpman RR, Gall EP, Pitt M: Spinal cord injury, spinal fracture, and spinal stenosis in ankylosing spondylitis, *J Neurosurg* 57:609, 1982.

Wilson MJ, Turkell JH: Multiple spinal wedge osteotomy: its use in a case of Marie-Strumpell spondylitis, *Am J Surg* 77:777, 1949.

Wilson PD: Surgical reconstruction of the arthritic cripple, *Med Clin North Am* 21:1623, 1937.

Wilson PD, Osgood RB: Reconstructive surgery in chronic arthritis, *N Engl J Med* 209:117, 1933.

Winfield J, Cooke D, Brook AS, Corbett M: A prospective study of the radiological changes in the cervical spine in early rheumatoid disease, *Ann Rheum Dis* 40:109, 1981.

Yonezawa T, Tsuji H, Matsui H, Hirano N: Subaxial lesions in rheumatoid arthritis: radiographic factors suggestive of lower cervical myelopathy, *Spine* 20:208, 1995.

Zanasi R, Fioretta G, Rotolo F, Zanasi L: "Open door" operation to raise the vertebral arch in myelopathy due to cervical spondylosis, *Ital J Orthop Traumatol* 10:21, 1984.

Zhang Z, Yin H, Yang K, et al: Anterior intervertebral disc excision and bone grafting in cervical spondylotic myelopathy, *Spine* 8:16, 1983.

Zeidman SM, Ducker TB, Raycroft J: Trends and complications in cervical spine surgery: 1989-1993, *J Spinal Disord* 10:523, 1997.

Zigler JE, Capen DA, Rothman SL: Spinal disease in the aged. *Clin Orthop* 316:70, 1995.

ANKYLOSING SPONDYLITIS

Biasi D, Carletto A, Caramaschi P, et al: Efficacy of methotrexate in the treatment of ankylosing spondylitis: a three-year open study, *Clin Rheumatol* 19:114, 2000.

Bradford DS, Tribus CB: Vertebral column resection for the treatment of rigid coronal decompensation, *Spine* 22:1590, 1997.

Brigham CD: Ankylosing spondylitis and seronegative spondyloarthropathies. In The Cervical Spine Research Society, Editorial Committee: *The cervical spine*, ed 3, Philadelphia, 1998, Lippincott-Raven.

Broom MJ, Raycroft JF: Complications of fractures of the cervical spine in ankylosing spondylitis, *Spine* 13:763, 1988.

Calabro JJ, Maltz BA: Current concepts: ankylosing spondylitis, *N Engl J Med* 282:606, 1970.

Collie DA, Smith GW, Merrick MV: 99mTc-MDP scintigraphy in ankylosing spondylitis, *Clin Radiol* 48:392, 1993.

Danisa OA, Turner D, Richardson WJ: Surgical correction of lumbar kyphotic deformity: posterior reduction "eggshell" osteotomy, *J Neurosurg* 92(suppl 1):50, 2000.

Detwiler KN, Loftus CM, Godersky JC, Menezes AH: Management of cervical spine injuries in patients with ankylosing spondylitis, *J Neurosurg* 72:210, 1990.

Duff SE, Grundy PL, Gill SS: New approach to cervical flexion deformity in ankylosing spondylitis: case report. *J Neurosurg* 93(suppl 2):283, 2000.

Fang D, Leong JCY, Ho EKW, et al: Spinal pseudarthrosis in ankylosing spondylitis: clinicopathological correlation and the results of anterior spinal fusion, *J Bone Joint Surg* 70B:443, 1988.

Freeman GE Jr: Correction of severe deformity of the cervical spine in ankylosing spondylitis with the halo device, *J Bone Joint Surg* 43A:547, 1961.

Graham B, Van Peteghem PK: Fractures of the spine in ankylosing spondylitis: diagnosis, treatment, and complications, *Spine* 14:803, 1989.

Hammerberg KW: Ankylosing spondylitis. In The Cervical Spine Research Society, Editorial Committee: *The cervical spine*, ed 3, Philadelphia, 1998, Lippincott-Raven.

Ho EK, Chan FL, Leong JC: Postsurgical recurrent stress fracture in the spine affected by ankylosing spondylitis, *Clin Orthop* 247:87, 1989.

Iplikcioglu AC, Bayar MA, Kokes F, et al: Magnetic resonance imaging in cervical trauma associated with ankylosing spondylitis: report of two cases, *J Trauma* 36:412, 1994.

Junghans H: Aufrichtoperation bei spondylitis ankylopoietica, *Dtsch Med Wochenschr* 93:1592, 1968.

Peh WC, Ho TK, Chan FL: Case report: pseudoarthrosis complicating ankylosing spondylitis—appearances on magnetic imaging, *Clin Radiol* 47:359, 1993.

Rowed DW: Management of cervical spinal cord injury in ankylosing spondylitis: the intervertebral disc as a cause of cord compression, *J Neurosurg* 77:241, 1992.

Simmons EH: Surgery of the spine in rheumatoid arthritis and ankylosing spondylitis. In Cruess RL, Mitchell NS, eds: *Surgery of rheumatoid arthritis*, Philadelphia, 1971, JB Lippincott.

Simmons EH: The surgical correction of flexion deformity of the cervical spine in ankylosing spondylitis, *Clin Orthop* 86:132, 1972.

Simmons EH: The cervical spine in ankylosing spondylitis. In The Cervical Spine Research Society, Editorial Committee: *The cervical spine*, ed 3, Philadelphia, 1998, Lippincott-Raven.

Taggard DA, Traynelis VC: Management of cervical spinal fractures in ankylosing spondylitis with posterior fixation, *Spine* 25:2035, 2000.

Thiranont N, Netrawichien P: Transpedicular decancellation closed wedge vertebral osteotomy for treatment of fixed flexion deformity of spine in ankylosing spondylitis, *Spine* 18:2517, 1993.

Trent G, Armstrong GW, O'Neil J: Thoracolumbar fractures in ankylosing spondylitis: high risk injuries, *Clin Orthop* 227:61, 1988.

Van Royen BJ, Slot GH: Closing-wedge posterior osteotomy for ankylosing spondylitis: partial corpectomy and transpedicular fixation in 22 cases, *J Bone Joint Surg* 77B:117, 1995.

Wade W, Saltzstein R, Maiman D: Spinal fractures complicating ankylosing spondylitis, *Arch Phys Med Rehabil* 70:398, 1989.

Wu PC, Fang D, Ho EK, Leong JC: The pathogenesis of extensive discovertebral destruction in ankylosing spondylitis, *Clin Orthop* 230:154, 1988.

TUMORS

Akbarnia BA, Rooholamini SA: Scoliosis caused by benign osteoblastoma of the thoracic or lumbar spine, *J Bone Joint Surg* 63A:1146, 1981.

Akiyama H, Tamura K, Takatsuka K, Kondo M: Spinal cord tumor appearing as unusual pain, *Spine* 19:1410, 1994.

Asnis SE, Lesniewski P, Dowling T Jr: Anterior decompression and stabilization with methylmethacrylate and a bone bolt for treatment of pathologic fractures of the cervical spine: a report of two cases, *Clin Orthop* 187:139, 1984.

Barlow IW, Archer IA: Brown tumor of the cervical spine, *Spine* 18:936, 1993.

Bas T, Aparisi F, Bas JL: Efficacy and safety of ethanol injections in 18 cases of vertebral hemangioma: a mean follow-up of 2 years, *Spine* 26:1577, 2001.

Bell GR: Surgical treatment of spinal tumors, *Clin Orthop* 335:54, 1997.

Biagini R, Orsini U, Demitri S, et al: Osteoid osteoma and osteoblastoma of the sacrum, *Orthopedics* 24:1061, 2001.

Bohlman HH, Sachs BL, Carter JR, et al: Primary neoplasms of the cervical spine: diagnosis and treatment of twenty-three patients, *J Bone Joint Surg* 68A:483, 1986.

Boriani S, Biagini R, DeIure F: Bone tumors of the spine and epidural cord compression: treatment options, *Semin Spine Surg* 7:317, 1995.

Boriani S, Biagini R, DeIure F, et al: En bloc resections of bone tumors of the thoracolumbar spine: a preliminary report on 29 patients. *Spine* 21:1927, 1996.

Boriani S, De Iure F, Campanacci L, et al: Aneurysmal bone cyst of the mobile spine: report on 41 cases. *Spine* 26:27, 2001.

Boriani S, Weinstein JN, Biagini R: Primary bone tumors of the spine: terminology and surgical staging, *Spine* 22:1036, 1997.

Calderoni P, Gusella A, Martucci E: Multiple osteoid osteoma in the seventh dorsal vertebra, *Ital J Orthop Traumatol* 10:257, 1984.

Capanna R, Albisinni U, Picci P, et al: Aneurysmal bone cyst of the spine, *J Bone Joint Surg* 67A:527, 1985.

Chabot MC, Herkowitz HN: Spine tumors: patient evaluation, *Semin Spine Surg* 7:260, 1995.

Chadduck WM, Boop WC Jr: Acrylic stabilization of the cervical spine for neoplastic disease: evolution of a technique for vertebral body replacement, *Neurosurgery* 13:23, 1983.

Clark CR, Keggi KJ, Panjabi MM: Methylmethacrylate stabilization of the cervical spine, *J Bone Joint Surg* 66A:40, 1984.

Conley RK, Britt RH, Hanbery JW, Silverberg GD: Anterior fibular strut graft in neoplastic disease of the cervical spine, *J Neurosurg* 51:677, 1979.

Constans JP, de Divitiis E, Donzell R, et al: Spinal metastases with neurological manifestations: review of 600 cases, *J Neurosurg* 59:111, 1983.

Cortet B, Cotton A, Boutry N, et al: Percutaneous vertebroplasty in patients with osteolytic metastases or multiple myeloma, *Rev Rhum Engl Ed* 64:145, 1997.

Cove JA, Taminiau AH, Obermann WR, Vanderschueren BM: Osteoid osteoma of the spine treated with percutaneous computed tomography–guided thermocoagulation, *Spine* 25:1283, 2000.

Cross GO, White HL, White LP: Acrylic prosthesis of the fifth cervical vertebra in multiple myeloma: technical note, *J Neurosurg* 35:112, 1971.

Cusick JF, Larson SJ, Walsh PR, Steiner RE: Distraction rod stabilization in the treatment of metastatic carcinoma, *J Neurosurg* 59:861, 1983.

DeCristofaro E, Biagini R, Boriani S, et al: Selective arterial embolization in the treatment of aneurysmal bone cyst and angioma of bone, *Skeletal Radiol* 21:523, 1992.

DeWald RL, Bridwell KH, Prodromas C, Rodts MF: Reconstructive spinal surgery as palliation for metastatic malignancies of the spine, *Spine* 10:21, 1985.

Doppman JL, Oldfield EH, Heiss JD: Symptomatic vertebral hemangiomas: treatment by means of direct intralesional injection of ethanol, *Radiology* 214:341, 2000.

Dunn EJ: The role of methyl methacrylate in the stabilization and replacement of tumors of the cervical spine, *Spine* 2:15, 1977.

Fidler MW: Pathological fractures of the cervical spine: palliative surgical treatment, *J Bone Joint Surg* 67B:352, 1985.

Fidler MW: Surgical treatment of giant cell tumors of the thoracic and lumbar spine: report of nine patients, *Eur Spine J* 10:69, 2000.

Fielding JW, Fietti VG, Hughes JEO, Gabrielian JZ: Primary osteogenic sarcoma of the cervical spine: a case report, *J Bone Joint Surg* 58A:892, 1976.

Flatley TJ, Anderson MH, Anast GT: Spinal instability due to malignant disease: treatment by segmental spinal stabilization, *J Bone Joint Surg* 66A:47, 1984.

Floman Y, Bar-On E, Mosheiff R, et al: Eosinophilic granuloma of the spine, *J Pediatr Orthop B* 6:260, 1997.

Fornasier VL, Czitrom AA: Collapsed vertebrae: a review of 659 autopsies, *Clin Orthop* 131:261, 1978.

Fountain SS: A single-stage combined surgical approach for vertebral resections, *J Bone Joint Surg* 61A:1011, 1979.

Fraser RD, Paterson DC, Simpson DA: Orthopaedic aspects of spinal tumours in children, *J Bone Joint Surg* 59B:143, 1977.

Ghelman B, Lospinuso MF, Levine DB, et al: Percutaneous computed tomography–guided biopsy of the thoracic and lumbar spine, *Spine* 16:736, 1991.

Gibson JNA, Reid R, McMaster MJ: Fibrocartilaginous mesenchymoma of the fifth lumbar vertebra treated by vertebrectomy, *Spine* 19:1992, 1994.

Gokaslan ZL, York JE, Walsh GL, et al: Transthoracic vertebrectomy for metastatic spinal tumors, *J Neurosurg* 89:599, 1998.

Gore DR, Mueller HA: Osteoid-osteoma of the spine with localization aided by 99m Tc-polyphosphate bone scan: case report, *Clin Orthop* 113:132, 1975.

Griffin JB: Benign osteoblastoma of the thoracic spine: case report with fifteen-year follow-up, *J Bone Joint Surg* 60A:833, 1978.

Guarnaschelli JJ, Wehry SM, Serratoni FT, Dzenitis AJ: Atypical fibrous histiocytoma of the thoracic spine: case report, *J Neurosurg* 51:415, 1979.

Hansebout RR, Blomquist GA Jr: Acrylic spinal fusion: a 20-year clinical series and technical note, *J Neurosurg* 53:606, 1980.

Harrington KD: Anterior decompression and stabilization of the spine as a treatment for vertebral collapse and spinal cord compression from metastatic malignancy, *Clin Orthop* 233:177, 1988.

Hart RA, Boriani S, Biagini R, et al: A system for surgical staging and management of spine tumors: a clinical outcome study of giant cell tumors of the spine, *Spine* 22:1773, 1997.

Hart RA, Weinstein JN: Primary benign and malignant musculoskeletal tumors of the spine, *Semin Spine Surg* 7:288, 1995.

Heiman ML, Cooley CJ, Bradford DS: Osteoid osteoma of a vertebral body, *Clin Orthop* 118:159, 1976.

Hejgaard N, Larsen E: Value of early attention to spinal compression syndromes, *Acta Orthop Scand* 55:234, 1984.

Hosono N, Yonenobu K, Fuji T, et al: Vertebral body replacement with a ceramic prosthesis for metastatic spinal tumors, *Spine* 20:2454, 1995.

Ingraham FD, Matson DD: *Neurosurgery of infancy and childhood,* Springfield, Ill, 1954, Charles C Thomas.

Jaffe HL: "Osteoidosteoma": benign osteoblastic tumour composed of osteoid and atypical bone, *Arch Surg* 31:709, 1935.

Jho HD: Posterolateral approach for anteriorly located cervical spine tumors: technical note, *Minim Invasive Neurosurg* 41:204, 1998.

Jones AAM, Rizzolo SJ, Cotler JM et al: Metastatic cystosarcoma phylloides associated with paraplegia: an uncommon complication of an uncommon tumor, *J Spinal Disord* 6:71, 1993.

Kagan AR: Diagnostic oncology case study: lytic spine lesion and cold bone scan, *Am J Roentgenol* 136:129, 1981.

Kahn DC, Malhotra S, Stevens RE, Steinfeld AD: Radiotherapy for the treatment of giant cell tumor of the spine: a report of six cases and review of the literature, *Cancer Invest* 17:110, 1999.

Kanayama M, Ng JT, Cunningham BW, et al: Biomechanical analysis of anterior versus circumferential spinal reconstruction for various anatomic stages of tumor lesions, *Spine* 24:445, 1999.

Kawabata M, Sugiyama M, Suzuki T, Kumano K: The role of metal and bone cement fixation in the management of malignant lesions of the vertebral column, *Int Orthop* 4:177, 1980.

Keggi KJ, Southwick WO, Keller DJ: Stabilization of the spine using methylmethacrylate, *J Bone Joint Surg* 58A:738, 1976 (abstract).

Keogh C, Bergin D, Brennan D, Eustace S: MR imaging of bone tumors of the cervical spine, *Magn Reson Imaging Clin North Am* 8:513, 2000.

Ker NB, Jones CB: Tumours of the cauda equina: the problem of differential diagnosis, *J Bone Joint Surg* 67B:358, 1985.

Kida A, Taniguichi S, Fukuda H, Sakai K: Radiation therapy for metastatic spinal tumors, *Radiat Med* 18:15, 2000.

King GJ, Kostuik JP, McBroom RJ, Richardson W: Surgical management of metastatic renal carcinoma of the spine, *Spine* 16:267, 1991.

Kirwan EOG, Hutton PAN, Pozo JL, Ransford AO: Osteoid osteoma and benign osteoblastoma of the spine: clinical presentation and treatment, *J Bone Joint Surg* 66B:21, 1984.

Kostas JP, Dailianna Z, Xenakis T, et al: Back pain caused by benign tumors and tumor-like lesions of the thoracolumbar spine, *Am J Orthop* 30:50, 2001.

Krakovits GE, Julow J, Illyes G: Desmoplastic fibroma in the spine: a case report, *Spine* 16:48, 1991.

Laing RJ, Jakubowski J, Kunkler IH, Hancock BW: Primary spinal presentation of non-Hodgkin's lymphoma, *Spine* 17:117, 1992.

Leeson MC, Zechmann JP: Metastatic carcinoma of the spine with neurologic complications: an autopsy review, *Orthopedics* 16:1119, 1993.

Leone A, Costantini A, Guglielmi G, et al: Primary bone tumors and pseudotumors of the lumbosacral spine, *Rays* 25:89, 2000.

Levine AM: Operative techniques for treatment of metastatic disease of the spine, *Semin Spine Surg* 2:210, 1990.

Lindholm TS, Snellman O, Osterman K: Scoliosis caused by benign osteoblastoma of the lumbar spine: a report of three patients, *Spine* 2:276, 1977.

Mammano S, Candiotto S, Balsano B: Cast and brace treatment of eosinophilic granuloma of the spine: long-term follow-up, *J Pediatr Orthop* 17:821, 1997.

Manabe S, Tateishi A, Abe M, Ohno T: Surgical treatment of metastatic tumors of the spine, *Spine* 14:41, 1989.

Marymont JV: Spinal osteoblastoma in an 11-year-old boy, *South Med J* 81:922, 1988.

Matsuura M, Nakamura H, Inoue Y, Yamano Y: Osteoid osteoma of the cervical spine depicted as dumbbell tumor by MRI, *Eur Spine J* 9:426, 2000.

Mayfield JK, Erkkila JC, Winter RB: Spine deformity subsequent to acquired childhood spinal cord injury, *J Bone Joint Surg* 63A:1401, 1981.

McAfee PC, Bohlman HH, Ducker T, Eismont FJ: Failure of stabilization of the spine with methylmethacrylate, *J Bone Joint Surg* 68A:1145, 1986.

Miszczyk L, Ficek K, Trela K, Spindel J: The efficacy of radiotherapy for vertebral hemangiomas, *Neoplasma* 48:82, 2001.

Nagashima C, Iwasaki T, Okada K, Sakaguchi A: Reconstruction of the atlas and axis with wire and acrylic after metastatic destruction: case report, *J Neurosurg* 50:668, 1979.

Nicholls PJ, Jarecky TW: The value of posterior decompression by laminectomy for malignant tumors of the spine, *Clin Orthop* 201:210, 1985.

O'Neil J, Gardner V, Armstrong G: Treatment of tumors of the thoracic and lumbar spinal column, *Clin Orthop* 227:103, 1988.

Osti OL, Sebben R: High-frequency radio-wave ablation of osteoid osteoma in the lumbar spine, *Eur Spine J* 7:422, 1998.

Ozaki T, Halm H, Hillmann A, et al: Aneurysmal bone cysts of the spine, *Arch Orthop Trauma Surg* 199:159, 1999.

Ozaki T, Liljenqvist U, Hillmann A, et al: Osteoid osteoma and osteoblastoma of the spine: experiences with 22 patients, *Clin Orthop* 397:394, 2002.

Palmer FJ, Blum PW: Osteochondroma with spinal cord compression: report of three cases, *J Neurosurg* 52:842, 1980.

Panjabi MM, Goel VK, Clark CR, et al: Biomechanical study of cervical spine stabilization with methylmethacrylate, *Spine* 10:198, 1985.

Papagelopoulos PJ, Currier BL, Shaughnessy WJ, et al: Aneurysmal bone cyst of the spine: management and outcome, *Spine* 23:621, 1998.

Parks PF Jr, Herkowitz HN: Spine tumors—patient evaluation, *Semin Spine Surg* 2:152, 1990.

Pena M, Galasko CSB, Barrie JL: Delay in diagnosis of intradural spinal tumors, *Spine* 17:1110, 1992.

Peyser AB, Makley JT, Callewart CC, et al: Osteoma of the long bones and the spine: a study of eleven patients and a review of the literature, *J Bone Joint Surg* 78A:1172, 1996.

Postacchini F, Urso S, Tovaglia V: Lumbosacral intradural tumours simulating disc disease, *Int Orthop* 5:283, 1981.

Raab P, Hohmann F, Kuhl J, Krauspe R: Vertebral remodeling in eosinophilic granuloma of the spine: a long-term follow-up, *Spine* 23:1351, 1998.

Ransford AO, Pozo JL, Hutton PAN, Kirwan EOG: The behaviour pattern of the scoliosis associated with osteoid osteoma or osteoblastoma of the spine, *J Bone Joint Surg* 66B:16, 1984.

Raycroft JF, Hockman RP, Southwick WO: Metastatic tumors involving the cervical vertebrae: surgical palliation, *J Bone Joint Surg* 60A:763, 1978.

Saengnipanthkul S, Jirarattanaphochai K, Rojviroj S, et al: Metastatic adenocarcinoma of spine, *Spine* 17:427, 1992.

Saifuddin A, White J, Sherazi Z, et al: Osteoid osteoma and osteoblastoma of the spine: factors associated with the presence of scoliosis, *Spine* 23:47, 1998.

Savini R, Martucci E, Prosperi P, et al: Osteoid osteoma of the spine, *Ital J Orthop Traumatol* 14:233, 1988.

Schaberg J, Gainor BJ: A profile of metastatic carcinoma of the spine, *Spine* 10:19, 1985.

Scoville WB, Palmer AH, Samra K, Chong G: The use of acrylic plastic for vertebral replacement or fixation in metastatic disease of the spine, *J Neurosurg* 27:274, 1967.

Seichi A, Kondoh T, Hozumi T, Krasawa K: Intraoperative radiation therapy for metastatic spinal tumors. *Spine* 24:474, 1999.

Sherk HH, Nolan JP, Mooar P: Treatment of tumors of the cervical spine, *Clin Orthop* 233:163, 1988.

Shin JH, Lee HK, Rhim SC, et al: Spinal epidural cavernous hemangioma: MR findings. *J Comput Assist Tomogr* 25:257, 2001.

Shinomiya K, Furuya K, Mutoh N: Desmoplastic fibroma in the thoracic spine, *J Spinal Disord* 4:229, 1991.

Shinomiya K, Mutoh N, Furuya K: Giant sacral cysts with neurogenic bladder, *J Spinal Disord* 7:444, 1994.

Shives TC, Dahlin DC, Sim FH, et al: Osteosarcoma of the spine, *J Bone Joint Surg* 68A:660, 1986.

Siegal T, Siegal T: Current considerations in the management of neoplastic spinal cord compression, *Spine* 14:223, 1989.

Siegal T, Tiqva P, Siegal T: Vertebral body resection for epidural compression by malignant tumors: results of forty-seven consecutive operative procedures, *J Bone Joint Surg* 67A:375, 1985.

Simmons EH, Grobler LJ: Acute spinal epidural hematoma: a case report, *J Bone Joint Surg* 60A:395, 1978.

Sonel B, Yagmurlu B, Tuncer S, et al: Osteoblastoma of the lumbar spine as a cause of chronic low back pain, *Rheumatol Int* 21:253, 2002.

Stambough JL, Reid JH, Ross MA, et al: Isolated intradural metastasis simulating lumbar disc disease, *Spine* 16:581, 1991.

Stauber MH: Tumors of the pediatric spine, *Semin Spine Surg* 4:258, 1992.

Stener B: Total spondylectomy in chondrosarcoma arising from the seventh thoracic vertebra, *J Bone Joint Surg* 53B:288, 1971.

Stener B, Gunterberg B: High amputation of the sacrum for extirpation of tumors: principles and technique, *Spine* 3:351, 1978.

Stener B, Johnsen OE: Complete removal of three vertebrae for giant-cell tumour, *J Bone Joint Surg* 53B:278, 1971.

Stevens WW, Weaver EN: Giant cell tumors and aneurysmal bone cysts of the spine: report of four cases, *South Med J* 63:218, 1970.

Stiles RG, Spottswood SE, Jolgren DL, et al: An unusual appearance of an aneurysmal bone cyst of the thoracic spine, *J Spinal Disord* 4:104, 1991.

Stillwell WT, Fielding JW: Aneurysmal bone cyst of the cervicodorsal spine, *Clin Orthop* 187:144, 1984.

Suit HD, Goitein M, Munzenrider J, et al: Definitive radiation therapy for chordoma and chondrosarcoma of base of skull and cervical spine, *J Neurosurg* 56:377, 1982.

Sundaresan N, Rosen G, Huvos AG, Krol G: Combined treatment of osteosarcoma of the spine, *Neurosurgery* 23:714, 1988.

Talac R, Yaszemski MJ, Currier BL, et al: Relationship between surgical margins and local recurrence in sarcomas of the spine, *Clin Orthop* 397:127, 2002.

Tigani D, Pignati G, Picci P, et al: Vertebral osteosarcoma, *Ital J Orthop Traumatol* 14:5, 1988.

Tolli TC, Cammisa FP, Lane JM, Martin TL: Metastatic disease of the spine, *Semin Spine Surg* 7:277, 1995.

Turner ML, Mulhern CB, Dalinka, MK: Lesions of the sacrum: differential diagnosis and radiological evaluation, *JAMA* 245:275, 1981.

Vahldiek MJ, Panjabi MM: Stability potential of spinal instrumentations in tumor vertebral body replacement surgery, *Spine* 23:543, 1998.

Venkateswaran L, Rodriguez-Galindo C, Merchant TE, et al: Primary Ewing tumor of the vertebrae: clinical characteristics, prognostic factors, and outcome, *Med Pediatr Oncol* 37:30, 2001.

Villas C, Martínez-Peric R, Barrios RH, Beguiristain JL: Eosinophilic granuloma of the spine with and without vertebra plana: long-term follow-up of six cases, *J Spinal Disord* 6:260, 1993.

Wada E, Yamamoto T, Furuno M, et al: Spinal cord compression secondary to osteoblastic metastasis, *Spine* 18:1380, 1993.

Wang G, Lewish GD, Reger SI, et al: Comparative strengths of various anterior cement fixations of the spine, *Spine* 8:717, 1983.

Wang G, Reger SI, McLaughlin RE, et al: The safety of cement fixation in the cervical spine: studies of a rabbit model, *Clin Orthop* 139:276, 1979.

Wang G, Wilson CS, Hubbard SL, et al: Safety of anterior cement fixation in the cervical spine: in vivo study of dog spine, *South Med J* 77:178, 1984.

White WA, Patterson RH Jr, Bergland RM: Role of surgery in the treatment of spinal cord compression by metastatic neoplasm, *Cancer* 27:558, 1971.

Whitehill R, Reger SI, Fox E, et al: Use of methylmethacrylate cement as an instantaneous fusion mass in posterior cervical fusions: a canine in vivo experimental model, *Spine* 9:246, 1984.

Wilkinson RH, Hall JE: The sclerotic pedicle: tumor or pseudotumor? *Radiology* 111:683, 1974.

Young RF, Post EM, King GA: Treatment of spinal epidural metastases: randomized prospective comparison of laminectomy and radiotherapy, *J Neurosurg* 53:741, 1980.

Zeidman SM, Ellenbogen RG, Ducker TB: Intradural tumors. *Semin Spine Surg* 7:232, 1995.

Zevgaridis D, Buttner A, Weist S, et al: Spinal epidural cavernous hemangiomas: report of three cases and review of the literature, *J Neurosurg* 88:903, 1998.

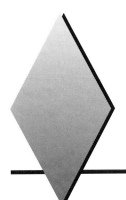

Index

Page numbers followed by *f* indicate figures, *t* indicate tables, and *b* indicate boxes.

I-1

Spinal Anatomy and Surgical Approaches

Fractures, Dislocations, and Fracture-Dislocations of Spine